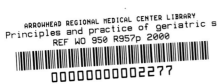

**Springer**
*New York*
*Berlin*
*Heidelberg*
*Barcelona*
*Hong Kong*
*London*
*Milan*
*Paris*
*Singapore*
*Tokyo*

Ronnie A. Rosenthal, MD
Associate Professor, Department of Surgery, Yale University School of Medicine, New Haven, and Chief, Surgical Service, VA Connecticut Healthcare System, West Haven, Connecticut

Michael E. Zenilman, MD
Associate Professor and Vice-Chairman, Department of Surgery, Montefiore Medical Center, Albert Einstein College of Medicine, Bronx, New York, and Chief of Surgery, Jack D. Weiler Hospital of the Albert Einstein College of Medicine, Bronx, New York

Mark R. Katlic, M.D.
Wyoming Valley Surgical Associates, Kingston, Pennsylvania, and Chief of Thoracic Surgery, Wyoming Valley Healthcare System, Wilkes-Barre, Pennsylvania

Editors

# Principles and Practice of Geriatric Surgery

With 393 Figures

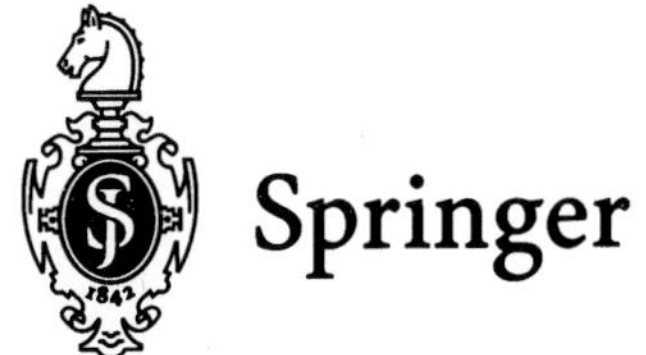

Ronnie A. Rosenthal, MD
Associate Professor
Department of Surgery
Yale University School of Medicine
New Haven, CT 06520
and
Chief, Surgical Service
Department of Veterans Affairs
VA Connecticut Healthcare System
West Haven, CT 06516, USA

Michael E. Zenilman, MD
Associate Professor and Vice-Chairman
Department of Surgery
Montefiore Medical Center
Albert Einstein College of Medicine
Bronx, NY 10461, USA
and Chief of Surgery
Jack D. Weiler Hospital of the Albert Einstein College of Medicine
Bronx, NY 10461, USA

Mark R. Katlic, MD
Wyoming Valley Surgical Associates
Kingston, PA 18704, USA
and Chief of Thoracic Surgery
Wyoming Valley Healthcare System
Wilkes-Barre, PA
18702, USA

*Chapter opening art:* From Gruman GJ (ed) Roots of Modern Gerontology and Geriatrics. New York: Ayer Company Publishers, 1979, with permission.

Library of Congress Cataloging-in-Publication Data
Principles and practice of geriatric surgery / editors, Ronnie A. Rosenthal, Michael E. Zenilman, Mark R. Katlic
p. cm.
Includes bibliographical references and index.
ISBN 0-387-98393-7 (alk. paper)
1. Aged—Surgery. 2. Surgery, Operative. I. Rosenthal, Ronnie A. II. Zenilman, Michael E. III. Katlic, Mark R., 1951–
[DNLM: 1. Surgical Procedures, Operative—Aged. WO 950 P957 2000]
RD145 .P75 2000
617.9′7—dc21
99-055303

Printed on acid-free paper.



Production coordinated by Chernow Editorial Services, Inc., and managed by Lesley Poliner; manufacturing supervised by Erica Bresler.
Typeset by Best-set Typesetters, Ltd., Hong Kong.
Printed and bound by Maple-Vail Book Manufcturing Group, York, PA.
Printed in the United States of America.

9 8 7 6 5 4 3 2 1

ISBN 0-387-98393-7 SPIN 10660226

Springer-Verlag New York Berlin Heidelberg
*A member of BertelsmannSpringer Science+Business Media GmbH*

*To Doris (Nana) and David (Poppa) Rosenthal*
*Karen (Rosenthal) Worchel*
*Lauren Andersen, Cori (Worchel) Novellion, Dana Worchel and Ashley Andersen.*
*Three generations that epitomize the most important consideration in the care of our elders—quality of life.*
*RAR*

*To Blanche Idoll, my late mother-in-law, who personified the need for focused, specialized surgical care of the geriatric patient.*
*MEZ*

*To my parents, Nancy and John Katlic, whose support of my grandparents—Frederick and Eva Nicely and Dorothy Deringer—is a model of compassionate care.*
*MRK*

# Preface

More than two decades ago, in response to the special healthcare needs of the aging American population, interest in the field of geriatric medicine began to grow and blossom in the United States. In 1984 and 1985, under the editorial leadership of Christine K. Cassel and William R. Hazzard, respectively, two major textbooks devoted to the medical care of aged patients were published. These scholarly, comprehensive texts provided insight into the principles of aging and guidance in the care of the geriatric patient. Three editions later, the need to understand the special issues involved in the medical care of the elderly is widely accepted by internists, primary care providers, and medical specialists.

For the editors of this book, the special issues involved in the surgical care of the elderly have been apparent for nearly as long. Although there have been a few scholarly texts on the subject, including one in 1990 by Mark R. Katlic, general acceptance of the concept of geriatric surgery by our surgical and medical colleagues has, however, lagged. This is not the result of a proportionately smaller number of older patients with surgical disease, because cancer, cardiovascular disease, and orthopedic problems are diseases, of the aged. It is rather the result of uncertainty about the value of surgery in the elderly and concerns about the risks of operations. In the past, such concerns prevented primary care givers from referring patients for surgical care and prevented surgeons from agreeing to operate. With the improvements in technology, monitoring, and anesthesia, we are now able to safely operate on most older patients, based on indications that are determined by the disease and the patient's overall health rather than by age. Since 1980, the percentage of operations performed in which the patient was over age 65 has nearly doubled to almost 40%. It is now estimated that approximately half of the patients in most general surgery practices, and even higher percentages in most cardiac and vascular surgery practices, are 65 years of age or older.

This recent rapid increase in the elderly surgical population has increased the awareness that older surgical patients are different from younger surgical patients and therefore require special consideration. In 1995, shortly before this text was conceived, the American College of Surgeons, with input from three well-respected senior surgeons, George E. Biock, Ben Eiseman, and Gerald O. Strauch, added a panel on Surgery in the Elderly to that year's program at the Annual Clinical Congress. Similar programs have since been presented at each of the last three Clinical Congresses. Also in 1995, the American Geriatrics Society in association with the Hartford Foundation began a program to increase geriatric expertise in nonprimary care specialties, including general surgery, orthopedics, urology, and gynecology. As part of this program, Drs. Walter Pories and Sherralyn Cox developed a geriatric syllabus that has now been added to the Surgical Resident Curriculum of the Association of Program Directors in Surgery. The field of "Geriatric Surgery" has begun to emerge.

Our goal in developing the present book was not to form the basis for a new surgical specialty because most surgeons, with the exception of our pediatric colleagues, will need to be "geriatric surgeons" soon. It was rather to provide a comprehensive collection of information that would allow all providers of healthcare to the elderly to understand the issues involved in choosing surgery as a treatment option for their patients. We have, by now, shown that we can operate on the elderly, the question is often whether we should. To help answer this question, we have divided the book into two parts. Part I, General Principles, describes general aspects of the physiology of aging and gives an overview of surgical management and important ethical considerations. Part II, Specific Issues, is organized by organ system. The first chapter in each section details the physiologic changes of that organ system with age. The subsequent chapters describe the pathophysiology, surgical treatment, and outcome of treatment for the disease of that organ system that are commonly encountered in elderly patients. With this information in hand, geriatricians, internists, and other primary care providers can better decide which of their patients will benefit from surgical referral; surgeons, surgical residents, and students can better understand how aging changes the assessment of risks, the choice of operation, the perioperative management, and treatment outcome.

Each section is also preceded by an invited commentary from well-known and widely respected senior members of each discipline. We have asked them to reflect on the changes they have seen in their area of expertise over the course of their careers and to comment on how they feel these changes have influenced the care of the elderly. We are extremely grateful to them for graciously agreeing to share their thoughts.

The road from concept to reality of this book has been long and somewhat bumpy, but throughout, there has been a genuine commitment to the importance of such a book by all involved. We are most grateful to our editor at Springer-Verlag, Laura Gillan, and her assistants for maintaining the high level of enthusiasm for the topic and commitment to the quality of the work. It has been a great pleasure to work with, and learn from, someone who understands so well why we embarked on this kind of journey and who so clearly shares our goal. Without her help, it would not have happened. We also thank Barbara Chernow and her associates for the very skillful copyediting done under considerable pressure. Finally we are extremely grateful to all of our authors, who have given so generously of their valuable time and effort to produce outstanding chapters in an era when rewards for such efforts are primarily internal. It is our belief that the information they have so carefully provided will bring significant improvements to the overall healthcare of our elderly patients.

# Contents

## Section 6 Gastrointestinal System

## Section 9 Soft Tissue and Musculoskeletal System



## Section 10 Nervous System



## Section 11 Transplantation



## Section 12 Applications of Minimal Access Techniques to the Surgical Case of the Elderly

# Contributors

*Steven A. Ahrendt, MD*
Division of Pancreatobiliary/Endocrine Surgery, Medical College of Wisconsin, Milwaukee, Wisconsin, 53226, USA

*Peter C. Albertsen, MD*
Division of Urology, The School of Medicine of the University of Connecticut Health Center, Farmington, CT 06030-3955, USA

*Dana K. Andersen, MD*
Section of Gastrointestinal Surgery, Department of Surgery Yale University School of Medicine, New Haven, CT 06520, USA

*Wilbert S. Aronow, MD*
Department of Geriatrics and Adult Development, Mount Sinai School of Medicine, New York, NY 10029, and Hebrew Hospital Home, Bronx and Valhalla, NY 10475, USA

*Nancy L. Ascher, MD*
Department of Surgery, University of California, San Francisco, San Francisco, CA 94143, USA

*Maryam M. Asgari, MD*
Dermatologic and Laser Surgery Unit, Department of Dermatology, Yale University School of Medicine, New Haven, CT 06520, USA

*Stanley W. Ashley, MD*
Department of Surgery, Harvard Medical School, Brigham and Women's Hospital, Boston, MA 02115, USA

*Lodovico Balducci, MD*
H. Lee Moffit Cancer Center, University of South Florida College of Medicine, Tampa, FL 33612-9497, USA

*Sancar Bayar, MD*
Department of Surgical Oncology, Yale University School of Medicine, New Haven, CT 06520, USA

*Palmer Q. Bessey, MD*
Department of Surgery, University of Rochester, Rochester, NY 14642-8410, USA

*Elisa H. Birnbaum, MD*
Division of Colon and Rectal Surgery, Department of Surgery, Washington University School of Medicine, St. Louis, MO 63110, USA

*Elizabeth Breen, MD*
Department of Surgery, Harvard Medical School, Brigham and Women's Hospital, Boston, MA 02115, USA

*F. Charles Brunicardi, MD*
Department of Surgery, Baylor College of Medicine, Houston, TX 77030, USA

*L. Michael Brunt, MD*
Department of Surgery, Washington University School of Medicine, St. Louis, MO 63110, USA

*Lauri Ellen Budnick, MD*
Department of Obstetrics and Gynecology, Montefiore Medical Center, Albert Einstein College of Medicine, Bronx, NY 10461, USA

*Edith A. Burns, MD*
Department of Medicine, University of Wisconsin Medical School, Milwaukee, WI 53233, USA

*Margarita T. Camacho, MD*
Department of Cardiothoracic Surgery, Montefiore Medical Center, Albert Einstein College of Medicine, Bronx, NY 10461, USA

*Edward J. Campbell, MD*
Department of Internal Medicine, University of Utah Health Sciences Center, Salt Lake City, Utah 84132, USA

*Marla J. Campbell, BS, Pharm. D.*
Faculty of Pharmacy, University of Connecticut, Bristol, CT 06010, USA

*Maria Torroella Carney, MD*
Division of Geriatrics, Department of Medicine, Winthrop-University Hospital, Mineola, NY 11501, USA

*Robert R. Cima, MD*
Department of Surgery, Harvard Medical School, Brigham and Women's Hospital, Boston, MA 02115, USA

*Elizabeth B. Claus, MD*
Departments of Epidemiology and Public Health and Neurosurgery, Yale University School of Medicine, New Haven, CT 06520, USA

*Brian Cohen, MD*
Department of Orthopaedic Surgery, The Mount Sinai Medical Center, New York, NY 10029, USA

*William F. Collins, MD*
Department of Neurosurgery, Yale University School of Medicine, New Haven, CT 06520, USA

*Michael Coomaraswamy, MD*
Division of Head and Neck Surgery, Department of Surgery, Montefiore Medical Center, Albert Einstein College of Medicine, Bronx, NY 10461, USA

*Leo M. Cooney, Jr., MD*
Section of General Internal Medicine, Yale University School of Medicine, New Haven, CT 06520, USA

*Christopher P. Coppola, MD*
Department of Surgery, Yale University School of Medicine, New Haven, CT 06520, USA

*Vincent Joseph Cristofalo, MD*
Lankenau Institute for Medical Research, Philadelphia, PA 19096, USA

*Charles W. Cummings, MD*
Department of Otolaryngology-Head and Neck Surgery, Johns Hopkins School of Medicine, Baltimore, MD 21287, USA

*J.C. de la Torre, MD, PhD*
Department of Neuroscience, University of California, San Diego, La Jolla, CA 92093, USA

*Joseph DiGiovanni, MD*
Department of Orthopaedic Surgery, The Mount Sinai Medical Center, New York, NY 10029, USA

*John B. Dossetor, MD, PhD*
Professor Emeritus, The Glebe, Ottawa, Ontario, K1S 2G7, Canada

*Margaret Drickamer, MD*
Department of General Internal Medicine, Yale University School of Medicine, New Haven, CT 06520, and Geriatric Care and Extended Care Section, VA Connecticut Healthcare System, West Haven, CT 06516, USA

*J. Chris Eagon, MD*
Department of Surgery, Washington University School of Medicine, St. Louis, MO 63110, USA

*Ben Eiseman, MD*
Department of Surgery, University of Colorado Health Science Center, Denver, CO 80262, USA

*Martine Extermann, MD*
H. Lee Moffit Cancer Center, University of South Florida College of Medicine, Tampa, FL 33612, USA

*L.A. Fay, MD*
Division of Neurosurgery, University of New Mexico, Albuquerque, NM 87151, USA

*Neal S. Fedarko, MD*
Division of Geriatrics, Department of Medicine, Johns Hopkins University, Baltimore, MD 21224, USA

*Sandy Feng, MD, PhD*
Department of Surgery, Harvard Medical School, Massachusetts General Hospital, Boston, MA 02114, USA

*Yuman Fong, MD*
Department of Surgery, Memorial Sloan Kettering Cancer Center, New York, NY 10021, USA

*Arlene A. Forastiere, MD*
Department of Surgery, Johns Hopkins School of Medicine, Baltimore, MD 21205, USA

*William H. Frishman, MD*
Department of Medicine, New York Medical College, Valhalla, NY 10595, USA

*Darlene Gabeau*
Yale University School of Medicine, New Haven, CT 06520, USA

*Timothy J. Gardner, MD*
Division of Cardiothoracic Surgery, University of Pennsylvania School of Medicine, Hospital of the University of Pennsylvania, Philadelphia, PA 19104, USA

*Ray F. Gariano, MD, PhD*
Department of Ophthalmology and Visual Science, Yale University School of Medicine, New Haven, CT 06520, USA

*Jayne N. Ge, MD*
Department of Ophthalmology and Visual Science, Yale University School of Medicine, New Haven, CT 06520, USA

*Bruce J. Giantonio, MD*
Department of Surgery, University of Pennsylvania School of Medicine, Philadelphia, PA 19104, USA

*Jeffrey P. Gold, MD*
Department of Cardiothoracic Surgery, Montefiore Medical Center, Albert Einstein College of Medicine, Bronx, NY 10461, USA

*James S. Goodwin, MD*
University of Texas Medical Branch, Sealy Center on Aging, Galveston, TX 77555, USA

*Ravi Goravalingappa, MD*
Department of Otolaryngology, Yale University School of Medicine, New Haven, CT 06520, USA

*Wilma Markus Greston, BS, MT*
Department of Obstetrics and Gynecology and Women's Health, Montefiore Medical Center, Albert Einstein College of Medicine, Bronx, NY 10461, USA

*Nora Hansen, MD*
John Wayne Cancer Institute, Santa Monica, CA 90404, USA

*Stephen N. Harris, MD*
Department of Anesthesiology, Yale University School of Medicine, and Department of Anesthesiology, VA Connecticut Healthcare System, West Haven, CT 06516, USA

*Leonard Hayflick, PhD*
Department of Anatomy, University of California, San Francisco, School of Medicine, The Sea Ranch, CA 95497, USA

*Richard F. Heitmiller, MD*
Department of Surgery, Johns Hopkins School of Medicine, Baltimore, MD 21205, USA

*David M. Hoenig, MD*
Department of Urology, Montefiore Medical Center, Albert Einstein College of Medicine, Bronx, NY 10461, USA

*Juana Hutchinson-Colas, MD*
Department of Obstetrics and Gynecology, Mount Sinai School of Medicine/Jersey City Medical Center, Jersey City, NJ 07304, USA

*Danny O. Jacobs, MD, MPH*
Department of Surgery, Division of General and Gastrointestinal Surgery, Brigham and Women's Hospital, Boston, MA 02115, USA

*Dennis W. Jahnigen, MD [deceased]*
Department of Medicine, University of Colorado Center on Aging, Denver, CO 50262, USA

*Jasleen Jasleen, MD*
Department of Surgery, Harvard Medical School, Brigham and Women's Hospital, Boston, MA 02115, USA

*Olga Jonasson, MD*
Education and Surgical Services Department, American College of Surgeons, Chicago, IL 60611, USA

*Kim U. Kahng, MD*
Department of Surgery, Medical College of Wisconsin, Milwaukee, WI 53226, and Department of Surgery, Clement Zavlocki VA Medical Center, Milwaukee, WI 53295, USA

*Hosam K. Kamel, MD*
Division of Geriatric Medicine, St. Louis University Health Sciences Center, St. Louis, MO 63104, USA

*Lewis J. Kaplan, MD*
Surgical Intensive Care Unit, MCP Hahnemann University School of Medicine, Philadelphia, PA 19129, USA

*Namir Katkhouda, MD*
Division of Emergency Non-Trauma Surgery, University of Southern California School of Medicine, Los Angeles, CA 90033, USA

*Mark R. Katlic, MD*
Wyoming Valley Surgical Associates, Kingston, PA 18704, and Department of Thoracic Surgery, Wyoming Valley Healthcare System, Wilkes-Barre, PA 18702, USA

*Fraser Keith, MD*
Cardiac Transplant Program, University of California, San Francisco, San Francisco, CA 94143, USA

*Barbara Kinder, MD*
Department of Surgery, Yale University School of Medicine, New Haven, CT 06520, USA

*David W. Kinne, MD*
Department of Surgery, Columbia Presbyterian Medical Center, New York, NY 10022, USA

*Kenneth J. Koval, MD*
Department of Orthopaedic Surgery, Hospital for Joint Diseases, New York, NY 10003, USA

*Loren Kroetsch, MD*
Department of Surgery, Montefiore Medical Center, Albert Einstein College of Medicine, Bronx, NY 10461, USA

*John F. Kveton, MD*
Department of Otolaryngology, Yale University School of Medicine, New Haven, CT 06520, USA

*Francis Kwakwa, MD*
Education and Surgical Services Department, American College of Surgeons, Chicago, IL 60611, USA

*Tirso Mark Lara, MD*
Department of Surgery, Harvard Medical School, Brigham and Women's Hospital, Boston, MA 02115, USA

*George Lazarou, MD*
Department of Obstetrics, Gynecology and Women's Health, Montefiore Medical Center, Albert Einstein College of Medicine, Bronx, NY 10461, USA

*David J. Leffell, MD*
Dermatologic and Laser Surgery Unit, Department of Dermatology, Yale University School of Medicine, New Haven, CT 06520, USA

*Joshua L. Levine, MD*
Department of Surgery, Montefiore Medical Center, Albert Einstein College of Medicine, Bronx, NY 10461, USA

*Roger N. Levy, MD*
Department of Orthopaedic Surgery, The Mount Sinai Medical Center, New York, NY 10029, USA

*Jonathan D. Lewin, MD*
Department of Orthopaedic Surgery, Montefiore Medical Center, Albert Einstein College of Medicine, Bronx, NY 10461, USA

*Keith D. Lillemoe, MD*
Department of Surgery, Johns Hopkins Hospital, Baltimore, MD 21287, USA

*Bernard Lytton, MD*
Department of Surgery, Yale University School of Medicine, New Haven, CT 06520, USA

*Thomas H. Magnuson, MD*
Johns Hopkins Bayview Medical Center, Baltimore, MD 21224-2780, USA

*Paolo L. Manfredi, MD*
Departments of Geriatrics, Anesthesia, and Neurology, Mount Sinai School of Medicine, New York, NY 10029, USA

*John A. Mannick, MD*
Department of Surgery, Harvard Medical School, Brigham and Women's Hospital, Boston, MA 02115, USA

*Richard A. Marottoli, MD*
Department of General Internal Medicine, Yale University School of Medicine, New Haven, CT 06520, and Medical Service/Geriatric Section, VA Connecticut Healthcare System, West Haven, CT 06516, USA

*D. LaRon Mason, MD*
Department of Surgery, Baylor College of Medicine, Houston, TX 77030, USA

*David McAneny, MD*
Department of General Surgery, Boston University Medical Center, Boston, MA 02118, USA

*George H. Meier, MD*
Northfolk Surgical Group, Brambleton Medical Center, Northfolk, VA 23510, USA

*Ronald C. Merrell, MD*
Department of Surgery, Medical College of Virginia, Richmond, VA 23298, USA

*Emery A. Minnard, MD*
Department of Surgery, Louisiana State University School of Medicine, New Orleans, LA 70112, USA

*John E. Morley, MD*
Division of Geriatric Medicine, Saint Louis University Health Sciences Center, St. Louis, MO 63104, USA

*R. Sean Morrison, MD*
Department of Geriatrics, Mount Sinai School of Medicine, New York, NY 10029, USA

*Monica Morrow, MD*
Department of Surgery, Lynn Sage Breast Center, Northwestern University Medical School, Chicago, IL 60611, USA

*John S. Najarian, MD*
Department of Surgery, University of Minnesota, Minneapolis, MN 55455, USA

*Pat O'Donnell, MD*
Department of Surgery, University of Arkansas for Medical Sciences, Little Rock, AR 72205, USA

*John Olsewski, MD*
Department of Orthopaedic Surgery, Montefiore Medical Center, Albert Einstein College of Medicine, Bronx, NY 10461, USA

*Jeffrey H. Peters, MD*
Section of General Surgery, USC University Hospital, University of Southern California School of Medicine, Los Angeles, CA 90033-4612, USA

*Joseph Piepmeier, MD*
Department of Neurosurgery, Yale University School of Medicine, New Haven, CT 06520, USA

*Roshini C. Pinto Powell, MD*
Department of Medicine, Dartmouth Hitchcock Medical Center, Lebanon, NH 03755, USA

*Konstadinos A. Plestis, MD*
Department of Cardiothoracic Surgery, Montefiore Medical Center, Albert Einstein College of Medicine, Bronx, NY 10461, USA

*Jeffrey M. Reilly, MD*
Vascular Surgical Associates, Marietta, GA 30060, USA

*Jeffrey H. Richmond, MD*
Department of Orthopaedic Surgery, Hospital for Joint Diseases, New York, NY 10003, USA

*Mark Roberts, MD*
Department of Political Economic and Health Policy, Harvard School of Public Health, Boston, MA 02115, USA

*Ronnie A. Rosenthal, MD*
Department of Surgery, Yale University School of Medicine, New Haven, CT 06520, and Surgical Service, Department of Veterans Affairs, VA Connecticut Healthcare System, West Haven, CT 06516, USA

*Daniel B. Rukstalis, MD*
Department of Surgery, Allegheny University of the Health Sciences, Philadelphia, PA 19129, USA

*Thomas J. Rutherford, MD*
Department of Obstetrics and Gynecology, Yale University School of Medicine, New Haven, CT 06520, USA

*John J. Ryan, MD*
Department of Surgery, University of South Dakota School of Medicine, Sioux Falls, SD 57105, USA

*Luis A. Sanchez, MD*
Department of Surgery, Montefiore Medical Center, Albert Einstein College of Medicine, Bronx, NY 10461, USA

*Thomas A. Santora, MD*
Department of Surgery, MCP Hahnemann University School of Medicine, Philadelphia, PA 19129, USA

*David S. Schrump, MD*
Department of Thoracic and Cardiovascular Surgery, University of Texas MD Anderson Cancer Center, Houston, TX 77030, USA

*Peter E. Schwartz, MD*
Section of Gynecologic Oncology, Department of Obstetrics and Gynecology, Yale University School of Medicine, New Haven, CT 06520, USA

*Seymour Schwartz, MD*
Department of Surgery, University of Rochester, School of Medicine and Dentistry, Rochester, NY 14642, USA

*Richard J. Scotti, MD*
Department of Obstetrics, Gynecology and Women's Health, Montefiore Medical Center, Albert Einstein College of Medicine, Bronx, NY 10461, USA

*Neal E. Seymour, MD*
Department of Surgery, Yale University School of Medicine, New Haven, CT 06520, USA

*Jay R. Shapiro, MD*
Department of Medicine, Uniformed Services University of the Health Sciences, Bethesda, MD 20814, USA

*K. Robert Shen, MD*
Department of Surgery, Harvard Medical School, Brigham and Women's Hospital, Boston, MA 02115, USA

*G. Tom Shires, MD*
Department of Trauma, University of Nevada, Las Vegas, NV 89102, USA

*Gregorio A. Sicard, MD*
Department of Surgery, Washington University School of Medicine, St. Louis, MO 63110-1093, USA

*William Silen, MD*
Department of Surgery, Beth Hospital, Boston, MA 02115, USA

*Nathaniel J. Soper, MD*
Section of Hepatobiliary, Pancreatic and Gastrointestinal Surgery, Department of General Surgery, Washington University School of Medicine, St. Louis, MO 63110, USA

*David I. Soybel, MD*
Department of Surgery, West Roxbury VA Medical Center, Harvard Medical School, West Roxbury, MA 02312, USA

*Seth A. Spector, MD*
Department of Surgery, Yale University School of Medicine, New Haven, CT 06520, USA

*Kathleen M. Stoessel, MD*
Department of Ophthalmology, Yale University School of Medicine, New Haven, CT 06520, USA

*William D. Suggs, MD*
Division of Vascular Surgery, Department of Surgery, Montefiore Medical Center, Albert Einstein College of Medicine, Bronx, NY 10461, USA

*Roby C. Thompson, Jr., MD*
Department of Orthopaedic Surgery, University of Minnesota, Minneapolis, MN 55455, USA

*Scott C. Thornton, MD*
Colon and Rectal Surgeons of Fairfield County, Bridgeport, CT 06606, USA

*Paola S. Timiras, MD*
Department of Molecular and Cell Biology, University of California, Berkley, Berkley, CA 04720-3202, USA

*Stephen J. Tomlanovich, MD*
Department of Surgery, University of California, San Francisco, San Francisco, CA 94143, USA

*Bruce Robert Troen, MD*
Lankenau Institute for Medical Research, Philadelphia, PA 19096, USA

*Stanley Z. Trooskin, MD*
Department of Surgery, MCP Hahnemann University School of Medicine, Philadelphia, PA 19129, USA

*Frank J. Veith, MD*
Division of Vascular Surgery, Department of Surgery, Montefiore Medical Center, Albert Einstein College of Medicine, Bronx, NY 10461, USA

*Barbara A. Ward, MD*
Department of Surgery, Yale University School of Medicine, New Haven, CT 06520, USA

*Jennifer A. Wargo, MD*
Department of Surgery, Massachusetts General Hospital, Harvard Medical School, Boston, MA 02114, USA

*James M. Watters, MD*
Department of Surgery, Loeb Health Research Institute at the Ottawa Hospital, Ottawa, Ontario K1Y 4K9, CANADA

*Craig L. Weinstein, MD*
Department of General Surgery, Boston University Medical Center, Boston, MA 02118, USA

*Samuel A. Wells, Jr., MD*
Center for Clinical Trials and Evidence-Based Medicine, American College of Surgeons, Chicago, IL 60611, USA

*Edward E. Whang, MD*
Division of General/Gastrointestinal Surgery, Harvard Medical School, Brigham and Women's Hospital, Boston, MA 02115, USA

*Earle W. Wilkins, Jr., MD*
Department of Surgery, Harvard Medical School, Massachusetts General Hospital, Boston, MA 02114, USA

*John R. Wilmoth, PhD*
Department of Demography, University of California, Berkeley, Berkeley, CA 94720, USA

*Bruce G. Wolff, MD*
Department of Colon and Rectal Surgery, Mayo Clinic, Rochester, Minnesota 55905, USA

*Tonia M. Young-Fadok, MD*
Department of Colon and Rectal Surgery, Mayo Clinic, Rochester, MN 55905, USA

*Edward T. Zawada, Jr., MD*
Department of Internal Medicine, The University of South Dakota School of Medicine, Sioux Falls, SD 57105, USA

*Peter D. Zdankiewicz, MD*
Department of Surgery, Yale University School of Medicine, New Haven, CT 06520, USA

*Michael E. Zenilman, MD*
Department of Surgery, Montefiore Medical Center, Albert Einstein College of Medicine, Bronx, NY 10461, and Department of Surgery, Jack D. Weiler Hospital of the Albert Einstein College of Medicine, Bronx, NY 10461, USA

*Joseph D. Zuckerman, MD*
Department of Orthopaedic Surgery, Hospital for Joint Diseases, New York, NY 10003, USA

# *Part I*
# *General Principles*

## Section 1
## Physiology of Aging

# Invited Commentary

Leonard Hayflick

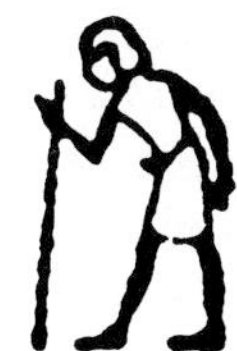

It seems strange that after performing the miracles that take us from conception to birth and then to sexual maturation and adulthood nature was unable to devise what would seem to be a more elementary mechanism that would simply maintain those earlier miracles forever. Nature has not done this, however, and the reason for her failure is an enigma.

This observation, made many years ago, is the central question in modern biogerontology. Although we do not yet have a complete answer, we do have several remarkable new insights. The common observation that there are as many theories of aging as there are biogerontologists is now thought to be nonsense. All theories of aging are derivative of one fundamental concept: Aging is simply an increase in molecular disorder.

Prior to discussing this idea, it is necessary to make clear the distinction between the concepts of aging and longevity determination. They are not the same. Failure to make this distinction has led us, and is leading us, into much confusion.

## Aging and Longevity Determination

Longevity determination, as distinguished from age changes, is indirectly determined by the genome. Aging in living systems is a stochastic process that occurs after reproductive maturity and results from increasing molecular disorder. Because age changes occur stochastically they are not directly programmed by the genome.

These conclusions are based on the following reasoning. Species survival depends on a sufficient number of members of that species living long enough to reproduce and, if necessary, to raise progeny to independence. The verity of this premise seems obvious because if a sufficient number of animals are unable to reach sexual maturity they do not reproduce and the species vanishes.

The best way to ensure survival to reproductive success is for natural selection to favor animals that have greater physiologic reserve in vital organs and are thus more capable of surviving predation, disease, accidents, and environmental extremes. Prey survival occurs by natural selection because as a predator becomes more skilled in capturing prey the surviving prey does so by developing better avoidance techniques. Animals that develop greater reserve capacity in their vital systems, such as faster repair processes, quicker sensory responses, or greater strength or speed, are better able to escape predators and survive disease, accidents, and harsh environmental conditions. The favored animals are selected for their greater redundant capacity or physiologic reserve.

Redundant physiologic capacity increases the chances for animals to survive long enough to achieve reproductive success, just as redundant vital systems in complex machines such as space vehicles better ensures that they will achieve their goals. Once animals achieve reproductive success, the excess physiologic capacity, like that engineered into a space vehicle, allows them to continue beyond their vital goal. Survival of the animal beyond reproductive success (and the space craft beyond its primary mission) is determined by the level of excess capacity present at the time each goal is reached.[1]

Because survival long beyond reproductive success has neutral or diminished value for survival of a species, the forces of natural selection diminish after animals reproduce. Energy is better spent on guaranteeing reproductive success than it is for increasing individual longevity. After reproductive success the forces of natural selection do not favor increased longevity. Animals and humans have the potential to survive for a time determined by the level of excess physiologic capacity reached at sexual maturation. The level reached determines the potential for continued longevity. This hypothesis is conceptually different from aging and is independent of aging processes.

The molecular order achieved from conception to sexual maturation becomes more disordered over time. Physiologic reserve does not renew at the same rate it incurs losses, thereby allowing molecular disorder to increase. Disorder increases despite the presence of repair processes because they themselves incur molecular disorder and are unable to keep vital processes in perfect repair. This increasing molecular disorder—the aging process—increases the vulnerability of an animal or human to predation, accidents, or disease.

Clearly, the developmental events that lead to survival of animals through reproductive success are determined genetically. Survival of animals beyond sexual maturation is determined only indirectly by the genome. The state of survival beyond reproductive success might be regarded as a period of "coasting" or "free-wheeling," when developmental processes have ended and the capacity to maintain vital systems declines. The length of this postreproductive period plus the time taken to reach sexual maturation can be viewed as the two components of an animal's longevity.[1]

The unrepaired molecular disorder that occurs after reproductive success and that fails to maintain the system produces what we recognize as age changes and increases the probability of dying. By this reasoning the aging of living things that are incapable of perfect repair is not unlike the aging of everything else in the universe including the universe itself. In the absence of perfect mechanisms for repair, molecular disorder increases in all animate and inanimate objects. The molecular disorder that we call aging might occur passively by simple decrements in the energy necessary to maintain molecular order or actively through, for example, the action of oxygen or its free radicals.

It is for these reasons that genes did not evolve to drive age changes directly. Furthermore, as is described subsequently, it is unlikely that feral animals live long enough for genes that govern age changes to have evolved. However, there are genes whose products increase physiologic capacity or survival skills and that are sustained through natural selection, thereby indirectly increasing the potential for greater longevity.

Nevertheless, there are animals whose age changes are so imperceptible the process occurs at the limits of our ability to detect them. I refer to that broad class of animals who do not reach a fixed size during adulthood. Examples include some turtles, many sport and deep sea fish, and the American lobster. The rate of aging in animals that continue to increase in size is low, and the measurements that have been made do not reveal easily detectable physiologic losses with age.

## Aging of Feral Animals

I mentioned earlier that aging is a peculiar human phenomenon.[1] There is a good argument for the belief that extreme manifestations of aging are unlikely to occur in wild animals because they rarely live long enough to experience them. Age changes do not cause sudden death after reproductive success because it would be prohibitively costly in energy to evolve a system in an animal that would cause it to die precisely on the day that its progeny become independent. That unnecessary cost in energy is equally applicable to complex machines where a system to destroy the machine after the guarantee period is unnecessary for similar reasons of economy. The machine continues to function after the guarantee period and the animal after reproductive success, with both experiencing age changes that were not part of the original design.

The class of animals generally referred to as "big bang animals," represented by the Pacific salmon and the marsupial male rat, may appear to be an exception to this notion. However, it is more likely that the deaths that occur after reproductive success in these animals is the result of their unique expenditure of enormous amounts of energy that precedes mating. It is questionable whether the biologic changes that precede their deaths are age changes. There is no reason why it is necessary for age changes to precede death.

## Redundancy, Trade-offs, and Repair

Redundant physiologic capacity is common in human vital organs, but there is a price to pay for that redundancy. The price is the expenditure of more energy during development to produce the redundant systems necessary to guarantee survival until reproductive success. This energy expenditure better ensures species survival but energy spent on increasing individual survival beyond reproductive success has little or no benefit.

There is a trade-off between reproductive effort and life-span. High reproductive capacity correlates with a short life-span, and low reproductive capacity correlates with a long life-span. Animals make a trade-off between growing up fast and then producing many offspring—a strategy that favors preservation of the organism's genes—versus survival of the animal for a longer time, which may or may not benefit reproductive success.

The energy costs of a perfect repair system would be so high it would put its possessor at an evolutionary disadvantage compared with an animal that puts less energy into repair and more into fueling greater fecundity. For example, if an animal has a high mortality rate in the wild, such as many species of birds, it is much better for the birds to invest their energy in growing up fast and producing many offspring than to invest the energy in strategies that might keep them alive for a longer time. This principle recently was observed in feral guppies.

A general rule-of-thumb is that the larger the proportion of resources allocated for reproduction, the lower is the chance that members of that species will live a long time. A high adult mortality rate favors evolution of a life style in which there is an early, high reproductive effort.

The opposite strategy, in which energy is invested in a later reproductive effort, has been adopted by humans and other animals (e.g., elephants) where resistance to environmental hazards or better adaptation to the environment has reduced the likelihood of death from accidents, disease, predation, or starvation. Using this strategy, a slow growth rate and a slow reproductive rate result in increased Darwinian fitness and, indirectly, in a longer life-span.

Stated another way, natural selection trades characteristics that favor longevity for those that favor enhanced early fecundity. The force of natural selection then declines with age, an idea first emphasized by the late Sir Peter Medawar.

## Aging: Artifact of Human Civilization

The engineer's term to describe the average period a mechanical device is expected to survive is the "mean time to failure." The mean time to failure of an inexpensive car might be 2 years before a major repair is needed, whereas with a more expensive car it might be 5 years. "Mean time to failure" refers to a future time when half of a group of identical objects stop functioning. It is identical to life expectation in humans where the "mean time to failure" of today's newborns is about 75 years.

If longevity is determined by our genes, albeit indirectly, and aging is not, why do we age? It is difficult to understand how evolution could select for a process such as aging when few if any animals have ever lived long enough to participate in the selection process.

Humans are the only species in which a large number of members usually experience aging. Aging of feral animals in numbers proportional to those seen in humans simply does not occur. It occurs only in animals humans choose to protect. Furthermore, animals that reach old age are not essential for survival of any species. For example, humans at birth had a life expectancy of 30 years or less for more than 99.9% of the time we have inhabited this planet. Prehistoric human remains have never revealed individuals older than about 50 years of age. There appears to be no selective advantage that favors survival of animals or humans whose physiologic capacities are in decline.

Finally, members of exotic wild animal species, who for millions of years have not experienced aging, reveal age changes when protected by humans who keep them as pets or house them in zoos. It would be difficult to explain how evolution could have selected for a process such as aging that could be made to appear in all members of a species after its expression was suppressed over millions of years of evolution.

The only animals among whom a large number of individuals experience significant age changes are humans or the animals we choose to protect. Indeed, biologic aging has been unmasked coincidentally with the recent evolution of the human species. Modern humans, unlike feral animals, have learned how to escape most causes of death not only during early life but long after reproductive success. In so doing, we have unmasked a process that, teleologically, was never intended for us to experience. One might properly conclude therefore that aging is an artifact of civilization.

It is for this reason that the late George Sacher proposed that biogerontologists have been asking the wrong question. Instead of asking "Why do we age?" the right question is "Why do we live as long as we do?" By asking that question we might reorder our thinking and design our experiments in a way in which more fundamental information is obtained.

## Disease and Aging

Another important conceptual distinction is between age changes and disease. Failure to recognize this distinction has not only blurred our understanding of aging but it has had, and is having, profound political and economic consequences.

There is a mistaken belief that an understanding, or even the resolution of, age-associated diseases can advance our knowledge of the fundamental aging processes. This belief is a result of the failure of many biogerontologists, geriatricians, and the public to distinguish between the diseases or pathologies that occur during aging and the aging process itself. There does not seem to be any difficulty for even the general public to distinguish between the diseases that occur during early life or embryogenesis and neonatal or childhood development. Similarly, it should be easy to distinguish between the diseases associated with old age and the aging process. It is not. This distinction is central to an understanding of why the resolution of, for example, Alzheimer's disease, can tell us little if anything about the fundamental biology of age changes. In fact, the resolution of all of the leading causes of death during old age—cardiovascular disease, stroke, cancer—also cannot advance our knowledge of the aging processes. Just as the virtual resolution of poliomyelitis, acute lymphocytic leukemia, Wilms' tumor, and iron deficiency anemia did not increase our knowledge of childhood development, the resolution of age-associated diseases will not advance our knowledge of the aging process.

Changes attributable to disease can be distinguished from age-related changes for at least four important reasons. First, unlike any known disease, age changes occur in every human given sufficient time. Second, unlike disease, age changes cross virtually all species barriers. Third, unlike disease, age changes occur in all members of a species only after the age of reproductive success. Fourth, unlike disease, aging occurs in all animals removed from the wild and protected by humans even when the species has not experienced aging for thousands or even millions of years.

## Policy Impacts

One example of the policy consequences that has resulted from failure to distinguish between research on age-associated diseases and the fundamental biology of age changes is that it is virtually impossible to raise funds for research on aging because in the minds of policymakers and the public no one suffers or dies from aging. The general belief is that we suffer and die from the diseases that occur during the aging process. Yet the diseases associated with old age occur because the underlying age changes increase vulnerability to what ultimately is written on death certificates.

Perhaps the best example of the policy results is the fact that more than 50% of the present budget of the National Institute on Aging in the United States is spent on Alzheimer's disease research. Yet elimination of Alzheimer's disease not only will have little effect on human life expectation, it will not advance our knowledge of the fundamental biology of aging. What we have failed to convey is that greater support must be given to a question that is rarely posed and is applicable to all pathologies and diseases of the elderly. And, it is a question whose resolution can advance our fundamental knowledge of aging. It is this: How do old cells differ from young cells, and why are they more vulnerable to pathology than are young cells?

## Normal Aging and Natural Causes

We frequently talk about aging as "normal aging," but to do so implies that there is a condition of "abnormal" aging. This, of course, is absurd. There are probably tens of thousands of age changes that occur at the molecular and cellular levels that do not compromise health or increase the likelihood of death. For example, no one has ever died of wrinkled skin, gray hair, or menopause.

To carry this argument to its logical conclusion, I would be willing to defend the position that no one over, say, 80 years of age has or will die from what is written on his or her death certificate. All persons over age 80 die from the usual increase in molecular disorder, or age changes, they have lived long enough to incur. Those changes simply have increased their vulnerability to whatever cause of death was written on their death certificates. This statement applies even to most accidental causes of death during old age, where diminished eyesight, hearing, or increased reaction time was the direct cause of the accident.

One must ask from what would we die if all causes of death currently written on death certificates were resolved. After all, that is the goal of biomedical research. Put more starkly, our goals should be to drive the National Institutes of Health and every biomedical research facility, hospital, and medical center out of business and to make our own jobs superfluous. I cannot imagine anyone disagreeing with that goal, although it is rarely discussed.

During the first half of the twentieth century many people died from natural causes. Few die from that cause today. One of the greatest triumphs over a leading cause of death during the twentieth century has become so marginalized that as we enter the twenty-first century no one has asked the obvious question: Who cured "natural causes," and how was it done?

Despite the magnitude of this achievement, I can find nowhere in the scientific literature a description of how "natural causes" were resolved. The extraordinary modesty of the discoverers of the cure if not the etiology of "natural causes" is awesome. The mystery deepens when one considers that this monumental achievement occurred without grant support.

The search for the etiology and resolution of deaths attributable to natural causes is not a silly exercise: It is one of the most important questions that can be asked in biogerontology: If all, or most, causes of death now written on the death certificates of the elderly are resolved, we will be faced with the reality of how death occurs in the absence of disease. The resolution of deaths attributable to the current causes appearing on the death certificates of the elderly will not result in immortality. It will result in the revelation of the true underlying causes of all such deaths. That is, the inexorable loss of physiologic capacity in vital organs that is the hallmark of aging. We must then invent a new vocabulary to describe these newly revealed causes of death.

The term "natural causes" represents a category of deaths attributable to the absence of disease and the presence of overwhelming age changes recognizable as loss in physiologic capacity. I suggest that the resolution of "natural causes" as a leading cause of death occurred because physicians have thought that to write "natural causes" on a death certificate, even when the cause of death is truly unknown, is an admission of ignorance and hence undesirable in an era of presumed scientific enlightenment. Thus in the United States cardiac arrest, stroke, pulmonary infarct, cancer, or some other, unproved cause is thought to be more acceptable professionally than to admit that the cause of death is natural or unknown. Moreover, the actual cause of death is almost always unknown for very old people. The impact of this nonmedically based, sociologically determined phenomenon on the statistics of true causes of death in the United States over the past 50 years can only be a matter of speculation. How much have we been misled to believe that some pathologies recorded as causes of death have increased merely because those causes have come to replace what was formerly called "natural causes"?

The resolution of all causes of death currently written on the death certificates of those over age 65 would result in an increase in life expectation at birth of only about 15 years. What needs to be better understood is that an increase in our knowledge of how age changes occur does not put a 15-year limit on what is possible.

## Reference

1. Hayflick L. How and Why We Age. New York: Ballantine, 1996.

# 1
# Cell and Molecular Aging

Bruce Robert Troen and Vincent Joseph Cristofalo

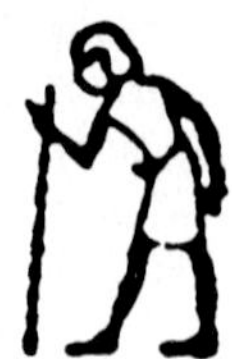

Discussions of aging invariably begin by establishing a satisfactory definition for the term *aging* and the related word *senescence*. Although the term aging is commonly used to refer to postmaturational processes that lead to diminished homeostasis and increased organismic vulnerability, the more correct term here is *senescence*. *Aging* can refer to any time-related process. In this chapter we use *senescence* and *aging* interchangeably. *Normal* aging involves inexorable and universal physiologic changes, whereas *usual* aging includes age-related diseases. For example, menopause and the decline in renal function represent aspects of normal aging. In contrast, coronary artery disease is an example of usual aging and is not found in all older persons. This approach to aging can utilize a conceptual framework that identifies intrinsic (developmental-genetic) versus extrinsic (stochastic) causes. Accumulating evidence increasingly stresses the importance of both. Indeed the altered homeostasis in older organisms is likely the result of a genetic program that determines the response to exogenous influences and thereby increases the predisposition to illness and death.

## Life-Span and Life Expectancy

The *average/median* life-span (also known as life expectancy) is represented by the age at which 50% of a given population survives, and *maximum* life-span potential (MLSP) represents the longest lived member(s) of the population or species. The average life-span of humans has increased dramatically over time, yet the MLSP has remained approximately constant and is usually stated to be 90–100 years (Fig. 1.1).[1] In 1900 the average life expectancy at birth for humans was 47 years; as of 1995 it was 76 years.[2] The longest lived human for whom documentation exists was Jeanne Calment, who died at the age of 122 in August 1997. As causes of early mortality have been eliminated through public health measures and improved medical care, more individuals have approached the maximum life-span. Between 1960 and 1994 the population of those aged 85 and over grew 274%, whereas the elderly population in general rose 100%. The entire U.S. population grew only 45%.[3]

The MLSP appears to be species-specific, implying a significant genetic component in the rate of aging. For example, humans have an MLSP 25- to 30-fold higher than that of mice. Some biodemographic estimates predict that elimination of most of the major killers such as cancer, cardiovascular disease, and diabetes would add no more than 10 years to the average life expectancy and would not affect the MLSP.[4,5] This implies an upper limit to the MLSP. Some models suggest that genes operate by raising or lowering the relative risk of death by making cancer, coronary disease, or Alzheimer's disease more likely, rather than by fixing the life-span. One mathematic model predicts that if participants in the Framingham Heart Study had been able to maintain the levels of 11 risk factors similar to those of a typical 30-year-old, the men and women would have survived to an average age of 99.9 and 97.0 years, respectively.[5]

Three known regimens can extend life-span. The first two involve lowering ambient temperature and reducing exercise; they are effective in poikilotherms (cold-blooded species). A 10°C drop or elimination of a housefly's capacity to fly extends the maximum life-span approximately 250%.[6] Each of these manipulations decreases the metabolic rate and is accompanied by a decrease in free radical generation and oxidative damage to protein and DNA. Dietary restriction without malnutrition can increase both the average and maximum life-spans of mice and rats by more than 50%.[7,8] In some studies, calories were severely restricted (up to 40%), but essential nutrients such as vitamins and minerals were maintained at levels equivalent to those found in ad libitum diets. The diet-restricted animals exhibited a delay in the onset of physiologic and pathologic changes with aging,[9] including hormone and lipid levels, female reproduction, immune function, nephropathy, cardiomyopathy, osteodystrophy, and malignancies. Size, weight, fat percentage, and some organ weights were markedly

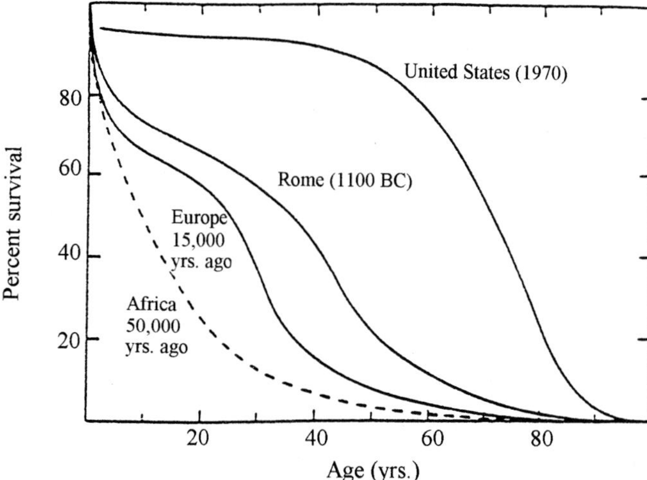


FIGURE 1.1. Human survivorship curve at different periods in history. The age at which 50% of the population is still alive has increased dramatically through time, yet the maximum life-span potential has remained essentially constant. (From Cutler,[1] with permission.)

less in calorically restricted animals.[10] The specific metabolic rate (the amount of oxygen consumed per gram of tissue) decreased in rats subjected to caloric restriction.[11,12] In one study, however, long-term food restriction did not alter the metabolic rate,[13] suggesting that the specific metabolic rate may not be a critical determinant of longevity. To date, the effect of dietary restriction on life-span has been convincingly demonstrated only in rodents. Caloric restriction in rhesus monkeys leads to reductions in body temperature and energy expenditure, consistent with changes seen in rodent studies in which aging is retarded by dietary restriction.[14,15] Calorie restriction also increases high-density lipoprotein[16] and retards the postmaturational decline in serum dehydroepiandrosterone sulfate in rhesus monkeys.[17]

## Characteristics of Aging

Evidence supports at least five common characteristics of aging in mammals.

1. *Increased mortality with age after maturation.* During the early nineteenth century Gompertz first described the exponential increase in mortality with aging due to various causes, a phenomenon that pertains today.[18] In 1995 the death rate for all causes between the ages of 25 and 44 was 189.5/100,000, and for ages 65 and over it was 5069/100,000, a more than 25-fold increase.[19]

2. *Changes in biochemical composition in tissues with age.* There are notable age-related decreases in lean body mass and total bone mass in humans.[20,21] Although the amount of subcutaneous fat remains unchanged or declines, total fat is the same.[21] Consequently, the percentage of adipose tissue increases with age. At the cellular level, many markers of aging have been described in various tissues from different organisms.[22] Two of the first to be described were increases in lipofuscin (age pigment)[23] and increased cross-linking in extracellular matrix molecules such as collagen.[24,25] Additional examples include age-related changes in the rate of transcription of specific genes, the rate of protein synthesis, and numerous age-related alterations in posttranslational protein modifications, such as glycation and oxidation.[26,27]

3. *Progressive decrease in physiologic capacity with age.* Many physiologic changes have been documented in cross-sectional and longitudinal studies. Examples include declines in the glomerular filtration rate, maximal heart rate, and vital capacity.[28] These decreases occur linearly from about the age of 30, however the rate of physiologic decline is heterogeneous from organ to organ and individual to individual.[29,30]

4. *Reduced ability to respond adaptively to environmental stimuli with age.* A fundamental feature of senescence is the diminished ability to maintain homeostasis.[31] It manifests not primarily by changes in resting or basal parameters but by the altered response to an external stimulus such as exercise or fasting. The loss of "reserve" can result in blunted maximum responses and delays in reaching peak levels and in returning to basal levels. For example, induction of hepatic tyrosine aminotransferase activity by fasting is both attenuated and delayed in old rodents.[31]

5. *Increased susceptibility and vulnerability to disease.* The incidence and mortality rates for many diseases increase with age and parallel the exponential increase in mortality with age.[32] For the five leading causes of death of people over age 65, the relative increases in the death rate compared to those for people ages 25–44 are as follows: heart disease, 92-fold; cancer, 43-fold; stroke, more than 100-fold; chronic lung disease, more than 100-fold; and pneumonia and influenza, 89-fold.[19] The basis for these dramatic rises in mortality is incompletely understood but presumably involves changes in the function of many cell types, leading to tissue/organ dysfunction and systemic illness.

## Theories of Aging

In an effort to explain the phenotype of aged organisms, many speculations about the cause(s) of aging have been proposed. What is known about the fundamental molecular mechanisms involved in aging remains controversial and largely unproved. A major reason is the obvious complexity of the problem. Aging changes manifest from the molecular to the organismic level; environmental factors affect experimental observations; secondary effects complicate elucidation of primary mechanisms; and precisely defined, easily measurable "biomarkers" are lacking. No single unifying theory exists, as the mechanisms of aging may be distinct in different organisms, tissues, and cells.

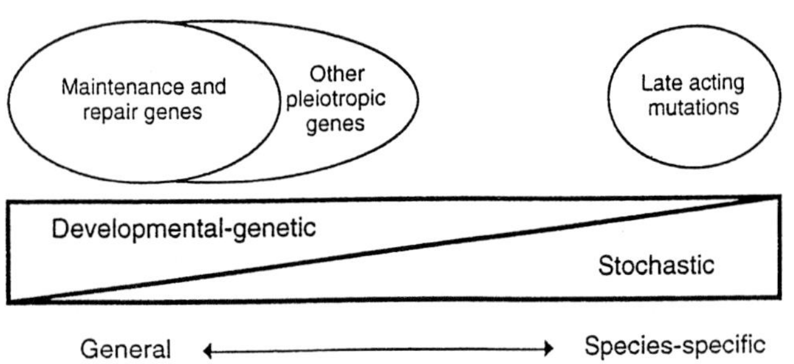


FIGURE 1.2. Genes and events regulating longevity and senescence. (Adapted from Kirkwood.[35])

A general framework for a plausible theory of aging begins with attempting to understand the evolutionary basis of senescence. Evolutionary pressures select for a minimum, successful life, including the ability to reach reproductive age, procreate, and then care for offspring until they are weaned (so they, in turn, will achieve reproductive age and continue the cycle).[33,34] Within this context, it is likely that the postreproductive/parental physiology of an organism is an epigenetic and pleiotropic manifestation of optimization for early fitness. Kirkwood proposed that three categories of genes may be involved in senescence[35]: (1) those that regulate somatic maintenance and repair; (2) negatively pleiotropic genes that enhance early survival but are disadvantageous later in life; and (3) harmful late-acting mutations on which little evolutionary selection is exerted. These genes may represent a spectrum from general to species-specific (Fig. 1.2). Genes involved in cell maintenance and repair are likely to be present in all (or most) organisms, as such essential processes are similar across species. Late-acting mutations are probably species-specific because they are likely to be individualistic and random. Nonmaintenance pleiotropic genes could be found universally within a population or species but may not be shared among species.

Theories of aging have historically been divided into two general categories: stochastic and developmental-genetic. The term "developmental-genetic" implies more active genetic control of senescence than likely exists (see above). In addition, as described below, these categories are not mutually exclusive, particularly when considering the free radical/mitochondrial DNA theory of aging. Indeed, there is likely a spectrum from birth to senescence that reflects a decreasing influence of active genetic influences and an increasing effect of stochastic events (Fig. 1.2). This spectrum would parallel the shift in importance in general versus species-specific genes.

## Stochastic Theories

### Somatic Mutation and DNA Repair

Stochastic theories propose that aging is caused by random damage to vital molecules. The damage eventually accumulates to a level resulting in the physiologic decline associated with aging, The most prominent example is the somatic mutation theory of aging, which states that genetic damage due to background radiation produces mutations that lead to functional failure and ultimately death.[37,38] Exposure to ionizing radiation does shorten the life-span.[39,40] However, analysis of survival curves of radiation-treated rodent populations reveals an increase in the initial mortality rate without an effect on the subsequent rate of aging.[41] Life-span shortening is probably due to the increased incidence of cancer and glomerulosclerosis rather than accelerated aging per se.[42]

The DNA repair theory is a more specific example of the somatic mutation theory. The ability to repair ultraviolet radiation-induced DNA damage in cell cultures derived from species with a variety of life-spans is directly correlated with the maximum life-span potential.[43] Unfortunately, there is not enough experimental support to conclude that these differences between species comprise a causative factor in aging. The cumulative evidence indicates that overall DNA repair capacity does not appear to change with age, although the site-specific repair of select regions of DNA appears to be important in several terminally differentiated cell types.[44] Studies are needed that focus on repair rates of specific genes rather than on indirect general measurements.

### Error-Catastrophe Theory

The error-catastrophe theory proposes that random errors in synthesis eventually occur in proteins that synthesize DNA or other "template" molecules.[45] Generally, errors in proteins are lost by natural turnover, and these molecules are simply replaced with error-free molecules. Error-containing molecules involved in the protein-synthesizing machinery, however, would introduce errors into the molecules they produce. This could result in an amplification such that the subsequent rapid accumulation of error-containing molecules results in an "error-catastrophe" that is incompatible with normal function and life. Although there are numerous reports of altered proteins during aging, no direct evidence of age-dependent protein mis-synthesis has yet been reported. The altered proteins that do occur in aging cells and tissues are, instead, due to posttranslational modifications such as oxidation and glycation.[46,47] The increases in altered proteins appear to be due to decreased clearance in old cells.[48]

### Protein Modification

In addition to age-related changes in the steady-state levels of proteins, qualitative alterations leading to changes in function occur. Aging is accompanied by decreased specific activity in many enzymes, altered heat stability, and increased carbonyl content of proteins.[47] These changes can be caused by direct oxidation of amino acid residues, metal-catalyzed oxidation, modification by lipid oxidation products, and glycation. Kohn[25] and Bjorksten[24] hypothesized that the accumulation of post-translationally altered proteins could impair cellular and, ultimately, organ function. Although collagen undergoes increased cross-linking with age,[49] such alterations can lead to improved function at some sites and impaired function at others.[50] The nonenzymatic reaction of carbohydrates with amino groups of proteins (glycation) can give rise to advanced glycosylation end-products (AGEs).[47] These AGEs increase with aging and are implicated in diabetes, eye disorders, and amyloid accumulation. Many extracellular matrix proteins exhibit increased cross-linking with age. Proper organ function depends on a normal extracellular matrix for processes such as diffusion of essential molecules. In addition, the extracellular matrix plays an important role in the regulation of gene expression. Both these processes could be altered by the cross-linking of macromolecules such as collagen, elastin, osteocalcin, and the eye lens protein crystallin, which may be responsible for cataract formation in both the diabetic and aged lens. These covalent protein–protein interactions likely play a role in the increased stiffness of vascular walls with aging.

### *Free Radical (Oxidative Stress)/Mitochondrial DNA*

Another potential cause of cross-linking—free radicals—forms the basis for a theory that has elements of both stochastic and developmental-genetic classes. Harman initially proposed that most aging changes are due to molecular damage caused by free radicals,[51,52] which are atoms or molecules that contain an unpaired electron and are therefore highly reactive chemical species. Aerobic metabolism generates the superoxide radical ($O_2^-$), which is metabolized by superoxide dismutases to form hydrogen peroxide ($H_2O_2$) and oxygen.[53] Hydrogen peroxide can go on to form the extremely reactive hydroxyl radical ($OH^-$). These oxygen-derived species can react with macromolecules in a self-perpetuating manner; they create free radicals from subsequently attacked molecules, which in turn create free radicals from other molecules, thereby amplifying the effect of the initial free radical attack.[6] Reactive oxygen species appear to play a role in regulating differential gene expression, cell replication, differentiation, and apoptotic cell death (in part by acting as second messengers in signal transduction pathways).[54,55] Production of free radicals in the heart, kidney, and liver of a group of mammals was found to be inversely proportional to the maximum life-span, although the activities of individual antioxidative enzymes were not consistently related to maximum life-span.[56] Overexpression of either superoxide dismutase or catalase alone in transgenic flies does not extend their life-span.[57] Some transgenic flies with increased expression of both Cu,Zn-superoxide dismutase and catalase, which act in tandem to remove $O_2^-$ and $H_2O_2$, respectively, exhibit up to one-third extension of average and maximum life-spans.[57] In addition, there was increased resistance to oxidative damage and an increase in the metabolic potential (total amount of oxygen consumed during adult life per unit body weight).

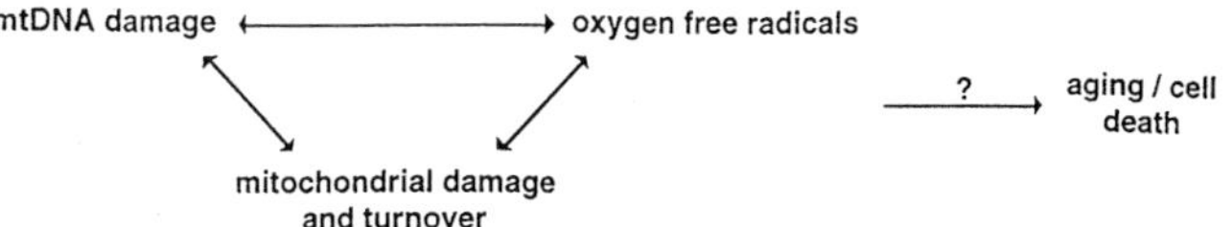


FIGURE 1.3. Mitochondrial DNA and free radical interaction.

The mitochondrial DNA (mtDNA)/oxidative stress hypothesis represents a synthesis of several theories and therefore comprises elements of both stochastic and developmental-genetic mechanisms of aging. It proposes that reactive oxygen species contribute significantly to the somatic accumulation of mtDNA mutations, leading to the gradual loss of bioenergetic capacity and eventually resulting in aging and cell death (Fig. 1.3).[58–60] Ozawa dubbed it the "redox mechanism of mitochondrial aging."[61] mtDNA undergoes a progressive age-related increase in oxygen free radical damage in skeletal muscle,[62–64] diaphragm,[65,66] cardiac muscle,[67–70] and brain.[71,72] This exponential increase in damage correlates with the increase in both point and deletional somatic mtDNA mutations seen with age. Interestingly, extrapolation of the curve to the point where 100% of cardiac mtDNA exhibits deletion mutations points to an age of 129.[61] Deleterious positive feedback results wherein mtDNA damage leads to defective mitochondrial respiration, which in turn enhances oxygen free radical formation, leading to additional mtDNA damage. Mitochondrial DNA is maternally transmitted; it continues to replicate throughout the life-span of an organism in proliferating and postmitotic (nonproliferating) cells and is subject to a much higher mutation rate than nuclear DNA. This is due, in large part, to inefficient repair mechanisms and its proximity to the mitochondrial membrane, where reactive oxygen species are generated. Defects in mitochondrial respiration are found with age not only in normal tissues[73] but also in the presence of diseases that increasingly manifest with age, such as Parkinson's disease,[74,75] Alzheimer's disease,[76,77] Huntington's chorea,[78] and other movement disorders.[79] Diseases for which mtDNA mutations have been found include Alzheimer's disease, Parkinson's disease,[72,80,82–84] and a large number of skeletal and cardiac myopathies.[36,66,85–88] Apoptosis has also been associated with mtDNA fragmentation.[84] Is the phenotype of aging in tissues due to mtDNA mutation? Specific mutations, although increasing with age, seldom account for more than several percent of the total mtDNA. Some studies suggest, however, that the total percentage of mtDNA affected by mutations is much higher, as much as 85%, and increases with age.[61] In addition, caloric restriction in mice retards the age-associated accumulation of mtDNA mutations.[90] Ongoing studies in Utah, utilizing extensive genealogic records of Mormons, are testing the hypothesis that longevity is maternally determined, given the inheritance of only maternal mtDNA.

Agents that bypass blocks in the respiratory chain such as coenzyme Q10, tocopherol, nicotinamide, and ascorbic acid would be predicted to ameliorate some of the effects of mitchondrial disease and aging. To date, results of studies on the treatment of patients with myopathies have been variably or only anecdotally successful.[61] This suggests that a complex interaction exists between prooxidant and antioxidant forces in the cell and that regulation of the balance between the two may be the critical determinant in mitochondrial and subsequently cellular and tissue integrity during aging.

## Developmental-Genetic Theories

Developmental-genetic theories consider the process of aging to be part of the genetically programmed and controlled continuum of development and maturation. Although this notion is attractive, the diverse expression of aging effects is in sharp contrast to the tightly controlled, precise processes of development. Also, evolution selects for the optimization of reproduction; the effects of genes expressed during later life probably do not play a large role in the evolution of a species. This class of theories is supported by the observation that the maximum life-span is highly species-specific. As noted above, the maximum life-span for humans is 30 times that of mice. In addition, studies comparing the longevity of monozygotic and dizygotic twins and nontwin siblings have shown a remarkable similarity between monozygotic twins that is not seen in the other two groups.

### *Longevity Genes*

There is ample evidence from multiple species that MLSP is under genetic control, though the degree of heritability is likely to be less than 35%.[91] Despite this apparently low figure, genetic mutations can significantly modify senescence. In yeast a number of genes affect the average and maximum life-spans.[92] The products of these genes act in diverse ways, including modulating stress response, sensing nutritional status, increasing metabolic capacity, and silencing genes that promote aging. In the nematode, mutants with increased life-spans have revealed various genes that appear to play a role:[93] *age*-1, altered aging rate; *daf*-2 and *daf*-23, activation of a delay in development; *spe*-26, reduced fertility; and *clk*-1, altered biologic clock. These genes alter stress resistance (particularly in response to ultraviolet light), development, signal transduction, and metabolic activity. The *daf*-2 gene has been isolated and appears to encode an insulin receptor family member.[94] Mutations in *daf*-2 can double the life-span but require the *daf*-16 gene.[95] A mutation in the *daf*-16 gene suppresses resistance to ultraviolet (UV) rays and increased longevity of the other gene mutants, suggesting that it acts at a critical point downstream of the other genes.[93] The *daf*-16 gene is a member of the hepatocyte nuclear factor-3/forkhead family of transcriptional regulators involved in a variety of signal transduction pathways, including insulin signaling.[96] Houseflies have been bred for longevity; but unlike yeast and nematodes, effects of single genes are difficult to find.[97] One group of long-lived flies is more resistant to oxidative stress,[98] whereas another group exhibits resistance to starvation and desiccation.[99] Genetic analysis of longevity in mammals has not been as revealing, although, immune loci in mice and humans have been implicated in long-lived subjects.[92] The epsilon 4 allele of apolipoprotein E (ApoE), which is associated with increased coronary disease and Alzheimer's disease, is inversely correlated with longevity.[100] In contrast, the epsilon 2 allele of ApoE and an angiotensin-converting enzyme (ACE) allele are found more frequently in French centenarians.[100] Interestingly, the ApoE2 allele is associated with type III and IV hyperlipidemia, and the ACE allele predisposes to coronary disease. These findings suggest that genes can exert pleiotropic age-dependent effects on longevity. They also again raise the question as to whether these genes affect susceptibility to disease rather than alter intrinsic aging.

### *Accelerated Aging Syndromes*

Although no genetic disease is an exact phenocopy of normal aging, several human genetic diseases, including Hutchinson-Guilford syndrome (the "classic" early-onset progeria seen in children), Werner syndrome ("adult" progeria), and Down syndrome (trisomy 21), display some features of accelerated aging.[101]

Werner syndrome (WS) is an autosomally recessive inherited disease.[102] Patients prematurely develop arteriosclerosis, glucose intolerance, osteoporosis, early graying, hair loss, skin atrophy, and menopause. The patients do not typically suffer from Alzheimer's disease or hypertension. WS patients have an increased incidence of sarcomatous tumors and develop cataracts in the posterior surface of the lens, not in the nucleus as is usually seen in old people. In addition, they develop laryngeal atrophy and ulcerations on the arms and legs. Most patients die before age 50. The gene responsible for WS has been localized to chromosome 8[103] and appears to be a helicase,[104] an enzyme involved in unwinding DNA. DNA helicases play a role in DNA replication and repair. Cells from WS patients display chromosomal instability, elevated rates of gene mutation, and nonhomologous recombination. However, there is no obvious defect in DNA repair mechanisms as evidenced by resistance to UV exposure or other DNA-damaging agents, similar to normal cells.

Hutchinson-Guilford syndrome is an extremely rare autosomal recessive disease in which aging characteristics begin to develop within several years of birth,[102] including wrinkled skin, stooped posture, and growth retardation. Progeria patients suffer from advanced atherosclerosis, and myocardial infarction is the usual cause of death by the age of 30. However, unlike those with WS, these patients do not typically suffer from cataracts, glucose intolerance, or skin ulcers.

People with Down syndrome have trisomy or a translocation involving chromosome 21.[101,102] They suffer from the early onset of vascular disease, glucose intolerance, hair loss, degenerative bone and joint disease, and increased cancer. The life-span is apparently 50–70 years (not as short as previously believed, as earlier mortality may have represented neglect of these individuals). Dementia occurs earlier and more often in patients with Down syndrome than in the general population. Patients develop neuropathologic changes similar to the changes seen with dementia of Alzheimer's type, including amyloid deposition and neurofibrillary tangles. This may be related to the presence of the β-amyloid gene on chromosome 21.

## Neuroendocrine Theory

The neuroendocrine theory proposes that functional decrements in neurons and their associated hormones are central to the aging process.[105] An important version of this theory holds that the hypothalamic-pituitary-adrenal (HPA) axis is the master regulator of aging in the organism. Because the neuroendocrine system regulates early development, growth, puberty, control of the reproductive system, metabolism, and many other aspects of normal physiology, functional changes in this system could exert effects throughout the organism. The decline in female reproductive capacity is an obvious neuroendocrine age-related change. Mounting evidence suggests that the ovary and the brain play key roles in menopause (rather than the previously held view of ovarian exhaustion).[106] The neuroendocrine theory of aging is supported by experiments showing that hypophesectomy, followed by replacement of known hormones, maintains (and may extend) the life-span of rodents.[107] In addition, reductions in brain dopaminergic neurotransmission are more prominent in a shorter-lived rat strain.[108] Levodopa, a dopaminergic drug, can prolong the mean life-span of mice.[109] Treatment of rats with deprenyl facilitates activity of the nigrostriatal dopaminergic neurons and protects these neurons from age-related decay.[110] Deprenyl also increases the average and maximum life-spans.[111,112] Many human studies have demonstrated gradually decreasing levels of peripheral hormones accompanied by normal levels of trophic hormones.[105] This finding suggests either an increased response to peripheral hormones by the HPA axis or inappropriately low expression of the stimulating hormone. Many organisms with aging phenotypes similar to those of higher vertebrates lack complex neuroendocrine systems. The changes that occur in the neuroendocrine system may be due to fundamental age-related changes in all cells and are therefore secondary manifestations of the aging phenotype.

## Intrinsic Mutagenesis Theory

The intrinsic mutagenesis theory advocated by Burnet attempts to reconcile stochastic theories of aging with the genetic regulation of maximum life-span by proposing that each species is endowed with a specific genetic constitution that regulates the fidelity of the DNA and its replication.[113] The degree of fidelity controls the appearance of mutations and thus the life-span. At present, there is little experimental support for this theory.

## Immunologic Theory

The immunologic theory of aging is based on two main observations: (1) The functional capacity of the immune system declines with age, as evidenced by a decreased response of T cells to mitogens and reduced resistance to infectious disease; and (2) autoimmune phenomena increase with age, such as an increase in serum autoantibodies.[114] There is a shift to increasing proportions of memory T cells accompanied by enhanced expression of the multidrug-resistance p-glycoprotein.[115] Humoral (B cell-mediated) immunity also declines with age, as evidenced by decreased antibody production and a disproportionate loss of the ability to produce high affinity immunoglotulin G (IgG) and IgA antibodies. In addition, differences in the MLSP of various strains of mice have been related to specific alleles in the major histocompatibility gene complex.[116] The genes in this region also contribute to the regulation of mixed-function oxidases (P-450 system), DNA repair, and free radical scavenging enzymes. Although the immune system obviously plays a central role in health maintenance and survival throughout the life-span, similar criticisms can be directed at the immunologic theory and the neuroendocrine theory. Complex immune systems are not present in organisms that share aspects of aging with higher organisms. In addition, the inability to distinguish between fundamental changes in many cells and tissues, not just those of the immune system, and the secondary effects mediated by the aging-altered immune system make interpretation of the theory difficult. Proposed mechanistic studies of the immune theory include producing transgenic mice carrying the histocompatibility complex from a longer-lived rodent species to determine the effects on disease incidence and life-span.

## Cellular Senescence

The complexity of studying aging in organisms has led to the use of well-defined cell culture systems as models for cellular aging or senescence. Hayflick and Moorhead[117] pioneered the model of replicative senescence and identified normal human diploid fibroblasts in culture as a model for aging by observing an initial period of rapid, vigorous proliferation invariably followed by a decline in growth rate and proliferative activity and finally a cessation of proliferation. This model proposed that aging is a cellular and an organismic phenomenon, and that the loss of functional capacity of the individual reflects the summation of the loss of critical functional capacities of individual cells. It is important to note that populations of senescent cells do not necessarily die; they can be maintained in culture for years in a postmitotic (nonproliferating) state with regular changes of culture medium.[118–120] The loss of proliferative capacity of human cells in culture is intrinsic to the cells and not dependent on environmental or culture conditions.[117] In addition, senescence is inevitable unless the cells undergo transformation and acquire a constellation of abnormal characteristics, such as multiple chromosomal abnormalities, genetic mutations, and changes in morphology and growth rate. The number of times the cells divide is also more important in determining proliferative life-span than the actual time the cells spend in culture.[121] Cells continuously passaged in culture until the end of their proliferative life-span achieve approximately the same number of population doublings as cells that are held in a stationary phase for an extended period (months) and then recultured until senescence. The cells therefore seem to have an intrinsic mechanism that "counts" the number of divisions and not the time that passes.

In addition to studies on fibroblasts, limited in vitro life-span has been reported for glial cells,[122] keratinocytes,[123] vascular smooth muscle cells,[124] lens cells,[125] endothelial cells,[126] and lymphocytes.[127] In vivo serial transplants of normal somatic tissues, such as skin and breast, from old donor mice to young genetically identical recipients show a decline in proliferative activity and eventual failure of the graft.[128] Similarly, skin from old donors retained an increased susceptibility to carcinogens whether transplanted to young or old recipients.[129] Do changes in cells in culture parallel changes in cells from aging organisms? The replicative life-span of fibroblasts in culture is inversely related to the maximum life-span of several diverse vertebrate species, as shown in Figure 1.4.[136] Studies suggest that the replicative life-span of cells in culture is inversely related to the age of the donor in both humans and rodents.[131–133] This in vivo/in vitro relation holds for several cell types, including

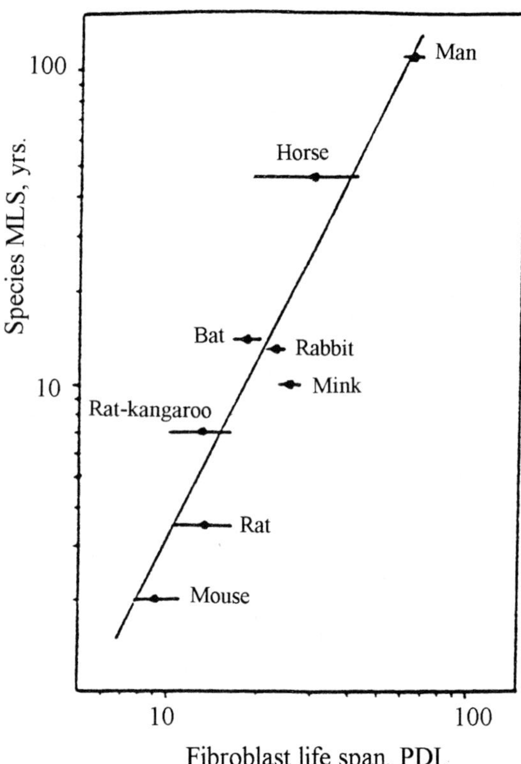


FIGURE 1.4. Correlation between fibroblast population doubling capacity and species maximum life-span potential. Fibroblasts derived from longer-lived species are able to undergo more cell divisions before senescence than cells derived from shorter-lived species. (From Rhome,[130] with permission.)

hepatocytes,[134] keratinocytes,[135] and arterial smooth muscle cells.[124] However, there is a great deal of variability in these cross-sectional studies; and the correlation coefficient, though statistically significant, is low. Cells cultured from healthy individuals do not appear to exhibit a consistent age-related proliferative capacity.[136] Cells from people with Werner syndrome do senesce more rapidly in culture than those from age-matched controls, although a consistently similar relation does not hold for cells from those with Hutchinson-Guilford syndrome.[102] Thus under some circumstances the in vivo proliferative characteristics of cells during aging are maintained in culture. Unfortunately, convincing evidence that senescent cells accumulate with age in vivo is lacking to date. A potential biomarker for aging, β-galactosidase, has been described that initially seemed to distinguish between senescent cells and either presenescent or quiescent cells.[137] However, subsequent data indicate that in situ expression of β-galactosidase exists in confluent quiescent presenescent cells and is not necessarily specific for senescence (e.g., possibly lysosomal damage) rather than senescence per se.[137a] Rubin proposed that the in vitro limit on replication is an artifact that reflects the cells' traumatic response to establishment in vitro and their subsequent maintenance in a foreign environment that is starkly different from their in vivo milieu.[138] He suggested that a decline in the *rate* of cellular proliferation more accurately correlates with aging in animals.

A major approach to studying regulation of cessation of replication in senescent cells has been to examine pathways at various levels that likely play significant roles in regulating cell proliferation and adaptive responses. Senescent cells are often less responsive to mitogens but can exhibit variable changes in growth factor and growth factor receptor expression compared to young cells. During senescence the Wistar-38 (WI-38) diploid fibroblast cell line displays a progressive loss of mitogenic response to platelet-derived growth factor (PDGF), epidermal growth factor (EGF), insulin, and dexamethasone[139] despite no change in the number and affinity of receptors for PDGF and EGF.[140,141] However, fibroblasts from a patient with Werner syndrome exhibit reduced PDGF receptors.[142] An altered form of the EGF receptor is present in extracts from senescent, but not young, cells.[143] Insulin-like growth factor-1 (IGF-1), in combination with other growth factors, can stimulate DNA synthesis and mitosis in young cells but cannot elicit such a response in senescent fibroblasts.[144] However, both young and senescent fibroblasts in culture express the IGF-1 receptors, which can be bound and activated by IGF-1.[144,145] In addition, senescent fibroblasts do not express the insulin-like growth factor-1 (IGF-1) gene.[146] Multiple other differentially expressed genes are found when comparing quiescent young to senescent fibroblasts or when comparing Werner syndrome fibroblasts to normal fibroblasts.[147–149] They include known transcripts such as procollagen, fibronectin, IGF binding protein-3, osteonectin, tissue plasminogen activator inhibitor type I, and thrombospondin in addition to transcripts with novel identities. Genes expressed predominantly in young quiescent cells include human *twist*, a transcription factor and EPC-1 (early population doubling cDNA-1), which is identical to the pigmented epithelial-derived factor and is related to a family of serine protease inhibitors.[147,150] The constitutive expression of interleukin-6 (IL-6) and its stimulation by serum, double-stranded RNA, and phorbol ester are diminished in senescent cells.[151] In contrast, forskolin elicits similar stimulation of IL-6 expression in both young and senescent cells.

Inducibility of the c-*fos* proto-oncogene by serum is repressed in late-passage senescent cells[152] and can be partially restored by pretreatment with phorbol ester.[153] Transient transfection of senescent cells with the c-*fos* gene increases by as much as sixfold the number of cells capable of initiating DNA synthesis,[154] although microinjection of the Harvey *ras* oncogenic protein leading to elevated c-*fos* did not enhance DNA synthesis.[155] In contrast, induction of c-*fos* expression in senescent fibroblasts from donors with Werner syndrome is similar to that in young cells.[156] Other studies also suggest that cellular senescence proceeds independent of c-*fos* suppression.[157,158] Expression of c-*ras* and c-*myc* proto-oncogenes is also diminished in senescent fibroblasts.[159,160]

Senescence-related alterations in signal transduction pathways and nuclear transcription factors have been documented. Arachidonic acid and prostaglandins are increased in late-passage human fibroblasts.[161] Extracellular calcium elicits less of a response (increased saturation density) in fibroblasts obtained from old donors than in cells from young donors.[162] Despite the absence of senescence-related changes in resting intracellular calcium levels and cytosolic calcium fluxes following growth factor stimulation,[163] calcium influx after bradykinin stimulation is reduced in senescent WI-38 cells.[164] Senescent cells contain normal or increased amounts of protein kinase A and protein kinase C (PKC).[165] Translocation of PKC following mitogen stimulation[153] and substrate phosphorylation by PKC[166] are decreased in senescent cells. Senescent cells exhibit decreased binding of nuclear transcription factors such as c-*fos*/AP-1, CREBP1 (cyclic AMP response element binding protein), ID1 (inhibitor of DNA binding 1), and ID2.[167,168] Levels of ceramide, a lipid second messenger derived from membrane sphingomyelin, are elevated in senescent fibroblasts.[169] In addition, exogenous ceramide induces a senescent phenotype, apparently via dephosphorylation of the retinoblastoma protein (see below).[170] Such findings indicate that senescent cells exist in a growth state that is quite distinct from that of young cells and hints at the complex alteration in cellular physiology during senescence.

The phenomenon of telomere shortening with aging represents a potential "clock" or counting mechanism for senescent cells.[171] Telomeres are structures at the end of chromosomes that prevent degradation and fusion with other chromosome ends.[172] The average length of the terminal restriction fragment of chromosomes decreases with both in vitro and in vivo aging of fibroblasts and peripheral blood lymphocytes.[171,173–177] Immortalized and transformed cells and germline cells express telomerase, which prevents shortening of the telomeres.[178,179] Some immortal cells do exist without detectable telomerase;[180] stem cells and some normal somatic cells express telomerase, yet continue to experience telomeric shortening.[181–183] These data suggest that the length of the telomeres per se, rather than the degree of telomerase activity, is the more important factor in cellular senescence. Experimental nonenzymatic elongation of telomeres extends the life-span of cells.[184] Furthermore, reactivation of telomerase, via introduction of the telomerase reverse transcriptase unit into normal human cells, increases telomere length and extends the life-span of both retinal epithelial cells and foreskin fibroblasts.[185] Cells that had exceeded their normal life-span by 20 population doublings exhibited normal karyotype and morphology, similar to their younger counterparts. The consequences of the absence of telomerase has been studied in the telomerase knockout mouse.[185a] Age-dependent telomere shortening in subsequent generations of mice is associated with a decreased life-span and a reduced homeostatic capacity in response to wound healing and hematopoietic ablation. Interestingly, telomerase null mice suffered an increase in spontaneous malignancies. This suggests that actions (or inaction) of telomerase at different stages in the life-span lead to pleiotropic effects.

Compelling evidence in support of a genetic basis for in vitro aging has been the finding that introduction of particular chromosomes into immortalized cells induces a senescent phenotype, including chromosomes 1,[186,187] 2,[188] 3,[189,190] 4,[191] 6,[192] 7,[193–195] 18,[196] and X.[197] Restoration of senescence by the introduction of chromosomes 3[190] and 7[193] resulted in loss of telomeric sequences via loss of telomerase (chromosome 3) and independent of effects on telomerase (chromosome 7). Cell fusion studies with immortal cells demonstrated four complementation groups, suggesting that at least four genes or gene pathways contribute to senescence, and that immortality results from recessive defects.[198,199] Chromosomes 1, 4, and 7 appear to contain senescence-related genes that segregate into three of these complementation groups, although, Ryan et al. were unable to obtain finite life-span hybrids via complementation with immortal cell lines.[200]

Products of the retinoblastoma (*Rb*) and *p53* tumor suppressor genes have also been implicated in replicative senescence.[201,202] Although similar levels of p53 are expressed in young and old cells in vitro, both DNA binding and transcriptional activity are increased in senescent cells.[203] The Rb gene product is not phosphorylated in senescent cells.[204] Simian virus 40 large T antigen, which is bound by the *p53* and *Rb* gene products, can facilitate escape from senescence.[205] T-antigen deletion mutants that lack either Rb or p53 binding domains are unable to mediate escape from senescence.[206] Furthermore, treatment with antisense oligonucleotides to the *Rb* and *p53* tumor suppressor genes can extend the in vitro life-span of human fibroblasts.[207] The p21[208–210] and p16[211–213] inhibitors of cyclin kinases (and therefore cell cycle progression) are overexpressed in senescent cells. The p21 protein appears to act by forming complexes with members of the family of E2F transcription factors in senescent cells (Rb/CDK2/cyclin E or with the Rb-related p107/CDK2/cyclin D), downregulating transcriptional activity and thereby inhibiting progression through the cell cycle.[208] Targeted disruption of the *p21* gene delays the onset of senescence in fibroblasts derived from human lung.[214] However, adrenocortical cells express high levels of p21 protein throughout their in vitro life-span, up to and including senescence.[215] Skin fibroblasts from patients with Li-Fraumeni syndrome are heterozygous for *p53*. These cells in culture lose the remaining *p53* allele and are subsequently unable to express p21, but still undergo in vitro aging,[216] suggesting that p53 and p21 are not required for senescence. In senescent cells, p16 complexes to and inhibits both the CDK4 and CDK6 cell cycle kinases.[211] The *ras* oncogene product can induce senescence accompanied by accumulation of p53 and p16.[217] This occurs only in nonimmortalized cells and may reflect a homeostatic response of the cell to a transforming stimulus. Induction of expression of p16 by demethylation-dependent pathways or of p21 by demethylation-independent pathways can induce senescence in immortal fibroblasts that do not express *p53*.[218] Of genes whose expression is required for $G_1$/S cell cycle progression, senescent fibroblasts express no cdk2 or cyclin A and reduced amounts of the $G_1$ cyclins C, D1, and E compared to young cells.[219] The expression of early $G_1$ markers, but not late $G_1$ markers, indicates that senescent cells may be blocked at a point during late $G_1$. These observations emphasize the presence of complex, incompletely understood overlapping networks regulating cell cycle progression and proliferation. Depending on the balance of positive and negative influences, cell proliferation can continue or senescence may ensue. These data are consistent with the theory that cellular senescence evolved as a mechanism of tumor suppression and that aging is a pleiotropic manifestation of evolutionary pressures to prevent malignant transformation.

## Cell Death

There are two distinct patterns of cell death: necrosis and apoptosis. Massive cell injury, often accompanied by inflammation, can lead to necrosis. Necrosis is essentially accidental and entails clumping of chromatin into ill-defined masses, swelling of organelles, and ultimately membrane and cell disintegration.[220] In contrast, apoptosis is an active gene-directed suicide in response to external or internal stimuli, usually in the absence of significant external injury.[220] In most circumstances, apoptosis is an important component that allows the organism to maintain homeostasis. Apoptosis initially involves compaction and segregation of chromatin adjacent to the nuclear membrane and condensation of the cytoplasm. The process progresses rapidly to nuclear/cellular pedunculation and fragmentation. The membrane-bound apoptotic bodies are then phagocytosed by adjacent cells. Although the terms "programmed cell death" and "apoptosis" are often used interchangeably, they are not synonymous. Lockshin and Zakeri[220] stressed that programmed cell death is a developmental event, whereas apoptosis is a mode of cell death. Programmed cell death often involves lysosomal enzyme increases and rarely exhibits the laddering of DNA seen during apoptosis. It is likely that programmed cell death is a type of apoptotic (controlled) cell death. Understanding the genetic basis of apoptosis initially depended on work conducted in the nematode *Caenorhabditis elegans*, which has been a useful model system because the developmental fate of every cell has been determined;[221] of the 1090 formed, 131 eventually die. Three genes (*ced-3, ced-4, ced-9*) play an important role in cell death in the nematode.[222,223] The *ced-3* gene is required for apoptosis in *C. elegans;* mammalian homologues include cysteine proteinases (ICE, CPP32, ICH-1).[224] The *ced-9* gene blocks apoptosis; mammalian homologues include *bcl-2* and *bcl-*$X_L$.[222] The *bcl-2* gene was originally identified as an oncogene because of its overexpression in a form of B cell lymphoma. Additional mammalian homologues of *bcl-2* that promote apoptosis include *bax, bad,* and *bak.*[225] The *bcl* gene family members can form homodimers or heterodimers, permitting a fine degree of control over cell survival. Heterodimerization with either *bcl-2* or *bcl-*$X_L$ prevents cell death.

Research is ongoing to elucidate the possible role of apoptosis in aging and diseases associated with aging. If cells are unable to repair DNA damage, apoptosis may ensue followed by replacement via division of another cell. Senescent fibroblasts in culture are resistant to apoptotic signals, being unable to downregulate *bcl-2* expression.[226] This raises the possibility that damaged senescent cells accumulate with increased organismal age, potentially compromising tissue function. Caloric restriction in rodents upregulates apoptosis in the liver via removal of preneoplastic cells.[227,228] Warner et al. suggested that this may counteract the diminished apoptosis during aging and explain life extension induced by caloric restriction.[229] Apoptosis plays a critical role in the immune system, where as many as 95% of T lymphocytes undergo cell death (presumably because they recognize self-antigens).[230] Lymphocyte apoptosis is mediated by a cell surface receptor, Fas. Mice lacking Fas exhibit increased autoimmune disease and are short-lived. Caloric restriction in such mice increases T lymphocyte apoptosis and extends the life-span.[231] Fas expression decreases in old mice, and transgenic overexpression maintains Fas-induced apoptosis.[232] Cell death is characteristic of a number of neurodegenerative diseases common in aging.[233] Specific neuronal loss is seen with Alzheimer's disease (hippocampus and cortex), Parkinson's disease (substantia nigra), Huntington's disease (striatum), and amyotrophic lateral sclerosis (motor neurons). β-Amyloid protein is cytotoxic to cultured neuronal cells, which then undergo apoptosis.

## References


1. Cutler RG. Evolutionary persective of human longevity. In: Hazzard WR, Andres R, Bierman EL, et al. (eds) Principles of Geriatric Medicine and Gerontology. McGraw-Hill, New York, 1985:16.
2. National Center for Health Statistics, Hyattsville, MD, 1997.
3. Bureau of the Census. Sixty-five Plus in the United States. Statistical Brief 95, 1995.
4. Greville TN, Bayo F, Foster R. United States Life Tables of Causes of Death: 1960–71, vol. 1, no. 5. Technical report.
5. Roush W. Live long and prosper? Science 1996;273:42–46.
6. Sohal RS, Weindruch R. Oxidative stress, caloric restriction, and aging. Science 1996;273:59–63.
7. Weindruch R, Walford RL. Dietary restriction in mice beginning at 1 year of age: effect on life-span and spontaneous cancer incidence. Science 1982;215:1415–1418.
8. Yu BP, Masoro EJ, McMahan CA. Nutritional influences on aging of Fischer 344 rats. I. Physical, metabolic, and longevity characteristics. J Gerontol 1985;40:657–670.
9. Masoro EJ. Dietary restriction and aging. J Am Geriatr Soc 1993;41:994–999.
10. Weindruch R, Sohal RS. Seminars in medicine of the Beth Israel Deaconess Medical Center: caloric intake and aging. N Engl J Med 1997;337:986–994.
11. Dulloo AG, Girardier L. 24-Hour energy expenditure several months after weight loss in the underfed rat: evidence for a chronic increase in whole-body metabolic efficiency. J Obestet Relat Metab Disord 1993;17:115–123.
12. Gonzales-Pacheco DM, Buss WC, Koehler KM, Woodside WF, Alpert SS. Energy restriction reduces metabolic rate in adult male Fisher-344 rats. J Nutr 1993;123:90–97.
13. McCarter R, Masoro EJ, Yu BP. Does food restriction retard aging by reducing the metabolic rate? Am J Physiol 1985;248:E488–E490.
14. Lane MA, Baer DJ, Rumpler WV, et al. Calorie restriction lowers body temperature in rhesus monkeys, consistent with a postulated anti-aging mechanism in rodents. Proc Natl Sci USA 1996;93:4159–4164.
15. Ramsey JJ, Roecker EB, Weindruch R, Kemnitz JW. Energy expenditure of adult male rhesus monkeys during the first 30 months of dietary restriction. Am J Physiol 1997;272:E901–E907.
16. Verdery RB, Ingram DK, Roth GS, Lane MA. Caloric restriction increases HDL2 levels in rhesus monkeys (Macaca mulatta). Am J Physiol 1997;273:E714–E719.
17. Lane MA, Ingram DK, Ball SS, Roth GS. Dehydroepiandrosterone sulfate: a biomarker of primate aging slowed by calorie restriction. J Clin Endocrinol Metab 1997;82:2093–2096.
18. Gompertz B. On the nature of the function expressive of the law of human mortality and a new mode of determining life contingencies. Philos Trans R Soc Lond 1825;115:513.
19. Rosenberg HM, Ventura SJ, Maurer JD, et al. Births and deaths: United States, 1995. Monthly Vital Stat Res 1996;45:31–33.
20. Riggs BL, Melton LD. Involutional osteoporosis. N Engl J Med 1986;314:1676–1686.
21. Shock NW, Greulich RC, Andres R, et al. Normal Human Aging: The Baltimore Longitudinal Study of Aging. U.S. Department of Human Services, Washington, DC, 1984.
22. Florini JR. Composition and function of cells and tissues. In: Handbook of Biolochemistry in Aging. CRC Press, Boca Raton, 1981.
23. Strehler BL. In: Time, Cells, and Aging. Academic, San Diego, 1977.

24. Bjorksten J. Cross linkage and the aging process. In: Rothstein M (ed) Theoretical Aspects of Aging. Academic, San Diego, 1974:43.
25. Kohn RR. Aging of animals: possible mechanisms. In: Principles of Mammalian Aging. Prentice-Hall, Englewood Cliffs, NJ, 1978.
26. Finch CE. Introduction: definitions and concepts. In: Longevity, Senescence, and the Genome. University of Chicago Press, Chicago, 1990.
27. Schneider EL, Rowe JW. Handbook of the Biology of Aging. Academic Press, San Diego, CA, 92101.
28. Shock NW. Longitudinal studies of aging in humans. In: Finch CE, Schneider EL (eds) Handbook of the Biology of Aging. Van Nostrand Reinhold, New York, 1985:721.
29. Lakatta EG. Changes in cardiovascular function with aging. Eur Heart J 1990;11(suppl C):22–29.
30. Lindeman RD, Tobin J, Shock NW. Longitudinal studies on the rate of decline in renal function with age. J Am Geriatr Soc 1985;33:278–285.
31. Adelman RC, Britton GW, Rotenberg S, et al. Endocrine regulation of gene activity in aging animals of different genotypes. In: Bergsma D, Harrison DE (eds) Genetic Effects on Aging. Liss, New York, 1978:355.
32. Brody JA, Brock DB. Epidemiological and statistical characteristics of the United States elderly population. In: Finch CE, Schneider EL (eds) Handbook of the Biology of Aging. Van Nostrand Reinhold, New York, 1985:3.
33. Rose MR, Graves JL Jr. What evolutionary biology can do for gerontology. J Gerontol 1989;44:1327–1329.
34. Kirkwood TB, Rose MR. Evolution of senescence: late survival sacrificed for reproduction. Philos Trans R Soc Lond B Biol Sci 1991;332:15–24.
35. Kirkwood TB. Human senescence. Bioessays 1996;18: 1009–1016.
36. Katsumata K, Hayakawa M, Tanaka M, Sugiyama S, Ozawa T. Fragmentation of human heart mitochondrial DNA associated with premature aging. Biochem Biophys Res Commun 1994;202:102–110.
37. Failla G. The aging process and carcinogenesis. Ann NY Acad Sci 1958;71:1124.
38. Szilard L. On the nature of the aging process. Proc Natl Acad Sci USA 1959;45:30.
39. Casarett GW. Concept and criteria of radiologic ageing. In: Harris RJ (ed) Cellular Basis and Aetiology of Late Somatic Effects of Ionizing Radiation. Academic, San Diego, 1963:189.
40. Walburg HE. Radiation-induced life-shortening and premature aging. Adv Radiat Biol 1975;5:145.
41. Sacher CA. Life table modification and life prolongation. In: Finch CE, Hayflick L (eds) Handbook of the Biology of Aging. Van Nostrand Reinhold, New York, 1977:582.
42. Lindop PJ, Rotblat J. Long-term effect of a single whole-body exposure of mice to ionizing radiations. Proc R Soc Lond 1961;154:350.
43. Hart RW, Setlow RB. Correlation between deoxyribonucleic acid excision—repair and life-span in a number of mammalian species. Proc Natl Acad Sci USA 1974;71:2169–2173.
44. Hanawalt PC, Gee P, Ho L. DNA repair in differentiating cells in relation to aging. In: Finch CE, Johnson TE (eds) Modecular Biology of Aging. UCLA Symposia on Molecular and Cellular Biology. Liss, New York, 1990:45.
45. Orgel LE. The maintenance of the accuracy of protein synthesis and its relevance to aging. Proc Natl Acad Sci USA 1963;49:517.
46. Kristal BS, Yu BP. An emerging hypothesis: synergistic induction of aging by free radicals and Maillard reactions. J Gerontol 1992;47:B107–B114.
47. Levine RL, Stadtman ER. Protein modifications with aging. In: Schneider EL, Rowe JW (eds) Handbook of the Biology of Aging. Academic, San Diego, 1996:184–197.
48. Gracy RW, Yuksel KU, Chapman MD, et al. Impaired protein degradation may account for the accumulation of "abnormal" proteins in aging cells. In: Adelman RC, Dekker EE (eds) Modern Aging Research, Modification of Proteins During Aging. Liss, New York, 1985.
49. Reiser KM, Hennessy SM, Last JA. Analysis of age-associated changes in collagen crosslinking in the skin and lung in monkeys and rats. Biochim Biophys Acta 1987;926:339–348.
50. Hall DA. Chemical and biochemical changes in aging connective tissues. In: The Aging of Connective Tissue. Academic, San Diego, 1976.
51. Harman D. Aging: a theory based on free radical and radiation chemistry. J Gerontol 1956;11:298.
52. Harman D. The aging process. Proc Natl Acad Sci USA 1981;78:7124–7128.
53. Fridovich I. Superoxide dismutases: an adaptation to a paramagnetic gas. J Biol Chem 1989;264:7761–7764.
54. Sen CK, Packer L. Antioxidant and redox regulation of gene transcription. FASEB J 1996;10:709–720.
55. Suzuki YJ, Forman HJ, Sevanian A. Oxidants as stimulators of signal transduction. Free Radic Biol Med 1997;22:269–285.
56. Sohal RS, Svensson I, Sohal BH, Brunk UT. Superoxide anion radical production in different animal species. Mech Ageing Dev 1989;49:129–135.
57. Orr WC, Sohal RS. Extension of life-span by overexpression of superoxide dismutase and catalase in Drosophila melanogaster. Science 1994;263:1128–1130.
58. Fleming JE, Miquel J, Cottrell SF, Yengoyan LS, Economos AC. Is cell aging caused by respiration-dependent injury to the mitochondrial genome? Gerontology 1982;28:44–53.
59. Linnane AW, Zhang C, Baumer A, Nagley P. Mitochondrial DNA mutation and the ageing process: bioenergy and pharmacological intervention. Mutat Res 1992;275: 195–208.
60. Wallace DC. Mitochondrial genetics: a paradigm for aging and degenerative diseases? Science 1992;256:628–632.
61. Ozawa T. Genetic and functional changes in mitochondria associated with aging. Physiol Rev 1997;77:425–464.
62. Katayama M, Tanaka M, Yamamoto H, Ohbayashi T, Nimura Y, Ozawa T. Deleted mitochondrial DNA in the skeletal muscle of aged individuals. Biochem Int 1991;25:47–56.
63. Lee CM, Chung SS, Kaczkowski JM, Weindruch R, Aiken JM. Multiple mitochondrial DNA deletions associated with age in skeletal muscle of rhesus monkeys. J Gerontol 1993;48:B201–B205.
64. Melov S, Shoffner JM, Kaufman A, Wallace DC. Marked increase in the number and variety of mitochondrial

DNA rearrangements in aging human skeletal muscle. Nucleic Acids Res 1995;23:4122–4126. Erratum Nucleic Acids Res 1995;23:493–498.

65. Hayakawa M, Torii K, Sugiyama S, Tanaka M, Ozawa T. Age-associated accumulation of 8-hydroxydeoxyguanosine in mitochondrial DNA of human diaphragm. Biochem Biophys Res Commun 1991;179:1023–1029.
66. Torii K, Sugiyama S, Tanaka M, et al. Aging-associated deletions of human diaphragmatic mitochondrial DNA. Am J Respir Cell Mol Biol 1992;6:543–549.
67. Hayakawa M, Hattori K, Sugiyama S, Ozawa T. Age-associated oxygen damage and mutations in mitochondrial DNA in human hearts. Biochem Biophys Res Commun 1992;189:979–985.
68. Hayakawa M, Katsumata K, Yoneda M, Tanaka M, Sugiyama S, Ozawa T. Age-related extensive fragmentation of mitochondrial DNA into minicircles. Biochem Biophys Res Commun 1996;226:369–377. Erratum. Biochem Biophys Res Commun 1997;232:832.
69. Hayakawa M, Sugiyama S, Hattori K, Takasawa M, Ozawa T. Age-associated damage in mitochondrial DNA in human hearts. Mol Cell Biochem 1993;119:95–103.
70. Sugiyama S, Hattori K, Hayakawa M, Ozawa T. Quantitative analysis of age-associated accumulation of mitochondrial DNA with deletion in human hearts. Biochem Biophys Res Commun 1991;180:894–899.
71. Corral-Debrinski M, Horton T, Lott MT, Shoffner JM, Beal MF, Wallace DC. Mitochondrial DNA deletions in human brain: regional variability and increase with advanced age. Natl Genet 1992;2:324–329.
72. Ikebe S, Tanaka M, Ohno K, et al. Increase of deleted mitochondrial DNA in the striatum in Parkinson's disease and senescence. Biochem Biophys Res Commun 1990;170: 1044–1048.
73. Trounce I, Byrne E, Marzuki S. Decline in skeletal muscle mitochondrial respiratory chain function: possible factor in ageing. Lancet 1989;1:637–639.
74. Schapira AH, Cooper JM, Dexter D, Clark IB, Jenner P, Marsden CD. Mitochondrial complex I deficiency in Parkinson's disease. J Neurochem 1990;54:823–827.
75. Schapira AH, Mann VM, Cooper IM, et al. Anatomic and disease specificity of NADH CoQ I reductase (complex I) deficiency in Parkinson's disease. J Neurochem 1990;55: 2142–2145.
76. Sims NR, Finegan JM, Blass JP, Bowen DM, Neary D. Mitochondrial function in brain tissue in primary degenerative dementia. Brain Res 1987;436:30–38.
77. Hoyer S. Senile dementia and Alzheimer's disease: brain blood flow and metabolism. Prog Neuropsychopharmacol Biol Psychiatry 1986;10:447–478.
78. Beal MF. Neurochemistry and toxin models in Huntington's disease. Curr Opin Neurol 1994;7:542–547.
79. Schulz JB, Beal MF. Mitochondrial dysfunction in movement disorders. Mech Dev 1996;57:3–20.
80. Shoffner JM, Brown MD, Torroni A, et al. Mitochondrial DNA variants observed in Alzheimer disease and Parkinson disease patients. Genomics 1993;17:171–184.
81. Lin FH, Lin R, Wisniewski HM, et al. Detection of point mutations in codon 331 of mitochondrial NADH dehydrogenase subunit 2 in Alzheimer's brains. Biochem Biophys Res Commun 1992;182:238–246.
82. Ikebe S, Tanaka M, Ozawa T. Point mutations of mitochondrial genome in Parkinson's disease. Brain Res Mol Brain Res 1995;28:281–295.
83. Ozawa T, Tanaka M, Ikebe S, Ohno K, Kondo T, Mizuno Y. Quantitative determination of deleted mitochondrial DNA relative to normal DNA in parkinsonian striatum by a kinetic PCR analysis. Biochem Biophys Res Commun 1990;172:483–489.
84. Ozawa T, Tanaka M, Ino H, et al. Distinct clustering of point mutations in mitochondrial DNA among patients with mitochondrial encephalomyopathies and with Parkinson's disease. Biochem Biophys Res Commun 1991;176:938–946.
85. Ionasescu VV, Hart M, DiMauro S, Morales CT. Clinical and morphologic features of a myopathy associated with a point mutation in the mitochondrial tRNA(Pro) gene. Neurology 1994;44:975–977.
86. Ozawa T. Mitochondrial cardiomyopathy. Herz 1994;19: 105–118, 125.
87. Ozawa T, Tanaka M, Sugiyama S, et al. Patients with idiopathic cardiomyopathy belong to the same mitochondrial DNA gene family of Parkinson's disease and mitochondrial encephalomyopathy. Biochem Biophys Res Commun 1991;177:518–525.
88. Poulton J, Deadman ME, Ramacharan S, Gardiner RM. Germ-line deletions of mtDNA in mitochondrial myopathy. Am J Hum Genet 1991;48:649–653.
89. Yoneda M, Katsumata K, Hayakawa M, Tanaka M, Ozawa T. Oxygen stress induces an apoptotic cell death associated with fragmentation of mitochondrial genome. Biochem Biophys Res Commun 1995;209:723–729.
90. Melov S, Hinerfeld D, Esposito L, Wallace DC. Multi-organ characterization of mitochondrial genomic rearrangements in ad libitum and caloric restricted mice show striking somatic mitochondrial DNA rearrangements with age. Nucleic Acids Res 1997;25:974–982.
91. Finch CE, Tanzi RE. Genetics of aging. Science 1997;278: 407–411.
92. Jazwinski SM. Longevity, genes, and aging. Science 1996; 273:54–59.
93. Murakami S, Johnson TE. A genetic pathway conferring life extension and resistance to UV stress in Caenorhabditis elegans. Genetics 1996;143:1207–1218.
94. Kimura KD, Tissenbaum HA, Liu Y, Ruvkun G. daf-2, an insulin receptor-like gene that regulates longevity and diapause in Caenorhabditis elegans. Science 1997;277: 942–946.
95. Kenyon C, Chang J, Gensch E, Rudner A, Tabtiang R. A C. elegans mutant that lives twice as long as wild type. Nature 1993;366:461–464.
96. Lin K, Dorman JB, Rodan A, Kenyon C. daf-16: An HNF-3/forkhead family member that can function to double the life-span of Caenorhabditis elegans. Science 1997;278: 1319–1322.
97. Fleming JE, Rose MR. Genetics of aging in Drosophila. In: Schneider EL, Rowe JW (eds) Handbook of the Biology of Aging. Academic, San Diego, 1996:74–93.
98. Dudas SP, Arking R. A coordinate upregulation of antioxidant gene activities is associated with the delayed onset of senescence in a long-lived strain of Drosophila. J Gerontol A Biol Sci Med Sci 1995;50:B117–B127.

99. Rose MR, Vu LN, Park SU, Graves JL Jr. Selection on stress resistance increases longevity in Drosophila melanogaster. Exp Gerontol 1992;27:241–250.
100. Schachter F, Faure-Delanef L, Guenot F, et al. Genetic associations with human longevity at the APOE and ACE loci. Natl Genet 1994;6:29–32.
101. Martin GM, Turker MS. Genetics of human disease, longevity, and aging. In: Hazzard WR, Andres R, Bierman EL, et al. (eds) Principles of Geriatric Medicine and Gerontology. McGraw-Hill, New York, 1990:22.
102. Brown WT. Genetic diseases of premature aging as models of senescence. Annu Rev Gerontol Geriatr 1990;10:23–42.
103. Goto M, Rubenstein M, Weber J, Woods K, Drayna D. Genetic linkage of Werner's syndrome to five markers on chromosome 8. Nature 1992;355:735–738.
104. Yu CE, Oshima J, Fu YH, et al. Positional cloning of the Werner's syndrome gene. Science 1996;272:258–262.
105. Mobbs CV. Neuroendocrinology of aging. In: Schneider EL, Rowe JW (eds) Handbook of the Biology of Aging. Academic, San Diego, 1996:234–282.
106. Wise PM, Krajnak KM, Kashon ML. Menopause: the aging of multiple pacemakers. Science 1996;273:67–70.
107. Denckla WD. A time to die. Life Sci 1975;16:31–44.
108. Gilad GM, Gilad VH. Age-related reductions in brain cholinergic and dopaminergic indices in two rat strains differing in longevity. Brain Res 1987;408:247–250.
109. Cotzias GC, Miller ST, Tang LC, Papavasiliou PS. Levodopa, fertility, and longevity. Science 1977;196:549–551.
110. Knoll J. (-)Deprenyl-medication: a strategy to modulate the age-related decline of the striatal dopaminergic system. J Am Geriatr Soc 1992;40:839–847.
111. Kitani K, Kanai S, Sato Y, Ohta M, Ivy GO, Carrillo MC. Chronic treatment of (-)deprenyl prolongs the life span of male Fischer 344 rats: further evidence. Sci 1993;52:281–288.
112. Milgram NW, Racine RJ, Nellis P, Mendonca A, Ivy GO. Maintenance on L-deprenyl prolongs life in aged male rats. Life Sci 1990;47:415–420.
113. Burnet M. Intrinsic Mutagenesis: A Genetic Approach for Aging. Wiley, New York, 1974.
114. Walford RL. Immunologic theory of aging: current status. Fed Proc 1974;33:2020–2027.
115. Miller RA. The aging immune system: primer and prospectus. Science 1996;273:70–74.
116. Yunis EJ, Salazar M. Genetics of life span in mice. Genetica 1993;91:211–223.
117. Hayflick L, Moorhead PS. The limited in vitro lifetime of human diploid cell strains. Exp Cell Res 1965;37:614–636.
118. Bayreuther K, Rodemann HP, Hommel R, Dittmann K, Albiez M, Francz PI. Human skin fibroblasts in vitro differentiate along a terminal cell lineage. Proc Natl Acad Sci USA 1988;85:5112–5116.
119. Matsumura T, Zerrudo Z, Hayflick L. Senescent human diploid cells in culture: survival, DNA synthesis and morphology. J Gerontol 1979;34:328–334.
120. Pignolo RJ, Rotenberg MO, Cristofalo VJ. Alterations in contact and density-dependent arrest state in senescent WI-38 cells. In Vitro Cell Dev Biol Anim 1994;30A:471–476.
121. Cristofalo VJ, Palaxxo R, Charpentier RL. Limited lifespan of human fibroblasts in vitro: metabolic time or replications? In: Adelman RC, Roberts J, Baker GT, et al. (eds) Neural Regulatory Mechanisms During Aging. Liss, New York, 1980:203.
122. Ponten J. Aging properties of glia. In: Bourliere F, Courtois Y, Macieira-Coelho A, et al (eds) Molecular and Cellular Mechanisms of Aging. INSERM, Paris, 1973:53.
123. Rheinwald JG, Green H. Serial cultivation of strains of human epidermal keratinocytes: the formation of keratinizing colonies from single cells. Cell 1975;6:331–343.
124. Bierman EL. The effect of donor age on the in vitro life span of cultured human arterial smooth-muscle cells. In Vitro 1978;14:951–955.
125. Tassin J, Malaise E, Courtois Y. Human lens cells have an in vitro proliferative capacity inversely proportional to the donor age. Exp Cell Res 1979;123:388–392.
126. Mueller SN, Rosen EM, Levine EM. Cellular senescence in a cloned strain of bovine fetal aortic endothelial cells. Science 1980;207:889–891.
127. Tice RR, Schneider EL, Kram D, Thorne P. Cytokinetic analysis of the impaired proliferative response of peripheral lymphocytes from aged humans to phytohemagglutinin. J Exp Med 1979;149:1029–1041.
128. Harrison DE. Cell and tissue transplantation: a means of studying the aging process. In: Finch CE, Schneider EL (eds) Handbook of the Biology of Aging. Van Nostrand Reinhold, New York, 1985:332.
129. Olsson L, Ebbesen P. Ageing decreases the activity of epidermal $G_1$ and $G_2$ inhibitors in mouse skin independent of grafting on old or young recipients. Exp Gerontol 1977;12:59–62.
130. Rohme D. Evidence for a relationship between longevity of mammalian species and life spans of normal fibroblasts in vitro and erythrocytes in vivo. Proc Natl Acad Sci USA 1981;78:5009–5013.
131. Martin GM, Sprague CA, Epstein CJ. Replicative life-span of cultivated human cells: effects of donor's age, tissue, and genotype. Lab Invest 1970;23:86–92.
132. Pignolo RJ, Masoro EJ, Nichols WW, Bradt CI, Cristofalo VJ. Skin fibroblasts from aged Fischer 344 rats undergo similar changes in replicative life span but not immortalization with caloric restriction of donors. Exp Cell Res 1992;201:16–22.
133. Schneider EL, Mitsui Y. The relationship between in vitro cellular aging and in vivo human age. Proc Natl Acad Sci USA 1976;73:3584–3588.
134. Le Guilly Y, Simon M, Lenoir P, Bourel M. Long-term culture of human adult liver cells: morphological changes related to in vitro senescence and effect of donor's age on growth potential. Gerontologia 1973;19:303–313.
135. Wille JJ Jr, Pittelkow MR, Shipley GD, Scott RE. Integrated control of growth and differentiation of normal human prokeratinocytes cultured in serum-free medium: clonal analyses, growth kinetics, and cell cycle studies. J Cell Physiol 1984;121:31–44.
136. Cristofalo VJ, Allen RG, Pignolo RJ, Martin BG, Beck JC. Relationship between donor age and the replicative lifespan of human cells in culture: a reevaluation. Proc Natl Acad Sci USA 1998;95:10614–10619.
137. Dimri GP, Lee X, Basile G, et al. A biomarker that identifies senescent human cells in culture and in aging skin in vivo. Proc Natl Acad Sci USA 1995;92:9363–9367.

137a. Severino J, Allen RG, Balin S, Balin A, Cristofalo VJ. Is beta-galactosidase staining a marker of senescence in vitro and in vivo? Exp Cell Res 2000;257:162–171.
138. Rubin H. Cell aging in vivo and in vitro. Mech Ageing Dev 1997;98:1–35.
139. Phillips PD, Kuhnle E, Cristofalo VJ. Progressive loss of the proliferative response of senescing WI-38 cells to platelet-derived growth factor, epidermal growth factor, insulin transferrin, and dexamethasone. J Gerontol 1984; 39:11–17.
140. Phillips PD, Kuhnle E, Cristofalo VJ. [$^{125}$I]EGF binding ability is stable throughout the replicative life-span of WI-38 cells. J Cell Physiol 1983;114:311–316.
141. Gerhard GS, Phillips PD, Cristofalo VJ. EGF- and PDGF-stimulated phosphorylation in young and senescent WI-38 cells. Exp Cell Res 1991;193:87–92.
142. Mori S, Kawano M, Kanzaki T, Morisaki N, Saito Y, Yoshida S. Decreased expression of the platelet-derived growth factor beta-receptor in fibroblasts from a patient with Werner's syndrome. Eur J Clin Invest 1993;23: 161–165.
143. Carlin C, Phillips PD, Brooks-Frederich K, Knowles BB, Cristofalo VJ. Cleavage of the epidermal growth factor receptor by a membrane-bound leupeptin sensitive protease active in nonionic detergent lysates of senescent but not young human diploid fibroblasts. J Cell Physiol 1994;160:427–434.
144. Sell C, Ptasznik A, Chang CD, Swantek J, Cristofalo VJ, Baserga R. IGF-1 receptor levels and the proliferation of young and senescent human fibroblasts. Biochem Biophys Res Commun 1993;194:259–265.
145. Phillips PD, Pignolo RJ, Cristofalo VJ. Insulin-like growth factor-1: specific binding to high and low affinity sites and mitogenic action throughout the life span of WI-38 cells. J Cell Physiol 1987;133:135–143.
146. Ferber A, Chang C, Sell C, et al. Failure of senescent human fibroblasts to express the insulin-like growth factor-1 gene. J Biol Chem 1993;268:17883–17888.
147. Doggett DL, Rotenbert MO, Pignolo RF, Phillips PD, Cristofalo VJ. Differential gene expression between young and senescent, quiescent WI-38 cells. Mech Ageing Dev 1992;65:239–255.
148. Linskens MH, Feng J, Andrews WH, et al. Cataloging altered gene expression in young and senescent cells using enhanced differential display. Nucleic Acids Res 1995;23:3244–3251.
149. Murano S, Thweatt R, Shmookler RR, Jones RA, Moerman EJ, Goldstein S. Diverse gene sequences are overexpressed in Werner syndrome fibroblasts undergoing premature replicative senescence. Mol Cell Biol 1991;11:3905–3914.
150. Pignolo RJ, Cristofalo VJ, Rotenbert MO. Senescent WI-38 cells fail to express EPC-1 gene induced in young cells upon entry into the $G_0$ state. J Biol Chem 1993;268:8949–8957.
151. Goodman L, Stein GH. Basal and induced amounts of interleukin-6 mRNA decline progressively with age in human fibroblasts. J Biol Chem 1994;269:19250–19255.
152. Seshadri T, Campisi I. Repression of c-fos transcription and an altered genetic program in senescent human fibroblasts. Science 1990;247:205–209.
153. De Tata V, Ptasznik A, Cristofalo VJ. Effect of the tumor promoter phorbol 12-myristate 13-acetate (PMA) on proliferation of young and senescent WI-38 human diploid fibroblasts. Exp Cell Res 1993;205:261–269.
154. Phillips PD, Pignolo RJ, Nishikura K, Cristofalo VJ. Renewed DNA synthesis in senescent WI-38 cells by expression of an inducible chimeric c-fos construct. J Cell Physiol 1992;151:206–212.
155. Rose DW, McCabe G, Feramisco JR, Adler M. Expression of c-fos and AP-I activity in senescent human fibroblasts is not sufficient for DNA synthesis. J Cell Biol 1992;119: 1405–1411.
156. Oshima J, Campis J, Tannock TC, Martin GM. Regulation of c-fos expression in senescing Werner syndrome fibroblasts differs from that observed in senescing fibroblasts from normal donors. J Cell Physiol 1995;162:277–283.
157. Afshari CA, Bivins HM, Barrett JC. Utilization of a fos-lacZ plasmid to investigate the activation of c-fos during cellular senescence and okadaic acid-induced apoptosis. J Gerontol 1994;49:13263–13269.
158. Lucibello FC, Brusselbach S, Sewing A, Muller R. Suppression of the growth factor-mediated induction of c-fos and down-modulation of AP-1-binding activity are not required for cellular senescence. Oncogene 1993;8:1667–1672.
159. Dean R, Kim SS, Delgado D. Expression of c-myc oncogene in human fibroblasts during in vitro senescence. Biochem Biophys Res Commun 1986;135:105–109.
160. Delgado D, Raymond L, Dean R. C-ras expression decreases during in vitro senescence in human fibroblasts. Biochem Biophys Res Commun 1986;137:917–921.
161. Cristofalo VJ, Phillips PD, Sorger T, Gerhard G. Alterations in the responsiveness of senescent cells to growth factors. J Gerontol 1989;44:55–62.
162. Praeger FC, Gilchrest BA. Influence of increased extracellular calcium concentration and donor age on density-dependent growth inhibition of human fibroblasts. Soc Exp Biol Med 1986;182:315–321.
163. Brooks-Frederich KM, Cianciarulo FL, Rittling SR, Cristofalo VJ. Cell cycle-dependent regulation of $Ca^{2+}$ in young and senescent WI-38 cells. Exp Cell Res 1993;205: 412–415.
164. Takahashi Y, Yoshida T, Takashima S. The regulation of intracellular calcium ion and pH in young and old fibroblast cells (WI-38). J Gerontol 1992;47:1365–1370.
165. Blumenthal EJ, Miller AC, Stein GH, Malkinson AM. Serine/threonine protein kinases and calcium-dependent protease in senescent IMR-90 fibroblasts. Mech Ageing Dev 1993;72:13–24.
166. Chang ZF, Huang DY. Decline of protein kinase C activation in response to growth stimulation during senescence of IMR-90 human diploid fibroblasts. Biochem Biophys Res Commun 1994;200:16–27.
167. Campisi J, Dimri G, Hara E. Control of replicative senescence. In: Schneider EL, Rowe JW (eds) Handbook of the Biology of Aging. Academic, San Diego, 1996:121–149.
168. Papaconstantinou J, Reisner PD, Lui L, Kuninger DT. Mechanisms of altered gene expression with aging. In: Schneider EL, Rowe JW (eds) Handbook of the Biology of Aging. Academic, San Diego, 1996:150–183.

169. Venable ME, Lee JY, Smyth MJ, Bielawska A, Obeid LM. Role of ceramide in cellular senescence. J Biol Chem 1995;270:30701–30708.
170. Dbaibo GS, Pushkareva MY, Jayadev S, et al. Retinoblastoma gene product as a downstream target for a ceramide-dependent pathway of growth arrest. Proc Natl Acad Sci USA 1995;92:1347–1351.
171. Harley CB. Telomere loss: mitotic clock or genetic time bomb? Mutat Res 1991;256:271–282.
172. Greider CW. Telomeres, telomerase and senescence. Bioessays 1990;12:363–369.
173. Allsopp RC, Vaziri H, Patterson C, et al. Telomere length predicts replicative capacity of human fibroblasts. Proc Natl Acad Sci USA 1992;89:10114–10118.
174. Chang E, Harley CB. Telomere length and replicative aging in human vascular tissues. Proc Natl Acad Sci USA 1995;92:11190–11194.
175. Harley CB, Futcher AB, Greider CW. Telomeres shorten during ageing of human fibroblasts. 1990;345:458–460.
176. Lindsey J, McGill NI, Lindsey LA, Green DK, Cooke HJ. In vivo loss of telomeric repeats with age in humans. Mutat Res 1991;256:45–48.
177. Vaziri H, Schachter F, Uchida I, et al. Loss of telomeric DNA during aging of normal and trisomy 21 human lymphocytes. Am J Hum Genet 1993;52:661–667.
178. Sugihara S, Mihara K, Marunouchi T, Inoue H, Namba M. Telomere elongation observed in immortalized human fibroblasts by treatment with $^{60}$Co gamma rays or 4-nitroquinoline 1-oxide. Hum Genet 1996;97:1–6.
179. Counter CM, Hirte HW, Bacchetti S, Harley CB. Telomerase activity in human ovarian carcinoma. Proc Natl Acad Sci USA 1994;91:2900–2904.
180. Bryan TM, Englezou A, Gupta J, Bacchetti S, Reddel RR. Telomere elongation in immortal human cells without detectable telomerase activity. EMBO J 1995;14:4240–4248.
181. Broccoli D, Young JW, de Lange T. Telomerase activity in normal and malignant hematopoietic cells. Proc Natl Acad Sci USA 1995;92:9082–9086.
182. Chin CP, Dragowska W, Kim NW, Vaziri H, et al. Differential expression of telomerase activity in hematopoietic progenitors from adult human bone marrow. Stem Cells 1996;14:239–248.
183. Counter CM, Gupta J, Harley CB, Leber B, Bacchetti S. Telomerase activity in normal leukocytes and in hematologic malignancies. Blood 1995;85:2315–2320.
184. Wright WE, Brasiskyte D, Piatyszek MA, Shay JW. Experimental elongation of telomeres extends the lifespan of immortal × normal cell hybrids. EMBO J 1996;15:1734–1741.
185. Bodnar AG, Ouellette M, Frolkis M, et al. Extension of life-span by introduction of telomerase into normal human cells. Science 1998;279:349–352.
185a. Rudolph KL, Chang S, Lee H-W, Blasco M, Gottlieb GJ, Greider C, DePinho RA. Longevity, stress response, and cancer in aging telomerase-deficient mice. Cell 1999;96: 701–712.
186. Karlsson C, Stenman G, Vojta PJ, et al. Escape from senescence in hybrid cell clones involves deletions of two regions located on human chromosome Iq. Cancer Res 1996;56:241–245.
187. Sugawara O, Oshimura M, Koi M, Annab LA, Barrett JC. Induction of cellular senescence in immortalized cells by human chromosome 1. Science 1990;247:707–710.
188. Uejima H, Mitsuya K, Kugoh H, Horikawa I, Oshimura M. Normal human chromosome 2 induces cellular senescence in the human cervical carcinoma cell line SiHa. Genes Chromosomes Cancer 1995;14:120–127.
189. Miyamoto S, Nishida M, Miwa K, et al. Increased actin cable organization after single chromosome introduction: association with suppression of in vitro cell growth rather than tumorigenic suppression. Mol Carcinog 1994;10:88–96.
190. Ohmura H, Tahara H, Suzuki M, et al. Restoration of the cellular senescence program and repression of telomerase by human chromosome 3. Jpn J Cancer Res 1995;86:899–904.
191. Ning Y, Weber JL, Killary AM, Ledbetter DH, Smith JR, Pereira-Smith OM. Genetic analysis of indefinite division in human cells: evidence for a cell senescence-related gene(s) on human chromosome 4. Proc Natl Acad Sci USA 1991;88:5635–5639.
192. Sandhu AK, Hubbard K, Kaur GP, Jha KK, Ozer HL, Athwal RS. Senescence of immortal human fibroblasts by the introduction of normal human chromosome 6. Proc Natl Acad Sci USA 1994;91:5498–5502.
193. Nakabayashi K, Ogata T, Fujii M, et al. Decrease in amplified telomeric sequences and induction of senescence markers by introduction of human chromosome 7 or its segments in SUSM-1. Exp Cell Res 1997;235:345–353.
194. Ogata T, Ayusawa D, Namba M, Takahashi E, Oshimura M, Oishi M. Chromosome 7 suppresses indefinite division of nontumorigenic immortalized human fibroblast cell lines KMST-6 and SUSM-1. Mol Cell Biol 1993;13: 6036–6043.
195. Ogata T, Oshimura M, Namba M, Fujii M, Oishi M, Ayusawa D. Genetic complementation of the immortal phenotype in group D cell lines by introduction of chromosome 7. Jpn J Cancer Res 1995;86:35–40.
196. Sasaki M, Honda T, Yamada H, Wake N, Barrett IC, Oshimura M. Evidence for multiple pathways to cellular senescence. Cancer Res 1994;54:6090–6093.
197. Wang XW, Lin X, Klein CB, Bhamra RK, Lee YW, Costa M. A conserved region in human and Chinese hamster X chromosomes can induce cellular senescence of nickel-transformed Chinese hamster cell lines. Carcinogenesis 1992;13:555–561.
198. Pereira-Smith OM, Smith JR. Genetic analysis of indefinite division in human cells: identification of four complementation groups. Proc Natl Acad Sci USA 1988;85: 6042–6046.
199. Smith IR, Pereira-Smith OM. Replicative senescence: implications for in vivo aging and tumor suppression. Science 1996;273:63–67.
200. Ryan PA, Maher VM, McCormick JJ. Failure of infinite life span human cells from different immortality complementation groups to yield finite life span hybrids. J Cell Physiol 1994;159:151–160.
201. Shay IW, Wright WE, Werbin H. Toward a molecular understanding of human breast cancer: a hypothesis. Breast Cancer Res Treat 1993;25:83–94.

202. Campisi J. Aging and cancer: the double-edged sword of replicative senescence. J Am Geriatr Soc 1997;45:482–488.
203. Atadja P, Wong H, Garkavtsev I, Veillette C, Riabowol K. Increased activity of p53 in senescing fibroblasts. Proc Natl Acad Sci USA 1995;92:8348–8352.
204. Stein GH, Beeson M, Gordon L. Failure to phosphorylate the retinoblastoma gene product in senescent human fibroblasts. Science 1990;249:666–669.
205. Ozer HL, Banga SS, Dasgupta T, et al. SV40-mediated immortalization of human fibroblasts. Exp Gerontol 1996;31:303–310.
206. Shay IW, Pereira-Smith OM, Wright WE. A role for both RB and p53 in the regulation of human cellular senescence. Exp Cell Res 1991;196:33–39.
207. Hara E, Tsurui H, Shinozaki A, Nakada S, Oda K. Cooperative effect of antisense-Rb and antisense-p53 oligomers on the extension of life span in human diploid fibroblasts, TIG-1. Biochem Biophys Res Commun 1991;179:528–534.
208. Afshari CA, Nichols MA, Xiong Y, Mudryj M. A role for a p21-E2F interaction during senescence arrest of normal human fibroblasts. Cell Growth Differ 1996;7:979–988.
209. Noda A, Ning Y, Venable SF, Pereira-Smith OM, Smith JR. Cloning of senescent cell-derived inhibitors of DNA synthesis using an expression screen. Exp Cell Res 1994;211: 90–98.
210. Tahara H, Sato E, Noda A, Ide T. Increase in expression level of p21 sdi I/cip I/wafl with increasing division age in both normal and SV40-transformed human fibroblasts. Oncogene 1995;10:835–840.
211. Alcorta DA, Xiong Y, Phelps D, Hannon G, Beach D, Barrett JC. Involvement of the cyclin-dependent kinase inhibitor p16 (INK4a) in replicative senescence of normal human fibroblasts. Proc Natl Acad Sci USA 1996;93: 13742–13747.
212. Palmero I, McConnell B, Parry D, et al. Accumulation of p161NK4a in mouse fibroblasts as a function of replicative sensecence and not of retinoblastoma gene status. Oncogene 1997;15:495–503.
213. Reznikoff CA, Yeager TR, Belair CD, Savelieva E, Puthenveettil JA, Stadler WM. Elevated p16 at senescence and loss of p16 at immortalization in human papillomavirus 16 E6, but not E7, transformed human uroepithelial cells. Cancer Res 1996;56:2886–2890.
214. Brown JP, Wei W, Sedivy JM. Bypass of senescence after disruption of p21CIP1/WAF1 gene in normal diploid human fibroblasts. Science 1997;277:831–834.
215. Yang L, Didenko VV, Noda A, et al. Increased expression of p21 Sdi I in adrenocortical cells when they are placed in culture. Exp Cell Res 1995;221:126–131.
216. Medcalf AS, Klein-Szanto AJ, Cristofalo VJ. Expression of p21 is not required for senescence of human fibroblasts. Cancer Res 1996;56:4582–4585.
217. Serrano M, Lin AW, McCurrach ME, Beach D, Lowe SW. Oncogenic ras provokes premature cell senescence associated with accumulation of p53 and p16INK4a. Cell 1997;88:593–602.
218. Vogt M, Haggblom C, Yeargin J, Christiansen-Weber T, Haas M. Independent induction of senescence by p16 1NK4a and p21 CIPI in spontaneously immortalized human fibroblasts. Cell Growth Differ 1998;9:139–146.
219. Afshari CA, Vojta PJ, Annab LA, Futreal PA, Willard TB, Barrett JC. Investigation of the role of GUS cell cycle mediators in cellular senescence. Exp Cell Res 1993;209: 231–237.
220. Lockshin RA, Zakeri Z. Programmed cell death and apoptosis. In: Tomei LD, Cope FO (eds) Apoptosis: The Molecular Basis of Cell Death. Cold Spring Harbor Laboratory Press, Plainview, NY, 1991:47–60.
221. Ellit SE, Yuan JY, Horvits HR. Mechanisms and functions of cell death. Annu Rev Cell Biol 1991;7:663–698.
222. Hengartner MO, Horvitz HR. C. elegans cell survival gene ced-9 encodes a functional homolog of the mammalian proto-oncogene bcl-2. Cell 1994;76:665–676.
223. Yuan JY, Horvitz HR. The Caenorhabditis elegans genes ced-3 and ced-4 act cell autonomously to cause programmed cell death. Dev Biol 1990;138:33–41.
224. Nagata S. Apoptosis by death factor. Cell 1997;88:355–365.
225. White E. Life, death, and the pursuit of apoptosis. Genes Dev 1996;10:1–15.
226. Wang E. Senescent human fibroblasts resist programmed cell death, and failure to suppress bcl2 is involved. Cancer Res 1995;55:2284–2292.
227. Grasl-Kraupp B, Bursch W, Ruttkay-Nedecky B, Wagner A, Lauer B, Schulte-Hermann R. Food restriction eliminates preneoplastic cells through apoptosis and antagonizes carcinogenesis in rat liver. Proc Natl Acad Sci USA 1994;91:9995–9999.
228. James SJ, Muskhelishvili L. Rates of apoptosis and proliferation vary with caloric intake and may influence incidence of spontaneous hepatoma in C57BL/6 × C3H F1 mice. Cancer Res 1994:5508–5510.
229. Warner HR, Fernandes G, Wang E. A unifying hypothesis to explain the retardation of aging and tumorigenesis by caloric restriction. J Gerontol 1995;50a:13017-13109.
230. Jacobson MD, Weil M, Raff MC. Programmed cell death in animal development. Cell 1997;88:347–354.
231. Luan X, Zhao W, Chandrasekar B, Fernandes G. Calorie restriction modulates lymphocyte subset phenotype and increases apoptosis in MRL/Ipr mice. Immunol Lett 1995;47:181–186.
232. Zhou T, Edwards CK, Mountz JD. Prevention of age-related T cell apoptosis defect in CD2-fas-transgenic mice. J Exp Med 1995;182:129–137.
233. Warner HR, Hodes RJ, Pocinki K. What does cell death have to do with aging? J Am Geriatr Soc 1997;45:1140–1146.

# 2
# Demography of Aging; Comparative, Differential, and Successful Aging; Geriatric Assessment

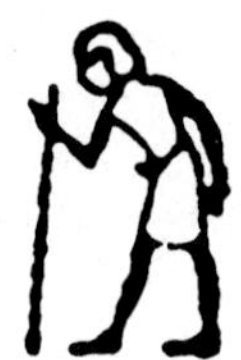

John R. Wilmoth and Paola S. Timiras

The first and most important purpose of this chapter is to describe the extraordinary demographic shifts that occurred during the twentieth century and that will probably extend into the next. The lengthening of life-span and the increasing proportions of the elderly (65 years and older) in human populations have brought continuing changes, not only in our medical education, specialties, and health services but also in the economic and cultural structure of our society. Indeed, this book is written to respond to these changes and to address the specialized requirements for surgery of the elderly.

To maximize the benefits of surgery at all ages—but particularly during old age, when physiologic competence may decline and pathology may increase—complete assessment of the individual is a prerequisite for any successful intervention. For this reason, a discussion of geriatric assessment is presented in this chapter. As for all aspects of medicine, cost-effectiveness is an important consideration. Although geriatric assessments are currently expensive, the potential benefits in terms of prevention and treatment of diseases associated with aging and in terms of good health and quality of life far outweigh diagnostic expenses. Such assessments are particularly useful in view of the considerable heterogeneity among individuals and the hope, made realizable by the current advances in genetics, of providing a health program and disease treatment tailored to the genetic makeup of each patient.

Heterogeneity of normal and abnormal function applies not only to body systems, organs, or cells of an individual within the same species but even more so between different species. Comparative and differential studies, described here briefly, have already provided some productive insights on aging and continue to help us obtain a better understanding of the aging processes.

## Demography of Aging

One of the greatest achievements in the history of our species is the increase in human life expectancy. From prehistoric levels, which were sometimes as low as 25 years, the average length of life has risen to around 75 or 80 years in most developed countries. The average baby born in the United States in 1900 could expect to live only about 50 years given the conditions of the time. Thus about half of the historic increase in life expectancy has taken place during the twentieth century.[1]

Many factors have contributed to this rapid and unprecedented change, which has benefited women much more than men. Although all parts of the world have enjoyed at least a modest reduction in mortality rates, the change occurred earliest and was most extreme in the wealthiest countries. One result of the rise in life expectancy has been the rapid aging of human populations. Now, individuals more frequently are surviving to become centenarians, approaching or even exceeding ages that were thought previously to represent the maximum potential life-span. Most importantly, these changes do not appear to have run their course, and future trends may bring more of the same.

### Life Tables

Demographers employ life tables to measure the level and pattern of human mortality. The columns of the life table describe numerically the life of a fictitious cohort of individuals (usually 100,000). Table 2.1 shows a life table for Japan (men and women together) during 1991–1995. The first column gives the age interval (from $x$ to $x + n$) followed by columns representing the number surviving to the beginning of the interval ($l_x$), the number dying

TABLE 2.1. Life Table for Japan, Both Sexes, 1991–1995

| Age (years) | $l_x$ | $_nd_x$ | $_nq_x$ | $_nL_x$ | $T_x$ | $e_x$ |
|---|---|---|---|---|---|---|
| 0 | 100,000 | 437 | 0.00437 | 99,597 | 7,953,416 | 79.5 |
| 1–4 | 99,563 | 165 | 0.00166 | 397,837 | 7,853,820 | 78.9 |
| 5–9 | 99,397 | 89 | 0.00090 | 496,764 | 7,455,982 | 75.0 |
| 10–14 | 99,308 | 71 | 0.00072 | 496,363 | 6,959,219 | 70.1 |
| 15–19 | 99,237 | 197 | 0.00199 | 495,692 | 6,462,856 | 65.1 |
| 20–24 | 99,040 | 256 | 0.00258 | 494,560 | 5,967,163 | 60.3 |
| 25–29 | 98,784 | 260 | 0.00263 | 493,271 | 5,472,604 | 55.4 |
| 30–34 | 98,524 | 310 | 0.00314 | 491,847 | 4,979,333 | 50.5 |
| 35–39 | 98,214 | 436 | 0.00444 | 489,982 | 4,487,486 | 45.7 |
| 40–44 | 97,778 | 708 | 0.00724 | 487,122 | 3,997,505 | 40.9 |
| 45–49 | 97,071 | 1,134 | 0.01168 | 482,519 | 3,510,382 | 36.2 |
| 50–54 | 95,937 | 1,746 | 0.01820 | 475,321 | 3,027,863 | 31.6 |
| 55–59 | 94,191 | 2,723 | 0.02891 | 464,148 | 2,552,542 | 27.1 |
| 60–64 | 91,468 | 4,185 | 0.04575 | 446,877 | 2,088,394 | 22.8 |
| 65–69 | 87,283 | 5,951 | 0.06818 | 421,536 | 1,641,517 | 18.8 |
| 70–74 | 81,332 | 8,733 | 0.10738 | 384,826 | 1,219,981 | 15.0 |
| 75–79 | 72,599 | 13,370 | 0.18417 | 329,567 | 835,156 | 11.5 |
| 80–84 | 59,228 | 18,207 | 0.30741 | 250,623 | 505,589 | 8.5 |
| 85–89 | 41,021 | 19,561 | 0.47686 | 156,201 | 254,966 | 6.2 |
| 90–94 | 21,460 | 14,038 | 0.65418 | 72,202 | 98,765 | 4.6 |
| 95–99 | 7,421 | 5,778 | 0.77863 | 22,660 | 26,563 | 3.6 |
| 100+ | 1,643 | 1,643 | 1.00000 | 3,902 | 3,902 | 2.4 |

*Source:* http://demog.berkeley.edu/wilmoth/mortality/

during the interval ($_nd_x$), the probability of death during the interval ($_nq_x$, which is $_nd_x/l_x$), the number of person-years lived during the interval ($_nL_x$), the total number of person-years remaining at the beginning of the interval ($T_x$), and the average number of remaining years of life ($e_x$, which is $T_x/l_x$). Thus the last column of the life table gives the estimated life expectancy at the beginning of each age interval.

From Table 2.1 we learn that the probability of death during the first year of life in Japan was only 0.44% during 1991–1995. The chance of surviving to age 70 was 81.3% (81,332/100,000), and the life expectancy at birth was 79.5 years. A common source of confusion is the population of individuals to whom these numbers apply. In general, a life table records the mortality experience of a population at a particular moment in time, not the mortality experience of a specific cohort of individuals. In this case, for example, no real group of individuals experience throughout their lives the mortality conditions recorded in Japan during 1991–1995. Therefore, statements about the expectation of life for a population refer to the average length of life for a hypothetic cohort if exposed to the mortality conditions affecting the population at that particular moment of time.

## Causes of the Mortality Decline

Life tables are used merely to record the pattern of mortality for some population at some moment. By computing life tables for different populations and time periods, demographers have been able to trace the long-term changes in human mortality that have taken place and to investigate hypotheses about the causes of change.

One general consensus is that most of the rise in human life expectancy has been due to several factors in addition to advances in the medical treatment of sick individuals.[2] For example, mortality due to infectious diseases had fallen markedly even before the advent of effective pharmaceutical interventions during the 1930s (sulfa drugs) and 1940s (antibiotics). In addition to antibacterial drugs, other important curative medicine contributions to the decline of mortality include the treatment of cardiovascular disease (heart disease and stroke) and the treatment of trauma (e.g., from motor vehicle accidents and gunshot wounds). Most of these developments have taken place during the past 50–60 years, however, after a considerable portion of the modern rise in life expectancy had occurred. For example, in Sweden by 1935 life expectancy at birth was already 65 years.

Probably the two most important causes of the historical decline of human mortality were (1) the general improvement in living conditions resulting from social and economic development during the past few centuries and (2) the extraordinary advances in organized public health efforts beginning in the latter half of the nineteenth century. An increase in the standard of living during the industrial era brought, first and foremost, a significant rise in the level and quality of human nutrition. The wonders of mechanized agriculture greatly increased the supply of food, and transportation networks improved the ability to move food around in times of local shortage. A higher standard of living meant that individuals were better protected from the hazards of nature through improvements in the quality and quantity of clothing and housing. Increasing wealth also contributed to decreasing mortality by financing the enormous medical and public health industries that have emerged during the past 150 years.

The modern public health movement began during the late nineteenth century with pioneers such as John Snow, who traced the transmission of cholera through the water pumps and pipes of London. When the germ theory of disease was confirmed by Koch's isolation of the tubercle bacillus in 1882, the public health movement blossomed. The upper classes of society came to realize that their health was linked to the health of even their poorest neighbors through the transmission of contagion or other environmental hazards. A sense of collective responsibility for the public's health has resulted in modern sanitation systems, water purification facilities, quarantine strategies, health education, antismoking and safe-sex campaigns, seat belt laws, and so forth. In the aggregate, these measures have probably been at least as effective as (and probably more effective than) the medical treatment of sick individuals in reducing mortality rates.[1–4]

## Sex Differences

The reduced mortality rates have not benefited men and women equally. Although the causes of the trend are only poorly understood, women have gained several more years of life expectancy than have men. Since 1900 in the United States, for example, life expectancy has risen by 30 years for women (from 49 to 79) but by only 26 years for men (from 46 to 72). These differential gains are typical of developed countries, where it is now usual for women to outlive men by about 6–7 years on average.[5]

Contrary to popular myth, the near-elimination of maternal mortality explains only a small fraction of this trend. It appears that women may have a natural advantage over men that should imply a difference of about 2 years in terms of life expectancy at birth. Other factors that may contribute to the much larger gap now commonly observed include differences between the sexes in several aspects of life: exposure to hazardous working conditions, personal habits such as drinking and smoking, utilization of medical care, and even the speed and strength of an individual's response in the face of serious illness.[6]

## Developing Countries

Mortality has fallen in most less developed countries, but usually not as far as in the wealthier countries. Today, some relatively poorer countries achieve advanced levels of life expectancy. For example, a newborn in China can expect to live 70 years (if mortality conditions remain constant). In Latin America as a whole, life expectancy is now 69 years. In sub-Saharan Africa, on the other hand, the average length of life is estimated to be only 45 years.[7] In almost all parts of the world, life expectancy has been increasing in recent decades partly because of economic growth but mostly as an infusion of modern public health and medical technologies. The reduction of malaria in tropical regions, the total eradication of smallpox, and the effective but simple treatment of childhood diarrhea through oral rehydration are notable successes. Prominent examples of deteriorating mortality conditions (with decreasing life expectancies) are found in the parts of Africa that have been most heavily affected by the acquired immunodeficiency syndrome (AIDS) epidemic[8] and some regions of the former Soviet Union.[9]

## Population Aging

One of the most significant consequences of the decline in mortality is the aging of human populations. The distribution of a population by age is affected not only by mortality, but also by fertility. Historically, the decline in mortality has been followed, in most regions of the world, by a significant reduction in average family size. These two sets of changes—the historical declines in both mortality and fertility over the past few centuries—are referred to jointly as the "demographic transition." The aging of human populations is a direct result of the demographic transition: The increase in longevity leads to more and more elderly persons, and the reduction in average family size leads to fewer and fewer children. Whether measured by the mean or median age of the population or by the percent of the population above age 65 or below age 18, an older population is the inevitable consequence of these grand historical changes.

In the United States and elsewhere, the process of population aging has been dramatic. In 1900 only about 4% of the total population was age 65 or older. Today that number has risen to around 13%, and it may rise as high as 22% by the middle of the twenty-first century.[10] The proportion of children (ages 0–17) in the population has fallen (and should continue to fall) in an almost symmetric fashion: 40% in 1900, 28% in 1990, and perhaps 20% in 2050. The United States is not unique in this regard. Italy provides an extreme example, as the number of persons age 60 and over should have surpassed the number under age 20 sometime during the 1990s, as shown in Figure 2.1.

The increasing social costs of caring for the elderly are thus balanced by the decreasing costs of raising children (for society as a whole). On the other hand, because of the greater economic independence of the elderly (compared to children) and because of their increasing consumption of health services, the rapid growth of the elderly population is a cause for serious concern among policy makers. In the long term, there are only two effective, yet reasonably acceptable solutions to the problem of old-age dependency. First, the average age of retirement must rise in tandem with increasing longevity and improving health conditions among persons in their sixties and seventies. Second, the skyrocketing costs of medical care for elderly individuals must somehow be restrained. Obvi-

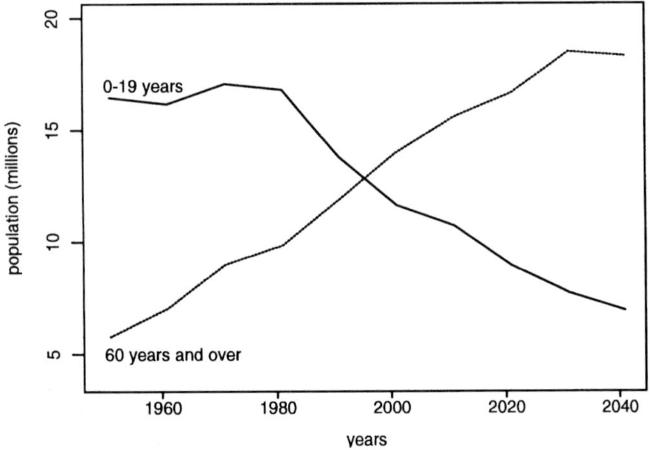


FIGURE 2.1. Number of persons ages 0–19 and ≥60 in Italy, 1951–2041. (From Lori A. Trends in Population Ageing. In: Pinnelli A, Golini A (eds) Population Ageing in Italy, United Nations—Malta: INIA, 1993:38, with permission.)

ously, neither of these goals can be easily achieved, but they should at least be acknowledged as desirable objectives in light of the large-scale demographic changes described here.

## Maximum Life-Span

One source of confusion in any discussion about decreasing mortality, population aging, and the increasing costs of caring for the elderly has been the idea that there is some maximum life-span that defines the outer limits of potential human longevity. If there is some age *x* beyond which no one can survive, arguably there must be some limit to the rise in life expectancy and thus to the "graying" of the population. The existence of such a maximal age is questionable, however.[11] First, if it is possible to survive to age *x*, surely it must also be possible to survive to age *x* plus 1 day. Following this logic, there may be no finite limit, even though survival to very old age is highly unlikely in a statistical sense.

The oldest individuals whose ages have been reliably documented are a Frenchwoman, Jeanne Calment, who died in 1997 at the age of 122, and a Danish-American immigrant, Christian Mortensen, who died in 1998 at the age of 115.[12] Because the chance of death is high at such ages, the probability of observing significantly older individuals in the near future is exceedingly small. Nevertheless, these records are likely to be broken eventually. For national populations with reliable data, the maximum age at death has been rising slowly but steadily for more than a century.[13] In Sweden, for example, the maximum age at death has been rising at a rate of about 1 year of age every two decades since the middle of the nineteenth century, as seen in Figure 2.2.

## Future Trends

Rather than converging to some biologic limit, it seems that mortality trends now point in the direction of further gains in human longevity. Mortality rates continue falling across the age range in most developed countries, where the pace of decline has accelerated among the elderly in particular. Like the trend of the maximum age at death in Sweden, there is no sign in most demographic data that humans are approaching a mortality plateau imposed by some fixed biologic limit.[14] The rapid increase in life expectancy witnessed during the first half of the twentieth century has slowed because the earlier increase resulted from the near-elimination of death during infancy and childhood. Saving a child, who may later die at age 70, yields a much larger increment in average life expectancy than saving a 70-year-old, who may eventually die at age 80. As measured by the chance of death at any given age, however, the reduction in mortality has been remarkably stable over the past century and shows no sign of decelerating.[15]

Current projections based on trend extrapolation anticipate that life expectancy at birth in developed countries will be around 85 years in 2050.[16,17] Given the long-term stability of mortality trends and the multiplicity of factors that have contributed to the historical change, it seems naive to believe that the pace of change in the future will be substantially different from that in the past. Thus it seems unlikely either that the increase in human longevity will end abruptly in the near future or that miracles of technology will lead to a significant acceleration in the pace of change. Rather, we should expect continued slow improvements in life expectancy, which will be accompanied by continued aging of the population and an associated increase in the demand for medical services for the elderly.

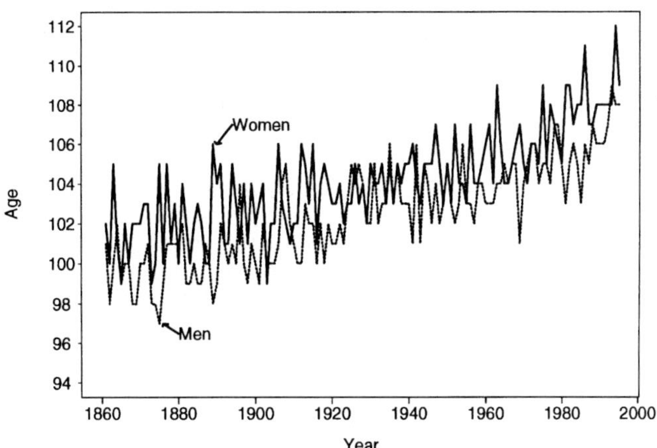


FIGURE 2.2. Maximum reported age at death, by sex, Sweden, 1861–1995. (From Wilmoth and Lundström,[13] with permission.)

# Comparative Physiology of Aging

Although the simple observation that some animal species live longer than others—humans being among the longer-living species—is convincing evidence for the usefulness of the comparative study of aging, such comparisons among a wide range of animal species have been relatively scarce when studying aging.[18–20] Most research on senescence in mammals has been done on laboratory rats and mice partly because of their biologic characteristics (e.g., well-known husbandry, physiology, pathology, genetics) but primarily for practical considerations (e.g., low cost, easy availability, high fecundity, relatively short life-span). If the comparative approach discloses how the various species differ from one another "in potentially instructive ways," comparative assessment of aging should have the following uses in aging research.[21]

1. Hypothesis formulation and evaluation (e.g., detailed information on a wide variety of species)
2. Generalization of putative aging mechanisms (e.g., selection of several distantly related animal models)

3. Isolation of key physiologic factors influencing the aging rate (e.g., evaluation of closely related species or populations with the hope that their aging rates may differ substantially)
4. Choice of the best animal models for particular research questions (e.g., identification and selection of appropriate species for specific studies)

The comparative approach is not without pitfalls despite its success in providing crucial information on principles of natural selection, ecology, and evolutionary biology. Attempts to find a link between a single variable (e.g., longevity, body size, enzyme activity) and species-specific aging processes may lead to invalid conclusions concerning interspecies differences.[22] Perhaps the more frequent use of multivariate analyses will allow "the comparative method not only to suggest hypotheses on aging processes, but also to test them."[23]

## Selective Longevity and Immortality

If senescence is viewed as a manifestation of the process of adaptation, in evolutionary terms the problem of adaptation is solved by the theory of natural selection: (1) the inherited, selected characteristics are those most favorable for survival and reproduction in a particular environment; and (2) the genes specifying these characteristics are passed to succeeding generations. In this sense, the aged (lacking direct reproductive function and characterized by accumulated damage) represent a declining force of natural selection, and the survival of the species would demand the aging and death of its members. Survival beyond the period of reproductive activity represents a luxury that few species can afford. Contrasting the immortality of the germ line with the mortality of somatic cells (the soma) suggests, at least in some species, that limiting the individual life-span may be a beneficial adaptation. The "disposable soma theory" estimates that the investment humans have made in protecting somatic cells (beyond the energy required for maximizing fertility) would provide enough energy for about 40 years; beyond that age, maintenance and repair of somatic cells would require greater energy expenditure than production of a new individual.[24,25] However, repeated injury during the life-span may enhance the normal level of repair (in worms) and result in rejuvenating the soma and prolonging the life-span.[26]

In certain life forms, particularly plants and invertebrates, aging may not occur at all.[27] Among unicellular organisms, protozoa have received considerable attention, but no one has definitively demonstrated or negated their immortality. Some strains of *Paramecium* in culture survive indefinitely without conjugation and cross-fertilization; other strains do not survive unless periodically cross-fertilized. What are the causes of this eventual immortality? Are specific genes involved? It is now evident that a large number of genes probably acting through a single or plural mechanism can influence how animals, specifically humans, age.[28] Given the linkage of genes to life-span, genetic manipulation may prolong life-span in some animals (e.g., fruit flies, nematodes); it is unclear if such observations have any relevance to humans.

Fruit flies can be made to live longer by selective breeding of long-lived progenitors.[29] The difference between long-lived and normal specimens might be the presence of a variant of a normal enzyme-specifying gene for the antioxidant superoxide dismutase. This enzyme is particularly active in the long-lived flies and provides stronger protection against the damage induced by accumulation of free radicals. Bacteria, yeast, and clones of many plants may not exhibit senescence. Similarly, metazoa (e.g., sea anemones) appear to be ageless; in these jellyfish the individual "jellies" have a fixed life-span, but the larval "stub" produces a constant supply of new blanks as old ones are removed; the specimens remain vigorous indefinitely. Even in some vertebrates, such as large fish and tortoises, the process of aging is so slow as to be almost undetectable. There does not seem to be an inherent factor common to all forms of life that automatically produces senescence. *Gerontogenes*, that is, genes inducing senescence, have been described; but firm evidence of their presence is not yet available. On the other hand, *longevity-determining genes*, or gene mutations responsible for lengthening the life-span, have been identified in worms and yeast.[30,31]

Senescence has been equated to a decline or even arrest of the proliferative ability of cells. For example, young human fibroblasts divide in vitro about 50 times and then stop.[32] This limit of cell proliferation is shortened with advancing age and with some forms of progeria (i.e., accelerated aging), such as Werner syndrome. Limitations in proliferative ability are associated with progressive shortening of the telomeres, which form the ends (i.e., the tails) of the chromosomes. With each division in normal cells, the telomeres shed a number of bases and shorten; thus their length reflects how young or old the cell is.[33–35] In contrast, in immortal cancer cells, telomeres do not shorten after each cell division owing to the presence of a special enzyme, telomerase, which enables the telomeres to replace lost DNA sequences, and cells divide indefinitely.

## Physiologic Correlates of Longevity

### *Brain Weight and Body Weight*

Brain weight and its relation to body weight is one of the factors that correlate with aging in animals. In placental mammals there is a highly significant relation between life-span and *body weight*: the larger the animal, the longer the life-span (Table 2.2). For example, the elephant may reach or exceed 70 years while in captivity, whereas the rat seldom lives more than 3 years. There are many excep-

TABLE 2.2. Physiologic Correlates with Longevity

| Index studied | Correlation |
|---|---|
| Body weight | Direct |
| Brain/body weight | Direct |
| Basal metabolic rate | Inverse |
| Stress | Inverse |
| Reproductive function/fecundity | Inverse |
| Length of growth period | Direct |
| Evolution | Uncertain |

*Source:* Timiras,[36] with permission.

tions to this generalization, however: Humans may reach 120 years of age, whereas larger mammals show a shorter potential longevity (horse, 60 years; hippopotamus and rhinoceros, 50 years; bear, 30 years; camel, 25 years). Among domestic animals, cats, although generally smaller than dogs, live longer. Bats live much longer than their body size would predict. The relation of body size to longevity may be influenced by environmental vulnerability: Large animals are less susceptible to the risk of predation (mice being more vulnerable than elephants and even than bats)[37] and are more resistant to food and water shortage.[38]

Another significant relation exists between life-span and *brain weight*. Insectivores, with smaller, simpler brains than ungulates, have a shorter life-span than the latter, which in turn have simpler brains and shorter life-spans than humans. Humans, with the longest life-span among vertebrates, have the heaviest brain in relation to body weight and also the most complicated structurally.[39] Of 12 major brain regions, the neocortex (the largest and most recently developed part of the cerebral cortex) shows the strongest correlation with life-span.[40] The higher the brain/body weight ratio and particularly the greater the degree of cerebral cortical expansion (i.e., the process of encephalization), the more precise are the physiologic regulations and thus the greater is the chance for longer survival.[41] Such an interpretation seems well justified in view of the key role of the nervous system in regulating vital physiologic adjustments, especially responses to environmental demands. Maintenance of the physiologic optimum and reduction of the magnitude of the fluctuations occurring over time diminish the probability of irreversible changes per unit time and thus the rate of aging and incidence of death. Although the brain is a functionally important organ, there is a similar positive relation between the size of other organs (e.g., adrenal, liver, spleen) and life-span.[42]

### Basal Metabolic Rate

The basal metabolic rate (BMR), another physiologic parameter, is inversely correlated with life-span. The rate-of-living theory states that the higher the metabolic rate, the shorter is the life-span.[43] BMR represents the energy expenditure per unit of time required to maintain an organism when it does no work against the environment—the cost of remaining alive in the basal state. Shrews, which have the highest metabolic rate of all mammals, have a life-span of 1 year compared with bats, which have a much lower metabolism and a life-span of more than 15 years.[24,44] The higher metabolic rate is thought to accelerate the accumulation of nuclear errors (DNA damage) or cellular damage (accumulation of damage by free radicals), thereby shortening the life-span. This rate-of-living hypothesis has stimulated a great deal of research on intracellular oxidative damage, the protective effects of antioxidants,[45] and the glycosylation of proteins and nucleic acid.[46]

The Pacific salmon and Atlantic eel are prime examples of the inverse relation between accumulation of damage, stress, and length of life-span. Both fish age rapidly at the time of spawning and die shortly thereafter. However, if spawning and its associated stress are prevented, the salmon continue to live several years. Lower body temperature in these animals increases longevity, perhaps by decreasing immune responsiveness and preventing autoimmune disorders.[47]

### Fecundity and Duration of Growth

Fecundity, an expression of reproductive function measured by the number of young born per year of mature life, appears to be inversely related to longevity. Shrews, with a short life-span, have a large litter size and produce two litters per year, whereas the longer-lived bats have only one young per year. *Duration of growth* also has been related to the life-span. For example, the chimpanzee has a growth period of approximately 10 years and a life-span of 40 years, whereas the human with a growth period of 20 years has a life-span of approximately 100 years.

The growth period has been prolonged experimentally in some animals, primarily rodents; and the onset of maturation can be delayed by restricting food intake in terms of total calories or some specific dietary components. Not only is the life-span thus prolonged, but some specific functions, such as reproduction and thermoregulation, are maintained until advanced age; also, the onset of aging-related pathology is delayed and its severity reduced.[48,49]

As discussed above, natural selection suggests that the individual member of a group must survive through at least the beginning of the reproductive period to contribute to the continuation of the species; thereafter survival of the individual becomes indifferent or detrimental (e.g., food competition) to the group. In this sense, a gene that acts to ensure a maximum number of offspring during youth but produces disease at later ages might be positively selected.

In modern times, not only is life expectancy increased, but humans live well beyond the reproductive years:

Women live some 30 years, on average, beyond the childbearing period. Aging then can be defined as a set of phenotypes that have escaped the force of natural selection.[50] Longevity of a species beyond the reproductive years must be unrelated to some earlier events, or the infertile individual must confer some advantage to the fertile. In our society, the latter must be the case, for increasing numbers of older members do contribute to the maintenance of the entire population structure and the development and progress of society.[51]

## Differential Aging among Humans

*Chronologic age* (age in number of years) and *physiologic age* (age in terms of functional capacity) do not always coincide, and often the physical appearance and health status belie the chronologic age; in many cases a person appears to be younger or older than his or her chronologic age. Disparities in the timetable of aging may occur among individuals or among selected populations. That is, some individuals "age" at a much slower or faster rate than others.

Changes with aging lack uniformity not only among individuals of the same species but also within the same individual. The onset, rate, and magnitude of the changes vary depending on the cell, tissue, organ, system, or laboratory evaluation of several parameters (Table 2.3).[52–54]

Traditionally, in humans the physiologic "norm" is represented by the sum of all functions in a 25-year-old man with weight 70 kg, height 170 cm, and free of disease. Comparison with this "ideal man" inevitably discloses a range of functional decrements with advancing age. Early studies were conducted in selected samples of "representative" elderly.[52] As the prevalence of chronic disease increases with age, functional loss with age in these studies may have been due to the effects of disease rather than the natural concomitants of aging itself. In these earlier studies, comparison of several functions from young to old age focused on a gradation of decrements with old age.

More recent research has challenged the inevitability of functional impairment with chronologic aging. Significant changes in laboratory evaluation of some physiologic functions may be erroneously attributed to aging, and normal aging changes may be misinterpreted as evidence of disease. Laboratory values are always stated within a normal range. Many of the age-related levels do not change on average, but the variance (i.e., the deviation from average) tends to increase.[53]

Regulation of certain functions may remain efficient until advanced age, whereas in others it declines at an early age. Examples of such differential aging may be inferred from fasting blood glucose levels and acid-base balance, which remain stable as late as 70–90 years of age. In contrast, the BMR declines continuously throughout the life-span. Certain sensory modalities, such as vision and hearing, show functional decrements beginning during early adulthood. A classic example of a unique timetable involving an organ that develops and ages during a specific period of the life-span is the ovary: It begins to function at adolescence (in humans at approximately 10–12 years of age) and ceases to function at menopause (in humans as much as 30 years before death).

Aging is a slow, continuous process. Therefore some of its effects can be observed only when they have progressed sufficiently to induce identifiable alterations

TABLE 2.3. Laboratory Values During Old Age

| |
|---|
| **Unchanged** |
| Hepatic function tests |
| Serum bilirubin |
| Aspartate aminotransferase (AST) |
| Alanine aminotransferase (ALT) |
| $\gamma$-glutamyltransferase (GGTP) |
| Coagulation tests |
| Biochemical tests |
| Serum electrolytes |
| Total protein |
| Calcium |
| Phosphorus |
| Serum folate |
| Arterial blood test |
| pH |
| $PaCO_2$ |
| Renal function tests |
| Serum creatinine |
| Thyroid function tests |
| $T_4$ |
| Complete blood count |
| Hematocrit |
| Hemoglobin |
| Red blood cells |
| Platelets |
| **Decreased** |
| Serum albumin |
| HDL-cholesterol (women) |
| Serum $B_{12}$ |
| Serum magnesium |
| $PaO_2$ |
| Creatinine clearance |
| $T_3$ (?) |
| White blood count |
| Insulin-like growth factor I (IGF-I) |
| **Increased** |
| Alkaline phosphatase |
| Uric acid |
| Total cholesterol |
| HDL-cholesterol (men) |
| Triglycerides |
| Thyroid-stimulating hormone (TSH) (?) |
| Glucose tolerance tests |
| Fasting blood glucose (within normal range) |
| Postprandial blood glucose |

*Source:* Adapted from Shock.[52]

that can be validated by available testing methods. An illustrative example is atherosclerosis, the consequences of which manifest during middle and old age even though the atherosclerotic lesion may start early in infancy. Whatever organ or tissue is considered, timetables of aging represent an approximation, as the onset of aging cannot be pinpointed precisely by a specific physiologic sign.

Although fasting blood glucose values are minimally affected by aging, when these levels are determined after increased physiologic demand (e.g., a glucose load as for the glucose tolerance test), the ability of the organism to maintain normal levels and the rate at which the levels return to normal are markedly different in mature and aged subjects. Similarly, conduction velocity in nerves, cardiac index [cardiac output/minute/body area ($m^2$)], renal function (filtration rate, blood flow), and respiratory function (vital capacity, maximum breathing capacity) can withstand less stress in the elderly than in young individuals. Such declining ability of the aging organism to withstand or respond adequately to stress reveals an age difference not otherwise detectable.

Some functions of the body begin to age relatively early during adult life and have minimum efficiency before age 65, officially heralding the stage of senescence. In the eye, accommodation begins to decline during the teens and regresses to a minimum during the mid-fifties. Auditory function begins to deteriorate at adolescence, and deterioration continues steadily thereafter. This auditory deterioration may be hastened by the environmental noise to which individuals in our civilization are continuously exposed from young age.

## Successful Aging

### Usual Versus Successful Aging

Undoubtedly, a number of functions decline in individuals 65 years and older compared with those in 25-year-old. As people live longer, the use of the classic profile of the 25-year-old man taken as the standard of optimal physiologic competence appears unrealistic and outdated. The extreme heterogeneity of functional status even in the oldest-old (80 years and older) supports the view that aging must be evaluated on an individual basis. In addition to genetic makeup, the elderly individual's health, social status, and economic and environmental conditions are responsible for his or her demographic and epidemiologic history.[55] Aging processes have been categorized as *usual aging*, referring to the average physiologic changes, and *successful aging*, referring to minimal physical decrements.[56]

Accordingly, individuals who age successfully are those who do not exhibit pathology and have minimal functional decrements. They represent a group clearly designated for successful surgery should the need arise. The concept of successful aging was formulated as "a reconceptualization of the aging process, one that provides a significant and necessary counterbalance to previous research that tended to emphasize age-related declines in functioning and health."[57] It distinguishes three modalities of aging: (1) disease/disabled, characterized by the presence of pathology, disability, or both; (2) "usual" (normal) aging, characterized by the absence of overt pathology but the presence of functional declines; and (3) "successful" aging, characterized by few or none of the physiologic losses seen in the usual aging group. The concept is based on: (1) the substantial heterogeneity among aged individuals; (2) the observation that aging is not a uniform or inevitable process of disease or disability; (3) the persistence of plasticity well into advanced age, that is, a continuing capacity for adaptive and compensatory rehabilitation; and (4) the identification of predictors of various patterns of aging, especially factors that contribute to more successful trajectories of aging.

### Evidence for Successful Aging

Current studies of successful aging (e.g., the MacArthur Research Network on Successful Aging) provide evidence for continuing good functional competence and recuperative plasticity during old age. This community-based longitudinal study, 2.5 years in duration, comprised men and women aged 70–79 years functioning in the top third of their age group in terms of physical and cognitive competence; nevertheless, significant differences in these parameters and with respect to other domains (e.g., leisure, social interactions) among participants led to further subdivision into high, medium, and low functioning groups.[58,59] Of the high functioning cohort only a few subjects showed a decline in physical or mental function over time.

The distinction among successful groups supports the hypothesis that extrinsic factors play an important role in age-associated functional decline. Factors promoting maintenance or improvement of functioning include younger age, higher income, being white, low body weight, good lung function, absence of diabetes or hypertension, higher education, and high cognitive performance. Other correlates of high functioning were absence of hospitalization during the 2.5-year study, participation in moderate/strenuous exercise, and receiving emotional support.[59] Taking all such factors into account, the prospects for avoidance, or eventual reversal, of functional loss with age are vastly improved, and the risks of adverse consequences are reduced.[56]

Many mechanisms emerge during later years that compensate for specific types of functional loss. Improvements in function are possible even among those who have shown a previous decline.[60–62] The potential for rehabilitation at advanced age is much greater than previously supposed,[54] and there is a significant probability of regaining function at all levels of disability.

## Consequences of Successful Aging

By focusing on the various modalities of aging, the heterogeneity of the aging process is emphasized and the validity of this concept is extended to all biomedical branches. Interventions may be beneficial at all ages provided they are customized (tailored) to the individual.[63,64] Physical exercise, hormone replacement or hormone therapy, and dietary, surgical, and pharmacologic interventions have proved successful in enhancing health even at older ages. Identification of "predictors" designed to maximize health and physiologic competence enhances the quality of life of the elderly, reduces their burden of disease and disability, and decreases the socioeconomic need for health care resources. Comparison of aging heterogeneity in humans and other animal species may also provide a better understanding of the aging process per se and its genetic and environmental correlates.

## Assessment of Physiologic Age in Humans

Assessment of physiologic competence in humans, at any age, is a multifactorial process. Given the heterogeneity of old individuals and the incomplete understanding of the fundamental processes of aging, it is difficult to identify biomarkers of aging that represent a valid, reliable measure of health or pathology during old age. The biomarkers or variables presented here are those found frequently in the recent literature and reflect a particular view of aging at a particular time in the history of this field. The choice of such variables will change as we acquire a better understanding of aging, and more meaningful and generally accepted biomarkers will emerge.[65]

At this relatively early stage of studies on aging, there is a broad diversity of putative markers, and assessment of aging requires quantitative measurements of numerous parameters selected as indices of physical, neurologic, and behavioral competence at progressive ages (Table 2.4).[66–69]

A number of criteria must be satisfied to establish an accurate profile that reflects the various age-related timetables for body systems and then combining them to represent the health status of the individual. These criteria should account for many variables, among which some of the prerequisites are as follows.

1. The variables must be indicative of a function important to the competence or general health of the individual and capable of influencing the rate of aging.
2. They must correlate with chronologic age.
3. They must change sufficiently and with discernible regularity over time to reveal significant differences over a 3- to 5-year interval between tests.
4. They must be practically measurable in an individual or cohort of individuals without hazard, discomfort, or expense to the participant or excessive labor or expense for the investigator.

TABLE 2.4. "Simple" Functional Assessment of Ambulatory Elderly

| |
|---|
| History physical examination |
| Neurologic and musculoskeletal evaluation of arm and leg; evaluation of vision, hearing, and speech |
| Urinary incontinence (eventually fecal incontinence): presence and degree of severity |
| Nutrition |
| Dental evaluation |
| Body weight |
| Laboratory tests depending on nutritional status and diet |
| Mental status |
| Folstein Mini-Mental Status Score |
| If score <24, search for causes of cognitive impairment |
| Depression: if Geriatric Depression scale is positive |
| Check for adverse medications |
| Initiate appropriate treatment |
| Activities of daily living and instrumental activities of daily living (see Table 2.5) |
| Home environment and social support |
| Evaluations of home safety |
| Family and community resources |

*Source:* Adapted from Rubenstein et al.[68]

The validity of any assessment lies in the choice of the proper test or battery of tests that best provide an overall picture of current health and serve eventually as a basis for predicting future health and the length of the life-span. Such a choice is complicated by the need to take into account the financial feasibility of, and the facilities available for, such testing. The relatively large number of tests for assessing physiologic competence and health status in the elderly reflects the current difficulty of reaching a consensus on the best parameters to be used and on the multitude of purposes for which the assessment is used. A global measure of physiologic status may be derived from many combinations of tests; selection depends on the purpose of the assessment and who is to use these data.

With respect to purpose of assessment, measurements may be expected to:

1. Describe the physiologic status of an individual at progressive chronologic ages
2. Screen a selected population for assessment of overall physiologic competence or competence of specific functions using cross-sectional or longitudinal sampling methods (see below)
3. Monitor the efficacy of specific treatments (e.g., drugs, exercise, diet)
4. Predict persistence or loss of physiologic competence, determine the incidence of disease, and evaluate life expectancy

With respect to the user, the choice of tests depends on whether he or she is a health provider, specialist, researcher, or case manager. Even with precise identification of the nature of the assessment needed and of the user who needs it, it is still difficult to choose the most significant and feasible tests.

Some tests, though relatively innocuous in young, healthy individuals, are potentially harmful to the elderly.[70–73] Yet it may be contrary to the interest of the elderly to assert that they represent a vulnerable group needing special protection. Benefits may accrue for the elderly from their participation in medical and psychosocial survey research. Such participation not only may lead to the discovery of an unsuspected illness and its eventual treatment, it may also provide altruistic commitment and mental satisfaction for the elderly.[74]

Assessment generally involves the entire organism, but it may also be limited to specific organs. Examples of this organ-specific assessment include studies on liver longevity in rats,[75] the relation of prostate volume to prostate-specific antigens,[76,77] measurements of lens transparency and the effects of irradiation thereon,[78] the degree of competence of thermogenesis,[79] and allometric description of organ weights versus body weight.[80] These organ-specific tests may be useful not only for giving information on the condition of the specific organ but may also indirectly represent an index of whole-organism health.

Assessment may also be directed toward the evaluation of risk factors, such as environmental smoke,[81] and to nutrition with respect to special functions, such as the glomerular filtration rate,[82] or to specific nutritional microelements.[83] During such an assessment selected techniques such as magnetic resonance imaging (MRI) for regional brain alteration[84] may be used; alternatively, the assessment may be designed to examine special medical conditions such as obesity[85] or specific medical/surgical preoperative interventions such as anesthesiology.[86]

## Geriatric Assessment

Geriatric assessment involves a multidimensional diagnostic process designed to evaluate an elderly individual not only in terms of functional capabilities and disabilities but also medical and psychosocial characteristics (Table 2.4). It is usually conducted by a multidisciplinary team with the intent of formulating a comprehensive plan for therapy and long-term follow-up. Its major purposes are to:

1. Improve the diagnosis (medical and psychosocial)
2. Plan appropriate rehabilitation and other therapy
3. Determine an optimal living location and arrange for high-quality follow-up care and case management
4. Establish baseline information useful for future comparison at later ages

Most of these assessment programs include several tests, which have been grouped into three categories.

1. Tests that examine general physical health, represented by physiologic competence and the absence of disease
2. Tests that measure the ability to perform basic self-care activities, the so-called activities of daily living (ADLs) (Table 2.5)

TABLE 2.5. Categories of Physical Health Index Measuring Physical Competence

**Physical health**
- Bed days
- Restricted-activity days
- Hospitalization
- Physician visits
- Pain and discomfort
- Symptoms
- Signs on physical examination
- Physiologic indicators (e.g., laboratory tests, radiography, pulmonary and cardiac function tests)
- Permanent impairment (e.g., vision, hearing, speech, paralysis, amputations, dental)
- Diseases/diagnosis
- Self-rating of health
- Physician rating of health

**Activities of daily living**
- Feeding
- Bathing
- Toileting
- Dressing
- Ambulation
- Transfer from bed
- Transfer from toilet
- Bowel and bladder control
- Grooming
- Communication
- Visual acuity
- Upper extremities (e.g., grasping and picking up objects)
- Range of motion of limbs

**Instrumental activities of daily living**
- Cooking
- Cleaning
- Using telephone
- Writing
- Reading
- Shopping
- Laundry
- Managing medications
- Using public transportation
- Walking outdoors
- Climbing stairs
- Outside work (e.g., gardening, snow shoveling)
- Ability to perform in paid employment
- Managing money
- Traveling out of town

*Sources:* Federoff and Botstein,[64] McClearn,[65] Kane and Kane,[66] and Rubenstein et al.[67,68]

Many of the items presented are components of several measures of physical and functional health as discussed in a number of geriatric screening and assessment programs.

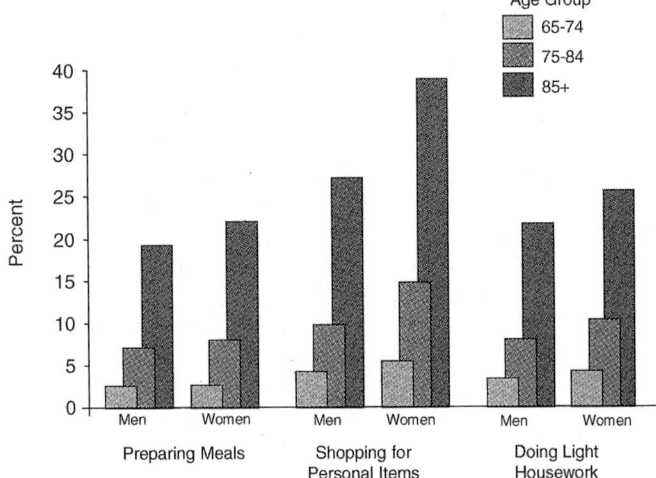


FIGURE 2.3. Percentage of community-dwelling population dependent for three instrumental activities of daily living, United States, 1994. Dependence is defined as needing help or supervision with the activity. (From Analyses of data from the National Health Interview Survey, Phase 1, 1994. Thanks to Dr. Suzanne G. Leveille for her analysis of the data.)

3. Tests that measure, in addition to basic activities, the ability to perform more complex instrumental activities daily living (IADLs) (Table 2.5)

The ADLs and IADLs are widely utilized in home-dwelling populations to determine capability for independent living or, vice versa, as indicators of disability (Fig. 2.3). *Disability is the inability to perform a specific function because of health or age, resulting in impaired functional performance.* With most testing the degree of wellness (i.e., the absence of disability/disease) is recorded, as is the presence and severity of disability/disease. According to one classification scheme (among many), the severity of the disability may be measured in terms of whether a person (1) does not perform the activity at all; (2) can perform it only with the help or in the presence of another person (but who does not actually give aid); or (3) can perform it with the help of special equipment. Disability is coded according to five degrees of severity: (1) no disability; (2) at least one IADL disability but no ADL; (3) one or two ADL disabilities; (4) three or four ADL disabilities; and (5) five or six ADL disabilities.[87]

With advancing age the intensity of disability increases (Fig. 2.3), with the highest disability at 85 years and older (85+). It is to be noted that the greater intensity of disability in women than in men manifests at the later ages of 74 to 85+ years. Thus women with a longer average life-span than men live longer with disability. The cause of this sex difference is unknown but may stem from the higher incidence of a number of chronic degenerative conditions (e.g., osteoporosis, diabetes, arthritis) in women that interfere with functions (e.g., walking, doing housework) necessary for independent living without being fatal. Some forms of disability, such as visual impairment, are equally prevalent in men and women.

## Evaluation of Geriatric Screening and Assessment Programs

Geriatric assessment has its origins in the pioneering work of British geriatricians during the 1930s and 1940s, who demonstrated that end-stage, bed-bound, geriatric patients could be dramatically mobilized, with many discharged to community settings following careful assessment and rehabilitation. Today, an increasing number of such assessment programs are available within a variety of health care structures, ranging from hospitals to nursing homes to outpatient clinics. Two basic tactics for the study of human aging using the tests discussed above are the cross-sectional study and the longitudinal study.

*Cross-sectional studies,* which compare characteristics among different age groups at one time, can be conducted with relative accuracy and rapidity in a large group of people. For example, a population with a broad span of ages, perhaps birth to 90 years, is sectioned into narrow, age-defined subsets, and measurements are made in identical fashion in each group. This type of study has been used in gerontologic research for such programs as short-term testing of new drugs or regimens capable of influencing some aspects of the aging process. It has also been used profitably in animal studies conducted in such species as rats and mice, which can be raised and maintained under special but standardized conditions (e.g., diet, drugs, exercise).

Human populations, however, live under widely different environmental conditions, and the same measurements obtained in cohorts of individuals of the same age are subject to multifactorial influences only one of which is aging per se. Thus the cross-sectional study, although less time-consuming than the longitudinal one, is subject to a number of errors. For example, because of the secular trend in stature (i.e., changes that occur in a population as a whole over time—in this case an increase in stature) the 20-year-old in 1980 is taller than was the 20-year-old in 1910. This difference must not be interpreted as an aging-related decrease in height because the oldest people were born when body height was lower. Similarly, differential survivorship depends on the selected survival only of those individuals with a particular trait. To continue with the example of stature, tall, lean individuals may tend to live longer than short, obese persons; if true, it would bias the outcome of the study.

The *longitudinal study,* which avoids some of these errors, is the preferred method of many gerontologists.

In the longitudinal study, in addition to comparison with a control group, the same individuals are examined at regular intervals throughout the life-span so the process of aging can be compared in a dynamic fashion, each individual being his or her own control between two or several ages. Longitudinal studies have been used with great success for studying growth processes. For aging, however, this method has many obvious disadvantages, especially when studying human populations: Not only is the human life-span relatively long, but in industrialized countries human populations are extremely mobile, and many of the components of the cohort are lost during the study.

A compromise approach combining cross-sectional and longitudinal studies is often used. With this type of study, initial data from cross-sectional studies are supplemented and corrected by data from longitudinal follow-ups. Another practical approach is to restrict the longitudinal survey to "critical" life periods (e.g., 5 years before and 5 years after menopause or retirement).

## References


1. Preston SH. Sources of variation in vital rates: an overview. In: Adams J, Lam D, Hermalin A, Smouse P (eds) Convergent Issues in Genetics and Demography. Oxford: Oxford University Press, 1990:335–350.
2. McKeown T. The Role of Medicine. Oxford: Basil Blackwell, 1979.
3. Johansson SR, Mosk C. Exposure, resistance and life expectancy: diseases and death during the economic development of Japan 1900–1960. Popul Stud 1987;41:207–235.
4. Szreter S. The importance of social intervention in Britain's mortality decline c. 1850–1914: a re-interpretation of the role of public health. Soc Hist Med 1988;1:1–38.
5. Waldron I. Recent trends in sex mortality ratios for adults in developed countries. Soc Sci Med 1993;36:451–462.
6. Vallin J. Social change and mortality decline: women's advantage achieved or regained? In: Federici N, Mason KO, Sogner S (eds) Women's Position and Demographic Change. Oxford: Clarendon, 1993:190–212.
7. 1997 World Population Data Sheet of the Population Reference Bureau: Demographic Data and Estimates for Countries and Regions of the World. Washington, DC: PRB, 1997.
8. Bongaarts J. Global trends in AIDS mortality. Popul Dev Rev 1996;22:21–45.
9. Haub C. Population Change in the Former Soviet Republics. Population Bulletin 49(4). Washington, DC: PRB, 1994.
10. Soldo BJ, Agree EM. America's Elderly. Population Bulletin 43(3). Washington, DC: PRB, 1988.
11. Gavrilov LA, Gavrilova NS. The Biology of Life Span: A Quantitative Approach. Chur, Switzerland: Harwood Academic, 1991.
12. Wilmoth JR, Skytthe S, Friou D, et al. The oldest man ever? A case study of exceptional longevity. Gerontolt 1996;36: 783–788.
13. Wilmoth JR, Lundström H. Extreme longevity in five countries: presentation of trends with special attention to issues of data quality. Eur J Popul 1996;12:63–93.
14. Kannisto, Väinö, Lauritsen J, et al. Reduction in mortality at advanced ages. Popul Dev Rev 1994;20:793–810.
15. Wilmoth JR. In search of limits. In: Wachter KW, Finch CE (eds) Between Zeus and the Salmon: The Biodemography of Longevity. Washington, DC: National Academy Press, 1997:38–64.
16. Lee RD, Carter LR. Modeling and forecasting U.S. mortality. J Am Stat Assoc 1992;87:659–675.
17. Wilmoth JR. Mortality projections for Japan: a comparison of four methods. In: Caselli G, Lopez A (eds) Health and Mortality among Elderly Populations. Oxford: Oxford University Press, 1996:266–287.
18. Comfort A. The Biology of Senescence, 3rd ed. New York: Elsevier, 1979.
19. Finch CE, Schneider EL. Handbook of The Biology of Aging, 2nd ed. New York: Van Nostrand Reinhold, 1985.
20. Strehler BL. Time, Cells and Aging, 2nd ed. San Diego: Academic, 1977.
21. Austad SN. Comparative aging and life histories in mammals. Exp Gerontol 1997;21:23–38.
22. Le Bourg E. Correlation analysis in comparative gerontology: an examination of some problems. Exp Gerontol 1996;31:654–653.
23. Stearns SC. The influence of size and phylogen on patterns of covariation among life-history traits in the mammals. Okios 1983;41:173–187.
24. Kirkwood TBL, Wolff SP. The biological basis of ageing. Age Ageing 1995;24:167–171.
25. Kirkwood TBL. Comparative life spans of species: why do species have the life spans they do? Am J Clin Nutr 1992; 55:1191s–1195s.
26. Martinez DE. Rejuvenation of the disposable soma: repeated injury extends lifespan in an asexual annelid. Exp Gerontol 1996;31:699–704.
27. Wolstenholme GEW, O'Connor M. The Lifespan of Animals. Ciba Foundation Colloquium on Ageing, vol 5. Boston: Little, Brown, 1959.
28. Herskind AM, McGue M, Holm NV, et al. The heritability of human longevity: a population-based study of 2872 Danish twin pairs born 1870–1900. Hum Genet 1996;97: 319–323.
29. Rose MR. Evolutionary Biology of Aging. Oxford: Oxford University Press, 1991.
30. Duhon SA, Murakami S, Johnson TE. Direct isolation of longevity mutants in the nematode Caenorhabditis elegans. Dev Genet 1996;18:144–153.
31. Johnson TE. Genetic influences on aging. Exp Gerontol 1997;32:11–22.
32. Hayflick L, Moorhead PS. The serial cultivation of human diploid cell strains. Exp Cell Res 1961;25:585–621.
33. Olovnikov AM. Telomeres, telomerase, and aging: origin of the theory. Exp Gerontol 1996;31:443–448.
34. Chiu C-P, Harley CB. Replicative senescence and cell immortality: the role of telomeres and telomerase. Proc Soc Exp Biol Med 1997;214:99–106.
35. Dahse R, Fiedler W, Ernst G. Telomeres and telomerase: biological and clinical importance. Clin Chem 1997;43:708–714.

36. Timiras PS. Physiological Basis of Aging and Geriatrics. Boca Raton, FL: CRC Press, 1994.
37. Stearns SC. The Evolution of Life Histories. Oxford: Oxford University Press, 1992.
38. Austad SN, Fischer KE. Primate longevity: its place in the mammalian scheme. Am J Primatol 1992;28:251–261.
39. Sacher GA. Relation of lifespan to brain weight and body weight in mammals. In: Wolstenholme GEW, O'Connor M (eds) The Lifespan of Animals, vol 5. Boston: Little, Brown, 1959:115–141.
40. Hofman MA. Energy metabolism, brain size and longevity in mammals. Q Rev Biol 1983;58:495–512.
41. Salk Y. The Survival of the Wisest. New York: Harper, 1973.
42. Finch CE. Longevity, Senescence, and the Genome. Chicago: University of Chicago Press, 1990.
43. Sacher GA. Life table modification and life prolongation. In: Finch CE, Hayflick K (eds) Handbook of the Biology of Aging. New York: Van Nostrand Reinhold, 1977:582–638.
44. Hart RW, Setlow RB. Correlation belween deoxyribonucleic acid excision-repair and life-span in a number of mammalian species. Proc Natl Acad Sci USA 1974;71:2169–2173.
45. Harman D. Role of free radicals in mutation, cancer, aging, and maintenance of life. Radiat Res 1962;16:752–763.
46. Cerami A. Hypothesis: glucose as a mediator of aging. J Am Geriatr Soc 1985;33:626–634.
47. Robertson OH, Wexler BC. Prolongation of the lifespan of Kokanec salmon (*Oncorhynkus nerka Kennerlyi*) by castration before beginning of gonad development. Proc Natl Acad Sci USA 1961;47:609–621.
48. Segall PE, Timiras PS. Patho-physiologic findings after chronic tryptophan deficiency in rats: a model for delayed growth and aging. Mech Ageing Dev 1976;5:109–124.
49. Segall PE, Timiras PS, Walton JR. Low tryptophan dietsdelay reproductive ageing. Mech Ageing Dev 1983;24:245–252.
50. Martin GM. Somatic mutagenesis and antimutagenesis in aging research. Mutat Res 1996;350:35–41.
51. De Beauvoir S. The Coming of Age, 1st American ed, translated by P O'Brien. New York: Putnam, 1972.
52. Shock NW. Age changes in physiological functions in the total animal: the role of tissue loss. In: Strehler BL, Ebert JD, Shock NW (eds) The Biology of Aging: A Symposium. Washington, DC: American Institute of Biological Science, 1960:258–264.
53. Cavalieri TA, Chopra A, Bryman PN. When outside the norm is normal: interpreting lab data in the aged. Geriatrics 1992;47:66–70.
54. Timiras PS. Physiology of aging: standards for age-related functional competence. In: Greger R, Windhorst U (eds) Human Physiology from Cellular Mechanisms to Integration. Berlin: Springer, 1996:2391–2405.
55. Suzman RM, Willis DP, Manton KG (eds) The Oldest Old. Oxford: Oxford University Press, 1992.
56. Rowe JW, Kahn RL. Human aging: usual and successful. Science 1987;237:143–149.
57. Seeman TE. Successful aging: reconceptualizing the aging process from a more positive perspective. In: Vellas BJ, Albarede JL, Garry PJ (eds) Epidemiology and Aging: Facts and Research in Gerontology. New York: Springer, 1994: 61–73.
58. Berkman LF, Seeman TE, Albert M, et al. High, usual and impaired functioning in community-dwelling older men and women: findings from the MacArthur Foundation Research Network on successful aging. J Clin Epidemiol 1993;46:1129–1140.
59. Seeman TE, Charpentier PA, Berkman LF, et al. Predicting changes in physical performance in a high-functioning elderly cohort; MacArthur studies of successful aging. J Gerontol Med Sci 1994;49:M97–M108.
60. Strawbridge WJ, Kaplan GA, Camacho T, et al. The dynamics of funtional change and disability in an elderly cohort: results from the Alameda County study. J Am Geriatr Soc 1992;40:799–806.
61. Strawbridge WJ, Camacho T, Cohen RD, et al. Gender differences in factors associated with change in physical funtioning in old age: a 6-year longitudinal study. Gerontologist 1993;5:603–609.
62. Kaplan GA, Wilson TW, Cohen RD, et al. Social funtioning and overall mortality: prospective evidence from the Kuopio Ischemic Heart Disease Risk Factor Study. Epidemiology 1994;5:495–500.
63. Martin GM. Genetic modulation of the senescent phenotype of homo sapiens. Exp Gerontol 1996;31:49–59.
64. Fedoroff N, Botstein D (eds) The Dynamic Genome: Barbara McClintock's Ideas in the Century of Genetics. Plainview, NY: Cold Spring Harbor Laboratory Press, 1992.
65. McClearn GE. Biomarkers of age and aging. Exp Gerontol 1997;32:87–94.
66. Kane RA, Kane RL. Assessing the Elderly. Lexington, MA: Lexington Books, 1981.
67. Rubenstein LV, Josephson KR, Nichol-Seamons M, et al. Comprehensive health screening of well elderly adults: an analysis of a communily program. J Gerontol 1986;41:342–352.
68. Rubenstein LV, Calkins DR, Greenfield S, et al. Health status assessment for elderly patients: report of the Society of General Internal Medicine Task Force on Health Assessment. J Am Geriatr Soc 1989;37:562–569.
69. Lachs MS, Feinstein AR, Cooney LM, et al. A simple procedure for general screening for functional disability in the elderly. Ann Intern Med 1990;112:699–706.
70. Colsher PL. Ethical issues in conductiong surveys of the elderly. In: Wallace RB, Woolson RF (eds) The Epidemiologic Study of the Elderly. New York: Oxford University Press, 1992:287–300.
71. Hendriksen C, Lund E, Stomgard E. Consequences of assessment and intervention among elderly people. BMJ 1984;289:1522–1524.
72. Annas GJ, Glantz LH. Rules for research in nursing homes. N Engl J Med 1986;315:1157–1158.
73. Harel Z, Ehrlich P, Hubbard R (eds) The Vulnerable Aged: People, Services, and Policies. New York: Springer, 1990.
74. Kaye JM, Lawton P, Kaye D. Attitudes of elderly people about clinical research on aging. Gerontologist 1990;30:100–106.
75. Sakai Y, Zhong R, Garcia B, et al. Assessment of the longevity of the liver using a rat transplant model. Hepatology 1997;25:421–425.
76. Aarnink RG, De La Rosette JJMCM, Huynen AL, et al. Standardized assessment to enhance the diagnostic value of prostate volume. Part II. Correlation with prostate-specific antigen levels. Prostate 1996;29:327–333.

77. Abrams P, Donova JL, De La Rosette JJMCM, et al. International Continence Society "benign prostatic hyperplasia" study: background, aims, and methodology. Neurourol Urodyn 1997;16:79–91.
78. Worgul BV, Kundiev Y, Likhtarey I, et al. Use of subjective and nonsubjective methodologies to evaluate lens radiation damage in exposed populations: an overview. Radiat Environ Biophys 1986;35:137–144.
79. Kirov SA, Talan MI, Kosheleva NA, et al. Nonshivering thermogenesis during acute cold exposure in adult and aged C57BL-6J mice. Exp Gerontol 1996;31:409–419.
80. Spencer RP. Organ-body weight loss with aging: evidence for coordinated involution. Med Hypotheses 1996;46:59–62.
81. Morawska L, Jamriska M, Bofinger ND. Size characteristics and ageing of the environmental tobacco smoke. Sci Total Environ 1997;196:43–55.
82. Kimmel PL, Lew SQ, Bosch JP. Nutrition, ageing and GFR: is age-associated decline inevitable? Nephrol Dial Transplant 1996;11:85–88.
83. Gardner EM, Bernstein ED, Dorfman M, et al. The age-associated decline in immune function of healthy individuals is not related to changes in plasma concentrations of beta-carotene, retinol, alpha-tocopherol or zinc. Mech Ageing Dev 1997;94:55–69.
84. Scheltens P, Pasquier F, Weerts JGE, et al. Qualitative assessment of cerebral atrophy on MRI: inter- and intra-observer reproducibility in dementia and normal aging. Eur Neurol 1997;37:95–99.
85. Grinker JA, Tucker K, Vokonas PS, et al. Overweight and leanness in adulthood: prospective study of male participants in the normative aging study. Int J Obes 1996;20:561–569.
86. McLeskey CH. Geriatric Anesthesiology. Baltimore: Williams & Wilkins, 1997.
87. Guralnik JM, Lacroix AZ. Assessing physical function in older populations. In: Wallace RB, Woolson RF (eds) The Epidemiologic Study of the Elderly. Oxford: Oxford University Press, 1992:159–181.

# 3
# Cancer, Carcinogenesis, and Aging

Lodovico Balducci and Martine Extermann

This chapter explores the biologic interactions of aging and cancer. In the process we review the epidemiology and clinical implications of cancer in the older-aged person.

## Epidemiology

Currently, 60% of all malignancies and 70% of all cancer deaths occur in persons aged 65 and older.[1–3] Both figures are likely to increase with the rapid expansion of the older population. Cancer is the second most frequent cause of death and one of the most common causes of morbidity for the aged.[2]

The incidence of most neoplasms increases with the age of the population (Fig. 3.1). This increment is noted in all countries for which data are available.[3] The incidence rate varies for different cancers. In the United States the Surveillance, Epidemiology and End Result (SEER) surveys shows that the incidence of breast cancer peaks at age 80 and plateaus until age 85; the incidence of colorectal cancer, prostate cancer, and malignant brain tumors[4] increases up to age 85; and the incidence of lung cancer peaks at age 68 and declines thereafter (Fig. 3.1).[1] The epidemiology of most neoplasms in the oldest-old (i.e., persons aged 85 and over) is poorly known, as data are scanty. Stanta et al. reviewed the experience of thousands of autopsies in older patients, 350 of whom were older than 95 years, and 99 were older than 100 years.[5] The authors concluded that the incidence of both clinical and occult cancer declined after age 95. The incidence of cancer-related deaths declined even more rapidly. This study suggests that cancer is a major management problem for the age window 65–95 years. Seemingly, most cancer patients over age 95 die *with* cancer rather than *of* cancer.

Another important aspect of cancer in the older person is the increasing prevalence of co-morbid conditions with age.[6–8] These conditions may affect cancer management in various ways: They may mask early signs of cancer, impair the tolerance to antineoplastic treatment, and shorten the life expectancy of the older person.[2,6–10]

## Carcinogenesis and Age

The association of cancer and aging may be accounted for by three nonmutually exclusive possibilities. First, cancer is more common in the older person because carcinogenesis is a time-consuming process. Second, cancer and aging share molecular changes that make older persons particularly susceptible to carcinogens. Third, the physiologic changes of senescence provide an environment that favors the development of cancer. To study these possibilities we review the molecular aspects of carcinogenesis and senescence.

Cancer entails progressive accumulation of a monoclonal population of cells capable of damaging adjacent tissues and spreading to distant organs.[11] Cancer involves disruption of the processes that regulate the life of a normal cell. Unlike normal cells, cancer cells are capable of unlimited proliferation and cannot undergo cellular differentiation and programmed cell death (apoptosis). Normal cellular processes are disrupted during carcinogenesis in a multistage process. Each carcinogenic stage involves genetic mutations, leading to activation of proto-oncogenes and loss of function of antiproliferative genes (anti-oncogenes). For example, many of the serial mutations leading to adenomatous polyps of the colon and eventually to colorectal cancer have been recognized (Fig. 3.2).[12] Seemingly, these mutations must occur in a precise serial order to give rise to cancer.

Oncogenes encode proteins involved in cell proliferation, such as growth factors, growth factor receptors, enzymes responsible for signal transduction, and DNA synthesis.[13] Antiproliferative genes encode proteins that block cell replication. One of the best defined of these genes is the *p53* anti-oncogene; located on the long arm of chromosome 17, it encodes a phosphoprotein that arrests the proliferation of mutated cells and allows

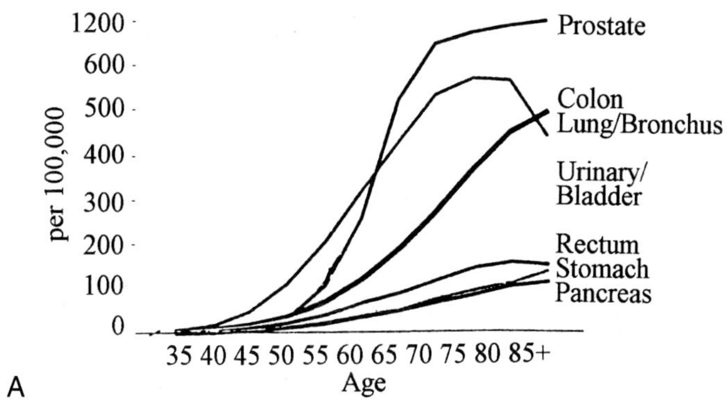


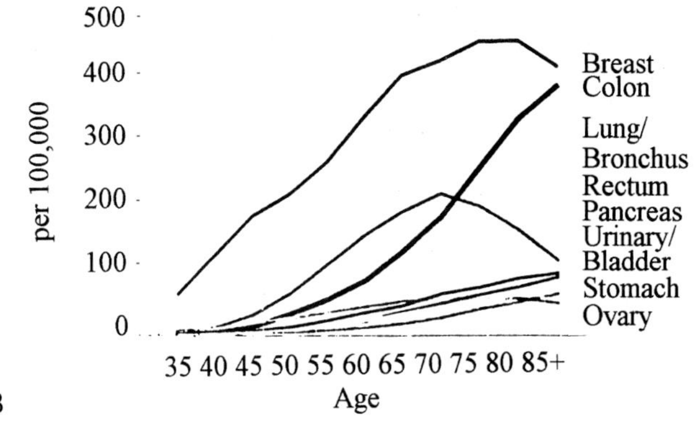


FIGURE 3.1. Age-related incidence of selected cancers in men (A) and women (B) according to SEER. (From Yancik and Ries,[1] with permission.)

repair of the genomic damage.[14] When the genomic damage is irreversible, the P53 phosphoprotein causes cell death. The importance of the *p53* anti-oncogene in carcinogenesis has been recognized in experimental and clinical studies. The incidence of spontaneous cancers has dramatically increased in *p53* knockout mice (J. Campisi, President Cancer Panel, Ann Arbor, MI, personal communication, July 31, 1997), a breed of mice deprived of the *p53* gene. In humans, Li-Fraumeni syndrome involves hereditary loss of one *p53* allele and is associated with a high incidence of multiple cancers at an early age.[15] Other genes that may play an important role in carcinogenesis are the c-*fas* and *Bc12* genes, which encode proteins capable of preventing apoptosis.[16]

The various stages of carcinogenesis are effected by different carcinogens classified as "early-stage carcinogens" (mutagens) and "late-stage carcinogens" (promoters). This distinction may have important clinical implications: The effects of early-stage carcinogens are generally irreversible, whereas those of late-stage carcinogens may be reversible by eliminating the carcinogen or by chemoprevention.[12,17]

Cellular senescence is associated with a number of mlecular changes, including DNA hypomethylation, point mutation, and translocations.[12] These changes are similar to those observed during early carcinogenesis. Thus age and carcinogenesis may involve similar early molecular changes, and these changes may prime the aging cell to the effects of late-stage carcinogens. Some studies have focused on proliferative senescence,[18] a special aspect of cellular senescence, and have provided new insights on the association of cancer and aging. All somatic cells, with the possible exception of stem cells, have limited ability to self-replicate in culture. Presumably, this limited ability is also present in vivo. The self-replicative ability of fetal fibroblasts is much higher than that of fibroblasts from young adults, and the latter is much higher than that of fibroblasts from old adults. The loss of self-replicative ability (proliferative senescence) is associated with a number of functional and molecular changes, including an inability to undergo apoptosis, loss of telomerase activity, extracellular matrix-degrading enzymes, and production of inflammatory cytokines. Of these changes, increased production of interleukin-1 (IL-1) is of special concern, as IL-1 stimulates production of epidermal growth factor receptors in surrounding cells.[19] Thus progressive accumulation of these senescent cells due to refractoriness to apoptosis

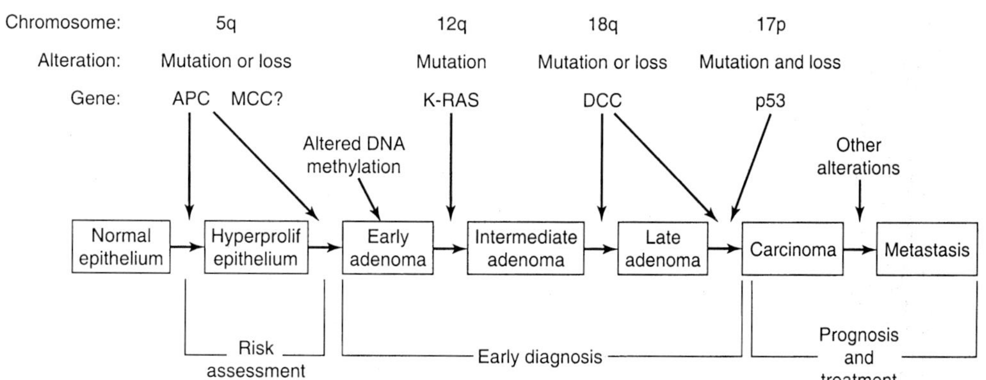


FIGURE 3.2. Model of colonic carcinogenesis. (From Fearon and Vogelstein,[12] with permission.)

may induce changes in surrounding tissues that favor carcinogenesis.

A number of physiologic changes in the aging organism may also favor the development of cancer. Of these changes, the best studied is immune senescence, which involves a progressive decline in immunologic function, especially cell-mediated immunity.[20] Another change that may favor cancer development is disruption of the extracellular stroma.[21]

Clearly, carcinogenesis is a time-consuming process whose length is roughly proportional to the number of carcinogenic stages involved. Accordingly, the cancers whose incidence increases late in age may also be those that involve more carcinogenic stages. For example, the incidence of malignant melanoma peaks at age 45 in women and 62 in men, whereas the incidence of nonmelanomatous skin cancer keeps increasing beyond age 85.[22] Presumably, fewer carcinogenic stages are involved in the pathogenesis of melanoma than in the pathogenesis of nonmelanomatous skin cancer.

Experimental and epidemiologic findings also support the possibility that older persons express increased susceptibility to environmental carcinogens. Certain rodent tissues, such as skin, fibroblasts, and hepatic and lymphatic tissue, are more likely to undergo malignant transformation after exposure to late-stage carcinogens when they are obtained from older rodents. This increased susceptibility to late-stage carcinogens is maintained even when tissues from older animals are transplanted into younger animals.[12] The incidence of some cancers, such as nonmelanomatous skin cancer, increases logarithmically with age,[23] a finding that suggests age is associated with increased sensitivity to late-stage carcinogens, not just with an increased opportunity for cancer to manifest. A study of environmental pollution in the Italian city of Trieste showed that the risk of lung cancer was directly related to the age of exposure to the pollutant; that is, old individuals had a higher risk of developing cancer than young individuals exposed to the same dose of carcinogen.[24]

The possibility that the aged organism favors the development of cancer is controversial.[25] The spontaneous development of some but not all tumors is more likely in immune suppressed animals and immune suppressed humans.[25,26] However, at least in some cases immune competence may also hasten and immune senescence may delay cancer growth, as mononuclear cells produce cytokines that stimulate cell proliferation.[27]

## Biology of Cancer in the Aged

The behavior of some cancers varies with the age of the patient. For example, the course of breast cancer[28–30] or non-small-cell lung cancer[31,32] is generally more indolent in older individuals, and age is a poor prognostic factor for acute myelogenous leukemia (AML),[33,34] non-Hodgkin's lymphoma,[35] and celomic ovarian cancer.[36] These variations may be explained by two not mutually exclusive mechanisms. First, the cancers developed by old and young persons are intrinsically different. Second, the old and young organisms modulate the growth of the same tumor in different ways. Experimental and clinical data support both possibilities.

In the case of breast cancer, the prevalence of tumors with indolent characteristics (high hormone receptor concentrations, low nuclear grade, low proliferation rate) increases with the age of the patient.[28–30] In the case of AML, the prevalence of leukemic cells expressing the multidrug resistance (*mdr1*) gene and the CD-34 antigen increases with the age of the patient. The *mdr1* gene is expressed in 67% of leukemics over 60 years of age and in 21% of those younger.[33] These changes account for the worst prognosis for AML in the elderly. The higher prevalence of more indolent tumors in old individuals may be explained by the fact that slower-growing tumors are more likely to manifest at more advanced ages (Fig. 3.3). The explanation for tumors with the worst prognosis, as is the case with AML, is elusive but may somehow be related to the molecular changes of aging.

The importance of the age of the tumor host in modulating tumor growth was demonstrated by the experiments of Erhsler,[25] who injected Lewis lung carcinoma and B16 melanoma from the same cell line in young and old syngeneic mice. The tumor growth and number of metastases were higher, and the survival shorter, in older mice.[25] Two reports have noted that the mononuclear cell reaction to primary breast cancer in humans varies inversely with the age of the patient.[27–29] These mononuclear cells release cytokine(s) that stimulate tumor growth. The factors modulating tumor growth in young and old individuals are only partially understood. In the

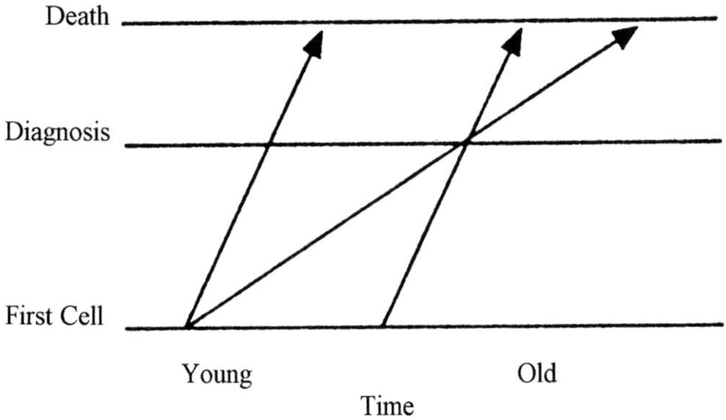


FIGURE 3.3. Explanation for varying tumor aggressiveness with age. If two tumors—one fast-growing and one slow-growing—arise at the same stage of life, the faster-growing one presents clinically at a younger age. This model may explain why tumors arising in younger patients tend to be more aggressive.

case of breast cancer, immune senescence appears to be associated with decreased tumor growth. Other factors may include increased concentrations of IL-6,[37] transforming growth factor-β (TGFβ),[38] and insulin-like growth factor-I (IGF-I) receptors[39] in the circulation of old individuals.

Although tumor biology may change with the age of the patient, age itself is a poor predictor of disease behavior in individual situations. For example, of the breast cancers occurring in women aged 80 and over, about 20% are aggressive, hormone receptor-poor tumors and deserve more aggressive treatment than the more common hormone receptor-rich tumors.[28] Clinical decisions should be based on the characteristics of individual tumors rather than the age of the tumor host.

## Cancer Prevention in the Old Person

Primary prevention of cancer involves elimination of environmental carcinogens and administration of substances that offset carcinogenesis (chemoprevention). As the susceptibility to late-stage carcinogens may increase with age, old individuals may benefit from primary prevention of cancer.[12] In view of this new insight, a nihilistic attitude toward cancer prevention in the aged is no longer justified. In other words, it is never too late to stop smoking and adopt healthy eating habits.

At least three groups of substances may have chemopreventive activity in humans.[17] Estrogen antagonists prevent contralateral breast cancer in women with a history of breast cancer; retinoids prevent second cancers of the upper airways; and nonsteroidal antiinflammatory drugs (NSAIDs) prevent death from cancer of the large bowel. Currently, there are no precise indications for the use of these agents outside of clinical trials weighing the benefits and risks of chemoprevention.

Secondary prevention of cancer involves early detection of cancer through screening asymptomatic individuals. Current screening approaches are outlined in Table 3.1. A number of screening guidelines have been issued by various bodies, including the American Cancer Society, the National Cancer Institute, and the United States Preventing Study Task Force (USPSTF).[40,41] The USPSTF guidelines are strictly evidence-based and were issued only after a demonstration that cancer-related mortality declined as a result of screening. We have adopted the same definition of effectiveness in Table 3.1.

Clearly, the benefits of cancer screening in older individuals are not established, even for interventions that clearly proved effective in young persons. There are reasons that both favor and disfavor cancer screening in the aged person. The positive predictive value (PPV) of screening tests is a function of the prevalence of the disease in the population screened. Thus the PPV may improve when screening old individuals in whom the prevalence of common cancers is increased. Also, early detection of cancer of the large bowel may prevent emergency surgery, which is particularly risky in the aged. On the other hand, the benefits of screening may be diminished as a result of previous screening and of reduced life expectancy.

In view of the fact that the benefits of screening interventions are first seen 3–7 years after the initial screening,[40] we recommend biennial mammography and yearly breast examination in women and yearly fecol occult blood examination in men and women whose estimated life expectancy is 3 years or longer. The adoption of other forms of screening should be tailored to the clinical situation.

The field of cancer screening is in continuous evolution, and we recommend that the reader keep abreast of the latest findings. A multiinstitutional study explored the value of screening individuals at risk for prostate, colorectal, lung, and ovarian cancer. The results of this study may modify current screening recommendations. As the populations at risk for certain cancers become better defined, screening efforts may become more focused and productive. Recognition of early carcinogenic changes with molecular techniques has opened a new era of cancer screening, as precancerous lesions may be recognized through molecular screening.

TABLE 3.1. Current Approaches to Cancer Screening

| Method | Age range (years) | Effectiveness |
|---|---|---|
| Breast | | |
| Mammography | 50–69 | Effective |
| CBE | 50–69 | Effective |
| BSE | All ages | Not established |
| Large bowel | | |
| FOB | 50–80 | Effective |
| Endoscopy | 50–80 | Not established |
| Uterine cervix | | |
| Cervical cytology | 18–60 | Effective |
| Liver | | |
| AFP and liver US[a] | — | Effective |
| Prostate | | |
| PSA | ≥50 | Not established |
| DRE | ≥50 | Not established |
| Endometrium | | |
| TVU | — | Not established |
| Pelvic examination | | Not established |
| Ovary | | |
| TVU | — | Not established |
| Pelvic examination | — | Not established |
| Ca-125 | — | Not established |

AFP, α-fetoprotein; BSE, breast self-examination; CBE, clinical examination of the breast; DRE, digital examination of the breast; FOB, fecal occult blood; US, ultrasonography; PSA, prostate-specific antigen; TVU, transvaginal ultrasonography.

[a] Limited to persons with a history of hepatitis B.

## Cancer Treatment

Treatment of cancer may involve surgery, radiation therapy, and systemic treatment, including cytotoxic chemotherapy and endocrine and biologic therapy. Surgical management of cancer in the old person is a major focus of this textbook and is dealt with in depth in other chapters.

The safety and effectiveness of radiation therapy in old individuals has been documented in several series of patients.[42–44] In these reports only a few patients (<10%) aged 70 and older were unable to complete the course of treatment because of toxicity. Radiation therapy was well tolerated even by individuals with a poor performance status who had been considered ineligible for other forms of cancer treatment. Tolerance of radiation therapy to the esophagus and the head and neck area was enhanced by early, aggressive nutritional intervention, involving feeding gastrostomy or jejunostomy.

Elderly cancer patients are at increased risk for some complications of cancer chemotherapy including myelotoxicity, mucositis, cardiotoxicity, and peripheral and central neurotoxicity.[45] Cytotoxic chemotherapy of old individuals has become safer because of a better understanding of the pharmacokinetic changes of aging, the development of safer agents and antidotes to the complications of chemotherapy, and the timely treatment of chemotherapy-related complications (Table 3.2).[45–48]

The most predictable physiologic change of aging is a progressive decline of the glomerular filtration rate (GFR).[47] The doses of agents excreted through the kidneys should be adjusted to the individual's GFR, measured with the formula of Cockroft and Gault.[49] Such agents include methotrexate, carboplatin, bleomycin, and fludarabine.

TABLE 3.2. Interventions That May Improve Tolerance to Cancer Chemotherapy by the Old Person

- Pharmacokinetic interventions
  - Dose adjustment of renally excreted drugs
  - Administration of doxorubicin by continuous infusion
- New and safer agents
  - Mitoxantrone
  - Gemcitabine
  - Vinorelbine
  - Liposomal anthracyclines
- Antidotes to drug-related toxicity
  - Hemopoietic growth factors
    - Granulocyte colony-stimulating factor (G-CSF)
    - Granulocyte/macrophage colony-stimulating factor (GM-CSF)
    - Erythropoietin
    - Thrombopoietin
  - Cardioprotectors
    - Dexrazoxane
  - Cytoprotectors
  - Amifostine
- Timely treatment of chemotherapy complications
  - Aggressive fluid replacement for mucositis
  - Prophylactic antibiotics for prolonged neutropenia
  - Discontinuance of neurotoxic drugs for peripheral weakness and decreased sensation

Another pharmacokinetic intervention of interest involves giving doxorubicin by continuous intravenous infusion. This method of administration reduces the cardiotoxicity of the drug but may be associated with enhanced mucositis and myelodepression.[45]

A number of new agents have a particularly favorable toxicity profile for old individuals.[50] Mitoxantrone is active in acute leukemia, lymphoma, and breast cancer and may represent a less toxic alternative to doxorubicin in frail patients. Gemcitabine has a broad spectrum of action, against many tumors including pancreatic cancer, breast cancer, non-small-cell lung cancer, and transitional cell carcinoma of the urothelium. Vinorelbine is active against breast cancer and non-small-cell lung cancer. Liposomal derivatives of doxorubicin and daunorubicin conserve the activity of the parent compound with minimal cardiotoxicity.

The development of antidotes to drug toxicity has been a major advance in cancer chemotherapy. Granulocyte- and granulocyte/macrophage colony-stimulating factors (G-CSF, GM-CSF) are comparable in terms of shortening the duration of neutropenia and reducing the risk of neutropenic infections.[46] Interleukin II effectively prevents chemotherapy-induced life-threatening thrombocytopenia.[51] Erythropoietin ameliorates anemia in about 50% of cancer patients.[45] One report suggested the effectiveness of erythropoietin in preventing chemotherapy-related anemia.[52]

Desrazoxane chelates the iron of the sarcomeres and prevents formation of the free radicals responsible for the cardiotoxicity of anthracyclines.[45–47] Amifostine is a thiol derivative with a broad spectrum of protection, including nephrotoxicity from platinum derivatives, cardiotoxicity of anthracyclines, and myelotoxicity of alkylating agents.[45–47] Currently, high cost, severe nausea, and hypotension make amifostine unfit for widespread use. Ongoing research is exploring the subcutaneous use of small doses of amifostine to enhance tolerance to this important agent.

Timely intervention for the treatment of chemotherapy-related complications is particularly important in old persons, who have a limited functional reserve and may succumb to treatment complications earlier than young individuals. Mucositis is a common complication of chemotherapy, especially that involving methotrexate and fluorinated pyrimidines.[45–47] Mucositis may cause volume depletion by preventing liquid intake and by causing severe diarrhea. Mucositis in old persons mandates early, aggressive fluid resuscitation. The prophylactic use of quinolones[45–47] and sulfamethoxazole/trimethoprim has reduced the risk of gram-negative septicemia in patients with prolonged neutropenia. It is used routinely in old individuals at risk for neutropenia of 1 week duration or longer. Neurotoxic drugs that should be discontinued at the appearance of symptoms of peripheral neuropathy include cisplatin, alkaloids, epipodophyllotoxins, and paclitaxel.

Hormonal treatment of cancer is generally safe for old patients. The estrogen antagonist tamoxifen is widely used to treat primary and metastatic breast cancer. Additional benefits of tamoxifen include prevention of contralateral breast cancer, osteoporosis, and possibly coronary artery disease. Complications are rare and are mostly confined to hot flushes and vaginal discharge. Deep vein thrombosis and endometrial cancer are rare. The new antiestrogen toremifene promises an even safer profile: It may have additional cardiovascular benefits and so far has not been associated with an increased risk of endometrial cancer.[53] The new aromatase inhibitors anastrozole, letrozole and etamestane have largely replaced the more toxic aminoglutethimide for managing breast cancer.[47] For management of prostate cancer, the luteinizing hormone releasing hormone (LH-RH) analogues offer a safe alternative to estrogen.[47] A number of androgen antagonists are available for use against prostate cancer, but the indications for these compounds are somewhat controversial.[54]

Biologic therapy of cancer involves interferon-α (IFNα) and IL-2. Experience with these compounds in old individuals is limited, however, and their safety in the aged is not proved.[48]

Of special interest to the old person is chemoradiation therapy in lieu of surgery for management of some tumors.[55] In the case of laryngeal cancer, treatment with chemotherapy and irradiation was found to be equivalent to radical laryngectomy in a randomized controlled trial. For squamous cell carcinoma of the anus and of the esophagus and for transitional cell carcinoma of the bladder, combined-modality treatment was found to be comparable to surgery in single-arm clinical trials. These results require validation in randomized clinical trials.

## Evaluation of the Elderly Cancer Patient

Clearly, elderly cancer patients may benefit from an array of treatment modalities. The practitioner is often faced with the vexing decision of whether to recommend a toxic treatment to patients with compromised functional status. Diversity is a unique characteristic of the population aged 75–90, and treatment decisions must be founded on an objective evaluation of this diversity. Basically, the questions involved in therapeutic decisions include the following: Is this elderly person likely to suffer (and die) of cancer during his or her limited life expectancy? Is the treatment likely to compromise the quality of life of the old individual? Is the treatment more likely than the cancer to cause the death of this old person?

For the first question, it is important to remember that the life expectancy of old persons is often underestimated. For example, the average life expectancy of an 85-year-old is in excess of 5 years, which is much longer than the expected survival for most patients with hematologic malignancies or metastatic cancers. The cancers that can be safely watched in persons as old as 85 include early-stage prostate cancer,[54] low-grade non-Hodgkin's lymphoma,[56] and chronic lymphocytic leukemia[57] at early stages.

The answers to the other questions are more complex. They involve personal values and an assessment of life expectancy, quality of life, and risk of therapeutic complications. At the Senior Adult Oncology Program of the H. Lee Moffitt Cancer Center and Research Institute we found that a comprehensive geriatric assessment may provide valuable assistance in treatment-related decisions. The comprehensive geriatric assessment involves (1) assessment of functional status as Activities of Daily Living (ADD)[58] and Instrumental Activities of Daily Living (IADL)[59]; (2) grading of co-morbidity with the Charlson[60] and CIRS-G[61] scales; (3) evaluation of cognition, nutritional status, depression, and living conditions; and (4) assessment of quality of life with the FACT-G instrument, which we have validated in elderly individuals.[62]

The comprehensive geriatric assessment provides (1) an estimate of life expectancy based on age, function, and co-morbidity; (2) information on treatment tolerance based on function and co-morbidity, as well as on family support and cognition (information of how treatment and cancer affect quality of life); and (3) a profile of potentially reversible conditions, such as malnutrition, limited mobility, and inadequate social support, which may compromise treatment outcome. Perhaps most importantly, the comprehensive geriatric assessment translates the diversity of the elderly population into objective categories that may be used when planning clinical trials of cancer treatment in old persons.

## References

1. Yancik R, Ries LA. Cancer in older persons: magnitude of the problem—how do we apply what we know? Cancer 1994;74:1995–2003.
2. Balducci L, Lyman GH. Cancer in the elderly: epidemiologic and clinical implications. Clin Geriatr Med 1997;13:1–14.
3. LaVecchia C, Levi F, Lucchini F, et al. International perspectives of cancer and aging. In: Balducci L, Lyman GH, Ershler WB (eds) Comprehensive Geriatric Oncology. Harwood Academic Publishers, London, 1998:19–94.
4. Fernandez PM, Brem S. Malignant brain tumors in the elderly. Clin Geriatr Med 1997;13:327–338.

5. Stanta G, Campagner L, Cavallieri F, et al. Cancer in the oldest old: what we have learned from autopsy studies. Clin Geriatr Med 1997;13:55–68.
6. Extermann M, Balducci L. Practical proposals for clinical protocols in elderly patients with cancer. In: Balducci L, Lyman GH, Ershler WB (eds) Comprehensive Geriatric Oncology. Harwood Academic Publishers, 1998:263–270.
7. Extermann M, Overcash J, Lyman GH, et al. Comorbidity and functional status are independent in older cancer patients. J Clin Oncol (in press); 1998;16:1582–1587.
8. Satariano WA, Ragland DR. The effect of comorbidity on 3-year survival of women with primary breast cancer. Ann Intern Med 1994;120:104–110.
9. Balducci L. Perspective on quality of life of older patients with cancer. Drugs Aging 1994;4:313–324.
10. Bennahum DA, Forman WB, Vellas B, et al. Life-expectancy, comorbidity, and quality of life: a framework of reference for medical decisions. Clin Geriatr Med 1997;13:33–53.
11. Bishop JM. The rise of the genetic paradigm. Genes Dev 1995;9:1309–1315.
12. Fearon ER, Vogelstein B. A genetic model for colorectal tumorigenesis. Cell 1990.
13. Anisimov VN. Age as a risk factor in multistage carcinogenesis. In: Balducci L, Lyman GH, Ershler WB (eds) Comprehensive Geriatric Oncology. Harwood Academic Publishers, London, 1998:157–178.
14. Arrowsmith CH: Structure and Function in the p53. Family Cell Death Differ, 1999;6:1169–1173.
15. Malkin D, Jolly KV, Barbier N, et al. Germline mutations of the p53 tumor-suppressor gene in children and young adults with second malignant neoplasms. N Engl J Med 1992;326:1309–1312.
16. Fisher DF. Apoptosis, chemotherapy and aging. In: Balducci L, Lyman GH, Ershler WB (eds) Comprehensive Geriatric Oncology. Harwood Academic Publishers, London, 1998: 237–246.
17. Minton SE, Shaw GL. Chemoprevention of cancer in the elderly. In: Balducci L, Lyman GH, Ershler WB (eds) Comprehensive Geriatric Oncology. Harwood Academic Publishers, London, 1998:307–324.
18. Campisi J. Aging and cancer: the double-edged sword of replicative senescence. J Am Geriatr Soc 1997;45:482–488.
19. Dinarello CA. Biologic basis for interleukin-1 in disease. Blood 1996;87:2095–2117.
20. Burns EA, Goodwin JS. Immunological changes of aging. In: Balducci L, Lyman GH, Ershler WB (eds) Comprehensive Geriatric Oncology. Harwood Academic Publishers, 1998: 213–222.
21. Wick M, Burger G, Brusselbach S, et al. A novel member of human tissue inhibitor of metalloproteinases (TIMP) gene family is regulated during $G_1$ progression, mitogenic stimulation, differentiation, and senescence. J Biol Chem 1994;269:18953–18960.
22. Marks R. An overview of skin cancer. Cancer 1995; 75(suppl):607–612.
23. Glass AG, Hoover RH. The emerging epidemic of melanoma and squamous cell cancer. JAMA 1989;262: 2097–2100.
24. Barbone F, Bovenzi M, Cavallieri F, et al. Air pollution and lung cancer in Trieste, Italy. Am J Epidemiol 1995;141: 1161–1169.
25. Erhsler WB. A gerontologist's perspective on cancer biology and treatment. Cancer Control JMCC 1994;1:103–107.
26. Levine AM. Lymphoma complicating immunodeficiency disorders. Ann Oncol 1994;5:29–38.
27. Kurtz JM, Jacquemier J, Amalric R, et al. Why are local recurrences after breast-conserving therapy more frequent in younger patients. J Clin Oncol 1990;10:141–152.
28. Balducci L, Silliman RA, Bakae P. Breast cancer in the older woman: an oncologic perspective. In: Balducci L, Lyman GH, Ershler WB (eds) Comprehensive Geriatric Oncology. Harwood Academic Publishers, London, 1998:629–660.
29. Nixon AJ, Neuberg D, Hayes DF, et al. Relationship of patient age to pathologic features of the tumor and prognosis of patients with stage I and II breast cancer. J Clin Oncol 1994;12:888–894.
30. Valentinis B, Silvestrini R, Daidone MG, et al. $^3$H thymidine labeling index, hormone receptors, and ploidy, in breast cancers from elderly patients. Breast Cancer Res Treat 1991;20:19–24.
31. O'Rourke MA, Feussner JR, Feigl P, et al. Age trends of lung cancer stage at diagnosis. JAMA 1987;258:921–926.
32. Antonia SJ, Robinson LA, Ruckdeschel JC, et al. Lung cancer. In: Balducci L, Lyman GH, Ershler WB (eds) Comprehensive Geriatric Oncology. Harwood Academic Publishers, London, 1998:611–627.
33. Willman CL: Molecular Evaluation of Acute Myeloid Leukemia. Semin Hemetol 1999;36:390–400.
34. Extermann M. Acute leukemia in the elderly. Clin Geriatr Med 1997;13:227–243.
35. International non-Hodgkin's lymphoma prognostic factors project: a predictive model for aggressive non-Hodgkin's lymphoma. N Engl J Med 1993;329:987–994.
36. Thigpen JT. Gynecologic cancers. In: Balducci L, Lyman GH, Ershler WB (eds) Comprehensive Geriatric Oncology. Harwood Academic Publishers, London, 1998, 721–732.
37. Ershler WB. Interleukin 6: a cytokine for gerontologists. J Am Geriatr Soc 1993;41:176–181.
38. Butta A, Maclennan K, Flanders KC, et al. Induction of transforming growth factor beta in human breast cancer "in vivo" following tamoxifen. Cancer Res 1992;52:4261–4264.
39. Yee D, Sharma J, Hilsenbeck SG. Prognostic significance of insulin-like growth factor binding protein expression in axillary lymph node-negative breast cancer. J Natl Cancer Inst 1994;86:1785–1789.
40. Balducci L, Barry P: A practical approach to the screening of asymptomatic older persons for cancer. Cancer Control JMCC 1994:1.
41. Robinson B, Beghe' C. Cancer screening in the older patient. Clin Geriatr Med 1997;13:97–118.
42. Olmi P, Ausili-Cefaro GP, Balzi M, et al. Radiotherapy in the aged. Clin Geriatr Med 1997;13:143–168.
43. Scalliet P, Pignon T. Radiotherapy in the elderly. In: Balducci L, Lyman GH, Ershler WB (eds) Comprehensive Geriatric Oncology. Hardwood Press, 1997.
44. Zachariah B, Balducci L. Radiation therapy of the older patient. Hematol Oncol Clin America 2000;14:131–168.
45. Balducci L, Extermann M. Cancer chemotherapy of the older patient: what the medical oncologist needs to know. Cancer (in press) 1997;80:1317–1322.
46. Zagonel V, Pinto A, Monfardini S. Strategies to prevent chemotherapy-related toxicities in older persons. In: Bal-

ducci L, Lyman GH, Ershler WB (eds) Comprehensive Geriatric Oncology. Harwood Academic Publishers, London, 1998:481–500.

47. Cova D, Berretta G, Balducci L. Cancer chemotherapy in the older patient. In: Balducci L, Lyman GH, Ershler WB (eds) Comprehensive Geriatric Oncology. Harwood Academic Publishers, London, 1998:429–442.
48. Balducci L. Medical therapy of solid tumors in the elderly: an update. Rays 1997;22:20–24.
49. Waller DG, Fleming JS, Ramsay B, et al. The accuracy of creatinine clearance with and withour urine collection as a measure of glomerular filtration rate. Postgrad Med J 1991;67:42–46.
50. Eckardt JR, Von Hoff DD. New antineoplastic agents of interest to the older patient. In: Balducci L, Lyman GH, Ershler WB (eds) Comprehensive Geriatric Oncology. Harwood Academic Publishers, London, 1998:443–470.
51. Vadhan-Raj S, Murray LJ, Bueso-Ramos C, et al. Stimulation of megakaryocyte and platelet production by a single dose of recombinant human thrombopoietin in patients with cancer. Ann Intern Med 1997:673–681.
52. DelMastro L, Venturini M, Lionetto R, et al. Randomized phase III trial evaluating the role of erythropoietin in the prevention of chemotherapy-induced anemia. J Clin Oncol 1997;15:2715–2721.
53. Saarto T, Blomqvist C, Enholm C, et al. Antiatherogenic effects of adjuvant antiestrogens: a randomized trial comparing the effects of tamoxifen and toremifene on plasma lipid levels in postmenopausal women with node-positive breast cancer. J Clin Oncol 1996;14:429–433.
54. Balducci L, Pow-Sang J, Friedland J, et al. Prostate cancer. Clin Geriatr Med 1997;13:283–306.
55. Balducci L, Trotti A. Organ preservation: an effective and safe form of cancer treatment. Clin Geriatr Med 1997; 13:203–219.
56. O'Reilly SE, Connors JM, Macpherson N, et al. Malignant lymphomas in the elderly. Clin Geriatr Med 1997; 13:251–264.
57. Rai K. Chronic lymphocytic leukemia in the elderly population. Clin Geriatr Med 1997;13:245–250.
58. Katz S, Ford AB, Moskowitz RW, et al. Studies of illness in the aged: the index on ADL. JAMA 1963;185:914–919.
59. Lawton MP, Brody EM. Assessment of older people: self-maintaining and instrumental activities of daily living. Gerontologist 1969;9:179–186.
60. Charlson M, Szatrowski TP, Peterson J, et al. Validation of a combined comorbidity index. J Clin Epidemiol 1994;47:1245–1251.
61. Conwell Y, Forbes NT, Cox C, et al. Validation of a measure of physical illness burden at autopsy: the cumulative illness rating scale. J Am Geriatr Soc 1993;41:38–41.
62. Cella D. The functional assessment of cancer therapy anemia (FACT-An) scale: a new tool for the assessment of outcome in cancer anemia and fatigue. Semin Hematol 1997;34(suppl 2):13–19.

# 4
# Effects of Aging on Immune Function

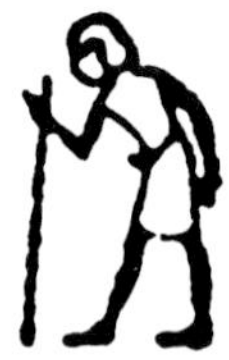

Edith A. Burns and James S. Goodwin

At first glance, a review of immune system changes with age may seem out of place in a surgical textbook. After stopping to consider for a few moments, however, it begins to make sense that such a topic be included. The traditional approach to describing immune function focuses on the role of cellular components in protection against infection and cancer and the diseases that result from hyper- or hypoactivity of these components. Proper function of the immune system is imperative if the body is to heal and protect itself properly, not only after microbial invasion or neoplastic transformation but after physical invasion, such as trauma and surgery. A well-functioning immune system helps ensure optimum wound healing and minimizes the risk of infection. As adults over age 85 years continue to be the fastest growing segment of the population, an increasingly larger proportion of patients taken to surgery will be in the geriatric age range. Age-related changes in immune function will assume greater significance during management of these patients surgically and in overall clinical practice.

In this chapter we describe changes in the immune system that are thought to be related to age per se. We then review the clinical implications of these changes, including the effects of surgical trauma on immune function. We close with a discussion of some of the latest research on ways to restore or stimulate immune function in the elderly. The combined effects of surgical stress and aging may be significant contributors to the increased surgical risk of older individuals. Future research may highlight interventions that reduce surgical risk and iatrogenic complications in the elderly through stimulation of immune function.

## Organization of the Immune System

The immune system is composed of a variety of cell populations that can be described by phenotype and function. Traditionally, the immune system has been divided into two "arms."

The cellular immune response is mediated primarily by thymus-derived lymphocytes (T cells), the major functions of which are to prevent autoimmunity, reject tissue grafts, kill virus-infected cells, protect against some intracellular parasites and bacteria, and maybe defend against growth of tumors. T cells are phenotypically identified as helper or suppressor cells based on the presence of specific cell surface receptors. Within the subpopulations of helper and suppressor cells there are unprimed, or "naive," T cells and primed, or "memory," T cells. Memory T cells are committed in terms of their ability to respond preferentially to a specific stimulus, or antigen.

The humoral arm of the immune system produces antibodies made by B cells, or differentiated bone marrow-derived lymphocytes. The antibodies produced by B cells can be polyclonal (with heavy-chain components of multiple classes, e.g., G, M, D) and "nonspecific" (i.e., not directed against a specific antigen). Many antibodies are antigen-specific, adhering to specific organisms or targets and causing cell lysis, or allowing ingestion and destruction by other cells.

As our knowledge expands, the distinction between cellular and humoral immunity has become somewhat artificial. Most immune cells do not fit exclusively into either the cellular or the humoral arm, playing roles in both components of the immune response. For example, although T cells are effectors of cellular immune responses, their help is required for most antibody responses (e.g., through elaboration of growth and differentiation factors for B cells). B cells function as antigen-presenting cells in some cellular immune responses. Antibodies are often major participants in specific cytotoxic responses, which typically are classified as functions of the cellular immune system. Natural killer cells are lymphocytes capable of lysing certain target cells without being sensitized to specific antigen. Cells of the monocyte/macrophage series can ingest or kill foreign material that may or may not have been previously coated, or "opsonized," with antibodies. They play an important role in regulating both humoral and cellular immune responses. Many of the mechanisms underlying age-related changes in immune function are unclear, in part because of the complexity of the immune system itself. For example, anergy to delayed-type hypersensitivity skin testing (common in adults over 60 years of age[1–3]) could represent problems with antigen recognition, vascular responses to inflammatory mediators, T cell proliferation, lymphokine production, lymphocyte chemotaxis, and a multitude of other steps that are required to produce induration after intradermal challenge with antigen. We describe age-related changes in immunity in terms of qualitative and quantitative changes in cell populations and the production of and response to macromolecules, rather than as changes in cellular versus humoral immunity.

## Changes in Immune Cell Function with Age

### T Lymphocytes

Quantitative changes in T cell populations in aging humans and experimental animals include declines in "virgin" (reactive) T cells and increases in "memory" (primed) T cells.[4–8] It is not clear which subpopulations account for the accumulation of memory cells. Some studies have described increases in the population of CD4+ T-helper memory cells,[9] and others reported increases in CD8+ T suppressor memory cells as well.[10] Although the number of naive T cells declines in old animals, they appear to produce larger amounts of interleukin-2 (IL-2) than naive cells from young animals.[11] Memory T cells normally produce IL-2; and although aged animals have larger proportions of memory cells, many studies have described decreased IL-2 production by aged memory lymphocytes. This paradox of low production of IL-2 despite increased proportions of IL-2-producing cells may be related to a lack of other regulatory cytokine signals, such as IL-4.[12]

A decrease in the proliferative response of lymphocytes to specific antigens or nonspecific mitogens was one of the earliest age-related changes in immune function to be reported.[1,13–15] Decreased responsiveness to mitogens is due to a number of variables, including reduced numbers of mitogen-responsive cells and decreased vigor of the proliferative response.[14] A smaller percentage of T splenocytes from old mice respond to mitogenic stimulation by entering active phases of cell replication, a defect noted with CD4+ T-helper cells and (to a lesser extent) with CD8+ T suppressor/cytotoxic cells.[16] Some studies suggest that the type of stimulus may affect the degree of decreased proliferation of lymphocytes from old animals.[17] T-helper cells from old mice generate fewer cytotoxic effector cells to participate in delayed hypersensitivity skin reactions.[18] Cytotoxic lymphocytes from old mice bind targets less efficiently, though they appear to be equally effective for destroying targets.[19]

The ability of T cells to support antibody production changes with increasing age. Lymphocytes from old subjects display increased helper activity in vitro for nonspecific antibody production,[20,21] and they proliferate more to nonspecific stimulation.[17] Studies comparing suppressor cells from young and old mice have shown that cells from aged animals have more difficulty recognizing and exerting suppressive effects against specific antigens from self and other old animals.[20,22–24] The increased incidence of autoantibodies seen during aging (antibodies directed against parts of the self) may be related to a failure of tonic inhibition by suppressor T cells[25] and has been correlated with the decreased proliferation of T cells to mitogen[26] (i.e., the lower the proliferation of T cells to mitogens, the higher was the level of autoantibodies).

When T cells are exposed to various stimuli the proliferative response is initiated by a complex set of interactions involving T cells and macrophages or other accessory cells. Mitogens or antigens are processed and presented by accessory cells, bind to T cell antigen receptors, and form cross-links that activate the receptors. This sequence results in activation of phospholipase C, cleavage of phosphatidylinositol phosphate components of the cell membrane, and liberation of inositol triphosphate and diacylglycerol. The inositol phosphates (triphosphate and perhaps tetrakisphosphate), stimulate elevation of intracellular free calcium and opening of calcium channels.[27–29] Diacylglycerol binds to and activates protein kinase C (PKC), a process enhanced by the intracellular free calcium levels. Other protein kinases have been identified and are believed to play a role in cell activation.

The cascade of events just described leads to increased transcription and subsequent translation of the gene coding for IL-2 (T cell growth factor) and of receptors for IL-2. IL-2 is thus an autocrine as well as a paracrine growth factor, produced by the same cells that respond to it. When T cells bearing IL-2 receptors are exposed to IL-2, they proliferate. Accessory cells such as monocytes can initiate the cascade by presenting antigen that then occupies and cross-links T cell receptors and stimulates IL-2 production. The accessory cells secrete IL-1 and other cytokines that provide additional signals necessary for complete activation of T cells.

The decreased proliferative response of lymphocytes seen with aging may be due to impairment of the membrane signal transduction pathways just described. Some murine studies have found defective proliferation associated with decreased calcium metabolism in old mice.[5,30] Stimulation with mitogen leads to smaller rises in intracellular calcium levels in old mouse T cells.[31] This correlates with a shift from naive to memory phenotype, with memory cells displaying more resistance to mitogens, decreased tyrosine phosphorylation of phospholipase

TABLE 4.1. Changes in T Cells with Age

| | |
|---|---|
| **Decreased** | |
| | Number of virgin (reactive) T cells |
| | Number of mitogen-responsive cells |
| | Proliferative response |
| | Expression of early activation genes |
| | Sensitivity to activating signals |
| | Activation of membrane protein kinases and phosphoproteins |
| | Cytotoxic cell target-binding |
| | Help for generation of cytotoxic effector cells |
| | T cell help for specific antibody production |
| **Increased** | |
| | Number of memory (primed) T cells |
| | T cell help for nonspecific antibody production |

Cγ1, and decreased ability to produce and respond to IL-2.[31] No changes in inositol triphosphate production were found in these studies.[31] In contrast, models utilizing human peripheral blood neutrophils found that inositol triphosphate formation was significantly reduced in old cells.[32]

Compared to lymphocytes from young animals, T lymphocytes from aged animals that retain the ability to proliferate to mitogens have normal or enhanced mobilization of calcium.[33] Similar results have been found with human peripheral blood lymphocytes and T cells. Decreased calcium mobilization was a factor in defective proliferation in some T cell subpopulations but not others.[4,34,35] Monocyte-depleted lymphocytes from old adults displayed decreased cell–cell binding (a calcium/magnesium-dependent reaction) compared to cells from young donors.[36] It was thought to be secondary to altered activation of the lymphocyte adhesion molecule [leukocyte function-associated antigen-1 (LFA-1)] in the cells from old adults.

The magnitude and duration of protein kinase activation by mitogens is significantly reduced in lymphocytes from old humans.[37] Levels of the isoenzyme protein kinase Cα are significantly reduced in old T cells, although functional properties are comparable to those in young cells.[38] In old mouse T cells, there is decreased phosphorylation of all 16 phosphoproteins that are vigorously phosphorylated in young mouse cells.[39] Moreover, phosphorylation of protein tyrosine kinases and protein phosphokinases is impaired in $CD4^+$ and $CD8^+$ T cells from old animals.[40] Decreased IL-2 production is correlated with decreased transcription of nuclear factors in old cells,[41] which is postulated to be due to impaired signal transduction, as expression of the nuclear factors is preserved with aging.[42] Changes in T cells related to age are summarized in Table 4.1.

## B Lymphocytes

Age-related quantitative changes in B cells have become apparent more recently than those described in T cells. The absolute number of B cells does not appear to change appreciably with age.[43] Studies in aged mice have shown a decrease in bone marrow B cell precursors[44–46] and structural changes in B cell membranes.[47] B cells from old individuals proliferate less efficiently in response to mitogen stimulation, similar to what has been described for T cells.[25] Also similar to T cells,[37] activation of PKC and protein tyrosine kinases is reduced in B cells from old humans.[48] The expression of PKC was not reduced in B cells in this study.[38]

The generation of antibody responses by B cells does change with age,[49] although much of it is related to changes in T cell function. The distinction between antibody responses to T cell-dependent and T cell-independent antigens is made on the basis of whether there is an absolute requirement for T cell help in the antibody response. The decrease in T cell-dependent antibody responses is obvious in experimental animals, with 80% fewer antibody-forming cells in older animals.[4] The accumulation of anti-idiotypes (antibodies directed against other antibodies) with increasing age may interfere with the production of specific antibody.[50,51]

The ability to respond to specific antigenic challenge with specific antibody production decreases with age.[49] This phenomenon has been described in studies of both primary and secondary antibody responses. When subjects of different ages were immunized with the primary antigen flagellin, similar levels of anti-flagellin antibody were found in both old and young subjects, but the older subjects were unable to maintain the response.[52] We studied a group of healthy old adults participating in a large study of emotions and health behavior. The old adults were less likely to mount an in vivo response to immunization with the primary antigen keyhole limpet hemocyanin than a group of healthy young control subjects (unpublished data). In contrast, De Greef et al. immunized old and young subjects with the primary antigen *Helix pomatia* hemocyanin. Compared to young subjects, old subjects had similar numbers of antibody-producing cells after in vitro stimulation with the antigen.[53]

Studies of the secondary antibody response to tetanus toxoid have found that B cells from old adults produce less anti-tetanus toxoid antibody when stimulated in vitro with tetanus than B cells from young adults, regardless of the source and the type of T cell help provided in the cultures.[54] We have examined changes in tetanus toxoid-specific antibody production by stimulating lymphocytes from old and young adults with tetanus toxoid and measuring anti-tetanus toxoid antibody production.[55] Significantly lower serum antibody levels of tetanus toxoid were found in old adults than young adults, even if they were recently immunized. Old adults had fewer numbers of B cells producing anti-tetanus toxoid antibody, and each B cell produced significantly less antibody on average. One reason for the decreased specific antibody production appeared to be a lack of

TABLE 4.2. Changes in B Cells with Age

| |
|---|
| Decreased surface major histocompatability complex (MHC) class II molecule expression |
| Decreased proportion of cells capable of clonal expansion |
| Decreased number of bone marrow precursors |
| Decreased number of T cell-dependent antibody-forming cells |
| Decreased specific antibody production to primary and secondary antigens |
| Decreased potency |
| Decreased antibody affinity |
| Increased anti-idiotypic antibodies |

precursor cells with the ability to respond to this specific antigen.[55] Immunizing the subjects with tetanus toxoid led to an increase in the number of specific antibody-producing B cells for both age groups, but the old adults still had significantly fewer B cells producing specific antibody.[56] Booster immunizations did not alter the mean amount of antibody produced per B cell regardless of the subject's age.[56]

Although most investigators agree that changes in antibody production with age are primarily the result of declines in T lymphocyte function, there is also evidence for a decline in intrinsic B cell function. Some studies suggest a diminished ability of purified human B cells to respond to purified T-helper cells, or to T cell-derived helper factors.[57,58] Studies with murine cells have shown that certain subsets of B cells from old animals function at a much lower level than the same cells from young mice, whereas other subsets produce comparable levels of antibody.[59] Cerny et al. found that the anti-phosphorylcholine antibody produced by aged mice did not protect animals against lethal doses of *Streptococcus pneumoniae*, although old animals produced levels of antibody comparable to those in young animals.[60] The genes encoding the variable heavy portions of the antibody molecule were different in the old mice. The resulting antibody had lower affinity for the bacterial antigen and conferred less protection.[60,61]

Some of the age-related changes in antibody production may be related to altered ability to recognize antigen due to changes in the manifestation of the major histocompatability receptor complex on the B cell surface.[24,62] Such changes result in an altered antibody repertoire of the B cells.[24,62] For example, immunization of mice with sheep red blood cells led to a significant rise in the proportion of immunoglobulin M (IgM)-secreting cells reacting with self antigens in the old animals, an effect not seen in the young animals.[63] Age-related changes in B cell function are summarized in Table 4.2.

## Macrophage Function

Macrophage function during aging is particularly relevant to the theme of this book, although it has been studied less intensively than other leukocyte populations. Early work suggested that "old" macrophages are comparable to "young" macrophages in terms of producing similar levels of cytokines.[64,65] Differences in function appeared to be modulated through changes in T and B cell responses to the cytokines. Studies of human monocytes have shown decreased secretion of IL-1 with mitogen stimulation.[66] Bone marrow stem cells from senescence-accelerated mice are defective in their ability to generate granulocyte/macrophage precursor cells.[67] In vivo function of macrophages illustrated by cutaneous wound healing in mice, showed that wounds in aged control animals took twice as long to heal as in young ones.[68] When peritoneal macrophages from animals of different ages were added to wounds on old mice, healing was accelerated regardless of the age of the source animal, although, macrophages from young mice accelerated the healing process to the greatest degree.[68]

Studies of macrophage function in aged mice and humans suggest defects in macrophage–T cell interactions. Antigen-sensitized macrophages from old mice stimulated significantly lower levels of T cell proliferation than sensitized macrophages from young mice.[17] Dendritic cells are tissue-fixed macrophages that stimulate formation of germinal centers in lymph follicles where B cell memory develops; they thus play an important role in the secondary immune response. Szakal et al. described serious age-related compromise in this pathway.[69] When macrophages were replaced with other sources for activation (e.g., IL-2, or an activator such as phorbol-12-myristate-13-acetate), T cells from old adults displayed enhanced responses.[70] Macrophages from young adults were able to restore old T cell responses to the level seen in young adults in 70% of the subjects studied. Because the "old" macrophages effectively supported "young" T cells, the authors postulated that the defect resulted from impaired macrophage–T cell communication.[70] In other studies, monocytes from old adults displayed less cytotoxicity against certain tumor cell lines, decreased production of reactive oxygen intermediates ($H_2O_2$ and $NO_2$), and lower IL-1 secretion than monocytes from young adults.[66,71]

## Natural Killer Cells

Natural killer (NK) cells are cytotoxic cells with the ability to lyse targets without the need for antigenic sensitization, a characteristic that distinguishes them functionally from cytotoxic T cells. Lymphokine-activated killer (LAK) cells, thought to be highly activated NK cells, are able to lyse certain cell lines that are resistant to NK cells. NK cells from mice display a declining ability to lyse spleen cells with increasing age.[72,73] Most studies using old human subjects have shown little or no change in NK cell cytotoxic ability.[74] There do appear to be differential requirements for maximal activation of NK cells by interferon-α (IFNα). Young NK cells show maximal responses when stimulated with low concentrations of

IFNα.[75] The activity of LAK cells from old humans appears to be reduced compared to that of LAK cells from young humans.[74,75]

### Lymphocyte DNA

The increased fragility of lymphocyte DNA with age may predispose to or compound immune senescence. For example, chromosomes of T cells from old adults are more fragile than those from young adults, and certain sites on the X chromosome appear to be more sensitive to chemical insults.[76] Atomic bomb survivors who were over age 55 when exposed to the bomb's radiation have lymphocytes that mount poorer cellular responses than survivors who were under age 15 at the time of exposure.[77] These results may reflect increased susceptibility of the aging immune system to irradiation. Although there are fewer breaks in double-stranded DNA in lymphocytes from old adults after in vitro exposure to radiation, the cells are unable to repair the breaks as effectively as lymphocytes from young donors.[78] Other measures of DNA damage are 10 times higher in lymphocytes from healthy old individuals than in those from newborns.[79]

## Changes in Production and Response to Regulatory Factors

### Prostaglandins

Prostaglandin $E_2$ ($PGE_2$), a metabolite of cell membrane arachidonic acid, is a feedback inhibitor of T cell proliferation in humans.[80] T cells from adults over 70 years of age are a magnitude more sensitive to inhibition by $PGE_2$ than those from adults less than 40 years of age.[15,81] Thus $PGE_2$ may interfere with expansion of antigen-specific T-helper cell clones. T cells from aged mice are not only more sensitive to inhibition by $PGE_2$, their splenocytes appear to produce more $PGE_2$ than splenocytes from young mice.[82] Meydani et al. have continued to provide evidence that macrophage production of excess $PGE_2$ is a significant mechanism in the suppression of T cell proliferation and IL-2 production in old mice.[83]

Delfraissey et al. found that $PGE_2$ suppressed the primary antibody response to trinitrophenylated polyacrylamide beads by lymphocytes from old adults.[64] Removing the monocytes that were the source of $PGE_2$ production or adding drugs that blocked production of $PGE_2$, partially reversed the depressed response.[15,64] Using a different system of lipopolysaccharide-stimulated versus unstimulated lymphocytes, other investigators have not found increased $PGE_2$ production in old versus young donors.[84] Polyclonal antibody production was not suppressed by $PGE_1$ when added to lymphocytes from donors of any age.[84]

The increased sensitivity to $PGE_2$ with age does not appear to be part of a general increase in sensitivity to all immunomodulators. Lymphocytes from subjects over 70 years of age are less sensitive to inhibition by substances such as histamine and hydrocortisone.[81]

### Interleukins

Interleukins-1 and -2 play a primary role in activation, recruitment, and proliferation of T lymphocytes. Activated T cells then go on to produce a variety of growth and differentiation factors. T-helper (Th) cells can be classified based on the profile of the cytokines they produce and by distinct surface receptors. Th1 cells elaborate IFN-γ, IL-2, IL-12, and tumor necrosis factor-β (TNF-β), leading to the induction of cytotoxic T cells and cellular immunity; Th2 cells elaborate IL-4, IL-5, IL-6, IL-10, and IL-13, which ultimately results in antibody production.[85,86]

A decreased response to IL-2 has been studied extensively as a potential mechanism underlying the age-related defect in cellular immunity. Work from various investigators has demonstrated decreased production of IL-2 after mitogen stimulation, decreased density of IL-2 receptor expression, and decreased proliferation of T cells in response to IL-2.[87–92] The picture is complicated by variable sensitivity to IL-2 depending on the activation signal.[6,93] Human memory T cells generally produce low levels of IL-2 when stimulated by mitogen, in contrast to high IL-2 production by young memory T cells.[12] However, production of IL-2 by old cells was greater when a different stimulus was employed.[12] Studies from Nagelkerken's group found no differences in T cell proliferation or IL-2 production when memory T cells from old and young humans were stimulated with a variety of activation signals.[6] $CD4^+$ T cells from old mice accumulate similar levels of IL-2 transcripts, though secretion of IL-2 is lower than that seen in cells from young mice.[94] Some studies have shown decreased expression of messenger RNA for IL-2 by lymphocytes from aged rats.[95]

Increasing evidence has been accumulating that there are age-related declines in lymphocyte production and response to cytokines other than IL-2.[4,96] Monocytes from aged humans produce levels of IL-1 precursor comparable to monocytes from young humans, although they secrete less IL-1.[67] Lymphocytes from old individuals produce higher levels of IL-1, IL-2, and TNF-α than those from healthy young individuals in mixed lymphocyte culture.[97] In some studies, lymphocytes from old animals are not stimulated by IL-4 to the same extent as lymphocytes from young mice[98] or by a combination of IL-4 and anti-IgM.[99]

Li and Miller found a threefold decline in IL-4 production with age when activated murine T cells were immobilized with antibody to the T cell receptor, CD3, and cultured with anti-CD3 and IL-2.[100] Memory T cells from old donors displayed a sixfold deficit in IL-4 production compared to cells from young donors.[100] In a similar system, $CD4^+$ T cells from young mice were more sensitive to stimulation with exogenous IL-4, producing much higher levels of IL-2 than old $CD4^+$ T cells.[12] Blocking endogenous IL-4 boosted "old" lymphocyte production of specific anti-influenza IgM and IgG1 to levels seen in young animals during a primary antibody response.[101] A similar effect was achieved by blocking endogenous IFNγ and IL-10.[101] We have shown that lymphocytes from old adults produce less IL-4 when stimulated with specific antigen than lymphocytes from young adults.[102] When IL-4 is added early during the course of stimulation, old lymphocytes are less inhibited to produce specific antibodies,[102] similar to findings described earlier in mice.[12]

Other investigators have found no differences between lymphocytes from old and young adults in terms of their ability to produce IL-4 or IL-6 when stimulated with the mitogen phytohemagglutinin.[103] In this system, lymphocytes from old adults produced significantly less IFN-γ.[103] With variation in the activating signals, old human T cells produce larger amounts of IL-4 and IFN-γ.[6,104]

Interferon-γ affects NK cell cytotoxicity differently depending on donor age.[75] When NK cells from old donors were incubated with IL-2 they secreted less IFN-γ than those from young adults, although cytotoxic activity was unchanged.[105] Contradictory findings of increased IFN-γ production by human lymphocyte[106] and $CD4^+$ T cell[104] cultures have been reported. Lymphocytes from old rats demonstrate increased IFN and decreased IL-2 production when stimulated with the mitogen concanavalin A.[92] Other investigators have found no correlation between the level of mitogen-stimulated proliferation and production of IFN.[107] Cells from old donors were more sensitive to a combination of IL-2 and IFN-γ than cells of young donors.[107] IFN-γ mRNA levels and synthesis of IFN-γ appear to increase in T cells from old donors.[108]

Several investigators have described elevated serum IL-6 levels in old mice, monkeys, and adult humans.[109–111] One investigation described elevated urinary IL-6 levels in old adults compared to that in young adults, although circulating levels were similar at both ages.[112] The authors thought these findings were due to either differential renal handling or production of IL-6 with age.[112] Peritoneal macrophages from old mice and B cells from old humans produced higher levels of IL-6 in vitro than did cells from young individuals.[25,113] IL-6 levels are higher in unstimulated cultures of murine lymphocytes and splenocytes or human lymphocytes compared to those in their young counterparts.[109] Other studies have failed to show any differences in IL-6 production by lymphocytes from old adults.[103]

Changes in production of the neutrophil chemoattractant IL-8 have been described in old adults compared with that in young adults. Lymphocytes from old men displayed lower levels of spontaneous IL-8 production.[114] Cells from the old men increased IL-8 production more than eightfold when stimulated with the mitogen lipopolysaccharide, whereas cells from old women showed no increase. Lymphocytes from young men and women increased production of IL-8 with the same stimulus but to a much smaller degree.[114] Age-related changes in interleukins are summarized in Table 4.3.

TABLE 4.3. Changes in Interleukins with Age

| |
|---|
| **Decreased** |
| Expression of IL-2 mRNA |
| Proportion of cells expressing IL-2R |
| T cell production of IL-2 |
| High-affinity binding sites for IL-2 |
| Memory T cell production of IL-2 |
| T cell proliferative response to IL-2 |
| Specific antigen-stimulated IL-4 production |
| B cell sensitivity to IL-4 |
| Nonspecific stimulation of lymphocyte-produced IL-8 |
| Monocyte secretion of IL-1 |
| IL-2-stimulated NK cell production of IFN |
| **Increased/unchanged** |
| In vivo levels of IL-6 |
| Nonspecific stimulation of T cell IL-4 and IL-6 |
| Nonspecific stimulation of T cell IFN-γ and IFN-γ mRNA |
| Lymphocyte production of IL-1 in MLC |

IL, interleukin; mRNA, messenger RNA; IL-2R, IL-2 receptor; IFN, interferon; MLC, mixed lymphocyte culture; NK, natural killer.

# Clinical Implications of Age-Related Immune Changes

## All-Cause Mortality

We have described a variety of immunologic changes with aging. What are the implications of these changes for the occurrence of disease and maintenance of health in older adults? There is little direct causal evidence linking specific changes in immunity to specific clinical diseases or mortality. Most authorities simply assume that a decline in immune function is deleterious or use theoretic arguments to support this belief. The question of whether decreased immune responses contribute to morbidity and mortality in elderly persons has been addressed mostly by cross-sectional studies looking for associations between a particular abnormal immune response and general health status.[115] For example, the Baltimore Longitudinal Aging Study found that declines in absolute lymphocyte counts predicted mortality after 3 years in aging men.[116] Ferguson et al. found that the presence of two or more suppressed immune parameters predicted poor 2-year survival in a group of adults over age 80.[117]

The response to delayed-type hypersensitivity skin tests has been associated with mortality in a number of studies. Delayed-type hypersensitivity skin testing is thought to be the in vivo correlate of in vitro mitogen-stimulated proliferation. Elderly subjects who respond poorly or not at all to a battery of antigens placed intradermally (anergy) have an increased risk of mortality compared to elderly subjects who respond well to one or more antigens.[1,118] We found a twofold higher mortality rate and incidence of pneumonia during 10 years of follow-up in the one-third of healthy elderly individuals who were anergic at initial testing.[2,118]

We and others have examined mitogen-stimulated lymphocyte proliferation in community-dwelling adults over age 65 years.[2,13,115,117] One study found that 18% of adults seen in an outpatient geriatric clinic had lymphocytes that did not respond to any of three mitogens.[13] These nonresponders had a 26% mortality rate at 3-year follow-up versus 13% mortality in those whose lymphocytes proliferated to at least one mitogen. The increase in all-cause mortality remained significant after controlling for medication use, an indirect indicator of health status. Our own studies showed slightly higher all-cause mortality in old adults with low proliferative responses to the mitogen phytohemagglutinin.[115]

## Response to Immunization and Infections

Adults over age 65 experience greater morbidity and mortality in association with common infections, providing a basis for targeting this population with preventive immunization. Unfortunately, elderly people respond less well to preventive immunizations against common infections compared with young individuals because of the waning of immunity. Epidemiologic evidence suggests that despite decreased efficacy in the elderly, immunizations do reduce morbidity and mortality. The next section focuses on influenza, pneumococcal pneumonia, tetanus, tuberculosis, and herpes zoster because information is available on disease epidemiology and aging immune responses specific to these entities. Because acquired immunodeficiency syndrome (AIDS) is an infectious process specifically involving the immune system, we also review the current literature on the occurrence and presentation of AIDS in the elderly.

### *Influenza*

Influenza is a common viral respiratory illness that becomes clinically important when complicated by bacterial pneumonia or when it occurs in debilitated or elderly patients (reviewed by Burns et al.[119]). Individuals who suffer from one or more chronic, systemic illnesses (e.g., chronic obstructive pulmonary disease, diabetes, chronic renal insufficiency) experience a 40- to 150-fold increase in the basal incidence rate for influenzal pneumonia of 4 cases per 100,000 persons per year. More than 80% of deaths related to influenza epidemics occur in the elderly,[120] and the risk of developing influenzal pneumonia or superimposed bacterial pneumonia increases with increasing age. Individuals living in long-term care facilities are at particularly high risk of morbidity and mortality.

After vaccination with influenza, old mice display impaired cytotoxic T cell function and ineffective antibody generation against the virus.[121] When an intranasal viral load is administered after vaccination, old animals are more likely to develop influenzal pneumonia than young animals.[121] Studies in humans have described impaired production of anti-influenza antibodies and impaired influenza-specific cytotoxic activity in old adults compared to that in young adults.[122] Some of the mechanisms mediating this response include reduced IL-2 production and T cell activation in vivo and in vitro.[88] NK cell cytotoxicity is unchanged in old adults after vaccination against influenza, in contrast to increased NK cell activity in young adults.[123] Elderly individuals who do display a significant response to influenza vaccine have increased numbers of T cells capable of responding to the specific viral stimulus, whereas nonresponders have low numbers of such cells.[124] After immunization, IgG and IgG1 antibody production and agglutinating ability were decreased in the elderly compared to that in young subjects.[125] The investigators were able to restore the responses of the elderly subjects to the levels seen in young subjects by doubling the dose of vaccine.[125]

Although influenza vaccination is less effective in the higher risk population of old adults, the incidence and severity of influenza infections is clearly reduced by annual usage of the standard preparation.[126,127] The vaccine confers the highest degree of protection when the epidemic strains are similar to those in the vaccine.[128] Even when the antigenic determinants of the wild virus have drifted over the course of a year, vaccine utilization can still have a substantial impact on morbidity and mortality.[126]

### *Pneumococcal Pneumonia*

An increased incidence of morbidity and mortality due to pneumonia has been recognized in the elderly for years.[119] Hospitalization necessitated by a diagnosis of pneumonia is most often caused by bacteria, primarily (about two-thirds of cases) *Streptococcus pneumoniae*. High mortality rates result from the increased incidence of bacteremia and meningitis seen in old adults. Similar to influenza, patients with one or more chronic systemic diseases are at increased risk of complications and mortality from pneumococcal infection.

Most of the information on the immunologic response to pneumococcal vaccination derives from murine studies. After vaccination with phosphocholine, old mice produce levels of antibody similar to those in young mice but with a molecular shift in the antibody repertoire.[60,129] The antibody produced by old animals has a lower affinity for its target and is less effective in preventing infection.[129] In old mice, many of the antibodies produced after pneumococcal vaccination cross-react with self-antigens.[130] In humans, serum antibody levels fade more rapidly in old individuals, prompting recommendations to repeat the vaccination after 6 years in elderly patients.[131] The vaccine has been estimated to be about 70% effective for reducing morbidity and mortality in the elderly.[132]

### Tetanus

Tetanus is relatively rare in the United States and other developed countries, with about 70–100 cases reported annually and an average annual incidence rate of 0.02/100,000 persons.[133,134] The disease occurs in individuals who have never been immunized, have not completed a primary series, or have not received booster immunization for many decades.[135,136] A large serosurvey found that fewer than 30% of adults over age 70 had protective levels of antibody against tetanus toxoid.[135] Adults older than age 80 have more than a 10-fold higher risk of contracting the illness than adults in their twenties. The mortality rate is three times higher in the older age group.[137] Changes in both T and B cells have been associated with the decreased response to the vaccine.[54–56]

Although older adults have diminished responses to tetanus immunization, the vaccine is virtually 100% effective in preventing illness.[135] Because of the low incidence rate some authorities have suggested that 10-year booster immunizations are not cost-effective for adults over age 65.[138] This attitude has sparked concern about future underutilization of this effective prevention and a potential increase in the incidence of the disease in the old population.[135–137,139]

### Tuberculosis and Intracellular Infections

For more than 20 years the risk of active tuberculosis in the Western world is increasingly confined to two populations: those with immunocompromising diseases (e.g., AIDS) and the very elderly.[140,141] Animal studies show that old mice display increased susceptibility to infection with *Mycobacterium tuberculosis*.[142] The infection containment rate in old mice is similar to that in young animals; but once pulmonary infection is established, there is increased hematogenous spread to other organs.[142] Old animals display decreased $CD4^+$ T cell function, significantly lower levels of IL-12 in the lung,[142] and delayed emergence of protective, IFN-$\gamma$-secreting $CD4^+$ T cells.[143] The protective cells from old animals were slower to express surface adhesion markers necessary for migration across endothelial linings to sites of active infection.[143] The increased spread of disease in old animals may also be related to alterations in other cytokine levels.[144] Orme has shown that $CD4^+$ cells from young mice protect old mice from infection, suggesting that old macrophages function adequately and the major defect lies in the T cell population.[145,146]

### Herpes Zoster

There is a clear positive correlation between age and the incidence of herpes zoster, with an annual incidence rate of 400 cases per 100,000 adults over age 75.[147] Other surveys suggest an even higher overall incidence.[148] The varicella-zoster virus is harbored in dorsal root ganglia for many decades following childhood illness; and when it is reactivated it causes a cutaneous, varicella-type vesicular eruption involving the dermatome of the involved dorsal root ganglion.

Cellular immunity, measured by cutaneous delayed hypersensitivity to varicella zoster, wanes with increasing age, although other factors may be involved in controlling viral latency.[149] Cutaneous zoster is often an indication of immune-compromised status in young persons and those with early recurrence[148] but is not associated with occult malignancy in old adults.[150]

### Acquired Immunodeficiency Syndrome

Acquired immunodeficiency syndrome is caused by the human immunodeficiency virus (HIV), which attacks the T4 epitope on helper lymphocytes, monocytes, and glial cells; these cells provide a reservoir for the virus.[151] Clinically, the syndrome is characterized by (1) infections with organisms that normally do not cause disease in immune-competent humans and (2) uncommon malignancies.

Since October 1995 more than 500,000 cases of AIDS have been reported in the United States.[152] Most are seen in individuals under age 40 years, but about 10% have occurred in adults older than age 50.[153] During the early 1990s most cases in older adults were probably related to transfusion with contaminated blood before national supplies were rigorously tested for HIV, though details are sketchy.[119] This pattern may shift to the more common route of sexual transmission. One survey found that significant numbers of adults over age 50 engage in high-risk sexual behaviors, and these individuals are much less likely to follow safe sexual practices than are young, at-risk adults.[154]

The syndrome can present atypically in the elderly, with symptoms such as arthralgia, wasting, and dementia, which are already common in this age group. The disease appears to progress more rapidly as a function of age,[155] and those who were more than 55 years at the time of the initial infection have a poor 10-year survival rate.[156]

## Stress, Immunity, and Aging

### Physical Stress

A number of studies have described the effects of physical stress on the immune system, although most have not analyzed outcomes by age. Time-limited physical stress, such as hypoxia, head-up tilt challenge (approximating conditions of acute hemorrhage), hyperthermia, and exercise, tend to enhance measures of immunity on a transient basis (e.g., increased lymphocyte numbers and increased NK cell activity).[157] Physical stress associated with tissue injury (e.g., trauma, burns, surgery) is generally characterized by suppressed immune function. $CD4^+$ and $CD8^+$ cells have been reported to decrease in number,[158–160] and T cell activation is decreased.[161] Mitogen-induced lymphocyte proliferation is decreased after surgery and trauma,[162–164] and anergy is increased.[165] The presence of anergy has been associated with an increased incidence of postoperative infection.[165] Neutrophil function is adversely affected by surgery, with decreased chemotaxis,[165,166] decreased intracellular killing,[167] and disruption of superoxide release.[166,167]

One of the most consistently demonstrated findings is decreased cytotoxicity of NK cells.[157,159,168–170] In murine studies, decreased NK activity following surgery is associated with increased tumor metastases.[171] Levels of IL-2, mRNA for IL-2, IFN IL-10, and IL-12 are decreased,[158,164,165,172] whereas IL-4 and IL-6 levels are generally increased,[158,161,162,165,172] although some investigators have reported decreased IL-6.[161,173] Of clinical relevance are observations that the degree of immune suppression correlates positively with the duration of surgery and volume of blood loss.[165,167]

The mechanisms underlying immune suppression with physical stress are slowly becoming elucidated. Tissue damage results in release of inflammatory substances, including TNF, IL-1, and IL-2.[174–176] Hypothalamic production of corticotropin-releasing hormone (CRF) and arginine vasopressin (AVP) is stimulated by the locally produced cytokines and by afferent nerve signals from the site of injury. CRF and AVP stimulate pituitary adrenocorticotropic hormone (ACTH) release and subsequent adrenal glucocorticoids, the latter two of which are also directly stimulated by the cytokines from the site of injury.[177,178] Activation of the hypothalamic-pituitary-adrenal (HPA) axis stimulates transformation of uncommitted Th cells to Th2 cells and inhibits transformation to Th1 cells.[179] The cellular immune responses are thus suppressed due partly to a lack of Th1 cells. The cytokines secreted by the Th2 cells (e.g., IL-1, IL-6, TNF-$\alpha$) further stimulate the HPA axis and glucocorticoid production[180] and subsequently cause immune suppression.[181,182] Given the extensive age-related changes in immunity, it is not surprising that old age in surgical patients has been associated with increased postoperative immune suppression and septic complications.[167] It is interesting to speculate that postsurgical immune suppression might be less pronounced in the elderly than expected because of decreased sensitivity to glucocorticoids,[80] as mentioned previously.

## Psychological Stress

In addition to physical stress from trauma or surgery, psychological stress can have a significant impact on immune system function. Complex and direct links have been described between the immune system and the perceptual capabilities of the central nervous system. Ader and Cohen demonstrated that it was even possible to condition specific immune responses with sensory cues.[183] In a series of taste-aversion learning experiments in rats, saccharin water was initially administered to the animals along with a dose of cyclophosphamide. The rats were subsequently injected with sheep red blood cells with or without readministration of the saccharin solution. Animals who received the saccharin along with the injection had profound suppression of the hemagglutinin response to sheep red blood cells.[183]

Carefully controlled experiments with rodents and primates have demonstrated the neurohumorally mediated effects of stress on the immune system.[184,185] Similar findings are seen in cross-sectional studies with humans, though it is impossible to achieve the same degree of control as in the animal studies. Clusters of illness, from the common cold to cancer, have been reported to occur around the time of major life changes.[186] Strong negative correlations have been seen between loneliness and the proliferative response of lymphocytes to mitogens, NK cell activity, and DNA splicing and repair.[186,187] We found that healthy old adults with a strong social support system had greater total lymphocyte counts and a stronger mitogen-induced proliferation of lymphocytes than those without a close confidant.[188]

Studies of individuals in "naturally occurring" stressful situations have also demonstrated links to suppressed immune function and illness. Mitogen-induced lymphocyte proliferation is suppressed after bereavement[35] and with depression.[189] The stress of taking final examinations has been correlated with recurrence of cold sores, rises in serum antibody titers against herpes simplex type I virus,[190] and decreased proliferation of memory T cells.[191] Caregiving for a demented spouse is associated with a poor response to influenza vaccination.[192] Lymphocytes from the caregivers produced less IL-1$\beta$ and IL-2 when stimulated with influenza virus in vitro compared to age-matched, non-care-giving controls.[192] Caregivers displayed slower wound healing after skin biopsy than did matched controls.[193]

## Reversal of Age-Related Declines in Immune Function

When considering physiologic changes of aging it is important to keep in mind that the changes described do not appear to be synchronized with each other.[4,51] Defects occur to varying degrees in different systems within a given individual, and immune modulatory substances may affect some systems and not others. It is increasingly clear that there are complex interactions between the nervous, endocrine, and immune systems, although no "global" mechanism has been found that might be the common underlying cause of immune senescence.[194] We conclude with a brief discussion of potential ways to stimulate a failing immune system in elderly persons and review a number of investigations reporting attenuation or reversal of surgically induced immune suppression in animals and humans.

One of the most obvious organ changes that occurs with aging is involution of the thymus, loss of thymic hormones, and a subsequent decline in T cell function.[195] In humans and experimental animals, involution begins during adolescence; and the lymphatic mass, particularly in the cortical area, decreases with age.[196] These observations stimulated a number of experiments attempting to enhance lymphocyte function by reestablishing "young" levels of thymic hormone. Exposing lymphocytes of old individuals to thymic hormones in vivo or in vitro or transplanting young thymic tissue into old animals has resulted in at least partial restoration of immunity on a temporary basis.[197–204] In old mice, administering thymopentin increased resistance to cutaneous infection with *Leishmania*.[205]

Other hormonal substances being studied for their potential to reverse age-related declines in immunity include melatonin, growth hormone, and adrenal androgens. The pineal hormone melatonin has free-radical-scavenging properties, and its production declines with age.[206] When melatonin has been administered to individuals with a variety of cancers, improved measures of immunity after surgery have been observed (increased number of lymphocytes, T cells, Th cells)[207] as have partial tumor regression and enhanced 1-year survival of patients with metastatic solid tumors.[208] When melatonin is injected into old mice, it enhances antibody production and increases Th cell activity and IL-2 production.[209]

Growth hormone (GH) and its precursor insulin-like growth factor-I (IGF-I) have immune-enhancing effects, including stimulation of phagocyte activity and cytokine production, both of which may help protect against bacterial infection.[210] Elderly patients with GH deficiency have low NK cell activity, but it can be at least partially restored in vitro by exposing NK cells to IGF-I.[211] However, healthy old women who were not GH-deficient did not display changes in immune parameters after receiving 6 months of daily supplements.[212] Vara-Thorbeck et al. gave hypocaloric parenteral nutrition with or without growth hormone supplements to patients undergoing the stress of open cholecystectomy.[213] Those receiving GH had improved responses to delayed hypersensitivity skin testing, a lower incidence of wound infection, and shorter duration of hospital stay than the nonsupplemented group.[213,214] In a series of experiments by Hinton et al., rats were given total parenteral nutrition with or without IGF-I and were subjected to the stress of a surgical incision or treatment with the synthetic glucocorticoid dexamethasone.[215] IGF-I treatment was associated with restoration of splenic B cell numbers in surgically stressed animals and increased mitogen-stimulated thymocyte proliferation and lymphyocyte-produced IL-6 in the dexamethasone-stressed animals.[215]

The adrenal androgen dehydroepiandrosterone (DHEA) has been evaluated as a potential immune stimulant because it antagonizes the actions of cortisol, stimulating increased production of IL-2 and IFN-$\gamma$.[182] In vivo administration also augments antibody production by up-regulating T cell subsets that are associated with increased antibody production.[216] When aged mice are primed with DHEA, the response to hepatitis B surface antigen vaccination and influenza vaccination is enhanced,[217,218] and the animals are more resistant to infection with influenza.[218] Old humans who received oral DHEA supplements before receiving influenza vaccine displayed a fourfold increase in hemagglutinin inhibition titers compared to elderly individuals who did not take supplements.[219]

A few studies in mice have explored the effect of administering cytokines to animals after surgical or burn trauma. In one study, administration of the recombinant cytokine IL-1$\alpha$ 20 hours after surgery showed restoration of suppressed NK and LAK cell activity.[220] In another study, mice with 20% burn injuries were treated in vivo with IL-12, which increased splenocyte production of IFN and significantly decreased mortality.[172]

The 1990s saw a rapid accumulation of studies investigating links between nutrition and immune function (reviewed by Chandra[221] and Burns and Goodwin[222]). Work on the effects of nutritional deprivation showed that starvation of experimental animals at young ages results in preservation of normal immune function into old age.[222] It is now known that caloric restriction rather than starvation can achieve the same results.[223,224] The possibility that lesser amounts of caloric restriction supplemented with essential nutrients might have similar beneficial effects in humans is being formally tested in primate models.[225]

In contrast to findings in the experimental setting, nutritional deficiencies in the clinical setting are generally associated with poor immune responses.[221] In both nutritionally deficient and healthy elderly adults caloric, vitamin, and trace element supplementation has been associated with enhanced immune responses, better responses to vaccines, and fewer days of infectious illness.[226,227] NK cell activity correlates negatively to the level of polyunsaturated fatty acids in the diet, but there was no effect on NK activity in men who ingested high levels of polyunsaturated fatty acids for 5 weeks.[228] Nutritional supplements given by the enteral or parenteral route have been associated with improved surgical outcomes, but the effects on immune function are not well characterized. Rats receiving total parenteral nutrition display deficits in gut immunity and lymphocyte proliferation.[229–233] In humans, most studies have focused on the role of lipid additives in depressing immune function.[232–237] In contrast to the immune suppression associated with surgery, patients with closed head trauma who receive early parenteral nutrition have preserved or increased $CD4^+$ cell counts and improved lymphocyte proliferation to mitogen stimulation.[238]

Antioxidants such as vitamins C (ascorbic acid) and E (tocopherol) have been studied intensively as potential "antiaging" treatments.[239,240] When healthy elderly subjects were supplemented with 400–800 IU of vitamin E, delayed-type hypersensitivity skin testing and in vitro lymphocyte production of IL-2 increased.[241,242] Vitamin E may cause these effects via inhibition of $PGE_2$ or other suppressive factors[239] (see below). In vitro exposure of T cells from mice to another antioxidant, glutathione, enhanced T cell proliferation at all ages owing at least in part to blockade of eicosanoid production.[243] A placebo-controlled, double-blind trial of vitamin E and β-carotene supplementation in healthy old adults was associated with marked increases in various parameters of immunity, 50% fewer days with infection, and 40% fewer days taking antibiotics during the 1-year trial.[227] Although there is concern over the findings of a higher incidence of lung cancer in heavy smokers taking β-carotene,[244,245] supplementation with vitamin E was not associated with an increased incidence of lung cancer.[245]

Administering drugs or vaccines that in one way or another stimulate immune function are other potential ways of preventing age-related declines in immunity. Nonsteroidal antiinflammatory drugs (NSAIDs) inhibit cyclooxygenase and reduce production of $PGE_2$, thus stimulating immune responses in vitro and in vivo.[80] For example, an early case report of two anergic patients with an acquired immunodeficiency state showed restoration of the response to delayed-type hypersensitivity skin testing after treatment with indomethacin.[246] The proportion of adults over age 75 displaying a fourfold rise in anti-A/Beijing antibody after influenza immunization was significantly increased by aspirin supplementation.[247] The use of NSAIDs might be especially relevant to elderly persons because their T cells are more sensitive to inhibition by $PGE_2$.[15] Cyclooxygenase inhibitors might also reduce the excess autoantibody production that occurs with age[248] and stimulate primary antibody responses to new antigens.[26] Unfortunately, the use of NSAIDs is not without risk, and older adults are at greater risk for experiencing the potential adverse effects of medications.

Many researchers are attempting to enhance immune responses of old adults by manipulating protective vaccines. Methods used have included increasing the strength of the vaccine,[249] using multiple boosters,[250] and adding coupling adjuvants to the original vaccine preparation,[251] with varying degrees of success. Other manipulations, such as use of split-virus vaccines versus whole virus vaccines[252] or live virus exposure with or without standard vaccination,[253] have resulted in increased responses in old adults.

The immune-suppressive effects of surgery have been affected by a number of surgically related variables. The use of epidural anesthesia was not associated with the reduction in NK cell toxicity seen with general anesthesia, and serum and urinary cortisol levels were significantly lower with the epidural approach.[254] Less invasive surgical approaches (e.g., laparoscopic cholecystectomy versus open cholecystectomy) result in a less pronounced shift toward Th2 activation,[255] less pronounced decrease in the $CD4^+/CD8^+$ ratio,[158] lower levels of locally released inflammatory substances (monocyte superoxide anion, TNF), less neutrophil chemotaxis, and lower postoperative white blood cell counts.[166]

Suppression of immunity due to psychological stress has been reversed with psychological interventions. Simple relaxation exercises and writing about traumatic events enhanced the measured immune response compared to that in control subjects.[256,257] The duration of these effects and the mechanisms that underlie them are not fully understood.

## Conclusions

The examples of immune restoration/stimulation discussed above are representative of the many therapies that have been proposed and sometimes tested to boost responses in the elderly. Although the few studies that link a disordered immune function with subsequent morbidity and mortality are suggestive, it is not clear that age-related declines in immunity are an independent risk factor for anything. It is difficult to justify medical intervention in an otherwise healthy individual with a disordered laboratory parameter (e.g., prescribing long-term NSAID therapy for an individual with low phytohemagglutinin response or skin test anergy). However, when an elderly individual undergoes the stress of surgery, benign interventions such as dietary manipulation or antioxidant supplementation may enhance immunity enough to improve the clinical outcome. Further research is needed to help clarify these important issues.

## References

1. Roberts-Thompson IC, Whittingham S, Young-Chaiyud U, et al. Aging, immune response and mortality. Lancet 1974; 2:368–370.

2. Goodwin JS, Searles RP, Tung KSK. Immunological responses of a healthy elderly population. Clin Exp Immunol 1982;48:403–410.
3. Hess EV, Knapp D. The immune system and aging: a case of the cart before the horse. J Chronic Dis 1978;31:647–649.
4. Miller RA. Aging and immune function. Int Rev Cytol 1991;124:187–215.
5. Philosophe B, Miller RA. Diminished calcium signal generation in subsets of T lymphocytes that predominate in old mice. J Gerontol 1990;45:B87–B93.
6. Nijhuis EW, Remarque EJ, Hinloopen B, et al. Age-related increase in the fraction of $CD27^-CD4^+$ T cells and IL-4 production as a feature of $CD4^+$ T cell differentiation in vivo. Clin Exp Immunol 1994;96:528–534.
7. Jackola DR, Ruger JK, Miller RA. Age-associated changes in human T cell phenotype and function. Aging 1994;6:25–34.
8. Xu X, Beckman I, Ahern M, Bradley J. A comprehensive analysis of peripheral blood lymphocytes in healthy aged humans by flow cytometry. Immunol Cell Biol 1993;71: 549–557.
9. Kudlacek S, Jahandideh-Kazempour S, Graninger W, et al. Differential expression of various T cell surface markers in young and elderly subjects. Immunobiology 1995;192:198–204.
10. Jackola DR, Ruger JK, Miller RA. Age-associated changes in human T cell phenotype and function. Aging 1994;6:25–34.
11. Dobber R, Tielemans M, Nagelkerken L. Enrichment for Th1 cells in the Mel-$14^+$ $CD4^+$ T cell fraction in aged mice. Cell Immunol 1995;162:321–325.
12. Dobber R, Tielemans M, de Weerd H, Nagelkerken L. $Mel14^+CD4^+$ T cells from aged mice display functional and phenotypic characteristics of memory cells. Int Immunol 1994;6:1227–1234.
13. Murasko DM, Weiner P, Kaye D. Association of lack of mitogen-induced lymphocyte proliferation with increased mortality in the elderly. Aging Immunol Infect Dis 1988;1: 1–6.
14. Inkeles B, Innes JB, Kuntz MM, et al. Immunological studies of aging. III. Cytokinetic basis for the impaired response of lymphocytes from aged humans to plant lectins. J Exp Med 1977;145:1176–1187.
15. Goodwin JS, Messner RP. Sensitivity of lymphocytes to prostaglandin $E_2$ increases in subjects over age 70. J Clin Invest 1979;64:434–439.
16. Ernst DN, Weigle WO, McQuitty DN, Rothermel AL, Hobbs MV. Stimulation of murine T cell subsets with anti-CD3 antibody: age-related defects in the expression of early activation molecules. J Immunol 1989;142:1413–1421.
17. Kirschmann DA, Murasko DM. Splenic and inguinal lymph node T cells of aged mice respond differently to polyclonal and antigen-specific stimuli. Cell Immunol 1992;139:426–437.
18. Vissinga C, Nagelkerken L, Sijlstra J, Hertogh-Huijbregts A, Boersma W, Rozing J. A decreased functional capacity of $CD4^+$ T cells underlies the impaired DTH reactivity in old mice. Mech Ageing Dev 1990;53:127–139.
19. Gottesman SRS, Edington J. Proliferative and cytotoxic immune functions in aging mice. V. Deficiency in generation of cytotoxic cells with normal lytic function per cell as demonstrated by the single cell conjugation assay. Aging Immunol Infect Dis 1990;2:19–29.
20. Kishimoto S, Tomino S, Mitsuya H, et al. Age-related changes in suppressor functions of human T cells. J Immunol 1979;123:1586–1592.
21. Crawford J, Oates S, Wolfe LA, Cohen HJ. An in vitro analogue of immune dysfunction with altered immunoglobulin production in the aged. J Am Geriatr Soc 1989;37:1141–1146.
22. Grossmann A, Ledbetter JA, Rabinovitch PS. Reduced proliferation in T lymphocytes in aged humans is predominantly in the $CD8^+$ subset and is unrelated to defects in transmembrane signaling which are predominantly in the $CD4^+$ subsets. Exp Cell Res 1989;180:367–382.
23. Doria G, Mancini C, Frasca D, Adorini L. Age restriction in antigen-specific immunosuppression. J Immunol 1987; 139:1419–1425.
24. Russo C, Cherniak EP, Wali A, Weksler ME. Age-dependent appearance of nonmajor histocompatibility complex-restricted helper T cells. Proc Natl Acad Sci USA 1993;90:11718–11722.
25. Hara H, Negoro S, Miyata S, Saiki O, et al. Age-associated changes in proliferative and differentiative response of human B cells and production of T cell-derived factors regulating B cell functions. Mech Ageing Dev 1987;38:245–258.
26. Hallgren H, Buckley C, Gilbertson V, et al. Lymphocyte phytohemagglutinin responsiveness, immunoglobulins, and autoantibodies in aging humans. J Immunol 1973;111: 1101–1107.
27. Lewis RS, Cahalan MD. Potassium and calcium channels in lymphocytes. Annu Rev Immunol 1995;13:623–653.
28. Jayaraman T, Ondriasova E, Ondrias K, Harnick DJ, Marks AR. The inositol 1,4,5-trisphosphate receptor is essential for T-cell receptor signaling. Proc Natl Acad Sci USA 1995;92:6007–6011.
29. Zweifach A, Lewis RS. Mitogen-regulated $Ca^{2+}$ current of T lymphocytes is activated by depletion of intracellular $Ca^{2+}$ stores. Proc Natl Acad Sci USA 1993;90:6295–6299.
30. Miller RA, Philosophe B, Ginis I, et al. Defective control of cytoplasmic calcium concentration in T lymphocytes from old mice. J Cell Physiol 1989;128:175–182.
31. Miller RA. Calcium signals in T lymphocytes from old mice. Life Sci 1996;59:469–475.
32. Fultop T Jr, Barabas G, Varga Z, Csongor J, et al. Transmembrane signaling changes with aging. Ann NY Acad Sci 1992;673:165–171.
33. Philosophe B, Miller RA. Calcium signals in murine T lymphocytes: preservation of response to PHA and to an anti-Ly-6 antibody. Aging Immunol Infect Dis 1990;2:11–18.
34. Kawanishi H, Ajitsu S, Mirabella S. Impaired humoral immune responses to mycobacterial antigen in aged murine gut-associated lymphoid tissues. Mech Ageing Dev 1990;54:143–161.
35. Lustyik G, O'Leary JJ. Aging and the mobilization of intracellular calcium by phytohemagglutinin in human T cells. J Gerontol 1989;44:B30–B36.
36. Jackola DR, Hallgren HM. Diminished cell-cell binding by lymphocytes from healthy elderly humans: evidence for altered activation of LFA-1 function with age. J Gerontol 1995;50:B368–B377.

37. Whisler RL, Newhouse YG, Bagenstose SE. Age-related reductions in the activation of mitogen-activated protein kinases p44mapk/ERK1 and p42mapk/ERK2 in human T cells stimulated via ligation of the T cell receptor complex. Cell Immunol 1996;168:201–210.
38. Whisler RL, Newhouse YG, Grants IS, Hackshaw KV. Differential expression of the alpha- and beta-isoforms of protein kinase C in peripheral blood T and B cells from young and elderly adults. Mech Aging Dev 1995;77:197–211.
39. Patel HR, Miller RA. Age-associated changes in mitogen-induced protein phosphorylation in murine T lymphocytes. Eur J Immunol 1992;22:253–260.
40. Shi J, Miller RA. Differential tyrosine-specific protein phosphorylation in mouse T lymphocyte subsets: effect of age. J Immunol 1993;151:730–739.
41. Whisler RL, Beiqing L, Chen M. Age-related decreases in IL-2 production by human T cells are associated with impaired activation of nuclear transcriptional factors AP-1 and NF-AT. Cell Immunol 1996;169:185–195.
42. Whisler RL, Liu B, Wu LC, Chen M. Reduced activation of transcriptional factor AP-1 among peripheral blood T cells from elderly humans after PHA stimulation: restorative effect of phorbol diesters. Cell Immunol 1993;152:96–109.
43. Makinodan T. Biology of aging: retrospect and prospect. In: Makinodan T, Yunis E (eds) Immunology and Aging. New York: Plenum, 1977:1–8.
44. Zharhary D. Age-related changes in the capability of the bone marrow to generate B cells. J Immunol 1988;141:1863–1869.
45. Ben-Yehuda A, Szabo P, Dyall R, Weksler ME. Bone marrow declines as a site of B-cell precursor differentiation with age: relationship to thymus involution. Proc Natl Acad Sci USA 1994;91:11988–11992.
46. Viale AC, Chies JA, Huetz F, Malenchere E, et al. VH-gene family dominance in ageing mice. Scand J Immunol 1994;39:184–188.
47. Callard R, Basten A, Blanden R. Loss of immune competence with age may be due to a qualitative abnormality in lymphocyte membranes. Nature 1979;281:218–221.
48. Whisler RL, Grants IS. Age-related alterations in the activation and expression of phosphotyrosine kinases and protein kinase C (PKC) among human B cells. Mech Ageing Dev 1993;71:31–46.
49. Delafuente JC. Immunosenescence: Clinical and pharmacologic considerations. Med Clin North Am 1985;69:475–486.
50. Arreaza EE, Gibbons JJ Jr, Siskind GW, Weksler ME. Lower antibody response to tetanus toxoid associated with higher auto-anti-idiotypic antibody in old compared with young humans. Clin Exp Immunol 1993;92:169–73.
51. Cinader B, Thorbecke GJ. "Aging and the Immune System." Report on Workshop #94 held during the 7th international congress of immunology in Berlin on August 3, 1989. Aging: Immunol Infect Dis 1990;2:45–53.
52. Whittingham S, Buckley JD, Mackay IR. Factors influencing the secondary antibody response to flagellin in man. Clin Exp Immunol 1978;34:170–178.
53. De Greef GE, Van Staalduinen GJ, Van Doorninck H, Van Rol MJ, Hijmans W. Age-related changes of the antigen-specific antibody formation in vitro and PHA-induced T cell proliferation in individuals who met the Seigneuret protocol. Mechs Ageing Dev 1992;66:1–14.
54. Kishimoto S, Tomino S, Mitsuya H, et al. Age-related decrease in frequencies of B-cell precursors and specific helper T cells involved in the IgG anti-tetanus toxoid antibody production in humans. Clin Immunol Immunopathol 1982;25:1–10.
55. Burns EA, Lum LG, Giddings BR, Seigneuret MC, Goodwin JS. Decreased Specific Antibody Synthesis by Lymphocytes from Elderly Subjects. Mechs Aging Dev 1990;53:229–241.
56. Burns EA, Lum LG, l'Hommedieu GD, Goodwin JS. Decreased humoral immunity in aging: in vivo and in vitro response to vaccination. J Gerontol 1993;48:B231–B236.
57. Ennist DL, Hones KH, St Pierre RL, Whisler RL. Functional analysis of the immunosenescence of the human B cell system: dissociation of normal activation and proliferation from impaired terminal differentiation into IgM immunoglobulin-secreting cells. J Immunol 1986;136:99–105.
58. Whisler RL, Williams JW, Newhouse YG. Human B cell proliferative responses during aging: reduced RNA synthesis and DNA replication after signal transduction by surface immunoglobulins compared to B cell antigenic determinants CD20 and CD40. Mech Ageing Dev 1991;61: 209–222.
59. Hu A, Ehleiter D, Ben-Yehuda A, et al. Effect of age on the expressed B cell repertoire: role of B cell subsets. Int Immunol 1993;5:1035–1039.
60. Nicoletti C, Yang X, Cerny J. Repertoire diversity of antibody response to bacterial antigens in aged mice. III. Phosphorylcholine antibody from young and aged mice differ in structure and protective activity against infection with Streptococcus pneumoniae. J Immunol 1993;150:543–549.
61. Miller C, Kelsoe G. Ig VH hypermutation is absent in the germinal centers of aged mice. J Immunol 1995;155: 3377–3384.
62. Schwab R, Russo C, Weksler ME. Altered major histocompatibility complex-restricted antigen recognition by T cells from elderly humans. Eur J Immunol 1992;22:2989–2993.
63. Zhao KS, Wang YF, Gueret R, Weksler ME. Dysregulation of the humoral immune response in old mice. Int Immunol 1995;7:929–934.
64. Delfraissey J, Galanaud P, Wallon C, et al. Abolished in vitro antibody response in the elderly: exclusive involvement of prostaglandin-induced T suppressor cells. Clin Immunol Immunopathol 1982;24:377–385.
65. Delfraissey JF, Galanaud P, Dormont J, Wallon C. Age-related impairment of the in vitro antibody response in the human. Clin Exp Immunol 1980;39:208–214.
66. McLachlan JA, Serkin CD, Morrey-Clark KM, Bakouche O. Immunological functions of aged monocytes. Pathobiology 1995;63:148–159.
67. Izumi-Hisha H, Ito Y, Sugimoto K, Oshima H, Mori KJ. Age-related decrease in the number of hemopoietic stem cells and progenitors in senescence accelerated mice. Mech Ageing Dev 1990;56:89–97.
68. Danon D, Kowatch MA, Roth GS. Promotion of wound repair in old mice by local injection of macrophages. Proc Natl Acad Sci USA 1989;86:2018–2020.
69. Szakal AK, Kapasi ZF, Masuda A, Tew JG. Follicular dendritic cells in the alternative antigen transport pathway:

microenvironment, cellular events, age and retrovirus related alterations. Semin Immunol 1992;4:257–265.
70. Beckman I, Dimopoulos K, Xaioning X, Bradley J, Henschke P, Ahern M. T cell activation in the elderly: evidence for specific deficiencies in T cell/accessory cell interactions. Mech Ageing Dev 1990;51:265–276.
71. McLachlan JA, Serkin CD, Morrey KM, Bakouche O. Antitumoral properties of aged human monocytes. J Immunol 1995;154:832–843.
72. Itoh H, Abo T, Sugawara S, Kanno A, et al. Age-related variation in the proportion and activity of murine liver natural killer cells and their cytotoxicity against regenerating hepatocytes. J Immunol 1988;141:315–323.
73. Ho S-P, Kramer KE, Ershler WB. Effect of host age upon interleukin-2-mediated anti-tumor responses in a murine fibrosarcoma model. Cancer Immunol Immunother 1990; 31:146–150.
74. Kutza J, Kaye D, Murasko DM. Basal natural killer cell activity of young versus elderly humans. J Gerontol 1995;50A:B110–B116.
75. Kutza J, Murasko DM. Effects of aging on natural killer cell activity and activation by interleukin-2 and IFN-alpha. Cell Immunol 1994;155:195–204.
76. Esposito D, Fassina G, Szabo P, et al. Chromosomes of older humans are more prone to aminopterin-induced breakage. Proc Natl Acad Sci USA 1989;86:1302–1306.
77. Akiyama M, Shou O-L, Kusunoki Y, et al. Age and dose related alteration of in vitro mixed lymphocyte culture response of blood lymphocytes from A-bomb survivors. Radiat Res 1989;117:26–34.
78. Mayer PJ, Lange CS, Bradley MO, Nichols WW. Age-dependent decline in rejoining of x-ray-induced DNA double-strand breaks in normal human lymphocytes. Mutat Res 1989;219:95–100.
79. Melaragno MI, De Arruda Cardoso Smith M. Sister chromatid exchange and proliferation pattern in lymphocytes from newborns, elderly subjects and in premature aging syndromes. Mech Ageing Dev 1990;54:43–53.
80. Goodwin JS, Webb DR. Regulation of the immune response by prostaglandins: a critical review. Clin Immunol Immunopathol 1981;15:116–132.
81. Goodwin JS. Changes in lymphocyte sensitivity to prostaglandin E, histamine, hydrocortisone, and X-irradiation with age: studies in a healthy elderly population. Clin Immunol Immunopathol 1982;25:243–251.
82. Hayek MG, Meydani S, Meydani M, et al. Age differences in eicosanoid production of mouse splenocytes: effects on mitogen-induced T cell proliferation. J Gerontol 1994;49: B197–B207.
83. Beharka AA, Wu D, Han SN, Meydani SN. Macrophage prostaglandin production contributes to the age-associated decrease in T cell function which is reversed by the dietary antioxidant vitamin E. Mech Ageing Dev 1997;93:59–77.
84. Riancho JA, Zarrabeitia MT, Amado JA, Olmos JM, et al. Age-related differences in cytokine secretion. Gerontology 1994;40:8–12.
85. Romagnani S. Induction of the Th1 and Th2 responses: a key role for the "natural" immune response? Immunol Today 1992;13:379–381.
86. Del Prete G, Maggi E, Romagnani S. Human Th1 and Th2 cells: functional properties, mechanisms of regulation, and role in disease. Lab Invest 1994;70:299–306.
87. Negoro S, Hara H, Miyata S, et al. Mechanisms of age-related decline in antigen-specific T cell proliferative response: IL-2 receptor expression and recombinant IL-2 induced proliferative response of purified Tac-positive T cells. Mech Ageing Dev 1986;36:223–241.
88. McElhaney JE, Beattie BL, Devine R, et al. Age-related decline in interleukin 2 production in response to influenza vaccine. J Am Geriatr Soc 1990;38:652–658.
89. Vissinga C, Hertogh-Huijbregts A, Rosing J, Nagelkerken L. Analysis of the age-related decline in alloreactivity of $CD4^+$ and $CD8^+$ T cells in CBA/RIJ mice. Mech Ageing Dev 1990;51:179–194.
90. Hara H, Tanaka T, Negoro S, et al. Age-related changes of expression of IL-2 receptor subunits and kinetics of IL-2 internalization in T cells after mitogenic stimulation. Mech Ageing Dev 1988;45:167–175.
91. Nagel JE, Chopra RK, Powers DC, Adler WH. Effect of age on the human high affinity interleukin 2 receptor of phytohaemagglutinin stimulated peripheral blood lymphocytes. Clin Exp Immunol 1989;75:286–291.
92. Goonewardene IM, Murasko DM. Age associated changes in mitogen induced proliferation and cytokine production by lymphocytes of the long-lived brown Norway rat. Mech Ageing Dev 1993;71:199–212.
93. Ajitsu S, Mirabella S, Kawanishi H. In vivo immunologic intervention in age-related T cell defects in murine gut-associated lymphoid tissues by IL-2. Mech Ageing Dev 1990;54:163–183.
94. Hobbs MV, Ernst DN, Torbett BE, et al. Cell proliferation and cytokine production by $CD4^+$ cells from old mice. J Cell Biochem 1991;46:312–320.
95. Wu W, Pahlavani M, Cheung HT, et al. The effect of aging on the expression of interleukin 2 messenger ribonucleic acid. Cell Immunol 1986;100:224–231.
96. Bradley SF, Vibhagool A, Kunkel SL, Kauffman CA. Monokine secretion in aging and protein malnutrition. J Leukoc Biol 1989;45:510–514.
97. Molteni M, Della Bella S, Mascagni B, et al. Secretion of cytokines upon allogeneic stimulation: effect of aging. J Biol Regul Homeost Agents 1994;8:41–47.
98. Udhayakumar V, Subbarao B, Seth A, Nagarkatti M, et al. Impaired T cell-induced T cell–T cell interaction in aged mice. Cell Immunol 1988;116:299–307.
99. Thoman ML, Keogh EA, Weigle WO. Response of aged T and B cells to IL-4. Aging Immunol Infect Dis 1988/1989; 1:245–253.
100. Li SP, Miller RA. Age-associated decline in Il-4 production by murine T lymphocytes in extended culture. Cell Immunol 1993;151:187–195.
101. Dobber R, Tielemans M, Nagelkerken L. The in vivo effects of neutralizing antibodies against IFN-gamma, IL-4, or IL-10 on the humoral immune response in young and aged mice. Cell Immunol 1995;160:185–192.
102. Burns EA, l'Hommedieu GD, Cunning J, Goodwin JS. Effects of interleukin 4 on antigen-specific antibody synthesis by lymphocytes from old and young adults. Lymphokine Cytokine Res 1994;13:227–231.
103. Candore G, Di Lorenzo G, Melluso M, et al. Gamma-interferon, interleukin-4 and interleukin-6 in vitro production in old subjects. Autoimmunity 1993;16:275–280.
104. Nagelkerken L, Hertogh-Huijbregts A, Dobber R, Drager A. Age-related changes in lymphokine production related

to a decreased number of CD45RBhi CD4+ T cells. Eur J Immunol 1991;21:273–281.
105. Krishnaraj R, Bhooma T. Cytokine sensitivity of human NK cells during immunosenescence. 2. IL-2-induced interferon gamma secretion. Immunol Lett 1996;50:59–63.
106. Caruso C, Candore G, Cigna D, et al. Cytokine production pathway in the elderly. Immunol Res 1996;15:84–90.
107. Faist E, Markewitz A, Fuchs D, Lang S, et al. Immunomodulatory therapy with thymopentin and indomethacin: successful restoration of interleukin-2 synthesis in patients undergoing major surgery. Ann Surg 1991;214:264–273.
108. Chopra RK, Holbrook NJ, Powers DC, et al. Interleukin 2, interleukin 2 receptor, and interferon-gamma synthesis and mRNA expression in phorbol myristate acetate and calcium ionophore A23187-stimulated T cells from elderly humans. Clin Immunol Immunopathol 1989;53:297–308.
109. Daynes RA, Araneo BA, Ershler WB, et al. Altered regulation of IL-6 production with normal aging. J Immunol 1993;150:5219–5230.
110. Ershler WB. Interleukin-6: a cytokine for gerontologists. J Am Geriatr Soc 1993;41:176–181.
111. Sothern RB, Roitman-Johnson B, Kanabrocki EL, et al. Circadian characteristics of circulating interleukin-6 in men. J Allerg Clin Immunol 1995;95:1029–1035.
112. Liao Z, Caucino JA, Schniffer SM, et al. Increased urinary cytokine levels in the elderly. Aging Immunol Infect Dis 1993;4:139–153.
113. Foster KD, Conn CA, Kluger MJ. Fever, tumor necrosis factor and interleukin-6 in young, mature and aged Fischer 344 rats. Am J Physiol 1992;262:R211–R215.
114. Clark JA, Peterson TC. Cytokine production and aging: overproduction of IL-8 in elderly males in response to lipopolysaccharide. Mech Ageing Dev 1994;77:127–139.
115. Goodwin JS. Decreased immunity and increased morbidity in the elderly. Nutr Rev 1995;53:S41–S46.
116. Bender BS, Nagel JE, Adler WH, Andres K. Absolute peripheral blood lymphocyte counts and subsequent mortality of elderly men. J Am Geriatr Soc 1986;34:649–654.
117. Ferguson FG, Wikby A, Maxson P, Olsson J, Johansson B. Immune parameters in a longitudinal study of a very old population of Swedish people: a comparison between survivors and nonsurvivors. J Gerontol 1995;50:B378–B382.
118. Wayne S, Rhyne R, Garry P, et al. Cell mediated immunity as a predictor of morbidity and mortality in the aged. J Gerontol 1990;45:45–49.
119. Burns EA, Goodwin JS. Immunology and infectious disease. In: Cassel CK, Riesenberg DE, Sorensen LB, Walsh JR (eds) Geriatric Medicine, 2nd ed. New York: Springer, 1990:312–329.
120. Sullivan KM, Monto AS, Longini IM Jr. Estimates of the US health impact of influenza. Am J Public Health 1993; 83:1712–1716.
121. Ben-Yehuda A, Ehleiter D, Hu AR, Weksler ME. Recombinant vaccinia virus expressing the PR/8 influenza hemagglutinin gene overcomes the impaired immune response and increased susceptibility of old mice to influenza infection. J Infect Dis 1993;168:352–357.
122. Fagiolo U, Amadori A, Cozzi E, et al. Humoral and cellular immune response to influenza virus vaccination in aged humans. Aging 1993;5:451–458.
123. Kutza J, Gross P, Kaye D, Murasko DM. Natural killer cell cytotoxicity in elderly humans after influenza immunization. Clin Diagn Lab Immunol 1996;3:105–108.
124. Swenson CD, Cherniack EP, Russo C, Thorbecke GJ. IgD-receptor up-regulation on human peripheral blood T cells in response to IgD in vitro or antigen in vivo correlates with the antibody response to influenza vaccination. Eur J Immunol 1996;26:340–344.
125. Remarque EJ, van Beek WC, Ligthart GJ, et al. Improvement of the immunoglobulin subclass response to influenza vaccine in elderly nursing home residents by the use of high-dose vaccines. Vaccine 1993;11:649–654.
126. Gross PA, Quinnan GV, Rodstein M, et al. Association of influenza immunization with reduction in mortality in an elderly population. Arch Intern Med 1988;148:562–565.
127. Arden NH, Patriarca PA, Kendal AP. Experiences in the use and efficacy of inactivated influenza vaccine in nursing homes. In: Kendal AP, Patriarca PA (eds) Options for the Control of Influenza. New York: Liss, 1986:155–168.
128. Advisory Committee on Immunization Practices. Prevention and control of influenza. MMWR 1997;46S:1–20.
129. Nicoletti C. Antibody protection in aging: influence of idiotypic repertoire and antibody binding activity to a bacterial antigen. Exp Mol Pathol 1995;62:99–108.
130. Borghesi C, Nicoletti C. Increase of cross(auto)-reactive antibodies after immunization in aged mice: a cellular and molecular study. Int J Exp Pathol 1994;75:123–130.
131. Stein BE. Adult vaccinations: protecting your patients from avoidable illness. Geriatrics 1993;48:46, 49–52, 55.
132. Sims RV, Steinmann WC, McConville JH, et al. The clinical effectiveness of pnemococcal vaccine in the elderly. Ann Intern Med 1988;108:653–657.
133. Sharma N, Trubuhovich R, Thomas MG. Tetanus in Auckland: a preventable disease. NZ Med J 1994;107:82–84.
134. Zuber PL, Schierz A, Arestegui G, Steffen R. Tetanus in Switzerland 1980–1989. Eur J Epidemiol 1993;9:617–624.
135. Gergen PJ, McQuillan TM, Kiely M, Ezzati-Rice TM, Sutter RW, Virella G. A population-based serologic survey of immunity to tetanus in the United States. N Engl J Med 1995;332:761–766.
136. Knight AL, Richardson JP. Management of tetanus in the elderly. J Am Board Fam Pract 1992;5:43–49.
137. Prevots R, Sutter RW, Strebel PM, Cochi SL, Hadler S. Tetanus surveillance—United States, 1989–1990. MMWR 1992;41:1–9.
138. Ballestra DJ, Littenberg B. Should adults tetanus immunization be given as a single vaccination at age 65? A cost-effective analysis. J Gen Intern Med 1993;8:405–412.
139. Lichtenhan JB, Kellerman RD, Richards JF. Tetanus: a threat to elderly patients. Postgrad Med 1992;92:59–60, 65–67, 70–72.
140. Stead WW, Lofgren JP, Warren E, et al. Tuberculosis as an endemic and nosocomial infection among the elderly in nursing homes. N Eng J Med 1985;312:1483–1487.
141. Stead WW, To T. The significance of the tuberculin skin test in elderly persons. Ann Intern Med 1987;107:837–842.
142. Cooper AM, Callahan JE, Griffin JP, et al. Old mice are able to control low-dose aerogenic infections with Mycobacterium tuberculosis. Infect Immun 1995;63:3259–3265.
143. Orme IM, Griffin JP, Roberts AD, Ernst DN. Evidence for a defective accumulation of protective T cells in old mice

infected with Mycobacterium tuberculosis. Cell Immunol 1993;147:222–229.
144. Orme IM. Mechanisms underlying the increased susceptibility of aged mice to tuberculosis. Nutr Rev 1995;53:S35–S40.
145. Orme IM. Aging and immunity to tuberculosis: increased susceptibility of old mice reflects a decreased capacity to generate mediator T lymphocytes. J Immunol 1988;140: 3589–3593.
146. Orme IM. The response of macrophages from old mice to Mycobacterium tuberculosis and its products. Aging Immunol Infect Dis 1993;4:187–195.
147. Ragozzino MW, Melton LJ III, Kurland LT, et al. Population-based study of herpes zoster and its sequelae. Medicine 1982;61:310–316.
148. Donahue JG, Choo PW, Manson JE, Platt R. The incidence of herpes zoster. Arch Intern Med 1995;155:1605–1609.
149. Burke BL, Steele RW, Beard OW, et al. Immune responses to varicella-zoster in the aged. Arch Intern Med 1982; 142:291–293.
150. Ragozzino MW, Melton LJ III, Kurland LT, et al. Risk of cancer after herpes zoster: a population-based study. N Engl J Med 1982;307:393–397.
151. Gallo RC, Wong-Staal F. A human T-lymphotrophic retrovirus (HTLV–III) as the cause of AIDS. Ann Intern Med 1985;103:679–689.
152. First 500,000 AIDS cases—United States, 1995. MMWR 1995;44:849–853.
153. Adler WH, Nagel JE. Acquired immunodeficiency syndrome in the elderly. Drugs Aging 1994;4:410–416.
154. Stall R, Catania J. AIDS risk behaviors among late middle-aged and elderly Americans. Arch Intern Med 1994;154:57–63.
155. Steel M. IVth international AIDS conference. Lancet 1988;2:54–55.
156. Darby SC, Ewart DW, Giangrande PL, Spooner RJ, Rizza CR. Importance of age at infection with HIV-1 for survival and development of AIDS in UK haemophilia population. Lancet 1996;347:1573–1579.
157. Pedersen BK, Kappel M, Klokker M, Nielsen HB, Secher NH. The immune system during exposure to extreme physiologic conditions. Int J Sports Med 1994;15:S116–S121.
158. Vallina VL, Velasco JM. The influence of laparoscopy on lymphocyte subpopulations in the surgical patient. Surg Endosc 1996;10:481–484.
159. Tønnesen E, Brinkløv MM, Christensen NJ, Olesen AS, Madsen T. Natural killer cell activity and lymphocyte function during and after coronary artery bypass grafting in relation to the endocrine stress response. Anesthesia 1987;67:526–533.
160. Zedler S, Faist E, Ostermeier B, von Donnersmarck GH, Schildberg FW. Postburn constitutional changes in T cell reactivity occur in CD8⁺ rather than CD4⁺ cells. J Trauma 1997;42:872–880.
161. Horgan AF, Mendez MV, O'Riordain DS, Holzheimer RG, Mannick JA, Rodrick ML. Altered gene transcription after burn injury results in depressed T lymphocyte activation. Ann Surg 1994;220:342–352.
162. Wlaszczyk A, Adamik B, Durek G, Kübler A, Zimeki M. Immunological status of patients subjected to cardiac surgery: serum levels of interleukin 6 and tumor necrosis factor $\alpha$ and the ability of peripheral blood mononuclear cells to proliferate and produce these cytokines in vitro. Arch Immunol Ther Exp 1996;44:225–234.
163. Keel M, Schregenberger N, Steckholzer U, et al. Endotoxin tolerance after severe injury and its regulatory mechanisms. J Trauma 1996;41:430–437.
164. Miller-Graziano CL, De AK, Kodys K. Altered IL-10 levels in trauma patients' M phi and T lymphocytes. J Clin Immunol 1995;15:93–104.
165. Meakins JL. Host defense mechanisms in surgical patients: effect of surgery and trauma. Acta Chir Scand Suppl 1988;550:43–53.
166. Redmond HP, Watson WG, Houghton T, Condron C, Watson RGK, Bouchier-Hayes D. Immune function in patients undergoing open vs laparoscopic cholecystectomy. Arch Surg 1994;129:1240–1246.
167. Shigemitsu Y, Saito T, Kinoshita T, Kobayashi M. Influence of surgical stress on bactericidal activity of neutrophils and complications of infection in patients with esophageal cancer. J Surg Oncol 1992;50:90–97.
168. Pollock RE, Lotzova, Stanford SD. Surgical stress impairs natural killer cell programming of tumor for lysis in patients with sarcomas and other solid tumors. Cancer 1992;70:2192–2202.
169. Pollock RE, Lotzova E, Stanford SD. Mechanism of surgical stress impairment of human perioperative natural killer cell cytotoxicity. Arch Surg 1991;126:338–342.
170. Blazar BA, Rodrick ML, O'Mahony JB, et al. Suppression of natural killer cell function in humans following thermal and traumatic injury. J Clin Immunol 1986;6:26–36.
171. Oka M, Hazama S, Suzuki M, et al. Depression of cytotoxicity of nonparenchymal cells in the liver after surgery. Surgery 1994;116:877–882.
172. O'Sullivan ST, Lederer JA, Horgan AF, Chin DH, Mannick JA, Rodrick ML. Major injury leads to predominance of the T helper-2 lymphocyte phenotype and diminished interleukin-12 production associated with decreased resistance to infection. Ann Surg 1995;222:482–490.
173. Trokel MJ, Bessler M, Treat MR, Whelan RL, Nowygrod R. Preservation of immune response after laparoscopy. Surg Endosc 1994;8:1385–1388.
174. Wilmore DW. Homeostasis: bodily changes in trauma and surgery. In: Sabiston DC (ed) Textbook of Surgery: The Biological Basis of Modern Surgical Practice, 14th ed. Philadelphia: Saunders, 1991:19–33.
175. Traynor C, Hall GM. Endocrine and metabolic changes during surgery. Br J Anaesth 1981;53:153–160.
176. Hauser CJ, Zhou X, Joshi P, et al. The immune microenvironment of human fracture/soft tissue hematomas and its relationship to systemic immnity. J Trauma 1997;42:895–903.
177. Besedovsky HO, Del Rey A, Klusman I, Furukawa H, Monge Arditi G, Kabiersch A. Cytokines as modulators of the hypothalamus-pituitary-adrenal axis. J Steroid Biochem Mol Biol 1991;40:613–618.
178. Gaillard RC. Neuroendocrine-immune system interactions: the immune-hypothalamo-pituitary-adrenal axis. Trends Endocrinol Metab 1994;5:303–309.
179. Rook GAW, Hernandez-Pando R, Lightman SL. Hormones, peripherally activated prohormones and regula-

tion of the Th1/Th2 balance. Immunol Today 1994;15:301–303.
180. Blalock JE. The syntax of immune-neuroendocrine communication. Immunol Today 1994;15:504–511.
181. Ottaviani E, Franceschi C. The neuroimmunology of stress from invertebrates to man. Prog Neurobiol 1996;48:421–440.
182. Hässig A, Wen-Xi L, Stampfli K. Stress-induced suppression of the cellular immune reactions: on the neuroendocrine control of the immune system. Med Hypotheses 1996;46:551–555.
183. Ader R, Cohen N. Conditioned immunopharmacologic responses. In: Ader R (ed) Psychoneuroimmunology. San Diego: Academic, 1981:281–317.
184. Borysenko M, Borysenko J. Stress, behavior and immunity: animal models and mediating mechanisms. Gen Hosp Psychiatry 1982;4:59–67.
185. Rosenberg LT, Coe CL, Levine S. Complement levels in the squirrel monkey. Lab Anim Sci 1982;32:371–372.
186. Minter RE, Patterson-Kimball C. Life events and illness onset: a review. Psychosomatics 1978;19:334–339.
187. Glaser R, Thorn BE, Tarr KL, et al. Effects of stress on methyltransferase synthesis: an important DNA repair enzyme. Health Psychol 1985;4:403–412.
188. Thomas PD, Goodwin JM, Goodwin JS. Effect of social support on stress-related changes in cholesterol level, uric acid level and immune function in an elderly sample. Am J Psychiatry 1985;142:735–737.
189. Bartoloni C, Guidi L, Antico L, et al. Psychological status and immunological parameters of institutionalized aged. Panminerva Med 1991;33:164–169.
190. Glaser R, Kiecolt-Glaser JK, Speicher CE, et al. The relationship of stress and loneliness and changes in herpes virus latency. J Behav Med 1985;8:249–260.
191. Glaser R, Pearson GR, Bonneau RH, et al. Stress and the memory T cell response to the Epstein-Barr virus in healthy medical students. Health Psychol 1993;12:435–442.
192. Kiecolt-Glaser JK, Glaser R, Gravenstein S, Malarkey WB, Sheridan J. Chronic stress alters the immune response to influenza virus vaccine in older adults. Proc Natl Acad Sci USA 1996;93:3043–3047.
193. Kiecolt-Glaser JK, Marucha PT, Malarkey WB, et al. Slowing of wound healing by psychological stress. Lancet 1995;346:1194–1196.
194. Fabris N. A neuroendocrine-immune theory of aging. Int J Neurosci 1990;51:373–375.
195. Song L, Kim YH, Chopra RK, et al. Age-related effects in T cell activation and proliferation. Exp Gerontol 1993;28:313–321.
196. Lewis V, Twomey J, Bealmear P, et al. Age, thymic function and circulating thymic hormone activity. J Clin Endocrinol Metab 1978;47:145–152.
197. Hirokawa K, Utsuyama M, Kasai M, et al. Aging and immunity. Acta Pathol Jpn 1992;42:537–548.
198. Effros RB, Casillas A, Walford RL. The effect of thymosin-1 immunity to influenza in aged mice. Aging Immunol Infect Dis 1988;1:31–40.
199. Goso C, Frasca D, Doria G. Effect of synthetic thymic humoral factor (THF-gamma 2) on T cell activities in immunodeficient ageing mice. Clin Exp Immunol 1992;87:346–351.
200. Frasca D, Adorini L, Doria G. Enhanced frequency of mitogen-responsive T cell precursors in old mice injected with thymosin alpha 1. Eur J Immunol 1987;17:727–730.
201. Cillari E, Milano S, Perego R, et al. Modulation of IL-2, IFN-gamma, TNF-alpha and IL-4 production in mice of different ages by thymopentin. Int J Immunopharmacol 1991;14:1029–1035.
202. Duchateau J, Servais G, Vreyens R, et al. Modulation of immune response in aged humans through different administration modes of thymopentin. Surv Immunol Res 1985;4(suppl 1):94–101.
203. Ershler WB, Moore AL, Hacker MP, et al. Specific antibody synthesis in vitro. II. Age-associated thymosin enhancement of anti-tetanus antibody synthesis. Immunopharmacology 1984;8:69–77.
204. Meroni PL, Barcellini W, Frasca D, et al. In vivo immunopotentiating activity of thymopentin in aging humans: increase of IL-2 production. Clin Immunol Immunopathol 1987;42:151–159.
205. Cillari E, Milano S, Dieli M, et al. Thymopentin reduces the susceptibility of aged mice to cutaneous leishmaniasis by modulating CD4 T-cell subsets. Immunology 1992;76:362–366.
206. Reiter RJ. Pineal function during aging: attenuation of the melatonin rhythm and its neurobiological consequences. Acta Neurobiol Exp 1994;54:31S–39S.
207. Lissoni P, Brivio O, Fumagalli L, et al. Immune effects of preoperative immunotherapy with high-dose subcutaneous interleukin-2 versus neuroimmunotherapy with low-dose IL-2 plus the neurohormone melatonin in gastrointestinal tract tumor patients. J Biol Regul Homeost Agents 1995;9:31–33.
208. Lissoni P, Barni S, Fossati V, et al. A randomized study of neuroimmunotherapy with low-dose subcutaneous interleukin-2 plus melatonin compared to supportive care alone in patients with untreatable metastatic solid tumour. Support Care Cancer 1995;3:194–197.
209. Caroleo MC, Frasca D, Nistico G, Doria G. Melatonin: an immunomodulator in immunodeficient mice. Immunopharmacology 1992;23:81–89.
210. Saito H, Inoue T, Fukatsu K, et al. Growth hormone and the immune response to bacterial infection. Horm Res 1996;45:50–54.
211. Auernhammer CJ, Feldmeier H, Nass R, et al. Insulin-like growth factor I is an independent coregulatory modulator of NK cell activity. Endocrinology 1996;137:5332–5336.
212. Bonello RS, Marcus R, Bloch D, Strober S. Effects of growth hormone and estrogen on T lymphocytes in older women. J Am Geriatr Soc 1996;44:1039–1042.
213. Vara-Thorbeck R, Guerrero JA, Rosell J, Ruiz-Requena E, Capitan JM. Exogenous growth hormone: effects on the catabolic response to surgically produced acute stress and on postoperative immune function. World J Surg 1993;17:530–538.
214. Vara-Thorbeck R, Ruiz-Requena E, Guerrero-Fernandez JA. Effects of human growth hormone on the catabolic state after surgical trauma. Horm Res 1996;45:55–60.
215. Hinton PS, Peterson CA, Lo H-C, Yang H, McCarthy D, Ney DM. Insulin-like growth factor-1 enhances immune response in dexamethasone-treated or surgically stressed

rats maintained with total parenteral nutrition. J Parenter Enteral Nutr 1995;19:444–452.

216. Swenson CD, Gottesman SR, Belsito DV, et al. Relationship between humoral immunoaugmenting properties of DHEAS and IgD-receptor expression in young and aged mice. Ann NY Acad Sci 1995;29:249–258.
217. Araneo BA, Woods ML II, Daynes RA. Reversal of the immunosenescent phenotype by DHEA: hormone treatment provides an adjuvant effect on the immunization of aged mice with recombinant hepatitis B surface antigen. J Infect Dis 1993;167:830–840.
218. Danenberg HD, Ben-Yehuda A, Zakay-Rones Z, et al. DHEA treatment reverses the impaired immune response of old mice to influenza vaccination and protects from influenza infection. Vaccine 1995;13:1445–1448.
219. Araneo B, Dowell T, Woods ML, et al. DHEA as an effective vaccine adjuvant in elderly humans: proof-of-principle studies. Ann NY Acad Sci 1995;774:232–248.
220. Shen R-N, Wu B, Lu L, Kaiser HE, Broxmeyer HE. Recombinant human interleukin-1 alpha: a potent bio-immunomodifier in vivo in immunosuppressed mice induced by cyclophosphamide, retroviral infection and surgical stress. In Vivo 1994;8:59–64.
221. Chandra RK. Nutrition is an important determinant of immunity in old age. Prog Clin Biol Res 1990;326:321–334.
222. Burns EA, Goodwin JS. Aging: nutrition and Immunity. In: Forse RA, Bell SJ, Blackburn GL (eds) Diet, Nutrition and Immunity. Boca Raton, FL: CRC Press, 1994:57–72.
223. Effros RB, Walford RL, Weindruch R, et al. Influences of dietary restriction on immunity to influenza in aged mice. J Gerontol 1991;46:B142–B147.
224. Ershler WB, Sun WH, Binkley N, et al. Interleukin-6 and aging: blood levels and mononuclear cell production increase with advancing age and in vitro production is modifiable by dietary restriction. Lymphoc Cytol Res 1993;12:225–230.
225. Kemintz JW, Weindruch R, Roecker EB, et al. Dietary restriction of adult male rhesus monkeys: design, methodology, and preliminary findings from the first year of study. J Gerontol 1993;48:B17–B26.
226. Chandra RK, Puri S. Nutritional support improves antibody response to influenza vaccine in the elderly. BMJ 1985;291:709.
227. Chandra RK. Effect of vitamin and trace-element supplementation on immune responses and infection in elderly subjects. Lancet 1992;340:1124–1127.
228. Rasmussen LB, Kiens B, Pedersen BK, et al. Effect of diet and plasma fatty acid composition on immune status in elderly men. Am J Clin Nutr 1994;59:572–577.
229. Alverdy JC, Aoys E, Moss GS. Total parenteral nutrition promotes bacterial translocation from the gut. Surgery 1988;104:185–190.
230. Alverdy JA, Eoys E, Weiss-Carrington P, et al. The effect of glutamine-enriched TPN on gut immune cellularity. J Surg Res 1992;52:34–38.
231. Mainous M, Dazhong X, Lu Q, et al. Oral-TPN-induced bacterial translocation and impaired immune defenses are reversed by refeeding. Surgery 1991;110:277–284.
232. Shou J, Lappin J, Daly JM. Impairment of pulmonary macrophage function with total parenteral nutrition. Ann Surg 1994;219:291–297.
233. Hamawy KJ, Moldawer LL, Georgieff M, et al. The effect of lipid emulsions on reticuloendothelial system function in the injured animal. J Parenter Enteral Nutr 1985;9: 559–565.
234. Sedman PC, Somers SS, Ramsden CW, et al. Effects of different lipid emulsions on lymphocyte function during total parenteral nutrition. Br J Surg 1991;78:1396–1399.
235. Gogos CA, Kalfarentzos FE, Zoumbos NC. Effect of different types of parenteral nutrition on T-lymphocyte subpopulation and NK cells. Am J Clin Nutr 1990;51:119–122.
236. Jensen GL, Mascioli EA, Seidner DL, et al. Parenteral infusion of long- and medium-chain triglycerides and reticuloendothelial system function in man. J Parenter Enteral Nutr 1994;18:35–39.
237. Salo M. Inhibition of immunoglobulin synthesis in vitro by intravenous lipid emulsion. J Parenter Enteral Nutr 1990;14:459–462.
238. Sacks GS, Brown RO, Teague D, Dickerson RN, Tolley EA, Kudsk KA. Early nutrition support modifies immune function in patients sustaining severe head injury. J Parenter Enteral Nutr 1995;19:387–392.
239. Meydani M. Vitamin E. Lancet 1995;345:170–175.
240. Meydani SN, Hayek M. Vitamin E and immune response. In: Chandra RK (ed) Proceedings of International Conference on Nutrition and Immunity. St. John's, Newfoundland: ARTS Biomedical, 1992:105–128.
241. Meydani SN, Meydani M, Blumberg JB, et al. Vitamin E supplementation and in vivo immune response in healthy elderly subjects: a randomized controlled trial. Am J Clin Nutr 1990;52:557–563.
242. Meydani SN, Leka L, Loszewski R. Long-term vitamin E supplementation enhances immune response in healthy elderly. FASEB J 1994;8:A274.
243. Wu D, Meydani SN, Sastre J, et al. In vitro glutathione supplementation enhances interleukin-2 production and mitogenic response of peripheral blood mononuclear cells from young and old subjects. J Nutr 1994;124:655–663.
244. Omenn GS, Goodman GE, Thornquist MD, et al. Risk factors for lung cancer and for intervention effects in CARET, the Beta Carotene and Retinol Efficacy Trial. J Natl Cancer Inst 1996;88:1550–1550.
245. Albanes D, Heinonen OP, Taylor PR, et al. Alpha-tocopherol and beta-carotene supplements and lung cancer incidence in the alpha-tocopherol, beta-carotene cancer prevention study: effects of base-line characteristics and study compliance. J Natl Cancer Inst 1996;88:1560–1570.
246. Goodwin JS, Bankhurst A, Murphy S, et al. Partial reversal of the cellular immune defect in common variable immunodeficiency with indomethacin. J Clin Lab Immunol 1978;1:197–199.
247. Hsia J, Tang T, Parrott M, Rogalla K. Augmentation of the immune response to influenza vaccine by acetylsalicylic acid: a clinical trial in a geriatric population. Methods Find Exp Clin Pharmacol 1994;16:677–683.
248. Cueppens J, Rodriguez M, Goodwin JS. Nonsteroidal anti-inflammatory drugs inhibit the production of IgM rheumatoid factor in vitro. Lancet 1982;1:528–531.
249. Levin MJ, Murray M, Zerbe GO, White CJ, Hayward AR. Immune responses of elderly persons 4 years after receiving a live attenuated varicella vaccine. J Infect Dis 1994;170:522–526.

250. Levine M, Beattie BL, McLean DM. Comparison of 1 and 2-dose regimens of influenza vaccine for elderly men. Can Med Assc J 1987;137:722–726.
251. Powers DC, Manning MC, Hanscome PJ, Pietrobon PJ. Cytotoxic T lymphocyte responses to a liposome-adjuvanted influenza A virus vaccine in the elderly. J Infect Dis 1995;172:1103–1107.
252. McElhaney JE, Meneilly GS, Lecheltk E, Bleackley RC. Split-virus influenza vaccines: do they provide adequate immunity in the elderly. J Gerontol 1994;49:M37–M43.
253. Gorse GJ, Campbell MJ, Otto EE, Powers DC, Chambers GW, Newman FK. Increased anti-influenza A virus cytotoxic T cell activity following vaccination of the chronically ill elderly with live attenuated or inactivated influenza virus vaccine. J Infect Dis 1995;172:1–10.
254. Koltun WA, Bloomer MM, Tilberg AF, et al. Awake epidural anesthesia is associated with improved natural killer cell cytotoxicity and a reduced stress response. Am J Surg 1996;171:68–73.
255. Decker D, Schöndorf M, Bidlingmaier F, Hirner A, von Ruecker AA. Surgical stress induces a shift in the type-1/type-2 T-helper cell balance, suggesting down-regulation of cell-mediated and up-regulation of antibody-mediated immunity commensurate to the trauma. Surgery 1996;119:316–325.
256. Pennebaker JW, Kiecolt-Glaser JK, Glaser R. Disclosure of traumas and immune function: health implications for psychotherapy. J Consult Clin Psychol 1988;56:239–245.
257. Kiecolt-Glaser JK, Glaser R, Williger D, et al. Psychosocial enhancement of immunocompetence in a geriatric population. Health Psychol 1985;4:25–41.

# 5
# Nutrition, Metabolism, and Wound Healing in the Elderly

Danny O. Jacobs and Tirso Mark Lara

## Nutrition in the Elderly

Throughout most of adult life our bodies maintain near-perfect metabolic balance interrupted only by disease. This equilibrium lasts a finite period—until the inevitable aging process begins. Aging is a complex phenomenon that includes molecular, cellular, physiologic, and psychological changes. Individual aging is influenced primarily by a person's genetic makeup, life style, and environment. Of these factors, the first is predetermined and constant; the other two are optional, variable, and therefore modifiable. Some very old individuals can stay healthy and have good nutritional status,[1,2] but physiologic decline and health problems are expected for most of us before death. Aging of cellular function results in a natural decline in physiologic performance and reserve capacity. Thus elderly individuals have increased susceptibility and are less resistant to illness.[3]

These factors contribute to an increased prevalence of illness and an increased risk for primary and secondary malnutrition. There is an estimated 5–10% prevalence of protein-calorie malnutrition among community dwelling elderly. In the United States approximately 85% of the noninstitutionalized elderly suffer from at least one condition that could be improved by proper nutrition.[1] Physicians often fail to recognize its presence. Malnutrition in this population may predispose the elderly to prolonged hospitalization.

Among the institutionalized elderly, the nutritional situation is much different. Many studies have documented a high prevalence of malnutrition among elderly residents of nursing homes. Although numbers vary, surveys have shown incidences of malnutrition that range from 30% to 85% and increased mortality rates.[4,5] Among these elderly, factors amenable to intervention include a dependence on others for feeding, poor appetite, slow eating, dysphagia, and energy and protein intake. Hypoalbuminemia may also be common: A 37% incidence of this disorder was documented in a Veterans Administration nursing home. Taking these factors into consideration, it seems that much of the malnutrition in nursing homes is preventable or reversible.[1]

Nutritional status during acute illness is a determinant of morbidity, length of stay in hospital, and mortality.[1,6] Surgery of the elderly is associated with high morbidity and mortality, particularly in the malnourished patient who requires an emergency operation. In addition, malnutrition negatively affects postoperative recovery and rehabilitation.[3] As approximately 30% of the health care budget is spent on this age group, nutritional screening and intervention in certain settings has been proposed as a cost-effective measure.[1]

### Physical and Psychosocial Issues in Nutrition

A combination of physical, social, and psychological factors contribute to primary malnutrition in the elderly. Physical deterioration with age can influence nutritional status. As years pass, the elderly become frail, have diminished visual function, increased cognitive impairment, and gait and balance disorders that affect mobility and decrease their ability to buy and prepare food.

Dental diseases are common in the elderly. There seems to be a relation between poor dentition and difficulty ingesting certain food items, such as meat and hard foods. This may result in changes in choice and the quality of food intake. Taste and smell are also affected (see Chapter 29). A progressive loss of taste buds occurs, predominantly affecting the anterior tongue, which contains the taste buds that detect sweet and salt. Because the remaining buds detecting bitter and sour are relatively increased with aging, elderly people have a greater sensitivity to these tastes.[7] Enhancing food flavors has been found to increase intake and nutritional status in elderly institutionalized patients.[1]

The presence of multiple diseases can also affect nutritional status. Disorders that interfere with eating include neurologic diseases, such as Parkinson's disease and cerebrovascular accidents, chronic obstructive pulmonary disease, congestive heart failure, and chronic renal insufficiency. Some of these diseases require dietary restrictions that affect the palatability or variety of the food offered. Swallowing disorders are not uncommon in the elderly and nutritional disorders are frequently associated with dysphagia in institutionalized persons.

Anorexia commonly occurs with aging. The decrease in appetite can be due to a decrease in basal metabolic rate, most likely secondary to a decrease in lean body mass and to a more sedentary life style. Drugs can also cause anorexia as well as interfere with the intake, absorption, and metabolism of nutrients. Because of their use of multiple medications, the elderly are at increased risk of drug interactions, which may interfere with nutrient assimilation.

Disturbances of mood and affect are common in the elderly. Cognitive impairments such as dementia may significantly decrease nutrient intake. Anorexia is a common symptom during depression, as these depressed patients often become malnourished. The prevalence of hospital malnutrition among the depressed elderly can be as high as 20–35%.[5] One of the most difficult situations in geriatric medicine is to determine if the refusal of food is due to a curable depression or is the will of a mentally healthy individual. In particular, the death of a spouse can dramatically influence appetite and food intake. Depressed patients may put less effort into caring for themselves and may lose the symbolism of warmth and sharing associated with eating.

Approximately 30% of elderly Americans live alone, and 25% of free-living elderly need assistance with daily life activities. Social isolation can lead to problems of obtaining and preparing food. An unsuitable meal environment is an important negative factor in institutional nutrition. Food intake of energy and protein can increase by 25% if the environment is changed to a familiar one. Timing of meals in hospitals and nursing homes may also be disadvantageous, as meals may be separated by short periods of time. Appetite may be poor for each meal when the times they are offered are too close together. Food presentation is key for patients to accept the meals offered. Pureed food is not readily accepted, so imaginative ways of presenting such meals should be tried.[8] Foreign or exotic dishes are less likely to be accepted than regional or known dishes. Last, financial problems may also affect diet quality and quantity and contribute to poor nutrition.

## Age-Related Changes in Body Composition

### *Lean Body Mass*

Presently, the most widely used body composition model is a two-compartment model in which the body is divided into lean body mass and fat. Aging is accompanied by a net loss of lean body mass. As a consequence, the elderly become debilitated and lose an important portion of their tissue amino acid and energy reserves. The lean body mass declines by approximately 6.3% every 10 years. Thus it decreases by an average of 0.45 kg/year after age 60. By age 70 muscle mass may be 20% less than that in young adults. This loss occurs disproportionately more from skeletal muscle than from viscera. Studies have suggested that changes in growth hormone metabolism may mediate age-related changes in body composition. People deficient in growth hormone have a decrease in lean body mass similar to that experienced by the healthy elderly.[9,10] In addition, treatment with growth hormone or insulin-like growth factor-I (IGF-I) increases lean body mass, nitrogen retention, and muscle strength in the elderly.[11,12] Androgens have also been proposed to play a role in the body composition changes of aging.[13] Plasma levels of testosterone may decrease with aging, and testosterone supplementation in aging individuals may increase their lean body mass.[14] Thus it is likely that an age-associated decline in growth hormone and androgen secretion contributes to the alterations in body composition and organ function seen during the normal aging process.[14] Despite all these changes, the elderly may continue to function adequately but may have decreased capacity to adapt and to mobilize endogenous protein stores during the catabolic stress imposed by infection or trauma.

### *Fiber Size Changes*

As alluded to earlier, aging is accompanied by a loss in muscle mass. Such muscle atrophy may result from a gradual, selective loss of muscle fibers. The decline in muscle mass is more marked in fast-twitch glycolytic red muscle fibers (type II), which decrease from an average of 60% in young men to less than 30% after age 80.[15] These changes are especially striking after age 70. Much of the reduction in muscle strength experienced during the aging process is accounted for by changes in muscle mass and fiber size.

Interestingly, these changes may be altered by exercise. A number of studies have described the beneficial effects of strength and resistance training. If done on a regular basis, strength training increases the cross-sectional area of slow twitch oxidative muscle fibers (type I) and increases muscle strength.[16] In addition, strength training reduces the loss of lean muscle mass as well as the increase and redistribution of body fat.[17]

### *Body Fat*

The proportion of body fat increases with age and is redistributed from subcutaneous to intramuscular sites. Body fat increases at a rate of 0.5–1.5% per year, beginning at around age 30. As with lean body mass, growth hormone and androgen administration appear to minimize alterations in body fat. The impact of testosterone supplementation on body fat is less dramatic and is controversial. Testosterone appears to decrease the uptake of triglycerides and increase triglyceride turnover while reducing lipoprotein lipase activity. Furthermore, growth hormone and androgens may act together in the regulation of fat metabolism during adult life.[14]

### *Energy Requirements*

The total energy expenditure (TEE) can be divided into three compartments. Resting energy expenditure (REE, the energy expended at rest after overnight fasting), thermic effect of feeding (TEF, the increase in energy expenditure above baseline due to the consumption and processing of food), and energy expenditure for physical activity and arousal (EEPAA). Daily energy expenditure declines progressively throughout adult life. REE is approximately 15% lower [7.35 vs. 6.20 megajoules (MJ)/day] in elderly subjects than that in the young. Changes in REE and EEPAA, which account for most of the energy consumed during daily activity, account for most (73%) of the decline in TEE observed in elderly individuals.[18] Interestingly, body weight, rather than fat-free mass, appears to best predict the REE (Fig. 5.1). Diet-induced thermogenesis decreases, along with the energy expenditure from physical activity. Nevertheless, controversy exists. Some authors have observed that the energy cost of physical activity increases, creating a less efficient system.[19] Aging is also associated with a significant decrease in energy expenditure per unit of fat-free mass and body weight. Changes in muscle mass affect energy consumption and utilization. Creatinine excretion, which is an index of muscle mass and is closely related to the basal metabolic rate, decreases with aging; thus the reduction in energy expenditure is in large part due to a decrease in lean body mass (fat-free mass) and to a more sedentary life style. These changes are reflected in a decreased total energy requirement in men from 2700 kcal/day at age 30 to 2100 kcal/day by age 80.[20] These observations suggest that preservation of muscle mass and prevention of muscle atrophy could help prevent the decrease in metabolic rate associated with advancing age.[16]

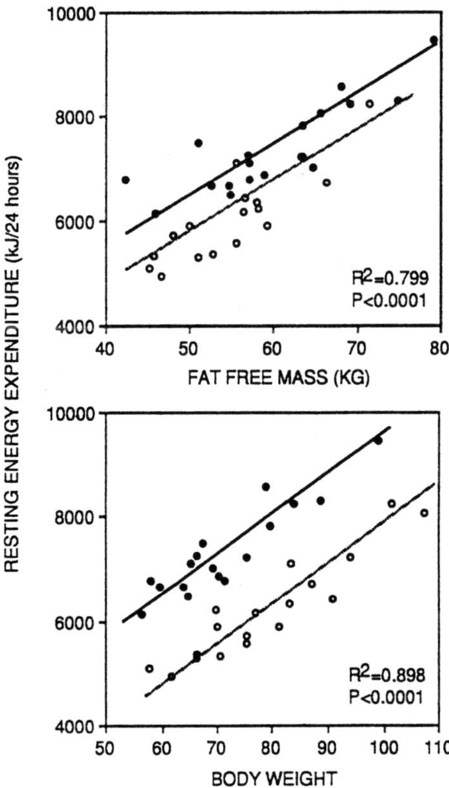


FIGURE 5.1. Resting energy expenditure in relation to fat-free mass and body weight in young men (filled circles) and elderly men (open circles). (From Roberts et al.,[18] with permission.)

## Nutritional Assessment

Nutritional assessment is a key aspect of elderly patient care. With so many physiologic changes due to aging that heighten the susceptibility to disease, the importance of proper nutrition grows. It is a challenge, however, to identify elderly persons who would benefit from dietary intervention. Not every elderly patient needs to undergo a cascade of anthropometric, dietary, and laboratory tests to assess their nutritional status. Nevertheless, knowledge of an elderly patient's nutritional status can improve a caregiver's perspective of the effects of a disease process and can drastically influence therapy and outcome.

### *History and Physical Examination*

A detailed social, nutritional, and medical history is an essential first step in assessing the nutritional status of the elderly. Particular attention should be paid to the presence of chronic diseases. Cancer by itself impairs nutritional status. Other diseases such as chronic obstructive pulmonary disease and congestive heart failure may make feeding difficult. Neurologic illnesses that interfere with the eating process place patients at particular risk. Swallowing function and absorptive capacity should be specifically assessed. Disturbances of mood and affect (e.g., depression) are not uncommon and should be considered during the evaluation.

A social history is equally important. The degree of independence can influence the capacity to purchase and prepare food. Information about who lives with the patient, cooking facilities, and income is also needed. Particular attention should be paid to patients who live in nursing homes and institutions. The physical and cognitive conditions of these patients and the eating environment and food presentation may be unsuitable, placing

TABLE 5.1. Drug Therapy That Interferes with Nutritional Support

| Drug therapy | Subject of interference or effect |
|---|---|
| Drugs that interfere with nutrient assimilation | |
| AlOH and MgOH | Phosphorus |
| $H_2$ antagonists | Vitamin $B_{12}$ |
| Cholesterol-binding agents | Fat-soluble vitamins, folate |
| Phenytoin | Vitamins D and K, folate |
| Drugs interfering with nutrient delivery | |
| Sucralfate | Forms clogs in the feeding tube |
| Digoxin, phenytoin, theophylline, potassium chloride | Diarrhea due to hyperosmolarity |
| Nutrients affecting drug therapy | |
| Calcium | Phenytoin absorption |
| Vitamin K | Anticoagulants |

*Source:* Data are from Rollandelli and Ullrich,[3] with permission.

them at risk of undernourishment. Elderly patients commonly take multiple medications. These drugs should be listed, as should alcohol use; and possible drug–nutrient interactions must be considered. Drugs that may interfere with nutrition are listed in Table 5.1.

The physical examination should always include body weight and height. Oral health, dentition, and swallowing capability should be assessed. Because dehydration may present subtly and atypically in the elderly, hydration status must be carefully evaluated. Orthostatic hypotension or tachycardia may indicate dehydration. Physical signs of malnutrition include muscle wasting and dermatitis associated with deficiency syndromes as well as perioral stomatitis and hair loss due to zinc deficiency. Cognitive impairments could indicate a deficiency of vitamin $B_{12}$, which should always be considered in the elderly if mentation is affected. The presence of decubitus ulcers is a common sign of malnutrition in institutionalized elderly and can indicate protein or vitamin C deficiency.

### *Nutrition Screening Initiative*

Evaluation of nutritional status is an especially important aspect of the surgical evaluation. Many attempts have been made to standardize nutritional risk assessment in the elderly. Perhaps the most important was the Nutrition Screening Initiative (NSI) that occurred in 1991. Three checklists were created. The first, called DETERMINE, is a self-assessment test that helps identify conditions that potentially place an older person at an increased nutritional risk. The second and third checklists are identified as levels 1 and 2. The level 1 screen was designed to be used in community settings where the availability of health care professionals may be limited. It consists of basic elements such as height, weight, body mass index, food intake and eating habits, income level, home environment questions, and a brief assessment of functional status. The level 2 screen includes all the elements contained in level 1 plus some additional parameters. Arm circumference and skinfold measurements are included and are compared with standard tables for older Americans. Serum albumin, cholesterol, medication use, and cognitive and emotional status are evaluated (Fig. 5.2). These tests do not have to be performed in sequence. The level 2 screen was designed as a first step in a formal screening process in institutionalized settings where multiple high-risk individuals reside. It can be used for the initial diagnosis of malnutrition and can facilitate selection of further diagnostic or therapeutic interventions.[21]

### *Anthropometrics*

Anthropometric measurements are a convenient tool for evaluating nutritional status. They are inexpensive, safe, and easily performed in any outpatient clinic or surgery ward. They do have some drawbacks. First, anthropometric data are affected by age and severity of illness more than any other index of nutritional status.[22] Second, they are subject to individual variation depending on who monitors the measurements. Third, they must be compared to normal standards; and in the case of the elderly, there are few normative anthropometric data. Lack of an appropriate reference group may influence the accuracy of anthropometric measurements, especially for different ethnic groups. Anthropometry can provide useful information about the nutritional status of patients with chronic disease. Nonetheless, in the severely ill, hospitalized patient who is subject to major shifts in body water, these measurements may be inaccurate.[23] Change of a specific parameter over time is generally more important than comparing it to standards. Various tables of weight per height that include elderly populations have been suggested by various investigators[24–26]; and a more valid ideal weight can be assigned using these age-specific tables. Weight loss of 5% over 4 weeks or 10% over 3 months is a sensitive indicator of malnutrition.[27]

If the patient is not able to stand upright, height can be calculated from knee-height measurements using a nomogram or the following height formulas.[28]

$$\text{Stature for men} = (2.02 \times \text{knee height}) - (0.04 \times \text{age}) + 64.19$$

$$\text{Stature for women} = (1.83 \times \text{knee height}) - (0.24 \times \text{age}) + 84.88$$

Calculation of ideal body weight provides a valid weight reference for the individual. Percent of ideal weight is calculated as:

$$\text{Actual weight/ideal weight} \times 100$$

An ideal body weight of less than 90% is an indicator of malnutrition. Weight/height ratios can be expressed as the body mass index (BMI): weight in kilograms/height in square meters. The Euronut-Seneca survey, which studied apparently healthy elderly individuals aged 70–75 years, found a mean BMI that ranged from 24.4 to 30.3 in men and from 23.9 to 30.5 for women. Results of the Third National Health and Nutrition Examination Surveys (NHANES III) include BMI data from men and women over 60 years of age in 10-year increments.[29] BMI, however, correlates more strongly with body fat than with lean body mass and may not be a sensitive index of muscle or body protein stores, except in the presence of emaciation.

Other anthropometric measures can determine body fat and lean body mass. Body fat can be assessed by measuring the triceps and subscapular skinfold thicknesses and at other sites.[30] Lean body mass can be estimated in women and men by measuring the mid-arm muscle circumference and by the creatinine height index. Equations that use these indexes have been developed to relate anthropometric measurements to body composition.[31] In 1989 Frisancho reported standards for the elderly 64–74 years of age[32]; the anthropometric data for European elderly over 90 years old were completed later.[33]

### *Biochemical Markers*

Use of serum laboratory values is an integral part of nutritional assessment in the adult population, although aging itself can affect test results. The most commonly used parameter, albumin, has been reported to be modified in the elderly. Albumin concentration decreases 3–9% each decade after age 70 in the community-dwelling elderly.[34,35] In these individuals the albumin loss is close to 0.8 g/L per decade,[34] and in institutionalized individuals albumin has been observed to decrease by 1.3 g/L per decade. Of course relative hypoalbuminemia may indicate poor nutritional status. Serum albumin is positively correlated with muscle mass in the elderly, and this relation may reflect shared changes with age in protein synthesis.[36] This decrease may be attributed to the decrease in skeletal muscle mass. Because of the minimal decline in albumin levels with age, hypoalbuminemia should not be ascribed solely to aging, and other causes should be considered.[1] Albumin is an important predictor of length of hospitalization, morbidity, and mortality among elderly people.[36] Severe hypoalbuminemia (<20 g/L) strongly predicts 90-day mortality and extended hospitalization in the elderly; it requires focused clinical attention regardless of the elderly patient's admitting diagnosis.[37] In the VA National Surgical Quality Improvement Program (a prospective analysis of surgical risk factors) low serum albumin was the single factor most predictive of poor postoperative outcome[38] (see Chapter 10).

Because of their shorter half-lives compared to that of albumin, prealbumin, transferrin, and retinol-binding protein are better markers for acute changes in nutritional status. The serum concentration of these proteins, especially prealbumin, are better maintained in the geriatric population.[38] Serum prealbumin protein appears to be a more sensitive marker of protein malnutrition than transferrin, although its use as a predictor of clinical outcome has yet to be determined.[38,39]

Iron stores (ferritin) usually increase with aging, which can cause circulating transferrin levels to diminish. Other conditions that may decrease transferrin levels include the anemia associated with chronic disease, acute inflammation, and chronic infection. High transferrin levels may be found with iron deficiency.

Total lymphocyte count is a nonspecific indicator of protein-energy malnutrition (PEM). An absolute lymphocyte count of less than 1500/mm$^3$ indicates malnutrition if other causes of lymphopenia can be excluded. The lymphocyte count appears to decrease in the elderly, although it remains above 1500/mm$^3$.[40]

Delayed hypersensitivity skin testing is a parameter used to assess relative immune competence. An anergic response has been linked to both increasing age and malnutrition. As yet it is unclear whether PEM-associated changes in immune competence can be distinguished from those due to aging alone. In general, anergy is a poor predictor of malnutrition in the elderly and may be less reliable than in younger patients.

Plasma IGF-I concentration is considered a valuable index of PEM in young and middle-aged adults. As mentioned previously, because IGF-I levels decrease with age, it may not be valid to extrapolate these results to the elderly. However, changes in IGF-I strongly predict the likelihood of life-threatening complications in the elderly.[41] Furthermore, in one study IGF-I was well correlated with markers of nutritional status, including: (1) serum albumin, transferrin, and cholesterol; (2) triceps skinfold thickness; and (3) percentage of ideal body weight. These changes may reflect the detrimental effects of low IGF-I concentrations. Despite these findings, the validity of IGF-I as a nutritional marker in the elderly still must be determined.

### *Functional Assessment*

Functional assessment of the elderly helps detect physical and cognitive alterations that may increase the risk of malnutrition. Nutritional well-being is related to the ability of elders to perform the activities of daily life. The BMI, used as a standard measure of overall nutrition, is related to the functional capabilities of community-dwelling elderly. Elderly individuals with a low BMI are at greater risk for functional impairment.[42] A relatively simple way to assess muscle strength is through handgrip dynamometry, which has been shown to correlate with body protein depletion and repletion.[43] Among other methods for evaluating capacity, direct measure-

# Level II Screen

Complete the following screen by interviewing the patient directly and/or by referring to the patient chart. If you do not routinely perform all of the described tests or ask all of the listed questions, please consider including them but do not be concerned if the entire screen is not completed. Please try to conduct a minimal screen on as many older patients as possible, and please try to collect serial measurements, which are extremely valuable in monitoring nutritional status. Please refer to the manual for additional information.

## Anthropometrics

Measure height to the nearest inch and weight to the nearest pound. Record the values below and mark them on the Body Mass Index (BMI) scale to the right. Then use a straight edge (paper, ruler) to connect the two points and circle the spot where this straight line crosses the center line (body mass index). Record the number below; healthy older adults should have a BMI between 22 and 27; check the appropriate box to flag an abnormally high or low value.

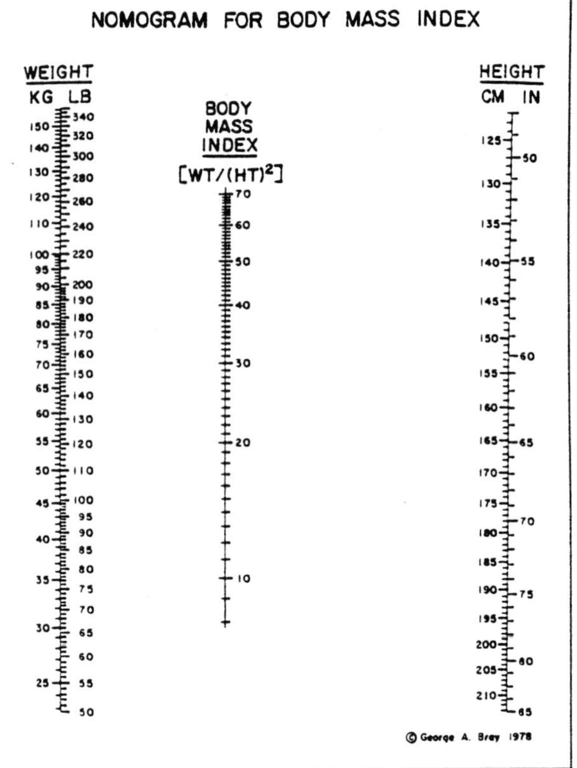


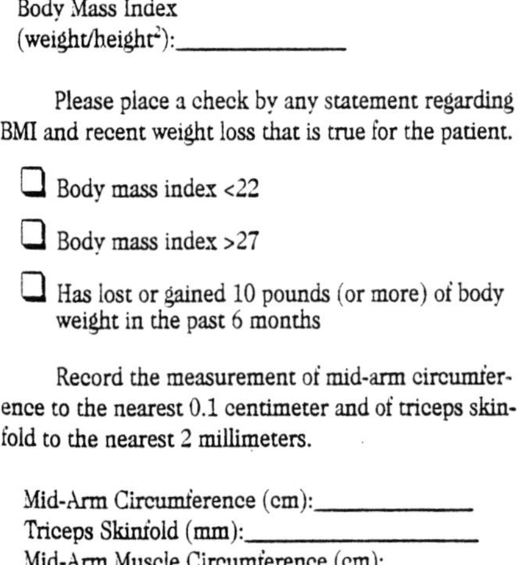

Height (in):________________
Weight (lbs):________________
Body Mass Index
(weight/height$^2$):______________

Please place a check by any statement regarding BMI and recent weight loss that is true for the patient.

- ❑ Body mass index <22
- ❑ Body mass index >27
- ❑ Has lost or gained 10 pounds (or more) of body weight in the past 6 months

Record the measurement of mid-arm circumference to the nearest 0.1 centimeter and of triceps skinfold to the nearest 2 millimeters.

Mid-Arm Circumference (cm):____________
Triceps Skinfold (mm):________________
Mid-Arm Muscle Circumference (cm):_______

Refer to the table and check any abnormal values:

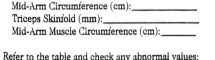

- ❑ Mid-arm muscle circumference <10th percentile
- ❑ Triceps skinfold <10th percentile
- ❑ Triceps skinfold >95th percentile

*Note:* mid-arm circumference (cm) - {0.314 x triceps skinfold (mm)}= mid-arm *muscle* circumference (cm)

For the remaining sections, please place a check by any statements that are true for the patient.

## Laboratory Data

- ❑ Serum albumin below 3.5 g/dl
- ❑ Serum cholesterol below 160 mg/dl
- ❑ Serum cholesterol above 240 mg/dl

## Drug Use

- ❑ Three or more prescription drugs, OTC medications, and/or vitamin/mineral supplements daily

**LEVEL II SCREEN**

**Name:**

**Date:**

FIGURE 5.2. Nomogram for body mass index. (From the Nutrition Screening Initiative, a project of the American Academy of Family Physicians, the American Dietetic Association, and the National Council on the Aging, with permission. Funded in part by a grant from Ross Products Division, Abbott Laboratories.)

ments of neuromuscular performance, including muscle strength, balance, and gait speed, are strongly related to disability.[44] In addition, many evaluation scales for cognitive and physical assessment that vary in simplicity have been developed.[45] A poor performance score on these tests should be carefully evaluated because deficits may result from malnutrition or may render the patient susceptible to malnutrition.

Other techniques that can be used to assess nutritional status mainly evaluate body composition. Among them are bioelectric impedance, dual x-ray absorptiometry scanning, computed tomography, and magnetic reso-

### Clinical Features

Presence of (check each that apply):

- ❑ Problems with mouth, teeth, or gums
- ❑ Difficulty chewing
- ❑ Difficulty swallowing
- ❑ Angular stomatitis
- ❑ Glossitis
- ❑ History of bone pain
- ❑ History of bone fractures
- ❑ Skin changes (dry, loose, nonspecific lesions, edema)

| | Men | | Women | |
|---|---|---|---|---|
| Percentile | 55-65 y | 65-75 y | 55-65 y | 65-75 y |
| *Arm circumference (cm)* | | | | |
| 10th | 27.3 | 26.3 | 25.7 | 25.2 |
| 50th | 31.7 | 30.7 | 30.3 | 29.9 |
| 95th | 36.9 | 35.5 | 38.5 | 37.3 |
| *Arm muscle circumference (cm)* | | | | |
| 10th | 24.5 | 23.5 | 19.6 | 19.5 |
| 50th | 27.8 | 26.8 | 22.5 | 22.5 |
| 95th | 32.0 | 30.6 | 28.0 | 27.9 |
| *Triceps skinfold (mm)* | | | | |
| 10th | 6 | 6 | 16 | 14 |
| 50th | 11 | 11 | 25 | 24 |
| 95th | 22 | 22 | 38 | 36 |

*From: Frisancho AR. New norms of upper limb fat and muscle areas for assessment of nutritional status. Am J Clin Nutr 1981; 34:2540-2545. © 1981 American Society for Clinical Nutrition.*

### Eating Habits

- ❑ Does not have enough food to eat each day
- ❑ Usually eats alone
- ❑ Does not eat anything on one or more days each month
- ❑ Has poor appetite
- ❑ Is on a special diet
- ❑ Eats vegetables two or fewer times daily
- ❑ Eats milk or milk products once or not at all daily
- ❑ Eats fruit or drinks fruit juice once or not at all daily
- ❑ Eats breads, cereals, pasta, rice, or other grains five or fewer times daily
- ❑ Has more than one alcoholic drink per day (if woman); more than two drinks per day (if man)

### Living Environment

- ❑ Lives on an income of less than $6000 per year (per individual in the household)
- ❑ Lives alone
- ❑ Is housebound
- ❑ Is concerned about home security
- ❑ Lives in a home with inadequate heating or cooling
- ❑ Does not have a stove and/or refrigerator
- ❑ Is unable or prefers not to spend money on food (<$25-30 per person spent on food each week)

### Functional Status

Usually or always needs assistance with (check each that apply):

- ❑ Bathing
- ❑ Dressing
- ❑ Grooming
- ❑ Toileting
- ❑ Eating
- ❑ Walking or moving about
- ❑ Traveling (outside the home)
- ❑ Preparing food
- ❑ Shopping for food or other necessities

### Mental/Cognitive Status

- ❑ Clinical evidence of impairment, e.g. Folstein<26
- ❑ Clinical evidence of depressive illness, e.g. Beck Depression Inventory>15, Geriatric Depression Scale>5

Patients in whom you have identified one or more major indicator (see pg 2) of poor nutritional status require immediate medical attention; if minor indicators are found, ensure that they are known to a health professional or to the patient's own physician. Patients who display risk factors (see pg 2) of poor nutritional status should be referred to the appropriate health care or social service professional (dietitian, nurse, dentist, case manager, etc.).

FIGURE 5.2. *Continued*

nance imaging. In general, these techniques are not useful for routine clinical evaluation.

## Nutritional Requirements of the Elderly

### *Fluid Requirements*

Dehydration is one of the main discharge diagnoses in patients over age 65.[46] Inadequate intake is one of the most common reasons for water and electrolyte disorders in this age group. Possible explanations include a decrease in the thirst sensation with increasing age. Age-related decreases in vasopressin secretion and an alteration in the opioid system may also impair fluid regulation.[47] Renal function decreases with age, as does the kidney's capacity to adapt to changes in hydration status and electrolyte intake, thereby interfering with regulatory mechanisms. Stress and infection are often associated with decreased fluid intake and dehydration. Fluid losses may be further increased by fever, vomiting, diarrhea, fistulas, and open surgical wounds; and they should be accounted for. In addition, fluid intake may be restricted owing to chronic renal insufficiency or congestive heart failure. The above factors predispose the elderly patient to dehydration and fluid overload. Thus a more gradual approach to fluid delivery is appropriate. It is essential to monitor fluid intake and output carefully in the elderly on a continuous basis.

Various formulas can be used to predict baseline fluid requirements, although some formulas do not account for obesity and low body weight and may give unrealistic estimates.[48] The following formula is appropriate for establishing fluid recommendations, as it adjusts for height and weight: 100ml fluid/kg for the first 10kg of body weight, 50ml/kg for the next 10kg of body weight, and 15ml/kg for the remaining kilograms of body weight. A goal of at least 1500–2000ml fluid is recommended. Given the reduced volume of formula required to meet the decreasing energy needs of the elderly, patients receiving tube feeding may need additional fluid to maintain adequate hydration.[1]

### Energy Requirements

Several formulas are available to estimate energy requirements of the elderly. The Harris and Benedict equations (HBEs), which take into consideration sex, age, height, and weight, can be used to estimate the resting energy expenditure (REE).

$$\text{Men} = 66.47 + [13.75 \times W\,(\text{kg})] + [5.0 \times H\,(\text{cm})] - [6.76 \times A\,(\text{years})]$$

$$\text{Women} = 66.51 + [9.6 \times W\,(\text{kg})] + [1.85 \times H\,(\text{cm})] - [4.68 \times A\,(\text{years})]$$

where $W$ = weight, $H$ = height, and $A$ = age. The REE obtained is expressed in kilocalories per day. Unfortunately, the HBEs are performed poorly in some instances, and they can underestimate the actual REE in malnourished and critically ill patients.[49] The same is true in undernourished nursing home residents.[50] In these instances, direct measurement of REE is more appropriate. Height is often difficult to obtain, and for this reason the World Health Organization (WHO) formulas may be preferable. For patients 60–80 years of age, the formulas are as follows.

$$\text{Men} = 8.8\,(W) + 1128\,(H) - 1071$$

$$\text{Women} = 9.2(W) + 637\,(H) - 302$$

WHO formulas should not be used to predict the REE for patients older than 80 years.[51] REE can also be predicted without height with only a minor loss of accuracy.[1]

$$\text{Men} = 13.5\,(W) + 487$$

$$\text{Women} = 10.5(W) + 596$$

A correction factor should be added to the REE depending on the degree of metabolic stress of the patient (Table 5.2). The REE can be assessed directly using indirect calorimetry. Indirect calorimetry provides reliable estimates of REE and can be performed at the patient's bedside. However, its use is not necessary in every patient because the use of predictive equations is usually satisfactory.[3] Judgment should always be exercised if a caloric level appears to overestimate needs. The doubly labeled water method measures total energy expenditure over a period of several days. It eliminates the need to add correcting factors and can be used to obtain data for free-living individuals. Unfortunately, because of its technical limitations it is not suitable for acutely ill patients.

Table 5.2. Adjustment Factors for Resting Energy Expenditure

| Correction factor | Stress |
|---|---|
| 1.0–1.1 | Postoperative |
| 1.1–1.3 | Multiple fractures |
| 1.2–1.5 | Weight gain/replenishment |
| 1.3–1.6 | Severe infection/bullet wounds |
| 1.6 | Sepsis |
| 1.5–2.1 | Third-degree burns |
| 1.2 | Confined to bed |
| 1.3 | Out of bed |
| 1.5 | Active |

*Source:* Data from Nelson and Franzi,[8] with permission.

Current recommendations for energy requirements in the elderly are based on assumed levels of physical activity relative to the basal metabolic rate (BMR). However, substantial error is found when total energy expenditure is derived from measurements or predictions of BMR.[52] Furthermore, current recommended daily allowances (RDAs) may significantly underestimate the energy requirements for physical activity in healthy elderly persons.[19] Accurate estimation of energy needs is important for delivering adequate nutritional care and preventing disability. Human aging has been associated with reduced ability to regulate energy balance. This might explain the vulnerability of older persons to unexplained weight gain and weight loss.[53] Thus in some older individuals, successful weight maintenance may require increased control over food intake and energy requirements.

### Protein Requirements

Studies of nitrogen metabolism in healthy elderly populations have shown that under basal conditions nitrogen balance is achieved with a protein intake of 0.8g/kg/day, which is the current RDA, although a recent reevaluation indicated a safe level of intake for most elderly people of 1.0g/kg/day.[50,54] A 24-hour urine urea nitrogen (UUN) can determine the amount of total nitrogen excreted and can be used to estimate protein requirements. The following formula accounts for insensible and fecal losses and can be used to estimate total nitrogen loss.

$$\text{Total nitrogen loss} = 24\text{ h UNN (g/day)} + (0.20 \times 24\text{ UNN}) + 2\text{ g/day}$$

$$\text{Nitrogen (N) balance} = \text{N intake} - [\text{urine N} + \text{stool N} + \text{insensible N losses}]$$

Generally a positive nitrogen balance of 4–6g is necessary for anabolism. During the metabolic response to trauma proteins are broken down to amino acids and are used for hepatic gluconeogenesis. The decrease in lean body mass that occurs with aging reduces tissue protein reserves and may diminish the body's capacity to resynthesize proteins. Whether the provision of adequate stores of protein and calories for the acutely ill elderly results in decreased protein breakdown under catabolic stress remains unanswered. However, excluding burn patients, it seems prudent that during periods of stress such as infection surgical trauma, or cancer the daily protein intake should be increased to 1.0–1.5g/kg/day.[7]

### *Vitamin Requirements*

As we have discussed, it is a combination of physical, social, and psychological factors that make the elderly population particularly susceptible to malnutrition. Aging alone might be accompanied by a decrease in some vitamin levels. These modifications may lead to an increased risk of vitamin deficiencies and disease. In the following sections we review the most important vitamins and the role their supplementation may play in the nutritional status of aged individuals.

#### Vitamin A

Special consideration should be given to vitamin A supplementation in elderly subjects. In contrast to other vitamin levels, serum concentrations of vitamin A are usually within the normal range in the elderly. The liver has a great capacity to store vitamin A, and hepatocellular levels of vitamin A are maintained throughout life. In addition, old individuals have an increased capacity to absorb vitamin A, and they have decreased renal excretion. Thus oversupplementation could predispose the elderly to vitamin A toxicity.[55] Increased vitamin A intake by the elderly can raise serum retinyl ester concentrations, which are an index of vitamin A overload. Elderly subjects with elevated fasting plasma retinyl esters were shown to have elevated liver function tests, indicative of liver damage. In view of the above findings, the current RDA for vitamin A of 5000IU for men and 4000IU for women may be too high for the elderly and should probably be reduced.[56]

#### Vitamin $B_6$

Vitamin $B_6$ appears to play an important role in the regulation of homocysteine metabolism. Vitamin $B_6$ plasma concentrations inversely correlate with homocysteine concentrations, and elevated levels of homocysteine are associated with the development of occlusive vascular disease.[57] In addition, plasma pyridoxal-5′-phosphate (the coenzyme of vitamin $B_6$) concentrations have been linked to stenosis.[58] At this time, it cannot be concluded that lowering plasma homocysteine by increasing vitamin intake reduces the risk of vascular disease. It is not uncommon to encounter low vitamin $B_6$ plasma levels among the elderly, so it is probable that vitamin $B_6$ requirements are insufficient.[58,59] Considering the above findings, a vitamin $B_6$ intake of 1.9–2.0mg/day is adequate.

#### Vitamin $B_{12}$

Serum vitamin $B_{12}$ levels decline with advancing age. Prevalence of vitamin $B_{12}$ deficiency varies among countries, from none in the United Kingdom up to 7.3% in the rest of Europe.[60] In the United States the prevalence of vitamin $B_{12}$ deficiency was shown to be more than 12% in a large sample of free-living elderly. By measuring serum homocysteine, a vitamin $B_{12}$ metabolite, many elderly people with normal serum vitamin concentrations were found to be metabolically deficient in cobalamin.[61] The reasons for the high prevalence of vitamin $B_{12}$ deficiency have not been established. Dietary vitamin $B_{12}$ deficiency is probably a major etiologic factor. The vitamin $B_{12}$ levels may also be affected by the high prevalence of atrophic gastritis (a partial decrease in fundic glands and of parietal cell mass) in the elderly population. There is a significant association between age and the prevalence of atrophic gastritis, which is as high as 24% after age 60 and 37% after age 80.[62] In addition, gastric and intestinal bacterial overgrowth may contribute to vitamin $B_{12}$ malabsorption.

In view of these findings, the current RDA may underestimate the need for vitamin $B_{12}$ in the elderly. Some authors have suggested that the RDA should be increased to 3.0μg/day and that serum cutoffs for vitamin $B_{12}$ deficiency should be raised to 258pmol/L.[63] Clinically, the hematologic changes typical of megaloblastic anemia can be absent in most subjects with evidence of deficiency.

Neuropsychiatric symptoms of vitamin $B_{12}$ deficiency may be present even with normal serum levels of vitamin $B_{12}$. Any elderly patient who is, or is suspected to be, vitamin $B_{12}$-deficient, based on the neurologic symptoms of vitamin $B_{12}$ deficiency, should receive a course of parenteral vitamin $B_{12}$ to replete stores.[1] Once the etiology of the deficiency is determined, appropriate maintenance therapy can be initiated.

#### Calcium and Vitamin D

With aging, serum vitamin D levels decline as a result of less efficient synthesis of vitamin D by the skin, less efficient intestinal absorption, and possibly reduced sun exposure and intake of vitamin D.[64] Sun exposure is essential for maintaining vitamin D levels. Home-bound or institutionalized elderly who do not receive enough sun are at particular risk of vitamin D deficiency.[65] Note that exposure of skin to sunlight that has passed through windowpane glass or Plexiglas does not produce cholecalciferol.[66] Sunscreen use and dark skin pigmentation can also substantially influence cutaneous production of vitamin D. Latitude influences the amount of vitamin D as well. In northern latitudes and during winter ultraviolet B rays do not reach the earth's surface. People in these regions are entirely dependent on dietary sources of vitamin D during this season. In the United States the major dietary source of vitamin D is milk. Elderly individuals with lactose intolerance may avoid milk products that contain vitamin D and may be dependent on endogenous synthesis of this vitamin.

Intestinal calcium absorption is independently reduced with age and after menopause as estrogen levels decrease.[67] This might be due to age-related changes in the metabolism of vitamin D. Although antifracture efficacy is of primary interest, change in bone mineral density (BMD) is widely used in clinical trials because it is a strong predictor of fracture risk; with its use, a far smaller number of patients are required for a study.[66] Data have shown that calcium supplements significantly reduce bone mineral loss and increase bone density. In addition, calcium combined with vitamin D supplements have reduced hip and other nonvertebral fracture rates in nursing home residents.[68] However, vitamin D supplements alone do not decrease the incidence of hip fractures, which suggests that only the combination of calcium and vitamin D is beneficial.[69] The current vitamin D RDA of 200 IU may not be sufficient to minimize bone loss. An intake of 400–800 IU/day appears to be needed for healthy postmenopausal women.[1,60,70] Calcium intakes of 1000 mg/day for postmenopauseal women taking estrogen and 1500 mg/day for women not taking estrogen are now considered optimal by many.[50,59,66] Calcium intake should not exceed 2400 mg/day, because of the risk of nephrolithiasis.[1]

### Nutrient Supplementation

Nutritional supplementation is useful in some instances. The consumption of a varied diet that includes foods from each of the major food groups should supply all of the essential nutrients in the recommended amounts. However, as discussed previously, nutrient insufficiencies resulting from impaired absorption and poor diets are commonly found in the elderly.

Adequate intakes of protein and energy may be ensured with the use of energy-dense foods or with nutritional supplements. The effect of a simple dietary intervention such as provision of a protein-energy supplement can increase the overall protein intake by as much as 60% and decrease morbidity of elderly patients with femoral fractures.[7] Supplement use is associated with weight gain in many nursing home patients and may improve their nutritional parameters.[71] In addition, daily vitamin and trace element supplementation may decrease the risk of infection in elderly subjects.[72] However, nutrient supplementation should not be provided routinely, as it may lead to clinically relevant vitamin toxicities.[73] In addition, the protective effects of supplementary vitamin intake on specific disease processes (i.e., vitamin E and β-carotene on lung cancer) have not yet been validated. Recommendations about supplementation with vitamin E and β-carotene might be premature.[74] Despite this reservation, early intervention to provide adequate energy and protein is likely to be beneficial.

Nutrient supplementation should always be guided by nutritional and clinical goals, and vitamin supplement prescription should be based on sound data and a judicious clinical assessment. More organized nutritional assessment protocols must be developed to determine who will benefit from nutritional supplementation, especially among the institutionalized population.[71]

## Wound Healing in the Elderly

Wound healing has been studied for a long time. The first publication that addressed this issue dates as far back as 1916. Many papers have since discussed this matter, but the issues remain controversial. The first major studies, done three decades ago, reported an increase in the incidence of wound dehiscence after laparotomy in old men.[75,76] Likewise, the incidence of anastomotic complications was reported to increase with age.[77,78] However, faulty studies have made it difficult to reach definite conclusions regarding poor wound healing in the elderly.

Wound healing is a continuous, complex process in which the various mechanisms involved are difficult to separate into clear stages. Knowledge of the particular events that occur during wound healing is important for understanding the overall process of healing and the effects that normal aging has on it.

### Physiology of Wound Healing

From the moment of injury, the body responds with a series of complex interactions that culminate in the restoration of integrity. Under normal conditions healing can be divided into four specific stages: coagulation, inflammation, fibroplasia, and remodeling. Although described in a sequential fashion, healing is an active, dynamic process that proceeds through a series of mechanisms that are often redundant and simultaneous.

#### *Coagulation*

Coagulation initiates the cascade that leads to healing. Injury disrupts tissue and cells and induces local hemorrhage. Vasoconstriction occurs almost immediately as a response to catecholamine release to limit blood loss. Tissue destruction induces mast cells to release various vasoactive compounds including bradykinin, serotonin, and histamine, which initiate the process of diapedesis. Platelets from the hemorrhage help form the hemostatic plug. They also release clotting factors that produce fibrin and form the fibrin mesh, onto which inflammatory cells migrate. Fibrin deposition is followed by fibrinolysis and release of chemoattractive peptides, particularly fibrinopeptide E, which attracts monocytes, and fibrinopeptide B, which is angiogenic. In addition, platelet degranulation releases platelet-derived growth factor (PDGF), platelet factor IV, transforming growth factor 1 (TGF-1), and IGF-I, all of which stimulate fibroblast replication. Platelets are important because they are the first to produce several essential cytokines thought to modulate many subsequent wound healing events.[80,81]

### *Inflammation*

The inflammation stage is characterized by an increased migration of mast cells, polymorphonuclear leukocytes (PMNs), and lymphocytes into the wound. Within 24 hours of injury, PMNs predominantly populate the wound area. Their role is more important for antibacterial defense than for repair. These cells are progressively replaced by macrophages, which are predominant by 48 hours after injury. Macrophages stimulate replication and movement of fibroblasts and vascular endothelial cells, which in turn regulate repair of the connective tissue. In addition, when stimulated by injured tissue, fibrin, foreign bodies, low oxygen, and high lactate concentrations, macrophages release a number of cytokines and growth factors. Among them, IL-1, IL-6, IL-8, tumor necrosis factor-$\alpha$ (TNF-$\alpha$), transforming growth factor-$\beta$ (TGF-$\beta$), IGF-I, and fibroblast growth factor-like molecules (LDGF) have been traced to macrophages. These factors regulate the cell growth and chemotaxis of inflammatory cells, new fibroblasts, and endothelial cells. Inflammation is aggravated by the release of free radicals. The damaging effect of free radicals is enhanced by reactive hyperemia.

### *Fibroplasia*

Fibroplasia is the stage where wound strength increases and integrity is restored. Fibroblasts originate locally, and replication rates are proportional to oxygen availability. By 72 hours fibroblasts migrate into the wound and synthesize collagen and proteoglycans. The latter are important extracellular compounds that stabilize and support cells and fibrous components of tissue. Collagen synthesis increases by 10 hours after injury, reaches a peak between 5 and 7 days, and then gradually decreases. The collagen during the first days following injury is comprised of large amounts of type III collagen but relatively little type I collagen. Collagen III provides strength during the late phase of wound healing by cross-linking. Vitamin C plays an important role in this process.

Production of ground substance in the matrix increases, and vessels proliferate. Neovascularization occurs along the steep oxygen gradient that characterizes wounds. Regrowth of sympathetic nerve fibers is associated with angiogenesis. Along with invading fibroblasts, fibronectin appears and promotes cell adhesion and phagocytosis, and it may be involved in matrix remodeling. Fibrinogen, laminin, and fibronectin constitute a framework from which new vessels can form and reepithelialization can occur. Reepithelialization is a complex phenomenon in which resting $G_0$ cells (cells in the inactive phase of mitosis) are recruited from the margins of the wound, followed by migration of epidermal cells. This process is essential for reconstitution of cutaneous barrier function.[82] It has been suggested that as the wound epithelializes, inflammation is downregulated owing to the presence of apoptotic cells at the advancing epithelial wound edge.[83]

### *Remodeling*

Remodeling is an extensive phase during which collagen is produced and remodeled, neovascularization regresses, and a mature scar is formed. Equilibrium is reached between collagen formation and destruction by collagenases, and the type III/type I collagen ratio decreases. Acute and chronic inflammatory cells gradually diminish, and fibroplasia ends. Fibronectin is removed within a few weeks.[84]

Fibroblasts reach their peak production of ground substance after 3 days; collagen concentration is maximal after 9 days; and the tensile strength of collagen reaches a maximum after 10–15 days. The first migration of epithelial cells has been observed 6–48 hours following an injury, and epidermal proliferation reaches maximum values at 12–48 hours.[7]

## Aging and Wound Healing

### *Inflammation*

There are specific age alterations in the coagulation and immune systems that can influence wound healing. Platelet and macrophage adhesion to substrates within the wound increases while macrophage function declines.[9] Old mice display a slower wound healing rate than young mice. Furthermore, wound healing is accelerated when macrophages from young mice are added locally to wounds of old mice. It is possible that the migratory capacity or some other macrophage function is affected by age, and the correction of such dysfunction might stimulate wound healing.[7,85] In accordance with the above reports, Ashcroft et al. observed a similar phenomenon. At 7 days after injury wounds of young animals consisted of mature granulation tissue and scattered inflammatory cells, whereas the wounds of middle-aged and old mice showed persistent inflammation and immature granulation tissue.[86]

T cell-mediated immune function also deteriorates during aging. There is a loss of T cell proliferative capacity, a decline in the synthesis and release of IL-2, and a decrease in IL-2 receptor expression. A major factor responsible for the loss of T cell function is an inability of the T cell to respond to activation signals transmitted through the membrane binding of specific stimulatory signals.[87] An IL-2 deficit alone cannot explain these effects because exogenous administration of IL-2 does not completely restore the decreased T cell proliferative response of the elderly.[88] A defect in IL-2 receptor expression or function may exist. In addition to IL-2, T cells have an increased ability to produce interferon-γ (IFN-γ), IL-4, IL-6, and TGF.[12,13] Aging is associated with a decrease in cytotoxic lymphocyte activity and a reduction in lytic capacity. A significant portion of the age-related decline in $CD8^+$ T cell-mediated cytotoxic activity is secondary to age-related alterations in the $CD4^+$ T cell subset. The well-documented diminution in IL-2 production with age may contribute to the defect seen in the $CD4^-$ cells[89] (see Chapter 4).

### Proliferation

Cell proliferation is affected by aging in a number of ways. Fibroblast migration in vitro is reduced, but the number of cells within an acute wound is not altered. Fibroblast proliferation declines as well. It seems that the mitogenic and stimulatory effects of growth factors, hormones, and other agents are significantly reduced during aging.[90] A loss of responsiveness in vitro to specific stimulatory cytokines also occurs, with no changes in response to inhibitors.[91] In addition, fibroblast cultures from premature aging syndromes such as Werner syndrome, show a significantly reduced mitogenic response to PDGF, fibroblast growth factor (FGF), and serum.[92] Nevertheless, these changes may occur only between youth and middle age. Production of cytokines is also altered with age. It is known that IL-1 increases, possibly affecting matrix remodeling, and PDGF decreases.[9]

There is general agreement that epidermal behavior in elderly subjects differs from that of young subjects. It has been found that reepithelialization is delayed in wounds of old mice.[11] The rate of epithelialization of open wounds is slowed in elderly patients compared to that in young individuals.[93,94] Moreover, in vitro studies have revealed a decline in keratinocyte responsiveness to stimulatory cytokines, an increased response to inhibitory cytokines, and a decline in IL-1 production in elderly patients.[9] This physiologic delay, when coupled with other factors that impair epithelial repair, may result in significant healing problems in the elderly.[18]

A few studies have described changes in angiogenesis during aging. Elements of the microvasculature in young rats are periodic acid-Schiff (PAS)-negative and become increasingly PAS-positive beyond the halfway life-span. This observation reflects an increase in the carbohydrate content of blood vessels with aging. During acute wound repair in old animals the microvasculature is PAS-negative after injury and intensely PAS-positive after 8 weeks, reproducing the process of aging in an accelerated manner.[95]

Aged endothelium may exhibit an increased adhesive response to leukocytes and an increased response and adhesion to TNF-α. Furthermore, IL-1 production is increased, and endothelial cell proliferation subsequently declines but vascular smooth muscle cell proliferation increases.[9] Despite a general consensus that aged endothelium has reduced the proliferative potential, an increased number of new vessels has been observed in mice and warrants further investigation.[11] Angiogenesis may itself influence the direction of fibroplasia. Orientation of vessels in wounds of aged mice may induce complex fibroblast (and subsequently collagen) orientation.

### Remodeling and Collagen Deposition

The structure of the extracellular matrix differs according to age. Aging is associated with significantly reduced levels of wound matrix constituents, including collagen, basement membrane components, glycosaminoglycans, and fibronectin.[11]

It is assumed that anastomotic strength and collagen metabolism is primarily determined by assessing collagen synthesis and content.[95] Collagen metabolism also seems to be altered by aging, although animal studies have reported conflicting findings and no general agreement has been reached.[11,97,98] Studies in healthy elderly individuals have concluded that age does not seem to have any effect on the collagen wound content.[18] Unfortunately, there is a paucity of information regarding collagen metabolism in humans, making it difficult to reach a conclusion with respect to collagen metabolism and aging.

Wound strength is an important property that has been reported to change with age. Tensile strength of the skin is positively correlated with collagen fiber diameter. During normal wound healing the tensile strength of wounds increases with time despite a decrease in the rate of collagen synthesis. The breaking strength of wounds in old animals has been found to be lower than that of young animals.[99,100] This difference has been hypothesized to be due to a less organized collagen fiber arrangement.[101] Tensile strength and energy absorption of abdominal incisional wounds are lower in old rats than in young rats by the fourth postoperative day.[22] In this same study age was found to have no influence on the healing of colonic anastomoses. Breaking strength remained unchanged in the older animals despite a higher collagen content in old rats. In a later study Stoop et al. also supported these findings. Breaking strength and bursting pressure of colonic anastomoses were unchanged in older rats despite a decrease in collagen production capacity.[102]

If wound healing is in fact impaired in the elderly, collagen might not be the only element involved in this phenomenon. A defect in the synthesis of noncollagenous proteins such as glycosaminoglycans, laminin, enzymes, and cytokines may affect the mechanical properties of wounds in the elderly.

Although various components of wound healing are impaired in the elderly, wound healing as a whole is essentially normal or slightly slower, provided no preexisting systemic or regional diseases complicate the recovery process.[7] It is likely that the vulnerability of the healing process in the elderly becomes evident only in the presence of certain conditions that exert their own, negative influence on wound repair.[103]

## Factors Affecting Wound Healing in the Elderly

A number of systemic and local factors can adversely affect wound healing in the elderly. Careful clinical evaluation of the patient can reveal the presence of disease processes that require intervention.

### *Nutrition*

As alluded to earlier, malnutrition is common in the elderly and has been associated with impaired wound healing in this age group.[104] Animal studies have helped us understand this relation. A commonly encountered degree of malnutrition, insufficient to affect nutritional indices used for clinical assessment, may interfere with colonic healing. Early reintroduction of nutrition during the postoperative period may be able to reverse this effect.[105] Daly et al. showed that rats deprived of protein for only 1 week exhibited a 17% reduction in mean bursting strength of colonic anastomoses compared to that of controls. They also observed a correlation between serum albumin and bursting strength with prolonged malnutrition.[106] These studies were later confirmed by Irving, who showed that severe protein deprivation reduced the breaking strength of abdominal wall wounds. A less pronounced effect was seen in colonic anastomoses. In this study, nutritional supplementation was associated with improved wound healing only in wounds severely affected by malnutrition.[107]

In humans the wound healing response has been assessed by measuring the collagen content (hydroxyproline) of subcutaneously inserted Gore-Tex tubes. In this respect, a delay in the wound healing response is also seen in malnourished elderly surgical patients; but contrary to what happens in animals, it occurs even with mild degrees of protein-calorie malnutrition.[108] In addition, low serum levels of nutritional markers such as albumin and transferrin correlate with a high incidence of wound complications in elderly patients undergoing vascular operations.[109]

The wound healing response, measured by hydroxyproline accumulation, is improved by intravenous nutrition in surgical patients. This improvement is seen after only 1 week of nutritional therapy and before indices of nutritional status are significantly changed.[110] However, preoperative food intake seems to have more influence on wound healing than acute losses of body protein and fat.[111] Accordingly, a review on nutrition support concluded that preoperative parenteral nutrition decreases postoperative complications by approximately 10% in moderately malnourished individuals.[112] To date, there is general agreement that malnutrition has a deleterious effect on wound healing. These negative effects can be diminished by providing optimal nutritional care.

### *Hypoxia and Hypoperfusion*

Local tissue perfusion and oxygenation are key elements in wound healing. Unfortunately, the elderly experience a progressive decline in health and are more prone to develop diseases that compromise tissue perfusion. Diabetes, arteriosclerosis, venous insufficiency, and cardiac failure are among the major diseases that can affect local oxygen delivery. It is even possible that a substantial portion of surgical patients are hypoperfused.[113] Healing of ischemic wounds in old animals is impaired by 40–65% (wound shrinkage) compared to similar wounds in young animals.[114] Tissues from older animals are less tolerant to ischemia with increasing age. Consequently, elderly patients may benefit if ischemia time is limited during surgical procedures.[115]

Collagen synthesis requires oxygen as a cofactor, especially during hydroxylation of proline. Oxygen tensions in surgical wounds are often below what is desirable.[116] Perfusion during the first postoperative days seems to be crucial for collagen accumulation. In fact, collagen deposition is directly proportional to wound oxygen tension and other measurements of perfusion[79] (Fig. 5.3). Interestingly, moderate anemia does not influence collagen deposition. Thus replacing fluid postoperatively based on the results of tissue oxygen tension measurements rather than clinical criteria may improve the overall wound healing response[116] (Fig. 5.4).

### *Infections*

Clinically, local wound infection represents the most frequent cause of defective wound healing. The mere presence of organisms in a wound is less important than the level of bacterial growth. Experimental data have shown

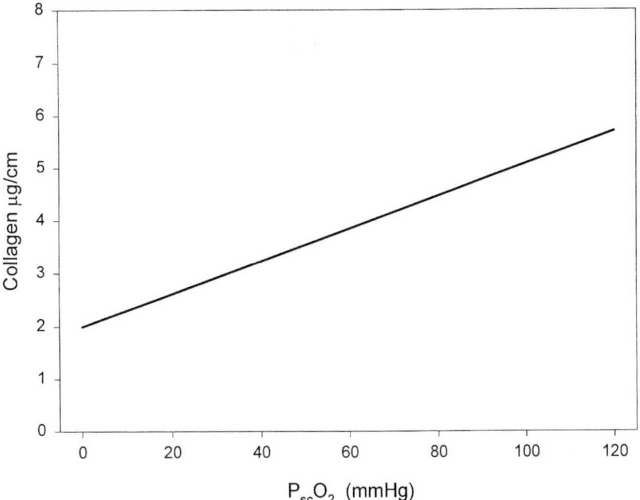


FIGURE 5.3. Relation between collagen accumulation and wound oxygen tension ($P_{sc}O_2$) 5 days after injury. (Modified from Jonsson et al.,[79] with permission.)

that bacterial growth of more than 100,000 organisms per gram of tissue is necessary to delay or inhibit wound healing. Generalized infections such as sepsis can also affect wound healing. The presence of fibrinopurulent exudate in the anastomotic space prevents fibroplasia, angiogenesis, and consequently primary anastomoses after a bowel resection.[117] In addition systemic sepsis, without intraabdominal bacterial infection, significantly alters collagen metabolism in colonic anastomoses. Collagen synthesis is reduced at both the transcriptional and protein levels with resultant impairment of anastomotic healing. Ultimately, this is reflected in a reduction in anastomotic bursting pressure.[118]

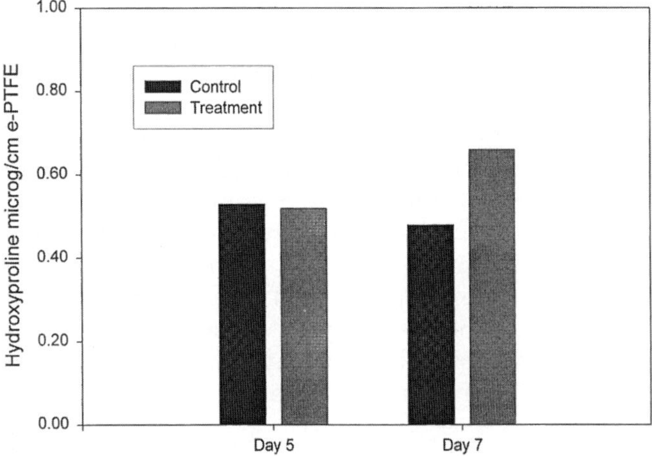


FIGURE 5.4. Effect of optimizing postoperative fluid replacement, according to $P_{sc}O_2$ measurements, on hydroxyproline accumulation 5 and 7 days after abdominal surgery. e-PTFE, expanded polytetrafluoroethylene. (From Hartmann et al.,[116] with permission.)

## Drugs

The major effect of steroids is to inhibit the inflammatory phase of wound healing. The stronger the antiinflammatory effect of the steroid used, the greater is the inhibitory effect on wound healing. Large doses of steroid hormones reduce collagen synthesis and wound strength.[119] Dexamethasone increases the frequency of anastomotic rupture at 5 days postoperatively.[120] In addition, long-term perioperative steroids have a deleterious effect on colonic anastomoses and skin healing.[121,122] Short-term high preoperative and postoperative steroid therapy does not decrease the strength of the anastomoses as measured by bursting pressure. Treatment with a single preoperative high dose of methylprednisolone may improve pulmonary function and reduce the inflammatory response without having a detrimental effect on collagen accumulation in the wound.[123]

Cancer therapies have long been known to affect wound healing adversely. Chemotherapeutic antimetabolite drugs inhibit early cell proliferation, which is crucial to the onset of successful wound repair. Radiation therapy also has unwanted effects, as it can induce fibrosis, strictures, and ischemia in adjacent tissues. It can also generate an early decrease in seromuscular blood flow in colorectal anastomoses, although single preoperative doses may not compromise healing.[44]

Other drugs may also have unexpected adverse effects on wound healing. Octreotide, a somatostatin analogue commonly used in surgical patients, has been shown to decrease wound breaking strength in experimental animals; these effects are comparable in magnitude to those caused by steroids.[124]

## Diabetes

Diabetes has been shown to impair wound healing and increase the potential for infection. Cruse and Foord demonstrated that diabetics have five times the risk of infection in a clean surgical wound compared to nondiabetics. Obesity, insulin resistance, and hyperglycemia all contribute significantly and independently to the wound impairment observed in diabetics.[125,126] In experimental animals, insulin restores collagen synthesis and granulation tissue formation to normal levels if given during the early phases of healing.[127,128] However, this is not the case in phenotypically obese mice. In humans with juvenile-onset diabetes, insulin treatment ensures normal wound collagen accumulation.[129] Specific phases of wound healing involving collagen metabolism and cellular proliferation as well as chemotactic, phagocytic, and adherence properties of neutrophils have been shown to improve with insulin administration or lowering of the blood glucose level below 200 mg/dl.[6] Careful preoperative correction of blood glucose levels can improve outcome of wounds in diabetic patients.[130]

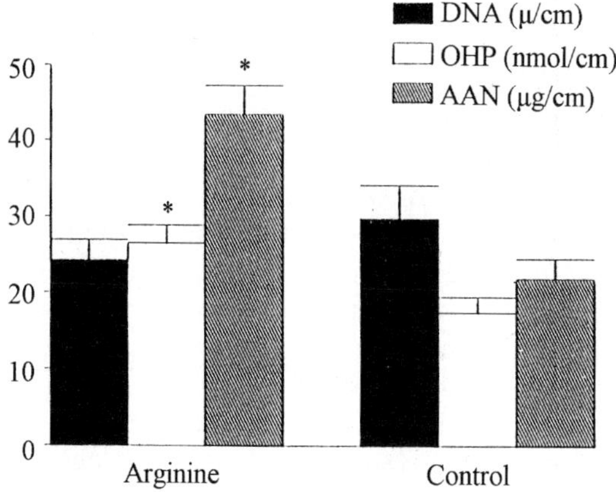


FIGURE 5.5. Arginine supplementation increased the amount of wound collagen deposition, as reflected by cathether hydroxyproline (OHP), and total protein content, as assessed by α-amino nitrogen (AAN). DNA did not change. *$p < 0.05$ vs. controls. (From Kirk et al.,[149] with permission.)

## Therapeutic Approaches

### *Growth Factors*

In wound healing studies, growth hormone (GH) has been shown to increase the strength of incisional wounds.[131] Rats treated with preoperative and postoperative GH experienced an increase in breaking strength and collagen content of colonic anastomoses. The increments of these parameters were accompanied by an increase in collagen deposition in the anastomotic segment. These effects were seen only when GH was given during the healing phase.[132] GH seems to stimulate structural organization of the anastomotic collagen fibrils into fibers.[133] In addition, GH administration significantly improves skin wound strength in malnourished rats.[134]

Growth hormone appears to exert its favorable effect in part by stimulating IGF-I synthesis; in turn, IGF-I mediates the anabolic effects of GH. IGF-I is released early during wound healing by the lysis of platelet alpha granules and later by fibroblasts. This molecule stimulates fibroblast and endothelial cell proliferation as well as collagen synthesis.[135] IGF-I stands out as critical for effective wound healing.[136]

Rats depleted of IGF-I experience a 50% decrease in wound protein, DNA, hydroxyproline, and macrophage concentrations. Moreover, infusion of IGF-I into the wounds restores these variables.[137] Similar to GH, IGF-I increases wound breaking strength in rats. However, its effect is evident only when it is combined with one of its specific binding proteins, such as IGFBP-1.[138,139]

Growth hormone can significantly reduce wound closure times and the length of hospitalization. In addition, it may accelerate donor site wound healing rates by 25%. With this increase in healing, patients with massive (>60% total body surface area) burn wounds can undergo further skin grafting procedures earlier.[140–143] The good results obtained with GH therapy in terms of the healing rates for donor sites and burn wounds are encouraging. Unfortunately, there is no published information on the use of this important growth factor in wound healing in elderly populations. Considering that aged individuals are reported to have a functional decline in the GH/IGF-I axis, it is probable that the same or even more significant effects might be observed in the elderly.[144,145]

### *Arginine*

There has been much interest in the use of arginine to stimulate immune responses and promote wound healing. In rodents arginine supplementation stimulates wound healing as assessed by wound breaking strength and reparative collagen synthesis.[146] In healthy adult humans arginine supplementation enhances wound collagen deposition and increases lymphocyte mitogenesis[147] (Fig. 5.5). Beneficial effects have also been observed in elderly individuals. Dietary supplementation with arginine for 14 days increases IGF-I concentrations, improves nitrogen balance, and reduces total cholesterol concentrations.[148] Furthermore, oral arginine supplementation in an elderly population has upregulated T cell activity and increased total protein and collagen deposition in an experimental wound model. Arginine does not increase the rate of epithelialization or DNA levels in wounds, suggesting that it acts solely by enhancing fibroblast synthetic responses.[149]

The mechanisms by which arginine achieves these effects are not known. Arginine may enhance wound healing by inducing growth hormone secretion. IGF-I is significantly increased in elderly human volunteers after 2 weeks of dietary arginine supplementation.[75,149] Arginine may also serve as a precursor for proline biosynthesis. Ornithine is a catabolite of arginine, which in turn can be converted to proline by wound cells. Arginine levels are low within the wound, which corresponds to high levels of arginase and ornithine.[38,75] However, no direct evidence of this has been shown. Finally, nitric oxide may be involved in these effects. Nitric oxide synthase catalyzes the conversion of arginine to citrulline and nitric oxide. At low concentrations this molecule may enhance wound collagen synthesis.[38,45] The above data show that arginine supplements have many beneficial effects, are well tolerated, and have few deleterious effects. These findings may lead to its routine use as a way to enhance wound healing and immune function safely in this age group.

### *Vitamin A*

Vitamin A has many beneficial effects in surgical patients. In particular, studies of its effects on wound healing and corticosteroids have proved to be of clinical value. Years ago Ehrlich and Hunt demonstrated that corticosteroids significantly impaired the healing of cutaneous wounds and that topical application of vitamin A partially reversed this effect. It did not have any effect, however, beyond the normal healing rate when cortisone was not given.[49] These reactions have been shown repeatedly.[150]

A similar protective effect of vitamin A is observed in intestinal anastomoses in steroid-treated animals. High-dose vitamin A increases bursting pressure in small and large bowel by 30% and 55%, respectively, compared to that in rats receiving corticosteroids.[151] Vitamin A may also be useful for preventing the loss of early anastomotic strength induced by the use of chemotherapeutic drugs such as fluorouracil and cyclophosphamide.[152,153] Vitamin A has been shown to improve cutaneous wound healing in situations where repair is suppressed by irradiation or tumor implantation. Furthermore, it helps in the healing of femoral fractures and tendon and arterial wall injuries in animals.[82,154]

The mechanism by which vitamin A improves wound healing is unclear. It is believed that the improvement is due to an early increase in the inflammatory response, which involves an influx of macrophages into the wound and enhanced fibroblast differentiation and collagen accumulation.[155] Speculation also exists regarding stimulation of collagen synthesis and inhibition of collagen degradation, but some authors have not found consistent data to support this idea.[152]

Vitamin A is a nutritional supplement that should be given perioperatively, especially to steroid-treated patients and those known to be immunocompromised. A recommended dose of 25,000 IU/day before and after elective surgery appears to be a safe, effective short-term dose, except in pregnant women. Special attention should be paid to patients in whom the antiinflammatory effect of steroids is essential, as it would be reversed by vitamin A.[156]

### Vitamin C

Vitamin C deficiency (scurvy) is the best example of the relation between nutrition and wound healing. The extensive literature on vitamin C and wound healing shows clearly that scurvy delays wound healing in humans. Ascorbate, the biochemically active form of vitamin C, is a cofactor for three enzymes required for proline and lysine hydroxylation in collagen biosynthesis.[157]

Vitamin C-deficient wounds are characterized by a decrease in angiogenesis and hemorrhage, decreased accumulation of extracellular matrix, and little collagen deposition. This combination results in a marked reduction in tensile strength. Wound remodeling is a continuous process during which collagen deposition and lysis are in equilibrium. With vitamin C deficiency, collagen lysis proceeds normally despite the decreased collagen deposition; thus it is no surprise that wounds break down in patients with scurvy. The effects of ascorbate deprivation on wound healing appear late. Healing of skin wounds can remain normal after 90 days of ascorbate depletion, and even longer times may be necessary for frank clinical signs of scurvy to appear. Normally, uninjured humans require about 10–20 mg of vitamin C daily to prevent the development of scurvy. Further supplementation does not seem to accelerate wound healing.[158]

Plasma concentration and urinary excretion of ascorbate are markedly decreased in injured humans. Tissue saturation of ascorbate is also reduced during the early hours after injury.[38] After trauma ascorbic acid levels in plasma and white blood cells fall immediately and in proportion to the severity of the injury; the predominant mechanism of this effect is unknown. Thus the daily requirement for vitamin C is increased in burned or trauma patients. The combination of injury or surgery with preexisting marginal vitamin C status may determine clinically relevant alterations of wound healing. Therefore supplementation with 100–200 mg of vitamin C per day, depending on the severity of the injury, may be beneficial in these patients.[5]

### Zinc

Zinc is the second most abundant trace metal in the human body and is present in all living cells and body scretions.[159] Approximately 300 enzymes are known to require zinc for their activities. In particular, it is an essential component of multiple metalloenzymes, including RNA- and DNA-polymerases. Zinc is required for DNA synthesis, cell division, and protein synthesis.

In humans zinc deficiency adversely affects lymphocyte proliferation, possibly related to the enzymatic role of zinc in DNA synthesis and cell division. Thymulin, a thymic hormone involved in T lymphocyte maturation, is known to be zinc-dependent and is adversely affected by zinc deficiency. Thus lymphocyte differentiation and maturity may also be affected by zinc deficiency. A decrease in IL-1 and IL-2 production by Th lymphocytes, as well as T cell lymphocyte subpopulation abnormalities, have been observed. All these changes are correctable with zinc supplementation.[160] It can be conceived that zinc deficiency is associated with poor wound healing.

Zinc supplementation has been reported to have positive effects on wound healing, but only in patients with a low pretreatment serum zinc level. Other studies have shown no effect.[38] A serum zinc level of <100 g/dl is associated with impaired wound healing.[5] Zinc supplementation seems reasonable in patients who are at particular high risk of zinc deficiency, including patients with decreased food intakes or increased fecal zinc losses such as diarrhea, gastrointestinal fistulas, or malabsorbtion syndromes.

## Conclusions

It is apparent that the wound healing response is altered in the elderly compared to that in young individuals. Inflammation, angiogenesis, epithelialization, and remodeling show changes that may consequently impair wound healing. However, in elderly patients not suffering from concomitant diseases, the rate of wound healing is normal or slightly reduced.[7] It is still difficult to reach definite conclusions in certain areas of this process, such as collagen metabolism, and about the influence the above alterations may have on morbidity and mortality.

Nonetheless, a clear relation is observed between wound healing and certain disease states (i.e., malnutrition, infections, hypoxia and reoxygenation, diabetes, and drug interactions). Patients with these conditions should be carefully evaluated and supplementation with growth factors and nutrient supplements considered. The potential uses of these factors may be of importance for surgeons who care for critically ill patients and their wound healing.

## References


1. Saltzman E, Mason JB. Enteral nutrition in the elderly. In: Rombeau JL, Rolandelli RH (eds) Enteral and Tube Feeding. Philadelphia: Saunders, 1997:385–402.
2. Garry PJ, Vellas BJ. Aging and nutrition. In: Ziegler EE, Filer LJ (eds) Present Knowledge in Nutrition. Washington, DC: ILSI Press, 1996:414–419.
3. Rolandelli RH, Ullrich JR. Nutritional support in the frail elderly surgical patient. Surg Clin North Am 1994;74:79–92.
4. Morley JE, Silver AJ. Nutritional issues in nursing home care. Ann Intern Med 1995;123:850–859.
5. Keller HH. Malutrition in institutionalized elderly: how and why? J Am Geriatr Soc 1993;41:1212–1218.
6. Giner M, Laviano A, Meguid MM. In 1995 a correlation between malnutrition and poor outcome in critically ill patients still exists. Nutrition 1996;12:23–29.
7. Rapin CH. Nutrition support and the elderly. In: Payne-James J, Grimble G, Silk D (eds) Artificial Nutrition Support in Clinical Practice. Boston: Little, Brown, 1995: 535–544.
8. Nelson RC, Franzi LR. Nutrition and aging. Med Clin North Am 1989;73:1531.
9. Toogood AA, Adams JE, O'Neill PA, et al. Body composition in growth hormone deficient adults over the age of 60 years. Clin Endocrinol (Oxf) 1996;45:339–405.
10. Boonen S, Lesaffre E, Aerssens J, et al. Deficiency of the growth hormone-insulin-like growth factor-I axis potentially involved in age-related alterations in body composition. Gerontology 1996;42:330–338.
11. Rudman D, Feller AG, Nagraj HS, et al. Effects of human growth hormone in men over 60 years old. N Engl J Med 1990;323:1–6.
12. Thompson JL, Butterfiel GE, Marcus R, et al. The effects of recombinant human insulin-like growth hormone on body composition in elderly women. J Clin Endocrinol Metab 1995;80:1845–1852.
13. Jorgensen J, Vahl N, Hansen TB. Influence of growth hormone and androgens on body composition in adults. Horm Res 1996;45:94–98.
14. Bhasin S, Storer TW, Berman N, et al. The effects of supraphysiologic doses of testosterone on muscle size and strength in normal men. N Engl J Med 1996;335:1–7.
15. Evans W. Functional and metabolic consequences of sarcopenia. J Nutr 1997;127:998S–1003S.
16. Taaffe DR, Pruitt L, Pyka G, et al. Comparative effects of high- and low-intensity resistance training on thigh muscle strength, fiber area, and tissue composition in elderly women. Clin Physiol 1996:16:381–392.
17. Fielding RA. The role of progressive resistance training and nutrition in the preservation of lean body mass in the elderly. J Am Coll Nutr 1995;14:587–594.
18. Roberts SB, Fuss P, Heyman M, et al. Influence of age on energy requirements. Am J Clin Nutr 1995;62(suppl): 1053S–1058S.
19. Voorrips LE, Van Acker TMCJ, Deurenberg P, et al. Energy expenditure at rest during standardized activities: a comparison between elderly and middle-aged women. Am J Clin Nutr 1993;58:15–20.
20. McGrandy RB, Barrows CH, Spanias A, et al. Baltimore Longitudinal Study. Nutrient intakes and energy expenditure in men of different ages. J Gerontol 1966;21:581–587.
21. White JV. The nutrition screening initiative: a 5 year perspective. Nutr Clin Practr 1996;11(3):89–93.
22. Jacobs DO, Scheltinga M. Metabolic assessment. In: Rombeau JL, Caldwell MD (eds) Clinical Nutrition: Parenteral Nutrition. Philadelphia: Saunders, 1993:245–274.
23. De Onis M, Hablicht JP. Anthropometric reference data for international use: recommendations from a World Health Organization expert committee. Am J Clin Nutr 1996;64: 650–658.
24. Weight by height by age for adults 18–74 years: U.S., 1971–74. DHEW Publ No (PHS)79-1656, September 1979.
25. Master AM, Lasser RP, Beckman G. Tables of average weight and height of Americans aged 65 to 94. JAMA 1960;172:658–662.
26. Frisancho AR. New standards of weight and body composition by frame size and height for assessment of nutritional status of adults and the elderly. Am J Clin Nutr 1984;40:808–819.
27. Mullen JL, Buzby GP, Matthews DC, et al. Reduction of operative morbidity and mortality by combined and postoperative nutritional support. Ann Surg 1980;192:604–613.
28. Chumlea WC, Roche AF, Steinbaugh ML. Anthropometric approaches to the nutritional assessment of the elderly. In: Munro HN, Danford DE (eds) Nutrition, Aging, and the Elderly. New York: Plenum, 1989:335.
29. Kuczmarski RJ, Flegal KM, Campbell SM, et al. Increasing prevalence of overweight among US adults: the national health and nutrition examination surveys, 1960 to 1991. JAMA 1994;272:205–211.
30. Durning JVGA, Womersley J. Body fat assessment from total body density and its estimation from skinfold thickness. Br J Nutr 1974;32:77–79.

31. Herrmann VM. Nutritional assessment. In: Torosian MH (ed) Nutrition for the Hospitalized Patient. New York: Marcel Dekker, 1995:233–253.
32. Frisancho AR. New norms of upper limb fat and muscle areas for assessment of nutritional status. Am J Clin Nutr 1989;34:2540–2545.
33. Ravaglia G, Morini P, Forti P, et al. Anthropometric characteristics of healthy Italian nonagenarians and centenarians. Br J Nutr 1997;77:9–17.
34. Salive ME, Cornoni-Huntley J, Phillips CL, et al. Serum albumin in older persons: relationship with age and health status. J Clin Epidemiol 1992;45:213.
35. Baumgartner RN, Koelher KM, Romero L. Serum albumin is associated with skeletal muscle in elderly men and women. Am J Clin Nutr 1996;64:552–558.
36. Sahyoun NR, Jacques PF, Dallal G, et al. Use of albumin as a predictor of mortality in community dwelling and institutionalized elderly populations. J Clin Epidemiol 1996;49:981–988.
37. Ferguson RP, O'Connor, Crabtree B, et al. Serum albumin and prealbumin as predictors of clinical outcomes of hospitalized elderly nursing home residents. J Am Geriatr Soc 1993;41:545–549.
38. Butters M, Straub M, Kraft K, et al. Studies on nutritional status in general surgery patients by clinical, anthropometric and laboratory parameters. Nutrition 1996;12:405–410.
39. Cals MJ, Devanlay M, Desveaux N, et al. Extensive laboratory assessment of nutritional status in fit, health-conscious, elderly people living in the Paris area. J Am Coll Nutr 1994;13:646–657.
40. McArthur WP, Taylor BK, Smith WT. Peripheral blood leukocyte population in the elderly with and without periodontal disease. J Clin Periodont 1996;23:846–852.
41. Sullivan DH, Carter WJ. Insulin-like growth factor I as an indicator of protein-energy undernutrition among metabolically stable hospitalized elderly. J Am Coll Nutr 1994;13:184–191.
42. Galanos AN, Pieper CF, Cornoni-Huntley JC. Nutritional and function: is there a relationship between functional capabilities of community-dwelling elderly? J Am Geriatr Soc 1994;42:386–373.
43. Hill GL. Body composition research: implications for the practice of clinical nutrition. J Parenter Enter Nutr 1992;16:197.
44. Ensrud KE, Nevitt MC, Yunis C, et al. Correlates of impaired function in older women. J Am Geriatr Soc 1994;42:481–489.
45. Applegate WB, Blass JP, Williams TF. Instruments for the functional assessment of older patients. N Engl J Med 1990;322:1207–1213.
46. Weinberg AD, Minaker KL, et al. Dehydration: evaluation and management in older adults. JAMA 1995;274:1552–1556.
47. Campbell WW, Evans WJ. Protein requirements of elderly people. Eur J Clin Nutr 1996;50(suppl 1):S180–S185.
48. National Research Council. Recommended Dietary Allowances, 10th ed. Washington, DC: National Academy Press, 1989.
49. Roza AM, Shizgal HM. The Harris Benedict equation reevaluated: resting energy requirements and the body cell mass. Am J Clin Nutr 1984;40:168–182.
50. Hoffman P, Richardson S, Giacoppe J. Failure of the Harris-Benedict equation to predict energy expenditure in undernourished nursing home residents. FASEB J 1995;9:A438.
51. Bell S. Current summaries: a practical equation to predict resting metabolic rate in older men. J Parenter Enteral Nutr 1994;44:741.
52. Fuller NJ, Sawyer MB, Coward WA. Components of total energy expenditure in free-living elderly men (over 75 years of age): measurement, predictability and relationship to quality-of-life indices. Br J Nutr 1996;75:161–173.
53. Roberts SB, Fuss P, Heyman MB. Control of food intake in older men. JAMA 1994;272:1601–1606.
54. Campbell WW, Evans WJ. Protein requirements of elderly people. Eur J Clin Nutr 1996;50(suppl 1):S180–S185.
55. Krasinski SD, Russell RM, Otradovec CL. Relationship of vitamin A and vitamin E intake to fasting plasma retinol, retinol-binding protein, retinyl esters, carotene, α-tocopherol, and cholesterol among elderly people and young adults: increased plasma retinyl esters among vitamin A-supplement users. Am J Clin Nutr 1989;49:112–120.
56. Russell RM. New views on the RDAs for older adults. J Am Diet Assoc 1997;97:515–518.
57. Selhub J, Jacques PF, Wilson PF, et al. Vitamin status and intake as primary determinants of homocysteinemia in an elderly population. JAMA 1993;270:2693–2698.
58. Ribaya-Mercado JD, Rusell RM, Sahyoun N. Vitamin B-6 requirements of elderly men and women. J Nutr 1991;121:1062–1074.
59. Bailey AL, Maisey S, Southon S, et al. Relationships between micronutrient intake and biochemical indicators of nutrient adequacy in "free-living" elderly UK population. Br J Nutr 1997;77:225–242.
60. Seneca Investigators. Changes in the vitamin status of elderly Europeans: plasma vitamins A, E, B-6, B-12, folic acid and caretenoids. Eur J Clin Nutr 1996;59(suppl 2):S32–S46.
61. Lindenbaum J, Rosenberg IH, Wilson P, et al. Prevalence of cobalamin deficiency in the Framingham elderly population. Am J Clin Nutr 1994;60:2–11.
62. Krasinski SD, Russell RM, Samloff M. Fundic atrophic gastritis in an elderly population: effect on hemoglobin and several serum nutritional indicators. J Am Geriatr Soc 1986;34:800–806.
63. Allen LH, Casterline J. Vitamin B-12 deficiency in elderly individuals: diagnosis and requirements. Am J Clin Nutr 1994;60:12–14.
64. Dawson-Hughes B. Calcium and vitamin D nutritional needs of elderly women. J Nutr 1996;126:1165S–1167S.
65. Webb AR, Pilbeam C, Hanafin N. An evaluation of the relative contributions of exposure to sunlight and of diet to the circulating concentrations of 25-hydroxyvitamin D in an elderly nursing home population in Boston. Am J Clin Nutr 1990;51:1075–1081.
66. Holick MF. McCollum award lecture, 1994: vitamin D—new horizons for the 21st century. Am J Clin Nutr 1994;60:619–630.
67. Lovat LB. Age related changes in gut physiology and nutritional status. Gut 1996;38:306–309.
68. Chapuy MC, Arlot E, Delmas PD, et al. Effect of calcium and cholecalciferol treatment for three years on hip fractures in elderly women. Br Med J 1994;308:1081–1082.

69. Lips P, Graafmans WC, Ooms ME, et al. Vitamin D supplementation and fracture incidence in elderly persons: a randomized, placebo controlled clinical trial. Ann Intern Med 1996;124:400–406.
70. Dawson-Hughes B, Harris SS, Krall EA. Rates of bone loss in postmenopausal women randomly assigned to one of two dosages of vitamin D. Am J Clin Nutr 1995;61:1140–1145.
71. Johnson LE, Dooley PA, Gleick JB. Oral nutritional supplementation use in elderly nursing home patients. J Am Geriatr Soc 1993;41:947–952.
72. Chandra RK. Effect of vitamin and trace element supplementation on immune response and infection in elderly subjects. Lancet 1992;340:1124–1127.
73. Mooradian AD. Nutritional modulation of life span and gene expression. Ann Intern Med 1988:109:890–904.
74. Alpha-tocopherol, Beta-carotene Cancer Prevention Group. The effect of vitamin E and beta carotene on the incidence of lung cancers in male smokers. N Engl J Med 1994;330:1029–1035.
75. Halasz NA. Dehiscence of laparotomy wounds. Am J Surg 1968;116:210–214.
76. Mendoza CB, Postlethwait RW, Johnson WD. Incidence of wound disruption following operation. Arch Surg 1970;101:396–398.
77. Irvin TT, Goligher JC. Aetiology of disruption of intestinal anastomoses. Br J Surg 1973;60:461–462.
78. Schrock TR, Deveney CW, Dunphy JE. Factors contributing to leakage of colonic anastomoses. Ann Surg 1973;177: 513–515.
79. Jonsson K, Jensen JA, Goodson WH, et al. Tissue oxygenation, anemia, and perfusion in relation to wound healing in surgical patients. Ann Surg 1991;214:605–613.
80. Hunt TK, Hopf HW. Nutrition in wound healing. In: Fischer JE (ed) Nutrition and Metabolism in the Surgical Patient. Boston: Little, Brown, 1996:423–441.
81. Cohen IK, Diegelmann RF, Crossland MC. Wound care and wound healing. In: Schwartz SI (ed) Principles of Surgery. New York: McGraw-Hill, 1994;279–303.
82. Van de Kerkhof PCM, Van Bergen B, Spruiit K, et al. Age-related changes in wound healing. Clin Exp Dermatol 1994;19:369–374.
83. Brown DL, Kao WWY, Greenhalgh DG. Apoptosis downregulates inflammation under the advancing epithelial wound edge: delayed pattern in diabetes and improvement with topical growth factors. Surgery 1997;121:372–380.
84. Ashcroft GS, Horan MA, Ferguson MW. The effects of ageing on cutaneous wound healing in mammals. J Anat 1995;187:1–26.
85. Danon D, Kowatch MA, Roth GS. Promotion of wound repair of old mice by local injection of macrophages. Proc Natl Acad Sci USA 1989;86:2018–2020.
86. Ashcroft GS, Horan MA, Ferguson MWJ. Aging is associated with reduced deposition of specific extracellular matrix components, an upregulation of angiogenesis, and an altered inflammatory response in a murine incisional wound healing model. J Invest Dermatol 1997;108:430–437.
87. Song L, Kim YH, Chopra RK, et al. Age-related effects in T cell activation and proliferation. Exp Gerontol 1993;28: 313–321.
88. Nagelkerken L, Hertogh-Huijbregts A, Dobber R, et al. Age-related changes in lymphokine production related to a decreased number of $CD45Rb^{hi}$ $CD4^{+}$ T cells. Eur J Immunol 1991;221:273–281.
89. Bloom ET. Functional importance of $CD4^{+}$ and $CD8^{+}$ cells in cytotoxic lymphocytes activity and associated gene expression: impact on the age-related decline in lytic activity. Eur J Immunol 1991;21:1013–1017.
90. Rattan SI, Derventzi A. Altered cellular responsiveness during ageing. Bioessays 1991;13:601–606.
91. Phillips PD, Kaji K, Cristofalo VJ. Progressive loss of the proliferative response of senescing WI-38 cells to platelet-derived growth factors, epidermal growth factor, insulin, transferrin, and dexamethasone. J Gerontol 1984;39:11–17.
92. Bauer EA, Silverman N, Busiek DF, et al. Diminished response of Werner's syndrome fibroblasts to growth factors PDGF and FGF. Science 1986;234:1240–1242.
93. Holt DR, Kirk SJ, Regan MC, et al. Effect of age on wound healing in healthy human beings. Surgery 1992;112:293–298.
94. Grove GL, Kligman AM. Age-associated changes in human epidermal cell renewal. J Gerontol 1983;38:137–142.
95. Sobin SS, Bernick S, Ballard KW. Acute wound repair in an aged animal: a model for accelerated aging of the microvasculature? J Gerontol 1992;47:B121–B125.
96. Shah M, Foreman DM, Ferguson MWJ. Control of scarring in the adult wounds by neutralizing antibody to transforming growth factor β. Lancet 1992;339:213–214.
97. Petersen TI, Kissmeyer-Nielsen P, Laurberg S, et al. Impaired wound healing but unaltered colonic healing with increasing age: an experimental study in rats. Eur Surg Res 1995;27:250–257.
98. Johnson BD. Effects of donor age on protein and collagen synthesis in vitro by human diploid fibroblasts. Lab Invest 1986;55:490–496.
99. Holm-Pedersen P, Zederfeldt B. Strength development of skin incisions in young and old rats. Scand J Plast Reconstr Surg 1971;5:7–12.
100. Sussman MD. Aging of connective tissue: physical properties of healing wounds in young and old rats. Am J Physiol 1973;224:1169–1171.
101. Holm-Pedersen P, Viidik A. Tensile properties and morphology of healing wounds in young and old rats. Scand J Plast Reconstr Surg 1972;6:25–35.
102. Stoop MJ, Dirksen R, Hendriks T. Advanced age alone does not suppress anastomotic healing in the intestine. Surgery 1996;119:15–19.
103. Stoop MJ, Dirksen R, Hendriks T. Advanced age alone does not suppress anastomotic healing in the intestine. Surgery 1996;119:15–19.
104. Solomon MP, Granick MS, Lau HC. Wound care in the elderly patient. Surg Clin North Am 1994;74:441–463.
105. Ward MWN, Danzi M, Lewin MR. The effects of subclinical malnutrition and refeeding on the healing of experimental colonic anastomoses. Br J Surg 1982;69:308–310.
106. Daly JM, Vars HM, Dudrick SJ. Effects of protein depletion on strength of colonic anastomoses. Surg Gynecol Obstet 1972;134:15–21.
107. Irving TT. Effects of malnutrition and hyperalimentation on wound healing. Surg Gynecol Obstet 1978;146:33–37.

108. Hydock DA, Hill GL. Impaired wound healing in surgical patients with varying degrees of malnutrition. J Parenter Enteral Nutr 1986;10:550–554.
109. Casey J, Flinn WR, Yao JST, et al. Correlation of immune and nutritional status with wound complications in patients undergoing vascular operations. Surgery 1983;93: 822–827.
110. Haydock DA, Hill GL. Improved wound healing response in surgical patients receiving intravenous nutrition. Br J Surg 1987;74:320–323.
111. Windsor JA, Knight GS, Hill GL. Wound healing response in surgical patients: recent food intake is more important than nutritional status. Br J Surg 1988;75:135–137.
112. Klein S, Kinney J, Jeejeebhoy K, et al. Nutrition support practice: review of published data and recommendations for future research directions. J Parenter Enteral Nutr 1997;21:133–156.
113. Stotts NA, Wipke-Tevis D. Nutrition, perfusion, and wound healing: an inseparable triad. Nutrition 1996;12: 733–734.
114. Quirina A, Viidik A. The influence of age on the healing of normal and ischemic incisional skin wounds. Mech Ageing Dev 1991;58:221–232.
115. Cooley BC, Gould JS. Influence of age on free flap tolerance to ischemia: an experimental study in rats. Ann Plast Surg 1993;30:57–59.
116. Hartmann M, Jonsson K, Zederfeldt B. Effect of tissue perfusion and oxygenation on accumulation of collagen in healing wounds. Eur J Surg 1992;158:521–526.
117. Thornton FJ, Barbul A. Healing in the gastrointestinal tract. Surg Clin North Am 1997;77:549–573.
118. Thornton FJ, Ahrendt GM, Schaffer MR, et al. Sepsis impairs anastomotic collagen gene expression and synthesis: a possible role for nitric oxide. J Surg Res 1997;69:81–86.
119. Barbul A, Regan MC. Biology of wound healing. In: Fischer JE (ed) Surgical Basic Science. St. Louis, Mosby-Year Book, 1997:67–89.
120. Eubanks TR, Greenberg JJ, Dobrin PB, et al. The effects of different corticosteroids on the healing colon anastomosis and cecum in a rat model. Am Surg 1997;63:266–269.
121. Del Rio JV, Beck DE, Opelka FG. Chronic perioperative steroids and colonic anastomotic healing in rats. J Surg Res 1996;66:138–142.
122. Hunt TK, Ehrlich HP, Garcia JA. Effect of vitamin A on reversing the inhibitory effect of cortisone on healing of open wounds in animals and man. Ann Surg 1969;170: 633–641.
123. Schulze S, Andersen J, Overgaard H, et al. Effect of prednisolone on the systemic response and wound healing after colonic surgery. Arch Surg 1997;132:129–135.
124. Wadell BE, Carlton WC, Steinberg SR, et al. The adverse effects of octreotide on wound healing in rats. Am Surg 1997;63:446–449.
125. Cruse PJ, Foord R. A five-year prospective study of 23,649 surgical wounds. Arch Surg 1973;107:206–210.
126. Israelsson LA, Jonssoon T. Overweight and healing of midline incisions: the impact of suture technique. Eur J Surg 1997;163:175–180.
127. Goodson WH, Hunt TK. Wound collagen accumulation in obese hyperglycemic mice. Diabetes 1986;35:491–495.
128. Goodson WH, Hunt TK. Studies of wound healing in experimental diabetes mellitus. J Surg Res 1977;22:221–227.
129. Goodson WH, Hunt TK. Wound healing in well-controlled diabetic men. Surg Forum 1984;35:614–616.
130. McMurry JF Jr. Wound healing with diabetes mellitus: better glucose control for better wound healing in diabetes. Surg Clin North Am 1984;64:769–778.
131. Belcher HJCR, Ellis H. Somatropin and wound healing after injury. J Clin Endocrinol Metab 1990;70:939–943.
132. Christensen H, Oxlund H. Growth hormone increases the collagen deposition rate and breaking strength of the left colonic anastomoses in rats. Surgery 1994;116:550–556.
133. Christensen H, Chemnitz J, Christensen BC, et al. Collagen structural organization of healing colonic anastomoses on the effect of growth hormone treatment. Dis Colon Rectum 1995;38:1200–1205.
134. Zaizen Y, Ford EG, Costin G, et al. Stimulation of wound bursting strength during protein malnutrition. J Surg Res 1990;49:333–336.
135. Herndon DN, Nguyen TT, Gilpin DA. Growth factors: local and systemic. Arch Surg 1993;128:1227–1233.
136. Steenfos H, Spencer EM, Hunt TK. Insulin-like growth factor I has a major role in wound healing. Surg Forum 1989;40:68–70.
137. Mueller RV, Hunt TK, Tokinaga A, et al. The effect of insulin-like growth factor I on wound healing variables and macrophages in rats. Arch Surg 1994;129:262–265.
138. Jyung RW, Mustoe TA, Busby WH, et al. Increased wound-breaking strength induced by insulin-like growth factor I in combination with insulin-like growth factor binding protein-1. Surgery 1994;115:233–239.
139. Meyer NA, Barrow RE, Herndon DN. Combined insulin-like growth factor-1 and growth hormone improves weight loss and wound healing in burned rats. J Trauma 1996;41:1008–1012.
140. Herndon DN, Barrow RE, Kunkel KR, et al. Effects of recombinant human growth hormone on donor-site healing in severely burned children. Ann Surg 1990;212: 424–431.
141. Sherman SK, Demling RH, Lanlonde C, et al. Growth hormone enhances re-epithelialization of human split-thickness skin graft donor sites. Surg Forum 1989;40:37–39.
142. Nguyen TT, Gilpin DA, Meyer NA, et al. Current treatments of severely burned patients. Ann Surg 1996;223:14–25.
143. Herndon DN, Pierre EJ, Stokes KN, et al. Growth hormone treatment for burned children. Horm Res 1996;45(suppl 1):29–31.
144. Toogood AA, Adams JE, O'Neill PA, et al. Body composition in growth hormone deficient adults over the age of 60 years. Clin Endocrinol (Oxf) 1996;45:339–405.
145. Boonen S, Lesaffre E, Aerssens J, et al. Deficiency of the growth hormone-insulin-like growth factor-I axis potentially involved in age-related alterations in body composition. Gerontology 1996;42:330–338.
146. Barbul A, Rettura G, Levenson S, et al. Wound healing and thymotrophic effects of arginine: a pituitary mechanism of action. Am J Clin Nutr 1983;37:786–794.

147. Barbul A, Lazarou SA, Efron DT, et al. Arginine enhances wound healing and lymphocyte immune responses in humans. Surgery 1990;108:331–337.
148. Hurson M, Regan MC, Kirk SJ, et al. Metabolic effects of arginine in a healthy elderly population. J Parenter Enteral Nutr 1995;19:227–230.
149. Kirk SJ, Hurson M, Regan MC, et al. Arginine stimulates wound healing and immune function in elderly human beings. Surgery 1993;114:155–160.
150. Haws M, Brown RE, Suchy H, et al. Vitamin A-soaked gelfoam sponges in wound healing steroid-treated animals. Ann Plast Surg 1994;32:418–422.
151. Phillips JD, Kin CS, Fonkalsrud EW, et al. Effects of chronic corticosteroids and vitamin A on the healing of intestinal anastomoses. Am J Surg 1992;163:71–77.
152. De Waard JWD, Wobbes T, Van Der Linden CJ, et al. Retinol may promote fluorouracil-suppressed healing of experimental intestinal anastomoses. Arch Surg 1995;130:959–965.
153. Petry JJ. Surgically significant nutritional supplements. Plast Reconstr Surg 1996;97:233–240.
154. Niu XT, Cushin B, Reisner A, et al. Effect of dietary supplementation with vitamin A on arterial healing in rats. J Surg Res 1987;42:62–65.
155. Demetriou AA, Jones LK. Vitamins. In: Rombeau JL, Caldwell MD (eds) Clinical Nutrition. Parenteral Nutrition. Philadelphia: Saunders, 1993:184–202.
156. Niu XT, Cushin B, Reisner A, et al. Effect of dietary supplementation with vitamin A on arterial healing in rats. J Surg Res 1987;42:62–65.
157. Levine M, Rumsey S, Wang Y, et al. Vitamin C. In: Ziegler EE, Filer LJ (eds) Present Knowledge in Nutrition. Washington, DC: ILSI Press, 1996:146–159.
158. Riet GT, Kessels AGH, Knipschild. Randomized clinical trial of ascorbic acid in the treatment of pressure ulcers. J Clin Epidemiol 1995;48:1453–1460.
159. Lansdown ABG. Zinc in the healing wound. Lancet 1996;346:706–707.
160. Prasad AS. Zinc: an overview. Nutrition 1995;11:93–99.

# *Part I*
# *General Principles*

## Section 2
## Surgical Management of the Elderly Patient

# Invited Commentary

Ben Eiseman

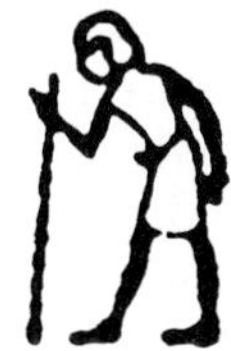

The Editors have invited commentaries by elder surgeons to provide historic perspective to the chapters that follow. Knowing the prolixity of the elderly, this is a perilous editorial risk, particularly as we are asked to compare the past with the present. The comments that follow are designed to serve as an aperitif of slightly outdated vintage wine designed to whet the appetite of readers before they plunge into the lean meat of the chapters that follow.

As the century ends, health care is in revolution. The elderly in particular suffer when the established order is overthrown. Their anticipated tranquil old age is upset by unanticipated violent change. Their major dissatisfactions therefore emphasize some of the more important changes in surgical management that have occurred under the new health care system. By identifying their causes it is intended that their correction be facilitated.

The philosophy of clinical health care has been changed from one of professionalism to one of commercialism. Clinical care is a highly expensive commodity. Those who undertake clinical care must use the skills of a politician: They must find the most acceptable compromise between what is best for the patient and what society can afford. Surgical care has been transformed—like politics—into finding the practice of the possible.

Physicians complain about this change, but the demands for economy are immutable. This adds a difficult new dimension to the decisions a physician must make when finding the best compromise between ideal clinical care, cost-effectiveness, and the satisfactions of the elderly patient. These powerful forces usually are competitive.

Physicians should use their diminishing personal and professional influence for achieving policy and operating changes in the evolving health care system. Such an active role not only can benefit the patients; it can serve to regain some of the prestige we physicians so irresponsibly squandered during the past quarter century. To ignore this responsibility hastens degradation of our diminishing public respect.

Both the elderly patients and their physicians should realize that no amount of hand wringing or lobbyist arm twisting can restore the remembered glories of the past. Universal unlimited health care will continue to be unaffordable in even the most affluent society. Changes are required in the organization and operation of the system, the education and performance of those who provide care, and the expectations of the patient.

The basis for such inexorable warnings are becoming increasingly evident. Clinical care emerged from an art form to an applied science during the twentieth century. It resulted in vastly improved clinical care but mostly at an unsupportable cost. There is a cruel irony that the dissatisfactions of the elderly peaks at the moment in history when the potential for clinical benefit has never been better. Life expectancy and the quality of the years up to approximately age 80 has in general improved dramatically compared to expectations of the past. The cause for this discrepancy provides a clue to its cause and its ultimate correction.

Health care has in the recent past emerged as one of the nation's largest industries not because of the machinations of a few entrepreneurial schemers or meddlesome government employees but because it has become so inherently expensive. Scientific clinical care is costly. It is no longer societally possible to provide more than basic care to everyone. Some form of rationing is inevitable. Such a stark statement evokes an uneasy un-American feeling among many. It is thought to be undemocratic and contrary to the philosophy of those who framed the Constitution. In fact, the framers had no intention of such limitless government entitlements when they created the Bill of Rights. For those of us in the twenty-first century to graft our own preconceptions onto a document drawn up two centuries ago is a misreading of history. Gradual acceptance of this notion by the general public has created a mismatch between the expectations of the elderly concerning their care and the realities of what can be afforded at government expense.

We in the medical profession must bear a significant share of responsibility for permitting overly optimistic claims of our potential for providing clinical benefits. Television anchormen and anchorwomen incessantly feed the aging public's appetite for a medical "breakthrough of the day." It is as much a part of the cocktail hour as a martini. Both presumably are designed to provide a temporary moral lift after a difficult day. Anyone wearing a borrowed white laboratory coat serves to confirm the exciting prospects of some obscure preliminary laboratory study on rats. Cancer, heart disease, and stroke are considered to be disappearing, just like polio. As a consequence, when an earnest clinician tries to explain to an aging patient sick with an incurable disease that there is little that can be done to prolong life or improve its quality, he or she is considered incompetent.

The sooner we correct such misperceptions, the better will the elderly learn to cope with the fact that they are not immortal. Human water pumps, power systems, and shock absorbers gradually fail, just as they do on aging automobiles.

In fact, most of the dissatisfactions of the elderly concerning their health care is with the style of its provision, not its content. Such complaints seem frivolous to those in less affluent countries where millions die of correctable diseases or of malnutrition. Valid or not, elderly Americans believe they spend such a disproportionate amount of their tax money and Gross National Product on health care that everyone deserves the best; and this conception equates in most people's minds with instant cure and unending vigorous life. We have forgotten we are mortal.

A major source of dissatisfaction by the elderly is their concern when they go to a doctor for management of an illness or complaint that they find their care is delegated to some lesser trained doctor-substitute. Such concern would be bearable if the person in charge were a registered nurse (RN), dressed as they remember these caring women of their youth. Such an image is indelibly associated in the minds of those of us who are elderly at the millennium with quiet efficiency, healing, and compassion. Also, the dignity of the RN uniform is passé and indeed is no longer politically acceptable. Slacks and even sandals are de rigueur so long as the "provider" has a stethoscope draped around his or her neck. Like the serpent of old this black tube coiled around the neck has become the symbol of healing. In fact, to the caregivers who ostentatiously display this symbol, a snake is just about as effective as a stethoscope in providing good care.

Like it or not, the elderly must adapt to paraprofessionals managing the care of their minor complaints most of which can be just as well cared for by less costly physician-substitutes. The problem is that the elderly do not consider any of their complaints to be minor.

Those in the baby boomer generation and their progeny will not feel such dissatisfaction. They will not anticipate seeing a "real, live physician" until their disease process has made them hemodynamically unstable. They will better accept the current graduated hierarchy of providers of health care. Meanwhile, the period of transition is irksome for the elderly.

Another frequent complaint of the elderly is poor communication with their doctors. The term doctor is of course an archaic or at least obsolescent sobriquet. It has been replaced by the currently more acceptable term "provider": one who provides care much as another professional delivers the mail or once delivered the family's milk.

Elderly patients often seek medical and surgical consultation not only to relieve the aches and pains of advancing bodily degeneracy—which they know are inevitable—but to discuss such complaints with a sympathetic physician who knows them and in whom they have trust. This is seldom possible in a cost-driven health care environment where every effort must be made to use expert talents efficiently so as to provide even basic care to the needy. Physicians, most of whom are now either directly or indirectly employed by corporations for providing care, cannot be afforded the luxury of prolonged discussion with patients. They are on as strict a time schedule for seeing patients as their fellow technicians are on an automobile assembly line. This is resented as much by the physician as by the patient. The unhurried chat with the doctor often is as therapeutic as prescription medications in terms of improving subsequent quality adjusted life years.

It is anachronistic that a breakdown in communication—in this case between the doctor and the elderly patient—is a major complaint in this age of the communication revolution. It is a complaint not correctable by eliminating a glitch in the software. Such perception confuses data transmission with true communication, which requires a free give-and-take discussion between two people. Improved health care requires better physician skills for communication and a change in existing corporate operating procedures to allow time for an unhappy patient to talk with his or her physician. The doctor must not be held to a frenetic appointment schedule. Such meaningful interpersonal communication is expensive but is in the best interests of patients, which, lest we forget, is the objective of health care.

The most obvious hard evidence of change between past and current surgical care of the elderly involves the corporate structure and operations of the institutions providing care. Commercialism has replaced professionalism in response to the demand for cost-effectiveness. It is irresponsibly simplistic to believe that the greed of any professional group (be they physicians or health care administrators) is solely to blame for this change. During the twentieth century war became too costly to be left in the hands of the generals and admirals. During the twenty-first century health care has became similarly too expensive to be left as the sole responsibility of physicians.

Following the disastrous attempt by the federal government to reorganize health care during the closing decade of the twentieth century, responsibility for change went by forfeiture to private industry. The powerful forces of the marketplace began to drive the revolution in care. As with every revolution, its course involved wide pendular swings from one extreme to another. We are currently in a period of chaotic transition. Every phase of health care support and provision is in a corporate feeding frenzy. Powerful owners of hospital chains, insurers, managed care organizations, and professional physician conglomerates, like some monster gone mad, are eating their young. Before digestion is complete, those who acquired those less financially viable are in turn acquired by a still more powerful organization that dominates an ever larger part of the national market. Such corporate behavior may be acceptable in a strictly entrepreneurial market where the product for sale is an automobile or dish-washing powder; but with health care the elderly in particular recognize it is not in the best interest of the public. How long the marketplace can go unregulated remains conjectural. All signs are that excess is driving the industry toward such regulation.

This brief commentary summarizing some of the more important complaints of the elderly with their current health care serves as a stark reminder of the enormous changes that have taken place during the past quarter century in their care. Twenty-five years ago not one of the cited dissatisfactions would have been conceivable. Each (and many more unmentioned) represents a major change in the health care system.

Those involved in providing surgical care have an awesome challenge. They must provide the best professional care possible at a cost affordable to society and must contrive ways to do so in a manner acceptable to the elderly patient. The leaders brave enough to find ways to improve this uncomfortable transition period will find a few important, powerful, responsible allies at every level of government and industry. As one who has unlimited confidence in the imagination of the younger generation of surgeons who follow, I am confident the challenge will be met; but it will not come easily—it never has.

At the bottom of every page in the chapters that follow might be written an invisible footnote: "Find a way to provide this care in the best interests of the patient, at an affordable price and in a manner as convenient and comfortable to the elderly as possible." Such a challenge would have been unthinkable a generation ago. What better way can there be to emphasize the historic changes that have taken place in the surgical care of the elderly?

# 6 Principles of Geriatric Surgery

Mark R. Katlic

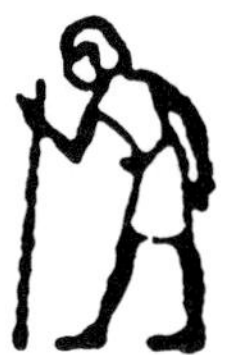

*An elderly patient is one older than his or her surgeon.*
—Anonymous

In the new millenium any surgeon who is not already a geriatric surgeon will become one. The population as a whole is aging, and the conditions that most frequently lead to surgery (e.g., atherosclerosis, cancer, arthritis, prostatism, cataract) increase in incidence with increasing years; surgeons have little influence on the age of patients referred for operation. Improving our overall care of the elderly surgical patient—the *raison d'etre* of this book—will yield great benefit.

Surgeons have always cared for the elderly, but the definition of "elderly" has changed. A threshold of 50 years was selected for the 167 patients described in a paper published in 1907,[1] and 20 years later prominent surgeons still taught that elective herniorrhaphy in this age group was not warranted.[2] Presently, complex operations are being performed in octogenarians and nonagenarians,[3–6] and elective herniorrhaphy is occasionally indicated in centenarians. In addition, the salutary results of such surgery can even influence general sentiment about medical care of the elderly. Lynn and Zeppa's study[8] of junior medical students reported that the surgery rotation, in contrast to other clerkships, positively influenced the students' attitudes about aging regardless of the students' career choices, as the elderly surgical patients were admitted and treated successfully.

Surgery therefore has much to offer the geriatric patient, but that patient must be treated with appropriate knowledge and attention to detail. Discussions of physiologic changes in the elderly and results of specific operations comprise the bulk of this book and are not presented here. A review of the extensive literature on surgery in the elderly, however, invites a distillate of several general principles (Table 6.1) which are relevant to all who care for the aged. These principles are worthwhile chiefly for propaedeutic purposes, as they cannot apply to every patient or every clinical situation. Some principles also apply to surgery in the young patient, but the quantitative differences in the elderly are significant enough to approach qualitative status. Risks of many emergency operations in the young, for example, are indeed greater than the risks of similar elective operations, but the differences are small compared to the threefold increase in the elderly. With respect to these principles the elderly need not be treated as a separate species but perhaps as a separate genus or order within the same larger group of surgical candidates.

Whether these differences in the elderly are due to age or to the medical conditions that often come with age is moot to the clinician. Lubin pointed out that the answer to the question, "Is age a risk factor for surgery?" is an unqualified "Yes." Unfortunately, the answer is not particularly useful. The real question is "What can we do as physicians to improve the patient's chances of surviving this surgical procedure?"[9] Although we become geriatric surgeons during our training, with sensitivity to these principles we can further improve the care of our grandparents, our parents, and (soon enough) our contemporaries.

## Principle I: Clinical Presentation

*The clinical presentation of surgical problems in the elderly may be subtle or somewhat different from that in the general population. This may lead to delay in diagnosis.*

The diagnosis of appendicitis becomes problematic at the extremes of age. Classic symptoms, for example, are present in a minority of elderly patients with appendicitis: in as few as 20% in Horattas et al.'s study.[10] Rebound tenderness was present in fewer than half the patients in two series[11,12] and leukocytosis in 42.9% in another.[13] To confound matters further, objective tests may point to alternative diagnoses: one of six patients has an elevated serum bilirubin level, and one of four has signs of ileus, bowel obstruction, gallstones, or renal calculi on abdom-

TABLE 6.1. Principles of Geriatric Surgery

I. The *clinical presentation* of surgical problems in the elderly may be subtle or somewhat different from that in the general population. This may lead to delay in diagnosis.
II. The elderly handle stress satisfactorily but handle severe stress poorly because of a *lack of organ system reserve.*
III. Optimal *preoperative preparation* is essential, because of principle II. When preparation is suboptimal, the perioperative risk increases.
IV. The results of elective surgery in the elderly are reproducibly good; the results of emergency surgery are poor though still better than nonoperative treatment for most conditions. The risk of *emergency surgery* may be many times that of similar elective surgery, owing to principles II and III.
V. Scrupulous *attention to detail* intraoperatively and perioperatively yields great benefit, as the elderly tolerate complications poorly, owing to principle II.
VI. A patient's age should be treated as a *scientific fact, not with prejudice.* No particular chronologic age, of itself, is a contraindication to operation (because of principle IV).

inal radiographs.[10] Unfortunately, rapid diagnosis is critical, as perforation is present in 42–60% of elderly patients despite operation within 24 hours of the onset of symptoms.[13–15]

Biliary tract disease is the most common abdominal problem leading to surgery in the aged, yet the diagnosis is often delayed. More than one-third of patients with acute cholecystitis are afebrile, one-fourth are nontender, and one-third are without leukocytosis.[16,17] Cholangitis may present only as confusion or fever of unknown origin,[18,19] and there is a normal age-related increase in sonographic common bile duct size with age.[20] Consequently, the elderly predominate in series of patients with severe complications of biliary tract disease, such as gallbladder perforation, empyema, gangrene, gallstone ileus, and cholangitis.[16–18,21,22] The first apparent symptom in many patients occurs with the complication.[23] Saunders et al.[24] reported that abdominal pain was a less prominent symptom and that the bilirubin level was nearly double in elderly patients presenting with bile duct carcinoma, compared to that of young patients seen during the same time period.

Peptic ulcer disease may present as confusion, malaise, weight loss, or anemia rather than pain.[25,26] Even with perforation pain may be absent (30% of patients in Coleman and Denham's series)[27] or minimal (84% of patients in Kane et al.'s series[28]). Objective signs of perforation, such as free intraperitoneal air on initial radiographs, are absent in as many as 50%.[29,30] Rabinovici and Manny[31] noted a discrepancy between "severe intraoperative findings" and objective parameters such as heart rate (mean 88/min), rectal temperature (37.2°C), white blood cell count (10,900/dl), and serum amylase (elevated in 3 of 41 patients). Delay in diagnosis beyond 24 hours led to increased mortality in Werbin's series[32]: 50% versus 0%.

Some have suggested that the elderly and possibly their physicians become tolerant over the years to abdominal pain, loss of energy, and other symptoms, leading to delay in diagnosis and more likely an emergency presentation. In Mulcahy et al.'s[33] series of patients with colorectal carcinoma, for example, elderly patients were nearly twice as likely (18%) as younger patients (11%) to present emergently. Old patients with perforated diverticulitis are three times more likely to have generalized peritonitis at operation than young patients.[34] Even gastroesophageal reflux disease may be diagnosed late because of decreased pain (visceral neuropathy, less gastric acidity) or its attribution to known coronary disease[35]; the elderly are more likely than their younger counterparts to present with dysphagia or wheezing.

Head and neck disease may also differ in the elderly. Sinusitis can cause subtle signs such as delirium or fever of unknown origin[36,37]; and head and neck cancers are less likely to be associated with smoking ($p < 0.01$),[38] alcohol use ($p < 0.001$),[38,39] or both ($p < 0.001$)[38,40] than in young individuals. Hyperparathyroidism is more likely to cause skeletal complaints or dementia and less likely to cause renal stones in the aged.[41–43] In Thomas and Grigg's series[44] of patients with carotid artery disease, stroke was the most common indication for surgery in octogenarians and was the least common indication in younger patients.

A few authors have reported no difference in clinical presentation between their young and old patients (e.g., Jougon et al.'s series[45] of patients with esophageal cancer and Maurice-Williams and Kitchen's[46] patients with meningioma). However, the clinician who understands that classic presentations of surgical disease occur in only a minority of elderly patients maintains the high index of suspicion necessary to minimize delay in diagnosis.

## Principle II: Lack of Reserve

*The elderly handle stress satisfactorily but handle severe stress poorly because of lack of organ system reserve.*

Functional reserve, representing the difference between basal and maximal function (Fig. 6.1), is the capacity to meet increased demands imposed by illness or trauma. Although there is variability among individuals, this organ system reserve inevitability declines in one's seventies, eighties, and nineties. With modern anesthetic and perioperative care, the elderly patient may tolerate the stress of even complex surgery, particularly if elective, but not the added stress of exceptional or emergency surgery.

The elderly patient with lung cancer, for example, can undergo routine pulmonary lobectomy with results

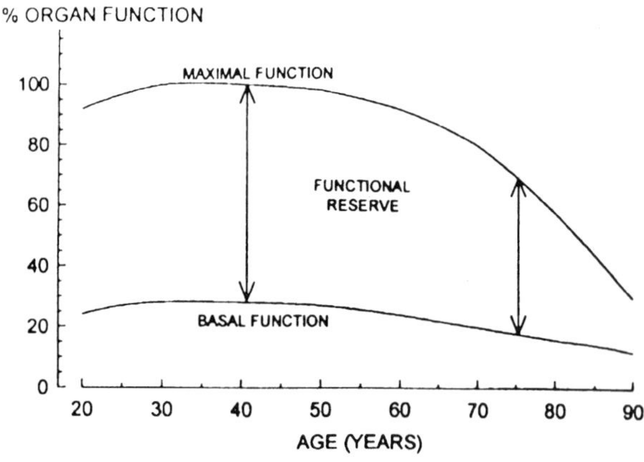


FIGURE 6.1. Organ system functional reserve is the difference between maximal function (e.g., maximal aerobic capacity in trained athletes) and basal function (e.g., basal metabolic rate). (From Muravchick,[47] with permission.)

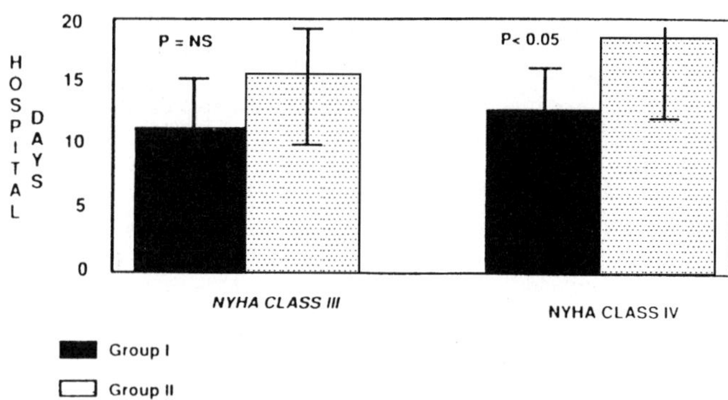


FIGURE 6.2. Hospital length of stay for aortic valve replacement patients based on New York Heart Association (NYHA) class. Group I, age less than 70 years; group II, age more than 70 years. (From Bergus et al.,[59] with permission.)

nearly indistinguishable from those of a young patient, but the added stress of concomitant chest wall resection leads to a disparate increase in risk.[48] In Keagy et al.'s series[49] the one death and two of the three respiratory failures were in patients who underwent the en bloc chest wall procedure. The aged patient, entering the operating room with decreased chest wall compliance and decreased elastic recoil as a baseline, may tolerate lung resection but lacks the reserve to handle an extended procedure. Other authors have reported increased mortality in septuagenarians and octogenarians following pneumonectomy, especially right pneumonectomy.[50–55] Approaching the other side of the spectrum, even more limited procedures, such as video-assisted thoracic surgery, may decrease stress further by preserving respiratory muscle strength.[56] Yim reported no deaths or pulmonary complications following thoracoscopic surgery in 22 patients over age 75 years, five with major resections[57]; and Jaklitsch et al. found decreased mortality, length of hospital stay, and postoperative delirium after 307 video-assisted procedures in patients aged 65–90 compared to that associated with open thoracotomy.[58]

Left ventricular functional reserve assumes critical importance in elderly patients undergoing cardiac surgery. In general, results in the elderly diverge from those of young age groups only in the worst functional classes. Bergus et al.,[59] for example, found that length of stay following aortic valve replacement was significantly longer ($p < 0.05$) in septuagenarians in New York Heart Association class IV but not in class III, compared to patients under age 70 (Fig. 6.2). Patients over age 75 in Salomon et al.'s large series[60] had significantly higher mortality after coronary artery bypass grafting if they had suffered a myocardial infarction less than 3 weeks preoperatively compared to more than 3 weeks (14.1% vs. 5.2%); there was much less difference in patients younger than age 75 (3.5% vs. 2.3%). When patients over age 70 years undergo a third coronary reoperation, only those in the worse Canadian Functional Class experience increased mortality, an increase not seen in young patients in a similar class.[61] Elayda et al.[62] reported that mortality for isolated aortic valve replacement in patients over age 80 was acceptable (5.2%), but addition of concomitant procedures increased this figure significantly (27.7%).

Similar findings pertain to major abdominal surgery. Fortner and Lincer[63] found that the increased number of deaths among elderly patients undergoing hepatic resection for liver cancer were nearly all in the extended-resection group (i.e., extended right hepatectomy or trisegmentectomy), among whom 60% of deaths were due to hepatic insufficiency. In another group of hepatic resections done for metastatic colon cancer, where cirrhosis and functional hepatic reserve are less important factors, there was no difference in mortality between young and old patients.[64] Even the addition of common duct exploration to open cholecystectomy significantly increased mortality in the elderly (3.5% vs. 1.8%, $p < 0.05$).[65] A more limited operation in the elderly (e.g., for gastric cancer) need not decrease survival.[66]

Overall, functional status as assessed by the American Society of Anesthesiologists (ASA) scoring system correlates with mortality and morbidity in the elderly as it does with younger patients (Fig. 6.3).[47,67] With modern anesthetic and critical care management, an elderly patient can tolerate the stress of even complex operations. However, if the most extended procedures are contemplated, a comprehensive preoperative evaluation of functional reserve is recommended.

## Principle III: Preoperative Preparation

*Optimal preoperative preparation is essential because of principle II. When preparation is suboptimal, the perioperative risk increases.*

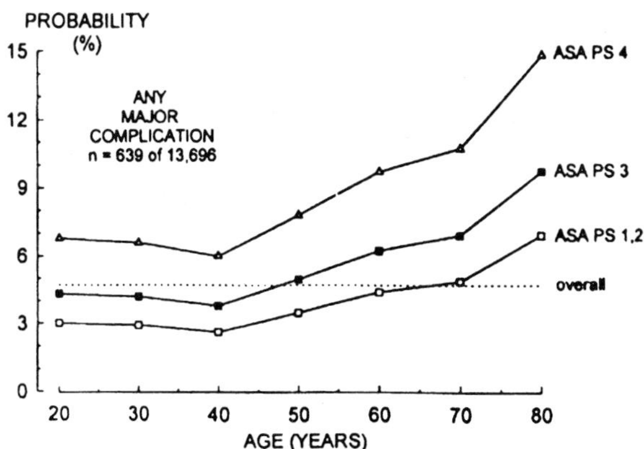


FIGURE 6.3. Probability of a major postanesthesia complication based on age and the American Society of Anesthesiologists Physical Status (ASA PS) system. (From Muravchick,[47] with permission.)

Unlike a patient's age, some factors can be improved preoperatively, with benefits in excess of those to a younger patient. No universal threshold of blood hemoglobin applies to every patient, but correction of anemia and dehydration do assume greater importance in the elderly because of their lack of system reserve. Seymour and Voz,[68] for example, found that for 288 elderly general surgical patients the most important predictors of postoperative respiratory morbidity were underlying respiratory disease, smoking, incision near the diaphragm, and volume depletion. Among the predictors of an overall good postoperative course in this series were a hemoglobin level of more than 11.0 g/dl and absence of volume depletion. Greenburg's group[69] thought that correction of anemia and dehydration contributed to their decreased incidence of cardiac complications following gastrointestinal operations in the elderly.

Pulmonary problems are among the most common perioperative complications in the elderly, in part due to decreased respiratory muscle strength. Nomori et al.[56] showed that following thoracotomy patients older than 70 years experience significant reductions in both maximum inspiratory and expiratory pressures, unlike their younger counterparts; this effect persists for 4 weeks (Fig. 6.4). Gerson et al.[70] found that the risk of pulmonary complications could be stratified in elderly surgical patients by objective measurement of exercise capacity via supine bicycle ergonometry. Nevertheless, few data exist to support the routine use of pulmonary conditioning or rehabilitation.[71] Most authors suggest smoking cessation and treatment of bronchitis and reactive airways disease such as asthma.[71,72] Prophylaxis against deep vein thrombosis and pulmonary embolism is also reasonable.[73]

The need for perioperative antibiotics for elective surgery differs with the type of surgery, though most researchers agree that advanced age is a risk factor for nosocomial infection.[74] Iwamoto et al.[75] studied 4380 patients who underwent general anesthesia for thoracic, abdominal, or neurologic surgery and concluded that advanced age is a risk factor for postoperative pneumonia, especially in patients who undergo thoracic surgery; only 1 of the 30 patients with pneumonia received preoperative antibiotics. Age over 70 years has been shown to be a risk factor for both positive bile cultures ($p < 0.001$) and septic complications of biliary surgery compared to that in younger patients[76]; antibiotic prophylaxis can reduce these complications.[77]

The value of preoperative optimization of cardiac function (e.g., via placement of a pulmonary artery catheter) is controversial. Some authors have shown clear benefit,[78] whereas others,[79,80] citing methodologic flaws in the former studies, reported no reduction in perioperative morbidity or mortality. These studies do not include exceptionally high risk or very elderly patients, who could well be helped by such treatment. Another unsettled issue concerns the value of aggressive preoperative

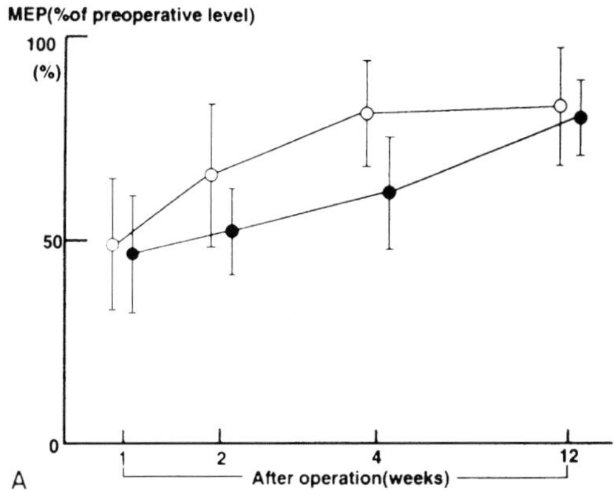


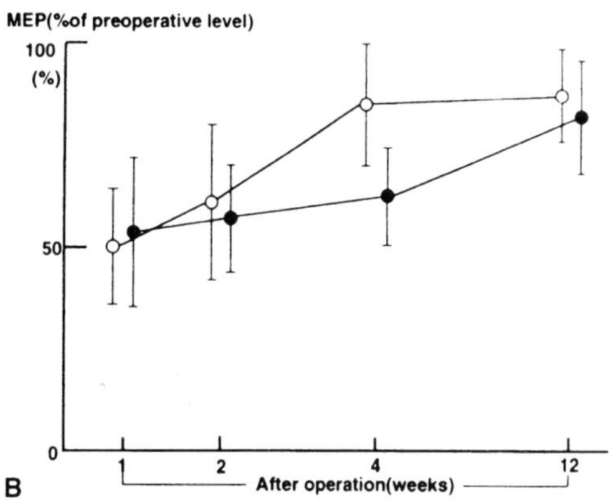


FIGURE 6.4. Postoperative changes in mean (A) maximum inspiratory pressure (MIP, percent of preoperative level) and (B) maximum expiratory pressure (MEP, percent of preoperative level) following pulmonary resection in 36 patients younger than 69 years (open circles) and 12 patients older than 70 years (closed circles). (From Nomori et al.,[56] with permission.)

screening for coronary and carotid artery disease, particularly in patients scheduled for peripheral vascular surgery. Bernstein et al.,[81] for example, believes that such screening contributed to his 0% mortality among 78 elective abdominal aortic aneurysm resections in patients over age 70. Leppo[82] considered age over 70 years one of several risk factors (the others being a history of angina, congestive heart failure, diabetes mellitus, prior myocardial infarction, and ventricular ectopy), which should trigger further cardiac assessment.

Striving for an optimal preoperative nutritional state also seems desirable, but the value of this parameter too is difficult to prove. Even active, community-dwelling older individuals are weaker preoperatively than younger ones, and they manifest impaired recovery of strength after major surgery.[83] It is unclear how to alleviate this problem. Souba[84] reviewed the literature on nutritional support and concluded that preoperative nutritional support should be reserved for severely malnourished patients scheduled to undergo major elective surgery and then should be provided for no more than 10 days.

A number of authors, in addition to those already cited, attribute their improved results in elderly patients to aggressive preoperative preparation. Bittner et al.[85] believed that the significant decrease in mortality after total gastrectomy in patients older than 70 years (32.0% in 1979 to 4.4% in 1996) was the result of standardized perioperative antibiotics, thromboembolic prophylaxis, "a systematic analysis of risk factors and their thorough preoperative therapy," and nutritional support for the malnourished. Lo et al.[86] noted that mortality for adrenal surgery in the elderly has fallen from 26% to 2–4% because of better preparation of patients before operation in order to avoid subsequent hormonal dysfunction.

Hypovolemia is tolerated poorly by the elderly patient, and it should be corrected. Treating other correctable aberrations such as bronchitis, anemia, and hypertension preoperatively increases the elderly patient's chance for a smooth postoperative course.

## Principle IV: Emergency Surgery

*The results of elective surgery in the elderly are reproducibly good; the results of emergency surgery are poor though still better than nonoperative treatment for most conditions. The risk of emergency surgery may be many times that of similar elective surgery because of principles II and III.*

For most common operations and many complex operations the results of elective surgery in the elderly are good, frequently indistinguishable from the results in younger counterparts. Coyle et al.[87] reported the results of carotid endarterectomy in 79 octogenarians at Emory University Hospital and summarized the results of five other series; morbidity and mortality were similar to those in a younger cohort (Table 6.2). Maehara et al.[88] reported 0% operative mortality in 77 patients over age 70 who underwent resection of gastric carcinoma; and Jougon et al.'s[45] results for esophagectomy in 89 patients aged 70–84 years were identical to those in 451 younger patients (Table 6.3). Although some researchers[50–55,89,90] found increased operative mortality for pneumonectomy in the elderly, others[72,91–94] have found that the risk of major complication or death is not related to age; in addition, long-term survival is identical to that in young patients (Fig. 6.5).[72]

Identical operations done emergently in the elderly, however, carry at least a threefold (and as much as a tenfold) increased risk.[69,95–97] Keller et al.,[97] for example, reported 31% morbidity and 20% mortality in 100 patients over age 70 who underwent emergency operation, which is significantly more ($p < 0.0005$) than the 6.8% morbidity and 1.9% mortality following elective operation in 513 similar patients. Length of stay was also dramatically increased following these emergency procedures (Fig. 6.6). A common procedure such as elective cholecystectomy can be performed in young and old with the risk of death approaching 0%; the risk of mortality for emergency cholecystectomy increases somewhat in the

TABLE 6.2. Reported Complication Rates for Patients Undergoing Carotid Endarterectomy

| Reference | Age range (years) | No. of patients | Stroke | Death | Stroke + death |
|---|---|---|---|---|---|
| Treiman et al.[a] | 80–91 | 183 | 3 (1.6%) | 3 (1.6%) | 6 (3.2%) |
| Pinkerton and Gholkar[b] | 75–91 | 115 | 0 | 1 (0.9%) | 1 (0.9%) |
| Rosenthal et al.[c] | 80–88 | 90 | 5 (6.0%) | 2 (2.2%) | 7 (8.2%) |
| Schultz et al.[d] | 80–93 | 90 | 1 (1.1%) | 2 (2.2%) | 3 (3.3%) |
| Ouriel et al.[e] | >75 | 77 | 3 (3.9%) | 0 | 3 (3.9%) |
| Present series | 80–89 | 79 | 0 | 1 (1.3%) | 1 (1.3%) |
| *Total* | | 634 | 12 (1.9%) | 9 (1.4%) | 21 (3.3%) |

*Source:* Coyle et al.,[87] with permission.

[a] Treiman RL et al., Carotid endarterectomy in the elderly. Ann Vasc Surg 1992;6:321–324.

[b] Pinkerton JA et al., Should patient age be a consideration in carotid endarterectomy? J Vasc Surg 1990;11:650–658.

[c] Rosenthal D et al., Carotid endarterectomy in the octogenarian: is it appropriate? J Vasc Surg 1986;3:782–787.

[d] Schultz RD et al., Carotid endarterectomy in octogenarians and nonagenarians. Surg Gynecol Obstet 1988;166:245–251.

[e] Ouriel K et al., Carotid endarterectomy in the elderly patient. Surg Gynecol Obstet. 1986;162:334–336.

TABLE 6.3. Esophagectory Morbidity and Mortality: Long-Term Results

| Result | Group 1 (≥70 years) | Group 2 (<70 years) | Statistical comparison |
|---|---|---|---|
| Morbidity | 22 (24.7%) | 121 (26.8%) | $\chi^2 = 0.10$; $p = 0.78$ (NS) |
| Hospital mortality | 7 (7.8%) | 24 (5.3%) | $\chi^2 = 0.82$; $p = 0.53$ (NS) |
| Mean postoperative hospital stay | 23.3 | 23.18 | ANOVA (NS) |
| Survival (1, 3, 5 years) | 59.1%, 23.3%, 13.3% | 64.0%, 25.9%, 20.7% | Log rank test, $p = 0.13$ (NS) |

*Source:* Jougon et al.,[45] with permission.
ANOVA, analysis of variance; NS, not significant.

younger group (1–2%) but increases a great deal in the elderly (5–15%).[21,64,98,99] More recently Lo et al.[100] reported no mortality following laparoscopic cholecystectomy for acute cholecystitis in the elderly, though only 13 patients underwent urgent operation; in addition, elderly patients had a significantly higher rate of conversion to open cholecystectomy (23.3% vs. 2.5%, $p < 0.05$).

The emergency nature of the operation is clearly a risk factor for cardiac surgery.[5,101–104] With respect to aortic valve replacement in the elderly, rare series[105] have reported no increased risk with emergency operation, but most[106–108] report that urgent or emergency status adversely influences early or late mortality (or both). Elective surgery for peptic ulcer disease in the elderly carries a risk of 0–10% in contrast to 20–30% for emergency surgery.[26,30,109] Elective operative mortality for colorectal surgery is as low as 1.5–3.0%, rising to over 20% for emergency operation[110–113] (Table 6.4).

Death is rare following elective inguinal herniorrhaphy[114] but occurs in 8–14% of elderly patients requiring emergency repair.[114,115] In Burns-Cox et al.'s series of operations in nonagenarians[116] three of the seven deaths following emergency surgery were in patients operated on for incarcerated hernia. The need for emergency hernia surgery also rises dramatically with age (Fig. 6.7).[117] Hernias, particularly in the elderly, should be repaired electively.

A patient's advanced age therefore weighs in favor of commencing rather than deferring needed elective surgery.

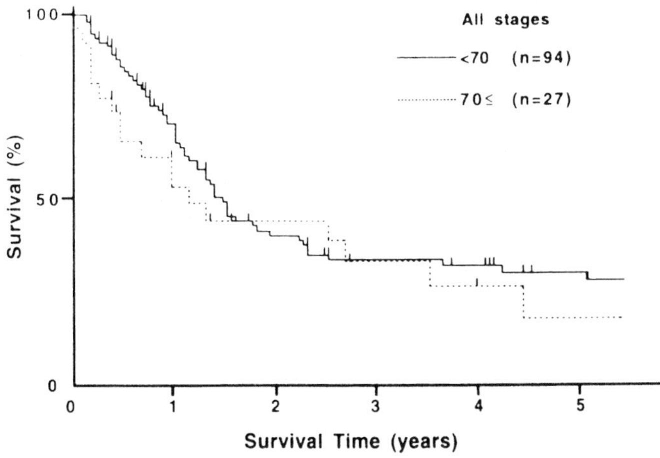


FIGURE 6.5. Pneumonectomy for bronchogenic carcinoma. Survival curves for patients under age 70 years (solid line) and over age 70 years (broken line). (From Mizushima et al.,[72] with permission.)

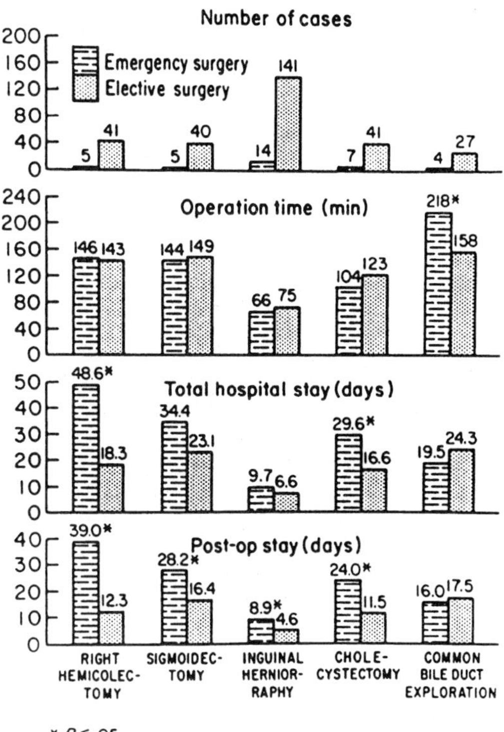


FIGURE 6.6. Emergency surgery resulted in significantly prolonged hospitalization when compared with similar elective procedures in patients older than 70 years. (From Keller et al.,[97] with permission.)

## Principle V: Attention to Detail

*Scrupulous attention to detail intraoperatively and perioperatively yields great benefit, as the elderly tolerate complications poorly (because of principle II).*

Perioperative blood loss is the *bête noire* of geriatric surgery, as the elderly lack the resilient compensatory mechanisms necessary to restore homeostasis. Fong et al.[64] found that the only independent predictor of postoperative complications in 138 patients over age 70 who underwent pancreatic resection was intraoperative blood loss of more than 2 liters. The need for meticulous hemostasis has also been promoted for elderly cardiac surgery

TABLE 6.4. Published Results of Colorectal Resection in the Elderly Population

| Study | Year | Age of patients (years) | Case (no.) | | Mortality (%) | |
|---|---|---|---|---|---|---|
| | | | Elective | Emergent | Elective | Emergent |
| Calabrese et al.*[ak] | 1973 | >80 | 107 | 49 | 22.0 | 41 |
| Kragelund et al.[b] | 1974 | >75 | 333[l] | — | 21.0[l] | — |
| Hobler[c] | 1985 | >80 | 61[l] | — | 2.2[l] | — |
| Greenburg et al.*[dk] | 1985 | >70 | 133 | 30 | 7.5 | 23 |
| Payne et al.[e] | 1986 | >75 | 310[l] | — | 9.0[l] | — |
| Waldron et al.[f] | 1986 | >70 | 197 | 242 | 18.0 | 38 |
| Keller et al.[g] | 1987 | >70 | 143 | 16 | 1.4 | 13 |
| Lewis and Khoury.[h] | 1988 | >80 | 92[l] | — | 19.0[l] | — |
| Morel et al.[ik] | 1989 | >80 | 93 | 22 | 18.0 | 27 |
| Wise et al.[jk] | 1991 | >80 | 56[l] | — | 7.0[l] | — |
| Current series | | | | | | |
| All cases[k] | | >80 | 104 | 36 | 3.8 | 22 |
| Colorectal resections | | >80 | 99 | 24 | 3.0 | 21 |
| Colorectal carcinoma[k] | | >80 | 86 | 17 | 4.7 | 29 |

*Source:* Spivak et al.,[110] with permission.
[a] Calabrese et al., Geriatric colon cancer. Am J Surg 1973;125:181–184.
[b] Kragelund et al., Resectability, operative mortality, and survival of patients in old age with carcinoma of the colon and rectum. Dis Colon Rectum 1974;17:617–621.
[c] Hobler et al., Colon surgery for cancer in the very elderly. Ann Surg 1985;203:129–131.
[d] Greenburg et al., Mortality and gastrointestinal surgery in the aged. Arch Surg 1981;116:788–789.
[e] Payne et al., Surgery for large bowel cancer in people aged 75 years and older. Dis Colon Rectum 1986;29:733–737.
[f] Waldron et al., Emergency presentation and mortality from colorectal cancer in the elderly. Br J Surg 1986;73:214–216.
[g] Keller SM et al., Emergency and elective surgery in patients over age 70. Am Surg 1987;53:636–640.
[h] Lewis AAM, Khoury GA. Resection for colorectal cancer in the very old: are the risks too high? BMJ 1988;296:459–461.
[i] Morel P et al., Results of operative treatment of gastrointestinal tract tumors in patients over 80 years of age. Arch Surg 1989;124:662–664.
[j] Wise et al., Abdominal colon and rectal operations in the elderly. Dis Colon Rectum 1991;34:959–963.
[k] All procedures including colostomies.
[l] Total cases.

patients. In Sisto et al.'s series[118] 6 of 23 octogenarians who required reexploration for bleeding died; and Logeais et al.[107] found that reoperation for tamponade after aortic valve replacement placed the elderly patient at exceptional risk of mortality ($p < 0.001$). Maurice-Williams and Kitchen[46] reported that postoperative intracranial bleeding following craniotomy for meningioma was especially age-related, occurring in 20% of 46 elderly patients and 0% of 38 young patients ($p < 0.05$); they observed that in the young patients there was a greater tendency for the brain to expand to obliterate deadspace left by removal of the mass.

Even if surgical bleeding in the elderly does not lead to reexploration, it may increase the risk of other complications such as infection. Chen et al.[119] recommended extra efforts to secure hemostasis and to facilitate bile drainage

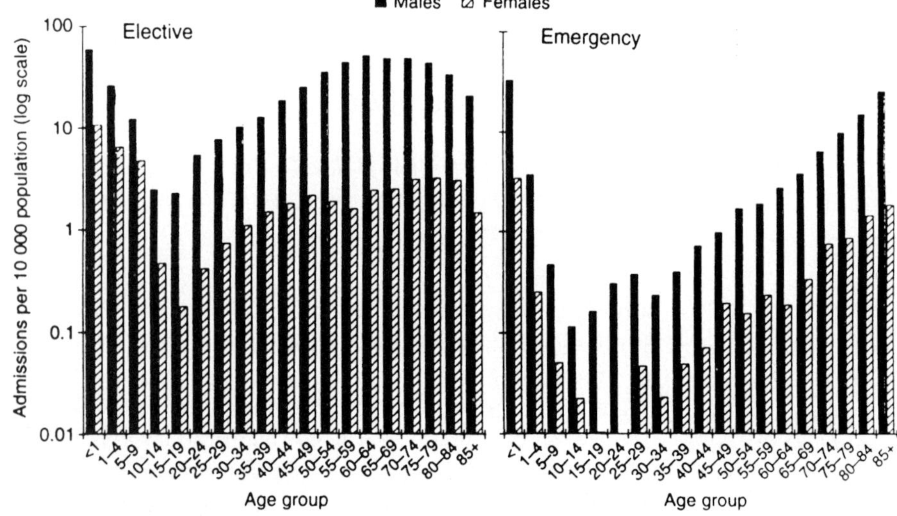


FIGURE 6.7. Age-specific and sex-specific admission rates for inguinal hernia repair in Oxford, UK, 1976–1986. (From Primatesta and Goldacre,[117] with permission.)

after hepatic resection in the aged to decrease the risk of intraperitoneal sepsis. Other measures to lower the risk of septic complications should be considered. Franko and Cohen[120] found that a general surgical problem occurring after vascular surgery carried a high risk of mortality; they suggested that intraoperative pathology should be treated prior to or at the same time as vascular surgery (e.g., cholecystectomy) or that the vascular procedure should be delayed (e.g., diverticulitis). Watenberg et al.,[121] in a series of patients over age 70 with gastrointestinal tumors, reported high rates of complications and death when a diseased gallbladder (symptomatic or not) was left in situ; they strongly recommended incidental cholecystectomy in the elderly. Huchcroft et al.,[122] however, reported that the presence of cancer per se was not an added risk factor for surgical wound infection in the elderly.

Careful surgical technique is important in any patient, but it becomes crucial in the very old. Anastomotic leak after gastric or esophageal resection, for example, carries a risk of death of 36–60%, which approaches 100% in the very elderly,[123–125] yet this complication can be minimized by careful technique.[126] Only one of Bandoh et al.'s[127] 60 elderly patients who underwent total gastrectomy for cancer suffered a leak, as did only 2 of 163 patients over age 70 in Bittner et al.'s series.[85] The elderly cardiac surgery patient may require extra care when they have a calcified aorta (e.g., epicardial echocardiography or modified clamping or cannulation techniques) or a fragile sternum (e.g., additional or pericostal wires).[128] Operative speed has become less important than technique: In Cohen et al.'s series[4] of 46 nonagenerarians undergoing major procedures the duration of the operation was not correlated with mortality.

Perioperative monitoring has also been credited with lowering risk in the elderly. Bernstein et al.[81] thought that the lack of mortality among 78 patients over age 70 who underwent abdominal aortic aneurysmectomy was promoted by intensive hemodynamic monitoring and the autotransfusion apparatus. Hemodynamic monitoring and intensive care were emphasized by Alexander et al.,[6] who reported excellent results for 59 octogenarians who underwent major upper abdominal cancer operations and by Lo et al.[86] for 85 elderly patients who underwent adrenal surgery at the Mayo Clinic.

Surgeons should continue to be taught the aphorism, "Elderly patients tolerate operations but not complications."

## Principle VI: Age Is a Scientific Fact

*A patient's age should be treated as a scientific fact, not with prejudice. No particular chronologic age, of itself, is a contraindication to operation (because of principle IV).*

Great biologic variability exists among the elderly, with some centenarians proving to be healthier than their sons and daughters. Nevertheless, advanced age can be prejudicial to optimal care, particularly when that care involves invasive procedures. Despite the fact that elderly patients treated for lung cancer have survivals equal to those of their younger matched counterparts[52,54,72,129–132] (Fig. 6.5), Nugent et al.[133] found that patients older than age 80 were significantly less likely ($p < 0.05$) to be treated surgically. Although operative mortality is increased in the elderly for extensive resections (e.g., en bloc chest wall resection), the 5-year survival of 27.7% is still better than that offered by any other treatment.[48] Dajczman et al.[134] found that elderly patients with small-cell lung carcinoma were more likely to have suboptimal therapy and were rarely entered into clinical trials, even when co-morbidity was taken into account; interestingly, their survival was comparable to that in younger age groups despite this less aggressive treatment.

A number of studies have shown that resection rates for colon cancer are lower in the elderly than in their younger counterparts,[135–137] although results of colon surgery are good, even in octogenarians and nonagenarians.[138,139] Survival rates following resection of colorectal carcinoma are comparable to those in younger patients (Fig. 6.8).[33,140,141] Elderly women with ovarian cancer are less likely to undergo definitive chemotherapy or surgery than younger patients.[142] Elderly women with breast cancer were less likely to have had screening mammograms[143,144] and were more likely to present in advanced stages than younger women[144]; once diagnosed, they tolerated surgery well[145,146] and received appropriate adjuvant therapy.[147] Selection bias in the elderly may also lead

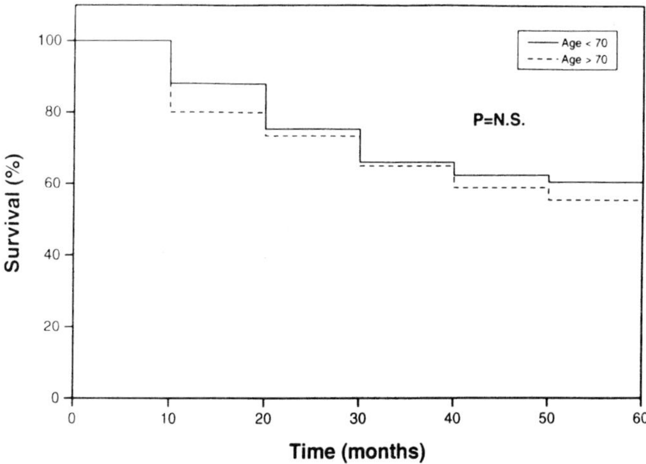


FIGURE 6.8. Crude survival following resection of colorectal cancer for two age groups: younger than 70 years (solid line) and older than 70 years (broken line). N.S., not significant. (From Avital et al.,[140] with permission.)

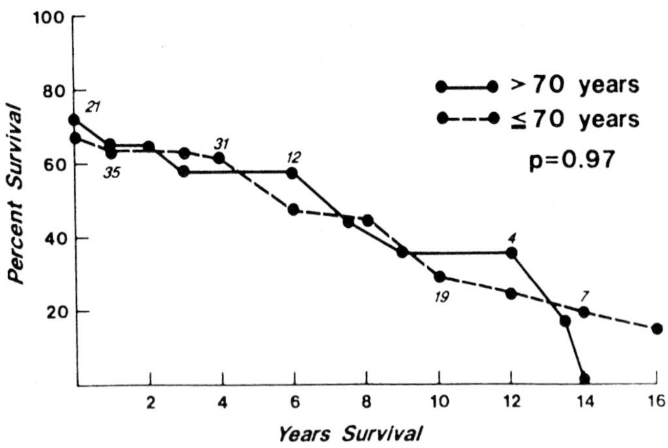


FIGURE 6.9. Postinfarction ventricular septal defect. Long-term survival in patients younger (solid line) and older (broken line) than 70 years. (From Muehrcke et al.,[160] with permission.)

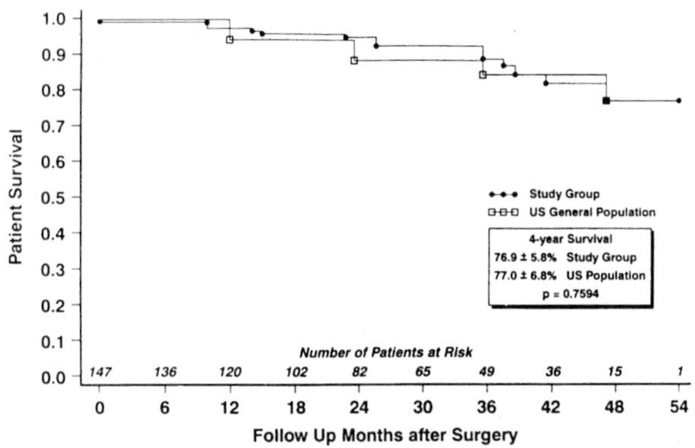


FIGURE 6.11. Cardiac valve surgery in patients over age 75 years. Kaplan-Meier analysis of survival, comparing the study group to an age-, race-, and gender-matched US general population. (From Shapira et al.,[161] with permission.)

to delay in referral for coronary artery bypass[5] or abdominal aortic aneurysm surgery.[148]

Some studies report increased rates of complications in the elderly, but overall results do not differ from those of younger patients for a wide of variety of procedures: neurosurgery[46,152,153]; head and neck surgery[38,39,41,149–151]; carotid endarterectomy[44,154–156] (Table 6.2); cardiac surgery[5,62,128,157–161] (Fig. 6.9); esophagectomy[45,162,163] (Table 6.3, Fig. 6.10); gastrectomy[6,88]; pancreatoduodenectomy[64,164]; radical hysterectomy[165–167]; total knee replacement[168,169]; microvascular free tissue transfer[170]; and hernia.[171]

For most patients, general medical condition and associated problems are more important than age (Fig. 6.3). Dunlop et al.[172] studied 8889 geriatric surgical patients in Canada and concluded that the severity of illness on admission was a much better predictor of outcome than age; Akoh et al.[67] presented similar findings in 171 octogenarians undergoing major gastrointestinal surgery. For elderly patients undergoing surgery for cancer, the stage of the malignancy influences outcome more than age.[149] Some geriatric surgery patients, even nonagenerarians,[3] have survival rates equal to those expected in the general age-matched population[158,161] (Fig. 6.11). As noted above, even the sobering results of emergency surgery in the elderly are better than the results of nonoperative treatment for most conditions.

A patient's age should be considered but not feared.

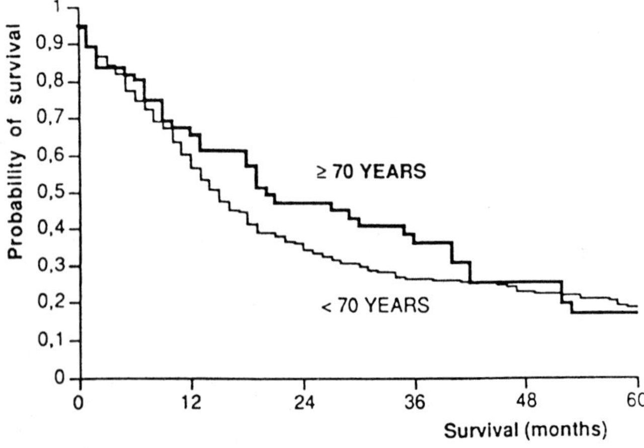


FIGURE 6.10. Survival (Kaplan-Meier) following resection of esophageal carcinoma. (From Thomas et al.,[163] with permission.)

## Conclusions

Surgical problems abound in the aged. However we define the elderly, they are increasing in number worldwide. Surgeons must become students of physiologic changes that occur with aging and then apply this knowledge, guided by a few general principles, to daily clinical care. The results of surgery in the elderly do not support prejudice against advanced age. We owe it to our elders to become good geriatric surgeons, and in so doing we will become better surgeons to patients of all ages.

## References

1. Smith OC. Advanced age as a contraindication to operation. Med Rec (NY) 1907;72:642–644.
2. Ochsner A. Is risk of operation too great in the elderly? Geriatrics 1967;22:121–130.
3. Warner MA, Hosking MP, Lobdell CM, et al. Surgical procedures among those >90 years of age. Ann Surg 1988;207:380–386.
4. Cohen JR, Johnson H, Eton S, et al. Surgical procedures in patients during the 10th decade of life. Surgery 1988;104:646–651.
5. Blanche C, Matloff JM, Denton TA, et al. Cardiac operations in patients 90 years of age and older. Ann Thorac Surg 1997;63:1685–1690.

6. Alexander HR, Turnball AD, Salamon J, et al. Upper abdominal cancer surgery in the very elderly. J Surg Oncol 1991;47:82–86.
7. Katlic MR. Surgery in centenarians. JAMA 1985;253:3139–3141.
8. Lynn BS, Zeppa R. Student attitudes about surgery in older patients before and after a surgical clerkship. Ann Surg 1987;205:324–328.
9. Lubin MF. Is age a risk factor for surgery? Med Clin North Am 1993;77:327–333.
10. Horattas MC, Guyton DT, Wu D. A reappraisal of appendicitis in the elderly. Am J Surg 1990;160:291–293.
11. Owens RJ, Hamit HF. Appendicitis in the elderly. Ann Surg 1978;187:392–396.
12. Elangovan SE. Clinical and laboratory findings in acute appendicitis in the elderly. J Am Board Fam Pract 1996;9:75–78.
13. Lan WY, Fan ST, Yiu TF, Chu KW, Lee JMH. Acute appendicitis in the elderly. Surg Gynecol Obstet 1985;161:157–160.
14. Hall A, Wright T. Acute appendicitis in the geriatric patient. Am Surg 1976;42:147–150.
15. Paajanen H, Kettunen J, Kostiainen S. Emergency appendectomies in patients over 80 years. Am Surg 1994;60:950–953.
16. Morrow DJ, Thompson J, Wilson SE. Acute appendicitis in the elderly. Arch Surg 1978;113:1149–1152.
17. Hafif A, Gutman M, Kaplan O, et al. The management of acute cholecystitis in elderly patients. Am Surg 1991;57:648–652.
18. Boey JH, Way LW. Acute cholecystitis. Ann Surg 1980;191:264–269.
19. Saharia PC, Cameron JL. Clinical management of acute cholecystitis. Surg Gynecol Obstet 1976;142:369–372.
20. Lygidakis NJ. Choledochoduodenostomy in calculus biliary tract disease. Br J Surg 1981;68:762–775.
21. Houghton PWJ, Jenkinson LR, Donaldson LA. Cholecystectomy in the elderly: a prospective study. Br J Surg 1985;72:220–222.
22. Kurtz RJ, Hermann TM, Bech AR, Kurz AB. Patterns of gallstone ileus over a 45 year period. Am J Gastroenterol 1985;80:95–98.
23. Roslyn J, Busuttel RW. Perforation of the gallbladder: a frequently mismanaged condition. Am J Surg 1979;137:307–312.
24. Saunders K, Tompkins R, Longmore W, Roslyn J. Bile duct carcinoma in the elderly. Arch Surg 1991;126:1186–1191.
25. Amberg JR, Zboralske FF. Gastric ulcers after 70. AJR 1966;96:393–399.
26. Clinch D. Baneji AK, Ostich G. Absence of abdominal pain in elderly patients with peptic ulcer. Age Ageing 1985;13:120–123.
27. Coleman JA, Denham MJ. Perforation of the peptic ulceration in the aged. Acta Chir Scand 1974;140:396–405.
28. Kane E, Fried G, McSherry CK. Perforated peptic ulcer in the elderly. J Am Geriatr Soc 1981;29:224–227.
29. Feyno G. Diagnostic problems of acute abdominal diseases in the aged. Acta Chir Scand 1974;140:396–405.
30. Narayana M, Steinhuber FU. Changing face of peptic ulcer in the elderly. Med Clin North Am 1976;60:1159–1172.
31. Rabinovici R, Manny J. Perforated duodenal ulcer in the elderly. Br J Surg 1991;157:121–125.
32. Werbin N, Kashton H, Wasserman I, Wiznitzer T. Perforated duodenal ulcer in the elderly patient. Can J Surg 1990;33:143–144.
33. Mulcahy HE, Patchett SE, Daly L, O'Donoghue DP. Prognosis of elderly patients with large bowel cancer. Br J Surg 1994;81:736–738.
34. Watters JM, Blakslee JM, March RJ, Redmond ML. The influence of age on the severity of peritonitis. Can J Surg 1996;39:142–146.
35. Gorman RC, Morris JB, Kaiser LR. Esophageal disease in the elderly patient. Surg Clin North Am 1994;74:93–112.
36. Knutson JW, Slavin RG. Sinusitis in the aged. Drugs Aging 1995;7:310–316.
37. Norman DC, Toledo DS. Infections in elderly persons: an altered clinical presentation. Clin Geriatr Med 1992;8:713–719.
38. Koch WM, Patel H, Brennan J, Boyle JO, Sidransky D. Squamous cell carcinoma of the head and neck in the elderly. Arch Otolaryngol Head Neck Surg 1995;121:262–265.
39. Ehlinger P, Fossion E, Vrielinck L. Carcinoma of the oral cavity in patients over 75 years of age. Int J Oral Maxillofac Surg 1993;22:218–220.
40. Nelson JF, Ship I. Intraoral carcinoma. J Am Diet Assoc 1971;82:564–568.
41. Ohrvall U, Akerstrom G, Lyringhall S, et al. Surgery for sporadic hyperparathyroidism in the elderly. World J Surg 1994;18:612–618.
42. Chigot JP, Menegaux F, Achrafi H. Should primary hyperparathyroidism be treated surgically in elderly patients older than 75 years? Surgery 1995;117:397–401.
43. Whitman ED, Norton JA. Endocrine surgical diseases of elderly patients. Surg Clin North Am 1994;74:127–144.
44. Thomas PC, Grigg M. Carotid artery surgery in the octogenarian. Aust NZ J Surg 1996;66:231–234.
45. Jougon JB, Ballester M, Duffy J, et al. Esophagectomy for cancer in the patient aged 70 years and older. Ann Thorac Surg 1997;63:1423–1427.
46. Maurice-Williams RS, Kitchen ND. Intracranial tumors in the elderly: the effect of age on the outcome of first time surgery for meningiomas. Br J Neurosurg 1992;6:131–137.
47. Muravchick S. Choosing an anesthetic for the elderly patient. Am Rev PAN 1997;19:117–124.
48. Piehler JM, Pairolero PC, Weinland LH, et al. Bronchogenic carcinoma with chest wall invasion; factor affecting survival following en bloc resection. Ann Thorac Surg 1982;34:684–691.
49. Keagy BA, Pharr WF, Bowes DE, Wilcox BR. A review of morbidity and mortality in elderly patients undergoing pulmonary resection. Am Surg 1989;211:141–145.
50. Naunheim KS, Kesler KA, D'Orazio SA, Fiore AC, Judd DR. Lung cancer surgery in the octogenarian. Eur J Cardiothorac Surg 1994;8:453–456.
51. Dalton ML, Warner RL, Feinberg E. The increased risk of right pneumonectomy in elderly patients. Contemp Surg 1992;41:81–82.
52. Pagni S, Federico JA, Ponn RB. Pulmonary resection for lung cancer in octogenarians. Ann Thorac Surg 1997;63:785–789.

53. Massard G, Moog R, Wihlm JM, et al. Bronchogenic cancer in the elderly: operative risk and long-term prognosis. Thorac Cardiovasc Surg 1996;44:40–45.
54. Yano T, Yokoyama H, Fukuyama Y, et al. The current states of postoperative complications and risk factors after a pulmonary resection for primary lung cancer: a multivariate analysis. Eur J Cardiovasc Surg 1997;71:445–449.
55. Morandi U, Stefani A, Golinelli M, et al. Results of surgical resection in patients over the age of 70 years with non small-cell lung cancer. Eur J Cardiovasc Surg 1997;11:432–439.
56. Nomori H, Horio H, Fuyuno G, Kobayaski R, Yashima H. Respiratory muscle strength after lung resection with special reference to age and procedures of thoracotomy. Eur J Cardiovasc Surg 1996;10:352–358.
57. Yim APC. Thoracoscopic surgery in the elderly population. Surg Endosc 1996;10:880–882.
58. Jaklitsch MT, DeCamp MM, Liptay MJ, et al. Video-assisted thoracic surgery in the elderly: a review of 307 cases. Chest 1996;110:751–758.
59. Bergus BO, Feng WC, Best AA, Singh AK. Aortic valve replacement (AVR): influence of age on operative morbidity and mortality. Eur J Cardiothorac Surg 1992;6:118–121.
60. Salomon NW, Page US, Bigelow JC, et al. Coronary artery bypass grafting in elderly patients: comparative results in a consecutive series of 469 patients older than 75 years. J Thorac Cardiovasc Surg 1991;101:209–218.
61. Lytle BW, Navia JL, Taylor PC, et al. Third coronary bypass operations: risks and costs. Ann Thorac Surg 1997;64: 1287–1295.
62. Elayda MA, Hall RJ, Reul RM, et al. Aortic valve replacement in patients 80 years and older: operative risks and long term results. Circulation 1993;88:11–16.
63. Fortner JG, Lincer RM. Hepatic resection in the elderly. Ann Surg 1989;211:141–145.
64. Fong Y, Blum TLH, Fortner JG, Brennan MF. Pancreatic or liver resection for malignancy is safe and effective for the elderly. Ann Surg 1995;222:426–437.
65. Escarce JJ, Shea JA, Chen W, Qian Z, Schwartz JS. Outcomes of open cholecystectomy in the elderly: a longitudinal analysis of 21,000 cases in the prelaparoscopic era. Surgery 1995;117:156–164.
66. Tsujitani S, Katano K, Oka A, et al. Limited operation for gastric cancer in the elderly. Br J Surg 1996;83:836–839.
67. Akoh JA, Matthew AM, Chalmers JWT, Finlayson A, Auld GD. Audit of major gastrointestinal surgery in patients aged 80 years or over. J R Coll Surg Edinb 1994;39:208–213.
68. Seymour DG, Voz FG. A prospective study of elderly general surgical patient. II. Postoperative complications. Age Ageing 1989;18:316–326.
69. Greenburg AG, Saik RP, Coyle JJ, Peskin GW. Mortality and gastrointestinal surgery in the aged. Arch Surg 1981;116:788–791.
70. Gerson MC, Hurst JM, Hertzberg VS, et al. Prediction of cardiac and pulmonary complications related to elective abdominal and noncardiac thoracic surgery in geriatric patients. Am J Med 1990;88:101–107.
71. Reilly JJ. Preparing for pulmonary resection: preoperative evaluation of patients. Chest 1997;112:2065–2085.
72. Mizushima Y, Noto H, Sugiyama S, et al. Survival and prognosis after pneumonectomy for lung cancer in the elderly. Ann Thorac Surg 1997;64:193–198.
73. Chagett GP, Anderson FA Jr, Heit J, Levine MN, Wheeler HB. Prevention of venous thromboembolism. Chest 1995; 108(suppl):3125–3345.
74. Celis R, Torres A, Gatell JM, et al. Nosocomial pneumonia: a multivariate analysis of risk and prognosis. Chest 1988;93:318–328.
75. Iwamoto K, Ichiyama S, Shimokata K, Nokashima H. Postoperative pneumonia in elderly patients: incidence and mortality in comparison with younger patients. Int Med 1993;32:274–277.
76. Landau O, Kott I, Deutsch AA, Stelman E, Reiss R. Multifactorial analysis of septic bile and septic complications in biliary surgery. World J Surg 1992;16:962–965.
77. Meyer WS, Schwartz PIM, Jeekel J. Meta-analysis of randomized controlled clinical trials of antibiotic prophylaxis in biliary tract surgery. Br J Surg1990;77:283–292.
78. Berlauk JF, Abrams JH, Gilmour IJ, et al. Preoperative optimization of cardiovascular hemodynamics improves outcome in peripheral vascular surgery. Ann Surg 1991;214: 289–299.
79. Bender JS, Smith-Meek MA, Jones CE. Routine pulmonary artery catheterization does not reduce morbidity and mortality of elective vascular surgery. Ann Surg 1997;226: 229–237.
80. Ziegler DW, Wright JG, Choban PS, Flancbaum L. A prospective randomized trial of preoperative "optimization" of cardiac function in patients undergoing elective peripheral vascular surgery. Surgery 1997;122:584–592.
81. Bernstein EF, Dilley RB, Randolph HF. The improving long term outlook for patients over 70 years of age with abdominal aortic aneurysms. Ann Surg 1988;207:318–322.
82. Leppo JA. Preoperative cardiac risk assessment for noncardiac surgery. Am J Cardiol 1995;75:42D–51D.
83. Watters JM, Clancey SM, Moulton SB, Briere KM, Zhu JM. Impaired recovery of strength in older patients after major abdominal surgery. Ann Surg 1993;218:380–393.
84. Souba WW. Nutritional support. N Engl J Med 1997; 336:41–48.
85. Bittner R, Butters M, Ulrich M, Uppenbrink S, Beger HG. Total gastrectomy: updated operative mortality and long-term survival with particular reference to patients older than 70 years of age. Ann Surg 1996;224:37–42.
86. Lo CY, Van Heerden JA, Grant CS, et al. Adrenal surgery in the elderly: too risky? World J Surg 1996;20:368–374.
87. Coyle KA, Smith RB, Salam AA, et al. Carotid endarterectomy in the octogenarian. Ann Vasc Surg 1994;8:417–420.
88. Maehara Y, Oshiro T, Oiwa H, et al. Gastric carcinoma in patients over 70 years of age. Br J Surg 1995;82:102–105.
89. Ginsberg RJ, Hill LD, Eagon RT, et al. Modern thirty-day operative mortality for surgical resections in lung cancer. J Thorac Cardiovasc Surg 1983;86:654–658.
90. Deneffe G, Locquet LM, Verbeken E, Vermant G. Surgical treatment of bronchogenic carcinoma: a retrospective study of 720 thoracotomies. Ann Thorac Surg 1988;45:380–383.
91. Ishida T, Yohoyama H, Kaneko S, Sugio K, Sugimachi K. Long term results of operation for non-small cell lung cancer in the elderly. Ann Thorac Surg 1990;50:919–922.
92. Breyer RH, Zippe C, Pharr WF, et al. Thoracotomy in patients over age seventy years. J Thorac Cardiovasc Surg 1981;81:187–193.

93. Berggren H, Ekroth R, Malmberg R, Naucler J, William-Olsson G. Hospital mortality and long-term survival in relation to preoperative function in elderly patients with bronchogenic carcinoma. Ann Thorac Surg 1984;38:633–636.
94. Kadri MA, Dussch JE. Survival and prognosis following resection of primary non-small cell bronchogenic carcinoma. Eur J Cardiothorac Surg 1991;5:132–136.
95. Linn BS, Linn MW, Wallen N. Evaluation of results of surgical procedures in the elderly. Ann Surg 1982;195:90–96.
96. Gengian KS, Nambiar R. Major surgery in the elderly—a study of outcome in 295 consecutive cases. Singapore Med J 1989;30:339–342.
97. Keller SM, Markovitz LJ, Welder JR, Aufses AH. Emergency and elective surgery in patients over age 70. Am Surg 1987;53:636–640.
98. Pigott JP, Williams JB. Cholecystectomy in the elderly. Am J Surg 1988;155:408–410.
99. Harnes JK, Stradeo EW, Talsma SE. Symptomatic biliary tract disease in the elderly patient. Am Surg 1986;8:442–445.
100. Lo CM, Lai ECS, Fan ST, Liu CLL, Wong J. Laparoscopic cholecystectomy for acute cholecystitis in the elderly. World J Surg 1996;20:983–987.
101. Tsai TP, Matloff JM, Chaux A, et al. Combined valve and coronary artery bypass procedures in septuagenarians and octogenarians: results in 120 patients. Ann Thorac Surg 1986;42:681–684.
102. Tsai TP, Chaux A, Matloff JM, et al. Ten-year experience of cardiac surgery in patients aged 80 years and over. Ann Thorac Surg 1994;58:445–451.
103. Peterson ED, Cowper PA, Jollis JG, et al. Outcomes of coronary artery bypass graft surgery in 24,461 patients aged 80 years or older. Circulation 1995;92(suppl 2):85–91.
104. Nauheim KS, Dean PA, Fiore AC, et al. Cardiac surgery in the octogenarian. Eur J Cardiovasc Surg 1990;4:130–135.
105. Bergus BO, Feng WC, Bert AA, Singh AK. Aortic valve replacement (AVR): influence of age on operative morbidity and mortality. Eur J Cardiothorac Surg 1992;6:118–121.
106. Tseng EE, Lee CA, Cameron DE, et al. Aortic valve replacement in the elderly: risk factors and long-term results. Ann Surg 1997;225:793–804.
107. Logeais Y, Langanay T, Roussin R, et al. Surgery for aortic stenosis in elderly patients: a study of surgical risk and predictive factors. Circulation 1994;90:2891–2989.
108. Galloway AC, Colvin SB, Grossi EA, et al. Ten-year experience with aortic valve replacement in 482 patients 70 years of age or older: operative risk and long-term results. Ann Thorac Surg 1990;49:84–93.
109. Watson RJ, Hooper TO, Ingram G. Duodenal ulcer disease in the elderly: a retrospective study. Age Ageing 1985; 14:225–229.
110. Spivak H, Vande Maele D, Friedman I. Colorectal surgery in octogenarians. J Am Coll Surg 1996;183:46–50.
111. Bender JS, Magnuson TH, Zenilman ME, et al. Outcome following colon surgery in the octogenarian. Am Surg 1996;62:276–279.
112. Vivi AA, Lopes A, Cavalconti SD, Rossi BM, Marques LA. Surgical treatment of colon and rectum adenocarcinoma in elderly patients. J Surg Oncol 1992;51:203–206.
113. Fabre JM, Rouanet P, Elc N, et al. Colorectal carcinoma in patients aged 75 years and more: factors influencing short and long term operative mortality. Int Surg 1993;78:200–203.
114. Deysine M, Grimson R, Sorrof HS. Herniorrhaphy in the elderly. Am J Surg 1987;153:387–391.
115. Nahme AE. Groin hernia in elderly patients: management and prognosis. Am J Surg 1983;146:257–260.
116. Burns-Cox N, Campbell WB, VanNimmen AJ, Vercaeren PMK, Lucarotti M. Surgical care and outcome for patients in their nineties. Br J Surg 1997;146:257–260.
117. Primatesta P, Goldacre MJ. Inguinal hernia repair: incidence of elective and emergency surgery, readmission and mortality. Int J Epidemiol 1996;25:835–839.
118. Sisto D, Hoffman D, Frater RWM. Isolated coronary artery bypass grafting in 100 octogenarian patients [letter]. J Thorac Cardiovasc Surg 1993;106:940–944.
119. Chen MF, Hivang TL, Jeng LB, Jan YY, Wang CS. Influence of age on results of resection of hepatocellular carcinoma. Eur J Surg 1991;157:591–593.
120. Franko E, Cohen JR. General surgical problems requiring operation in postoperative vascular surgery patients. Am J Surg 1991;162:247–250.
121. Watemberg S, Landau O, Avrahami R, Nudelman IL, Reiss R. Incidental cholecystectomy in the over 70 age group. Int Surg 1997;82:102–104.
122. Huchcroft SA, Nicolle LE, Cruse PJE. Surgical wound infection and cancer among the elderly: a case control study. J Surg Oncol 1990;45:250–256.
123. Adam DJ, Craig SR, Sang CTM, Cameron EWJ, Walker WS. Esophagectomy for carcinoma in the octogenarian. Ann Thorac Surg 1996;61:190–194.
124. Inberg MN, Heinonen R, Lauren P, Rantakokko V, Vikkau SJ. Total and proximal gastrectomy in the treatment of gastric carcinoma: a series of 305 cases. World J Surg 1981;5:249–257.
125. Paolini A, Tosato F, Cassese M, et al. Total gastrectomy in the treatment of adenocarcinoma of the cardia. Am J Surg 1986;151:238–243.
126. Mathisen DJ, Grillo HC, Wilkins EW, Moncure AC, Hilgenberg AD. Transthoracic esophagectomy: a safe approach to carcinoma of the esophagus. Ann Thorac Surg 1988;45:137–143.
127. Bandoh T, Osyama T, Toyoshima H. Total gastrectomy for gastric cancer in the elderly. Surgery 1991;109:136–142.
128. Katz NM, Chase GA. Risks of cardiac operations for elderly patients: reduction of the age factor. Ann Thorac Surg 1997;63:1309–1314.
129. Duque JL, Ramos G, Castrodeza J, et al. Early complications in surgical treatment of lung cancer: a prospective multicenter study. Ann Thorac Surg 1997;63:944–950.
130. Sherman S, Gaudot CE. The feasibility of thoracotomy for lung cancer in the elderly. JAMA 1987;258:927–930.
131. Gebitekin C, Gupta NK, Martin PG, Saunders NR, Walker DR. Long-term results in the elderly following pulmonary resection for non-small cell carcinoma. Emerg J Cardiovasc Surg 1993;7:653–656.
132. Thomas P, Sielezenff I, Rajni J, Giridicilli R, Fuentes P. Is lung cancer resection justified in patients aged over 70 years? Eur J Cardiovasc Surg 1993;7:246–251.
133. Nugent WC, Edmund MT, Hammerness PG, et al. Non-small cell lung cancer at the extremes of age: impact on diagnosis and treatment. Ann Thorac Surg 1997;63:193–197.

134. Dajczman E, Fa LY, Small D, Wolkove N, Kreisman H. Treatment of small cell lung carcinoma in the elderly. Cancer 1996;77:2032–2038.
135. Samet J, Hunt WC, Hey C, Humble CG, Goodwin JS. Choice of cancer therapy varies with age of patient. JAMA 1986;255:3885–3390.
136. Irvin TT. Prognosis of colorectal cancer in the elderly. Br J Surg 1988;75:419–421.
137. Waldron RP, Donovon IA, Drumm J, Mottram SN, Tedman S. Emergency presentation and mortality from colorectal cancer in the elderly. Br J Surg 1986;73:214–216.
138. Wise WE, Padmonabhan A, Meesig DM, et al. Abdominal colon and rectal operations in the elderly. Dis Colon Rectum 1991;34:959–963.
139. Ondrula DP, Nelson RL, Prasad ML, Coyle BW, Abcarian H. Multifocal index of preoperative risk factors in colon resections. Dis Colon Rectum 1992;35:117–122.
140. Avital S, Kashton H, Hadad R, Werbin N. Survival of colorectal carcinoma in the elderly. Dis Colon Rectum 1997;40:523–529.
141. Hobler KE. Colon surgery for cancer in the very elderly; cost and 3 year survival. Ann Surg 1986;203:129–131.
142. Moore DH. Ovarian cancer in the elderly patient. Oncology 1994;8:21–29.
143. Singletary SE, Shallenberger R, Guinee VF. Breast cancer in the elderly. Ann Surg 1993;218:6667–6671.
144. Wanebo HJ, Cole B, Chung M, et al. Is surgical management compromised in elder patients with breast cancer? Ann Surg 1997;225:579–589.
145. Swanson RS, Sawicka J, Wood WC. Treatment of carcinoma of the breast in the older geriatric patient. Surg Gynecol Obstet 1991;173:465–469.
146. Van Dalsen AD, DeVries JE. Treatment of breast cancer in elderly patients. J Surg Oncol 1995;60:80–82.
147. Guadagnoli E, Shapiro C, Gurwitz JH, et al. Age-related patterns of care: evidence against ageism in the treatment of early-stage breast cancer. J Clin Oncol 1997;15:2338–2344.
148. Chalmers RTA, Stonebridge PA, John TG, Murie JA. Abdominal aortic aneurysm in the elderly. Br J Surg 1994;80:1122–1123.
149. Barzan L, Veronesi A, Caruso G, et al. Head and neck cancer and ageing: a retrospective study in 438 patients. J Laryngol Otol 1990;104:634–640.
150. McGuirt WF, Davis SP. Demographic portrayal and outcome analysis of head and neck cancer surgery in the elderly. Arch Otolaryngol Head Neck Surg 1995;121:150–154.
151. Kowalski LP, Alcantara PSM, Magrin J, Parise O. A case-controlled study on complications and survival in elderly patients undergoing major head and neck surgery. Am J Surg 1994;168:485–490.
152. Smith EB, Honigan WC. Surgical results and complications in elderly patients with benign lesions of the spinal cord. J Am Geriatr Soc 1992;40:867–870.
153. Samii M, Tatagiba M, Matthies C. Acoustic neuroma in the elderly: factors predictive of operative outcome. Neurosurgery 1992;31:615–620.
154. Schroe H, Suy R, Nevelsteen A. Carotid artery endarterectomy in patients over seventy years of age. Ann Vasc Surg 1990;4:133–137.
155. Favre JP, Guy JM, Frering V, Boissier C, Barral X. Carotid surgery in the octogenarian. Ann Vasc Surg 1994;8:421–426.
156. Treiman RL, Wagner WH, Forin RF, et al. Carotid endarterectomy in the elderly. Ann Vasc Surg 1992;6:321–324.
157. Canver CC, Nichols RD, Coller SD, Heisey DM, Murray EL, Cronke GM. Influence of increasing age on long-term survival after coronary artery bypass grafting. Ann Thorac Surg 1996;62:1123–1127.
158. Akins CW, Daggett WM, Vlahakes GJ, et al. Cardiac operations in patients 80 years old and older. Ann Thorac Surg 1997;64:606–615.
159. Chocron S, Rude N, Dussaucy A, et al. Quality of life after open-heart surgery in patients over 75 years old. Age Ageing 1996;25:8–11.
160. Muehrcke DD, Blank S, Daggett WM. Survival after repair of postinfarction ventricular septal defects in patients over the age of 70. J Cardiac Surg 1992;7:290–300.
161. Shapira OM, Kelleher RM, Zelingher J, et al. Prognosis and quality of life after valve surgery in patients older than 75 years. Chest 1997;112:885–894.
162. Adam DJ, Craig SR, Sang CTM, Cameron EWJ, Walker WS. Esophagectomy for carcinoma in the octogenarian. Ann Thorac Surg 1996;61:190–194.
163. Thomas P, Doddoli C, Neville P, et al. Esophageal cancer resection in the elderly. Eur J Cardiothorac Surg 1996;10:941–946.
164. O'Sullivan KL, Hart MJ. Pancreaticoduodenectomy in the elderly: a ten year experience. Contemp Surg 1996;48:265–269.
165. Matthews CM, Morris M, Burke TW, et al. Pelvic exenteration in the elderly. Obstet Gynecol 1992;79:773–777.
166. Levrant SG, Fruchter RG, Maiman M. Radical hysterectomy for cervical cancer: morbidity and survival in relation to weight and age. Gynecol Oncol 1992;45:317–322.
167. Geisler JP, Geisler HE. Radical hysterectomy in patients 65 years of age and older. Gynecol Oncol 1994;53:208–211.
168. Zicat B, Rorabeck CH, Bourne RB, Devane PA, Nott L. Total knee arthroplasty in the octogenarian. J Arthroplasty 1993;8:395–400.
169. Anderson JG, Wixson RL, Tsai D, Stulberg SD, Chang RW. Functional outcome and patient satisfaction in total knee patients over the age of 75. J Arthroplasty 1996;11:831–840.
170. Malata CM, Cooper RD, Batchelor AGG, et al. Microvascular free-tissue transfers in elderly patients: the Leeds experience. Plast Reconstr Surg 1996;98:1234–1241.
171. Gianetta E, DeCian F, Cuneo S, et al. Hernia repair in elderly patients. Br J Surg 1997;84:983–985.
172. Dunlop WE, Rosenblood L, Lawrason L, Birdsall L, Rusnak CH. Effects of age and severity of illness on outcome and length of stay in geriatric surgical patients. Am J Surg 1993;165:577–580.

# 7 Aging of America: Implications for the Surgical Workforce

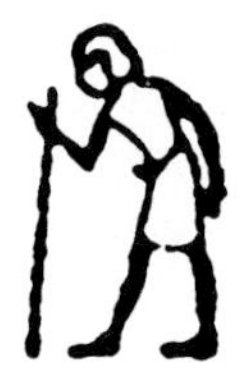

Olga Jonasson and Francis Kwakwa

Aging of the American population will have a major impact on the surgical workload for most surgical specialties. During the next two decades it is estimated that the total population will grow by nearly 13%, even though the proportion of the population under the age of 20 will decline.[1] The dramatic rise in the number of persons 65 years old and older is documented in many population studies,[2,3] as is the increase in the number of the very old, 85 years and older.[2]

Largely as a result of these population changes and the typical diseases of the elderly, surgical specialties such as general surgery will experience an increase in workload as high as 33%,[1,4,5] and workloads for the specialties of pediatrics and obstetrics will decrease. In addition to general surgery, other surgical specialties affected are thoracic, orthopedic, and vascular surgery, reflecting the likely increases in diseases of the elderly needing surgical attention: cardiovascular, cancer, arthritis, and peripheral vascular disease. Heart disease, cancer, and stroke are responsible for three-fourths of deaths in the elderly; of these, heart disease is by far the leading cause of mortality, far outpacing cancer and other conditions, and arthritis is the leading cause of disability and morbidity.[2]

The demand, as well as the need, for surgical services is also driven upward by a predominantly elderly population whose use of health care services is greater than that of the general population. On average, elderly persons visit a physician more often, are hospitalized three times the rate of the general population, and stay in the hospital 50% longer, most often as a consequence of cardiac, vascular, and gastrointestinal conditions and cancer.[2] Many of these visits and hospitalizations are surgical in nature (Table 7.1, Fig. 7.1). Of all surgical disciplines, the impact on general surgery has been most studied and is the focus of our discussion.

## Needs Analysis for General Surgery

Although it is difficult to determine the number of practicing general surgeons and their geographic distribution,[6–8] it is even more difficult to forecast the number and distribution of surgeons needed for future years.[9–13] Unpredicted changes in disease occurrence and manifestations, improvements in medical care, new technologies, new methods of health care delivery, changing life styles, and the development of nonsurgical treatments for surgical diseases combine to confound predictions of future needs and demands.[14,15]

### GMENAC Study

The "needs-based" method has been used extensively in large studies of future workforce requirements. This method is based on the assumption that full services will be provided to the entire population. An "adjusted" needs-based model was used by the Graduate Medical Education National Advisory Committee (GMENAC)[16]; the adjustment accounted for the proportion of persons in each category of medical condition *likely to seek medical care*. Delphi panels of experts in each specialty were asked to review and revise data on the incidence and prevalence of disease, the norms of care, and physician productivity in the specialty. A mathematic model then concentrated on workforce planning. Technical panels of experts studied the financing of graduate medical education (with the aim of influencing specialty selection through payment mechanisms), the availability of physician extenders for the specialty (e.g., nurse practitioners, physician's assistants), the geographic distribution of physicians, and the influence of the educational environment on the practice of the specialty. These thorough studies were conducted during 1977–1980, and needs for

TABLE 7.1. Operative Procedures for Patients Discharged from Short-Stay Hospitals: Patients ≥65 Years Old Versus All Ages

| Year and patient age | No. of operations (thousands) | Rate per 1000 population | Average length of stay (days) |
|---|---|---|---|
| 1983 | | | |
| ≥65 | 6,192 | 226.1 | 9.7 |
| All ages | 26,220 | 112.9 | 6.9 |
| 1985 | | | |
| ≥65 | 5,969 | 209.2 | 8.7 |
| All ages | 24,800 | 104.6 | 6.5 |
| 1987 | | | |
| ≥65 | 6,425 | 215.4 | 8.6 |
| All ages | 25,655 | 106.2 | 6.4 |
| 1989 | | | |
| ≥65 | 6,736 | 217.4 | 8.9 |
| All ages | 23,370 | 94.8 | 6.5 |
| 1991 | | | |
| ≥65 | 6,960 | 219.2 | 8.6 |
| All ages | 23,403 | 93.4 | 6.4 |
| 1993 | | | |
| ≥65 | 7,039 | 214.7 | 7.8 |
| All ages | 22,766 | 88.8 | 6.0 |

*Source:* Socio-Economic Factbook for Surgery, 1996–1997. American College of Surgeons, Socioeconomic Affairs Department, Chicago, with permission.

physicians in the various medical specialties in 1990 were projected based on panel integration of data regarding disease occurrence, the population, and characteristics of the health care workforce.

Based on this methodology, GMENAC concluded that there would be an excess of nearly 12,000 general surgeons by the year 1990; this figure was derived from the number of currently practicing general surgeons plus the number entering the workforce each year minus those leaving each year, their work performance, and projections of the need for surgical services. On review of the GMENAC assumptions about the workforce during 1975–1980, it is clear that errors were made when estimating the number of general surgeons and the number of residents entering general surgery each year, no doubt related to the consistent errors in classification and overcounting perpetuated by the American Medical Association's (AMA) Physician Masterfile,[6] the basic source of the data used by the Bureau of Health Professions. The misconception that an excess of general surgeons would exist in 1990 has colored much of the workforce planning and recommendations to reduce the number of general surgery residency positions by national committees and individual health care policy experts.[14,17,18]

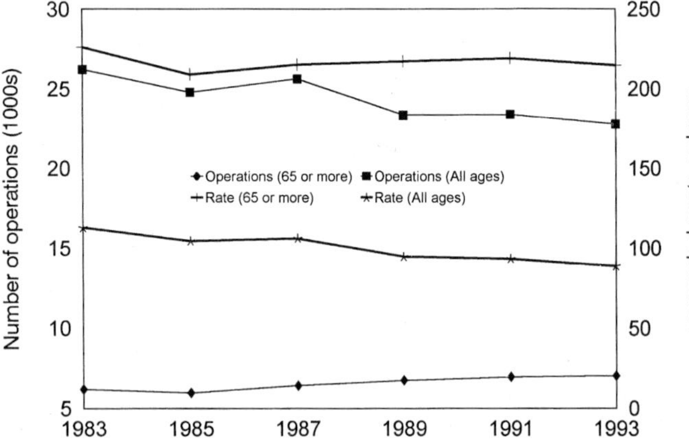


FIGURE 7.1. Data on operative procedures between 1983 and 1993 for patients discharged from short-stay hospitals show that the rate per 1000 population for patients 65 years and older is more than twice that of the general population (all ages). There is a small upward trend in the number of operative procedures for the patients 65 years and older compared to a small downward trend for the general population. (From Socio-Economic Factbook for Surgery, 1996–1997. American College of Surgeons, Socioeconomic Affairs Department, Chicago, with permission.)

## GMENAC Update: Abt Report, 1991

Because of the inaccuracies in GMENAC's projections for some specialties, in 1991 the Council on Graduate Medical Education (COGME), organized to advise the government on workforce issues in the nation's graduate medical education programs, commissioned Abt Associates to perform an update of the GMENAC study. This report, submitted to and used by COGME but never published separately, updates the GMENAC model for seven medical specialties, including general surgery and obstetrics/gynecology.[1]

As in the GMENAC study, the Abt study was derived from the medical need model rather than a demand forecast. It forecasts the number of physicians required to serve the needs of the nation if ideal levels and types of medical care are provided to meet the expected morbidity and health care needs of the population without regard to barriers such as ability to pay, access to care, availability of care, or ignorance. Expert panels again were used to (1) analyze data about incidence and prevalence of diseases and procedure rates, (2) recommend adjustments to the need for services, (3) provide information on the norms of care, and (4) indicate when care could be delegated to a physician extender or required additional physicians. The time needed for procedures and visits was calculated and a factor introduced about the work performance of the physician specialists involved. Finally, a summary of the physician specialty workforce in seven selected specialties was derived for general family practice, general internal medicine, general pediatrics, obstetrics/gynecology, general surgery, psychiatry, and child psychiatry.

The Abt report was especially informative in its analysis of the general surgery workload and supply projections for the years spanning 1990–2010. When projecting the annual supply of general surgeons (those currently practicing plus entry-level general surgeons minus those leaving general surgery) and the increased workload expected as the population ages, the study found that, unique among the seven specialties analyzed, the supply of general surgeons falls far short of need by the year 2010. Updated supply figures suggested that the supply of general surgeons was in approximate balance in 1990 and 2000, a conclusion supported by our analysis of the general surgery workforce in 1994.[6,8] The projected discrepancy for the year 2010 is the result of the aging population generating an increased requirement for general surgeons and the constrained growth in surgical residency positions, limiting the supply of new general surgeons. In fact, there has been a steady state of general surgery residency graduates since 1982 (approximately 1000 graduates each year), and the number of graduates continuing on to surgical subspecialties with completion of a general surgery residency as a prerequisite (thoracic surgery, vascular surgery, surgical oncology, pediatric surgery, transplantation) has progressively increased, producing a decline in the number of graduates who practice general surgery[19] (Fig. 7.2). If anything, the Abt projections of a deficit of 15% for general surgeons by 2010 may be optimistic and the actual deficit much larger.[20] Other specialties included in the Abt study, such as internal medicine, also will experience an increase in need for services; residency programs in internal medicine, however, have regularly expanded so the supply of internists will be adequate for the anticipated increased need (Fig. 7.3). Obstetrics/gynecology, in contrast, will be affected by the inversion of the population age characteristics and is projected to be in large oversupply (44%) by 2010 if the supply of current and new obstetricians remains as predicted by the Abt report.[1]

The General Surgery Review Panel in the Abt study

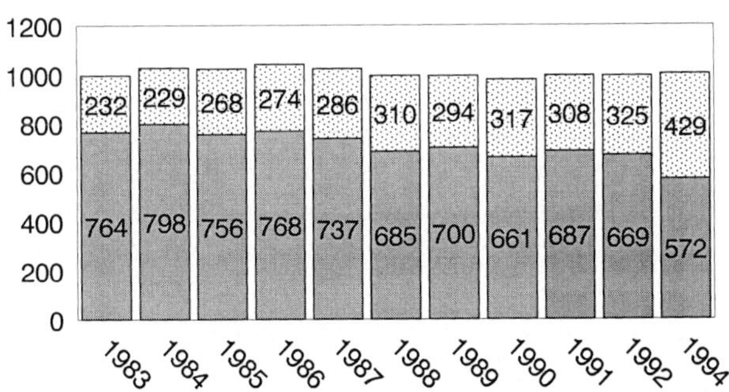


FIGURE 7.2. General surgery graduates entering accredited subspecialty residency, 1983–1994. There has been a steady state of general surgery residency graduates since 1982 (approximately 1000 graduates each year), and the number of graduates continuing to surgical subspecialties with completion of a general surgery residency as a prerequisite (thoracic surgery, vascular surgery, surgical oncology, pediatric surgery, transplantation) has increased progressively, producing a decline in the number of graduates who practice general surgery. Gray portion of bars, graduates not continuing in general medical education; dotted portion of bars, graduates entering accredited subspecialty residency.

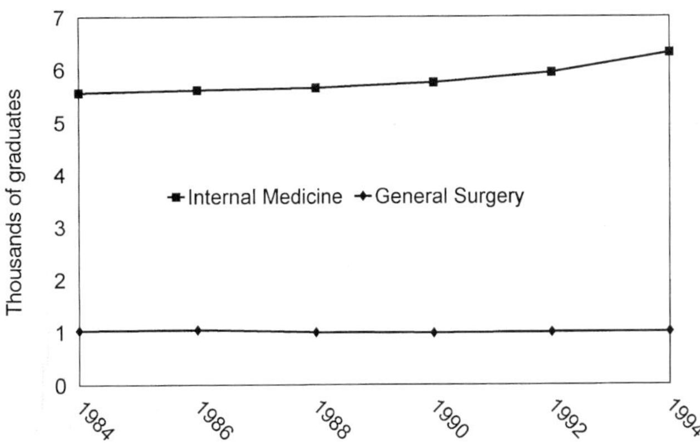


FIGURE 7.3. Graduates of general surgery and internal medicine residencies, 1984–1994. Compared to the steady state of general surgery residency graduates since 1982, residency programs in internal medicine have regularly expanded, and graduates of internal medicine have increased. (Data are from the American College of Surgeons' Longitudinal Study of Surgical Residents and from the Directory of Training Programs in Internal Medicine Residency and Subspecialty Fellowship in 1995, prepared by the University of Chicago Center for Health Administration Studies.)

analyzed only the surgical care provided to patients and did not review office visits separate from those associated with preoperative and postoperative visits. Both inpatient and outpatient surgical procedures were reviewed, with the list of procedures including about 85% of the total general surgical volume. The panel assigned a percent of the procedures that should be done by a general surgeon rather than a subspecialist. All time needed for pre- and postoperative visits and the total procedure time (including scrubbing, preparation, anesthesia induction, dictating, and writing postoperative orders) was calculated as total minutes per procedure. Procedures requiring more than one surgeon were identified.

Procedure rates in general surgery vary greatly by age subgroups of the population. Surgical procedures were grouped into 16 broad categories (ICD9-CM) used by the National Health Discharge Survey. As the population ages, projected increases of 9% (nervous system) to 26% (cardiovascular) are seen in 12 categories. Showing zero change (gynecology) or a decline (obstetrics 15%; ear 4%; nose and throat 1%) are the procedures most commonly needed in young patients. Based on these calculations, the Abt report concluded that general surgery should add 6000 general surgeons from year 2000 to year 2010 to provide the services needed.

## Changes in Surgical Care

The weaknesses of these predictions, sophisticated though the methodology may be, are clearly evident in the detailed lists of procedures used for the Abt study.

Advances in surgical technology, especially in minimal access surgery techniques and the predominance of outpatient procedures, were not anticipated even in 1991. Some of these advances have lessened the need for operation; for example, acid-reducing procedures for peptic ulcer disease have rarely been needed since the introduction of effective pharmacologic agents to reduce acid production and the identification of *Helicobacter pylori* as a treatable causative agent.[21–23] Other developments have increased the need for procedures; for example, acceptance of the laparoscopic approach for cholecystectomy has broadened its indications and increased its utilization in older patients and those with co-morbidities who were not considered for operation in past years.[24,25]

The practice of general surgeons has evolved considerably since the GMENAC study in 1980; the 10 most common procedures for general surgeons in 1980 account for less than half of the workload of general surgeons in 1991. Review of the 10 leading general surgery procedures in the Abt report in 1991 shows that it is already out of date; for example, breast conservation procedures, now the dominant treatment modality for breast cancer, are not even listed; and modified radical mastectomy appears on the top 10 list.

Advances in surgical and nonoperative techniques have many implications for the aging population. Abdominal and thoracic surgeons, and even neurosurgeons, have embraced minimal access techniques for certain procedures and have lowered the threshold for many elective surgery procedures in elderly patients. Although requiring general anesthesia, the postoperative convalescence of patients who have had surgery with a minimal access approach is often improved, and patient acceptance of needed therapy has been disproportionately enhanced by the aura of a kinder, gentler surgical method. Evidence to this effect exists for certain surgical procedures, notably cholecystectomy. [25,26] The minimal access approach is used now for many abdominal surgery procedures; and of these advanced techniques, some are clearly being applied extensively in the elderly. They include laparoscopic antireflux procedures for esophageal reflux disease, gastric stapling procedures for morbid obesity, abdominoperineal resections for rectal cancer, staging for prostate cancer, and others.[26] Because of continued improvements in instrumentation and experience among general surgeons, more applications of minimal access procedures in the abdomen are inevitable.

Of considerable importance to the elderly population is that the emphasis on screening for colon cancer and the use of colonoscopy and other screening measures have resulted in early detection of many colon cancers. More widespread use of screening for colon cancer will reduce the need for extensive colon resections by replacing them with endoluminal or local resection procedures and lessen the mortality from this disease.[27] New information about the genetic associations of colon cancer and the ability to identify and screen for the genes involved may eventually have an effect on identification and early preventive surgical measures; it raises the prospect of gene therapy for some premalignant or malignant conditions.[28] The practicing general surgeon has participated in these changes by increasing the use of fiberoptic endoscopy, a procedure that now ranks highest on the list of procedures performed by general surgeons.[29] These surgeons must keep abreast of molecular strategies as they develop, incorporating them into clinical practice.

Age of course is the most important risk factor for the development of breast cancer[30] (Table 7.2), and the widespread acceptance of screening mammography has facilitated early detection of minimal breast cancer. Image-guided technology, both stereotactic and ultrasonographic, has begun to replace open biopsy of suspicious findings on screening mammograms.[31] The treatment of minimal breast cancer may also be evolving; techniques using image-guided core excisions, laser treatment delivered through image-guided fiberoptics, and image-guided cryotherapy of minimal lesions are in the investigational phases of clinical application.[32]

New technology in the form of endovascular prostheses and stents is widely applied for peripheral vascular occlusive disease. Transfemoral placement of aortic prostheses for abdominal and thoracic aortic aneurysms is in early clinical trials; and despite technical problems apparent at long-term follow-up, the use of these endovascular prostheses is increasing and indications for their use are expanding.[33,34]

Similar advances are taking place in all surgical specialties. Notably, minimal access cardiac surgery for revascularization and valve replacement, general improvements in coronary artery surgical procedures and myocardial preservation, and laser revascularization of the myocardium have been interesting developments with a potential for improving outcomes and making cardiac surgery procedures more accessible for the elderly. Implanted ventricular assist devices have improved the treatment of severe cardiac failure in selected patients.[35]

TABLE 7.2. Risk of Breast Cancer

| Age (years) | Risk per year |
|---|---|
| 30 | 1:5900 |
| 35 | 1:2300 |
| 40 | 1:1200 |
| 50 | 1:590 |
| 60 | 1:420 |
| 70 | 1:330 |
| 80 | 1:290 |

*Source:* Henderson,[30] with permission.

In summary, surgical advances in technology, pharmacology, molecular physiology, and cell biology have greatly enhanced and altered surgical practices. Many of these advances have improved surgical care for the elderly. Surgeons must continue to require appropriate evaluation and testing of new technology so evidence of its worth is available before it is disseminated into practice. The next step is to learn the new skills before applying new techniques to patients. Keeping abreast of the rapidly evolving field of surgery provides the surgeon with constant opportunities to serve the needs of the changing demographics of the population.

## Changes in Health Care Delivery

The advent of the Medicare and Medicaid systems provided access to medical care for most elderly Americans who could seek care from the doctor of their choice in the hospital of their choice. In attempts to control the costs of these public programs, elderly patients and Medicaid recipients are being encouraged to leave traditional fee-for-service medical care and enroll in managed care organizations.[36] These organizations focus on obtaining maximum efficiency in the delivery of health care; one of the consequences of this agenda has been a reduced need for physicians in the specialties of medicine and surgery. Managed care organizations employ only the number of physicians needed to serve their enrollees; this number is smaller than the workforce available for many medical specialties and several surgical specialties.

How many surgeons will be needed, and where should they locate to ensure quality surgical care for the population? Are there special factors related to the elderly that affect this equation? These questions are difficult, and many factors influence the answers. It is apparent from the corrected count of general surgeons that the need and the supply was in near-balance during the 1990s; it is also apparent that although the supply is stable, need is increasing as the population ages. Data on supply and distribution of surgeons are available or are being gathered by other surgical specialties, taking into account the impact of the aging population.[37] These studies are needed for rational planning of graduate surgical education programs.

Studies conducted by the American College of Surgeons during the 1970s[9] and more recently[8] have shown that general surgeons are well distributed in the United States. Although most general surgeons are located in metropolitan areas and few are found in the federally designated Primary Care Health Professions Shortage Areas (PC-HPSAs), especially in rural locales, few geographic areas lack general surgeons.

The relative lack of general surgeons in rural locations may have implications for the care of the elderly. The proportion of the elderly is higher in rural areas and small towns than in nonrural areas. In 1988 people older than 65 years comprised 12% of the total U.S. population and 25% of rural populations; some of these elderly people did not qualify for Medicare or Medicaid, and a disproportionately high number were uninsured.[2,38–40] Managed care has not been established in rural areas to a great extent, and access to surgical care for these rural elderly persons may be limited. The increased need and demand for surgical services found for elderly patients is the same for rural and urban populations, and adjustments in health care delivery systems and personnel to provide surgical care to the rural populations may become necessary. New surgical residency graduates may be well advised to seek practice positions in rural areas and small towns.

## References


1. Abt Associates. Reexamination of the Adequacy of Physician Supply Made in 1980 by the Graduate Medical Education National Advisory Committee for Selected Specialties. Final Report. BHPr, DHHS. Publ. No. HSRA 240-89-0041, 1991.
2. Aging America: Trends and Projections. An information paper to the Special Committee on Aging, United States Senate 101st Congress 2nd Session, Committee print S.PRT 101-80, February 1990. 1994.
3. Projections of the Population of the United States, by Age, Sex, and Race: 1983 to 2080. Washington, DC: US Department of Commerce, Series P-25, No. 952, 1984.
4. Marder WD, Kletke PR, Silberger AB, Willke RJ. Physician Supply and Utilization by Specialty: Trends and Projections. Chicago: American Medical Association, 1988.
5. Council on Long Range Planning and Development: Report on the future of general surgery. JAMA 1989;262:3178–3183.
6. Jonasson O, Kwakwa F, Sheldon GF. Calculating the workforce in General Surgery. JAMA 1995;274:731–734.
7. Kwakwa F. Unpublished data on certified general surgeons as of March 1993 extracted from the database of the American Board of Medical Specialties (ABMS), 1994.
8. Kwakwa F, Jonasson O. The general surgery workforce. Am J Surg 1997;173:59–62.
9. Surgery in the United States: A Summary Report of the Study on Surgical Services for the United States (SOSSUS). Baltimore: American College of Surgeons and the American Surgical Association, 1975.
10. Donaldson WF. GMENAC, the numbers game. ACS Bull 1981;March:12–18.
11. Harris JE. How many doctors are enough. Health Aff (Millwood) 1986 Winter;5(4):73–83.
12. Hart LG, Wagner E, Pirzada S, Nelson AF, Rosenblatt RA. Physician staffing ratios in staff-model HMOs: A cautionary tale. Health Aff (Millwood) 1997;16:55
13. Weiner JP. The demand for physician services in a changing health care system: A synthesis. Med Care Rev 1994;50: 412–449.

14. Feil EC, Welch HG, Fisher ES. Why estimates of physician supply and requirements disagree. JAMA 1993;269:2659–2663.
15. Iglehart JK. From physician shortage to patient shortage: The uncertain future of medical practice. Health Aff (Millwood) 1986 Fall;5(3):142–151.
16. Graduate Medical Education National Advisory Committee: Summary Report to the Secretary, Department of Health and Human Services, vol 1. Publ. No. (HRA) 81–651. Hyattsville, MD: Health Resources Administration, 1980.
17. Perry HB, Detmer DE, Buchanan-Davidson DJ. Policy proposal for correcting the imbalance in general surgical manpower. Surgery 1984;95:243–248.
18. Kindig DA, Libby D. How will graduate medical education reform affect specialties and geographic areas? JAMA 1994; 272:37–42.
19. Kwakwa F, Jonasson O. The longitudinal study of surgical residents, 1993–1994. J Am Coll Surg 1996;183:425–433.
20. Jonasson O, Kwakwa F. Retirement age and the work force in general surgery. Ann Surg 1996;224:574–582.
21. Witte CL. Is vagotomy and gastrectomy still justified for gastroduodenal ulcer? J Clin Gastroenterol 1995;20:2–3.
22. Labenz J, Borsch G. Highly significant change of the clinical course of relapsing and complicated peptic ulcer disease after cure of Helicobacter pylori infection. Am J Gastroenterol 1994;89:1785–1788.
23. Axon A. Helicobacter gastroduodenitis: a serious infectious disease. Br Med J 1997;314:1430–1431.
24. Escarce JJ, Chen W, Schwartz JS. Falling cholecystectomy thresholds since the introduction of laparoscopic cholecystectomy. JAMA 1995;273:1581–1585.
25. Milheiro A, Castro Sousa F, Oliveira L, Joao Matos M. Pulmonary function after laparoscopic cholecystectomy in the elderly. Br J Surg 1996;83:1059–1061.
26. Johnson A. Laparoscopic surgery. Lancet 1997;349:631–635.
27. Winawer SJ, Fletcher RH, Miller L, Godlee F, et al. Colorectal cancer screening: clinical guidelines and rationale. Gastroenterology 1997;112:594–642.
28. Giardiello FM, Brensinger JD, Petersen GM, et al. The use and interpretation of commercial APC gene testing for familial adenomatous polyposis. N Engl J Med 1997;336: 823–827.
29. Health Care Financing Administration, Bureau of Data Management and Strategy. 1995 Medicare Part B Procedure Summary File. Washington, DC: US Department of Health and Human Services, June 30, 1996.
30. Henderson IC. Risk factors for breast cancer development. Cancer 1993;71(suppl):2127–2140.
31. Bassett L, Winchester DP, Caplan RB, et al. Stereotactic core-needle biopsy of the breast: a report of the joint task force of the American College of Radiology, American College of Surgeons, and College of American Pathologists. CA Cancer J Clin 1997;47:171–190.
32. Staren ED, Sabel MS, Gianakakis LM, et al. Cryosurgery of breast cancer. Arch Surg 1997;132:28–33.
33. Yusuf SW, Baker DM, Chuter TAM, Whitaker SC, Wenham PW, Hopkinson BR. Transfemoral endoluminal repair of abdominal aortic aneurysm with bifurcated graft. Lancet 1994;344:650–651.
34. Parodi JC. Endovascular repair of aortic aneurysms, arteriovenous fistulas, and false aneurysms. World J Surg 1996; 20:655–663.
35. Perry MO. What's new in vascular surgery. J Am Coll Surg 1997;184:223–232.
36. Ginzberg E, Ostow M. Managed care: a look back and a look ahead. N Engl J Med 1997;336:1018–1020.
37. Bureau of Health Professions, U.S. Department of Health and Human Services. National Conference, Estimating Medical Specialty Supply and Requirements in a Changing Health Care Environment: The Technical Challenge. Washington, DC: DHHS, March 27–28, 1995.
38. National Health Policy Reform: The Rural Perspective. Kansas City, MO: National Rural Health Association, 1992.
39. Health Care in Rural America. Office of Technology Assessment (OTA), Publ. No. OTA-H-434. Washington, DC: Government Printing Office, 1990.
40. Staff Report, Special Committee on Aging, United States Senate. The Rural Health Care Challenge. Washington, DC: Government Printing Office, 1988:100–145.

# 8
# Should Surgery Be Rationed for the Elderly on Cost-Effectiveness Grounds?

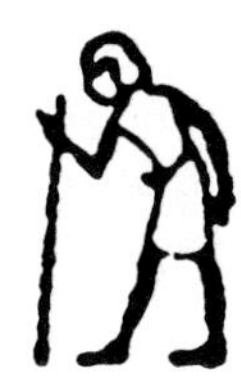

Mark Roberts

We live in a world in which health care costs continue to rise, even as society's willingness to pay those costs does not. As a result, the issue of how to limit health care expenditures is becoming increasingly salient and controversial. The suggestion has sometimes been made that one way to limit costs would be to limit care for the elderly. Such "age rationing" is often justified by the argument that care for the aged yields less benefit than care for the young. Sometimes the claim is made that such care is less likely to be successful because older people's underlying health status is often compromised by comorbidity. Alternatively, some contend that, even if successful, care for the elderly yields less benefit than care for the young, because older individuals' life expectancy is less.

I propose to critically explore such arguments, focusing especially on their underlying basis in ethics and moral philosophy. This question is important because health care resources will become increasingly scarce in the years ahead. I begin by describing the long-term, systemic forces that will produce that result. Next, I turn to the ethics of cost-effectiveness and to the assumptions one would have to make to justify certain kinds of age rationing. Then I propose an alternative perspective—namely, the argument that there are "rights" to health or health care apart from cost-effectiveness considerations. I explore one particular argument for such rights and analyze some of its implications. Finally, I argue that these questions are not resolvable within a merely technical framework. Instead, the amount and kind of care we provide for the elderly will, and should, reflect an act of national, moral, and ethical self-definition. We have a choice about what kind of society to be and to become; and care for the elderly is one arena in which that choice will be most crucially and starkly revealed.

## Why Is Some Sort of Health Care Rationing Inevitable?

Health care rationing is inevitable exactly because health care costs are increasing faster than society's capacity or willingness to pay for them. First, there is the continuing development of new technology, including new pharmaceuticals. In medical schools, teaching hospitals, research institutes, and corporate laboratories, many of humanity's most talented members are busily at work advancing biomedical technology. Such new technology, in some cases, does lower costs, but the largest professional and financial gains come from being able to do something now that was previously unachievable and charging a large fee for it. No one can make much money from a cost-reducing innovation because then it would not reduce costs, but individuals and societies will pay a great deal for a new drug or device that saves those who were about to die. With the products of modern molecular biology and genetic engineering just beginning to reach the pharmaceutical market, recent trends in the availability of new and expensive technology will only accelerate.

Demographic trends are also raising health care costs. In industrial countries the population is becoming older and sicker. Some of the change is the result of the baby boom, but much is due to the "failures of success." Thanks to good medical care, more and more of our older fellow citizens are now still living and using substantial heath care resources. With the important exception of the human immunodeficiency virus (HIV), in industrial societies death does not come from infectious diseases. Instead, our problems are cardiovascular disease, stroke, cancer, and diabetes, all of which are chronic or degenerative conditions (or both). Therefore all of these diseases offer the opportunity for years of expensive care before they finally kill us. Indeed, HIV too is becoming a chronic disease. Pharmaceutical companies, well aware of the profit potential of compounds that can be marketed to millions of people for decades of use, are focusing their research efforts on such possibilities.

The third cost driver involves changes in consumer demand. Economically, health care is a luxury. The rich not only spend more than the poor, they spend a higher proportion of their income on health care. As all industrial societies become richer, they demand more health care as a result. In addition, a worldwide cultural evolution is taking palace. Older religious values, including stoic resignation in the face of death, are fading in the face of a relentlessly youth-oriented, media-driven popular culture. Everyone now wants to be young and active for as long as possible. Retirees take up golf, volunteer, start second careers, and travel around the world; and the demands for everything from joint replacements, to Rogaine, to Viagra go up accordingly.

None of these forces is going to stop or reverse. On the contrary, they all seem poised to accelerate in coming decades. The willingness and ability of societies to pay for the higher medical costs these forces will produce is clearly in doubt.

## Who Will Pay the Piper?

Improvements in transportation and communication have been truly phenomenal. Business travelers now check their voice mail and e-mail from any decent hotel anywhere in the world. Jet transport and containerized freight mean that my local liquor store in Boston, Massachusetts sells beer made everywhere from the shores of the South China Sea to the heart of the Amazon basin. The technologic gap between the advanced and developing societies narrows continually. Much computer programming is now done in Bangladesh and India; and U.S. airlines fly sleek, modern jet aircraft from Embair in Brazil.

As a result, business around the world increasingly focuses on controlling costs for competitive purposes. In the United States in recent years many industrial disputes about downsizing or outsourcing reflect corporate efforts to escape high labor costs, including the high health care costs of their union contracts. The fact that the percentage of the workforce without health insurance has increased in recent years, despite unprecedented growth, only shows how effective and widespread such efforts have been.

Public payers are encountering parallel pressures. Disillusionment with government is widespread. Negative campaign advertising, official misconduct, poor service from government organizations, and the post-Watergate boom in investigative reporting have all played a role. As a result, lowering, or not raising, taxes is the political platform with the greatest popular appeal. Even left-leaning leaders such as Tony Blair in the United Kingdom or Gerhard Schröder in Germany—not to mention Bill Clinton—espouse a "third way" of lowering taxes. It involves less government, greater individual responsibility, and private sector economic growth. The volatility of international capital markets places additional limits on governments' ability to pay for health care with deficit spending and increased inflation. Even the impending budget surplus in the United States is not touching off any stampede among politicians to increase payments to doctors and hospitals through Medicare and Medicaid. Instead, most of the talk is of spending on education, police, and defense; of tax cuts; and of taking care of the demographic burden implicit in Social Security. Thus even though many citizens want improved health care, they are also not willing to pay for it.

## Special Problems of the United States

The United States is the only industrial country to finance most of its health care through insurance premiums. Every other country uses broad-based taxes (often payroll taxes) so upper income groups pay more than, and hence cross-subsidize, lower income groups. In the United States, perhaps 20% of the under-65 population has no health insurance, exactly because they are too poor to afford it.

The lack of coverage in the United States is exacerbated by our competitive insurance industry and the increasingly predictable nature of health care costs. In a world of chronic disease we know too well who will be a high cost user of care next year: someone who is already sick. With 5% of a typical insurance pool consuming up to 60% of the resources, insurance companies have a great incentive to not cover sick people. At the same time, individuals and small groups have every incentive to engage in "adverse selection"—buying insurance only when someone becomes sick. As a result, many insurance markets are unstable. Government tries to require companies to cover sick people, not charge them too much, or both, whereas private companies seek to avoid doing so. Given adverse selection, the costs of covering those in the small group and individual markets are often high and so are premium levels. This discourages even more low income workers, who often work in small firms or have seasonal employment, from becoming insured.

The problem this situation poses for coverage for the elderly is clear. So long as many Americans *under* 65 have no health insurance, how far can we expand coverage to those *over* 65? What seems fair and doable in the political process? If we ever do create a system to cover everyone, will the costs of doing so not make the need for some explicit rationing even more critical?

These arguments have led at least some commentators to recommend one form or another of age rationing of care on the grounds of cost-effectiveness. As we have seen, the problems at which such proposals are directed are real, but how appealing are these ideas as a solution?

## Why Cost-Effectiveness?

At first glance the cost-effectiveness argument seems so appealing that many find it difficult to see any alternative. The idea of getting the "biggest bang for the buck" seems to be the very definition of *rational resource allocation*. An enormous amount of literature in medicine and public health is based on this framework; clinical cost-effectiveness studies suggest that we must set priorities based on maximizing the number of disability adjusted life years (DALYs) saved per dollar expended. Moreover, this approach underlies the entire intellectual apparatus of modern economics.

From a philosophic perspective, cost-effectiveness is a form of the doctrine known as *consequentialism*. This is the view that decisions are not intrinsically good or bad but, rather, that such an evaluation depends on the decision's consequences. Although appealing, many individuals intuitively limit the scope of such arguments. Each parent who tells children they should not lie, regardless of what happens, is saying that morally correct behavior is not just a matter of consequences.

The cost-effectiveness rationale for age rationing draws on a particular form of consequentialism known as *utilitarianism*. This doctrine, originally propounded during the nineteenth contury by Jeremy Bentham in England, argued that the correct way to think about consequences was to ask about the effect of a decision on the *well-being* of each and every individual. Moreover, Bentham took the quite radical view that people could and should decide for themselves what improved their own level of well-being. Bentham called that level *utility*, hence the name of the theory. The idea was to add up all the gains and losses from a decision and base the choice on "the greatest good of the greatest number."

This tactic, of relying on indivuduals' *subjective* evaluations of their own circumstances, is now only one of two utilitarian schools of thought. The other school insists that individuals are too erratic, emotional, and uninformed to make such choices. Instead, this school requires that experts devise an *objective* index that describes different levels of each person's well-being. This sort of *objective utilitarianism* is what lies behind most cost-effectiveness arguments in health policy.

Philosophers by no means universally accept utilitarianism, in part because it can lead to almost unlimited ruthlessness. If ten people on a lifeboat need to eat some of their number to survive, utilitarianism seems to justify doing so. Similarly, if we need to quarantine those with infectious disease or withdraw care from those most expensive to save, utilitarianism says we should do so with a clear conscience. Before I explore where such objections might take us, I want to look inside the method a bit more deeply. For even those attracted by the idea of cost-effectiveness must still resolve some formidable practical and philosophic difficulties if they are to try to use it to make real decisions.

## Age Rationing Through Cost-Effectiveness: Some Serious Problems

There are both ethical and scientific problems facing those who would implement age rationing on the basis of cost-effectiveness. The critical ethical problem concerns how to measure effectiveness for such purposes. The key scientific problem is to forecast the consequences of all possible actions. Both of these tasks are needed if one is to translate the principle into action.

The measure of effectiveness we choose is of critical importance in shaping the implications of any cost-effectiveness program. Possible measures include number of lives saved, years of life saved, quality adjusted life years (QALYs) saved, potential economic benefit, and potential social benefit. Obviously, if we choose number of lives instead of years of life as our measure of effectiveness, the age distribution of those treated will be quite different. Similarly, using QALYs implies that there is less value in saving the life of someone who is physically disabled or mentally ill than someone who is not. Using economic gain as an index implies that those with higher incomes from their own labor are more valuable than those who produce less. If we want to use the parameter "benefit to society," who is to decide on a measure that compares, in exact numeric terms, the social benefit of rock stars, mothers, surgeons, basketball players, ditch diggers, welders, bond traders, used car salesmen, and day care workers?

A particularly difficult conceptual problem lies in the task of reducing morbidity and mortality gains to a single index. One objection to using a measure of gains such as lives saved (or if we were more terminologically honest, deaths postponed) is that it takes no account of the alleviation of suffering and disability. Nor does it account for how long any given death was in fact postponed. Those who argue for using an index such as QALYs or DALYs thus claim that only their approach takes these considerations into account.

Yet the QALY or DALY methods operate in a particular and controversial way. They calibrate changes in quality of life on a zero-to-one scale and then multiply such gains by the number of years the gain persists. The value of life-saving is calculated in a similar fashion. The quality of life saved is multiplied by the expected number of years produced by treatment. Thus lifesaving is not treated as something special, but just as another way of producing years of life lived at various quality levels.

This approach runs counter to the widespread sentiments of many individuals. They want to treat *life-saving* as somehow special or different from improving life *quality*. Saving someone from death so he or she can live 5 years of life at moderate quality, yielding, for example, a total of 3 QALYs, is seen as more valuable than a modest gain in quality over 20 years that also yields a total of 3 QALYs. The citizens of Oregon rejected the first draft of the state's proposed priority-setting scheme for its Medicaid program—done with the QALY method—exactly because it failed to make this distinction.

Even once one computes a number such as QALYs or DALYs, there is yet another age-related issue. Are additional DALYs or QALYs gained at different ages equally valuable? In fact, the DALY method used by the World Heath Organization (WHO) values gains during the middle of life more highly than gains for the young or the old.

The point of raising all these questions is to highlight just how difficult and ethically challenging it is to implement a cost-effectiveness program. Such an enterprise does not avoid difficult ethical choices. On the contrary, it forces us to make a series of such choices and to do so explicitly before we begin even to use the method in question.

## Markets as an Alternative to Cost-Effectiveness Calculations

Having experts construct an index to value health gains is controversial. Can experts tell us how valuable less morbidity is versus less mortality? Economists believe that all values are set by individuals so they want to retreat from such centralized valuation into a decentralized *subjective* process. Rather than have experts weigh quality versus quantity of life or compare the value of gains in added life years at different ages, they want to let individuals decide all this for themselves. There is no one "rationed" basis for preferences, they say. Instead, everyone must decide for themselves how important the various kinds of health gain are. This is why economists want to use markets to allocate health care resources. In a market, each person gets what they personally want. They buy only those goods or services whose value to them exceeds their cost of production.

One difficulty with markets, of course, is that the pattern of resource use they produce reflects the distribution of income and wealth. The rich get more, and their tastes have a greater impact on what gets consumed. For that reason, in 1966, the United States decided (when Medicare was established) that it was unfair to provide care for the elderly purely through market mechanisms. Make no mistake, competitive markets do allocate resources effectively, which is why economists like them; but individual ability and willingness to pay determines the outcome.

Still, in the United States the political lure of markets is considerable. The new "Medicare + Choice" program has been explicitly justified on the grounds of using markets to set priorities. The goal is to let recipients make some of the decisions about what coverage to buy (or not) for themselves.

Medical savings accounts go even further in the direction of relying on personal choice. These accounts would allow individuals to put money into a tax-free savings account and then buy health care from that account with a catastrophic insurance plan to protect them against exhausting their funds. This scheme would radically exacerbate problems of adverse selection, especially if funds left in the accounts could ever be used for other purposes. The healthiest would opt out of Medicare and establish such funds, expecting to be able eventually to collect the leftovers, leaving only the sickest individuals in the regular insurance pool.

Even the most radical market-oriented proposals for Medicare reform do not do away with the need to confront the age-rationing issue. Such proposals generally retain some tax-supported minimum package of care. The content of that minimum is yet to be decided. That decision again raises the age-rationing problem in an unavoidable way.

## Some Practical Problems with Cost-Effectiveness

Suppose society could agree on an index to be used to evaluate the relative cost-effectiveness of various procedures? We would still be faced with the need to predict both the costs and the effects of treatment in order to decide what to do, and neither of those predictions is easy to make.

Medical knowledge about the effects of many treatments is surprisingly limited. Although the clinical trials literature is expanding steadily, we often still do not know how much benefit each treatment would yield for each condition. Cost information is also often rudimentary or even nonexistent. Many available studies have used insurance records (based on bills) to measure cost, which is not what economists mean by cost. For economists, the correct measure is "opportunity cost." This refers to the value of the goods and services that could have been produced elsewhere in the economy if a given activity were not undertaken. This determination requires an investigation of the costs that would be saved or incurred if a given activity were subtracted from, or added to, the health care system. In reality, the practical problems are so substantial that well-justified cost numbers are seldom available.

Perhaps most troublesome is the fact that in any real health care system the costs and the gains from any one treatment are highly variable. Patients vary in level of co-morbidity and overall health status. As a result, the effect of treatments vary greatly. Transplants, for example, work best on those who are healthiest. Costs are lower, and life expectancy is longer. Costs and gains not only vary across patients but across providers. Some doctors and hospitals have much better results than others, lower costs, or both; the two are seldom correlated.

Thus, sophisticated coherent advocates of cost-effective rationing, unlike the Oregon plan, would not make judgments about whether to pay for a whole category of treatments for all patients cared for by all providers. Instead, they might well say that certain transplants are acceptable but only for sufficiently healthy recipients (the reverse of current "sickest first" organ transplant rules). In another case, the rule might be that certain cancer treatments may be done, but only for those whose disease had not progressed beyond a certain stage. Certain treatments might be funded only to providers with the best demonstrated cost-effectiveness. Once one started down the cost-effectiveness road, as a matter of intellectual consistency, it would be difficult to stop until the decision rules were as nuanced and finely tuned as possible.

## Can Cost-Effectiveness Be Used to Justify Age Rationing of Surgical Care to the Elderly?

Now that we see where cost-effectiveness analysis would lead, can it be used to justify age rationing for surgical care for the elderly? The first and most obvious point is that it very much depends on how the measure of "effectiveness" is defined, for example, effectiveness as lives versus life years versus quality adjusted life years. It would also matter how gains at different ages and to individuals at different levels of functioning were valued. The ultimate effect of such a program also would depend on the actual scientific state of medicine. Some interventions for elderly patients might well seem appropriate provided they were inexpensive enough and provided enough gain.

Indeed, a rational priority setter might well believe that the use of age criteria in a rationing scheme was a manifestation of scientific failure. After all, treatment gains for patients of the same age, with the same disease, are typically variable. Using just age to predict outcomes leaves too much variance unaccounted for. As a result, some patients who could be treated cost-effectively would not receive care, and some who would not benefit sufficiently would be treated. Aggressive advocates of cost-effectiveness would work to refine their list of predictors so age itself would play less and less of a role.

However, let us not fool ourselves. On average, our bodies do become more decrepit with age; and it is often less expensive to improve the health conditions of the healthier than the sick. Hence, even sophisticated cost-effectiveness-based rationing schemes that used predictive indicators other than age would, on average, tend to limit care to the old because that is what those other criteria would tell us to do. Expensive, low payoff interventions would be the first to go under such a scheme, and some of these would surely be certain surgical interventions in the elderly.

This conclusion makes many observers uneasy. Are we really prepared, critics ask, to abandon our elderly simply because their care is less cost-effective? Is that not a violation of their rights and dignity and a failure on our part to respect our obligations? This question leads us to the broader issues of whether there are rights to health care, and if so what rights in particular should the elderly have?

## Does Anyone, Including the Elderly, Have Health Care Rights?

The question is whether anyone, including the elderly, has a right to health or health care. If so, what those rights are has been the subject of much debate. Philosophically, the position most often used to justify such rights is called *liberalism*. (In most of the world, that term does not mean on the political left, as it does in the United States.) Following the work of the great German thinker Immanual Kant, philosophical liberalism begins from the premise that because all humans are capable of making responsible moral choices they are all worthy of some measure of basic respect. The question then is: What does such respect require of us?

For *libertarian liberals*, all that is required is that we leave other people alone to do what they want. We must respect their "negative rights" to noninterference. Thus libertarians oppose even such minimal government actions as physician licensing or drug regulation. They see these actions as illegitimate infringements on individuals' freedom to obtain whatever care, from whatever source, they want.

To justify rights to health care one must go beyond negative rights to "positive rights." This is the position of *egalitarian liberals*, who say that respect for other persons as "moral actors" requires us to provide them with the prerequisites for making meaningful choices. Those prerequisites include not only basic political and personal freedom but also, egalitarians argue, minimum levels of those goods and services that make real choice possible.

To claim that there are specific rights to health or health care, then, one must believe that health is different from other goods or services: If health is just another good, then all egalitarian liberal "respect" would require of us would be to give everyone a reasonable income and let them buy whatever they wanted, including health care services.

In contrast, some writers argue that health itself is a prerequisite to being able to exercise meaningful choice. They conclude that, like political liberty, a certain level of health should be provided by the state to all, quite apart from the workings of the marketplace. Note that the right in question is not to health care but to health itself, because it is health itself that is the prerequisite to choice. Does this mean that there is not a right to health care that is ineffective? Care that does not improve someone's health does not help satisfy our moral obligations. This theory, then, does not require us to offer maximum care for everyone.

This line of analysis does not tell us how much health to which we are entitled or who exactly is obligated to pay for it. Those questions must be resolved if we are to conclude that the elderly have rights, even to relatively less cost-effective care.

## To What Health Are We Entitled?

The egalitarian liberal analysis we are exploring suggests that our health entitlement consists of whatever health status we must have to exercise meaningful life choices. The specific implications of that argument are not easy to determine.

One way to proceed would be to say that everyone is entitled to some minimum quality and quantity of life, because only if someone lives long enough, and at a high enough functional level, can they make meaningful life choices. This implies that society is obligated to get every person up to those minimum levels. This requires priority treatment for those who were the worst off in health terms on a lifetime basis. It would be especially important for the health care system to avoid early deaths or the effects of chronic illness that prevented effective life choices (e.g., early onset mental illness). Such a scheme would not imply any particular social obligation to the elderly, however. From this particular egalitarian point of view, they would be seen as having made their choices and lived their lives. Society might choose to spend money to alleviate their suffering out of charity or empathy, but individuals beyond the socially guaranteed life expectancy would not have a rights-based claim to have society support their medical care.

Of course, as resources expand, society could decide to raise the minimum quantity and quality of life it wanted to provide for everyone. It could decide that ensuring a fit, productive old age was part of the meaning of mutual respect. That decision would have to carry with it a commitment to whatever care citizens needed early in life, so all would have the opportunity to get old enough to benefit from support once they were elderly.

Once we realize that resource limits could require even those who believe in health rights to set priorities, we confront a basic question. How much should a society spend on health given that all the resources used for such activities do come, ultimately, from other citizens? Can we tax some, even against their will, to benefit others; and if so, to what extent? Why does such coercion not violate the principle of mutual respect? Within this framework, the answers to such questions determine just how much care for the elderly (and everyone else) society can provide.

The standard egalitarian liberal answer to this question is that much of the existing distribution of income and wealth is fundamentally illegitimate. High incomes due to natural talent, social advantages, superior education, or inheritance are not a product of a person's own level of effort. Hence such income is not deserved by those who earn it, and so it can legitimately be taxed and redistributed. Of course, society would be foolish to raise taxes so high that even those it was trying to help suffered as a result. This could happen if, for example, economic growth were so injured by high taxes that the beneficiaries of redistribution got less, even if they got a larger share, because the economy had shrunk. In addition, it would be inconsistent, even for the most radical egalitarian, to tax the rich and healthy to the point that their life chances became less extensive than those of the sick who were being helped. The healthy and successful are themselves worthy of liberal respect and cannot be pushed below whatever level of opportunity we establish as the baseline for all.

Still, these constraints seem not to be highly restrictive. The egalitarian liberal argument seems to require the United States to make more efforts to provide the health care needed to ensure health for all than we do today. One qualification to this conclusion, however, is raised by the fact that U.S. health care spending is already high compared with that of all other industrial countries. It is possible that we could use existing resources much more efficiently and perhaps come close (or certainly closer) to meeting the goal of the egalitarian liberal argument without large spending increases.

On the other hand, the extent of redistribution that is politically possible may be substantially less than the egalitarian ideal. When it comes right down to it, many citizens of industrial countries do not consider income due to superior talent and skill totally undeserved. Instead, they view someone's talents as a constituent part of that person and hence deserving of respect. Thus they place some limits on the extent to which the fruits of those talents can be appropriated by the state.

There are yet two more concerns that tend to limit political support for the health care redistribution the egalitarian liberal argument appears to require. One issue is raised by the possibility that bringing everyone up to some minimum level would be extremely costly in some cases. Are we prepared to spend whatever it takes to bring even the sickest up to some minimum quantity and quality of life? The second issue has to do with incentives. In a world of chronic disease, where diet, exercise, and smoking have such an effect on health status, if society pays for everyone's care, does that undermine individuals' accountability for their own health-promoting behavior?

Those who advocate egalitarian liberal rights to health are thus left in a difficult position. The available arguments become inexact just at the point they are most needed. What exactly does it mean to say that we are obligated to provide the prerequisites for moral choice when we face expensive care for an elderly individual? Does that claim tell us to fund such care? Does the principle in question mean that medical care for those too demented to make moral choices is not required? If age limits to our entitlements are required by resource limits, what then is the correct level of resources to devote to health care? The egalitarian liberal program of rights to health has not been developed fully enough to resolve many of these issues.

## A Postmodern Way Found?

Both utilitarians and liberals generally believe that moral questions have correct answers. They believe that some combination of intuition, logic, and empiric analysis can be said to justify some particular philosophic position. They are generally what philosophers call *moral realists*.

The broad intellectual movement called *postmodernism* provides an alternative perspective. Postmodernists reject the idea that morality can be based on some compelling, transcendent justification. Instead, they believe that morality is not found, but created, that it is a form of art rather than of science. This means that moral arguments can, at the most basic level, be judged only by criteria that have evolved *within* the traditions that give rise to them. Just as Renaissance portraiture and abstract expressionism are forms of painting with different rules and criteria, so too are different schools of moral argument. No foundational or universal justification is available, any more than it is for choosing among various schools of painting or music.

This argument implies that the question of rights to care for the elderly and of the use of cost-effectiveness to define those rights cannot be solved by looking to philosophy for some single provable "right answer." For postmodernists there is no one authoritative source whose self-evident correctness demands our intellectual and moral deference. Instead, establishing a particular set of rights is an act of collective cultural creativity. It is one means by which a society defines itself, just as struggles over racial and gender equality have defined us. Such an act of collective self-definition is a matter of poetry and prophecy, worked out in the arena of democratic politics.

The great contemporary liberal philosopher John Rawls has argued that humans, in fact, have two moral powers. One enables us to develop and work out our private life plans. The other enables us to participate in the collective processes of defining common institutions and reciprocal civic rights and obligations. It is the exercise of this second moral power that is, I believe, at stake in this debate.

Personally, I am most concerned with extending effective health care to those who, unlike senior citizens who are already covered by Medicare, now have no publicly financed access to care. I also believe that helping those who are worst off from a lifetime perspective should be a compelling priority. I also believe that in a world of scarce resources spending money on care that is not genuinely helpful is foolish. I do believe, however, that our older citizens are entitled to a certain kind of mutual respect. That respect (now too often denied) includes taking seriously their own preferences about end-of-life treatment, including withdrawal of treatment when that is their wish. Such respect also, for me at least, involves providing surgical care even for relatively elderly patients when there is a reasonable chance of reasonable benefit.

The philosopher Bernard Williams has argued that when faced with difficult moral choices we should engage in "reflective criticism." We should not only argue from theory to practice, as I have done in this chapter; we should also use our intuitions about specific cases to illuminate our theory. Therefore, allow me to discuss a specific case: A 93-year-old woman had undergone surgery for a bowel obstruction due to cancer 5 years ago. That surgery has given her, to date, five more years of good, if imperfect, quality of life. She has had two trips abroad with her grandchildren and several trips to the opera with her friends. I believe that in a country as rich as ours, we must try to organize our health care system so that such care is available to all. That concept is appropriate social poetry.

# 9 Interacting with the Elderly Patient, Family, and Referring Physicians

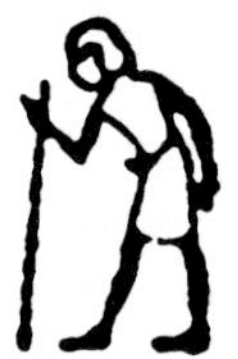

Dennis W. Jahnigen

The relationship of the physician with an elderly patient involves more than simple application of the most current diagnostic and therapeutic information. Knowing this is necessary but not sufficient to ensure an optimum outcome. It also requires recognition of the differences and similarities between the patient and the physician. It requires sensitivity to age-related changes that may increase the anxiety associated with illness for the patient and that may increase the difficulty of obtaining accurate historical and physical information for the physician. It also involves appreciation of differences in the values among elderly patients and a willingness to negotiate what may be medically indicated or medically possible, with what is most desirable from the patient's frame of reference. The goals of therapy for an elderly person may lie in relief of symptoms rather than a cure, preservation of independent living rather than returning to employment, and easing suffering at the end of life rather than fighting death.

The relationship an elderly person has with a primary care physician can be important to his or her overall health. It is here where there is opportunity for preventive services, accurate assessment and treatment of existing conditions, and planning for the eventual need for end-of-life medical treatment. The primary care physician has the opportunity to come to know the elderly patient as an individual, as a part of his or her family and community, and to learn something about the individual's past and hopes for the future. This type of information can be invaluable when making the decisions commonly required of the physician.

Elderly persons make high use of health services in virtually all care settings. Although the use of long-term care services such as home care and nursing homes is usually recognized as common among elderly populations, these persons require acute services as well, including emergency care, surgery, hospital care, and intensive care. The emergency department (ED) is a common point of entry to the hospital for elderly patients. Although elderly patients rarely use the ED as a source for primary care, when they do come to the ED they are more seriously ill than younger patients. In a multicenter study, patients over 65 years of age were 4.4 times more likely to arrive at the ED by ambulance, 5.6 times more likely to be admitted to the hospital, and 5.5 times more likely to require intensive care on admission than were younger patients.[1–3]

## Diagnosis

Identification of disease and disability in an elderly patient can be difficult. Many common geriatric conditions do not fit as discrete diseases but are better thought of as syndromes (Table 9.1). The presentation of disease may be atypical. As many as one-third of elderly patients with a myocardial infarction have no chest pain; shortness of breath is one of the most common presenting symptoms. Pneumonia without fever, peritonitis without abdominal pain, and hyperthyroidism without tachycardia are but a few atypical presentations (Table 9.2). Many of the symptoms of elderly patients are nonspecific, such as weakness, weight loss, incontinence, tiredness, dizziness, and falling (Table 9.3). A sudden change in mental function is an important clue to underlying acute illness. Likewise, a sudden decrease in functional status, such as loss of competence for carrying out tasks associated with a given level of independence, is often the only sign of a serious underlying event. Parsimony of diagnosis, which attempts to use a single disease process to explain all symptoms, often fails with elderly patients because of the presence of multiple co-morbidities that interact. For example, depression can lead to anorexia and malnutrition. Tachycardia associated with sepsis can unmask coronary artery disease.

The concept of functional status is often more important than the presence of a specific disease. Functional ability is the combined effect of disease and disability on the person's ability to carry out a task associated with everyday living (Table 9.4). Functional ability can be eval-

TABLE 9.1. Common Geriatric Problems

| |
|---|
| Loss of autonomy |
| Inactivity |
| Gait instability |
| Decreased functional level |
| Cognitive impairment |
| Malnutrition |
| Polypharmacy |
| Incontinence |
| Infections |
| Decreased hearing / vision |
| Depression |
| Inadequate social support |
| Iatrogenesis |
| Substance abuse |

uated in a number of ways. Two simple screens are the Activities of Daily Living (ADLs) and Instrumental Activities of Daily Living (IADLs) (Table 9.5). The items are arranged in a hierarchic order, from basic skills to more complex skills. These skills tend to be lost sequentially. Each function can be rated on degree of independence and an overall score developed, which can then help determine the type of assistance needed, appropriate living arrangements, and changes over time.

## Role of the Primary Care Physician

In the office setting, the role of the primary care physician is obvious, but it is equally important in the hospital.[5] Even though the patient may ultimately become the primary responsibility of a surgeon, medical specialist, or intensivist, the primary care physician can provide reassurance to the patient, participate in difficult decisions, and offer continuity of medical care later in the hospital stay and after discharge. The hospital environment poses unique threats to the health of elderly patients, such as adverse outcomes from diagnosis and therapy, medication side effects, malnutrition, infections, falls, pressure ulcers, and functional decline, all of which are potentially preventable by careful medical and nursing oversight.

The first encounter a patient has with the physician is especially important.[6] In addition to establishing confidence in the physician's concern and competence, it conveys the degree of respect and style of communication that will characterize future interactions. The extent to which the physician succeeds in this effort will have a major effect on patient trust and willingness to consider and follow recommendations in the future.[7–10] Although geriatric patients typically take for granted physician competence initially, they are able to judge physician concern themselves. Elderly patients usually wish to be fully included in the medical decision-making process.[11, 12] They want to be informed in terms they can understand but are reliant on physician authority for making medical decisions; they are less likely to challenge the physician's recommendations than younger patients. Contrary to popular belief, older patients are less inclined to report symptoms than younger patients.[13] Such hesitation may be due to embarrassment about a symptom such as incontinence or because they believe that a symptom such as joint pain or memory loss are normal with old age. Frequently an older patient has a friend or family member accompany them to the office or hospital to help understand and remember discussions. The setting in which this initial meeting occurs clearly influences both the manner and urgency with which information is obtained. If the first meeting is in the context of an acute or life-threatening event, a focused, rapid assessment is needed. On most occasions, there is

TABLE 9.2. Clinical Conditions with Atypical Presentations in the Elderly

| Condition | Atypical presentation |
|---|---|
| Myocardial infarct | No chest pain |
| Pulmonary embolism | No shortness of breath |
| Acute abdomen | No abdominal pain |
| Hyperthyroidism | No tremor or tachycardia |
| Cancer | Depression |
| | Mass without symptoms |
| Hypothyroidism | Cognitive impairment |
| Depression | Masked, no sadness |
| Alcohol abuse | Falls, weight loss |
| Drug reaction | Confusion |
| Endocarditis | Confusion |
| Congestive heart failure | Confusion |
| Pneumonia | No fever |

TABLE 9.3. Nonspecific Symptoms of Illness in Elderly Persons

| |
|---|
| Confusion |
| Weight loss |
| Weakness |
| Incontinence |
| Dizziness |
| Falling |
| Self-neglect |
| Functional decline |
| Apathy |
| Anorexia |

TABLE 9.4. Diseases Causing Difficulty with Physical Tasks

| Disease | Men (%) | Women (%) | Total % |
|---|---|---|---|
| Arthritis | 39 | 55 | 49 |
| Old age | 13 | 11 | 12 |
| Heart disease | 16 | 13 | 14 |
| Injury | 10 | 13 | 12 |
| Lung disease | 7 | 5 | 6 |
| Stroke | 5 | 2 | 3 |

*Source:* Modified from Ettinger et al.,[4] with permission.

TABLE 9.5. Activities of Daily Living and Instrumental Activities of Daily Living

| |
|---|
| **Activities of daily living (ADLs)** |
| Feeding |
| Ambulation |
| Bathing |
| Continence |
| Communication |
| Dressing |
| Toileting |
| Transferring |
| Grooming |
| **Instrumental activities of daily living (IADLs)** |
| Writing |
| Cooking |
| Shopping |
| Climbing stairs |
| Managing medication |
| Ability to do outside work |
| Reading |
| Cleaning |
| Doing laundry |
| Using telephone |
| Managing money |
| Ability to use public transportation |

sufficient time for the physician to interview and examine the patient deliberately, frequently checking to make sure the patient understands and is comfortable with what is occurring. Several practical "pointers" can assist in this process.

1. As a sign of respect an older patient should be addressed as Mr., Mrs., Ms., etc. Avoid using the patient's first name unless invited to do so. Many elderly persons resent being treated in an overly familiar fashion, especially by a much younger person. Speak facing the person, and with a slow cadence and medium voice volume. Do not shout, as it rarely improves understanding and can actually be painful owing to the sudden transmission of a loud noise. An inexpensive headset amplifier can be easily obtained at electronics stores and made available in any office or hospital setting to assist in communication. If the patient uses a hearing aid, make sure it is turned on and functioning. Examine the patient in a well-lit area free of extraneous noises, if possible. Check to verify that the patient is able to understand what is being said. This is best done by asking them to repeat back their understanding of what they were just told. The choice of words used is important, as the educational range of elderly patients can range from elementary school through graduate level. The physician must attempt to use appropriate language and avoid complex medical terminology unless the patient is familiar with it.

Elderly patients are usually most comfortable with ambient temperatures of 75°–78°F. They are less efficient at maintaining comfortable body temperatures and should be provided with a blanket if they are in a hospital gown for any length of time. Few geriatric patients are able to lie flat on a standard office examination table because of nearly universal kyphosis and cervical osteoarthritis, which limits neck extension. A pillow is almost always required for comfort. Electric tables are safer and easier than standard tables for frail patients. As they can be lowered to approximately 20 inches, they allow a short patient to sit without undue assistance.

2. In an ambulatory setting, patients should initially be dressed in their own clothing rather than a gown, which most people find embarrassing and certainly undignified.[14] Examine patients in a position of equality, addressing them at the same level. Sit facing the patient rather than looking down over them.

If in a hospital setting, the patient's head should be elevated, and the physician should sit to communicate. Hospitals are unsettling to most people because of the uncertainty of the illness that requires them being there. Explaining each step of the examination can be reassuring. Do not sit on a patient's bed or remove the bedclothes without asking the patient's permission first. The inpatient environment can be particularly frightening to elderly patients because of the rapid pace, numerous encounters with hospital personnel at all hours of the day, and loss of privacy and personal control. Small gestures such as drawing the curtain to offer a degree of privacy is appreciated. Although a medical team in a teaching institution often includes several physicians in training, the senior physician should ask the patient's permission for others to watch or participate in the examination. In teaching hospitals during rounds when a team of several individuals may participate, only one person should ask questions and examine the patient at a time.

Be aware that differences in age, race, sex, or cultural background may influence interpretation of symptoms, expectations from medical care, communication, and the attitude of the patient toward the physician. Some are significant barriers to overcome. A youthful-appearing physician may seem "too young to know anything." An elderly man may be reticent with a female physician, and a similar disparity may occur between doctor and patient of a different race or cultural background. Although there is no single way to overcome these issues, clearly conveying interest in the person and acknowledging and respecting the differences usually leads to satisfactory communication. The few minutes of socializing with the patient can help to accomplish this. It helps put the patient at ease, and the physician can learn about their level of comfort, method of expression, affect, and even mental status.

3. Treat family members as important allies but focus on the patient.[15] Speak directly to the patient, not to adult children who may be present. Competent adult children with a frail parent, with good intentions, may speak as

though the patient is not present. Furthermore, they may have their own agenda for the physician, such as having the doctor "insist" the patient relocate to a "safer" environment or prohibiting the physician from telling the patient about their medical condition. Family members usually have important information for the physician and should be included in all discussions,[16] but the patient should remain the primary decision maker. When a patient is of questionable competence, courtesy is still essential, although historical information is suspect and questioning is often abbreviated.

4. Be culturally sensitive. Patients from Middle Eastern cultures may be extremely modest and may need to be examined while partially or completely clothed. A native American Indian may insist on having their room in a nursing home "smudged" before they agree to move in. It involves the use of burning sweetgrass to bless the area. When this occurred in a nursing home, the staff initially refused owing to fear of setting off the fire alarm. Eventually it was turned off and the ceremony performed. Allow for variations in patient beliefs and expectations of the physician. Family members can help provide translation when needed for interpretation of symptoms and reinforcement of medical cooperation.

5. Pace the examination based on time available and tolerance by the patient. Rarely is it necessary or even feasible to obtain a "complete history and physical examination" from an elderly frail person in a single setting. The lifelong volume of information, large number of past or current problems, and a sometimes endless series of complaints in the "review of systems" can be draining on patient and physician alike and calls for a different method of information gathering. The urgency of the apparent problem and the time allocated are the first determinants of the depth and extent of questioning. For complex patients a complete examination can be performed over two or three visits, so long as one has a good medical record of what needs to be done. For patients with stable chronic diseases who visit every 3–4 months, part of a complete examination can be performed at each encounter, a practice known as a "rolling physical."[17] Limit the number of problems dealt with at one visit to three of four. It is difficult for patients to keep track of multiple plans. Schedule more visits as needed to deal with multiple problems. Write down instructions, changes in medications, and follow-up visits for the patients.

6. Use a team approach. Frail elderly persons typically have need for professional assistance beyond simple medical care. Where available, an interdisciplinary team can benefit the patient by offering a more thorough evaluation, and access to a wider range of services, including social services, community-based nursing, physical and occupational therapy, and psychological, nutritional, dental, and other types of support. Most of these services are available in a hospital setting, but in an office setting arrangement for community referral may be necessary.

7. Support the caregiver. Providing physical and emotional support for a frail, dependent person is stressful. Caregivers of persons with Alzheimer's disease, for example, have greater physical and mental illness than age-matched controls. Even immunologic function is diminished under the stress of caregiving. Caregivers may delay or ignore their own health needs. The physician should monitor the vigor of the support system and the apparent health needs of any primary caregivers. Respite programs can be advised to allow caregivers a period of rest.

## Competence

All persons are assumed to be competent unless demonstrated to be otherwise. Although the legal determination of incompetence is made by a court, the clinical definition of competence is the ability to understand the implications of medical decisions and a willingness to participate in one's care. The patient known to have dementia may still be medically competent. Many patients with moderate or severe dementia are unable to participate in their own care, and other persons to assist in decision making must be sought. States' laws vary regarding surrogate decision makers. A call to the state medical society can lead to accurate regional information in this regard. Most accept a family member as a surrogate spokesperson for the incompetent patient, but some require a court-appointed guardian. The use of advanced directives, such as the Durable Power of Attorney for Health Care Matters may be useful. The primary care physician should become familiar with such guidelines in his or her state of practice.

If the competence of the patient is questionable, detailed mental status testing may be necessary. This must be approached gently as it can be a great source of anxiety and frustration to an elderly person, confused or not. When competence is still uncertain, a detailed evaluation by a psychiatrist or psychologist may be needed.

## Truth Telling

A widely held value in Western medicine is the right of patients to know the truth regarding their medical conditions and their options. Adult family members wishing to spare their elderly relative anxiety may request that the physician not inform the patient of the facts about their illness. If patients are competent, they should have the option of knowing as much as they wish about their condition. This situation can be handled by discussing the findings of the examination with the patient and the family, asking the patient first, "What do you wish to know about your illness?" and "If this is a serious or life-threatening illness, would you want to know about it?" The response to the first question allows the patient to specify the type of information and level of detail they seek. Most patients answer in the affirmative to the second question and, in so doing, help the physician speak honestly to the patient but still respect the family's concern. For patients with Alzheimer's or other dementing illnesses, arguments both for and against telling the patient the diagnosis have been made.[18] For patients with early disease who have insight into their cognitive deficits, the offer of information should be made, as some patients may wish to organize their activities and future plans accordingly. For patients with more severe cognitive impairment, the ability to retain new information may be lost, and individuals may forget each time they are told the diagnosis. In such circumstances, constantly telling persons they have a progressive illness of thinking seems to have little value.

## Office Visit

The office visit with an elderly person is a time-limited encounter. Likewise, few physicians in the context of a busy office can devote hours to a medical assessment. Initial data collection can be obtained during two or three visits, rather than during a single one. Typically, one or more family members wish to participate in the interview. This is important, as the patient may forget or mitigate important historical facts. The patient should clearly be the center of attention, faced by the physician, with family members in the background. The shaking of heads in opposite directions by the patient and family in response to a question can be an early clue that memory loss is the reason for the evaluation.

After allowing the patient to describe the reason for the visit and to answer focused questions, the physician can encourage the patient with multiple complaints to prioritize those that are most bothersome. This list can be limited by the physician to those that can be addressed on the first visit and others to be pursued at a future time. This approach can be useful for the patient with 10 or more complaints.

Next, the physician can invite the patient to change into a gown while the physician and family members step out of the room. At this juncture the family can be asked what they wish to add to the patient's statement. This part of the interview often reveals essential information the patient was unwilling or unable to recount. Family members may reveal functional deficits, self-neglect, depression, recent physical decline, or alcohol abuse. This brief encounter allows the family to participate but preserves the patient as the focal point. If there are serious family stresses under way at the time of the first visit, and social services are available on site, the family can be immediately interviewed by a social worker technician, psychologist, or nurse practitioner while the patient is examined. During this family interview urgent needs can be identified and addressed (safety, legal guardianship, meals, living arrangements, and supportive home services, to name but a few).

During this same time the physician can examine the patient, performing as much of a complete examination as practical in the time available. Rarely is a complete examination practical or essential. Major components omitted are documented with a plan for completing them. During the examination, the physician can ask additional questions to verify or elaborate the patient's earlier responses. Touching the patient during every visit is important, as it creates a physical bond with the patient and is reassuring. The patient's affect and responses to questions may be different when alone than with a caregiver in the room. The physician can develop a problem list and planned actions during the examination.

At completion of this part of the visit, the patient can dress while the physician finishes notes, visits the family, or sees another patient. The physician then briefly reconvenes with the patient and family to discuss findings and recommendations. The initial visit may be just the start of the evaluation of a complex patient; but plans for diagnostic testing, initial therapy, referral for additional evaluations (audiology, physical therapy, dental, social services, and others) can be made and arrangements for follow-up visits established. This initial evaluation can be done in 1 hour or less. An important point to allow for this expeditious evaluation is the use of a minimum data set, with nonduplicative information collected.

## Follow-Up Visits

Subsequent visits can be used to monitor therapy, discuss the results of tests, and pursue new or additional problems. Weight is obtained at each visit, as a decline may be a marker for underlying illness that otherwise goes unnoticed. Patients are requested to bring all medications to each visit. The medication, dosage, and how the patient is taking it are verified at each visit to help improve compliance and reduce errors. Unnecessary or ineffective medications can be discontinued. The patient and family can relate whether the therapy has led to the desired result. In addition to attending to active problems, at least one other preventive issue should be covered at each visit, which can be any of a number of items (Table 9.6). This type of visit should require only 20–30 minutes even for the very old patient. Another member of the health care team, such as a nurse, can visit with the patient, assist with dressing as needed, reinforce information to the patient, and help bring the visit to a close. Patients with multiple problems or with extensive frailty should be seen as often as their condition dictates but usually at intervals of no longer than 3–4 months.

TABLE 9.6. Preventive Issues

| |
|---|
| Immunization status |
| Counseling on exercise and accident risks |
| Counseling on diet and alcohol use |
| Mental status screening |
| Mammogram |
| Pelvic/Papanicolaou smear |
| Rectal examination |
| Screen of gait, vision, hearing |
| Advance directive discussion |

This permits the physician to do a "rolling physical" (a partial physical at each visit) and to monitor for functional decline.

## Medical Decision Making

Medical decision making with elderly patients can be perplexing, especially to the physician in training. The volume of complaints, nonspecificity of symptoms, and large number of potential diseases a typical review of symptoms identifies, can be challenging to approach in a systematic fashion. Knowing the conditions on which to focus one's attention, how aggressive to be, and when to shift from attempting cure to palliation can challenge the physician. A five-step process described below can be used to rate disabilities or complaints in a fashion that appreciates individual wishes and values while selectively using medical diagnostic and therapeutic techniques. It provides a way to avoid unwanted care but to offer beneficial interventions when judged appropriate by both patient and physician. In this way a unique "best" answer can emerge by which the patient's objectives define the desired outcome and the physician uses the best available technology to achieve this goal, rather than the symptom or the disease defining the "best" treatment. This process can be incorporated into a primary care relationship and accomplished over a series of visits. If necessary, this process can be used during a single visit to plan strategies. Generally, it is preferable for it to occur in an ambulatory environment, free from the stress of acute illness, thereby allowing issues to be raised and considered by patient and family in a deliberative fashion. The goals of medicine for the patient can be dynamic and change over time to reflect the response to therapy or a change in the patient's goals.

## "Geriatric-Sensitive" Model of Medical Decision Making

### Learn about the Patient's Values

Old persons differ from each other about what is important in their lives and differ as a group from young populations. Young persons typically fear death more than any other event, whereas the elderly rate loss of independence and autonomy, long-term disability, being a financial burden on others, and loss of mental faculties as more important than death.[19] Few very old persons have not considered death, and many approach it with calm resignation or even welcome it as an end to suffering. Some older persons are "fighters" and are willing to undergo great discomfort and risk for possible extension of any amount of life. The current quality of life as perceived by the person is important for the physician to determine. Health professionals often project their own perceptions on quality-of-life judgments of patients and frequently undervalue current quality perceived by patients. How do they feel about their present life? Have they thought about circumstances under which they would not want to live? Does their religion, if any, provide comfort or guidance to them as they approach the end of life? Have they talked to others about their wishes, or have they prepared an advance directive or durable power of attorney? What do they enjoy in life—running a marathon, caring for a beloved pet? This information helps set the stage on which medical decisions can be made.

### Determine the Person's Objectives from the Medical Encounter

The response from the patient to the question "Why are you here today?" may range from "because my daughter made me come" to "I just don't feel good." The person may be seeking one or more outcomes from the medical encounter, which may include the following.

| Patient objective | Example |
|---|---|
| Cure of the condition | "Please fix my painful hip." |
| Relief of symptoms | "Help me tolerate the pain of my arthritis." |
| Reassurance | "Do I have cancer?" "Do I have Alzheimer's disease?" |
| Preservation of function | "Help me control my falling so I can stay in my own home." |
| Explanation | "What's happening to me?" "What can I expect in the future?" |
| Sympathy | "I want someone to listen to me." |
| Validation | "I am important because you treat me with respect and take my concern seriously." |
| Secondary gain | "I want my family to care more about me." |

Failure to recognize what the person is seeking can lead to major miscommunication and dissatisfaction to patient, physician, and family.

TABLE 9.7. Estimated Versus Actual Survival after In-Hospital CPR in Elderly Persons

| Patients | Survival (%) Actual | Estimated |
|---|---|---|
| All | 13 | 62 |
| Healthy 80-year-olds | No data | 51 |
| From nursing homes | 1 | 41 |
| With severe infections | 1 | 40 |
| With widespread cancer | 1 | 28 |

*Source:* Miller et al.,[20] with permission. Copyright 1992. American Medical Associates.

## Determine the Medical Facts

Using the patient's values and objectives as guides, the physician now becomes diagnostician, determining the most likely disease(s), conditions, disabilities present, along with an assessment of prognosis, therapeutic options, and risk/benefit estimates. The physician must have the most current information on the utility of potential interventions, as elderly persons may overestimate their utility. Many elderly patients (and their families) have greatly inflated expectations of the success of many medical interventions. For example, in one study, community dwelling elderly persons believed that in-hospital cardiopulmonary resuscitation (CPR) leads to a more than 60% rate of discharge alive from hospital, whereas the actual rate is 13% (Table 9.7).[20] This overestimation is due in part to the fact that the primary source of health information for elderly persons is television (Table 9.8). This and similar misconceptions emphasize the need for education on accurate prognosis and utility of interventions. Elderly persons are discerning regarding the use of interventions based on perceived utility and adjust their preference when presented with accurate information.[21] The relative utility of many interventions for elderly persons needs to consider cohort and more importantly, estimates of life expectancy (Table 9.9). Many interventions near the end of life may have minimal or no impact on either quantity of life or relief of symptoms. In some circumstances the use of artificial feedings or even antibiotics may be of no benefit to the patient.[22,23] A study

TABLE 9.8. Elderly Persons' Source of Knowledge about CPR

| Source | % |
|---|---|
| Television | 66 |
| Books and magazines | 53 |
| First aid or CPR class | 35 |
| Family and friends | 35 |
| Other health professionals | 23 |
| Never heard of CPR | 9 |
| Family physician | 6 |
| Religious teachings | 2 |

*Source:* Miller et al.,[20] with permission, Copyright 1992. American Medical Association.

TABLE 9.9. Life Expectancy for Elderly Persons

| Age (years) | Men (%) | Women (%) |
|---|---|---|
| 65 | 14.7 | 18.6 |
| 75 | 9.1 | 11.7 |
| 85 | 5.2 | 6.4 |

*Source:* 1986 National Center for Health Statistics. Vital Statistics of the US, Vol II: Mortality Part A. Washington, DC, US Public Health Service.

of hospice patients demonstrated that the symptoms associated with thirst and hunger could be well managed by offering small amounts of water.[24,25] Physicians must exercise their judgment about the likely benefit of any proposed interventions.[26] Part of what patients expect from their doctors is a recommendation. Every option possible need not be presented. Interventions that, in the physician's opinion, are futile need not be presented. Physicians can offer several courses of action they believe are reasonable.

## Recommend/Negotiate

In this step the physician recommends a course of diagnosis or therapy to the patient and family and "tests" it for acceptance. This step is to check how well the physician understands the patient's values and wishes. Negotiation may be needed. If the patient wants something other than what the physician recommends, the reasons should be explored. If the family wants something other than what the patient wants or the physician recommends, it must be discussed and reconciled.

## Agree on a Strategy and Measure of Success

The final step in this process is to agree on an overall strategy for medical care and the expected outcome. In this way the patient, physician, and family can understand the expected outcome and the measure of success. Some examples of explicit strategies include:

| Strategy | Expected outcome |
|---|---|
| Cure | Total resolution of the problem |
| Rehabilitation | Recovery of lost function |
| Prevention | Avoidance of disease |
| Diagnosis | Obtain needed information for subsequent decision |
| Experimental valuation | High risk/low likelihood of benefits |
| Acute care | Aggressive treatment of illness/stabilization |
| Symptom-based therapy | Relief of discomfort without cure |
| Palliation | Preservation of patient control; comfort during death |

This process is dynamic, and the outcome may change depending on response to therapy or other factors.

Agreement on the goals of medical care for a specific patient ahead of time helps everyone understand what is occurring and to judge the success of the care plan. Physicians must keep in mind that the success of their care is best judged in the patient's own terms of achieving the most with what life offers them. Physicians who knowingly accept this challenge are rewarded with the satisfaction of using their best skills: "To cure when possible, to comfort often, to care always."

## References


1. Strange GR, Chen EH, Sanders AB. Use of emergency departments by elderly patients: projections from a multicenter data base. Ann Emerg Med 1992;21:819–824.
2. Singal BM, Hedges JR, Rousseau EW, et al. Geriatric patient visits. Part I. Comparison of visits by geriatric and younger patients. Ann Emerg Med 1992;21:802–807.
3. Sanders A, Morley J. The older person in the emergency department. J Am Geriatr Soc 1993;41:880–882.
4. Ettinger W, Fried L, Harris T, et al. Self-reported causes of physical disability in older people. J Am Geriatr Soc 1994;42:1035–1044.
5. Fahs M. Primary medical care for elderly patients II. J Commun Health 1989;14:89–99.
6. Gastel B. Working With Your Older patient: A Clinician's Handbook. Bethesda, MD: National Institute on Aging, National Institutes of Health, 1994.
7. Adelman R. Green M, Charon R. Issues in physician–elderly patient interaction. Ageing Soc 1991;2:127–148.
8. Anderson L, Zimmerman M. Patient and physician perceptions of their relationship and patient satisfaction: a study of chronic disease management. Patient Educ Counsel 1993;20:27–36.
9. Beisecker A, Beisecker T. Patient information-seeking behaviors when communicating with doctors. Med Care 1990;28:19–28.
10. Green M, Adelman R, Charon R, Friedman E. Concordance between physicians and their older and younger patients in the primary care medical encounter. Gerontologist 1989;29:808–813.
11. Haug MR (ed). Elderly Patients and Their Doctors. New York: Springer, 1981.
12. Beisecker AE. Aging and the desire for information and input in medical decisions: patient consumerism in medical encounters. Gerontologist 1988;28:330–335.
13. Branch L, Nemeth K. When elders fail to visit physicians. Med Care 1990;23:11.
14. Carlson M, Jahnigen D. The hospital gown. J Am Geriatr Soc 1991;38(8):A30.
15. Glasser M, Prohaska T, Roska J. The role of the family in medical case-seeking decisions of older adults. Family Commun Health 1992;15:59–70.
16. Haley W, Clair J, Saulsberry K. Family caregiver satisfaction with medical care of their demented relatives. Gerontologist 1992;32:219–226.
17. Jahnigen DW, Schrier RW. The doctor/patient relationship in geriatric care. In: Jahnigen D, Schrier RW (eds) Issues in the Care of the Elderly, vol 2. Philadelphia: Saunders, 1986:457–464.
18. Drickamer MA, Lachs MS. Should patients with Alzheimer's disease be told their diagnosis? N Engl J Med 1992;326:947–951.
19. Americans View Aging. Alliance for Aging Research, 1991.
20. Miller D, Jahnigen D, Gorbien M, Simbartl L. Cardiopulmonary Resuscitation: how useful? Attitudes and knowledge of an elderly population. Arch Intern Med 1992;152: 578–582.
21. Murphy D, Burrows P, Santilli S, et al. The influence of the probability of survival on patients' preferences regarding cardiopulmonary resuscitation. N Engl J Med 1994;330: 545–549.
22. Fabiszewski K, Volicer B, Volicer L. Effect of antibiotic treatment on outcome of fevers in institutionalized Alzheimer's patients. JAMA 1990;263:3168–3172.
23. Quill T. Utilization of nasogastric feeding tubes in group of chronically ill, elderly patients in a community hospital. Arch Intern Med 1989;149:1937–1941.
24. McCann R, Hall W, Groth-Juncker A. Comfort care for terminally ill patients: the appropriate use of nutrition and hydration. JAMA 1994;274:1263–1268.
25. Fabiszewski K, Volicer B, Volicer L. Effect of antibiotic treatment on outcome of fevers in institutionalized Alzheimer patients. JAMA 1990;263:3168–3172.
26. Miller D, Gorbien M, Simbart L, et al. Factors influencing physicians in recommending in-hospital cardiopulmonary resuscitation. Arch Intern Med 1993;153:1999–2003.

# 10
# Preoperative Evaluation of the Elderly Surgical Patient

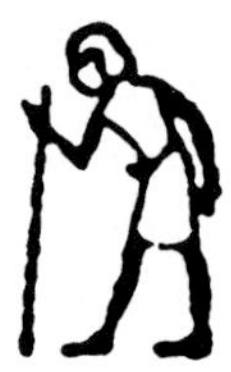

Darlene Gabeau and Ronnie A. Rosenthal

The aging of the American population has created the need to provide surgical care to an ever-increasing number of older persons. In the United States over the short period from 1980 to 1996 the percentage of operations for which the patient was over age 65 increased from 19% to 36%; when obstetrical procedures are excluded this portion rises to 43%.[1] It is now estimated that at least half of the patients in most general surgical practices are over age 65. During the next 50 years the portion of the population over age 65 is expected to continue to grow from the present 12.5% to 20%, or nearly 80 million people. Those over age 85 are the most rapidly growing segment of this population, and their number is expected to increase sixfold to 18 million by the year 2050[2] (Fig. 10.1).

Over the past several decades, advances in surgical and anesthetic techniques have led to an overall decline in operative mortality in older patients (Fig. 10.2).[3] The "risk" of surgery therefore has become somewhat less of a concern, whereas the need and ability to provide maximal disease management has increased. It is not appropriate, however, to assume that age should be ignored during the process of selecting patients for surgical care. Although considerable variation exists among individuals, aging confers certain limitations that must be carefully assessed and addressed if surgical therapy is to be successful. As the number of persons reaching old age continues to grow, it will become increasingly important for all surgeons to understand the special issues involved in the selection and evaluation of older patients for surgical care.

Before discussing the process of selecting and evaluating elderly patients, it is important to note that the pattern of surgical disease in the elderly is not always superimposable on the pattern seen in younger patients. The indication for surgery therefore may not be apparent until a complication has occurred. The absence of the classic signs and symptoms often leads to delays in treatment and errors in diagnosis. As a result, emergency surgical intervention is frequently necessary. In the elderly patient with gallstone disease, for example, the classic progression of worsening biliary symptoms leading to elective cholecystectomy is often absent. Instead, many elderly patients who undergo cholecystectomy present with a complication of gallstone disease with no antecedent symptoms. As many as two-thirds of the cholecystectomies in patients over age 65 are performed under urgent or emergent circumstances compared to fewer than one of five in patients less than age 65.[4]

Although the decision to operate and the process of evaluation is simplified by the urgency of the situation, the outcome from emergency surgery is far from satisfactory. Emergency surgery is associated with at least a threefold increase in mortality and morbidity. In one series of patients over age 70 years, emergency operation carried a mortality rate 10 times higher than that for elective procedures.[5] Emergency surgery is also associated with a higher rate of long-term hospital stay (>30 days), more need for postoperative intensive care, larger decline in functional status, and increased need for postoperative nursing home placement.[6]

With these issues in mind, the decision to proceed with surgery in old persons should include the following considerations: How clear is the indication for surgery, *including the likelihood of progression of the disease*? What are the practical limitations imposed on the patient by the disease process? What degree of improvement can be expected after the procedure? What quality of life can be expect with *or without* the surgery? Does the patient and his or her family understand the problem and the proposed solution? What is the risk of a negative outcome as determined by the nature of the procedure and the presence of co-morbid conditions?

Once the decision to proceed with surgery has been made, planning for the postoperative period should begin. A thorough assessment of psychosocial support structure is necessary to identify existing resources and anticipate the need for additional rehabilitation and home nursing care. A robust individual living with involved family members, for example, requires far less

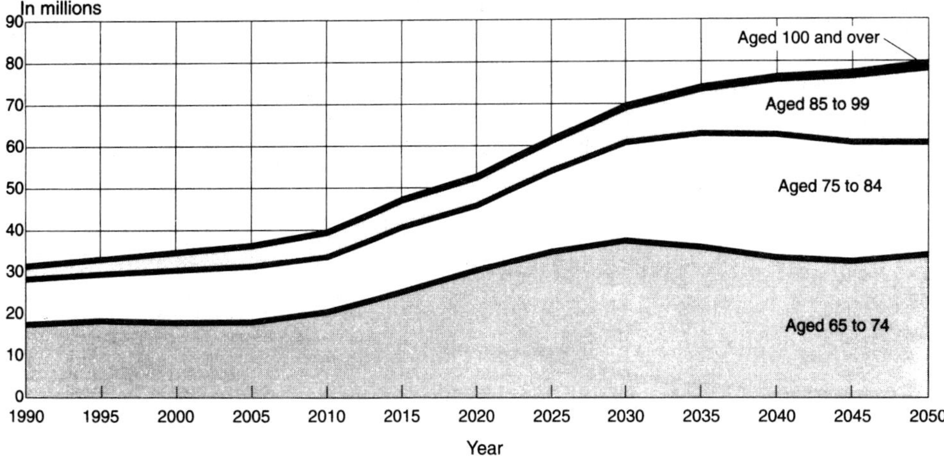


FIGURE 10.1. Projected growth in the population over age 65. The most rapidly growing portion of this population are persons over age 85. (From Day[2], with permission.)

ancillary support than a frail individual living alone. Determining the level of additional support required and preparing for this support prior to surgery helps shorten the hospital stay and speeds functional recovery.

Although all of these issues must be addressed, the main thrust of the preoperative evaluation is to identify, and improve when possible, any coexisting disease processes or decline in physiologic reserve. With this information, an accurate risk/benefit determination can be made for each surgical intervention in each elderly patient. Although we refer to risk primarily as the chance of postoperative mortality and morbidity, risk in the elderly should also be assessed in terms of restoration of preoperative functional status and quality of life (see Chapter 14). For the elderly patient, survival is not necessarily the only important outcome measure.

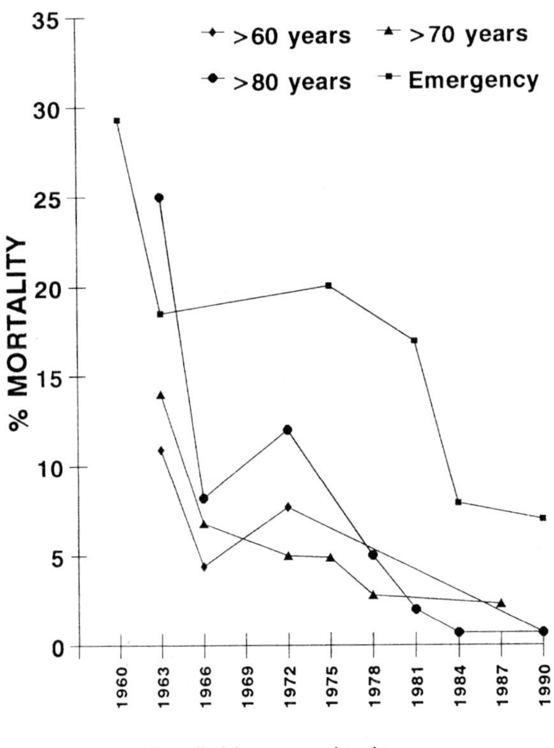


FIGURE 10.2. Decline in surgical mortality over the past four decades. (The data for this figure were obtained by the authors from several unreferenced studies.) (From Thomas and Ritchie[3], with permission.)

## General Evaluation

The general approach to the preoperative assessment is directed toward identifying those factors that place the patient at increased risk for postoperative complications or death. Although some of these factors are related to the surgical disease itself and to the type of operation required, the two most important factors in the determination of risk are related to the overall health and physiologic status of the patient. As discussed throughout this text, the physiologic changes that accompany aging are myriad but extremely variable among individuals and among organ systems. Discussion of the specific nature and magnitude of this decline can be found in the physiology chapter for each organ system. For this discussion, it suffices to say that in most cases the impact of these changes on the outcome of uncomplicated elective surgery in otherwise healthy, functional older patients is minimal. However, declining physiologic reserves may significantly impair the ability of the elderly patient to compensate appropriately for the additional stress of complicated or emergency surgery.

The more important determinant of all surgical outcome is the presence of pathologic processes other than the primary surgical disease, termed co-morbid conditions. Age as an isolated factor has minimal effect on postoperative morbidity or mortality. The sections that follow further define the importance of co-morbidity and describe methods for evaluating the potential impact of this co-morbidity on surgical outcome.

TABLE 10.1. Prevalence of Preoperative Co-morbid Conditions in Percent

| | Prevalence (%), by age in years | | | | |
|---|---|---|---|---|---|
| Condition | 50–59 | 60–69 | 70–79 | >80 | Total |
| Cardiovascular | 36 | 52 | 57 | 85 | 53 |
| Pulmonary | 8 | 17 | 20 | 17 | 16 |
| Renal | 5 | 8 | 24 | 15 | 13 |
| Hepatic | 7 | 10 | 16 | 20 | 12 |
| Nutritional | 2 | 7 | 10 | 22 | 8 |
| Other | 13 | 18 | 21 | 20 | 18 |

*Source:* Boyd et al.,[7] with permission.

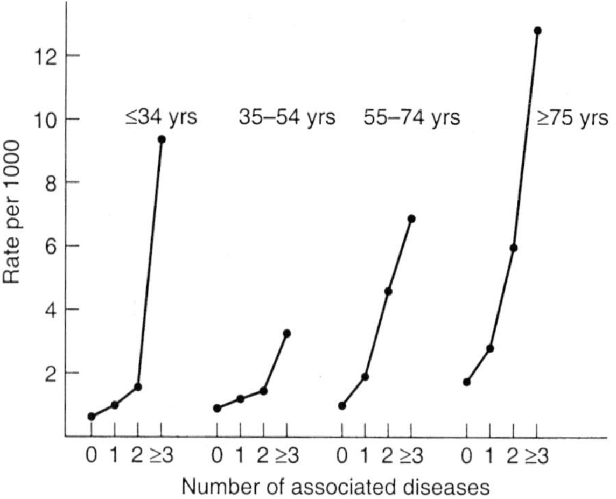


FIGURE 10.4. Perioperative complications as a function of the number of co-morbid conditions for several age groups. There is a clear rise in the incidence of perioperative complications with increasing number of co-morbid conditions in all age groups, but the effects are most pronounced in the youngest and oldest groups. (From Tiret L et al.[9] with permission.)

## Co-morbidity

The prevalence of co-morbid diseases clearly rises with increasing age. Boyd et al. documented the age-related increase of various co-morbid conditions in a study involving surgery for colon cancer in patients over age 50 years (Table 10.1).[7] In a larger, more detailed review of co-morbidity in elderly patients with colon cancer, Yancik et al. explored the increase in the number of additional conditions with age.[8] By age 75 patients with colon cancer had a mean of five disorders in addition to the primary cancer. The cumulative distribution of co-morbidity in these patients is shown in Figure 10.3.

As the number of associated illnesses increases, so does the rate of perioperative complications. In a study on the effect of increasing co-morbidity on outcome, Tiret and colleagues demonstrated a strong correlation between the number of conditions and the rate of perioperative complications. This effect was seen in all age groups but was most pronounced in the youngest and oldest patients (Fig. 10.4).[9] Only a minimal increase in mortality and morbidity was seen in old patients who lacked coexisting disease. Such minimal increases were insignificant when compared to the threefold increase associated with as few as two additional co-morbidities. Other studies of outcome for both surgical and medical treatment demonstrate a similar correlation between co-morbidity and poor treatment outcome.[8,10]

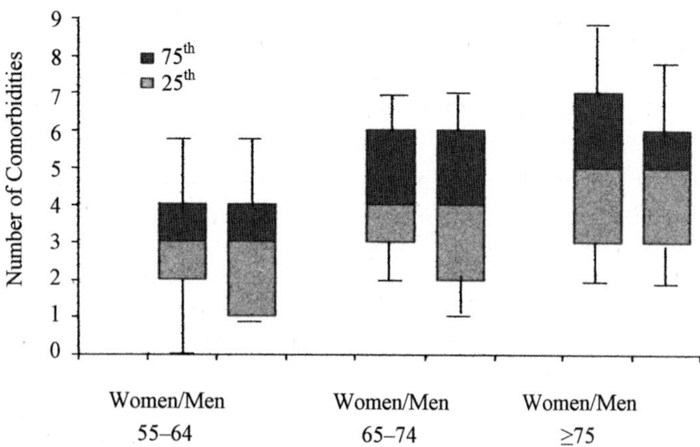


FIGURE 10.3. Number of co-morbid conditions as a function of age of men and women with colon cancer. Tails are 10th and 90th percentiles, and the bars are 25th and 75th percentiles. By age 75, 50% of both male and female patients have at least five other disorders in addition to the cancer. (From Yancik R et al.[8] with permission.)

Unfortunately, as is the case with the surgical disease itself, the manifestations of co-morbid illnesses in the elderly are frequently less specific and less "typical" than they are in younger patients. The search for co-morbid illness must therefore be diligent. In the Framingham heart study for example, myocardial infarction was unrecognized or silent in more than 40% of persons age 75–84 compared to fewer than 20% of those ages 45–54.[11] Apathetic hyperthyroidism, cognitive impairment, and malnutrition are among the many other coexisting disorders that may not be apparent from the initial history and physical examination. For example, one study of hospitalized patients over age 70 years revealed that 72% of moderate to severe cognitive deficits and 46% of moderate to severe nutritional deficits identified during admission had been previously unrecognized by the primary caregiver in the community (Fig. 10.5).[12]

Extensive testing for co-morbidity in every organ system is neither cost-effective nor necessary for every patient. A thorough history and physical examination provide information that can direct further workup, if necessary. It is important, however, to adjust the history and physical examination to look for risk factors and signs and symptoms of the more common co-morbid disorders. The addition of simple tools for assessing

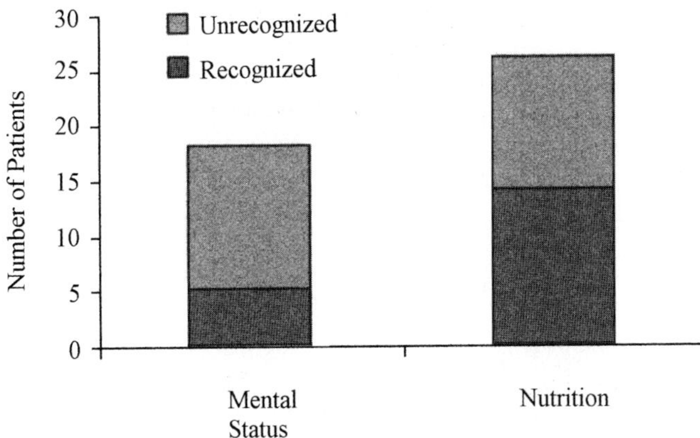


FIGURE 10.5. Patients found to have nutritional and mental status deficits during formal geriatric assessment at admission to the hospital compared to those identified by the primary caregiver in the community. Lighter bars indicate the results of formal assessment. It is seen that most of the nutritional deficits and a large percentage of mental status deficits were not recognized prior to admission to the hospital, indicating that these deficits are subtle and may not be appreciated without purposeful attempts to identify them. (From Pinholt[12] with permission, Copyright 1987. American Medical Association.)

functional, cognitive, and nutritional status significantly enhances understanding the individual elderly patient's true operative risk. When initial evaluation identifies disease or risk factors for disease, further workup may be indicated (see specific organ systems below).

## Functional Status Evaluation

Assessment of functional status, by a variety of methods, is the most useful means for predicting postoperative outcome. For decades, the American Society of Anesthesiologists (ASA) Physical Status Classification has been one of the most reliable and accurate predictors of surgical mortality. This simple classification ranks patients according to the functional limitations imposed by coexisting disease (see Table 11.1). Curves for mortality versus ASA class in old patients are superimposable on those of young patients, demonstrating that coexisting disease rather than chronologic age has the most profound impact on surgical outcome.[13] Even in patients over age 80, ASA classification has been shown to predict postoperative mortality accurately.[14]

The value of the ASA classification is further demonstrated by the results of a large, multicenter Department of Veterans Affairs (VA) study begun in 1991, in which surgical patients were assessed prospectively for operative risk. Risk-adjusted models were then created to allow comparison of the quality of surgical care among institutions.[15] Sixty-eight preoperative and intraoperative variables were collected, and nine models for mortality and morbidity (one for each subspecialty and one overall) were created.[16,17] Table 10.2 shows the 12 most significant risk factors for mortality and morbidity and the average rank of each factor in the models for fiscal year 1997.[18] The ASA Functional Classification was the second most predictive factor for mortality and the most predictive for morbidity. A discussion of the predictive value of serum albumin is found under Nutritional Assessment, below.

Other standard measures of functional status have proven to be predictive of postoperative outcome as well. The ability to perform activities of daily living (ADLs) or the simple tasks of life (e.g., feeding, continence, transferring, toileting, dressing, bathing) has been correlated with postoperative mortality and morbidity.[19] In one study, patients identified as inactive were shown to have a higher incidence of all major surgical complications (Fig. 10.6).[20] Inactivity was defined as the inability to leave home by one's own efforts at least twice a week. In another study of noncardiac surgical cases, mortality in patients with severely limited activity was 9.7 times higher than in active patients.[21] In this study limited activity was defined as confined to bed or, at maximum, able to transfer from bed to chair. Of all the risk factors studied, inactivity was found to be the single strongest predictor of death.

Preoperative functional deficits may contribute to postoperative immobility, with associated complications such

TABLE 10.2. Order of Entry of the Most Predictive Preoperative Risk Factors in Mortality and Morbidity Models

| Risk factor | Fiscal year 1997 | Average rank[a] |
|---|---|---|
| **Mortality** | | |
| Serum albumin | 1 | 1 |
| ASA class | 2 | 2 |
| Disseminated cancer | 3 | 3.3 |
| Emergency operation | 5 | 4.3 |
| Age | 6 | 5 |
| BUN > 40 mg/dl | 9 | 7 |
| DNR | 4 | 7.3 |
| Operation complexity | 13 | 11 |
| SGOT > 40 IU/ml | 17 | 11.3 |
| Weight loss >10% | 10 | 11.5 |
| Functional status | 8 | 12.3 |
| WBC > 1000/mm$^3$ | 11 | 14 |
| **Morbidity** | | |
| Serum albumin | 2 | 1.3 |
| ASA class | 1 | 2 |
| Operation complexity | 3 | 3.3 |
| Emergency operation | 4 | 4 |
| Functional status | 5 | 5 |
| History of COPD | 6 | 7.5 |
| Age | 10 | 8.3 |
| Hematocrit ≤ 38% | 7 | 9.5 |
| WBC > 11,000/mm$^3$ | 9 | 10 |
| Weight loss > 10% | 8 | 13.3 |
| Ventilator-dependent | 38 | 16.5 |
| BUN > 40 mg/dl | 29 | 20.3 |

[a] Average rank of 419,944 cases from October 1991 to September 1997.

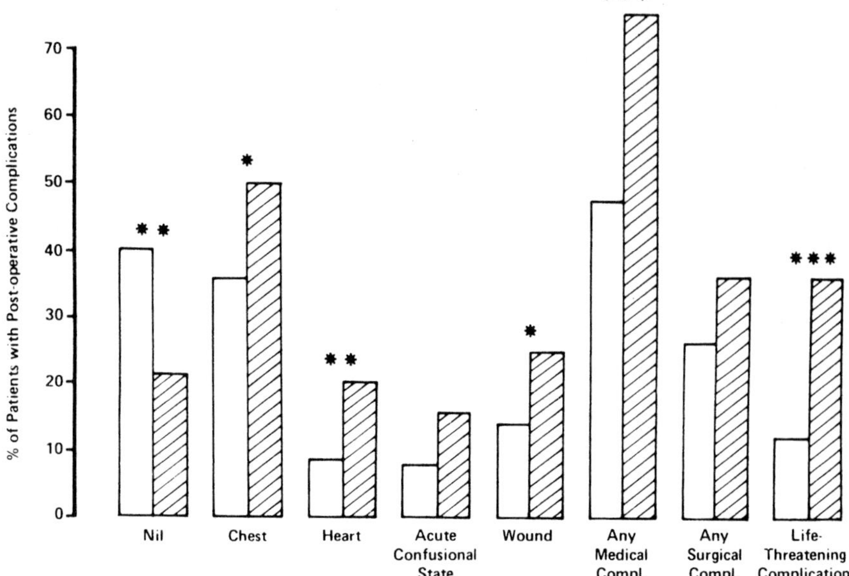


FIGURE 10.6. Incidence of postoperative complications in active and inactive patients. Inactivity was defined in this study as the inability to leave home by one's own effort at least twice a week. (From Seymour and Pringle,[20] with permission.)

as atelectasis and pneumonia, venous stasis and pulmonary embolism, and multisystem deconditioning. Deconditioning is an important clinical entity that leads to further functional decline despite improvement in the acute illness.[22] The recovery period from deconditioning can be three or more times as long as the period of immobilization that led to the decline.

Even for patients with less obvious limitations, functional capacity or exercise tolerance is the single most important predictor of cardiac and pulmonary complications following noncardiac surgery. In a study comparing Dripps Criteria (ASA), Goldman Clinical Criteria, pulmonary function tests, exercise tolerance, and several other variables, Gerson et al. demonstrated that the inability to raise the heart rate to 99 beats/min while doing 2 minutes of supine bicycle exercise was the most sensitive predictor of postoperative cardiac and pulmonary complications, and death.[23,24]

The physiologic basis for this finding has been further clarified by a study in which elderly patients performed supine ergometry while connected by mouthpiece to a metabolic cart.[25] The authors identified an anaerobic threshold—defined as the level of oxygen consumption above which circulatory supply could not meet metabolic demand—and correlated this threshold with surgical outcome. For those patients able to reach an anaerobic threshold of 11 ml/kg/min or more, the mortality was 0.8% compared to 18% for those unable to reach this threshold. Even in patients who experienced ischemia at the time of exercise testing, threshold levels were highly predictive of postoperative mortality (Table 10.3).

Should all preoperative elderly patients therefore be subjected to this type of exercise testing? Clearly this is neither practical nor necessary. The metabolic requirements for many routine activities have already been determined and are quantitated as metabolic equivalents (METs). One MET, defined as 3.5 ml/kg/min, represents the basal oxygen consumption of a 70-kg, 40-year-old man at rest. Estimated energy requirements for various activities are shown in Table 10.4.[26] The inability to func-

TABLE 10.3. Mortality in Relation to Anaerobic Threshold

| Anaerobic threshold (ml/min/kg) | All patients | | Patients with ischemia | |
|---|---|---|---|---|
| | No. | % Mortality | No. | % Mortality |
| <11 | 55 | 18 | 19 | 42 |
| >11 | 132 | 0.8 | 25 | 4 |
| | | $p < 0.001$ | | $p < 0.01$ |

*Source:* Older et al.,[25] with permission.

TABLE 10.4. Estimated Energy Requirements for Various Activities

**1–4 Metabolic equivalents (METs)**
- Can you take care of yourself?
- Eat, dress, or use the toilet?
- Walk indoors around the house?
- Walk a block or two on level ground at 2–3 mph or 3.2–4.8 km/hr?
- Do light work around the house such as dusting or washing dishes?

**4–10 Metabolic equivalents (METs)**
- Climb a flight of stairs or walk up hill?
- Walk on level ground at 4 mph or 6.4 km/hr?
- Run a short distance?
- Do heavy work around the house such as scrubbing floors or lifting or moving heavy furniture?
- Participate in moderate recreational activities such as golf, bowling, dancing, doubles tennis, or throwing a baseball or football?
- Participate in strenuous sports such as swimming, singles tennis, football, basketball, or skiing?

*Source:* Eagle et al.,[26] with permission.

tion above 4 METs has been associated with increased perioperative cardiac events and long-term risk. By asking appropriate questions about the level of activity or using a standardized self-assessment tool such as the Duke's Activity Status Index, functional capacity can be determined accurately without the need for additional testing.[27] Some assessment of functional capacity should be a routine component of the preoperative evaluation.

## Nutritional Assessment

The impact of poor nutrition as a risk factor for pneumonia, poor wound healing, and other postoperative complications has long been appreciated. The variety of psychosocial issues, physiologic dysfunctions, and comorbid conditions common to the elderly places this population at high risk for nutritional deficits. Malnutrition, defined as a decrease in nutrient reserves, occurs in approximately 0–15% of community dwelling elderly persons, 35–65% of older patients in acute care hospitals, and 25–60% of institutionalized elderly[28] (refer also to Chapter 5).

The assessment of nutritional status begins by understanding the risk factors for nutritional deficiency in this age group (Table 10.5).[29] Factors that may lead to inadequate intake and utilization of nutrients include the ability to get food (e.g., financial constraints, availability of food, limited mobility), the desire to eat food (e.g., living situation, mental status, chronic illness), the ability to eat and absorb food (e.g., poor dentition, chronic gastrointestinal problems such as gastroesophageal reflux disease or diarrhea), and medications that interfere with appetite or nutrient metabolism.

Measuring nutritional status in the elderly, however, is difficult. Standard anthropomorphic measures do not take into account the change in body composition and structure that accompanies aging. Immune measures of nutrition are influenced by age-related changes in the immune system in general. Furthermore, criteria for the interpretation of biochemical markers in this age group have not been well established.

Table 10.5. Historical Findings Associated with an Increased Risk of Nutritional Deficiency

| |
|---|
| Recent weight loss |
| Restricted dietary intake (limited variety): limited variety, food avoidances |
| Psychosocial situation: depression, cognitive impairment, isolation, economic difficulties |
| Problems with eating, chewing, swallowing |
| Previous surgery |
| Increased losses due to gastrointestinal disorders such as malabsorption and diarrhea |
| Systemic disease interfering with appetite or eating (chronic lung, liver, heart and renal disease, abdominal angina, cancer) |
| Excessive alcohol use |
| Medications that interfere with appetite or nutrient metabolism |

*Source:* Rosenberg,[29] with permission.

Serum albumin, however, has been implicated as a strong predictor of outcome. Evidence demonstrates that low serum albumin in elderly patients correlates with increased length of stay, increased rates of readmission, unfavorable disposition, and increased all-cause mortality.[30] In surgical patients, low albumin has also been shown to correlate with postoperative morbidity and mortality.[31] As mentioned above, in the VA NSQIP study a low serum albumin level was the most important preoperative predictive risk factor, suggesting that low serum albumin is an important marker of outcome, regardless of whether it is related to poor nutritional status or an unidentified complex chronic illness.

Complicated markers of malnutrition exist[28] but are not necessary in the routine surgical setting. Subjective assessment by history and physical examination, in which risk factors and physical evidence of malnutrition are assessed, has been shown to be as effective as objective measures of nutritional status.[32]

The Subjective Global Assessment (SGA) is one relatively simple reproducible tool for assessing nutritional status from the history and physical exam.[33] SGA ratings are most strongly influenced by loss of subcutaneous tissue, muscle wasting, and weight loss. In a study of patients undergoing elective gastrointestinal surgery, both SGA and serum albumin were predictive of postoperative nutrition-related complications.[34]

## Cognitive Assessment

The perioperative cognitive assessment tends to be undervalued and underapplied as a predictor of postoperative outcome. However, cognitive dysfunction as either a presurgical condition or postoperative complication can interfere with surgical treatment and postsurgical recovery. The lack of standard guidelines for effectively assessing perioperative cognitive function undermines the importance of such observation to surgical outcome. The relative incidence of delirium following a variety of procedures is shown in Table 10.6.[35]

Delirium, also called acute confusional state, is defined as a transient organic mental syndrome characterized by a global disorder of attention and cognition, reduced level of consciousness, abnormal levels of psychomotor activity, and disturbed sleep–wake cycles.[36] Delirium in the hospitalized elderly patient is often unrecognized because of physician uncertainty about patient confusion. Inouye, a leading scholar of delirium in hospitalized medical patients, has contrasted the myths of delirium in this population to the realities (Table 10.7).[37] Common findings frequently accepted as routine in older patients are often important indicators of serious underlying disturbances. Inouye and colleagues have added greatly to the understanding of delirium by developing the Confu-

TABLE 10.6. Incidence of Delirium Following Various Procedures

| Procedure | No. of patients | No. with delirium (%) |
|---|---|---|
| Colectomy | 21 | 3 (14.3) |
| Exploratory laparotomy | 26 | 3 (11.5) |
| Mastectomy | 12 | 0 |
| Hysterectomy | 11 | 1 (9.1) |
| Radical prostatectomy | 30 | 0 |
| Thoracotomy | 43 | 3 (7.0) |
| Thoracoscopic lung resection | 22 | 3 (13.6) |
| Total hip replacement | 66 | 4 (6.1) |
| Total knee replacement | 58 | 9 (15.5) |
| Laminectomy | 11 | 2 (18.2) |
| Peripheral vascular | 18 | 4 (22.2) |
| Abdominal aortic aneurysm | 17 | 1 (5.9) |
| Aortobifemoral bypass | 7 | 0 |
| Carotid endarterectomy | 19 | 1 (5.3) |
| *Total* | 361 | 34 (9.4) |

*Source:* Modified from Lynch et al.,[35] with permission.

sion Assessment Method (CAM), an easy-to-use, validated instrument with specificity and sensitivity higher than 90%.[38] The four key features of the CAM are (1) acute onset and fluctuating course of mental status change; (2) inattention; (3) disorganized thinking; and (4) altered level of consciousness (Table 10.8).

Delirium must be distinguished from dementia, the more chronic type of baseline cognitive impairment. Dementia, a preoperative cognitive impairment, is a major risk factor for delirium in the postoperative period. There are several methods for evaluating baseline cognitive function in the elderly. Among them, the Folstein Mini Mental Status test has become widely accepted for its ease of administration and reliability (Appendix 1).[39]

TABLE 10.7. Myth and Reality about Delirium in the Hospitalized Elderly

| Myth | Reality |
|---|---|
| "Older people get confused during the postoperative period, it is to be expected." | Delirium is a potential medical emergency, and may be the sole manifestation of a life-threatening complication. |
| "Oriented times one . . . this patient must have Alzheimer's disease." | Delirium is often misdiagnosed as dementia or depression or misattributed senescence. Cognitive function is rarely assessed pre- or postoperatively. |
| "The hallmarks of delirium are agitation, disorientation, hallucinations, and inappropriate behavior." | In older persons delirium often presents with lethargy and decreased activity—the hypoactive form of delirium, which is easily overlooked. |
| "The nurse says the patient got confused last night, but (s)he's totally with-it now. I don't think anything's going on." | Lucid intervals are characteristic of delirium. A fluctuating course is one of the key features. |

*Source:* Inouye,[37] with permission.

This instrument gives a total of 30 points to four areas: (1) orientation, (2) registration, (3) attention/calculation, and (4) language. A score below 24 is an indication of cognitive impairment. The Telephone Interview for Cognitive Status (TICS) is a validated, reliable modification of the Mini Mental Status Examination (MMSE), which can be administered over the telephone.[40] Both of these instruments, although extremely informative, are time-consuming and may not be practical in the preoperative clinic. Simple clinical strategies for assessing mental

TABLE 10.8. Confusion Assessment Method: Diagnostic Algorithm

| Feature | Description |
|---|---|
| **1: Acute onset and fluctuating course** | This feature is usually obtained from a family member or nurse and is shown by positive responses to the following questions: Is there evidence of acute changes in mental status from the patient's baseline? Did the (abnormal) behavior fluctuate during the day; that is, did it tend to come and go or fluctuate in severity? |
| **2: Inattention** | This feature is shown by a positive response to the following question: Did the patient have difficulty focusing attention, for example, being easily distractible or having difficulty keeping track of what has been said? |
| **3: Disorganized thinking** | This feature is shown by a positive response to the following question: Was the patient's thinking disorganized or incoherent, such as exhibiting rambling or irrelevant conversation, unclear or illogical flow of ideas, or unpredictable switching from subject to subject? |
| **4: Altered level of consciousness** | This feature is shown by the answer other than "alert" to the following question: Overall how would you rate this patient's level of consciousness [alert (normal), vigilant (hyperalert), lethargic (drowsy, easily aroused), stupor (difficult to arouse), or coma (unarousable)]? |
| ***Diagnosis of delirium*** | |
| **Feature 1**: must be present | |
| **Feature 2**: must be present | |
| **Feature 3**: must be present | |
| **Feature 4**: must be present | |

*Source:* Modified from Inouye et al.,[38] with permission.

TABLE 10.9. Etiology of Delirium

| |
|---|
| **D**enemtia |
| **E**lectrolytes |
| **L**ungs, liver, heart, kidney, brain |
| **I**nfection |
| **R**x |
| **I**njury, pain, stress |
| **U**nfamiliar environment |
| **M**etabolic |

*Source:* Inouye,[37] with permission.

TABLE 10.10. Drugs Associated with Delirium in the Elderly

| | |
|---|---|
| **Minor tranquilizers** | **Analgesics** |
| Diazepam | Meperidine |
| Flurazepam | Acetylsalicylic acid |
| Meprobamate | Naproxen |
| Oxazepam | |
| Chlorazepate | **Antibiotics** |
| Droperidol | Ciprofloxacin |
| | Tobramycin |
| **Major tranquilizers** | Chloramphenicol |
| Haloperidol | |
| Thorazine | **Anticholinergics** |
| Thioridazine | Atropine |
| Amitriptyline | Scopolamine |
| | |
| **Antihypertensives** | **Others** |
| Methyldopa | Cimetidine, ranitidine |
| Reserpine | Insulin |
| Nitroprusside | Digoxin |
| | Amantidine |
| **β-Adrenergic blockers** | |
| Propanolol | |
| | |
| **Diuretics** | |
| Hydrochlorothiazide | |

*Source:* Modified from Larson et al.,[42] with permission.

status may suffice for elucidating a patient's baseline function. They include (1) orienting to person, place, and time; (2) the ability to list five items (e.g., cities, fruits, vegetables); and (3) the ability to remember and recall three objects after a short delay.[41]

The etiology of delirium in hospitalized patients is multifactorial (Table 10.9).[35] In surgical patients, postoperative delirium may be the manifestation of unrecognized preexisting disease or the result of intra- or postoperative events. Among the many factors studied, the use of multiple medications, termed "polypharmacy," stands out as both a common and important cause of delirium. Many individual medications are known to impair cognitive function (Table 10.10).[42] When used together, the likelihood of precipitating delirium is enormous.

Over the past several years several studies have attempted to identify risk factors for delirium in hospitalized elderly surgical and medical patients. Although the results vary somewhat with the reasons for hospitalization, type of surgery, and the variables studied, age, polypharmacy, preoperative cognitive impairment, and poor functional status are among the most frequently associated factors. The results of several of these studies are shown in Table 10.11.[43–50]

A "predictive rule" for postoperative delirium has been developed from a large prospective study of major

TABLE 10.11. Risk Factors for Delirium in Hospitalized Elderly Patients

| Study | Type of patients | Age (years) | No. | Type of study | Independent predictors |
|---|---|---|---|---|---|
| Williams[43] (1985) | Hip fracture | ≥60 | 170 | Prospective daily rating by nurses | Age; preop cognitive deficit; low preop activity |
| Gustafson[44] (1988) | Hip fracture | ≥65 | 111 | Prospective daily observ. | Age; dementia |
| Rogers[45] (1989) | Elective orthopedic | ≥60 | 46 | Prospective pre and post | Use of scopolamine, propranolol, flurazepam |
| Francis[46] (1990) | Medical | ≥70 | 229 | Prospective q 48 h | Severe illness; chronic cognitive deficit; fever/hypothermia; psychoactive drugs; azotemia; low serum $Na^+$ |
| Schor[49] (1992) | Medical and surgical | ≥65 | 291 | Prospective daily observ. | Age ≥ 80; chronic cognitive deficit; fracture on admission; neuroleptic or narcotic; infection; male gender |
| Inuoye[48] (1993) | Medical | ≥70 | 107 | Prospective daily observ. | Vision impairment; severe illness; cognitive impairment; high BUN/Cr ratio |
| Marcantonio[47] (1994) | Major elective noncardiac | ≥50 | 1341 | Prospective daily interview | Age ≥70; self-reported alcohol abuse; poor cognitive status; poor functional status, markedly abnormal preop $Na^+$, $K^+$, glucose; thoracic/aortic surgery |

*Source:* Modified from Inouye,[50] with permission.

elective noncardiac surgery patients over age 50 years.[47] Independent correlates for postoperative delirium in this study included age over 70 years; self-reported alcohol abuse; poor cognitive function; poor functional status; markedly abnormal serum sodium, potassium, or glucose levels; aortic aneurysm surgery; and noncardiac thoracic surgery. A point system was devised to quantify these factors. Postoperative delirium developed in 2% of patients with 0 points, 8% with 1 point, 13% with 2 points, and 50% with ≥3 points.

Intraoperative and postoperative factors have also been studied. No association has been found with the route of anesthesia (epidural versus general[51,52]) or the occurrence of intraoperative hemodynamic complications. Intraoperative blood loss, the need for blood transfusion, and postoperative hematocrit <30%, however, are associated with a significantly increased risk of postoperative delirium.[52] Alterations in the wake–sleep cycle following surgery has also been associated with delirium.[53] In nonsurgical hospitalized elderly patients, independent precipitating factors for delirium include malnutrition, the use of physical restraints, the use of bladder catheters, the need for more than three medications, and any iatrogenic event during hospitalization.[54]

The negative impact of postoperative delirium on other surgical outcomes is clear. Mortality, major morbidity, length of hospital stay, and discharge to long-term care or rehabilitation facilities are significantly increased in patients who develop postoperative delirium (Table 10.12).[47] In addition, cognitive dysfunction during the postoperative period has been shown to persist for as long as 3 months after operation in a significant percentage of elderly patients.[55]

It is most important to recognize that mental status changes in the elderly surgical patient are often the earliest signs of a postoperative complication. Therefore tests for cognitive impairment are essential components of the routine postoperative evaluation. The postoperative mental status evaluation is mostly based on knowing what to recognize in the particular patient and acting on observed changes. If an adequate preoperative mental status examination, as described above, is recorded and the patient's baseline cognitive status is known, postoperative assessment should entail brief observations of behavior with a comparison to baseline. Observations such as changes in the patient's sleep cycle, the inability to remember names, and so on are easily detectable and serve as informative indicators of the postoperative cognitive state.

TABLE 10.12. Association of Postoperative Delirium with Other Surgical Outcomes

| Outcome | Delirium ($n$ = 117) | No delirium ($n$ = 1224) | $p$ |
|---|---|---|---|
| Major complication[a] | 18 (15%) | 28 (2%) | <0.001 |
| Death | 5 (4%) | 3 (0.2%) | <0.001 |
| Length of stay | 15 ± 20 | 7 ± 5 | <0.001 |
| Discharge to LTC or rehabilitation facility | 43 (36%) | 136 (11%) | <0.001 |

*Source:* Marcantonio et al.,[47] with permission.
LTC, long-term care.
[a] Cardiac arrest, ventricular tachycardia or fibrillation, myocardial infarction, pulmonary edema, respiratory failure requiring intubation, renal failure requiring dialysis, and stroke.

### Gender

In developed countries women typically outlive men by 6–7 years. Despite the clear gender differences in longevity, conflicting gender-based differences in the patterns of postoperative morbidity and mortality have been observed. Of eight complications studied in one report on postoperative morbidity in elderly general surgical patients, only cognitive impairment exhibited a statistically significant gender difference.[20] The incidence of postoperative morbidity was similar between women and men on all other parameters. However, in another report on the perioperative morbidity, mortality, and long-term outcome of 795 consecutive surgical patients aged 90 years and over, there was a significantly poorer long-term postoperative survival for men.[56] Men exhibited 3.9% higher 30-day mortality, 8.5% higher 1-year mortality, and 10.5% higher 5-year mortality.

## Specific Evaluations

In the elderly patient both cardiac and pulmonary complications are common during the postoperative period. These complications prolong hospital stay and increase the likelihood of functional decline and the need for postoperative rehabilitation. History or physical examination findings suggestive of cardiac or pulmonary disease should therefore prompt a more extensive preoperative evaluation.

### Cardiovascular Assessment: Algorithmic Approach

Of all co-morbid conditions, cardiovascular disease is the most prevalent. Cardiovascular events are a leading cause of severe perioperative complications and death. For this reason, preoperative evaluation of cardiac risk has been studied extensively. The American College of Cardiology (ACC) and the American Heart Association (AHA) Task Force on Practice Guidelines has published an in-depth set of guidelines for perioperative cardiovascular evaluation that addresses all the current major concerns.[26] The Guidelines provide a stepwise bayesian strategy for optimally determining which patients will need extensive tests to clarify cardiac risk or additional therapy to diminish long-term risks (Appendix 2). Stratification of risk based on clinical and operative factors is discussed. For elderly patients with known cardiac disease, rigorous workup may be necessary (see below). For most other elderly patients, assessments of functional status, exercise tolerance, and general health are accurate predictors of adequate cardiac reserves.

The general scheme of the strategy relies on assessment of: (1) indication and urgency of the surgery; (2) prior coronary evaluation and treatment; (3) clinical predictors of increased perioperative cardiovascular risk; (4) functional capacity; and (5) surgery-specific risks. These factors are discussed in sequence.

### *Indication and Urgency of the Surgery*

Emergent situations do not allow time for careful preoperative cardiac evaluation. Given a surgical emergency, rapid assessment of cardiovascular vital signs, volume status, and an electrocardiogram suffice as the preoperative evaluation. Postoperative risk stratification and management may be justified to decrease the likelihood of perioperative cardiac failure in such cases.

### *Prior Coronary Evaluation and Treatment*

Patients who have received a favorable report on a coronary evaluation within 2 years prior or who have undergone successful coronary revascularization during the past 5 years without new or recurrent signs/symptoms generally do not require repeat cardiac testing. According to the Guidelines, these patients may usually proceed with surgery.

### *Clinical Predictors of Increased Perioperative Risk*

The Guidelines' strategy categorizes clinical predictors of risk into major, intermediate, and minor predictors (Table 10.13).[57,58] The presence of any major clinical predictors indicates that cancellation or delay of elective noncardiac surgery is in order. The patient's major problems should be identified and treated before proceeding with the surgery. In the presence of intermediate and minor predictors of cardiac risk, the need for further testing may be determined by assessing the patient's functional capacity and determining the level of surgery-specific risk. The choice of noninvasive versus invasive tests depends on the cardiac risk stratification of the planned surgical procedure (see below).

### *Functional Capacity*

Functional capacity estimates functional status based on the ability of the patient to perform certain activities of daily living. It is expressed in metabolic equivalent (MET) levels, where 1 MET equals the oxygen consumption of a 70-kg man at rest (a numeric value of 3.5 ml/kg/min).

TABLE 10.13. Clinical Predictors of Increased Perioperative Cardiovascular Risk

**Major predictors**
- Unstable coronary syndromes
  - Recent myocardial infarction (>7 days but <30 days) with evidence of important risk based on clinical symptoms or noninvasive study
  - Unstable or severe angina (Canadian class III or IV)[58]
- Decompensated congestive heart failure
- Significant arrhythmias
  - High-grade atrioventricular block
  - Symptomatic ventricular arrhythmias in the presence of underlying heart disease
  - Supraventricular arrhythmias with uncontrolled ventricular rate
- Severe valvular disease

**Intermediate predictors**
- Mild angina pectoris (Canadian class II or II)
- Prior myocardial infarction based on history or pathologic waves
- Compensated or prior congestive heart failure
- Diabetes mellitus

**Minor predictors**
- Advanced age
- Abnormal electrocardiographic findings
  - Left ventricular hypertrophy
  - Left bundle branch block
  - ST-T abnormalities
- Rhythm other than sinus
  - Atrial fibrillation, for example
- Low functional capacity
  - Unable to climb one flight of stairs while carrying a bag of groceries
- History of stroke
- Uncontrolled systemic hypertension

*Source:* Eagle et al.,[57] with permission.

Questioning patients on their ability to perform daily physical activities for which the estimated MET values are known provides individual scoring of functional capacity (Table 10.4). Functional capacity of more than 7 METS is considered excellent; between 4–7 METS indicates moderate functional capacity. Patients unable to meet a 4-MET demand during most normal daily activities are at increased risk for perioperative cardiopulmonary and long-term dysfunction.

### *Surgery-Specific Risk*

Surgery-specific risk for noncardiac surgery is stratified as high, intermediate and low risk (Table 10.14). This classification is related to the type of surgery and the degree of hemodynamic stress associated with the procedure. High risk surgery in a patient with intermediate clinical predictors and poor functional capacity indicates the need for invasive tests, such as coronary angiography. In a patient with moderate to excellent functional capacity, adequate performance on noninvasive tests, such as electrocardiography and stress tests, should suffice as clearance for high risk surgery. Cardiac assessment for low

TABLE 10.14. Cardiac Risk[a] Stratification for Noncardiac Surgical Procedures

| |
|---|
| **High (risk > 5%)** |
| Emergency major operation, particularly in the elderly |
| Aortic or other major vascular surgery |
| Peripheral vascular surgery |
| Anticipated prolonged surgical procedure associated with large fluid shifts, blood loss, or both |
| **Intermediate (risk < 5%)** |
| Carotid endarterectomy |
| Head and neck surgery |
| Intraperitoneal and intrathoracic surgery |
| Orthopedic surgery |
| Prostate surgery |
| **Low (risk < 1%)** |
| Endoscopic procedures |
| Superficial procedures |
| Cataract surgery |
| Breast surgery |

*Source:* Eagle et al.,[26] with permission.
[a] Combined incidence of cardiac death and nonfatal myocardial infarction.

risk surgery, such as endoscopic or superficial procedures, requires noninvasive testing only when the patient's functional capacity is poor; usually such procedures do not call for extensive testing.

## Pulmonary Assessment

Although the thrust of preoperative risk assessment has been to define cardiac risk factors, pulmonary complications are at least as common, if not more so, following noncardiac surgical procedures.[59] The incidence of pulmonary complications cited in the literature varies depending on the methodology and the criteria used to define the complications. Frequently, cardiac and pulmonary complications occur together. This is probably an indication of the poor general health of the patient rather than the result of a specific or single perioperative variable. As with all adverse surgical outcomes, pulmonary complications are more common following emergency operations. This is particularly important in the elderly because of the high incidence of emergency presentation in this age group.

### *Risk Factors*

Many preoperative, intraoperative, and postoperative factors have been implicated in the development of postoperative pulmonary complications. In a review, Smetana[60] identified five preoperative potential risk factors: ASA class >II, chronic obstructive pulmonary disease (COPD), smoking, obesity and age >70 years. The incidence of complications when each of these factors was present or absent is shown in Table 10.15.

The ASA classification, as an indication of functional status and overall co-morbidity, is a sensitive predictor of both cardiac and pulmonary postoperative complications.[61] In the study by Gerson et al. cited above,[24] inability to perform 2 minutes of supine exercise was the best predictor of both cardiac and pulmonary events. Poor exercise tolerance was predictive of 79% of the pulmonary complications. In another recent multivariate analysis of preoperative risk factors, other indicators of general health status (the Charleston co-morbidity index[62] and the Goldman cardiac risk index,[63]) were also found to be predictive of postoperative pulmonary events.[64]

The relative risk of developing postoperative pulmonary problems in patients with obstructive pulmonary disease varies from 2.7 to 4.7. In the multivariate analysis referred to above,[64] the degree of obstructive disease (none to mild versus moderate to severe) did not contribute to the multivariate model. However, an abnormal chest examination and abnormal chest radiograph, as an indication of underlying lung disease, were significantly associated with complications. Preoperative treatment with bronchodilators, antibiotics, aggressive physical therapy, and if necessary corticosteroids has been shown to decrease the incidence of postoperative pulmonary problems.[65,66]

Smoking is a well-established risk factor, with smokers having a 1.4–4.3 relative risk of developing a pulmonary complication. Although smoking cessation should be a routine recommendation prior to surgery, a decrease in the relative risk of complications is seen only after at least 8 weeks of cessation.

Although obesity is widely thought to be associated with postoperative pulmonary complications and changes in pulmonary physiology with age should predispose to complications,[67] there are few data in the literature to support this assumption. A prospective study from Spain found that obesity, defined as a body mass index higher than the 90th percentile, was associated with an increased risk of postoperative pneumonia.[68] Another study reported that obese patients were twice as likely to have acute respiratory events during the postoperative

TABLE 10.15. Potential Patient-Related Risk Factors for Postoperative Pulmonary Complications

| | Incidence of complications (%) | |
|---|---|---|
| Risk Factor | Factor present | Factor absent |
| Smoking | 15–46 | 6–21 |
| ASA class ≥ II | 26–44 | 13–19 |
| Age >70 years | 9–22 | 4–21 |
| Obesity | 11–36 | 9–27 |
| COPD | 6–26 | 2–8 |

*Source:* Modified from Smetana,[60] with permission © Massachusetts Medical Society.
COPD, chronic obstructive pulmonary disease.

period.[69] The incidence of pulmonary complications following surgery for morbid obesity, however, is no higher than would be expected in a group of procedure-matched nonobese patients.

Chronologic age, as an isolated factor, is not associated with an increased risk of pulmonary complications in most studies. However, many co-morbid conditions commonly found among the elderly can increase the risk of postoperative pneumonia and atelectasis. Preexisting pulmonary disease, malnutrition, immunologic decline, subtle swallowing disorders, oropharyngeal colonization with gram-negative bacteria, and impaired mobility have been implicated as possible explanations for the high rate of postoperative pulmonary problems seen among old patients.[12,70]

Intraoperative factors implicated in the development of postoperative pulmonary complications include the site of incision, type of anesthesia, duration of the procedure, amount of blood loss, and use of devices that traverse the oropharynx, such as nasogastric tubes and possibly transesophageal echocardiograph probes.

The proximity of the surgical incision to the diaphragm has long been known to influence the rate of postoperative pulmonary complications. Upper abdominal incisions are accompanied by a 13–33%[65,71] pulmonary complication rate, compared to a 0–16%[71,72] rate for incisions in the lower abdomen. Rates as high as 40% are reported with thoracic incisions.[73] Minimally invasive procedures, such as laparoscopic cholecystectomy, are associated with little risk of pulmonary complications. In several large series rates as low as 0.3–0.4% were reported.[74,75]

The importance of the type of anesthesia and the length of operation in terms of the incidence of postoperative pulmonary complications is less clear. Although most studies support the lower complication rate following regional anesthesia compared to general anesthesia, these results are not uniform. Duration of anesthesia of more than 3 hours has been shown to be significant by some[60,76] but not all.[70]

In one retrospective analysis, intraoperative blood loss of more than 1200 ml was an independent predictor of postoperative pneumonia.[70] This may be an indication of the complexity of the procedure or of underlying comorbidity. Although multiple transfusions are known to be immunosuppressive, the relation of transfusion to postoperative infection is not clear.[77] However, when combined with the declining immunologic competence associated with aging, a transfusion-related alteration in host defenses may facilitate the development of pneumonia in the elderly.

Subtle nasopharyngeal dysfunction is frequently unrecognized in the elderly but is known to be a factor predisposing to aspiration pneumonia. Devices that traverse the oropharynx may further disrupt the normal swallowing process and further increase the risk of aspiration. In one multivariate analysis, postoperative nasogastric intubation was the single most important variable associated with postoperative pulmonary complications.[76] In another study of cardiac surgery patients, the use of transesophageal echocardiography probes intraoperatively was significantly associated with the development of postoperative aspiration.[78]

During the postoperative period the basic strategies to reduce pulmonary complications are deep breathing with incentive spirometry, early ambulation, and adequate pain control. Lung-expanding maneuvers, when done properly, can decrease pulmonary complications by 50%.[79] Early ambulation can decrease the incidence of atelectasis and venous thrombosis with pulmonary embolus. Unfortunately, owing to co-morbidity or declining reserves, elderly patients are frequently unable to accomplish these two seemingly simple maneuvers.

Adequate pain control is particularly important for encouraging patients to deep-breathe. In the elderly, however, oversedation can worsen rather than improve compliance with incentive spirometry. Epidural anesthesia is particularly effective in reducing postoperative pain without sedation and decreasing the rate of pulmonary complications.[80]

### *Preoperative Assessment of Pulmonary Function*

Although previous guidelines for preoperative pulmonary function testing suggested that spirometry was indicated for every patient over age 70 years,[81] more recent data refute that claim. In the few studies that have compared clinical findings to pulmonary function tests, clinical findings have proved more predictive than spirometry results.[82–84] Abnormal chest findings on physical examination and chest radiography have been shown to be highly associated with postoperative pulmonary complications, whereas spirometry results have not.[64]

Present guidelines from the American College of Physicians for the use of preoperative pulmonary function tests are shown in Table 10.16.[86] There is consensus that all patients undergoing lung resection should have pul-

TABLE 10.16. ACP Guidelines for Preoperative Spirometry

| |
|---|
| Lung resection |
| Coronary artery bypass graft and smoking history or dyspnea |
| Upper abdominal surgery and smoking history or dyspnea |
| Lower abdominal surgery and uncharacterized pulmonary disease,[a] particularly if the surgical procedure is prolonged or extensive |
| Other surgery and uncharacterized pulmonary disease,[a] particularly in those who might require strenuous postoperative rehabilitation programs. |

*Source:* Hnatiuk et al.,[86] with permission.

[a] Uncharacterized pulmonary disease defined as pulmonary symptoms or history of pulmonary disease and no pulmonary function tests within 60 days.

monary function tests. Those with uncharacterized pulmonary disease and those having high risk incisions with a history of smoking probably should also be tested. However, those patients with normal physical examinations and good exercise tolerance do not benefit from additional studies.

## Improving Outcome

Adverse outcomes in elderly hospitalized populations include mortality, longer hospital stays, and discharge to nursing homes. Geriatric intervention programs to improve adverse outcomes of hospitalized medical patients are concerned with targeting "at risk" patients for geriatric services. Although these intervention programs have not yet been thoroughly studied in relation to surgical patients, the results may offer some important insights.

In a prospective cohort study of 507 acutely hospitalized male veterans aged 65 years or more, Satish et al. assessed the ability of 12 geriatric targeting criteria to predict adverse outcomes of hospitalization[87]: socioeconomic problems, polypharmacy, vision impairment, hearing impairment, appetite loss, weight loss, incontinence, confusion, depression, dementia, falls, and prolonged bed rest. Of these criteria, only confusion was associated with all three adverse outcomes: longer hospital stays, increased likelihood of nursing home placement, or death. Weight loss was the strongest predictor of death, although appetite loss, depression, falls, and socioeconomic problems were also significantly associated. Polypharmacy and prolonged bed rest predicted nursing home placement. Falls and prolonged bed rest were associated with increased total hospital stay. Efforts to minimize the effect of hospitalization on patients at risk have led to the design of special geriatric care units. Such units are based on a multidisciplinary approach to assessment and treatment. Studies indicate that units of this kind can have a significant and positive effect on the maintenance of independence and discharge to home.[88]

## Appendix 1: Folstein Minimental Status Test

| Maximum Score | Score | |
|---|---|---|
| | | **Orientation** |
| 5 | ( ) | What is the (year) (date) (day) (month) (season)? |
| 5 | ( ) | Where are we: (state) (county) (town) (hospital) (floor) (clinic)? |
| | | **Registration** |
| 3 | ( ) | Name 3 objects: 1 second to say each. Then ask patient all 3 after you have said them. |
| | | **Attention and Calculation** |
| 5 | ( ) | Serial 7's backward from 100 [1 point for each correct] *Stop after 5*<br>Alternatively spell "world" backwards (or if limited education try repeating the months backwards, or serial 10's from 100's to 50. |
| 3 | ( ) | Ask for 3 objects repeated above. Give 1 point for each correct. |
| | | **Language** |
| 2 | ( ) | Name a pencil, and watch (2 points) |
| 1 | ( ) | Repeat the following "No ifs, ands or buts." (1 point) |
| 3 | ( ) | Follow a 3-stage command: "Take a paper in your hand, fold it in half, and put it on the floor." (3 points) |
| 1 | ( ) | Read and Obey the following: "Close your eyes" (1 point) see back |
| 1 | ( ) | Write a sentence (1 point) on back |
| 1 | ( ) | Copy design (1 point) (see back) |
| Total score* | | |

* Decrease denominator for items missed due to noncognitive disabilities (e.g., vision).

# Appendix 2A: Stepwise Approach to Preoperative Cardiac Assessment: Initial Tests

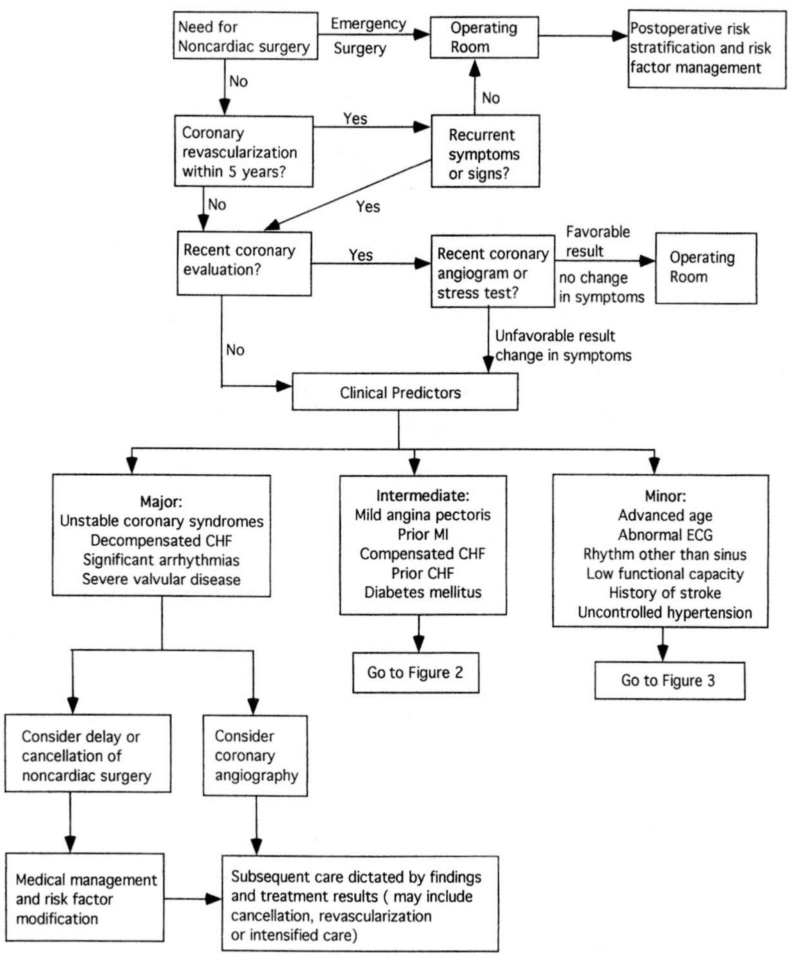

# Appendix 2B: Stepwise Approach to Preoperative Cardiac Assessment: Intermediate Clinical Predictors

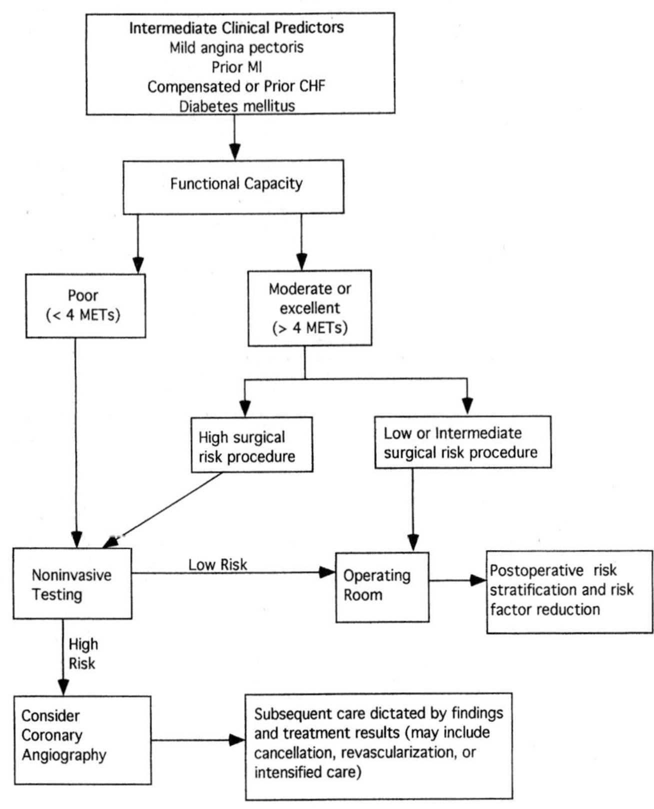


MET = Metabolic Equivalents

# Appendix 2C: Stepwise Approach to Preoperative Cardiac Assessment: Minor or No Clinical Predictors

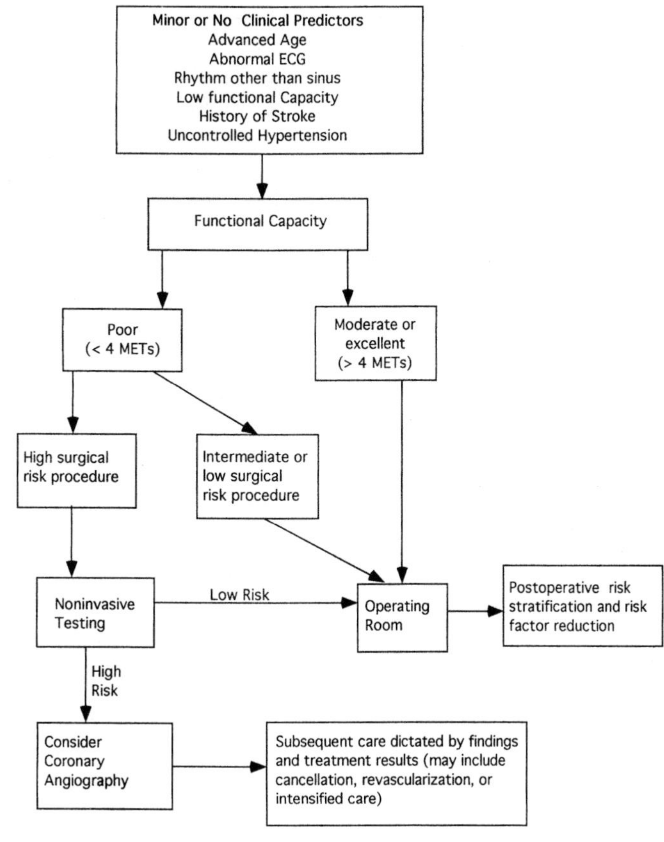


MET: Metabolic Equivalents

## References

1. Peebles RJ, Schneidman DS (eds). Socio-economic Factbook for Surgery 1997, Chicago: American College of Surgeons, 1997.
2. Day JC. Population projections of the United States by age, sex, race and Hispanic origin: 1993–2050. In: Current Population Reports, US Department of Commerce Bureau of the Census, P25–1104. 1993.
3. Thomas DR, Ritchie CS. Preoperative assessment of older adults. J Am Geriatr Soc 1995;43:811–821.
4. Rosenthal RA, Andersen DK. Surgery in the elderly: observations on the pathophysiology and treatment of cholelithiasis. Exp Gerontol 1993;28:459.
5. Keller SM, et al. Emergency and elective surgery in patients over age 70 years. Am Surg 1987;53:636.
6. Zenilman ME. Considerations in surgery in the elderly. In: Master Series in Surgery 2. Advances in Surgery in the Elderly. New York: World Medical Press, 1993.
7. Boyd BJ, et al. Operative risk factors of colon resection in the elderly. Ann Surg 1980;192:743.
8. Yancik R, et al. Comorbidity and age as predictors of risk for early mortality of male and female colon carcinoma patients: a population based study. Cancer 1998;82: 2123–2134.
9. Tiret L, et al. Complications associated with anaesthesia—a prospective survey in France. Can Anaesth Soc J 1986;33: 336–344.
10. Escarce JJ, et al. Outcomes of open cholecystectomy in the elderly: a longitudinal analysis of 21,00 cases in the prelaparoscopic era. Surgery 1995;117:156.
11. Kannel WB, Dannenberg AV, Abbott RD. Unrecognized myocardial infarction and hypertension: Framingham Study. Am Heart J 1985;109:581.
12. Pinholt EM, et al. Functional assessment of the elderly: a comparison of standard instruments with clinical judgement. Arch Intern Med 1987;147:484.
13. Buxbaum JL, Schwartz AJ. Perianesthetic considerations for the elderly patient. Surg Clin North Am 1994;74:41–61.
14. Djokovic JL, Hedley-White J. Prediction of outcome of surgery and anesthesia in patients over 80. JAMA 1979; 242:2301.
15. Khuri SF, et al. The National Veterans Administration Surgical Risk Study: risk adjustment for the comparative assessment of the quality of surgical care. J Am Coll Surg 1995;180:519–531.

16. Khuri SF, et al. Risk adjustment of the postoperative mortality rate for the comparative assessment of quality of surgical care: results of the National Veterans Affairs Surgical Risk Study. J Am Coll Surg 1997;185:315–327.
17. Daley J, et al. Risk adjustment of the postoperative morbidity rate for the comparative assessment of the quality of surgical care: results of the National Veterans Affairs Surgical Risk Study. J Am Coll Surg 1997;185:341–351.
18. Khuri SF, et al. The Department of Veterans Affairs' NSQIP. Ann Surg 1998;228:491–507.
19. Narain P, et al. Predictors of immediate and 6-month outcomes in hospitalized elderly patients. The importance of functional status. J Am Geriatr Soc 1988;36(9):775–783.
20. Seymour DG, Pringle R. Post-operative complications in the elderly surgical patient. Gerontology 1983;29:262.
21. Browner WS, Mangano DT. In hospital and long-term mortality in male veterans following non-cardiac surgery: the study of perioperative ischemia research group. JAMA 1992;268:228.
22. Shahar A, Powers KA, Black JS. The risk of postoperative deconditioning in older adults. J Am Geriatr Soc 1996;44:471.
23. Gerson MC, et al. Cardiac prognosis in noncardiac geriatric surgery. Ann Intern Med 1985;103:832.
24. Gerson MC, Hurst JM, Hertzberg VS, et al. Prediction of cardiac and pulmonary complications related to elective abdominal and noncardiac thoracic surgery in geriatric patients. Am J Med 1990;88:101–107.
25. Older P, et al. Preoperative evaluation of cardiac function and ischemia in elderly patients by cardiopulmonary exercise testing. Chest 1993;103:701.
26. Eagle KA, Brundage BH, Chaitman BR, et al. ACC/AHA task force report: guidelines for perioperative cardiovascular evaluation for noncardiac surgery. Circulation 1996;93: 1278.
27. Hlatky MA, et al. A brief self-administered questionnaire to determine functional capacity (the Duke's Activity Status Index). Am J Cardiol 1989;64:651.
28. Reuben DB, Greendale GA, Harrison GG. Nutrition screening in older persons. J Am Geriatr Soc 1995;43:415.
29. Rosenberg IH. Nutrition and aging. In: Hazzard WR, Bierman EL, Blass JP, Ettinger WH, Halter JB (eds). Principles of Geriatric Medicine and Gerontology, 3rd ed. New York: McGraw-Hill, 1994.
30. Corti M, et al. Serum albumin level and physical disability as predictors of mortality in older persons. JAMA 1994;272: 1036.
31. Gibbs J, Cull W, Henderson W, Daley J, Hur K, Khuri SF. Preoperative serum albumin level as a predictor of operative mortality and morbidity. Arch Surg 1999;134:36.
32. Detsky AS, et al. What is subjective global assessment of nutritional status? JPEN 1987;11:8–13.
33. Detsky AS, et al. Predicting nutrition-associated complications for patients undergoing gastrointestinal surgery. JPEN 1987;11:440–446.
34. Souba WW. Nutritional support. N Engl J Med 1997;336:41.
35. Lynch EP, et al. The impact of postoperative pain on the development of postoperative delirium. Anesth Analg 1998;86:781–785.
36. Fisher BW, Flowerdew G. A simple model for predicting postoperative delirium in older patients undergoing elective orthopedic surgery. J Am Geriatr Soc 1995;43:175.
37. Inouye SK. Delirium in hospitalized elderly patients: recognition, evaluation and management. Conn Med 1993;57: 309–312.
38. Inouye S, van Dyck CH, Alessi CA, Balkin S, Siegal AP, Horwitz RI. Clarifying confusion: the confusion assessment method; a new way for detecting delirium. Ann Intern Med 1990;113:941.
39. Folstein MF, Folstein SE, McHugh PR. The Mini-mental State Examination: a practical method for grading the cognitive state of patients for the clinician. J Psychiatr Res 1975;12:189.
40. Brandt J, Spencer M, Folstein MF. The telephone interview for cognitive status. Neuropsychiatry Neuropsychol Behav Neurol 1988;1:111.
41. Galazka SS. Preoperative evaluation of the elderly surgical patient. J Fam Pract 1988;27:622.
42. Larsen EB, Kukull WA, Buchner D, Reifler BV. Adverse drug reactions with global cognitive impairment in elderly persons. Ann Intern Med 1987;107:169.
43. Williams MA, Campbell EB, Raynor WJ, et al. Predictors of acute confusional states in hospitalized elderly patients. Res Nurs Health 1985;8:31–40.
44. Gustafson Y, Berggren D, Brannstrom B, et al. Acute confusional states in elderly patients treated for femoral neck fracture. J Am Geriatr Soc 1988;36:525–530.
45. Rogers MR, Liang MH, Daltroy LH, et al. Delirium after elective orthopedic surgery: risk factors and natural history. Int J Psychiatry Med 1989;19:109–121.
46. Francis J, et al. A prospective study of delirium in hospitalized elderly. JAMA 1990;263:1097–1101.
47. Marcantonio ER, Goldman L, Mangione CM, et al. A clinical prediction rule for delirium after elective noncardiac surgery. JAMA 1994;271:134.
48. Inouye SK, et al. A predictive model for delirium in hospitalized medical patients based on admission characteristcs. Ann Intern Med 1993;119:474–481.
49. Schor JD, et al. Risk factors for delirium in hospitalized elderly. JAMA 1992;267:827–831.
50. Inouye SK. The dilemma of delirium: clinical and research controversies regarding diagnosis and evaluation of delirium in hospitalized elderly medical patients. Am J Med 1994;97:278–288.
51. Williams-Russo P, et al. Post-operative delirium: predictors and prognosis in elderly orthopedic patients. J Am Geriatr Soc 1992;40:759–777.
52. Marcantonio ER, Goldman L, Orav JE, Cook FE, Lee TH. The association of intraoperative factors with the development of postoperative delirium. Am J Med 1998; 105:380.
53. Kaneko T, Takahashi S, Naka T, Hirooka Y, Inoue Y, Kaibara N. Postoperative delirium following gastrointestinal surgery in elderly patients. Surg Today 1997;27:107.
54. Inouye SK, Charpentier PA. Precipitating factors for delirium in hospitalized elderly persons: predictive model and interrelationship with baseline vulnerability. JAMA 1996; 275:852–857.
55. Moller JT, Cluitmans P, Rasmussen LS, et al. Long-term postoperative cognitive dysfunction in the elderly: ISPOCD1 study. Lancet 1998;351:857.
56. Hosking MP, et al. Outcomes of surgery in patients 90 years of age and older. JAMA 1989;261:1909–1912.

57. Eagle KA, et al. Guidelines for perioperative cardiovascular evalution for noncardiac surgery: an abridged version of the American College of Cardiology/American Heart Association task force on practice guidelines. Mayo Clin Proc 1997;72:524–531.
58. Campeau L. Grading of angina pectoris. Circulation 1976; 54:522–523.
59. Lawrence VA. Incidence and hospital stay for cardiac and pulmonary complications after abdominal surgery. J Gen Intern Med 1995;10:67–68.
60. Smetana GW. Current concepts: preoperative pulmonary evaluation. N Engl J Med 1999;340:937–944.
61. Hall JC, et al. A multivariate analysis of the risk of pulmonary complications after laparotomy. Chest 1991;99: 923–927.
62. Charlson ME, et al. A new method of classifying prognostic comorbidity in longitudinal studies: development and validation. J Chron Dis 1987;40:373–383.
63. Goldman L, et al. Multifactorial index of cardiac risk in noncardiac surgical procedures. N Engl J Med 1997;297:845–850.
64. Lawrence VA, et al. Risk of pulmonary complications after elective abdominal surgery. Chest 1996;110:744–750.
65. Tarhan S, et al. Risk of anesthesia and surgery in patients with bronchitis and chronic obstructive pulmonary disease. Surgery 1973;74:720–720.
66. Stein M, Cassara EL. Preoperative pulmonary evaluation and therapy for surgery patients. JAMA 1970;211:787–790.
67. Varon J, Marik P. Letter to editor. N Engl J Med 1999;341:613.
68. Delgado-Rodriguez M, et al. Usefulness of intrinsic wound infection risk indices as predictors of postoperative pneumonia. J Hosp Infect 1997;35:269–276.
69. Rose DK, et al. Critical respiratory events in the postanesthesia care unit: patient, surgical and anesthetic factors. Anesthesiology 1994;81:410–418.
70. Fujita T, Sakurai K. Multivariate analysis of risk factors for postoperative pneumonia. Am J Surg 1995;169:304–307.
71. Pedersen T, et al. A prospective study of risk factors and cardiopulmonary complications associated with anaesthesia and surgery: risk indicators of cardiopulmonary morbidity. Acta Anaesthesiol Scand 1990;34:144–155.
72. Gracey DR, et al. Preoperative pulmonary preparation of patients with chronic obstructive pulmonary disease: a prospective study. Chest 1979;76:123–129.
73. Garibaldi RA, et al. Risk factors for postoperative pneumonia. Am J Med 1981;70:677–680.
74. Philips EH, et al. Comparison of laparoscopic cholecystectomy in obese and nonobese patients. Am Surg 1994;60: 316–321.
75. Southern Surgical Club. A prospective analysis of 1518 laparoscopic cholecystectomies. N Engl J Med 1991;324: 1073–1078.
76. Mitchell CK, et al. Multivariate analysis of factors associated with postoperative pulmonary complications following general elective surgery. Arch Surg 1998;133: 194–198.
77. Alexander JW. Transfusion-induced immunomodulation and infection. Transfusion 1991;31:195–196.
78. Hogue CW Jr, et al. Swallowing dysfunction after cardiac operations: associated adverse outcomes and risk factors including intraoperative transesophageal echocardiography. J Thorac Cardiovasc Surg 1995;110:517–522.
79. Brooks-Brunn JA. Postoperative atelectasis and pneumonia. Heart Lung 1995;24:94–115.
80. Cushieri RJ, et al. Postoperative pain and pulmonary complications: comparison of three analgesic regimens. Br J Surg 1985;72:495–498.
81. Tisi GM. Preoperative evaluation of pulmonary function. Am Rev Respir Dis 1979;119:293–310.
82. Kroenke K, et al. Postoperative complications after thoracic and major abdominal surgery in patients with or without obstructive lung disease. Chest 1993;104:1445–1451.
83. Williams-Russo P, et al. Predicting postoperative pulmonary complications: is it a real problem? Arch Intern Med 1992;152:1209–1213.
84. Cain HD, et al. Preoperative pulmonary function and complications after cardiovascular surgery. Chest 1979;76: 130–135.
85. Preoperative pulmonary function testing. American College of Physicians position statement. Ann Intern Med 1990; 112:793–794.
86. Hnatiuk MOW, et al. Adherence to established guidelines for preoperative pulmonary function testing. Chest 1995; 107:1294–1297.
87. Satish S, Winograd CH, Chavez C, Bloch DA. Geriatric targeting criteria as predictors of survival and health care utilization. J Am Geriatr Soc 1996;44:914.
88. Landefeld CS, et al. A randomized trial of care in a hospital medical unit especially designed to improve the functional outcome of acutely ill older patients. N Engl J Med 1995; 332:1338.

# 11
# Anesthetic Considerations for Geriatric Surgery

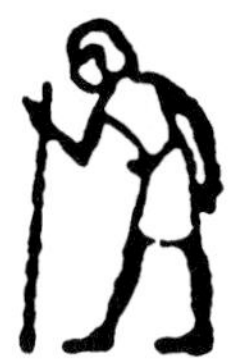

Stephen N. Harris

Is a healthy geriatric patient different from a healthy 20-year-old? If so, how should one approach the elderly from an anesthetic standpoint when assessing them prior to surgery? Are there some basic differences that affect anesthetic management? Understanding the physiologic and pharmacologic changes associated with aging give us insight to help discern the effects of aging and the consequences of age-related disease. Other chapters of this book cover preoperative risk assessment and specific organ systems in great detail; this chapter addresses the geriatric patient from the anesthesiologist's viewpoint. Pertinent organ systems are taken into consideration in terms of their impact on the perioperative anesthetic plan. In addition, recommendations concerning perioperative care of the geriatric patient focus on how commonly used anesthetics, techniques, and management affect the perioperative care of the geriatric patient.

The anesthesiologist and surgeon must be aware of two distinct processes when encountering a geriatric patient. This patient has undergone *direct effects of aging* as a result of a gradual physiologic process common to all. This universal effect progresses as chronologic age increases and manifests as distinct changes in the structure and function of vital organs. In addition to the direct effects of aging on the human body, the effects of *age-related disease* might be present in varying degrees. This is best described as end-organ disease that has developed out of proportion to the patient's age. When describing a geriatric patient to a colleague, a comparison is often made between the patient's chronologic age and biologic age. For example, an active 70-year-old patient who has refrained from smoking and drinking and whose parents are still alive must be viewed in terms of the direct effects of aging when undergoing a preoperative assessment for surgery. His biologic age may equal his chronologic age. In contrast, the 65-year-old man whose alcohol intake has rivaled his two-pack-per-day smoking habit is viewed in terms of direct effects of aging in addition to the age-related disease of accelerated atherosclerosis and pulmonary dysfunction due to his lifelong abuse of tobacco and alcohol. In this situation, his biologic age may surpass his chronologic age.

It is difficult, if not impossible, to separate the effects of aging from the effects of disease and life style changes. The latter may dramatically affect both the incidence of disease and the normal physiology of aging.[1] All three factors must be simultaneously addressed when evaluating a patient: the effect of aging, life style, and the presence of coexisting disease.[2] In addition, it is important to understand how the geriatric patient views his or her aging process. For many older adults health problems may be attributed to the inevitable consequence of the aging. Such attribution to aging has been shown to be associated with a tendency to delay seeking health care, less compliance, and denial of the severity of problems.[3] This may be a factor during the preoperative assessment. Symptoms attributed to the belief that old age is the cause of health problems may be underestimating the severity of a disease or disease process.

## Preoperative Assessment

Prior to surgery the geriatric patient must undergo a preoperative anesthetic assessment. The anesthesiologist should be aware of two major facts. Geriatric patients are at increased risk for perioperative morbidity and mortality compared to their younger counterparts partly owing to the higher incidence of coexisting disease. Perioperative mortality rates of geriatric patients are largely dependent on three factors: elective versus emergency surgery, the operative site, and the physical status of the patient at the time of surgery.

The purpose of the preoperative assessment is to: (1) educate the patient about anesthesia and perioperative care; (2) inform about the available perioperative pain relief options; (3) grasp an idea of the patient's overall physical and mental status through a directed interview and review of available preoperative data; (4) order additional tests or consultations regarding the patient's physical status if needed; and (5) obtain informed consent.[4]

The morbidity associated with surgery may be reduced through this process. With the knowledge of increased morbidity and mortality concerning geriatric patents, one may be tempted to order "shotgun" laboratory testing for all patients over the age of 65 years prior to elective surgery. The controversy concerning the number of preoperative laboratory tests ordered may be avoided by performing a thorough, directed history and physical examination prior to scheduling any needed preoperative tests. Two standards published in the American Society of Anesthesiologists (ASA) Directory of Members, 1994 state that "The routine use of laboratory or diagnostic screening tests is *not* an essential part of the preanesthetic screening of patients." However, "the history, physical, and chart review *are essential* when obtaining tests as a part of preoperative care."[5] When properly done, a detailed, focused history and physical examination may yield far more information than laboratory tests and give the clinician areas on which to focus when preoperative tests are indicated. In this same direction, Roizen suggested that for an asymptomatic patient 65 years or older undergoing peripheral surgery with minimal blood loss only a hematocrit (Hct), electrocardiogram (ECG), blood urea nitrogen (BUN), and serum glucose be obtained. Addition of a preoperative chest radiograph to the previously mentioned tests may be indicated only for an asymptomatic patient more than 75 years of age.[6] Close communication between surgeon and anesthesiologist prior to surgery enables the most appropriate tests to be ordered, eliminating unnecessary testing and costs.

Advances in treatment of hypertension and coronary artery disease have contributed to an increased percentage of patients surviving past the age of 65 years. It has been stated that the number of persons older than 65 years in the United States will increase by 25–35% over the next 30 years.[3] This same age group will also undergo the largest number of surgical procedures. The prevalence of cardiovascular disease increases with age, reflected in autopsy studies revealing that as many as 60–70% of an unselected group of old patients have some evidence of coronary disease, even though clinical manifestations of coronary disease were present in only half of them.[2] When encountering a geriatric patient with a history of cardiac disease who presents for noncardiac surgery, one must realize that the occurrence of a perioperative cardiac event (myocardial infarction, congestive heart failure) leads to increased morbidity and mortality.[7,8]

The preoperative examination of the patient should not only identify the presence of preexisting cardiac disease but also define the disease severity, stability, and responses to prior treatment. Questions arising during consultation with the patient should be aimed toward determining the patient's current and previous physical health, identification of significant medical problems and their history, and response to treatment. Is the patient compliant about taking medications? A current list of medications is ideal and may aid in determining the physical status of the patient. It has been shown that continuance of preoperative medications for hypertension may result in a more stable perioperative period.[4] Consultation with the patient's primary care physician is aimed at determining if the patient is in the best medical condition as possible. Questions are directed about specific organ systems and the past and current treatment regimens for any abnormalities. For example, is the patient's chronic stable angina well managed with sublingual nitroglycerine tablets PRN? Is the hypertension well controlled with a β-blocker and an angiotensin-converting enzyme (ACE) inhibitor? Did the dye load from the angiogram increase the creatinine from 1.2 to 2.2 mg/dl? Will additional manipulation of the medications significantly improve the preoperative status?

The ASA preoperative patient assessment has no consideration for age (Table 11.1). The assignment of a patient status number from 1 to 5 depends on the number and severity of preexisting medical diseases. The assignment of a certain number (e.g., ASA 3 or ASA 4) is subjective at times but has been shown to be a reliable indicator of perioperative morbidity and mortality.[9,10] The clinician must be aware of the progression of age-related diseases and diminished physiologic reserve in the elderly and refrain from treating an active, healthy 80-year-old similarly to a 35-year-old smoker. When evaluated, both may be assigned ASA physical status 2.

The presence of emergency surgery in the geriatric patient may be the largest predictor of perioperative morbidity and mortality. The geriatric patient presenting for emergent surgery has been shown to have at least a three- to fourfold greater incidence of mortality than younger, healthy patients.[11,12] This may due to a number of factors. The normal sequence of preoperative preparation for surgery may be accelerated or even omitted. Such deficiencies in assessment of preoperative status may not be addressed until during or after the surgery.[2] Take, for example, the 80-year-old hypertensive on Coumadin for atrial fibrillation with active upper gastrointestinal

TABLE 11.1. American Society of Anesthesiologists Physical Status Classification

| ASA class | Description |
|---|---|
| 1 | No gross organic disease, healthy patient |
| 2 | Mild or moderate systemic disease without functional impairment |
| 3 | Organic disease with definite functional impairment |
| 4 | Severe disease that is life-threatening |
| 5 | Moribund patient, not expected to survive |

ASA, American Society of Anesthesiologists.

bleeding. The preoperative intravascular volume may be severely diminished owing to concomitant diuretic therapy superimposed on nausea, vomiting, and blood loss. Attempts to correct electrolyte, hematologic, and coagulation deficiencies rapidly may result in congestive heart failure, myocardial infarction, and arrhythmias.

In addition to lack of time for preoperative preparation, the staff on call for emergencies may not be oriented to the special needs of the geriatric patient. A cursory preoperative evaluation in addition to decreased perioperative vigilant attention to organ systems, which have diminished physiologic reserve, may occur. Risk of bacteremia, sepsis, or systemic anticoagulation may preclude the use of regional anesthesia for perioperative pain control, leaving parenteral or intramuscular opioids as the only option for postoperative pain relief. In this population, undesirable side effects (i.e., nausea, vomiting, psychosis, excessive somnolence) may be encountered with the use of intramuscular or patient controlled analgesia administration of narcotics.

The location and nature of the surgery contributes to perioperative risk.[12–14] For example, an emergent retinal detachment does not have major fluid shifts, significant postoperative pain, and risk for postoperative pulmonary dysfunction. In contrast, a large bowel obstruction, an acutely inflamed gallbladder, or a dissecting abdominal aortic aneurysm places greater physiologic demand on the patient. Emergent operations superimposed on an elderly person who may have delayed seeking health care with advanced disease processes, places unnecessary stress on their diminished physiologic reserve, resulting in less tolerance for deviations from baseline.

## Body Composition and End-Organ Changes

Traditional methods of dosing and administering drugs are based on body weight (milligrams or micrograms per kilogram body weight). These normalized data enable the anesthesiologist to calculate and administer a specific dose of drug with a predictable effect in a safe fashion for a wide range of the population. Aging, however, results in perturbations of total body weight, percent lean body mass, and adipose tissue, which differ between the sexes. These changes have a significant effect on the geriatric patient and must be taken into consideration.

Men universally gain body mass in the form of fat during middle adulthood (40–55 years), and lean body mass decreases steadily from age 30, then more rapidly from age 60. Men lose stature and body weight with proportional decreases in percent lean body mass and adipose tissue. Women similarly lose stature but may maintain body weight. This is at the expense of greater losses in lean body mass offset by proportional increases in percent adipose tissue as aging progresses. The decrease in total body water during the aging process is probably due to a decrease in intracellular water because of the progressive loss of lean body mass. It is due to progressive atrophy of skeletal muscle and vessel-rich organs (i.e., liver and kidney). The total body water may decrease to 50% of total body weight. Plasma volume is not reduced with aging.[12]

Age-related decreases in the size and metabolic activity of vital organs, notably the liver and kidney, directly affect the anesthesiologist. Drug dosing may need to be modified as a result of changes observed in hepatic and renal structure and function. Altered mechanisms of drug metabolism and elimination may result in a pharmacokinetic profile other than what is expected. A working understanding of the age-related effects on liver and kidney function is critical when anesthetizing elderly patients.

As a result of the aging process, total liver mass may be decreased to 40% of its original size. Total liver blood flow and percent derived from cardiac output parallels the decrease in size. Hepatic microsomal function is preserved, not paralleling the loss of liver mass. Oxidative mechanisms and enzyme activity do not exhibit age-related changes.[2] However, the loss of hepatic mass and blood flow is important to the anesthesiologist in that there is a progressive decrease in hepatic functional reserve. The hepatic biotransformation rate may be significantly decreased compared to that in younger individuals. Compounds undergoing phase 1 reactions, the cytochrome $P_{450}$ oxidation or mixed function oxidase system, result in oxidation or hydroxylation of the compound for hepatic elimination. This phase of metabolism may be severely affected by decreased liver mass and blood flow associated with aging. Typical drugs affected by this pathway are barbiturates, warfarin, propanolol, ibuprofen, benzodiazepines, lidocaine, meperidine, and Benadryl. Phase 2 pathways, synthetic in nature, forming a more water-soluble drug or metabolite, result in conjugation, acetylation, or methylation. These pathways appear to be relatively unaffected by the effects of decreased hepatic tissue mass and blood flow.[15]

Renal mass is reduced 10–20% as a direct effect of aging. It results from renal tissue atrophy, decreasing the number of nephrons by 30% at the end of the fifth decade. By the eighth decade, elderly patients may have as few as 700,000 nephrons, even in the absence of overt renal disease.[12] Remaining glomeruli may be dilated, sclerosed, or hyalinized, rendering them less efficient. Decreased renal blood flow may be the major factor acting on global renal function. Renal cortical perfusion decreases from 500 ml/min/100 g tissue to less than 325 ml/min/100 g between the ages of 20 and 80 years. Renal medullary perfusion is preserved, decreasing only 20% in elderly patients. The sum of all the previously mentioned effects—fibrosis, atrophy, loss of glomerular and tubular structures—results in a severe reduction in renal blood flow, which may approach 50% reduction by age 80. The glomerular filtration rate (GFR) decreases by 6–8% per decade up to age 70.[12]

Preoperative assessment of renal function in the elderly is not straightforward. Serum creatinine alone is not an adequate predictor of the decline in GFR. Total creatinine clearance is determined by the balance of production and tubular secretion of creatinine. Loss of skeletal muscle mass in elderly patients decreases creatinine production and the load on the kidney. Plasma creatinine may not increase until the GFR falls below 50 ml/min. A "normal" plasma creatinine of 1.4 mg/dl in a cachectic elderly patient may not adequately reflect a severely decreased GFR (see Chapter 58).

The effect of aging and age-related disease on the liver and kidney greatly affect the surgeons' and anesthesiologists' decisions. Even in an otherwise healthy elderly patient, administration of anesthesia decreases hepatic and renal perfusion. One can expect a decrease in urine flow of approximately 20–30% during anesthetic administration. Situations that result in elevated levels of renin, angiotensin II, and aldosterone (hemorrhage, high levels of catecholamines and overall increased surgical stress) initiate salt and water retention and perpetuate an overall state of vasoconstriction, which predisposes to perioperative oliguria. High levels of circulating catecholamines induce renal vasoconstriction via α-adrenergic stimulation or renin release. Patients taking ACE inhibitors may benefit from suppression of renal reflex vasoconstrictor mechanisms. Adequate levels of anesthesia result in lesser amounts of circulating catecholamines. Patients who develop perioperative renal dysfunction (acute tubular necrosis) exhibit increased in-hospital mortality.[16] Rational intraoperative management is to avoid prerenal causes of decreased renal blood flow via adequate hydration, resulting in a stable circulating blood volume, maintenance of cardiac output, and renal perfusion. The addition of pharmacologic adjuncts to improve renal perfusion may assist in renal protection in the elderly patient.

## Intraoperative Temperature Management

The *Morbidity and Mortality Weekly Report* from the Centers for Disease Control (CDC) titled "Hypothermia related deaths—Georgia, January 1996–December 1997," states that each winter hundreds of elderly die as a result of hypothermia. The report goes further to define hypothermia as an unintentional lowering of the core body temperature to less than or equal to 35°C. Environmental hypothermia results from a combination of heat loss by convection, conduction, and radiation to the surrounding ambient air. According to the CDC, risk factors for hypothermia-related deaths are directly related to age, preexisting disease, and nutritional status.[17] The elderly are at highest risk for death because of physiologic changes that manifest as impaired vasoconstrictive activity in a cold environment, decreased basal metabolic rate, impaired shivering mechanisms, and underlying disease. Interestingly, the CDC did not aim these statements toward surgeons and anesthesiologists. The focus group for their warnings was the elderly and those caring for the elderly *outside* the hospital and operating room. Is it no wonder that once geriatric patients enter the operating room they have an even greater incidence and severity of hypothermia and resultant perioperative morbidity and mortality due to hypothermia.

Thermoregulation in humans is a complex relation utilizing central mechanisms within the hypothalamus in concert with cutaneous thermosensors. Responses to a cold environment activate a series of reflexes designed to maintain a stable core temperature. Such responses to a cold environment include peripheral vasoconstriction and shivering in the awake, unanesthetized individual. However, core body temperature poorly reflects the mean body temperature because peripheral tissues are normally 2°–4°C cooler.[18] The normal core/peripheral tissue temperature gradient is maintained by tonic thermoregulatory vasoconstriction. All anesthetics significantly inhibit thermoregulation, decreasing the thresholds for vasoconstriction and shivering. Following the induction of anesthesia, tonic vasoconstriction is inhibited, enabling a prompt core to peripheral redistribution of body heat. This disruption of autonomic homeostasis occurs as a result of interrupted afferent information from peripheral chemoreceptors and thermosensors. The situation is further complicated by a decrease in hypothalamic responsiveness. After the initial rapid decrease in core temperature, there is a slower, more gradual decrease in core temperature due to heat loss in excess of metabolic heat production.[19] How does this affect perioperative management of the geriatric patient?

Admission of geriatric patients to the hospital creates stress they have not encountered in their everyday activities. As humans age, there is a progressive decline in metabolic heat production through loss of lean tissue mass. Shivering less effectively raises the core temperature, and the thresholds for initiating cutaneous vasoconstrictor responses are higher. Extrinsic forces act on the elderly patient, as preoperative bowel preparation in a cold hospital room and wearing minimal clothing contribute to preoperative volume deficit and lowering of core temperature.[20] These factors work synergistically to predispose the elderly patient to develop hypothermia during the preoperative period.

Inadvertent hypothermia in the operating room should be of concern to the entire operative team. The usual temperature in the operating room ranges from 20° to 25°C, which feels much colder to a geriatric patient wearing, at best, a hospital gown. All patients, including the elderly, exhibit an impaired threshold for thermoregulatory vasoconstriction in response to hypothermia while receiving anesthesia. Body heat is redistributed from central to peripheral compartments as a result of loss of peripheral vasoconstriction. Core temperature drops intraoperatively, and the elderly patient may not be able to initiate thermoregulatory responses until the core temperature has fallen to as low as 34°C. Compared to young patients, elderly patients in the operating room experience a more rapid drop of body temperature, have a greater degree of temperature loss, and remain colder for a longer time when active rewarming is initiated in the recovery room.[20]

Concern about intraoperative hypothermia has prompted investigators to determine an association between perioperative morbidity and the occurrence of intraoperative hypothermia. Frank et al. clearly demonstrated in elderly patients with cardiac risk factors that intraoperative hypothermia was an independent predictor of morbid cardiac events.[19] In 100 patients undergoing lower extremity vascular surgery, hypothermic patients (<35°C) had an increased incidence of postoperative angina, ECG changes consistent with myocardial ischemia, and an arterial $PaO_2 < 80$ mmHg. The same investigators documented, in a similar population of elderly patients, that perioperative maintenance of normothermia is associated with a reduced incidence of morbid cardiac events and ventricular tachycardia.[21]

In addition to the cardiovascular concerns regarding unintentional perioperative hypothermia, it has been brought to light that hypothermia affects the immune system and wound healing. It has been documented that the elderly exhibit an impaired immune response, evidenced by decreased lymphocyte proliferation as a result of decreased release of interleukin-2 (IL-2) and soluble IL-2 receptor.[22] This decreased immune response has also been demonstrated in patients whose core temperature decreased by only 1°C while undergoing abdominal surgery. These hypothermic patients demonstrated decreased mitogenic responses as well as decreased IL-2 production, while normothermic patients had significantly higher production of IL-1β 24 hours after surgery.[23] In a population undergoing colorectal surgery, hypothermic patients had a significantly higher incidence of surgical wound infections and significantly longer duration of hospitalization.[24] Clearly, intraoperative hypothermia affects all major organ systems, the elderly being even more susceptible than younger individuals.

In light of this information, how can one minimize decreases in core temperature in elderly patients during surgery? Anesthetic technique may be a factor, as there may be less autonomic dysfunction with regional anesthesia (i.e., epidural anesthesia, upper extremity block) than with a general anesthetic.[20] Administration of certain intravenous anesthetics (propofol) and systemic vasodilators (nifedipine and sodium nitroprusside) may result in significant vasodilation, causing a decrease in the core/peripheral temperature gradient.[18,25] Intraoperative management of the geriatric patient should be aimed at minimizing heat loss by convection, conduction, and radiation. Preoperative skin surface warming of the patient prior to entering the operating room has been shown to reduce the initial postinduction hypothermia, preventing intraoperative hypothermia and postoperative shivering in patients undergoing procedures lasting longer than 3 hours.[25] Ambient room temperature should remain high until the patient is draped. Warming prep and irrigation solutions may minimize heat loss. Warmed intravenous fluids in addition to heat- and moisture-exchanging filters should be routinely placed in the breathing circuit. The application of forced-air heating blankets to unprepped portions of the patient's body have been shown to be beneficial to keep the core temperature from decreasing below 35°C.[26]

Whenever a geriatric patient presents for an extensive abdominal operation, the use of combined lower and upper body forced-air heating blankets is recommended. The use of the heating blankets should be continued into the recovery room postoperatively. Lower extremity revascularization and orthopedic cases may benefit from epidural anesthesia and upper body forced-air blankets. Attention to maintenance of normothermia in the geriatric population may have a far greater impact on perioperative morbidity and mortality than previously imagined.

## Anesthetic Considerations for the Cardiovascular System

The changes in cardiac function observed during the aging process in the absence of disease are similar to those seen in the laboratory. Humans parallel animals in that there is evidence of modest left ventricular hypertrophy with age because of a chronic pressure load, which produces a number of effects. Cardiac relaxation is prolonged, and decreases in early left ventricular diastolic filling and maximum diastolic filling rates are similarly observed. These age-related decreases in the rate and magnitude of relaxation have no effect on overall left ventricular function and the capacity to augment cardiac performance during exercise in euvolimic individuals.[27] Data from exercise studies reveal lower peak heart rates in healthy aging individuals. However, responses to exercise may not be an entirely accurate representation of what will happen in the operating room. Understanding known data concerning the cardiac and vascular responses to aging and exercise furthers our understanding of these responses and helps us propose treatment modalities to manage perioperative responses.[28]

The age-associated increase in left ventricular load (afterload) results from stiffening of the central arterial system resulting from changes in the structure and composition of the collagen and ground substances. The pulse wave velocity increases with age in a linear fashion because of the loss of compliance of the central arteries. A stiff, dilated central aorta develops, resulting in the higher systolic blood pressure. The increase in left ventricular load may also, in part, be due to diminished arterial vasodilatation induced by β-adrenergic-mediated receptors.[27,29]

A universally accepted consequence of aging is that there is diminished response to exercise. Compared to that of young individuals, there is an increase in impedance to left ventricular ejection during exercise in elderly patients. This point is of particular concern to the anesthesiologist, who must ask patients about their exercise capacity and rely upon this history to construct an adequate assessment of their physical or cardiopulmonary reserve. Based on this evaluation, we come to conclusions regarding the person's physical status. An understanding of the mechanisms controlling the responses of elderly patients to exercise is an important key to understanding the patient's preoperative status.[28]

The decrease in maximum work capacity and oxygen consumption is a reflection of diminished cardiovascular performance and decreased ability of the heart to augment cardiac output during exercise. The maximum obtainable heart rate decreases with age. Additional factors contribute to the age-related decline in exercise capacity. Skeletal muscle may be more easily fatigued (or perceive to be), and there may be increased work of breathing. These two factors may contribute to an earlier sense of muscle fatigue and dyspnea. Cardiac output is maintained in the elderly population by a number of compensatory mechanisms. In contrast to younger individuals, stroke volume is maintained by end-diastolic dilation. End-systolic volumes remain elevated in the elderly because of the lack of β-adrenergic-mediated vasodilation during exercise.[29] This age-associated decrease in the sympathetic modulation to exercise may contribute to decreased heart rate and rate of relaxation, increased left ventricular end-diastolic and end-systolic volumes, and decreased ejection fraction and contractility. Therefore, during exercise there are larger end-diastolic volumes and probably higher end-diastolic pressures. Cardiac output is maintained consistent with the Frank-Starling mechanism. Increased afterload to the left ventricle results in an increased end-systolic volume, which in turn results in a larger volume at the start of diastolic and consequently a larger end-diastolic volume. Thus the elderly ventricle functions on a higher position of the Frank Starling curve in order to maintain cardiac output in the face of an increased afterload, and decreased heart rate and left ventricular compliance.[29] All compensatory mechanisms available to maintain forward flow are being used when exercising or during stress. These points are important to remember when elderly patients present for surgery who are hypovolemic or manifest disturbances in atrial conduction, atrial fibrillation, or frequent premature atrial contractions (PACs) due to electrolyte imbalance. The elderly patients are much more dependent on preload for normal cardiac function than are younger individuals. Alterations in ventricular filling diminish ventricular preload producing adverse hemodynamic responses when anesthetics are administered.

The elderly patient is also more sensitive to the vasodilating properties of nitroglycerin (NTG) and sodium nitroprusside (SNP). Cahalan et al. studied 30 patients older than 70 years and infused NTG in a standardized protocol. They reported that patients more than 70 years of age could be predicted to experience a twofold greater decrease in systolic arterial pressure (approximately 33 mmHg) than patients in their fifties.[30] Wood et al. similarly reported an increased sensitivity to SNP in elderly patients undergoing surgery requiring deliberate hypotension.[31]

As a consequence of greater need and less responsiveness to catecholamine release and stimulation, elderly patients are highly susceptible to abrupt decreases in circulating catecholamine levels. This is due to a diminished responsiveness to β-adrenergic-mediated stimulation due to a decrease in the affinity of the molecule and receptor.[12] The generalized age-related decline in β-adrenergic-mediated end-organ function and decreased ventricular function render the elderly patient dependent on adequate preload and maintenance of the atrial contraction to preserve end-diastolic volume.

Perioperative management of an elderly patient undergoing a surgical procedure in which large fluid shifts are encountered may require some means of central monitoring, for example, by a central venous pressure (CVP) catheter or pulmonary artery (PA) catheter. Realizing that the elderly heart is less compliant and more preload-dependent, information gained from placement of central venous monitors can assist in optimizing cardiac and renal performance through the directed administration of fluid. A "normal" CVP of 3–5 mmHg or pulmonary capillary wedge pressure (PCWP) of 8–12 mmHg may reflect inadequate intravascular volume and left ventricular preload in this patient population. Operating on a higher portion of the Frank-Starling curve, the elderly patient may need a CVP of 8–10 mmHg or a wedge pressure of 14–18 mmHg for adequate cardiac output. Optimal central pressures for the individual patient can be determined by measuring of and maximizing cardiac output during fluid administration. If cardiac output is maintained with adequate fluid therapy, prerenal causes of low urine output should be all but eliminated. Renal function always benefits from adequate perfusion and preload.[16] Placement of a central line may not be critical for patient management in the operating room, but the information obtained may assist in directing postoperative management, when significant fluid shifts have occurred.

Accurate diagnosis of hypovolemia may be difficult during extensive operations and may require serial measurements of CVP, PCWP, and cardiac output. During abdominal operations, preexisting pulmonary disease or intraabdominal packing may contribute to elevations in intrathoracic pressure, falsely elevating the central filling pressures through the increase in transmural pressure.[32] The clinician may be presented with an elevated CVP or PCWP, in the setting of decreased urine output. If the clinical numbers are equivocal and fluid challenges do not produce expected results, additional diagnostic measures may be indicated. If available in the operating room, determination of left ventricular performance and end-diastolic volume may be obtained with the use of transesophageal echocardiography (TEE).[33] TEE images enable the anesthesiologist to measure the left ventricular end-diastolic area, and the ejection fraction, determine cardiac output,[34] and estimate intracardiac filling pressures.[35] Once this information is obtained, proper resuscitation could proceed, knowing exactly how the patient is responding to fluid and inotropic therapy. If the anesthesiologist has the training, experience, and equipment to perform TEE, it can be invaluable for management of elderly patients undergoing extensive abdominal and thoracic operations.

Because of reliance on the Frank-Starling mechanism, any losses of preload caused by inadequate perioperative hydration, diuretic therapy, and blood loss leave the elderly patient without further compensatory mechanisms to rely on for maintenance of cardiac output. This point is especially important in the operating room, where it is not uncommon to encounter an elderly patient who has been NPO for 8–12 hours and who has had a bowel prep the night before. Rational preoperative management of the geriatric inpatient is aimed toward maintenance of the intravascular volume by either increased oral intake or intravenous hydration. In a same-day admission setting, optimal management is to establish intravenous access as soon as possible and infuse fluids at a maintenance rate (i.e., 75–125 ml/hr). NPO status may be modified to enable less iatrogenic preoperative dehydration. Clear liquids may be tolerated up to 3 hours prior to surgery and solid food no sooner than 6 hours prior to surgery unless severe gastroesophageal reflux is present. Geriatric patients should be encouraged to continue taking their antihypertensive, antiarrhythmic, and antianginal medications, especially β-adrenergic receptor blocking drugs. If patients take sublingual nitroglycerin, they should bring it with them. Nitropaste preparations should be continued. Diuretics should be held unless heart failure management dictates daily adherence to such dosing.[4]

## Perioperative β-Adrenergic Receptor Blockade

The medical literature has shown many benefits to the administration of β-adrenergic blocking agents during episodes of myocardial ischemia.[36,37] The rationale for using β-blockers during acute myocardial ischemia is based on improving the oxygen supply and demand through a decrease in heart rate and inotropic state. Their use also prevents the deleterious actions of increased sympathetic tone by attenuating the actions of endogenous catecholamines on β-adrenergic receptors. The antiischemic benefits of β-blocker administration in ambulatory, nonsurgical patients have been clearly demonstrated in multicenter investigations.[38] Compared to other antiischemic drugs, β-blockers have been the only drugs shown to decrease mortality during myocardial infarction. Even in the failing heart, β-blockade has been shown to be beneficial, improving filling parameters and providing favorable systemic effects.[39]

The risk factors for adverse perioperative outcomes are preexisting congestive heart failure, myocardial infarction within 6 months, unstable angina, left ventricular hypertrophy, age ≥65 years, male sex, and preoperative myocardial ischemia.[40–42] Interventions aimed at preventing or modifying these risk factors are not always possible. Because of the high morbidity and mortality associated with intraoperative myocardial ischemia, prevention of this potentially avoidable risk may affect the long-term survival of high-risk patients.[41]

Reports have brought to light the impact of administering β-blockers to an at-risk population during surgery. In these studies, patients with cardiac risk factors undergoing noncardiac surgery were randomized to receive atenolol (15 mg IV prior to surgery, continued with PO dosing postoperatively) or placebo throughout the perioperative period. Wallace et al. concluded that perioperative administration of atenolol for 1 week significantly reduced the incidence of postoperative myocardial ischemia.[43] Mangano et al. reported reduced mortality and incidence of cardiovascular complications for as long as 2 years in the atenolol-treated group.[44] Both studies utilized the same patient population ($n$ = 200), exclusively men with a mean age of 68 years. However, two methodologic deficiencies were present concerning patient selection. For patients with bradycardia, hypotension, and other contraindications to β-blockers, atenolol was withheld after entry into the study, rather than excluding these patients from participation in the study. Second, no women participated in the studies. Despite these issues, the studies demonstrate that patients with coronary artery disease who are treated with β-blockers during the perioperative period may exhibit a decreased incidence of morbidity and mortality.[45] In addition, prophylactic administration of atenolol for 1 week did not increase the incidence of bronchospasm, hypotension, severe bradycardia, or dysrhythmia. The reduced incidence of postoperative myocardial ischemia, may have been due to a decrease in intraoperative ischemic events through improvement of myocardial supply and demand or modulation of the effects of circulating catecholamines. These investigations, along with previous trials of β-blockers in nonsurgical patients, demonstrate the efficacy of this class of drugs in a high risk population: the elderly with cardiovascular disease. If perioperative use of β-blockers is being considered, therapy should be initiated prior to anesthetic induction and continued during the postoperative period. Long-term survival may be ultimately attributed to an increased awareness of attenuation of intraoperative hemodynamic responses and aggressive management of blood pressure and heart rate during the perioperative period.

## Pharmacologic Concerns for the Anesthesiologist

As aging occurs, other age-related diseases are superimposed on the direct effects of aging on the human heart and circulatory system. The presence of age-associated changes previously discussed lowers the extent of disease severity required to manifest clinical symptoms. The age-associated changes alter the responsiveness to interventions and medical therapy. Initial effects of intravenous drugs may have a delayed onset due to a longer circulation time or volume of distribution. Their duration of action may be prolonged in the setting of diminished hepatic or renal function.[46]

In pharmacokinetic terms, reduced drug clearance is often associated with old age. Reduced clearance implies that after any specific dose of a drug is given, an elderly person has a greater area under the curve than a corresponding young control subject. Therefore, for some or all of the time following a single dose, plasma drug concentrations are higher in the elderly. During long-term dosage, steady-state plasma concentration ($C^{ss}$) is inversely proportional to the clearance. Therefore, the elderly person receiving an infusion at a specific rate has a higher $C^{ss}$ than the younger person; with this comes the possibility of greater drug response in the elderly.[46] In pharmacodynamic terms the elderly may have greater drug "sensitivity" than a younger person. For the elderly, any given plasma concentration, or target organ concentration, produces a greater clinical effect compared to that in a young control. In everyday practice, increased pharmacodynamic sensitivity observed in the elderly may coexist with or be independent of pharmacokinetic changes. Therefore conscious sedation or anesthetic induction may have to be initiated in a slower, more specific fashion, reflecting the above-mentioned principles. The anesthetic plan must be precise in terms of administration of premedication and titration of volatile anesthetics.

The backbone of many general anesthetics is an inhalation agent. Addition of these agents to the anesthetic technique facilitates the ease of attaining adequate anesthesia and analgesia without dependence on organ elimination or biotransformation. The depth of anesthesia can be easily titrated to the degree of surgical stimulation. Inhalation anesthetics are commonly combined with intravenous agents, narcotics, to produce a "balanced" technique. The currently used inhalation anesthetics include nitrous oxide, isoflurane, desflurane, sevoflurane, and to a lesser extent halothane and enflurane. This section focuses on the newer inhalation and intravenous agents and their impact on the geriatric patient. A brief review of the uptake and distribution of inhalation anesthetics and our current understanding of the effect of inhalation anesthetics on the geriatric patient are discussed.

### Inhalation Anesthetics

The most important aspect of delivery of inhalation anesthetics is that they must be delivered through the lungs via ventilation. Following the initial administration, further uptake and distribution are determined by the blood solubility of the drug (blood/gas partition coefficient), blood flow through the lungs, blood flow to organs, solubility of the gas in tissue (tissue/blood partition coefficient), and the mass of the tissue. The greater the blood/gas partition coefficient, the more soluble the drug is in the blood. The smaller the blood/gas partition coefficient, the less drug is dissolved in the blood (less soluble) and the higher is the alveolar/inspired ratio in the blood. As the anesthetic partial pressure in all tissues approaches that in the alveoli, development of high brain partial pressures with a more soluble agent (halothane) takes longer than less soluble agents (isoflurane, desflurane, sevoflurane). This results in a longer induction of anesthesia.[47]

One may control the alveolar partial pressure by increasing inspired anesthetic concentrations and alveolar ventilation. Inhalation agents with low blood/gas partition coefficients (desflurane, sevoflurane) are less dependent on ventilation to augment their uptake. Anesthetic uptake by the pulmonary circulation is rapid. The vessel-rich group of organs (brain, heart, liver, kidney, endocrine glands) equilibrate rapidly because they receive approximately 75% of the cardiac output,[47] A high cardiac output results in greater pulmonary blood flow, thereby lowering the alveolar concentration and prolonging the induction. A low cardiac output acts in the opposite fashion. In the setting of diminished cardiac function, high concentrations of inhalation anesthetics may result in severe depression of an already low cardiac output and may precipitate cardiovascular collapse.

Anesthetic potency is based on the minimum alveolar concentration (MAC) of an agent that produces immobility in 50% of subjects exposed to noxious (skin incision) stimuli. The MAC concentration, once equilibrated, directly represents the partial pressure of the anesthetic in the brain. The MAC decreases with decreasing temperature and increasing age.[12] The MAC for an octogenarian is approximately half that of an infant.[2,12,47] The increase in potency, or decreased MAC, seen with increasing age is consistent for all inhalation anesthetics.[48] A change in norepinephrine availability significantly influences anesthetic requirements. Drugs that decrease central levels of norepinephrine result in a dose-related decrease in MAC. In contrast, agents that increase central levels of norepinephrine increase the anesthetic requirement. Use of $\alpha_2$-receptor blocking drugs (dexmetomidine and clonidine) significantly decrease the MAC.[47]

Emergence from an inhalation-based anesthetic occurs in the exact opposite fashion as induction. Emergence is most rapid with increased ventilation, sustained cardiac output, and agents of low solubility. Because of the speed of induction and emergence associated with poorly soluble agents, development of drugs with these properties has been a priority. Ideally the agent does not irritate the airway, and has rapid onset and termination of effect with minimal cardiovascular changes. This is most important when dealing with geriatric patients, who may present with diminished cardiac function and diminished physiologic reserve. Enflurane and halothane result in myocardial depression and peripheral vasodilation. Isoflurane causes less myocardial depression, but hypotension resulting from its use is due primarily to vasodilation. It had also been implicated in contributing to myocardial ischemia in patients with "steal-prone" coronary anatomy. Ventricular dysrhythmias are more prevalent with the use of halothane, which sensitizes the myocardium to catecholamines to a much greater extent than enflurane and isoflurane.

Desflurane and sevoflurane are the most recent inhalation agents approved for use in the United States. Desflurane and sevoflurane have blood/gas partition coefficients similar to that of nitrous oxide: 0.42, 0.69, and 0.47, respectively.[47] Sevoflurane has a pleasant odor and is nonirritating to the airway, making it ideal for mask induction when intravenous access is not available. Desflurane, on the other hand, has a pungent odor, which precludes its use for mask induction; it has also been associated with cardiovascular stimulation. The cardiovascular stimulatory properties seen with desflurane administration are a decrease in systemic vascular resistance and an increase in heart rate, thus maintaining the cardiac index. However, there have been reports of desflurane precipitating myocardial ischemia when used as the sole induction agent in at-risk populations. Helman et al. examined the use of desflurane compared to sufentanil in patients presenting for cardiac surgery.[49] ECG signs of myocardial ischemia were present during induction in 9% of the patients receiving desflurane compared to 0% of the sufentanil group. This result was confirmed by a similar increase in myocardial ischemia determined by precordial echocardiography. The pre-bypass incidence of hypotension and tachycardia was greater in the desflurane group than in the sufentanil group. Clearly, desflurane is not a first choice for use as the sole agent of induction. This deficiency is far outweighed by its benefits of low solubility, making it ideal for rapid elimination and emergence at the end of long operations.

Sevoflurane has not shown any signs of increasing the heart rate or blood pressure during inhalation induction. Ebert et al. compared sevoflurane to isoflurane in a population with known risk factors for coronary disease undergoing noncardiac surgery.[50] They found no differences between the two agents with respect to hemodynamic deviations from baseline and adverse cardiac outcomes. Controversy has arisen concerning the degradation of sevoflurane with $CO_2$ absorbents to produce a potentially nephrotoxic by-product, compound A. This compound has been found to cause renal proximal tubule injury in rats but has had no effect on the BUN or creatinine concentrations in humans. Kharasch et al. and Bito et al. examined the production of compound A when comparing isoflurane and sevoflurane low-flow anesthesia in humans over periods of 3.7 hours and 6.1 hours, respectively.[51,52] They found no difference in renal function between the two groups, as determined by BUN, creatinine, and other sensitive markers of renal tubule injury. They concluded that although compound A formation does occur, a sevoflurane, based anesthetic is as safe as a low-flow isoflurane anesthetic.

Overdose of inhalation anesthetics may cause severe hypotension, diminish end-organ perfusion, and result in delayed emergence from anesthesia. The importance of titratability, speed of removal from the circulation, and cardiovascular stability are critical during management of geriatric patients. This is why the newer inhalation anesthetics, desflurane and sevoflurane, are useful adjuncts in the induction and maintenance of the geriatric patient. These drugs have a rapid onset and effect with a rapid offset and emergence from anesthesia. In view of the fact that MAC requirements are decreased in the elderly, the properties of desflurane and sevoflurane make them ideal to "titrate to effect" in this population. A meta-analysis of six studies comparing desflurane and isoflurane to propofol revealed that patients who received propofol were discharged home more quickly than those who received desflurane as their main anesthetic.[53] Patients who received desflurane responded to

TABLE 11.2. Properties of Commonly Used Inhalational Agents

| Agent | Vapor pressure at 20°C (mmHg) | Blood/gas partition coefficient[a] | MAC[b] | | Structure |
|---|---|---|---|---|---|
| | | | With $N_2O$ | With $O_2$ only | |
| $N_2O$ | 39,000 | 0.47 | | 104 | N≡N=O |
| Isoflurane | 238 | 1.46 | 0.50 | 1.15 | $CF_3$—O—CHCl—$CF_3$ |
| Sevoflurane | 160 | 0.69 | 0.66 | 1.71 | $CFH_2$—O—CH[$CF_3$]$_2$ |
| Desflurane | 664 | 0.42 | 2.83 | 6.0 | $CF_2$H—O—CFH—$CF_3$ |

[a] Blood/gas partition coefficient: solubility of the drug in the blood. Less-soluble agents have a lower value and therefore more rapid equilibration between inspired and alveolar concentrations. The addition of fluorine to the inhalational anesthetic provides greater molecular stability and lower tissue solubility. An inspired $N_2O$ concentration of more than 60% generally decreases the MAC by 1%.

[b] MAC, or minimum alveolar concentration, is expressed as a percent of 1 atmosphere required to prevent movement in 50% of subjects in response to a painful stimulus. In practice, MAC must be exceeded by a factor of 1.25–1.30 to prevent skeletal muscle movement in response to a surgical stimulus.

commands sooner than those who received isoflurane. Juvin et al. examined recovery from prolonged anesthesia (mean 199 minutes) using desflurane, isoflurane, or propofol anesthesia in an elderly population.[54] They found that patients undergoing desflurane anesthesia had significantly shorter immediate recovery times (time to eye opening) and time to extubation than isoflurane or propofol. Time to discharge from the postanesthesia recovery unit was similar in all three groups. The use of desflurane may facilitate more rapid emergence and may afford earlier tracheal extubation in the geriatric patient and facilitate exit from the operating room without the need for additional airway support. In the geriatric population where concern about diminished MAC, end-organ reserve, and cardiovascular stability are of great concern, it appears that sevoflurane and desflurane both possess properties making them attractive options in the induction and maintenance of general anesthesia (Table 11.2).

## Intravenous Anesthetics

The routine use of hypnotics/sedatives for induction and narcotics for maintenance of anesthesia are the mainstay of the modern-day anesthetic technique. An elderly patient requires less hypnotic and narcotic than a young person for the desired effect. Similarly, administration of the drug may result in a delayed onset of action. These two points may result in the anesthesiologist wondering, "When is this drug going to work?" A second dose may follow because of fear of underdosing. As time passes, the drug has had time to reach the desired receptor, and a prolonged effect is seen. Delayed emergence for short procedures and sustained hypotension are not uncommon. An awareness of the dependence on end-organ metabolism for termination of the effects of narcotics and barbiturates has led to the development of agents having increased potency and decreased duration of action. The attributes of the newer drugs are ideally suited for the geriatric population. This section reviews the use of propofol, diazepam, midazolam, fentanyl, sufentanyl, and the newest narcotic, remifentanil, in the geriatric population.

Propofol, or 2,6-diisopropyl phenol was first introduced in 1977 and may be the most commonly used hypnotic for anesthetic induction and conscious sedation in or out of the operating room. Propofol is insoluble in aqueous solution, so it is formulated as a 1.0% egg lecithin emulsion consisting of 10% soybean oil, 2.25% glycerol, and 1.2% egg phosphatide.[55] This formulation does not cause the serious hypersensitivity reactions or histamine release seen with early formulations. Because of its widespread use, it is important to understand how the pharmacokinetics and pharmacodynamics are altered in the elderly population. Dosing of propofol for induction, 2.0 mg/kg, commonly produces a duration of anesthesia of about 4 minutes in healthy adults. There is extensive tissue distribution of propofol, and plasma protein binding is approximately 98%. Hepatic cirrhosis, renal failure, sex, and obesity do not affect the pharmacokinetic parameters of propofol.[56]

Dosage and administration of propofol was studied by Kirkpatrick et al., who revealed that there were higher blood propofol concentrations in the elderly population (65–80 years) than in their younger counterparts (18–35 years) after a 2.0 mg/kg induction dose versus 2.5 mg/kg for the younger population. The elderly group had a significantly smaller central compartment, and total body clearance of propofol was significantly lower in this group.[55] Zamacora et al. found serum propofol levels were significantly elevated in elderly patients compared to levels in control patients when serum albumin levels were decreased. [57] Observed decreases in serum albumin diminished the amount of protein binding, resulting in higher levels of unbound propofol. This is of concern because elderly patients may present to the operating room with a reduction in serum protein due to disease or deficient nutrition. Propofol has the potential to produce a more pronounced effect when administered to a critically ill elderly patient. Long-term infusions of propofol might produce higher concentrations because of decreased clearance.

Schnider et al. reported extensive evaluations of propofol in elderly subjects, finding intercompartmental drug distribution to be influenced by age and the metabolic clearance of the drug to be under the influence of weight, lean body mass, and height.[58] In the elderly, pharmacokinetic data predict a faster initial decrease in the plasma concentration. However, the pharmacodynamic data concerning elderly patients reveal that as age increases, the sensitivity of the brain to the drug similiarly increases. There is also a tendency for a longer time to peak effect following a small bolus in the elderly. During an infusion of propofol, the steady-state plasma levels necessary for sleep in a 25-year-old are twice that needed for a 75-year-old to maintain sleep, further exhibiting greater sensitivity to propofol in the elderly population.[58]

Diazepam is widely used for intravenous administration for conscious sedation and anesthetic induction. Approximately 50% of the clearance of diazepam in humans is accounted for by the oxidative reaction of *N*-demethylation, yielding desmethyldiazepam (DMDZ) as the principal metabolite. The other major component of clearance is hydroxylation with the formation of temazepam. The appearance of DMDZ after oxidative metabolism contributes minimally to the pharmacodynamic actions of a single dose of diazepam. However, during long-term therapy, DMDZ and diazepam accumulate in plasma. The clearance of temazepam is higher than that of diazepam or DMDZ, so long-term therepy shows low plasma concentrations of this drug.[46] Following single intravenous doses of diazepam in elderly volunteers and patients, diazepam clearance has been found to decrease with age. Both the beta elimination half-time ($t_{1/2\beta}$) and volume of distribution (Vd) have been found to be significantly increased in the elderly. Clearance of diazepam is slower in the elderly than in young subjects regardless of sex despite the fact that elderly women have a larger Vd for diazepam (in part because of greater adipose tissue) than their elderly male counterparts. In the elderly with decreased albumin levels, the Vd of the unbound fraction of diazepam was found to be higher. This, along with increased Vd and decreased clearance, leads to a marked prolongation of diazepam $t_{1/2\beta}$ in the elderly.[59]

Midazolam, a water-soluble benzodiazepine available for intravenous or intramuscular injection, is used extensively for its anxiolytic, hypnotic, and amnestic properties. Midazolam is primarily metabolized via hepatic hydroxylation to yield its major metabolite 1-hydroxymidazolam. It is then conjugated and excreted in the urine. This metabolite normally does not contribute to the pharmacologic effect of midazolam, but it may accumulate in patients with renal insufficiency and produce sedation. The unbound fraction of midazolam is not influenced by age or sex.[59] Among elderly men, the $t_{1/2\beta}$ of midazolam was found to be significantly prolonged and the clearance significantly reduced compared to younger controls; elderly women did not exhibit the changes in clearance and $t_{1/2\beta}$ observed in men. Jacobs et al. found that the steady-state plasma midazolam concentrations required to ablate responsiveness to verbal commands were significantly reduced in an elderly population.[60] Although no hard data exist concerning age-related changes in receptor affinity or number, age-related increases in pharmacodynamic sensitivity to midazolam have been reported consistently in the literature, explaining the age-related decreases in dose requirements for midazolam sedation.[61]

Fentanyl, a synthetic opioid of the phenylpiperidine family, is 50–100 times more potent than morphine. The rapid onset and brief duration of lower doses are ideally suited for the operating room and conscious-sedation locations. Singleton et al. evaluated the pharmacokinetics in the elderly, comparing doses of 15 μg/kg for an elderly group to 20 μg/kg for a young group.[62] In this population, fentanyl concentrations were significantly higher in the elderly at 2 and 4 minutes after starting the infusion. Fentanyl exhibited a smaller Vd in elderly patients compared to that of young cohorts. Scott et al. evaluated the sensitivity of the brain (a pharmacodynamic evaluation) to fentanyl dosing in both young and elderly patients. Sensitivity was established by comparing electroencephalographic (EEG) responses after administered doses of fentanyl. They concluded that the decrease in fentanyl dose response seen with age is due to an increase in brain sensitivity to the drug.[63]

Sufentanil is another derivative of fentanyl, with a potency 5–10 times that of fentanyl. Sufentanil produces excellent cardiovascular stability during cardiac surgery with fewer incidences of hemodynamic responses to noxious stimuli. It has a slightly smaller Vd and $t_{1/2\beta}$ than fentanyl, yet both have similar clearances and hepatic extraction ratio. When sufentanil was compared to fentanyl-based general anesthetics in geriatric patients undergoing major abdominal surgery, no significant hemodynamic difference was seen. However, there was a significant difference in the potency ratios of the two drugs. Sufentanil was found to be six times as potent as fentanyl (6.6 : 1.0) in this patient population.[64] In a population of elderly patients undergoing anesthesia for neurosurgical procedures, Matteo et al. found that a lower initial Vd was the only significant difference in pharmacokinetic parameters seen between the elderly and young patients.[65] However, six of seven of the elderly patients required naloxone at the termination of the surgery to achieve an adequate respiratory rate. The use of sufentanil in the elderly population is influenced by pharmacodynamic differences (i.e., decreased MAC, brain sensitivity to narcotics), rather than pharmacokinetic differences.

Remifentanil is a new, highly potent opioid with rapid onset and a short duration of action because of its rapid hydrolysis by esterases in blood and tissue. It is of the class of 4-anilidopiperidines, which act at the mu opioid receptor. The introduction of a methyl ester group onto the *N*-acyl side chain of the piperidine ring confers increased susceptibility to hydrolytic metabolism by esterases and thereby rapid termination of effect. Its systemic half-life is 9–11 minutes.[66] The "context-sensitive" half-time (CSHT), or the time required for a 50% decrease in drug concentration, for remifentanil is 3 minutes and is independent of the duration of the infusion. Fentanyl, sufentanil, and alfentanil have longer CSHTs; and they are prolonged when administered by an infusion.[67] This pharmacokinetic profile of remifentanil makes it an ideal drug for outpatient procedures, conscious sedation, and other areas where rapid recovery is essential. Jhaveri and colleagues have determined that remifentanil is 15 times more potent than alfentanil.[68] Dosing at 1 μg/kg for intubation and 0.25–0.50 μg/kg/min for maintenance produces stable operating conditions. At these doses, however, significant bradycardia, hypotension, chest wall rigidity, and respiratory depression may occur during induction.

Remifentanil has been compared to propofol in an outpatient setting, with propofol-treated patients having significantly higher sedation scores than the remifentanil-treated patients. The remifentanil-treated patients exhibited a higher incidence of respiratory depression, determined by a respiratory rate of <8 breaths/min or oxygen desaturation <90% and a longer time to home readiness. These pharmacodynamic properties of remifentanil may be undesirable in the geriatric population. Minto et al. evaluated the influence of age and sex on the pharmacokinetics and pharmacodynamics of remifentanil in the young and adults to 84 years by determining the changes in the spectral edge ($SE_{95}$) of the EEG to a programmed remifentanil infusion.[67,69] Age was found to be an important covariant in the pharmacokinetics of remifentanil. A reduced central Vd was evident and resulted in higher initial blood concentrations after a given bolus than in young persons. Slower equilibration between blood and brain concentrations in the elderly offset their higher initial blood concentrations. They recommended cutting the initial bolus dose in half because of pharmacodynamic, not pharmacokinetic, differences. Delays are seen at the onset of the peak effect following a bolus dose. Clearance of remifentanil is decreased by 33% compared to that in younger persons,[67] which has an effect on the infusion rate; it is recommended that the infusion rate in the elderly be one-third that of a similar infusion in a young person. Because of the short duration of action of remifentanil, the anesthesiologist must be aware of postoperative pain and its treatment. Proper timing and titration of the remifentanil infusion with longer-acting analgesics play a critical role in the transition from the operating room to recovery and ultimately to home (Table 11.3).

TABLE 11.3. Pharmacokinetic and Pharmacodynamic Alterations of Commonly Used Intravenous Anesthetics in the Elderly

| Drug | CL | $t_{1/2\beta}$ | Metabolism | Other |
|---|---|---|---|---|
| Propofol | ↓ | ↑ | Hepatic | Delayed peak effect, ↑ pharmacodynamic effect |
| Diazepam | ↓ | ↑ | Hepatic | Active metabolites, ↑ pharmacodynamic effect |
| Midazolam | ↔ | ↔ | Renal | Water soluble, ↑ pharmacodynamic effect |
| Fentanyl | ↓ | ↓ | Hepatic | ↑ Pharmacodynamic effect |
| Sufentanil | ↓ | ↔ | Hepatic | ↑ Pharmacodynamic effect |
| Remifentanil | ↓ | ↑ | Plasma esterases | Greater bolus dose; lower infusion rate; ↑ pharmacodynamic effect |

CL, plasma clearance of the drug; $t_{1/2\beta}$, beta elimination half-life of the drug; ↑, increased; ↓, decreased; ↔, unchanged.

## Neuromuscular Blocking Agents

Anesthesiologists commonly employ neuromuscular blocking agents to achieve muscle relaxation for laryngoscopy, intubation, and surgical exposure as an adjunct to volatile and intravenous anesthetics. Advances in pharmacology have resulted in drugs that exhibit minimal cardiovascular effects in addition to decreased dependence on organ elimination for removal from the circulation.

Neuromuscular blocking drugs are quaternary ammonium compounds. The positive charges at these sites mimic the quaternary nitrogen of acetylcholine and are the main reason for the attraction of these drugs to the cholinergic receptor. Succinylcholine produces a depolarizing neuromuscular blockade at the motor endplate by imitating acetylcholine, acting as an agonist at the cholinergic receptor. After lowering the transmembrane potential through binding at the cholinergic receptor, depolarization of the postsynaptic membrane occurs, which prevents a propagated action potential by acetylcholine. The muscle is then unresponsive to further stimulation. The duration of action of succinylcholine is determined by the plasma concentrations of pseudocholinesterase.[70]

The principal action of nondepolarizing neuromuscular blocking drugs is competitive antagonism of acetylcholine at the nicotinic receptor on the postjunctional membrane of the neuromuscular junction. All muscle relaxants are highly water-soluble. The ester linkages of

TABLE 11.4. Neuromuscular Blocking Agents and the Elderly

| Drug | Metabolism | Onset of block | Recovery of block | Comments |
|---|---|---|---|---|
| Succinylcholine | Plasma cholinesterase | ↔ | ↔ | Depolarizing, muscle fasciculations |
| Pancuronium | 80% Renal, 20% hepatic | ↔ | ↑ | Vagolytic effect, longest lasting |
| Vecuronium | 80% Hepatic, 20% renal | ↑ | ↑ | Nonvagolytic |
| Rocuronium | Similar to vecuronium | ↑ | ↑ | More rapid onset than vecuronium |
| Atracurium | Hofmann + ester hydrolysis | ↔ | ↔ | Dose-related histamine release |
| Cisatracurium | Hofmann reaction | ↑ | ↔ | No histamine release |

Decreased temperature, inhalational anesthetics, and antibiotics (neomycin, streptomycin, clindamycin, aminoglycosides) potentiate neuromuscular blockade.
↑, increased duration (longer); ↓, decreased duration (shorter); ↔, unchanged.

succinylcholine and atracurium, the acetate groups of pancuronium, vecuronium, rocuronium, and the methoxy groups of mivacurium and atracurium assist in the hydrophilic nature of the compounds. The steroidal compounds of pancuronium, vecuronium, and rocuronium exhibit high potency and no histamine release on administration. The benzylisoquinolinium compounds doxacurium, atracurium, and cisatracurium have no vagolytic effect and, with the exception of cisatracurium, exhibit a tendency to cause histamine release.[71–73]

In the elderly patient decreases in total body water and hepatic and renal function along with increases in body fat help account for alterations in the response to neuromuscular blocking agents. Acetylcholine receptor sensitivity to nondepolarizing muscle relaxants is unaltered by old age.[74,75] Pancuronium, vecuronium, and rocuronium all exhibit decreased clearance from the plasma, resulting in increased duration of action.[76–78] Lien et al. revealed that spontaneous recovery from a vecuronium-induced neuromuscular blockade was significantly longer in the elderly.[77] In addition, the elimination half-life of vecuronium was significantly prolonged. The onset of action of rocuronium, a structural relative of vecuronium, was shown to be significantly longer in an elderly population than in young patients.[78]

Mivacurium, atracurium, and cisatracurium exhibit metabolism independent of hepatic or renal blood flow. Mivacurium is hydrolyzed by plasma cholinesterases at a rate roughly 85% that of succinylcholine and causes significant histamine release when administered at intubating doses, limiting its use in the hemodynamically unstable patient. Should plasma pseudocholinesterase activity be decreased because of a genetic deficiency in the enzyme quantity or an atypical form of the enzyme, the duration of action of mivacurium (and succinylcholine) is prolonged. Maddineni et al. demonstrated no differences in onset of neuromuscular blockade but a significantly longer time to recovery from the blockade in elderly patients treated with mivacurium 0.15 mg/kg.[79] Atracurium depends on Hofmann elimination, a pH- and temperature-dependent reaction that acts on a cyclic quaternary nitrogen grouping, opening it to a tertiary amine, facilitating clearance. In the elderly population, atracurium was shown to exhibit clearance similar to that in young patients, but it had a larger volume of distribution and longer elimination half-life. However, the pharmacokinetic differences were not reflected by a significant difference in pharmacodynamics. Cisatracurium, one of 10 stereoisomers of atracurium, is three to four times as potent as atracurium without the histamine-releasing side effects. The onset time at a 0.1 mg/kg dose in an elderly population was delayed by at least 1 minute compared to that in young persons.[72] Other pharmacokinetic parameters revealed no significant difference. The benefits of cisatracurium in the geriatric population are its metabolism, Hofmann elimination, which is not affected by hepatic or renal disease. This drug is ideal for an elderly patient because of its lack of hemodynamic side effects, no vagolytic or histamine release, and its unique pathway of metabolism, Hofmann degradation[80] (Table 11.4).

## Conclusions

The unifying theme throughout this chapter is the overwhelming presence of a decrease in physiologic reserve seen in the elderly population. This decrease is a consistent finding when it comes to dealing with the major organ systems, all of which affect decisions made by the anesthesiologist and surgeon when managing geriatric patients in the perioperative setting. The geriatric patient is at increased risk for perioperative complications as a result of aging and age-related disease. Successful perioperative management of a geriatric patient requires an understanding of physiologic differences between young and old as well as meticulous attention to detail.

## References

1. Seeman TE, Singer BH, Rowe JW, Horwitz RI, McEwen BS. Price of adaptation and allostatic load and its health conse-

quences: MacArthur studies of successful aging. Arch Intern Med 1997;157:2259–2268.
2. McLeskey CH. Anesthesia for the geriatric patient. In: Barash P, Cullen B, Stoelting R (eds) Clinical Anesthesia, 2nd ed. Philadelphia: Lippincott, 1992.
3. Rakowski W, Hickey T. Mortality and the attribution of health problems to aging among older adults. Am J Public Health 1992;82:1139–1141.
4. Fleisher LA. Preoperative evaluation. In: Barash P, Cullen B, Stoelting R (eds) Clinical Anesthesia, 3rd ed. Philadelphia: Lippincott, 1997.
5. American Society of Anesthesiologists. The ASA Directory of Members 1994. Park Ridge, IL: American Society of Anesthesiologists, 1994.
6. Roizen MF. Preoperative evaluation. In: Miller RD (ed) Anesthesia. New York: Churchill Livingstone, 1994:827.
7. Goldman L, Caldera DL, Nussbaum STR, et al. Multifactorial index of cardiac risk in non-cardiac surgical procedures. N Engl J Med 1997;297:845.
8. Mangano DT. Perioperative cardiac morbidity. Anesthesiology 1990;72:153–184.
9. Vacanti CJ, Van Houten RJ, Hill RC. A statistical analysis of the relationship of physical status to postoperative mortality in 68,388 cases. Anesth Analg 1970;49:564.
10. Owens WD, Felts JA, Spitznagel EL. ASA physical status classifications: a study of consistency of ratings. Anesthesiology 1978;49:239.
11. Grenburg AG, Saik RP, Pridham D. Influence of age on mortality of colon surgery. Am J Surg 1985;150:65–70.
12. Muravchick S. Geroanesthesia: Principles for Management of the Elderly Patient. St. Louis: Mosby, 1997.
13. Tiret L, Desmonts JM, Hatton F, et al. Complications associated with anaesthesia: a prospective survey in France. Can Anaesth Soc J 1986;33:336.
14. Dripps RD, Lamont A, Eckenhoff JE. The role of anesthesia in surgical mortality. JAMA 1961;178:261.
15. Greenblatt DJ, Harmatz JS, Shader RI. Clinical pharmacokinetics of anxiolytics and hypnotics in the elderly: therapeutic considerations. Part 2. Clin Pharmacokinet 1991;21:262–273.
16. Sladen R, Prough D. Perioperative renal protection. Probl Anesth 1997;9:314–331.
17. Hypothermia related deaths—Georgia, January 1996–December 1997, and United States, 1979–1995. MMWR 1999;47(48):1037–1041.
18. Matsukawa T, Sessler D, Sessler A, et al. Heat flow and distribution during induction of general anesthesia. Anesthesiology 1995;82:662–673.
19. Frank SM, Beattie C, Christopherson R, et al. Unintentional hypothermia is associated with postoperative myocardial ischemia: the perioperative ischemia randomized anesthesia trial study group. Anesthesiology 1993;78:468–476.
20. Frank SM, Shir Y, Raja SN, Fleisher LA, Beattie C. Core hypothermia and skin surface temperature gradients, epidural versus general anesthesia and the effects of age. Anesthesiology 1994;80:502–508.
21. Frank SM, Fleisher LA, Breslow MJ, et al. Perioperative maintenance of normothermia reduces the incidence of morbid cardiac events: a randomized clinical trial. JAMA 1997;277:1127–1134.
22. Beilin B, Shavit Y, Razumovsky J, Wolloch Y, Zeidel A, Bessler H. Effects of mild perioperative hypothermia on cellular immune responses. Anesthesiology 1998;89:1133–1140.
23. Rink L, Cakman I, Kirchner H. Altered cytokine production in the elderly. Mech Ageing Dev 1998;102:199–209.
24. Kurz A, Sessler DI, Lenhardt R. Perioperative normothermia to reduce the incidence of surgical-wound infection and shorten hospitalization. N Engl J Med 1996;334:1209–1215.
25. Just B, Trevien V, Delva E, Lienhardt A. Prevention of intraoperative hypothermia by preoperative skin-surface warming. Anesthesiology 1993;79:214–218.
26. Hynson J, Sessler D. Intraoperative warming therapies: a comparison of three devices. J Clin Anesth 1992;4:194–199.
27. Lakatta EG. Aging effects on the vasculature in health: risk factors for cardiovascular disease. Am J Geriatr Cardiol 1994;6:11–17.
28. Lakatta EG. Cardiovascular regulatory mechanisms in advanced age. Physiol Rev 1993;73:413–467.
29. Braunwald E. Heart Disease: A Textbook of Cardiovascular Medicine, 5th ed. Philadelphia: Saunders, 1997.
30. Cahalan MK, Hashimoto Y, Aizawa K, et al. Elderly, conscious patients have an accentuated hypotensive response to nitroglycerin. Anesthesiology 1992;77:646–655.
31. Wood M, Hyman S, Wood AJ. A clinical study of sensitivity to sodium nitroprusside during controlled hypotensive anesthesia in young and elderly patients. Anesth Analg 1987;66:132–136.
32. Harris SN, Ballantyne GH, Luther MA, Perrino AC Jr. Alterations of cardiovascular performance during laparoscopic colectomy: a combined hemodynamic and echocardiographic analysis. Anesth Analg 1996;83:482–487.
33. Perrino AC Jr. Cardiac output monitoring by echocardiography: should we pass on Swan-Ganz catheters? Yale J Biol Med 1993;66:397–413.
34. Perrino AC Jr, Harris SN, Luther MA. Intraoperative determination of cardiac output using multiplane transesophageal echocardiography: a comparison to thermodilution. Anesthesiology 1998;89:350–357.
35. Nishimura RA, Tajik AJ. Evaluation of diastolic filling of left ventricle in health and disease: Doppler echocardiography is the clinician's Rosetta stone. J Am Coll Cardiol 1997;30:8–18.
36. Frishman WH, Furberg CD, Friedwald WT. Beta-adrenergic blockade for survivors of acute myocardial infarction. N Engl J Med 1984;310:830–837.
37. First International Study of Infarct Survival Collaborative Group. Randomised trial of intravenous atenolol among 16,027 cases of suspected acute myocardial infarction: ISIS-1. Lancet 1986;2:57–66.
38. Pepine CJ, Cohn PF, Deedwania PC, et al. Effects of treatment on outcome in mildly symptomatic patients with ischemia during daily life, The Atenolol Silent Ischemia Study (ASIST). Circulation 1994;90:762–768.
39. Cleland J, Bristow M, Erdman E, Remmes W, Swedberg K, Waagstein F. Beta blocking agents in heart failure. Eur Heart J 1996;17:1629–1639.
40. Eagle KA, Rihal CS, Mickel MC, et al. Cardiac risk in non cardiac surgery: influence of coronary disease and type of surgery in 3368 operations. Circulation 1997;96:1882–1887.

41. Fleisher LA, Eagle KA. Screening non cardiac surgery patients for cardiac disease. Ann Intern Med 1996;124:767–772.
42. Fleisher LA, Nelson AH, Rosenbaum SH. Postoperative myocardial ischemia: etiology of cardiac morbidity or manifestation of underlying disease? J Clin Anesth 1995;7:97–102.
43. Wallace A, Layug E, Tateo I, et al. Prophylactic atenolol reduces postoperative myocardial ischemia. Anesthesiology 1998;88:7–17.
44. Mangano D, Layug E, Wallace A, Tateo I. Effect of atenolol on mortality and cardiovascular morbidity after noncardiac surgery. N Engl J Med 1996;335:1713–1720.
45. Waltier D. β-Adrenergic blocking drugs: incredibly useful, incredibly underutilized. Anesthesiology 1998;88:2–5.
46. Hammerlein A, Derendorf H, Lowenthal DT. Pharmacokinetic and pharmacodynamic changes in the elderly. Clin Pharmacokinet 1998;35:49–64.
47. Stevens WC, Kingston HG. Inhalational anesthesia. In: Barash P, Cullen B, Stoelting R (eds) Clinical Anesthesia, 3rd ed. Philadelphia: Lippincott, 1997.
48. Strum D, Eger EI II, Unadakat J, Johnson B, Carpenter R. Age affects the pharmacokinetics of inhaled anesthetics in humans. Anesth Analg 1991;73:310–318.
49. Helman JD, Leung J, Bellows W, et al. The risk of myocardial ischemia in patients receiving desflurane versus sufentanil anesthesia for coronary artery bypass graft surgery. Anesthesiology 1992;77:47–62.
50. Ebert TJ, Kharasch ED, Rooke GA, Shroff A, Muzi M. Myocardial ischemia and adverse cardiac outcomes in cardiac patients undergoing noncardiac surgery with sevoflurane and isoflurane. Anesth Analg 1997;85:993–999.
51. Kharasch ED, Frink EJ Jr, Zager R, Bowdle TA, Artu A, Nogami WM. Assessment of low flow sevoflurane and isoflurane effects on renal function using sensitive markers of tubular toxicity. Anesthesiology 1997;86:1238–1253.
52. Bito H, Ikeuchi Y, Ikeda K. Effects of low-flow sevoflurane anesthesia on renal function: comparison with high flow sevoflurane anesthesia and low-flow isoflurane anesthesia. Anesthesiology 1997;86:1231–1237.
53. Dexter F, Tinker JH. Comparisons between desflurane and isoflurane or propofol on time to following commands and time to discharge: a metaanalysis. Anesthesiology 1995;83:77–82.
54. Juvin P, Servin F, Giraud O, Desmonts JM. Emergence of elderly patients from prolonged desflurane, isoflurane, or propofol anesthesia. Anesth Analg 1997;85:647–651.
55. Kirkpatrick T, Cockshott ID, Douglas EJ, Nimmo WS. Pharmacokinetics of propofol (diprivan) in elderly patients. Br J Anaesth 1988:60:146–150.
56. Schnider TW, Minto CF, Gambus PL, et al. The influence of method of administration and covariates on the pharmacokinetics of propofol in adult volunteers. Anesthesiology 1998;88:1170–1182.
57. Zamacora MK, Suarez E, Aguilera L, Rodriguez-Sasiann, Aguirre C, Calvo R. Serum protein binding of propofol in critically ill patients. Acta Anaesthesiol Scand 1997;41:1267–1272.
58. Schnider TW, Minto CF, Shafer SL, et al. The influence of age on propofol pharmacodynamics. Anesthesiology 1999;90:1502–1516.
59. Greenblatt DJ, Harmatz JS, Shader RI. Clinical pharmacokinetics of anxiolytics and hypnotics in the elderly. Part 1. Clin Pharmacokinet 1991;21:165–177.
60. Jacobs JR, Reves JG, Marty J, White WD, Bai SA, Smith LR. Aging increases the pharmacodynamic sensitivity to the hypnotic effects of midazolam. Anesth Analg 1995;80:143–148.
61. Albrecht S, Ihmsen H, Hering W, et al. The effect of age on the pharmacokinetics and pharmacodynamics of midazolam. Clin Pharmacol Ther 1999;65:630–639.
62. Singleton MA, Rosen JI, Fisher DM. Pharmacokinetics of fentanyl in the elderly. Br J Anaesth 1988;60:619–622.
63. Scott JC, Cooke JE, Stanski DR. Electroencephalographic quantitation of opioid effect: comparative pharmacodynamics of fentanyl and sufentanil. Anesthesiology 1991;74:34–42.
64. Helmers JH, van Leeuwen L, Zuurmond WW. Sufentanil pharmacokinetics in young and elderly surgical patients. Eur J Anaesthesiol 1994;11:181–185.
65. Matteo RS, Schwartz AE, Ornstein E, Young WL, Chang WJ. Pharmacokinetics of sufentanil in the elderly surgical patient. Can J Anaesth 1990;37:852–856.
66. Burkle H, Dunbar S, Van Aken H. Remifentanil: a novel, short acting, mu-opioid. Anesth Analg 1996;83:646–651.
67. Minto CF, Schnider TW, Egan TD, et al. Influence of age and gender on the pharmacokinetics and pharmacodynamics of remifentanil. Anesthesiology 1997;86:10–23.
68. Jhaveri R, Joshi P, Batenhorst R, Baughman V, Glass PS. Dose comparison of remifentanil and alfentanil for loss of consciousness. Anesthesiology 1997;87:253–259.
69. Minto CF, Schnider TW, Egan TD, et al. Influence of age and gender on the pharmacokinetics and pharmacodynamics of remifentanil. Anesthesiology 1997;86:24–33.
70. Bevan David R, Donati F. Muscle relaxants. In: Barash P, Cullen B, Stoelting R (eds) Clinical Anesthesia, 3rd ed. Philadelphia: Lippincott, 1997.
71. Kitts JB, Fisher DM, Canfell PC, et al. Pharmacokinetics and pharmacodynamics of atracurium in the elderly. Anesthesiology 1990;72:272–275.
72. Ornstein E, Lien CA, Matteo RS, Ostapkovich ND, Diaz J, Wolf KB. Pharmacodynamics and pharmacokinetics of cisatracurium in geriatric surgical patients. Anesthesiology 1996;84:520–525.
73. Sorooshian SS, Stafford MA, Eastwood NB, Boyd AH, Hull CJ, Wright PM. Pharmacokinetics and pharmacodynamics of cisatracurium in young and elderly adult patients. Anesthesiology 1996;84:1083–1091.
74. Vanlinthout LE, van Egmond J, de Boo T, Lerou JG, Wevers RA, Booij LH. Factors affecting magnitude and time course of neuromuscular block produced by suxamethonium. Br J Anaesth 1992;69:29–35.
75. Koscielniak-Nelson Z, Bevan J, Baxter M, Donati F, Bevan D. Onset of maximum neuromuscular block following succinylcholine or vecuronium in four age groups. Anesthesiology 1993;79:229–234.
76. Rupp SM, Castagnoli KP, Fisher DM, Miller RD. Pancuronium and vecuronium pharmacokinetics and pharmacodynamics in younger and elderly patients. Anesthesiology 1987;67:45–49.

77. Lien CA, Matteo RS, Ornstein E, Schwartz AE, Diaz J. Distribution, elimination, and action of vecuronium in the elderly. Anesth Analg 1991;73:39–42.
78. Bevan DR, Fiset P, Balendran P, Law-Min JC, Ratcliffe S, Donati F. Pharmacodynamic behavior of rocuronium in the elderly. Can J Anaesth 1993;40:127–132.
79. Maddineni VR, Mirakhur RK, McCoy EP, Sharpe TD. Neuromuscular and haemodynamic effects of mivacurium in elderly and young adult patients. Br J Anaesth 1994;73:608–612.
80. Atherton DP, Hunter JM. Clinical pharmacokinetics of the newer neuromuscular blocking drugs. Clin Pharmacokinet 1999;36:169–189.

# 12
# Pain Management

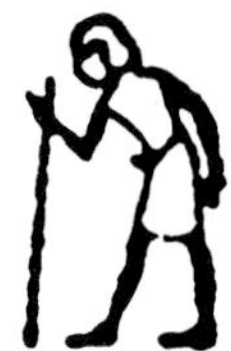

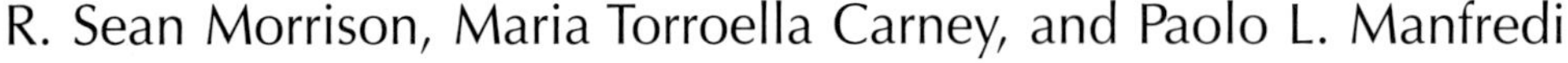

R. Sean Morrison, Maria Torroella Carney, and Paolo L. Manfredi

Whereas postoperative pain was once thought to be an inevitable, albeit severely unpleasant, consequence of surgery, it is now clear that appropriate analgesic therapies can result in effective pain management for nearly all surgical patients. Nevertheless, despite recent efforts to improve management of pain in the United States, undertreatment of pain, particularly postoperative pain, remains a persistent problem.[1,2] This undertreatment appears to be dramatically worse in the elderly.[3] Untreated or undertreated pain may have a substantial impact on patients' postoperative recovery and may exacerbate underlying co-morbidities and normal age-related physiologic changes. Pain can induce tachycardia, increase myocardial oxygen requirements, and produce cardiac ischemia. Pain, or the fear of pain, may lead to limited postoperative physical activity, which may further increase the risk of thromboembolism, urinary retention, fecal impaction, ileus, and atelectasis. For all these reasons, control of postoperative pain in the elderly surgical patient is of critical importance.

## Pathophysiology

Pain is an unpleasant sensory and emotional experience associated with actual or potential tissue damage, or it is described in terms of such damage.[4] No matter how dextrous the surgeon, operations cause tissue trauma, which results in direct activation of free nerve terminals (nociceptors). Additionally, surgical trauma causes the release of inflammatory mediators such as prostaglandins, bradykinin, serotonin, histamine, and hydrogen ions. These mediators activate or sensitize (or both) nociceptors that enhance and prolong the painful state. Primary afferent nerve fibers have also been shown to contribute to the pain response by releasing substance P and other neuropeptides that play a role in nociception and "neurogenic inflammation." Prolonged noxious stimuli can alter sensory processing in the spinal cord by lowering the firing threshold of dorsal horn neurons (sensitization).

Nociceptive signals travel via primary afferent fibers (A-delta for thermal and mechanical nociceptors and C fibers for polymodal nociceptors) and form ascending nociceptive tracts (spinothalamic and spinohypothalamic tracts). Pain signals then reach the thalamus and cortex. From midbrain centers, descending pathways modulate transmission of pain signals at the level of the dorsal horn. The inflammation caused by the surgical trauma also evokes "stress hormone responses" and triggers the "flight or fight response." Persistent pain promotes continuation of these responses, which can result in increased metabolic rate, blood clotting, and water retention—all of which can be harmful to the elderly patient.

The question as to whether age-related changes occur with regard to the perception of pain has yet to be fully answered. Degenerative changes occur in areas of the central and autonomic nervous systems that mediate pain, although the clinical relevance of these changes has yet to be determined.[3] Clinical observations from elderly patients who report minimal pain and discomfort despite the presence of cardiac ischemia or intraabdominal catastrophe suggest that pain perception may be altered in the elderly. However, experimental data suggest that significant age-related changes in pain perception probably do not occur.[5] Until further studies conclusively demonstrate that the perception of pain decreases with age, the consequences of stereotyping most elderly patients as experiencing less pain may be inaccurate clinical assessments and needless suffering.[3]

## Classification of Pain Syndromes

Pain syndromes may be classified by their temporal course (acute versus chronic) and their underlying etiology (somatic versus visceral versus neuropathic). Acute pain follows a straightforward course with a well-defined cause, typical behavior (grimacing, sobbing, splinting), sympathetic nervous system hyperactivity (tachycardia, tachypnea, diaphoresis), and anxiety. Postoperative pain is the prototype of acute pain.

Chronic pain may coexist with surgically induced acute pain or may develop as a complication of the surgery itself. Chronic pain, defined as pain present for more than three months,[6] typically has a different constellation of symptoms and requires a more complex approach to treatment. The autonomic changes (tachycardia, diaphoresis, hypertension) seen with acute pain syndromes are absent with chronic pain; instead, changes in personality, functional status, life style, and affect (particularly depression and dysphoria) become more prominent. Successful therapy requires an interdisciplinary, multidimensional approach that focuses on the physical and psychological aspects of the pain syndrome. Prototypical examples of chronic pain include postherpetic neuralgia, phantom limb pain, and postthoracotomy pain.

In addition to assessing the temporal course of the pain syndrome, it is important to determine the type of pain the patient is experiencing. Pain may be categorized into three types—somatic, visceral, neuropathic—and each type of pain may be seen in surgical patients.

*Somatic pain* refers to the activation/stimulation of peripheral nociceptors in cutaneous and deep tissues. This type of pain is often described as well localized, aching, or gnawing in sensation. Examples of somatic pain include pain secondary to bone metastases or fractures and incisional pain.

*Visceral pain* results from infiltration, compression, or distension of abdominal or thoracic viscera. Visceral pain can be poorly localized and is described as pressure or squeezing; it may be accompanied by nausea, vomiting, and diaphoresis; and it can be associated with referred pain sites. Examples of visceral pain are biliary colic with or without referred shoulder pain, right upper quadrant pain due to hepatic tumors, or back pain due to pancreatic cancer.

*Neuropathic pain* results from injury to the peripheral or central nervous system due to compression, infiltration, or degeneration of peripheral nerves or the spinal cord. The pain is typically severe and constant; and it is described as burning, aching, or vise-like. Patients may also complain of radiating shock-like sensations. Examples of neuropathic pain include diabetic peripheral neuropathy, tumor infiltration of the lumbar plexus, or pain due to spinal stenosis.

Correctly categorizing the type of pain is important in terms of selecting the appropriate analgesic therapy. Somatic and visceral pain syndromes typically respond well to standard opioid and nonopioid therapies. Conversely, neuropathic pain is more resistant to conventional analgesic techniques. Although some studies suggest that neuropathic pain responds to high doses of opioids,[7] the side effects associated with these doses often limit therapy. For most patients, so-called adjuvant analgesic agents (tricyclic antidepressants, anticonvulsants, corticosteroids, oral local anesthetic agents) may be the most efficacious therapy for neuropathic pain. Alternatively, anesthetic blocks and neurosurgical procedures may be needed if pharmacotherapies fail.

## Pain Assessment

The appropriate management of pain begins with a careful and detailed assessment. The goal of this assessment should be to assess the location and character (temporal pattern, quality, exacerbating and alleviating factors, associated symptoms, and severity) of the pain(s), define the etiology(ies), and develop a plan of care. Although typically the focus of this assessment is centered on pain resulting from the surgical procedure, it should be noted that pain is highly prevalent in the geriatric population,[8,9] and a detailed pain assessment is likely to elucidate a number of pain syndromes and etiologies (e.g., osteoarthritis, osteoporosis, neuropathies, postherpetic neuralgia, vascular disease). The principles of pain assessment and management described below, although targeted toward surgical pain, can also be applied to other pain syndromes discovered during the assessment.

The guiding principle of pain assessment is to ask the patient and believe the patient's complaint of pain. All too often, unfortunately, a patient's pain is treated based on the nurses' or physicians' perceptions of that pain. Several studies show that physicians' and nurses' estimates of patients' pain severity are significantly lower than the patients' self-reports.[10,11] The initial interview should focus on the location of the pain and its quality, severity, temporal location, and exacerbating and alleviating (including analgesic agents) factors. Multiple pains should be considered individually and attempts made to determine the underlying etiologies. Several studies have observed a general bias among older persons against expressing pain.[12–14] Hence, older patients should be encouraged to express their experience of pain, and these reports should be believed and acted on.

Assessment tools may be of assistance to evaluate, measure, and follow a patient's pain complaint. These tools were initially developed for research purposes but have evolved for clinical use. The assessment instruments for pain include visual analogue scales, numerical rating scales, and verbal descriptor scales. Visual analogue scales typically consist of a 10-cm line on a piece of paper with "no pain" labeled on the left and "most severe pain" on the right. Patients are to indicate on the line the severity of their pain. Numeric rating scales are similar to visual analogue scales except that the line is replaced with a series of numbers, typically 1 (no pain) through 10 (worst pain imaginable). The patient is asked to select a number representing their level of pain. Verbal Descriptor Scales (VDS) consist of words or numbers representing different levels of pain (e.g., none, moderate, severe, very severe). Patients select the word that best describes their level of pain.

There currently exist a number of validated instruments for the comprehensive assessment of pain. Although not designed specifically for use in the surgical population, these instruments can provide valuable, comprehensive information about the patient's pain syndrome(s) if used routinely. The McGill Pain Questionnaire is the most comprehensive instrument and assesses the location of pain, its pattern over time, and miscellaneous components of the pain and its intensity. It includes both visual analogue and verbal descriptor scales.[15] A short form of this instrument is available and is probably easier to use in the clinical setting.[16] The Wisconsin Brief Pain Inventory,[17] although relatively short, was developed primarily for use with cancer patients and may be less applicable to the surgical patient. It consists of a combination of numeric rating and verbal descriptive scales. The Memorial Pain Assessment Card measures pain intensity, pain relief, and mood.[18] It is the simplest, the shortest, and the easiest to use of the instruments listed and consists of visual analogue and verbal descriptive scales. Whenever possible, patients should be instructed as to the use of assessment tools prior to surgery.

Pain assessment in the elderly is often complicated by the coexistence of cognitive impairment. The assessment and management of pain in cognitively impaired patients presents special challenges. The cognitively impaired patient is often unable to express pain adequately, request analgesics, or operate patient-controlled analgesia (PCA) medications and thus may be at substantial risk for undertreatment of the pain. The fear of exacerbating a delirious episode or precipitating delirium in an otherwise stable postoperative elderly patient by employing opioids in the management of pain may also lead to inadequate pain management. As with cognitively intact patients, the initial step when assessing pain in the demented individual is to ask the patient. Although patients with severe dementia may be incapable of communicating, many with moderate degrees of impairment can accurately localize and grade the severity of their pain,[19] and these self-reports should be regarded as valid.

In the noncommunicative patient, pain self-reports are impractical, and alternative means of assessment are needed. Pain assessment in this population of patients is of particular importance given tentative evidence suggesting that medical professionals undertreat pain in the presence of cognitive impairment,[20] and that pain is aggravated in the presence of cognitive deficits.[21] Untreated pain can result in agitation or disruptive behavior, and it may worsen or precipitate a delirious episode.

Until further research is performed, the best means of assessing pain in the noncommunicative patient is probably through the use of nonverbal cues such as facial expressions (grimacing, frowning) and motor behavior (bracing, restlessness, agitation) and through the use of verbal cues such as groaning, screaming, or moaning. Data from cognitively intact individuals suggest that these nonverbal behaviors appear to correlate with self-reported pain in nondemented patients recovering from surgery.[22,23] Pharmacologic therapy should be titrated upward in small incremental doses until the nonverbal/verbal behavior disappears or side effects become apparent. This approach is particularly useful in the agitated postoperative patient whose agitation may well stem from untreated or undertreated pain. The risk of undertreating severe pain is generally more concerning, both medically and ethically, than the risk of worsening delirium with medications.

## Pharmacologic Management of Pain

### Nonopioid Analgesic Agents

Nonopioid analgesic agents [acetaminophen, aspirin, nonsteroidal antiinflammatory drugs (NSAIDs)] are useful for treatment of mild pain. The antipyretic properties of these agents, however, may limit their use during the early postoperative period, when masking a febrile response may be clinically inadvisable.

#### *Acetaminophen*

Acetaminophen is a peripheral analgesic agent that does not affect the enzyme cyclooxygenase. Acetaminophen has no antiinflammatory properties, and its analgesic potency is equivalent to that of aspirin. Although generally considered to have an excellent safety profile, problems related to hepatic toxicity can develop in patients who are taking products that combine acetaminophen with opioids. For example, patients taking two tablets of Percocet (650 mg acetaminophen) every 4 hours in combination with two 325 mg tablets of acetaminophen every 4 hours ingest 7.8 g during a 24-hour period (almost twice the recommended daily dose of 2.6–3.9 g). Concerns about overdosage are magnified in patients with memory disorders who may not remember how much medication they have been taking.

#### *Oral NSAIDs*

The NSAIDs are useful primarily for treating mild pain. NSAIDs reduce inflammation and nociception by inhibiting cyclooxygenase and preventing the production and release of endogenous prostaglandins. Additionally, NSAIDs appear to act centrally by binding to spinal and supraspinal sites.[24] All NSAIDs can result in renal insufficiency; and with the exception of salicylate and choline magnesium trisalicylate, for which the risk is minimal, they can inhibit platelet aggregation and cause dyspepsia and gastric ulceration.

Clinically, there is a ceiling of analgesia associated with NSAIDs and acetaminophen. That is, there is a fixed dose at which no further dose escalation results in increased analgesia. Although this analgesic ceiling varies among individuals for the same NSAID, it typically occurs at or below the manufacturer's recommended maximal dose; therefore exceeding this dose rarely results in enhanced analgesia.[25] In general, for elderly patients agents with short half-lives (e.g., ibuprofen) are most appropriate; for patients with a history of dyspepsia, ulcer disease, or bleeding diatheses, either salicylate or choline magnesium trisalicylate should be used if an NSAID is indicated. NSAIDs can be combined with opioids to enhance analgesia.

### *Parenteral NSAIDs*

Parenteral NSAIDs (e.g., ketorolac) are being used increasingly for postoperative pain as sole analgesic agents and in conjunction with opioids as opioid-sparing agents. The efficacy of ketorolac, currently the only available parenteral NSAID in the United States, has been well established with 30mg being equianalgesic with 12mg of parenteral morphine. Intravenous ketorolac has been shown to reduce opioid requirements for knee and hip replacement surgery by 35–44%[26] and by 50–75% for thoracotomy and upper abdominal surgery.[27] Peak analgesia from ketorolac is typically seen 1–2 hours after administration, and the half-life is approximately 6 hours, although it may be prolonged in patients with reduced renal function or in the elderly. The manufacturer's recommended dose for elderly individuals or those with renal insufficiency is 15mg every 6 hours following a 30mg loading dose. Ketorolac has a side effect profile similar to those of other NSAIDs. There appears to be a significantly increased risk of gastrointestinal bleeding in the elderly, particularly with high doses and with duration of use of more than 5 days.[28–30]

## Opioid Analgesic Agents

Exogenous opioids mimic the action of naturally occurring opioid peptides (enkephalins, dynorphins, β-endorphin, α-neoendorphin) through recognition of common receptors. Each of these endogenous peptides is derived from a genetically distinct precursor polypeptide and has a characteristic anatomic distribution.

The development of specific radioligands and selective antagonists allowed recognition of different classes of receptors implicated in the production of analgesia. Mu receptors, subdivided into mu1 and mu2, are the binding sites responsible for morphine-induced analgesia. Mu1 receptors predominate at the supraspinal level and in particular in the periaqueductal gray matter, the locus ceruleus, the nucleus raphe magnum, and the nucleus reticularis gigantocellularis. In the dorsal horns of the spinal cord morphine analgesia is mediated by mu2 receptors. There is a synergistic analgesic effect from the concomitant activation of supraspinal and spinal systems. Morphine also interacts with two other classes of receptors that mediate analgesia—kappa and delta—although the degree of affinity for these receptors is much lower. Other actions of morphine are related to its interaction with these specific receptors. For example, respiratory depression is mediated by mu2 receptors in the brain stem,[31] and constipation is mediated by mu2 receptors within the brain[32] and intestinal plexus.[33]

Activation of mu and delta receptors by exogenous opioids results in the production of a guanine nucleotide regulatory protein (G-protein), which then couples the receptors to effector proteins resulting in hyperpolarization of the neuronal membranes. G-proteins can also decrease neuronal excitability by inhibiting the synthesis of cyclic adenosine monophosphate (cAMP) through their binding to adenylate cyclase.

Drugs that bind to opioid receptors are classified as agonists (e.g., morphine) if they produce analgesia, antagonists (e.g., naloxone) if they block the action of an agonist (i.e., they possess affinity but not efficacy), and agonist-antagonists (e.g., pentazocine) if they produce analgesia by interacting with a specific receptor (e.g., kappa) but also bind to other receptors (e.g., mu receptors) where they can block the action of an agonist. Partial agonists (e.g., buprenorphine) bind to receptors and produce analgesia but, unlike agonists, exhibit a ceiling effect.[34] The clinical use of mixed agonist-antagonists is limited by the increased incidence of the kappa and nonopioid sigma receptor-mediated side effects of dysphoria and hallucinations.[35,36] Mixed agonist-antagonists and partial agonists cause a withdrawal syndrome when administered to patients on chronic opioid therapy.

Opioids are the closest thing we have to an ideal analgesic. They exhibit no ceiling effect and can produce profound analgesia by progressive dose escalation. They are the most effective agents for the relief of any type of acute pain because of their predictable dose-dependent response. Opioids have no significant long-term organ toxicity and can be used for years. Addiction is negligible when opioids are used in the context of medical care.[37]

It is clinically useful to classify opioids as weak or strong depending on their relative efficacy (Table 12.1). Weak opioids are used for moderate or less severe pain, and their efficacy is limited by an increased incidence of side effects at higher doses [e.g., nausea and constipation with codeine, central nervous system (CNS) excitation with propoxyphene]. When opioids are used in a fixed oral dose mixed with a nonopioid analgesic, their efficacy is limited by the maximal safe dose for the acetaminophen or aspirin. Strong opioids are used for more

TABLE 12.1. Oral and Parenteral Opioid Analgesic Equivalences and Relative Potency of Opioids

| | Equivalence/relative potency, by route of administration | | | |
|---|---|---|---|---|
| Opioid agonist | Parenteral | Oral | Conversion (IV to PO) | Duration of effect (hours) |
| Morphine | 10 | 30 | 3 | 3–4 |
| Long-acting morphine | | 30 | NA | 8–12 |
| Oxycodone | | 20 | NA | 3–4 |
| Long-acting oxycodone | | 20 | NA | 8–12 |
| Hydromorphone | 1.5 | 7.5 | 5 | 3–4 |
| Levorphanol[a] | 2 | 4 | 2 | 4–6 |
| Meperidine[b] | 100 | 300 | 3 | 3 |
| Fentanyl | 0.1 | | NA | 1–2 |
| Codeine | 130 | 200 | 1.5 | 3–4 |

[a] Long half-life: When multiple doses are administered the risk of accumulation is high, especially in the elderly.
[b] Meperidine *should not be used* long term or in high doses because of central nervous system toxic metabolites. It is contraindicated with monoamine oxidase inhibitors.

severe pain. They have a wide therapeutic window and no ceiling effect, with higher doses producing an increasing level of analgesia. They are the agents of choice for parenteral administration. Patients experiencing moderate pain should be started on a weak opioid. Patients whose pain is severe or whose pain persists despite the use of a weak opioid should be administered a strong opioid.

### Weak Opioid Agents

Codeine, an alkaloid of opium, is the prototype "weak" analgesic. Although a parenteral preparation is available, it is nearly always given orally and often in a fixed mixture with a nonopioid analgesic. A 200 mg dose is equipotent to 30 mg of morphine. The half-life of codeine is 2.5–3.0 hours.

Hydrocodone is a codeine derivative, available in the United States only in combination with acetaminophen, aspirin, or ibuprofen. It is more potent than codeine, although good data are lacking.

Oxycodone is a semisynthetic derivative of thebaine, an opium alkaloid. Because of its high bioavailability (>50%) it is suitable for oral administration and is 105 times more potent than morphine by this route and 10 times more potent than codeine.[38,39] When administered parenterally, its intensity and duration of analgesia are 25% less than those of morphine.[39] Oxycodone has a half-life of 2–3 hours and a duration of action of 4–5 hours. It is metabolized like codeine: demethylated and conjugated in the liver and excreted in the urine.[39] Oxycodone has been considered a "weak" analgesic because of its use in a fixed combination with acetaminophen and aspirin, which limits its dose to 10 mg every 4 hours. When oxycodone is used alone it has no ceiling effect for analgesia. It is more potent than morphine, and there are reports suggesting it might have fewer side effects.[40,41] Its availability in 5 mg tablets permits careful titration in patients with a narrow therapeutic margin. Oxycodone is a versatile and flexible oral medication that can be used to treat pain of any intensity requiring an opioid analgesic.

Propoxyphene is a synthetic analgesic structurally related to methadone. It is approximately equipotent to codeine as an analgesic but lacks its antitussive properties. Its analgesic activity lasts 3–5 hours, its half-life is 6–12 hours, and its major metabolite is norpropoxyphene, which has a half-life of 30–36 hours and may be responsible for some of the observed toxicity.[42] Norpropoxyphene has local anesthetic effects similar to those of lidocaine, and high doses may cause arrhythmias. Seizures occur more often with propoxyphene intoxication than with other opioids. It is more difficult to manage and offers no advantage over other opioids.

Tramadol is a weak opioid analgesic that also inhibits the reuptake of serotonin and norepinephrine. Tramadol has been recently released in the United States and may be useful for mild to moderate pain. A tramadol dose of 50 mg appears to be equianalgesic with 60 mg of codeine.[43] Unlike other opioids, tramadol exhibits an analgesic ceiling, which limits its use for severe pain syndromes. Tramadol appears not to be associated with physical dependence but does have a relatively high incidence of associated nausea compared to that of other opioids.[44]

### Strong Opioid Agents

Morphine is the prototype strong opioid agonist. All other opioids are compared to morphine when determining their relative analgesic potency. Like other "strong" opioids, there is no ceiling to the analgesic effect, although side effects, particularly sedation and confusion, may intervene before optimal analgesia. Morphine is metabolized in the liver, where it undergoes glucuronidation at the 3- and 6-positions. Morphine-3-glucuronide (M3G) and morphine-6-glucuronide (M6G) accumulate with chronic morphine administration.[45] M6G binds to mu receptors with affinity similar to morphine[46] but also binds to delta receptors, which may account for its higher analgesic potency.[37] M6G appears to be 20 times more analgesic than morphine when administered directly in the periaqueductal gray,[46] but only 0.077% of this metabolite crosses the intact blood–brain barrier following oral or parenteral administration.[47] With single-dose morphine studies, the relative parenteral/oral potency ratio is 1:6.[48] After chronic use the ratio changes to 1:3[49] as a result of the accumulation of active metabolites. There is experimental[50] and clinical[51] evidence that M3G, which has negligible affinity for opioid receptors and does not produce analgesia,[46] has excitatory effects on neurons and can cause myoclonus and rarely a hyperalgesic state. It is thought that the myoclonus and hyperalgesia precipitated by M3G are mediated by different receptor mechanisms.[52] The half-life of morphine is about 2 hours, and the half-life of M6G is slightly longer.[53] The duration of analgesia is 4 hours. Slow-release preparations, which permit a twice-a-day regimen, are safe and effective.[54] Slow-release mechanisms should be used only after dose titration with morphine sulfate and only if the pain is expected to continue. Morphine metabolites are eliminated by glomerular filtration and can accumulate in patients with renal insufficiency, leading to an increased incidence of side effects.[55] Morphine should be used with caution in the presence of renal failure; and if utilized, the dosing interval should be increased.

Hydromorphone is a potent semisynthetic phenanthrene-derivative opioid agonist. When single doses are administered parenterally, 1.3 mg of hydromorphone is equipotent to 10 mg of morphine. Hydromorphone is somewhat shorter-acting than morphine but has a higher peak effect. Its bioavailability is 30–40% with an oral to parenteral ratio of 5:1.[56] It has a half-life of 1.5–2.0 hours, and active metabolites may accumulate during renal failure.[57] Continuous subcutaneous infusion and intravenous infusions of hydromorphone result in similar analgesia and side effects.[58]

Fentanyl is a synthetic phenylpiperidine-derivative opioid agonist that interacts primarily with mu receptors.[53] It is 80–100 times more potent than morphine and highly lipophilic. The latter properties make it a suitable candidate for administration via the epidural route. It is also available in a transdermal form. The transdermal form is not recommended, however, for the treatment of postoperative pain because the titration is lengthy and it lacks the flexibility, which is the cornerstone of treatment for acute and evolving pain. Oral transmucosal fentanyl is used for anesthesia induction in pediatric patients and will probably be useful for postoperative pain control, although to date studies are lacking. In studies with children, initial pain relief was noted within a few minutes with a maximum effect seen within 20–30 minutes.[59]

Levorphanol is a synthetic opioid agonist structurally related to the phenanthrene-derivative opiates. It is a potent mu agonist but also binds delta and kappa receptors.[60] When administered parenterally 2 mg of levorphanol are equianalgesic to 10 mg of morphine.[61] Because it has a half-life of 12–30 hours and a duration of analgesia of 4–6 hours, dose reduction may be required 2–4 days after starting the drug to avoid side effects resulting from drug accumulation. Levorphanol should not be used in patients with impaired renal function or encephalopathy because of the dangers of drug accumulation and the development of toxic serum levels. It should be used only for patients who cannot tolerate other opioids because of the combination of inadequate analgesia and intolerable side effects.

Methadone is a synthetic diphenylheptane-derivative opiate mu agonist. It is an inexpensive and effective analgesic, but its use is limited by the need for a carefully individualized dose and interval titration. When administered to opioid-naive patients, especially the elderly, the risk of overdose is high. It should therefore be used only for selected patients and only by individuals experienced with its use. The oral bioavailability is high, ranging from 41% to 99%,[62] and it is rapidly absorbed from the gastrointestinal tract with measurable plasma concentrations within 30 minutes after oral administration.[62] When administered in single parenteral doses it is equipotent to morphine, with a duration of analgesia of 4–6 hours.[63] Its plasma level declines in a biexponential manner with a half-life of 2–3 hours during the initial phase and 15–60 hours during the terminal phase.[64] This biexponential decline accounts for the relatively short analgesic action and the tendency for drug accumulation with repeated dosing. A reduction in dose and interval frequency is often needed during the first few days of treatment to prevent side effects from overdosage.[65] The rare patient allergic to morphine and intolerant fentanyl might benefit from methadone because of its different chemical structure. Furthermore, as methadone is cleared almost exclusively by the liver, it can be a useful medication in patients with renal failure.[66]

Meperidine, a synthetic phenylpiperidine derivative mu agonist with anticholinergic properties, is the most commonly prescribed analgesic for acute pain and is widely used for chronic pain. The reasons for this enthusiasm are unclear and irrational. Although in animal models meperidine causes less biliary spasm than morphine,[53] this property has not been shown to be clinically advantageous. The CNS excitatory effects that appear after chronic use, particularly in the elderly and in patients with renal insufficiency, are well substantiated and the accumulation of its metabolite normeperidine causes multifocal myoclonus and grand mal seizures[67,68] that are not reversed by naloxone. The half-life of meperidine is 3 hours. Short-term treatment with meperidine has been associated with mild negative alterations in various elements of mood.[68] Severe respiratory depression or excitation, delirium, hyperpyrexia, and convulsions can occur when meperidine is administered to patients also receiving monoamine oxidase (MAO) inhibitors. The equianalgesic dose to 10 mg of parenteral morphine is 75–100 mg. The oral/parenteral ratio is 1:4. Its use by either route is rarely if ever justified.

## Principles of Dosing and Delivery Methods

Onset, peak, and duration of analgesia vary with the drug, route of administration, and individual patient. The recognition of this variability allows the appropriate choice of drug, route, and scheduling. The elderly exhibit a more pronounced pharmacologic effect after any weight-adjusted opioid dose. The analgesia is more intense, but the cognitive and respiratory effects and perhaps constipation are more severe. This enhanced effect is likely due to a lesser volume of distribution (approximately half that of younger patients), decreased clearance, and diminished target organ reserve (CNS, pulmonary function, and bowel function). Age is the single most important predictor of initial opioid dose requirements for postoperative pain.[69] The following formula, based on a review of records of more than 1000 adults between age 20 and 70 years, provides a rough estimate of the appropriate starting dose for adult patients (with the exception of the old–old).[69]

Average first 24-hour morphine (mg) requirement for patients over 20 years of age = 100 − age

Other factors that influence opioid effects, but to a lesser degree than that of age, are body weight, severity of pain, abnormal renal function, nausea/vomiting, and cardiopulmonary insufficiency. After the initial dose determination, drugs are titrated based on the analgesic effect.

For patients with severe acute pain, such as postoperative pain, parenteral morphine is the opioid of choice. When morphine is not well tolerated, other useful agents are hydromorphone and fentanyl. Opioids should be titrated until one of two endpoints is reached: adequate analgesia or the development of intolerable side effects. Dose titration can be best accomplished with the use of an intravenous pump with a device for self-administration of medication every few minutes [patient-controlled analgesia (PCA)].

### *PCA and Intravenous Infusions*

Patient-controlled analgesia is a safe, effective modality for delivery of opioids for pain that is expected to resolve (e.g., postoperative pain). The patient self-delivers fixed doses of an opioid by pressing a button. An overdose is infrequent because the patient must be alert to press the button and there is a lock-out time between delivered doses during which pressing the button does not result in delivery of medication. The usual PCA starting doses for the average adult are shown in Table 12.2. All of these agents should be given at 10- to 15-minute intervals (lock-out time on the PCA pump). Even while PCA is in effect, continuous infusion of a low dose of opioid can be given at night (e.g., morphine 0.5 mg/hr) to avoid frequent awakenings because of pain, especially for the first 2–3 nights after surgery. PCA has been compared to the more traditional "as-needed" administration of intramuscular opioids in a randomized trial involving elderly men, and PCA was found to result in better analgesia, fewer complications, less sedation, and higher patient satisfaction than intramuscular opioids.[70]

For patients unable to operate PCA or in situations where PCA is not available, a continuous opioid infusion (e.g., morphine 0.5–1.0 mg/hr or hydromorphone 0.10–0.25 mg/hr) should be started and the patient observed for excessive sedation (reduce dose) or behavioral cues of pain (increase dose). Frequent assessments focusing on face and body language that may indicate pain are essential, particularly during the first 24 hours following surgery.

TABLE 12.2. Starting Dose Ranges for Opioid Intravenous Infusions, PCA, and Epidural Infusions

| |
|---|
| **Intravenous infusions (hourly)** |
| Morphine 0.5–1.0 mg |
| Hydromorphone 0.10–0.25 mg |
| Fentanyl 5–20 μg |
| **Intravenous PCA (lock-out time 15 minutes)** |
| Morphine 0.5–1.0 mg |
| Hydromorphone 0.10–0.25 mg |
| Fentanyl 5–20 μg |
| **Dose range for epidural opioid infusions (3–10 ml/hr)** |
| Fentanyl 3–10 mg/ml |
| Sufentanil 1–3 mg/ml |
| Bupivacaine 0.05–0.25% |

Use lower doses for older patients, low body weight, low pain score, abnormal renal function, presence of nausea/vomiting, or cardiopulmonary insufficiency.

The ranges are for starting doses, after which the drugs are titrated based on the analgesic effect.

Higher concentrations of bupivacaine are associated with orthostatic hypotension.

When venous access is problematic the subcutaneous route can be used. The infraclavicular area is generally the best site when a continuous infusion, PCA, or both are used. A 27-gauge butterfly needle is well tolerated and can be maintained for 3–5 days, after which the site must be rotated. When intermittent dosing is required, an insulin syringe is used to minimize trauma. Doses for subcutaneous administration are equal to intravenous doses, and hydromorphone is the agent of choice because of its high potency and lipid solubility. It is best to avoid the intramuscular route because of erratic absorption and pain from the injection.

Initial opioid doses are much higher for patients on chronic opioid therapy. For these patients the presurgical opioid dose must be converted to a continuous infusion, and the as-needed PCA dose should be set equal to the hourly infusion dose. When converting oral opioids to parenteral opioids refer to an opioid conversion chart (Table 12.1). A patient receiving 180 mg of oral morphine every 24 hours prior to surgery during the postoperative phase, for example, should be started on 60 mg of morphine intravenously in 24 hours (2.5 mg/hr) and a PCA dose of 2.5 mg every 15 minutes. If the pain is severe, the continuous infusion rate should be increased. Patients on chronic opioid therapy have almost always developed tolerance to the respiratory suppressant and cognitive side effects of opioids, and so it is rare for these patients to develop these symptoms, even after receiving doses substantially higher than their baseline.

### *Intraspinal Administration*

Discovery of opioid receptors in the spinal cord provided a rationale for the administration of opioids into the epidural and subarachnoid spaces for the treatment of pain.[31,71] Reports have documented the efficacy and safety of this approach in a variety of patient populations.[32] The subarachnoid route is useful intraoperatively and for the management of chronic pain but is not recommended for treatment of acute pain. For postoperative pain and acute pain in general, the epidural route is highly effective, especially if a combination of opioid plus local anesthetic is used.[72] When epidural analgesia was compared to parenteral opioid anesthesia in a randomized study of high risk surgical patients, epidural anesthesia was associated with significantly less postsurgical mortality and morbidity.[72] The epidural route is used for continuous infusion with or without PCA.

When choosing the opioid for epidural infusion, it is important to consider the lipid solubility of the drug. Lipid-soluble drugs (fentanyl, sufentanil) are absorbed rapidly, resulting in a fast onset of analgesia. Additionally, lipid-soluble agents concentrate at the spinal level where the tip of the epidural catheter is positioned. Thus, the tip of the catheter should be positioned, if possible, at the segmental level of the surgery. Hydrophilic drugs (e.g., morphine) have a slower absorption rate and, upon entering the cerebrospinal fluid (CSF), have more rostral distribution. Morphine causes more sedation and respiratory depression than fentanyl because of its ability to reach brain stem centers.

Various combinations of opioid and local anesthetic can be used to meet the needs of individual patients. Local anesthetic side effects include orthostatic hypotension, numbness/weakness, and urinary retention. Opioid side effects include sedation, urinary retention, and pruritus. The local anesthetic/opioid ratio is adjusted based on the type and severity of side effects that develop. Complications of epidural infusions include inadvertent subarachnoid puncture with postdural puncture headache (generally benign and self-limiting), epidural hematoma, and epidural abscess. Side effects and complications are minimal if the catheters are inserted and monitored by those experienced with the technique.

For frail, elderly patients undergoing painful procedures (thoracotomy, extensive abdominal and pelvic surgery) and particularly for those with cognitive impairment, the epidural route is probably the best option for pain management because of its better analgesic efficacy/side effect profile (sedation/delirium, constipation, and postoperative complications). Concomitant use of the epidural and parenteral routes is not recommended because (1) it makes titration of drugs overly complicated, and (2) it becomes difficult to determine the origin of side effects if they develop. It is generally not advisable to maintain an epidural catheter for more than 8 days even if the site of insertion is without evidence of inflammation or infection. If the epidural route is still needed, the catheter can be replaced with a new one at the segmental level above or below the insertion of the old catheter.

### *Oral Administration*

Once pain is controlled and bowel function restored, analgesics should be changed to the oral route. Depending on individual variability and the type of surgery, this transition should occur 3–8 days after the surgery. Occasionally patients require parenteral or epidural opioids for a more prolonged period, usually because of intervening complications. Typically, patients require oral opioids for 5–10 days after parenteral or epidural opioids are discontinued. A certain percentage of patients, especially after more painful surgeries, require oral opioids for 2 weeks or longer. Oral analgesics such as oxycodone or codeine are appropriate choices for a patient with mild to moderate pain.[73] Fixed combinations with nonopioid analgesics can be useful, but they sometimes limit the careful individualized titration that is the basis of therapeutic success. The oral transmucosal route may prove effective for rescue doses, but absorption is probably inadequate for more sustained relief. This latter statement also holds for the rectal route, which, additionally, is often uncomfortable for the patient and the caregiver.

So long as the pain is continuous, the opioid should be administered regularly, including waking the patient from sleep at intervals based on the duration of analgesia for the given drug.[74] This approach keeps the patient's pain at tolerable levels and often results in a reduction in the total amount of medication taken during a 24-hour period. When the pain is present only during particular activities (e.g., physical therapy) or at particular times of the day, the opioid should be administered on an as-needed basis. It must be remembered that it takes approximately 1 hour to reach peak serum levels after oral administration.

### *Regional and Local Blockade*

The most useful form of blockade for treatment of postoperative pain is administration of epidural local anesthetic, usually combined with a lipophilic opioid. For the blockade to be effective the tip of the catheter should be at or above the segmental level of the surgical incision. Bupivacaine 0.1% is usually adequate to provide significant pain relief and is complementary to the effect of the opioid. Higher concentrations (0.25%), useful in selected patients, are likely to cause some sensory block and less commonly motor block. When the epidural infusion contains local anesthetic only, additional opioids can be administered systemically.

The intrapleural administration of an infusion of local anesthetic can provide some relief for postthoracotomy pain, but its effectiveness is hampered by the loss of local anesthetic via the chest tube. Intercostal nerve blocks are useful in selected patients (e.g., relief of postthoracotomy pain not responding to epidural or systemic analgesia). Although the effect of the local anesthetic is limited to a few hours, the pain relief sometimes extends for a longer time, especially if a cycle of pain–muscle spasm–more pain is interrupted.

### *Preemptive Analgesia*

Preemptive analgesia is administration of an analgesic agent prior to application of a painful stimulus. The rationale for preemptive analgesia stems from basic science research demonstrating noxious stimuli-induced changes in neural function such as hyperexcitability in the spinal cord.[75] Subsequent studies suggested that analgesia given before the nociceptive stimulus began were more effective than the same dose given after the stimulus.[76] Few randomized controlled trials have explored this question, and of the ones that have, many have lacked adequate statistical power. A systematic review by McQuay[76] summarized the existing literature and examined the value of preemptive nonsteroidal antiinflammatory drugs (NSAIDs), epidural analgesia, nerve blocks, and preemptive opioids. Three studies in oral surgery patients revealed no significant preemptive effect from NSAIDs.[76] All but one of seven studies examining local anesthetic techniques failed to reveal a preemptive effect.[76] With respect to preemptive opioids, data from three studies suggest that opioids may have a preemptive effect resulting in decreased postoperative pain and decreased postoperative analgesic use.[76] Given the limitations of these studies, their lack of inclusion of elderly subjects, and the paucity of data regarding the side effects and complications associated with preemptive analgesia compared to traditional therapy, it is inadvisable at this time to recommend this analgesic technique for geriatric surgical patients.

Table 12.3 summarizes options for postoperative pain management. Table 12.2 notes the appropriate opioid starting doses for the elderly.

TABLE 12.3. Choosing the Best Option for Postoperative Pain Control in the Elderly

| Cognitively intact | Cognitively impaired |
|---|---|
| **More painful procedures (e.g., thoracotomy, complex abdominal/pelvic surgery)** | |
| *Epidural*: lipophilic opioid (e.g., fentanyl) plus local anesthetic as a continuous infusion with or without epidural PCA *or* | *Epidural*: opioid plus local anesthetic as a continuous infusion without PCA *or* |
| *Intravenous*: strong opioid as an intravenous infusion with intravenous PCA | *Intravenous*: strong opioid as a continuous infusion without PCA |
| **Less painful procedures (e.g., lower abdominal surgery, hip/knee replacement)** | |
| *Intravenous*: strong opioid via PCA or given intravenously every 4–6 hours | *Epidural*: opioid plus local anesthetic as a continuous infusion without PCA *or* |
| | *Intravenous*: strong opioid as a continuous infusion without PCA |

When intravenous access is not available and the oral route cannot be used, the subcutaneous route is better than the intramuscular route. When the subcutaneous route is used, the absorption is less erratic with hydromorphone (more lipid-soluble) than with morphine. For intermittent dosing it is best to use an insulin syringe. For continuous infusion a 27-gauge butterfly needle can be used. Postoperative orders for pain medication should be standing rather than PRN. The remarks "hold for excessive sedation" and "patient may refuse" adds a safety valve to the order.

PCA, patient-controlled analgesia.

## Management of Opioid Side Effects

The use of opioid analgesics is complicated in the elderly because of the high prevalence of constipation, cognitive impairment, and polypharmacy seen in this population. Successful management of pain in the elderly requires both a comprehensive knowledge of the side effect profile of opioids and the ability to administer appropriate prophylactic measures and manage side effects if they develop. The most common side effects seen with opioids are constipation, nausea, and sedation. Less common, although still seen with measurable frequency, are delirium (hallucinations, agitation, dysphoria, euphoria), urinary retention, respiratory depression, dry mouth, and the syndrome of inappropriate secretion of antidiuretic hormone. Fortunately, tolerance to most of the side effects—with the exception of constipation—develops rapidly in patients started on opioids.

### *Gastrointestinal Side Effects*

Constipation is universally seen in all patients given opioids and necessitates the use of prophylactic laxatives. In the elderly surgical patient, opioid-precipitated constipation is further exacerbated by patients' limited mobility and limited oral fluid intake. Constipation may present as urinary retention/incontinence, diarrhea (resulting from oozing of liquid stool around an impaction), and delirium. Given its frequency, constipation should always be ruled out in any elderly patient receiving opioids and demonstrating a change in their clinical condition. Untreated and unrecognized constipation can rapidly evolve into fecal impaction resulting in serious, life-threatening complications. Prophylaxis of constipation should begin as soon as the patient is started on an opioid. Appropriate regimens should combine a stool softener (e.g., docusate sodium) with a stimulant laxative (e.g., senna or biscadoyl) with the addition of a hyperosmotic agent (e.g., milk of magnesia, lactulose, sorbitol) or tap water enemas for resistant constipation. Patients who cannot yet take oral medications can be managed with biscadoyl suppositories or enemas.

Postoperative nausea and vomiting occurs in approximately 20–50% of patients.[77] The etiology of this complication is multifactorial but appears to be related to anesthetic agents, preoperative anxiety, type of surgery, pain, and use of opioids.[77] Standard antiemetic agents are typically effective and include metoclopramide, perchlorperazine, haloperidol, hydroxyzine, and ondansetron. The anticholinergic and extrapyramidal side effects of the phenothiazine derivatives may limit their use in the elderly; ondansetron, although more expensive, may be better tolerated. Antiemetics should be administered on a regular basis, rather than as-needed dosing, if nausea or vomiting develops. Some patients' symptoms may respond to a change in the opioid agent itself (e.g., substituting oxycodone for codeine) or a change to a nonopioid analgesic agent for cases of mild pain.

### *Urinary Tract Side Effects*

The anticholinergic properties of opioids can result in urinary retention, particularly in patients with coexisting fecal impaction or prostatic hypertrophy, or as a result of a drug interaction with other medications with anticholinergic properties. Urinary retention is more common in patients receiving spinal opioids. Phenoxybenzamine has been shown to be useful for ameliorating opioid-induced urinary retention, although the orthostatic hypotension associated with it mandates caution when using it in the elderly.

### *CNS Side Effects*

Cognitive side effects may prove troublesome in the surgical patient treated with opioids. Sedation is a common early side effect and should be managed by close observation and a reduction in subsequent opioid doses. Opioid antagonists (e.g., naloxone) are not indicated unless sedation is accompanied by respiratory compromise. For patients in whom adequate analgesia cannot be obtained without troublesome sedation, small doses of psychostimulants (e.g., 2.5 mg methamphetamine) may be utilized if it is not contraindicated by other medical conditions. Agitation, hallucinations, and dysphoria may also be seen with the administration of opioids, particularly those with agonist–antagonist properties. As with all cases of delirium, other contributing factors should first be ruled out (e.g., infection, metabolic disturbances, anemia, hypoxia). If no other contributing factors can be identified, the delirium can be managed by reducing the opioid dose or increasing the dosing frequency (if analgesia is adequate) or, if analgesia is inadequate, by switching to a different opioid or administering a low dose of a major tranquilizer (e.g., haloperidol or resperidol). It is important to recognize that pain itself may result in delirium, and that in some patients increasing the dose of analgesia may be the most appropriate symptomatic intervention. Again, as with all cases of pain management, therapy should be guided by an assessment of the patient's pain and analgesic requirements.

### *Respiratory Side Effects*

Respiratory suppression is the most feared and serious side effect of opioid therapy. Factors predisposing patients to respiratory suppression include age, medication dose, frequency of administration, and the concurrent administration of other centrally acting medications.[78] Respiratory suppression is universally preceded by sedation, and the presence of respiratory compromise in the absence of sedation should prompt a search for another inciting factor (e.g., pulmonary embolus, myocardial ischemia, infection). Conversely, patients who experience sedation should be monitored carefully for respiratory compromise. Respiratory suppression typically occurs when peak serum levels are reached. Although peak serum levels develop fairly early following oral or parenteral administration, peak levels may be significantly delayed following spinal administration.[79] Although the incidence of respiratory suppression following spinal opioid administration is reportedly low, the potential for this complication mandates that patients who receive spinal opioids be monitored for extended periods.[78] Patients who develop respiratory depression can be treated with naloxone. As naloxone typically reverses all opioid effects, including analgesia, it should be titrated slowly to avoid the recurrence of pain and the precipitation of opioid withdrawal in patients who have been receiving prolonged opioid therapy. It is important to remember that the half-life of naloxone is typically shorter than that of most opioids, particularly intraspinal opioids; and repetitive doses of naloxone may be required to prevent the recurrence of respiratory compromise.

## Addiction, Tolerance, and Dependence

Concerns and misunderstanding surrounding the terms of addiction (psychological dependence), tolerance, and dependence contribute significantly to the inadequate management of pain. Physical dependence is a pharmacologic property of a medication and is defined as the development of a withdrawal state following abrupt discontinuation of the drug or following administration of an antagonist. This problem usually is not of clinical significance in patients receiving short courses of opioid therapy as is typically the case in the postoperative patient. For patients receiving prolonged courses, dependence should not be problematic if patients are tapered off the opioid and are warned not to discontinue the medication abruptly.

Tolerance is also a pharmacologic property of the medication and may be defined as the requirement for increased doses of a medication over time to maintain the same effect. Clinical tolerance develops at varying rates to the different properties of opioids. For example, tolerance develops fairly rapidly to the respiratory suppression and sedation associated with opioids (typically within days) but appears not to develop at all with respect to constipation.[74] Analgesic tolerance is rarely an issue that should concern the physician caring for the postoperative patient for several reasons. First, and most importantly, data from cancer patients and other patients suffering from chronic pain suggest that patients maintain adequate analgesia on relatively stable opioid doses and that patients who develop pain on stable doses should be assessed first for worsening pathology rather than tolerance.[80,81] Second, during the postoperative period, nociceptive stimuli typically decrease as healing occurs such that patients' analgesic requirements diminish. If tolerance does develop in the postoperative patient, it should be addressed by simply increasing the analgesic dose or dosing frequency. This usually restores analgesia without increasing the side effects. Tolerance should not be managed by limiting the amount of analgesia the patient receives.

Tolerance and physical dependence can become clinically relevant issues in the elderly cancer patient who is on chronic opioid therapy and subsequently undergoes surgery. Such patients may develop symptoms of acute opioid withdrawal if they are not maintained on their regular amount of opioid (i.e., if opioids are stopped inadvertently prior to surgery or re-started postoperatively at a lower dose). Similarly, administration of a mixed opioid agonist–antagonist (e.g., butorphanol, pentazocine) or naloxone (i.e., for the reversal of opioid-induced respiratory suppression) during the postoperative period likely will precipitate a withdrawal state in these patients. Mixed agonist–antagonists should be avoided in all patients who have been receiving prior opioid therapy and indeed should probably be avoided in all elderly postoperative patients for reasons stated earlier. Finally, it should be noted that patients on chronic opioid therapy may require doses considerably higher than those typically used postoperatively to control their superimposed surgical pain.

The fear of addiction or psychological dependence is one of the major barriers to the appropriate management of pain in the United States. Psychological dependence is the development of drug-seeking behavior that persists despite harm to the patient or others. Such drug-seeking behavior includes the hoarding of medication, use of medication for purposes other than control of pain, and obtaining opioids from multiple sources. It is important to distinguish true psychological dependence from "pseudoaddiction,"[82] which can develop in patients who are undermedicated for their level of pain. Pseudoaddiction is drug-seeking behavior motivated by a need to obtain enough analgesia to control pain. When pain is appropriately managed and adequate analgesia provided, the behavior disappears. Although further research is needed, it appears that the incidence of psychological addiction in patients without a history of substance abuse and treated with opioids for control of pain is rare.[37] Fear of addiction should never limit the use of opioids for pain control in the elderly patient who has no history of substance abuse.

## Nonpharmacologic Approaches to Pain Management

Several nonpharmacological measures may be useful as adjunctive therapy to improve pain management in the surgical patient. Transcutaneous electrical nerve stimulation (TENS) had been advocated as a means of reducing opioid dose requirements. The rationale for the use of TENS stems from the belief that by increasing input through large-diameter myelinated peripheral nerve fibers one inhibits the transmission of nociceptive impulses in the dorsal horn of the spinal cord.[83] There are no well-controlled trials involving TENS and placebo, and the studies that exist suggest a modest benefit at best. TENS may be useful for stimulating peristalsis following surgery[84,85] in addition to its analgesic effects.

Acupuncture is insertion of hair-thin needles into specific points of the body to prevent or treat illness. Acupuncture has been used for centuries for the treatment of pain in traditional Chinese medicine, although few randomized placebo (sham acupuncture)-controlled trials involving this technique have been performed. Acupuncture appears to be effective for a variety of pain syndromes [86–89] including postoperative pain.[90] It is hypothesized that the analgesic effects of acupuncture result from its stimulation of natural endorphins.

Psychological techniques including relaxation therapy, distraction techniques, guided imagery, and hypnosis may also be beneficial in reducing pain. Hypnosis, with and without imagery, has been shown to improve chronic pain syndromes,[91] cancer pain,[92,93] pain associated with procedures,[94] and postoperative pain.[95] Three randomized controlled trials, one of which involved elderly hip fracture patients, have demonstrated that preoperative training in relaxation techniques can significantly reduce postoperative pain and analgesic requirements.[96–98] Although studies in the elderly are lacking, age should not be seen as a barrier to the use of these techniques, and the cognitively intact older adult should be strongly considered for psychological interventions.[78] Whenever possible, training in these techniques should occur prior to surgery. Finally, several studies[99,100] have demonstrated that informing patients about the nature and character of postoperative pain and providing appropriate assurances that pain can be effectively relieved are often enough to reduce postoperative pain and analgesic requirements.

## Conclusions

Good pain management in the elderly surgical patient is a complex, challenging undertaking of critical importance. Ensuring adequate analgesia requires an understanding of age-related changes in pharmacokinetics and pharmacodynamics, pain physiology, the appropriate use of analgesic agents, and knowledge of these agents' limitations and side effects. Unfortunately, few studies have focused on the assessment and treatment of pain in elderly individuals, and guidelines for analgesic therapy are often based on the experiences of young and middle-aged adults. Further research involving pain in the elderly is critically needed given the evolving changes in population demographics (persons over 65 represent the most rapidly growing segment of the U.S. population) and the increasing rates of surgery in this population. Until such research is completed, clinicians must continue to interpret the available data in the context of their knowledge of age-related physiologic changes, medication effects, side effect profiles, and clinical experience. This approach results in appropriate pain management for most elderly surgical patients.

## References


1. Lynch E, Lazor M, Gellis J, Orav J, Goldman L, Marcantonio E. Patient experience of pain after elective noncardiac surgery. Anesth Analg 1997;85:117–123.
2. Oates J, Snowdon S, Jayson D. Failure of pain relief after surgery. Anaesthesia 1994;49:775–758.
3. Ferrell B. Pain management in elderly people. J Am Geriatr Soc 1991;39:64–73.
4. World Health Organization (WHO). Cancer Pain Relief. Geneva: WHO, 1986.
5. Harkins S. Pain perceptions in the old. Clin Geriatr Med 1996;12:435–459.
6. IASP Subcommittee on Taxonomy Pain Terms. A list with definitions and notes on usage. Pain 1979;6:249.
7. Portenoy R, Foley K, Inturrisi C. The nature of opioid responsiveness and its implications for neuropathic pain: new hypotheses derived from studies of opioid infusions. Pain 1990;43:273–286.
8. Ferrell B, Ferrell B, Osterweil D. Pain in the nursing home. J Am Geriatr Soc 1990;38:409–414.
9. Roy R, Michael T. Survey of chronic pain in an elderly population. Can Fam Physician 1986;32:513.
10. Camp L. A comparison of nurses' record assessment of pain with perceptions of pain as described by cancer patients. Cancer Nurs 1988;11:237–243.
11. Teske K, Daut R, Cleeland C. Relationships between nurses' observations and patients' self-reports of pain. Pain 1983;16:289–296.
12. Leventhal E, Prohaska T. Age, symptom interpretation and health behavior. J Am Geriatr Soc 1986;34:185–191.
13. Greenlee K. Pain and analgesia: considerations for the elderly in critical care. AACN Clin Issues Crit Care Nurs 1991;2:720–728.
14. Clinton P, Eland J. Pain. In: Maas M, Buckwalter K (eds) Nursing Diagnoses and Intervention for the Elderly. Reading, MA: Addison-Wesley, 1990:348–368.
15. Melzack R. The McGill Pain Questionnaire: major properties and scoring methods. Pain 1975;1:277–299.
16. Melzack R. The short-form McGill Pain Questionnaire. Pain 1987;30:191–197.
17. Daut R, Cleeland C, Flanery R. The development of the Wisconsin Brief Pain Questionnaire to assess pain in cancer and other diseases. Pain 1983;17:197–210.
18. Fishman B, Pasternak S, Wallenstein S, Houde R, Holland J, Foley K. The Memorial pain assessment card: a valid instrument for the evaluation of cancer pain. Cancer 1987;60:1151–1158.
19. Ferrell B, Ferrell B, Rivera L. Pain in cognitively impaired nursing home patients. J Pain Symptom Manage 1995; 10:591–598.
20. Sengstaken E, King S. The problem of pain and its detection among geriatric nursing home residents. J Am Geriatr Soc 1993;41:541–544.
21. Parmelee P. Pain in cognitively impaired older persons. Clin Geriatr Med 1996;12:473–487.
22. Mateo O, Da K. A pilot study to assess the relationship between behavioral manifestations and self-report of pain in post-anesthesia care unit patients. J Post Anesth Nurs 1992;7:15–21.
23. Le Resche L, Dworkin S. Facial expressions of pain and emotions in chronic TMD patients. Pain 1988;35:71–78.
24. Ferreira S. Prostaglandins: peripheral and central analgesia. In: Bonica J, Lindblom U, Iggo A (eds) Advances in Pain Research and Therapy. New York: Raven Press, 1983.
25. Jacox A, Carr DB, Payne R, et al. Management of Cancer Pain. Clinical Practice Guideline No. 9. AHCPR Publication No. 94-0592. Rockville, MD: Agency for Health Care Policy and Research, U.S. Department of Health and Human Services, Public Health Service; 1994:257.
26. Etches RC, Warriner CB, Badner N, et al. Continuous intravenous administration of ketorolac reduces pain and morphine consumption after total hip or knee arthroplasty. Anesth Analg 1995;81:1175–1180.
27. Stouten E, Armbuster S, Houmes R, et al. Comparison of ketorolac and morphine for post operative pain after major surgery. Acta Anesthesiol Scand 1992;336:716–721.
28. Strom BL, Berlin JA, Kinman JL, et al. Parenteral ketorolac and risk of gastrointestinal and operative site bleeding: a postmarketing surveillance study. JAMA 1996;275:376–382.

29. Camu F, Lauwers MH, Vandersberghe C. Side effects of NSAIDs and dosing recommendations for ketorolac. Acta Anaesthesiol Belg 1996;47:143–149.
30. Maliekal J, Elboim CM. Gastrointestinal complications associated with intramuscular ketorolac tromethamine therapy in the elderly. Ann Pharmacother 1995;29:698–701.
31. Reynolds D. Surgery in the rat during electrical anaesthesia induced by focal brain stimulation. Science 1969;164: 444–445.
32. Akil H, Mayer D, Liebeskind J. Antagonism of stimulation-produced analgesia by naloxone, a narcotic antagonist. Science 1974;191:961–962.
33. Evans C, Hammond D, Frederickson R. The opioid peptides. In: Pasternak G (ed) The Opiate Receptors. Clifton Park, NJ: Humana Press, 1988:23–71.
34. Ling G, Spiegel K, Nishimura S, Pasternak G. Dissociation of morphine's analgesic and respiratory depressant actions. Eur J Pharmacol 1983;86:487–488.
35. Ling G, Spiegel K, Nishimura S, Pasternak G. Separation of opioid analgesia from respiratory depresion: evidence for different receptor mechanisms. J Pharmacol Exp Ther 1985;232:149–155.
36. Heiman JS, Williams CL, Burks TF, Mosberg HI, Porreca F. Dissociation of opioid antinociception and central gastrointestinal propulsion in the mouse: studies with naloxazine. J Pharmacol Exp Ther 1988:238.
37. Fishbain D, Rosomoff H, Rosomoff R. Drug abuse, dependence, and addiction in chronic pain patients. Clin J Pain 1992;8:77–85.
38. Beaver W, Wallenstein S, Rogers A, Houde W. Analgesic studies of codeine and oxycodone in patients with cancer. 1. Comparison of oral with intramuscular codeine and oral with intramuscular oxycodone. J Pharmacol Exp Ther 1978;207:92–100.
39. Beaver W, Wallenstein S, Rogers A, Houde R. Analgesic studies of codeine and oxycodone in patients with cancer. 2. Comparison of intramuscular oxycodone with intramuscular morphine and codeine. J Pharmcol Exp Ther 1978;207:101–108.
40. Kantor T, Hopper M, Laska E. Adverse effects of commonly ordered oral narcotics. J Clin Pharmacol 1981;21: 1–8.
41. Kalso E, Vanio A. Hallucinations during morphine but not during oxycodone treatment. Lancet 1987;2:912.
42. Chan G, Matzke G. Effects of renal insufficiency on the pharmacokinetics and pharmacodynamics of opioid analgesics. Drug Intell Clin Pharm 1987;21:773–783.
43. Sunshine A. New clinical experience with tramadol. Drugs 1994;47:8–18.
44. Moore R, McQuay H. Single-patient data meta-analysis of 3453 postoperative patients: oral tramadol versus placebo, codeine, and combination analgesics. Pain 1997;69:287–294.
45. Sawe J, Svensson J, Rane A. Morphine metabolism in cancer patients on increasing oral doses—no evidence of autoinduction or dose-dependence. Br J Clin Pharmacol 1983;16:85–93.
46. Pasternak G, Bodnare R, Clarke J, Inturrisi C. Morphine-6-glucuronide, a potent mu agonist. Life Sci 1987;41:2845–2849.
47. Portenoy R, Khan E, Layman M, et al. Chronic morphine therapy for cancer pain: plasma and cerebrospinal fluid morphine and morphine-6-glucuronide concentrations. Neurology 1991;41:1457–1461.
48. Houde R, Wallenstein S, Beaver W. Evaluation of analgesics in patients with cancer pain. In: Lasagna L (ed) International Encyclopedia of Pharmacology and Therapeutics. New York: Pergamon, 1966:59–67.
49. Twycross R. The use of narcotic analgesics in terminal illness. J Med Ethics 1975;1:10–17.
50. Labella F, Pinsky C, Havlicek V. Morphine derivatives with diminished opiate receptor potency show enhanced central excitatory activity. Brain Res 1979;174:263–271.
51. Morley J, Miles J, Wells J, Bowsher D. Paradoxical pain. Lancet 1992;340:1045.
52. Smith M, Watt J, Cramond T. Morphine-3-glucuronide: a potent antagonist of morphine analgesia. Life Sci 1990;47: 579–585.
53. Jaffe J, Martin W. Opioid analgesics and antagonists. In: Gillman A, Rall T, Nies A, Taylor P (eds) Goodman and Gilman's The Pharmacological Basis of Therapeutics. New York: Pergamon, 1990:485–521.
54. Kaiko R. Controlled-release oral morphine for cancer-related pain: the European and North American experiences. Adv Pain Res Ther 1990;14:171–189.
55. Osborne R, Joel S, Slevin M. Morphine intoxication in renal failure: the role of morphine-6-glucuronide. BMJ 1986;292: 1548–1549.
56. Houde R. Clinical analgesic studies of hydromorphone. Adv Pain Res Ther 1986;8:129–135.
57. Babul N, Darke A, Hagen N. Hydromorphone metabolite accumulation in renal failure. J Pain Symptom Manage 1995;10:184–186.
58. Moulin D, Kreeft J, Murray-Parsons N, Bouquillon A. Comparison of continuous subcutaneous and intravenous hydromorphone infusions for management of cancer pain. Lancet 1991;337:465–468.
59. Fine P, Marcus M, Just De Boer A, Van der Oord B. An open label of oral transmucosal fentanyl citrate (OTFC) for the treatment of breakthrough cancer pain. Pain 1991;45:149–153.
60. Pasternak G. Pharmacological mechanisms of opioid analgesia. Clin Neuropharmacol 1993;16:1–18.
61. Houde E, Wallenstein S, Beaver W. Clinical measurement of pain. In: Analgesics. San Diego: Academic, 1975:75–122.
62. Faisinger R, Schoeller T, Bruera E. Methadone in the management of chronic pain: a review. Pain 1993;52:137–147.
63. Beaver W, Wallenstein S, Houde R, Rogers A. A clinical comparison of the analgesic effects of methadone and morphine administered intramuscularly and of oral and parenterally administered methadone. Clin Pharmacol Ther 1967;8:415–426.
64. Sawe J. High dose morphine and methadone in cancer patients: clinical pharmacokinetic consideration of oral treatment. Clin Pharmacol 1986;11:87–106.
65. Morley J, Watt J, Wells J, Miles J, Finnegan M, Leng J. Methadone in pain uncontrolled by morphine. Lancet 1993;342:1243.
66. Kreek M, Schecter A, Gutjahr C, Hecht M. Methadone use in patients with chronic renal disease. Drug Alchohol Depend 1980;5:195–205.

67. Szeto H, Inturrisi C, Houde R, et al. Accumulation of normeperidine, an active metabolite of meperidine, in patients with renal failure and cancer. Ann Intern Med 1977;86:738–740.
68. Kaiko R, Foley K, Grabinski P, et al. Central nervous system excitatory effects of meperidine in cancer patients. Ann Neurol 1983;13:180–185.
69. Macintyre P, Jarvis D. Age is the best predictor of postoperative morphine requirements. Pain 1995;64:357–364.
70. Egbert A, Parks L, Short L, Burnett M. Randomized trial of postoperative patient-controlled analgesia vs intramuscular narcotics in frail elderly men. Arch Intern Med 1990;150:1897–1903.
71. Stjernsward J, Teoh N. Current status of the Global Cancer Control Program of the World Health Organization. Pain Symptom Manage 1993;8:340–347.
72. Yeager M, Glass D, Neff R, Brinck-Johnsen T. Epidural anesthesia and analgesia in high risk surgical patients. Anesthesiology 1987;66:729–736.
73. World Health Organization. Cancer Pain Relief and Palliative Care. Geneva: WHO, 1990.
74. Foley KM. The treatment of cancer pain. N Engl J Med 1985;313:84–95.
75. Woolf C. Evidence for a central component of post-injury hypersensitivity. Nature 1983;306:686–688.
76. McQuay H. Pre-emptive analgesia: a systematic review of clinical studies. Ann Med 1995;27:249–256.
77. Quinn A, Brown J, Wallace P, Asbury A. Studies in postoperative sequelae: nausea and vomiting—still a problem. Anaesthesia 1993;49:62–65.
78. Yang K, Portenoy R. Pain management in the geriatric surgical patient. In: Katlic M (ed) Geriatric Surgery. Baltimore: Urban & Schwarzenberg, 1990:329–348.
79. Knill R, Clement J, Thompson W. Epidural morphine causes delayed and prolonged respiratory depression. Can Anaesth Soc J 1981;28:537.
80. Kanner R, Foley K. Patterns of narcotic use in a cancer pain clinic. Ann NY Acad Sci 1981;362:161–172.
81. Brescia F, Portenoy R, Ryan M, Krasnoff L, Gray G. Pain, opioid use, and survival in hospitalized patients with advanced cancer. J Clin Oncol 1992;10:149–155.
82. Weissman D, Haddox J. Opioid pseudoaddiction: an iatrogenic syndrome. Pain 1989;36:363–366.
83. Melzack R, Wall P. Pain mechanism: a new theory. Science 1965;150:971–979.
84. Hymes A, Yonegiro E, Raab D, Nelson G, Printy A. Electrical stimulation for the treatment and prevention of ileus and atelectasis. Surg Forum 1974;25:222–224.
85. Richardson R, Cerullo L. Transabdominal neurostimulation in the treatment of neurogenic ileus. Allp Neurophysiol 1979;42:375–382.
86. Coan R, Wong G, Coan P. The acupuncture treatment of low back pain: a randomized controlled trial. Am J Chin Med 1980;8:181–189.
87. Coan R, Wong G, Coan P. The acupuncture treatment of neck pain: a randomized controlled study. Am J Chin Med 1980;9:362–332.
88. Vincent C. A controlled trial of the treatment of migraine by acupuncture. Clin J Pain 1990;1989:305–312.
89. Helms J. Acupuncture for the management of primary dysmenorrhea. Obstet Gynecol 1987;69:51–56.
90. Christensen P, Noreng M, Andersen P, Nielsen J. Electroacupuncture and postoperative pain. Br J Anaesth 1989; 62:258–262.
91. Haanen H, Hoenderdos H, van Romunde L, et al. Controlled trial of hypnotherapy in the treatment of refractory fibromyalgia. J Rheumatol 1991;18:72–75.
92. Spiegel D, Bloom J. Group therapy and hypnosis reduce metastatic breast carcinoma pain. Psychosom Med 1982;45: 333–339.
93. Syrjala K, Cummings C, Donaldson G. Hypnosis or cognitive behavioral training for the reduction of pain and nausea during cancer treatment: a controlled clinical trial. Pain 1992;48:137–146.
94. Zeltzer L, LeBaron S. Hypnosis and non-hypnotic techniques for reduction of pain and anxiety in children and adolescents with cancer. Behav Pediatr 1982;101:1032–1035.
95. Brown D. Transurethral resection under self-hypnosis. Am J Clin Hypn 1973;16:132–134.
96. Lawlis G, Selby D, Hinnant D, McCoy C. Reduction of postoperative pain parameters by presurgical relaxation instructions for spinal pain patients. Spine 1985;10:649–651.
97. Ceccio C. Postoperative pain relief through relaxation in elderly patients with fractured hips. Orthop Nurs 1984;3:11–19.
98. Flaherty C, Fitzpatrick J. Relaxation technique to increase comfort level of postoperative patients: a preliminary study. Nurs Res 1978;27:352–355.
99. Langer E, Janis I, Wolfer J. Reduction in psychological stress in surgical patients. J Exp Soc Psychol 1975;11:155–165.
100. Weis O, Sriwatanakul K, Weintraub M, Lasagna L. Reduction of anxiety and postoperative analgesic requirements by audiovisual instruction. Lancet 1983;1:43–44.

# 13 Drug Usage in Elderly Persons

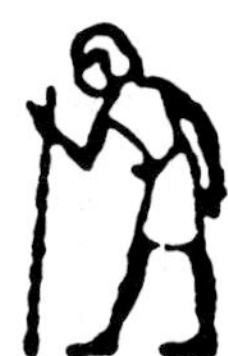

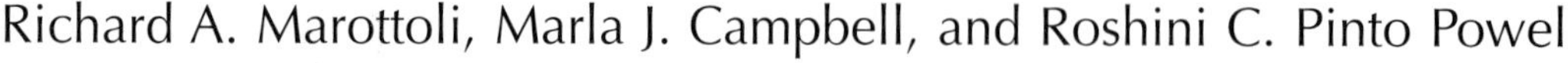

Richard A. Marottoli, Marla J. Campbell, and Roshini C. Pinto Powell

Although elderly persons tend to be more sensitive to the effects and side effects of medications, most drugs are well tolerated if used judiciously. This chapter reviews some of the factors that contribute to this sensitivity, general approaches to prescribing, signs and symptoms to monitor, and highlights of certain drug categories that are commonly used or have substantial potential to cause side effects.

## Biology of Aging

A number of changes occur as we age that can potentially affect the effectiveness of medications and the development of side effects. These changes are reviewed here in general terms to provide a background for the discussion of individual drug classes (Table 13.1).

All organ systems decline in function to some extent with advancing age, but they decline at varying rates, independently of each other. In the absence of disease, these declines are not sufficient to impair daily function, but the reserve capacity of an organ system diminishes. Thus the ability to withstand even a minor insult is decreased, and recovery may be delayed.

On a cellular level, the numbers of cells decrease with advancing age, with a compensatory increase in size. Total body and intracellular water decrease, as does muscle mass, whereas body fat increases.[1,2] These changes have important implications for pharmacokinetics.

Pharmacokinetics can be defined as the delivery of a drug to its site of action. (Pharmacodynamics, which encompasses the drug–receptor interaction and postsynaptic events, is beyond the scope of this chapter and is not discussed.) There are four elements of pharmacokinetics: absorption, distribution, metabolism, and excretion. Some changes occur in the gastric environment, but for the most part absorption is not appreciably changed with aging.[3]

The distribution of drugs is altered by the aging process.[4] Water-soluble drugs tend to have an increased level per unit dose because of the decreased total body and intracellular water described above. Similarly, the volume of distribution for lipid-soluble drugs tends to be higher because of increased fat stores, resulting in prolonged and less predictable half-lives. Another factor that must be considered for protein-bound medications is that in the case of low albumin levels the relative proportion of free or unbound drug may be increased, enhancing the pharmacologic and toxic properties of the drug. Thus it is important to consider drug toxicity if the symptoms are consistent with this situation, even in the setting of a drug level within the therapeutic range. One such example is phenytoin, where what is usually measured is the total drug level.[5] In the setting of low albumin, however, the free drug concentration may be high, resulting in toxicity despite a total level in the therapeutic range. In contrast, the carrier protein $\alpha_1$-acid glycoprotein may increase with age, as it does with illness, so drugs that bind to this protein may have a lower proportion unbound; an example is propranolol.[6] Another caveat with drug levels is that normal ranges are often established on young persons, so it may be worth aiming for the lower end of that range if clinically feasible to minimize the risk of toxicity.

The metabolism of most drugs is handled by the liver. Because liver size and blood flow tend to decrease with age, drugs that depend on extensive first-pass metabolism may have higher levels.[7–10] In addition, drugs metabolized via pathways involving microsomal oxidation are slowed with aging and often have active metabolites.[4,11,12] Consequently, drugs metabolized through these pathways, including benzodiazepines such as diazepam and chlordiazepoxide, tend to have longer and less predictable half-lives. In contrast, metabolism via glucuronide conjugation is slowed little or not all with advancing age, and metabolites tend to be inactive. Thus drugs metabolized through these pathways, including benzodiazepines such as lorazepam, oxazepam, and temazepam, have shorter, more predictable half-lives and are therefore preferred for elderly patients. In addition,

TABLE 13.1. Age-Related Changes Affecting Pharmacokinetics

| Body component or function | Direction of change | Drugs affected by this change | Result of change |
|---|---|---|---|
| Serum albumin | ↓ | Phenytoin, naproxen, valproate, warfarin | Increased free (active) fraction of drug; increased effects |
| $\alpha_1$-Acid glycoprotein | ↑ | Propranolol, antidepressants, lidocaine, methadone, quinidine | Decreased free (active) fraction of drug; decreased effects. |
| Body fat | ↑ | Fat-soluble drugs (e.g., benzodiazepines) | Increased volume of distribution; increased half-life and potential for accumulation |
| Lean muscle mass | ↓ | Digoxin | Decreased volume of distribution; increased concentration; lower loading dose is needed |
| Body water | ↓ | Water-soluble drugs (e.g., lithium) | Decreased volume of distribution; increased concentration and effects |
| Hepatic blood flow | ↓ | High hepatic extraction ratio drugs (e.g., morphine, meperidine, lidocaine, isosorbide) | Decreased first-pass metabolism; increased effects |
| Hepatic metabolism (phase 1: reduction, oxidation, hydroxylation, demethylation) | ↓ | Diazepam, alprazolam, triazolam, theophylline, quinidine, propranolol, phenytoin, imipramine | Decreased metabolism; increased half-life and concentration |
| Renal function | ↓ | Aminoglycosides, digoxin, ciprofloxacin, allopurinol | Decreased clearance; increased effects, toxicity, or both |

metabolism can be affected by diet, smoking, enzyme induction or inhibition, and alcohol intake.[3]

The kidney is the main route of excretion for most drugs. On average, there are declines in glomerular filtration rate and renal blood flow with advancing age, although up to one-third of elderly persons have no substantial changes in renal function.[13,14] Because of decreases in muscle mass and therefore creatine production, serum creatinine levels are not the best measure of renal function; creatinine clearance is preferred. Thus an elderly person with a seemingly normal serum creatinine level may actually have decreased creatinine clearance. This can be measured with a 24-hour urine collection or estimated using the Cockcroft-Gault formula.[15]

$$\frac{[(140-\text{age})\times(\text{lean body weight in kilograms})]}{(72\times\text{serum creatinine})}[\times 0.85 \text{ for women}]$$

The dosage or interval of primarily renally excreted drugs should be adjusted accordingly. It is also helpful to keep in mind that drugs with active metabolites may have prolonged durations of action during renal insufficiency. An example is the tertiary amine tricyclics (amitriptyline, imipramine), which are metabolized to secondary amine tricyclics (nortriptyline and desipramine, respectively). Thus it is preferable to prescribe the metabolites themselves, which are available as medications, if a tricyclic is indicated given their shorter and more predictable half-lives.

## General Prescribing Approaches

With this background in mind, several underlying principles can help minimize the occurrence of medication side effects and maximize compliance with prescribed drug regimens. Although they may seem rudimentary, they are nonetheless helpful to review (Table 13.2).

First, it is important on admission to the hospital and on outpatient visits to obtain a full medication history, ideally having the patient or a family member bring all medications with them. It is important to include over-the-counter, herbal, or alternative medications as well,

TABLE 13.2. Principles of Safe Geriatric Prescribing

1. Take a detailed medication history (including over-the-counter and herbal/alternative preparations).
2. Establish clear, feasible therapeutic endpoints.
3. Know the clinical pharmacology of drugs prescribed; use a few drugs well; balance safety with efficacy.
4. Begin with a low dose of a drug and titrate up to achieve the desired response.
5. Keep the regimen as simple as possible.
6. Review medications regularly and discontinue those no longer needed.
7. Remember that new symptoms (and illness) can be caused by a drug as well as by a new illness.
8. Select the least costly alternative whenever possible.
9. Encourage compliance. Utilize available pharmacy resources for counseling, written information, special packaging, and other reminder devices.

given that many drugs with potential toxicity and interactions are available without a prescription. The clinical pharmacist, if available, is a valuable resource for conducting the medication history/review.[16]

When prescribing medications it is helpful to have a specific target sign or symptom before initiating therapy and use that to gauge effectiveness. When dosing, the maxim "start low, go slow" is applicable to determine how well a patient tolerates the medication. During the course of treatment, the patient should be monitored closely and regularly for effects and side effects. Once the desired effect has been achieved and maintained, or the inciting event has passed, taper and discontinue the medication. Many drugs can be discontinued directly, but others (e.g., benzodiazepines and β-blockers) should be tapered to avoid rebound phenomena. Periodically, monitor the medications and discontinue if there is no clear need to continue. If new symptoms develop, suspect medications as the cause. If they are, change the dose, discontinue entirely, or switch to a medication with a different side effect profile.

In general, it is best to avoid prescribing more than one drug in the same class or with overlapping side effects. For agents used less frequently, such as some psychotropics, it is useful to become familiar with a few drugs in each class, including their side effect profiles and dosing schedules, rather than trying to use the full spectrum of drugs available. For outpatients or those about to be discharged from the hospital, keep medication regimens simple. Many hospitals have clinical pharmacists available for comprehensive medication counseling and to assist in streamlining regimens. If a complicated regimen is necessary, the hospital pharmacist can arrange for the patient's retail pharmacy to dispense the medication in a pill box or to have them blister packed. These approaches may enhance compliance with the regimen.

## Delirium

Although seemingly a deviation from the topic, a discussion of delirium is warranted at this point because it is prevalent, potentially serious, and potentially reversible, and because medications are leading contributors. This point is of particular significance in the hospital and during the perioperative period because a number of factors may contribute to the onset and propagation of delirium, including underlying cognitive impairment, change in environment, co-morbid illnesses, underlying illness prompting hospitalization or surgery, complications of that illness or procedures, anesthesia, the surgery itself, and a variety of medications, many of which are described below. The major issues about delirium focus on looking for and recognizing its appearance and then moving quickly to identify and correct the inciting factors.

Delirium is the acute or subacute development of an alteration in mental state that fluctuates during the course of the day. Standardized assessment instruments such as the Confusion Assessment Method can be helpful for its detection.[17] Risk factors can be thought of as "predisposing factors," making one vulnerable to developing delirium, and "precipitating factors," which directly or indirectly lead to it. Among the predisposing factors are cognitive impairment, visual impairment, severe illness, and renal insufficiency.[18] Precipitating factors include the use of physical restraints, malnutrition, bladder catheterization, iatrogenic events, and a number of medications.[19] Certain medications have been linked to a particular risk of postoperative delirium (e.g., meperidine and benzodiazepines).[20] However, one study noted that the simultaneous addition of three or more medications to a drug regimen in the hospital was a significant contributing factor to delirium, suggesting that the sheer volume of new medications in certain hospitalized patients may be sufficient to overwhelm their reserve capacity (it should be noted that as the number of prescribed medications increased there was a greater likelihood of at least one of the medications being psychoactive).[19]

A number of strategies may be employed to try to decrease the risk of delirium, including attention to underlying illness and complications. The general prescribing principles outlined above may also be helpful along with specific examples detailed below when discussing individual drug categories. Another factor that is particularly problematic in the hospital setting is the scheduling of medications or treatments at night that require patients to be awakened, sometimes repeatedly. Although it may be necessary for acutely or severely ill patients or during the immediate postoperative period, it is helpful to attempt to minimize the occurrence later in the hospital course.

## Antipsychotics

Antipsychotics are used to treat hallucinations, delusions, paranoia, and extreme agitation or physical violence.[21] They tend to not be useful for pacing or wandering; and because of potential serious side effects they should not be used to treat insomnia. It is important to look for delirium as the potential cause of a new-onset behavioral disturbance or thought disorder, so the underlying etiology can be determined and treatment of the primary process initiated.

Once a target sign or symptom is identified to gauge the effectiveness of treatment, the choice of agent largely depends on the desired side effect. For the most part, neuroleptics are essentially equally effective so the choice of agent depends on which side effect profile fits the characteristics of the patient or is best tolerated by the patient. Low potency agents, such as thioridazine and chlorpromazine (starting dose 10 mg/day, maximum daily dose 100 mg), are more likely to produce sedation, orthostatic hypotension, and peripheral anticholinergic effects such as dry mouth, urinary retention, constipation, and increased intraocular pressure in patients with narrow-angle glaucoma. Central anticholinergic effects include delirium with altered mental status and agitation early and seizures and coma in the extreme. Of these two agents, thioridazine is the more widely used, but chlorpromazine has the advantage of having a parenteral (intramuscular) form that can be useful for acute extreme agitation.

High potency agents, such as haloperidol (starting dose 0.5 mg/day, maximum daily dose 2.0 mg), are more likely to produce extrapyramidal side effects but are less likely to cause sedation, orthostasis, and anticholinergic effects than are the low potency agents. A parenteral form is available. Among the extrapyramidal effects are parkinsonian features including tremor, bradykinesia, and masked fascies. Although these symptoms may fade over time, they have in the past also been treated with anticholinergic agents such as benztropine and trihexyphenidyl. Caution should be used with this approach because of the increased potential for delirium with concomitant therapy; a wiser approach might be to decrease the dose or switch to a low potency agent. Akathisia is manifested as motor restlessness, pacing, or disturbed sleep and may be reported as discomfort or anxiety. A danger is that these features may be misinterpreted as increasing psychosis, with the neuroleptic dose then being increased, resulting in worsened symptoms. As a result, it is often better to decrease the dose as an initial response to such symptoms to see if they are alleviated.

Tardive dyskinesia is one of the potentially more serious side effects of neuroleptic use and one of the reasons their use should be limited to the indications described above. Tardive dyskinesia starts as fine movement of the tongue, a facial tic, or lip smacking but may progress in the extreme to affect speech, eating, and breathing. Furthermore, it may be irreversible. Elderly persons and women are most likely to develop tardive dyskinesia, and it is more likely to be severe and less likely to be reversible in the elderly. It is less clear that treatment duration and type of agent are important contributors to risk.[22,23] The primary treatment is to taper and discontinue the drug.

The choice of a low or high potency agent depends in part on the characteristics of the patient and the side effect profile of the agent. For patients with a thought disorder and disturbed sleep, the sedative properties of the low potency agents are advantageous. For patients who are ambulatory and already orthostatic, a high potency agent may be preferred.

Although there are a number of agents with intermediate potency, being familiar with one or two high or low potency agents is sufficient to treat most patients. A number of newer agents are purported to have fewer extrapyramidal effects, although risperidone can have such effects if used at high enough doses. Although clozapine may indeed be less likely to cause extrapyramidal effects, its potential for causing agranulocytosis and the associated cost of monitoring limit its use to individuals requiring long-term treatment or who are unable to tolerate other agents.

A number of precautions can be taken to minimize the risk or extent of side effects. Once the desired effect is achieved and the target symptom is alleviated, or the inciting event is resolved, the drug should be tapered and discontinued. Many of the problems with neuroleptic use result from patients being left on the drug long after the inciting event has resolved and after discharge from the hospital. If patients are discharged to a rehabilitation or long-term care facility it is helpful to indicate a time limit to treatment with these agents, much as one would do with a course of antibiotics. If agents are prescribed on an as-needed, or pro re nata (PRN), basis, the indication for use and maximum daily dose should be clearly stated in the orders. The maximum daily doses provided for agents outlined above are guidelines; while they may be exceeded, this should be done cautiously and under close supervision because of the increased risk of side effects.

## Antidepressants

The cardinal features of depression are the "vegetative" or depressive signs and symptoms, including increased or decreased sleep, decreased activity level, fatigue, decreased concentration, increased or decreased appetite or weight, motor slowing or agitation, guilt, suicidality, chronic somatic complaints, and pain.[24] Although standardized instruments such as the Geriatric Depression Scale,[25] can be useful adjuncts, diagnosis still often relies on the recognition of depressive signs and symptoms. It is important to rule out underlying medical illnesses contributing to depression, such as stroke, myocardial infarction, congestive heart failure, thyroid disorders, uremia, and certain cancers. Medications may contribute as well, including central-acting antihypertensives and β-blockers, narcotics, neuroleptics, benzodiazepines, antihistamines, and sedative/hypnotics.[26]

Once these contributing factors have been ruled out and target signs or symptoms identified, the choice of agent again depends in part on the characteristics or features of the patient and the desired side effect profile.[24,27]

Tertiary amine tricyclics (e.g., amitriptyline, imipramine, doxepin) were among the early agents used. Although still effective, their side effects are poorly tolerated by elderly persons. Their metabolites (secondary amine tricyclics such as nortriptyline and desipramine) are available and are preferred. Like the low potency neuroleptics, tricyclics have as potential side effects sedation, orthostasis, and anticholinergic effects. In addition, they have the potential to contribute to arrhythmias. While nortriptyline and desipramine have relatively low arrhythmogenicity, they should be used cautiously in persons with underlying conduction disorders, and PR and QRS intervals should be monitored periodically while on treatment. Desipramine (starting dose 25 mg/day) is an activating agent and is preferable for persons who are apathetic, withdrawn, and anhedonic. Nortriptyline (starting dose 10 mg/day) is a sedating agent and is preferred in individuals who are anxious or have sleep difficulties as well as depression. Blood levels are available for both agents and can be used to adjust doses depending on effect and side effects (nortriptyline has a therapeutic window—a level beyond the upper limit may lead to less effectiveness and more side effects).[28]

There has been a veritable explosion of new antidepressants during the past few years, particularly in the serotonin reuptake inhibitor class of medications. Many of these agents, particularly the early ones, have been studied in the elderly and found to be safe and effective, albeit somewhat costly. Agents such as fluoxetine (starting dose 10 mg/day), paroxetine (starting dose 10 mg/day), and sertraline (starting dose 50 mg/day) can be used once daily and appear to lack the arrhythmogenicity of tricyclics. For the most part they are activating agents and should be dosed in the morning. Paroxetine is the most sedating agent in the class. Among the potential side effects are gastrointestinal upset and anorexia, so such drugs should be used cautiously in elderly persons with decreased appetite or weight loss as a feature of their depression.

Other agents are available that may be useful in certain situations, such as trazodone (starting dose 25 mg/day) and nefazodone; these drugs are alternative sedating antidepressants (trazodone can cause priapism in men).[29] All the agents described above take several weeks to achieve an effect, and patients should be so warned. Methylphenidate (starting dose 5 mg/day), which often exhibits an effect within 24–48 hours, may be used as a bridging activating agent for particularly anhedonic or apathetic patients until other agents exert their effect, with its primary side effects being excessive arousal, gastrointestinal upset, and tachycardia.[30] Monoamine oxidase (MAO) inhibitors are used infrequently because of their potential serious interactions with certain medications and tyramine-containing foods. For life-threatening depression or patients refractory to medications, electroconvulsive therapy can be used safely and effectively in elderly persons.[26]

## Anxiolytics

Pharmacologic intervention for anxiety is warranted if symptoms are sufficiently severe to interfere with daily coping or enjoyment of life. In general, treatment should be short term: for a grief reaction or as an adjunct to supportive therapy to develop coping strategies. It is again important to rule out contributing disorders such as congestive heart failure and chronic obstructive pulmonary disease.

The mainstays of anxiolytic therapy are the benzodiazepines.[21,31] Given the metabolic changes that occur with aging, described above, short-acting agents such as lorazepam (starting dose 0.5 mg/day) and oxazepam (starting dose 7.5 mg/day) are preferred because of their more predictable half-lives and duration of action. All benzodiazepines share potential side effects, including sedation, dizziness, depression, confusion, agitation, and disinhibition. Dependence can develop, and tolerance to their effects often occurs after 2–4 weeks of continuous use. Consequently, it is best to use these agents short term. Because a withdrawal reaction or "rebound" characterized by tremor and agitation can occur after abrupt withdrawal, benzodiazepines should be tapered prior to discontinuing. Buspirone (starting dose 5 mg twice a day) is a nonbenzodiazepine anxiolytic that is less likely to cause dependence, sedation, or psychomotor retardation. However, it has a delayed onset of action (several weeks) and lacks the soporific and muscle relaxant effect of benzodiazepines. Its primary side effects are dizziness and nausea. Barbiturates should be avoided because they are less effective and have greater addictive potential than other available agents.[31,32]

## Sedative/Hypnotics

Disturbed sleep is a common complaint among older persons, particularly in the hospital.[21,33] Part of this is due to changes that occur in sleep patterns with aging, including a phase shift (falling asleep and waking up earlier than in prior years) and more disruptions to sleep. Disturbed sleep may manifest as difficulty falling asleep, difficulty staying asleep, or early morning awakening. A variety of medical factors contribute to sleep difficulties, including anxiety, depression, pain, itching, nocturia, and congestive heart failure. Medications that may contribute include amphetamines, steroids, decongestants, caffeine, and alcohol. A number of other factors may play a role among hospitalized patients, including daytime naps, intravenous lines, catheters, traction, and frequent wakings for medications or treatments. After establishing by history if sleep is disturbed, the mainstay of treatment should be nonpharmacologic interventions directed at potential contributing factors.

If drug treatment is indicated, there are several potential choices that can be used safely and effectively short term (suggested maximum duration of use is 7–10 days). Among the benzodiazepines, short-acting agents are preferred because they are less likely to cause carryover sedation the following day. Temazepam (starting dose 7.5 mg) has a reasonable duration of action but a delayed onset of action and so must be given approximately 1–2 hours before bedtime. Triazolam (starting dose 0.0625–0.125 mg at bedtime) has a short duration of action and so is best for persons who have difficulty falling asleep.[34] Chloral hydrate (starting dose 250 mg at bedtime) is safe, effective, and inexpensive, with its primary side effects being gastrointestinal upset, although its use should be avoided in patients with a creatinine clearance less than 50 ml/min or with severe hepatic dysfunction. Zolpidem (5 mg starting dose) is a newer agent that also appears relatively safe in elderly persons.[35,36] Again, if persons are depressed and have sleep difficulties, treatment with a sedating antidepressant is preferable to separate treatment with two different medications. Similarly, if someone has a thought disorder and disturbed sleep, a sedating neuroleptic is preferred, but neuroleptics should not be used for sleep alone.

## Pain Management

Pain is a common complaint among elderly persons and can have a substantial impact on affect and physical functioning. Adequate treatment is thus important, but caution must be exercised because of the strong potential for adverse effects with many of these agents. As such, it is helpful to follow the stepwise approach defined above for assessing the nature and extent of pain, determining its etiology, and starting with lower doses of less potent agents. A variety of instruments are available to help gauge the current severity of pain and the effectiveness of treatment.[37,38]

The first line of therapy often consists of acetaminophen, aspirin, or nonsteroidal antiinflammatory agents (NSAIDs).[38,39] Although all three possess analgesic and antipyretic properties, acetaminophen lacks the antiinflammatory properties of the other two classes. Acetaminophen is safe, effective, inexpensive, and well tolerated by older persons. Caution should be exercised in the setting of liver disease or alcohol use, and there may be an increased risk of end-stage renal disease with high-dose long-term use.[38,40] Aspirin and the nonsteroidals can cause gastrointestinal bleeding or renal insufficiency and can interfere with platelet function. A variety of central nervous system (CNS) side effects may also be seen with nonsteroidals. Given that these three classes provide roughly equipotent analgesic effects, acetaminophen may be the safer choice in the absence of inflammation.

If pain is not controlled with these agents, opioid analgesics are the next line of treatment.[38,39] They are often characterized as mild or strong. Mild opioids, such as codeine and oxycodone, may provide relief alone or in conjunction with the nonopioid analgesics described above. Strong opioids, such as morphine, are used if pain remains unrelieved. All opioids have similar potential side effects, among which are respiratory depression, constipation, urinary retention, nausea and vomiting, delirium, and myoclonus. The patient should be monitored closely and appropriate dose adjustments made when these side effects appear. Prophylactic bowel regimens are often necessary and should be initiated when the narcotic is started. Tolerance to some of the effects may appear and may be facilitated by continuous, rather than as-needed, administration schedules. For respiratory depression, the opiate antagonist naloxone may be helpful. Meperidine should be used with caution in patients with renal insufficiency; and its metabolite, normeperidine, may cause seizures. Topical analgesics such as capsaicin may be helpful for conditions such as herpes zoster. Nonpharmacologic modalities such as heat, cold, massage, biofeedback, and transcutaneous electrical nerve stimulation (TENS) help in certain situations. Nerve blocks are another potential option for certain types of refractory pain.

## Antihypertensives

Given the prevalence of hypertension among elderly persons and its potential consequences, treatment is warranted in most cases. Again, most agents can be used safely and effectively, but caution is required because of the potential side effect profile of certain classes of agents. Nonpharmacologic interventions such as salt intake reduction, exercise, and stress reduction remain valuable components of treatment.[41,42]

Evidence continues to mount regarding the benefit of treating systolic or diastolic hypertension.[43–49] The current mainstays of therapy are thiazide diuretics, β-blockers, angiotensin-converting enzyme (ACE) inhibitors, and long-acting calcium-channel blockers.[41,50] Each class of agents effectively controls hypertension in elderly persons.

Diuretics and β-blockers have been shown to reduce mortality and a number of important cardiovascular and cerebrovascular endpoints.[43–49] Thiazide diuretics (hydrochlorothiazide 12.5–25.0 mg/day starting dose, maximum dose 50 mg) remain the cornerstone of therapy and are safe, inexpensive, and well tolerated by elderly patients. They are not efficacious in patients with a creatinine clearance below 30 ml/min. Potassium loss should be monitored periodically and replacement added if needed. Longer-acting β-blockers (metoprolol 25 mg/day starting dose) are also effective and reasonably well tolerated; they are particularly helpful in the setting of recent myocardial infarction or coronary artery disease.[51–53] The patient should be monitored for orthostasis, dizziness, and bradycardia. β-Blockers should be used cautiously or avoided in patients with bronchospastic disease, congestive heart failure, depression, diabetes, heart block, or peripheral vascular disease.[41]

The ACE inhibitors are particularly useful for patients with concomitant congestive heart failure, diabetes with proteinuria, or renal insufficiency. They should be used cautiously or avoided in those with renovascular disease.[41,54]

Although there has been some concern regarding the potential safety of short-acting calcium channel blockers, long-acting agents appear to be safe and may be helpful in the setting of underlying coronary artery disease.[55] Constipation and peripheral edema are common annoying side effects of these agents.

Other agents may be advantageous in certain situations.[41,50] α-Blockers may be helpful with concomitant prostatic hypertrophy or dyslipidemia; orthostatic hypotension is a prominent side effect that should be monitored closely. Vasodilators may be used with concomitant congestive heart failure. Central-acting agents, such as clonidine and α-methyldopamine, should be used cautiously because they can contribute to altered mental status and depression.[56]

## Antihistamines

Histamine $H_1$ receptor blockers are commonly used for treatment of allergies and allergic reactions; occasionally they are used as sedative/hypnotics. Because of their prominent anticholinergic properties, they should be used cautiously in the elderly. Agents with relatively low anticholinergic properties, such as chlorpheniramine, are preferred. Their use as sleep medications should be limited given the availability of safer agents.

The nonsedating antihistamines terfenadine and astemizole can interact with erythromycin, ketoconazole, and itraconazole resulting in life-threatening arrhythmias. This combination is absolutely contraindicated, and terfenadine has been removed from the U.S. market.[57] If a nonsedating antihistamine is required, loratadine may be preferred.

Histamine $H_2$ receptor blockers, used to inhibit gastric acid secretion, can be safely used in elderly persons. All of these agents can cause alterations in mental status.[58] In general, the dose and duration of use should be kept to a minimum and always adjusted for renal function. If used prophylactically during the perioperative period, the dose should be decreased and ultimately discontinued as soon as possible.

## Antibiotics

There are two major clinical categories of antibiotic usage among surgical inpatients: perioperative prophylaxis and the treatment of postoperative infections. Although this chapter does not deal with specific antibiotic recommendations, it addresses the general principles of antibiotic dosing in the geriatric patient. With the expansive antibiotic armamentarium now available, it is imperative that the proper choice of antibiotic be made by taking into account possible drug interactions (Table 13.3), the side effect profile of a particular drug, and the appropriate dose in a given patient.

Proper dosing of antibiotics and other drugs in the elderly reduces the incidence of adverse drug reactions (ADRs). This point is especially important in light of the fact that the incidence of ADRs increases with advancing age and the effects are more serious in the frail elderly patient than in their younger counterparts.[60] In general, improper dosing is a more frequent cause of error in therapy than is the use of an inappropriate drug.[61]

Some of the factors that may contribute to the need for drug/dosage alterations in the elderly, as outlined above,

TABLE 13.3. Selected Antibiotics and Their Drug Interactions

| Antibiotic | Other drug | Effect |
|---|---|---|
| Ampicillin | Anticoagulants | ↑ Anticoagulation |
| Aminoglycosides | Amphotericin B | ↑ Nephrotoxicity |
| | Cyclosporine | ↑ Nephrotoxicity |
| | Loop diuretics | ↑ Ototoxicity |
| | Neuromuscular blockers | ↑ Respiratory paralysis |
| | NSAIDs | ↑ Nephrotoxicity |
| | Vancomycin | ↑ Nephrotoxicity |
| Cefoperazone, cefotetan | Anticoagulants | ↑ Anticoagulation |
| Clindamycin | Theophylline | ↑ Theophylline level |
| Ciprofloxacin | Antacids/sucralfate | ↓ Absorption of ciprofloxacin if taken within 2 hours |
| | Theophylline | ↑ Theophylline level |
| | Anticoagulants | ↑ Anticoagulation |
| Erythromycin | Astemizole/ terfenadine | ↑ Cardiotoxicity |
| | Cyclosporine | ↑ Cyclosporine level |
| | Digoxin | ↑ Digoxin level (10%) |
| | Lovastatin | Rhabdomyolysis |
| | Theophylline | ↑ Theophylline level |
| Metronidazole | Alcohol | Disulfiram-like reaction |
| | Oral anticoagulants | ↑ Anticoagulation |
| Imipenem-cilastatin | Cyclosporine | ↑ Cyclosporine level |
| Trimethoprim-sulfamethoxazole | Anticoagulants | ↑ Anticoagulation |

*Source:* Data from Sanford et al.[59]

include (1) decreased creatinine clearance; (2) low serum albumin levels; (3) increased proportion of body fat; (4) achlorhydria; and (5) increased number of concomitantly prescribed drugs. Of these factors, the one with the most direct clinical relevance to antibiotic dosing is the decline in renal function. Many disease processes, including most notably hypertension and diabetes, contribute to and accelerate this decline.[60]

Most clinicians are aware of the need to decrease the dose of certain nephrotoxic antibiotics such as aminoglycosides in the setting of renal insufficiency. However, other commonly used drugs such as quinolones and most cephalosporins, including ceftriaxone, also need to be dose-adjusted for a creatinine clearance of less than 30 ml/min.[62] Table 13.4 lists selected antibiotics whose dosages need to be adjusted.

Although aminoglycosides remain important drugs for treatment of serious infections, alone or in combination with other drugs, the availability of newer agents (quinolones, monobactams, carbapenems) with broad-spectrum coverage and less nephrotoxicity make the use of aminoglycosides less attractive in elderly persons. In addition to nephrotoxicity, aminoglycosides also cause ototoxicity. This is more likely to occur in elderly patients especially if given in high dose or for prolonged periods because ototoxicity is cumulative. Furthermore, the risk of ototoxicity is greater in patients concomitantly taking a loop diuretic.[65–67]

TABLE 13.4. Selected Antibiotics Requiring Dose Adjustment During Renal Insufficiency

| Antibiotic | Usual dose | Dose for CrCl <30 ml/min |
|---|---|---|
| Cefazolin | 1–2 g q8h | 1–2 g q12h |
| Cefuroxime | 0.75–1.50 g q8h | 0.75–1.50 g q12h |
| Ceftazidime | 1–2 g q8h | 1–2 g q24h |
| Ceftriaxone | 1–2 g q24h | 0.5–1.0 g q24h |
| Penicillin G | 0.5–4.0 million units q4h | 75% of dose |
| Ampicillin | 1–2 g q6h | 1–2 g q6–12h |
| Nafcillin | 1–2 g q4–6h | 1–2 g q6–8h |
| Piperacillin | 3–4 g q4–6h | 4 g q8h |
| Ticarcillin clavulanate | 3.1 g q4h | 2 g q8h |
| Aztreonam | 1–2 g q8h | 50–75% of dose |
| Erythromycin | 250–500 mg q6h | 50–75% if CrCl <10 |
| Imipenem-cilastatin | 0.5–1.0 g q8h | 0.25 g q6–12h |
| Metronidazole | 250–500 mg q6–8h | 50% of dose if CrCl <10 |
| Vancomycin | 1 g q12h | 1 g q1–4 days |
| Gentamicin | 1.7 mg/kg q8h | 30–70% of dose q12h |
| Amikacin | 7.5 mg/kg q12h | 30–80% of dose q12–18h |
| Amphotericin B | 0.3–0.8 mg/kg q24h | 0.3–0.8 mg/kg q24–36 when CrCl <10 |
| Fluconazole | 200–400 mg q24h | 50% of dose |
| Ciprofloxacin (IV) | 200–400 mg q12h | 50–75% of dose |

*Source:* Data are from McCue[63] and Sanford et al.[64]
CrCl, creatinine clearance.

TABLE 13.5. Selected Antibiotics Requiring Dose Adjustment in the Presence of Severe Hepatic Dysfunction

| |
|---|
| Nafcillin |
| Cefoperazone |
| Clindamycin |
| Erythromycin |
| Ketoconazole |
| Isoniazid |
| Rifampin |

Evidence suggests that once-daily dosing of an aminoglycoside is at least as effective as, and less toxic than, conventional dosing regimens of multiple daily dosages. Several analyses of pooled data from randomized controlled studies in adults found that once-daily aminoglycoside dosing may be associated with less nephrotoxicity and no greater ototoxicity than with conventional dosing.[68–70] Although this may be attractive in the elderly it is important to note that few studies have included patients with life-threatening infections or patients with renal dysfunction. In general, once-daily aminoglycoside dosing is not appropriate for, or recommended in, any patient with a creatinine clearance less than 30 ml/min. Thus although once-daily dosing of aminoglycosides is not contraindicated in older patients, pending further studies, it cannot be recommended without reservation, especially in patients who are seriously ill or immunocompromised or who have substantial renal dysfunction.

As mentioned above, although liver size and blood flow tend to decrease with age, in the absence of serious liver disease and subsequent hepatic dysfunction, antibiotic dosages do not need to be adjusted. Drug-induced hepatitis in patients treated with antituberculous agents, especially isoniazid, increases in incidence from 2.8/1000 in patients <35 years old to 7.7/1000 in patients ≥55 years old.[65,71] Therefore liver function tests must be performed frequently prior to and during the course of antituberculous therapy. Antibiotics that require dose adjustments in patients with hepatic dysfunction include cefoperazone, clindamycin, erythromycin, isoniazid, ketoconazole, nafcillin, and rifampin (Table 13.5).

β-Lactam antibiotics (penicillins, cephalosporins, cephamycins, carbapenems, monobactams) have varying characteristics of absorption, peak concentration, bioavailability, and metabolism. These subjects have been elucidated in detail in standard texts and are not covered here. In general, bioavailability is relatively poor after oral administration, which has implications for the switch from intravenous to oral preparations; and pharmacokinetics are similar after intramuscular or intravenous administration.[63]

Cephalosporins are relatively safe drugs to use in older persons. Dosages for certain cephalosporins need adjustment for renal insufficiency (Table 13.4). The broad spectrum of activity of ceftriaxone together with its convenient daily dosing make it an ideal drug for empiric use in a variety of clinical infections in the elderly.[72,73] In addition, it has both renal and biliary excretion and as a result, needs little adjustment for renal insufficiency. A lesser known side effect of ceftriaxone is the formation of biliary sludge with prolonged use.[74]

Cefoperazone, another commonly used third-generation cephalosporin, has primarily biliary excretion and needs no adjustment for renal insufficiency[75]; however, it can cause elevation of the prothrombin time. There are three proposed mechanisms of cephalosporin-associated hypoprothrombinemia, two of which involve the *N*-methylthiotetrazole (NMTT) moiety. The most plausible mechanism is NMTT inhibition of vitamin K epoxide reductase in the liver. Patients at increased risk for this adverse event include those with low vitamin K stores, specifically patients who are malnourished with low albumin concentrations and poor food intake. The elderly and patients with liver or renal dysfunction are examples of populations at potential risk. The manufacturer therefore recommends concomitant use of vitamin K once a week during cefoperazone administration, although epidemiologic studies suggest that bleeding complications with antibiotics in general may have more to do with other risk factors than the specific antibiotic.[76–79] It should also be noted that cefoperazone causes a mild disulfiram-like reaction when given within 72 hours of alcohol ingestion.

As the only widely available carbapenem in the United States, imipenem-cilastatin has a broader spectrum of activity (gram-positive, gram-negative, aerobic, and anaerobic) than most cephalosporins; and its use is restricted in most hospitals. Its pharmacokinetics are similar to that of cephalosporins, and it requires dose adjustment for renal insufficiency because it is excreted renally. The cilastatin component has no antibacterial activity but is used to inhibit renal tubular metabolism of imipenem, thereby increasing the urinary concentration of the active drug. Its major adverse effects are related to the CNS, including seizures, somnolence, and confusion.[80]

Aztreonam is a monobactam that has only aerobic gram-negative bacterial coverage. Its pharmacokinetics are similar to that of the cephalosporins. It is frequently used in patients with renal insufficiency as a substitute for aminoglycosides, although it too needs dose adjustment in such patients. Its use in combination with β-lactam antibiotics for synergy (as with aminoglycosides for enterococcal or pseudomonal infections), however, has not been validated. It lacks cross-reactivity with other β-lactam antibiotics and can be used safely in patients with severe allergy to penicillin or cephalosporins.[81,82]

The fluorinated quinolones are a relatively new class of drugs that have gained wide usage during the past few years. They have a broad spectrum of aerobic gram-positive and gram-negative bacterial activity with excellent pharmacokinetic profiles. The gram-positive coverage, especially in vitro activity against *Streptococcus pneumoniae*, of the earlier quinolones (ciprofloxacin) is not as good as that of the new generation of quinolones, such as sparfloxacin and ofloxacin. In addition, they are active against intracellular organisms such as *Legionella*, *Mycoplasma*, *Chlamydia*, and *Mycobacteria*. They are well absorbed orally, with a high degree of bioavailability that makes them especially useful drugs in the transition from intravenous to oral dosing. They also have excellent tissue penetration. Care should be taken with the oral administration of these drugs to ensure that they are administered 2 hours before or after antacids, sucralfate, or other multivalent metallic cations lest their absorption be severely impaired.[83,84]

## References


1. Shock NW, Watkin DM, Yiengst MJ, et al. Age differences in the water content of the body as related to basal oxygen consumption in males. J Gerontol 1963;18:1–8.
2. Forbes GB, Reina JC. Adult lean body mass declines with age: some longitudinal observations. Metabolism 1970;19: 653–663.
3. Mayersohn MB. Special pharmacokinetic considerations in the elderly. In: Evans WE, Schentag JJ, Jusko WJ (eds) Applied Pharmacokinetics: Principles of Therapeutic Drug Monitoring, 3rd ed. Vancouver, WA: Applied Therapeutics, 1992.
4. Greenblatt DJ. Sellers EM, Shader RI. Drug disposition in old age. N Engl J Med 1982;306:1081–1088.
5. Tozer TN, Winter ME. Phenytoin. In: Evans WE, Schentag JJ, Jusko WJ (eds) Applied Pharmacokinetics: Principles of Therapeutic Drug Monitoring, 3rd ed. Vancouver, WA: Applied Therapeutics, 1992.
6. Paxton JW, Briant RH. Alpha one-acid glycoprotein concentrations and propranolol binding in elderly patients with acute illness. Br J Clin Pharmacol 1984;18:806–810.
7. Robertson DRC, Wood ND, Everest H, et al. The effect of age on the pharmacokinetics of levodopa administered alone and in the presence of carbidopa. Br J Clin Pharmacol 1989;28:61–69.
8. Castleden CM, George CF. The effect of ageing on the hepatic clearance of propranolol. Br J Clin Pharmacol 1979;7:49–54.
9. Cusack B, O'Malley K, Lavan J, et al. Protein binding and disposition of lignocaine in the elderly. Eur J Clin Pharmacol 1985;29:323–329.
10. Jaillon P, Gardin ME, Lecocq B, et al. Pharmacokinetics of nalbuphine in infants, young healthy volunteers, and elderly patients. Clin Pharmacol Ther 1989:46:226–233.
11. Greenblatt DJ, Shader RI, Harmatz JS. Implications of altered drug disposition in the elderly: studies of benzodiazepines. J Clin Pharmacol 1989;29:866–872.
12. Greenblatt DJ, Harmatz JS, Shader RI. Clinical pharmacokinetics of anxiolytics and hypnotics in the elderly: therapeu-

tic considerations. Part I. Clin Pharmacokinet 1991;21:165–177.

13. Rowe JW, Andres R, Tobin JD, et al. The effect of age on creatinine clearance in men: a cross-sectional and longitudinal study. J Gerontol 1976;31:155–163.
14. Lindeman RD, Tobin J, Shock NW. Longitudinal studies on the rate of decline in renal function with age. J Am Geriatr Soc 1985;33:278–275.
15. Cockcroft DW, Gault MH. Prediction of creatinine clearance from serum creatinine. Nephron 1976;16:31–41.
16. Hanlon JT, Weinberger M, Samsa GP, et al. A randomized, controlled trial of a clinical pharmacist intervention to improve prescribing in elderly outpatients with polypharmacy. Am J Med 1996;100:428–437.
17. Inouye SK, van Dyck CH, Alessi CA, et al. Clarifying confusion: the confusion assessment method: a new method for detection of delirium. Ann Intern Med 1990;113:941–948.
18. Inouye SK, Viscoli CM, Horwitz RI, et al. A predictive model for delirium in hospitalized elderly medical patients based on admission characteristics. Ann Intern Med 1993;119:474–481.
19. Inouye SK, Charpentier PA. Precipitating factors for delirium in hospitalized elderly persons: predictive model and interrelationship with baseline vulnerability. JAMA 1996;275:852–857.
20. Marcantonio ER, Juarez G, Goldman L, et al. The relationship of postoperative delirium with psychoactive medications. JAMA 1994;272:1518–1522.
21. Jenike MA. Psychoactive drugs in the elderly: antipsychotics and anxiolytics. Geriatrics 1988;43(9):53–65.
22. Task Force on Late Neurological Effects of Antipsychotic Drugs. Tardive dyskinesia: summary of a task force report of the American Psychiatric Association. Am J Psychiatry 1980;137:1163–1172.
23. Smith JM, Baldessarini RJ. Changes in prevalence, severity, and recovery in tardive dyskinesia with age. Arch Gen Psychiatry 1980;37:1368–1373.
24. Jenike MA. Psychoactive drugs in the elderly: antidepressants. Geriatrics 1988;43(11):43–57.
25. Yesavage JA, Brink TL, Rose TL, et al. Development and validation of a geriatric depression screening scale: a preliminary report. J Psychiatr Res 1983;17:37–49.
26. Stimmel GL, Gutierrez MA. Psychiatric disorders. In: Delafuente JC, Stewart RB (eds) Therapeutics in the Elderly, 2nd ed. Cincinnati: Harvey Whitney Books, 1995:324–343.
27. Tourigny-Rivard MF. Pharmacotherapy of affective disorders in old age. Can J Psychiatry 1997;42(suppl 1):10S–18S.
28. Perry PJ, Pfohl BM, Holstad SG. The relationship between antidepressant response and tricyclic antidepressant plasma concentrations: a retrospective analysis of the literature using logistic regression analysis. Clin Pharmacokinet 1987;13:381–392.
29. Gitlin MJ. Psychotropic medications and their effects on sexual function: diagnosis, biology, and treatment approaches. J Clin Psychiatry 1994;55:406–413.
30. Wallace AE, Kofoed LL, West AN. Double-blind, placebo-controlled trial of methylphenidate in older, depressed, medically ill patients. Am J Psychiatry 1995;152:929–931.
31. Schneider LS. Overview of generalized anxiety disorder in the elderly. J Clin Psychiatry 1996;57(suppl 7):34–45.
32. Shuckit MA. Current therapeutic options in the management of typical anxiety. J Clin Psychiatry 1981;42(11, sect 2):15–26.
33. Flamer HE. Sleep problems. Med J Aust 1995;162:603–607.
34. Greenblatt DJ, Harmatz JS, Shapiro L, et al. Sensitivity to triazolam in the elderly. N Engl J Med 1991;324:1691–1698.
35. Roger M, Attali P, Coquelin JP. Multicenter, double-blind, controlled comparison of zolpidem and triazolam in elderly patients with insomnia. Clin Ther 1993;15:127–136.
36. Fairweather DB, Kerr JS, Hindmarch I. The effects of acute and repeated doses of zolpidem on subjective sleep, psychomotor performance and cognitive function in elderly volunteers. Eur J Clin Pharmacol 1992;43:597–601.
37. Herr KA, Mobily PR. Pain assessment in the elderly: clinical considerations. J Gerontol Nurs 1991;17(4):12–19.
38. Ferrell BA. Pain management in elderly people. J Am Geriatr Soc 1991;39:64–73.
39. Ferrell BA. Pain evaluation and management in the nursing home. Ann Intern Med 1995;123:681–687.
40. Barrett BJ. Acetaminophen and adverse chronic renal outcomes: an appraisal of the epidemiologic evidence. Am J Kidney Dis 1996;28(suppl 1):S14–S19.
41. Sixth Report of the Joint National Committee on Prevention, Detection, Evaluation, and Treatment of High Blood Pressure. Arch Intern Med 1997;157:2413–2446.
42. Messerli FH, Schmieder RE, Weir MR. Salt: a perpetrator of hypertensive target organ disease? Arch Intern Med 1997;157:2449–2452.
43. Curb JD, Pressel SL, Cutler JA, et al. Effect of diuretic-based antihypertensive treatment on cardiovascular disease risk in older diabetic patients with isolated systolic hypertension. JAMA 1996;276:1886–1892.
44. Collins R, Peto R, MacMahon S, et al. Blood pressure, stroke, and coronary heart disease. Lancet 1990;335:827–838.
45. Dahlof B, Lindholm LH, Hansson L, et al. Morbidity and mortality in the Swedish Trial in Old Patients with Hypertension (STOP–Hypertension). Lancet 1991;338:1281–1285.
46. Hypertension Detection and Follow-up Program Cooperative Group. Five-year findings of the Hypertension Detection and Follow-up Program. I. Reduction in mortality of persons with high blood pressure, including mild hypertension. JAMA 1979;242:2562–2571.
47. SHEP Cooperative Research Group. Prevention of stroke by antihypertensive drug treatment in older persons with isolated systolic hypertension: final results of the Systolic Hypertension in the Elderly Program (SHEP). JAMA 1991;265:3255–3264.
48. Gueyffier F, Boutitie F, Boissel JP, et al. Effect of antihypertensive drug treatment on cardiovascular outcomes in women and men: a meta-analysis of individual patient data from randomized, controlled trials. Ann Intern Med 1997;126:761–767.
49. MacMahon S, Rodgers A. The effects of blood pressure reduction in older patients: an overview of five randomized controlled trials in elderly hypertensives. Clin Exp Hypertens 1993;15:967–978.
50. Kaplan NM, Gifford RW. Choice of initial therapy for hypertension. JAMA 1996;275:1577–1580.
51. Yusuf S, Peto R, Lewis J, et al. Beta blockade during and after myocardial infarction: an overview of the randomized trials. Prog Cardiovasc Dis 1985;27:335–371.

52. Hennekens CH, Albert CM, Godfried SL, et al. Adjunctive drug therapy of acute myocardial infarction: evidence from clinical trials. N Engl J Med 1996;335:1660–1667.
53. Smith SC, Blair SN, Criqui MH, et al. Preventing heart attack and death in patients with coronary disease. J Am Coll Cardiol 1995;26:292–294.
54. Gansevoort RT, Sluiter WJ, Hemmelder MH, et al. Antiproteinuric effect of blood-pressure-lowering agents: a meta-analysis of comparative trials. Nephrol Dial Transplant 1995;10:1963–1974.
55. Ad Hoc Subcommittee of the Liaison Committee of the World Health Organisation and the International Society of Hypertension. Effects of calcium antagonists on the risks of coronary heart disease, cancer and bleeding. J Hypertens 1997;15:105–115.
56. National High Blood Pressure Education Program Working Group. National High Blood Pressure Education Program Working Group report on hypertension in the elderly. Hypertension 1994;23:275–285.
57. Du Buske LM. Introduction: risk management in asthma and allergic diseases. J Allergy Clin Immunol 1996;98(6, part 3):S289–S290.
58. Cantu TG, Korek JS. Central nervous system reactions to histamine-2 receptor blockers. Ann Intern Med 1991;114: 1027–1034.
59. Sanford JP, Gilbert DN, Moellering RC, Sande MA (eds). Anti-infective drug–drug interactions. In: The Sanford Guide to Antimicrobial Therapy, 27th ed. Vienna, VA: Antimicrobial Therapy, 1997:123–126.
60. Gleckman RA. Antibiotic concerns in the elderly. Infect Dis Clin North Am 1995;9:575–590.
61. Lesar TS, Lomaestro BM, Pohl H. Medication-prescribing errors in a teaching hospital: a 9-year experience. Arch Intern Med 1997;157:1569–1576.
62. Gilbert DN, Bennett WM. Use of antimicrobial agents in renal failure. Infect Dis Clin North Am 1989;3:517–531.
63. McCue JD. Antimicrobial therapy. Clin Geriatr Med 1992;8:925–945.
64. Sanford JP, Gilbert DN, Moellering RC, Sande MA (eds). Dosage of antimicrobial drugs in adult patients with renal impairment. In: The Sanford Guide to Antimicrobial Therapy, 27th ed. Vienna, VA: Antimicrobial Therapy, 1997:116–120.
65. Posner JD. Particular problems of antibiotic use in the elderly. Geriatrics 1982;37(8):49–54.
66. Tablan OC, Reyes MP, Rintelmann WF, et al. Renal and auditory toxicity of high-dose, prolonged therapy with gentamicin and tobramycin in Pseudomonas endocarditis. J Infect Dis 1984;149:257–263.
67. Moore RD, Smith CR, Lietman PS. Risk factors for the development of auditory toxicity in patients receiving aminoglycosides. J Infect Dis 1984;149:23–30.
68. Marra F, Partovi N, Jewesson P. Aminoglycoside administration as a single daily dose. Drugs 1996;52:344–370.
69. Barza M, Ioannidis JPA, Cappelleri JC, et al. Single or multiple daily doses of aminoglycosides: a meta-analysis. BMJ 1996;312:338–345.
70. Hatala R, Dinh T, Cook DJ. Once-daily aminoglycoside dosing in immunocompetent adults: a meta-analysis. Ann Intern Med 1996;124:717–725.
71. Van den Brande P, van Steenbergen W, Vervoort G, et al. Aging and hepatotoxicity of isoniazid and rifampin in pulmonary tuberculosis. Am J Respir Crit Care Med 1995; 152:1705–1708.
72. Mandell LA, Bergeron MG, Ronald AR, et al. Once-daily therapy with ceftriaxone compared with daily multiple-dose therapy with cefotaxime for serious bacterial infections: a randomized, double-blind study. J Infect Dis 1989;160:433–441.
73. Barriere SL, Flaherty JF. Third-generation cephalosporins: a critical evaluation. Clin Pharm 1984;3:351–373.
74. Michielsen PP, Fierens H, Van Maercke YM. Drug-induced gallbladder disease: incidence, etiology and management. Drug Saf 1992;7:32–45.
75. Brogden RN, Carmine A, Heel RC, et al. Cefoperazone: a review of its in vitro antimicrobial activity, pharmacological properties and therapeutic efficacy. Drugs 1981;22:423–460.
76. Rockoff SD, Blumenfrucht MJ, Irwin RJ, et al. Vitamin K supplementation during prophylactic use of cefoperazone in urologic surgery. Infection 1992;20:146–148.
77. Goss TF, Walawander CA, Grasela TH, et al. Prospective evaluation of risk factors for antibiotic-associated bleeding in critically ill patients. Pharmacotherapy 1992;12:283–291.
78. Grasela TH, Walawander CA, Welage LS, et al. Prospective surveillance of antibiotic-associated coagulopathy in 970 patients. Pharmacotherapy 1989;9:158–164.
79. Schentag JJ, Welage LS, Williams JS, et al. Kinetics and action of N-methylthiotetrazole in volunteers and patients: population-based clinical comparisons of antibiotics with and without this moiety. Am J Surg 1988;155(5A):40–44.
80. MacGregor RR, Gibson GA, Bland JA. Imipenem pharmacokinetics and body fluid concentrations in patients receiving high-dose treatment for serious infections. Antimicrob Agents Chemother 1986;29:188–192.
81. Neu HC. Aztreonam activity, pharmacology, and clinical uses. Am J Med 1990;88(suppl 3C):2S–6S.
82. Fillastre JP, Leroy A, Baudoin C, et al. Pharmacokinetics of aztreonam in patients with chronic renal failure. Clin Pharmacokinet 1985;10:91–100.
83. Davies BI, Maesen FPV. Drug interactions with quinolones. Rev Infect Dis 1989:11(suppl 5):S1083–S1090.
84. Norrby SR, Ljungberg B. Pharmacokinetics of fluorinated 4-quinolones in the aged. Rev Infect Dis 1989;11(suppl 5)S1102–S1106.

# 14
# Postoperative Outcome and Rehabilitation

Leo M. Cooney, Jr.

Successful aging means, for most individuals, that they remain as independent and as functional as possible. Independence means that they can maintain themselves at home with little or no human assistance. The independent old person must be able to bathe, groom, dress, feed, and toilet herself or himself without assistance. The ability to carry out these functions allows old individuals to remain in their own home, limits the care burden on their family, and is a strong indicator of long-term mortality.

Physicians and surgeons should strive, therefore, to keep old individuals as independent as possible. The desired outcome from a surgical procedure must exceed the traditional mortality and morbidity of the procedure. A successful surgical outcome means that the patient returns to a desired level of function and can live as independently as possible. Achievement of this goal requires careful assessment of the surgical candidate, interventions to prevent functional decline, and direction of a rehabilitative program to return the patient to as high a level of function as possible.

The process of hospitalization itself often causes a decline in function in old individuals. Thirty-five to fifty percent of patients over age 65 experience a decline in function during a hospitalization.[1] This decline is often unrelated to the reason for hospital admission. Functional decline is associated with a prolonged hospital length of stay, increased need for nursing home placement, and increased mortality.[2] The following case illustrates how this decline can occur:

> An 80-year-old man enters the hospital for a colectomy for adenocarcinoma of the colon. The surgery goes well, but the patient becomes acutely confused for several days after surgery. He pulls out his intravenous line and his dressing and requires both sedation and physical restraints. An indwelling bladder catheter is left in place to monitor urine output. One week after surgery the patient's wound has healed well, his white blood cell count and temperature are normal, but the patient is now confused, incontinent of urine, and unable to dress, bathe, feed, and toilet himself. He requires transfer to a nursing home.

Although this patient had technically successful surgery, the outcome was poor. This patient may or may not ultimately be able to return to independent living. How can these poor outcomes be avoided, and what can be done to return this patient to independent living?

The final functional outcome of a patient is, in the final analysis, the responsibility of the attending surgeon. The surgeon must now include an assessment of a patient's function prior to hospital admission, attempt to prevent any decline in function during hospitalization, and take responsibility for the maintenance and recovery of function following surgery. As the rehabilitation of surgical patients now often occurs in a setting outside the acute hospital (subacute centers, skilled nursing facilities, rehabilitation hospitals or units, home care), the surgeon must ensure that this activity is carried out in a coordinated, competent fashion.

When a surgeon is contemplating emergent or elective surgery on an old individual, he or she must evaluate:

1. How will the proposed surgery affect this individual's ability to live independently?
2. How might hospitalization itself affect this person's independence?
3. Does this individual have risk factors that might result in loss of independence after surgery?
4. Can any interventions prevent loss of function with surgery?
5. How can an old individual best regain function after surgery?

## Functional Independence

The ability of old individuals to care for themselves is essential to the dignity, independence, and quality of their life. In 1963 Katz et al. described the basic activities

Table 14.1. Activities of Daily Living

| |
|---|
| Transfer |
| Bathe |
| Dress |
| Feed |
| Go to toilet |
| Continent of urine and stool |

of daily living (ADLs) (Table 14.1) as the ability to bathe, dress, groom, feed, and toilet oneself; to transfer in and out of a chair and walk independently; and to have control of urination.[3] To live independently, one must be able to perform these tasks without human assistance.

The ability to carry on these tasks is highly dependent on a patient's mental status. Altered mental status is the most common cause of functional decline in older individuals. Many patients with mild or moderate dementia can continue to function independently in a familiar environment but lose their ability to function during the stress of hospitalization and surgery.

The development of delirium, or acute confusional state, during a hospitalization has a major impact on a patient's function and long-term outcome. Delirium occurs most frequently in patients with underlying dementia.[4] Dementia is common in older individuals. Approximately 1.5% of individuals between the ages of 65 and 70 have some degree of dementia. The prevalence of dementia doubles during each 5-year period after that. Thus nearly 25% of individuals over age 85 have some degree of dementia, and this number reaches 50% for those aged 90 and above. Many patients with mild or moderate cognitive losses still have good social graces and do not appear, on casual observation, to have any major problems with their mental function. It is essential to identify patients with cognitive deficits as one plans for hospitalization and surgical interventions.

## How Patients Lose Function

Old individuals are at much higher risk for the complications of hospitalization and medical and surgical interventions than young people.[5] Hospitalization is often a crucial period for frail elderly individuals with little mental or physiologic reserve and limited social support.[6] The elderly have a high incidence of complications with therapy, including drug reactions, adverse effects of procedures, hospital-acquired infections, and other iatrogenic events. Elderly individuals in acute hospitals often have significant functional problems. Warshaw et al. studied a cross section of patients over age 70 in a community hospital. At one point in time, 50% of these individuals had mild or moderate confusion, 47% were incontinent of urine or catheterized, 65% could not ambulate independently, and 40% needed help with eating.[7]

The path to loss of function can be identified by problems with the "geriatric vital signs": confusion, incontinence, immobility, skin breakdown, and poor nutrition (Table 14.2).

Acute confusion is often caused by medications. Sedatives, hypnotics, narcotic analgesics, and drugs with anticholinergic effects frequently cause confusion in old patients. The stressful environment of the intensive care unit (ICU) and the use of physical restraints often produce delirium. Lack of sleep caused by in-room intercoms, administration of medication, and the measuring of vital signs often results in acute confusion.[8]

Continence of bladder and bowel is essential to an individual's independence. Indwelling bladder catheters should be removed as soon as possible after surgery. Transient urinary incontinence is common following surgery. The management of this problem can affect its chronicity. If the nursing staff manages the incontinent patient with diapers and external catheters, it may be difficult to regain bladder control. Reassurance and frequent toileting on the part of the nursing staff is more likely to result in the return of continence.

The very nature of nursing care can contribute to a loss of function for older hospitalized patients. Such activities as providing a bed pan, bathing, dressing, feeding, and administering medications may decrease a patient's ability to care for himself or herself. The nursing staff can better prepare the patient for discharge if they assist patients with various tasks and ensure that they can carry them out independently, rather than performing the task for the patient.

Physicians have a major role in the development of patient dependence. Sedatives and sleeping pills should be used with extreme caution in old individuals. These medications often have a prolonged half-life in the elderly and can cause lethargy and confusion. The use of indwelling or external bladder catheters to monitor urine output often results in at least temporary loss of bladder control. The role of early postoperative ambulation is now well recognized. The ability to transfer out of a bed or chair, however, is a more difficult task than walking and requires more attention during rehabilitation.

The use of physical restraints to prevent patients from removing dressings, intravenous lines, and other devices is associated with many adverse effects. Use of these devices produces an increased incidence of delirium or acute confusion.[4] The surgeon must work in close partnership with the nursing and rehabilitative staff of each

Table 14.2. Geriatric Vital Signs

| |
|---|
| Confusion |
| Incontinence |
| Immobility |
| Skin breakdown |
| Poor nutrition |

TABLE 14.3. Factors Associated with Hospital Decline

| |
|---|
| Bed rest |
| Sedating or hypnotic drugs |
| Anticholinergic drugs |
| Prolonged use of bladder catheters |
| Use of physical restraints |

TABLE 14.4. Predictors of Hospital Decline

| |
|---|
| Altered mental status |
| Physical function prior to admission |
| Social function prior to admission |
| Frequency of going out of home |

hospital unit to ensure that the patients are as mobile as possible, have no trouble with bladder and bowel control, are not confused or delirious, and are able to care for their own basic daily needs (see Table 14.3).

## Predictors of Functional Decline

The most important predictors of functional outcome following surgery are a patient's preexisting mental status, physical function, and social activities. Such measures of independence as how often one goes outside one's home or participates in outside social activities are excellent predictors for return of function following surgery for hip fractures.[9] Patients who are socially active have a much better outcome than individuals who stay in their own home or apartment and have limited social contacts. It is important to determine prior to hospitalization not only whether a patient can get out of bed and walk independently, but whether that individual is socially active outside of his or her own home setting (Table 14.4).

Altered mental status is an extraordinarily important predictor of outcome following surgical interventions. It is often difficult to assess the role of mental status in surgical outcomes, as this factor is so rarely evaluated carefully prior to surgery. When prospective studies are done, however, alterations in mental status have a profound impact on the results of surgery. Dementia increases the mortality for hip fracture almost threefold.[10] The most important predictor of delirium or acute confusion during a hospitalization is preexisting dementia. In many instances, however, the surgeon is unaware of the early signs of dementia in their patients such as loss of recent memory, world-finding difficulty, visuospatial difficulty, or difficulty with calculations. Patients with significant dementia can still be oriented to time and place and thus pass many physicians' screens. The consensus of studies that have evaluated decline during hospitalizations conclude that the factors that predict functional decline are dementia, decreased mobility, decreased social interaction, and infrequent trips outside the home.[1,11]

## Prevention of Functional Decline

Interventions are most effective and efficient if they are applied to people in most need of assistance. It is thus important to identify patients who are apt to lose function in order to intervene in the care of those most at risk for problems. The surgeon must be fully aware of a patient's physical and mental status prior to admission for surgery. Tests of memory are the best screens for dementia. It is unusual that patients with significant dementia can remember three of three objects after 2 minutes. The most appropriate mental status screen for old patients is the Folstein Mini-Mental Status Test (see Chapter 10, Appendix 1). This 30-point test takes only 5 minutes to administer. It has been well studied and validated in a number of populations. Patients with more than an eighth-grade education who score 24 or less on this test should be evaluated for the presence of dementia. Scores of 24 and less are associated with an increased incidence of acute confusion during hospitalization.

The first screening evaluation for a patient's physical function should be to watch the patient get in and out of a chair and walk short distances. In addition, the surgeon should determine whether the patient can climb stairs, is still driving an automobile, and does his or her own shopping, meal preparation, house cleaning, and other such activities. It is, of course, important to know with whom the patient lives and if the patient will have family or other assistance at home following hospital discharge.

## Postoperative Rehabilitation

Returning a patient to a higher level of function requires a concerted effort on the part of a number of health care providers. The nursing staff and the patient's family are usually the best observers of a patient's mental status. The physician must know whether the patient had nighttime confusion; any problems recognizing family members, following commands, or attending to daily tasks; or difficulty with memory or orientation. Although temporary confusion is common following anesthesia, any alterations in mental status that persist beyond 24 hours after surgery should be evaluated. Medications should be reviewed and a search undertaken to ensure that there are no acute medical problems causing the patient's delirium (see Table 14.3). Returning the patient to his or her usual mental function is an essential first step in the rehabilitative process.

Although physicians have long recognized the importance of early postoperative mobilization, they must also realize that a patient's ability to transfer in and out of a bed or chair is more important to independent function than walking. The patient should be able to go from a supine to sitting position and then transfer independently out of a bed or chair. If patients are unable to carry out this task independently, a physical therapy consultation is appropriate.

Older individuals must use their upper extremities to go from a supine to a sitting position. Intravenous lines and restraints may limit their ability to do so. Upper extremity problems such as shoulder disease or a hemiparesis may limit this maneuver. Before returning home, the patient should be able to go from a supine to sitting position in bed without assistance of a bed rail or trapeze.

There are several maneuvers a patient can use to go from a sitting position to a wheelchair or standing. A patient with significant lower extremity weakness or pain can be taught how to maneuver from a bed to a wheelchair using a "side to side" transfer or using a "sliding board" to move one's body from the bed to a wheelchair. The most common method to transfer from a bed to a standing or chair position is to use a "stand-pivot" transfer. The patient needs good lower extremity strength, the absence of lower extremity pain, and good balance to perform this maneuver. He or she should push off with the upper extremities from the bed, using a walker to balance oneself during this maneuver.

While physical therapists can be essential to help with transfers, the nursing staff must also focus on this maneuver. It is best if the nursing staff works with the patient several times every day to ensure that he or she is frequently attempting to transfer out of a bed or chair independently.

The following questions must be answered before determining whether a patient can return home and how much help that patient may need in his or her own home environment.

1. Can the patient go from lying to sitting by oneself?
2. Can the patient go from a bed to a standing position by oneself?
3. Can the patient walk independently?
4. Is the patient continent of urine and stool?
5. Can the patient feed oneself?
6. Can the patient toilet oneself?
7. Can the patient bathe, groom, and dress oneself?

Patients who know their limitations and when to ask for help when they cannot perform a task independently are considered to have good "safety awareness." The absence of this awareness often makes it unsafe for such individuals to be left alone (Table 14.5).

A rough guide to the need for care at home would provide 24-hour-a-day help for patients who cannot transfer in and out of bed independently, are incontinent of urine or stool, or have poor safety awareness. Those patients who need help only with feeding can be given 8 hours of care per day. Those who need help only with dressing and grooming usually need approximately 4 hours of care a day. Those patients who need help only with bathing can be provided with help several times per week.

TABLE 14.5. Returning Home from Subacute Facilities

| |
|---|
| Good mental status |
| Good daily living function |
| Integrated medical care |
| Intensity of rehabilitative services |
| Intensity of discharge planning |
| Good social support |

Patients who have significant care needs at the time of hospital discharge and insufficient help at home to provide these needs may be candidates for a short period of rehabilitation in a subacute or skilled nursing facility. It is essential that the patient's care be well coordinated between the physicians and staff at the acute-care hospital and the physician and staff at the subacute-care facility.

## Subacute Care

Medicare diagnosis-related group (DRG) reimbursement policies and the push to limit hospital lengths of stay have moved a great deal of the rehabilitation of older individuals into skilled nursing facilities. A number of these facilities have set up special units for "subacute care." Some acute-care hospitals have subacute-care units.

Although it may be logical and reasonable to use lower-acuity facilities for rehabilitation, overuse of these facilities without careful coordination of care between the acute and chronic care providers can lead to adverse outcomes. Fitzgerald et al. reported two important studies that demonstrated the problems associated with early transfers to skilled nursing facilities.[12,13] These studies pointed out that the frequency of transfer of patients from acute hospitals to skilled nursing facilities for rehabilitation of a fractured hip more than doubled with introduction of the Medicare DRG-based reimbursement system. The greatest concern, however, was the increase of permanent nursing home placement from 13% to 39% after the introduction of prospective payments. These studies should caution the surgeon to ensure that temporary nursing home placements do not become permanent.

Bonar et al. studied the factors associated with permanent nursing home placement for patients transferred from hospitals to skilled nursing facilities for rehabilitation following hip fractures. She found that patients who were oriented, younger, could bathe independently, could transfer and walk independently, and had increased family involvement were more likely to be discharged from the nursing home to home.[14] In addition, the number of physical therapy hours available in the nursing home predicted discharge home.

Two studies have evaluated the outcome of older patients transferred from hospitals to rehabilitation hospitals, subacute nursing homes, and traditional nursing homes. Kramer et al. found that after adjusting for patients' admission cognitive and physical functions, stroke patients admitted to rehabilitation hospitals were more likely to return to the community and recover function in ADLs. For patients with fractured hips, however, there was no difference in outcome for patients admitted to rehabilitation hospitals, subacute nursing homes, or traditional nursing homes.[15] Kane et al. also found that stroke patients fared better when treated in rehabilitation hospitals and rehabilitative nursing homes. Although healthier hip fracture patients who received rehabilitative nursing home care fared better, the functional change for sicker hip fracture patients was not different between regular and rehabilitative nursing homes.[16]

Fitzgerald et al., in their studies, found one interesting fact about hip fracture patients who were able to return to their own home: Patients followed by their own health maintenance physicians in the nursing home had a better chance of returning home than those who had a separate nursing home physician.[13]

Although subacute-care facilities and traditional nursing homes may have a role in the rehabilitation of old surgical patients, it is important to ensure that the care given in these facilities is as coordinated as possible with the acute-care facility. Surgeons should recognize that patients with altered mental status, substantial deficits in their ability to carry out ADLs, complex medical conditions, and limited social support at home are at substantial risk for permanent nursing home placement. The most complex aspect of returning an old person to his or her own home is the discharge planning process. The surgeon must ensure that the subacute-care facility has all the requisite resources and skills to carry out this complex process.

The integration of care between the acute-care and chronic-care facility requires, first and foremost, that the physicians caring for the patient in the nursing home setting be closely integrated with the acute-care physician. Communication between the acute-care providers must be close. Systems in which there is integrated physician coverage appear to have better rehabilitative outcomes and a higher frequency of patients returning home. An integrated system of care, in which the staff of the nursing home facility have complete access to the laboratory, diagnostic imaging, and other reports of the acute hospital, also increases the potential for improved care.

As surgeons and health care systems are evaluating nursing homes and subacute-care facilities, they must determine the following facts.

1. Does the facility devote a substantial part of its resources to restorative care?
2. What percentage of patients admitted to the facility for short-term care return to their own homes?
3. What percentage of patients are be transferred back to the acute-care hospital?
4. What are the rehabilitative resources available in this facility, including physical therapy, occupational therapy, speech therapy, respiratory therapy, social work, and discharge planning?
5. What level of diagnostic imaging and laboratory support is available at the facility?
6. Is there integration between physicians caring for the patient in this facility and both the acute-care hospital and the community physicians and systems responsible for the patient?

## Conclusions

The ultimate outcome for an old patient who survives his or her surgical procedure is a return to as high a level of daily function as possible. This function means that this individual can carry out daily tasks without human assistance. Many older patients lose these abilities during hospitalization.

The most important predictor of a patient's potential to lose function and to experience long-term decline in function is a patient's preadmission mental status. It is essential for the surgeon to assess this mental status before contemplating an elective surgical procedure. Although many patients with altered mental status can have good outcomes from surgical procedures, a substantial percentage of these patients develop acute confusion or delirium during a hospitalization. Identifying patients at high risk for delirium allows the surgeon to ensure that every effort is made to avoid this important complication of hospitalization and surgery.

Patients who are independent prior to hospitalization have the highest potential of returning to full independence. This independence not only means the ability to take care of one's ADLs but the amount of social interaction the patient has outside of the home.

The surgeon should ensure that the patient's "geriatric vital signs" (confusion, incontinence, mobility, skin breakdown, poor nutrition) are monitored daily. Any deficits in these domains should be addressed promptly.

Patients must be able to transfer in and out of a bed or chair independently before returning home. They must be aware of their own deficits and when they need assistance. They must have full control of their bladder and bowel and be able to take in adequate nutrition.

Subacute-care facilities and nursing homes have taken on an increased role in the rehabilitation of old individuals following surgery. The use of these facilities can be associated with increased risk of permanent nursing home placement. Patients with altered mental status, decreased ADL function, and limited social support are at increased risk for long-term nursing home placement. It is essential that the medical, rehabilitative, and nursing care at these facilities be closely linked with the acute-care system and the community resources that will provide for the patient after discharge.

With the careful identification of presurgical risk factors, attention to preventing decline during hospitalization, and a coordinated surgical rehabilitative process, the outlook for returning old patients to a high level of independence and function can be quite good.

## References


1. Inouye SK, Wagner DR, Acampora D, et al. A predictive index for functional decline in hospitalized elderly medical patients. J Gen Intern Med 1993;8:645–652.
2. Hirsch CH, Sommers L, Olsen A, et al. The natural history of functional morbidity in hospitalized older patients. J Am Geriatr Soc 1990;38:1296–1303.
3. Katz S, Ford A, Moskowitz R, et al. Studies of illness in the aged: the index of ADL; a standardized measure of biological and psychosocial function. JAMA 1963;185:94–99.
4. Inouye SK, Charpentier PA. Precipitating factors for delirium in hospitalized elderly persons: predictive model and interrelationship with baseline vulnerability. JAMA 1996; 275:852–857.
5. Creditor MC. Hazards of hospitalization of the elderly. Ann Intern Med 1993;11:219–223.
6. Gillick MR, Serrell NA, Gillick LS. Adverse consequences of hospitalization in the elderly. Soc Sci Med 1982;16:1033–1038.
7. Warshaw GA, Moore JT, Friedman SW, et al. Functional disability in the hospitalized elderly. JAMA 1982;248:847–850.
8. Inouye SK. The dilemma of delirium: clinical and research controversies regarding delirium in hospitalized elderly medical patients. Am J Med 1994;97:278–288.
9. Cobey J, Cobey J, Conant L, et al. Indicators of recovery from fractures of the hip. Clin Orthop 1976;117:258–262.
10. Miller CW. Survival and ambulation following hip fracture. J Bone Joint Surg Am 1978;60:930–933.
11. Pompei P, Foreman M, Rudberg M, et al. Delirium in hospitalized older persons: outcomes and predictors. J Am Geriatr Soc 1994;42:809–815.
12. Fitzgerald J, Fagan L, Tierney W, et al. Changing patterns of hip fracture care before and after implementation of the prospective payment system. JAMA 1987;258:218–221.
13. Fitzgerald J, Moore T, Dittus R. The care of elderly patients with hip fracture: changes since implementation of the prospective payment system. N Engl J Med 1988;319:1392–1397.
14. Bonar S, Tinetti M, Speechley M, et al. Factors associated with short- versus long-term skilled nursing facility placement among community-living hip fracture patients. J Am Geriatr Soc 1990;38:1139–1144.
15. Kramer A, Steiner J, Schlenker R, et al. Outcomes and costs after hip fracture and stroke: a comparison of rehabilitation settings. JAMA 1997;277:396–404.
16. Kane R, Chen Q, Blewett L, et al. Do rehabilitative nursing homes improve the outcomes of care? J Am Geriatr Soc 1996;44:545–554.

# *Part I*
# *General Principles*

## Section 3
## Ethical Considerations

# Invited Commentary

Michael E. Zenilman

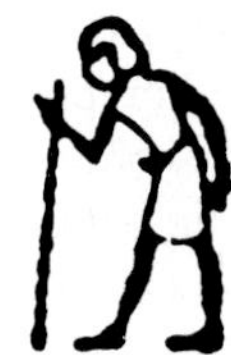

The following section deals with ethical issues encountered with elderly patients. This is a relatively young topic in surgery and its subspecialties and is currently being addressed at the resident education level. A point of introduction is that elderly patients really are different from younger ones. A prominent cardiac surgeon—a geriatric patient—outlined a number of unique facts about the elderly patient (*Bull Am Coll Surg* 1996;81:8–11, 65). First, communication by the physician with the elderly patient should be approached in a much different way from the younger one. Aside from the need to speak loudly to overcome the usual loss of hearing, important conversations should occur with family members in attendance so they can later help clarify issues and communicate with other family members. Second, elderly persons usually do not like being told what to do, even when they are frightened by their illness. Third, elderly patients have long-term goals that are different from those of younger individuals. They are frequently unimpressed with concepts such as 5-year survival rates and focus on shorter-term goals, such as getting home to their families. Finally, elderly patients tolerate major surgery differently from younger ones. Aside from the basic physiologic differences in the aged person, easy fatigability commonly occurs after surgery, and it may last for weeks following discharge.

As our technical ability to maintain life by artificial means has become more available and affordable, ethical issues have arisen regarding the care of elderly patients. Planning the use of "do not resuscitate" (DNR) orders and withdrawing or withholding medical treatment should be addressed with all geriatric patients. The issues particular to surgeons are (1) when to withdraw life support in critically ill intensive care patients, (2) the definition of futility of care, and (3) the issue of DNR orders for patients on the wards and undergoing operative procedures.

Studies have shown that although 80–90% of patients who die in tertiary care centers eventually do have DNR orders written, the orders are usually written within days of the patient's death. My interpretation of this is that writing DNR orders is still considered by many tantamount to delivering a patient's last rites. This problem can be changed with adequate, open, proactive communication by us with the patients and their families.

Liberalization of the use of DNR orders in very ill and terminally ill patients has led to surgical consultation for many patients who are terminally ill and have signed active DNR orders. There is even debate about honoring such orders in the operating room: Some argue that DNR orders *should be honored* intraoperatively. Although some hospitals have policies that DNR orders be *temporarily rescinded* in the operating room and reinstated after the procedure, this is not the norm.

With respect to ethical questions in medical futility, the American Medical Association issued a statement that there is "no ethical distinction between withdrawing and withholding life-sustaining treatment" (*JAMA* 1992;267:2229–2233). The problem lies in identifying the patients for whom medical care will be futile. Prognostic indicators are being developed similar to the APACHE scoring system. These objective estimates for survival correlate better with survival than estimates by even experienced clinicians. Studies have also shown that witholding care from such patients does not decrease health care expenditures significantly, but aggressive interventions in these patients have adverse effects on patients, physicians, and family members.

The Patient Self-Determination Act requires that hospitals and other health care facilities inform patients of their rights to appoint a proxy (or surrogate) decision-maker to act on their wishes regarding life-sustaining care should they become incompetent. This practice usually results in advance directives, living wills, documents that appoint a durable power of attorney, and accurate documentation of the patient's wishes. Currently only 3–15% of the population employ such documents. Interventions by nurse clinicians to enhance communication has been shown to increase the utilization of advance directives. Unfortunately, even when signed, advance directives are sometimes left behind when patients are transferred from nursing homes to the hospital, missed by house staff, or simply overridden by the patient's family. Whether any real benefit comes from the use of advance directives or a health care proxy is still unclear.

All these issues—DNR status, medical futility, and self-determination—should be discussed with all elderly patients with a surgical illness. In our quest to maximize the human life-span, it is our obligation to do so while maintaining our patients' dignity of life and to maximize self-esteem.

# 15
# Ethics in Clinical Practice

Margaret Drickamer

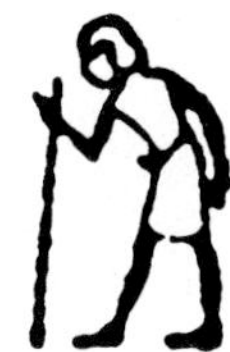

The physician-patient relationship is based on several sequential and interlocking principles that guide the process by which decision-making occurs. If everything is going well, these processes are hardly noticed; but in difficult situations and times of crisis it is important to be able to structure one's response and actions on the basis of accepted principles and guidelines. The process of medical decision-making is grounded in the ethical principles of truth-telling, informed consent, autonomy, professionalism, competence, and confidentiality.

## Truth-Telling

*Patients have a right to have explained to them, in reasonable terms, what is known about their condition.*

Since the time of Hippocrates, *primum non nocere*, first do no harm, has been the principle cited to justify the withholding of "bad news" from patients. What was lacking was the proof that withholding information does less harm than would full disclosure. This edict was little challenged until the 1950s when the question began to arise as to the validity of this assumption. In surveys conducted during the late 1950s and early 1960s,[1,2] fewer than one-third of physicians responding stated that they always tell the truth to their patients about the diagnosis of cancer; and in one survey 69% stated that they usually do not or never tell the patient the diagnosis of cancer. By 1979 a similar survey revealed that 97% of responding physicians thought that a patient should be told the diagnosis of cancer.[3]

This shift in attitude may, at least in part, be due to the increase in treatment options available for cancer patients. Patients cannot be offered chemotherapy or irradiation unless they consent to the treatment. Patients cannot give informed consent for chemotherapy or radiation unless they have been told their diagnosis. Even when treatment options are still limited or nonexistent, as is the case with patients diagnosed with Alzheimer's disease, the weight of the argument is in favor of truth-telling.[4] As we place an increasing emphasis on advance health care planning, the obligation to inform patients while they are capable of making decisions about their own future has become imperative. This is especially true when there is a risk of the patient becoming incapable of participating in decision-making, whether the patient is in the early stages of cognitive decline or facing the possibility of complications during surgery.

On occasion, because of cultural values or other personal reasons patients may wish not to be told a diagnosis.[5] They may then waive their right to being informed, but this must be an explicit decision between the patient and the physician.[6]

## Informed Consent

*Patients have the right to know available treatment options and to understand the implications of their choice. Each patient can then make choices consistent with their own values and goals.*

Every adult patient who has decisional capacity has the right to refuse any treatment.[7] Informing the patient of the benefits, side effects, and alternatives of even common and simple therapies (e.g., a diet change for hypercholesterolemia) is the first step toward the patient's consent to or compliance with that therapy. Elderly patients may base their decision to undertake a particular course of therapy on different values and goals or a different perception of their quality of life than a younger patient would or that their physician might assume.[8,9]

The process of informed consent when obtaining consent for invasive procedures is much more complex, but the same principles hold true (Table 15.1). The patient must understand the benefits of the procedure and the possible risks and burdens associated with it. The patient should also be informed of the benefits, risks, and

TABLE 15.1. Principles of Informed Consent

| |
|---|
| Assess the patient's ability to understand consequences of the decision. |
| If the patient is incapable, identify an appropriate surrogate. |
| Document the goals/values of the patient (or surrogate) expressed as the most important for the decision. |
| Explain how the goals would be affected by the benefits/burdens/risks of the intervention. |
| Document the decision and those present for the discussion. |

burdens of all alternative therapies, including doing nothing. The quality of this discussion is as important as the content.[10] Long lists of unlikely complications may not serve any useful purpose. The discussion should be based on patients' values, fears, and goals and should inform them of risks that either are common or, although rare, devastating. Documentation of the discussion should reflect the entire discussion, including the basis on which patients agreed or declined intervention and their ability to make the decision.[11]

Many interventions other than those traditionally referred to as invasive are now requiring formal consent. The use of physical and chemical restraints in psychiatric and long-term care settings require documentation of acceptance either by the patient or a surrogate. Similar requirements in the acute setting are likely in the near future. Appropriately informing patients of the meaning (i.e., positive and negative predictive value) of screening tests has been a recent focus, especially for such conditions as human immunodeficiency virus (HIV) infection or cancer screening.

## Refusal of Treatment

*Patients have a right to decline any and all medical interventions while they are capable of making a decision and to refuse by advance directive or proxy when they are no longer capable of decision-making.*

The corollary to a patient's right to informed consent is their right to refuse treatment. In 1991 the Supreme Court of the United States ruled in the case of *Cruzan v. the State of Missouri*: The right of a patient to refuse intervention was confirmed and expanded to the right to refuse treatment for future care. Chief Justice William H. Rehnquist wrote that a competent patient has a "constitutionally protected liberty interest in refusing unwanted treatment."[7] The physician has an obligation to ensure that the patient has an opportunity to make a fully informed decision and that the patient is capable of understanding the consequences of that decision.

Refusal of treatment may occur before an intervention has been initiated or after it has been instituted. Withdrawal of an intervention has no legal or ethical difference from not initiating (i.e., withholding) the same intervention, although frequently it has a stronger emotional component.[12,13] If a patient has end-stage kidney disease and opts to forgo dialysis, he or she will die from uremia. If patients who have been on dialysis for a period of time decide to stop dialysis, they too will die from their kidney disease.

Two areas often present problems in the clinical setting: the withdrawal of ventilatory support and the withdrawal or withholding of artificial food or hydration. The withdrawal of ventilatory support parallels that of dialysis. An intervention has been instituted that is maintaining the patient through artificial means because of failure of a vital organ to function. The patient will die from the effects of the underlying disease and resultant organ failure. The difficulties cited in the case of withdrawal of ventilatory support are threefold: (1) the active act (an act of commission) versus a passive act (act of omission) causing the demise of the patient; (2) the proximity of the action/inaction to the death of the patient; and (3) our comfort level with palliation of the symptoms that may occur as ventilatory support is withdrawn.

Much has been made of the arguments of "passive" versus "active" acts. Neither the legal nor the ethical literature support it as a valid distinction, but it can make a major difference in the practitioner's level of comfort. The proximity of an action to the patient's death is discomforting, but the need to discontinue invasive treatments for a patient who does not desire them is the more compelling duty. Being familiar with a routine of dignity and comfort care at the time of withdrawal of ventilatory support is crucial.[14]

Withholding or withdrawing artificial food or hydration in a dying patient also may cause some discomfort on the part of the physician. Neither nutrition nor fluid support is necessary for comfort care, and there is evidence that fluids near the end of life cause discomfort by increasing secretions and suppressing the patient's endogenous endorphin responses.[15] The duty to withhold artificial food and hydration if it is the patient's wish has been upheld in both state and federal courts and was confirmed in the Cruzan case.

## Advanced Care Planning

*Patients may participate in health care decisions when they no longer have decisional capacity through advance care directives.*

The term Advance Directives may refer to either of two documents; a Living Will and a Durable Power of Attorney for Health Affairs. The Living Will is a document in which patients indicate what medical interventions would or would not be desirable under circumstances where they can no longer speak for themselves. The Durable Power of Attorney for Health Affairs (also called

Health Care Proxy or Health Care Agent) is a document in which patients can name a person who they believe is best able to represent their wishes and make health care decisions for them once they are incapable of doing so.

There are several important points to remember about Living Wills.

1. If patients are still capable of making decisions, all treatments must still be discussed with them even if they have a Living Will. A Living Will is not in effect until the patient has lost decisional capacity. Patients capable of making decisions can always change their mind, and their current decision would take precedence over the Living Will.

2. The Living Will is a "what if" statement—a hypothetical situation. The patient is saying, "*If* one of these conditions occurs to me (e.g., permanent coma), *then* do not attempt resuscitation." It does not necessarily mean that the patient does not desire this intervention in the present state of health. For example, if a preoperative patient has a Living Will stating that he or she would decline resuscitation if in a vegetative state but fully capable of decision-making prior to surgery and without declining resuscitation, when such a patient suffers a cardiac arrest intraoperatively resuscitation should be attempted. If after the resuscitation the patient is found to be vegetative, the Living Will would take effect and no further resuscitation attempts should be made if the patient arrests again.

3. In emergency situations, when either the specifics of the Living Will are unknown (i.e., under what circumstances would this person wish to forgo which interventions) or it is unclear whether the conditions of the Living Will are satisfied (e.g., one does not know if the patient has a terminal illness), one should initiate treatments until these issues can be clarified.[16] Once they have been clarified the Living Will should be honored, and any unwanted interventions that had been instituted should be discontinued.

Living Wills may be formal documents executed by a lawyer, but they may also be readily available forms completed by the patient with or without assistance or simply a written statement or narrative. Living Wills cannot cover all circumstances that may arise, and most patients wish to have a proxy decision-maker to interpret their intent.[17] State laws vary as to whether the Living Will or the proxy decision-maker takes precedence when there is a conflict with the decisions.

## Special Case of "DNR in the OR"

*As for all other instances of decision-making, the decision to uphold or rescind a "do not resuscitate" order in the operating room rests with the utility of the intervention and the goals of the patient.*

Let us look at the example of a patient who has metastatic prostate cancer. This patient may decide that if his heart were to stop or his condition were to worsen to the point where a respirator would be needed he would forgo these interventions. This does not mean that the patient does not have other goals that could best be served by an operative procedure requiring intubation (e.g., cecostomy). The important element of the decision is not the intervention per se but whether the goal to be achieved by the intervention in this particular situation is one the patient desires. Therefore it is reasonable to rescind an order not to intubate to perform such a surgery. The same may apply to resuscitation; a cardiac arrest that occurs under general anesthesia where an immediate response is possible and where the cause may be readily reversible is different from an arrest under other circumstances.

If a decision is made to reverse a do-not-resuscitate or do-not-intubate order during surgery, there must be a clear understanding prior to surgery of how postoperative events should be handled in case the patient postoperatively is not capable of making these decisions. How long should an intubation continue if the patient is not quickly able to be extubated? If the patient does arrest and is resuscitated but has lost decisional capacity, what other treatment modalities become an unwanted burden? Discussions with the patient, surgeon, anesthesiologist, and primary care physician can help safeguard against confusing and distressful situations.[18]

## Assessment of Decisional Capacity

*All patients should have their decisional capacity assessed; and if they are incapable of making the decision, an appropriate surrogate decision-maker must be identified.*

Decisional capacity refers to the patient's ability to understand the consequences of the decision they are making.[19] Ability to understand may be impaired because of temporary conditions such as delirium, transient coma, intoxication, or depression; or it may be permanently impaired by cognitive damage or psychiatric illness. Whatever the cause of the impairment, the key to the determination of capacity is the patient's ability to comprehend the advantages and disadvantages of treatment options and to make a decision. It is imperative that communication is done in such a way that the individual's ability to fully understand the options is maximized. Whether we believe that the patient's decision is rational is not a determinant of capacity. Our society has decided that people are allowed to be what most would label "irrational"; for example, we cannot prohibit alcoholics from drinking, even when it has been shown to impair their health or shorten their longevity.[20]

Patients' religious or ethnic beliefs may conflict strongly with our own beliefs, but they have the right to refuse any treatment option they believe is in conflict with their beliefs.

Every physician obtaining informed consent should be able to do a basic assessment of decisional capacity, at least in regard to the specific decision being made. If the physician is unsure of a patient's capacity, a psychiatric consultation may be requested if the question arises from psychiatric problems; or a neuropsychologist or other specialist may be consulted about other problems. The decisional capacity of the patient at the time of any decision, be it to accept or to refuse treatment, should be recorded in the medical record.

Competence is a term that has legal implications beyond what a physician judges on examination. Physicians should avoid using this term unless a court has ruled on the patient's competence. The court recognizes many levels of competence; and only if they have ruled the indivdual to be incompetent *of person* should the indivdual be assumed to lack decisional capacity for medical decisions.

## Decision-Making for Incapacitated Patients

> *Patients who are incapable of making decisions should, to the best of everyone's ability, have their wishes honored directly or by substituted judgment. When this is not possible, a decision should be based on beneficence.*

If a patient is judged to lack the capacity to make an informed decision, a surrogate decision-maker must be identified. The principle behind identifying a surrogate is that that individual should be the person most capable of representing the patient's wishes. If the patient has completed an Advance Directive that names a proxy decision-maker, this is the person to whom questions should be deferred if the patient has lost decisional capacity. A patient may also choose a person in a less formal manner, and documentation of such a choice should help to guide the decision. If the patient's choice of surrogate is not available, usually the next-of-kin are utilized. The heirarchy of authority is spouse, adult children, parents, adult siblings. Adult friends may sometimes be able to act as surrogate if the relationship with the patient is such that they can act on his or her behalf. If it is thought that the person identified by this procedure cannot, in fact, act as an appropriate surrogate (see below), if there is conflict about identifying a decision-maker, or if there is a lack of consensus among individuals, alternative arrangements should be made. If there is no one to act for the patient and it is not an emergent situation, a legal conservator should be sought. In all emergent situations where the decision-making process is unclear, physicians should err on the side of saving a life or preserving function until the situation is clarified. Each institution may have different procedures for obtaining such permission to act.

Beyond the mechanics of identifying surrogate decision-makers, the task of making the decision for the incapacitated patient should follow a procedure meant to maximize the individual's continued influence on the ultimate decision. If a patient gave explicit directives that apply to the situation at hand at a time when he or she was capable of decision-making, they must be followed. For example, if patients with a terminal illness who know they are entering the terminal phases of their illness request that no further interventions be done, including artificial food and hydration, a family member cannot reverse this directive once the patient is in a coma.

If patients have not been explicit about their wishes, the surrogate decision-maker and the physician are then obliged to apply substituted judgment. This term is defined as "the application of the patient's preferences and values . . . trying to choose as the patient would have wanted."[21] Helping a family to understand that their obligation is to do what their relative would have wanted often relieves them of some of the burden of decision-making and helps clarify their thinking. Living Wills are usually most useful in this context. Frequently the exact circumstances outlined in a Living Will are not met, but it can give a good indication of the patient's preferences and values, which then can be applied to the current situation. Encouraging the family to remember other health care decisions or comments the patient made when other family members were ill is often helpful.

If there is no information that helps the surrogate decision-maker to reconstruct what the patient would have said, the guiding principle becomes that of beneficence (or best interest), defined as weighing the benefits, risks, and burdens of an intervention in the context of the individual. The best-interest standard and the reasonable-person standard are similar but differ in important ways. The reasonable-person standard bases health care decisions on categorizing the individual's situation (i.e., is the patient "terminal," "gravely disabled," "vegetative"), and states that the decision should reflect what a reasonable person would want under these circumstances. Beneficence is more individualized, making the person involved the center of the decision. With beneficence, although a patient may no longer be fully capable of making a decision, his or her voice can still be an important one. Their stated preferences and fears can be used to guide the decision about relative benefits and burdens. This can be true for even markedly demented patients.

For example, the relative burden of an intervention in two patients, equally cognitively impaired, can be quite different. One patient may not become agitated when an intravenous line is started, and intravenous treatment would not be a great burden. Another patient may fight such an intervention, pulling it out, needing restraints, and so on. Although the second patient is not making an informed decision to forgo intravenous therapy, the relative burden of the intervention is greater in this patient and therefore the relative benefit would need to be greater for the burden/benefit ratio to be the same.

## Limits of Autonomy

*The individual's autonomy may be limited by the futility of the intervention, the availability of resources, professional judgment, and other societal interests.*

The previous sections have dealt heavily with the respect for and safeguards of the patient's right to exercise autonomy. There are circumstances where this autonomy is tempered by other forces.[22] Professional judgment is a major player in decision-making. Although patients have a right to refuse treatment, they do not have a right to demand a treatment if, in the opinion of the professional, the intervention is not indicated. On the other hand, professionals should seek to understand the patient's goals of treatment and respect patient's own assessment of their quality of life.

There are two aspects of futility discussed here, often labeled quantitative and qualitative. An intervention is said to be quantitatively futile if it cannot achieve its physiologic objective. An example is not offering resuscitation to a patient who is in the terminal phases of metastatic cancer. A therapy is said to be qualitatively futile if it is unlikely to help patients achieve their primary goal even if it has a physiologic effect. An example is the forgoing of antibiotic therapy in a patient who is in the terminal phase of an illness. Although the antibiotics might have the physiologic effect of treating the infection, it would have no effect on comfort and a negative effect in prolonging the person's death.

If a procedure is judged futile, the physician does not have to offer to carry out that therapy to the patient or the surrogate. The very act of offering conveys the sense that there must be some benefit, some chance of success. Why else would it be offered? Therapies the patient and family might expect to have performed but that have become futile, such as an attempt to resuscitate a patient when circumstances clearly demonstrate that it would be futile,[14] should be discussed in the context of their futility. For example, the patient or family should be told that were the patient's heart to stop, attempts to restart it would be futile and therefore would not be initiated. Simply ignoring the subject may engender mistrust of judgment, as most individuals are aware of the spectrum of treatments available.

Other examples of defining a therapy as futile is simple under some circumstances and more difficult under others. The decision that someone is "not a surgical candidate" is frequently made when the relative risks and benefits clearly demonstrate that the treatment is not indicated. The decision to stop a therapy may also be made on the grounds of professional judgment; that is, if a tumor is not responding to chemotherapy, that chemotherapy could be unilaterally stopped by the clinician. The difficulty seems to lie in defining which therapies near the end of life still hold enough of an advantage for the patient that they should be offered. This remains an area where clinical experience is the gold standard, although there are now a few clinical instruments (e.g., APACHE III[23]) that can guide these decisions.[24] These instruments use a combination of diagnosis, cause of illnes, and a scale for physiologic parameters to predict mortality risk.

Autonomy can also be limited by the lack of availability of a treatment or the patient's access to that treatment. Insurance companies, health maintenance organizations, or other forms of managed care may limit the reimbursement for specific procedures or have a cap on the amount that can be spent for certain services. A physician has an obligation to explain all accepted medical options to a patient but cannot always make the options available.[25] This may seem cruel, but having the knowledge is the only way a patient may take the option to pursue access if they so desire. The existence of "gag rules," explicit or implicit, is not considered professionally acceptable.

## Principles of Palliative Care

*When the goals of treatment are for comfort above all else, the intent of all therapies should be that of relief of symptoms.*

When a patient's disease process is at such a stage where cure is not possible and even those therapies that might prolong the person's life are a greater burden than the prolongation of existence would justify to that individual, therapies should be intended to enhance the quality of the time that is left. This may be to the detriment of the quantity of time; certain therapies may shorten life while relieving symptoms. An example is when the dose of morphine needed for pain control is near the same dose that could cause suppression of respiratory drive. This is considered an acceptable risk to take if that is the agreement between physician and patient and the medication or treatment is given with the *intention* of relieving symptoms. This is often referred to as the "rule of double effect." A treatment has two effects (to relieve symptoms and to shorten life), but so long as the intended effect is the relief of symptoms, it is considered acceptable.[21]

Physician-assisted suicide and euthanasia are instances when a therapy is prescribed, provided, or administered with the *intention* of ending that patient's life. The acceptability of such actions from both a moral and a practical point of view is under wide debate within the profession and in society in general.[26] Those who argue for the practice of assisted suicide point out that there are some symptoms that cannot be alleviated short of death (e.g., the discomfort and indignity of destructive head and neck cancer), and individuals should have the right to determine the time and mode of their death. Arguments against physicians assisting in suicide point out that the medical profession's obligation is to "care and to cure" and not to destroy life. Public opinion polls and surveys of physicians show that most individuals in and out of the profession probably do support a role for at least physician-assisted suicide.[27,28]

## Confidentiality

> *Patients have a right to privacy and to confidentiality in matters pertaining to their health and medical care.*

Although this principle seems the most self-evident of the principles discussed here, it is probably the one that is most often broken. From discussions in the elevators to the publication of psychiatric encounters, the breaches in patient's confidentiality and right to privacy abound. A few specific areas that are breached most often bear mentioning.

Sharing of information with patients' relatives or friends is appropriate in only two circumstances: when patients have specifically stated that the physician may discuss their condition with the individual or when the patient has lost decisional capacity and a surrogate decision must be made. It is advisable to ask patients well in advance who they wish to have informed and how much they wish to have told.

The sharing of information among colleagues should be done in private and with respect for the patient's right to confidentiality. Casual conversations in public places, rounds in the hallways, and discussions in lobbies or waiting rooms with multiple families present can be a breach of a patient's right to privacy.[29] Our sensitivity to this issue must be heightened, and the policing of each other should become everyone's responsibility.

Sharing medical information among health care providers without the patient's explicit authorization, if the clinical circumstances so require, is permitted. The use of clinical material for teaching purposes can be done only with sufficient safeguards to anonymity so the individuals involved are not identifiable. Other information can be released only with the patient's or surrogate's authorization unless it is required by law (as in the case of public health reporting of communicable and sexually transmitted diseases).

## References


1. Fitts, WT, Ravdin IS. What Philadelphia physicians tell patients with cancer. JAMA 1953;153:901–904.
2. Oken D. What to tell cancer patients: a study of medical attitudes. JAMA 1961;175:1120–1128.
3. Novack DH, Olumer R, Smith RL, Ochitill H, Morrow GR, Bennett JM. Changes in physicians' attitudes toward telling the cancer patient. JAMA 1979;241:897–900.
4. Drickamer MA, Lachs LS. Should patients with Alzheimer's disease be told their diagnosis? N Engl J Med 1992; 336:947–951.
5. Blackhall LJ, Murphy ST, Frank G, Michel V, Azen S. Ethnicity and attitudes toward patient autonomy. JAMA 1995; 274:820–825.
6. Drickamer MA, Lachs LS. Telling the diagnosis of Alzheimer's disease. N Engl J Med 1993;328:442.
7. Lo B, Steinbrook R. Beyond the Cruzan case: the U.S. Supreme Court and medical practice. Ann Intern Med 1991;114:895–901.
8. Uhlmann R, Pearlman R, Cain KL. Physicians' and spouses' predictions of elderly patient's resuscitation preferences. J Gerontol 1988;43:M115–M121.
9. Mazur D, Merz JF. How older patients' treatment preferences are influenced by disclosures about therapeutic uncertainty: surgery versus expectant management for localized prostate cancer. J Am Geriatr 1996;44:934–937.
10. Mazur DJ, Hickam DH. Patients' preferences for risk disclosure and role in decision making for invasive medical procedures. J Gen Intern Med 1997;12:14–17.
11. Meisel A, Kuczewski M. Legal and ethical myths about informed consent. Arch Intern Med 1996;156:2521–2526.
12. President's Commission for the Study of Ethical Problems in Medicine and Biomedical and Behavioral Research. Summing up: final report on studies of the ethical and legal problems in medicine and biomedical and behavioral research, March 1983. Government Printing Office: Washington, DC, 1983:65–81.
13. American Thoracic Society. Withholding and withdrawing life-sustaining therapy. Ann Intern Med 1991;115: 478–485.
14. Schneiderman LJ, Spragg RG. Ethical decisions in discontinuing mechanical ventilation. N Engl J Med 1988;318: 984–988.
15. Sullivan RJ. Accepting death without artificial nutrition or hydration. J Gen Intern Med 1993;8:220–224.
16. Annas GJ. The health care proxy and the living will. N Engl J Med 1991;324:1210–1213.
17. Sehgal A, Galbraith A, Chesney M, Schoenfeld P, Charles G, Lo B. How strictly do dialysis patients want their advance directive followed? JAMA 1992;267:59–63.
18. Walker RM. DNR in the OR: resuscitation as an operative risk. JAMA 1991;266:2407–2412.
19. Appelbaum PS, Grisso T. Assessing patients' capacities to consent to treatment. N Engl J Med 1988;319:1635–1638.
20. Brock DW, Wartman SA. When competent patients make irrational choices. N Engl J Med 1990;322:1595–1599.
21. Hastings Center. Guidelines on the Termination of Life-sustaining Treatment and the Care of the Dying. Indiana University Press: Indianapolis, 1987.

22. Quill TE, Brody H. Physician recommendations and patient autonomy: finding a balance between physician power and patient choice. Ann Intern Med 1996;125:763–769.
23. Knaus WA, Wagner DP, Draper EA, et al. The APACHE III prognostic system: risk predication of hospital mortality for critically ill hospitalized adults. Chest 1991;100:1619–1636.
24. Lynn J, Teno JM, Harrell FE Jr. Accurate prognostication of death: opportunities and challenges for clinicians. West J Med 1995;163:250–257.
25. Sugarman J, Powers M. How the doctor got gagged: the disintegrating right to privacy in the physician patient relationship. JAMA 1991;266:3323–3327.
26. Drickamer MA, Lee MA, Ganzini L. Practical issues in physician-assisted suicide. Ann Intern Med 1997;126: 146–151.
27. Blendon RJ, Szalay US, Knox RA. Should physicians aid their patients in dying? The public perspective. JAMA 1996;267:2229–2233.
28. Bachman JG, Alcser KH, Doukas DJ, Lichtenstein RL, Corning AD, Brody H. Attitudes of Michigan physicians and public toward legalizing physician-assisted suicide and voluntary euthanasia. N Engl J Med 1996;334:303–309.
29. Ubel PA, Zell MM, Miller DJ, Fischer GS, Peters-Stefani D, Arnold RM. Elevator talk: observational study of inappropriate comments in a public space. Am J Med 1995; 99:190–194.

# 16 Surgery in the Frail Elderly: Nursing Home Patients

Michael E. Zenilman

As our population ages, survivors will approach the limit of aging, or the life-span. As a result of primary and preventive medicine, heathier life styles, and decreased health risk, the population of the United States and other Western societies is trending toward this limit. A comparative study performed on life expectancy of 80-year-old persons in Western countries showed that American octogenarian men and women are expected to live 7.0 and 9.1 more years, respectively. In England the survival of octogenarians was 6.2 and 8.1 years, respectively; in France 6.7 and 8.6 years, respectively; in Sweden 6.5 and 8.3 years, respectively; and in Japan, 6.5 and 8.9 years, respectively.[1]

In 1983, Katz et al. showed that the predicted active life expectancy for patients aged 65–70 years is 10 years, and for those over age 85 it is 2.9 years.[2] More recently others have shown that the life expectancy of a person already aged 65 years was 17 years, a person aged 75 years 11 years, a person aged 85 years 7 years, and a person aged 95 years 3 years. Today, even a person aged 100 years is expected to live an additional 2.5 years. Many of these patients will, no doubt, need chronic nursing care.

It is predicted that the overall average life expectancy in the United States will increase to 83 by the year 2050,[3] and by 2030 there will be 8.8 million persons over the age of 85.[3] The increased survival of the human population is graphically evidenced by "rectangularization" of the Gompertz survival curve, whereupon members of the population survive closer to the limit of aging.

As the limit of life expectancy is reached, a significant percentage of elderly persons become debilitated and become increasingly dependent on others for care. We already known that at age 65 about 10–20% of persons become dependent on others for one or more basic activities of daily living (ADLs). This proportion has been shown to increase to 25% at age 75 and to 50% at age 85.[2]

Old age per se does not necessarily mean disability and helplessness. Age-related morbidity/disability has been associated with life style patterns, which can be changed. In 1980 Fries postulated the theory of "compression of morbidity."[4] The theory states that primary prevention of disease and decreased health risk delay substantially the development of disability by increasing the age of initial disability. It does not result in much gain in years of life, though. This net result is fewer years of disability and a lower level of cumulative lifetime disability. Investigators have since shown that higher socioeconomic status, higher educational level, and regular aerobic exercise are better overall long-term health and independence factors than others,[4,5] suggesting that the hypothesis has some validity.

Fries' group has moved toward proving the hypothesis of compression of morbidity. In a follow-up study of 1741 elderly university alumni, they compared health risk and cumulative disability.[6,7] Health risk was measured by life style issues: obesity, smoking, and exercise (Table 16.1).[8,9] They found that decreased health risk results in decreased morbidity later in life; persons with increased health risk have increased morbidity (Fig. 16.1). Importantly, the onset of minimal disability was postponed by 5 years by the presence of a low risk life style; and progression to a specific level of disability (i.e., based on the delayed rate of rise of the curves) was delayed 7 years.

A population with increased disability must have care, which is typically undertaken in nursing homes. Other options include home care and hospice care, but the present chapter deals exclusively with nursing homes. One study forecast that of the 2.2 million persons who turned 65 in 1990, 43% (900,000) will enter a nursing home before they die: 32% are expected to spend more than 3 months under such care, 24% more than 1 year, and 9% more than 5 years (Figs. 16.2, 16.3).[10] The impli-

Portions of this chapter have appeared previously in the following publication: Zenilman ME. Surgery in the elderly patient. *Current Problems in Surgery* 1998; 35:99–178.

TABLE 16.1. Health Factors Important for Determining Risk from Disability

| Score[a] | BMI | No. cigarettes/day | Exercise (min/week) |
|---|---|---|---|
| 0 | <22.5 | 0 | >240 |
| 1 | 22.5 to ≤24 | 1–20 | 120–239 |
| 2 | 24 to ≤26 | 21–30 | 1–119 |
| 3 | ≥26 | >30 | 0 |

*Source:* Adapted from Vita et al.[6]
[a] 0–2, low risk; 3–4, moderate risk; 5–9, high risk.
BMI, body mass index.

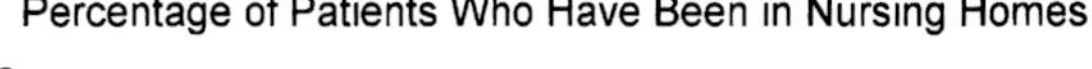


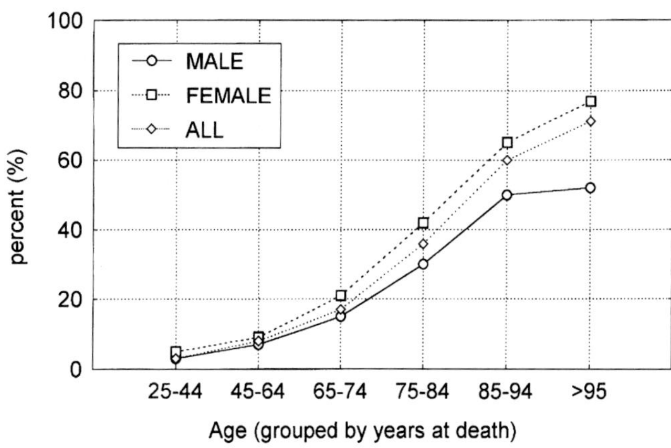


FIGURE 16.2. Lifetime use of nursing homes for persons who died in 1986. Nursing home use increases with increasing age of death. Overall, only 7% of people who were under the age of 65 entered a nursing home at some point in their lives, whereas 37% of those over age 65 entered. (Adapted from Kemper and Murtaugh.[10])

cations for medical management of these patients is obvious, and there is a definite need for good surgical care, as delineated below.

## Focusing Surgical Care on the Frail Elderly: Development of a Dedicated Consult Service for Nursing Home Patients

A number of studies have addressed the utility of focused medical care for frail elderly patients in the inpatient setting. The establishment of an aggressive medical geriatric assessment service for frail elderly populations has been shown to increase patient survival, quality of life, and ability to return to independence.[11–13] In these studies, rehabilitation, independence in self-care, detailed discharge planning, and avoidance of iatrogenic illness were stressed. The interventions resulted in 10% improvement in function on discharge (34% vs. 24%) and decreased need for long-term care (14% vs. 22%).[13]

One study, however, found no real benefit of focused geriatric assessment in the hospital,[14] but in this study the geriatrician was used only as a consultant, not the coordinator of care. There is little argument about the fact that the only person capable of dealing with the complicated elderly patient is one who coordinates the medical, social, rehabilitatative, and surgical care.

Little has been reported about the surgical care of nursing home patients. There are a fair number of reports on the treatment and outcomes of care for decubiti[15–17] but little else. Most studies on this population have been

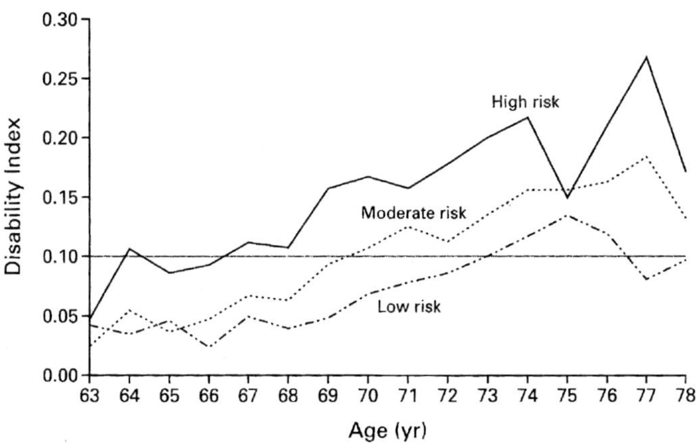


FIGURE 16.1. Disability index by age, stratified by health risk. Health risk for this group was determined as outlined in Table 16.1. Although disability increases in all groups with respect to age, progression to a specific level is achieved earlier in the population of individuals with high health risk. A disability index of 0.1 corresponds to minimal disability. (From Vita et al.,[6] with permission © Massachusetts Medical Society.)

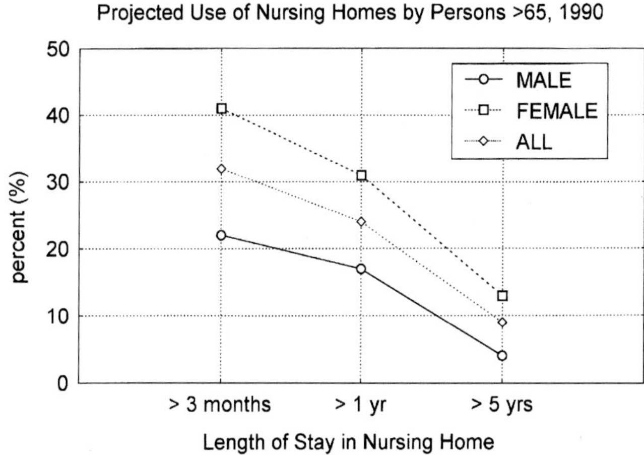


FIGURE 16.3. Projected use of nursing homes by persons turning 65 years of age in 1990. About 33% of men, 52% of women, and overall 43% of this population need some use of a nursing home prior to death. (Adapted from Kemper and Murtaugh.[10])

limited to addressing risk factors for death and survival. As a result, little is known about the utility of aggressive surgical care for the hospitalized or nursing home frail elderly patient. Moreover, some surgeons are reluctant to deal with common surgical illnesses in nursing homes because the patients are usually chronically sick, there is a question about its utility, and some patients have active "do not resuscitate" (DNR) orders.

It is reasonable to assume that a service devoted to the surgical care of chronically ill elderly patients would have a positive impact on their survival and quality of life. I therefore developed a geriatric surgery consult service at the Johns Hopkins Bayview Medical Center, whose goal was to improve surgical care of the frail elderly resident at home, in the hospital, and in the nursing home. Below, the author present data from the effect of this service on the nursing home patient.

The consult service was established on August 1, 1991. We were in a unique position to establish such a service and study its effect. The Johns Hopkins Bayview Medical Center campus had an active general surgery service and geriatric medicine service. The Geriatric Medicine Department has an active acute medical care facility in the hospital, and they control the Johns Hopkins Geriatric Center as well, a 240-bed chronic care facility/nursing home on campus for patients who require both simple and complex chronic nursing home care. The consult service therefore established a close association with the geriatric division, giving exclusive surgical care for the patients residing in this nursing home facility. Using this service, with subsequent expansion to care for patients in other nursing homes affiliated with our institution, we planned to answer the following questions.

1. What is the typical makeup of the patient population referred to this service?
2. What is the incidence and severity of specific general and vascular surgical problems in this patient population?
3. What are the risks of surgical intervention, specifically the complication and morbidity rates?

Patients needing elective surgical consultation were consecutively referred to this service. All patients evaluated and treated by our service were enrolled, along with specific demographic data, into a computer database. All patients were followed in a prospective manner until June 1, 1994. We subsequently reported the results elsewhere.[18]

Altogether 153 patients were enrolled, and 117 of them required intervention. The admission diagnoses to the nursing home and reasons for the surgical consultation are shown in Table 16.2. While maintenance care (decubitus, stoma, and enteral tube care) made up a substantial percentage of referrals, common surgical diseases of the abdomen, breast, and vascular systems were routinely encountered (55%). The actuarial 18-month survival of all patients referred was 35%.

A total of 117 patients underwent 168 surgical procedures. The distribution of cases is shown in Table 16.3. In patients subjected to surgery, the 30-day mortality rate was 8.5% and complication rate 9.4%. Interestingly, the 30-day mortality of the 36 patients not undergoing any intervention was 11.4%; this translated into *absolutely no difference* in overall survival for patients who underwent surgery compared to those who did not (Fig. 16.4).

TABLE 16.2. Diagnoses for Geriatric Surgery Consult Service

| Diagnosis | % |
|---|---|
| **At admission** | |
| Dementia | 20.9 |
| Stroke | 19.4 |
| ADL | 14.2 |
| Peripheral vascular disease | 9.0 |
| Infection | 7.5 |
| Abdominal | 6.7 |
| Cancer | 6.7 |
| Chronic renal failure | 6.0 |
| Coronary artery disease | 4.5 |
| Chronic obstructive pulmonary disease | 3.7 |
| Diabetes | 1.5 |
| *Total* | 100 |
| **At consult** | |
| Maintenance | 32.5 |
| Abdominal/rectal | 27.7 |
| PVD | 16.0 |
| Breast | 10.6 |
| Hernia | 4.6 |
| HD access | 1.2 |
| *Total*[a] | 92.6 |

*Source:* Adapted from Zenilman et al.[18]
Maintenance, decubitus care, chronic intravenous lines, enterostomy, and enteral tubes.
[a] Others included gynecologic problems, lymph node biopsy, trauma, posttransfusion hepatitis.

TABLE 16.3. Operations in Nursing Home Patients

| Procedure | No. | % |
|---|---|---|
| **Adbominal** | | |
| Total biliary | 11 | 6.5 |
| Endoscopy/gastrostomy tube | 12 | 7.1 |
| Laparotomy | 26 | 15.5 |
| *Total* | 56 | 29.1 |
| **Nonabdominal** | | |
| Débridement of decubitus | 42 | 25.0 |
| Amputations | 22 | 13.1 |
| Intravenous access | 25 | 15.0 |
| Breast | 14 | 8.3 |
| Hernia | 5 | 3.0 |
| Other | 11 | 6.5 |
| *Total* | 119 | 70.9 |

*Source:* Adapted from Zenilman et al.[18]

FIGURE 16.4. Survival of nursing home patients referred electively to a geriatric surgical consult service. There was no difference in survival between those for whom surgical intervention was unnecessary and those for whom surgical intervention was necessary. (Adapted from Zenilman et al.[18])

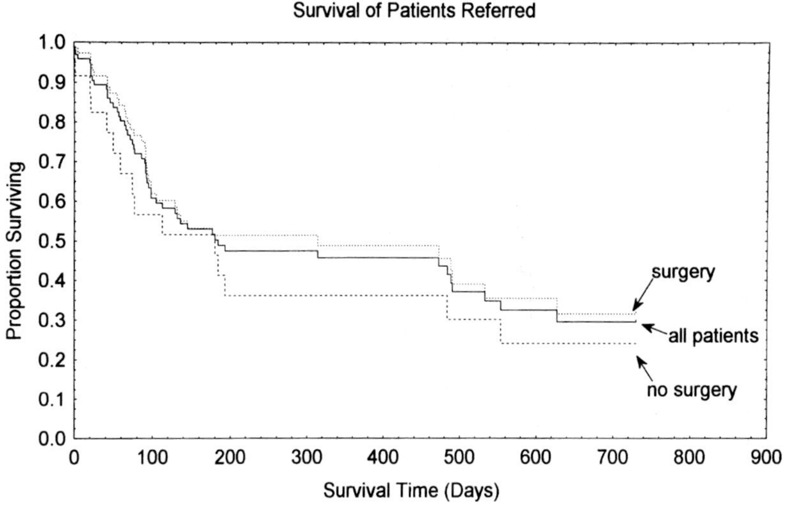


Although those undergoing major abdominal and vascular procedures had a higher complication rate (17.6%) than those undergoing lesser procedures (6.3%, $p = 0.05$), there was no difference in 30-day mortality (9.8% vs. 6.3%, respectively) or 18-month actuarial survival (33% vs. 32%, respectively). Univariate analysis showed that age, length of stay in the nursing home, the presence of coronary artery disease, and dementia had a negative impact on survival (Fig. 16.5). Multivariate analysis of survival using the Cox regression model showed that survival was adversely affected by the presence of the co-morbid conditions of coronary artery disease [relative risk (RR) 3.27, $p = 0.01$] and dementia (documented by a Mini-Mental Score less than 24) (RR 2.39, $p = 0.04$), and age greater than 70 (RR 2.03, $p = 0.06$). It is interesting that the significance value of age was low compared to that of

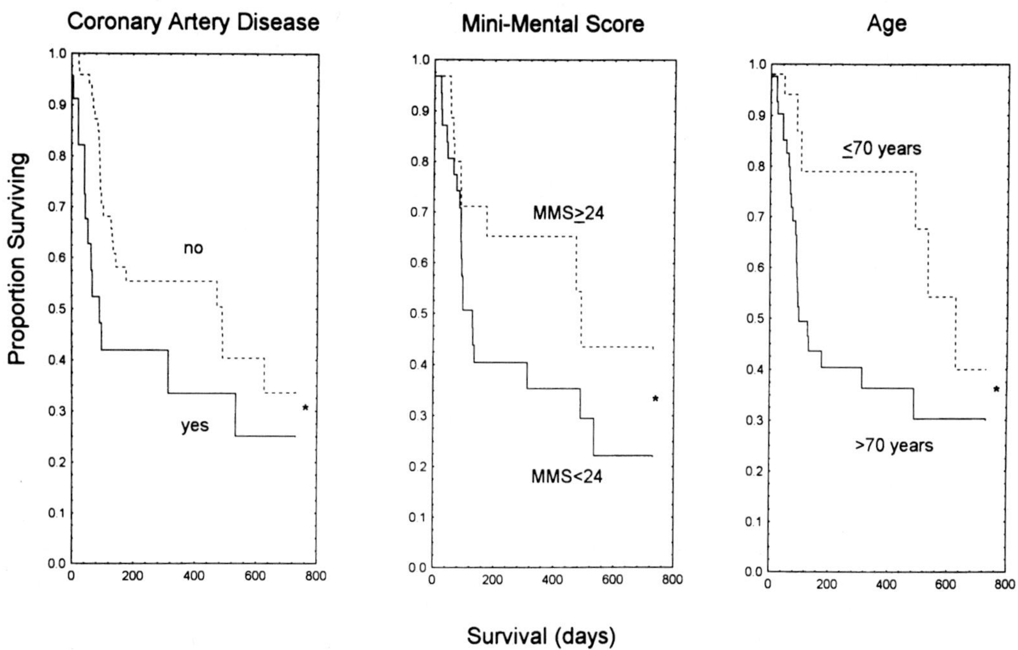


FIGURE 16.5. Survival of patients subjected to surgery when sorted by the co-morbid condition of coronary artery disease (CAD), admission Mini-Mental Score, and age. Univariate analysis revealed that each was a predictor of survival in this population of frail elderly persons. Multivariate regression analysis showed that CAD was the most significant predictor of survival and age the least. Unlike the "healthier" elderly population, the absolute number of co-morbid diseases was not a statistically significant factor (see text). $^{*}p < 0.05$. (Adapted from Zenilman et al.[18])

the other variables. Although univariate analysis showed age to be significant, multivariate analysis put it right on the edge of significance when compared to the co-morbid conditions of cardiac disease and dementia. Overall survival was unaffected by the need of surgery, the magnitude of the procedure performed, sex, number of co-morbid conditions or medications, and whether a preoperative DNR order was present.

From this study, we concluded that general surgical disease is routinely found in the geriatric population, and, therefore, proper surgical care by a general surgeon is necessary. We also showed that routine surgical procedures can be performed safely in residents of nursing homes. Unfortunately, the overall survival of residents of nursing homes referred for surgical intervention is poor, even worse than the published survival of patients in geriatric inpatient units, which is approximately 77.2% (1-year survival).[19]

## Analysis of Data from the Geriatric Surgery Consult Service: Role of Dementia, Age, and Coronary Artery Disease in the Nursing Home Patient

In the population of patients we encountered, the relative risk of death was increased by the presence of cardiac disease and dementia (determined by a Mini-Mental Score less than 24) (Fig. 16.5). Age, as described above, only approached statistical significance. Studies have shown that the presence of dementia adversely affects survival rates of nursing home patients.[20–22] The reported survival of nursing home patients with dementia is 68% at 1 year, 55% at 2 years, and 28% at 3 years.[22] The diagnosis alone increases the relative risk of mortality in these patients by a factor of 2.7.[23,24]

Dementia is prevalent among not only the nursing home patient[20,22–25] but also the "healthy elderly." Skoog et al.[26] showed that in a cohort of 494 nonhospitalized or institutionalized subjects aged 85 and older the prevalence of dementia was 29.8%. The dementia was mild in 8.3%, moderate in 10.3%, and severe in 11.1%. Interestingly 43.5% of the dementia was Alzheimer's type, 46.9% was vascular (multiinfarct)-related, and 9.5% was due to other causes. As in our study and others, the presence of dementia was a risk factor for death: The 3-year mortality was 23.1% in normal persons, 42.2% in those with Alzheimer's dementia, and 66.7% in those with vascular dementia.

Dementia can be assessed rapidly by the Mini-Mental examination.[20,25] Although in our study we used only the Mini-Mental Score obtained on admission to the nursing home, in the future it might be useful to obtain a score at the time of the surgical consult to see if it can be an accurate predictor of short-term survival.

Contrary to what others have shown, survival in our nursing home population was also not dependent on the absolute number of concomitant medical diseases. This result is in contrast to those of other studies, which showed that in the general hospitalized elderly patient co-morbid illness significantly increased the relative risk of death.[20–22]

Univariate analysis showed that our patients' survival was related to age, which is both intuitive and in agreement with the observations of others.[24] No difference was noted between sexes, whereas other studies have shown that instutionalized women survive longer.[22]

The absence of difference in survival in nursing home patients who required surgical intervention compared to those who did not is interesting. Although one might infer that surgery in this population had no effect on survival because most of the procedures performed were life-saving (e.g., amputation for infected or gangrenous limbs, gallbladder removal for acute cholecystitis) or life-maintaining (e.g., long-term intravenous access for nutrition or antibiotics, wound débridement to prevent systemic infection, mastectomy for local control of breast cancer), surgery in these patients actually improved their chances and brought their survival curve back to the downward sloping baseline.

## Case Examples

Three cases highlight the utility of a geriatric-oriented surgical service and the need for surgical leadership in this arena.

### Case 1

We were consulted to evaluate a 92-year-old arthritic woman who had had symptomatic gallstones for more than a year. She was maintained on chronic antibiotics and pain medications after eating. Her only other medications were nonsteroidal antiinflammatory drugs (NSAIDs) for the arthritis. After evaluation by our service, elective removal of the gallbladder was recommended. It was performed laparoscopically without incident. Postoperatively, she remained intubated overnight but was discharged back to the nursing home on postoperative day 2. Almost immediately after discharge she noted only minimal symptoms after eating, her appetite improved, and she gained weight. She expired from unrelated illness 3 months later. She, her family, her geriatrician, and the nurses caring for her thought that she was much more comfortable after removal of the inflamed gallbladder.

Prior to our evaluation, all thought she was too old and frail for even elective surgery. She was a good surgical candidate; forthermore, because of the significant complication of the biliary system that had developed from the gallstones, I believe she would have expired rapidly. This patient was clearly helped by seemingly aggressive, but appropriate, surgical management. The patient, her family, and her health care providers had to be educated about the benefit of elective surgery, as all were basically uninformed prior to the surgical consult. Her DNR order, in effect during her nursing home stay, was rescinded during her procedure and her short stay in the intensive care unit (ICU).

## Case 2

We were consulted to evaluate a malfunctioning percutaneously placed gastrostomy in an 85-year-old man. An endoscopic photograph of the stomach showed that the tube had migrated out of the stomach and into the prefascial space. Under local anesthesia with intravenous sedation, the tube was removed, the stomach was identified, and a new gastrostomy was placed (Fig. 16.6). This procedure was performed as an outpatient operation, and the feeding tube was used the next day.

## Case 3

A 78-year-old woman was a nursing home resident for 8 months after emergency subtotal colectomy due to septic colitis complicated by respiratory and cardiac problems. After a remarkable but prolonged recovery, she began to tolerate oral food well. Over a 2-week period she developed right upper quadrant pain, nausea and vomiting, anorexia, and fevers. Her white blood cell (WBC) count was 15,000 cells/mm$^3$; alkaline phosphatase was 400 IU/L; and other liver function tests and amylase were normal. Ultrasonography revealed a large gallstone and normal common bile duct. To convert this urgent situation to an elective one, a percutaneous cholecystostomy tube was placed, 250cc of pus was removed, and the patient was placed on intravenous antibiotics. The WBC count normalized, and a diet was started the next day. Cholangiography was performed through the cholecystostomy 3 days later due to persistently elevated alkaline phosphatase, and a stone was noted in the common bile duct (Fig. 16.7). Endoscopic retrograde cholangiopancreatography was performed 3 days later, and the stone was removed successfully. The patient did well and underwent elective open cholecystectomy 1 month later.

## Comment

These three cases illustrate the need for surgical involvement in the care of nursing home patients. We must educate the patient, family, and even primary physician

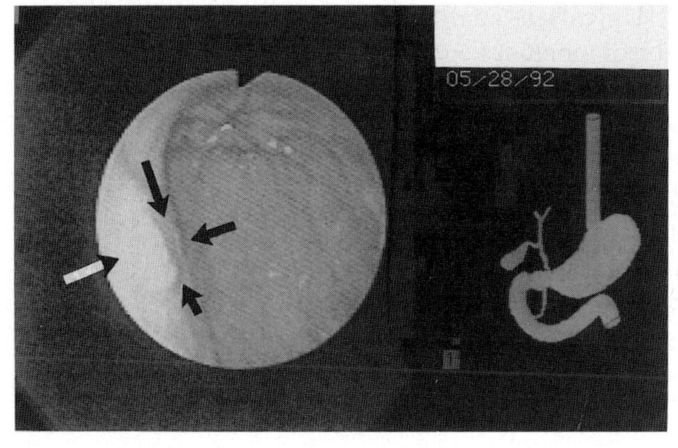


A

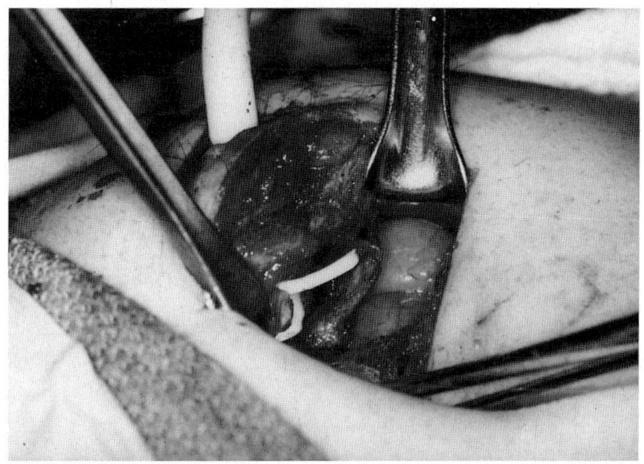

B

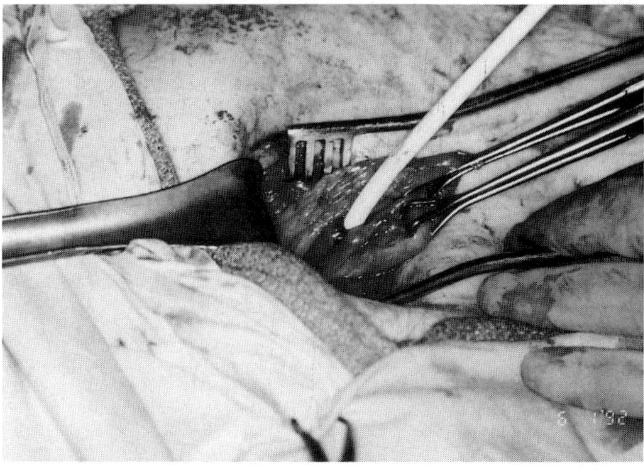

C

FIGURE 16.6. Late complication of percutaneous endoscopic gastrostomy. A. Endoscopic photograph of the stomach in an 85-year-old man in whom the flanged catheter of a percutaneous endoscopic gastrostomy (PEG) had migrated out of the stomach and into the prefascial space. Arrows point to the gastric mucosa overlying the end of the catheter. B. Operative approach was via a paramedian incision away from the PEG site. The catheter and stomach were identified, and a new gastrostomy using a 24F Foley catheter and Stamm technique were performed and the incision closed about the catheter (C).

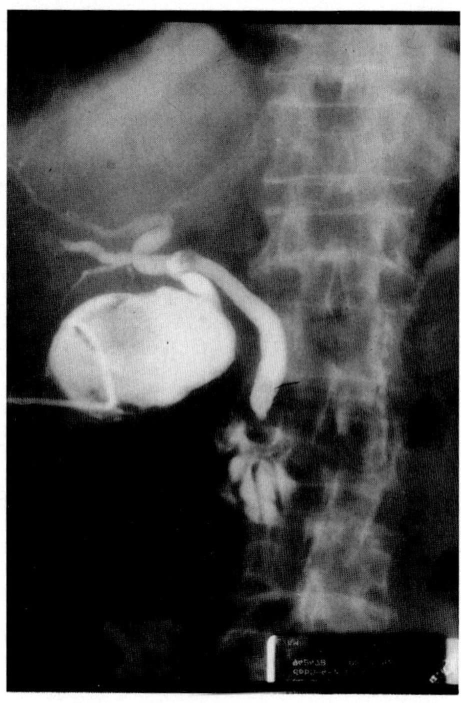

FIGURE 16.7. Cholangiogram after percutaneous drainage of the gallbladder. A stone is noted in the common bile duct (line). Endoscopic retrograde cholangiopancreatography (ERCP) was performed 3 days later, successfully removing the stone. Elective open cholecystectomy was performed later.

about the utility of an invasive procedure for palliation of the patient's illness. We also must coordinate the multidisciplinary care these patients frequently need.

## Development of a Second Geriatric Surgery Consult Service: Decubitus Care

An issue raised by the aforementioned study[18] is that the nursing home studied was situated near a tertiary care center and hence may have had a different population of patients from the "community nursing home." Furthermore, it dealt with a multitude of surgical illnesses, and conclusions about individual types of illness cannot be drawn from such studies.

To evaluate factors determining survival in residents of community nursing homes suffering from a single disease, we retrospectively studied 105 patients consecutively referred for surgical débridement of decubiti in a nursing home in the Bronx, New York.[27] The mean (±SD) age of the patients was 75 ± 1.3 years, and 70% were women. Patients were followed for 10.9 ± 1.0 months. The 1- and 2-year actuarial survivals were 60% and 42.7%, respectively, somewhat higher than what we previously observed. This survival is similar to that of the general nursing home population. It is probable that persons with decubiti are not as ill as others who develop surgically treatable illness.

Univariate analysis showed that the patient's sex and the diagnosis of coronary artery disease had a statistically significant effect on survival (Fig. 16.8). Whereas the diagnosis of dementia appeared not to matter (Fig. 16.9),

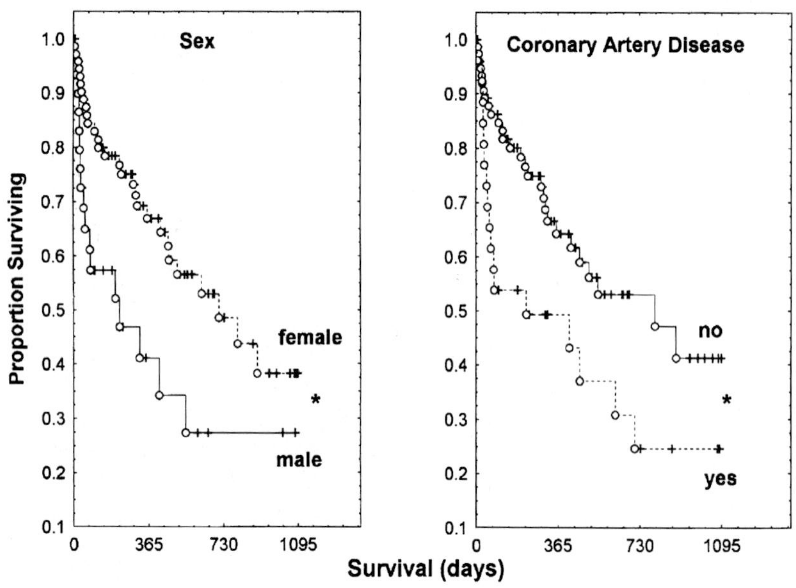


FIGURE 16.8. Survival of nursing home patients referred for care of decubiti, sorted by sex and the presence of coronary artery disease (CAD). Multivariate analysis showed that CAD was the most important factor for predicting survival. $^{*}p < 0.05$.

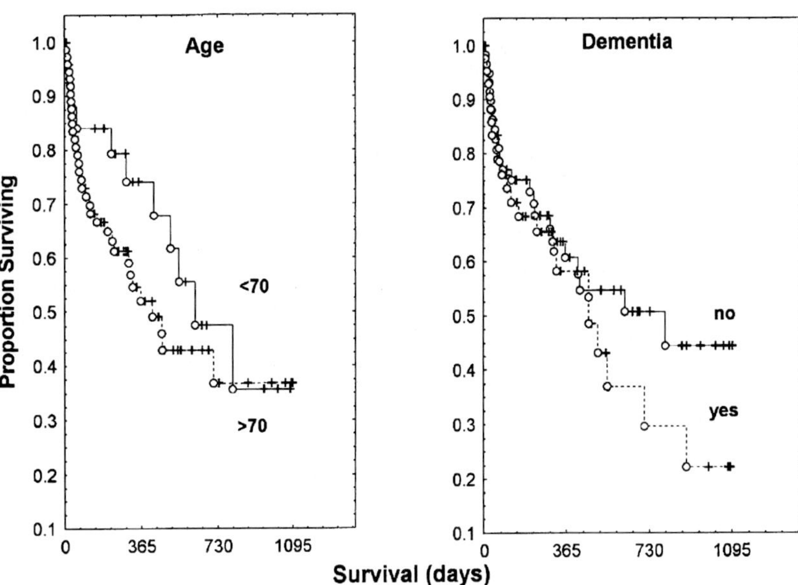


FIGURE 16.9. Survival of nursing home patients referred for the care of decubiti, sorted by age and the presence of dementia. In this patient population, neither factor was a significant predictor of mortality.

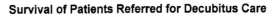

neither dementia nor age factored into survival in this study. Interestingly, these two factors were identified as significant in the previous study. There were differences between the two studies. The first was a prospective analysis in a nursing home associated with a tertiary care center and dealt with all surgical problems. The second (present) study is retrospective, in a community nursing home, and dealt only with surgically managed decubitus ulcers.

Cox regression analysis revealed the relative risk of death for male patients was 2.56 ($p = 0.004$) and for patients with coronary artery disease, 2.2 ($p = 0.008$). We concluded that survival of nursing home patients referred for surgical intervention for decubiti is similar to that of the overall nursing home population. The presence of decubiti in these patients does not adversely affect outcome, and their treatment should be aggressive. Obviously, a dedicated decubitus service in this setting may even improve patient quality of life.

## Hospice: More Palliative Care

We have expanded our palliative care focus to include hospice patients. This population is also growing, and unfortunately they include a number of patients with surgical illnesses. Patients are eligible for admission to hospice programs when there is a life expectancy of less than 6 months. Eighty percent have cancer. In a review of 6451 hospice admissions, Christakis and Escarce[28] noted that a fair number were admitted because of noncorrectable surgical illnesses: 10.5% colorectal cancers, 4.5% pancreatic cancers, 3.2% hepatobiliary cancers, 3.4% upper gastrointestinal cancers; and 1.6% breast cancers. Male and female urogenital cancers made up 15%, half of which were cancers of the prostate.

My experience with hospice patients is small, but the patients have been similar to the frail nursing home patient. Patients are typically referred for help with maintaining enteral feedings, for parenteral feedings, and for superficial abscesses. Interestingly, even though the survival of many these patients is on the order of days, if not months, we still see very stable patients and help with their long-term palliation. In the aformentioned study, 28.5% of patients died within 14 days of enrollment, but 14.9% lived more than 180 days. The latter group do have surgical issues, and it is our responsibility to help these patients approach death in a comfortable, dignified manner.

## Conclusions

The population of nursing homes is going to increase over the next few decades, resulting from the increased population of elderly patients and the increased disability that accompanies the normal aging process. Common surgical illnesses are encountered in nursing home patients, and surgical leadership is needed to guide the care of such patients. We presented here two studies, one prospective and one retrospective. They both showed that the frail nursing home patient can undergo surgical treatment with reasonable results.

TABLE 16.4. Goals of Medical and Surgical Care for Elderly Patients

| |
|---|
| Maximize or maintain potential life-span |
| Maintain dignity of life, maximize self-esteem |
| Maximize independent function, minimize dependence |
| Relieve suffering, with particular attention to pain |
| Cure might not be possible; palliation and comfort are just as important |

In this patient population, quality of life, patient dignity, and relief of suffering take precedence over curative therapy. Care in this population is generally not curative, but it is not futile either.[18] The goals delineated in Table 16.4 should be followed to allow our elders dignity and comfort in their final days.

## References


1. Manton DG, Vaupel JW. Survival after the age of 80 in the United States, Sweden, France, England and Japan. N Engl J Med 1995;333:1232–1235.
2. Katz S, Branch LG, Branson MH, Papsidero JA, Beck JC, Greer DS. Active life expectancy. N Engl J Med 1983;309: 1218.
3. Roush W. Live long and prosper? Science 1996;273:42–46.
4. Fries JF. Aging, natural death and the compression of morbidity. N Engl J Med 1980;303:130–135.'
5. Duffy ME, Macdonald E. Determinants of functional health of older persons. Gerontologist 1990;30:503–509.
6. Vita AJ, Terry RB, Hubert HB, Fries JF. Aging, health risks and cumulative disability. N Engl J Med 1998;338:1035–1041.
7. Campion EW. Aging better. N Engl J Med 1998;338: 1064–1066.
8. Fiatarone MA, O'Neill EF, Ryan ND, et al. Exercise training and nutritional supplementation for physical frailty in very elderly people. N Engl J Med 1994;330:1769–1775.
9. Stevens J, Cai J, Pamuk ER, Williamson DF, Thun MJ, Wood JL. The effect of age on the association between body mass index and mortality. N Engl J Med 1998;338:1–7.
10. Kemper P, Murtaugh CM. Lifetime use of nursing home care. N Engl J Med 1991;324:595–600.
11. Appelgate WB, Miller ST, Graney MJ, Elam JT, Burns R, Akins DE. A randomized controlled trial of a geriatric assessment unit in a community rehabilitation hospital. N Engl J Med 1990;322:1572–1578.
12. Gracey DR, Viggiano RW, Naessens JM, Hubmayr RD, Silverstein MD, Koenig GE. Outcomes of patients admitted to a chronic ventilator-dependent unit in an acute care hospital. Mayo Clin Proc 1992;67:131–136.
13. Landefeld CS, Palmer RM, Kresevic DM, Fortinsky RH, Kowal J. A randomized trial of care in a hospital medical unit especially designated to improve the functional outcomes of acutely ill older patients. N Engl J Med 1995;332:1338–1344.
14. Reuben DB, Borok GM, Wolde-Tsadik G, et al. A randomized trial of comprehensive geriatric assessment in the care of hospitalized patients. N Engl J Med 1995;332: 1345–1350.
15. Ferrell BA, Osterweil D, Christenson P. A randomized trial of low-air-loss beds for treatment of pressure ulcers. JAMA 1993;269:269–494.
16. Inman KJ, Sibbald WJ, Rutledge FS, Clark BJ. Clinical utility and cost effectiveness of an air suspension bed in the prevention of pressure ulcers. JAMA 1993;269:1139–1143.
17. Granick MS, McGowan E, Long CD. Outcome assessment of an in-hospital cross-functional wound care team. Plast Reconstr Surg 1998;101:1243.
18. Zenilman ME, Bender JS, Magnuson TH, Smith GS. General surgical disease in the nursing home patient: results of a dedicated geriatric surgery consult service. J Am Coll Surg 1996;183:361–370.
19. Rubenstein LZ, Wieland D, English P, Josephson K, Sayre JA, Abrass IB. The Sepulveda VA geriatric evaluation unit: data on four year outcomes and predictors of improved patient outcomes. J Am Geriatri Soc 1984;32:503–512.
20. Keller BK, Potter JF. Predictors of mortality in outpatient geriatric evaluation and management clinic patients. J Gerontol A Biol Sci Med Sci 1994;49:M246–M251.
21. Winograd CH, Gerety MB, Chung M, Goldstein MK, Dominquez F Jr, Vallone R. Screening for frailty: criteria and predictors of outcomes. J Am Geriatr Soc 1991;39: 778–784.
22. Van Dijk PTM, van de Sande HJ, Dippel DWJ, Habbema JDF. The nature of excess mortality in nursing home patients with dementia. J Gerontol A Biol Sci Med Sci 1992;47: M28–M34.
23. Perls TT, Morris JN, Ooi WL, Lipsitz LA. The relationship between age, gender and cognitive performance in the very old: the effect of selective survival. J Am Geriatr Soc 1993;41:1193–1201.
24. Brodaty H, McGilchrist C, Harris L, Peters KE. Time until institutionalization and death in patients with dementia: role of caregiver training and risk factors. Arch Neurol 1993;50:643–650.
25. Folstein MF, Folstein SE, McHugh PR. The Mini Mental State: a practical method for grading the cognitive skills of patients for the clinician. J Psychiatr Res 1975;12:189–198.
26. Skoog I, Nilsson L, Palmertz B, Andreasson LA, Svanborg A. A population-based study of dementia in 85 year olds. N Eng J Med 1993;328:153–158.
27. Levine J, Michalski SA, Patel K, Kalemian M, Nelson M, Zenilman ME. Survival of patients in nursing homes referred for surgery. Surg Forum (*in press*).
28. Christakis NA, Escarce JJ. Survival of Medicare patients after enrollment in hospice programs. N Engl J Med 1996;335:172–178.

# 17
# Surgery in Centenarians

Mark R. Katlic

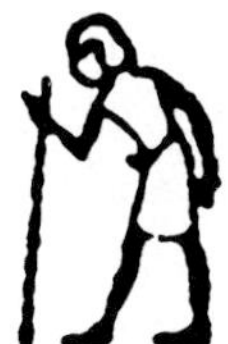

*Ninety years is old, but 100 is news.—Belle Boone Beard*[1]

The 100th anniversary of an individual's birth still bestows an aura, a mystique, as the centenarian is as close to immortality as a human can be. This special prestige has been afforded the imprimatur of scientific study by Baker,[2] who found that centenarians represented a striking exception to the inverted U curve of status across the life-span in Western culture. Baker's data, derived from factorial survey analysis, fit the postulate that there is an "American arc of life" that gives maximum prestige to middle age and least prestige to young and old persons. Centenarians, however, were given unique status nearly equal to that of middle-aged individuals (Fig. 17.1), because "like four leaf clovers or quintuplets, centenarians are rare." Webb and Williams described a case of acute tenosynovitis of the right wrist and hand (centenarian hand syndrome) resulting from the congratulatory handshakes of many friends and relatives on a man's 100th birthday.[3]

We have an inherent curiosity about our oldest old. What does he eat? What is her secret? Can it be bottled and sold? Decades ago one entrepreneur, Dr. Marie Davenport, became a professional centenarian, offering to teach her secrets of longevity to others for a fee.[1] Jeanne Calment, the world's presumed oldest person when she died at 122 years, was interviewed weekly by the foreign press who sought her out in Arles, France.[4] In 1997 a popular magazine devoted its cover story to "How to Live to 100."[5]

The mystique may wane, however, as more of us reach this milestone. The present paucity of centenarians results from high mortality rates and a much smaller overall population a century ago. Over the past 40–50 years the number of centenarians has nearly doubled every decade owing chiefly to improved survival from age 80 to 100 years.[6] When Beard began her monumental, sedulous study of centenarians in 1940 there were 3700 possible subjects living in the United States; when she ended it during the late 1970s there were at least 14,000.[7] This number may reach 100,000 by the year 2000,[5] over 200,000 by 2020,[8] and 500,000 to 4 million in 2050.[9] Some authors argue that even these projections are too conservative because they discount the possibility of future baby booms and assume slow rates of mortality decline and low levels of immigration.[10] Vaupel and Gowan calculated that if mortality is reduced 2% per year by the year 2080 the number of centenarians in the United States would approach 19 million.[11]

Surgical problems do not end on a person's centennial. Surgeons will become increasingly familiar with these most senior citizens.

## History

Surgeons have written with increasing frequency about operations in the elderly, but the definition of "elderly" has changed. A report in 1907 listed 167 operations performed on patients older than 50 years,[12] and even 20 years later Ochsner taught that "an elective operation for inguinal hernia in a patient older than 50 years was not justified."[13] Brooks used a limit of 70 years as "advanced age" in his series of 293 operations reported in 1937,[14] and over the next few decades most authors considered patients above age 60–70 years to be elderly. More recent studies show that good results can be expected in octogenarians and nonagenarians,[15,16] even in those undergoing complex vascular,[17,18] cardiac,[19] and cancer operations.[20]

An occasional centenarian is included in these series, but most papers devoted to centenarians per se are case reports, some written 40 years ago. Welch and Whittemore[21] in 1954 presented a 100-year-old woman who recovered well from abdominoperineal resection of the rectum for carcinoma. The next year Maycock and Burns[22] discussed prostate surgery in two patents in this age group, and in 1957 Childress[23] successfully treated three femoral fractures under spinal anesthesia. In 1971

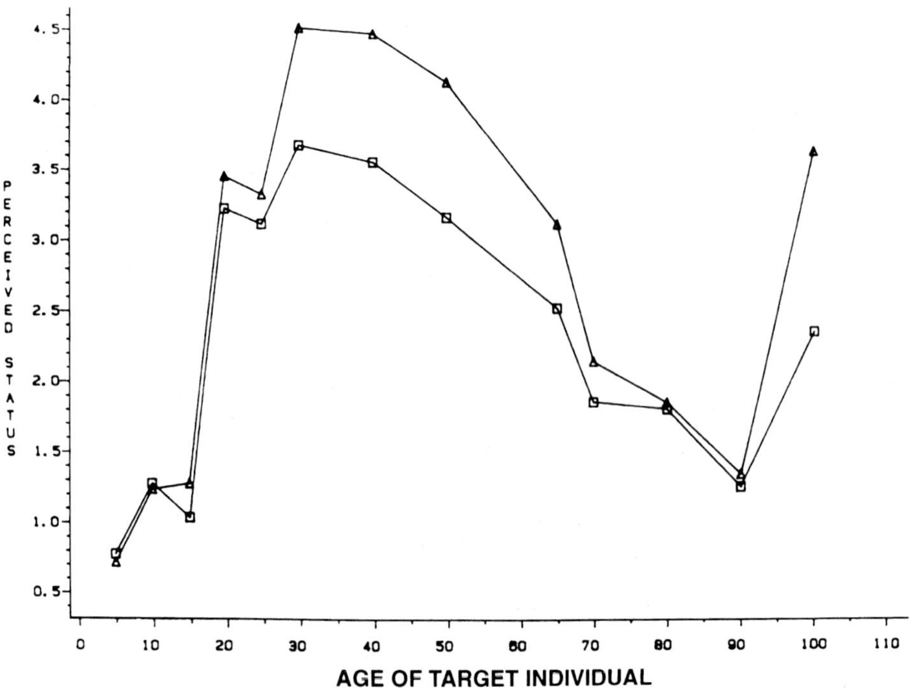


FIGURE 17.1. Perceived status by age and sex of target individual. Triangles, men; squares, women. (From Baker,[2] with permission.)

isolated cases of pacemaker placement[24] and below-knee amputation[25] were reported. A basket-size ovarian leiomyoma was excised from a 103-year-old woman because of bowel obstruction in 1979, allowing her to live at least two additional years.[26] Six patients aged 100–106 underwent pacemaker procedures with good results in the 1989 report of Cobler et al.[27]

During the 1990s a somewhat larger number of patients were reported. There were three deaths (12.5% mortality) in McCann and Smith's series of 24 patients undergoing a variety of operations, such as colon resection, ruptured aortic aneurysm repair, and hip prosthesis placement.[28] Cogbill et al.'s 1992 series of 16 patients reported perioperative mortality of 6% and a 1-year survival of 69% after a variety of small operations.[29] This author reported a series of major and minor procedures in 6 patients aged 100–104 years, all of whom survived (Table 17.1).[30] The illustrative cases below are from that series.

## Case Studies

### Case 1

A 100-year-old woman fractured her right hip in a nursing home fall. She had a history of myocardial infarction, congestive heart failure, aortic stenosis, arthritis, and hiatus hernia. She had previously undergone cataract surgery, cystocele repair, and open reduction/internal fixation of a left hip fracture. Open reduction/internal fixation of her new fracture was performed under general anesthesia. During her second postoperative week she developed acute gangrenous cholecystitis, requiring emergency cholecystectomy. This episode was complicated by left lower lobe pneumonia, which resulted in antibiotic treatment, and by a localized intraabdominal abscess, which was successfully treated with percutaneous drainage and antibiotics. Six weeks after admission she returned to her nursing home. Protruding Enders rod pins in her right leg led to pin removal under local anesthesia 8 months later.

At 101 years of age, she underwent elective endoscopic resection of a rectal villous adenoma containing carcinoma in situ. Postoperative bleeding from the resection site mandated suture ligation under general anesthesia. She returned to her nursing home, where she later died, 2 weeks before her 103rd birthday.

### Case 2

A 100-year-old retired laborer was ambulatory at his nursing home until his toes became painful. He had a history of hypertension, chronic lung disease, and severe peripheral vascular disease and had undergone prostatectomy. On examination, he had a gangrenous right foot with *Proteus* cellulitis extending to the calf and an absence of leg pulses below the femoral arteries. He underwent amputation of the right leg above the knee while under general anesthesia (spinal anesthesia was aborted because of the patient's agitation) and was discharged 11 days later. He had one later 4-day admission for bronchitis and died at age 101 years of "old age."

## Case 3

A 101-year-old woman was ambulatory and independent at home but suffered from a large right inguinal hernia. Her past history included congestive heart failure, atrial fibrillation, adult-onset diabetes mellitus, blindness, and a resected basal cell carcinoma of the face. Elective right inguinal herniorrhaphy was completed under local anesthesia in the outpatient surgical unit. Postoperatively, stating that she would "rather wear out than rust out," she took a 3-month cruise around the world and later lectured at a local college geriatric course. On the penultimate day of her life she completed a political poll. She died of congestive heart failure at age 102.

## Discussion

Centenarians recover surprisingly well from surgery, leading one to speculate that the 100-year-old patient who has not already succumbed to a myocardial infarction or pulmonary embolus is less likely to do so, even in the perioperative milieu. The Mayo Clinic study of

TABLE 17.1. Clinical Summary of Centenarians Undergoing an Operation

| Patient No./sex | Age (years) | Medical problems | Operation | Status | Anesthesia | Complications | Death | Follow-up |
|---|---|---|---|---|---|---|---|---|
| 1/M | 100 | Old MI, sick sinus syndrome with pacemaker, CHF, prostatectomy, cataract extraction, gout, arthritis, chronic renal failure | Pacemaker generator replacement | Urgent | Local | None | No | Died, age 102 years of CHF |
| 2/F | 100 | Old MI, left radical mastectomy (13 years), arthritis | Excision of right femoral head, cemented Moore prosthesis | Urgent | General | None | No | Died, age 102 years of cerebrovascular disease |
| 3/M | 100 | Hypertension, severe peripheral vascular disease, prostatectomy, chronic lung disease | Above-knee amputation | Urgent | General | None | No | Died, age 101 years of "old age" |
| 4/F | 100 | Old MI, CHF, aortic stenosis, cataract extraction, cystocele repair, left hip open reduction internal fixation, arthritis, hiatus hernia | Open reduction, internal fixation of right hip fracture | Urgent | General | Acute gangrenous cholecystitis, protruding Enders rod pins | No | Died, age 102 years of "old age" |
| | | | Cholecystectomy | Emergency | General | Pneumonia, resolved; abdominal abscess, percutaneously drained | | |
| | | | Removal of Enders rod pins | Elective | Local | None | | |
| | 101 | | Colonoscopic resection of villous adenoma | Elective | Local | Bleeding at excision site | | |
| | | | Suture ligation of bleeding rectal polypectomy site | Emergency | General | None | | |
| 5/F | 101 | CHF, atrial fibrillation, blind, basal cell carcinoma of face excised, adult-onset diabetes | Right inguinal herniorrhaphy | Elective | Local | None | No | Died, age 102 years of CHF |
| 6/M | 104 | Squamous cell carcinoma of neck excised, basal cell carcinoma of nose excised and irradiated | Gastroscopy with biopsy | Emergency | Local | None | No | Died, age 105 years of gastric carcinoma |

*Source:* Katlic,[30] with permission.
MI, myocardial infarction; CHF, congestive heart failure.

surgery in nonagenarians supports this finding, as neither pneumonia nor atherosclerosis with myocardial infarction was a major cause of postoperative death.[15]

Certainly all that has been learned about surgery in the elderly should be applied to the centenarian. Clinical presentation of surgical problems may be subtle, preoperative preparation is essential, and scrupulous attention to detail intraoperatively and perioperatively yields great benefit. Virtually all studies of surgery in the elderly have also shown an up to threefold greater risk for emergency surgery than elective surgery.[31] The worst complications in the author's series, pneumonia and intraabdominal abscess, did occur after emergency surgery, but the patients generally tolerated even urgent operations well.

Centenarians may be considered a natural model of successful aging. What is it about the 100-year-old that allowed him or her to enter this select age group?

## Physiologic Changes in Centenarians

The oldest-old manifest low frequencies of the E4 form of gene coding for apolipoprotein E, a protein linked to an increased risk of acquiring Alzheimer's disease. Among healthy subjects age 90–103 years, 14% had at least one E4 gene, in contrast to 25% of subjects younger than age 65.[9] It may be that many of those with E4 suffer early Alzheimer's disease and do not survive to become centenarians. This *cohort effect* may explain some of the other physiologic and pathologic changes in centenarians described below.

Morphologic changes occur in the brain with age—decreased brain weight, atrophy of the cerebral hemispheres, fall in the number of Purkinje cells in the cerebellum—but healthy aged subjects show little difference from young adults with respect to cerebral blood flow and oxygen uptake.[32] Hubbard et al. studied electroencephalograms in centenarians and found slowing of the posterior dominant rhythm, but there was no evidence of a progressive decrease in frequency between the ages of 80 and 100 years.[33] Well-preserved mucociliary clearance in the lung of a centenarian was documented by Pavia and Thomson despite 80 years of smoking history.[34]

An even more paradoxical finding was described by Mari's group.[35] They found that a high proportion of 25 healthy centenarians had laboratory evidence of activation of the coagulation system, shown by high levels of enzymes, activation peptides, and enzyme–inhibitor complexes. Levels of factor X activation peptide were equal to those found in patients with disseminated intravascular coagulation. Even procoagulant proteins such as fibrinogen and factor VIII—predictors of cardiovascular disease in young adults—were elevated in centenarians; yet these individuals had no current or past thrombotic events. The authors concluded that significant alterations of these markers are still compatible with health and long life. A more recent study by this group found that the 4G allele and 4G 4G genotype associated with elevated levels of plasminoe activator inhibitor 1 (PAI-1), which predicts recurrence of myocardial infarction in young men, were even more frequent in centenarians than young adults. The homozygous genotype for the deletion of polymorphism of the angiotensin-converting enzymes, which predisposes to coronary artery disease, is also paradoxically more frequent in centenarians than in adults age 20–70 years.[36] Mannucci et al. speculated that occult factors compensate for these putatively unfavorable genotypes in centenarians (e.g., linkage dysequilibrium with a locus counteracting the bad effect of elevated PAI-1 levels offsets the risk of hypofibrinolysis). It may be that if an elderly person has already escaped thrombotic disease it is advantageous to have decreased fibrinolysis.[37] A different genetic finding in centenarians—decreased frequency of the E4 allele of the gene, which encodes apolipoprotein E—would go along with decreased risk of ischemic heart disease.[36]

Laboratory values in healthy centenarians may differ even from those of younger elderly adults: widening of the range for sodium levels to 132–146 mmol/L, slightly higher potassium and chloride, decreased total calcium, slight increase in ionized calcium, increased blood glucose, increased alkaline phosphatase and lactate dehydrogenase, slightly decreased bilirubin and total protein, increased amylase likely due to decreased renal function, increased serum urea nitrogen and slightly increased creatinine, increased urinary albumin, elevated urate, decreased albumin, elevated carcinoembryonic antigen, decreased cholesterol and triglycerides, decreased vitamin $B_{12}$, decreased zinc, slightly decreased thyroxine, increased prolactin, no change in corticotropin, decreased testosterone and estradiol, marked decrease in dehydroepiandrosterone, decreased progesterone, unchanged cortisol, slightly higher gastrin, lower erythrocyte, leukocyte, and platelet counts, and slight decreases in hemoglobin, hematocrit, and iron.[38] Discussion of possible mechanisms for these findings is beyond the scope of this chapter.

Franceschi et al. asserted that a complex remodeling of the immune system occurs in healthy centenarians in contrast to the presumed progressive deterioration (especially with the T cell branch).[39] Peripheral blood T cells and major T cell subsets are only slightly decreased despite age-related thymic involution. B lymphocytes are deceased despite data that several immunoglobulin classes are elevated in the serum. Interestingly, peripheral blood lymphocytes in centenarians appear resistant to the oxidative stress that causes irreversible cell damage in younger individuals; such stress may retard entrance into the cell cycle rather than cause permanent damage.[40]

Centenarians are more likely to have low body weight,[41] possibly due to loss of muscle and fat[42]; a number of investigators have reported short stature even when the effects of aging are considered. Both male and female centenarians are more likely to have feminine or androgynous personality traits, rather than masculine ones and are more likely to have a type B behavior pattern (easygoing).[44]

## Pathology in Centenarians

Although atherosclerosis has been found in coronary, cerebral, femoral, and abdominal aortas of centenarians,[44] the ascending aorta may be spared.[41,45] Myocardial fibrosis is located chiefly in the left ventricle and septum, and cardiac amyloid deposition is characteristic.[43] Pneumonia was found in 15 of 23 patients in Ishii and Sternby's series and was also the most common cause of death.[43] Alveolar ectasia and decreased elastic fiber were also seen in the lungs. Interestingly, recent or old thromboembolism in the pulmonary arterial tree was common at autopsy despite the absence of clinical pulmonary emboli during life.[43]

In the kidney, chronic pyelonephritis and atherosclerosis are usually pronounced; and the testes, ovaries, and uterus show atrophic changes.[46] In the gastrointestinal tract the liver also shows atrophy, and colonic diverticula are common. Gallstones are common (13/23 patients), and peptic ulcer is rare.[46] Osteoporosis is common.[47]

Cancer as a cause of death was unusual in Ishii and Sternby's autopsy series[47]; it represented 7.1% of Santo et al.'s 99 autopsies in centenarians,[48] and 31% of Klatt and Meyer's 32 patients.[49] The 7.1% rate in Santo et al.'s series was significantly different ($p < 0.001$) from that in age groups 75–90 years (25%) and 95–99 years (9.5%). Metastases in this series were found in 23.5% of the centenarians with cancer and 63.2% of those 75–90 years old; local infiltration did not differ among groups. Many of the cancers in centenarians (70%) were undiagnosed during life, a fact that may explain the exceptionally low incidence of cancer (4%) as a cause of death in epidemiologic studies.[50] Of all the types of cancer, only the prevalence of gallbladder adenocarcinoma was increased in Santo et al.'s series.[48] In summary, cancer in the oldest-old is less frequent and less aggressive.

## Determinants of Extreme Longevity

Despite our fascination with centenarians, little is known about the influences—genetic, environmental, medical—on their longevity. Vaupel's group, in extensive studies of nearly 3000 Danish twin pairs born during 1870–1900 estimated the heritability of longevity to be 0.26 for men and 0.23 for women; the sex difference resulted from the greater impact of unshared environmental factors in the women.[51] Earlier family studies had shown weak correlations for life-span between parents and offspring (0.01–0.05) and somewhat higher correlations between siblings (0.15–0.35),[52] suggesting either that the genetic factors are nonadditive (genetic intralocus interaction) or there is a higher degree of shared environmental influences among siblings than parents.

TABLE: 17.2. Determinants of Extreme Life-span in the Industrialized World

| |
|---|
| **Genetics: genes coding for** |
| Human leukocyte antigens HLA-DR (?) |
| Apolipoprotein E (?) |
| Angiotensin-converting enzyme (ACE) (?) |
| **Environment** |
| Year of birth |
| Smoking (?) |
| Alcohol (?) |
| Diet (?) |
| **Medicine** |
| Dehydroepiandrosterone (DHEA) (?) |

Several specific genetic factors have been associated with extremely long life. In a study of Japanese centenarians, Takata et al.[53] showed a significantly lower frequency of HLA-DRw9 and a higher frequency of HLA-DR1 among centenarians compared to younger adults; these antigens are negatively associated with autoimmune diseases in Japan, suggesting mediation of the genetic influence through a lower incidence of disease. The low prevalence of the E4 allele of apolipoprotein E and increased prevalence of the DD genotype for angiotensin-converting enzyme have been mentioned above.[37] The mediation of genetic influences on longevity via genetic influences on smoking and body mass index—two factors associated with longevity in epidemiologic studies—was disproved by Herschind et al.[54] Even smoking status has shown no definite association with extreme longevity, nor has alcohol consumption, diet, or exercise.[55] Environmental factors such as socioeconomic status and early life nutrition appear to have little influence.[56] Although no "fountain of youth" medicine has been discovered, the inverse correlation of blood levels of dehydroepiandrosterone (DHEA) with mortality has prompted ongoing clinical trials of its administration.[57]

In summary, it is likely that a large number of factors interact to determine longevity, three-fourths of them environmental (Table 17.2). The involvement of a number of genes, each contributing a little, might influence longevity directly or, more likely, through determining susceptibility to disease at different ages.

## Selective Survival Hypothesis

*A 100-year-old is as likely to survive surgery as are his sons and daughters, and one may speculate that he is even more likely to do so. The man or woman who has endured ten decades of life's labors enters a select*

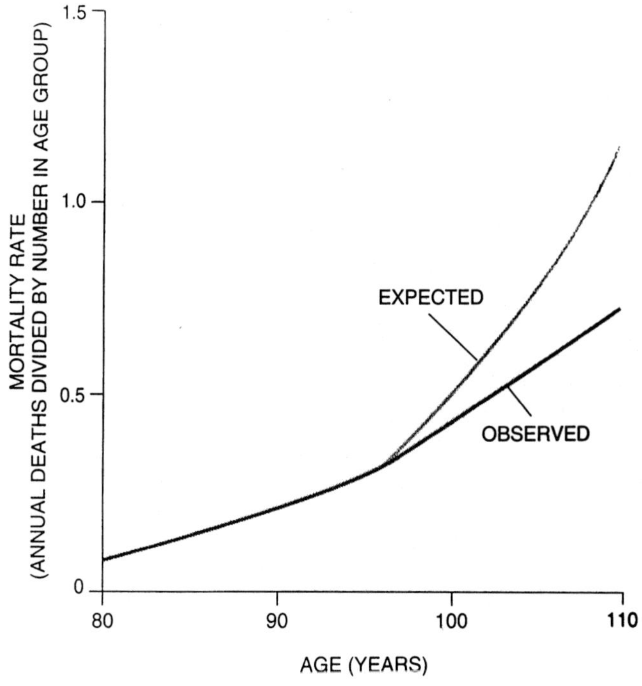


FIGURE 17.2. Observed mortality rate slows after age 97 years compared to the expected mortality rate. (From Perls,[10] with permission.)

*group whose physiological resilience is greater than that of many who are chronologically younger.—M.R. Katlic, 1985*[30]

This selective survival concept was discussed by Thomas Perls, principal investigator with the New England Centenarian Study.[9] Perls postulated, supported by his research and that of others, that certain individuals are resistant to the diseases that cripple and kill most people before age 90. These individuals not only live longer lives, they also live relatively free of infirmities.

Mortality rates for centenarians, for example, are lower than would be anticipated by extrapolating the death rates of younger adults. Mortality can be reasonably predicted up to approximately age 80, but the linear decline in health not only slows at advanced age but varies more among individuals, thus selecting the most fit.[58] Selection is more than sufficient to overcome the effects of aging and is greater in men, probably because of their higher mortality at younger ages.[59,60] This "gender crossover" resulting from the selection of fit men can be seen as early as age 80 but is more evident in centenarians: men make up 20% of 100-year-olds and 40% of 105-year-olds. Age 95–97 years appears to be the age at which a person's chance of dying increases in a linear rather than an exponential manner with time (Fig. 17.2).[9] Carey et al. found the same phenomenon in medflies.[61] Whether due to compositional change in the cohort (selection of the fittest) or better intrinsic cellular defense mechanisms (see peripheral blood lymphocyte data above), the very old have a higher threshold for acquiring disease and a decreased mortality rate, allowing them not only to survive but to do so in relatively good health (Fig. 17.3). In 1990 the Medicare costs for those who died at age 70 was $6475 during each of the last 5 years of life compared to $1800 per year for those who died at age 100.[62] In 1995 medical expenses for the last 2 years of life average $22,600 for people who died at age 70 and $8300 for those who died after age 100.[5]

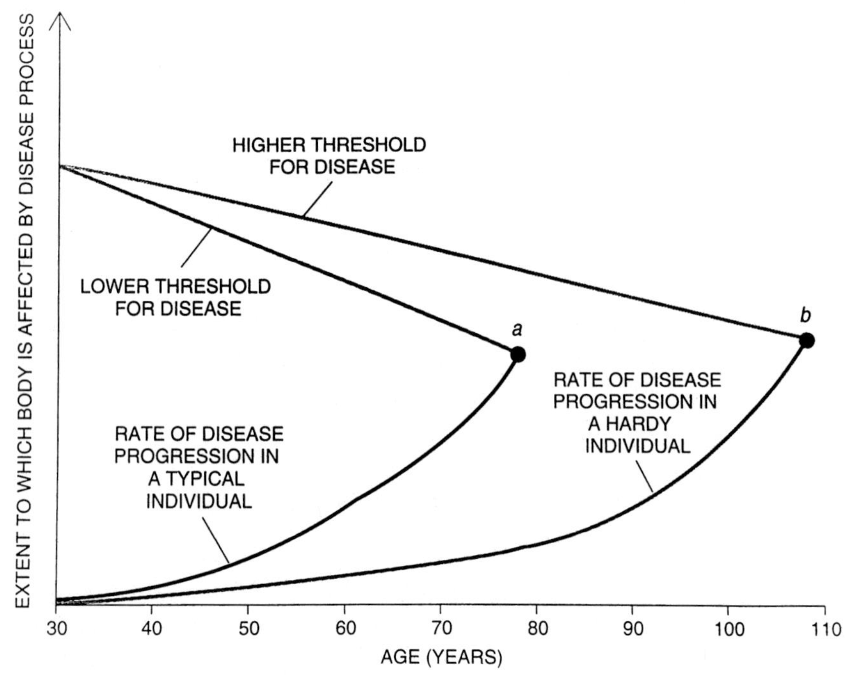


FIGURE 17.3. High threshold for acquiring disease and slow aging process may promote survival because of the good health of centenarians. (From Perls,[9] with permission.)

## Conclusions

Certainly all that has been learned about surgery in the elderly should be applied to the centenarian: clinical presentation of surgical problems may be subtle, preoperative preparation is essential, emergency surgery carries high risk compared to elective operation, and scrupulous attention to detail intraoperatively and perioperatively yields great benefit. It is not unreasonable to speculate that the 100-year-old who has not already succumbed to a myocardial infarction or pulmonary embolus is unlikely to do so, even during the perioperative period. Survival to the centenary indicates that one has been tested by life and has been found exceptionally fit. Elective surgery should not be deferred nor emergency surgery denied the centenarian on the basis of chronologic age.

## References


1. Beard BB. Centenarians: The New Generation. Greenwood Press: Westport, CT, 1991:3.
2. Baker PM. The status of age: preliminary results. J Gerontol 1985;40:506–508.
3. Webb R, Williams LM. Centenarian hand syndrome [letter]. N Engl J Med 1985;313:188.
4. Matalon JM (Associated Press). World's oldest person dies. The Times Leader: Wilkes Barre, PA, August 5, 1997.
5. Cowley G. How to live to 100. Newsweek, June 30, 1997:56–67.
6. Vaupel JW, Jeune B. The emergence and proliferation of centenarians. In: Jeune B, Vaupel JW (eds) Exceptional Longevity: From Prehistory to the Present. Odense University Press: Odense, Denmark, 1995.
7. United States Bureau of the Census. America's Centenarians. Current Population Reports. Series P-23, No 153. US Government Printing Office: Washington, DC, 1987.
8. Windom RE. From the assistant secretary for health. JAMA 1988;259:2201.
9. Perls TT. The oldest old. Sci Am 1995;January:70–75.
10. Ahlburg DA, Vaupel JW. Alternative projections of the U.S. population. Demography 1990;27:639–651.
11. Vaupel JW, Gowan AE. Passage to Methuselah: some demographic consequences of continued progress against mortality. Am J Public Health 1986;76:430–433.
12. Smith OC. Advanced age as a contraindication to operation. Med Rec (NY) 1907;72:642–644.
13. Ochsner A. Is risk of operation too great in the elderly? Geriatrics 1967;22:121–130.
14. Brooks B. Surgery in patients of advanced age. Ann Surg 1937;105:481–495.
15. Warner MA, Hosking MP, Lobdell CM, et al. Surgical procedures among those ≥90 years of age. Ann Surg 1988;207: 380–386.
16. Cohen JR, Johnson H, Eton S, et al. Surgical procedures in patients during the 10th decade of life. Surgery 1988;104: 646–651.
17. Coyle KA, Smith RB, Salam AA, et al. Carotid endarterectomy in the octogenarian. Ann Vasc Surg 1994;8:417–420.
18. Chalmers RTA, Stonebridge PA, John TG, Murie JA. Abdominal aortic aneurysm in the elderly. Br J Surg 1993;80: 1122–1123.
19. Blanche C, Matloff JM, Denton TA, et al. Cardiac operations in patients 90 years of age and older. Ann Thorac Surg 1997;63:1685–1690.
20. Alexander HR, Turnball AD, Salamon J, et al. Upper abdominal cancer surgery in the very elderly. J Surg Oncol 1991;47:82–86.
21. Welch CE, Whittemore WS. Carcinoma of the rectum in a centenarian. N Engl J Med 1954;250:1041–1042.
22. Maycock PP, Burns CM. Prostatic surgery in centenarians. J Urol 1955;74:546–548.
23. Childress HM. Hip fractures in patients over 100 years of age. New York J Med 1957;57:1604–1606.
24. Grayzel J. Pacemaker in a centenarian [letter]. JAMA 1971;218:95.
25. Milliken RA, Milliken GM. Centenarian surgery [letter]. JAMA 1971;218:1435.
26. Sapala JA, Sapala MA. Excision of a large ovarian leiomyoma in a centenarian. Henry Ford Hosp Med J 1983;31: 37–39.
27. Cobler JL, Akiyama T, Murphy GW. Permanent pacemakers in centenarians. J Am Geriatr Soc 1989;37:753–756.
28. McCann WJ, Smith JW. The surgical care of centenarians. Curr Surg 1990;47:2–3.
29. Cogbill TH, Strutt PJ, Landercasper J. Surgical procedures in centenarians. Wisc Med J 1992;91:527–529.
30. Katlic MR. Surgery in centenarians. JAMA 1985;253:3139–3141.
31. Linn BS, Linn MW, Wallen N. Evaluation of results of surgical procedures in the elderly. Ann Surg 1982;195:90–96.
32. Brody H. Aging of the vertebrate brain. In: Rockstein M, Sussman ML (eds) Development and Aging in the Nervous System. Academic: San Diego, 1973:121–133.
33. Hubbard O, Sunde D, Goldensohn ES. The EEG in centenarians. Electroencephalogr Clin Neurophysiol 1976;40: 407–417.
34. Pavia D, Thomson ML. Unimpaired mucociliary clearance in the lung of a centenarian smoker. Lancet 1970;663:101–102.
35. Mari D, Mannucci PM, Coppola R, et al. Hypercoagulability in centenarians: the paradox of successful aging. Blood 1995;85:3144–3149.
36. Schacter F, Faure-Delanef L, Guenot F, et al. Genetic associations with human longevity at the APOE and ACE loci. Nat Genet 1994;6:29–32.
37. Mannucci PM, Mari D, Merati G, et al. Gene polymorphism predicting high plasma levels of coagulation and fibrinolysis proteins: a study in centenarians. Arterioscler Thromb Vasc Biol 1997;17:755–759.
38. Tietz NW, Shuey DF, Wekstein DR. Laboratory values in fit aging individuals: sexagenarians through centenarians. Clin Chem 1992;38:1167–1185.
39. Franceschi C, Monti D, Sansoni P, Cossarizza A. The immunology of exceptional individuals: the lesson of centenarians. Immunol Today 1995;16:12–16.
40. Franceschi C, Monti D, Cossarizza A, et al. Aging, longevity and cancer: studies in Down's syndrome and centenarians. Ann NY Acad Sci 1991;621:428–440.

41. Lowbeer L. Autopsy pathology in centenarians [letter]. Arch Pathol Lab Med 1987;111:784.
42. Ravaglia G, Morini P, Forti P, et al. Anthropometric characteristics of healthy Italian nonagenarians and centenarians. Br J Nutr 1997;77:9–17.
43. Ishii T, Sternby NH. Pathology of centenarians. I. The cardiovascular system and lungs. J Am Geriatr Soc 1978;26:108–115.
44. Shimonalia Y, Nakazato K, Homma A. Personality, longevity and successful aging among Tokyo metropolitan centenarians. Int J Aging Hum Dev 1996;42:173–187.
45. Klatt EC, Meyer PR. Autopsy pathology in centenarians [letter]. Arch Pathol Lab Med 1987;111:784.
46. Ishii T, Sternby NH. Pathology of centenarians. II. Urogenital and digestive systems. J Am Geriatr Soc 1978;26:391–396.
47. Ishii T, Sternby NH. Pathology of centenarians. III. Osseous system malignant lesions, and causes of death. J Am Geriatr Soc 1978;26:529–533.
48. Santa G, Campagna L, Cavallieri F, Giarelli L. Cancer of the oldest old: what have we learned from autopsy studies. Clin Geriatr Med 1997;13:55–68.
49. Klatt EC, Meyer PR. Geriatric autopsy pathology in centenarians. Arch Pathol Lab Med 1987;111:367–369.
50. Smith DWE. Cancer mortality at very old ages. Cancer 1996;77:1367.
51. Herschind AM, McGue M, Holm NV, et al. The heretability of human longevity: a population-based study of 2872 Danish twin pairs 1870–1900. Hum Genet 1996;97:319–323.
52. Wyshuk G. Fertility and longevity in twins, sibs, and parents of twins. Soc Biol 1978;25:315–330.
53. Takata H, Suzuki M, Ishii T, et al. Influence of major histocompatibility complex region on human longevity among Okinawan Japanese centenarians and nonagenarians. Lancet 1987;2:824–826.
54. Herschind AM, McGue M, Iachive IA, et al. Untangling genetic influences on smoking, body mass index and longevity: a multivariate study of 2464 Danish twins followed for 28 years. Hum Genet 1996;98:467–475.
55. Christensen K, Vaupel JW. Determinants of longevity: genetic environmental and medical factors. J Intern Med 1996;240:333–341.
56. McGue M, Vaupel JW, Holm N, Harvald B. Longevity is moderately heritable in a sample of Danish twins from 1870–1880. J Gerontol 1993;48:37–244.
57. Herbert J. The age of dehydroepiandrosterone. Lancet 1995;345:1193–1194.
58. Economos AC. Rate of aging, rate of dying and the mechanism of mortality. Arch Gerontol Geriatr 1982;1:3–27.
59. Barrett JC. Longevity of selected centenarians. Lancet 1984;Nov 2;1:1032.
60. Barrett JC. The mortality of centenarians in England and Wales. Arch Gerontol Geriatr 1985;4:211–218.
61. Carey JR, Liedo P, Orozio D, Vaupel JW. Slowing of mortality rates at older ages in large medfly cohorts. Science 1992;258:457–461.
62. Lubitz J, Beebe J, Baker C. Longevity and Medicare expenditures. N Engl J Med 1995;332:999–1003.

# *Part II*
# *Specific Issues in Geriatric Surgery*

## Section 1
## Critical Care and Trauma

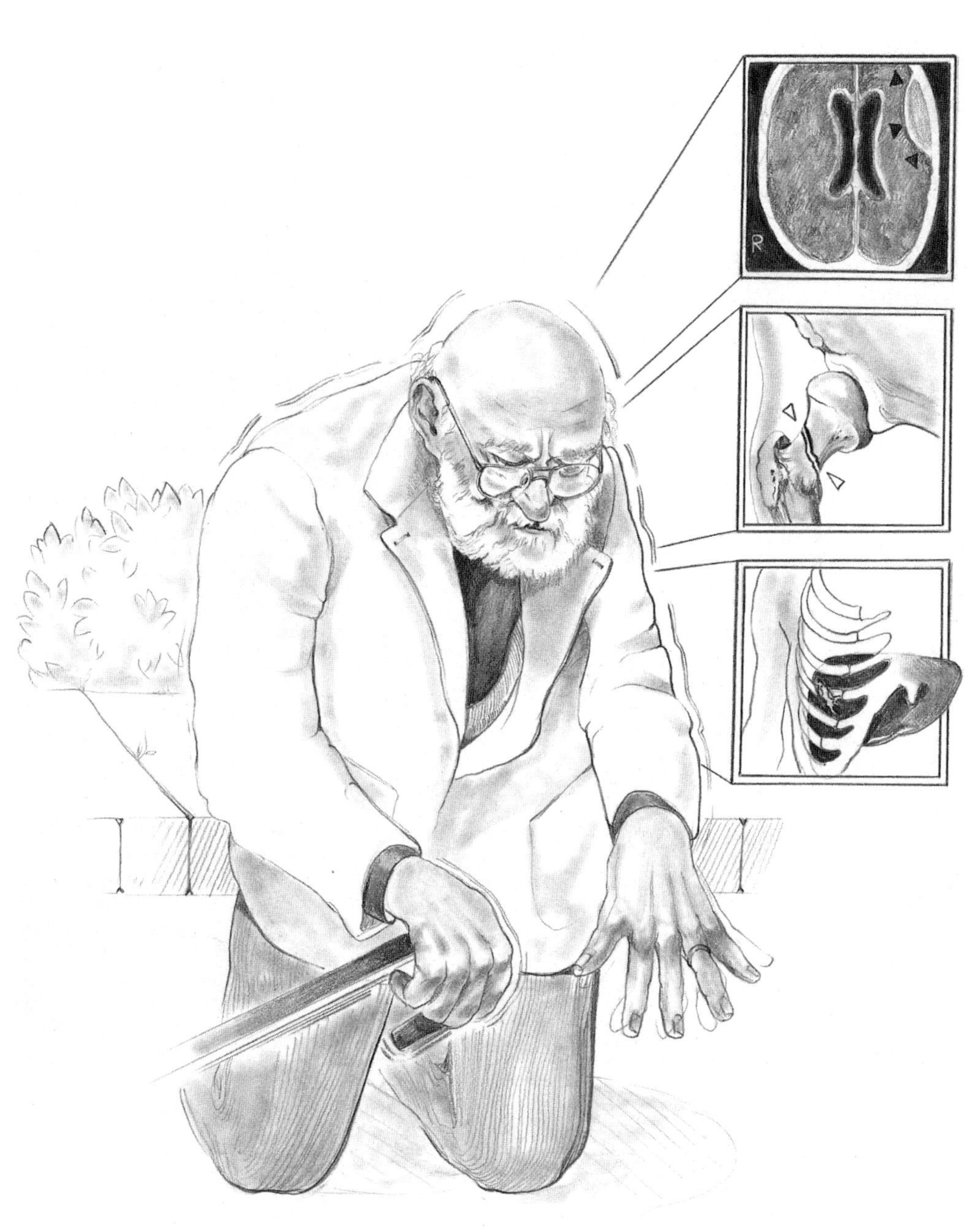

# Invited Commentary

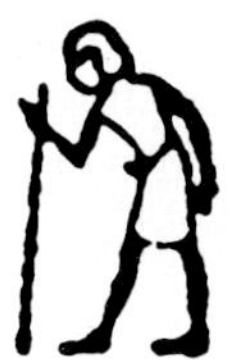

G. Tom Shires

The development of intensive care and modern trauma care has progressed remarkably since 1960. These advances in patient care have been produced by several disciplines over the past 30–40 years.

A number of developments occurred during the twentieth century that were essential to the development of care of the traumatized patient and critical care.[1] Some of those necessary advances include the following.

1900 Blood typing (Landsteiner)
1901 Imaging (Roentgen)
1923 Intensive care unit (ICU; neurologic), first ICU
1940 Ventilation (Denmark), developed originally to manage the polio epidemic
1940 Dialysis (Kolff)
1940 Antibiotics
1953 Open heart surgery
1956 Defibrillator (Zoll)
1960 Cardiopulmonary resuscitation (CPR) (Kouivenhoven)
1960 Adult ICU and cardiac care unit (CCU)
1965 95% Hospital ICU
1970 Triage, resuscitation, fluids, acute respiratory distress syndrome diagnoses (ARDS)
1971 Ultrasonography
1972 Computed tomography (CT) scanning
1973 Magnetic resonance imaging (MRI)
1980 Thrombolytic therapy
1981 Organ transplantation

As technologic advances in many fields, including biology occur, success becomes difficult to measure. In a milestone study reported in 1976, Comroe and Dripps described the scientific basis for the support of biomedical research.[2] These respected investigators examined clinical advances since the early 1940s, specifically in the field of cardiovascular and pulmonary diseases. The top 10 clinical advances in cardiovascular and pulmonary medicine and surgery during the past 30 years were evolved by asking 40 physicians to list the advances they considered the most important for their patients. These selections were then divided and sent to another 50 specialists in each field asking each to vote on the list and add additional advances they believed belonged on the list. Their votes selected the top 10 advances. With the help of 140 consultants, Comroe and Dripps identified the essential bodies of knowledge that had to be developed before each of the 10 clinical advances could reach their current state of achievement.

As their study pointed out, general anesthesia was first put to use in 1846, and it was not until 107 years later that John Gibbon performed the first successful operation on an open heart with complete cardiopulmonary bypass. For all 10 advances they identified 137 essential bodies of knowledge. To arrive at these conclusions they examined 4000 published articles; 2500 specific scientific reports were particularly important to the development of one or more of the 137 essential bodies of knowledge. From this, 529 key articles were selected as prerequisite background to this one significant clinical advance.

## Funding

A major reason for success in research by the surgical biologist relates to funding of biomedical research. Prior to World War II research played a relatively minor role in the nation at large and certainly in academic institutions. The total national expenditure for medical research in 1940 was $45 million of which more than half was expended by and within industry, mainly for privately oriented research. The federal government's investment in biomedical research amounted to only $3 million; today that figure is more than $16 billion. Although a number of important advances resulted from medical research during the pre-World War II era, particularly in regard to control of infectious diseases by immunization, the rate of discovery was slow by recent standards. The 25-year period between 1945 and 1970 was a golden era in biomedical research during which substantial financial support and enormous advances in the prevention and treatment of disease were accomplished. James A. Shannon,[3] the remarkable director of the National Institutes of Health (NIH) at this time, developed the support and the peer review system that persists today.

## Clinical Advances

Similarly, in the previously noted 1976 report, Comroe and Dripps stated, "it is easy to select examples in which basic undirected nonclinical research led to dramatic advances in clinical medicine and equally easy to give examples in which either clinically oriented research or development was all important." In that study, 41% of all work to be judged essential for later clinical advance was not clinically oriented at the time it was done. Consequently, it seems clear that patient care-initiated basic or applied research will be the future cutting edge for advances in care, as 60% of all such work was clinically related.

When turning to specific injuries and patient care, obviously a large number of factors have led to improved survival. One could list such items as improvement in early diagnosis, early use of restoration of body fluids with blood and electrolyte solutions, early presumptive use of antibiotics, intensive care modes of respiratory, renal, and hepatic support, and improvement in operative techniques themselves. Some examples of specific improvements can be cited.

The concept of a constant internal environment was first articulated by the great French physiologist Claude Bernard. Bernard stated, "the stability of the milieu intérieur is the primary condition for freedom and independence of existence: the mechanism which allows of this is that which insures in the milieu intérieur the maintenance of all the conditions necessary to the life of the elements." The constancy of the internal environment is protected by multiple intrinsic mechanisms, including renal, pulmonary, hepatic, and even cell membrane function.[4] Walter Cannon, a professor of physiology at Harvard, subsequently evolved the term homeostasis, which led to the concept that fitness for survival is directly related to the capacity of an organism to maintain homeostasis.[5] From this concept evolved the biologic precept that extracellular fluid, including the circulation, is the true milieu of life because it enables the cells of the body to function.

One of the earliest attempts at resuscitation was carried out by administering large volumes of salt solutions intravenously. Latta[6] and O'Shaughnessy[7] treated cholera victims by giving them large volumes of salt solutions intravenously in 1831. This was one of the first documented attempts to replace and maintain the extracellular internal environment.

During World War I, a variety of theories existed concerning the cause of vascular collapse in injured patients. It was assumed that vascular collapse was caused primarily by toxins. In a unique set of experiments begun by Blalock,[8] it was determined that almost all acute injuries are associated with changes in fluid and electrolyte metabolism. These studies showed that the alterations were primarily the result of reductions in the effective circulating blood volume. However, reduction in the effective circulating volume following injury may be the result of loss of blood, as with hemorrhage; loss of vascular tone, as with sepsis or neurogenic shock; pump failure as with cardiac tamponade or myocardial infarction; or loss of large volumes of extracellular fluid (ECF), as in patients with diarrhea, vomiting, or fistula drainage. Blalock's studies clearly showed that fluid loss in injured tissues was loss of extracellular fluid, which was now unavailable to the intravascular space for maintenance of circulation. The original concept of a "third space" in which fluid would be sequestered and therefore unavailable to the intravascular space evolved from those studies.

By the time World War II occurred, plasma became the favored resuscitative solution in addition to whole-blood replacement. The concept that a limited amount of salt and water should be given to a patient after surgical or other injuries, however, prevailed through the Korean War. This was largely due to the work of Coller and Moyer in experiments at the University of Michigan.[9] These capable surgical investigators showed what was called, "salt intolerance in response to operative trauma." We reproduced these data but overcame the "intolerance" by adequate replacement of ECF with a saline mimic.[10] These patients had developed ECF volume deficit due to the trauma; consequently, renal retention of sodium and water was physiologically a desirable response to surgery. The mechanism of this response was later shown to be mediated via aldosterone for sodium retention and antidiuretic hormone (ADH) for water retention.

The exact mechanism for the electrolyte changes and the marked diminution in extracellular water that follows hemorrhagic shock is now better understood. It appears that they may well represent a reduction in the efficiency of an active ionic pump mechanism at the cellular level, a selective increase in muscle cell membrane permeability to sodium, or both.[11]

Detailed reviews of resuscitation after thousands of civilian injuries have been reported with excellent results. Similarly, large numbers of battle casualties have been resuscitated using newer forms of resuscitation. A review of Vietnam battle casualty resuscitations led Hardaway to write, "Intravenous blood and fluid administration is the single most important factor in the treatment of shock."[12]

Although the mortality rate of seriously injured patients in Vietnam approximate those in Korea (2.5%), the wounded-to-killed ratio was very different. In

Vietnam the ratio was 6:1, whereas in Korea it was 3:1. This dramatically indicates that better resuscitation methods resulted in more patients surviving combat injuries.

It is only recently that the concept of maintaining adequate homeostasis by volume resuscitation beyond replacement of shed blood became an acceptable practice. During World War II acute tubular necrosis was a common consequence of hypovolemic shock, but because of the liberal use of fluid resuscitation during the Vietnam War, the incidence of acute tubular necrosis dramatically decreased.[13] Data have shown that posttraumatic renal failure in Vietnam was approximately 1 in every 1867 combat casualties, whereas in Korea the incidence of posttraumatic renal failure was approximately 1 per 200 casualties.

With advances in the management of hemorrhagic shock and support of circulatory and renal function in injured patients, more patients survived and 1–2% of significantly injured patients (with previously normal lungs) developed acute respiratory failure during the postinjury period. Initially this lung injury was thought to be related specifically to the shock state and its resuscitation. It was called "shock lung" and "traumatic wet lung," which have been applied to acute respiratory insufficiency following injury. It is now recognized that there are many similarities in the pathophysiology and clinical presentation of acute lung injury following a variety of insults, resulting in the realization that the lung has a limited number of ways to react to injury. Several different causes of acute diffuse lung injury are the result of similar pathophysiologic response. The common denominator of this response appears to be damage at the alveolar–capillary interface, with resulting leakage of proteinaceous fluid from the intravascular space into the interstitium and subsequently into alveolar spaces. A variety of factors have subsequently been implicated as capable of producing adult respiratory distress syndrome (ARDS) or pulmonary failure following injury and resuscitation: (1) sepsis syndrome (80%); (2) aspiration (5%); (3) pulmonary contusion (5%); (4) multiple fractures; (5) multiple transfusions; and (6) drowning or near-drowning (factors 4–6 combined, 10%).[14]

For burn injuries many specific factors can be reasonably assessed. The mortality, by percent of body surface burn, before and after the use of topical chemotherapy has been reviewed. In the salvageable burn category, the mortality rate (which was as high as 50%) was essentially halved by the introduction of topical chemotherapy.[15] The development of the Parkland formula by Baxter and Shires[16] clearly resulted in reduced mortality from the initial shock phases of burn injury with adequate fluid replacement in an orderly fashion.

As Donald Trunkey pointed out, the facts remain that one-half of all trauma deaths occur before hospitalization, and many are from fatal multiple injuries, including head injury.[17] This situation emphasizes the urgent need for injury prevention. The remaining half of trauma deaths occur in the hospital; and of these, 62% occur within the first 4 hours of hospitalization, emphasizing the peak of necessity for early, adequate correction of fluid and electrolyte balance as well as supportive care and prompt surgical intervention. The third death peak after trauma occurs late in the remaining approximately 20% of all trauma deaths. Most of these deaths are due to sepsis and multiple organ failure. Consequently, it is clear that the need to prevent and control sepsis is a major issue for improvement of survival following injury.

The isolation and characterization of bacterial endotoxin/lipopolysaccharide (LPS) by Shear and Turner (1943) led to the subsequent delineation of pathophysiologic responses attributable to LPS. Wide derangements of organ function and cellular homeostasis characterized by acute inflammatory responses, altered energy metabolism, and lethal tissue injury are observed after LPS administration. It is now known that many (if not all) of these effects are mediated by humoral factors released in response to endotoxemia. Our laboratory was the first to show the role of tumor necrosis factor (TNF) in vivo. The role of the macrophage-secreted protein TNF-$\alpha$ as an early or proximal mediator of the deleterious event induced by LPS was the first of the cytokines to be incriminated when in excess. Subsequently, many proinflammatory and antiinflammatory cytokine receptors have been described. Antiinflammatory cytokines have also been identified.

During the mid-to-late 1990s, a number of articles have examined the effects of intensive care and critical care on injured elderly patients. One such study was reported by Battistella et al. at the University of California-Davis, in which they examined, with long-term follow-up, patients who had sustained trauma and who were 75 years and older.[18] As the authors pointed out, patients at this age represent one of the fastest growing subsegments of the geriatric population. Although trauma ranks only seventh among the leading causes of death in patients 75 years and older, it is well known and documented that these patients face higher mortality rates, longer hospital stays and more complications after trauma, thereby consuming more trauma dollars than their younger counterparts. The UC-Davis study was long term and compared the results following trauma and critical care in these patients. It revealed that despite the higher expected mortality after discharge, aggressive management of patients 75 years and older was justified by their favorable long-term outcome. On a Kaplan-Meier survival curve, the comparison for survival up to 90 months was comparable to the actuarial survival curve. The authors summarized their study by saying that aggressive treatment in the oldest subgroup of trauma patients was justified based on their favorable long-term survival and functional outcome. At least 42% of the patients were still living more than 4 years after discharge, and they were living and thriving in independent settings.

A better definition of availability of care for old patients is developing. Godley et al.[19] from Harvard, indicated that nonoperative management of adults with blunt splenic injury failed in old patients independent of other clinical and radiographic variables. Their conclusions from this large study was that patients over the age of 55 should not be treated nonoperatively in the presence of blunt splenic injury. This is in opposition to the current trend of nonoperative therapy in the young patient.

Another interesting study was that by van der Sluis et al. in The Netherlands. They evaluated the differences in mortality and long-term outcome between young and elderly patients with multiple injuries.[20] As in other studies, mortality for a given level of trauma was higher in the elderly patients, but they experienced multiple organ failure far less commonly. This study also showed that the elderly could be discharged home. Their functional outcome at the 2-year follow-up in this study did not differ from that of patients with comparable degrees of trauma in the younger age group. These authors concluded that there was no valid argument to support the idea that severely injured elderly patients should be treated any differently from their younger counterparts despite the early increased care costs.

Other studies have looked at the incidence of trauma recidivism or recurrent trauma in the elderly patient[21] and showed clearly that trauma is more recurrent in the older patient. Consequently, epidemiologic studies were undertaken and more are certainly needed to define the recidivism in the age 66 and older patient. Of the nearly 10,000 patients in this study matched for gender and age strata,[21] the injured elderly were almost twice as likely to be readmitted for injury, and this figure increased with age.

When looking at the subset of patients considered to be at risk for recurrent injury, it appears there is a discrete group of patients for whom the single most likely predictor of subsequent admission is previous injury. This obviously is an important indication of the need to develop injury prevention programs for the elderly patient.

In conclusion, care of the injured patient has advanced dramatically during the past 3 decades. More attention is being directed to the salvageability of the geriatric patient. Early studies indicate that such work would be extremely fruitful.

## References


1. Calvin JE, Habert K, Parrillo JE. Critical care in the United States: who are we and how did we get there? Crit Care Clin 1997;13:373–376.
2. Comroe JH, Dripps RD. Scientific basis for the support of biomedical science. Science 1976:192–105.
3. Shannon JA. Research in the service of man: biomedical knowledge, development and use. Document 55, US Senate, 90th Congress, 1st Session 1967:72.
4. Bernard C. An Introduction to the Study of Experimental Medicine, Green HC (transl). Macmillan: New York, 1927.
5. Cannon WB. The Wisdom of the Body. WW Norton: New York, 1937.
6. Latta R. Quoted by Weatherhill I. Case of malignant cholera in which 480 ounces of fluid were injected into the vein with success. Lancet 1831–1832;2:688.
7. O'Shaughnessy WB. Experiments on the blood in cholera. Lancet 1831–1821;1:490.
8. Blalock A. Experimental shock: the cause of low blood pressure caused by muscle injury. Arch Surg 1930;20:959.
9. Coller FA, Iob V, Vaughn HH, et al. Translocation of fluid produced by intravenous administration of isotonic salt solutions in man postoperatively. Ann Surg 1945;122:663.
10. Shires T, Jackson DE. Postoperative salt tolerance. Arch Surg 1962;84:703–706.
11. Shires GT. Current status of resuscitation: solutions including hypertonic saline. Adv Surg 1995;28:133–170.
12. Hardaway RM. Care of the wounded of the US army from 1775 to 1991. Surg Gyn Obstetrics 1992;175(1):74–88.
13. Whelton A, Doinadiq JV Jr. Post-traumatic acute renal failure in Vietnam. Johns Hopkins Med J 1969;124:95–105.
14. Shires GT III, Shires GT, Carrico CJ. Shock in Principles of Surgery, 5th ed. McGraw-Hill: New York, 1989.
15. Curreri PW, Luterman A, Braun DW Jr, et al. Burn injury: analysis of survival and hospitalization time for 937 patients. Ann Surg 1980;192:472–478.
16. Baxter CR, Shires GT. Physiological response to crystalloid resuscitation of severe burns. Ann NY Acad Sci 1968; 150:875–894.
17. Trunkey DM. What's wrong with trauma care? Bull Am Coll Surg 1999;188(3):315–316.
18. Battistella FD, Din AM, Perez L. Trauma patients 75 years and older: long-term follow-up results justify aggressive management. J Trauma 1998;44(4):618–623.
19. Godley CD, Warren RL, Sheridan RL, et al. Nonoperative management of blunt splenic injury in adults: age over 55 years as a powerful indicator for failure. J Am Coll Surg 1996;183:133–139.
20. Van der Sluis CK, Klasen HJ, Eisma WH, et al. Major trauma in young and old: what is the difference? J Trauma 1996;4:78–82.
21. Gubler KD, Maier RV, Davis R, et al. Trauma recidivism in the elderly. J Trauma 1996;4:952–956.

# 18
# Critical Care

James M. Watters and Palmer Q. Bessey

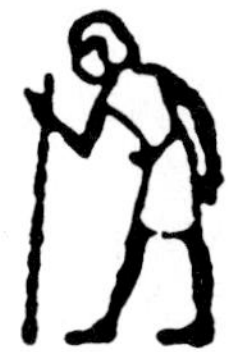

Care of the elderly patient with critical illness is frequently more challenging than that of younger patients for several reasons. Co-morbidity is more frequent and may complicate the primary problem. Treatment goals may differ markedly from those of younger patients, and the likelihood that they can be achieved may be less. Normal, age-related declines in maximal organ system function limit the ability of the elderly patient to respond to and recover from critical illness, even in the absence of chronic medical conditions. Every effort must be made to minimize unnecessary physiologic and metabolic stresses. Homeostatic mechanisms are predictably less sensitive and effective in the elderly patient, and our clinical care must be meticulous. It is the purpose of this chapter to examine how elderly patients with critical illness differ from younger patients in terms of altered physiologic and metabolic responses, clinical outcomes, decision-making, and specific therapies. Although our knowledge base is incomplete, these concepts should guide an integrated, multidisciplinary approach to the care of the elderly surgical patient who is critically ill.

Generalizations about the problems and care of the elderly surgical patient must be tempered by an appreciation of the heterogeneity of the elderly population. For example, the physiologic changes associated with normal aging are variable and are presumed to reflect genetic factors, long-term patterns of physical activity, and dietary and environmental exposures. The heterogeneity of the elderly population is even more marked when age-associated medical problems are considered as well. Some elderly persons have maintained high levels of physical, social, and intellectual activity and function independently in their communities, whereas others are frail, institutionalized, have multiple co-morbidities and limited functional status, and may be unable to recover from acute illnesses of even mild severity. Variability in the elderly population also arises simply from continued aging: The elderly population is often considered to be comprised of persons aged 65 years or more, but the physiologic reserve of a healthy individual 85 years old is substantially less than that of a 65-year-old.

Interpreting clinical reports and judging their relevance for one's own practice requires a clear description of the elderly patients studied, including the policies and criteria by which patients are accepted for intensive care unit (ICU) admission. In some studies patients or subjects are screened for clinical or occult disease, whereas in others all those who meet an age criterion are included. The specific purpose of the study or research question usually determines the extent of screening. Studies of the effects of aging or old age in surgical patients are, of necessity, most often cross-sectional in design (i.e., they examine both young and old patients at a single point in time). Such studies risk selection bias in that the older patients are "selected" as survivors; that is, patients in the older group differ from younger patients studied at the same point in time by having demonstrated an ability to survive to an older age. Bias may also occur in that elderly patients referred for consideration of a major surgical procedure or for ICU admission may be relatively fit representatives of the larger population of elderly patients with the same problems. Similarly, reports of outcomes of elderly patients cared for in single institutions may not accurately reflect the outcomes that would be identified in population-based data. The risks identified in the experience of a single institution can be underestimated or overestimated relative to the broader population, depending on the patterns of referral.[1] A further consideration is that individuals obviously cannot be randomly assigned to being young or old: Thus variables other than age that can influence the outcomes of interest may be unbalanced among groups, unrecognized, or unmeasured. These factors and others must be considered when interpreting for one's own use clinical reports of elderly patients with critical illness, but important age-associated information can nonetheless be derived and applied to the clinical care of elderly patients.

## Physiology of Aging and Critical Illness: Basis for Therapy

Much of the supportive care we provide to critically ill patients is physiologically based. The physiologic changes that accompany normal aging are generally predictable and have important consequences during critical illness. These changes occur in virtually every organ system and integrated homeostatic mechanism. They reflect a gradual, more or less linear decline that begins during young adulthood, although they may vary considerably in magnitude among individuals.[2] In this section, age-related changes in physiologic function are discussed in terms of their impact on host responses to critical surgical illness and their implications for clinical care. In general, maximal levels of physiologic function are diminished, and the "reserve" between resting and maximal levels of function is reduced. Physiologic "sensors" are less sensitive to perturbations from homeostatic norms; and once evoked, the mechanisms for restoring physiologic norms are less efficient in the elderly. As a result, deviations from those norms are more marked, and the elderly require close attention and meticulous care to avoid physiologic abnormalities and to identify and rapidly correct those that are present. The elderly patient may have difficulty initiating and sustaining adequate responses to severe, prolonged, or complicated illness: Every opportunity to minimize avoidable stresses mut be taken.

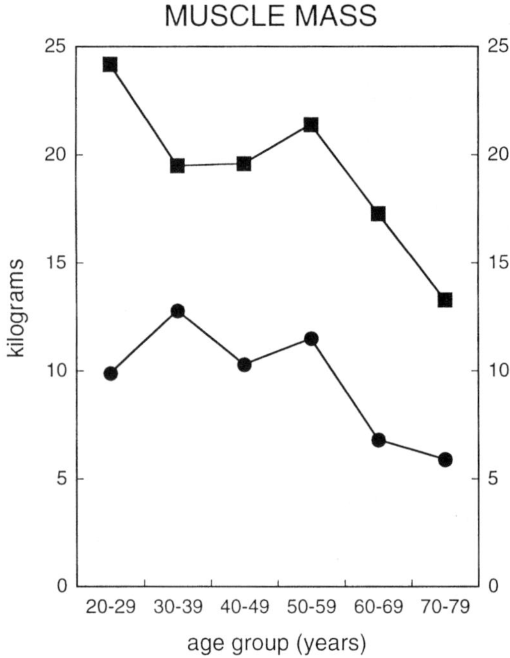


FIGURE 18.1. Muscle mass (kg) as a function of age in men (squares) and women (circles). (From the data of Cohn SH, Vartsky D, Yasumura S, et al. Compartmental body composition based on total-body nitrogen, potassium, and calcium. Am J Physiol 1980;239:E524–E530.)

## Body Composition, Muscle Mass, Strength

Age-related changes in body composition are substantial, have important consequences, and have major implications for clinical care. In general, body weight remains relatively unchanged, as body fat tends to increase and lean body mass to decrease. Lean body mass is comprised of the extracellular mass and the cellular mass of the body, or "body cell mass." Body cell mass is the work-performing, energy-consuming, potassium-rich tissue compartment; and muscle represents its largest constituent.[3] Decreased muscle mass accounts to a large extent for age-related decreases in body cell mass. Muscle mass may decrease as much as 40% from young adulthood to age 80 (Fig. 18.1), and there are more or less parallel declines in muscle strength and power.[4] Age-related decreases in maximal strength measures are even more profound than the changes in the mass of the corresponding muscles, presumably as a result of changes in the relative proportions of muscle fiber types.

Decreased strength in the elderly is reflected in a diminished ability to perform specific tasks or maneuvers. For example, the average 80-year old woman in good health is at the threshold of quadriceps muscle strength required to rise from sitting in an armless chair.[5] Periods of relative immobility or inadequate nutrition (or both) are common during critical illness and, in the elderly patient, result in losses from an already diminished muscle mass. Moreover, the catabolic nature of acute surgical illness is characterized by the rapid net breakdown of skeletal muscle protein. Thus muscle mass and strength, including that of the respiratory muscles, may quickly fall below clinically important threshold levels in the critically ill elderly patient.[6] For example, even with the limited stress of elective abdominal surgery, vital capacity falls to significantly lower levels in old than in young patients, approaching values of 10 ml/kg in some individuals (Fig. 18.2).[7] In addition, the recovery of strength in elderly patients is markedly impaired relative to the rapid recovery in young patients.

The accelerated metabolic demands that accompany acute illness must be minimized if losses of muscle mass and strength are to be limited. The primary illness must be treated promptly and effectively. Pain, exposure to a cool environment, and other factors that impose additional metabolic demands must be avoided. Bed rest and relative inactivity are usual for patients in an ICU. The adverse consequence of immobility are numerous and exacerbate many of the effects of acute illness. Muscle mass and strength decline. The inability to move about

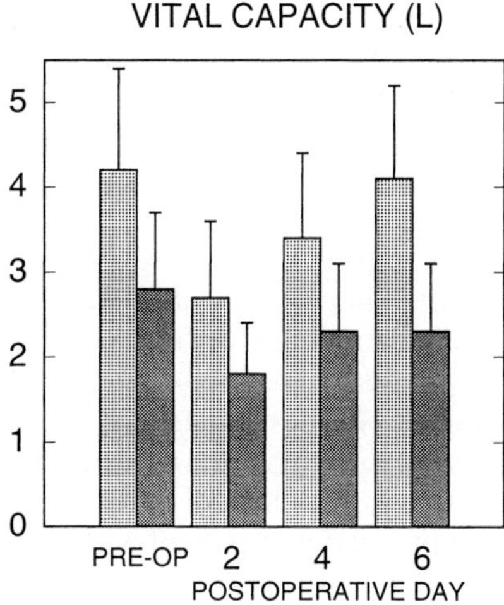


FIGURE 18.2. Preoperative and postoperative vital capacity (liters) in young (open bars) and old patients (black bars) following major elective abdominal surgery (mean ± standard deviation). (From Watters et al.,[7] with permission.)

and cough effectively results in atelectasis, ventilation/perfusion mismatch, and pneumonia. The latter is the most frequent serious postoperative complication in the elderly.[8] Cardiovascular deconditioning results from immobility and may lead to orthostatic hypotension and tachycardia when an upright posture and physical activity are resumed. Maximal oxygen consumption, cardiac index, and stroke volume also decline. Tissue sensitivity to insulin decreases, exaggerating age-related and illness-related glucose intolerance. Constipation and fecal impaction may occur, and the potential for decubitus ulcers is greatly increased in immobile patients. The incidence of deep venous thrombosis is also increased. Unfortunately, many of these changes compound those that accompany normal aging and further predispose the elderly patient to important clinical complications. Strength has been demonstrated to be a significant predictor of complications following a variety of surgical procedures.

Functional status and the ability to conduct activities of daily living are related to muscle strength and power: the greater the loss of strength in the elderly patient during an acute illness, the longer his or her convalescence is likely to be and the greater the potential for needing long-term institutional care. Strength and function are best restored and maintained by early resumption of physical activity, as allowed by the constraints of acute illness and the opportunities available in the ICU and on the ward. Elderly patients require greater assistance in their return to activity, at least initially, and benefit from their glasses and hearing aids if they require them. Effective pain management and adequate nutrition are essential.

## Oxygen Transport, Energy Expenditure

Assessment of oxygen transport is central to the care of critically ill patients, and there are several considerations pertinent to the elderly. Resting energy expenditure (REE) and oxygen consumption are strongly correlated with lean body mass and body cell mass (BCM), and their decline with age can be accounted for to a considerable extent by age-related changes in body composition.[9–11] REE and oxygen consumption (expressed as a function of body surface area) decline consistently with age in healthy individuals (Fig. 18.3). Resting energy expenditure can be estimated as $37\,\text{kcal/m}^2\text{/hr}$ at age 20 years, less $1\,\text{kcal/m}^2\text{/hr}$ for each 10 years of age above 20.[13] The empirically derived standards of Fleisch (Table 18.1) and the equations derived by Harris and Benedict for REE reflect the dependence on age, gender, and body size.[13,14]

$$\begin{aligned}&\text{Heat production in men (kcal/day)}\\&\quad = 66.473 + 13.7516 \times \text{weight (kg)} + 5.003 \times \text{height (cm)}\\&\qquad - 6.775 \times \text{age (years)}\end{aligned}$$

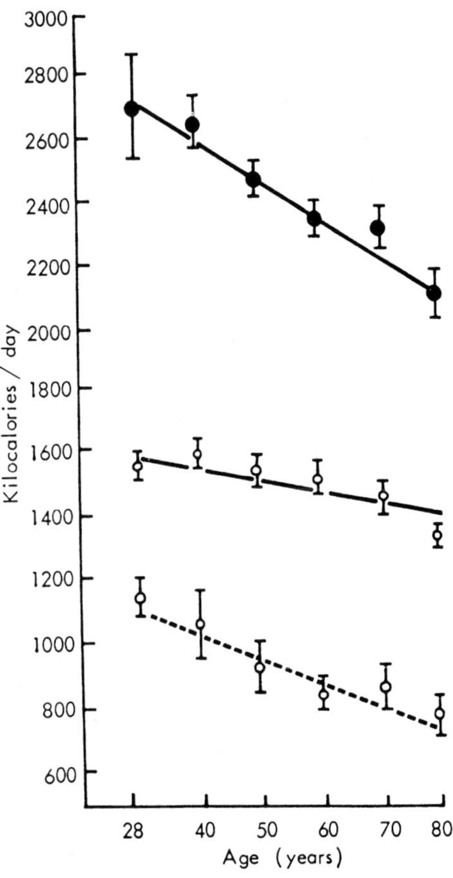


FIGURE 18.3. Daily energy expenditure (kcal/day) attributable to resting metabolism (open circles, solid line) and activity (open circles, broken line) and total daily energy intake as a function of age in healthy men. (From Shock,[12] with permission.)

TABLE 18.1. Basal Energy Expenditure

| Age (years) | Energy expenditure (kcal/m²/hr) Women | Men |
|---|---|---|
| 20 | 35.3 | 38.6 |
| 25 | 35.2 | 37.5 |
| 30 | 35.1 | 36.8 |
| 35 | 35.0 | 36.5 |
| 40 | 34.9 | 36.3 |
| 45 | 34.5 | 36.2 |
| 50 | 33.9 | 35.8 |
| 55 | 33.3 | 35.4 |
| 60 | 32.7 | 34.9 |
| 65 | 32.2 | 34.4 |
| 70 | 31.7 | 33.8 |
| 80 | 30.9 | 33.0 |

*Source:* Adapted from Fleisch A. Le metabolisme basal standard et sa determination au moyen du metabocalculator. Helv Med Acta 1951;18:23–44.

$$\text{Heat production in women (kcal/day)} = 655.0955 + 9.5634 \times \text{weight (kg)} + 1.8496 \times \text{height (cm)} - 4.6756 \times \text{age (years)}$$

Energy expended during physical activity is a major contributor to total daily energy expenditure in healthy individuals, and substantial age-related reductions have been described here as well.[15,16] The average decrease in total daily energy expenditure with age in healthy adult men has been estimated, using dietary records, to be 12.4 kcal/day/year.[15]

Acute surgical illness also influences REE. After resuscitation, oxygen consumption and REE are typically increased above predicted values presumably to support the increased cardiopulmonary work and accelerated transport and synthetic processes necessary for host defense and wound repair. The magnitude of the increase is thought to be a proportional one based on the predicted basal energy expenditure (BEE). In this way, age-related changes in BEE are reflected in the REE of critically ill patients. Old patients are less hypermetabolic than young ones.[17] Although a 40% body surface area (BSA) burn would be expected to increase the REE 50% in both young and old patients alike, the REE of a 70-year-old would be lower than that of a younger patient with the same injury.

Age-related changes in maximal energy expenditure during exercise may provide some insight into these responses. Maximal oxygen consumption during exercise is manyfold greater than resting levels, at least in young individuals. Although oxygen consumption may increase substantially during acute surgical illness, it is usually less than 50% above resting values and rarely double.[13] Maximal oxygen consumption ($VO_2$max) decreases consistently with age and does so as a function of the habitual level of physical activity.[18,19] The rate of decline in $VO_2$max has been reported to be approximately 12% per decade in sedentary men and 5.5% per decade in master athletes[20] (Fig. 18.4). These observations suggest that there are major reductions in maximal energy expenditure when young adults are compared with octogenarians, for example. It is not known, however, if increases in oxygen consumption during severe, acute illness are

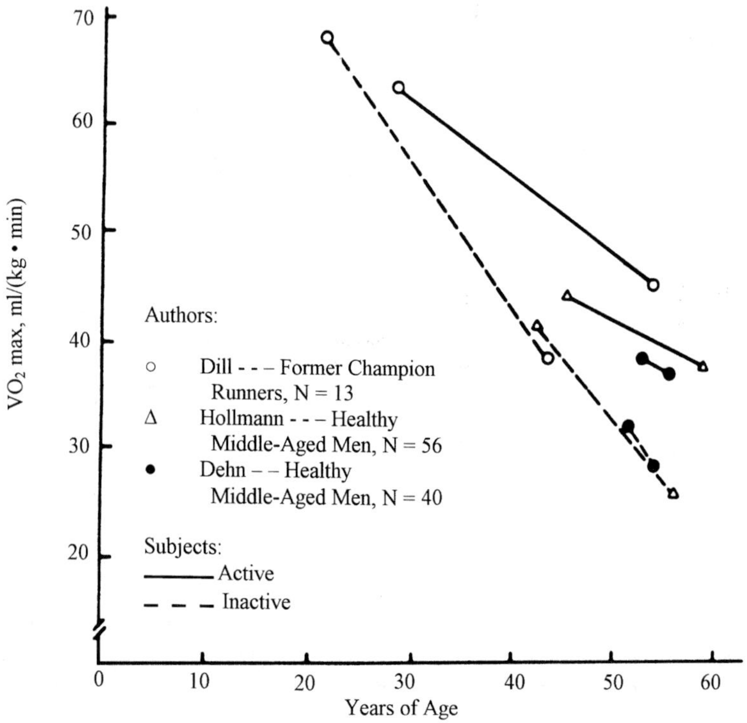


FIGURE 18.4. Decline in maximal oxygen consumption ($VO_2$max) with age in healthy active (solid lines) and inactive (broken lines) men during exercise, studied longitudinally. (From Dehn and Bruce,[19] with permission.)

limited to a different degree in the elderly than in the young. Nor is it known whether there are any clinical consequences of a much lower maximal energy expenditure in older patients. Setting similar "supraphysiologic" targets for oxygen transport variables in the young and the old is likely ill-advised. Several avoidable factors contribute to increased metabolic demands and oxygen consumption, including pain, shivering, aggressive weaning from ventilatory support, and overfeeding. These problems should be sought and corrected in all patients to reduce the catabolic effects of their critical illness. In patients receiving nutritional support, estimates of caloric requirements (see below and Chapter 5) must take into account the effects of age-related changes in body composition and other factors.

## Cardiovascular Function

The changes in cardiovascular physiology described as accompanying aging depend to a considerable degree on the screening measures used to select the elderly subjects studied. When subjects are not screened for cardiovascular disease, deterioration is observed in many resting cardiovascular variables. By contrast, in old subjects who have been demonstrated to be free of cardiovascular disease, resting cardiac function seems to be well maintained. Unscreened subjects may well be representative of old patients presenting to us with surgical problems and critical illness, but understanding the changes in cardiovascular physiology attributable to normal aging requires that some screening be conducted to exclude subjects with significant disease.

A consistent age-related decrease in maximal cardiac output, together with changes in the mechanisms by which increases in cardiac output are achieved, are of particular importance for the critically ill elderly patient (Fig. 18.5). Critical illness typically increases cardiac performance in proportion to its effect on oxygen consumption and REE. Maximal cardiac index during exercise, which presumably is relevant to responses during surgical illness, is on the order of 10 L/min/m$^2$ in healthy young adults; it is 30–40% less in individuals in their eighties.[20] Increases in both heart rate and stroke volume contribute to increases in cardiac output during exercise in subjects of all ages. However, in young subjects the ejection fraction (EF) and stroke volume (SV) increase, end-systolic volume (ESV) declines, and end-diastolic volume (EDV) is little changed. Healthy old subjects differ in that the maximal heart rate is substantially reduced; and increases in stroke volume, but not the ejection fraction, contribute to increased cardiac output. By contrast with young subjects, the EDV in old subjects increases as cardiac output increases, whereas the ESV decreases relatively little (Fig. 18.6). As a result, old subjects are particularly dependent on efficient ventricular filling to achieve higher end-diastolic volumes and to maintain increased cardiac output. However, myocardial relaxation tends to be prolonged in the old subject, early diastolic filling is slowed and delayed, and ventricular filling is more dependent on the contribution of atrial contraction. Thus, hypovolemia in the elderly patient must be corrected promptly, and volume loading must be sufficient to support optimal ventricular filling. Tachyarrhythmias and atrial fibrillation also compromise the ability of the elderly patient to maintain an increased cardiac output and should be corrected whenever feasible.

Stiffening of the aorta and peripheral vessels generally leads to increased peripheral vascular resistance, another age-related phenomenon. In normal individuals there is a modest age-related increase in left ventricular wall thickness that is exaggerated in those with hypertension and coronary artery disease. Age-related decreases in chronotropic, inotropic, and arterial vasodilatory responses to given doses of β-agonists (e.g., dobutamine and isoproterenol) and lower maximal responses are well recognized.[21–23] When inotropic support is indicated, a

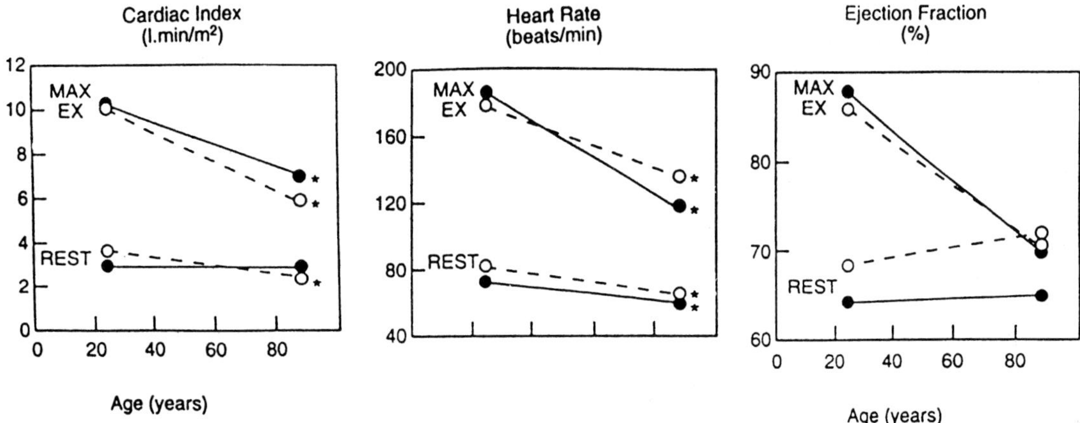


FIGURE 18.5. Linear regression of age on cardiac output, heart rate, and ejection fraction at rest and during maximal cycle ergometry in healthy sedentary men (solid lines) and women (dotted lines). All subjects are healthy, community-dwelling volunteers screened to exclude hypertension and occult coronary artery disease. (From Lakatta,[20] with permission.)

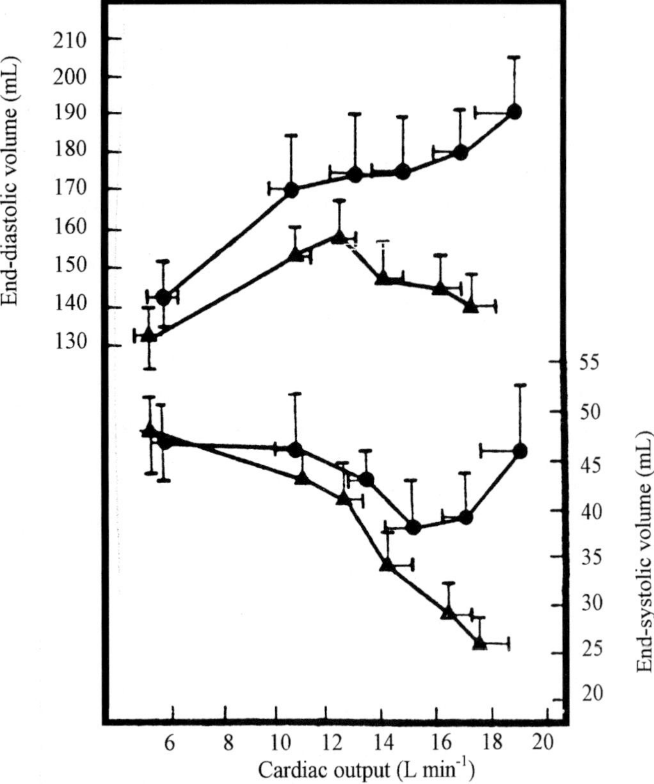


FIGURE 18.6. Relation of end-diastolic and end-systolic volumes to a given cardiac output at rest and during graded exercise in healthy young (triangles) and old (circles) subjects. (From Lakatta EG. Changes in cardiovascular function with aging. Eur Heart J 1990;11(suppl C):22–29, with permission.)

combination of nonvasoconstricting inotropes, agents with nonadrenergic mechanisms, and afterload reduction may be most helpful in the elderly.

Coronary artery disease is common in the elderly when evaluated by clinical history and resting electrocardiogram (ECG), and even more so when exercise or other stress testing is used. During exercise, the likelihood of ECG and ventricular wall motion abnormalities is significantly higher in old, unselected subjects.[24,25] Coronary artery disease and its sequelae may limit the increases in cardiac output that can be achieved and can put the elderly patient at risk for acute ischemic events. The increased demands of critical illness on the oxygen transport system of the elderly patient may not be readily met and may, in the presence of coronary artery disease, precipitate myocardial ischemia.

## Respiratory Function

The aging process affects virtually every aspect of respiratory physiology and oxygen transport, with important consequences for the elderly patient with critical illness.[26] Pulmonary complications and adverse pulmonary events (e.g., episodes of oxygen desaturation and periods of apnea) are relatively common following even elective surgical procedures, and old age is a strong predictor of them.[27–30] The age-related changes that are most clinically familiar include declines in vital capacity, forced expiratory volume in one second, alveolar-arterial oxygen gradient, arterial oxygen tension, and maximal oxygen consumption. Also relevant for the elderly surgical patient are decreased sensitivity of the airways to noxious stimuli, increased chest wall stiffness, and increased closing volumes. Alveolar oxygen tension does not vary significantly with age, but arterial oxygen tension declines progressively and can be estimated by the regression equation: $PaO_2 = 109 - 0.43 \times \text{age (years)}$.[31] Diminished airway sensitivity to stimuli such as refluxed gastric fluid and impaired mucociliary transport and cough render the elderly patient at increased risk of silent pulmonary aspiration.[32] Ventilatory responses to hypoxia and hypercarbia are blunted (Fig. 18.7), another example of an impaired homeostatic mechanism in the elderly.[33,34]

Closing volume is the lung volume at which closure of small airways begins. Even in good health, small airways may begin to close during tidal respiration, when the functional residual capacity (FRC) falls below the closing volume. Closing volume increases with aging as a result of the loss of elastic lung recoil and other factors and exceeds the FRC during tidal respiration in seated, normal subjects aged 65 years or older and in supine subjects aged 45 years or older (Fig. 18.8).[35] The result is that closure of small airways occurs to a greater extent in the elderly, resulting in decreased ventilation of dependent lung zones, ventilation/perfusion mismatch, impaired gas exchange, and a predisposition to atelectasis. Abdom-

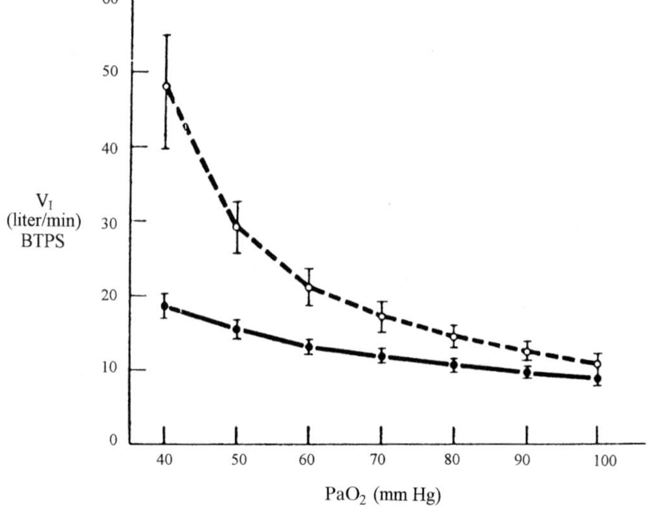


FIGURE 18.7. Ventilatory responses to isocapnic hypoxia in eight young (broken line) and eight older (solid line) healthy men (mean ± standard error of mean). BTPS, body temperature and ambient pressure. (From Kronenberg and Drage,[33] with permission.)

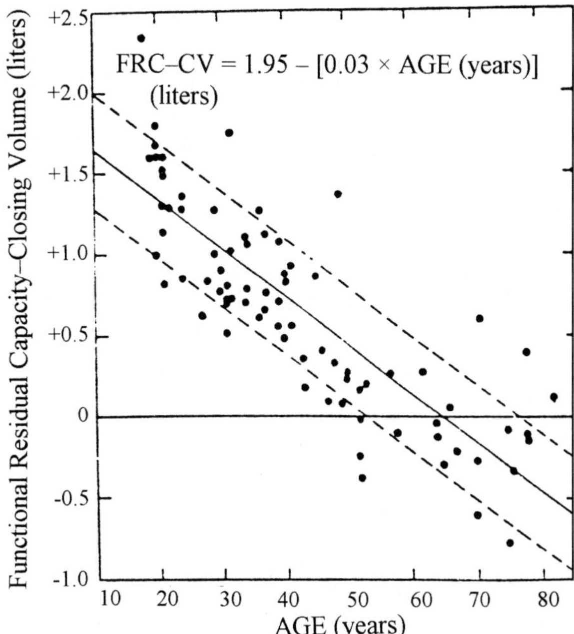


FIGURE 18.8. Difference between functional residual capacity (FRC) and closing volume as a function of age in healthy seated subjects, with the regression line ±1 SD shown. Negative values indicate that small airway closure is occurring during normal tidal respiration. IC, inspiratory capacity; VC, ventilatory capacity; ERV, expiratory reserve volume; RV, residual volume; CC, closing capacity. (From Leblanc et al.,[35] with permission.)

inal and thoracic surgery, supine positioning, and other circumstances in which the FRC is diminished promote closure of small airways. Several other age-related changes affect respiratory function and reserve, including (1) an increase in the volume of alveolar ducts and respiratory bronchioles resulting in decreased alveolar volume; (2) increased number and size of interalveolar fenestrae and decreased alveolar surface area; (3) thickening of the intima and media of larger pulmonary arteries resulting in a tendency to greater pulmonary vascular resistance; and (4) a blunted vasoconstrictor response to alveolar hypoxia. Diminished elastic lung recoil, increased stiffness of the chest wall, increased anteroposterior diameter of the thorax, and a shorter thorax, contribute to an increased dependence of the elderly patient on diaphragm function. The impairment of diaphragm function that occurs following abdominal and thoracic surgery thus predisposes the elderly patient to respiratory compromise. The forced vital capacity decreases progressively with age, leaving old patients with less "reserve" before levels associated with adverse clinical effects are reached.

Assuming an upright position increases the FRC and should lessen the closure of small airways that is promoted in the supine position. Oxygen consumption following thoracotomy is lower in the sitting than the supine position, suggesting that the work of breathing may be lessened when upright.[36] Parenteral narcotics have been associated with more frequent respiratory disturbances following surgery, and epidural techniques for pain management and nonnarcotic analgesics may therefore be particularly valuable in the elderly patient.[28] In the patient who is not mechanically ventilated, measures such as incentive spirometry, positive-pressure breathing, and regular breathing exercises may complement the basic measures of pain management and mobilization. The techniques of mechanical ventilation and weaning do not differ in the elderly, although they may require a longer period of support, given the impairments imposed by age, co-morbidity, and acute illness. Parameters used to predict successful weaning from mechanical ventilation in young patients appear less reliable in the elderly.[37]

## Renal Function, Fluids, Electrolytes

Age-related changes in renal physiology have important implications for the fluid and electrolyte management of elderly surgical patients and for the selection and use of drugs. Declines in glomerular filtration rate (GFR) and creatinine clearance are substantial and relatively consistent among individuals (Fig. 18.9). Serum creatinine con-

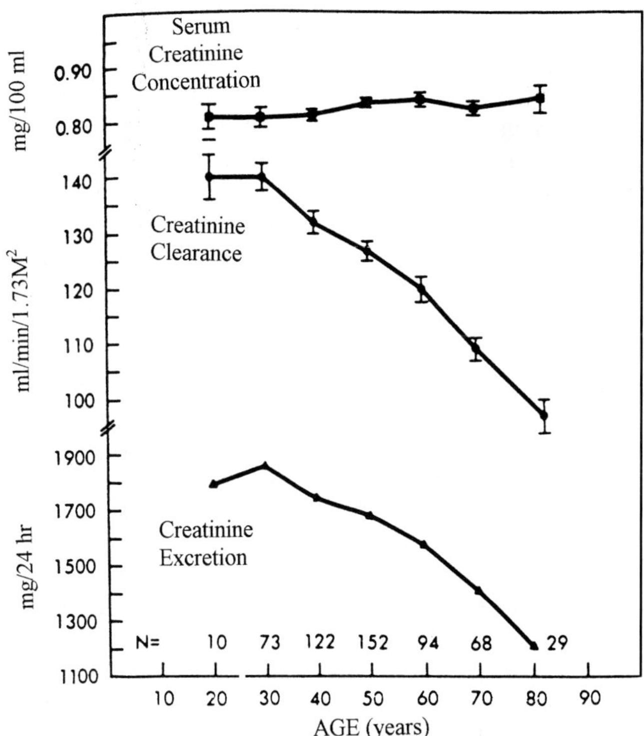


FIGURE 18.9. Serum creatinine, creatinine clearance, and creatinine excretion as a function of age in healthy subjects. (From Meakins JL, McClaran JC (eds) Surgical Care of the Elderly. Mosby–Year Book: Chicago, 1988:129–148, with permission.)

centration does not change to any marked extent as a function of age, despite the decline in creatinine clearance, as muscle mass and creatinine production decrease as well. Thus normal serum creatinine in an old patient, particularly a frail elderly woman in whom muscle mass is markedly reduced, does not mean that her renal function is preserved relative to that of a young individual but, rather, that it has declined more or less in parallel with her muscle mass. Creatinine clearance should be measured or estimated when knowledge of the GFR is important for determining therapy, rather than simply using serum creatinine as a guide.[38] A widely used formula for men in estimating (milliliters per minute) GFR is:

$$\text{GFR} = \frac{(140 - \text{age in years}) \times \text{weight in kg}}{72 \times \text{serum creatinine in mg/dl}}$$

This result is multiplied by 0.85 to derive the value for women.[38]

Dosages of drugs that are cleared renally must be adjusted in the elderly, and drugs with potential nephrotoxic effects should be avoided when possible (see Chapter 13). For example, nonsteroidal antiinflammatory drugs (NSAIDs) can have a number of detrimental effects on renal function in the elderly and should be used with caution. Unopposed vasoconstriction and marked decreases in renal blood flow and GFR in hypovolemic states may result from inhibition of prostaglandin synthesis.[39]

Alterations in renal, cardiovascular, and endocrine function make close attention to fluid and electrolyte management mandatory in the elderly patient. Homeostatic mechanisms in young patients are effective in maintaining a relatively constant internal milieu despite a wide range of physiologic insults and varied approaches to fluid therapy. In contrast, the physiologic sensors of the elderly are less sensitive to perturbations of electrolyte, fluid, and acid–base status; and the compensatory mechanisms evoked are less effective. For example, old subjects are less able to decrease urine flow and increase urine osmolarity in response to water deprivation, and the time required to achieve sodium equilibrium in the face of sodium restriction is prolonged. With increased insensible fluid losses through thinned skin in addition, the net result of these changes is an increase in the minimum requirement for water in the elderly. Because sodium and water conservation are impaired, hypovolemic states are likely to be exacerbated in the elderly, and the onset of oliguria as a marker of hypovolemia is delayed. Vasoconstrictor responses and increases in heart rate are also less robust in the elderly individual. The result is that cardiac output is less well maintained before adequate fluid therapy is administered, as increases in cardiac output are especially dependent on effective ventricular filling in the elderly.

The elderly also have decreased ability to excrete acute loads of water or salt and thus experience relatively prolonged extracellular fluid volume expansion during and subsequent to acute illness.[40] They are prone to excessive secretion of antidiuretic hormone, especially during the stress of acute surgical illness, and to hyponatremia. Hyponatremia and water intoxication can manifest as lethargy, confusion, weakness, and if severe, as seizures or coma. Respiratory mechanisms for regulating acid–base status are probably little affected by age; however, renal regulation may be significantly impaired by reduced renal mass and GFR, inefficient elimination of bicarbonate, and an impaired ability to deaminate glutamine. The renal threshold for glucose excretion is elevated in the elderly, placing them at risk of extreme hyperglycemia and an associated hyperosmolar state, particularly when glucose-rich nutritional support is being given. Thus, old patients are much more reliant on meticulous, ongoing clinical and laboratory assessment, and on the administration of appropriate fluid solutions and volumes if they are to avoid extreme abnormalities of their fluid, electrolyte, and acid–base status.

## Thermoregulation

The elderly are, in general, less sensitive to changes in ambient temperature and have less effective mechanisms of heat conservation and production. They are less well able to maintain core temperature and tend to sustain more marked declines when exposed to a cool environment if preventive measures are not taken, during surgical procedures for example.[41] Hypothyroidism and diabetes may also predispose the elderly to hypothermia. The potential adverse effects of hypothermia include a predisposition to cardiac arrhythmias, elaboration of catecholamines and other counterregulatory hormones, reduced cardiac output, altered oxyhemoglobin dissociation, vasoconstriction, impaired hemostasis, and increased blood loss.[42] Maintenance of normothermia during surgical procedures has been accompanied by a reduced wound infection rate and shortened length of stay following major elective surgery in one study, and a reduced incidence of morbid cardiac events in another.[43,44]

Acutely ill patients have an elevated endogenous temperature setpoint and invoke heat conservation and production mechanisms to attempt to raise and maintain the core temperature to match the setpoint. Metabolic heat production requires energy expenditure, which, in burn patients, has been demonstrated to increase as a function of decreasing ambient temperature. When shivering occurs, the muscular work involved is accompanied by oxygen consumption that is increased several-fold above nonshivering levels, and it may make cardiopulmonary demands the elderly patient is unable to meet. For all these reasons, hypothermia is a physiologic and metabolic burden for the elderly patient that is morbid and unnecessary. It may be avoided by minimizing exposed surfaces, administering warm intravenous fluids and blood products, using heated and humidified gases, and maintaining an appropriate ambient temperature.

Blunting of the febrile response to infection probably occurs in only a small proportion of the elderly, specifically those who are frail or malnourished and those at extreme old age.[45] Diminished temperature perception in the elderly, less robust vasomotor responses, and altered central nervous system regulation of temperature may each contribute. Infection in such patients may manifest in nonspecific ways, such as weakness and confusion, either of which may contribute to a blunted febrile response by impairing appropriate behavioral regulation of temperature (e.g., covering exposed surfaces). Although fever is usually well tolerated and serves as a guide to the course of illness, it can have deleterious effects. The rates of chemical reactions tend to increase with temperature ($Q_{10}$ effect) and an average increase in the metabolic rate of 10–13% per degree centigrade elevation in temperature has been described.[46] Cardiac output rises as well, and heart rate increases approximately 10 beats per minute per degree centigrade.[13] If fever is associated with patient discomfort, reaches extreme levels, or places major demands on the cardiopulmonary reserve of the elderly patient, treatment is appropriate. Surface cooling should be initiated only after administration of antipyretic agents because, unless the endogenous temperature setpoint is lowered pharmacologically, cooling only stimulates further vasoconstriction and heat production.

# Clinical Care

## Physiologic Monitoring

Routine clinical assessment, particularly of cardiovascular performance, may be insensitive to the physiologic derangements of the injured or acutely ill elderly patient.[47] By the time clinical manifestations of disturbed homeostasis become apparent, the disturbances are likely to be well advanced and thus less amenable to correction in the elderly patient. For example, old patients with relatively good trauma scores at admission have much greater mortality than do young patients.[48] Planned physiologic monitoring of elderly patients at risk (e.g., following moderate or severe trauma) should provide earlier information about such derangements than does routine clinical assessment, ideally at a time when therapy may be simpler and clinical outcomes can be favorably affected. Institution of early, invasive monitoring of hemodynamic and oxygen transport variables has been advocated in older trauma patients with one or more risk factors for mortality: pedestrian-motor vehicle mechanism, initial systolic blood pressure <150 mmHg, acidosis, multiple fractures, and head injury.[47] Although there is a rationale for such an approach, its influence on outcomes following trauma and other critical illnesses in elderly patients has not been well tested. Invasive monitoring carries risks, which are at least as great in the elderly as in younger patients.[49] Noninvasive technologies hold considerable appeal and should be employed routinely in the acutely ill elderly patient. In concept, real-time measures of molecular markers of cellular function and injury hold the potential of providing therapeutic direction well before end-organ, physiologic, and clinical effects are apparent.

## Cardiovascular Support

Many studies have documented a favorable association between outcome and the ability to increase cardiac performance following operation, trauma, and shock.[50–52] The data are limited, but it appears as though this observation is also true for elderly patients. Thus continuing resuscitation in an attempt to achieve robust cardiac performance may be beneficial in the older patient, as it is in the young. Moore and colleagues studied patients during resuscitation from severe trauma and shock.[51] Those who achieved a cardiac index of 4.5 L/min/m$^2$ during the first 12 hours had a much lower incidence of subsequent multiple organ failure and death than did those who achieved a mean index of only 3.5 L/min/m$^2$, even though that value is within the "normal" range. Because the cardiac index in the favorable group (mean age 32 years) was approximately half of their expected, age-adjusted maximal output, a parallel value in an older group—one-half the estimated, age-adjusted maximal cardiac output of a normal individual (see above and Appendix)—might serve as a reasonable marker and goal of satisfactory resuscitation. Other parameters should also be used to assess resuscitation efficacy, such as clearance of lactate, correction of base deficit, and improvements in markers of regional organ perfusion (e.g., gastric mucosal $PCO_2$ or intermucosal pH [pHI].[53]

## Nutrition Support

Optimal care of the elderly patient in the ICU requires careful attention to metabolic and nutritional issues from the time of first assessment (see Chapter 5). The elderly are at increased risk for preexisting nutritional deficiencies, both micronutrient (e.g., vitamins and trace elements) and protein–calorie. Dietary intake in hospitalized patients, especially the elderly, is often inadequate to meet requirements; and caloric demands and micronutrient requirements increase during acute illness. Acute illness is accompanied by the rapid breakdown of skeletal muscle protein and a concomitant loss of muscle mass and strength. The elderly typically have a much smaller muscle mass than young patients, and it erodes rapidly during the catabolism of acute illness with consequences as described above.

A structured clinical assessment (e.g., Subjective Global Assessment[54]) provides a useful template for nutritional assessment and can be completed rapidly. The value of weight loss as a marker of nutritional status in acutely ill patients is limited because of the rapid changes that can occur in body water compartments. In the elderly patient with moderate to severe malnutrition, and when the clinical scenario is not simply that of a straightforward elective surgical procedure, full nutritional support aimed at meeting energy and protein requirements should be considered early. The enteral route is superior to the parenteral route in most situations.

The provision of macronutrients to elderly patients should be modified from that in young patients in several ways. Energy expenditure, and therefore requirements, reflect metabolic body size among other factors. Resting energy expenditure is approximately 15% lower in 80-year-old men than in 40-year-old men.[12] Elderly patients are less tolerant of glucose loads than younger patients, so nutritional support should be initiated gradually and with regular monitoring of blood glucose levels. Alternate calorie sources such as lipid may be useful. Glucose intolerance reflects impaired pancreatic insulin release in elderly patients and may result from more marked tissue insensitivity to the effects of insulin than is seen in younger patients.[55] Renal clearance of glucose is a defense mechanism against hyperglycemia. The renal glucose threshold increases with age, however, predisposing the elderly patient to hyperglycemia and hyperosmolarity. Hyperglycemia adversely affects polymorphonuclear leukocyte function, promotes wound infection, and impairs wound healing.[56] It should be avoided by initiating nutritional support at a modest level and increasing the rate with regular monitoring of blood glucose, administering exogenous insulin to maintain consistent blood glucose levels, and including alternate calorie sources such as lipid in the nutrient prescription.[57]

Protein prescriptions are generally similar to those in young patients. However, age-related decreases in the GFR are significant. Such changes may lead to azotemia in elderly patients receiving protein in amounts that would be well tolerated in younger patients.[58] Blood urea nitrogen levels should be measured on a regular basis.

Elderly patients may well have preexisting, subclinical micronutrient deficiencies and, as a result of their acute illness, experience both increased losses and increased requirements to support their immune function, wound repair, and defenses against free radical injury. Multivitamin and mineral supplementation should be considered in the elderly ICU patient in all but the most routine situations, regardless of nutritional status. Daily supplementation of healthy, community-dwelling, elderly subjects with a multiple vitamin and trace element combination improves immune function and lowers the incidence of clinical infections.[59] Comparable findings have been reported in institutionalized elderly subjects.[60]

## Clinical Pharmacology

Age-related changes in gastrointestinal absorption, hepatic and renal metabolism, body composition, and protein binding may each contribute to alterations in pharmacokinetics and necessitate changes in drug selection and dosing in the elderly patient. Decreased hepatic "first-pass" metabolism, reflecting altered liver mass, blood flow, and enzyme activity, may result in increased systemic drug availability following oral administration. Similarly, the renal blood flow and GFR decline consistently with age. Decreased protein binding may increase both therapeutic and toxic effects for a given drug dose or circulating concentration. Relatively low initial blood levels of lipophilic drugs would be anticipated because of age-related increases in the proportion of body fat, whereas the levels of hydrophilic drugs are likely to be high relative to those in younger individuals, who have greater lean body mass. Age effects on pharmacodynamics (i.e., the interaction of drugs with receptors and the resulting physiologic effects) have not been studied extensively. Polypharmacy is common in the elderly, and consideration must be given to the potential for drug interactions, especially during acute illness and when medications are prescribed in hospital in addition to a patient's existing drug profile.

Age-related reductions in the GFR are not well reflected in serum creatinine values, which tend to remain constant after the muscle mass (and therefore creatinine production) decline. Such predictable alterations in renal function have implications for the selection and dosing of drugs. Alternatives to drugs with potential nephrotoxicity (e.g., aminoglycosides and NSAIDs) should be sought, particularly when renal function may be compromised by other factors such as hypovolemia. Measurement of drug levels is appropriate in some circumstances. Advanced age is a recognized risk factor for nephropathy due to intravenous contrast agents, as are diabetes mellitus and dehydration. Protective measures that have been employed include prior hydration and the use of mannitol, furosemide, or dopamine.

## Maintaining Cognitive Function

Acute confusion is relatively common in the elderly patient in hospital, and its occurrence in the ICU can be promoted by a number of factors,[61,62] including sleep deprivation, loss of day–night cues, repeated and unfamiliar visual and auditory stimuli, lack of familiar stimuli, immobility, loss of speech because of intubation, and the use of sedative, anticholinergic, and other medications. Preexisting visual and auditory impairments may be unmasked by removing eyeglasses and hearing aids. Acute confusion usually corresponds to delirium, characterized by the acute onset of fluctuating inattentiveness, cognitive impairment, and psychomotor changes that may include agitation, retardation, or both. Confusion may be the initial manifestation of a surgical complication, particularly an infectious or respiratory complication.[63] Once delirium is diagnosed, a thorough evaluation is required to identify specific complications, physiologic derangements, and any underlying organic etiologic factors. Focal neurologic deficits and potential sources of sepsis must be sought during a complete physical examination.

Close supervision is needed to ensure that confused patients do not inadvertently harm themselves, and the need for behavior control with medication, such as haloperidol, must be determined. Reassurance, explanation, and reorientation provided on a repeated basis in a calm, well-lit environment with family present may be of considerable help to the delirious patient. Long-term cognitive dysfunction following surgery is more common in the elderly and is associated with a decline in the ability to conduct activities of daily living.[63] Whether similar long-term effects occur in elderly patients following critical illness is not known.

### Prophylaxis

Old age is a risk factor for deep vein thrombosis and pulmonary embolism. Prophylaxis with subcutaneous heparin or other measures should be routine in elderly patients in the absence of specific contraindications.

Osteoporosis, osteoarthritis, and prosthetic joints are common in elderly patients, and care must be taken when moving and positioning them, especially when obtundation or sedation allow positioning that would be uncomfortable or beyond the usual range of motion in the alert patient. Padding of pressure points is essential. Maintaining a neutral head position minimizes compromise of cerebral blood flow in unconscious patients with cervical arthritis.

The skin of elderly patients is often fragile and prone to bruising and injury from pressure and even from adhesive tape and dressings. Age-related changes in skin and other organs, malnutrition, incontinence, and other factors predispose the elderly ICU patient to decubitus ulcers.[64] Such lesions can develop significant infection, and measures to prevent them should be routine.

## Outcomes of Intensive Care in the Elderly

### Determinants

Mortality in the ICU or in hospital are outcomes of intensive care that are commonly evaluated, although others such as long-term survival, functional recovery, postdischarge placement status, and health-related quality of life, are relevant for the elderly patient. There are reasonably consistent conclusions that can be drawn from published reports of outcomes from intensive care in the elderly, despite a number of factors that make direct comparisons between studies difficult. Such factors include (1) varying assessments of acute severity of illness; coexisting or chronic illness and prior functional status; (2) inclusion of heterogeneous diagnostic groups; (3) evaluation of outcomes using various methods and at various times; and (4) potential selection bias arising from criteria or policies for ICU admission.[65] Studies usually evaluate convenience samples of patients admitted to an ICU; information about potentially eligible patients who are not admitted is uncommon. In addition, patient groups are most often unit- or institution-based rather than population-based and thus are subject to referral and other biases.

A relation between age and hospital mortality in patients who have received intensive care has been identified by univariate analysis in many studies.[26,66–74] Variables such as co-morbidity, functional status, and physiologic reserve vary with age, and factors other than age are at least as important for predicting clinical outcomes. For example, mortality is frequently identified as being a function of the severity of the acute illness.[66,67,69,71,75,76] Severity of illness is commonly described as an Acute Physiology Score (APS), which is determined from the most abnormal values of 12 physiologic variables during the first 24 hours of ICU admission, which is thus a measure of physiologic derangement.[77] For all of the reasons already discussed, the elderly are less able to maintain homeostasis in the face of physiologic stresses than are young patients, even in the absence of any co-morbidity. It is to be expected, therefore, that they will have more marked derangements for a given "insult" (e.g., injury, infection, or surgical procedure) than the young, so the APS reflects their responses and the severity of illness. In one study, the impact of age on outcome weakened as the severity of the acute illness (or physiologic derangement) increased.[72] ICU mortality among surgical patients in another study was related to severity of illness (evaluated as Simplified APS, or SAPS) and did not differ significantly between nonagenarians and younger patients when stratified for SAPS.[78] In two reports of patients admitted to medical ICUs, old age no longer predicted mortality when acute severity of illness, diagnosis, and prior health were taken into account.[68,71] Failure of two or more organ systems was accompanied by mortality rates of 88% and 100% at 30 days and 1 year following hospital discharge, respectively, in a series of medical and surgical ICU patients aged 85 years or more.[79]

The relation of age and severity of illness to mortality is further modified by specific diagnosis. In one study, patients admitted following trauma had the highest long-term survival compared to other diagnostic groups in a mixed ICU.[67] Old age, a history of cancer, and medical rather than surgical service were identified as the most important factors associated with reduced long-term survival in another study of mixed ICU patients.[80] Age, severity of illness (APS), and diagnosis were independent predictors of 1-year survival in a recent study of medical and surgical patients aged 70 years or older.[74]

The interaction of prior functional status and age may also influence mortality. In one study patients aged 75 years or more who had functional limitations were six times more likely to die in hospital than those aged 50–64 years without limitations.[66] Among patients without functional limitation, there was no difference in mortality between the youngest and oldest groups. Physical activity status and quality of life prior to admission were significant predictors of survival in a mixed ICU population with large proportions of older and chronically ill patients.[81] Of note, the quality of life of long-term survivors was comparable to that prior to their acute illness. Others have also observed that age does not distinguish the degree of recovery among survivors, most older patients having regained their prior health status 1 year following admission.[70] Eighty percent of patients aged 65 years or older who survived 1 year following ICU admission had returned home in one report.[82] Seventy-one percent of the patients would choose to receive intensive care again if the need were to arise. In another study, increasing age was inversely related to patients' assessments of quality of life following discharge but not to objective scores of physical and psychosocial disability.[75] These observations are consistent with the concept that individual and societal views of quality of life do not necessarily coincide in older patients, who may be more accepting of health-related limitations in life style than young patients.[75,76] In addition, patients' assessments of their quality of life do not necessarily correlate with their wishes regarding life-sustaining therapy.[83]

Outcomes of patients who have required mechanical ventilation have been the focus of a number of reports. A hospital mortality of 52% and 1-year mortality of 63% have been identified in data compiled from multiple studies.[65] Age, severity of illness, co-morbidity, and diagnosis are predictors in ventilated patients, as they are in critically ill patients in general.[65,84] In some studies, prolonged ventilation (defined as 15 days in one study and a total score of more than 100 for the number of days of ventilation and age in years in another) has been accompanied by poor outcomes,[85,86] whereas in others the duration of mechanical ventilation has not been significantly related to outcome.[87,88] In a study of patients with acute respiratory distress syndrome (ARDS), age over 60 was associated with a fivefold increase in mortality, presumably because of age-related impairments in cardiopulmonary regulatory mechanisms.[26]

Mortality among elderly patients may be substantial during the year following hospital discharge. The 5-year survival of patients discharged alive from hospital was significantly lower than that predicted in an age- and gender-matched normal population (58% vs. 92%).[80] In a study of medical and surgical patients aged 70 years or more, the 1-year survival was 56% in patients aged less than 85 years and 27% in those 85 years or older—rates markedly lower than in a matched population (93%).[74] Others have reported mortality rates of 30%, 43%, and 64% at ICU discharge, at 30 days posthospital discharge, and at 1-year follow-up, respectively, in patients aged 85 years or older admitted to a mixed unit.[79] The long-term survival of critically ill patients of extreme old age appears limited.

The specific diagnosis also affects long-term survival.[68,80] In a study in which many of the patients were admitted to the ICU following surgery or trauma, the subsequent survival of those who were alive 6 months following hospital discharge approached that of an age-, year-, and gender-matched general population.[70] Elderly patients admitted to the ICU following cardiac arrest have a poor long-term outcome.[82,89]

## Goals of Therapy and Decision-Making

Outcomes from critical illness in the elderly are strongly influenced by prior health and functional status, the severity of the acute illness as manifested in the degree of physiologic derangement, and the specific diagnosis. There is no justification for using chronologic age alone to predict the benefit to be obtained from intensive care or to exclude individuals from such care.

Discussions with patients and their families regarding appropriate management must address several age-related factors. At the outset, it is important for health care personnel to seek to understand patients' premorbid functional status and their perceptions regarding quality of life. These considerations, in addition to objective physiologic data reflecting organ system performance, appreciation of the demands and potential hazards during recovery from the patient's specific critical illness, and thoughtful appraisal of the likely short-term and long-term outcomes, should inform our discussions. Other factors, such as maximum potential life-span and independent function, dignity, self-esteem, and likely pain and suffering associated with intensive care, also commonly must be considered in the elderly. Critically ill patients are often unable to participate in these discussions because of their critical illness or its treatment. More commonly, the patient's family or some other spokesperson must serve as surrogate decision-maker. See Chapter 7 for additional discussion on interacting with families.

After thoughtful consideration of these factors, consensus about appropriate critical care management should be sought. Although some patients may have an advanced directive or a "living will," these documents usually apply to conditions that are irreversible. Most critical illness, especially in surgical patients, is not irreversible, at least at the outset. The advanced directive, however, may provide a context for setting limits on care if the patient's status were to deteriorate. Limits on care may be appropriate if the likelihood of an outcome that the patient would value seems remote. Such limits might exclude certain interventions if the patent develops specific complications, such as cardiopulmonary resuscitation in the event of cardiac arrest or hemodialysis in the event of acute renal failure. In those cases, the development of the complications would indicate a worse prognosis than was originally apparent, and therapy could be considered futile. Alternatively, a trial of therapy (e.g., hemodialysis for renal failure or antifungal therapy for fungemia) might be initiated for a limited time and the patient's response monitored. A decision to continue the intervention or discontinue it could then be based on the patient's response. See Chapter 16 for a fuller discussion of futility and end of life care.

## Conclusions

Critical care of elderly patients is both the same and quite different from that of younger patients. It is different in that age has multifarious effects on all organ systems, and these age-related changes influence the way elderly patients respond to their critical illness and to treatment. It is similar in that the principles, procedures, techniques, and devices used to support organ system insufficiency or failure are the same. It is also similar in that with a comprehensive approach to care and close attention to detail many can survive their critical illness and resume a valued and enjoyable life.

## Appendix: Estimates of Age-Related Effects on Measures of Normal Physiologic Function in Adults

**Resting energy expenditure (REE)**

$$\text{REE (kcal/m}^2\text{/hr)} = 37 - [0.1 \times (\text{age} - 20)]$$

(See Table 18.1 for more exact values of BEE)

$$\text{REE}_{\text{men}} \text{ (kcal/day)} = 66.47 + [13.75 \times \text{weight (kg)}] + [5.0 \times \text{height (cm)}] - [6.78 \times \text{age}]$$

$$\text{REE}_{\text{women}} \text{ (kcal/day)} = 655.1 + [9.56 \times \text{weight (kg)}] + [1.84 \times \text{height (cm)}] - [4.68 \times \text{age}]$$

**Maximum oxygen consumption ($VO_2max$)**

$$VO_2\text{max (ml/kg/min)} = 35.6 - [0.55 \times (\text{age} - 50)]$$

sedentary (men)

$$VO_2\text{max (ml/kg/min)} = 55.6 - [0.32 \times (\text{age} - 50)]$$

master athlete (men)

**Maximum cardiac index (CImax)**

$$\text{CImax (L/m}^2\text{/min)} = 10.0 - [0.06 \times (\text{age} - 20)]$$

**Arterial oxygen tension ($PaO_2$)**

$$PaO_2 \text{ (mmHg)} = 109 - [0.43 \times \text{age}]$$

**Glomerular filtration rate (GFR)**

$$\text{GFR}_{\text{men}} \text{ (ml/min)} = \frac{(140 - \text{age}) \times \text{weight (kg)}}{72 \times \text{serum creatinine (mg/dl)}}$$

$$\text{GFR}_{\text{women}} \text{ (ml/min)} = 0.85 \times \text{GFR}_{\text{men}}$$

These mathematic relations were empirically determined in studies on apparently normal subjects. They may be useful for approximating expected "normal" organ system performance in aging subjects. See the text for further discussion and references.

## References


1. Warner MA, Hosking MP, Lobdell CM, Melton LJ III. Effects of referral bias on surgical outcomes: a population-based study of surgical patients 90 years of age or older. Mayo Clin Proc 1990;65:1185–1191.
2. Shock NW, Greulich RC, et al. (eds). Normal Human Aging: The Baltimore Longitudinal Study of Aging. NIH Publ. no. 84-2450. Washington, DC: US Government Printing Office, 1984.
3. Moore FD, Olesen KH, McMurrey JD, Parker HV, Ball MR, Boyden CM. The Body Cell Mass and Its Supporting Environment. Philadelphia: Saunders, 1963.
4. Metter EJ, Conwit R, Tobin J, Fozard JL. Age-associated loss of power and strength in the upper extremities in women and men. J Gerontol 1997;52A:B267–B276.
5. Young A. Exercise physiology in geriatric practice. Acta Med Scand 1986;(suppl. 711):227–232.
6. Griffiths RD. Muscle mass, survival, and the elderly patient. Nutrition 1996;12:456–458.
7. Watters JM, Clancey SM, Moulton SB, Briere KM, Zhu J-M. Impaired recovery of strength in older patients after major abdominal surgery. Ann Surg 1993;218:380–393.
8. Seymour DG, Vaz FG. Aspects of surgery in the elderly: preoperative medical assessment. Br J Hosp Med 1987;37: 102–112.
9. Kinney JM, Lister J, Moore FD. Relationship of energy expenditure to total exchangeable potassium. Ann NY Acad Sci 1963;110:711–722.
10. Tzankoff SP, Norris AH. Effect of muscle mass decrease on age-related BMR changes. J Appl Physiol 1977;43:1001–1006.
11. Watters JM, Redmond ML, Desai D, March RJ. Effects of age

and body composition on the metabolic responses to elective colon resection. Ann Surg 1990;212:89–96.
12. Shock NW. Energy metabolism, caloric intake and physical activity of the aging. In: Carlson LA (ed) Nutrition in Old Age. 10th Symposium of the Swedish Nutrition Foundation. Uppsala: Almqvist & Wiksell, 1972:12–23.
13. Wilmore DW. The Metabolic Management of the Critically Ill. New York: Plenum, 1977:22, 28, 169.
14. Harris JA, Benedict FG. Standard basal metabolism constants for physiologists and clinicians. In: A Biometric Study of Basal Metabolism in Man. Philadelphia: Lippincott, 1919:233–250.
15. McGandy RB, Barrows CH Jr, Spanias A, Meredith A, Stone JL, Norris AH. Nutrient intakes and energy expenditure in men of different ages. J Gerontol 1966;21:587.
16. Verbrugge LM, Gruber-Baldini AL, Fozard JL. Age differences and age changes in activities: Baltimore Longitudinal Study of Aging. J Gerontol 1996;51B:S30–S41.
17. Frankenfield DF, Cooney RN, Smith JS, Rowe WA. Age-related differences in the metabolic response to injury. J Trauma 2000;48:49.
18. Rogers MA, Hagberg JM, Martin WH III, Ehsani AA, Holloszy JO. Decline in $VO_2max$ with aging in master athletes and sedentary men. J Appl Physiol 1990;69:2195–2199.
19. Dehn MM, Bruce RA. Longitudinal variations in maximal oxygen intake with age and activity. J Appl Physiol 1972; 33:805–807.
20. Lakatta EG. Cardiovascular reserve capacity in healthy older humans. Aging Clin Exp Res 1994;6:213–223.
21. Lakatta EG. Cardiovascular regulatory mechanisms in advanced age. Physiol Rev 1993;73:413–467.
22. Stratton JR, Cerqueira MD, Schwartz RS, et al. Differences in cardiovascular responses to isoproterenol in relation to age and exercise training in healthy men. Circulation 1992;86:504–512.
23. Rich MW, Imburgia M. Inotropic response to dobutamine in elderly patients with decompensated congestive heart failure. Am J Cardiol 1990;65:519–521.
24. Strandell T. Circulatory studies on healthy old men with special reference to the limitation of the maximal physical working capacity. Acta Med Scand 1964;175:1–44.
25. Port S, Cobb FR, Coleman RE, Jones RH. Effect of age on the response of the left ventricular ejection fraction to exercise. N Engl J Med 1980;303:1133–1137.
26. Gee MH, Gottlieb JE, Albertine KH, Kubis JM, Peters SP, Fish JE. Physiology of aging related to outcome in the adult respiratory distress syndrome. J Appl Physiol 1990;69: 822–829.
27. Hall JC, Tarala RA, Hall JL, Mander J. A multivariate analysis of the risk of pulmonary complications after laparotomy. Chest 1991;99:923–927.
28. Catley DM, Thornton C, Jordan C, Lehane JT, Royston D, Jones JG. Pronounced, episodic oxygen desaturation in the postoperative period: its association with ventilatory pattern and analgesic regimen. Anesthesiology 1985;63:20–28.
29. Lawrence VA, Hilsenbeck SG, Mulrow CD, Dhanda R, Sapp J, Page CP. Incidence and hospital stay for cardiac and pulmonary complications after abdominal surgery. J Gen Intern Med 1995;10:671–678.
30. Smetana GW. Preoperative pulmonary evaluation. N Engl J Med 1999;340:937–944.
31. Sorbini CA, Grassi V, Solinas E, Muiesan G. Arterial oxygen tension in relation to age in healthy subjects. Respiration 1968;25:3–13.
32. Pontoppidan H, Beecher HK. Progressive loss of protective reflexes in the airway with the advance of age. JAMA 1960;174:77–81.
33. Kronenberg RS, Drage CW. Attenuation of the ventilatory and heart rate responses to hypoxia and hypercapnia with aging in normal men. J Clin Invest 1973;52:1812–1819.
34. Peterson DD, Pack AI, Silage DA, Fishman AP. Effects of aging on ventilatory and occlusion pressure responses to hypoxia and hypercapnia. Am Rev Respir Dis 1981;124: 387–391.
35. Leblanc P, Ruff F, Milic-Emili J. Effects of age and body position on "airway closure" in man. J Appl Physiol 1970;28: 448–451.
36. Brandi LS, Bertolini R, Janni A, Gioia A, Angeletti CA. Energy metabolism of thoracic surgical patients in the early postoperative period: effect of posture. Chest 1996;109: 630–637.
37. Krieger BP, Ershowsky PF, Becker DA, Gazeroglu HB. Evaluation of conventional criteria for predicting successful weaning from mechanical ventilatory support in elderly patients. Crit Care Med 1989;17:858–861.
38. Cockcroft DW, Gault MH. Prediction of creatinine clearance from serum creatinine. Nephron 1976;16:31–41.
39. Garella S, Matarese RA. Renal effects of prostaglandins and clinical adverse effects of non-steroidal anti-inflammatory agents. Medicine 1984;63:165–181.
40. Hill GL. Implications of critical illness, injury, and sepsis on lean body mass and nutritional needs. Nutrition 1998;14: 557–558.
41. Vaughan MS, Vaughan RW, Cork RC. Postoperative hypothermia in adults: relationship of age, anesthesia, and shivering to rewarming. Anesth Analg 1981;60: 746–751.
42. Sessler DI. Mild perioperative hypothermia. N Engl J Med 1997;336:1730–1737.
43. Kurz A, Sessler DI, Lenhardt R. Perioperative normothermia to reduce the incidence of surgical-wound infection and shorten hospitalization. N Engl J Med 1996;334:1209–1215.
44. Frank SM, Fleisher LA, Breslow MJ. Perioperative maintenance of normothermia reduces the incidence of morbid cardiac events: a randomized clinical trial. JAMA 1997;227: 1127–1134.
45. Jones SR. Fever in the elderly. In: Mackowiak P (ed) Fever: Basic Mechanisms and Management. New York: Raven, 1991:233–242.
46. DuBois EF. Fever and the Regulation of Body Temperature. Springfield, IL: Charles C Thomas, 1948.
47. Scalea TM, Simon HM, Duncan AO, et al. Geriatric blunt multiple trauma: improved survival with early invasive monitoring. J Trauma 1990;30:129–134.
48. Finelli FC, Jonsson J, Champion HR, Morelli S, Fouty WJ. A case control study for major trauma in geriatric patients. J Trauma 1989;29:541–548.
49. McDaniel DD, Stone JG, Faltas AN, et al. Catheter-induced pulmonary artery hemorrhage. J Thorac Cardiovasc Surg 1981;82:1–4.

50. Clowes GHA Jr, Del Guercio LR. Circulatory response to trauma of surgical operations. Metabolism 1960;9:67.
51. Moore FA, Haenel JB, Moore EE, Whitehill TA. Incommensurate oxygen consumption in response to maximal oxygen availability predicts postinjury multiple organ failure. J Trauma 1992;33:58–67.
52. Shiozaki T, Kishikawa M, Hiraide A, et al. Recovery from postoperative hypothermia predicts survival in extensively burned patients. Am J Surg 1993;165:326–330.
53. Porter JM, Ivatury RR. In search of the optimal end points of resuscitation in trauma patients: a review. J Trauma 1998;44:908–914.
54. Detsky AS, McLaughlin JR, Baker JP, et al. What is subjective global assessment of nutritional status? JPEN 1987;11: 8–13.
55. Watters JM, Moulton SB, Clancey SM, Blakslee JM, Monaghan R. Aging exaggerates glucose intolerance following injury. J Trauma 1994;37:786–791.
56. Bessey PQ, Watters JM. Glucose metabolism following trauma and sepsis. In: Burke PA, Forse RA (eds) Clinical Responses to Injury and Sepsis: Mechanisms of Survival and Repair. New York: Marcel Dekker (in press).
57. Walker J, Cole M, Bessey PQ. Insulin protocol provides rapid, safe, and effective glucose control and saves time (in press).
58. Clevenger FW, Rodriguez DJ. Demarest GB, Osler TM, Olson SE, Fry DE. Protein and energy tolerance by stressed elderly patients. J Surg Res 1992;52:135–139.
59. Chandra RK. Effect of vitamin and trace-element supplementation on immune responses and infection in elderly subjects. Lancet 1992;340:1124–1127.
60. Girodon F, Lombard M, Galan P, et al. Effect of micronutrient supplementation on infection in institutionalized elderly subjects: a controlled trial. Ann Nutr Metab 1997;41: 98–107.
61. Parikh SS, Chung F. Postoperative delirium in the elderly. Anesth Analg 1995;80:1223–1232.
62. Creditor MC. Hazards of hospitalization of the elderly. Ann Intern Med 1993;118:219–223.
63. Moller JT, Cluitmans P, Rasmussen LS, et al. Long-term postoperative cognitive dysfunction in the elderly: ISPOCD1 study. Lancet 1998;351:857–861.
64. Shannon ML, Lehman CA. Protecting the skin of the elderly patient in the intensive care unit. Crit Care Nurs Clin North Am 1995;8:17–28.
65. Chelluri L, Grenvik A. Intensive care for critically ill elderly: mortality, costs, and quality of life. Arch Intern Med 1995; 155:1013–1022.
66. Mayer-Oakes SA, Oye RK, Leake B. Predictors of mortality in older patients following medical intensive care: the importance of functional status. J Am Geriatr Soc 1991;39: 862–868.
67. Ridley S, Jackson R, Findlay J, Wallace P. Long term survival after intensive care. BMJ 1990;301:1127–1130.
68. Wu AW, Rubin HR, Rosen MJ. Are elderly people less responsive to intensive care? J Am Geriatr Soc 1990;38: 621–627.
69. Heuser MD, Case LD, Ettinger WH. Mortality in intensive care patients with respiratory disease: is age important? Arch Intern Med 1992;152:1683–1688.
70. Zarén B, Bergström R. Survival compared to the general population and changes in health status among intensive care patients. Acta Anaesthesiol Scand 1989;33:6–12.
71. McClish DK, Powell SH, Montenegro H, Nochomovitz M. The impact of age on the utilization of intensive care resources. J Am Geriatr Soc 1987;35:983–988.
72. Nicolas F, Le Gall JR, Alperovitch A, Loirat P, Villers D. Influence of patients' age on survival, level of therapy and length of stay in intensive care units. Intensive Care Med 1987;13:9–13.
73. McLauchlan GJ, Anderson ID, Grant IS, Fearon KCH. Outcome of patients with abdominal sepsis treated in an intensive care unit. Br J Surg 1995;82:524–529.
74. Djaiani G, Ridley S. Outcome of intensive care in the elderly. Anaesthesia 1997;52:1130–1136.
75. Sage WM, Rosenthal MH, Silverman JF. Is intensive care worth it? An assessment of input and outcome for the critically ill. Crit Care Med 1986;14:777–782.
76. Rockwood K, Noseworthy TW, Gibney RTN, et al. One-year outcome of elderly and young patients admitted to intensive care units. Crit Care Med 1993;21:687–691.
77. Knaus WA, Draper EA, Wagner DP, et al. APACHE II: a severity of disease classification. Crit Care Med 1985;13: 818–829.
78. Margulies DR, Lekawa ME, Bjerke S, Hiatt JR, Shabot MM. Surgical intensive care in the nonagenarian: no basis for age discrimination. Arch Surg 1993;128:753–758.
79. Kass JE, Castriotta RJ, Malakoff F. Intensive care unit outcome in the very elderly. Crit Care Med 1992;20:1666–1671.
80. Dragsted L, Qvist J, Madsen M. Outcome from intensive care. IV. A 5-year study of 1308 patients: long-term outcome. Eur J Anaesthesiol 1990;7:51–62.
81. Yinnon A, Zimran A, Hershko C. Quality of life following intensive medical care. Q J Med 1989;264:347–357.
82. Chelluri L, Pinsky MR, Donohoe MP, Grenvik A. Long-term outcome of critically ill elderly patients requiring intensive care. JAMA 1993;269:3119–3123.
83. Uhlmann RF, Pearlman RA. Perceived quality of life and preferences for life-sustaining treatment in older adults. Arch Intern Med 1991;151:495–497.
84. Cohen IL, Lambrinos J. Investigating the impact of age on outcome of mechanical ventilation using a population of 41,848 patients from a statewide database. Chest 1995;107: 1673–1680.
85. Cohen IL, Lambrinos J, Fein IA. Mechanical ventilation for the elderly patient in intensive care: incremental charges and benefits. JAMA 1993;269:1025–1029.
86. Swinburne AJ, Fedullo AJ, Bixby K, Lee DK, Wahl GW. Respiratory failure in the elderly: analysis of outcome after treatment with mechanical ventilation. Arch Intern Med 1993;153:1657–1662.
87. Pesau B, Falger S, Berger E, et al. Influence of age on outcome of mechanically ventilated patients in an intensive care unit. Crit Care Med 1992;20:489–492.
88. Dardaine V, Constans T, Lasfargues G, Perrotin D, Ginies G. Outcome of elderly patients requiring ventilatory support in intensive care. Aging Clin Exp Res 1995;7:221–227.
89. Murphy DJ, Murray AM, Robinson BE, Campion EW. Outcomes of cardiopulmonary resuscitation in the elderly. Ann Intern Med 1989;111:199–205.

# 19 Care of the Injured Elderly

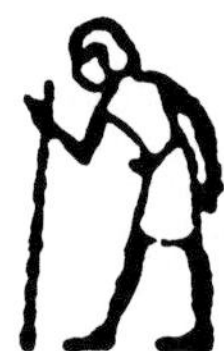

Thomas A. Santora, Stanley Z. Trooskin, and Lewis J. Kaplan

Not only is trauma a difficult disease to combat, it is difficult to recognize as a disease at all. Although injuries affect people of all ages, gender, and race, because of its unpredictable onset most people believe that it cannot or will not affect them. No one plans for trauma; they may buckle their seat belts when they get into their car, but they never expect to crash. They might even shovel and salt their front steps in the winter when it snows, but they never expect anyone to have a serious fall. Therefore it is difficult for anyone to plan for the consequences of an unexpected injury-induced, life-altering experience. Any sudden change in an individual's independence not only significantly affects the patient, it has a widespread effect on the family as a whole. Injury creates these unexpected, unplanned, unwanted consequences for hundreds of individuals each day. Such injuries can have cataclysmic effects in terms of loss of life, limb, income, and sense of self-worth. The portion of the health care team that treats the victims of trauma are intimately aware of the magnitude of this problem; however, other disciplines in the medical profession, legislators, funding agencies, and the lay public have not recognized injury and its consequences as a *plague* on modern-day living.

Review of the following statistics from the National Safety Council indicate that even if the pain and suffering of traumatic injury is not personally experienced, each American suffers the consequences of this disease by how it affects our health care delivery system. It is estimated that one in four Americans are injured each year.[1] In 1994 the National Health Interview Survey conducted personal interviews of approximately 46,000 households, representing 116,000 persons, to catalog the occurrence and consequences of the extent of (intentional and unintentional) injuries on the health status of the nation. This survey documented the incidence of an injury during the 2 weeks prior to the survey in this select population; extrapolation from these results estimated that approximately 60 million persons sustained injuries that resulted in 215.6 million days of bed confinement and 709.5 million days of restricted activity.[2] In the United States trauma accounts for approximately 40% of all emergency room visits, 10% of all hospital admissions, and 17% of hospital days. Independent of age, injury is the leading cause of all physician contacts.[3]

Death due to injury has been classified for epidemiologic reasons into five etiologies: unintentional, suicide, homicide, undetermined, and the result of operations of war. In 1995 death from unintentional injury increased in the United States for the third consecutive year: 93,300 Americans died, for a death rate of 35.5 per 100,000 population.[1] Unintentional injury comprised the largest cause of death due to injury mechanisms and is the fifth leading cause of death in America, independent of age. Based on 1993 U.S. National Center for Health Statistics data, after combining all causes of injury-related deaths (unintentional, 90,523, suicides, 31,102, homicides, 25,653, undetermined, 3419, operations of war, 8), injury became the fourth leading cause of death across all age categories.

The future of health care is projected to be affected to an even greater extent by this burgeoning plague. Murray and Lopez[4] developed a regression analysis of vital statistics from 47 countries for the years 1950–1990 to project the impact of various diseases on world health through the year 2020. This Global Burden of Disease Study correlated nine disease processes (including injury) with four independent variables (income per person, average years of schooling per adult, smoking intensity, time). They projected that deaths from injuries will increase worldwide by 65% during the 30 years between 1990 and 2020 (from 5.1 million to 8.4 million). Road traffic accidents are projected to be the third leading cause of death worldwide behind ischemic heart disease and unipolar major depression. Using a parameter called disability-adjusted life-years to reflect the percentage of overall disease disability attributed to a specific disease or class of diseases, injury is predicted to cause 20% of the overall disability due to disease by the year 2020. Though these projections are based on assumptions that may not materialize, the likelihood that injury and its management will

TABLE 19.1. Contribution of Unintentional Injury to Overall Mortality, Stratified by Age

| Age (years) | Death rate (%)[a] |
|---|---|
| <14 | 14.1 |
| 15–24 | 39.4 |
| 25–44 | 17.5 |
| 45–64 | 3.9 |
| >64 | 1.7 |

Total deaths due to unintentional injury for 1995 was 93,300.
[a] Number of deaths due to unintentional injury for the specific age group/all causes of death in that age group.

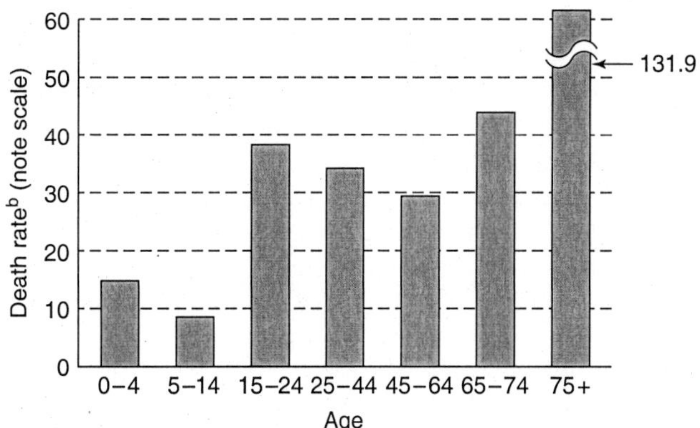


FIGURE 19.2. Mortality due to unintentional injury, all causes included, stratified by age. The elderly have the greatest death rate due to unintentional injury, especially the oldest-old. Death rate is given per 100,000 population within each age category. (From National Safety Council,[1] with permission.)

represent a significant "burden" for the health care provider of the early twenty-first century is high.

## Injured Elderly

Trauma is the most frequent cause of death in persons less than 38 years of age.[1] Based on 1993 death statistics, unintentional injury caused only 1.7% of the deaths in the elderly population (Table 19.1). Consequently, some consider this medical crisis to be an exclusively young persons' "problem." However, the elderly population comprise a large portion of the injured population and contribute disproportionally to the fatality of unintentional injury. In 1995 the elderly, defined as age >65, comprised 12.8% of the population but were responsible for 30% of the deaths due to unintentional injury (Fig. 19.1). In fact, the population-based death rate for unintentional injuries, all causes included, is greatest for the group >65 years (Fig. 19.2). The elderly, especially the oldest-old, have population-based mortality rates that exceed their younger cohort for most of the common causes of unintentional injury (Table 19.2).

The elderly increasingly are becoming victims of trauma. The 1994 National Health Interview Survey revealed that 9.9% of injuries or approximately 6 million, involved persons who were >65 years of age. Other reports have shown the rate of elderly involvement in trauma to vary between 4.4% and 29.0%, with the most recent studies showing the highest percentage of elderly victims.[1,5–8] Contributing to this increased volume of injury in the elderly is the disproportionate growth of the U.S. population since the turn of the twentieth century. During the past 90 years, the U.S. population has tripled, from 76 million to more than 250 million. During the same interval the elderly population has increased 10-fold, from 3.1 million to 31.1 million.[9] In 1991 the elderly represented 12.7% of the population; by the year 2050 Spencer[10] projects this proportion will reach 23%. Using Spencer's predictions, MacKenzie and coworkers[8] projected that the elderly will comprise 40% of the trauma population by the mid-twenty-first century. In this projection, MacKenzie et al. assumed a constant age-specific rate of hospitalization for trauma; however, this assump-

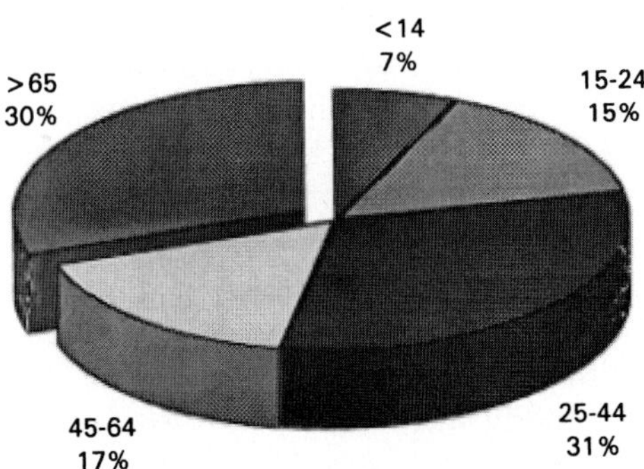


FIGURE 19.1. Percentage of deaths due to unintentional injury stratified for age. Unintentional injury is responsible for only a small percentage of the overall deaths in the elderly population, (1.7%, see text), but they comprise the second largest age group that experiences mortality from unintentional injury.

TABLE 19.2. Causes and Mortality of Unintentional Injury

| Cause | Overall death rate[a] (%) | Death rate in the Elderly[b] (%) Age 65–74 | Age > 75 |
|---|---|---|---|
| All | 35.5 | 43.0 | 13.2 |
| Motor vehicle crash | 16.7 | 18.0 | 29.0 |
| Falls | 4.8 | 8.2 | 54.8 |
| Poisoning (liquids) | 3.8 | 1.1 | 2.4 |
| Drowning | 1.7 | 1.1 | 1.5 |
| Burns | 1.6 | 2.2 | 4.8 |
| Suffocation | 1.1 | 2.2 | 8.4 |
| Firearms | 0.5 | 0.5 | 0.26 |
| Poisoning (gas) | 0.2 | 0.2 | 0.5 |

Data based on extraction from Census estimates of the 1995 population.
[a] Death rate per 100,000.
[b] Death rate per 100,000 in each age group.

tion may not be valid due to changing behavioral characteristics of the elderly.

Contemporary elders are living longer and in better health during their late years owing to advances in the treatment of such debilitating processes as cardiovascular diseases, diabetes, and arthritis. A healthier longevity allows them to be more physically active and mobile than their predecessors.[11] This increased activity exposes the elderly to more opportunities for injury. An active life style has been increasingly reported as a risk factor for falls and motor vehicle crashes.[12–14] Therefore the projection made by MacKenzie et al. should be considered an underestimation, but it may serve as a reference point to measure the efficacy of future injury prevention programs.

The elderly are predisposed to injuries because of the inevitable consequences of aging and the accumulation of diseases common to the aged population (Table 19.3). Age-related deterioration of the senses (diminution in hearing, presbyopia) along with changes in coordination, balance, motor strength, and postural stability reduce the elders' ability to avoid or react to environmental hazards. Diseases such as dementia, congestive heart failure, postural hypotension, and arthritis further exacerbate these limitations. Osteoporosis, a common process in elderly women, has been cited as a major factor contributing to the high incidence of fractures seen in elderly trauma patients.[3] The effect of osteoporosis is exemplified by the threefold increase in fractures seen in women following low-energy falls compared with those in elderly men.[12] Once injured, the elderly are predisposed to complications because of the co-morbidities of cardiovascular disease, diabetes, chronic obstructive pulmonary disease, liver disease, and renal insufficiency.

TABLE 19.3. Factors Predisposing the Elderly to Injury

**Reduced ability to react to environmental hazards**
- Reduced hearing
- Presbyopia
- Significant degenerative joint disease
- Vertigo

**Elderly placed in potentially dangerous situations**
- Dementia
- Cardiovascular accident
- Coronary artery disease
  - Dysrhythmias
  - Myocardial infarction
  - Postural hypotension

**Increased consequences of injury**
- Osteoporosis
- Cirrhosis
- Chronic obstructive pulmonary disease
- Coronary artery disease
- Disabling central nervous system disorders

The elderly may have chronic ailments that increase the likelihood and the consequences of injury.

The elderly trauma population experience the same injuries as their younger cohorts, but the cause of the injury, its physiologic effects, gender dominance, duration of disability, and outcome (Fig. 19.3) differs considerably. Understanding these differences between young and old patients better prepares physicians to handle the special challenges presented by the injured elder.

## Characteristics of Injury in the Elderly

Many of the differences between the age groups can be seen by reviewing the results of the Major Trauma Outcome Study (MTOS).[5] The MTOS, an American College of Surgeons cooperative study, established a database of 46,613 patients (3833 elderly) representing all trauma activity in 111 trauma centers in the United States and Canada during 1982–1986. Though this database contains patient care records from more than 10 years ago, the trends recorded for that period have not changed appreciably and illuminate the grave consequences injury frequently imposes on the elderly.

Falls, usually from level surfaces, are the most common mechanism leading to injury in the elderly population.[5,15] In contrast, topping the list of injury mechanisms for the younger cohort is motor vehicle crashes, which is the second most common mechanism in the elderly and the leading cause of trauma-related death in the elderly age 65–75.[13,16]

The MTOS results showed that mortality increased directly with age >55 years, regardless of the injury mechanism (Fig. 19.3), severity of the anatomic injury as measured by the Injury Severity Score (ISS) (Fig. 19.4), or the body region injured. Numerous other studies have similarly shown that injury in the elderly is associated with a higher mortality despite less severe anatomic injuries. For example, Evans[17] found the fatality rate for motor vehicle crash occupants over the age of 70 was three times that of those age 20. Oreskovich and coworkers[18] profiled the nonsurviving elderly patient as one who required prehospital intubation, had shock physiology more than 15 minutes, required mechanical ventilation more than 5 days, or who later developed pulmonary sepsis.

Elderly trauma patients more frequently die from their injuries than do these in any other age group (Table 19.2); and within the elderly group the mortality rate increases directly with age (Fig. 19.2).[5,7] Morris et al.[19] attributed the higher elderly mortality to the effects of associated diseases, specifically cirrhosis, ischemic heart disease, obstructive lung disease, and diabetes. Other studies[15] have refuted the significance of chronic illnesses.

Similar extent of anatomic injury, as measured by the ISS, leads to increased complications and death in the elderly group when compared to younger trauma

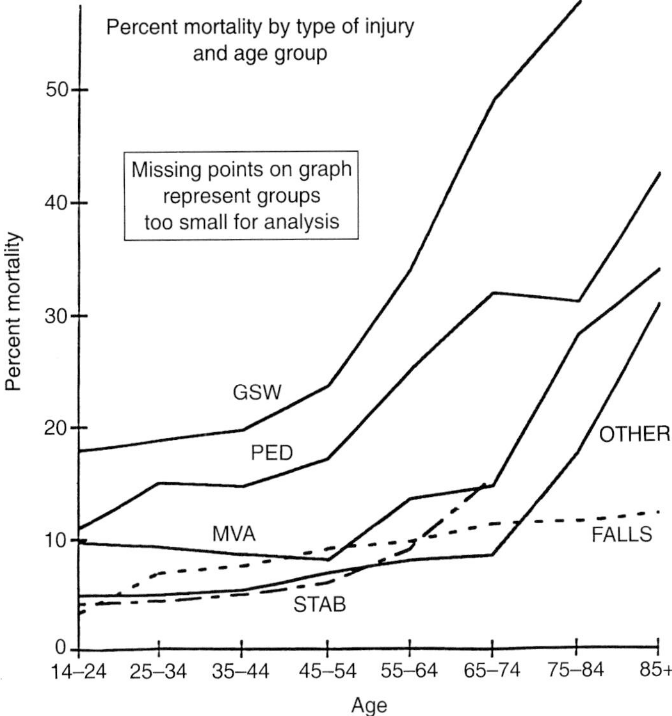


FIGURE 19.3. Major Trauma Outcome Study (MTOS) data from 1982 to 1986 that show the age-related increases in mortality due to injury, regardless of cause. Dashed lines represent the mortality rates for the categories of stab wounds and "other" mechanisms. Missing points on the graph represent groups too small for analysis. GSW, gunshot wounds; PED, pedestrian accidents; MVA, motor vehicle accidents. (From Finelli et al.,[7] with permission.)

patients (Fig. 19.4).[5,7,15,20] In a study by Smith and coworkers,[15] the ISS at which the probability of death was 10% was found to be 17.3 in those over 65 years of age and 24.9 in the younger cohort. In 1989 Finelli et al.[7] used the MTOS data to show a marked difference in mortality between the young and the old (9.8% vs. 19.0%, respectively) despite similar scores on the ISS and Revised Trauma Score (RTS). Within the elderly group, the ISS directly correlated with mortality (survivors' ISS, 10.6 vs. nonsurvivors' ISS, 23.9). All patients with an ISS of more than 55 had a universally poor outcome, regardless of age (Fig. 19.4). Oreskovich and coworkers[18] showed insensitivity of the ISS to predict mortality in 100 elderly patients (age >70). Despite a similar ISS for survivors and nonsurvivors (19 vs. 17, respectively), 15% died; whereas an ISS of 19 would have predicted a mortality of 3%.[21] The apparently conflicting results of the predictive utility of the ISS in the elderly population between the latter two studies has been attributed to the small number of nonsurviving patients in the Oreskovich et al. study. Whether the ISS can discriminate outcome within the elderly trauma population may be debatable, but it seems clear that adjustments of the ISS-predicted mortality are necessary to obtain accurate outcome predictions for the elderly population.

Physiologic derangements have been used to explain mortality following traumatic injury in the elderly. In a study from Cedars-Sinai Medical Center in Los Angeles,[22] outcome following trauma was specifically analyzed for the effect of age in 2166 patients, 289 of whom were more than 65 years of age. Three important points were illustrated in this retrospective review. The elderly, when compared to the <65 age group, had significantly more physiologic derangement measured by the Simplified Acute Physiological Score (SAPS) (average 12.3 vs. 7.9, respectively; $p < 0.0005$) despite similar anatomic injuries (ISS 14.2 vs. 12.3, respectively; $p = 0.06$). There was no difference in SAPS in nonsurviving patients regardless of age (18.2 vs. 19.9, respectively). The significant difference in mortality seen in the elderly group (16.3% vs. 5.3%) was eliminated when the two age groups were stratified by SAPS, except in the mildly deranged SAPS group (range 5–14), where the elderly died significantly more often than their younger cohort with similar mild physiologic derangements.

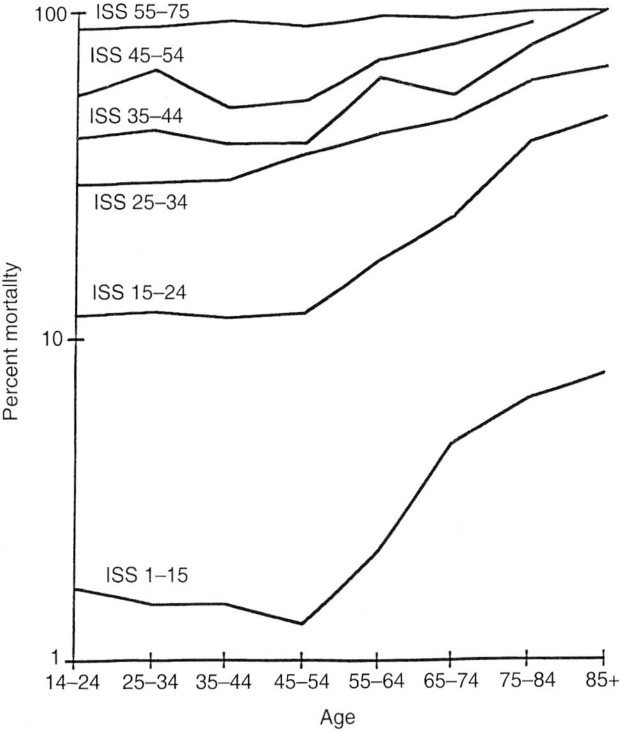


FIGURE 19.4. MTOS data from 1982 to 1986 show the age-dependent variation in mortality stratified for injury severity. Notice the increase in mortality for the age group more than 55 years old; this increase is especially marked in the lower Injury Severity Score (ISS) ranges. For any ISS, the difference in mortality between the young and old diminishes as the ISS increases such that any patient with an ISS > 55, regardless of age, had nearly universal mortality. (From Finelli et al.,[7] with permission.)

It seems logical that the presence of significant co-morbidities predispose the elderly to the development of complications following injury. This logic is consistent with the proposed "two-hit" theory of organ dysfunction: addition of injury-induced physiologic stress imposed on impaired organ function due to preexisting co-morbid medical conditions should lead to increased morbidity and mortality. Smith and coworkers[15] showed that complications occurred in 26% of their elderly population, the most common being infection in 14.5%, followed by pulmonary in 10.7%, cardiac in 5.5%, and renal in 3.7%. In this study, more than one complication following trauma was associated with a mortality of 30%. Complications following injury increase the potential for death, regardless of age. As an illustration, Bellemare et al.[23] reviewed 10,001 trauma patients to correlate complications to outcome. The elderly who developed pneumonia had significantly increased mortality compared to the younger pneumonia cohort (54% vs. 27.8%; $p < 0.01$). Mortality in complicated cases was significantly higher than in cases without complications (45.6% vs. 5.8%; $p < 0.01$), independent of age.

## Effect of Substance Abuse on Elder Trauma

### Alcohol

Alcohols are central nervous system (CNS) depressants and as such impair the brain's ability to process incoming stimuli and integrate data to formulate and implement an appropriate response. It is intuitive that the elder with age-compromised brain function such as diminished vision, audition, or cognition may be more severely hampered by a CNS depressant at equipotent doses than would a younger person. To support such a hypothesis, an analogy is drawn to the use of clinically important sedatives in elderly ICU patients; the elderly generally require considerably smaller doses to achieve the desired response than do younger patients. Fortunately, alcohol intake appears to play a lesser role in trauma in the elderly than it does in the younger patient population. Accordingly, Rhem and Ross[24] documented that of the drivers judged to be at fault for their respective crash, only 4 of 84 elderly drivers compared to 19 of 130 younger drivers were legally intoxicated. Similarly, Wolf and Rivara stated that the elderly are approximately one-fifth as likely to operate a motor vehicle while intoxicated as youthful drivers.[16]

Moderate to heavy alcohol use by the elderly was found to be statistically associated with concomitant malignancy and to be independently predictive of elder suicide.[25] Curiously, alcohol has not been associated with falls in the elderly population;[26] instead, failure of balance mechanisms as predicted by the one-leg balance test are statistically associated with fall injuries in the elderly.[27] It should be noted that the incidence of alcohol use in the elderly may be underrepresented in current studies, as most rely on self-reporting instead of objective testing methods. Additionally, the practitioner should be aware that substances other than alcohol may influence the predilection for injury as well as the resultant anatomic injury patterns.

### Substance Abuse

For the purposes of this discussion, substance abuse is loosely defined in both the traditional manner (substances used for pleasure or to satisfy chemical dependence) and as the inappropriate use of prescription medications or improper intake of an appropriate medication with a subsequent untoward effect. There are few data to address the effect of illicit drug use on trauma in the elderly, possibly because users of illicit drugs only infrequently survive to 65 years of age.

The "abuse" potential in the elderly is great for a variety of factors, some of which are: multiple co-morbid conditions treated with multiple medications, impaired mentation due to organic causes or side effects of medications, and unrecognized drug–drug or nutrient–drug interactions due to the use of multiple physicians, pharmacies, or both. Whether substance "abuse" is because of pleasure-seeking behavior or is a consequence of polypharmacy, abusive practices predispose the elderly to injury. Ryynanen et al.[28] found that both advanced age and benzodiazepine use were independently predictive of falls requiring medical therapy. These same authors noted that digitalis use in men but not women correlated with falls.

Most substance abuse aside from alcohol in the elderly stems from physician-prescribed medications to treat ailments such as chronic pain syndromes, herniated nucleus pulposus, osteoarthritis, migraine headache, and myriad disorders whose hallmark is somatic complaints or neuropsychological disturbances (i.e., anxiety syndromes). Health care professionals treating elderly trauma victims must maintain a high index of suspicion for substance abuse as a contributing factor to the injury and rigorously evaluate the potential of drug–drug interactions that may have unexpected consequences. Recognition of these "abuses" may allow behavior modification to reduce the potential for subsequent injury.

## Epidemiology of Injury in the Elderly

### Falls

The elderly account for 70%[29] of all falls. These falls are rarely from great heights, as they are in younger patients; rather, they occur on steps or, most commonly, from flat surfaces as the elder fails to navigate environmental hazards or simply drops owing to a syncopal episode or loss of balance. Approximately one-third of the population over 65 years of age who live in the community sustain a fall each year.[30] Estimates from hospital records suggest that 3.8% of the group over age 65 suffer a significant fall each year,[31] and the incidence of falls increases directly with age.[1,32] Most falls occur in or about the home, with the greatest number during winter months.[33] Once fallen, up to 50% of the elderly cannot get up without assistance because of weakness or limited range of motion due to underlying musculoskeletal disabilities.[30] In the latter situations, if the fall is unwitnessed, the elder may be "down" for long enough periods of time to develop decubiti, rhabdomyolysis, and even dehydration. Serious injury has been reported with 12–47% of falls. Fractures of the hip or upper extremity are the most common serious sequelae of falls in the elderly. Though elderly women are no more likely to fall, they sustain serious injury, usually fractures, more commonly than men.[12,34] Compared to age-matched women, elderly men incur more CNS injuries and have higher mortality following falls.[32,35] Sattin and coworkers[12] attributed it to higher risk-taking and underreporting of less severe fall-injuries in men.

Numerous studies[12,29,36–39] have outlined the risk factors for falls among the elderly (Table 19.4). Debilitating chronic diseases such as parkinsonism, stroke, arthritis, dementia, and anemia are more prevalent in the population of elderly who sustain falls.[40,41] Among the other factors are older age; Caucasian race; history of previous falls; polypharmacy (especially psychotropic agents, diltiazem, laxatives, and diuretics); dependence for activities of daily living; low body mass; and impaired mobility, muscle strength, gait, balance, vision, hearing, and cognition. These factors have all been correlated with an increased risk of falls and fall-related injury. The role of exercise as a risk factor is not clear. Though exercise may lead to increased coordination and strength, which some studies have shown significantly decreases the incidence of falls,[41] exercise also increases the exposure of the elderly to possible fall scenarios.

TABLE 19.4. Risk Factors for Falls and Fall-Related Injuries

| |
|---|
| Chronic debilitating diseases |
| Parkinson's |
| Strokes |
| Arthritis |
| Anemia |
| Dementia |
| Neuromuscular disorders |
| Acute illnesses |
| Advanced age |
| Sensory impairments |
| Unsteady gait |
| Lower extremity weakness |
| Low body mass |
| Caucasian |
| Exercise[a] |
| Previous falls |
| Dependence for ADLs |
| Postural hypotension |
| Syncope |
| Dysrhythmias |
| Seizure |
| Carotid stenosis |
| Aortic stenosis |
| Medications |
| Benzodiazepines |
| Phenothiazines |
| Antidepressants |
| Diuretics |
| Laxatives |
| Diltiazem |

[a] Exercise has an inconsistent effect on the incidence of falls and fall-related injuries (see text).
ADLs, activities of daily living.

Falls among the elderly result from a complex interaction of structural and physiologic disabilities resulting from the aging process, alterations in safe behavioral practices, and environmental hazards (Fig. 19.5). The consequences of a fall depend on such factors as the kinetic energy generated during the falling process, the ability of the body structures to absorb the energy, the capacity of the fall surface to accept the kinetic energy transfer, the protective responses and the garments of the faller, and the direction and body location of the impact.[34] Functional consequences of the aging process such as diminished visual, vestibular, and somatosensory sensation that adversely affect gait, balance, and coordination along with an alteration in cognition due to dementia, which may lead to increased risk-taking or just lack of realization of their limitations, predispose the elderly to falls with potential serious consequences. In addition, the aging process frequently leads to loss of muscle mass and changes in body composition that results in reductions in strength; combined with a limited range of motion due to degenerative joint diseases, the elderly are less able to

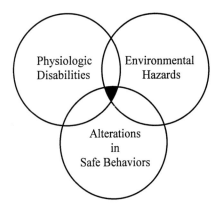


FIGURE 19.5. Major forces leading to falls in the elderly population. Elders with the greatest risk for falls are represented in the shaded area, where all three conditions are operative.

absorb the kinetic energy transferred during a fall without injurious consequences.

Many elderly have more than one of the above risk factors that predispose them to falls. Duthie[29] suggested that approximately 25% of falls by the elderly were caused by an underlying medical problem. Therefore in addition to treating the resultant injuries, management of the elderly fall victim must include an investigation into the cause of the fall, which can frequently be determined from a thorough history.

Falls by the elderly lead to life-altering consequences. Approximately 8% of the elderly population seek emergency room care as a result of a fall; 40% of these visits lead to hospital admission, with an average length of stay of 11.6 days.[12] According to Nelson and Amin,[37] 50% of the elderly hospitalized for falls die within a year. Alexander et al.[42] showed that patients hospitalized for falls were discharged to a nursing facility more frequently than patients hospitalized for other conditions: 43% versus 13%, respectively. In a self-reporting national survey, the elderly reported falls and fall-related injury as the largest cause of restricted activity of all health-altering conditions.[43] Fear of falling has been shown to cause poor motivation in the elderly, which can lead to a reduction in activities and isolation.[37,40,44]

The economic impact of falls among the elderly population has been estimated by Englander and coworkers.[45] Using the same methodology as the only detailed cost analysis on the effect of injury performed by Max et al. in 1990,[46] adjustments were made to account for demographic and price level changes to project cost of care in terms of 1994 dollars. The elderly were projected to consume $20.2 billion of health care as a result of falls and resultant injury. This expenditure would constitute approximately one-third of the total cost of care for falls in all age groups. This projection was taken to the year 2020, where care of the elderly fall victim was estimated to cost $32.4 billion in 1994 dollars. This 60% increase in cost is explained by the projected increases in the elderly population as the "baby-boomers" reach their twilight years.

## Motor Vehicle Crashes

Elderly drivers appear to have low crash rates compared with younger drivers, but they drive much less often. When the groups are normalized for the number of miles driven, the >65 years group has the second highest crash rate after new drivers. The >85 years group has the highest per-mile-driven crash rate of all age groups. In contrast to the young cohort, the elderly are more likely to be involved in vehicle–vehicle crashes, usually during daylight hours and frequently at intersections. The elderly are less likely to crash because of reckless driving, driving while intoxicated, or driving at excessive speeds; rather, they are more likely to crash because of failure to yield the right of way, during turns, or while reversing direction. The elderly have the highest crash-related mortality of all age groups. The National Accident Sampling System data have shown that of all elderly occupants killed, 25% are involved in side-impact crashes. Of those, nearly 50% are due to elderly driver error.[14] Other studies[16,47,48] have shown the elderly are likely to be responsible for the crash in which they are involved. Driver error in these instances is frequently the result of inattention or misjudgment at intersections.

Altered perception due to reduced vision or hearing, impaired judgment, and reduced reaction times are well recognized as factors leading to vehicular crashes in the elderly. Investigation into the influence of chronic diseases on the capacity of the elderly motorist has been undertaken. In a case–control study, Koepsell and coworkers[48] showed that diabetes, especially when insulin-dependent and with a disease duration of more than 5 years, significantly increased the risk of a vehicular crash with injury. Though this population-based study did not report on the incidence of hypoglycemia in these diabetic victims, it suggested that diabetes with or without hypoglycemia can lead to transient alterations in cognition that may adversely effect operation of a motor vehicle. Rehm and Ross[47] showed that elderly crash victims had a significantly higher incidence of underlying disease(s) such as cardiac, hypertension, diabetes, or neurologic diseases than did victims in the young cohort. Whether these diseases led to causation of the crash is not clear from this study; however, the authors stated that these diseases were more commonly found in the elderly drivers found at fault for their crash than in the no-fault elderly drivers.

In a study that involved more than 6000 crashes, 312 of which involved an elderly occupant, McCoy and coworkers[3] found that the resultant injury pattern was independent of age with the exception that the elderly suffered more sternal fractures than the younger cohort (11.0% vs. 1.5%, respectively). In general, the elderly are more seriously injured than the young cohort for any given crash, have longer hospital stays, and are significantly more likely to succumb as a direct result of the crash or its consequences.

## Pedestrian–Motor Vehicle Crashes

McCoy et al.[3] showed the elderly were more likely to be involved in a pedestrian crash as a result of walking directly into the path of oncoming vehicles, often due to confusion or impairment of visual or auditory acuity. Reduced gait speed of the elderly pedestrian may be inadequate to complete the crosswalk at time-controlled traffic intersections, thus leaving the elder in the street and exposed to inattentive drivers. The elderly pedestrian victim is more likely to have significant lower extremity and head injuries than the younger group. The

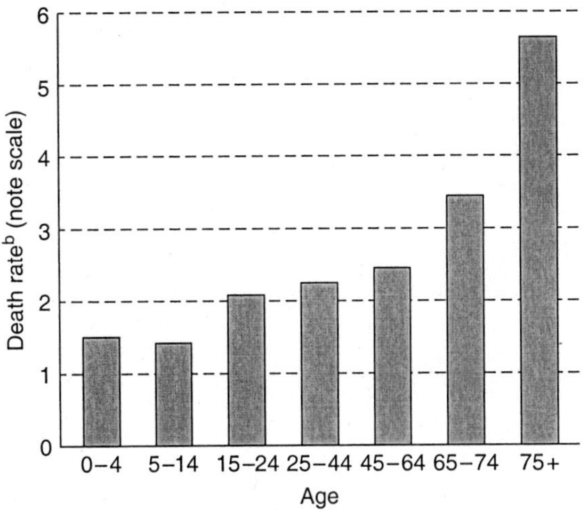


FIGURE 19.6. Mortality rates for pedestrians struck by motor vehicles, stratified by age. The elderly experience the greatest mortality of all victims of pedestrian–motor vehicle collisions. The death rate is per 100,000 population within each age category. (From National Safety Council,[1] with permission.)

elderly pedestrian has higher mortality rates after motor vehicle collisions than any other age group, including children (Fig. 19.6).

## Burns

As with all age groups, most burn injuries sustained by the elderly occur in the residential setting. Though the elderly comprise a small portion of the total population injured by burns, they have the highest case-fatality rate of any age group. The oldest-old have the highest mortality. Men have a higher mortality in all age groups and make up a larger proportion of the elderly group. The elderly have a higher fatality rate than young adults for the same extent of burn.[13] In general, burn mortality varies directly with increasing age and the size of the burn. Risk factors for burn injury in the elderly are the same as in younger adults; they include use of cigarettes or alcohol (or both) and living in poverty.

## Elder Abuse

When the elderly suffer abuse, it is usually at the hands of their care providers: spouses, children, other family members, nursing-facility employees. This abuse may take many forms, such as psychological, financial, or merely neglect of the duties of elder care. Such injuries are considerably more subtle in their presentation than the physical wounds of the elder who suffers from a physical assault. The health care provider must have a keen insight into the possibility of elder abuse to make the diagnosis, keeping in mind that this subtle presentation could be compounded by the episodic, though chronic, nature of most forms of domestic abuse. The incidence of elder abuse has been reported to be 3.2%,[49] but this surely underestimates the magnitude of the problem owing to the victim's reluctance to admit abuse for fear of loss of care, retribution from the abuser, or being ashamed to be in an abusive relationship. In addition, there is considerable variation of what is considered abuse among ethnic groups.

TABLE 19.5. Risk Factors for Elder Abuse

| |
|---|
| Increased frailty of the victim |
| Cognitive impairment of the victim |
| Mental illness of the abuser |
| Substance abuse by the abuser |
| Family history of violence or antisocial behavior |
| Victim and abuser live together |
| Isolation of the victim |
| Recent life stress |

Risk factors[49,50] have been recognized to alert the health care provider to the diagnosis of abuse (Table 19.5). Once suspicion of abuse has been raised, the victim should be interviewed one-on-one to increase the likelihood of frank disclosure of the extent and details of the abuse without the victim's fear of embarrassment often imposed by revealing such details to a group of health care personnel. The details of the abuse should be documented completely in the medical record for the possibility of subsequent legal action. The physician who documents or suspects elder abuse is ethically obligated, and in most states legally bound, to report the case to an adult protective service agency. The reader is cautioned about the potential liability for the physician who does not recognize or report elder abuse.

The most important intervention is to protect the victim from dangerous situations. Often the victim is reluctant to leave the care of their abuser because of ambivalent feelings regardless of the perceived danger. Unless the victim lacks the cognitive skills to make informed decisions, the individual liberty of the victim to make decisions must not be compromised. Under these circumstances, the physician should interview the abuser in a nonconfrontational fashion to better understand the situation from another perspective. The physician should be careful to acknowledge and empathize with the difficulty of shouldering the burden of elder care. Armed with this additional information, the physician is better prepared to intervene to break the cycle of abuse.

## Suicide

The rates of self-inflicted injury and suicide are increasing in the elderly population.[51] Caucasian men, with modest monetary assets, have the highest incidence of suicide in the elderly population. A factor potentially contributing to this increased suicide rate may be the apparent "resigned acceptance" by factions of the medical profession of suicide as an answer to the pain and suffering of the consequences of aging. This "ageism" view does not take into consideration potentially correctable factors that contribute to the elder's despair. Factors such as a sense of hopelessness, the anniversary of a bereavement, or impending relocation from their usual living environment may fuel these feelings of despair. Risk factors for suicide in the elderly population include psychiatric disorders, especially depression; medical conditions, especially cancer or chronic lung disease; moderate to large alcohol use; and social isolation. Family members and the health care professional should recognize that changes in behavior such as altering a will, new preoccupation with religion, or giving away life possessions may be warning signs of impending suicide in the at-risk elder. The elderly frequently use overmedication, or poisons ingestion to effect their suicidal gesture.[52]

## Influence of Senescence

Understanding how co-morbid disease states affect elderly trauma victims hinges on an appreciation of the diminished physiologic reserve that accompanies aging. Senescence affects all organ systems but does so to varying degrees and at variable times during the aging process of any individual person. At times the decline in function that occurs in all organ systems with increasing age may be difficult to decipher from the impact of co-morbid diseases with specific end-organ damage. For example, in the CNS the cerebral atrophy and small-vessel microocclusion that occur with aging are easily identified on a cerebral computed tomography (CT) scan as decreased brain volume and periventricular leukodystrophic changes. The functional correlate of these anatomic changes is identified as impaired cognition, with decreased short-term memory. This same presentation may be due to many of the dementia-producing disease processes. Less ambiguous are the appreciable decreases in vision and audition that "normally" accompany aging.

With increasing age, cardiopulmonary function declines in specific ways. Myocardial contractility is depressed, and ventricular compliance falls for any given preload. The aged myocardium also fails to respond briskly to heightened endogenous or exogenous catecholamine challenge. There is a fall in the maximum oxygen utilization and maximum attainable heart rate. The incidence of dysrhythmia is increased, probably as a result of ischemic changes to the conduction system.[53] Ventriculoarterial coupling is hampered by progressive arteriolar stiffening and loss of arterial elastance, leading to an increased frequency of orthostatic hypotension.

Lung elastance also progressively declines, and the time constants for individual lung units progressively lengthen. The net effect is a diminished total lung volume and alveolar surface area available for gas exchange. Furthermore, the aging mucociliary elevator functions less well and with fewer cilia per square centimeters of surface area, which leads to impaired secretion clearance and a predisposition to pulmonary infection. Gram-negative organisms predominate in the oral flora of the elderly, and this altered flora increases the risk of pulmonary infection from aspiration.[54]

Decreased renal function, as measured by the glomerular filtration rate, creatinine clearance, renal blood flow (decreased 40% by age 65), and maximal renal tubular solute-concentrating function (decreased 35% by age 65), inexorably accompanies aging.[55] The physician must bear in mind that renal function may be underestimated by evaluating the serum creatinine alone. Because this biochemical marker is directly influenced by muscle mass, as elders undergo loss of lean body mass, their serum creatinine for a given level of renal function is falsely low.

Endocrine dysfunction accompanies aging as well. The most notable endocrinopathy of aging is glucose intolerance, stemming primarily from impaired insulin release to a given glucose load rather than enhanced peripheral insulin resistance.[56] Desai et al.,[57] investigating the effect of age on blood glucose, insulin, and cortisol responses after mild and moderate trauma, noted that increasing age was associated with an increase in serum glucose but not an increase in insulin. Serum cortisol responses were increased in old patients and then decreased with time after injury. This finding suggests that the endocrine stress response to trauma in the elderly may be blunted, making resuscitation more complicated. Growth hormone levels, protein turnover, and urinary nitrogen loss are decreased in geriatric trauma patients compared to that in younger patients, suggesting reduced metabolic responsiveness to trauma in the elderly.[58] Rudman et al.[59] documented that half of the 12 healthy individuals between the ages of 60 and 79 years of age showed evidence of impaired growth hormone release. In the geriatric population, in contrast to the young, there was significant sodium, phosphorus, and potassium retention in response to exogenous growth hormone administration. These observations suggest that the elderly may have difficulty in handling fluid shifts associated with major injuries. There are also age-related changes in the hypothalamic-pituitary axis and decreases in the robustness of thyroid function and responsiveness to metabolic stress. Similarly, adrenal insufficiency is more commonly diagnosed in the elderly, perhaps related to diminished reserve, which may be recognized only when failure to respond to the stress of acute illness or injury is realized.

Nutritional reserve is depressed in the elderly population owing to the potential combination of poor intake (caused by lack of adequate care or reduced appetite due to chronic diseases) and active debilitating chronic diseases (e.g., the cachexia of severe cardiac dysfunction or malignancy).[60] The precise impact of defective immunologic function is not well understood for the aging process but would undoubtedly adversely affect host defenses against a microbial challenge or evolution of a neoplastic process.

## Consequences of Co-Morbid Diseases

Clearly, senescence-induced decrements in physiologic function and reserve predisposes the elderly to a variety of injuries and may seriously hinder an elder's ability to weather the consequences of the trauma. In addition to senescence, the physiologic and anatomic capabilities of the elderly are adversely affected by an increased prevalence of chronic diseases. Milzman and coworkers identified that co-morbidities increased with age such that approximately three-fourths of injured patients aged 75 years or greater have at least one preexisting major organ system dysfunction.[61] This same group documented that mortality rose from 6.1% with one preexisting condition to 24.7% with three or more preexisting diseases. Other workers found that gender and the presence of preexisting conditions enhanced the predictive value of the Trauma and Injury Severity Score (TRISS) and A Severity Characterization of Trauma (ASCOT) methodologies to predict survival from low falls.[62] Co-morbid conditions must be identified in the injured elder not only because knowledge of the co-morbidities may offer insight to the cause of the injury but these co-morbidities frequently require treatment for adequate recovery to be made from the resultant injury. Once recovered, knowledge of the co-morbidities may allow interventions that can prevent recidivism.

In addition, understanding the gravity of the underlying diseases may allow the physician treating the injured elder to stratify the risk of mortality.[63] Because these analyses deal with probabilities and not certainties, application to an individual patient may be problematic but can allow the physician a context from which to refer when discussing care plans with patients and their families. It is hoped that through frank discussions such as these, patient care can proceed with clear, realistic goals that are consistent with the individual's self-determined care plan.

### Neurologic Disease

It is important to recall that neurologic injury is influenced by the housing structures of the CNS in addition to the well-recognized transfer of kinetic energy to the neural parenchyma. Age-related brain atrophy lengthens the distance between the inner table of the skull and the outer surface of the brain. The bridging veins are thus pulled taut and are more likely to sustain a shear-type injury during rotational stress, such as during a deceleration force in a motor vehicle crash. This geometric arrangement results in a higher proportion of subdural extraaxial hematomas in the elderly than in the young. Similarly, degenerative disease of the bony cervical spine narrows the central spinal canal and leads to an increased frequency of central cord syndrome, especially with extension-type forces.[64] Thromboembolic cerebral ischemic events, demyelinating processes, and sequelae of CNS infections predispose the elderly to gait abnormalities, incoordination, and physical and mental disability. The cumulative result of such impairments and the prevalence of CNS abnormalities in the elderly makes even the simplest tasks a potential setup for injury. In fact, largely due to CNS dysfunction, navigation of stairways has been cited as a major cause of fall injuries in the elderly.[65] The Global Burden of Disease Study projects cerebrovascular disease to be the fourth leading cause of disability-adjusted life years in 2020, so the elderly population of the future will face similar challenges for even the simplest activities of daily living (ADLs).[4]

As the population ages, the proportion of elderly individuals progressively increases and so does the proportion of elderly with "physically functional but cognitively impaired" disorders such as Alzheimer's disease. In fact, one community-based study documented 58.4 injuries per 100 person-years in patients with Alzheimer's disease.[66] More than 50% of those injured required medical treatment, and the likelihood of injury was statistically associated with cognitive impairment and limitation in ADLs.

### Cardiovascular Disease

The well-described progression of coronary artery disease with aging contributes greatly to problems faced by the injured elder. Wilson described a 13.7% incidence of hypertension and 5.6% occurrence of symptomatic coronary artery disease (CAD) in a series of trauma patients over the age of 65 years.[67] In the population of patients older than 75 years, complications of symptomatic CAD rose to 12.9%. Accordingly, Wilson recommended aggressive use of invasive hemodynamic monitoring to avoid myocardial stress due to hypoperfusion and hypoxemia. Despite the known cardiovascular changes that accompany aging, there is no consensus regarding the use of invasive hemodynamic monitoring in the elderly. A collective review of the literature from the United Kingdom detailed no fewer than 10 reviews of trauma in the elderly that cited cardiovascular disease, complications of cardiovascular disease, or cardiac medications as important etiologic factors.[68] Syncope was a frequently (14%) cited etiologic factor in motor vehicle crashes involving "at fault" elderly motorists.[24,28] Syncope has been associated with dysrhythmias (primarily ventricular) and medications or their side effects (most notably β-blockade). Directly and indirectly, syncope frequently stems from underlying CAD or therapy for that condition.

The treating physician must be aware that medications and CAD (especially right-sided coronary lesions) may blunt or inhibit the expected tachycardic response to acute intravascular loss and cloud the anticipated pattern of response to injury. Reported mortality rates for geriatric trauma patients admitted to the ICU are approximately 22%[69] and stem from cardiovascular failure as a primary event or due to delay in diagnosis of secondary cardiovascular dysfunction. Secondary cardiovascular failure may arise as a consequence of underresuscitation, or it may be an accompaniment to sepsis or the systemic inflammatory response syndrome (SIRS). Advanced age (>65 years), preexisting conditions such as CAD or hypertension, and malnutrition were among the important independent predictors of multisystem organ failure in one study of trauma patients.[70]

## Pulmonary Disease

Aging clearly has a deleterious effect on pulmonary function, as detailed earlier. Injury induces pulmonary dysfunction while simultaneously increasing the work necessary for gas exchange; coupling these changes with the known maximal frequency of pulmonary dysfunction during the sixth decade[13] may cripple a severely injured elder. Chronic obstructive pulmonary disease (COPD), bronchiectasis, and bronchitis promote pulmonary infection following blunt thoracic injury. Intubated elders with these disease processes demonstrate a higher ventilator-associated pneumonia rate than their more youthful cohort. Osteopenia of the thoracic cage may contribute to pulmonary contusion, the frequency of rib fractures, and pneumo- and hemopneumothoraces by failing to allow the bony thorax to absorb and recover from transmitted kinetic energy. Accordingly, flail chest in the elderly correlates with prolonged mechanical ventilation.[54]

Because COPD is so prevalent in the elderly population, we consider it in some detail as it relates to promotion of complications following traumatic injury. COPD is a disease process characterized by nonreversible airflow impedance, deranged gas exchange with subsequent development of secondary pulmonary hypertension, and increased work of breathing. Reduced synthesis of nitric oxide (NO) has been implicated in the pathogenesis of pulmonary hypertension associated with COPD and may be related to chronic tissue hypoxia.[71] In addition to being constitutively synthesized by pulmonary vascular endothelium where it acts as a vasodilator, NO is released by macrophages and neutrophils as a cytotoxic agent,[72] and as a neurotransmitter for nonadrenergic, noncholinergic inhibitory nerves of the human bronchial tree where it serves as a bronchodilator.[73] It has also been suggested that the toxic products of inhaled tobacco smoke damages the NO-producing bronchial mucosal cells and subsequently reduces the exhaled NO concentration and impairs desirable bronchial dilatation.[74] Thus reduced endovascular and epithelial NO production from a complex interplay of factors renders the elder with COPD less able to reduce intrapulmonary shunting, augment pulmonary blood flow, and induce bronchial dilatation in response to pulmonary trauma. This constellation of deleterious effects may be responsible for the difficulty weaning some elderly patients from mechanical ventilation. Clinical trials with inhaled NO are under way to determine its role in the treatment of acute lung injury.

## Renal Disease

Preexisting renal dysfunction may promote injuries in the elderly. Chronic renal failure with secondary uremia may lead to mental obtundation and confusion; both of these states can promote falls and other unintentional harm. The platelet dysfunction commonly seen with renal failure may lead to prolonged bleeding after even minor trauma and may necessitate blood product transfusion with its attendant problems, ranging from minor febrile reactions to massive transfusion-related acute lung injury (TRALI) or blood-borne viral infections. All forms of chronic renal replacement therapy carry the risk of infection and sepsis, which may lead to muscular weakness, altered mentation, and dysfunctional thermoregulation; and all of these consequences may lead to injury. Electrolyte disorders, most notably hyponatremia, hypo- or hyperkalemia, hypomagnesemia, and hypocalcemia may result in dysfunctional neural transmission, cardiac dysrhythmias, seizures, mental confusion, muscular weakness, or syncope.

Chronic renal insufficiency predisposes the elderly patient to a number of iatrogenic injuries during their trauma care. Owing to impaired thirst, the elderly may be chronically volume-depleted intravascularly. Compounding this dehydration with acute volume loss may precipitate acute tubular necrosis and fulminant renal failure. Furthermore, extensive imaging procedures may challenge an impaired renal parenchymal and tubular system with iodinated contrast and induce contrast-mediated nephropathy. Nonsteroidal antiinflammatory drugs (NSAIDs) have been employed frequently in the elderly to avoid the sedative effects of the narcotic analgesics, but they carry a significant risk of interstitial nephritis. Life-threatening infections with gram-negative organisms may require aminoglycoside therapy for cure, but such therapy may induce renal dysfunction despite seemingly acceptable drug levels. Despite the availability of renal replacement therapies, acute renal failure in a trauma patient results in a mortality rate of approximately 50% regardless of cause.[75] Thus the physician must remain acutely aware of the impact of diagnostic and therapeutic interventions on renal function in the elderly patient.

## Musculoskeletal Disease

It is immediately obvious that when degenerative joint diseases of any etiology results in diminished range of motion around a major axial joint such as the hip, the individual suffering from that impairment is at high risk for a fall. Furthermore, the diminished muscle mass that frequently accompanies aging lessens patients' potential to rescue themselves from the initial postural instability. Osteopenia, as reviewed earlier, results in more fractures following a given load than would occur in a young patient. Kyphosis is accentuated in the elderly owing to loss of intervertebral disc spaces and a greater potential for neuraxis devastation. Furthermore, the kyphotic posture reduces the field of vision, thereby making avoidance of obstacles in one's path more difficult; this limitation may contribute to the fact that pedestrian injury is the third most common form of elder trauma in the United States.[76] The well-known sequelae of primary or secondary skeletal malignancy may result in pathologic fractures and life-threatening hypercalcemia from bone lysis.

## Resuscitation of the Elderly

The obvious aim of resuscitation is to identify life-threatening injuries in a prioritized manner and to restore adequate perfusion as early as possible. A number of studies have suggested that there is survival benefit for patients who develop a hyperdynamic cardiovascular response, as evidenced by generating supranormal oxygen delivery and consumption after sepsis and major general surgical procedures. Studies have offered some evidence that after major trauma even young patients require a hyperdynamic response for optimal recovery. A series of retrospective studies from the Kings County Hospital[77] demonstrated that young patients, under the age of 40, who attained predetermined hyperdynamic goals, had a higher than predicted survival rate. Other studies[78,79] correlated the rate of serum lactate clearance after trauma with survival. They demonstrated that patients had a mortality rate over 75% if they required more than 48 hours for the serum lactate to return to normal. The ability to respond to the stress of injury can also be assumed to have even greater importance for the ability of the elderly to survive major injuries.

Horst et al.[80] investigated multiple factors with the potential to influence survival of elderly trauma patients. Elderly survivors had a higher hemoglobin level, lower systemic vascular resistance, and higher oxygen delivery than nonsurvivors. These differences in survival were attributed to the inadequacy of the initial resuscitation. Based on these observations, these authors postulated a link between adequate perfusion in the elderly after trauma and subsequent mortality. They underscored the concept that perfusion should be maximized in the elderly by optimizing the red blood cell mass, which would positively affect survival. In the MTOS study, Champion et al.[5] showed that geriatric patients had four times the incidence of cardiovascular complications as the young cohort, supporting the importance of trying to improve cardiovascular response of the elderly trauma patient to maximize survival potential. Possibly as a result of suboptimal resuscitation, the complication rate in the elderly population was 33.4%, whereas it was 19.4% for the younger group.

There are some special considerations for managing the acutely injured elderly patient. Demarest et al.[81] pointed out that the amount of fluid to be administered should be corrected for the reduced lean body mass of the elderly. The elderly are frequently prescribed diuretics that cause chronic volume contraction and total body potassium depletion; therefore the elderly trauma patient who takes a diuretic may require more volume and more potassium supplementation than would be anticipated otherwise. The widespread use of β-blocking agents and calcium channel blockers used to treat hypertension and angina cause slowing of the heart rate and interfere with conduction through the atrioventricular node. The injured elders' heart rate response to stress may be limited by the effects of these medications or the conduction abnormalities that accompany senescence; therefore absence of tachycardia in elderly trauma patients may not be indicative of adequate perfusion as it usually is in the younger cohort. In fact, these conduction abnormalities, whether intrinsic or medication-induced, may make restoration of adequate perfusion after injury more difficult.

Given the discussion above, our approach to resuscitation has focused on restoration of adequate perfusion in the elderly trauma patient as soon as possible. It includes liberal use of the ICU along with early invasive hemodynamic monitoring, in addition to the routine use of continuous pulse oximetry, capnography, electrocardiographic (ECG) monitoring, recording hourly urine output, and frequent blood pressure determinations. Early insertion of a pulmonary artery catheter allows calculation of oxygen transport variables; the latter cardiopulmonary variables may be the only indicators of an inadequate perfusion state. Our standard approach to resuscitation involves frequent patient evaluations. In patients with cool extremities plus a base deficit >5 or a serum lactate >3.0 mmol/L that does not respond to a simple fluid challenge, we advocate insertion of a pulmonary artery catheter to allow measurement of cardiac output and mixed venous oxygen saturation and calculation of oxygen transport variables. If suboptimal oxygen parameters are obtained early and are corrected, the cellular oxygen debt can be minimized and the potential for favorable outcome optimized.

The algorithm for resuscitation of the injured elder that we employ is shown in Figure 19.7. All patients are resuscitated in the manner described by the American College of Surgeons Committee on Trauma's Advanced Trauma Life Support (ATLS) course. Specifically for the initial resuscitation, we advocate volume loading of both the young and the elderly with 2 liters of Ringer's lactate followed by packed red blood cells as needed. In general, trauma patients should receive only the amount of fluid necessary to have vital signs return to normal. At this point in time, treatment of the young and elderly diverges. Young patients suffering injuries requiring less than 5 units of blood during resuscitation do not routinely undergo invasive monitoring. All patients with transfusion requirements of more than 5 units of blood and all patients >65 years of age (unless sustaining minimal trauma) or patients of any age who exhibit signs of hypoperfusion as evidenced by cool extremities, calculated base deficit >5 or elevated serum lactate >3.0 mmol/L undergo invasive monitoring. If hypoperfusion persists after volume-loading the elderly trauma patient to a pulmonary artery occlusion pressure of 15 mmHg, vasodilating inotropes are used to achieve mixed venous oxygen saturation of more than 70% and a normal serum lactate level. Scalea et al.[82] at the Kings County Hospital, described their experience utilizing early invasive monitoring for management of the geriatric trauma patient who suffered nonpenetrating injuries. They noted that despite normal vital signs the initial cardiac output and mixed venous saturation were low in most elderly patients. Surviving patients were able to increase their cardiac output and normalize the mixed venous oxygen saturation. Although invasive monitoring is associated with potential complications such as errant insertions resulting in pneumothorax or hemothorax, dysrhythmias, catheter-related sepsis, and infrequently catheter-associated pulmonary artery rupture, the risks of this intervention seem to be outweighed by the possible benefit of improved survival in high risk patients. In the Kings County Hospital experience, resuscitation management with a pulmonary artery catheter improved survival from 7% to 53%.

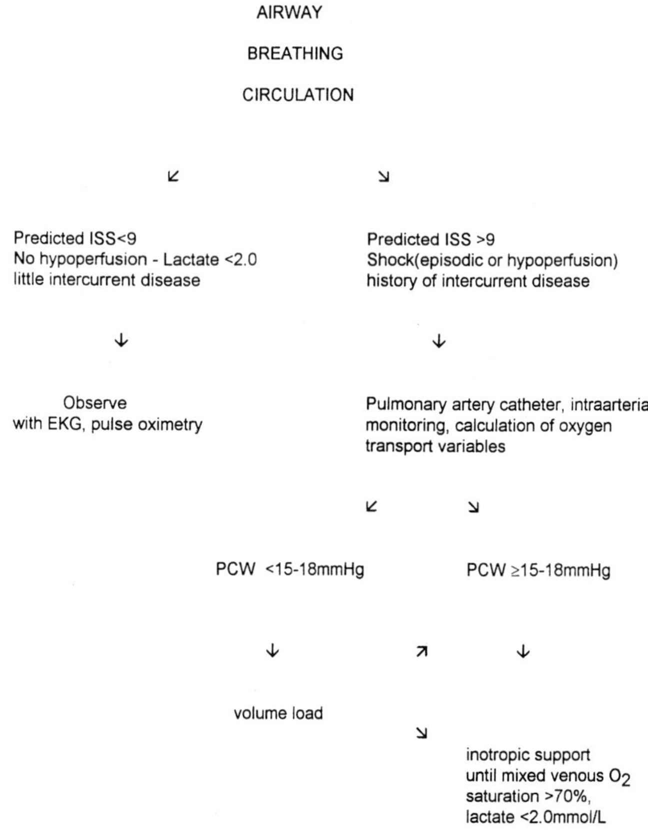


FIGURE 19.7. Algorithm for initial resuscitation of elderly trauma victims. ISS, injury severity score; PCW, pulmonary capillary wedge pressure.

## Management Considerations for Specific Injuries in the Elderly

### Head Injuries

Kirkpatrick and Pearson in 1978 reviewed a medical examiner's series of fatal head injuries. The elderly group showed fewer severe cerebral contusions but had a higher incidence of subdural and intraparenchymal hematomas when compared to the younger cohort. Falls were the most common cause of injury in the elderly and appear to be precipitated by physical illness or alcohol ingestion. Others have also identified an association of head injury with alcohol use in the elderly.

Amacher and Bybee[83] reported a high incidence of intracranial hematomas after falls in the home in those older than 80 years. Howard et al.[84] reported on the outcome of treatment after subdural hematoma in the elderly. They noted that the most frequent mechanism of injury in the elderly were falls, whereas for the young it was motor vehicle accidents. Injury Severity Scores (ISSs) and Glasgow Coma Scores (GCSs) were similar in the young and the old. Compared to young patients with subdural hematomas, the mean volume of the subdural hematoma was larger in the elderly as was the degree of midline shift. The mortality of the elderly approached 75% in this series, which was four times higher than for the younger cohort. Jamjoom et al.[85] confirmed that there was poor survival after trauma in the elderly who underwent craniotomy for evacuation of intracranial hematomas, particularly if papillary dilatation or extensor muscle reflexes were present preoperatively. Ross et al.[86] noted 100% 6-month mortality for elderly head-injured patients remaining comatose for more than 3 days and 90% mortality for those who developed increased intracranial pressure. Most recently, in a study of patients with severe head injury identified by a GCS between 3 and 5, the group from Allegheny General Hospital in Pittsburgh,[87] noted that there was an absence of survivors in the advanced-age groups. The oldest survivor of a head injury who presented with GCS 3 was chronologically in his thirties; another GCS 4 was in his forties, and another with GCS 5 was in his fifties. There were no functional survivors older than 60 years in this series, demonstrating that the elderly have decreased survival in the presence of severe head injuries. Pentland et al.[88] reported that elderly patients experienced higher mortality, died more frequently from secondary organ failure, and consumed more resources per favorable outcome than younger patients.

Since 1968 it has been appreciated that cognitive recovery is linked to the duration of coma and that this phenomenon is affected by age. Carlsson et al.[89] reported that patients older than 51 years had virtually no chance of mental restitution if the coma lasted 5.5 days, whereas patients who were younger than 51 who remained in a coma 7 days continued to have a 50% chance of mental recovery. Patients less than 20 years of age had a reasonable chance of good cognitive recovery regardless of the duration of coma. Lehman[90] suggested that the severity of head trauma may be greater in the elderly because of preexisting brain diseases such as hydrocephalus, Alzheimer's, or microvascular disease. Elderly patients frequently suffer from severe concurrent medical problems such as cardiovascular disease or pulmonary disease with hypoxemia and may use medications such as anticoagulants that can worsen the head injury. Goldstein et al.[91] noted that the elderly had more cognitive defects during the early stages of recovery. These deficiencies included word fluency, verbal and visual memory, and ability to infer similarities.

Management of the head-injured elder is generally similar to that of the head-injured young patient: specifically, maintenance of perfusion and early diagnosis of the specific neurologic injury using head CT scans. Special consideration should be given to monitoring the adequacy of systemic perfusion through the use of a pulmonary artery catheter and the adequacy of intracranial perfusion with an intracranial pressure monitoring device. During the postinjury period, the usual prophylactic measures to avoid complications such as thromboembolism and decubiti should be undertaken in addition to early nutritional support. During the recovery stage, the elderly patients frequently require intensive rehabilitative efforts.

When managing elderly patients with severe head injury it is important to involve the family in the decision to continue aggressive management. This is particularly true for patients who remain in a coma for more than 5 days and those showing signs of increased intracranial pressure. Elderly patients with GCS $< 6$ should also have the family involved early in the decision process. The decision to withhold aggressive support should be discussed with the family in terms of the previously stated desires of the patient. Involvement of clergy or the hospital's ethics committee may also help with these difficult decisions.

## Spinal Injuries

The general principles for managing spinal injuries hold for both young and geriatric trauma patients. Spivak et al.[92] found that cervical spine injury occurs commonly after relatively minor trauma in older patients. This susceptibility to injury is related to the high incidence of degenerative disease of the bony cervical spine, which reduces the flexibility in the cervical region and limits the available space for the spinal cord in this region. They cautioned that odontoid fractures must be carefully considered in older patients with neck pain even after minor trauma, as this injury is frequently occult in the elderly. Identifying these injuries in the elderly requires high quality cervical spine radiographs (which include three standard films: lateral view through T1, anteroposterior view, and odontoid view) and a radiologist experienced in evaluating the cervical spine. In the patient with extensive degenerative changes of the cervical spine, additional studies such as flexion-extension views or a CT with lateral reconstructions are frequently necessary to evaluate the stability of the cervical spine. Until the status of the cervical spine is defined, the axial skeletal alignment must be maintained with a cervical collar. Spivak et al. reported a mortality rate of 26% after spinal cord injury and noted a delay in functional motor recovery in elderly patients with incomplete deficits.[92]

DeVivo et al.[93] compared patients with spinal cord injury who were older than age 61 with those 16–30 years of age to investigate the influence of age on long-term outcome. The elderly were more likely to have sustained the spinal injury after a fall, and the young patients were more likely to have been injured as a result of a motor vehicle crash. Elderly patients were 2.1 times more likely to develop pneumonia, 2.7 times more likely to develop gastrointestinal bleeding, and 5.6 times more likely to have pulmonary emboli. The 2-year survival for the elderly was 59% compared with 95% for the younger group. Penrod et al.[94] reviewed the effect of age on functional recovery after acute, traumatic central cord syndrome. They found that 97% of the younger patients were ambulatory, whereas only 41% of the elderly were able to walk. In addition, the younger patients with central cord syndrome achieved independence in self-care of bladder and bowel function more frequently than did the older group. Few studies have attempted specifically to improve the management of spinal cord injuries in the elderly. In one study Pepin et al.[95] reported on patients with odontoid fractures. They noted that a halothoracic jacket was poorly tolerated in patients more than 75 years of age and led to an increased rate of pneumonia and decubiti. They suggested that C1–2 fusion and an appropriate brace was superior to halo stabilization alone in these patients. Clearly, much work is needed to create specific strategies for the management of spinal injuries in the elderly, as the prognosis remains poor.

## Torso Injuries

The strategy for managing chest and abdominal injuries in the geriatric population is the same as that for trauma patients of all ages. Only a few studies have specifically examined chest trauma in the elderly. Allen and Schwab[54] reviewed 48 patients who were over the age of 60 who had suffered blunt chest trauma. Nearly one-half of the patients suffered these injuries after falls, and slightly less than half had motor vehicle crashes. Most of the patients did well and were discharged home, although 8.3% required a nursing home after discharge. They found that severe chest trauma did not, therefore, automatically lead to a poor prognosis. The Maryland Institute for Emergency Medical Services[96] reported that significant differences could be identified between the old and young patients who suffer blunt thoracic trauma. In this series, most of the chest injuries (87%) resulted from motor vehicle crashes or pedestrian collisions. The young and the elderly suffered a similar pattern of injuries; both groups most commonly sustained rib fractures and hemothoraces. The mortality rate was higher for the elderly patients, even though a smaller number presented in shock. More elderly patients with chest trauma presented in cardiac arrest than the younger group with blunt chest trauma. The authors interpreted this as a failure of cardiopulmonary reserve. The incidence of complications was not affected by age. They suggested that management of the geriatric trauma patient with chest trauma should include careful fluid management, aggressive pulmonary toilet, prophylaxis against thromboembolic events, cardiac rhythm monitoring, and measurement of cardiac hemodynamic parameters. In addition, we recommend ICU monitoring for the elder with evidence of chest injury to facilitate pulmonary toilet, thereby preventing pneumonia, a life-threatening complication in the elderly trauma victim.[23]

## Burns

The risk of death from thermal injuries has decreased over the past several decades, attributed to improved treatment of burn-induced shock, management of burn wounds, nutritional support, and overall improvement in the care delivered to the acutely ill in the ICU. Merrell et al.[97] revealed that survival after burns was adversely affected by advanced age. The burn size correlating with a 50% survivorship was approximately 67% total body surface area (TBSA) for victims between the ages of 21 and 40, but only 25% for patients older than 71 years of age. Hunt and Purdue[98] reported on their 16-year experience with burn patients age 64 and older. The overall mortality was 50%. They reported no survivors among patients sustaining burns of more than 47% TBSA. The leading cause of death in this series was pulmonary sepsis. Anous and Heimbach[99] examined factors associated with death after burns in the elderly. Patients more than 60 years of age have special problems that increased mortality and morbidity. Many of these elderly burn victims live alone and have impaired senses and a slow reaction time; they therefore are exposed to the burning substrate for longer times and suffer deeper burns. The elderly tend to have atrophic skin with a thin dermis, which may lead to deep burns. Epidermal proliferation rate has been shown to be inversely proportional to age. Geriatric patients with more than 70% TBSA burns do not survive even with the most aggressive management. Anous and Heimbach suggested that elderly patients be treated only with adequate pain medication and be allowed to die peacefully.[99] Smith et al.[15] noted that the most important factor when predicting mortality was the percent TBSA burn or a combination of percent TBSA burn and patient age.

Although the elderly have a reduced rate of survival with less-severe burns than their younger counterparts, the long-term outlook for those who do survive is somewhat optimistic. Manktelow et al.[100] reported that 53% of those burned elders who survived did not have a more dependent living status on discharge. Another 8% of patients achieved independent status within 5 years of the burn. Discharged patients did not have an accelerated death rate compared to that of the unburned population.

In addition to the standard management of burn victims, the elderly present other challenges. The elderly burn victim may suffer hypoperfusion in the face of normal vital signs and adequate urine output. Bowser-Wallace et al.[101] advocated hemodynamic monitoring for routine management of severe life-threatening burns in the elderly. They noted excellent survival in the elderly who were resuscitated with hypertonic lactated saline. Early wound closure has been viewed as a major advance in the management of young burn patients, resulting in decreased length of hospitalization and decreased mortality. Kara et al.[102] noted that early excision and grafting in the elderly yielded fewer episodes of infection, resulting in a reduction in hospital stay, but it did not improve survival. Deitch and Clothier[103] and Scott-Conner et al.[104] noted improvement in survival of elderly burn patients by employing early excision and grafting after major burns.

## Fractures

Hip fractures remain the most frequent cause of hospital admission after trauma in the elderly. Responsible for this epidemic are the combined effects of increased bone fragility, loss of bone density, and the propensity for the elderly to fall. Myers et al.[105] investigated factors associated with in-hospital mortality for fractures in patients 65 years of age and older. Men died 60% more often than women. Factors associated with in-hospital death included sepsis, pneumonia, and gastrointestinal disorders. The risk of dying after hip fracture was doubled in patients with cardiac disease, cancer, or cerebrovascular disease. These authors concluded that the most important complication leading to in-hospital deaths after hip fracture was sepsis.

General guidelines for management of the multiinjured trauma patient include early fracture fixation and early mobilization to decrease pulmonary complications. Laskin et al.[106] presented a management scheme for intertrochanteric fractures in the elderly. This protocol included early rigid fixation using compression hip screws to allow early mobilization and immediate weight-bearing. It also employed vigorous pulmonary toilet, prophylactic antibiotics, and anticoagulation. Gustafson et al.[107] developed a specific geriatric anesthesia program designed to reduce the postanesthetic confusional state in the elderly with hip fractures. It consisted of preoperative and postoperative geriatric assessment, oxygen therapy, early surgery, and prevention and treatment of perioperative hypotension. They found that this protocol reduced perioperative acute confusional states in the elderly and the length of hospital stay.

Few studies have investigated management of other specific fractures in the elderly. Roumen et al.[108] found that external fixation for unstable Colles' fractures was no more effective than nonoperative management in the elderly. Ritchie et al.[109] noted good limb salvage for type III open tibial fractures in patients over 60 years of age. Age alone should not represent a contraindication to limb salvage in patients with severe open fractures and concomitant vascular injuries. Helfet et al.[110] reported excellent results employing the technique of an open reduction and repair of acetabular fractures in the elderly, which may obviate total hip arthroplasty at a later date.

## Consequences of Injury in the Elderly

Probably the greatest consequence of injury in the elderly is the fear of injury itself. The elderly, who often suffer from limitations of activity due to chronic debilitating diseases, best understand the impact of injury—that being further alteration in their independence. The elderly learn of these consequences by the experience of their peers. This fear frequently restricts the activity of the elderly, sometimes resulting in potentially dangerous living conditions. As an illustration, during a recent ice storm in Philadelphia that resulted in widespread power outages, an 86-year-old widowed neighbor who lives alone chose to remain in her home without heat or electricity for 5 days rather than chance a fall in the process of leaving to seek more livable conditions. This seemingly irrational behavior from this educated woman was based on her past experience with trauma: Her husband died as a direct consequence of a hip fracture sustained in a fall.

Compared to the young cohort, the injured elderly have a more protracted recovery; and if hospitalized, as many as 40–65% require nursing home placement upon discharge.[42,101] Among 100 elderly patients following trauma, 96% of whom were independent before injury, Oreskovich et al.[18] showed at a 1-year follow-up that only 7 (8%) of the 85 surviving patients were independent and 61 (72%) remained institutionalized. In contrast to these dismal results, the 1989 report of Ross et al.[111] showed a return to independence in 29% of surviving elderly trauma patients. The high rate of continued institutionalization of the elderly has been attributed to "dumping" them into nursing homes by family members who are unable or unwilling to care for their recuperating elder family member. Although this is a distinct possibility, determination of the extent of this phenomenon is unknown and probably not obtainable.

In addition to having disproportionately high representation in the volume of trauma victims, the elderly consume an even greater portion of the cost of trauma care. MacKenzie et al.[8] used data from the National Hospital Discharge Surveys to estimate the cost of trauma care for 1985. They showed that the elderly, who represented approximately 12% of the population in 1985, comprised 23% of the trauma volume and consumed 28% of the $11.4 billion spent on trauma care. Max et al.[46] used similar methodology to estimate the lifetime cost of trauma sustained in 1985. Using all injuries regardless of severity, the total cost for the 56.9 million injuries totaled $156.7 billion. This total cost was then divided into two components: (1) direct costs, which represent the actual cost of providing medical care; and (2) indirect costs, which represent monies lost because of partial or total workforce disability as a consequence of the trauma. Direct costs were $44.8 billion (29%), indirect costs due to premature death were $47.9 billion (30%), and indirect costs due to loss of survivor's workmanship—the highest proportion at 41%—represented $64.9 billion. The direct costs for the elderly were 2.5–6.0 times higher than for any other age group due largely to the protracted hospital stays and the need for specialized care upon discharge. The elder's indirect costs were appropriately less than for the younger cohort, as most of the elderly had retired from the workforce. The total costs of elderly trauma care were found to be $14.2 billion, or 9%, of the total trauma care expenditures.

The total cost of unintentional injury in 1995 was $434.8 billion[1] (Fig. 19.8). A detailed breakdown of these costs

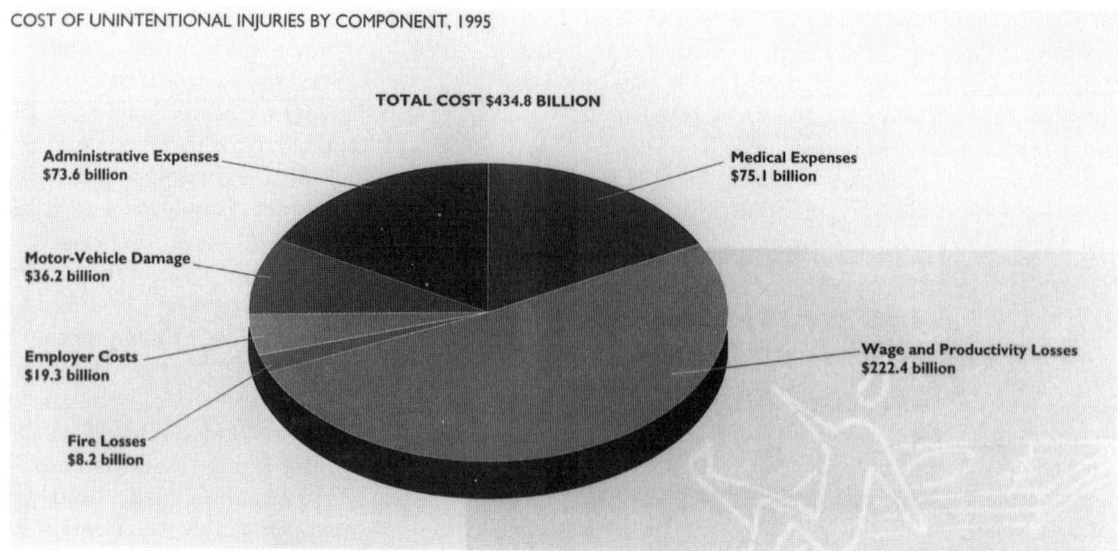


FIGURE 19.8. Cost of unintentional injury in 1995. The elderly consume a disproportionate amount of the direct costs (administrative and medical expenses) and lesser amounts of the indirect costs. (From National Safety Council,[1] with permission.)

are not yet available for the various age groups. If the proportion of costs incurred by the elderly are assumed to remain at the same 9% found in the study by Max et al.,[46] which is probably an underestimation due to the increased volume of elders in the traumatized population, the elder trauma care cost $39.1 billion in 1995. Though this calculation does not take into account the difference in the value of money between these two periods, the nearly 300% increase in costs during the 10-year interval illustrates the staggering economic burden of injury management.

Trauma costs are not adequately reimbursed under the federal prospective payment system, which is based on Diagnosis-Related Groups (DRGs), for patients of any age.[112] In a study of 82 elderly hospitalized trauma patients, DeMaria et al.[6] compared the cost of acute trauma care, exclusive of professional fees, to projected reimbursement if each patient was covered under the Medicare system. This study showed a significant under-reimbursement for patients more than 80 years of age, those with severe injuries (ISS > 25), and those with more than two complications. With predictions that the elderly will make up 40% or more of the trauma population in the future, the implication of this study for hospitals and physicians who care for injured elders is obvious: the conflict of continuing to provide care despite diminishing revenues.

The issue of diminishing revenues has ramifications far exceeding the care of the injured elder. For example, it appears that diminished revenues also play a role in the trend of newly trained surgeons choosing not to participate in trauma care or pursue careers in the field of trauma surgery. It may be controversial how much diminished revenues play in limiting the manpower to provide adequate trauma care. What is irrefutable is that many hospitals are opting out of the delivery of trauma care due to the financial imbalances. Trauma care requires large expenditures, and the revenues generated often are unable to achieve a break-even point. Sometimes the costs threaten the solvency of the hospital as a whole. It is unclear where the solution to unreimbursed or underreimbursed care is to be found: perhaps larger DRG reimbursement for trauma care delivered at a trauma center, a trauma center-directed tax on tobacco and alcohol, or institution of a federally funded national health insurance program.

## Rehabilitation

The aim of rehabilitation is "to restore an individual to his/her former functional environmental status or, alternatively, to maintain or maximize remaining function."[113] Recovery of potential function requires special treatment efforts in the geriatric patient. Unlike the younger population, in whom rehabilitative outcomes are more apt to be dramatic, the geriatric patient is likely to realize more subtle progress. The degree of independence the patient is able to attain is dictated by these modest achievements and can mean the difference between living at home and living in a long-term care facility.[113] For many elders, independence is their ongoing reason to live. The physician caring for the injured elder must understand the importance of attaining or maintaining independence for their elderly patients and do whatever is necessary to achieve this endpoint. The elderly with chronic debilitating disease more frequently require rehabilitative interventions following trauma because of the limitations imposed by injury. The interested reader should refer to Chapter 14 for the specific rehabilitative interventions for the elderly.

## Prevention

The National Safety Council, which has been tabulating data on injuries since 1921, has shown that Americans are faced with many of the same risks that faced our predecessors in the twentieth century (Table 19.3). Prevention has the greatest impact on problems presented by the trauma population in general but especially in the elderly. The first step toward prevention of injury is to recognize the individuals who are most likely to suffer injuries. Many of the factors that predispose the elderly to injury (Table 19.4) can and should be discovered on routine history-taking in the elderly patient. There are three injury-prevention approaches: (1) pre-event strategies, which focus on increasing public awareness through educational programs, some of which may influence legislation; (2) event strategies, which involve interventions to reduce energy transfer during the injury process; and (3) post-event strategies, which deal with efforts to improve resuscitation and reduce complications. In the elderly trauma population, the first two strategies hold the most promise for success.

As an example of pre-event educational promotion, geriatric care groups have developed interventions such as home safety inspections, modifying medications known to affect balance adversely, gait training, and improving any correctable sensory deficits in an effort to reduce the incidence of falls. Though early prevention programs to reduce falls sought to modify factors shown to affect elderly fall victims, these programs have reported little or no reduction in the incidence of falls and fall-related injury.[40,114–116]

Realizing the complexity of the problem of falls in the elderly population, in April 1989 the National Institute on Aging in cooperation with the National Center for Nursing Research and the Centers for Disease Control, began coordinating a series of clinical trials designed to study the relation of biomedical, behavioral, and environmental factors that contribute to falls in the elderly population. These coordinated clinical trials, collectively called Frailty and Injuries: Cooperative Studies of Intervention Techniques (FICSIT), are independent trials at eight medical centers across the United States that are investigating various aspects of falls in the elderly. Though looking at slightly different factors that influence falls, the studies can be divided into two general categories: (1) studies that aim to increase the physical capabilities of the elder, and (2) studies that optimize healthy behaviors or environmental conditions that may lead to a reduction in either the incidence or the consequences of falls. The results of these coordinated studies are emerging presently.

Motor vehicle crashes may potentially be avoided by identifying and reporting individuals who are unfit drivers. This includes persons with visual or hearing deficits, dementia, or disabling musculoskeletal disorders, and those using medications that decrease driving skills. In an effort to refresh skills and update traffic knowledge, driver education courses for adults over age 55 have been established by the American Association of Retired Persons (AARP) and the National Retired Teachers Association. In the short term, such programs have been shown to reduce fatal and injury-associated collisions.[117]

Retting et al.[118] showed that a pedestrian accident-prevention program significantly reduced the fatal and serious injury occurrence by 43% and 86%, respectively. This program implemented prolongation of traffic light times to accommodate the decreased gait of the elderly, modifications of road and crosswalk signs, tighter speed limit enforcement, and safety education presentations at senior centers.

The elderly can be expected to benefit from vehicular modifications, promulgated by Federal Motor Vehicle Safety Standard 208, which provide "passive" protection by either automatic shoulder restraints or airbags. These restraint systems can potentially reduce crash fatalities 60–77%[119]; whether the elderly, who are more susceptible to injury, will realize this extent of protection is yet to be shown.

## References


1. National Safety Council. Accident Facts, 1996 ed. NSC: Itasca, IL, 1996.
2. Adams PF, Marano MN. Current estimates from the NHIS, 1994: National Center for Health Statistics. Vital Health Stat 1995;10:193.
3. McCoy GF, Johnston BA, Duthie RB. Injury to the elderly in road traffic accidents. J Trauma 1989;29:494.
4. Murray CJL, Lopez AD. Alternative projections of mortality and disability by cause 1990–2020: global burden of disease study. Lancet 1997;349:1498–1504.
5. Champion HR, Copes WS, Buyer D, et al. Major trauma in geriatic patients. Am J Public Health 1989;79:1278.
6. DeMaria EJ, Merriam MA, Casanova LA, et al. Do DRG payments adequately reimburse the costs of trauma care in geriatric patient? J Trauma 1988;28:1244.
7. Finelli FC, Jonsson J, Champion HR, et al. A case control study for major trauma in geriatric patients. J Trauma 1989;29:541.
8. MacKenzie EJ, Morris JA, Smith GS, et al. Acute hospital costs of trauma in the United States: implications for regionalized systems of care. J Trauma 1990;30:1096.

9. US Bureau of the Census. Current Population Reports, Special Studies, P 23–178, Sixty-Five Plus in America. US Government Printing Office: Washington, DC, 1992.
10. Spencer G. Projections of the Population of the United States by Age, Sex, and Race: 1988 to 2080, Current Population Reports, Series p. 25, no. 1018, US Government Printing Office, Washington, DC, 1989.
11. Rosenbloom S. The morbidity needs of the elderly. In: Transportion in an Aging Society. Special Report 218. Transportation Research Board, National Research Council: Washington DC, 1988:21.
12. Sattin RW, Lambert DA, DeVito CA, et al. The incidence of fall injury events among the elderly in a defined population. Am J Epidemiol 1990;131:1028.
13. Schwab CW, Kauder DR. Trauma in the geriatric patient. Arch Surg 1992;127:701.
14. Viano DC, Culver CC, Evans L, et al. Involvement of older drivers in multivehicle side-impact crashes. Accid Anal Prev 1990;22:177.
15. Smith DP, Enderson BL, Maull KL, et al. Trauma in the elderly: determinants of outcome. South Med J 1990;83:171.
16. Wolf ME, Rivera FP. Nonfall injuries in older adults. Annu Rev Public Health 1992;13:509.
17. Evans L. Risk of fatality from physical trauma versus sex and age. J Trauma 1988;28:368.
18. Oreskovich MR, Howard JD, Copass MK, et al. Geriatric trauma: injury patients and outcome. J Trauma 1984;24: 565.
19. Morris JA, MacKenzie EJ, Edelstein SL. The effect of preexisting conditions on mortality in trauma patients. JAMA 1990;263:1942.
20. Osler T, Hales K, Baack B, et al. Trauma in the elderly. Ann J Surg 1988;156:537.
21. Baker SP, O'Neill B. The injury severity score: an update. J Trauma 1976;16:882.
22. Johnson CL, Margulies DR, Kearney TJ, et al. Trauma in the elderly: an analysis of outcomes based on age. Am Surg 1994;60:899–902.
23. Bellemare JF, Tepas JJ, Imami ER. Complications of trauma care: risk analysis pneumonia in 10,001 adult trauma patients. Am Surg 1996;62:207–211.
24. Rhem CG, Ross SE. Elderly drivers involved in road crashes: a profile. Am Surg 1995;61:435–437.
25. Grabbe L, Demi A, Camann MA, Potter L. The health status of elderly persons in the last year of life: a comparison of deaths by suicide, injury, and natural causes. Am J Public Health 1997;87:434–437.
26. Nelson RC, Sattin RW, Langlois JA, et al. Alcohol as a risk factor for fall injury events among elderly persons living in the community. J Am Geriatr Soc 1992;40:658.
27. Vellas BJ, Wayne SJ, Romero L, Baumgartner RN, Rubenstein LZ, Garry PJ. One-leg balance test is an important predictor of injurious falls in older persons. J Am Geriatr Soc 1997;45:735–738.
28. Ryynanen OP, Kivela SL, Honkanen R, Laippala P, Saano V. Medications and chronic diseases as risk factors for falling injuries in the elderly. Scand J Soc Med 1993; 21:264–271.
29. Duthie EH. Falls. Med Clin North Am 1989;73:1321.
30. King MB, Tinetti ME. A multifactorial approach to reducing injurious falls. Clin Geriatr Med 1996;12:745–759.
31. Ryynanen OP, Kivela SL, Honkanen R, et al. Incidence of Falling Injuries Leading to Medical Treatment in the Elderly. Public Health 1991;105:373–386.
32. Campbell AJ, Borrie MJ, Spears GF, et al. Circumstances and consequences of falls experienced by a community population 70 years and over during a prospective study. Age Ageing 1990;19:136.
33. Sjogren H, Bjornstig U. Injuries to the elderly in the traffic environment. Accid Anal Prev 1991;23:77.
34. Tinetti ME, Doucette J, Claus E. Risk factors for serious injury during falls by older persons in the community. J Am Geriatr Soc 1995;43:1214–1221.
35. Sattin RW, Lambert DA, DeVito CA, et al. The incidence of fall injury events among the elderly in a defined population. Am J Epidemiol 1990;131:1028.
36. Myers AH, Baker SP, Van Natta ML, et al. Risk factors associated with falls and injuries among elderly institutionalized persons. Am J Epidemiol 1991;133:1790.
37. Nelson RC, Amin MA. Falls in the elderly. Emerg Med Clin North Am 1990;8:309.
38. Tinetti ME, Speecley M, Ginter SF. Risk factors for falls among elderly persons living in the community. N Engl J Med 1988;319:1701.
39. Gubler KD, Maier RV, David R, et al. Trauma recidivism in the elderly. J Trauma 1996;41:952–956.
40. Tinetti ME. Prevention of falls and falls in elderly persons: a research agenda. Prevent Med 1994;23:756–762.
41. Herndon JG, Helmick CG, Sattin RW, et al. Chronic medical conditions and risk of fall injury events at home in older adults. J Am Geriatr Soc 1997;45:739–743.
42. Alexander BH, Rivara FP, Wolf ME. The cost and frequency of hospitalization for fall-related injuries in older adults. Am J Public Health 1992;82:1020.
43. Kosorok MR, Omenn GS, Diehr P, et al. Restricted activity days among the elderly. Am J Public Health 1992;82: 1263–1267.
44. Zylke JW. As nation grows older, falls become greater source of fear, injury, death. JAMA 1990;263:2021.
45. Englander F, Hodson TJ, Terregrossa RA. Economic dimensions of slip and fall injuries. J Forensic Sci 1996; 41:733–746.
46. Max W, Rice DP, MacKenzie EJ. The lifetime cost of injury. Injury 1990;27:332.
47. Rehm CG, Ross SE. Elderly drivers involved in road crashes: a profile. Am Surg 1995;61:435–437.
48. Koepsell TD, Wolf ME, McCloskey L, et al. Medical conditions and motor vehicle collision injuries in older adults. J Am Geriatr Soc 1994;42:695–700.
49. Lachs MS, Pillemer K. Abuse and neglect of elderly persons: current concepts. N Engl J Med 1995;332:437–443.
50. Cammer Parris BE, Meier DE, Goldstein T, et al. Elder abuse and neglect: how to recognize warning signs and intervene. Geriatrics 1995;50(4):47–51.
51. Grabbe L, Demi A, Camann MA, et al. The health status of elderly persons in the last year of life: a comparison of deaths by suicide, injury, and natural causes. Am J Public Health 1997;87:434–437.
52. Duffy D. Suicide in later life: how to spot the risk factors. Nurs Times 1997;93(11):56.

53. Watters JM, McClaran JC. The elderly surgical patient. In: The American College of Surgeons: Care of the Surgical Patient, vol 1. Scientific American: New York, 1991.
54. Allen JE, Schwab CW. Blunt chest trauma in the elderly. Am Surg 1985;51:687.
55. Kenney RA. Physiology of aging. Clin Geriatr Med 1985; 1:37.
56. Watters JM, Moulton SB, Clancey SM, et al. Ageing exaggerates glucose intolerance following injury. J Trauma 1994;37:786–791.
57. Desai D, March R, Watters JM. Hyperglycemia after trauma increases with age. J Trauma 1989;28:719.
58. Jeevanadam M, Petersen SR, Shamos RF. Protein and glucose fuel kinetics and hormonal changes in elderly trauma patients. Metabolism 1993;42:1255–1262.
59. Rudman D, Kutner MH, Rogers CM, et al. Impaired growth hormone secretion. J Clin Invest 1981;67:1361.
60. Robinson A. Age, physical trauma and care. Can Med Assoc J 1995;152:1453.
61. Milzman DP, Boulanger BR, Rodriguez A, et al. Preexisting disease in trauma patients: a predictor of fate independent of age and ISS. J Trauma 1992;32:236.
62. Hannan EL, Mendelhoff J, Farrell LS, Cayten CG, Murphy JG. Multivariate models for predicting survival of patients with trauma from low falls: the impact of gender and preexisting conditions. J Trauma 1995;38:697–704.
63. Kraus WA, Draper EA, Wagner DP, et al. APACHE II: a severity of disease classification system. Crit Care Med 1985;13:818.
64. McGoldrick JM, Marx JA. Traumatic central cord syndrome in a patient with os ondontoideum. Ann Emerg Med 1989;18:1358.
65. Hemenway D, Solnick SJ, Koeck C, Kytir J. The incidence of stairway injuries in Austria. Accid Anal Prevent 1994; 26:675.
66. Oleske DM, Wilson RS, Bernard BA, Evans DA, Terman EW. Epidemiology of injury in people with Alzheimer's disease. J Am Geriatr Soc 1995;43:741–746.
67. Wilson RF. Trauma in patients with pre-existing cardiac disease. Crit Care Clin 1994;10:461–506.
68. Lilley JM, Arie T, Chilvers CED. Special review: accidents involving older people; a review of the literature. Age Ageing 1995;24:346–365.
69. Shapiro MB, Dechert RE, Colwell C, Bartlett RH, Rodriguez JL. Geriatric trauma: aggressive intensive care unit management is justified. Am Surg 1994;60:695–698.
70. Tran DD, Cuesta MA, van Leeuwen PA, Nauta JJ, Wesdorp RI. Risk factors for multiple organ system failure and death in critically injured patients. Surgery 1993;114:21–30.
71. Dinh-Xuan AT, Higenbottam TW, Clelland CA, et al. Impairment of endothelium-dependent pulmonary artery relaxation in chronic obstructive pulmonary disease. N Engl J Med 1991;324:1539–1547.
72. Mancada S, Higgs A. The L-arginine-nitric oxide pathway. N Engl J Med 1993;329:2002–2012.
73. Belvisi MG, Stretton CD, Yacoub M, Barnes PJ. Nitric oxide is the endogenous neurotransmitter of bronchodilator nerves in humans. Eur J Pharmacol 1992;210:221–222.
74. Schilling J, Holzer P, Guggenbach M, Gyurech D, Marathia K, Geroulanos S. Reduced endogenous nitric oxide in the exhaled air of smokers and hypertensives. Eur Respir J 1994;7:467–471.
75. Muther RJ. Acute renal failure: acute azotemia in the critically ill. In: Civetta JM, Taylor RW, Kirby RR (eds) Critical Care, 2nd ed. Lippincott: Philadelphia, 1992.
76. McMahon DJ, Schwab CW, Kauder D. Comorbidity and the elderly trauma patient. World J Surg 1996;20:1113–1120.
77. Abou-Khalil, Scalea T, Trooskin SZ, et al. Hemodynamic responses to shock in young trauma patients: need for invasive monitoring. Crit Care Med 1994;22:633–639.
78. Abramson D, Scalea TM, Hitchock R, et al. Lactate clearance and survival following injury. J Trauma 1993;35: 584–589.
79. Rady MY, Rivers EP, Nowak RM. Resuscitation of the critically ill in the ER: responses of blood pressure, heart rate, shock index, central venous oxygen saturation, and lactate. Am J Emerg Med 1996;14:218–225.
80. Horst HM, Obeid FN, Sorensen VJ, et al. Factors influencing survival of elderly trauma patients. Crit Care Med 1986;14:681.
81. Demarest GB, Turner MO, Clevenger FW. Injuries in the elderly: evaluation and initial response. Geriatrics 1990; 45:36.
82. Scalea TM, Simon HW, Duncan AO, et al. Geriatric blunt multiple trauma: improved survival with early invasive monitoring. J Trauma 1990;30:129.
83. Amacher AL, Bybee DE. Toleration of head injury by the elderly. Neurosurgery 1987;20:954.
84. Howard MA, Gross AS, Dacey RG, et al. Acute subdural hematomas: an age-dependent clinical entity. J Neurosurg 1989;71:858.
85. Jamjoom A, Nelson R, Stranjalis G, et al. Outcome following surgical evacuation of traumatic intracranial haematomas in the elderly. Br J Neurosurg 1992;6:27.
86. Ross AM, Pitts LH, Kobayashi S. Prognosticators of outcome after major head injury in the elderly. J Neurosci Nurs 1992;24:88.
87. Quigley MR, Vidovich D, Cantella D, et al. Defining the limits of survivorship after very severe head injury. J Trauma 1997;42(1):7.
88. Pentland B, Jones PA, Roy CW, et al. Head injury in the elderly. Age Ageing 1986;15:193.
89. Carlsson CA, Essen CV, Lofgren J. Factors affecting the clinical course of patients with severe head injuries. J Neurosurg 1968;29:242.
90. Lehman LB. Head trauma in the elderly. Postgrad Med 1988;83:140.
91. Goldstein FC, Levin HS, Presley RM, et al. Neurobehavioral consequences of closed head injury in older adults. J Neurol Neurosurg Psychiatry 1994;57:961–966.
92. Spivak JM, Weiss MA, Cotler JM, et al. Cervical spine injuries in patients 65 and older. Spine 1994;19:2302–2306.
93. DeVivo MJ, Kartus PL, Rutt RD, et al. The influence of age at time of spinal cord injury on rehabilitation outcome. Arch Neurol 1990;47:687.
94. Penrod LE, Hedde SK, Ditunno JF. Age effect on prognosis for functional recovery in acute, traumatic central cord syndrome. Arch Phys Med Rehabil 1990;71:963.
95. Pepin JW, Bourne RB, Hawkins RJ. Odontoid fractures, with special reference to the elderly patient. Clin Orthop 1985;193:178.

96. Shorr RM, Rodriquez A, Indeck MC, et al. Blunt chest trauma in the elderly. J Trauma 1989;29:234.
97. Merrell SW, Saffle JR, Sullivan JJ, et al. Increased survival after major thermal injury. Am J Surg 1987;154:623.
98. Hunt JL, Purdue GF. The elderly burn patient. Am J Surg 1992;164:472.
99. Anous MM, Heimbach DM. Causes of death and predictors in burned patients more than 60 years of age. J Trauma 1986;20:135.
100. Manktelow A, Meyer AA, Herzog SR, et al. Analysis of life expectancy and living status of elderly patients surviving a burn injury. J Trauma 1989;29:203.
101. Bowser-Wallace BH, Cone JB, Caldwell FT. Hypertonic lactated saline resuscitation of severely burned patients over 60 years of age. J Trauma 1985;25:22.
102. Kara M, Peters WJ, Douglas LG, et al. An elderly surgical approach to burns in the elderly. J Trauma 1990;30:430.
103. Deitch EA, Clothier J. Burns in the elderly: an early surgical approach. J Trauma 1983;23:891.
104. Scott-Conner CEH, Love R, Wheeler W. Does rapid wound closure improve survival in older patients with burns? Am Surg 1990;56:57–60.
105. Myers AH, Robinson EF, Van Natta JL, et al. Hip fractures among the elderly: factors associated with in-hospital mortality. Am J Epidemiol 1991;134:1128.
106. Laskin RS, Gruber MA, Zimmerman AJ. Intertrochanteric fractures of the hip in the elderly. Clin Orthop 1979;141:188.
107. Gustafson Y, Brannstrom B, Berggren D, et al. A geriatric-anesthesiologic program to reduce acute confusional states in elderly patients treated for femoral neck fractures. J Am Geriatr Soc 1991;39:655.
108. Roumen RM, Hesp WL, Bruggink ED. Unstable Colles' fractures in elderly patients. J Bone Joint Surg 1991;73:307. British Volume.
109. Ritchie AJ, Small JO, Hart NB, et al. Type III tibial fractures in the elderly: results of 23 fractures in 20 patients. Br J Accid Surg 1991;22:267.
110. Helfet DL, Borrelli J, DiPasquale T. Stabilization of acetabular fractures in elderly patients. J Bone Joint Surg 1992; 74:753. American Volume.
111. Ross N, Timberlake GA, Rubino LJ, et al. High cost of trauma care in the elderly. South Med J 1989;82: 857.
112. Jacob LM. The effect of prospective reimbursement on trauma patients. Am Coll Surg Bull 1985;70:17.
113. Williams TK. Rehabilitation in the aging: philosophy and approaches. In: Williams TK (ed) Rehabilitation in the Aging. Raven: New York, 1984:xiii.
114. Rubenstein LZ, Robbins AJ, Josephson KR. The value of assessing falls in an elderly population: a randomized trial. Ann Intern Med 1990;113:308–316.
115. Velter NJ, Lewis PA, Ford D. Can health visitors prevent fractures in elderly people. Br Med J 1992;308:889–890.
116. Hornbrook MC, Stevens VJ, Wingfield DS, et al. Preventing falls among community-dwelling older persons. Gerontologist 1994;34:16–23.
117. Stylos L, Janke MK. Annual tabulations of mature driving program driving record comparisons, 1989. CAL-DMV-RSS-89–119. State California Department of Motor Vehicles: Sacramento.
118. Retting R, Schwartz SI, Kulewiicz M, et al. Queens Boulevard pedestrian safety project, New York City. MMWR 1989;38:61.
119. National Technical Information Services. Evaluation of the Effectiveness of Occupant Protection. Federal Motor Vehicle Safety Standard 208. Interim Report June 1992. US Department of Transportation, National Highway Traffic Safety Administration.

# *Part II*
# *Specific Issues in Geriatric Surgery*

## Section 2
## Endocrine System

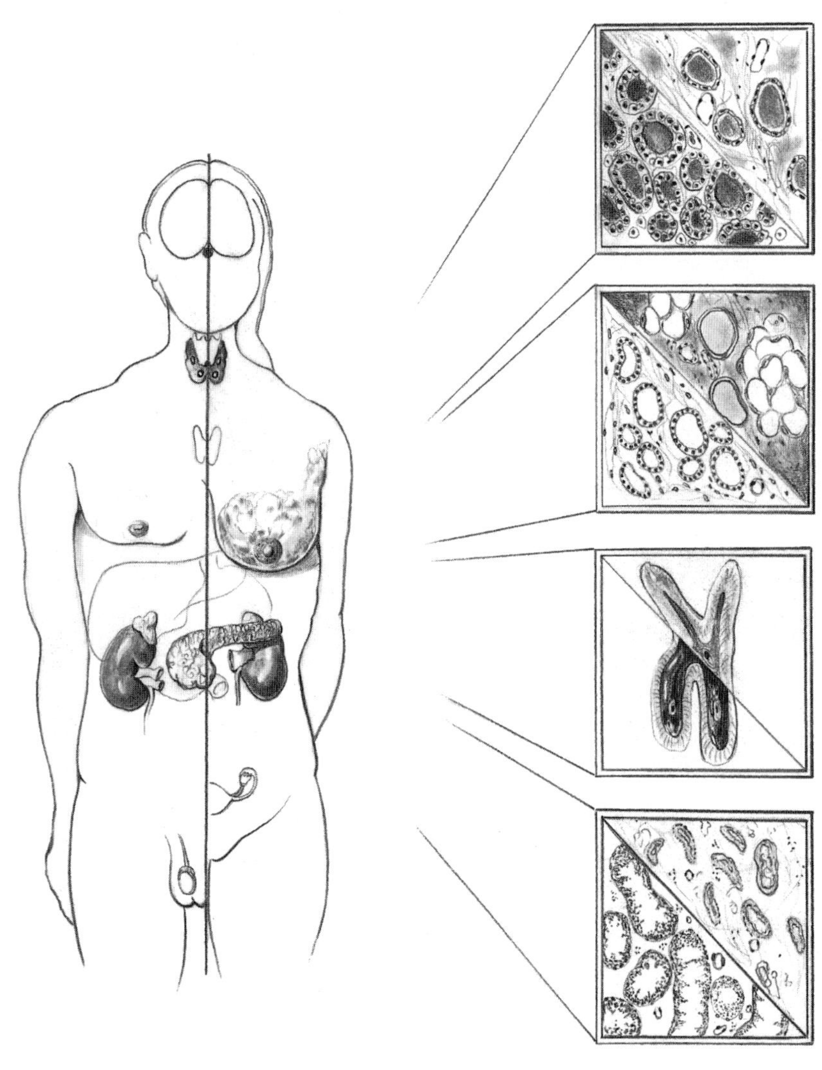

# Invited Commentary

Samuel A. Wells, Jr.

The average length of human life may increase from 75 years to more than 85 years during the next two decades, but the prolongation will not necessarily be paralleled by an increase in good health. It is known that admissions to hospitals, nursing homes, and extended care facilities increase with advancing age. Throughout adult life humans experience a gradual decline in a number of physiologic functions, characterized by decreases in cellular protein synthesis, immune function, muscle mass and strength, and bone mineral density. Even though most elderly individuals die from cancer, cardiovascular disease, or dementia, the loss of muscle strength primarily determines their ability to live independently. It has been shown by several studies that the frailty associated with aging can be reversed by proper diet and exercise, but the attrition of elderly people from structured exercise programs is high. It is important to note that the loss of muscle mass and strength, decrease in bone mineralization, and increase in fat mass may also relate to an aging endocrine system, and there have been attempts to treat elderly patients with hormone replacement to restore their endocrine milieu to that of a younger adult. It is important to examine some of the more significant changes in endocrine function associated with aging and to define opportunities where endocrine therapy has proven benefit.

Age-related alterations in endocrine function are important considerations in the surgical patient and must be considered when planning operative intervention. Because the endocrine system is integrally related to the nervous system, the immune system, renal function, skeletal function, and the cardiovascular and pulmonary systems, it is not reasonable to think of the singular effects of a specific hormone deficiency. It is impossible to cover all aspects of the endocrinology of aging, and in this introduction we address the changes that are most significant.

Perhaps the most important endocrine change associated with aging arises in the pancreas and relates to the decreased availability of insulin. Forty percent of individuals 65–75 years of age have impaired glucose tolerance, the incidence of which increases directly with age. The abnormality is undetected in many elderly patients, and they are at risk for developing vascular, ocular, and neurologic complications at an accelerated rate. It is not only the decreased insulin secretion from the pancreatic beta cell that leads to the diabetic state; additional contributing factors are physical inactivity, poor diet, increased abdominal fat, and decreased lean body mass. If glucose intolerance is detected in patients being considered for elective surgery, priority should be given to improving their physical state and to introducing proper treatment before proceeding with an operation.

Thyroid abnormalities, including autoimmune thyroiditis, thyroid nodules, and the metabolic states of hypothyroidism and hyperthyroidism, also increase with age; and the physician must be aware of occult thyroid disease in the elderly. It should particularly be noted that the incidence of thyroid nodules exceeds 80% in patients over 70 years of age and is higher in women than men. More importantly, the presence of thyroid disease (hypothyroidism and hyperthyroidism) may be occult and unsuspected by the surgeon who is caring for an elderly patient with an acute surgical problem. It should be noted that whether hyperthyroid, or hypothyroid, the patient being treated with thyroid medication is at increased risk for cardiac failure.

Physiologically, the significant metabolic change in thyroid function relates to a decrease in peripheral degradation of thyroxine ($T_4$) to triiodothyronine ($T_3$), but this alteration has not been associated with any detectable clinical change in the aging process. Nevertheless, some clinicians have suggested that $T_3$ replacement therapy is indicated in the elderly.

There are significant changes in the skeleton as one ages, primarily characterized by a decrease in bone density in both its cortical and trabecular segments. The decrease in bone mineralization is particularly problematic in women, where trabecular bone loss accelerates at menopause and reaches a rate of 4% per year. Estrogen deficiency accounts for a 15–20% decrease in skeletal density, which is increased further in the presence of hyperparathyroidism, a disease that occurs primarily in postmenopausal women. Understandably, there is an increase in fracture rate in elderly patients due not only to decreased bone density, but to a decrease in muscle strength and impaired coordination.

Menopause, one of the most dramatic age-related changes, is primarily associated with the loss of cyclic estradiol production. Menopause appears to be brought on by changes in both the ovarian follicles and the hypothalamus and pituitary. Long-term estrogen replacement therapy has benefits, not only on the skeleton but on the cardiovascular system, reproductive tract, skin, and central nervous system. A serious consideration is the fact that there is a modest but definitely increased incidence of breast cancer in patients on estrogen replacement therapy. Recent studies have shown that chronic administration of the antiestrogen tamoxifen reduces the incidence of new breast cancers in patients previously treated for the disease, while demonstrating a protective effect on the cardiovascular system and the skeleton. This is due to the fact that tamoxifen, and perhaps related compounds, have antagonistic effects on breast cancer cells yet agonistic effects on other tissues.

In aging men there is a decline in serum testosterone levels and an accompanying reduction in the number of Leydig cells. Studies show that testosterone replacement in elderly men is associated with increased muscular strength, cognition, and red blood cell mass. However, testosterone administration has a stimulatory effect on the prostate, and the risk of enhancing the growth of an occult prostate cancer is a definite perceived risk.

Hormonal changes also occur in the adrenal cortex, characterized by a decrease in circulating levels of dehydroepiandrosterone (DHEA), and in the pituitary gland, characterized by a reduction in growth hormone and insulin-like growth factor. It seems plausible that replacement of the deficient hormones during and after menopause, the andropause, and the somatopause would be beneficial in elderly patients, but the data published to date are controversial. There have been prospective randomized placebo-controlled trials where DHEA was administered to old, but not elderly, adults for several months. In subjects receiving DHEA, compared to those receiving placebo, circulating levels of DHEA and androgen were restored, and there was a sense of improved well-being. The risk of administering these agents relates to the stimulatory effect they have, directly or indirectly, on the breast and prostate gland and perhaps other tissues. Similarly, growth hormone, administered in prospective randomized placebo-controlled trials, has been associated with increased muscle strength and bone mineral content. It has already been shown in acutely injured patients, particularly those with fractures or burns, that administration of growth hormone has clear benefit in wound healing and return to independent living. As with DHEA, the question remains whether adverse effects will become evident with long-term administration of growth hormone. There is the possibility that administration of selected hormones would have a beneficial effect on the elderly surgical patient, as minimal adverse effects have been seen with their short-term administration.

The surgeon must understand that both profound and subtle changes occur in the endocrine system with aging and that these alterations influence the response of the surgical patient to the disease. Therapeutic correction of diagnosed endocrine deficiencies is clearly indicated in the elderly patient whether in the emergent or the elective setting. Hormonal replacement in older persons may also help prevent some of the complications of aging, particularly those associated with changes in muscle, bone, and the central nervous system. However, much work remains to be done on the evaluation of hormonal administration in healthful elderly persons to clarify whether the benefits outweigh the risks. The question is important, as the results will influence how elderly patients respond to surgical treatment and their underlying disease process.

# 20 Endocrinology and Aging

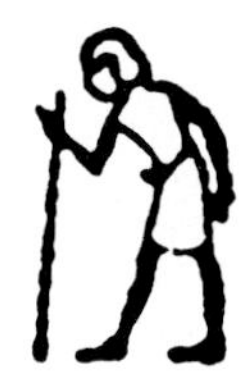

Hosam K. Kamel and John E. Morley

In 1889 C.E. Brown-Sequard, a noted French scientist, claimed that a water-soluble extract of dog testes gave him an "astonishing degree of rejuvenation" and improved his long-standing problems with impotence.[1] Although we now know that there was minimal testosterone or other sex steroids in this water-soluble extract, the link between hormones and aging was clearly postulated. Over the past century our understanding of hormonal changes with age and the effect of hormonal repletion in elderly individuals has increased dramatically. It is now well established that aging is associated with a host of changes in the endocrine system (Table 20.1). At present, it is not completely clear whether these age-related changes aggravate the alterations in various biologic functions that accompany aging or are compensatory events that minimize tissue damage and conserve organ vitality. This chapter reviews the age-related changes in the endocrine system. The diagnosis and management of several endocrine disorders that are frequent during later life are discussed, and the current status of hormones as antiaging agents is explored.

## Thyroid

Aging is associated with several changes in the anatomy of the thyroid gland. The gland volume has been reported to decrease in some studies,[2] and to increase in others,[3] probably reflecting regional differences in the amount of dietary iodine intake. Thyroid follicles decrease in number, and its lining cells become flattened. Aging is also associated with a variety of changes in the physiology of the hypothalamic-pituitary-thyroid axis (Table 20.2). The half-life of serum L-thyroxine ($T_4$) increases from 4.0 days during youth to 9.3 days during later life,[4] although serum levels of free $T_4$ and free triiodothyronine ($T_3$) remain constant throughout life. This is due to the decreased production of $T_4$ by the aging thyroid gland.[5] The serum concentration of thyroid-stimulating hormone (TSH) does not change with normal aging. The TSH response to the thyrotropin-releasing hormone (TRH), however, may be reduced with age, especially in men.[6]

### Hypothyroidism

The prevalence of hypothyroidism in old adults varies widely with the population studied. Hypothyroidism was reported in 5.9% of a population of active elderly Americans,[7] in 7% of old women residents of Worcester, Massachusetts, and in 0.9% of a group of old women in Italy.[8] Regardless of the population studied, however, the prevalence of hypothyroidism is significantly increased in the elderly population.

Hypothyroidism in old adults is most commonly due to chronic autoimmune thyroiditis. Treatment of prior Graves' disease is another frequent cause.[9] Hypothyroidism may also be iatrogenic resulting from exposure to certain drugs. Of particular importance are iodine-containing drugs such as radiographic contrast agents, the antiarrhythmic drug amiodarone, and certain cough medicines. Hypothyroidism caused by pituitary or hypothalamic disease is rare and is usually the result of tumors or surgery in these regions.

The clinical features of hypothyroidism in old adults are similar to that in young adults and include hyponatremia, anemia, myopathy, pericardial effusion, and rheumatologic findings.[10] In addition, some old patients with hypothyroidism have delusional and hallucinatory phenomena, leading to the syndrome "myxedema madness." In old adults, other age-related disorders and normal age-related findings frequently confound the diagnosis of hypothyroidism. Many of the normal manifestations of aging, such as dry skin, poor skin turgor, slowed mentation, constipation, and cold intolerance, are features of hypothyroidism. The delay in relaxation of the ankle jerk is less reliable in the elderly, and the ankle jerk cannot be elicited in 40% of elderly patients.[11]

Primary hypothyroidism, the most common form of hypothyroidism, is best diagnosed by finding elevated levels of circulating serum TSH and low serum $T_4$ levels.

TABLE 20.1. Age-Related Changes in Serum Hormone Levels

| Hormone | Change with aging[a] |
|---|---|
| Growth hormone | N in men; ↓ in women |
| Somatomedin C (insulin-like growth factor 1) | ↑ |
| ACTH | N |
| Cortisol | N or ↑ |
| Dehydroepiandrosterone | ↓ |
| Renin | N |
| Aldosterone | ↓ |
| Thyroid-stimulating hormone | N or ↑ |
| Thyroxine | N |
| Triiodothyronine | ↓ |
| Parathyroid hormone | ↑ |
| Calcitonin | ↓ |
| $1,25(OH)_2D$ | ↓ |
| Luteinizing hormone | ↑ or N in men; ↑ in women |
| Follicle-stimulating hormone | ↑ or N in men; ↑ in women |
| Testosterone | ↓ |
| Bioavailable testosterone | ↓ |
| Atrial natriuretic factor | ↑ |
| Insulin | ↑ |
| Glucagon | ↓ |

$1,25(OH)_2D$, 1,25-dihydroxyvitamin D.
[a] N, no change; ↑, increase; ↓, decrease.

Finding low levels of both TSH and free $T_4$ suggests pituitary dysfunction.[4] Measurements of total serum $T_4$ or serum $T_3$ are less useful for diagnosing hypothyroidism because of the variety of factors that can affect protein binding of thyroid hormones and thus total hormone values. Using clinical findings as a guide to identify a group of old patients in whom these tests should be ordered is clearly not adequate. Lioyd and Goldberg[12] noted that the clinical examination established a definite diagnosis of hypothyroidism in only 10% of patients with laboratory-confirmed hypothyroidism. Thus biochemical screening for hypothyroidism should be undertaken in old patients. A high yield may be expected by screening people with a history of autoimmune disease, Graves' disease, or Hashimoto's thyroiditis and from people with a family history of thyroid disease. The presence of dementia, taking medications known to affect thyroid function, or unexplained lethargy also mandates screening.[13]

TABLE 20.2. Age-Related Changes in Thyroid Physiology

| |
|---|
| **Decreased** |
| Serum $T_3$ |
| $T_4$ clearance |
| $T_3$ degradation |
| $T_4$ production |
| $T_3$ production |
| Radioactive iodine uptake |
| TSH response to TRH (men) |
| TSH sensitivity to $T_4$ |
| Circadian TSH variation |
| **No change** |
| $T_4$ |
| TSH |
| TSH response to TRH (women) |
| Reverse $T_3$ |
| **Increased** |
| TSH (women) |

$T_3$, triiodothyronine; $T_4$, thyroxine; TSH, thyroid-stimulating hormone; TRH, thyrotropin-releasing hormone.

Many patients with a clearly elevated serum TSH level have neither specific symptoms nor a clearly low value of serum $T_4$.[14] These patients are said to have subclinical hypothyroidism. The subclinical disorder is common in old persons, more so in women than in men.[15] Studies from the United Kingdom and the United States have reported rates of 4–8% in persons more than 60 years of age.[16–18] Parle et al.[17] followed 73 patients with elevated TSH and normal free $T_4$ and reported that 17.8% developed low free $T_4$ levels after a year of follow-up. The progression to overt hypothyroidism was more common in those with positive anti-thyroid peroxidase antibodies. The presence of subclinical hypothyroidism may not be as benign as was once thought. Studies have confirmed an increased systolic time interval associated with subclinical hypothyroidism and improvement in quality of life following thyroid hormone replacement compared with placebo.[19] For these reasons, many clinicians advocate starting these individuals on thyroid hormone replacement therapy, especially those with positive anti-thyroid antibodies and TSH values of more than 10mU/L.

Hypothyroidism is treated with thyroid hormone replacement using L-thyroxine preparations. When treating the elderly with L-thyroxine, it is important to "start low and go slow." The usual starting dosage is 25μg daily, which is increased by 25μg increments after equilibration has been reached (approximately five half-lives, or 4–6 weeks). In patients with severe cardiac disease it may be prudent to begin with 12.5μg daily and increase the dosage by similar increments. In general, old patients require a lower total replacement dosage of L-thyroxine (110 ± 8μg/day) than young patients (158 ± 6μg/day).[20] Patients on thyroid hormone replacement require periodic monitoring of their serum TSH levels (every 6–12 months). The replacement dose should be carefully titrated to maintain the serum TSH concentration within the normal range.

## Hyperthyroidism

The exact prevalence of hyperthyroidism in the general elderly population is not known. A study from New Zealand reported a prevalence of 0.47% in a population of community-based elderly.[21] It is estimated that 15–25% of all persons with hyperthyroidism are aged 65 years and over.[22] The preponderance of women having hyperthyroidism decreases with age, such that by the seventh decade men and women are affected almost equally.

The most common cause of hyperthyroidism in the elderly is a toxic nodular goiter. Unlike young adults, Graves' disease (diffuse toxic goiter) or toxic nodules appear to be less common causes of hyperthyroidism in old adults. Occasionally, patients develop transient hyperthyroidism secondary to subacute thyroiditis. Thyrotoxicosis may also be iatrogenic, resulting from excessive intake of thyroid hormone or following administration of iodine-containing contrast dye or certain drugs such as amiodarone and lithium.

The clinical manifestations of hyperthyroidism in old adults are different from those encountered in young adults. Goiter may be absent in up to 37% of patients.[5] Tremors occur at a lower frequency, and ophthalmologic findings are rarer in elderly persons with hyperthyroidism. The occurrence of frequent, loose bowel movements is less common in old hyperthyroid patients, although it is not infrequent that old patients with hyperthyroidism note correction of preexisting constipation. Tachycardia is not as prominent as it is in the young patients. In one series, 11% of old patients with hyperthyroidism had a normal heart rate.[22] An estimated 60% of old patients with hyperthyroidism present with new or worsening congestive heart failure.[22] Atrial fibrillation occurs in one-third of old patients with hyperthyroidism, and new or worsening angina is noted in 20% of old patients with this condition. Myopathy is a consistent finding in elderly hyperthyroid patients. It is usually more proximal and may result in an inability to rise from a seated position and so be independent in toileting and walking.[22] One presentation that occurs almost exclusively in the elderly is apathetic hyperthyroidism. Patients with apathetic hyperthyroidism are usually apathetic or depressed, have lost weight, and lack the signs or symptoms of adrenergic hyperstimulation. Atrial fibrillation and blepharoptosis are frequent findings with this syndrome.[22]

Elderly persons with hyperthyroidism may have an excess of either $T_4$ alone, $T_3$ alone, or both. The isolated finding of excessive amounts of circulating serum $T_3$ is known as $T_3$ thyrotoxicosis, an entity almost exclusively noted in the elderly.[22] Individuals with $T_3$ thyrotoxicosis may have suppressed $T_4$ levels. Because total $T_4$ and $T_3$ levels may be affected by changes in serum iodothyronine-binding proteins, free thyroid hormone determination is recommended for an assessment of the thyroidal state.[23] The new supersensitive TSH assay cannot distinguish between normal (euthyroid) and hyperthyroid levels of TSH in old persons.[24] A high value suggests either primary thyroid gland failure or the presence of a TSH-secreting pituitary nodule. A low value suggests a hyperthyroid state resulting from endogenous overproduction of thyroid hormone or ingestion of excessive exogenous hormone or pituitary gland failure.[4] As experience grew with these methods of assessing serum TSH, a new clinical entity was identified. These individuals have suppressed or low serum TSH values despite normal levels of free $T_4$ and free $T_3$. This condition is now known as subclinical hyperthyroidism.[22] Data are too preliminary at the present time to specify the prevalence or the prognosis of this condition. However, low levels of TSH may be spurious, and old persons with hyperthyroidism may have normal levels.

Hyperthyroidism can be a life-threatening disease in the elderly and deserves prompt attention. Ablative therapy with radioactive iodine (RAI) is the treatment of choice for those with toxic thyroid nodules (adenoma or multinodular goiter). The long-term treatment of Graves' disease remains controversial. Some experts advocate use of propylthiouracil (PTU) or methimazole to block thyroid hormone biosynthesis in the hope that the disease will resolve spontaneously. This is usually not the case, however, and RAI is often ultimately required.[25] An euthyroid state, which must be induced before using RAI, can be achieved by using PTU or methimazole. As these medications may take weeks to begin working, the use of adrenergic blocking medications or even iodine as adjunctive therapy may be required to control symptoms. Antithyroid drugs should be discontinued for 1 week before administration of RAI to allow uptake of RAI by the gland; they may be restarted 1 week after treatment and continued until the RAI becomes effective.[25] After treatment these patients should be followed closely for the emergence of hypothyroidism.

## Thyroid Nodules

Thyroid nodules increase in frequency with age such that by age 80 virtually 100% of glands examined postmortem show microscopic nodularity, and 10–15% of patients have nodules larger than 1 cm.[25] Most thyroid nodules are benign, with 90% being either colloid or benign adenomas. Thyroid scanning is done to evaluate nodules with either iodine 123 or technetium 99. Although all thyroid cancers are cold on scan, only 5% of cold nodules prove to be malignant. The fine-needle biopsy is the most cost-effective method to diagnose a thyroid carcinoma. If the biopsy is nondiagostic, a solitary nodule that is cold on scan should be surgically removed. Multinodular goiters have the same rate of malignancy as solitary nodules, and physicians evaluating multinodular goiters are advised to biopsy several nodules, targeting those that are large, hard on palpation, or cold on scans.[25]

## Thyroid Cancer

Anaplastic carcinoma is the most common variety of thyroid carcinoma in the elderly. This carcinoma usually arises from a previously existing papillary or follicular carcinoma and so should be considered in patients with a history of a well-differentiated tumor who present with a recurrent, rapidly enlarging neck mass or widely metastasizing disease.[26] The biologic behavior of well-differentiated thyroid cancers is more aggressive in the elderly than in the young. Thus it is essential that elderly patients with thyroid cancer are given the full benefit of total thyroidectomy coupled with postoperative ablation of the remnant thyroid tissue with RAI.[5] Medullary tumors are uncommon in the elderly population.

## Calcium Metabolism

Despite the lack of dramatic change in serum calcium, alterations in calcium metabolism with age are significant. The capacity of the intestine to absorb calcium declines with age,[27] and net resorption of calcium from bone increases. In addition, there are large age-related changes in serum 1,25($OH_2$)-vitamin D [1,25($OH_2$)D] and parathyroid hormone (PTH). The actions of these hormones on their target tissues also change. Such changes in calcium metabolism in old persons may contribute to the loss of bone mass that occurs with advancing age.[28]

### Vitamin D and Aging

Serum 1,25$(OH)_2$D levels have been shown to decline with advancing age. The magnitude of this decline has been reported to be as large as 75% of the levels of young adults.[29] This decline has been attributed largely to diminished renal response to PTH with advancing age.[30] There is also a decrease in renal 1$\alpha$-hydroxylase enzyme activity with age. Armbrecht et al.[31] demonstrated a loss in 1$\alpha$-hydroxylase enzyme in cortical renal slices in older rats, even in the absence of appreciable renal disease. The effect of 1,25$(OH)_2$D on the intestine decrease with age. This has been documented in the rat[32] but has not yet been studied systematically in humans.

There have been conflicting reports as to whether serum levels of 25-hydroxyvitamin D [25(OH)D] change with age. Studies from Europe have reported decreased 25(OH)D levels in the elderly,[33] whereas studies in the United States have tended to find no age-related changes in serum 25(OH)D.[34] There are, however, reports of a longitudinal decline in 25(OH)D in old persons in New Mexico. These conflicting findings may reflect differences in diet and sunlight exposure between the two populations. Nursing home populations seem to be especially at risk of low serum 25(OH)D levels.[35,36] Decreased serum 25(OH)D levels may be due to a combination of decreased exposure to sunlight, decreased capacity to synthesize vitamin D in the skin with age,[37] and decreased vitamin D in the diet. The effect of age on the conversion of vitamin D to 25(OH)D by the liver has not been studied.

### Hyperparathyroidism

With hyperparathyroidism, PTH is inappropriately secreted by the parathyroid glands. The disease is considered primary when the increased secretion of PTH is not in response to other systemic abnormalities.[38] Secondary hyperparathyroidism occurs when there is a prolonged hypocalcemic stimulus, as in cases of vitamin D deficiency or chronic renal failure. Tertiary hyperparathyroidism occurs in patients with secondary hyperparathyroidism who develop autonomous hypersecretion of PTH.[39] Here we limit our discussion to primary hyperparathyroidism (PHP).

The diagnosis of PHP increased substantially with the introduction of routine multiphasic serum calcium studies. A study in Rochester, Minnesota, reported an incidence of 27.7 per 100,000 per year.[40] The incidence of PHP increases with age. In those over the age of 60 the annual incidence is reported to be as high as 1.5%.[41] PHP is caused by a solitary adenoma in 80% of patients. Other causes include hyperplasia (15%), "double" adenomas (2%), and carcinoma (<1%).[42] A history of irradiation to the neck and upper chest area during childhood is obtained in as many as 15–25% of patients with PHP.[40] PHP has been reported following administration of radioactive iodine for thyroid disease.[43]

Most patients with PHP are asymptomatic and are identified based on the hypercalcemia that is accidentally discovered on a routine serum calcium determination. In some series as many as 80% can be classified as without symptoms.[44] One organ frequently affected in patients with PHP is the kidney. Nephrolithiasis occurs in as many as 20% of patients with PHP.[45] Renal stones due to PHP are usually composed of calcium oxalate or calcium phosphate.[44] Deposition of calcium-phosphate crystals throughout the renal parenchyma, a process also known as nephrocalcinosis, is another form of kidney disorder in PHP that may cause reduction in renal function.[44]

Bone is also affected by PHP. The classic bone disease of PHP is osteitis fibrosa cystica, which may be experienced by patients as bone pain. Local destructive lesions, bone cysts, and "brown tumors" in long bones and the pelvis constitute other skeletal manifestations of the disease. Brown tumors are collections of osteoclasts intermixed with poorly mineralized woven bone.[40] Bone involvement in PHP is associated with several typical radiographic signs. Subperiosteal bone resorption of the distal phalanges is the most sensitive radiologic sign of PHP. It is appreciated best on the radial side of the middle phalanges.[40] Tiny "punched-out" lesions may cause the so-called salt-and-pepper appearance in the skull.[44] The distal one-third of the clavicles may appear to be tapered.

Most other signs and symptoms of PHP can be attributed to the resultant hypercalcemia. Although mild hypercalcemia is often asymptomatic, extreme hypercalcemia may lead to coma and even death. Less severe cases often present with manifestations related to the nervous system, the gastrointestinal tract, or both. Neurologic manifestations may include confusion, lethargy, weakness, and hyporeflexia. Gastrointestinal manifestations include constipation, anorexia, nausea, and vomiting. Acute pancreatitis and hypertension have also been reported to be associated with hypercalcemia. Hypercalcemia, by interfering with antidiuretic hormone, often results in polyuria and polydipsia. Finally, calcium may precipitate in the cornea causing band keratopathy or in soft tissue causing calciphylaxis.

Demonstrating elevated PTH levels associated with hypercalcemia indicates the biochemical diagnosis of PHP. Earlier PTH assays could not reliably distinguish individuals with PHP from those with cancer. More recently, improved assays have been able to detect intact PTH molecules (at both the N-terminal and the C-terminal) with immunoradiometric techniques, making it possible to diagnose hyperparathyroidism directly rather than by exclusion, as was done previously.

Symptomatic hypercalcemia can usually be managed with intravenous saline and furosemide. Pamidronate (an intravenously administered second-generation bisphosphonate), calcitonin, or plicamycin may be added in more severe cases.[46] At the present time, there is no ideal long-term medical treatment for patients with PHP. The best studied treatment has been estrogen, which remains an excellent option for selected postmenopausal women.[47] $\alpha$-Adrenergic blockers, phosphate supplementation with potassium phosphate, etidronate disodium, or oral cellulose phosphate with dietary calcium restriction may lower calcium levels, although other aspects of the disease may progress. No data are available regarding the use of the oral bisphosphonate (alendronate) to treat primary hyperparathyroidism.

When treated operatively by an experienced surgeon, PHP is curable in more than 95% of cases.[48] Surgical treatment is indicated for all patients with biochemical evidence of PHP (elevated serum calcium and PTH) and documented signs or symptoms of the disease. Surgical treatment is also indicated for young asymptomatic patients with PHP because these patients may be at high risk for developing significant symptoms with time. In asymptomatic old patients, careful observation and follow-up are recommended, with surgery reserved for patients who develop signs and symptoms.[49] Postoperatively, patients should be monitored closely for development of hypocalcemia.

## Osteoporosis

Osteoporosis is a disease characterized by low bone mass and microarchitectural deterioration of bone tissue leading to increased bone fragility and fracture risk.[50] It can be classified as primary or secondary, depending on the absence or presence of an associated medical condition known to cause bone loss (Table 20.3). Secondary causes of osteoporosis are identified in 20% of women and 40% of men presenting with vertebral fractures and should always be sought.[51] If no secondary cause is identified, osteoporosis is termed primary. A form of primary osteoporosis that occurs in children or young adults of both genders with normal gonadal function is frequently termed idiopathic osteoporosis. The other two forms of primary osteoporosis are known as type I and type II osteoporosis.[52]

Type I osteoporosis affects mainly trabecular bone and results in fractures primarily in vertebral bodies and the distal forearm. It occurs more frequently in women than in men (6:1) and is related to the accelerated bone loss in women found during the first two decades after menopause.[53] The precise mechanism involved in the pathogenesis of bone loss due to estrogen deficiency is not completely understood. There is evidence to indicate that estrogen governs skeletal cytokine activity and that with the depletion of this hormone, upregulation of several key cytokines result in accelerated bone

TABLE 20.3. Causes of Osteoporosis

| |
|---|
| **Primary osteoporosis** |
| Idiopathic osteoporosis (juvenile) |
| Type I osteoporosis (postmenopausal) |
| Type II osteoporosis (senile) |
| **Secondary osteoporosis** |
| Hypogonadism |
| Hyperadrenocorticism |
| Chronic glucocorticoid administration |
| Hyperparathyroidism |
| Thyrotoxicosis |
| Malabsorption |
| Scurvy |
| Calcium deficiency |
| Immobilization |
| Chronic heparin administration |
| Systemic mastocytosis |
| Adult hypophosphatemia |
| Associated with other metabolic bone diseases |
| Rheumatoid arthritis |
| Malnutrition |
| Alcoholism |
| Epilepsy |
| Primary biliary cirrhosis |
| Diabetes mellitus |
| Chronic obstructive pulmonary disease |
| Heritable connective tissue disorders (osteogenesis imperfecta, homocystinuria, Ehlers-Danlos syndrome, Marfan syndrome) |

resorption.[54] The cytokines most often implicated are interleukin-1 (IL-1), IL-6, IL-11, and tumor necrosis factor (TNF).[55–57]

Type II osteoporosis affects both trabecular and cortical bone and is associated with fractures of the femoral neck, proximal humerus, proximal tibia, and pelvis. The primary pathogenesis is related to be impaired production of $1,25(OH)_2D$. This low vitamin D state, in turn, results in decreased calcium absorption from the gut leading to hypocalcemia, which stimulates the release of PTH, causing calcium to be mobilized from the skeleton to restore serum levels.

Measurement of bone mineral density (BMD) is probably the most useful means of diagnosing osteoporosis and stratifying people by level of fracture risk.[58] There is a 1.5- to 3.0-fold increase in the fracture rate for each standard deviation of decrease in BMD.[59] Currently, a variety of techniques are available for assessing bone density noninvasively, including single-energy x-ray absorptiometry, dual-energy x-ray absorptiometry (DEXA), quantitative computed tomography (CT), and quantitative ultrasonography. DEXA is currently the most frequently used method for evaluating bone density in clinical practice. It has a high rate of precision and exposes the subjects to a low dose of radiation.

Laboratory studies (Table 20.4) are used mainly to exclude other diseases that can cause osteopenia, such as multiple myeloma, endocrinopathies, and osteomalacia. In recent years it became possible to identify high rates of bone turnover by measuring biochemical products of resorption and formation. Bone-specific alkaline phosphatase and osteocalcin are two sensitive serum markers for bone formation. Osteocalcin has been demonstrated to be an independent determinant of BMD of the hip in elderly women, and its level is a sensitive predictor of the subsequent risk of hip fracture.[52] Markers of bone degradation (e.g., urinary hydroxyproline), on the other hand, are nonspecific. Recently, however, two markers of bone degradation that are highly specific to bone have become available: deoxypyridinoline and *N*-telopeptides.[60] These markers not only indicate patients with active bone turnover likely to increase bone loss but also have been shown to predict fracture risk.[61]

TABLE 20.4. Laboratory Evaluation of Patients with Osteopenia

| |
|---|
| **Serum** |
| Calcium |
| Phosphorous |
| Magnesium |
| Alkaline phosphatase |
| 25(OH)D |
| PTH |
| Thyroid function tests |
| Serum protein electrophoresis |
| Testosterone (men) |
| **Urine** |
| Calcium/creatinine |
| Hydroxyproline/creatinine |
| Deoxypyridinoline/creatinine |
| *N*-Telopeptides/creatinine |

TABLE 20.5. Drugs Used for Prevention and Treatment of Osteoporosis

| |
|---|
| **Hormone therapy** |
| Estrogen |
| Partial estrogen agonists (tamoxifen, tibilone, raloxifene) |
| Androgens (testosterone) |
| **Calcium** |
| **Vitamin D** |
| Cholecalciferol (vitamin $D_3$) |
| $1,25(OH)_2D$ |
| Calcitriol analogues (alfacidol) |
| **Bisphosphonates** |
| Etidronate |
| Alendronate |
| **Calcitonin** |
| Salmon calcitonin (subcutaneous, intramuscular, intranasal) |
| Human calcitonin |
| **Sodium fluoride** |
| **Future agents** |
| PTH analogues |
| Anabolic agents |

Currently, several therapeutic modalities are available for management of osteoporosis (Table 20.5). These modalities can be grouped into those that decrease bone resorption and those that increase bone formation. Drugs that inhibit bone resorption do not generally affect bone mass. They are most effective when bone turnover is increased, and their effect is greater on cancellous bone than on cortical bone, in which the rate of turnover is lower. The agents from this group currently approved in the United States include estrogen, calcitonin (both nasal spray and parenterally administered), calcium, vitamin D, and alendronate.[62] Drugs that increase bone formation, on the other hand, increase bone mass. At this time these agents remain relatively experimental. The side effects of the regimens used to date appear to prevent their widespread use. One drug in this group, slow-release sodium fluoride, has been available in Europe for this indication for many years and is likely to be available soon in the United States.

## Sex Steroids

### Testosterone

As early as 1948 it was found that bioassayable urinary androgens were decreased in older men.[63] Subsequently, circulating testosterone was shown to decrease with advancing age, with the difference becoming apparent by the fifth decade.[64] Testosterone exists in the circulation bound to sex hormone-binding globulin (SHBG), bound

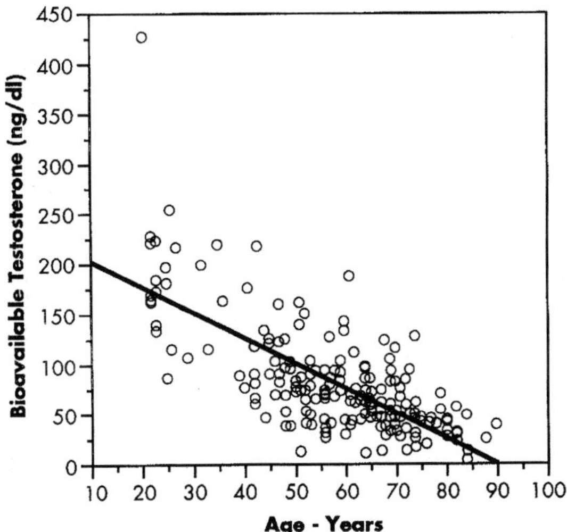


FIGURE 20.1. Demonstration of age-related decrease in bioavailable testosterone. (From Morley and Kaiser[65], with permission.)

to albumin, or as "free" testosterone. Non-SHBG-bound testosterone, or bioavailable testosterone, represents that which is "free" and that which is bound to albumin, and it appears to predict more accurately the testosterone available to tissues than does "free" testosterone alone.[65] Both "free" (1.2% per year) and albumin-bound (1% per year) testosterone levels decline at a faster rate than total serum testosterone (0.4% per year).[66] The circadian rhythm of both "free" and bioavailable testosterone is markedly blunted with age.[67] Plasma levels of bioavailable testosterone have been shown to decrease dramatically with advancing age (Fig. 20.1). Between the ages of 50 and 70 years, half of healthy men have a bioavailable testosterone level below the lowest level seen in healthy men who are 20–40 years of age.[69] Whether the older men who have bioavailable testosterone levels within the normal limits represent those who originally had high levels when younger is not yet clear. Our longitudinal study has demonstrated a clear decline in testosterone over a 14-year period in older men.

With aging there is a general decline in the mass and weight of the testicles. The tubules undergo some atrophy, and the number of Leydig cells decrease.[70] This observation led investigators initially to believe that primary hypogonadism was the most likely cause of the decline in serum testosterone. To support this possibility, most of the early studies[71–73] reported an increase in luteinizing hormone (LH) levels with age. Since the early 1980s, however, this consensus appears to have disappeared. In 1982 Zummoff et al.[74] were the first to report that they did not detect age-related increases in 24-hour mean plasma LH levels despite a decline of the 24-hour mean plasma testosterone level. Similar findings were later reported by other investigators.[75] Furthermore, the increased LH level demonstrated in earlier studies occurs predominantly in the very old, with only small increases being seen in middle-aged and young-old men.[76] It should be also noted that with aging, there is increased secretion of the $\alpha$-subunit of the LH glycoprotein. This raised the possibility that in some studies LH may be falsely higher because some anti-LH antibodies cross-react with the $\alpha$-subunit. Thus, contrary to the previous belief that primary hypogonadism is the most likely change seen in older men, it appears that the initial factor that results in a decline in testosterone with advancing age resides in the hypothalamic-pituitary unit.[76]

The exact mechanism(s) underlying these age-related changes in the hypothalamic-pituitary unit have not been clearly elucidated. In the Baltimore study,[77] as in several other studies,[78–80] a delay in the time and the peak of LH concentration after LH-releasing hormone administration, was reported in older men. There is also evidence that increased "sensitivity" of the hypothalamic-pituitary axis to exogenous androgens occurs with aging, with testosterone producing more inhibition of LH secretion in older individuals than in the young.[81] In addition, there is a decrease in the gonadotropin-releasing hormone (GnRH) pulse generator resulting in altered LH pulses with aging.

The most common predictor of low testosterone syndrome is a decrease in libido. Another predictor is loss of axillary and pubic hair. A "low testosterone syndrome" checklist has been developed at St. Louis University (Fig. 20.2). In the absence of depression, a positive response to questions 1 and 7 or any three of the other questions indicate a need to evaluate for hypogonadism.[82]

Testosterone therapy in older men has been shown to enhance lean body mass,[83] decrease body fat,[84] increase muscle strength,[85,86] and improve visuospatial memory.[87] The effects of testosterone on bone have been less clearly

**St. Louis University**
**ADAM: Androgen Deficiency in Aging Males**
**questionnaire**

____ 1. Do you have a decrease in libido (sex drive)?
____ 2. Do you have a lack of energy?
____ 3. Do you have a decrease in strength and/or endurance?
____ 4. Have you lost height?
____ 5. Have you noticed a decreased "enjoyment of life"?
____ 6. Are you sad and/or grumpy?
____ 7. Are your erections less strong?
____ 8. Have you noted a recent deterioration in your ability to play sports?
____ 9. Are you falling asleep after dinner?
____ 10. Has there been a recent deterioration in your work performance?

Please answer yes or no to the above questions.

FIGURE 20.2. ADAM (Androgen Deficiency in Aging Males) questionnaire for evidence of hypogonadism. A positive answer is yes to 1, 2 or any 3 others.

TABLE 20.6. Forms of Testosterone Replacement Therapy

| |
|---|
| **Intramuscular** |
| Testosterone enanthate |
| Testosterone cypionate |
| **Transdermal** |
| Testoderm (scrotal patch) |
| Androderm (nonscrotal skin) |
| **Oral** |
| Testosterone undeconate[a] |
| **Slow release** |
| Testosterone pellets |

[a] Not available in the United States.

delineated. A number of options are now available for the administration of testosterone (Table 20.6). The major side effect of testosterone administration is an increase in the hematocrit level. In one study, approximately 25% of patients developed an elevated hematocrit. Testosterone may increase the prostate-specific antigen (PSA) level slightly but usually not progressively.[86] Concerns regarding stimulation of benign prostatic hypertrophy (BPH) and prostatic carcinoma have not been supported experimentally. Other side effects include gynecomastia, fluid retention, and hepatic toxicity. If testosterone is prescribed, careful prostate examination and laboratory testing for hematocrit level, liver function, and PSA level should be performed every 3–6 months.

## Dehydroepiandrosterone

Dehydroepiandrosterone (DHEA) and its sulfated conjugate, DHEA sulfate (DHEAS), are the most abundant steroid hormones in the human body. DHEA is a key hormone early in steroid hormone biosynthesis (Fig. 20.3). DHEA with DHEAS serve as precursors for both androgenic and estrogenic steroids. Most DHEA is produced in the adrenal cortex from cholesterol under the influence of the adrenocorticotrophic hormone (ACTH). The testes and ovaries are responsible for 5% of the total DHEA production.[88] The DHEAs circulate in the blood in a free nonbound form as well as bound to albumin and SHBG.

Cross-sectional[89] and longitudinal[90] studies have demonstrated the decline of DHEA and DHEAS levels with advancing age (Fig. 20.4). It has been shown conclusively that, with age, levels of DHEA and DHEAS in both sexes, decrease at a relatively constant rate of 2% per year. Hence, at age 80 levels are only about 20% of those at age 25. Some researchers have attributed this decline to a decrease in the number of functional zona reticularis cells, whereas others attributed it to intra-adrenal changes in 17α-hydroxylase activity.[92] The

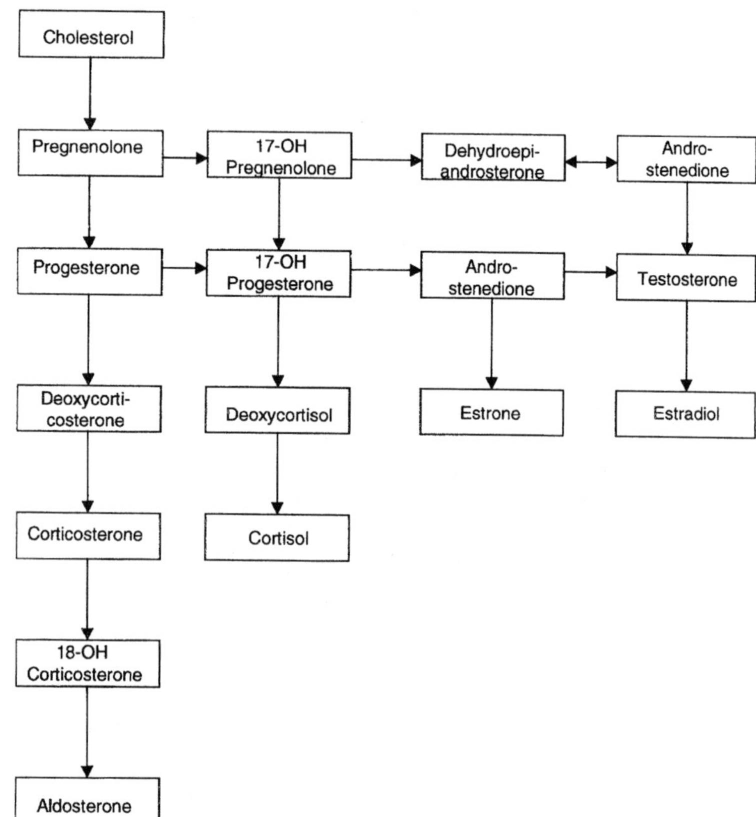


FIGURE 20.3. Synthesis and metabolism of DHEA and related steroids.

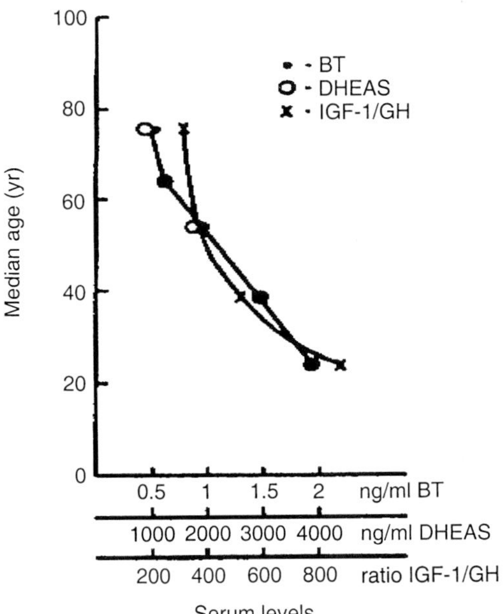


FIGURE 20.4. Age-related decline in dehydroepiandrosterone sulfate (DHEAS) blood levels in humans. BT, bioavailable testosterone; IGF-1/GH, insulin-like growth factor-1/growth hormone. (From Morley et al.[91] with permission.)

decline in serum DHEA levels with age parallels the development of decreased immunity, physical frailty, decreased muscle mass, increased fat mass, decreased ability to cope, disturbed sleep patterns, and increased incidence of disease. Thus DHEA can be viewed as a marker of aging in humans.[93] More importantly, low levels of DHEA and DHEAS are associated with a variety of morbidities and increased mortality. A low serum DHEAS level has been correlated with increased all-cause and cardiovascular mortality in men,[94] premenopausal breast cancer,[95] and gastric cancer.[96] Low DHEA levels may also be a risk factor for osteoporosis.[97]

Numerous animal studies have demonstrated that DHEA has multiple antiaging effects. It remains to be established, however, whether any of the beneficial consequences of DHEA administration demonstrated in animal models are relevant in humans. Small-scale human studies have demonstrated a possible cardiovascular protective effect[98,99]; possible positive immunomodulatory effects in older patients[100] and in patients with the acquired immunodeficiency syndrome (AIDS)[101]; possible insulin sensitivity-enhancing effects in patients with diabetes[102]; and possible positive effects on mood, memory,[103] and length and quality of sleep in old patients and those with psychiatric disorders.[104] These effects, however, must be confirmed by large-scale controlled studies. At the present time, the side effects of chronic DHEA administration are virtually not known.

## Estrogen

Menopause is defined as that point in time when permanent cessation of menstruation occurs following the loss of ovarian activity.[105] With the onset of menopausal amenorrhea, there is a rapid fall in ovarian estrogen production. The decreased serum estradiol occurs over a 1-year interval; and once the atretic process is complete the serum estradiol concentration in postmenopausal women may eventually resemble that of premenopausal individuals who have undergone oophorectomy.[106] During the menopausal transition, women may experience hot flashes, sweats, prolonged menstrual irregularities, vaginal dryness, and a host of other symptoms including depression, irritability, weight gain, insomnia, and dizziness. Development of osteoporosis[107] and increased cardiovascular disease morbidity[108] and mortality[109] are the main long-term effects of estrogen deficiency. Estrogen deficiency is also related to a decrease in muscle strength and an increasing risk of falling.[110]

Estrogen replacement therapy is indicated to alleviate hot flashes and other perimenopausal symptoms, delay bone loss, and prevent cardiovascular disease (Table 20.7). More recent data indicate that estrogen replacement therapy may help prevent or delay the onset of Alzheimer's disease in postmenopausal women.[111,112] Estrogen is most commonly administered as conjugated equine estrogen at a dose of 0.625 mg/day given orally for the first 25 days or daily each month. Estrogen can also be administered in a percutaneous patch of gel for transdermal absorption. Transdermal estrogen is as effective as orally administered estrogen in preventing postmenopausal bone loss.[113] Transdermal estrogen, however, lacks the favorable effects of orally administered estrogen on high density lipoprotein (HDL) levels.[114]

Estrogen replacement therapy is not without complications. It increases the risk of endometrial cancer,[115] an effect that can be eliminated by concurrent administration of a progestogen.[116] Following hysterectomy, a progestogen (e.g., medroxyprogesterone 5 mg/day) may be added for the first or last 12–14 days of estrogen administration. Estrogen and a low dose of progestogen (e.g., medroxyprogesterone 2.5 mg/day) may also be

TABLE 20.7. Clinical Indications for Estrogen Replacement Therapy

| |
|---|
| Hot flashes |
| Dysphoric mood |
| Atrophic urethritis |
| Stress incontinence |
| Urge incontinence |
| Atrophic vaginitis |
| Dyspareunia |
| Decreased sexual motivation |
| Osteoporosis prevention |
| Cardiovascular prevention |

administered continuously. Whether estrogen therapy increases the incidence of breast cancer has not been settled. Some evidence suggests that administration of estrogen for 15 years or more slightly increases the risk of breast cancer.[117] Selective estrogen receptor modulators, such as raloxifene, affect predominantly bone and may decrease the development of breast cancer. Tibolone is a mixed testosterone/estrogen/progesterone product that has positive effects on bone, causes uterine bleeding in fewer than 10% of women, and has a higher compliance rate than classic hormone replacement therapy.

## Diabetes Mellitus

Diabetes mellitus is a disorder of carbohydrate metabolism that results from a relative or absolute deficiency of insulin. It affects 18% of persons aged 65–75 years and as many as 40% of persons older than 80 years of age.[118] Most of the older diabetics have type II diabetes mellitus. It is estimated that nearly half of elderly diabetics are undiagnosed.[119]

The criteria for the diagnosis of diabetes mellitus in old adults are similar to that in young adults. The Diabetes Expert Committee of the American Diabetes Association (ADA) has published new diagnostic criteria.[120] They state that diabetes mellitus can be diagnosed if the fasting plasma glucose level is ≥126 mg/dl. When the fasting plasma glucose level is <126 mg/dl in suspected cases, a standardized oral glucose tolerance test (OGTT) is performed (Table 20.8). The 1997 ADA recommendations also identified another category of altered glucose metabolism called impaired glucose tolerance (IGT). Patients falling in this category are at a greater risk of developing overt diabetes mellitus with time. The diagnosis of IGT is based on the result of an OGTT with a 2-hour postchallenge glucose level ≥140 mg/dl but <200 mg/dl. The 1997 ADA recommendations also described a new category called impaired fasting glucose (IFG) to include those persons who have a fasting glucose ≥110 mg/dl but <126 mg/dl. The IFG category allows identification of many individuals who would meet the criteria for IGT based on measurement of the fasting blood glucose levels.[121]

TABLE 20.8. 1997 American Diabetes Association Diagnostic Criteria for Diabetes Mellitus

**Diabetes mellitus**
- A random serum glucose level ≥200 mg/dl plus classic diabetes symptoms
- Fasting glucose level ≥126 mg/dl
- Glucose level ≥200 mg/dl at 2 hours during a standard oral glucose tolerance test OGTT

**Impaired glucose tolerance (IGT)**
- Glucose level ≥140 mg/dl and <200 mg/dl at 2 hours during a standard OGTT

**Impaired fasting glucose (IFG)**
- Fasting glucose ≥110 mg/dl and <126 mg/dl

TABLE 20.9. Currently Available Oral Hypoglycemic Agents

| Drug | Mechanism of action |
|---|---|
| **Sulfonylureas** | Enhance insulin secretion |
| *First generation* | |
| Acetohexamide | |
| Chlorpropamide | |
| Tolazamide | |
| Tolbutamide | |
| *Second generation* | |
| Glimepiride | |
| Glipizide, sustained release | |
| Glyburide | |
| Glyburide, micronized | |
| Glimepiride | |
| **α-Glucosidase inhibitor** | |
| Acarbose | α-glucosidase inhibitor |
| Miglitol | α-glucosidase inhibitor |
| **Biguanide** | |
| Metformin | Decreases hepatic glucose production |
| **Thiazolidenedione** | |
| Rosiglitazone | Enhances insulin sensitivity |
| Pioglitazone | Enhances insulin sensitivity |
| **Nonsulfonylurea** | |
| Repaglinide | Enhances insulin secretion |

The ADA has set a target fasting glucose <120 mg/dl and a hemoglobin $A_{1c}$ level within 1% of the upper limit of normal as a therapeutic goal of diabetes management.[120] Although the ADA has indicated that age per se should not be an excuse for suboptimal control of blood glucose,[122] it may be neither feasible nor appropriate to attempt to achieve such tight control in many old patients with diabetes. Thus the goals of diabetes management in old adults should be individualized. Factors such as patient's estimated life expectancy, coexistent medical conditions, economic issues, and availability of support services should always be considered when setting therapeutic goals in elderly diabetics.[121]

Several therapeutic interventions are available for old patients with diabetes. Dietary intervention is the cornerstone of diabetes management in young patients. The ADA recommends a diet low in fat (less than 30% of total calories) to decrease the rate of atherosclerosis-related complications.[123] Caloric restriction is recommended in patients with a body mass index (BMI) greater than 27 kg/m$^2$. However, many old diabetics are not overweight, and dietary restriction may result in malnutrition. No patients in nursing homes should be given diabetic diets. Patients treated with insulin should maintain consistency of dietary intake in terms of meal composition and timing. An exercise program may have beneficial effects on glucose intolerance, blood pressure control, weight control, lipid profile, and cardiovascular status.[119] Physical activity has been shown to enhance insulin sensitivity and improve glucose intolerance in diabetic subjects.[124]

Currently, a number of oral medications are available for management of old adults with diabetes (Table 20.9).

Sulfonylurea drugs are the most widely used. They act initially by increasing pancreatic insulin secretion and later enhance insulin sensitivity, probably via a postreceptor mechanism.[125] Hypoglycemia is the main side effect associated with sulfonylurea drugs. Repaglinide, a non-sulfonylurea that must be given before each meal, has been used successfully in the elderly. The α-glucosidase inhibitor acarbose works by inhibiting glucose absorption from the gut. Acarbose is particularly helpful for reducing postprandial hyperglycemia and may be a useful adjunct to therapy with other agents.[125] Metformin works primarily by suppressing hepatic glucose production and to a lesser extent by improving insulin sensitivity. Metformin may result in loss of appetite and weight loss, a desirable side effect in obese diabetics. It should be avoided in persons over 80 years of age. The thizolidenediones is the most recently introduced group of oral antidiabetic agents.[126] They appear to work primarily by enhancing peripheral tissue sensitivity to insulin. In addition to being the most expensive oral agent on the market, there have been several reports of patients developing idiosyncratic hepatic toxicity, which in a few cases led to hepatic failure and patient death particularly with troglitazone.[127,128] However, these drugs do not cause hypoglycemia and are ideal drugs in old persons. Because of their different modes of action, combining agents from different classes may result in synergistic therapeutic efficacy.

If patients fail to respond to oral agents, insulin is indicated. Physicians should not refrain from initiating insulin therapy in older diabetic patients simply because of age. Most elderly diabetics do well on insulin injection,[129] but physicians should regularly check the ability of their elderly patients to draw the insulin into the syringe. One study[130] estimated that elderly diabetics, in general, err by 10–20% when filling their syringes.

In most elderly patients requiring insulin therapy, a single daily injection of an intermediate-acting insulin (NPH or lente) is usually sufficient. When the required total daily insulin dose exceeds 50 units, a split-dose regimen is usually preferred. An oral agent, such as a thiazolidenedione or metformin, may be added to an insulin regimen to enhance insulin sensitivity in patients with insulin resistance, thereby avoiding such high doses of insulin, which may have adverse cardiovascular effects.[131,132]

Substantial education and continuously monitoring for the degree of diabetic control and the development of chronic complications are key to the management of elderly diabetics. In addition to home glucose monitoring and regular assessments of glycosylated hemoglobin, ongoing care should include annual eye examinations, monitoring of renal function, and regular foot care.[25]

## Pituitary

Aging is associated with several anatomic and histologic changes in the pituitary gland. Both the weight of the gland and its blood supply have been reported to decrease. Adenomas occur at a high frequency. The hypothalamic-pituitary function remains intact in older adults, and the circadian rhythms are usually unaffected.[4] The sensitivity of the gland to hormonal feedback is diminished, which results in higher baseline levels of pituitary hormone secretion. ACTH and TSH feedback loops becomes less responsive to cortisol and to $T_4/T_3$, respectively. LH and follicle stimulating hormone (FSH) levels increase in postmenopausal women as a result of loss of ovarian function. LH and FSH may be normal or lightly elevated in men. Serum prolactin levels increase in both men and women as a function of age.[133]

Levels of growth hormone (GH) and insulin-like growth factor-1 (IGF-1) decrease with aging in both genders.[134] The response of pituitary secretion of GH to provocative stimulation, such as insulin-induced hypoglycemia, intravenous arginine, or intravenous growth hormone-releasing hormone (GHRH), also declines.[135] There are many similarities between the syndrome associated with the lack of GH in adults and the characteristics of normal old adults. Hence it is uncertain whether these changes represent a deficiency state in need of correction, or they reflect necessary adaptation in response to aging. Rudman and colleagues[136] demonstrated that administering recombinant human GH to a small group of elderly men with low GH levels reversed some signs of aging, resulting in increased lean body mass, decreased excess fat, and increased skin thickness. In addition, administering GH to a subset of malnourished frail elderly men resulted in positive nitrogen balance and enhanced weight gain.[137] Prolonged administration of GH is complicated by the development of carpal tunnel syndrome, gynecomastia, and hyperglycemia.[138] At best, GH increases muscle mass without increasing strength.

## Adrenals

There is a slight decline in the weight of the adrenal gland with age. The amount of fibrous tissue in the adrenal cortex increases, and the number of epithelial cells decreases. Nodular hyperplasia occurs at a higher frequency in old individuals, with 50% of adrenals at autopsy showing mild cortical nodularity. Basal, circadian, and ACTH-stimulated secretion of cortisol in old individuals is similar to that of young individuals. Metabolic clearance of cortisol decreases with age, but it is compensated by a similar decrease in production resulting in plasma cortisol levels staying stable with aging.[139] Aldosterone and renin secretion decrease with age, placing old persons at risk of developing iatrogenic hyporeninemic hypoaldosteronism when receiving drugs such as β-blockers or nonsteroidal antiinflammatory agents.[140]

Cushing syndrome is rare in elderly persons, occurring most frequently as an iatrogenic reaction in chronic corticosteroid users. Malignant adrenal tumors and ectopic ACTH syndrome occur at a higher frequency in old patients. The presence of centripetal obesity, striae, buffalo hump, hypertension, and glucose intolerance demands a diagnostic screen. The workup should include analysis of cortisol and adrenal androgen production, measurement of serum ACTH levels, and a dexamethasone suppression test. A CT scan of the abdomen is indicated if there is chemical evidence of hypercortisolism. Elevated adrenal androgen levels suggest an adrenal tumor. Bilateral adrenal enlargement on CT scan suggests pituitary Cushing's disease or an ACTH-secreting tumor. Unilateral enlargement with contralateral suppression suggests an adrenal tumor. Therapy is primarily surgery.[133]

The principal cause of primary adrenal insufficiency (Addison's disease) in the elderly is autoimmune disease. It is important to rule out other causes such as tuberculosis, metastatic involvement of the adrenal glands, and adrenal hemorrhage especially in elderly patients on anticoagulants. Iatrogenic adrenal suppression due to prolonged steroid administration should always be sought in patients taking chronic steroids for conditions such as rheumatoid arthritis or obstructive airway disease. Sudden withdrawal of steroids can precipitate such symptoms as fever, abdominal pain, and hypotension. Low early morning levels of plasma cortisol suggest the presence of adrenocortical insufficiency. The diagnosis can be confirmed by performing a cosyntropin stimulation test. Treatment involves replacement with cortisol. Fludrocortisone is added in patients who remain weak or hypotensive while on cortisol replacement therapy.

## Conclusions

The biologic bases of endocrine alterations that accompany aging have been identified. It is well recognized that aging is associated with progressive decline in the levels of several hormones, notably estrogen, testosterone growth hormone, and insulin-like growth factor. Glucose tolerance is impaired, and insulin resistance is increased in both genders. Preliminary data on hormone replacement therapy in aging adults indicate a possible positive effect on reversing various signs of aging. With the exception of estrogen replacement therapy in postmenopausal women, experience with other hormones remains in the experimental stage. Although short-term human studies suggest a possible salutary effect of testosterone, growth hormone, and DHEA administration, controlled placebo studies are needed to define the risks and benefits of long-term administration of these hormones. At the present time, with the exception of estrogen in postmenopausal women, the generalized use of hormone replacement therapy cannot be recommended.

## References


1. Brown-Sequard CE. Du role physiologique et therapeutique d'un sue extrait de testicules d'animaux d'apres nombre de faits observes chez l'homme. Arch Physiol Norm Pathol 1889;1:739–746.
2. Gregerman RI, Davis PJ. Effects of intrinsic and extrinsic variables on thyroid economy. In: Werner SC, Ingbar SH (eds) The Thyroid, 4th ed. Harper & Row: Hagerstown, MD, 1978:223.
3. Hegedus L, Perrild H, Poulsen LR, et al. The determination of thyroid volume by ultrasound and its relationship to body weight, age, sex in normal subjects. J Clin Endocrinol Metab 1983;56:260.
4. Gambert SR. Endocrinology and aging. In: Reichel W (ed) Care of The Elderly, 4th ed. Williams & Wilkins: Baltimore, 1995:365–372.
5. Mooradian AD, Morley JE, Korenman SG. Endocrinology in aging. Dis Mon 1998;34:398–461.
6. Kaiser FE. Variability of response to thyroid-releasing hormone in normal elderly. Age Ageing 1987;16:345–354.
7. Sawin CT, Geller A, Kaplan MM, et al. Low serum thyrotropin (thyroid-stimulating hormone) in older persons without hyperthyroidism. Arch Intern Med 1991;151:165.
8. Meyers B, Gionet M, Abreau C, et al. Iodine intake probably affects the incidence of hypothyroidism and Hashimoto's thyroiditis in elderly women [abstract]. J Nucl Med 1986;27:909.
9. Okamoto T, Fujimoto Y, Obara T, et al. Retrospective analysis of prognostic factors affecting the thyroid function status after subtotal thyroidectomy for Graves' disease. World J Surg 1992;16:690.
10. Davis PJ, Davis FB. Hyperthyroidism in patients over the age of 60 years: clinical features in 85 patients. Medicine 1974;53:161–181.
11. Cropper CFJ. Hypothyroidism in psycho-geriatric patients: ankle jerk reaction time as a screening technique. Gerontol Clin 1973;15:15–24.
12. Lioyd WH, Goldbeg IJL. Incidence of hypothyroidism in the elderly. Br Med J 1961;2:1256.
13. Morley JE. The aging endocrine system. Postgrad Med 1983;73:107.
14. Barnett DB, Greenfield AA, Howlett PJ, et al. Discriminant value of thyroid function tests. Br Med J 1973;2:144.
15. Sawin CT. Subclinical hypothyroidism in older persons. Clin Geriatr Med 1995;11:231–238.
16. Bagchi N, Brown TR, Parish RF. Thyroid dysfunction in adults over age 55 years: a study in an urban US community. Arch Intern Med 1990;150:785.
17. Parle JV, Franklyn JA, Cross KW. Prevalence and follow-up of abnormal thyrotropin (TSH) concentrations in the elderly in the United Kingdom. Clin Endocrinol (Oxf) 1991;34:77.
18. Sawin CT, Chopra D, Azizi F, et al. The aging thyroid increased prevalence of elevated serum thyrotropin levels in the elderly. JAMA 1979;242:247.

19. Ridgway EC, Cooper DS, Walker H, et al. Peripheral responses to thyroid hormone before and after L-thyroxine therapy in patients with subclinical hypothyroidism. J Clin Endocrinol Metab 1981;52:1238–1242.
20. Rosenbaum RL, Barzel US. Levothyroxine replacement dose for primary hypothyroidism decreases with age. Ann Intern Med 1982;144:175.
21. Tunbridge WMG, Evered DC, Hall R, et al. The spectrum of thyroid disease in a community: the Wickham survey. Clin Endocrinol (Oxf) 1997;7:481.
22. Davis PJ, Davis FB. Hyperthyroidism in patients over the age of 60 years: clinical features in 85 patients. Medicine 1974;53:161–181.
23. Dabon-Almirante CM, Surks M. Clinical and laboratory diagnosis of thyrotoxicosis. Endocrinol Metab Clin North Am 1998;27:25–35.
24. Nicoloff JT, Spencer CA. Clinical review. 12. The use and misuse of the sensitive thyrotropin assay. J Clin Endocrinol Metab 1990;71:553.
25. Gambert SR. Endocrine and metabolic disorders. In: Reubin D, et al. (eds) Geriatric Review Syllabus, 3rd ed. AGS, Washington DC 1996:296–303.
26. Mooradian AD, Allan CR, Khalil MF, et al. Anaplastic transformation of thyroid cancer: report of two cases and review of the literature. J Surg Oncol 1983;23:95–98.
27. Bullamore JR, Gallagher JC, Wilkinson R, et al. Effect of age on calcium absorption. Lancet 1970;2:535–537.
28. Armbrecht HJ. Calcium, vitamin D, and aging. In: Morley JE, Korenman SG (eds) Endocrinology and Metabolism in the Elderly. Blackwell Scientific: Boston, 1992:170–182.
29. Lund B, Clausen N, Laund B, et al. Age-dependent variations in serum 1,25-dihydroxyvitamin D in childhood. Acta Endocrinol (Copenh) 1980;94:426–429.
30. Tsai KS, Heath H, Kumar R, et al. Impaired vitamin D metabolism with aging in women: possible role in pathogenesis of senile osteoporosis. J Clin Invest 1984;73: 1668–1672.
31. Armbrecht H, Zenser T, Davis B. Effect of age on the conversion of 25(OH)D to 1,25-(OH)2 D by kidney of rat. J Clin Invest 1980;66:1118.
32. Elbeling PR, Yergey AL, Viera NE, et al. Influence of age on effects of endogenous 1,25(OH)2D on calcium absorption in normal women. Calcif Tissue Int 1994;55: 330–334.
33. Chapuy M-C, Durr F, Chapuy P. Age-related changes in parathyroid hormone and 25-hydroxycholecaciferol levels. J Gerontol 1983;38:19–22.
34. Clemems TL, Zhou X-Y, Myles M, et al. Serum vitamin D2 and vitamin D3 metabolite concentrations and absorption of vitamin D2 in elderly subjects. J Clin Endocrinol Metab 1986;63:656–660.
35. Goldray D, Mizzrahi-Sasson E, Merdler C, et al. Vitamin D deficiency in elderly patients in a general hospital. J Am Geriatr Soc 1989;37:589–592.
36. Bullamore JR, Gallagher JC, Wilkinson R, et al. Effect of age on calcium absorption. Lancet 1970;2:535–537.
37. Maclaughlin J, Holick MJ. Aging decreases the capacity of human skin to produce vitamin D. J Clin Invest 1985;76: 1536–1538.
38. Kamel H. Primary hyperparathyroidim: clinical presentation and diagnosis. Clin Geriatr 1997;5(3):72–77.
39. Lyles KW. Hyperparathyroidism and Paget's disease of bone. In: Hazzard WR, et al (eds) Principles of Geriatric Medicine and Gerontology. pp. 1085–1096, McGraw-Hill: New York, 1998:1085–1096.
40. Bilezikian JP, Silverberg SJ, Horwitz MJ. Clinical presentation of primary hyperparathyoidism. In: Bilezikian JP, Marcus R, Levine MA (eds) The Parathyroids. Raven: New York, 1994:457–469.
41. Chigot J, Menagaux F, Achrafi H. Should primary hyperparathyoidism be treated surgically in elderly patients older than 75 years. Surgery 1995;117:397–401.
42. Whitman ED, Norton JA. Endocrine surgical diseases of elderly patients. Surg Clin North Am 1994;74:127–144.
43. Bondenson AG, Bondenson L, Thompson NW. Hyperparathyroidsm after treatment with radioactive iodine: not only a coincidence? Surgery 1989;106:1025–1027.
44. Holick MF, Krane SM, Potts JT. Disorders of bone and mineral metabolism. In: Isselbacher KJ, et al. (eds) Harrison's Principles of Internal Medicine, 13th ed. McGraw-Hill: New York, 1994:2137–2171.
45. Bilezikian JP, Silverberg SJ, Shane E, et al. Characterization and evaluation of asymptomatic primary hyperparathyroidism. J Bone Miner Res 1991;4:283–291.
46. Kamel H. Primary hyperparathyroidism: management. Clin Geriatr 1997;5(6):71–81.
47. Grey AB, Stapleton JP, Evans MC, Tatnell MA, Reid IR et al. Effects of hormone replacement therapy on bone mineral density in postmenopausal women with mild primary hyperparathyoidism. Ann Intern Med 1996;125: 360–368.
48. Norton JA. Controversies and advances in primary hyperparathyroidism. Ann Surg 1992;215:297.
49. Norton JA, Brennan MF, Well SA. Surgical management of hyperparathyroidism. In: Bilezikian JP, Marcus R, Levine MA (eds) The Parathyroids. Raven: New York, 1994:531–551.
50. Report of a WHO study group: assessment of fracture risk and its application to screening for postmenopausal osteoporosis. WHO Techn Rep Ser 1994;843:3–5.
51. Riggs BL. Osteoporosis. In: Wyngaarden JB, Smith LH, Bennet JC (eds) Cecil Textbook of Medicine, 19th ed. Saunders: Philadelphia, 1992:1426–1431.
52. Kamel HK. Osteoporosis and aging: etiology and current diagnostic strategies. Ann Long Term Care 1998;6:352–357.
53. Beatriz JE, Perry M III. Age-related osteoporosis. Clin Geriatr Med 1994;10:575–587.
54. Rosen C, Kessenich CR. The pathophysiology and treatment of postmenopausal osteoporosis. Endocrinol Metab Clin North Am 1997;26:295–311.
55. Passeri G, Girasole G, Jilka RL, Manalagas SC. Increased interleukin-6 production by murine bone marrow and bone cells after estrogen withdrawal. Endocrinology 1993;133:295–311.
56. Girasole G, Passeri G, Jilka RL, et al. Interleukin-11: a new cytokine critical for osteoclast development. J Clin Invest 1994;93:1516–1524.
57. Bellido T, Stahl N, Farruggella TJ, et al. Detection of receptors for interleukin-6, interleukin-11, leukemia inhibitory factor, oncostatin M, and ciliary neutrophilic factor in bone marrow stromal/osteoclastic cells. J Clin Invest 1996;97: 431–437.

58. World Health Organization. Assessment of Fracture Risk and Its Application to Screening for Postmenoapusal Osteoporosis. WHO: Geneva, 1994. Nical Report Series 843.
59. Cummings SR, Black DM, Nevitt MC, et al. Bone density at various sites for prediction of hip fractures: the study of the osteoporotic fracture research group. Lancet 1993;341: 72–85.
60. Bettica P, Taylor AK, Talbot J, et al. Clinical performance of galactosyl hydroxylisine, pyridinoline, and deoxypyridoniline in postmenopausal osteoporosis. J Clin Endocrinol Metab 1996;81:542–546.
61. Markers of bone resorption predict hip fracture in elderly women: the EPIDOS prospective study. J Bone Miner Res 1996;11:1531–1538.
62. Kamel HK. Pharmacological management of osteoporosis: current trends and future prospects. Ann Long Term Care 1998;6:382–388.
63. Pedersen-Bjerggard K, Tonnesen M. Sex hormone analysis. II. The excretion of sexual hormones by normal males, impotent males, polyathritics, and prostitics. Acta Med Scand 1948;213:284–297.
64. Plymate SR, Tenver JS, Bremner WJ, Circadian variation in testosterone, sex hormone-binding globulin, and calculated non-sex hormone-binding globulin bound testosterone in healthy young and elderly men. J Androl 1989;10: 366.
65. Morley JE, Kaiser FE. Hypogonadism in the elderly man. Adv Endocrinol Metab 1993;4:241–262.
66. Gray A, Feldman HA, Mckenlay JB, et al. Age, disease and changing sex hormone levels in middle-aged men: results of the Massachusetts Male Aging Study. J Clin Endocrinol Metab 1991;73:1016–1025.
67. Korenman SG, Morley JE, Mooradian AD, et al. Secondary hypogonadism in older men: its relationship to impotence. J Clin Endocrinol Metab 1990;71:963–969.
68. Morley JE, Kaiser FE. Hypogonadism in the elderly man. Adv Endocrinol Metab 1993;4:241.
69. Plymate SR, Tenover JS, Bremner WJ. Circadian variation in testosterone, sex hormone binding globulin and calculated non-sex-hormone binding globulin bound testosterone in healthy young and elderly men. J Androl 1989; 10:366–371.
70. Kaiser FE, Morley FE. Gonadotropins, testosterone, and the aging male: neurobiology of aging. Horm Res 1995;43 (1–3):25–28.
71. Baker HWG, Brenner WJ, Burger HG, et al. Testicular control of follicle stimulating hormone secretion. Recent Prog Horm Res 1976;32:429.
72. Rubens RM, Dhont M, Vermeulen A. Further studies on Leydig cell function in old age. J Clin Endocrinol Metab 1974;39:40.
73. Stearns EL, MacDonald JA, Kaufman BJ, et al. Declining testicular function with age, hormonal and clinical correlates. Am J Med 1974;57:761.
74. Zummoff B, Strain GW, Kream J. Age variation of the 24-hour mean plasma concentrations of androgens, estrogens and gonadotropins in normal adult men. J Clin Endocrinol Metab 1982;54:534.
75. Korenman SG, Morley JE, Mooradian AD, et al. Secondary hypogonadism in older men: its relation to impotence. J Clin Endocrinol Metab 1990;71:963–969.
76. Morley JE, Kaiser FE, Sih R, et al. Testosterone and frailty. Clin Geriatr Med 1997;13:685–695.
77. Harman SM, Tsitouras PD, Costa PT, et al. Reproductive hormones in aging men. II. Basal pituitary gonadotropins and gonadotropin responses to luteinizing hormone-releasing hormone. J Clin Endocrinol Metab 1982;54:547.
78. Ceda GP, Enti L, Cerseini G, et al. The effects of aging on the secretion of the common alpha-subunit of the glycoprotein hormones in men. J Am Geriatr Soc 1991;39:353.
79. Pontiroli AE, Ruga S, Maffi P, et al. Pituitary reserve after repeated administration of releasing hormones in young and in elderly men: reproducibility on different days. J Endocrinol Invest 1992;15:559.
80. Winters SJ, Troen P. Episodic luteinizing hormone (LH) secretion and the response of LH and follicle-stimulating hormone to the LH-releasing hormone in aged men: evidence for coexistent primary testicular insufficiency and an impairment in gonadotropin secretion. J Clin Endocrinol Metab 1982;55:560.
81. Winters SJ, Sherins RJ, Troen P. The gonadotropin-suppressive activity of androgen is increased in the elderly men. Metabolism 1984;33:1052–1059.
82. Kamel H, Kaiser FE, Morley JE. Erectile dysfunction (impotence). In: Hazzard W, et al (eds) Principles of Geriatric Medicine and Gerontology, 4th ed. McGraw-Hill: New York, 1998:1585–1594.
83. Tenover JS. Effects of testosterone supplementation in the aging male. J Clin Endocrinol Metab 1992;75:1092–1098.
84. Reid IR, Wattie DJ, Evans MC, et al. Testosterone therapy in glucocorticoid-treated men. Arch Intern Med 1996;156: 1173–1177.
85. Morley JE, Perry HM III, Kaiser FE, et al. Longitudinal changes in testosterone luteinizing hormone and follicle stimulating hormone in healthy older males. Metabolism 1997;46:410–414.
86. Sih R, Morley JE, Kaiser FE, et al. Testosterone replacement in older hypogonadal men: a 12 month randomized controlled trial. J Clin Endocrinol Metab 1997;82:1661–1667.
87. Jankowsky JS, Oviatt SK, Orwoll ES. Testosterone influences spatial cognition in older men. Behav Neurosci 1994;108:325–332.
88. Watson RR, Huls A, Araghinikuam M, Chung S. Dehydroepiandrosterone and diseases of aging. Drugs Aging 1996;9:274–291.
89. Vermeulen A. Adrenal Androgens. Raven: New York, 1980:207–217.
90. Orentreich N, Brind JL, Vogelman JH, Andres R, Baldwin H. Long-term longitudinal measurements of plasma dehydroepiandrosterone sulfate in normal men. J Clin Endocrinol Metab 1992;75:1002–1004.
91. Morley JE, Kaiser F, Raum WJ, et al. Potentially predictive and manipulable blood serum correlates of aging in the healthy human male: progressive decreases in bioavailable testosterone, dehydroepiandrosterone sulfate. Proc Natl Acad Sci USA 1997;94:7537–7542.
92. Liu CH, Laughlin GA, Fischer UG, Yen SS. Marked attenuation of ultradian and circadian rhythms of dehydroepiandrosterone in postmenopausal women: evidence for a reduced 17,20-desmolase enzymatic activity. J Clin Endocrinol Metab 1990;71:900–906.

93. Vermeulen A. Dehydroepiandrosterone sulfate and aging. Ann NY Acad Sci 1995;774:121–127.
94. Barrett-Connor E, Khaw KT, Yen SS. A prospective study of dehydroepiandrosterone sulfate, mortality, and cardiovascular disease. N Engl J Med 1986;315:1519–1524.
95. Helzouer KJ, Gordon GB, Alberg AJ, Bush TL, Comstock GW. Relationship of prediagnostic serum levels of dehydroepiandrosterone and dehydroepiandrosterone sulfate to the risk of developing premenopausal breast cancer. Cancer Res 1992;52:1–4.
96. Gordon GB, Helzouer KJ, Alberg AJ, Comstock GW. Serum levels of dehydroepiandrosterone and dehydroepiandrosterone sulfate and the risk of developing gastric cancer. Cancer Epidemiol Biomarkers Prev 1993;2:33–35.
97. Szathmari M, Szucs J, Feher T, Hollo I. Dehydroepiandrosterone sulfate and bone mineral density. Osteoporosis Int 1994;4:84–88.
98. Jesse RL, Lesser K, Eich DM, et al. Dehydroepiandrosterone inhibits human platelet aggregation in vitro and in vivo. Ann NY Acad Sci 1995;774:281–290.
99. Beer NA, Jakubowicz DJ, Matt DW, Beer RM, Nestler JE. Dehydroepiandrosterone reduces plasma plasminogen activator inhibitor type 1 and tissue plasminogen activator antigen in men. Am J Med Sci 1996;311:205–210.
100. Yen SSC, Morales AJ, Khorram O. Replacement of DHEA in aging men and women: potential remedial effects. Ann NY Acad Sci 1995;774:128–142.
101. Jakubowicz D, Beer N, Rengifo R. Effect of dehydroepiandrosterone on cyclic-guanosine monophosphate in men of advancing age. Ann NY Acad Sci 1995;774:312–315.
102. Bates GW Jr, Egerman RS, Umstor ES, Buster JE, Casson PR. Dehydroepiandrosterone attenuates study-induced declines in insulin sensitivity in postmenopausal women. Ann NY Acad Sci 1995;774:291–293.
103. Wolkowitz OM, Reus VI, Roberts E, et al. Antidepressant and cognition: enhancing effects of DHEA in major depression. Ann NY Sci 1995;774:337–339.
104. Morales AJ, Nolan JJ, Nelson JC, et al. Effects of replacement dose of dehydroepiandrosterone in men and women of advancing age. J Clin Endocrinol Metab 1994;78: 1360–1367.
105. Kamel H, Kaiser FE. The menopause: clinical aspects and current trends in therapy. In: Vellas B, Albarede JL, Garry PJ (eds) Women, Aging and Health. Serdi: Paris, 1998:105–143.
106. Longcope C. Hormone dynamics at the menopause. Am J Obstet Gynecol 1980;13:564.
107. Utian WH. The place of estriol therapy after menopause. Acta Endocrinol Suppl (Copenh) 1980;233:51–56.
108. Kuller LH, Meilahn EN, Gutai J, et al. Lipoproteins, Estrogen, and the Menopause: Biological and Clinical Consequences of Ovarian Failure: Evolution and Management. Serono Symposia USA: Norwell, MA, 1990:179–197.
109. Sarrel PM, Lufkin EG, Ousler MJ, Keefe D. Estrogen actions in arteries, bone, and brain. Sci Am Sci Med 1994;1: 44–53.
110. Winner SJ, Morgan CA, Evans JG. Perimenopausal risk of falling and incidence of distal forearm fracture. BMJ 1989; 298:1486–1488.
111. Paganini-Hill A, Henderson VW. Estrogen replacement therapy and risk of Alzheimer disease. Arch Intern Med 1996;28:156:2213–2217.
112. Tabg MX, Jacobs D, Stern Y, et al. Effect of estrogen during menopause on risk and age at onset of Alzheimer's disease. Lancet 1996;348:429–432.
113. Lufkin EG, Riggs BL. Three-year follow-up on effects of transdermal estrogen [letter]. Ann Intern Med 1996;125: 77.
114. Haines CJ, Chung TK, Masarei JR, et al. The effect of percutaneous estrogen replacement therapy on Lp(a) and other lipoproteins. Maturitas 1995;22:219–225.
115. Walsh BW, Li H, Sacks FM. Effect of postmenopausal hormone replacement with oral and transdermal estrogens on high density lipoprotein metabolism. J Lipid Res 1994;35:2083–2089.
116. Whitehead MI, Townsend PT, Pryse-Davies J, et al. Effects of estrogens and progestins on the biochemistry and morphology of the postmenopausal endometrium. N Engl J Med 1981;305:1599–1605.
117. Voigt LF, Eeiss CSC, Chu J, Dalling JR. Progestagens supplementation of exogenous estrogens and risk of endometrial cancer. Lancet 1991;338:274–277.
118. Harris MI, Hadden WC, Knowler WC, et al. Prevalence of diabetes and impaired glucose tolerance and plasma glucose levels in US populations, ages 20–74 years. Diabetes 1987;36:523–534.
119. Singh I, Marshall MC. Diabetes mellitus in the elderly. Endocrinol Metab Clin North Am 1995;24:255–272.
120. American Diabetes Association. Clinical practice recommendation 1998. Diabetes Care 1998;21(suppl 1):S1–S98.
121. Halter JB. Diabetes mellitus. In: Hazzard W, et al. (eds) Principles of Geriatric Medicine and Gerontology, 4th ed. McGraw-Hill: New York, 1998:991–1011.
122. American Diabetes Association. Nutritional principles for the management of diabetes and related complications [technical review]. Diabetes Care 1994;17:490–518.
123. American Diabetes Association. Nutritional recommendations and principles for people with diabetes mellitus [position statement]. Diabetes Care 1994;17:519–522.
124. LeBlanc J, Nadeau A, Richard D, et al. Studies on the sparing effect of exercise on insulin requirements in human subjects. Metabolism 1981;30:1119–1124.
125. Gerich JE. Oral hypoglycemic agents. N Engl J Med 1989;321:1231–1245.
126. Fonseca VA, Valiquett TR, Huang SM, et al. Troglitazone monotherapy improves glycemic control in patients with type 2 diabetes mellitus: a randomized controlled study: the Troglitazone Study Group. J Clin Endocrinol Metab 1998;83:3169–3176.
127. Neuschwander-Teri BA, Isley WL, Oki JC, et al. Troglitazone-induced hepatic failure leading to liver transplantation: a case report. Ann Intern Med 1998;129:38–41.
128. Watkins PB, Wintcomb RW. Hepatic dysfunction associated with troglitazone [letter]. N Engl J Med 1998;338: 916–917.
129. Morley JE, Kaiser FE. Unique aspects of diabetes mellitus in the elderly. Clin Geriatr Med 1990;6:693–702.
130. Kerson CM, Baile GR. Do diabetic patients inject accurate doses of insulin? Diabetes Care 1981;4: 333–337.
131. Peters AL, Davidson MB. Insulin plus a sulfonylurea agent for treating type 2 diabetes. Ann Intern Med 1991;115: 45–53.

132. Morley JE, Kaiser FE. Unique aspects of diabetes mellitus in the elderly. Clin Geriatr Med 1990;6:693–702.
133. Hornick T, Kowal J. Endocrine disorders in the elderly. In: Jahnigen DW, Schrier RW (eds) Geriatric Medicine, 2nd ed. Blackwell Science: Boston, 1996:754–767.
134. Maheshwari H, Sharma L, Baumann G. Decline of plasma growth hormone binding protein in old age. J Clin Endocrinol Metab 1996;81:995–997.
135. Vermeulen A. Nyctohemeral growth hormone profiles in young and aged men: correlation with somatomedin C levels. J Clin Endocrinol Metab 1987;64:884.
136. Rudman D, Feller AG, Cohn L. Effects of human growth hormone binding protein in old age. J Clin Endocrinol Metab 1996;81:995–997.
137. Kaiser FE, Silver AJ, Morley JE. The effect of recombinant human growth hormone on malnourished older individuals. J Am Geriatr Soc 1991;39:235–240.
138. Cohn L, Feller AG, Draper MW, et al. Carpal tunnel syndrome and gynecomastia during human growth hormone treatment of elderly men with low circulation IGF-1. Clin Endocrinol (Oxf) 1993;39:417–425.
139. Wolfsen AR. Aging and the adrenals. In: Korenman SG (ed) Endocrine Aspects of Aging. Elsevier-North Holland: New York, 1982:55–74.
140. Tuck ML, Williams GM, Cain JP. Relation of age, diastolic pressures and known duration of hypertension to presence of low renin essential hypertension. Am J Cardiol 1973; 32:632–637.

# 21 Surgical Diseases of the Thyroid and Parathyroid Glands

Barbara Kinder

As Olshansky et al. pointed out,[1] senescence is the product of evolutionary neglect, not design. The laws of natural selection favor those whose genetic makeup ensures that they survive long enough to reproduce successfully. Expression of other, also genetically linked traits that emerge after reproductive age (certain cancers, cardiovascular disease, degenerative conditions such as osteoarthritis) are not susceptible to evolutionary pressure. Thus medical and technologic advances have permitted more people to reach and move beyond the reproductive age into senescence, where they encounter disabling and life-threatening diseases that have escaped evolutionary scrutiny. A major challenge for geriatric medicine includes the recognition, treatment, and ultimately prevention of these processes to provide an acceptable quality of life for aging citizens.

## Thyroid

All endocrine systems are tightly regulated by homeostatic mechanisms. With aging, changes in hormone metabolism and receptor number and function may be offset by the substantial reserves that exist in most endocrine systems. Ultimately, however, stress and other illness may overwhelm the system.

### Epidemiology and Diagnosis

The usual biochemical measures of thyroid function, such as triiodothyronine ($T_3$), thyroxine ($T_4$), and thyroid-binding protein levels change little with advancing age in the absence of systemic illness. Similarly, thyrotropin (TSH) levels and the production of TSH in response to thyrotropin-releasing hormone (TRH) administration are also relatively constant with increasing age. Although 5–10% of elderly women may have decreased thyroxine and increased TSH levels, it usually relates to autoimmune thyroid disease and is not a consequence of the aging process per se.[2] In healthy elderly subjects there is also normal diurnal variation of TSH secretion. The half-life of $T_4$ does increase from approximately 6.7 days in young adults to 9.3 days in those aged 80–90 years.[3] This change in the half-life of $T_4$ is thought to be due to decreases in both fractional turnover rate and distribution space of $T_4$. Peripheral conversion of $T_4$ to $T_3$ is decreased but intrathyroidal conversion is increased, resulting in fairly stable $T_3$ levels in the elderly. The Wickham survey documented the prevalence of thyroid disorders in a sample of 2779 adults representative of the British population, and the 20-year follow-up study was published in 1995.[4,5] The annual incidence of hypothyroidism was found to increase with age and correlated with the presence of anti-thyroid antibodies or elevated TSH levels, and especially with both present.

#### Assessment of Thyroid Function

A decision analysis reported that screening for thyroid disease by TSH determination was particularly cost-effective in elderly female patients[6]; and because the clinical symptoms of thyroid dysfunction may be atypical in this age group, a low threshold for testing is appropriate in the elderly. Thyroid function can be evaluated by several laboratory tests[7,8]: total $T_4$ and $T_3$, free $T_4$, free $T_3$, $T_3$ resin uptake, and TSH. Total $T_4$ and $T_3$ levels may appear elevated if the thyroid-binding proteins are increased, or lowered in the presence of decreased binding capacity. Factors that increase serum TBG levels are estrogens, acute hepatitis, and chronic liver disease. Significant protein loss, cortisol, and anabolic steroids decrease TBG concentrations (Table 21.1). In these cases measurement of $T_3$ uptake, which varies inversely with available TBG binding sites, may be necessary. When interpreting the results of thyroid function tests it is important to recognize that elderly patients are more likely than young adults to have other medical conditions or to be on medications that may influence test data. Nonthyroidal illness (any systemic illness, acute psychiatric condition, or post-operative state) may modify the metabolism of thyroid

TABLE 21.1. Causes of Altered Binding of Thyroxine to TBG

**Increased binding**
- Drugs
  - Estrogens
  - Tamoxifen
- Medical conditions
  - Liver disease
  - Genetic factors
  - HIV infection

**Decreased binding**
- Drugs
  - Androgens
  - Corticosteroids
- Medical conditions
  - Acromegaly
  - Nephrotic syndrome
  - Major systemic illness
  - Genetic factors

TBG, thyroxine-binding globulin; HIV, human immunodeficiency virus.

hormones without implying thyroid dysfunction. These results are grouped under the rubric "euthyroid sick syndrome" and may display a variable pattern, although $T_3$ is generally low, $T_4$ is usually normal or low, and TSH is low normal or slightly elevated (Fig. 21.1). In addition to medical conditions, common medications affecting thyroid function include amiodarone, lithium, glucocorticoids, and dopamine. In many instances measurement of TSH, which in the presence of normal pituitary function is a sensitive indicator of free thyroid hormone concentration, may be all that is required as a screening test. The

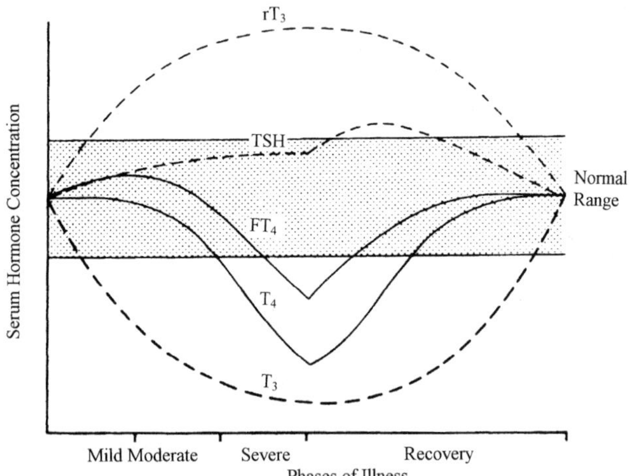


FIGURE 21.1. Effect of illness on thyroid function tests. The most common finding is a decrease in serum $T_3$ concentration and elevation in $rT_3$ levels. The total $T_4$ level may fall, but the free $T_4$ is usually within the normal range unless the patient is seriously ill. Serum TSH usually remains normal. With recovery, the thyroid function tests return to normal. (From Brent,[22] with permission.)

levels of free hormones determine what is available for cellular metabolic regulation. In addition to the usual tests of thyroid function, measurement of anti-thyroid antibodies may be diagnostically useful. Antibodies to the TSH receptor (TSHRAb) are diagnostic of Graves' disease and may also be seen with other forms of autoimmune thyroid disease such as Hashimoto's thyroiditis. Anti-thyroid peroxidase antibodies (TPOAb) and anti-thyroglobulin antibodies (TgAb) are seen with all forms of autoimmune thyroid disease and in some patients with goiter, thyroid nodules, or thyroid carcinoma.

### *Hypothyroidism*

Hypothyroidism results from a deficiency of thyroid hormone and may be primary (due to thyroid failure) or secondary (a result of lack of TSH stimulation of the gland from the pituitary). Symptoms of hypothyroidism include weight gain, cold intolerance, dry skin and hair loss, fatigue, lethargy, depression, constipation, and muscle cramps. On physical examination a patient may exhibit bradycardia, diastolic hypertension, a deepened voice, puffy face and hands, and a delay in the relaxation phase of the deep tendon reflexes. Many features of hypothyroidism can be found as a result of other conditions and, because of their insidious development, may be incorrectly attributed to aging. The prevalence of hypothyroidism in the elderly ranges between 2.5% and 3.0% in different studies.[8,9] The major cause of hypothyroidism in all studies is autoimmune disease. In addition to Hashimoto's thyroiditis, previous treatment of hyperthyroidism by radioiodine or surgery or thyroid resection for benign or malignant thyroid disease are common causes of hypothyroidism. Subacute thyroiditis and drugs such as lithium and amiodarone should also be considered in the hypothyroid patient.

Treatment of hypothyroidism is achieved by thyroid hormone replacement, usually with levothyroxine ($T_4$) because of its longer half-life and therefore more stable serum concentrations. In old patients therapy should be initiated with caution, particularly in the severely hypothyroid patient, to avoid precipitating anginal events. The usual starting dose is 25 μg/day, which is increased by 25 μg every 4–6 weeks until a euthyroid state (manifested by a TSH level within the normal range) is achieved.[8] It is important to exclude secondary hypothyroidism prior to beginning thyroid hormone replacement to avoid adrenal crisis in patients with underlying adrenal insufficiency. Subclinical hypothyroidism is characterized by normal total $T_4$ and free $T_4$ levels but elevated TSH levels. As many as 17% of elderly patients progress to frank hypothyroidism, especially if the TSH level is higher than 10 μU/ml and anti-thyroid antibodies are elevated. The decision whether to treat subclinical hypothyroidism must be made on an individual basis. Although early treatment prevents the development of symptomatic hypothyroidism, not all patients progress to a clinical status, and treatment may exacerbate underlying coronary disease.

### Hyperthyroidism

Hyperthyroidism results from an increase in circulating thyroid hormones. Classic symptoms include heat intolerance, tachycardia, weight loss, nervousness, and weight loss despite increased appetite. Physical findings are tachycardia, particularly atrial fibrillation, warm moist skin, exophthalmos, lid lag, goiter, tremor, proximal muscle weakness, hyperreflexia, and systolic hypertension. Elevated thyroid hormone levels and suppressed TSH are the usual laboratory findings. Rarely, TSH is elevated in TSH-secreting pituitary adenomas or thyroid hormone resistance syndromes.

The prevalence of hyperthyroidism in the elderly ranges from 0.5% to 2.3% in different series.[10,11] In the Whickham study, hyperthyroidism did not increase in frequency with age or with positive antibody status, and it was rare in men. In old patients the classic symptoms may be absent; and depression, fatigue, and hypokinesis characterize the "apathetic" type of hyperthyroidism.[12] Often the clinical presentation is dominated by exacerbation of a patient's underlying medical condition. Atrial fibrillation and heart failure are common manifestations of hyperthyroidism in patients with cardiac disease, and cognitive changes are frequent findings in patients with dementia.

The most common cause of hyperthyroidism in patients of all ages is Graves' disease, closely followed by toxic multinodular goiter. Other etiologies include overtreatment with thyroid hormone, subacute thyroiditis, and iodine overload due to administration of contrast agents for radiographic studies and use of amiodarone as an antiarrhythmia treatment. Amiodarone, a potent class II antiarrythmia agent, contains 75 mg iodine per 200 mg active substance, resulting in a daily iodine intake in the range of 200–600 mg. Treatment may cause both hypo- and hyperthyroidism.[13] Hypothyroidism is easily managed by discontinuing the drug, thyroid hormone replacement, or both. Amiodarone-induced thyrotoxicosis (AIT) is a much more complex clinical problem, especially if continued use of the medication is required to control refractory arrhythmias (see below). Rarely, hyperthyroidism is due to TSH-secreting pituitary adenoma, to struma ovarii, or to metastatic follicular thyroid carcinoma.

Treatment of symptomatic hyperthyroidism has two features: prompt attention to the symptoms, particularly cardiac, of thyroid toxicity and definitive treatment of the underlying cause. Thyrotoxicosis due to endogenous hormone production is treated initially, regardless of etiology, with antithyroid medications. The thionamides (propylthiouracil, methimazole, carbimazole) decrease thyroid hormone production by inhibiting the oxidation and binding of iodine in the thyroid gland. Propylthiouracil (PTU) has the additional advantage of decreasing peripheral conversion of $T_4$ to $T_3$, the active form of thyroid hormone, and may more promptly alleviate the symptoms of thyrotoxicosis. These drugs can cause allergic reactions and other side effects such as granulocytopenia, hepatitis, and agranulocytosis. Agranulocytosis is seen in fewer than 1% of patients and usually occurs during the initial weeks or months of treatment. The presenting symptoms of agranulocytosis are fever and sore throat, and patients should be cautioned to report such symptoms immediately. Granulocytopenia may be an adverse reaction to thionamide treatment or may be associated with thyrotoxicosis. The total white blood cell (WBC) count and differential should be determined prior to treatment and monitored serially. If a downward trend is seen, treatment should be discontinued and other methods of treatment considered. Allergic reactions such as a rash or hives are seen in as many as 10% of patients. Substitution of another thionamide may be considered, but because there may be cross-reactivity between these agents, the patient must be closely monitored. Less frequent reactions include arthralgia, myalgia, and hepatitis (with propylthiouracil), including hepatic necrosis requiring transplantation. Baseline liver function tests should be obtained prior to instituting treatment and repeated periodically.[7]

In patients allergic to thionamides, administration of iodine may be used to control thyroid hormone release temporarily during an impending thyrotoxic crisis, with acute surgical emergencies, or during preparation for definitive surgical treatment. The inhibitory effect of iodine is lost after 10–14 days (iodine escape), and so iodine cannot be used alone long term.

In addition to preventing further synthesis of thyroid hormone, blockade of the catecholamine effects of thyroid hormone is required and is particularly important in the elderly with limited cardiac reserve. β-Adrenergic antagonists such as propranolol promptly reduce tremulousness, palpitations, diaphoresis, and tachycardia. Propranolol also decreases peripheral $T_4$-to-$T_3$ conversion. Propranolol is contraindicated in patients with asthma or chronic obstructive pulmonary disease (COPD) and in those with heart block and congestive heart failure because of its myocardial depressant action. Calcium channel blockers may be used in patients in whom β-blockade is contraindicated.

Thyrotoxic crisis or thyroid storm is a rare occurrence today given the availability of the effective antithyroid drugs noted above.[14] It occurs in patients usually with Graves' disease but also rarely with multinodular goiter who have unrecognized or inadequately treated hyperthyroidism. Thyrotoxic crisis is precipitated by intercurrent infection, trauma, surgical emergencies, or diabetic ketoacidosis; it is characterized by acute exacerbation of the hyperthyroid hypermetabolic state. Fever is invariably present and extreme (>104°F); and tachycardia progressing to congestive heart failure and pulmonary edema are expected sequelae in untreated cases. Neurologic findings beginning with nervousness and tremulousness and progressing to stupor and coma are characteristic of the syndrome. Nausea, vomiting, and abdominal pain are prominent early features and may confuse the diagnostic picture and complicate treatment. The diagnosis of thyrotoxic crisis is made on a clinical basis, and treatment must be implemented immediately. Supportive measures designed to reduce fever (including ice packs and iced saline gastric lavage if necessary), correct dehydration and hyponatremia, and provide adequate energy substrates with intravenous glucose are critical. Large doses of antithyroid drugs are given, by nasogastric tube if necessary. Iodine to inhibit further hormone release and β-adrenergic antagonist to block receptor response are administered intravenously. Steroids are administered, both because of their ability to inhibit peripheral $T_4$-to-$T_3$ conversion and to treat potential relative adrenal insufficiency. Adequate oxygen delivery may require intubation and mechanical ventilation. Even with aggressive treatment, the mortality rate for thyroid storm is about 20%. Given the atypical clinical appearance of hyperthyroidism in some old patients, thyrotoxic crisis should be suspected in the elderly patient who develops an acute, fulminant hypermetabolic state without obvious cause.

Perhaps 5% of patients in an elderly outpatient population have what is termed subclinical hyperthyroidism. This is defined as normal $T_4$ and $T_3$ levels but low or suppressed TSH. As few of these patients progress to clinical hyperthyroidism and many see their TSH values normalize during a serial follow-up, no treatment is necessary. Because of the potential for thyroid-induced cardiac disease in this group, however, close monitoring is required to exclude the development of overt hyperthyroidism. Sawin et al. reported a threefold increase in the risk of atrial fibrillation over a 10-year period in patients with suppressed TSH and a 1.6-fold increase in those with low levels.[10]

In addition to the cardiovascular risk of hyperthyroidism, it is clear that prolonged elevation of thyroid hormone levels has a deleterious effect on the skeleton. Hyperthyroidism is associated with decreased absorption of dietary calcium, increased calcium excretion, and ultimately decreased bone mineral density due to the stimulation of bone resorption by osteoclasts.[15] These effects are seen most clearly in postmenopausal patients. Whether subclinical hyperthyroidism carries a similar risk over the long term is unknown, but certainly bone mineral density should be followed in such patients; treatment may be necessary if serial studies show progressive bone loss in the absence of other causes. These data also have implications for treatment with thyroid hormone for patients with benign and malignant thyroid nodules, as discussed below.

Definitive treatment of thyrotoxicosis may require antithyroid medications, radioactive iodine, or surgery, depending on the etiology of the hyperthyroidism and on patient and physician preference. With Graves' disease, as noted above, the first line of treatment is medical, aimed at preventing release of additional hormone and blocking the effects of secreted hormone on target tissues. Antithyroid medications are usually given for 6–12 months in the hope of effecting a lasting remission, which occurs in about one-third of patients.

Those most likely to achieve lasting remission are patients with low and decreasing titers of anti-thyroid receptor antibody, the initial presence of $T_3$ toxicosis, a small thyroid, a decrease in the size of the thyroid during treatment, and return of TSH to normal levels during treatment.

Radioactive iodine is the standard treatment for thyrotoxicosis of Graves' disease, toxic multinodular goiter, and toxic adenoma. Because radiation thyroiditis may occur 10–14 days after iodine administration, antithyroid drugs are usually given for several weeks to patients with diffuse disease to deplete the gland of its hormone stores. The drugs are discontinued 3–5 days prior to treatment but may be resumed, if necessary, the following week. Although avoiding surgery and anesthesia in the elderly patient with hyperthyroidism is appealing, the effects of radioactive iodine may require weeks to months to become evident; and in patients with antithyroid drug allergies, large goiters, or pressing cardiac issues, surgical ablation may be preferable. In patients with multinodular goiter, the size of the gland and other issues such as local symptoms and evidence of airway compromise, particularly if the goiter has a substernal component, may also recommend surgery as definitive therapy. In these instances, although radioactive iodine controls the hypermetabolic state, it may have little effect on the overall size of the gland; hence the transient edema associated with radiation thyroiditis may be problematic.

In an elderly population, the use of amiodarone to treat a variety of cardiac arrhythmias may be associated with the development of thyrotoxicosis. There appear to be two types of AIT. The first type occurs in an abnormal thyroid, such as one with a nodular goiter or Graves' disease, and is due to increased thyroid hormone synthesis induced by iodine. This (type I) thyrotoxicosis is usually treated by antithyroid drugs (see below) and occasionally by iodine washout using perchlorate. The second type (type II) occurs in a normal thyroid gland and appears to represent destruction of thyroid tissue by iodine or amiodarone.[16] Glucocorticoids are used in these patients to counteract the inflammatory response. Sometimes surgical resection is required to permit continued antiarrhythmic therapy.[17]

Finally, there is evidence that radioiodine treatment of Graves' disease can exacerbate ophthalmopathy in patients with preexisting eye findings. In such individuals treatment with surgery or antithyroid medications may be preferable.[18,19]

Because it is impossible to calculate the dose of radioactive iodine that will render the patient permanently euthyroid, most iodine treatment for diffuse thyroid disease results in eventual hypothyroidism. Patients must understand that they will likely be on lifelong thyroid hormone replacement regardless of the type of definitive therapy elected.

Patients with toxic adenoma and suppression of the surrounding thyroid tissue are ideal candidates for radioactive iodine, as function of the normal thyroid tissue is protected. Again, large nodules may not entirely regress despite resolution of the thyrotoxic state.

## Thyroid Nodules and Neoplasia

### *Diagnostic Evaluation*

In addition to the occurrence of hypo- and hyperfunctioning thyroid states, elderly patients are frequently found to harbor thyroid nodules. Many studies have shown that the incidence of thyroid nodules, as detected by physical examination, ultrasonography, or autopsy evaluation, increases throughout life. Nodules are four times more common in women than in men, so members of a demographic group consisting of postmenopausal women are likely to require evaluation and perhaps treatment for nodular disease. Thyroid nodules may be solitary colloid nodules, part of a diffuse process of multinodular goiter that is often asymmetric, benign adenomas, cysts, or areas of thyroiditis. Thyroid carcinomas are rare, representing only about 5% of all thyroid nodules.[20]

Treatment options in patients with thyrotoxicosis have been reviewed above. The other issues posed by the presence of a thyroid nodule are whether it is malignant and if it causes local mechanical problems such as pain or difficulty swallowing or breathing, which would make treatment necessary even in the absence of metabolic abnormalities. Cosmetic concerns and patient anxiety may also influence the decision to proceed with further treatment.

The patient's history and physical examination are important first steps when investigating the possibility of malignancy in the patient presenting with a new thyroid nodule. The incidence of carcinoma is increased in male patients and in those presenting at the extremes of age. A history of previous radiation exposure or treatment increases the risk for both benign and malignant thyroid nodules. Nodules associated with the development of hoarseness suggest malignant involvement of the recurrent laryngeal nerve. On physical examination, nodules that are hard, poorly circumscribed, or fixed and those associated with cervical adenopathy are also more likely to be malignant. Thyroid function tests are important to establish the metabolic status of the patient being evaluated for thyroid disease, but they are usually normal even in patients with extensive thyroid malignancies. Patients with Hashimoto's thyroiditis may have firm nodular glands suspicious for papillary carcinoma, and measurement of anti-thyroid peroxidase and anti-thyroglobulin antibodies may clarify the autoimmune nature of the thyroid process. Hashimoto's thyroiditis and well-differentiated thyroid cancer may coexist, and the presence of autoimmune thyroid disease increases the risk of developing thyroid lymphoma.[21]

Fine-needle aspiration cytology (FNA) of thyroid nodules has had a major impact on patient management. An algorithm (Fig. 21.2) illustrates the role of FNA in evaluating the thyroid nodule. FNA is readily carried out at the initial office visit. The skin is prepared with alcohol and a 23- to 25-gauge needle is inserted into the palpable nodule. While maintaining gentle suction on the syringe, the needle is moved forward and backward through the nodule to introduce tissue into the needle. Suction is released, and the needle is withdrawn. The contents of the needle are expelled onto a frosted microscope slide and smeared using a second slide. It is usually possible to determine whether an adequate specimen has been obtained by gross examination of the compressed tissue between the slides prior to pathologic evaluation.

Assessment of tissue by an experienced thyroid cytologist can reliably identify the characteristic nuclear features of papillary carcinoma, such as nuclear grooves or intranuclear cytoplasmic inclusions. Psamomma bodies and papillary structures may also be seen. Aspiration cytology of a benign nodule reveals bland follicular cells, hemosiderin-laden macrophages, and admixed small lymphocytes typical of a degenerative process. Many benign nodules (and some papillary carcinomas) have a substantial cystic component, which makes obtaining an adequate cellular sample difficult. Performing FNA under ultrasound guidance enhances the chances of retrieving a representative cellular specimen in these circumstances.

The cells of medullary thyroid cancer have a characteristic plasmacytoid appearance and can be immunostained for the presence of calcitonin if clinical suspicion warrants. Thyroid lymphoma and anaplastic carcinoma are more common in old patients and present in a similar manner, with a history of rapid growth of a thyroid nodule and often accompanying subjective respiratory compromise and stridor. Prompt differential diagnosis is critical here, as immediate chemotherapy is rapidly beneficial in the case of lymphoma, whereas surgery is usually required to establish an adequate airway in the patient with anaplastic carcinoma. Fortunately, the cytologic data can resolve this diagnostic dilemma and can

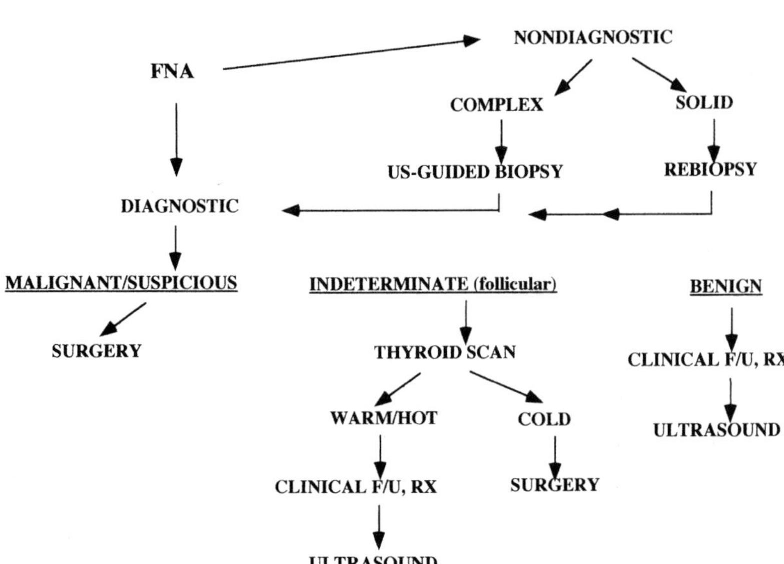


FIGURE 21.2. Evaluation of the patient with a thyroid nodule: role of fine-needle aspiration (FNA) cytology. Following the clinical history and physical examination, cytologic evaluation of a thyroid nodule directs the diagnostic process. US, ultrasonography; F/U, follow-up; RX, therapy.

also differentiate large-cell lymphomas from the less common lymphoplasmacytic lymphomas, though the latter may require additional studies to subtype.

A major limitation in the usefulness of FNA lies in the management of follicular neoplasms. The cells comprising follicular adenomas and carcinomas rarely have distinctive cytologic features, and the final differential diagnosis depends on identifying capsular or vascular invasion of surrounding normal thyroid on permanent section assessment of the resected lobe containing the nodule. When a cytologic diagnosis of follicular neoplasm has been rendered, a thyroid scan may be useful, as a warm or hot nodule is much less likely to be malignant. In addition, because the likelihood of a hot nodule causing clinical hyperthyroidism over time is a function of its size, an elderly patient with a large, hot nodule should be considered for treatment if there is evidence of autonomous function to prevent the development of atrial fibrillation or other cardiac complications so common in this population.

Several studies have indicated that the use of FNA to identify thyroid lesions that can be safely followed clinically has reduced purely diagnostic thyroid surgery by 50% and increased the yield of thyroid cancers removed at surgery twofold.[23] If the cytologic evaluation is consistent with a benign process, a trial of thyroid hormone may be undertaken. If the nodule remains unchanged or shrinks, as measured by comparing it at baseline and at 6-month follow-up by thyroid ultrasonography, suppression may be discontinued or continued for some defined period. Permanent suppressive therapy of presumed benign thyroid nodules is probably unwise in elderly women, given the potential long-term skeletal and cardiac effects of thyroid hormone. If an adequate cytologic specimen has been obtained and there has been no clinical change in the nodule, repeated FNA examinations do not usually contribute additional management information.[23] Data gathered using the algorithm can be used to calculate the probability of significant disease according to Bayes' theorem (Fig. 21.3).[24]

In addition to resolving questions regarding malignancy, thyroid surgery may be indicated because the thyroid mass causes local symptoms related to the aerodigestive system. Depending on the location of the nodule, patients may have difficulty swallowing, chronic cough, or in the case of a substernal goiter, difficulty breathing, particularly when supine or with exertion.[25] In most series of substernal goiter, the patients are generally older than 60 years. Patients with substernal goiter are at risk for acute airway decompensation with respiratory infections or of spontaneous hemorrhage into a nodule.[26] Frequently, older patients with long-standing goiter and respiratory complaints are diagnosed as having asthma or COPD when the extent of airway narrowing caused by the goiter is not recognized. A routine chest radiograph is probably the most cost-effective initial study, as it can demonstrate the presence of a mediastinal soft tissue mass or tracheal deviation. Computed tomography (CT) or magnetic resonance imaging (MRI) are useful for determining the extent of the goiter and the status of the patient's airway (see below). The utility of radioiodine scanning of intrathoracic goiters is limited by the heterogeneous uptake of radionuclide by most goiters and by the image being obscured by overlying vascular structures in the mediastinum. Pulmonary function tests with flow–volume loops can help differentiate intra- and

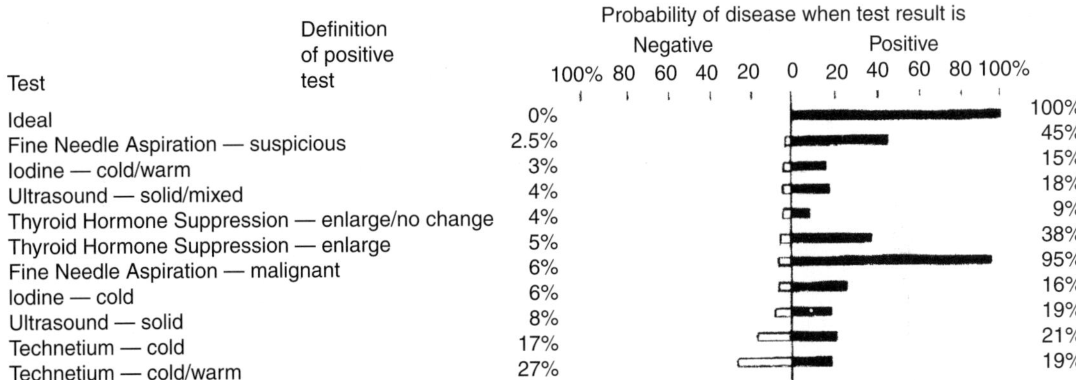


FIGURE 21.3. Probability of malignant disease based on test results calculated according to Bayes' theorem. Solid bars represent the percentage of surgeries during which malignancies were found. The significance of suspicious or malignant cytology are shown. Growth of a nodule in a patient on hormone suppression is associated with a significant risk of malignancy. (From Burrow,[24] with permission.)

extrathoracic causes of airway obstruction and lend additional support to a decision to pursue surgical resection. In almost all cases, substernal goiters can be removed through the usual cervical thyroid incision, even in reoperative circumstances.[27] Surgery for thyroid and parathyroid disease, using modern anesthetic techniques, is well tolerated even by the frail elderly (see below).

### *Follow-up of Benign Nodules*

Thyroxine has been widely used for treatment of solitary, clinically benign thyroid nodules. The rationale for the treatment is based on the assumption that nodule development and growth is dependent on TSH stimulation of thyroid tissue and that suppressing TSH secretion results in a decrease in the size of the nodule. There have been several randomized prospective trials of thyroxine treatment of solitary nodules, but in only one of them was there a significant difference in nodule shrinkage between thyroxine-treated and untreated control patients over a 12-month period. Moreover, only nodules with a volume of 10 ml or less decreased by 50% or more.[28] It is also unclear what level of TSH suppression is necessary to achieve growth control or over what period of time treatment should continue.[20] In an elderly population, especially postmenopausal women, long-term thyroxine therapy with its potential for cardiac and skeletal complications is unappealing. Using ultrasonic monitoring, a trial of thyroxine therapy in doses designed to reduce TSH levels to the low-normal range for a defined period of 6–12 months is probably reasonable. If the nodule grows, even with a benign cytologic report, surgery should be considered.

### *Management of the Irradiated Thyroid*

Exposure to radiation results in the continuing occurrence of thyroid nodules and thyroid carcinoma over the lifetime of the individual. Optimal follow-up and treatment of these patients is still unclear. Thyroid ultrasonography is more sensitive than radionuclide scanning and physical examination for detecting nodular disease. In one study[29] of irradiated patients, only 50% of nodules 1.5 cm or larger detected by ultrasonography were palpable, and these nodules were anteriorly positioned in the gland; 25% of those 1.0 cm or larger were not detected by nuclear scan.

The sensitivity of ultrasonography for detecting nodular disease raises the possibility that unnecessary procedures are undertaken. The role of thyroid hormone replacement in patients with radiation exposure is a matter of some debate. Follow-up of patients using serial thyroglobulin determinations has shown that both high and rising thyroglobulin levels correlate with an increased risk of developing thyroid nodules. Although thyroid hormone administration has been shown to decrease the incidence of recurrent thyroid nodules in irradiated patients undergoing partial thyroid resection, it has not clearly been shown that hormone treatment prevents the development of nodular disease or limits the increase in size of an existing nodule in this patient population.[29] Overall, thyroid hormone suppression should be considered in higher risk individuals (elevated thyroglobulin levels, significant nodular disease, old age) with a history of radiation exposure and thyroidectomy undertaken with evidence of progression by ultrasonography or thyroglobulin determination.

### *Thyroid Carcinoma*

Thyroid carcinoma is classified as shown in Table 21.2. Well-differentiated thyroid carcinoma consists of tumors of follicular cell origin that fall into two main groups based on histologic appearance and biologic behavior. The most common and most favorable prognostically are

TABLE 21.2. Classification of Thyroid Neoplasms

**Primary epithelial tumors**
- Tumors of follicular cells
  - Benign: follicular adenoma
  - Malignant: carcinoma
    - Differentiated
      - Papillary
      - Follicular
    - Poorly differentiated
      - Insular
      - Others
    - Undifferentiated
- Tumors of C cells
  - Medullary carcinoma
- Tumors of follicular and C cells
  - Mixed medullary-follicular carcinomas

**Primary nonepithelial tumors**
- Malignant lymphomas
- Sarcomas
- Others
- Metastatic tumors

*Source:* Larsen et al.,[7] with permission.

the papillary carcinomas, which have a papillary or frond-like appearance histologically and exhibit characteristic nuclear features, including nuclear grooves and folds and cleared nuclear chromatin ("Orphan Annie" nuclei) on paraffin sections. These neoplasms tend to exhibit intra- and extraglandular lymphatic spread; but the presence of lymphatic metastases, unlike other cancers, generally does not adversely influence prognosis. Recognized variants of papillary carcinomas include encapsulated, follicular, tall cell, columnar cell, clear cell, and diffuse sclerosing carcinomas.[30] Follicular carcinomas do not show the nuclear features of papillary neoplasms but form follicles and exhibit the capacity for vascular and capsular invasion. Lesions with capsular invasion only have a much more favorable prognosis. Follicular carcinomas are more aggressive than papillary neoplasms and metastasize hematogenously, particularly to the lung. The Hurthle cell (oxyphylic or oncocytic) carcinoma is a variant of follicular carcinoma. The follicular variant of papillary carcinoma does not form papillae but does exhibit the typical nuclear features noted above. Importantly, this tumor behaves biologically like papillary carcinoma and should be considered under that heading.

Hurthle cell neoplasms are oncocytic tumors which, like other follicular lesions, are diagnosed as carcinoma when there is evidence of capsular or vascular invasion. Although considered well-differentiated, Hurthle cell carcinomas have a significantly worse prognosis than papillary or follicular carcinomas. Follicular malignancies tend to occur in older patients, with the mean age of patients with pure follicular carcinoma being 50 years and that of patients with Hurthle cell carcinoma about 60 years.

"Insular" or poorly differentiated carcinoma occupies a histologic and clinical niche between well-differentiated and anaplastic carcinomas. This entity is identified by the presence of nests, or "insulae," of monotonous round cells, sometimes forming follicles. Tumor necrosis is common. The presence of insular carcinoma, even if focal within an otherwise well-differentiated neoplasm, portends a more aggressive course. Although the mean age at diagnosis of this tumor is 55 years, insular carcinoma may account for many of the "low risk" young patients who have aggressive papillary and follicular tumors.[31]

Appropriate treatment of well-differentiated thyroid cancer remains a matter of debate. Proponents of lobectomy and isthmusectomy alone point to the usually excellent prognosis for most patients with these tumors and stress the importance of protecting the recurrent laryngeal nerve and parathyroids on the contralateral side by limiting surgical dissection. Disadvantages of a unilateral approach include the inability to use radioactive iodine diagnostically or therapeutically because of the remaining normal thyroid tissue, and to follow serum thyroglobulin as a tumor marker. These issues become of critical importance in the few patients (usually older or with tumors exhibiting locally invasive behavior) who have more aggressive tumors and contribute to the overall recurrence rate for all well-differentiated carcinomas of slightly more than 20% and the overall mortality rate of 10%. Evidence suggests that the clinical course in high risk patients may be improved by aggressive initial therapy.[19,32,33]

A number of clinical scoring systems have been developed to identify these high risk patients prospectively. The AGES (age, grade, extent, size), MACIS (metastasis, age, completeness of resection, invasion, size), and AMES (age, metastases, extent, size, sex) systems applied by the Mayo Clinic (AGES and MACIS) and Lahey Clinic (AMES) to their thyroid cancer patients can distinguish patients at greatest risk of dying of well-differentiated thyroid cancer.[7] Risk stratification of patients using these staging systems is comparable to that derived using the TMN system adopted by the International Union Against Cancer (UICC) and the American Joint Committee on Cancer (AJCC) for predicting prognosis and guiding therapy. The AJCC TNM staging criteria for thyroid cancer are shown in Table 21.3. The importance of age

TABLE 21.3. TMN Staging for Thyroid Cancer

| Stage | Papillary or follicular | | Medullary | Anaplastic |
|---|---|---|---|---|
| | Age <45 | Age ≥45 | (any age) | (any age) |
| I | M0 | T1 | T1 | — |
| II | M1 | T2–T3 | T2–T4 | — |
| III | — | T4 or N1 | N1 | — |
| IV | — | M1 | M1 | Any |

*Source:* Larsen et al.,[7] with permission.

and invasiveness, but not nodal status, for predicting the prognosis of patients with well-differentiated thyroid malignancies has been reported.

The molecular pathogenesis of thyroid neoplasms is the subject of extensive research. Chromosomal structural abnormalities have been identified in up to 33% of patients with papillary carcinoma but no history of irradiation and in 60–80% of tumors occurring in a setting of radiation exposure.[30] The abnormalities most commonly involve intrachromosomal inversions and translocations of the *ret* proto-oncogene locus on chromosome 10. These rearrangements convert the *ret* proto-oncogene, a member of the receptor tyrosine kinase family, into several oncogenes (*ret/PCT* 1–3). Such oncogenes have been found to be expressed even in occult papillary carcinomas, suggesting that their activation may be a critical part of oncogenesis.[7] Mutational activation of *ret* is also the genetic abnormality underlying the multiple endocrine neoplasia type II (MEN-II) and familial medullary thyroid cancer syndromes.

For follicular carcinoma, the following evidence suggests a multistep mutational evolution from adenoma to carcinoma similar to that for colon carcinoma. Most follicular adenomas and all follicular carcinomas are monoclonal in origin. Oncogene activation, especially of *ras*, is common in both benign and malignant follicular neoplasms and suggests that these events are important in oncogenesis. Finally, cytogenetic abnormalities and evidence of genetic loss are seen in both follicular carcinomas and adenomas and are distinctly more common in these neoplasms than in papillary lesions. Loss of tumor suppressor function may be important in the development of follicular neoplasms.[7]

The treatment of papillary carcinoma in most patients, particularly those with clinical features suggesting a less favorable prognosis by the AGES or AMES systems (essentially all older patients), is total lobectomy on the side of the lesion and intracapsular resection of the contralateral lobe. All parathyroids should be preserved if this is consistent with gross removal of tumor. Parathyroids with doubtful viability should be locally autotransplanted. The incidence of permanent hypoparathyroidism is less than 1% in experienced hands. Nodes in the central compartment are removed, and a functional neck dissection is performed if there are palpable jugular chain nodes.

Follicular carcinoma is often not diagnosed until permanent sections can be scrutinized for evidence of vascular or capsular invasion. Capsular invasion alone carries a favorable prognosis, so treatment may involve only TSH suppression and clinical observation. If there is evidence of significant vascular invasion and the patient has other criteria that indicate a more aggressive course, a decision must be made about whether and when to ablate the remaining lobe. Ablation can be accomplished either surgically or with iodine 131 ($^{131}$I). Radioiodine ablation of a whole lobe is associated with an increased incidence of complications compared to remnant or tumor ablation. Complications include neck edema syndrome, pain, radiation thyroiditis, and transient hyperthyroidism. Because reoperation is an unattractive option, a near-total thyroidectomy should be considered the primary procedure for large (>4 cm) follicular lesions, particularly in the older or male patient, as the incidence of malignancy increases with increasing size of the tumor. Because of its aggressive behavior, Hurthle cell carcinomas should be treated with near-total thyroidectomy with $^{131}$I ablation. Although these tumors often do not take up radioiodine, some elements of the tumor, perhaps more well-differentiated, may do so and can be treated.

Postoperative ablation with $^{131}$I is carried out in patients who are judged to be at risk of recurrence based on clinical criteria or who present with bulky local or nodal disease. Thyroid replacement is withheld after surgery for 3 weeks. After ensuring an increased TSH level, the patient undergoes a scan with 400 μCi of $^{123}$I to confirm the presence and determine the amount of residual thyroid tissue. The ablative dose of $^{131}$I is based on the scan profile and the patient's clinical status (usually between 30 and 200 mCi). A treatment scan is performed at 1 week on an outpatient basis to visualize the treated tissue and see if metastatic uptake can be identified.

Ablation of all thyroid tissue permits the use of serum thyroglobulin as a tumor marker. In the absence of antithyroglobulin antibodies, thyroglobulin levels, when elevated, correlate with residual and metastatic disease. Scanning with $^{123}$I and $^{131}$I or thallium 201 can be used to identify recurrent disease, which is then treated after thyroid hormone withdrawal with doses of 150–200 mCi of $^{131}$I with the goal of delivering approximately 20,000 rad to the tumor tissue. Recently, intramuscular administration of human recombinant TSH (rTSH) has been used in lieu of thyroid hormone withdrawal.[34] This is a promising development in that it avoids a lengthy period of hypothyroidism with its unpleasant clinical sequelae and potential for stimulating tumor growth.

Medullary carcinoma arises from the parafollicular, or C (calcitonin-secreting), cells, which are derived from the neural crest and populate the thyroid in mammals during embryologic development. The tumor occurs sporadically or as part of the MEN-II or familial medullary thyroid carcinoma (FMTC) syndromes. MTC exhibits locally invasive characteristics and an ability to spread by both lymphatic and vascular routes. Sporadic medullary thyroid carcinoma usually occurs after age 40. In familial contexts, the process begins as C cell hyperplasia and progresses to carcinoma in situ before becoming frankly invasive. Historically, C cell hyperplasia was identified in individuals at risk in a kindred by an inappropriate rise of serum calcitonin following a calcium-pentagastrin infusion. Advances in molecular biology now permit presymptomatic identification and treatment of gene carriers by screening peripheral blood leukocyte DNA for the presence of mutations of the *ret* proto-oncogene.[35]

Total thyroidectomy is the procedure of choice for this often aggressive neoplasm. Central lymph nodes should be removed and a modified neck dissection performed if there are palpable jugular chain nodes. Postoperatively, calcitonin remains a highly sensitive tumor marker and may remain elevated in patients who present with bulky disease. Even when biochemical cure is not achieved, many patients do well clinically with no foci of tumor clinically identifiable. It is important to realize that MTC can secrete other peptide hormones, notably adrenocorticotrophic hormone (ACTH), serotonin, and vasoactive intestinal peptide (VIP), which may cause clinical symptoms. Radiation therapy may be useful for controlling nonresectable disease. The best results are achieved in kindreds where patients can be identified presymptomatically and treated.

Anaplastic carcinoma is seen primarily in older patients. This is among the most malignant tumors known. It is unencapsulated and invades surrounding structures. Cervical lymphadenopathy and pulmonary metastases are common. Elements of papillary or follicular carcinoma are often found, suggesting that these tumors may be precursors of anaplastic carcinoma. Mutations of the *p53* gene are present in many undifferentiated tumors but are not found in the residual well-differentiated foci, indicating that *p53* loss may be in part responsible for the anaplastic transformation.[7] The clinical presentation is usually dramatic with the history of rapid growth of a hard, diffuse neck mass and local symptoms of difficulty swallowing and dyspnea. Diagnosis can be made by FNA, as noted above.

Although the prognosis is dismal, with most patients dying of pulmonary metastases within months, local control should be attempted with surgery and radiation therapy. In the rare patient who has a late recurrence with local disease alone, re-resection may be indicated. Local control in highly selected long-term survivors may be achieved by laryngectomy, pharyngectomy, and gastric pull-up. Such cases are distinctly unusual.

Thyroid lymphoma is uncommon, representing perhaps 5% of all thyroid malignancies; most cases of primary thyroid lymphoma are seen in middle-aged to elderly patients. The most common type of thyroid lymphoma is the diffuse large-cell type, with immunoblastic lymphoma next in frequency. Thyroid lymphoma is more common in women, and there is a recognized association with Hashimoto's thyroiditis, which in 80% of instances is found elsewhere within the gland. Most low-grade lymphomas of the thyroid appear to belong to the mucosa-associated lymphoid tissue (MALT) category, and nearly all are of B cell origin.[7] Clinical presentation may be indistinguishable from that of anaplastic carcinoma. FNA is critical for making this differential diagnosis. Although the diagnosis of large-cell lymphoma is usually straightforward, the differential diagnosis of lymphoma and extensive Hashimoto's thyroiditis may be problematic. In such cases, immunophenotypic evidence of immunoglobulin light-chain restriction is conclusive evidence of lymphoma, as lymphocytes in Hashimoto's thyroiditis should express both types of light chains.[31]

Unless the process is clearly confined to the thyroid, lymphoma is not primarily a surgical disease. The use of multimodality chemotherapy and radiation therapy results in dramatic tumor shrinkage and rapid resolution of airway compromise. Overall, the 5-year survival is around 70%, with variability based on stage and histologic type.

## Hyperparathyroidism

### Epidemiology and Diagnosis

Hyperparathyroidism was first recognized during the 1920s and was thought to be a relatively uncommon condition, presenting usually as renal lithiasis or as a result of the complications of severe bony demineralization. With the application of multiphasic blood testing revealing elevated serum calcium concentrations and the availability of accurate parathyroid hormone (PTH) determinations, hyperparathyroidism is now recognized to be a common diagnosis, particularly in aging populations.

Unlike the early patients with hyperparathyroidism, those identified today are often seen as relatively "asymptomatic." To address the issue of appropriate management of this large group of patients, the U.S. National Institutes of Health (NIH) convened a consensus conference in 1990 to review indications for surgical intervention in hyperparathyroidism. Table 21.4 lists the current indications for parathyroidectomy in patients with hyperparathyroidism. The conference also recommended that patients not treated operatively be followed semiannually to annually for symptoms, blood pressure measurement, serum and urinary calcium determination, abdominal radiographs, and bone density measurement. Although there is some difference of opinion as to frequency and specifics of nonoperative follow-up, it is clear that over time such scrutiny becomes tedious and expensive. There is also considerable debate about whether patients with even mild hyperparathyroidism are truly asymptomatic.[36] Burney et al. at Michigan, used a sensitive test of global functioning, the SF-36 questionnaire, to evaluate the outcome of parathyroidectomy. A radar plot of their data shows improvement in the 6 domains of health (Fig. 21.4) months after correction of hyperparathyroidism. Because the SF-36 instrument was not

TABLE 21.4. Indications for Parathyroidectomy in Patients with Primary Hyperparathyroidism: NIH Consensus Statement

| |
|---|
| Symptomatic patients |
| Serum calcium >3.0 mmol/L |
| Reduction in creatinine clearance by 30% |
| Urinary calcium excretion >400 mg/24 hr |
| Bone mass >2 SD below age-matched controls |
| Age <50 years |

*Source:* Diagnosis and management of asymptomatic primary hyperparathyroidism: consensus development conference statement. *Ann Intern Med* 1991;114:593, with permission.

TABLE 21.5. Questionnaire Items for Hyperparathyroid Patients

| |
|---|
| Pain in the bones |
| Feeling tired easily |
| Mood swings |
| Feeling "blue" or depressed |
| Pain in the abdomen |
| Feeling weak |
| Feeling irritable |
| Pain in the joints |
| Being forgetful |
| Difficulty getting out of a chair or car |
| Headaches |
| Itchy skin |
| Being thirsty |

*Source:* Pasieka and Parsons,[37] with permission.

validated specifically for an elderly population, it is possible that these data underestimate the benefit of surgery for this group. Pasieka and Parsons developed a prospective visual analogue scale (VAS) questionnaire specific for hyperparathyroidism; it can be used to document the impact of surgical intervention on the patient's symptoms.[37] Table 21.5 lists symptoms addressed by the questionnaire; many of which fall into the "vague," or neuropsychiatric, category and might be dismissed in an elderly population as part of the aging process. Figure 21.5 depicts the improvement in symptom scoring in a study population undergoing parathyroidectomy compared to a control group having thyroid surgery.[37] Other studies have supported the contention that parathyroidectomy can be of dramatic benefit in the elderly with symptoms of dementia[38] and can be accomplished with minimal morbidity, negligible morbidity, and low cost.[39]

Although hyperparathyroidism has a number of physiologic consequences, in an aging, especially elderly female population, the skeletal impact of the disease becomes of paramount importance. The prevalence of osteoporosis in women in the United States is depicted in Figure 21.6[40] as a function of age. Bone remodeling is a continuous and coupled process consisting of bone resorption and new bone formation. At remodeling sites, the time lag between bone resorption and completion of new bone formation represents a period of skeletal

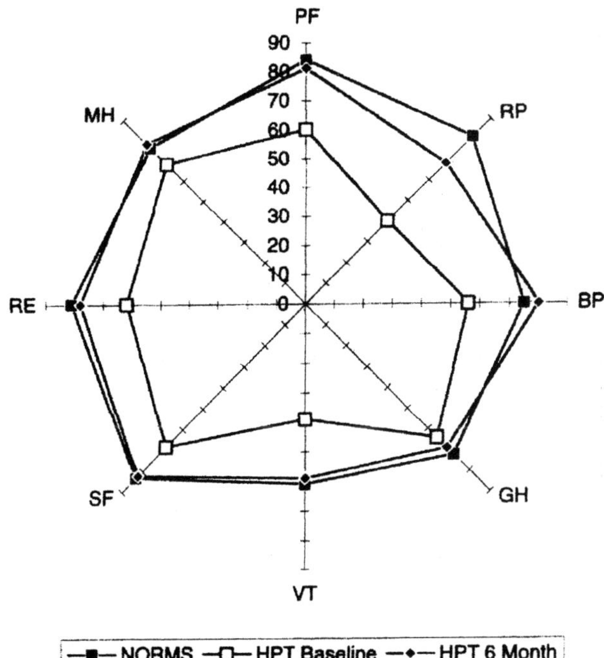


FIGURE 21.4. Assessing outcome of surgery in patients with hyperparathyroidism: use of the SF-36 questionnaire. Radar plot of SF-36 scores of patients with hyperparathyroidism at baseline and 6 months after surgery compared with a normal population. Improvement is seen for all six domains of health. (GH, general health perception; PF, physical function; RP and RE, physical and emotional role limitation; SF, social function; MH, mental health; BP, bodily pain; VT, energy/fatigue or vitality. (From Burney et al.,[36] with permission.)

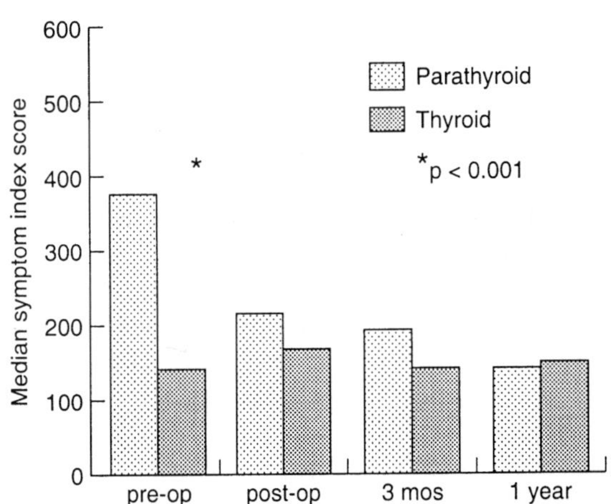


FIGURE 21.5. Assessment of outcome of parathyroid surgery: use of a parathyroid-specific visual analogue scale. Median symptom index scores using a visual analogue scale in patients treated for hyperparathyroidism are compared with those from thyroid surgical patients. (From Pasieka and Parsons,[37] with permission.)

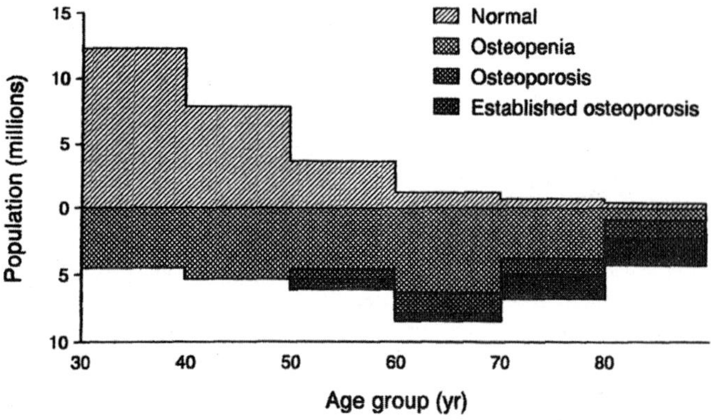


FIGURE 21.6. Estimate of the current prevalence, by age, of osteoporosis in the United States. Based on World Health Organization criteria, more than 9 million women have osteoporosis. Another 17 million postmenopausal women have osteopenia and are at risk for the development of osteoporosis. (From Melton,[40] with permission.)

deficit. With hyperparathyroidism, because PTH stimulates both resorption and new bone formation, the number of bone remodeling units is increased, and a new equilibrium is reached; but this deficit or remodeling space represents a larger fraction of the skeleton than occurs under normal circumstances and is detectable as decreased bone mineral density.

Although osteitis fibrosa cystica, the classic form of parathyroid bone disease is rarely seen today with primary hyperparathyroidism, even patients with mild disease can be seen to have biochemical or histologic evidence of bone involvement if it is carefully sought. Measurement of bone density by dual-energy x-ray absorptiometry (DEXA) shows a decrease in bone mass compared to that of age-matched controls in probably most patients with primary hyperparathyroidism.[41]

Hyperparathyroidism, unlike osteoporosis, primarily affects cortical bone sites, leaving trabecular bone (e.g., that in the lumbar spine) relatively preserved. In addition, the connectivity of the trabeculae, a key determinant of mechanical strength, is maintained to a greater degree in hyperparathyroidism than in other forms of osteoporosis.[42,43] Studies have shown that bone density remains relatively stable in patients with mild primary hyperparathyroidism during medical follow-up. On the other hand, follow-up of patients selected for parathyroidectomy based on the NIH criteria, revealed continued and substantial improvement in bone density measurements at the lumbar spine, femoral neck, and radius 4 years after surgery.[44] Thus the advantageous effect of parathyroidectomy on bone in patients with moderate primary hyperparathyroidism seems well established. The development of increasingly more accurate means of assessing bone strength may help to determine the role for parathyroidectomy in patients with mild disease.

## Treatment

Medical treatment of osteoporosis primarily involves the use of agents that limit further loss of bone by reducing the activation of new remodeling units in the skeleton. Estrogens, salmon calcitonin, and the bisphosphonates, notably alendronate, have been used to treat hyperparathyroidism in patients not undergoing surgery. Interestingly, because PTH increases both resorption and new bone formation, a 3-year trial of daily subcutaneous PTH administration in osteoporotic postmenopausal women, showed an improvement in bone mineral density in the group receiving PTH and hormone replacement therapy but no change in a control group on hormone replacement therapy (HRT) alone.

A new calcimimetic drug, R-568, which is an agonist at the recently sequenced calcium sensor, has shown promise by reducing serum parathyroid hormone levels and ionized calcium concentration in postmenopausal women with primary hyperparathyroidism.[45] The feasibility of long-term administration of this agent and its effect on bone have yet to be determined.

One of the most interesting areas of clinical research is in the possibility of preventing postmenopausal hyperparathyroidism. It has long been recognized that immunoreactive PTH levels increase with aging, concomitant with a decline in vitamin D levels, gastrointestinal calcium absorption, and renal calcium conservation. At the same time, dietary surveys have shown that the median intake of calcium by elderly women is less than 700 mg per day. This group of patients is thus in essentially negative calcium balance, much like the patient with early uremia who develops secondary hyperparathyroidism. McKane et al. showed that consumption of a high calcium diet (>2000 mg/day) by elderly women was able to prevent the increase in circulating PTH and biochemical markers of bone resorption, whereas women on a "usual" calcium diet were not. In fact, the biochemical profiles of the postmenopausal high calcium diet group were indistinguishable from those of a control group of premenopausal women.[46] Widespread application of such dietary regimens, if successful, has the capacity to alter the epidemiology of hyperparathyroidism substantially.

## Surgical Approaches to Thyroid and Parathyroid Disease

Successful thyroid and parathyroid surgery requires an appreciation for the normal anatomic relations of the thyroid and parathyroid glands, the recurrent and supe-

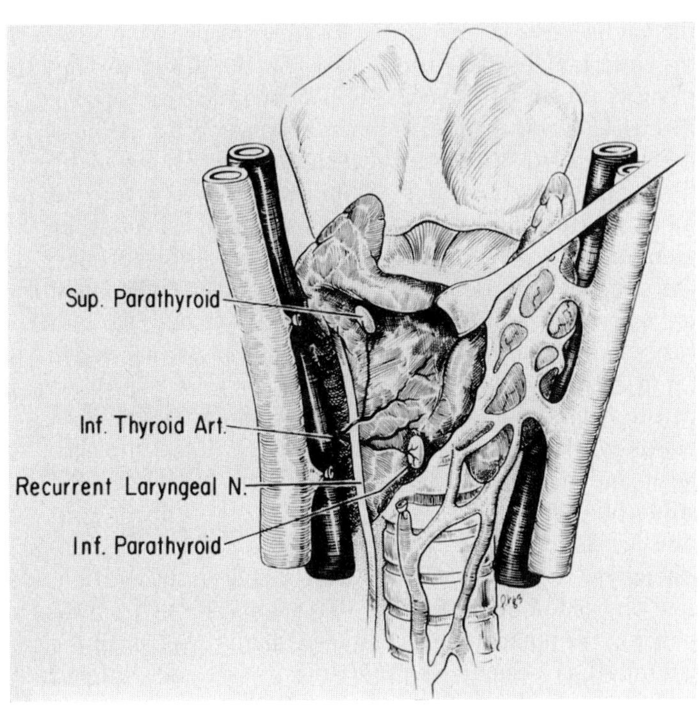


FIGURE 21.7. Surgical anatomy of the thyroid gland. The recurrent laryngeal nerve and inferior thyroid artery are closely related. The inferior and superior parathyroid glands are shown, with the superior gland positioned more posteriorly, often within the surgical capsule of the thyroid gland at the superior pole.

rior laryngeal nerves, and the inferior thyroid arteries as well as their common embryologic variations.[47] Critical to the success of the operation is the maintenance of meticulous homeostasis throughout to visualize the anatomic structures depicted in Figure 21.7.

In most cases, thyroid and parathyroid surgery are performed using general anesthesia. The relatively short duration of these procedures and the lack of significant fluid shifts and hemodynamic changes aid in making them well tolerated even in an elderly population. General endotracheal anesthesia is most commonly used, although laryngeal mask anesthesia (LMA)[48] is an excellent choice as well, particularly in cases where functional identification of the recurrent laryngeal nerves is required, and in instances where it is desirable to avoid local trauma to the cords of intubation, such as in vocalists. Neuromuscular blockade should be avoided until the external branch of the superior laryngeal nerve has been identified or, in the case of LMA, the identity of the recurrent nerve is demonstrated. Locoregional anesthesia may also be used, although there is much less experience with this approach. LoGerfo recently reported a personal series of 1275 patients over a 9-year period who underwent thyroid surgery using a bilateral C2–3 superficial cervical block and conscious sedation.[49] A postoperative patient questionnaire revealed a high level of satisfaction with this technique.

For thyroid and parathyroid surgery, a transverse skin incision is made along defined skin lines to maximize the cosmetic outcome of the procedure. Dissection proceeds through the platysma muscle, and subplatysmal skin flaps are raised to the level of the superior aspect of the thyroid cartilage and inferiorly to the sternal notch. In most cases the strap muscles do not need to be divided, although sectioning the sternothyroid muscle alone may provide easier access to the superior thyroidal vessels.

The strap muscles are dissected off the thyroid gland, and the middle thyroid vein is divided to mobilize the thyroid lobe out of the tracheoesophageal groove. In cases of malignancy, if the lesion appears to be invading the strap muscles, these are resected en bloc with the thyroid lobe. During mobilization of the gland the inferior parathyroid is often identified close to the inferolateral border of the thyroid gland or in the thyrothymic tissue inferiorly. As the potential space between the carotid sheath and the thyroid gland is further developed, the inferior thyroid artery is sought. This anatomic landmark aids in identification of the recurrent laryngeal nerve, and visualization of a large branch of the artery may direct the surgeon to a parathyroid adenoma. Figure 21.7 depicts the typical anatomic relations between the parathyroids, recurrent laryngeal nerve, and interior thyroid artery.

The recurrent laryngeal nerve is most easily identified in the low neck, where it is more laterally located. The nerve frequently divides above the level of the inferior thyroid artery and sends a sensory branch superiorly to anastomose with the internal branch of the superior laryngeal nerve. Both branches must be protected, as it is usually not clear which is the motor branch. The nerve may be nonrecurrent on the right, passing directly from the vagus nerve in the carotid sheath or recurring around the inferior thyroid artery. Use of the LMA airway permits functional identification of the recurrent nerve: Electrical stimulation of the nerve causes contraction of the vocal cord apparatus, which can be visualized by fiberoptic bronchoscopy.[48] Mobilization of the thyroid lobe continues superiorly, freeing the lateral aspect of the gland at the level of the superior pole vessels by entering the surgical capsule of the thyroid gland. At this point the superior parathyroid gland often is visualized; and further dissection of the superior pole is not necessary for parathyroid exploration. During thyroid resections, before dividing the superior pole vessels, care should be taken to preserve the external branch of the superior laryngeal nerve, which may be intertwined with the superior thyroidal vessels en route to the cricothyroid muscle. Its identity can be confirmed by observing contraction of the cricothyroid muscle on nerve stimulation. The thyroid lobe is further dissected off the trachea, keeping the recurrent nerve in view at all times, until the isthmus has been freed. The isthmus is cross-clamped and the specimen sent to pathology for touch preparation and frozen section evaluation. It is advantageous for the surgeon to review the gross and microscopic data with the pathologist intraoperatively, as the additional clinical perspective may be helpful in arriving at a working diagnosis, which determines whether the other lobe must be resected. The procedure is completed by achieving meticulous hemostasis. Drains are rarely used unless a neck dissection has been performed or a large or substernal goiter has been resected. Considerable attention is paid to attaining a superior cosmetic closure. Patients are usually discharged on the day following surgery.[49]

LoGerfo reported his experience with outpatient management of patients undergoing thyroidectomy. In his protocol, patients are observed for 6 hours following surgery and discharged if there is no evidence of swelling in the neck that suggests postoperative bleeding. He found that 85% of patients who were operated on early in the day could be discharged after the 6-hour observation period. There were no readmissions to the hospital, but two patients required reoperation while in hospital.[49]

Although most patients who experience a significant bleeding episode have evidence of it within 6 hours, there are some who bleed later during a 24-hour period and who might experience substantial morbidity or mortality if the condition were not treated immediately. The exact role of outpatient management for thyroid and parathyroid conditions is still unclear,[50] and its application in an elderly population should probably be limited.

The surgical approach to the large multinodular and substernal goiters commonly seen in an elderly patient population is similar in most respects to that for other thyroid conditions. Most substernal goiters can be removed via a cervical incision, even in the reoperative situation, as they are only secondarily intrathoracic and their blood supply is cervical, from the superior and inferior thyroidal vessels. Primary intrathoracic goiters, derived from accessory thyroid parenchyma developing embryologically in association with the aortic sac are rare (0.2–0.3% of cases)[26] and require thoracotomy, as their blood supply is from intrathoracic vessels.[51]

Establishment of an adequate airway by endotracheal intubation is of paramount importance for safe performance of surgery for large goiters. Although tracheal deviation may be impressive in these circumstances, it does not usually pose a problem for intubation. Of more potential consequence is the tracheal narrowing that characteristically occurs at the thoracic inlet as the goiter descends into the mediastinum. Patients who exhibit stridor in the supine position or flushing of the skin and dilation of the external jugular veins on elevating the arms above the head (Pemberton's sign) should be suspected of having significant tracheal narrowing. The diameter of the airway and the extent and location of the goiter should be assessed by CT scan with contrast in patients undergoing surgery for substernal goiter. MRI should be used instead of CT scan if the goiter is suspected of harboring a malignancy that might require postoperative $^{131}$I therapy.

Figure 21.8 shows a typical substernal goiter with tracheal deviation and maximal tracheal narrowing at the level of the thoracic inlet. Awake fiberoptic intubation is rarely necessary. Division of the middle and superior thyroidal vessels bilaterally permits mobilization of the gland. An intracapsular dissection is carried out, following the course of the gland as it descends into the mediastinum. In this way, the recurrent laryngeal nerves and parathyroids are usually excluded from the dissection compartment, though care should be taken to identify them. Intrathoracic goiters that descend into the posterior mediastinum derive from the lateral and posterior aspects of the thyroid, displacing the recurrent nerves and inferior thyroid arteries anteriorly and the esophagus medially; the recurrent nerves are particularly vulnerable in this setting.[51] Even large intrathoracic goiters can be coaxed out of the mediastinum, although rarely a goiter must be removed piecemeal (morcellization).

Tracheomalacia, or softening of the tracheal cartilage, can be detected intraoperatively and provisions for more prolonged intubation (24–48 hours) or rarely tracheostomy instituted. In most series, tracheomalacia is rare, even in patients with long-standing, circumferential goiters.

Postoperative mortality is close to zero, as are instances of hypoparathyroidism and vocal cord paresis. These procedures are well tolerated by the elderly and afford often dramatic improvement in symptoms related to obstruction of the aerodigestive systems.

The surgical approach to the parathyroids is essentially identical to that outlined above for thyroid resection. Although there are no data to indicate that preoperative

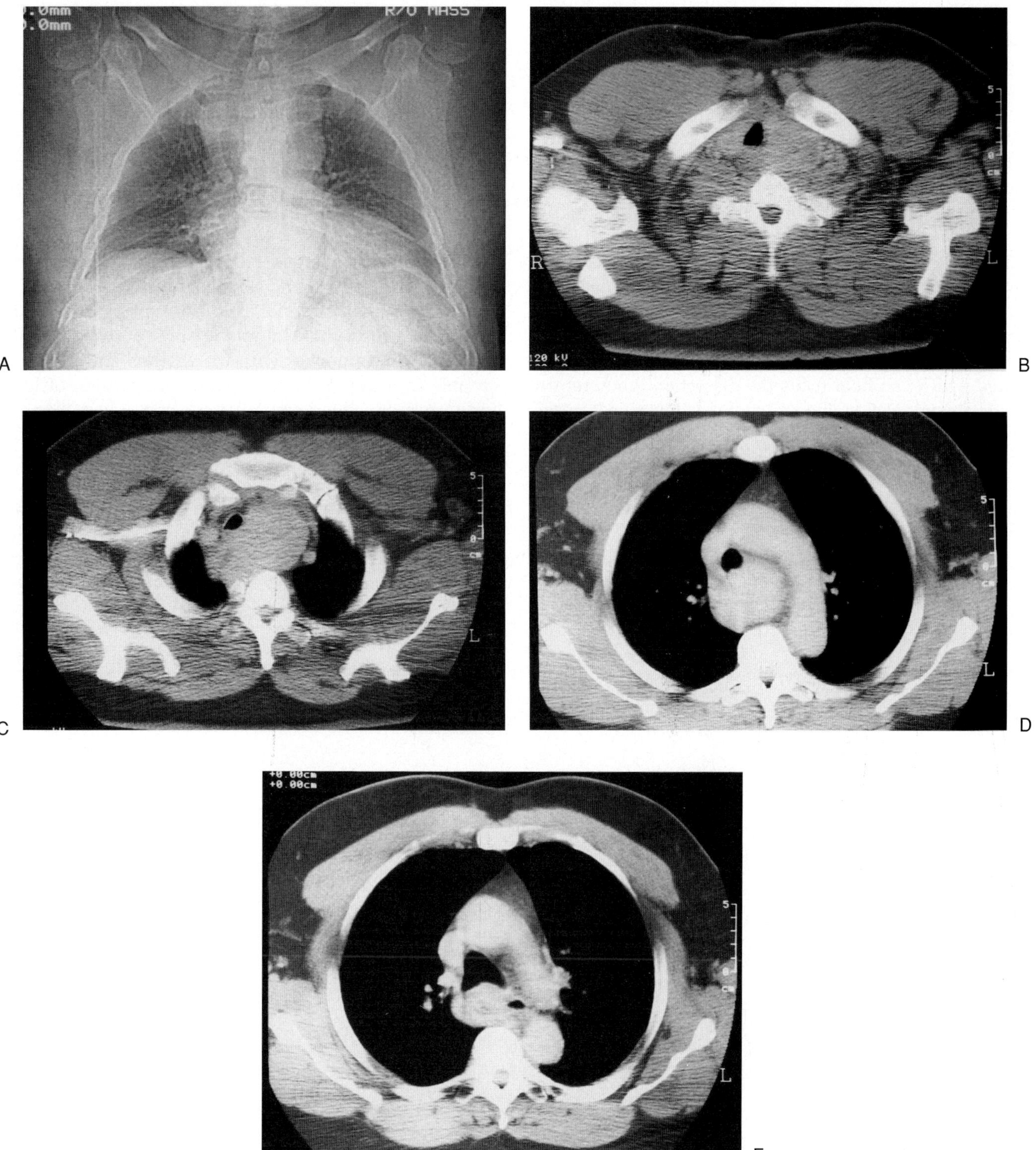

FIGURE 21.8. Substernal goiter. Preoperative imaging studies of a 60-year-old man with dyspnea and a substernal goiter. A. Chest film shows a mediastinal mass and tracheal narrowing and deviation. B. CT scan of the neck at the level of the clavicles reveals predominantly left-sided goiter. C. Retrosternal component of goiter with tracheal deviation and compression. D. Posterior mediastinal component at the level of the aortic arch. E. Goiter ends at the level of the carina. This goiter was removed intact through the usual transverse cervical incision with resolution of the patient's dyspnea.

imaging increases the success of parathyroid exploration in experienced hands, localization probably does decrease the operative time (and potentially permits unilateral exploration) (see below).[52] In most cases (85–90%) an adenoma is present, and the initial goal is identification of an enlarged, normal-appearing gland on the affected side. If imaging data are available, the suspected side is explored first.

After visual identification of the inferior and superior glands on one side, the other side is then explored in the same manner. If, after cursory dissection on the initial side, one or both parathyroids have not been identified, exploration of the contralateral side is undertaken. Often dissection of the contralateral side reveals an adenoma and helps clarify the anatomic positions of the parathyroids, which can help focus the dissection when returning to the initial side. If an adenoma is identified grossly and three other apparently normal glands are visualized, one may be biopsied to confirm the presence of parathyroid tissue. In general, pathologists are unable to differentiate between normal, hyperplastic, and adenomatous parathyroid tissue, as histologic criteria (including the absence of intracellular or extracellular fat) have not reliably predicted hormonal hyperactivity.[53,54]

If an adenoma is not found, attention is directed to identifying the normal parathyroids. Clarification of whether an inferior or superior gland is missing provides direction for a focused dissection of the appropriate side. Whether a gland is superior or inferior is determined more reliably based on its anteroposterior orientation than its craniocaudal position. Superior glands derive embryologically[55] from the fourth branchial pouches and are usually more posterior in location, typically resting behind the superior pole and within the capsule of the thyroid gland. Enlarged superior glands frequently descend inferiorly in the tracheoesophageal groove to rest in the posterosuperior mediastinum or behind the trachea or esophagus. Inferior glands derive from the third branchial pouches with the thymus and are more variable in location. Inferior glands, regardless of location, are more anteriorly situated, and when separate from the inferior pole of the thyroids, are usually to be found in association with thymic remnants along the thyrothymic tract in the anterior mediastinum, almost always anterior to the recurrent laryngeal nerve.[53] Cervical thymectomy can frequently disclose a missing inferior gland, which has extended its embryologic migration. Figure 21.9 illustrates the various routes of descent of

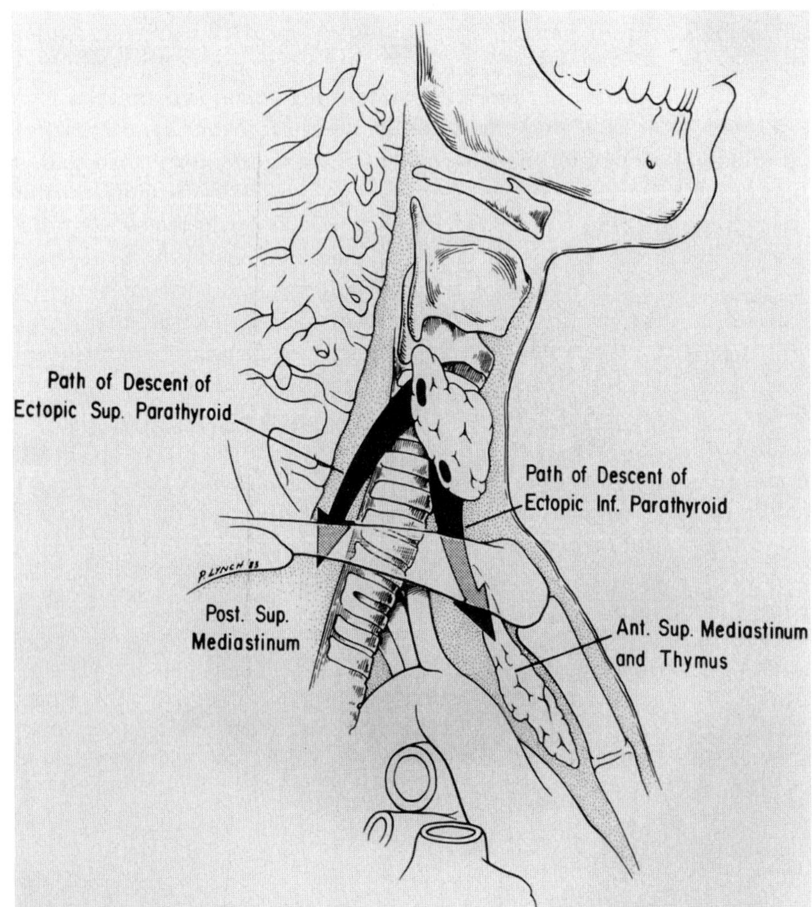


FIGURE 21.9. Descent patterns of ectopic parathyroids. The superior (Sup.) glands remain posterior (Post.), and the inferior (Inf.) glands track anteriorly (Ant.) in association with thymic tissue.

superior and inferior parathyroid glands.[52] Arrested descent of the third branchial pouch complex leaves the inferior parathyroid at or above the level of the carotid bifurcation. In the National Institutes of Health series, such cases accounted for 17 of their 225 (7%) of reoperative cases.[56]

The most common cause of unsuccessful parathyroid surgery is failure to find an adenoma, and in most cases the adenoma is ultimately found in the common sites of embryologic derivation described above. Shown in Figure 21.10 are the locations of adenomas found in Wang's series of reoperated cases.[57] If an adenoma is not found despite identification of the other glands and focused dissection, the thyroid should be carefully palpated, as enlarged parathyroids are often palpable within a normal thyroid lobe. About 3–5% of parathyroid adenomas are intrathyroidal and may be removed by thyroidotomy or partial lobe resection, taking care to avoid disruption of the capsule of the parathyroid and implantation of parathyroid cells. If preoperative studies have not been performed, intraoperative ultrasonography[58] may be useful in this instance, especially if the thyroid gland is nodular. Finally, the carotid sheath should be explored on the side of the missing gland. In this instance, biopsy of the parathyroids found is indicated to document which glands have been positively identified. At this point, neck exploration should be abandoned and the patient reevaluated. There is no place for a blind median sternotomy searching for an ectopic adenoma at the time of initial surgery.

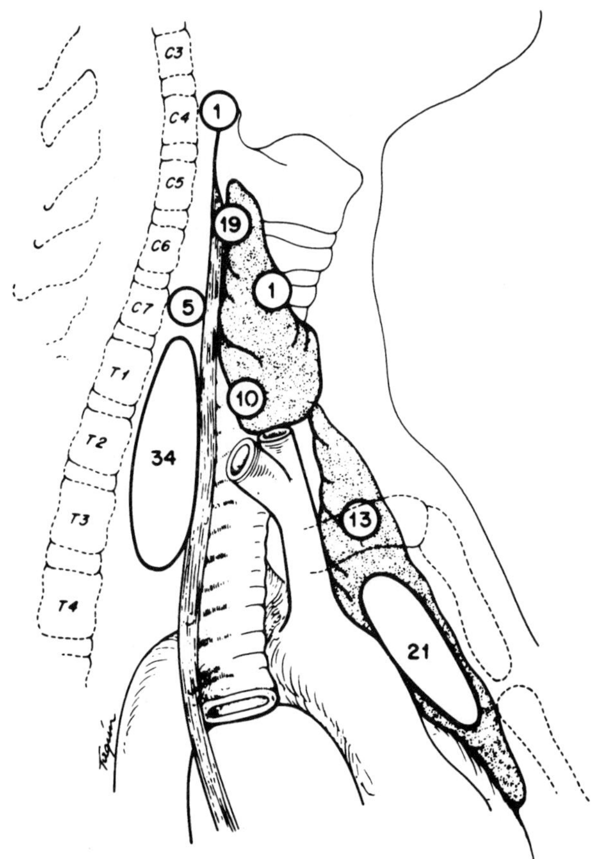


FIGURE 21.10. Location of 104 parathyroid adenomas found at reoperation for persistent or recurrent hyperparathyroidism. The location of the adenomas in Wang's series documents the fact that most missed adenomas are in embryologically predictable locations. (From Wang,[60] with permission.)

Several experienced endocrine surgeons have reported good results with a unilateral exploration when an enlarged and a normal gland are found on one side.[59,60] Laparoscopic techniques have been applied to parathyroid surgery with some preliminary success. Carbon dioxide insufflation underneath the strap muscles is accomplished via a 5 mm incision at the sternal notch. Trocars (2 mm) permit introduction of instruments and retractors, enabling the rest of the operation to be carried out using a gasless technique. Visualization is excellent, and specimens are easily retrieved via the insufflation site.[61]

Technetium sestamibi has also been used as a radiolabel for intraoperative detection of parathyroid tissue.[62] In the patient who has not had prior neck surgery, it is not clear that radioguided surgery offers an additional advantage over the information already conferred by the sestamibi scan. However, in reoperative situations where scarring may be extensive, intraoperative and preoperative localization may be invaluable. The availability of convincing preoperative localization studies and "quick" intraoperative PTH assays, which confirm that all abnormal parathyroid tissue has been removed, may make this a more accepted approach in future.[63,64] Currently, most endocrine surgeons favor bilateral exploration.[53]

If multiple abnormal glands are encountered, the decision must be made as to how much tissue is to be removed. Although controversial, double adenomas have been reported in 2–5% of the general population and in perhaps 9% of older patients. The presence of multiple enlarged glands more often implies a diagnosis of hyperplasia, which may be asymmetric in nature. Complete evaluation of all glands is mandatory. Clarification of the status and location of all parathyroids should be carried out before any gland is resected.

Absent a family history of parathyroid or endocrine disease or a specific etiology for secondary hyperparathyroidism, subtotal parathyroidectomy is the most straightforward approach to parathyroid hyperplasia. If all four glands are enlarged, one may resect three to three and one-half glands, depending on the size of the glands. If one of the glands is small and close to normal size, we would leave that gland intact. The goal is to leave a well-vascularized remnant of about 50–80 mg. It is optimal if an inferior gland or portion of an inferior gland can be left in situ, as the relatively anterior location of the inferior glands leaves them more accessible in the event that reexploration is required for recurrent disease in future. Even when four glands have been identified, the cervical thymus should be resected (see above), as the incidence of supernumerary glands appears to be higher in the hyperplasias, particularly with MEN-I syndrome.[65,66] In patients with water-clear cell hyperplasia, a larger amount of parathyroid tissue may need to be left in place (150 mg) to prevent postoperative hypocalcemia, as the hormonal activity of these cells appears less reliable.[67]

Wells et al. developed the technique of total parathyroidectomy and autotransplantation because they were dissatisfied with their long-term results of subtotal parathyroidectomy in patients with secondary hyperparathyroidism.[68] After total parathyroidectomy, minced fragments of parathyroid tissue are placed in separate sites of the brachioradialis muscle in the forearm and secured with nonabsorbable suture material. Additional tissue may be cryopreserved against the unlikely event of graft failure.[68,69] The advantage of this approach is that if recurrent (graft-dependent) hyperparathyroidism occurs, treatment requires only removal of some of the grafts under local anesthesia rather than neck reexploration. Successful application of the technique, of course, depends on identification and removal of all parathyroid tissue from the neck (including supernumerary glands). In addition to patients with secondary hyperparathyroidism, other groups at risk for recurrent hyperparathyroidism who may be candidates for this procedure include patients with hyperplasia, given the fact that remnant tissue is abnormal. The risk of recurrence appears to be greatest in patients with MEN-I syndrome, possibly because of the presence of a circulating parathyroid mitogenic factor.[70]

Comparison of the results of subtotal versus total parathyroidectomy and autotransplantation in patients with secondary hyperparathyroidism suggest that both are reliable techniques. Recurrence after subtotal parathyroidectomy in recent series appears to be substantially less than 10%. This is most likely due to improved medical management of patients on chronic renal dialysis, particularly the use of $1,25(OH)_2$ vitamin $D_3$ to enhance calcium absorption and regulate parathyroid growth and function. Most recurrences have been due to remnant hypertrophy, which can be treated with simple excision with no morbidity.[71–73] Less commonly, recurrent hyperparathyroidism is due to a missed fourth or supernumerary gland or progressive growth of originally microscopic embryologic rests. Postoperative hypocalcemia is less severe and protracted in the subtotal resection group.[72,73] Permanent hypoparathyroidism due to functional failure of the partially resected remnant can be avoided by careful attention to creation of the remnant. Prior to removal of any parathyroid tissue, we identify and trim (if necessary) the gland to be left in situ. If there is any question about vascularization of the remnant, one of the other glands is used instead. Once a viable remnant has been constructed, the other glands may be removed.

Postoperatively, all patients who have undergone bilateral thyroid resection or parathyroid exploration must be evaluated for hypocalcemia. Patients should be carefully instructed about the symptoms of hypocalcemia (perioral numbness and tingling, muscle cramping, and muscular rigidity). To facilitate early discharge, patients are started on oral calcium supplements, 1500–3000 mg of elemental calcium a day in divided doses, and encouraged to increase their intake of dairy products (often not possible in the lactose-intolerant elderly). If patients remain symptomatic on the higher calcium intake, calcitriol (Rocaltrol) or 1,25-dihydroxyvitamin D is added to increase calcium absorption. Intravenous calcium should be avoided except in those with incipient tetany, as it suppresses parathyroid function. Intravenous supplements are rarely required except in patients operated on for renal osteodystrophy. Oral calcium supplements are continued indefinitely in patients with evidence of bone loss.

## Conclusions

Diseases of the thyroid and parathyroid glands are present with increased prevalence in an aging population. Although modern imaging techniques, the use of fine-needle aspiration for cytologic diagnosis, and a variety of medical treatments are available, in many instances, surgery becomes necessary for diagnosis or treatment of these conditions. Fortunately, surgical procedures and anesthetic techniques for the thyroid and parathyroid are well tolerated, even by the frail elderly.

## References

1. Olshansky SJ, Carnes BA, Grahn D. Confronting the boundaries of human longevity. Am Sci 1998;86:52–61.
2. Lamberts SWJ, VandenBald AW, VanderLely AJ. The endocrinology of aging. Science 1997;278:419–423.
3. Gambert SR. Environmental and physiologic variables. In: Braverman LE, Utiger RD (eds) The Thyroid, 6th ed. Lippincott: Philadelphia, 1991:347–357.
4. Tunbridge WMG, Evered DC, Hall R, et al. The spectrum of thyroid disease in the community: the Wickham survey. Clin Endocrinol (Oxf) 1977;7:481–493.
5. Vanderpump MPJ, Tunbridge WMG, French JM, et al. The incidence of thryoid disorders n the community: a twenty-year follow-up of the Wickham survey. Clin Endocrinol (Oxf) 1995;43:55–68.
6. Powe NR, Danese MD, Ladenson PW. Decision analysis in endocrinology and metabolism. Epidemiol Clin Decis Making 1997;26:89–111.

7. Larsen PR, Davies TF, Hay ID. The thyroid gland. In: Wilson JD, Foster DW, Kronenberg HM, Larsen PR (eds) Williams Textbook of Endocrinology, 9th ed. Saunders: Philadelphia, 1998:389–517.
8. Wallace K, Hofmann MT. Thyroid dysfunction: how to manage overt and subclinical disease in older patients. Geriatrics 1998;53:32–41.
9. Chuang CC, Wang ST, Wang PW, et al. Prevalence study of thyroid dysfunction in the elderly of Taiwan. Gerontology 1998;44:162–167.
10. Sawin CT, Geller A, Wolf PA, et al. Low serum thyrotropin concentrations as a risk factor for atrial fibrillation in older persons. N Engl J Med 1994;331:1249–1252.
11. Parle JV, Franklyn KW, Jones SC, et al. Prevalence and follow up of abnormal thyrotropin (TSH) concentrations in the elderly in the United Kingdom. Clin Endocrinol (Oxf) 1991;34:77–83.
12. Lahey FA. Non-activated (apathetic) type of hyperthyroidism. N Engl J Med 1981;204:747–748.
13. Iervasi G, Clerico A, Bonini A, et al. Acute effects of amiodarone on thyroid function in patients with cardiac arrhythmia. J Clin Endocrinol Metab 1997;82:275–280.
14. Gavin L. Thyroid storm. Med Clin North Am 1991;75: 179–191.
15. Burman KD. Thyroid disease and osteoporosis. Hosp Pract 1997;32:71–86.
16. Bartalena L, Marcocci C, Bogazzi F, et al. Relation between therapy for hyperthyroidism and the course of Graves' ophthalmopathy. N Engl J Med 1998;338:73–78.
17. Hamoir E, Meurisse M, Defechereux T, et al. Surgical management of amiodarone-associated thyrotoxicosis: too risky or too effective? World J Surg 1998;22:537–543.
18. Torring O, Tallstedt L, Wallin G, et al. Graves' hyperthyroidism: treatment with antithyroid drugs, surgery, or radioiodine: a prospective, randomized study. J Clin Endocrinol Metab 1996;81:2986–2993.
19. DeGroot LJ, Gorman CA, Pinchera A. Radiation and Graves' ophthalmopathy. J Clin Endocrinol Metab 1995;90: 339–349.
20. Hermus AR, Huysmans DA. Treatment of benign nodular thyroid disease. N Engl J Med 1998;388:1438–1447.
21. Dayan CM, Daniels GH. Chronic autoimmune thyroiditis. N Engl J Med 1996;338:297–306.
22. Brent GA. In: Van Middlesworth L (ed) The Thyroid Gland: A Practical Clinical Treatise. Year Book: Chicago, 1986: 83–110.
23. Ghareib H. Fine needle aspiration biopsy of thyroid nodules: advantages, limitations, and effect. Mayo Clin Proc 1994;69:44–49.
24. Burrow GN. The thyroid: nodules and neoplasia. In: Felig P, Baxter JD, Gishman LA (eds) Endocrinology and Metabolism, 3rd ed. McGraw Hill: New York, 1995:521–553.
25. Melliere D, Scada F, Etienne G. Goiter with severe respiratory compromise: evaluation and treatment. Surgery 1988; 103:368–373.
26. Newman E, Shah A. Substernal goiter. J Surg Oncol 1995;60:207–212.
27. Hsu B, Reeve TS, Guinea AI, et al. Recurrent substernal nodular goiter: incidence and management. Surgery 1996; 120:1072–1075.
28. LaRosa GL, Lupo L, Giuffrida D, et al. Levothyroxine and potassium iodide are both effective in treating benign solitary cold nodules of the thyroid. Ann Intern Med 1995;122:1–8.
29. Schneider AB, Bekerman C, Leland J, et al. Thyroid nodules in the follow up of irradiated individuals: comparison of thryoid ultrasound with scanning and palpation. J Clin Endocrinol Metab 1997;82:4020–4027.
30. Schlumberger KJ. Papillary and follicular thyroid carcinoma. N Engl J Med 1998;338:297–306.
31. Rosai J, Carcangiu ML, Dellelis RA. Tumors of the Thryoid Gland. Armed Forces Institute of Pathology: Washington, DC, 1992:1–343.
32. Mazzaferri EL, Jhiang SM. Long-term impact of initial surgical and medical therapy on papillary and follicular thyroid cancer. Am J Med 1994;97:418–428.
33. DeGroot LJ, Kaplan EL, McCormick M, et al. Natural history, treatment, and course of papillary carcinoma. J Clin Endocrinol Metab 1990;71:414–424.
34. Ladenson PW, Braverman LE, Mazzaferri EL, et al. Comparison of administration of recombinant human thyrotropin with withdrawal of thryoid hormone for radioactive iodine scanning in patients with thyroid carcinoma. N Engl J Med 1997;337:888–896.
35. Lips CJM, Lansvater RM, Hoppener JWM. Clinical screening as compared with DNA analysis I of families with multiple endocrine neoplasia. N Engl J Med 1994;331:828–835.
36. Burney RE, Jones KR, Coon JW, et al. Assessment of patient outcomes after operation for primary hyperparathyroidism. Surgery 1996;120:1013–1019.
37. Pasieka JL, Parsons LL. Prospective surgical outcome study of relief of symptoms to following surgery in patients with primary hyperparathyroidism. World J Surg 1998;22:513–519.
38. Ohrvall U, Lundgren H, Eriksson E, et al. Dementia-like symptoms related to primary hyperparathyroidism in the elderly. Presented at 30th World Congress of Surgery, Acapulco, Mexico, August 1997.
39. Chen H, Parkerson J, Udelsman R. Parathyroidectomy in the elderly: do the benefits outweigh the risks? World J Surg 1998;22:531–536.
40. Melton LJ. How many women have osteoporosis now? J Bone Miner Res 1995;10:175–177.
41. Kleerekoper M. Clinical course of primary hyperparathyroidism. In: Bilezikian JP, Levine MA, Marcus R (eds) The Parathyroids. Raven: New York, 1994:471–483.
42. Muir JW, Baker LR. Hypercalciuria and recurrent urinary stone formation despite successful surgery for primary hyperparathyroidism. Br Med J 1978;738:1–3.
43. Maschio G, Vecchioni R, Tessitore N. Recurrence of autonomous hyperparathyroidism in calcium nephrolithiasis. Am J Surg 1980;68:607–609.
44. McGeown MG. Effect of parathyroidectomy on the incidence of renal calculi. Lancet 1961;1:586–587.
45. Silverberg SJ, Bone HG, Marriott TB, et al. Short term inhibition of parathyroid hormone secretion by a calcium receptor agonist in patients with primary hyperparathyroidism. N Engl J Med 1997;337:1506–1510.
46. McKane WR, Khosla J, Egan KS, et al. Role of calcium intake in modulating age-related increases in parathyroid function

and bone resorption. J Clin Endocrinol Metab 1996;81: 1699–1703.

47. Thompson N, Eckhauser F, Harness J. The anatomy of primary hyperparathyroidism. Surgery 1982;92:297–299.
48. Hobbiger HE, Allen JG, Greatorex RG, et al. The laryngeal mask airway for thyroid and parathyroid surgery. Anesthesia 1996;51:972–974.
49. LoGerfo P. Local/regional anesthesia for thyroidectomy: evaluation as an outpatient procedure. Presented at the American Association of Endoscopic Surgery, 19th Annual Meeting, 1998, paper 9.
50. Schwartz AE, Clark OH, Itnarle P, et al. Thyroid surgery: the choice. J Clin Endocrinol Metab 1998;83:1097–1105.
51. Mack E. Management of patients with substernal goiter. Surg Clin North Am 1995;75:377–395.
52. Mitchell BK, Merrell RC, Kinder BK. Localization studies in patients with hyperparathyroidism. Surg Clin North Am 1995;75:483–498.
53. Kaplan E, Yashiro T, Salti G. Primary hyperparathyroidism in the 1990s. Ann Surg 1992;215:300–317.
54. Bondeson A, Bondeson L, Ljungberg O, et al. Surgical strategy in nonfamilial primary parathyroid hyperplasia: long-term follow-up of thirty-nine cases. Surgery 1985;97:569–573.
55. LiVolsi V. Embryology, anatomy, and pathology of the parathyroids. In: Bilezikian JP, Levine MA, Marcus R (eds) The Parathyroids. Raven: New York, 1994:1–14.
56. Billingsley K, Fraker D, Doppman J, et al. Localization and operative management of undescended parathyroid adenomas in patients with persistent primary hyperparathyroidism. Surgery 1994;116:982–990.
57. Wang C. Parathyroid re-exploration. Ann Surg 1987;186: 140–145.
58. Kern KA, Shawker TH, Doppman JL, et al. The use of high-resolution ultrasound to locate parathyroid tumors during reoperations for primary hyperparathyroidism. World J Surg 1987;11:579–583.
59. Worsey MJ, Carty SE, Watson CG. Success of unilateral neck exploration for sporadic primary hyperparathyroidism. Surgery 1993;114:1024–1030.
60. Wang CA. Unilateral neck exploration for primary hyperparathyroidism. Arch Surg 1990;125:985–990.
61. Miccoli P, Bendinelli C, Vignali C, et al. Endoscopic parathyroidectomy: report of an initial experience. Surgery 1998;124:1077–1079.
62. Denham DW, Norman J. Cost-effectiveness of preoperative sestamibi scan for primary hyperparathyroidism is dependent solely upon the surgeon's choice of operative procedure. J Am Coll Surg 1998;186:293–305.
63. Irvin GL, Dembrow VD, Prudhomme DL. Clinical usefulness of an intraoperative "quick parathyroid hormone" assay. Surgery 1993;114:1019–1023.
64. Nussbaum S, Thompson A, Hutcheson A, et al. Intraoperative measurement of parathyroid hormone in the surgical management of hyperparathyroidism. Surgery 1988;194: 1121–1127.
65. Metz D, Jensen R, Allen B, et al. Multiple endocrine neoplasia type I: clinical features and management. In: Bilezikian J, Levine M, Marcus R (eds) The Parathyroids. Raven: New York, 1994:591–646.
66. Thompson N. The surgical management of hyperparathyroidism and endocrine disease of the pancreas in the multiple endocrine neoplasia type I patient. J Intern Med 1995;238:269–280.
67. Tissel L, Hedman I, Hansson G. Clinical characteristics and surgical results in hyperparathyroidism caused by water-clear hyperplasia. World J Surg 1981;5:565–571.
68. Wells S, Gunnells J, Shelbourne J, et al. Transplantation of the parathyroid glands in man: clinical indications and results. Surgery 1975;78:34–44.
69. Niederle B, Roka R, Brennan M. The transplantation of parathyroid tissue in man: development, indications, technique, and results. Endocr Rev 1982;3:245–279.
70. Brandi ML, Aurbach GD, Fitzpatrick LA, et al. Parathyroid mitogenic activity in plasma from patients with familial multiple endocrine neoplasia type 1. N Engl J Med 1986; 314:1287–1293.
71. Punch J, Thompson N, Merion R. Subtotal parathyroidectomy in dialysis-dependent and post-renal transplant patients. Arch Surg 1995;130:538–543.
72. Neonakis E, Wheeler MH, Krishana H, et al. Results of surgical treatment of renal hyperparathyroidism. Arch Surg 1995;130:643–648.
73. Koonsman M, Hughes K, Dickerman R, et al. Parathyroidectomy in chronic renal failure. Am J Surg 1994;168: 631–634.

# 22
# Neoplasms of the Adrenal and Endocrine Pancreas in the Elderly

Christopher P. Coppola and Ronald C. Merrell

## Adrenal Neoplasms

With the variety of functions served by the adrenal glands and their deep location inaccessible to direct physical examination, it is no surprise that the management of adrenal neoplasm is a fascinating and challenging venture. An age-dependent increase in both malignant adrenal disease and concomitant medical disease, further complicates treatment decisions in elderly patients. Because nearly every type of adrenal tumor occurs more frequently in women, women over the age of 64 represent a disproportionate share of patients with adrenal tumors. Some patients seek medical attention secondary to symptoms caused by abnormal adrenal secretion. Adrenocortical tissue can produce excess mineralocorticoids, glucocorticoids, or sex steroids; and medullary tissue can overproduce catecholamines.

Autopsy series have identified that clinically silent adrenal adenomas are common. As the use of computed tomography (CT) increases, more of these tumors are identified during life and present a therapeutic dilemma. Due to increased life expectancy, it is projected that 22% of the population will be 64 years or older in 2031.[1] As the population ages, more surgical procedures are needed by elderly patients who can experience increased perioperative morbidity and mortality. Age is not a contraindication to adrenal resection in the proper setting with adequate preoperative preparation. Various surgical approaches to the adrenal glands are available and the recent application of minimally invasive laparoscopic adrenalectomy may benefit elderly patients with decreased surgical risk.

## Anatomy

The adrenals are paired flat glands with a triangular shape, each weighing about 5g. They take their name from their position above the kidneys. Each gland is comprised of an inner dark gray medulla, an outer golden yellow cortex, and a fibrous capsule. The medulla is of ectodermal origin and is derived from the neural crest. It contains homogeneous sheets of cells organized into nests. Cells have large varied nuclei and abundant cytoplasm packed with numerous secretory granules containing catecholamines and other substances specific to chromaffin cells. The cortex is of mesodermal origin and is derived from the adrenogenital ridge. The cortex is organized into three layers, each with a different function. The most superficial layer is the zona glomerulosa, a thin layer of ovoid clusters of cells responsible for aldosterone production. Next is the zona fasciculata with radial colums of lipid-laden cells that produce cortisol and adrenal sex hormones. The deepest layer is the zona reticularis with irregular sheets of cells that store cholesterol for steroidogenesis and secrete cortisol and sex hormones.

The blood supply to the adrenal is threefold; via the superior adrenal arteries from the inferior phrenic arteries, the middle adrenal from the aorta, and the inferior adrenal artery from the renal arteries. Blood passes from the cortex to the medulla, and the gland is drained by a single central vein emptying into the vena cava on the right and the renal vein on the left.

There is little macroscopic change in the normal adrenal over the course of life. Autopsy studies show that microscopic hyperplastic adrenocortical nodules develop in up to half of patients.[2]

## Physiology

### *Adrenocortical Function*

Steroid end-products secreted by the adrenal cortex are metabolites of cholesterol. The common pathway is conversion of cholesterol to δ5-pregnenolone and then progesterone. In the zona glomerulosa, progesterone is converted through several steps to the mineralocorticoid aldosterone. In the other layers of the cortex, progesterone is converted first to 17-hydroxyprogesterone and then to either the 17-hydroxysteroid cortisol or the 17-ketosteroid sex hormones. Each day the adrenal glands secrete 15–20 mg of cortisol, 25–30 mg of androgens, and 75–125 µg of aldosterone.[3]

The zona fasciculata and zona reticularis are responsible for glucocorticoid production. Secretion of cortisol is controlled via the hypothalamic-pituitary-adrenal (HPA) axis. Neural stimulation of the anterior hypothalamus controls release of corticotropin-releasing hormone (CRH). CRH reaches the anterior pituitary via the pituitary portal circulation and causes release of corticotropin (adrenocorticotrophic hormone, ACTH), which stimulates the adrenal cortex to release cortisol. As cortisol concentration achieves the physiologic range of 15–20 µg/dl, it exerts a negative feedback on both hypothalamus and anterior pituitary secretion. Corticotropin has a plasma half-life of 25 minutes and cortisol has a plasma half-life of 90 minutes.[4] Corticotropin and cortisol production are constant over life in normal, unstressed individuals.

Adrenal androgens are also produced in the zona fasciculata and zona reticularis. Adrenal androgen release is regulated by corticotropin, whereas gonadal release of testosterone and estrogen are under a separate pathway of pituitary control. Androgen production peaks at puberty and progressively declines with advancing age.[5]

The mineralocorticoid aldosterone is produced in the outermost layer of the adrenal cortex, the zona glomerulosa. Aldosterone secretion is primarily controlled through a renal pathway. Decreased arterial pressure or decreased serum sodium concentration is sensed by the juxtaglomerular apparatus and the macula densa, respectively. The result is production and release of renin, a renal peptidase. Renin cleaves renin substrate, a circulating hepatic protein, to produce the decapeptide angiotensin I. Within the lung, the carboxypeptidase angiotensin-converting enzyme converts most of the angiotensin I to the octapeptide angiotensin II. Circulating angiotensin II stimulates aldosterone secretion from the zona glomerulosa. To a lesser degree, aldosterone secretion is stimulated by direct effects of corticotropin and elevated serum potassium. With aging, there is decreased production of aldosterone.[6]

### *Adrenomedullary Function*

Stimulation of the adrenal medulla is via preganglionic sympathetic fibers. Stimulation results in migration of secretory granules to the cell membrane and degranulation, with release of dopamine, norepinephrine, and epinephrine. Sympathetic neural outflow is increased by the fight-or-flight response, fear, emotional stress, upright posture, pain, cold, hypotension, hypoglycemia, and other stress. Norepinephrine exerts negative feedback at the preganglionic sympathetic fibers via $\alpha_2$ receptors and within the adrenal medulla by concentration-dependent inhibition of tyrosine hydroxylase activity. Interruption of the signals transmitted via the sympathetic nervous system secondary to injury or medications results in autonomic dystrophy with loss of the adrenergic response to change in position, stress, or hypotension. With increasing age, there is no change in epinephrine levels, but norepinephrine and total plasma catecholamine are increased.[6] However, this does not seem to be associated with hypertension in the elderly, which is probably due to an increased incidence and severity of atherosclerosis.[7] This change in the cardiovascular system may also be responsible for the attenuated response to sympathetic stimuli seen in the elderly.

## Pathology

Disorders of the adrenal gland are being evaluated in an increasing number of elderly patients, most notably because of the increased application of tomographic imaging. Any of the substances normally produced by the adrenal gland can be secreted in excess. Signs and symptoms at presentation are determined by the substance being abnormally secreted. Some tumors secrete multiple products. At times, functional tumors are discovered incidentally through imaging studies performed for other conditions, before they cause symptoms. Their abnormal function can be subsequently detected through laboratory tests. It is important to differentiate benign from malignant disease and unilateral from bilateral disease, as these distinctions guide treatment and prognosis counseling. These characteristics can sometimes be deduced from the appearance of the lesion in preoperative imaging studies. In particular, the size of a tumor has diagnostic significance (Table 22.1). The relative frequencies of diagnoses in unselected or elderly patients requiring adrenalectomy are listed in Table 22.2. Notably, as age increases there is a percentage increase in nonfunctioning adenomas and a decrease in pheochromocytomas. The distribution of age at diagnosis for some adrenal lesions is illustrated in Figure 22.1.

### *Cushing Syndrome*

The classic constellation of signs and symptoms associated with hypercortisolism were first described by

TABLE 22.1. Mean Diameter of Adrenal Lesions

| Pathology | Mean diameter (cm) |
| --- | --- |
| Cortisol-producing adenoma | 4 |
| Aldosteronoma | 2 |
| Pheochromocytoma | 7 |
| Incidentaloma | 3 |
| Adrenocortical carcinoma | 13 |
| Myelolipoma | 5 |

*Source:* Merrell,[8] Herrera et al.,[9] Lucon et al.,[10] van Heerden et al.,[11] Han et al.[12]

TABLE 22.2. Indications for Adrenalectomy

| Diagnosis | % Unselected patients | % Elderly patients |
|---|---|---|
| Pheochromocytoma | 22–43 | 19 |
| Adrenocortical carcinoma | 18 | 8 |
| Cushing syndrome | 17–18 | 22 |
| Nonsecreting adenoma | 16–18 | 31 |
| Conn's disease | 11–19 | 20 |
| Virilizing/feminizing tumor | 6 | <1 |
| Myelolipoma | 4 | <1 |
| Cyst | 2–5 | <1 |
| Metastasis | 1 | <1 |

*Source:* Data from Linos et al.,[13] Proye et al.,[14] Lo et al.[15]

Harvey W. Cushing in 1932.[28] Signs and symptoms, which develop after an extended period of time, can be difficult to discriminate from some normal changes of aging. The most common complaint of patients with Cushing syndrome is weight gain. This symptom becomes less diagnostic owing to increased incidence of obesity in the elderly and evidence that adipose tissue becomes less responsive to glucocorticoids.[29] The skin can become fragile, resulting in violaceous striae over the abdomen and proximal extremities, easy bruisability, and telangiectasias, but these also are less discernible in the elderly. Muscle wasting and weakness is more likely to be present in elderly patients,[7] but are difficult to assess. Hypertension and oligomenorrhea or glucose intolerance can occur. Depression, loss of libido, and insomnia are common. Old patients have an increased tendency to suffer osteoporosis and thin, papery skin.

The cause of Cushing syndrome in each patient must be determined before treatment can be initiated (Table 22.3). Hypercortisolism must be verified through measurement of 24-hour urinary free cortisol; more than 100 µg (275 nmol) in 24 hours is considered abnormal.[30] When cortisol secretion is only mildly elevated, pseudo-Cushing syndrome due to alcoholism or depression, which is common in the elderly, must be ruled out with a dexamethasone suppression test. Dexamethasone

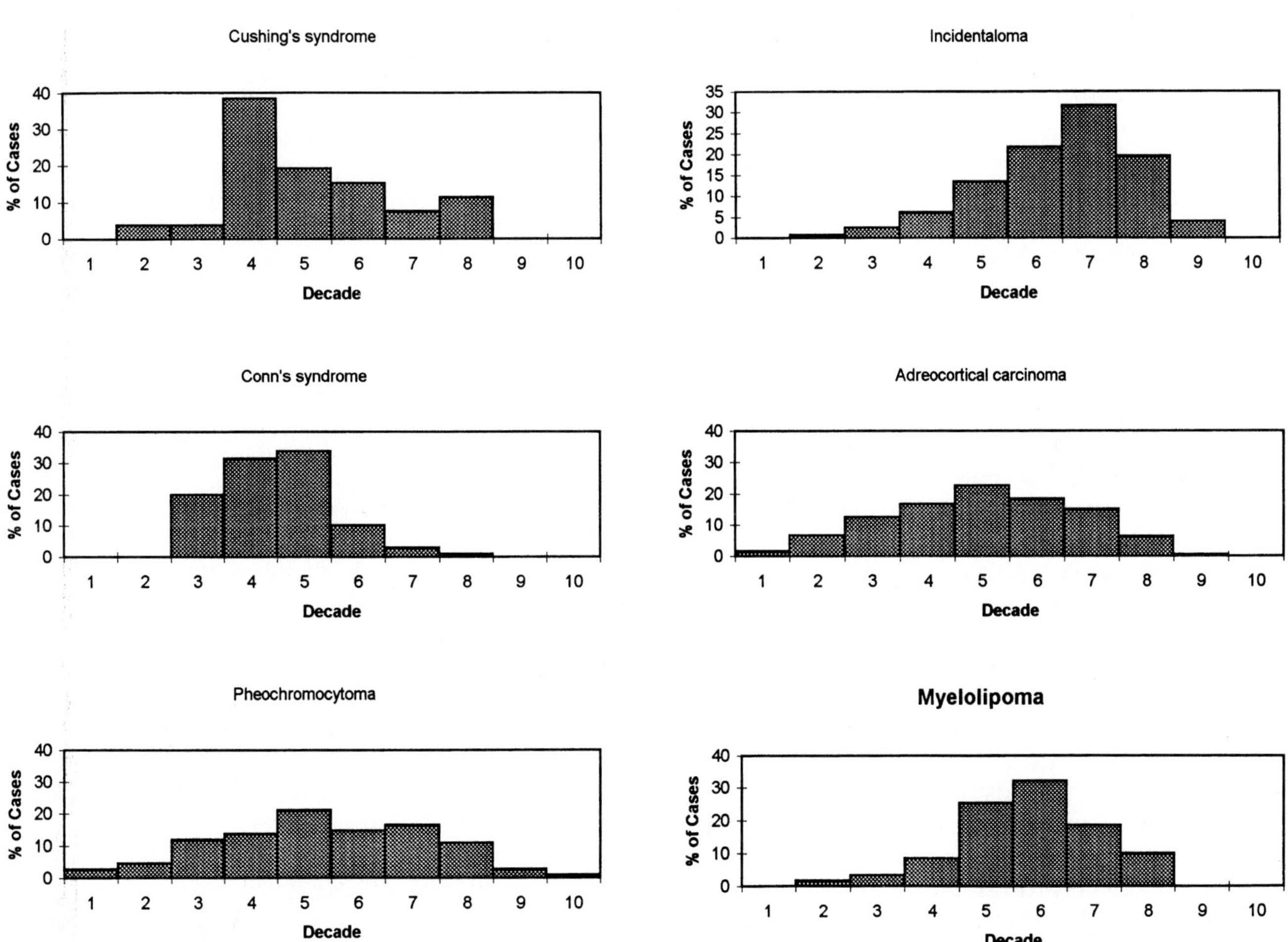


FIGURE 22.1. Distribution of age at diagnosis for adrenal lesions. (Data from Doherty et al.,[16] Brunicardi et al.,[17] Sjöberg et al.,[18] Obara et al.,[19] Peplinski and Norton,[20] Sutton et al.,[21] Samaan et al.,[22] Herrera et al.,[9] Terzolo et al.,[23] Henley et al.,[24] Pommier and Brennan,[25] Luton et al.,[26] Dieckmann et al.[27])

TABLE 22.3. Recative Prevalence of Various Types of Cushing Syndrome Among 630 Patients Studied at Different Times

| Diagnosis | Percentage of patients |
|---|---|
| Corticotropin-dependent Cushing syndrome | |
| Cushing's disease (pituitary adenoma) | 68 |
| Ectopic corticotropin syndrome | 12 |
| Ectopic corticotropin releasing hormone syndrome | <1 |
| Corticotropin-independent Cushing syndrome | |
| Adrenal adenoma | 10 |
| Adrenal carcinoma | 8 |
| Micronodular hyperplasia | 1 |
| Macronodular hyperplasia | <1 |
| Pseudo-Cushing syndrome | |
| Major depressive disorder | 1 |
| Alcoholism | <1 |

*Source:* Orth,[30] with permission. © Massachusetts Medical Society.

suppression testing can be hindered in the elderly by increased metabolism while on anticonvulsants or rifampicin[7] or owing to resistance to the negative feedback effect of glucocorticoids.[31] Further tests to rule out pseudo-Cushing syndrome are combining dexamethasone suppression with corticotropin stimulation and stimulation of corticotropin release with naloxone or hypoglycemia.

Once Cushing syndrome is diagnosed, the next step is to determine if the hypercortisolism is corticotropin-dependent or corticotropin-independent. Plasma cortisol and corticotropin are measured simultaneously after 4 P.M. (preferably at the midnight nadir of secretion). With corticotropin-dependent Cushing syndrome, corticotropin is >15 pg/ml, whereas with corticotropin-independent Cushing syndrome, it is <5 pg/ml with cortisol >15 μg/dl.[30] Patients with corticotropin-independent hypercortisolism have primary adrenal Cushing syndrome and require CT imaging of the adrenal glands.

Abnormal elevated corticotropin can be due to Cushing's disease (a corticotropin-secreting pituitary adenoma) or ectopic corticotropin secretion. A high-dose dexamethasone suppression test can be used to differentiate between these two causes. Almost no cases of ectopic corticotropin secretion are suppressible by high-dose dexamethasone. Stimulation with metyrapone, which inhibits conversion of 11-deoxycortisol to cortisol, increases serum 11-deoxycortisol concentration and urinary 17-hydroxysteroids in 71% of patients with Cushing syndrome but not those with ectopic corticotropin secretion.[32] When these tests fail to elucidate the source of the excess corticotropin, petrosal venous sinus catheterization with corticotropin-releasing stimulation can demonstrate a pituitary tumor through an increased pituitary venous blood/systemic venous blood corticotropin concentration ratio. Petrosal catheterization should not be performed until after searching for an abdominal or thoracic mass suspicious for ectopic corticotropin secretion with CT scanning.

### *Cushing's Disease*

Patients with a pituitary tumor require CT or magnetic resonance imaging (MRI) of the brain to guide surgery. If a tumor is seen, patients should undergo transsphenoidal resection. When no tumor is seen, an 85–90% resection of the anterior pituitary should be performed. Initial surgery results in a cure rate as high as 80% if patients of all ages are considered.[30] When surgery is not curative, irradiation of the pituitary with 4200–4500 cGy can be performed.[30] This can be applied in the elderly, but patients under the age of 40 have a better response.[33] If these measures fail to reduce cortisol production, patients should undergo bilateral total adrenalectomy.

### *Ectopic Corticotropin Production*

Ectopic corticotropin production is the cause of 12–23% of hypercortisolism.[11,30] Most patients with an ectopic source of corticotropin are over 50 years of age[34] and have a poor prognosis. Thoracic tumors represent most of the cases. They include small-cell lung cancer and bronchial or thymic carcinoid tumors. Other sources are pancreatic islet cell tumors, medullary thyroid carcinoma, pheochromocytoma, and prostate cancer. In addition to CT and MRI,[111] In-octreotide scintographic scanning can detect many of these tumors. Curative resection can be performed for 10% of tumors.[30] Others should be treated with medications that reduce cortisol, such as ketoconazole, metyrapone, or aminoglutethimide or with mifepristone (RU-486), which blocks peripheral cortisol action.[30] When there is no response to this therapy, bilateral adrenalectomy should be performed.

### *Cortisol-Producing Adrenal Adenomas*

Patients with adrenal adenomas comprise 10% of all cases of Cushing syndrome and are the most common cause of corticotropin-independent hypercortisolism, approximately 50–72% (Table 22.3).[4,11,30,35] In one series of 85 elderly patients, cortisol-secreting adenomas represented 37% of patients undergoing adrenalectomy for Cushing syndrome and 8% of patients undergoing adrenalectomy for any reason.[15] The female/male ratio for adrenal Cushing syndrome is as high as 9:1.[11] The etiology of adrenal adenoma is unknown, but it does not seem to follow chronic corticotropin excess.

Cortisol-producing adenomas produce cortisol autonomously and efficiently without excess release of cortisol precursors. Tumors have a mean diameter of 3.9 cm.[11] Often the surrounding and contralateral normal adrenocortical tissue has atrophied.

Clinical diagnosis should follow the protocol for evaluating Cushing syndrome, outlined above. Adrenal CT or MRI identifies adrenal lesions 1 cm or larger and can differentiate adrenal adenoma from adrenocortical carcinoma and bilateral adrenal hyperplasia.

Treatment of cortisol-producing adenoma is unilateral adrenalectomy.[36] Resection is curative and results in a good prognosis.[16,37] The laparoscopic approach should be used if available and the posterior approach if not. Perioperative mortality is similar for all methods, but the laparoscopic approach has been shown to result in less morbidity and postoperative pain.[13] Possible contraindications to the laparoscopic approach are a large tumor, suspicion of adrenocortical carcinoma, or the need for concurrent intraabdominal procedures.[38] Tumor characteristics, not age, should determine the approach.

Patient's with Cushing syndrome are at risk for increased morbidity and mortality due to thromboembolism, suppression of immune function, and delayed wound healing.[18,39] In recent series, postoperative mortality rates are 0–14% and the rate of wound infection has been 1.1–10.0%.[11,17,40–43] Elderly patients should not be excluded from surgery based on their age alone, but the increased prevalence of associated medical problems during old age is associated with more perioperative morbidity and mortality.

Following resection, patients require glucocorticoid replacement therapy until endogenous production resumes in the atrophied contralateral gland. Recovery of the HPA axis occurs in a median of 15 months and can take as long as 2 years.[16] Perioperatively, patients should be given 40 mg methylprednisolone IV or IM during the morning before surgery and again that evening; alternatively, 100 mg hydrocortisone may be given every 6 hours starting before or during surgery.[11] The steroid dose should be tapered over the following days, and the patient can be discharged on prednisone 5 mg PO bid or hydrocortisone 12 mg/m$^2$ daily. Therapy should be titrated to avoid signs of Cushing syndrome or Addison's disease. The corticotropin stimulation test can be used to detect the return of normal adrenal function.

Nonoperative therapy should be reserved for patients who are unable to undergo surgery. Metyrapone and aminoglutethimide can decrease cortisol production by inhibiting steroid synthesis. Metyrapone inhibits 11β-hydroxylase, which converts 11-deoxycortisol to cortisol.

### Adrenal Hyperplasia

Primary bilateral nodular adrenocortical hyperplasia is a form of adrenal Cushing syndrome where no solitary adenoma or carcinoma is identified but there is diffuse hyperplasia of both glands with unregulated excess secretion of cortisol. Adrenal hyperplasia is responsible for approximately 1% of Cushing syndrome.[30] Hyperplasia can be divided into macronodular and micronodular. The average age at diagnosis for patients with macronodular hyperplasia is 48 years with a wide range from the fourth to the seventh decade.[44] Patients with this type of hyperplasia usually have markedly enlarged adrenal glands bilaterally (an average combined adrenal weight of 120 g in one series).[11] Oversecretion of cortisol in response to meals or gastric inhibitory polypeptide has been described in two patients with macronodular hyperplasia, which may represent a rare variant.[45,46] Micronodular disease is referred to as primary pigmented nodular adrenal disease (PPNAD) and is essentially limited to patients younger than 30 years.

Imaging the adrenal glands by CT or MRI can diagnose hyperplasia. The treatment for hyperplasia is bilateral total adrenalectomy.[47,48] The surgical approach is bilateral posterior incisions unless the gland is large or concomitant intraabdominal procedures mandate an anterior approach. Bilateral laparoscopic adrenalectomy is an emerging possibility. Perioperative morbidity and mortality are low, and surgery results in uniformly successful resolution of Cushing syndrome.[43] Patients require perioperative and lifelong glucocorticoid and mineralocorticoid steroid replacement tailored to each patient through serial monitoring.[49] Patients require physiologic boluses of steroids during periods of stress and should wear medical alert bracelets to indicate this need. No late mortality is described, but fatigue, nausea, hypotension, or syncope occur at some time in most patients and are probably due to periods of insufficient adrenocortical steroid replacement.[49]

### Conn Syndrome

Excessive secretion of aldosterone results in the syndrome of hypertension and hypokalemia. Conn syndrome, due to a benign aldosterone-secreting adenoma, is rare and is responsible for 0.5–1.0% of hypertension.[8] Its incidence increases with age, and the peak occurrence is during the fourth and fifth decades. In a series of elderly patients, aldosteronoma was the indication for 18% of adrenal resections.[15] The female/male ratio is 5:1.[8]

Aldosterone-secreting adenomas must be differentiated from other causes of aldosteronism (Table 22.4).

TABLE 22.4. Hyperaldosteronism

| | Percentage |
|---|---|
| **Primary aldosteronism** | |
| Aldosterone-producing adenoma | 65 |
| Bilateral adrenal glomerulosa hyperplasia or idiopathic hyperaldosteronism | 30 |
| Primary adrenal hyperplasia | <1 |
| Aldosterone-producing carcinoma | <1 |
| **Secondary aldosteronism** | |
| Physiologic | |
| Glucocorticoid-suppressible aldosteronism | |

*Source:* Melby,[52] with permission.

Patients require potassium repletion, adequate sodium intake, and discontinuation of antihypertensive medication prior to laboratory evaluation for Conn syndrome. Primary aldosteronism is suggested by a serum potassium level <3.5 mEq/L, 24-hour urinary potassium excretion >30 mEq, plasma renin activity <3 ng/ml/hr, and a ratio of plasma aldosterone/renin activity of >20.[50] The diagnosis is confirmed by 24-hour urinary aldosterone secretion >14 μg after 5 days of a high-sodium diet with a serum potassium level of ≥3 mEq/L. Plasma renin is elevated in patients with secondary aldosteronism.

Adrenal CT should be performed to diagnose the cause of primary aldosteronism. In 90% of cases CT can localize an aldosterone-secreting adenoma.[51] The presence of a solitary adrenal lesion >1 cm and aldosteronism is diagnostic of an aldosterone-secreting adenoma. Aldosterone-secreting adrenal adenomas account for 65–70% of primary aldosteronism.[52] Normal adrenal glands, solitary lesions smaller than 1 cm, or multiple nodules should prompt testing for the presence of idiopathic adrenal hyperplasia. Adenomas exhibit diurnal variation because they are corticotropin-sensitive; in contrast, hyperplasia responds to angiotensin. A posture study is performed by measuring serum aldosterone, cortisol, renin, and potassium at 8 A.M. after being supine overnight and then at 12 P.M. after being upright for 4 hours. With an adenoma, aldosterone secretion parallels the drop in cortisol levels. With hyperplasia, aldosterone increases ≥33% in response to upright posture. Accuracy is improved by measuring supine 8 A.M. serum 18-hydroxycorticosterone, which is >100 ng/dl with an adenoma and <100 ng/dl with hyperplasia.[50] $^{131}$I-6-β-iodomethylnorcholesterol (NP-59) scintigraphy can help differentiate adenomas from hyperplasia. In cases where a tumor cannot be localized by radiographic studies, bilateral adrenal venous sampling is useful. The normal adrenal venous aldosterone concentration is 100–400 ng/dl, whereas on the side of an adenoma the aldosterone concentration is 1000–10,000 ng/dl with a side-to-side ratio of at least 10:1.[52]

For treatment, the two options of adrenalectomy and medical therapy with the aldosterone antagonist spironolactone both result in excellent resolution of symptoms and a good prognosis. Medical therapy is preferable in elderly patients with an unacceptable perioperative risk profile. This approach is available because the tumor is uniformly benign. Enucleation of aldosteronomas with a favorable result has been reported.[53] The availability of laparoscopic adrenalectomy may allow patients who would have traditionally received medical therapy to undergo resection safely. Preoperatively, patients should be given the spironolactone to control hypertension and potassium to correct hypokalemia. The laparoscopic approach should be used unless the tumor is very large, suspicious for carcinoma, or a concomitant intraabdominal procedure is planned. The laparoscopic approach may enable elderly patients to be treated surgically earlier and with decreased morbidity. Perioperative morbidity and mortality are low. Resection is curative in >90% of patients and has a success rate of 70–90%.[50,54] After surgery patients require mineralocorticoid support with oral fludrocortisone until the suppressed zona glomerulosa resumes endogenous aldosteronism secretion. Better prognosis is associated with female sex, short duration of hypertension, normal kidneys, and favorable response to spironolactone preoperatively.[19] Age over 50 is associated with persistent hypertension after resection.[19]

### Sex Steroid-Secreting Tumor

Androgen-secreting adrenal adenomas are rare. Virilization or feminization in the setting of an adrenal mass are most likely due to an adrenocortical carcinoma, especially in the elderly. Androgens secreted by the adrenal cortex are dehydroepiandrosterone, dehydroepiandrosterone sulfate, and androstenedione.[55] They exert a direct effect and can also serve as precursors for testosterone and estrogen. Boys and men with androgen excess can exhibit precocious puberty or feminization, and girls and women can experience hirsutism or virilization. Screening is done only when clinical signs are present. Signs of sex steroid excess are investigated in all such patients by measuring urinary 17-ketosteroids. Urinary testosterone should be measured in women with virilization, as cases have been reported where testosterone but not 17-ketosteroids were elevated.[56] Estrogens are measured in men with feminization, as some patients with sex steroid-secreting adrenocortical carcinoma have had normal 17-ketosteroids but elevated estrogens.[57] When a tumor secreting androgens is detected, treatment is unilateral adrenalectomy, taking care to perform an adequate resection should the tumor prove to be a carcinoma (see Adrenocortical Carcinoma, below).

### Pheochromocytoma

Pheochromocytomas are tumors developing from the adrenal medulla that produce catecholamines. They are rare, with an incidence of 1–2 per 100,000.[21,22,58,59] Peak incidence occurs during the ages of 30–50 years. The male/female ratio is approximately 1:1, and most patients are white. Hypertensive patients have an increased incidence of 0.01–1.00%.[60] Of patients undergoing adrenalectomy, pheochromocytoma is the indication for surgery in 22–43% of all patients and in 19% of elderly patients.[13–15,38,40] Clinically silent pheochromocytomas are discovered in 1–9% of patients with incidentally diagnosed adrenal masses.[9,23,61]

Although pheochromocytoma is associated with the multiple endocrine neoplasia type II (MEN-II) syndromes, the early age of presentation makes the syndromes highly unlikely to be present in an elderly patient

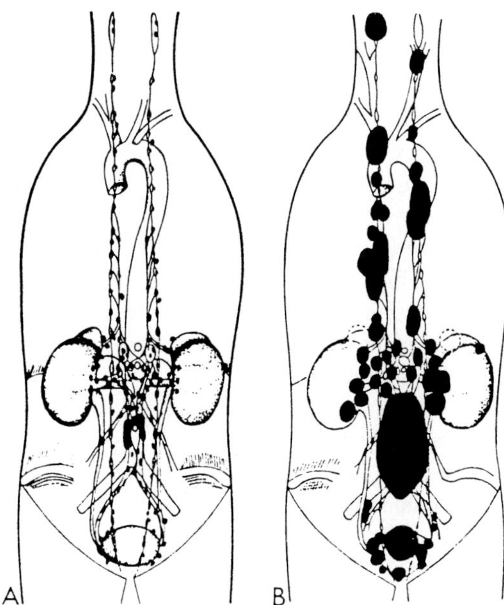


FIGURE 22.2. Sites of extraadrenal neuroendocrine tissue. (From Olson et al.,[66] with permission.)

diagnosed with pheochromocytoma. For both MEN-II subtypes, the onset of pheochromocytoma is earlier, with the peak incidence from 10 to 30 years of age; and 80% have bilateral tumors.[62] Pheochromocytoma is also associated with neuroectodermal dysplasia syndromes such as von Recklinghausen's neurofibromatosis, von Hippel-Lindau disease,[63] tuberous sclerosis, and Sturge-Weber syndrome, but most patients presenting in this manner are young. Genetic abnormalities detected in patients with pheochromocytoma are deletions from chromosomes 1p, 3p, 17p, or 22q.[64]

The term pheochromocytoma, derived from Greek for dusky-colored cell mass, was coined in 1912 based on the finding that chromium salts stain these tumors a deep rust red.[65] Tumors have a median diameter of 7 cm and a median weight of 100 g but can grow as large as 20 cm and weigh 2 kg.[10] Pheochromocytomas can occur in any focus of neuroendocrine tissue including the adrenal medulla and the ganglia of the heart, aorta, or bladder (Fig. 22.2). The most common extraadrenal site is the organ of Zuckerkandl, paired bodies of chromaffin tissue associated with the origin of the superior mesenteric artery, first described in 1901.[67,68] Almost all tumors are intraabdominal, but 2–3% are in the chest and 1% are in the neck. Tumors of the right adrenal are more common.

Malignant pheochromocytoma occurs in 10–20% of cases and is three times as common in women. Extra-adrenal tumors are two to three times as likely to be malignant.[69] Malignancy is proven by invasion of adjacent structures, nodal involvement, or metastasis. Sites of metastasis are bone, liver, lymph nodes, lungs, and brain. Histologic differentiation between benign and malignant tumors is unreliable.

Most pheochromocytomas produce symptoms. However, in an elderly patient with an adrenal mass and hypertension, adrenocortical carcinoma must remain the most significant possibility in the differential diagnosis. In this population, a medullary lesion on CT, not hypertension, should be the impetus for an evaluation for pheochromocytoma. Patients commonly present with episodes of a varied constellation of signs and symptoms that can mimic refractory hypertension, panic disorder, myocardial infarct, or stroke (Table 22.5). Symptoms are due to the effects of circulating catecholamines and hypertension. These complaints can be severe and alarming, and they cause patients to seek care; but unless hormonal screening is performed, the diagnosis is missed. Some patients present with a hypertensive episode during unrelated surgery. The most consistent sign, hypertension, is present in approximately 80% of patients; and paroxysmal hypertension is present in 30–40%.[70,72] Malignant tumors usually exhibit persistent, not paroxysmal, hypertension. Exposure to elevated catecholamines can result in orthostatic hypotension, ileus, arrhythmia, myocardial infarction, stroke, or sudden death.

Diagnosis is reliably made by demonstrating elevated levels of catecholamines and their metabolites in a 24-hour urine sample. Urinary levels of epinephrine, norepinephrine, dopamine, metanephrines, and vanillylmandelic acid (VMA) can be measured. Measurement of urinary metanephrines is the most accurate single

TABLE 22.5. Symptoms of Pheochromocytoma

| Manifestation | % Patients |
|---|---|
| Headache | 52–57 |
| Palpitation | 45–73 |
| Vomiting | 23 |
| Abdominal discomfort | 20–26 |
| Pallor | 20 |
| Anxiety attack | 0–60 |
| Nausea | 15–43 |
| Weakness | 15–38 |
| Diaphoresis | 14–75 |
| Angina | 12–18 |
| Dyspnea | 11–18 |
| Tremor | 10–51 |
| Dizziness | 3–43 |
| Visual disturbance | 3–21 |
| Convulsion | 3–5 |
| Polyuria after crises | 5 |
| Flushing | 3 |
| Itching | 3 |
| Paresthesia | 0–11 |

*Source:* Orchard, et al.,[70] Peplinski and Norton,[20] Lucon et al.,[10] Gifford et al.[71]

test, with a sensitivity of 100% and specificity of 80%.[20] Urinary VMA testing can be falsely elevated secondary to ingesting coffee, tea, or raw fruits or after methyldopa administration. Elevated urinary epinephrine, norepinephrine, and dopamine levels do not differentiate pheochromocytoma from essential hypertension. Plasma epinephrine, norepinephrine, and dopamine can be measured but detect only 75% of pheochromocytomas; and samples must be obtained at the time of the attack in a controlled environment.

When urinary catecholamine metabolites test results are equivocal, adrenergic stimulation or suppression can diagnose a pheochromocytoma. Glucagon 1–2 mg IV bolus precipitates a rise in plasma catecholamines to above 2000 pg/ml (more than three times baseline) in the presence of pheochromocytoma. If free plasma catecholamines are elevated, clonidine 0.3 mg PO decreases them to <500 pg/ml within 3 hours in the presence of essential hypertension but not pheochromocytoma. Accuracy decreases if patients are dehydrated or have taken adrenergic antagonists within 2 days of testing.

Prior to surgery, CT or MRI must be performed to localize the tumor. With MRI, an intensity three times greater than that of the liver is highly specific for pheochromocytoma and can detect some tumors missed on CT.[131] I-metaiodobenzylguanidine scintigraphic scanning is highly specific for pheochromocytoma and is especially useful for extraadrenal lesions.

Surgical resection offers the only chance of cure for pheochromocytoma. The erratic release of catecholamines from these tumors, especially during manipulation, makes perioperative hemodynamic management dangerous and difficult. The key to safe surgery is effective preoperative blood pressure control, rigid intraoperative pressure management, and clear communication between surgeon and anesthesiologist. Elderly patients with concomitant cardiovascular disease may benefit from perioperative pulmonary artery catheter monitoring. After diagnosis, maintenance $\alpha$-adrenergic blockade should be undertaken for 1–3 weeks before surgery. Options for therapy are (1) phenoxybenzamine 10–40 mg PO bid or tid, increasing 10–20 mg/day to effect; (2) phentolamine 5–15 mg IV bolus or 0.5–1.0 mg/min IV continuous infusion. Terazosin 1–20 mg/day PO and doxazosin 1–16 mg/day PO, which are $\alpha_1$-adrenergic antagonists, or calcium channel blocking agents such as nifedipine 10–20 mg PO tid and nicardipine 20–40 mg PO tid can also be used for hypertension.[71] Patients must be hydrated adequately to fill the expanded intravascular space to normal volume. Patients with tachycardia or other arrhythmias should receive $\beta$-blockers, but propranolol should be avoided because it can enhance the norepinephrine effect.

Traditionally, the anterior transperitoneal approach has been used for pheochromocytoma. As pheochromocytomas can be multicentric and bilateral, many perform a thorough exploration of both adrenal beds and the intraabdominal ganglia. With improved diagnostic imaging techniques, the benefits of a unilateral exploration via the laparoscopic or posterior approach outweigh the small chance of discovering a contralateral mass not detected preoperatively.

During surgery arterial blood pressure should be constantly monitored through a radial artery catheter. Aggressive volume replacement is used to compensate for rapid decreases in blood pressure. Pheochromocytomas can be stimulated to release catecholamines by anesthetic agents or morphine.[73] A sodium nitroprusside drip and a short-acting $\beta$-blocker such as esmolol should be used to provide rapid adjustments in blood pressure and heart rate. Lidocaine can be used for arrhythmias. Elderly patients and patients with existing ischemic or congestive heart disease may require more meticulously regimented fluid administration, so a pulmonary artery catheter should be used to guide therapy. Patients may experience hemodynamic instability postoperatively and should have their blood pressure monitored in an intensive care unit (ICU). With these measures the perioperative mortality rate has been 0–3%.[10] Prognosis is good after resection of benign tumors, although some patients continue to have hypertension.

With malignant pheochromocytoma, patients are at risk for recurrence as much as 20 years after resection. Ablation with $^{131}$I-metaiodobenzylguanidine or combination chemotherapy with cyclophosphamide, vincristine, and dacarbazine may give a response. Palliative irradiation of bony metastases can reduce symptoms. The 5-year survival is 36–60%.[60]

### Incidentaloma

Incidentally discovered adrenal masses are a significant therapeutic dilemma in the elderly because the risks of adrenalectomy must be weighed against the remote chance that the mass is malignant. It has long been known from autopsy studies that there is a 1.4–8.7% incidence of unsuspected adrenal adenomas.[74–79] They occur with increasing frequency in the elderly and may be secondary to episodes of focal ischemia secondary to atherosclerotic disease followed by compensatory regeneration.[9] Adrenal masses are incidentally discovered in 0.4–4.3% of CT scans performed for other complaints and are referred to as incidentalomas.[2,9,38,74,80–85] Elderly patients are more likely to experience a disease requiring a CT scan and therefore are diagnosed with an incidentaloma more often than the young. There is much controversy over the course of evaluation and treatment to follow for patients with incidentalomas. In groups of patients with adrenal lesions, 13–30% are diagnosed incidentally.[9,74] The female/male ratio is 1.5:1.0, and most patients are 50–70 years old.[9]

TABLE 22.6. Pathology of Resected Incidentalomas

| Pathology | % Patients |
|---|---|
| Benign adenoma | 26–61 |
| Cortisol-producing adenoma | 3–11 |
| Adrenocortical carcinoma | 4–13 |
| Myelolipoma | 3–12 |
| Pheochromocytoma | 0–9 |
| Conn's disease | 0–7 |
| Neuronal | 3–7 |
| Cyst | 6–9 |
| Hyperplasia | 3 |
| Metastasis | 1–4 |
| Granuloma | 1 |
| Pseudocyst | 7 |
| Hematoma | 4 |
| Echinococcal cyst | 4 |

*Source:* Data from Terzolo et al.,[23] Bastounis et al.,[61] Gajraj and Young,[83] Abecassis et al.,[74] Ross and Aron.[84]

Most incidentalomas are presumed to be benign, nonfunctioning adrenal adenomas. Resected incidentalomas vary widely in pathologic diagnosis and even include subclinical hormonally active tumors (Table 22.6).

The average incidentaloma size is 2.9 cm; the tumors were located on the right in 49–57% of cases, were on the left in 35–42%, and were bilateral in 6–9%.[9,23,61,74] Size correlates with risk of adrenocortical carcinoma. For lesions <6 cm, fewer than 1 in 10,000 are malignant; but for lesions ≥6 cm, 92% contain malignancy.[84] Adenomas have an average size of 2.4 cm; only 0.025% of adenomas achieve a size ≥6 cm, with the largest seen being 11 cm.[81,85] The average size of incidentally discovered adrenocortical carcinomas is 9.4 cm, and tumors smaller than 3 cm are rare.[9,23,86]

Metastasis to the adrenal gland can occur, with the most common sources being lung, breast, colon, kidney, and melanoma.[87–89] Bilateral adrenal lesions visualized on CT are consistent with metastasis. Adrenal cysts can be echinococcal parasitic, lymphangiomatous, or angiomatous endothelial, cystic degenerative adenomas or embryonal retention cysts.[90] Pseudocysts result from hemorrhage into normal glands or pathologic lesions such as pheochromocytoma. Benign cysts typically have a thin wall with no soft tissue component. Malignancy can be associated with cysts, with some containing bloody fluid.

Common presentations resulting in discovery of an incidentaloma are abdominal pain, back pain, and known abdominal, thoracic, or renal disease. An organized protocol helps guide therapy for elderly patients with incidentalomas (Fig. 22.3). Evaluation should begin with a thorough history and physical to detect evidence of an extraadrenal malignancy or hormonal excess. A breast and skin examination, fecal occult blood testing, or a chest roentgenogram may reveal an undiscovered primary cancer. CT-guided fine-needle aspiration (FNA) is useful for diagnosing metastasis from an extraadrenal source but is of little value for differentiating benign from malignant primary tumors because of their great histologic similarity.

If the incidentaloma was found on ultrasonography or contrast pyelography, CT of the adrenal glands with thin cuts should be performed. The features of myelolipomas, lipomas, and cysts are characteristic. Features suggestive of malignancy are heterogeneity, necrosis, hemorrhage, irregularity, and invasion. Irregular borders and bilateral locations are features associated with metastasis. The diameter should be measured in three orthogonal planes and the greatest diameter used when selecting treatment. Some advocate percutaneous aspiration for cysts, but others recommend no treatment for benign-appearing cysts.[74] Aspiration of cyst contents can be informative, as virtually all cysts containing clear fluid are benign, whereas a portion of those yielding bloody fluid are malignant.[81] Contrast cystography is a diagnostic option to define the contours of the cyst wall.

Judicious use of MRI or $^{131}$I-6-β-iodomethylnorcholesterol (NP-59) scintography in selected patients has the potential to identify malignant lesions. Uptake of NP-59 on the same side as a tumor is typical of benign lesions processing steroid precursors, whereas discordant laterality suggests a space-occupying lesion with little steroidogenic activity and is consistent with a malignancy or cyst.

Recommendations for evaluating the biochemical activity of incidentalomas varies widely, from no screening to a full battery of endocrine laboratory tests. A rational approach to selecting tests should take into consideration abnormal features in the history and physical examination, adrenal dysfunction that would increase perioperative morbidity, the relative frequency of biochemically active tumors in incidentalomas, and a modicum of restraint. A basic battery of tests includes a 1 mg overnight dexamethasone suppression test, serum potassium level with adequate dietary potassium, and a 24-hour urinary metanephrine measurement.[9] Inconclusive results can be pursued with further testing. Evaluation of sex-steroid excess should be reserved for patients with signs of virilization or feminization.

During the few decades that incidentalomas have been diagnosed with frequency during life, no consensus has been reached over their treatment. If concomitant illness in elderly patients makes adrenalectomy excessively risky, further evaluation may be moot. The most hotly debated aspect of care is the problem of nonfunctioning masses smaller than 6 cm, weighing the risk of surgery against the risk of a rare, undetected carcinoma. When an incidentaloma is first detected, an attempt should be made to rule out etiologies for which clear treatment protocols exist. All patients should undergo the basic screening for abnormal adrenal function outlined above, and

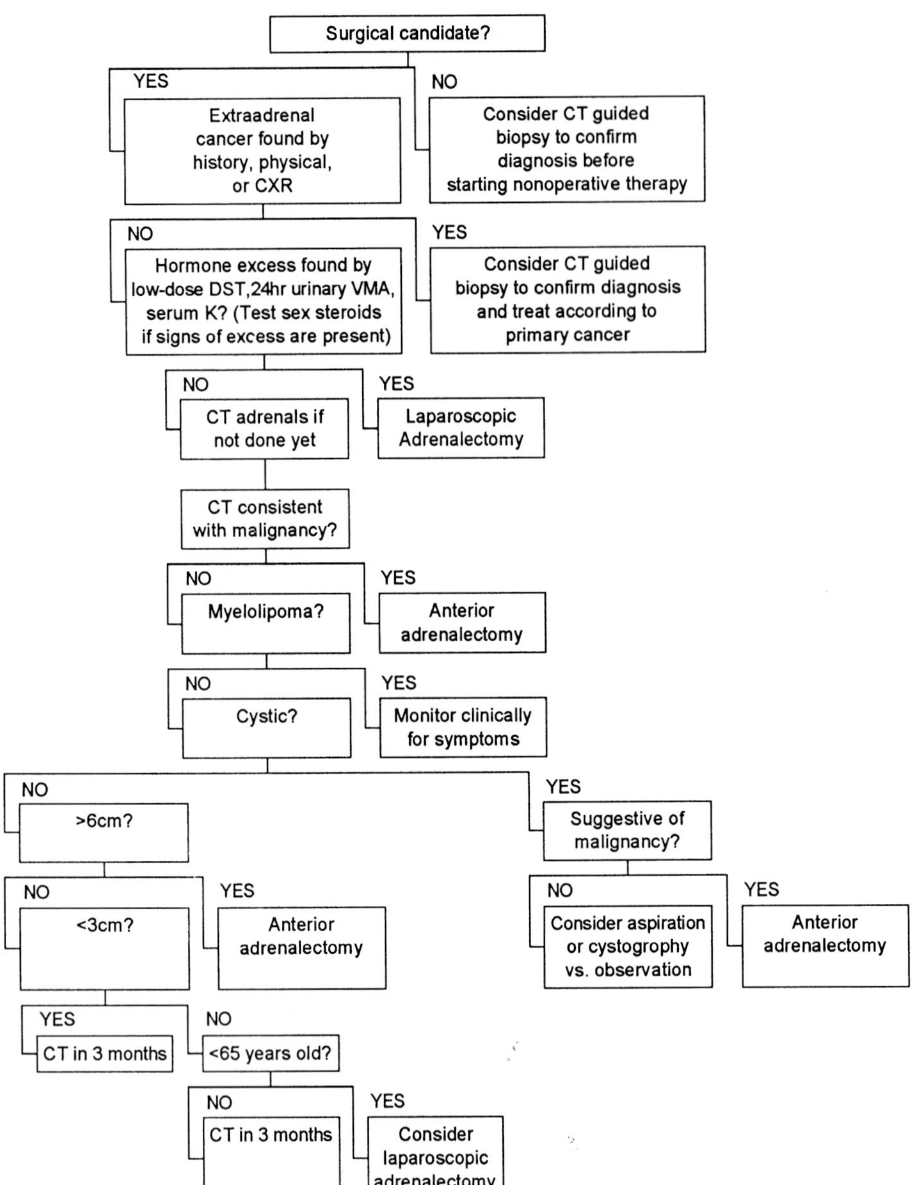


FIGURE 22.3. Evaluation of patients with incidentalomas. CT, computed tomography; CXR, chest roentgenogram; DST, dexamethasone suppression test; VMA, vanillylmandelic acid.

functional tumors should be removed. Patients with pheochromocytomas require cautious intraoperative hemodynamic management, and patients with cortisol excess require postoperative corticosteroid replacement. If metastasis from an extraadrenal malignancy is found, care is guided by the nature of the primary tumor. Benign cysts require no treatment. Lesions with suspicious features such as a thick wall, soft tissue wall irregularity, or bloody aspirate fluid require resection. Myelolipomas require no treatment unless symptoms develop. There is much controversy about the tumors that remain. Any with radiographic features suggestive of malignancy should be removed. The best prognostic indicator of malignancy is tumor size, as described above. Recommendations for adrenalectomy in this group of patients has ranged from all incidentalomas to only those >6cm. Using a cutoff of 3–6cm leads to resection of most carcinomas but also a high number of adrenalectomies in older patients, in whom most tumors are benign. The reduced morbidity of laparoscopic adrenalectomy may allow this threshold to be lowered safely. If nonoperative therapy is elected, patients should undergo routine surveillance for tumor enlargement or development of signs of steroid excess, either of which is an indication for adrenalectomy. Suggested schedules of surveillance range from a single CT scan 3 months after diagnosis to scans every 3 months for a year and then yearly for 2 years.[9,74]

## *Adrenocortical Carcinoma*

Adrenocortical carcinomas are rare, with a yearly incidence of about 200–300 new cases in the United States, which is 0.5–2.0 cases per million inhabitants.[81] It represents 0.05–0.20% of all cancers.[81] It is highly aggressive and has a poor prognosis. Some tumors are clinically silent, and others secrete adrenocortical hormones. Age at diagnosis ranges from 0 to 70 years (mean 46 years), and there is a bimodal distribution with peaks during the first and fifth decades.[23] There is increased incidence in the elderly of primarily hormonally inactive tumors.[81] The female/male ratio ranges from 1:1 to 2:1.[26,91–93] Most patients with secreting tumors are female, but the opposite is true for nonsecreting tumors.[94] The prevalence of adreneocortical carcinoma in cohorts of patients undergoing adrenalectomy is 8% in patients ≥64 years, 13% in those with incidentally diagnosed adrenal masses, and 18% in unselected patients.[13,15,23]

Carcinomas have an average diameter of 12.9 cm but can range up to 40 cm with weights of more than 100 g.[15,23,85] They typically have heterogeneous regions with necrosis and hemorrhage, are of irregular shapes, and can invade the adrenal capsule, surrounding structures, or the inferior vena cava. Tumors are unilateral and occur in either adrenal with equal frequency. Histologic findings are large hyperchromatic nuclei, more than 20 mitoses per high power field, and invasion of adjacent structures. Approximately half (36–60%) of adrenocortical carcinomas secrete hormones and can produce the signs and symptoms of Cushing syndrome, virilization, feminization, or rarely aldosteronism.[15,23,95] Some secrete cortisol in response to a variety of agonists that do not normally stimulate glucocorticoid regulation.[96] Hormonally active tumors are characteristically inefficient at cortisol production and can secrete a variety of androgen precursors resulting in virilization.[35] Adrenocortical carcinoma is responsible for 8% of Cushing syndrome and <1% of Conn syndrome.

Presentation is hormone excess, an abdominal mass, or incidental discovery. Elevated levels of 17-ketosteroids and dehydroepiandrosterone sulfate are often present along with hypercortisolism. Patients with hormonally inactive tumors present with abdominal pain or distension; and they may have paraneoplastic syndromes of weight loss, weakness, anorexia, or nausea. A mass is palpable in 50% of these patients, and 25% have hepatomegaly.[26]

Therapy is guided by CT or MRI. Features suggestive of carcinoma are a hyperdense heterogeneous mass, irregular shape or borders, and invasion of surrounding structures.[97,98] Carcinomas have more intensity than liver on T2-weighted MRI scans. The probability of a lesion being malignant is directly related to its size. Utilizing a threshold of 5 cm carries 93% sensitivity and 64% specificity for adrenocortical carcinoma.[23] Imaging studies can also reveal tumor extension into surrounding tissue. Staging follows the TNM classification (Table 22.7). Local extension is present in 65% and metastasis in 25% of patients at diagnosis.[23] Common sites of metastasis are lymph nodes, lung, liver, and bone; therefore preoperative evaluation should include abdomen and chest CT, a chest roentgengram, and a bone scan. Function in the contralateral kidney should be verified prior to surgery. If findings are equivocal or if operative treatment is to be deferred and the diagnosis of carcinoma needs to be confirmed, a CT-guided FNA biopsy can be performed.

TABLE 22.7. Staging of 69 Patients with Adrenocortical carcinoma

| Stage | Criteria | N (%) |
|---|---|---|
| I | Tumor <5 cm<br>Negative nodes<br>No local invasion<br>No metastasis | 3 (4) |
| II | Tumor <5 cm<br>Same | 22 (32) |
| III | Positive nodes or<br>Local invasion | 20 (29) |
| IV | Positive nodes and local invasion<br>Distant metastases | 24 (35) |

*Source:* Pommier and Brennan,[25] with permission.

All lesions suspicious for adrenocortical carcinoma by radiographic appearance, biopsy specimen features, or diameter ≥5–6 cm should be resected by anterior transperitoneal adrenalectomy with en bloc resection of all involved tissue. Curative resection can be attempted in 80% of cases. The anterior open approach is favored because these lesions tend to be large and vascular invasion is a possibility, which makes the laparoscopic approach tenuous.

Patients should be screened for excess secretion of cortisol or aldosterone preoperatively. Those with cortisol-secreting carcinomas require perioperative glucocorticoid steroid replacement as per adenomas. Treatment can be tapered as the atrophied contralateral adrenal cortex resumes steroid production.

Operative mortality is 9.7% in most patients.[24] Patients with Cushing syndrome may experience increased morbidity in the form of wound infection, thromboembolism, and delayed healing. Elderly patients had a mortality rate of 43% in one study, compared to 4% for those with other adrenal disorders.[15] Length of hospitalization can be longer for patients with carcinoma, 11 days in one study, but this may be related to the need for oncologic consultation or treatment.[13]

Recurrences are common and are refractory to nonoperative treatment resulting in a 5-year survival of 16–35% for all patients,[24,25,92,99] 50% for stage I, and 10% for stage II.[24,93] Adjuvant therapy with the adrenocortical-specific cytolytic mitotane (4 g/day PO) after curative resection may decrease recurrence.[93,100,101] Surgical debulking may increase survival, so patients should be monitored for recurrences.[25]

Treatment for patients with unresectable disease is chemotherapy or irradiation. Mitotane gives a response rate of 34% or less and no survival benefit.[25] In cases of Cushing syndrome, adrenal enzyme inhibitors such as metyrapone or aminoglutethimide can palliate symptoms, albeit gradually. Side effects are adrenal insufficiency requiring glucocorticoid and mineralocorticoid replacement as well as anorexia, nausea, fatigue, ataxia, and other central nervous system (CNS) symptoms.

### *Myelolipoma*

Adrenal myelolipoma, a rare benign tumor, was first described in 1905[102] and named in 1929.[103] It consists of ectopic growth of lipomatous and myelogenous tissue in a discrete mass within the adrenal gland.[27] The incidence from autopsy series ranges from 0.08% to 0.40%.[104–106] The tumor seems to affect men and women with equal frequency, although in one series 60% of the patients were women.[12] It has been diagnosed in patients from age 12 to 93[107] but occurs with the highest frequency during the fifth to seventh decades.[108,109] Most of the patients reported have been white.

Tumors locate in either gland with equal frequency and are occasionally bilateral.[12] The tumors are smooth, spherical, soft masses and are contained within a pseudocapsule of compressed normal adrenal tissue.[110] On cut section, they have dark red areas corresponding to myelogenous tissue and yellow fatty areas. Histologic examination reveals large vacuolated lipomatous cells and hematopoietic cells.[107] Myelolipomas do not invade surrounding tissues but can compress adjacent organs.

Most myelolipomas are hormonally inactive, but association with Cushing syndrome, primary aldosteronism, virilization, and feminization has been reported.[12,104] Renal vascular hypertension secondary to renal artery compression has been seen.[12] A myelolipoma can undergo necrosis or rarely can result in retroperitoneal hemorrhage.[111,112] The natural history is benign, and tumors can grow, shrink, or remain the same size.[12] Some patients with asymptomatic myelolipomas later develop symptoms. The most widely accepted theory of pathogenesis of myelolipoma is that adrenocortical metaplasia in response to necrosis, infection, or stress results in metaplastic change.

Previously myelolipomas were most frequently discovered on autopsy, but with the advent of tomographic imaging many are encountered as asymptomatic lesions detected incidentally. A few present as abdominal pain or discomfort. Rare modes of presentation are hypertension, hormone excess, and shock, as described above. The lesion has a characteristic appearance on CT, which is usually diagnostic.[12] MRI can be used to clarify tissue planes, and FNA biopsy should be performed if there is suspicion of carcinoma. Laboratory investigations for hormone excess are reserved for patients who exhibit characteristic signs.

Because of the benign nature of the disease, treatment is mostly expectant. Myelolipomas that should be removed are those associated with syndromes of hormone excess, symptomatic lesions, and masses that could be consistent with carcinoma. Patients treated nonoperatively should undergo clinical surveillance for the onset of symptoms and repeat CT.[12]

### Operative Strategy

There is varied opinion over the optimum strategy for adrenal resection, and progress in laparoscopy has stirred the debate. Adrenalectomy is the extent of resection for all unilateral lesions, with the possible exception of aldosteronoma.[53] Bilateral adrenalectomy is performed for bilateral lesions or refractory adrenocortical oversecretion.

The first approach to adrenalectomy was anterior transperitoneal, as described in 1927.[113] Anterior adrenalectomy continues to be used today. Indications used by some authors who advocate the anterior approach are large tumors, adrenocortical carcinoma, extraadrenal tumor extension, concomitant intraabdominal procedures, pheochromocytoma with possible multicentric disease, and bilateral adrenalectomy.[13,38,114]

The posterior approach, which is most widely used today, consists of a curvilinear (Hugh-Young)[115] or hockey-stick-shaped (Moyer)[14] incision with or without removal of the 12th and 11th ribs. Studies have shown quicker return of gastrointestinal function and shorter postoperative stay after posterior adrenalectomy than after using the anterior approach.[13,116,117] Complications specific to this approach are flank hernia after injury of the subcostal nerve and chronic back pain.[13,117]

Laparoscopic adrenalectomy[118] is rapidly gaining popularity and carries the benefits of decreased pain and speedier recovery.[13,38,114] It is useful in cases of incidentaloma, aldosteronoma, cortisol-secreting adenoma, and small pheochromocytomas when multiple lesions have been excluded. Contraindications to the laparoscopic approach are tumors larger than 7 cm and adrenocortical carcinoma. There are variations in technique including transperitoneal and retroperitoneal approaches. Bilateral laparoscopic adrenalectomy has also been performed successfully (B.K. Kinder and J.C. Rosser, New Haven, CT, personal communication). As development continues, laparoscopic adrenalectomy will become the procedure of choice.

## Tumors of the Endocrine Pancreas

Tumors of the endocrine pancreas are rare, with an incidence of about five cases per one million.[119] They are rare in the elderly population; but when they do occur,

TABLE 22.8. Endocrine Tumors of the Pancreas

| Parameter | Insulinoma | Zollinger-Ellison | Verner-Morrison | Glucagonoma | Somatostatinoma | Nonfunctioning |
|---|---|---|---|---|---|---|
| Cell type | β | G | $\delta_2$ | α | δ | Variable |
| Hormone | Insulin | Gastrin | VIP, prostaglandins | Glucagon | Somatostatin | PP, NSE |
| Incidence (per million) | 1–4 | 0.4 | 0.1 | 0.025 | 0.025 | 0.2 |
| Mean age and range (years) | 42 (20–78) | 59 (7–90) | 47 (5–79) | 52 (19–73) | 53 (30–84) | 56 (20–79) |
| Extrapancreatic (%) | 1–5 | 10–38 | 10–15 | <1 | 15–50 | <1 |
| Malignant (%) | 10–15 | 50–70 | 40 | Most | Most | Most |
| Metastatic (%) | 5 | 50 | 30–40 | 70 | 70 | 60 |
| Multiple (%) | 10 | 70 | Rare | Rare | 0 | Variable |
| Resectable (%) | >90 | Pancreatic <20<br>Duodenal 100 | 70 | 25 | 60 | Variable |
| MEN-I-associated (%) | 4–5 | 70 | Occasional | Occasional | 0 | Most |

VIP, vasoactive intestinal peptide; PP, pancreatic peptide; NSE, neuron-specific enolase; MEN, multiple endocrine neoplasia.

they are associated with increased morbidity and mortality owing to the frequency of coexisting medical disease. Therefore a brief discussion of these tumors is warranted.

The tissue of the pancreas can be divided into the exocrine pancreas, producing products secreted into the gastrointestinal tract, and the endocrine pancreas, which elaborates hormones secreted directly into the bloodstream. In one series of pancreatic tumors, 36% arose from the endocrine pancreas.[120] Pancreatic endocrine function is responsible for homeostasis of glucose and other energy source production, storage, and availability as well as aspects of gastrointestinal function. The cells comprising this system are clustered in the islets of Langerhans, which are nestled between the exocrine structures throughout the pancreas. These cells are members of the amine precursor uptake and decarboxylation (APUD) cell type, a varied group of cells scattered throughout the body but sharing common metabolic pathways and the presence of cytosolic neuron-specific enolase and chromogranin. The salient features of the better characterized endocrine tumors of the pancreas are summarized in Table 22.8.

Tumors of the endocrine pancreas can be physiologically active or nonfunctioning. The effect of active tumors is determined by the substance secreted. About half of the tumors produce more than one hormone,[120] but usually only one is secreted into the circulation and predominates in the clinical presentation.[119] The endocrine tumors of the pancreas are best organized based on the substance they secrete to excess. Most tumors secrete glucagon, insulin, somatostatin, VIP, gastrin, or pancreatic peptide. Insulinomas and gastrinomas are most common. Often systemic manifestations of hormone excess herald the presence of a neoplasm before the effects of local progression are apparent. Malignancy is not defined by the histology of individual cells but, rather, by the presence of metastases. There is a correlation between increased size and malignancy.[120] There is a definite association between endocrine tumors of the pancreas and MEN-I syndrome,[121] and there may be increased frequency in von Recklinghausen's disease,[122] von Hippel-Lindau syndrome,[123] and tuberous sclerosis.[124] Surgical excision offers the best chance for cure for all types.

## Insulinoma

Insulinoma, a neoplasm that overproduces insulin, occurs at a rate of 4 per million people, with a female/male ratio of 3:2.[125] It usually occurs between the ages of 20 and 50, but it has been seen in patients as old as 78 years and 40% of patients are older than age 60.[126] It is caused by a solitary adenoma of beta islet cells in 90% of cases. Ten percent of cases are associated with MEN-I syndrome, and these patients are more likely to have multiple lesions.[127] Some controversy exists over whether nesidioblastosis (diffuse nodular pancreatic enlargement) is a cause of hyperinsulinemia. Most tumors are less than 2 cm at the time of diagnosis, and most are benign.[125] Tumors occur with equal frequency throughout the pancreas, and fewer than 5% are ectopic.[125] Beta cells of an insulinoma exhibit an abnormal pattern of secretion in that insulin continues to be secreted after blood glucose levels have fallen. In some cases of insulinoma, increased levels of the insulin precursor, proinsulin, are detected.

Clinical symptoms of insulinoma are due to fasting hypoglycemia secondary to increased insulin. Occasionally, presentation can be confused with reactive hypoglycemia because the onset of symptoms can be as soon as 4 hours after the last meal. Symptoms can also follow periods of exercise. Symptoms are neuroglycopenic or adrenergic in nature. The neuroglycopenic symptoms are apathy, dizziness, decreased awareness, behavior change, seizure, stroke, and coma. Focal neurologic deficits can also occur. Adrenergic symptoms are anxiety, tremor, tachycardia, palpitations, nausea, vomiting, chest pain, and diarrhea.

The classic requirement for diagnosis of insulinoma is the presence of Whipple's triad: (1) symptoms after fasting or exercise; (2) simultaneous hypoglycemia; (3) relief of symptoms after glucose administration. The first step in diagnosis is to document hypoglycemia at the time of symptoms. If patients present emergently, the blood glucose level should be measured before glucose administration; and blood obtained at the time of presentation should be reserved for measuring insulin, C-peptide, proinsulin, and cortisol if necessary. Blood glucose nadirs vary widely, and levels as low as 22 mg/dl have been measured in healthy young women without symptoms. An acceptable level for diagnosing hypoglycemia is probably less than 40 mg/dl,[119] with the requirement that blood is drawn during hypoglycemic symptoms. In patients who present asymptomatically but have a history suspicious for insulinoma, a 72-hour fast in a monitored hospital setting is the most reliable diagnostic test. A 5-hour glucose tolerance test has low reliability for diagnosing or excluding insulinoma, but it can detect cases of early diabetes mellitis presenting with paradoxic hypoglycemia. During a 72-hour fast, serum glucose, insulin, and C peptide should be measured every 6 hours. The fast should continue until the onset of symptoms, and blood levels should be checked at that time before administering glucose.

Insulinoma is diagnosed by detecting hypoglycemia with the persistent presence of insulin. When the blood glucose level falls, insulin levels should become undetectable. An insulin level of 5 μU/ml or more during symptomatic hypoglycemia is abnormal.[119] The insulin/glucose ratio should also be calculated, and a level of 0.4 (when calculated as microunits per milliliter divided by milligrams per deciliter) or more is indicative of insulinoma.[128] In some patients C peptide or proinsulin levels (or both) are elevated. The possibility of surreptitious insulin or sulfonylurea administration should be evaluated by ensuring that insulin and C peptide levels correspond, and that sulfonylureas are not present in the serum or urine at the conclusion of the fast.[129]

Imaging studies should be performed only after a biochemical diagnosis of insulinoma is secured. Abdominal ultrasonography, CT, and MRI can detect some insulinomas, but many are too small to be visualized. Angiography, $^{131}$I-octreotide scintigraphy, portal venous sampling,[130] endoscopic ultrasonography,[131] or selective angiography with calcium stimulation[132] can be useful for localizing small tumors. Treatment is surgical resection. Preoperatively, symptoms can be avoided by increasing meal frequency, adding cornstarch to the diet to slow absorption, and administering diazoxide.[119] Many insulinomas can be removed by enucleation. Tumors associated with the pancreatic duct or too large for enucleation can be treated by distal pancreatectomy or pancreaticoduodenectomy depending on location. Tumors not localized during surgery can sometimes be detected by intraoperative pancreatic ultrasonography.[130] If a tumor cannot be identified at the time of surgery, the options are to perform a blind distal pancreatectomy or abort the resection and perform portal venous sampling postoperatively. In nearly all patients with insulinoma, the tumor can be identified and resected for cure.[133]

For the few insulinomas that are malignant, resection of the primary tumor and accessible metastases or tumor debulking, can alleviate symptoms in some patients. Hypoglycemic symptoms are sometimes alleviated with diazoxide, 600–1000 mg/day, along with a thiazide diuretic. Some clinicians treat with streptozotocin or octreotide.

## Gastrinoma

Gastrinomas are rare in the general population, occurring at a rate of 0.5–1.0 per million.[134,135] Hypersecretion of gastrin, or Zollinger-Ellison syndrome (ZES),[136] is thought to cause 0.1% of peptic ulcer disease[137] and 0.2% of recurrent ulcer disease. The mean age at presentation is 45 years (range 7–90 years),[138] and it occurs more frequently in men than women at a ratio of 3:2. Twenty percent of gastrinomas are associated with the MEN-I syndrome.[127,139] Most gastrinomas are located in the gastrinoma triangle (Fig. 22.4), which includes the cystic duct, duodenal curve, and junction of the body and neck of the pancreas. In recent series, about half of the gastrinomas have been intramural duodenal lesions.[141,142] More than three-fourths of patients have multiple lesions, and patients with MEN-I have a high incidence of multiple tumors. Within the pancreas, gastrinomas are most commonly found in the head or tail and less frequently

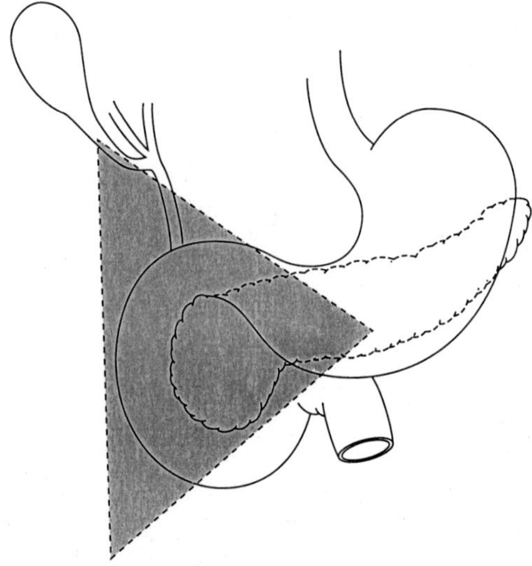

FIGURE 22.4. Most gastrinomas are found within the gastrinoma triangle, which includes the cystic duct, duodenal curve, and junction of the body and neck of the pancreas. (From Stabile et al.,[25] with permission.)

in the body. In some, the entire pancreas is diffusely involved. More than 60% of gastrinomas exhibit malignant behavior, and half of patients have metastases at the time of diagnosis; these figures may drop with earlier screening.

The normal site of gastrin production is G-cells of the gastric antrum. They are stimulated by dietary protein and gastric distension. Gastrin acts to increase acid and pepsin production by the parietal and chief cells of the gastric fundus. With gastrinoma there is unregulated production of gastrin resulting in hypersecretion of acid. Pathologic changes are peptic ulceration, sometimes in an atypical pattern, such as postbulbar duodenal ulcers, multiple duodenal ulcers, jejunal ulcers, or marginal ulcers. In addition, exaggerated gastric rugal folds have been observed. As a result of the trophic effect of gastrin, there is often an increased parietal cell mass.

Patients with gastrinoma present with epigastric pain, weight loss, nausea, vomiting, hematemesis, or melena. Approximately 50% of patients experience diarrhea, sometimes as their only symptom. Diarrhea is due to acid hypersecretion and responds well to nasogastric suction. Some patients have esophagitis with dysphagia. Peptic ulcer disease occurs in 90% of patients with ZES. A high degree of suspicion is necessary to discriminate patients with ZES from the many patients with ulcer disease. Patients presenting with atypical ulceration, hypertrophied gastric mucosal folds, young age of onset, poor medical control, or rapid disease progression should be evaluated for gastrinoma. Prior to the development of a test for serum gastrin, the diagnosis rested on the presence of a triad of an unusual pattern of peptic ulcers, acid hypersecretion while on medical therapy, and an islet cell tumor. More recently, with earlier diagnosis, 30–40% of patients do not have peptic ulcer disease when diagnosed.[142,143] A fasting serum gastrin level of more than 200 pg/ml is suggestive of gastrinoma, and a level over 1000 pg/ml is nearly diagnostic. Hypersecretion can be episodic, so multiple measurements should be made. A basal acid secretion rate of more than 15 mEq/hr (5 mEq/hr after acid-reducing surgery)[144] and a basal/maximal acid output ratio of more than 0.6 is suggestive of gastrinoma. An intravenous secretin stimulation test is performed by administering 2 U/kg and measuring the serum gastrin level at 2, 5, 10, and 20 minutes. Gastrinoma is associated with a more than 100% or an absolute 200 pg/ml increase over baseline.[145] Hypergastrinemia due to other causes must be excluded. Gastric outlet obstruction, G-cell hyperplasia, and retained excluded gastric antrum also result in high acid output (ulcerogenic) hypergastrinemia. Conditions with low acid output hypergastrinemia are pernicious anemia, chronic atrophic gastritis, chronic renal insufficiency, vagotomy, and short gut syndrome.

Patients with gastrinoma should undergo CT or MRI scanning to search for primary and metastatic tumor. Additional tumor masses may be detected with selective angiography, with or without secretin stimulation.[146] Liver lesions suspicious for metastases should be evaluated with percutaneous biopsy. If no distant metastases are detected, an attempt is made to locate and clear all tumor tissue. Preoperatively, acid secretion is controlled with the proton pump inhibitors omeprazole 40–160 mg/day or lansoprazole 30–90 mg/day. Malnutrition must be corrected. Pancreatic lesions less than 2 cm and not associated with the pancreatic duct can be removed by enucleation, whereas larger tumors can be removed by distal pancreatectomy or pancreaticoduodenectomy, depending on location. All suspicious lymph nodes and nodules should be removed, and some surgeons recommend systematic sampling. If no tumor is located initially, intraoperative ultrasonography can be used to detect nonpalpable lesions[147] and duodenotomy[148] or endoscopic transillumination[149] can be performed to search for duodenal lesions. In the few patients in whom no tumor is found, parietal cell vagotomy or gastrectomy can be performed. In one series, tumor could be identified in 78% of patients and resected in 58%.[142] Many patients have a recurrence. Total gastrectomy should be considered for patients in whom tumor is left behind or who have peptic ulcer complications while on maximal therapy.

There is little effective therapy for unresectable gastrinoma. Death occurs secondarily to the direct progression of tumor, not ulcer disease, because the stomach, which is the target organ for gastrin, can be removed. Chemotherapy with streptozotocin and 5-fluorouracil has been used but has a poor response rate. Both octreotide and interferon have been shown to reduce serum gastrin, and interferon can reduce tumor size. Essentially, surgery remains the only hope for cure.

## VIPoma

VIPomas, tumors secreting excess vasoactive intestinal peptide (VIP), bear the name Verner-Morrison syndrome, after the two who described the phenomenon in 1958.[150] They occur at a rate of 1 in 10 million people. The range of age at presentation is 5–79 years (mean 47 years).[138] Hypersecretion of prostaglandins and peptide-histidine-isoleucine (PHI) may also be involved in the symptoms produced. Of tumors secreting VIP, 90% are found in the pancreas; most of the others are in the retroperitoneum. Most tumors are larger than 3 cm. About 80% of the tumors are solitary, and 80% are located in the body or tail of the pancreas.[151] The syndrome is a result of diffuse islet cell hyperplasia in a few cases. Extrapancreatic tumors secreting excess VIP that have also been seen are bronchogenic carcinomas, pheochromocytomas, ganglioneuromas, and ganglioneuroblastomas. Most of these tumors are malignant.[151]

VIP secretion results in transfer of water and electrolytes into the lumen of the gastrointestinal tract.[152] Unregulated secretion of VIP results in watery diarrhea, hypokalemia, and achlorhydria (WHDA syndrome).[153] Diarrhea is often intermittent, and patients may have hypochlorhydria, not achlorhydria.[154] The high-volume diarrhea, usually more than 3 liters, is refractory to treatment. The term pancreatic cholera is also used to describe Verner-Morrison syndrome because of the characteristic diarrhea. Cutaneous flushing is observed in 20% of patients.[151] Dilated gallbladder secondary to inhibitory effects of VIP can be seen. The diagnosis is made by the presence of a serum VIP level elevated above the normal range of 0–170 pg/ml.[151] Multiple measurements should be made, as secretion can be episodic.

An attempt should be made to localize the tumor preoperatively using tomographic imaging, ultrasonography, or angiography. Imaging studies should be carefully evaluated for signs of metastasis. Preoperatively, patients require correction of fluid and electrolyte losses. Octreotide can reduce VIP levels and symptoms. For nearly all tumors, treatment is operative resection for attempted cure or reduction of tumor burden. For advanced disease, debulking, octreotide, or indomethacin may reduce symptoms.

## Glucagonoma

Glucagon-producing tumors, or glucagonomas, are rare, occurring in about 1 of 20 million people. Most occur in patients during the fourth to sixth decade of life, but patients as old as 73 years have been reported. Typically, tumors are solitary, are larger than 5 cm, and are usually in the body and tail of the pancreas.[155] In most cases, tumors have metastasized at the time of diagnosis.

Glucogonomas can present with diabetes, severe dermatitis, malnutrition, anemia, glossitis, hypocholesterolemia, hypoproteinemia, or venous thrombosis. Diagnosis is often delayed until the disease is at a late stage, mostly because the clinical signs are subtle and commonly confused with other conditions. The hallmark of glucagonoma is necrolytic migratory erythema, a rash typically occurring in the perineum, lower abdomen, perioral area, or feet. When properly identified, it is pathognomic for glucagonoma. Patients often report diarrhea, nausea, and vomiting. Because excess glucagon results in hyperglycemia, patients can have polyuria, polydipsia, and blurred vision secondary to hyperglycemia; and some patients have been diagnosed with diabetes mellitis. A history of frequent infections may be present. If suspected, serum glucagon, normally below 120 pg/ml, should be measured; levels higher than 500 pg/ml are diagnostic. Insulin is often secondarily elevated. Localization via CT or MRI is usually feasible owing to the large size of these tumors.

Preoperatively, dermatitis should be treated, diabetes controlled, and malnutrition corrected. Steroids, zinc, octreotide, and total parenteral nutrition (TPN) have been shown to improve skin lesions. Heparin therapy should be considered for the prevention of thrombosis. The treatment is surgical excision, and nearly all patients should be explored for possible curative resection. Curative resection is possible in only about 30% of patients. All tumor and metastases detected should be removed, as debulking can reduce symptoms. For unresectable disease streptozotocin and dacarbazine have been used as chemotherapy; octreotide can alleviate symptoms.

## Somatostatinoma

Somatostatin-secreting tumors occur in about 1 per 40 million people annually. The typical age at presentation is 50 years (range 30–84 years). Approximately half are associated with the MEN syndrome. Most tumors are larger than 5 cm in diameter at the time of presentation.[156] Intrapancreatic tumors are usually located in the head of the pancreas. In a series of 48 cases 44% were in the duodenum or jejunum.[156] Hepatic metastasis is observed in most cases. The tumors exhibit unregulated secretion of somatostatin.

Somatostatin has a broad effect on many components of the gastrointestinal tract. It causes a clinical syndrome of steatorrhea, diabetes, and gallstones. Liver metastases are often present at the time of diagnosis. As this disease is rare and the presentation can mimic more common processes, the diagnosis may be overlooked. If somatostatinoma is suspected, serum somatostatin should be measured. Normal somatostatin levels are less than 100 pg/ml, and tumors can be associated with levels as high as 10 ng/ml. Tomographic imaging should be employed to search for tumors and metastases, and the gallbladder should be examined for stones ultrasonographically. Preoperatively, diabetes should be controlled and malnutrition corrected. Most tumors cannot be resected for cure, but resection of all accessible disease can alleviate symptoms. If hypersomatostatinoma cannot be corrected, cholecystectomy should also be performed.

## Nonfunctioning Islet Cell Tumors

About 80% of pancreatic endocrine tumors removed are clinically active; the remainder cause no detectable hormone excess or clinical syndrome and so are described as nonfunctional.[157,158] Nonfunctional islet cell tumors are diagnosed at a frequency of 1 case in 5 million of the general population. It is interesting to note that one autopsy series reported that approximately 1% of cadavers harbored nonfunctioning islet cell tumors.[159] The median age in one series of 20 patients was 44 years (range 22–76 years).[160] Some nonfunctional islet cell tumors secrete pancreatic peptide, which can be detected in the blood. Nonfunctional tumors commonly present at a size larger than 5 cm[161,167] and can be clinically silent until they cause a mass effect,[163] similar to a pancreatic adenocarcinoma. The favored location is the head of the pancreas.[164] It has long been thought that nonfunctional tumors have a higher rate of malignancy and a worse prognosis than functional tumors,[164] but a retrospective review did not find this to be true.[165] They can present with pain, jaundice, mass, hemorrhage, and weight loss.[161,166] After preoperative evaluation with tomographic imaging and angiography if necessary, resectable lesions should be managed with distal pancreatectomy or pancreaticoduodenectomy. Biliary and gastric bypass should be performed in patients who become obstructed or are found to have unresectable disease on exploration. Chemotherapy with 5-fluorouracil and streptozotocin has been used with symptomatic response in as many as 60% of patients.[167,168]

## Other Endocrine Tumors of the Pancreas

A variety of active substances not usually seen in islet cells can be secreted by rare islet cell tumors. Syndromes of excess secretion of calcitonin, neurotensin,[169] growth hormone-releasing factor,[170] ACTH,[171] parathyroid hormone-like factor, and peptide-histidine-methionine have been seen. Carcinoids secreting serotonin or substance P can arise in islet cells.

## References


1. US Bureau of the Census: Population Projections. Government Printing Office: Washington, DC, 1993.
2. Glazer HS, Weyman PJ, Sagel SS, et al. Nonfunctioning adrenal masses: incidental discovery on computed tomography. AJR 1982;139:81–85.
3. Newsome HH. Adrenal glands. In: Greenfield LJ, Mulholland MW, Oldham KT, et al. (eds) Surgery: Scientific Principles and Practice. Lippincott: Philadelphia, 1993: 1209–1224.
4. Carpenter PC. Cushing's syndrome: update of diagnosis and management. Mayo Clin Proc 1986;61:49–58.
5. Tsagarakis S, Grossman A. The hypothalamic-pituitary-adrenal axis in senescence. In: Morley JE, Dorenman SG (eds) Endocrinology and Metabolism in the Elderly. Blackwell Scientific: Boston, 1992:70–93.
6. Morley JE. Hormones, aging, and endocrine disorders in the elderly. In: Felig P, Baxter JD, Frohman LA (eds) Endocrinology and Metabolism, 3rd ed. McGraw-Hill: New York, 1995:1813.
7. MacLennan WJ, Peden NR. Pituitary and adrenal disorders. In: MacLennan WJ, Peden NR (eds) Metabolic and Endocrine Problems in the Elderly. Springer: Berlin, 1989: 124–135.
8. Merrell RC. Aldosterone-producing tumors (Conn's syndrome). Semin Surg Oncol 1990;6:66–70.
9. Herrera MF, Grant CS, van Heerden JA, et al. Incidentally discovered adrenal tumors: an institutional perspective. Surgery 1991:110:1014–1021.
10. Lucon AM, Pereira MAA, Mendonça BB, et al. Pheochromocytoma: study of 50 cases. J Urol 1997;157:1208–1212.
11. Van Heerden JA, Young WF Jr, Grant CS, Carpenter PC. Adrenal surgery for hypercortisolism—surgical aspects. Surgery 1995;117:466–472.
12. Han M, Burnett AL, Fishman EK, et al. The natural history and treatment of adrenal myelolipoma. J Urol 1997;157: 1213–1216.
13. Linos DA, Stylopoulos N, Boukis M, et al. Anterior, posterior, or laparoscopic approach for the management of adrenal diseases? Am J Surg 1997;173:120–125.
14. Proye CAG, Huart JY, Cuvillier XD, et al. Safety of the posterior approach in adrenal surgery: experience in 105 cases. Surgery 1993;114:1126–1131.
15. Lo CY, van Heerden JA, Grant CS, Söreide JA, Warner MA, Ilstrup DM. Adrenal surgery in the elderly: too risky? World J Surg 1996;20:368–374.
16. Doherty GM, Nieman LK, Cutler GB Jr, et al. Time to recovery of the hypothalamic-pituitary-adrenal axis after curative resection of adrenal tumors in patients with Cushing's syndrome. Surgery 1990;108:1085–1090.
17. Brunicardi FC, Rosman PM, Lesser KL, et al. Current status of adrenalectomy for Cushing's disease. Surgery 1985; 98:1127–1133.
18. Sjöberg HE, Blombäck M, Granberg PO. Thromboembolic complications, heparin treatment and increase in coagulation factors in Cushing's syndrome. Acta Med Scand 1976;199:95–98.
19. Obara T, Ito Y, Okamoto T, et al. Risk factors associated with postoperative persistent hypertension in patients with primary aldosteronism. Surgery 1992;112:987–993.
20. Peplinski GR, Norton JA. The predictive value of diagnostic tests for pheochromocytoma. Surgery 1994;116:1101–1110.
21. Sutton MG St J, Sheps SG, Lie JT. Prevalence of clinically unsuspected pheochromocytoma: review of a 50-year autopsy series. Mayo Clin Proc 1981;56:354–360.
22. Samaan NA, Hickey RC, Shutts PE. Diagnosis, localization, and management of pheochromocytoma: pitfalls and follow-up in 41 patients. Cancer 1988;62:2451–2460.
23. Terzolo M, Ali A, Osella G, et al. Prevalence of adrenal carcinoma among incidentally discovered adrenal masses: a retrospective study from 1989 to 1994. Arch Surg 1997;132: 914–919.
24. Henley DJ, van Heerden JA, Grant CS, et al. Adrenal cortical carcinoma: a continuing challenge. Surgery 1983;94:926–931.
25. Pommier RF, Brennan MF. An eleven-year experience with adrenocortical carcinoma. Surgery 1992;112:963–971.
26. Luton JP, Cerdas S, Billaud L, et al. Clinical features of adrenocortical carcinoma, prognostic factors, and the effect of mitotane therapy. N Engl J Med 1990;322:1195–1201.
27. Dieckmann K-P, Hamm B, Pickartz H, et al. Adrenal myelolipoma: clinical, radiologic, and histologic features. Urology 1987;29:1–8.
28. Cushing H. The baasophil adenomas of the pituitary body and their clinical manifestations (pituitary basophilism). Bull Johns Hopkins Hosp 1932;50:137–195.

29. Roth GS, Livingston JN. Reductions in glucocorticoid inhibition of glucose oxidation and presumptive glucocorticoid receptor content in rat adipocytes during aging. Endocrinology 1976;99:831–839.
30. Orth DN. Cushing's syndrome. N Engl J Med 1995;332: 791–803.
31. Rosenbaum AH, Schatzberg ÑF, MacLaughlin RA, et al. The dexamethasone suppression test in normal control subjects: comparison of two assays and effect of age. Am J Psychiatry 1984;141:1550–1555.
32. Avgerinos PC, Yanovski JA, Oldfield EH, Nieman LK, Cutler GB Jr. The metyrapone and dexamethasone suppression tests for the differential diagnosis of the adrenocorticotropin-dependent Cushing syndrome: a comparison. Ann Intern Med 1994;121:318–327.
33. Schteingart DE. The diagnosis and medical management of Cushing's syndrome. In: Thompson NW, Vinik AW (eds) Endocrine Surgery Update. Grune & Stratton: Orlando, 1983:87.
34. Neville AM, O'Hare MJ. Aspects of structure, function and pathology. In: James VHT (ed) The Adrenal Gland. Raven: New York, 1979:1–66.
35. Bertagna C, Orth DN. Clinical and laboratory findings and results of therapy in 58 patients with adrenocortical tumors admitted to a single medical center (1951 to 1978). Am J Med 1981;71:855–875.
36. Salassa RM, Laws ER, Carpenter PC, et al. Cushing's disease: 50 years later. Trans Am Clin Climatol Assoc 1982;94:122–129.
37. Valimaki M, Pelkonen R, Porkka L, et al. Long-term results of adrenal surgery in patients with Cushing's syndrome due to adrenocortical adenoma. Clin Endocrinol (Oxf) 1984;20:229–236.
38. Prinz RA. A comparison of laparoscopic and open adrenalectomies. Arch Surg 1995;130:489–494.
39. McLeod MK. Complications following adrenal surgery. J Natl Med Assoc 1990;83:161–164.
40. Malmaeus J, Markæs A, Oberg K, et al. Adrenal gland surgery: preoperative location of lesions, histologic findings and outcome of surgery. Acta Chir Scand 1986;152: 577–581.
41. Grabner P, Jauer-Jensen M, Jervell J, et al. Long-term results of treatment of Cushing's disease by adrenalectomy. Eur J Surg 1991;157:461–464.
42. Blichert-Toft M, Bagerskov A, Lockwood K, et al. Operative treatment, surgical approach, and related complications in 195 operations upon the adrenal gland. Surg Gynecol Obstet 1972;135:261–266.
43. Sarkar R, Thompson NW, McLeod MK. The role of adrenalectomy in Cushing's syndrome. Surgery 1990;108:1079–1084.
44. Zeiger MA, Fraker DL, Pass HI, et al. Effective reversibility of the signs and symptoms of hypercortisolism by bilateral adrenalectomy. Surgery 1993;114;1138–1134.
45. Lacroix A, Bolté E, Tremblay J, et al. Gastric inhibitory polypeptide-dependent cortisol hypersecretion: a new cause of Cushing's syndrome. N Engl J Med 1992;327; 974–980.
46. Reznik Y, Allali-Zerah V, Chayvialle JA, et al. Food-dependent Cushing's syndrome mediated by aberrant adrenal sensitivity to gastric inhibitory polypeptide. N Engl J Med 1992;327:98–99.
47. Priestley JT, Sprague RG, Walters W, Salassa RM. Subtotal adrenalectomy for Cushing's syndrome: a preliminary report of 29 cases. Ann Surg 1951;134:464–472.
48. Bennett AH, Cain JP, Dluhy RG, Tynes WV, Harrison JH, Thorn GW. Surgical treatment of adrenocortical hyperplasas: 20-year experience. J Urol 1973;109:321–324.
49. O'Riordain DS, Farley DR, Young WF Jr, Grant CS, van Heerden JA. Long-term outcome of bilateral adrenalectomy in patients with Cushing's syndrome. Surgery 1994;116:1088–1094.
50. Young WF Jr, Hogan MJ, Klee GG, et al. Primary aldosteronism: diagnosis and management. Mayo Clin Proc 1990;65:96–110.
51. Dunnick NR, Leight GS Jr, Roubidoux MA, et al. CT in the diagnosis of primary aldosteronism: sensitivity in 29 patients. Am J Radiol 1993;160:321–324.
52. Melby JC. Diagnosis of hyperaldosteronism. Endocrinol Metab Clin North Am 1991;20:247–255.
53. Nakada T, Kubota Y, Sasagawa I, et al. Therapeutic outcome of primary aldosteronism: adrenalectomy versus enucleation of aldosterone-producing adenoma. J Urol 1995;153:1775–1780.
54. Schenker Y. Medical treatment of low-renin aldosteronism. Endocrinol Metab Clin North Am 1989;18:415–442.
55. Meikle AW, Daynes RA, Araneo BA. Adrenal androgen secretion and biologic effects. Endocrinol Metab Clin North Am 1991;20:381–400.
56. Gabrilove JL, Seman AT, Sabet R, et al. Virilizing adrenal adenoma with studies. 1981;2:462–470.
57. Gabrilove JL, Sharma DC, Wotiz HH, Dorfman RI. Feminizing adrenocoartical tumors in the male: a review of 52 cases including a case report. Medicine 1965;44:37–79.
58. Cryer PE. Phaeochromocytoma. Clin Endocrinol Metab 1985;14:203–220.
59. Sheps SG, Jiang N-S, Klee GG. Diagnostic evaluation of pheochromocytoma. Endocrinol Metab Clin North Am 1988;17:397–414.
60. Van Heerden JA, Sheps SG, Hamberger B, et al. Pheochromocytoma: current status and changing trends. Surgery 1982;91:367–373.
61. Bastounis EA, Karayiannakis AJ, Anapliotou MLG, et al. Incidentalomas of the adrenal gland: diagnostic and therapeutic implications. Am Surg 1997;63:356–360.
62. Cance WG, Wells SA Jr. Multiple endocrine neoplasia type IIa. Curr Probl Surg 1985;22:7–56.
63. Richard S, Beigelman C, Duclos J-M, et al. Pheochromocytoma as the first manifestation of von Hippel-Lindau disease. Surgery 1994;116:10076–10081.
64. Khosla S, Patel VM, Hay ID, et al. Loss of heterozygosity suggests multiple genetic alterations in pheochromocytomas and medullary thyroid carcinomas. J Clin Invest 1991;87:1691–1699.
65. Pick L. Das ganglioma embryonale sympathicum, eine typische bosartige geschwuestform des sympathischen nerven systems. Berl Klin Wochenschr 1912;49:16–22.
66. Olson JA Jr, Wells SA Jr. In: Sabiston DC Jr, Lyerly HK, (eds). Textbook of Surgery the Biological Basis of Modern Surgical Practice, 15th ed. Saunders, Philadelphia, 1997:694, with permission.

67. Zuckerkandl E. Ueber neben organe des sympathicus in retroperitonaealraum des menschen. Anat Anz 1901;15:97.
68. Altergott R, Barbato A, Lawrence A, et al. Spectrum of catecholamine-secreting tumors of the organ of Zuckerkandl. Surgery 1985;98:1121–1126.
69. Remine WH, Chong GC, van Heerden JA, et al. Current management of pheochromocytoma. Ann Surg 1974;179: 740–748.
70. Orchard T, Grant CS, van Heerden JA, et al. Pheochromocytoma: continuing evolution of surgical therapy. Surgery 1993;114:1153–1159.
71. Gifford RW Jr, Manger WM, Bravo EL. Pheochromocytoma. Endocrinol Metab Clin North Am 1994;23:387–404.
72. Bravo EL, Gifford RW Jr. Pheochromocytoma. Endocrinol Metab Clin North Am 1993;22:329–341.
73. Shapiro B, Fig LM. Management of pheochromocytoma. Endocrinol Metab Clin North Am 1989;18: 443–481.
74. Abecassis M, McLoughlin MJ, Langer B, et al. Serendipitous adrenal masses: prevalence, significance and management. Am J Surg 1985;149:783–788.
75. Hedeland H, Östberg G, Hökfelt B. On the prevalence of adrenocortical adenomas in an autopsy material in relation to hypertension and diabetes. Acta Med Scand 1968; 184:211–214.
76. Kokko JP, Brown TC, Berman MM. Adrenal adenoma and hypertension. Lancet 1967;1:468–470.
77. Russi S, Blumenthal HT. Small adenomas of the adrenal cortex in hypertension and diabetes. Arch Intern Med 1945;76:284–290.
78. Russell RP, Mas AT, Richter ED. Adrenal cortical adenomas and hypertension: a clinical pathologic analysis of 690 cases with material controls and a review of the literature. Medicine 1972;51:211–225.
79. Commons RR, Callaway CP. Adenomas of the adrenal cortex. Arch Intern Med 1948;81:37–41.
80. Hensen J, Stark S, Pavel M, et al. Non-functioning adrenocortical adenomas (ACA): age and sex dependency. Presented at the 76th Annual Meeting of the Endocrine Society, June 15, 1994, Anaheim, CA.
81. Copeland PM. The incidentally discovered adrenal mass. Ann Intern Med 1983;98;940–945.
82. Belldegrun A, Hussain S, Seltzer SE, et al. Incidentally discovered mass of adrenal gland. Surg Gynecol Obstet 1986;163:203–208.
83. Gajraj H, Young AE. Adrenal incidentaloma. Br J Surg 1993:80:422–426.
84. Ross NS, Aron DC. Hormonal evaluation of the patient with an incidentally discovered adrenal mass. N Engl J Med 1990;323:1401–1405.
85. Bitter DA, Ross DS. Incidentally discovered adrenal masses. Am J Surg 1989;158:159–161.
86. Didolkar MS, Bescher RA, Elias EG, et al. Natural history of adrenal cortical carcinoma: a clinicopathologic study of 42 patients. Cancer 1981;47:2153–2161.
87. Zornoza J, Bernardino ME. Bilateral adrenal metastasis: "head light" sign. Urology 1980;15:91–92.
88. Pagani JJ, Bernardino ME. Incidence and significance of serendipitous CT findings in the oncologic patient. J Comput Assist Tomogr 1982;6:268–275.
89. Candel AG, Gattuso P, Reyes CV, et al. Fine-needle aspiration biopsy of adrenal masses in patients with extraadrenal malignancy. Surgery 1993;114:1132–1137.
90. Abeshouse GA, Goldstein RB, Abeshouse BS. Adrenal cysts: review of the literature and report of three cases. J Urol 1959;81:711–719.
91. Zografos GC, Driscoll DL, Karakousis CP, et al. Adrenal adenocarcinoma: a review of 53 cases. J Surg Oncol 1994;55:160–164.
92. Icard P, Chapuis Y, Andreassian B, et al. Adrenocortical carcinoma in surgically treated patients: a retrospective study on 156 cases by the French Association of Endocrine Surgery. Surgery 1992;112:972–980.
93. Bodie B, Novick AC, Pontes JE, et al. The Cleveland Clinic experience with adrenal cortical carcinoma. J Urol 1989; 141:257–260.
94. Gross MD, Shapiro B, Boufard AJ, et al. Distinguish benign from malignant euadrenal masses. Ann Intern Med 1988; 109:613–618.
95. Kloos RT, Gross MD, Francis IR, et al. Incidentally discovered adrenal masses. Endocr Rev 1995;16:460–484.
96. Schorr I, Tathnam, Saxena BB, et al. Multiple specific hormone receptors in the adenylate cyclase of an adrenocortical carcinoma. J Biol Chem 1971;246:5806–5811.
97. Reznek RH, Armstrong P. Imaging in endocrinology: the adrenal gland. Clin Endocrinol (Oxf) 1994;40:561–576.
98. Falke THM, Sandler MO. Classification of silent adrenal masses: time to get practical. J Nucl Med 1994;35: 1152–1154.
99. Kvols LK, Buck M. Chemotherapy of endocrine malignancies: a review. Semin Oncol 1987;14:343–353.
100. Schteingart DE, Motazedi A, Noonan RA, et al. Treatment of adrenal carcinomas. Arch Surg 1982;117:1142–1146.
101. Vassilopoulou-Sellin R, Guinee VF, Klein MJ, et al. Impact of adjuvant mitotane on the clinical course of patients with adrenocortical cancer. Cancer 1993;71:3119–3123.
102. Gierke E. Über Knochenmarksgewebe in der nebenniere. Bietr Z Pathol Anat 1905;37(suppl 7):311.
103. Oberling C. Les formations myelo-lipomateuses. Bull Assoc Fr Etude Cancer 1929;18:234.
104. Plaut A. Myelolipoma in the adrenal cortex. Am J Pathol 1958;34:487.
105. McDonnell WV. Myelolipomas of adrenal. Arch Pathol 1956;61:416.
106. Olsson CA, Krane RJ, Klugo RC, et al. Adrenal Myelolipoma. Surgery 1973;73:665–670.
107. Meaglia JP, Schmidt JD. Natural history of an adrenal myelolipoma. J Urol 1992;147:1089–1090.
108. Cyran KM, Kenney PJ, Memel DS, et al. Adrenal myelolipoma. AJR 1996;166:395–400.
109. Oliva A, Duarte B, Hammadeh R, et al. Myelolipoma and endocrine dysfunction. Surgery 1988;103:711–715.
110. Filobbos SA, Seddon JA. Myelolipoma of the adrenal 1980. Br J Surg 1980;67:147–148.
111. Albala DM, Chung CJ, Sueoka BL, et al. Hemorrhagic myelolipoma of adrenal gland after blunt trauma. Urology 1991;38:559–562.
112. Medeiros LJ, Wolf BC. Traumatic rupture of an adrenal myelolipoma [letter]. Arch Pathol Lab Med 1983;107:500.
113. Mayo CW. Paroxysmal hypertension with tumor of retroperitoneal nerve. JAMA 1927;89:1047.

114. Vargas HI, Davoussi LR, Bartlett DL, et al. Laparoscopic adrenalectomy: a new standard of care. Urology 1997; 49:673–678.
115. Young HH. A technique for simultaneous exposure and operation on the adrenals. Surg Gynecol Obstet 1936; 54:179–188.
116. Russell CF, Hamberger B, van Heerden JA, et al. Adrenalectomy: anterior or posterior approach? Am J Surg 1982;144:322–324.
117. Buell JF, Alexander HR, Norton JA, et al. Bilateral adrenalectomy for Cushing's syndrome: anterior versus posterior surgical approach. Ann Surg 1997;225:63–68.
118. Gagner M, Lacroix A, Prinz RA, et al. Early experience with laparoscopic approach for adrenalectomy. Surgery 1993; 114:1120–1125.
119. Norton JA. Neuroendocrine tumors of the pancreas and duodenum. Curr Probl Surg 1994;31:79–156.
120. Kloppel G, Heitz PU. Pancreatic endocrine tumors. Pathol Res Pract 1988;183:155–168.
121. Larsson C, Skogseid B, Öberg K, et al. Multiple endocrine neoplasia type 1 gene maps to chromosome 11 and is lost in insulinoma. Nature 1988;332:85–87.
122. Burke AP, Sobin LH, Shekitka KM, et al. Somatostatin-producing duodenal carcinoids in patients with von Recklinghausen's neurofibromatosis: a predilection for black patients. Cancer 1990;65:1591–1595.
123. Binkovitz LA, Johnson CD, Stephens DH. Islet cell tumors in von Hippel-Lindau disease: increased prevalence and relationship to multiple endocrine neoplasia. AJR 1990; 155:501–505.
124. Davoren PM, Epstein MT. Insulinoma complicating tuberous sclerosis [letter]. J Neurol Neurosurg Psychiatry 1992; Y5:1209.
125. Doherty GM, Doppman JL, Shawker TH, et al. Results of a prospective strategy to diagnose, localize and resect insulinoma. Surgery 1991;110:989–997.
126. Mozell E, Stenzel P, Woltering EA, et al. Functional endocrine tumors of the pancreas: clinical presentation, diagnosis, and treatment. Curr Probl Surg 1990:309–383.
127. Sheppard BC, Norton JA, Doppman JL, et al. Management of islet cell tumors in patients with multiple endocrine neoplasia; a prospective study. Surgery 1989;106:1108–1118.
128. Pasieka JL, McLeod MK, Thompson NW, et al. Surgical approach to insulinomas assessing the need for localization. Arch Surg 1992;127:442–447.
129. Grunberger G, Weiner JL, Silverman R, et al. Factitious hypoglycemia due to surreptitious administration of insulin: diagnosis, treatment and long-term follow-up. Ann Intern Med 1988;188:252–257.
130. Norton JA, Shawker TH, Doppman JL, et al. Localization and surgical treatment of occult insulinomas. Ann Surg 1990;212:615–620.
131. Rosch T, Lightdale CJ, Botet JF, et al. Localization of pancreatic endocrine tumors by endoscopic ultrasonography. N Engl J Med 1992;172:1721–1726.
132. Doppman JL, Miller DL, Chang R, et al. Insulinomas localization with selective intraarterial injection of calcium. Radiology 1991;178:327–241.
133. Rothmund M, Angelini L, Brunt LM, et al. Surgery for benign insulinoma: an international review. World J Surg 1990;14:393–399.
134. Buchanan KD, Johnston CF, O'Hare MMT, et al. Neuroendocrine tumors: a European view. Am J Med 1986;81(suppl 68):14–23.
135. Eriksson B, Oberg K, Skogseid B. Neuroendocrine pancreatic tumors: clinical findings in a prospective study of 84 patients. Acta Oncol 1989;28:373–377.
136. Zollinger RM, Ellison EH. Primary peptic ulcerations of the jejunum associated with islet cell tumors of the pancreas. Ann Surg 1955;142:709–723.
137. Jensen RT, Gardner JD. Zollinger-Ellison syndrome: clinical presentation, pathology, diagnosis and treatment. In: Dannenberg A, Zakim D (eds) Peptic Ulcer and Other Acid-Related Diseases. Academic Research Association: New York, 1991:117–121.
138. Delcore R, Friesen SR. Gastrointestinal neuroendocrine tumors. J Am Coll Surg 178:187–211.
139. Pipeleers-Marichal M, Somers G, Willems G, et al. Gastrinomas in the duodenums of patients with multiple endocrine neoplastic type 1 and the Zollinger-Ellison syndrome. N Engl J Med 1990;322:723–727.
140. Stabile BE, Morrow DJ, Passaro E. The gastrinoma triangle: operative implications. Am J Surg 1984;147:25–31, with permission.
141. Thom AK, Norton JA, Axotis CA, et al. Location, incidence and malignant potential of duodenal gastrinomas. Surgery 1991;110:1086–1093.
142. Norton JA, Doppman JL, Jensen RT. Curative resection in Zollinger-Ellison syndrome: results of a 10 year prospective study. Ann Surg 1992;215:8–18.
143. Anderson DK. Current diagnosis and management of Zollinger-Ellison Syndrome. Ann Surg 1989;210:685–703.
144. Maton PN, Frucht H, Vinayek R, et al. Medical management of patients with Zollinger-Ellison syndrome. Gastroenterology 1988;94:924–929.
145. Frucht H, Howard JM, Slaff JF. Secretin and calcium, provocative tests in patients with Zollinger-Ellison syndrome: a prospective study. Ann Intern Med 1989;111: 713–722.
146. Imamura M, Takahashi K, Adachi H, et al. Usefulness of selective arterial secretin injection test for localization of gastrinoma in the Zollinger-Ellison syndrome. Ann Surg 1987;205:230–239.
147. Norton JA, Cromack DT, Showker TH, et al. Intraoperative ultrasonographic localization of islet cell tumors. Ann Surg 1988;207:160–168.
148. Thompson NW, Vinik AI, Eckhauser FE. Microgastrinomas of the duodenum. Ann Surg 1989;209:396–404.
149. Sugg SL, Norton JA, Fraker DL, et al. A prospective study of intraoperative methods to diagnose and resect duodenal gastrinomas. Ann Surg 1993;218:138–144.
150. Verner JV, Morrison AB. Islet cell tumor and a syndrome of refractory watery diarrhea and hypokalemia. Am J Med 1958;25:374–380.
151. Mekhjian HS, O'Dorisio TM. VIPoma syndrome. Semin Oncol 1987;14:282–291.
152. Rambaud JR, Modigliani R, Matuchansky C, et al. Pancreatic cholera: studies on tumoral secretion and pathophysiology of diarrhea. Gastroenterology 1975;69: 110–122.

153. Marks IN, Bank S, Louw JH. Islet cell tumor of the pancreas with reversible watery diarrhea and achlorhydria. Gastroenterology 1967;53:695–708.
154. Verner JV, Morrison AB. Endocrine pancreatic islet disease with diarrhea: report of a case due to diffuse hyperplasia of nonbeta islet tissue with a review of 54 additional cases. Arch Intern Med 1974;133:492–500.
155. Boden G. Glucagonomas and insulinomas. Gastroenterol Clin North Am 1989;18:831–845.
156. Boden G, Shimoyama R. Somatostatinoma. In: Cohen S, Soloway RD (eds) Hormone-Producing Tumors of the Gastrointestinal Tract. Churchill Livingstone: New York, 1985:85.
157. Dent RB, van Heerden JA, Weiland LJ. Nonfunctioning islet cell tumors. Ann surg 1981;193:185–193.
158. Broughan TA, Leslie JD, Soto JM, et al. Pancreatic islet cell tumors. Surgery 1986;99:671–678.
159. Weil C. Gastroenteropancreatic endocrine tumors. Klin Wochenschr 1985;63:433–459.
160. Cheslyn-Curtis S, Sitaram V, Williams RCN. Management of non-functioning neuroendocrine tumours of the pancreas. Br J Surg 1993;80:625–627.
161. Legaspi A, Brennan MF. Management of islet cell carcinoma. Surgery 1988;104:1018–1023.
162. Langstein HN, Norton JA, Chaiang HCV, et al. The utility of circulating levels of human pancreatic polypeptide as a marker of islet cell tumors. Surgery 1990;108: 1109–1116.
163. Dial PF, Braasch JW, Rossi, RL, et al. Management of nonfunctioning islet cell tumors of the pancreas. Surg Clin North Am 1985;65:291–299.
164. Eckhauser FE, Chung PS, Vinik AI, et al. Nonfunctioning malignant neuroendocrine tumors of the pancreas. Surgery 1986;100:978–988.
165. White TJ, Edney JA, Thompson JS, et al. Is there a prognostic difference between functional and nonfunctional islet cell tumors? Am J Surg 1994;168:627–630.
166. Thompson GB, van Heerden JA, Grant CS, et al. Islet cell carcinomas of the pancreas: a twenty-year experience. Surgery 1988;104:1011–1017.
167. Broder LE, Carter SK. Pancreatic islet cell carcinoma: clinical features of 52 patients. Ann Intern Med 1973;79:101–107.
168. Moertel CF, Hanley JA, Johnson LA. Streptozocin alone compared with streptozocin plus fluorouracil in the treatment of advanced islet-cell carcinoma. N Engl J Med 1980;292:941–945.
169. Blackburn AM, Bryant MG, Adrian TE, et al. Pancreatic tumors produce neurotensin. J Clin Endocrinol Metab 1981;52:820–822.
170. Bostwick DG, et al. Growth hormone-releasing factor immunoreactivity in human endocrine tumors. Am J Pathol 1984;117:167–170.
171. Corrin B, et al. Oat cell carcinoma of the pancreas with ectopic ACTH secretion. Cancer 31:1523–1527.

# Invited Commentary: Breast Cancer

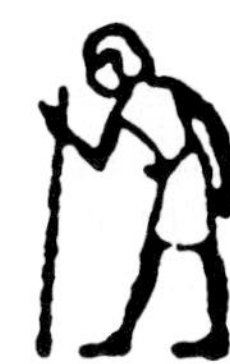

David W. Kinne

Thirty years ago, when I was a surgical house officer at Columbia-Presbyterian Medical Center, the approach favored for breast cancer management was monolithic. Under the leadership of Cushman Haagensen, patients who were deemed operable (and thus potentially curable) according to the Columbia Clinical Classification he had developed, were advised to undergo radical mastectomy. It included a wide skin margin around the primary tumor and a split-thickness skin graft taken from the thigh for closure of the wound. No two-step procedures were advised; it was believed that as soon as the tumor was biopsied, potential systemic spread occurred. The preferred approach was biopsy (incisional for large tumors, excisional for small ones), frozen section, and once the diagnosis of breast cancer was confirmed, radical mastectomy. The commitment to wide excision was such that after the diagnosis had been established the breast, axilla, and a thigh were prepared and draped after gowns, gloves, and instruments had been changed. The initial procedure was to take the skin graft from one thigh—a skin graft was always necessary.

This approach was favored for elderly patients as well, so long as their medical condition permitted it. In Haagensen's analysis of 181 patients over the age of 65 years, all but three underwent radical mastectomy. These three, because of poor medical conditions, underwent modified radical mastectomy, a procedure he believed to be unsatisfactory and unlikely to produce cure rates equal to the radical mastectomy. In his words, "neither old age nor moderate cardiovascular disease is a contraindication to radical mastectomy."

Other surgical leaders at Columbia during that period questioned the need for this procedure. Following the lead of Patey and others, and responding to patients' objections to the cosmetic deformity caused by the radical surgery, Auchincloss reported a series of breast cancer patients upon whom he had performed modified radical mastectomy. He believed the axillary dissection to be just as complete as with the radical, with far better cosmetic results due to pectoral muscle preservation and a more oblique incision without a skin graft.

As a senior resident during the late 1960s, well trained to do the Haagensen radical mastectomy, I was helped by Dr. David Habif to do a modified radical mastectomy. I was unfamiliar with and puzzled by the procedure, but I helped him do it. As was the custom of the day, all surgical attending physicians saw the patients and their wounds at weekly surgical grand rounds. I can still recall the shocked looks on the faces of these senior, respected surgeons when they saw this patient's wound. Clearly, they believed we had done an inadequate procedure and doomed her to die of breast cancer.

During the past three decades, there have been dramatic changes in our understanding of the biologic behavior of breast cancer, the means of improved, earlier diagnosis, and therapeutic options, both locoregional and systemic. These changes have been brought about by prospective, randomized trials. The radical mastectomy is no longer done except in rare circumstances. These changes have had an impact on all patients with breast cancer, the elderly included.

One of the major facts, leading no doubt to the publication of this book, is that fortunately women (and men) are living to greater ages and in healthier conditions than in the past. Life style changes, such as better diets, exercise, avoiding tobacco, and consuming alcohol in moderation, may be partly responsible. Improved methods of diagnosis and management of medical conditions have contributed to greater longevity as well. Despite this healthier old population, it is well recognized that the risk of breast cancer increases with each decade of life. Thus, the diagnosis and management of breast cancer in the elderly has become extremely important. I believe we should emphasize that old patients be evaluated and managed according to their physiologic age (or performance status), not their chronologic age. An 85-year-old woman may be perfectly healthy (and even athletic); her physiologic age is much "younger" than her chronologic age, and she should be managed just like a younger woman. To put it another way, if she is undertreated because of a philosophy that says "why put this nice old lady through all that treatment," her main health threat is likely to be breast cancer, and the reason for failure would likely be due to inadequate treatment.

It used to be thought that breast cancer was more virulent in young women and more slow-growing in the elderly. Such interpretation may lead to undertreatment of the elderly. In studies where young and old breast cancer patients are matched for stage of disease, specifically the sizes of primary tumors and axillary lymph node status, few or no differences are seen. Furthermore, when investigators analyze breast cancer survival in the elderly, it is not uncommon to observe that mammography is done less often than in young women, and less treatment is offered, with poorer outcomes seen.

Some differences of breast cancer in the elderly may lead to different treatment from that in young patients. Some observations suggest that outpatient breast radiotherapy for 6 weeks after breast-conservation therapy is associated with more morbidity in old women, especially in terms of fatigue. When options of breast conservation versus mastectomy are discussed with these patients, it is not uncommon for them to pick mastectomy, as they perceive it to be a quicker therapy with less morbidity. This is especially true when an older patient verbalizes "I don't need this breast." Mastectomy (without reconstruction) is clearly faster and less expensive than breast conservation with radiotherapy. In studies reporting less breast conservation in old patients than in their young counterparts, this particular sentiment is probably a major reason.

Some point out that in studies where breast irradiation is not undertaken, breast tumor recurrence is more prevalent compared to that in the irradiated group, but no difference in survival is seen. Thus, breast irradiation is necessary to increase chances of saving the breast, but has no survival benefit. In old patients, perhaps with comorbid illnesses, omitting breast radiotherapy may be acceptable; and it seems even more appropriate if the tumor extirpation is by quadrantectomy. In Veronesi's series, treated by quadrantectomy without irradiation, breast recurrences in old patients was much lower than in young women.

Furthermore, most breast cancers in old women are hormone receptor-positive. The use of adjuvant tamoxifen in this group has been shown not only to improve distant disease-free and overall survival but to reduce ipsilateral breast recurrence and contralateral breast cancer. The use of wide excision such as quadrantectomy and tamoxifen affords two reasons to considering omission of breast irradiation in elderly patients.

In patients who develop cancer in the nonirradiated breast, a second chance for breast conservation is possible. Some have tumors too large for conservation, however, and so should be, or may elect to be, managed by mastectomy.

The need for axillary dissection in this age group has been questioned. If primary tumor-related factors (size and hormone receptor status) indicate that tamoxifen should be given, the prognostic information provided by nodal status is not particularly important. If it is judged that even with many positive nodes no aggressive chemotherapy is to be given, perhaps nodal irradiation at the time of breast radiotherapy is advisable to control disease in the nodal bed. The use of a sentinel node biopsy in this age group spares many a nodal dissection. Axillary lymph node dissection should be done in patients with suspicious axillary nodes who are otherwise healthy. Randomized studies are under way and more are needed to indicate optimal ways of managing breast cancer in the older population.

# 23
# Physiologic Changes and Benign Perimenopausal Breast Disease

Sancar Bayar and Barbara A. Ward

Familiarity with breast microanatomy and physiology aids in understanding benign breast physiology. The female breast is composed of ductal and lobular units. The main breast ducts arise from lactiferous sinuses in the nipple and divide several times to form small ducts and then the smallest ductal elements, or "ductules," which in fact form the lobular unit of the breast. The ductules also divide and terminate blindly with club-shaped endings. The ductules are sensitive to hormonal stimulation; during pregnancy they proliferate and form the alveolar components of the breast.[1]

Ductal and lobular units of female breasts can be seen as early as during the neonatal period. Maternal estrogen, progesterone, mammotrophic peptides including prolactin, and human placental lactogen promote growth and development of the fetal breasts. During the neonatal period, the ductal system shows evidence of secretory epithelium and surrounding myoepithelial cells, although these findings involute and a latent phase starts from childhood to puberty.[2]

During puberty, hypothalamic synthesis of gonadotropin-releasing hormone (GnRH) begins. This hormone stimulates release of follicle-stimulating hormone (FSH) and luteinizing hormone (LH) from the pituitary gland. The FSH then stimulates the ovaries, and estradiol synthesis begins. During the first years of puberty, anovulatory cycles are common. Because of this, estradiol is the primary stimulant of the breast during this period. It promotes the elongation and branching of the ductal system and increases the volume of the breasts with fat deposition. When the luteal phase begins, progesterone stimulates dilatation of the ductal system and differentiates the alveolar cells to secretory cells.

The most dramatic alterations in the anatomy and physiology of the breasts occur during pregnancy. Estrogen, progesterone, prolactin, growth hormone (GH), cortisol, and insulin prepare the female breast to lactate, its primary role. Ductal and lobular units of the breast increase in size and complexity. Endings of the ductules become secretory alveoli during this period. Lactogenesis occurs throughout gestation, but lactopoiesis begins after delivery of the child. Estrogen and progesterone are believed to inhibit secretion of milk during gestation.[3]

With the beginning of menopause, ovarian secretion of estrogen and progesterone cease, resulting in breast involution. Lobules are mostly affected in this process. With the progression of involution, glandular epithelium is disrupted and phagocytized. Main ductal systems are least affected; they survive, but their number decreases and some develop cystic changes. Alterations occur in the elastic and collagen fibers, resulting in loss of supporting tissue, and fat deposition increases. The duration of involution of the breast is generally incomplete and variable. Although most of the lobular structures disappear, remnants and mature lobular structures can remain; patient variability is significant.[1,4,5]

## Perimenopausal Benign Breast Disease

Although uncommon, we are faced more frequently with benign breast problems in an aging population. Benign breast disorders are most common in the young population and are again exacerbated by menopause; the frequency of problems declines sharply after menopause.[6]

### Mastalgia and Nodular Breasts

Mastalgia is a term applied to various conditions where pain is present in one or both breasts. This entity can be divided into cyclic and noncyclic pain. Mastalgia and nodular breasts are a common problem in young women during their reproductive period. The most common form of mastalgia in these young patients is cyclical mastalgia and constitutes 67% of the cases. The pain typically occurs during the premenstrual period, accompanied by an increase in breast nodularity. This type of cyclic mastalgia usually resolves after menopause. Noncyclic mastalgia generally starts at the fourth decade. In 50% of persons affected it resolves after menopause, but in the other half it persists.[7] Breast nodularity with or without mastalgia is a common benign breast disorder in the elderly. Devitt reported a 23% incidence in breast nodularity with or without pain in 581 patients with benign breast disorders, a percentage similar to that in young patients.[6]

Although cyclic breast pain generally resolves after menopause, the use of hormone replacement therapy (HRT) may cause these symptoms to persist. HRT is widely used in menopausal women because it reduces the risk of heart attack, stroke, hot flashes, osteoporosis, and other symptomatology. Some patients on HRT suffer from mastalgia and breast nodularity despite the absence of these problems prior to menopause. Although this tenderness is transient and usually resolves in 6 months, it may cause a patient to discontinue therapy. Ryan et al. showed a 5% discontinuation rate in patients treated with HRT for osteoporosis. To prevent mastalgia it is wise to start with a low-dose regimen and increase it gradually.[7–9A]

Many drugs currently used for breast pain relieve symptoms of cyclic mastalgia more effectively than those of noncylic mastalgia. Vitamin E, evening primrose oil, bromocriptine, danazol, tamoxifen, and goserelin are used to treat mastalgia. Vitamin E and evening primrose oil are simple first-line agents with few side effects. Vitamin E capsules provide a dose of 400–800IU per capsule, and typically 1200IU per day is required to achieve an effect. Despite the lack of proven efficacy in randomized clinical trials, some patients report significant benefit. Similarly, evening primrose oil has been shown to produce a good response in 58% of patients with cyclic mastalgia and 38% of those with noncyclic mastalgia. As a dietary manipulation, 4 months of treatment should be endorsed before a therapeutic failure is accepted. If a good response is seen, therapy is continued for a year.

Bromocriptine, a dopamine agonist, when used at a dose of 5mg daily, relieves pain in 47–54% of patients with cyclic mastalgia and in 20–33% of patients with noncyclic mastalgia. Side effects occur in up to one-third of patients and include nausea, headache, postural hypotension, and constipation. These problems may be less severe if the treatment is initiated at 1.25mg/day and increased by 1.25mg increments over 2 weeks until a dosage of 5mg/day is reached. Danazol, a gonadotropin releasing inhibitor, is the most potent agent for inhibiting mastalgia. When used at 200mg daily, it is effective in 70–79% of patients with cyclic mastalgia and 30–40% of those with noncyclic mastalgia. Many patients are unwilling to accept the possible side effects, which include menstrual irregularity, body weight gain, hirsutism, greasy hair and skin, acne, headache, and nausea. To minimize these bothersome side effects, the dosage can be reduced to 100mg per day after 2 months of therapy and then to an every-other-day routine. Treatment may be discontinued after 6 months. Danazol is contraindicated in women with a history of thromboembolic disease.

Tamoxifen at doses of 10–20mg daily may relieve mastalgia as well. Higher doses were no more effective, and hot flashes and menstrual irregularity were common side effects. It can be used in patients resistant to bromocriptine, danazol, and evening primrose oil.

Goserelin, an LH-releasing hormone analogue, can be quite effective. It is given as a subcutaneous depot injection monthly over 6 months and has an overall efficacy of 81% for both cyclic and noncyclic mastalgia. Again, there are unwanted side effects, which include menopausal symptoms and bone mass reduction, so it is reserved for short-term use in severe refractory cases.

Testosterone, gestrinone, and cabergoline are additional agents under investigation. Some other agents were used in the past to treat mastalgia, but current studies do not support their continued use. They include diuretics, vitamin $B_6$ (pyridoxine), and medroxyprogesterone.[7,10]

## Fibroadenoma

Fibroadenomas are rare in the elderly, although they are the most common benign solid lesion of the breast in the young. They constitute 12% of all breast masses in postmenopausal women. There are two classic structural types: intracanalicular or pericanalicular. Generally, the clinical examination, radiologic studies, and fine-needle aspiration (FNA) cytology or core biopsy confirm the diagnosis.[11–13]

Fibroadenomas involute after menopause and calcify. They are frequently seen on the mammogram associated with central heavy amorphous or peripheral coarse calcifications.[14]

Fibroadenomas are considered an aberration of normal development. They arise not from a single cell but from a single lobule and resemble hyperplastic lobules in the breast. They grow and lactate during pregnancy and degenerate during menopause, exhibiting their hormone dependence.[1,13,14]

Sandison, in a surgical series, found 51.4% of cases in those 20–29 years of age and only 5.6% in those 40–49 years. He reported six giant fibroadenomas in those 60–69 years of age among the 110 fibroadenomas found in 1010 women.[15] Frantz et al. also described four gross fibroadenomas after age 40 in 225 postmortem cases studied.[16]

In the elderly, there may be two reasons for the low incidence of fibroadenoma. One is that fibroadenomas generally become less cellular and hyalinized, and sometimes they become fibrotic or disappear in the breast without the influence of estrogen. The other factor may be high resection rates of these masses during reproductive years in women for fear of malignancy. The latter cause is generally less accepted.[11]

Once the diagnosis is established, excision and observation are the two main options. Patients generally prefer excision, although the risk of their becoming malignant is no different from that of normal breast tissue. The problem in general is being certain of the diagnosis of a fibroadenoma, especially in the elderly where the level of suspicion for breast cancer is justifiably high.[13] Calcified involuting fibroadenomas in the elderly do not deserve excision if they have been serially followed mammographically. Spiculation, architectural distortion, and fine and irregular calcifications are signs of coincidental cancer in a fibroadenoma, so further workup and therapy are needed in these patients.[17]

## Ductal Ectasia

Ductal ectasia, or dilatation of the ductal system, is frequently discovered by chance during autopsy or surgery. Grossly, the specimen consists of firm breast tissue with prominent ducts containing pasty or granular secretions. These secretions are white to brown. The walls of the dilated ducts are firm as a result of periductal fibrosis, and sometimes calcium is noted in the ducts.[18] The commonest clinical finding is spontaneous nipple discharge, although nipple retraction may also be seen. The disease may be bilateral. Once it was thought that ductal ectasia and periductal mastitis were related diseases. In the latter situation periductal inflammation and fibrosis destroy the elastic lamina of the ducts and cause ductal dilatation, or possibly true leakage of ductal components from the dilated ducts causes the periductal inflammation.[19,20]

Currently these two conditions are considered to be different diseases because previous and some present studies show that periductal mastitis is most commonly seen in young patients and ductal ectasia in the elderly. Although there is a strong correlation between smoking and periductal mastitis (90%), the correlation between smoking and ductal ectasia is weak (30%). Also, many patients with ductal ectasia do not have a history of periductal mastitis. These data suggest that they are different disease entities.[21]

On mammography ductal ectasia may be seen as dilated ducts underneath the areola that are fairly symmetric. Asymmetric and solitary ducts may be pathologic. Intraductal papilloma and carcinoma must be ruled out in these cases.[22]

Because ductal ectasia increases with age, it is diagnosed more frequently in the elderly. Frantz et al. based a study on 225 postmortem examinations and showed that 52 of 54 patients with ductal ectasia were postmenopausal at the time of death, and most of the patients were older than 50 years. Eleven percent of these patients had nipple retraction.[16]

Sandison reviewed the association of cystic disease and ductal ectasia and found that 574 of 800 cases were affected (71.4%). He found that by the fourth decade, more than 60% of women were affected. The maximum incidence was noted between ages 76–80 and 81–85. They were rare in patients age 21–25 and 86–90.[23]

Patients suffering from nipple discharge may gain benefit from surgery. Major duct excision with removal of the central nipple ducts is performed. If a fistula is present, it may be opened or excised. Pathology demonstrates prominent ductal dilatation and mild to moderate periductal chronic inflammation. Recurrence may be seen in patients when excision is incomplete. Also, reconnection of the divided ducts may cause this problem, and reoperation is needed in these cases.[19]

## Cystic Disease of the Breast

Cysts of the breast are common in those 40–50 years of age. Patients with cysts suffer from breast pain or a lump in their breast. Frequently cysts are discovered incidentally during radiologic screening.

There are two types of cysts. One is lined with apocrine epithelium and the other with flattened epithelium. Simple cysts, lined with flattened epithelium, arise from dilatation of terminal portions of ductules and are generally too small to palpate. Sometimes they coalesce and form larger cysts, and they are regarded as physiologic changes of involution during menopause. Cysts that are palpable are generally apocrine cysts, and they may grow to 4–5 cm. The highest percentage are generally small and cannot be detected clinically. Apocrine cysts also originate from lobular units; and like simple cysts, they are thought to be physiologic changes of the breast because they are common during the involutional phase of lactation and menopause. They may be considered pathologic if found in young women and in excessive quantity.[1,13]

There is a relation between development of the cysts and HRT. Devitt showed that nearly half of the patients with cysts were taking HRT.[6]

Cysts surrounded by fatty tissue appear as round or oval, well-circumscribed masses on the mammogram. If they are surrounded by breast parenchyma, some of the contour may be obscured by dense breast tissue; generally the posterior parts of the cysts are indistinct. Because some malignancies of the breast appear as smoothly contoured and round masses, it is wise to undertake further diagnostic workup especially in elderly patients. Sonography usually detects whether the lesion is cystic or solid. If the cyst is not a simple cyst or is simple but causing discomfort in the patient, the next step is to aspirate the cyst. Simple cysts generally have smooth margins on sonography, and the contents of the cyst are anechoic. If echoes are detected in the cyst, it can be the result of inflammation, intracystic papilloma, an extremely hypoechoic fibroadenoma, or a malignancy; Medullary carcinoma, in particular, must be considered in the differential diagnosis. Aspiration biopsy aids in the diagnosis. If the aspirated fluid is green to brown and the lesion completely disappears after aspiration, it is probably a simple cyst, and no further workup is needed. Cyst fluid of this nature need not be sent for cytology. If a patient is postmenopausal and not on HRT, the fluid should be analyzed. Additionally, if the fluid is bloody, it may indicate an intracystic papilloma or carcinoma and should be examined. Rapid refilling of cysts a short time after aspiration may be an unusual sign of cancer.[24] A residual mass after cyst aspiration, rapid refilling of the cyst, solid papillary components in a cyst confirmed by ultrasonography, and atypical cells or papillary cells in a cyst aspirate are all reasons to perform an open biopsy to rule out malignancy.[24]

## Hormone Replacement Therapy and Mammographic Findings

It is helpful for the surgeon to be familiar with abnormal-appearing but benign mammographic lesions of the breast. In general, with the start of menopause the overall density of the breast decreases owing to glandular atrophy and fatty replacement. According to the Wolfe classification, there are four types of breast parenchymal patterns seen on mammography. In order of increasing densities are N1, P1, P2, and DY patterns. N1 breasts are fatty and radiolucent and are commonly detected in the elderly, whereas DY breasts are composed of patchy plaques of homogeneous densities and are most commonly encountered in the young. P1 breasts contain prominent ducts in the subareolar areola, involving less than one-fourth of the breast; and P2 breasts contain a prominent ductal pattern occupying more than one-fourth of the breast volume. Fatty breasts (N1 breasts according to the Wolfe classification) are more easily interpreted by radiologists. New masses, benign or malignant, can be more easily detected than in a dense breast.[25,26]

Although the subject is still controversial, continuous HRT may increase mammographic densities in the elderly. Peck and Lowman first reported that HRT increases benign changes in the breast with involution after discontinuing treatment.[27] The mammographic changes attributed to HRT may be diffuse, symmetric, asymmetric, multifocal, or cystic densities; and their degree of increased density is reported as a quantitative density percentage increase or upward change according to Wolfe's classification. Roughly, it is accepted that one-fourth of patients receiving HRT show evidence of increased breast density (Figs. 23.1, 23.2).

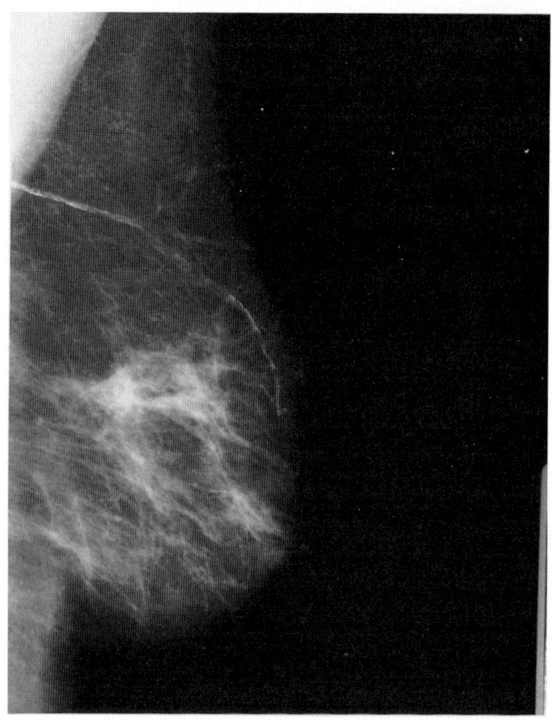

FIGURE 23.1. Baseline mammographic appearance in patient without estrogen.

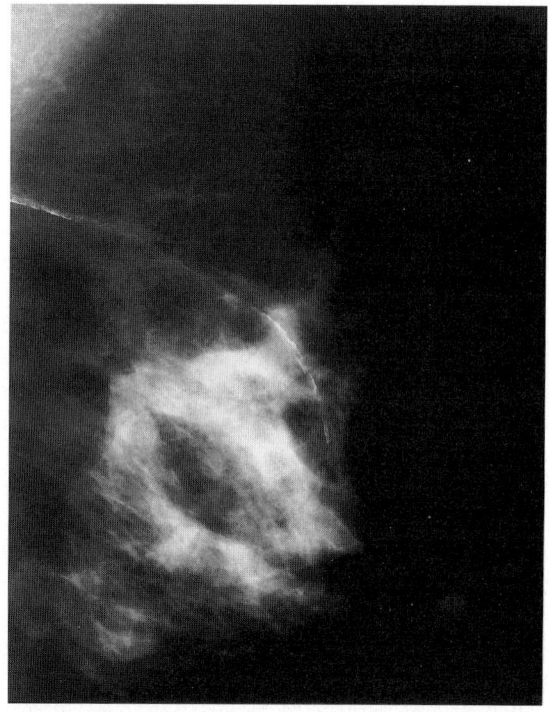

FIGURE 23.2. Increasing mammographic breast density in patient on estrogen.

Combination regimens with estrogen and progesterone are believed to produce this effect much more commonly than estrogen replacement therapy alone. Tissue edema, proliferation of periductal connective tissue, or ductal and lobular units may be responsible for these increased densities. Patients older than 50 years of age and those who have lower baseline density percentages are more likely to develop breast densities with treatment. Generally, it takes months to years for these densities to develop. Persistence of breast densities in the elderly may alter the sensitivity of the mammogram, and some masses that occur during menopause may go undetected. Low-dose regimens may be helpful in patients with increased density of the breast. Temporary discontinuation of the HRT for a few months before mammography may be useful in severe cases.[28–30]

## Abnormal but Benign Calcifications in the Elderly

Cysts can calcify, giving an eggshell appearance; and fibroadenomas may calcify as mentioned earlier. Calcifications may also be present secondary to fat necrosis, postsurgical scar, and suture calcification. Arteriosclerotic calcification is common in the elderly and is typically seen as large tubular structures that appear hollow[31] (Fig. 23.3).

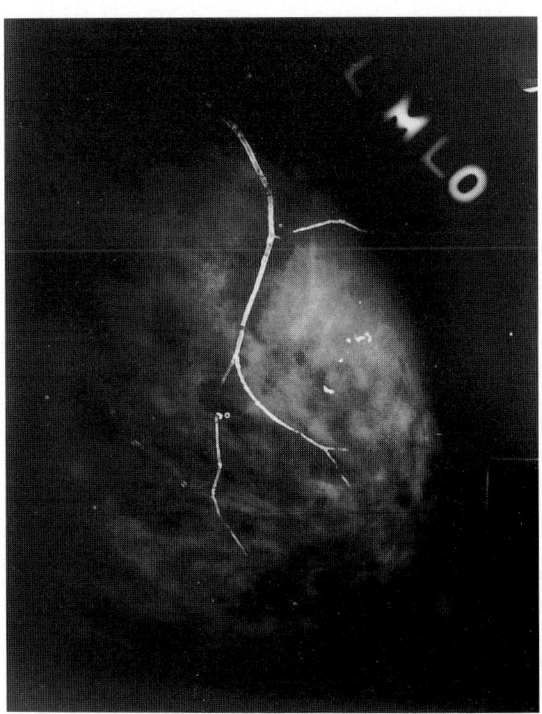


FIGURE 23.3. Mammogram with marked vascular calcifications.

## Gynecomastia

Although this chapter is primarily dedicated to breast ailments that affect women, gynecomastia can be troublesome to the male patient, who presents with enlarged or tender breasts. On physical examination, breast swelling or a discrete mass may be noted. Gynecomastia can be divided into two main histopathologic types: Type 1 consists of florid and stromal proliferation, and Type 2 consists of dilated ducts and increased amount of homogenous stroma. According to the distinct age groups, gynecomastia can be detected in the neonatal, pubertal, or adult age groups. Neonatal and pubertal gynecomastias are generally physiologic and disappear within 4–6 months. The incidence of gynecomastia increases with age. Williams found it most commonly during the seventh decade of life in an autopsy series. The reason for this increase is attributed to progressive testicular failure due to aging.[32–34]

There are many etiologic factors in the formation of gynecomastia. Although most causes are physiologic or idiopathic, some chronic illnesses, tumors, and drugs (Table 23.1) must be considered in the differential diagnosis. Careful history taking and physical examination with regard to patient age is mandatory. Further endocrinologic workup is needed in some patients when testicular atrophy is invoked.[34]

One must consider the possibility of male breast cancer in the aged population, although the clinical presentation

TABLE 23.1. Drugs Causing Gynecomastia and Their Mechanisms

| Drug | Mechanism |
|---|---|
| $H_2$-receptor blockers | Competitively displaces dihydrotestesterone from androgen receptor |
| Spironolactone | Decreases testosterone biosynthesis; increases testosterone clearance |
| Phenytoin<br>Ketoconazole | Enhances conversion of testosterone to estradiol; inhibits enzymes needed for testosterone synthesis |
| Digoxin | Has estrogen-like properties |
| Isoniazid | Has estrogen-like properties |
| Cannabis | Mimics estrogen effects because of contamination by plant phytoestrogens |
| Diethylstilbestrol | Directly stimulates breast tissue |
| Flutamide, cyproterone | Block androgens at target tissue |
| Leuprolide | Inhibits testosterone by pituitary suppression |
| Finasteride | Prevents conversion of testosterone to active form |
| Diazepam, tricyclic antidepressants, phenothiazines | Increase prolactin levels |
| Alcohol | Metabolic product inhibits testosterone biosynthesis, increases estrogen levels, increases estrogen receptors, decreases testicular gonadotropin receptors |

*Source:* Data from Neuman,[34] with permission.

is different from that of gynecomastia. Male breast cancer is a disease of elderly men (>50 years of age), and it presents clinically with skin and nipple retraction or ulceration or bloody nipple discharge; or it may appear as a hard, immobile, fixed mass in the breast. If the physical findings are equivocal, mammography may aid in the diagnosis. Gynecomastia is apparent as a triangular or a round area of increased density with flame-shaped margins. Male breast cancer presents as a well-defined mass eccentric to the nipple, with associated spiculation and calcification. Generally, biopsy is not needed for the differential diagnosis of gynecomastia and breast cancer; physical examination and mammography are sufficient.[32,34]

Gynecomastia can be treated with hormonal therapy or surgery. Tamoxifen, clomiphene, danazol, or testolactone may be used for hormonal therapy. Large (>6cm) and chronic (present for more than 4 years) gynecomastias are less likely to regress with hormonal therapy, and surgery is indicated in these cases if the patient is symptomatic.[34]

## References


1. Parks AG. The microanatomy of the breast. Ann R Coll Surg 1959;25:235–251.
2. Anbazhagan R, Bartek J, Monaghan P, Gusteron BA. Growth and development of the human infant breast. Am J Anat 1991;192:407–417.
3. Reyniak JV. Endocrine physiology of the breast. J Reprod Med 1979;22:303–309.
4. Vorherr H. Menopausal mammary involution. In: The Breast. Morphology, Physiology and Lactation. Academic: San Diego, 1974:215–217.
5. Tavossoli FA. Postmenopausal involution (atrophy). In: Pathology of the Breast. Elsevier: New York, 1992:20.
6. Devitt JE. Benign disorders of the breast in older women. Surg Gynecol Obstet 1996;162:340–342.
7. Gateley CA, Mansel RE. Management of the painful and nodular breast. Br Med Bull 1991;47:284–294.
8. Bengtsson C. Aspects of hormone replacement therapy in the post menopause. Maturitas 1989;11:35–41.
9. Marsh MS, Whitcroft S, Whitehead MI. Paradoxical effects of hormone replacement therapy on breast tenderness in postmenopausal women. Maturitas 1994; 19:97–102.

9A. Ryan PJ, Harrison R, Blake GM, Fogelman I. Compliance with hormone replacement therapy (HRT) after screening for postmenopausal osteoporosis. Br J Obstet Gynaecol 1992;99:325–328.

10. Holland P, Gateley C. Drug therapy of mastalgia: what are the options? Drugs 1994;48:709–716.
11. Kern WH, Clark RW. Retrogression of fibroadenomas of the breast. Am J Surg 1973;126:59–56.
12. Hunter TB, Roberts CC, Hunt R, Fajardo LL. Occurrence of fibroadenomas in postmenopausal women referred for breast biopsy. J Am Geriatr Soc 1996;44:61–64.
13. Dixon JM. Cystic disease and fibroadenoma of the breast: natural history and relation to breast cancer risk. Br Med Bull 1991;47:258–271.
14. Egan R. Fibroadenoma. In: Breast Imaging. Diagnosis and Morphology of Breast Diseases. Saunders: Philadelphia, 1988:178–182.
15. Sandison AT. Fibroadenoma: an autopsy study of the adult human breast. Natl Cancer Inst Monogr 1962;8:30.
16. Frantz VK, Pickren JW, Melcher GW, Auchincloss H. Incidence of chronic cystic disease in so-called "normal breasts": a study based on 225 postmortem examinations. Cancer 1951;4:762–783.
17. Kopans DB. Benign and probably benign lesions. In: Breast Imaging. Lippincot-Raven: Philadelphia, 1998:351– 373.
18. Rosen PP. Mammary duct ectasia. In: Rosen's Breast Pathology. Lippincot-Raven: Philadelphia, 1997:29–32.
19. Hughes LE. Nonlactational inflammation and duct ectasia. Br Med Bull 1991;47:272–283.
20. Dixon JM, Anderson TJ , Lumsden AB, Elton RA, Roberts MM, Forrest APM. Mammary duct ectasia. Br J Surg 1983; 70:601–603.
21. Dixon JM, Ravisekar O, Chetty U, Anderson TJ. Periductal mastitis and duct ectasia: different conditions with different aetiologies. Br J Surg 1996;83:820–822.
22. Martin JE. Benign diseases of the breast. In: Harris JH Jr (ed) Atlas of Mammography. Histologic and Mammographic Correlations. Williams & Wilkins: Baltimore, 1982:192–195.
23. Sandison A. Atrophy, duct ectasia and cyst formation: an autopsy study of the adult human breast. Natl Cancer Inst Monogr 1962;8:11–16.
24. Heywang–Kobrunger SH, Scherer I, Dershaw DD. Benign Breast Disorders. Thieme: Stuttgart, 1997:141–165.
25. Laya MB, Gallagher JC, Schreiman JS, Larson EB, Watson P, Weinstein L. Effect of postmenopausal hormonal replacement therapy on mammographic density and parenchymal pattern. Radiology 1995;196:433–437.
26. Wolfe JN. Breast parenchymal patterns and their changes with age. Radiology 1976;121:545–552.
27. Peck DR, Lowman RM. Estrogen and the postmenopausal breast: mammographic considerations. JAMA 1978;240: 1733–1735.
28. Stomper PC, Voorhis BJV, Ravnikar VA, Meyer JE. Mammographic changes associated with postmenopausal hormone replacement therapy: a longitudinal study. Radiology 1990;174:487–490.
29. Persson I, Thurfjell E, Holmberg L. Effect of estrogen and estrogen-progestin replacement regimens on mammographic breast parenchymal density. J Clin Oncol 1997;15: 3201–3207.
30. Berkowitz JE, Gatewood OMB, Goldblum LE, Gayler BW. Hormonal replacement therapy: mammographic manifestations. Radiology 1990;174:199–201.
31. Martin JE. Benign calcifications. In: Harris JH Jr (ed) Atlas of Mammography. Histologic and Mammographic Correlations. Williams & Wilkins: Baltimore, 1982:196–209.
32. Cooper RA, Gunter BA, Ramamurthy L. Mammography in men. Radiology 1994;191:651–656.
33. Williams MJ. Gynecomastia. Am J Med 1963;34:103–112.
34. Neuman JF. Evaluation and treatment of gynecomastia. Am Fam Physician 1997;55:1835–1844.

# 24 Breast Cancer in Elderly Women

Nora Hansen and Monica Morrow

Breast cancer is the most common malignancy in American women and the second leading cause of cancer death. It was estimated that there would be 180,300 new breast cancer cases diagnosed in the United States in 1998 and 43,500 deaths.

The incidence of breast cancer increases with age; and despite competing causes of mortality, breast cancer remains a significant cause of death in elderly women. Cancer is the leading cause of death in those 55–74 years of age and is second only to heart disease in the 75+ age group.[1] As life expectancy increases and the elderly population continues to grow, there will be an increasing number of elderly women diagnosed with breast cancer in the future. Despite the high prevalence of this disease in the elderly, they largely have been excluded or discouraged from participating in clinical trials and often are not given the same therapeutic options as their younger counterparts.[2–4]

The goal of this chapter is to review the important issues related to the management of breast cancer in the elderly. They include age-specific issues regarding the value of mammographic screening, the selection of local surgical therapy, the need for adjuvant radiotherapy, the efficacy and toxicity of systemic therapy, and the effect of mortality due to breast cancer in this population. Because there is no standard definition of "elderly," for the purpose of this chapter an elderly patient is one who is older than 70 years of age.

## Epidemiology

Breast cancer incidence and mortality increase with age, with the greatest increase observed during the childbearing years. In Western countries, a continued increase in incidence is seen after menopause, whereas in Asian countries the incidence decreases in elderly women.[5,6] Approximately one-half of the breast cancers in the United States are diagnosed among women age 65 and over.[7] For women in this age group, an incidence rate of 322 cases per 100,000 population was noted in the SEER database,[8] compared with 60 cases per 100,000 for women younger than age 65. The incidence rate for women aged 85 or more rose to 375 cases per 100,000 population.

Breast cancer incidence rates in the United States increased by 32% from 1980 to 1987[9] (Fig. 24.1) largely due to an increase in incidence in women over age 40, and this increase was noted in elderly women as well as their younger counterparts. During this time period, a marked increase in the incidence of in situ and localized disease was observed in all age groups, with a decrease in regional disease and a stable metastatic disease rate.[9] This stage shift is reflected in a 6.8% decrease in overall breast cancer mortality from 1989 through 1993. Decreased mortality was observed for every decade of age under 80 years and probably reflects both the increased utilization of screening mammography and improvements in therapy (Fig. 24.2).

As in young women, infiltrating ductal carcinoma is the most common histologic tumor type in the elderly, accounting for 77–85% of cases.[8,10–13] The relatively favorable subtypes of colloid and papillary carcinoma are observed more frequently in elderly women but still account for less than 10% of mammary carcinomas even in women aged 85 or more,[8,11,14,15] whereas inflammatory and medullary carcinoma are seen less commonly in old women than in their young counterparts.[8,14,15] Breast cancers in old women are more likely to be moderately to well differentiated, contain estrogen receptors, and have a low thymidine labeling index.[15–17]

## Screening

Screening mammography in women age 50 and older reduces breast cancer mortality by approximately one-third.[18–23] However, only two of the major screening trials included women over age 65, and the upper age limit for the benefit of screening has not been determined. A small case–control study from the Nijmegen screening program

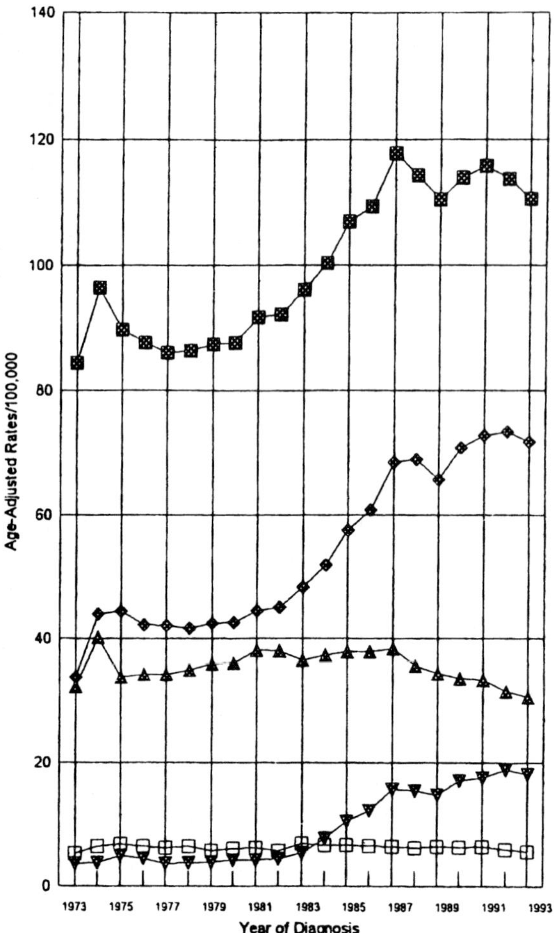


FIGURE 24.1. Age-adjusted breast cancer incidence rates per 100,000 population by extent of disease at diagnosis for white women. Filled squares, totally invasive; diamonds, localized; triangles, regional; inverted triangles, in situ; open squares, distant. (Data from Chu et al.[9])

demonstrated a relative risk of breast cancer death of 0.26 [95% confidence interval (CI) 0.05–1.32] for women continuing screening after age 65 and 0.38 (95% CI 0.03–4.15) for those age 70 and older. However, no benefit was observed for screening after age 74.[18] Van Dijck et al.[24] reported the results of a nonrandomized trial of screening in 6773 women aged 68–83 enrolled during 1977–1978 and followed through 1990. Women from the same birth cohort in a neighboring city without a screening program served as controls. Over the entire study period, the cumulative mortality rate ratio was 0.80 (95% CI 0.53–1.22) for the screened women; and 9–13 years after the start of screening it had decreased to 0.53 (95% CI 0.27–1.04).

Other data support the use of screening in older women. Faulk et al.[25] compared the results of screening in 6701 women age 65 and older to those in women age 50–64. The two groups had similar rates of nonpalpable breast tumors, but the positive predictive value for cancer was higher in the older group, and the nodal status was more frequently negative. Wilson et al.[26] retrospectively compared cancers detected in women undergoing screening to those in unscreened women in a study of 60 patients aged 75 and older. Tumors in the screened group were smaller and had fewer nodal metastases than those in the unscreened group. Because randomized trials have demonstrated the benefit of screening in women aged 50–64, it is reasonable to assume that similar benefits will be observed in older women. However, the potential cost-benefit ratio and the effect of co-morbid conditions on the benefits of mammographic screening in women over age 65 remain areas of concern.

Mandelblatt et al.[27] used a decision analysis model to determine whether mammographic screening extends life for women age 65 and over in the presence and absence of co-morbid conditions. Patients were stratified into age groups of 65–69, 70–74, 75–79, 80–84, and 85 years or more. In each age category, women were further stratified into those with average health, those with mild diastolic hypertension, and women with symptomatic congestive heart failure to determine the effect of co-morbid conditions on screening benefit. Screening was found to save lives for all ages of elderly women, although the magnitude of benefit decreased as the severity of the co-morbidity increased. For a woman with breast cancer, screening prolonged life 617 days for the woman of average health aged 65–69 and 311 days for women in the same age group with congestive heart failure. The prolongations of survival for women over age 85 in the same health groups were 178 and 126 days, respectively. The cost-effectiveness of annual screening ranged from $13,200 to $34,600 per year of life saved. In comparison, the cost per year of life saved by treating mild to moderate hypertension in the nonelderly is $16,000 to $72,000.[27] These estimates of cost are based on the use of annual screening mammograms. Moskowitz[28] calculated that owing to the longer lead times seen with breast cancer in older women, most of the benefits of screening could be obtained with a 2- to 3-year interval between studies.

Boer et al.[29] used a model incorporating the natural history of breast cancer and the known effect of screening to identify the optimum upper age limit for screening. Using a model in which preclinical duration of breast cancer was assumed not to increase after age 65, no upper limit for screening benefit was identified. If the duration of the preclinical phase was "pessimistically" assumed to increase in the elderly, screening up to age 80 was found to be of benefit. These findings suggest that mammographic screening is a beneficial technique in the elderly. The current U.S. Preventive Services Task Force guidelines recommend screening mammography for women ages 50–75[30]; however, a number of studies indicate that breast cancer screening in the elderly, whether

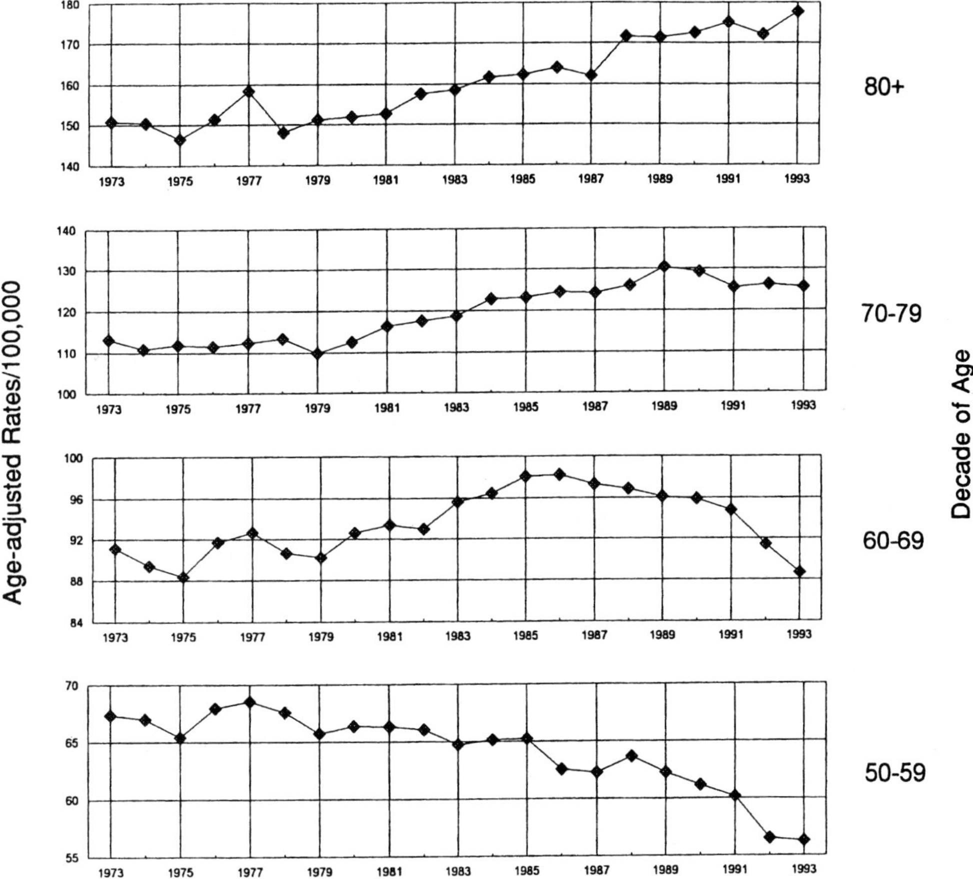


FIGURE 24.2. Age-adjusted breast cancer mortality rates for U.S. white women per 100,000 population. (Data from Chu et al.[9])

by mammography or clinical breast examination, is underutilized.

Brown and Hulka[31] attempted a case–control study to determine the effect of mammographic screening on the incidence of metastatic breast cancer in women older than age 60. Fewer than 6% of either the cases or the controls had ever had a screening mammogram. The National Cancer Institute Breast Cancer Screening Consortium[32] reported the results of seven population-based surveys of women aged 50–74. In five of the seven studies, the rates of breast screening by mammography and breast examination in the 70- to 74-year age group were lower than those reported for other ages. This occurred despite the fact that more than 90% of women surveyed had a regular source of medical care. Similarly, Hayward and coauthors[33] analyzed data from a 1986 nationwide telephone survey of 4659 women. Information regarding the frequency of physician breast examination and screening mammography was collected. The proportion of women undergoing physician breast examination decreased from 60% for women aged 40–49 to 49% for women aged 65 or older ($p < 0.0001$), a difference that was significant after adjustment for confounding variables. The decreased use of screening measures was not thought to be due to the existence of major co-morbid conditions in the older patient group because the results remained unchanged even after controlling for health status. Harris et al.[34] noted that only 37% of women in their seventies had ever had a mammogram, compared with 52% of women in their fifties ($p < 0.01$).

Weinberger and colleagues[35] gathered data from 576 primary care physicians in Indiana regarding attitudes toward age and breast cancer screening. More than 90% of physicians surveyed were aware of the benefits of screening mammography and believed that mammography could detect early cancer in women over 65 years of age. However, annual breast examination was conducted less often in elderly women than in their younger counterparts, and this was true even for elderly women with a personal history of breast cancer. Screening mammography was performed less frequently in the elderly regardless of the patient's risk of breast cancer development. Barriers to screening, including confusion regarding guidelines, physician forgetfulness, belief that breast examination was sufficient, concern over co-morbidity, and patient refusal were all greater for older women.

Lack of awareness of breast cancer risk and screening procedures in elderly women is another factor contributing to the underutilization of these techniques. Leather

TABLE 24.1. Utilization of Mammography in Elderly U.S. Women

| | 1987 | | 1990 | | 1992 | |
|---|---|---|---|---|---|---|
| Age (years) | % Past year | % Ever | % Past year | % Ever | % Past year | % Ever |
| 50–59 | 26.3 | 46.3 | 46.6 | 68.4 | 51.8 | 75.9 |
| 60–69 | 21.5 | 39.1 | 42.0 | 62.5 | 48.4 | 69.7 |
| 70–79 | 17.7 | 32.0 | 34.5 | 54.5 | 39.8 | 63.5 |
| ≥80 | 9.9 | 20.4 | 20.9 | 35.1 | 21.6 | 48.5 |

*Source:* Adapted from Chu et al.[9]

and Roberts[36] identified a lack of knowledge among elderly women about breast cancer, a pessimistic attitude toward disease outcome, and embarrassment about being examined as major barriers to screening. Fox et al.[37] conducted a telephone survey of 724 women age 65 and older to assess factors influencing the use of mammography. Only physician recommendation predicted a recent mammogram, with age, race, and health status found to be insignificant factors. Harris et al.[34] surveyed 1163 female residents of North Carolina regarding breast cancer screening practices. The women ranged in age from 30 to 74, with 161 in their seventies. Overall, only 20% knew that breast cancer risk increased with age, and a significantly smaller percentage of women in their seventies reported being worried about developing breast cancer than in the younger age groups. Only 37% of women in this study thought that a mammogram was a better cancer screening test than a clinical breast examination. These data indicate that education of elderly women by health care providers regarding their level of breast cancer risk and the benefits of screening is critical. Improvements in mammographic utilization have been noted since 1987 (Table 24.1), suggesting a greater awareness of benefits on the part of both physicians and patients.

## Local Therapy of Breast Cancer

What constitutes appropriate local treatment for the elderly woman with breast cancer is probably the most controversial issue in the management of these women. In the past, when mastectomy was the standard surgical therapy for breast cancer, the major debate in older women centered on dissection of the axillary nodes. The emergence of breast-conserving surgery as an accepted modality for the local therapy of breast cancer and the development of tamoxifen, an antitumor agent with significant efficacy and limited toxicity, have increased the available options for local treatment in this population. When evaluating therapeutic options, it is important to consider not only the immediate morbidity and mortality of treatment but also the efficacy of the therapy in maintaining local control for the duration of the woman's life. Current options for the local management of breast carcinoma in the elderly include mastectomy, breast-conserving therapy consisting of excision and irradiation or excision alone, and tamoxifen.

### Mastectomy

Mastectomy is the most common treatment option utilized in the elderly patient. A modified radical mastectomy includes removal of breast tissue, the underlying pectoralis fascia, and the axillary lymph nodes. The 30-day operative mortality rate is uniformly low, and the procedure is physically well tolerated. In a review of the SEER data from 1960–1973, Schneiderman and Axtell reported a 30-day operative mortality rate of 0.4% for the 37,745 patients treated during that period. For women aged 75 or older the operative mortality was 0.8% during 1960–1966 and 0.9% during 1967–1973.[38] Similar results have been noted in other studies. Singletary et al. reported an operative mortality rate of 1.6% in a study of 184 women diagnosed after the age of 69, 82% of whom underwent modified radical mastectomy.[39] Davis et al. reported a 3% mortality rate for women aged 80 or older treated by mastectomy and a 7% incidence of major complications.[40] Hunt et al., in a study of 94 patients, reported a complication rate of 20% in elderly patients, but the operative mortality was still only 1%.[41] Wound problems accounted for most of the complications in this series. Kessler and Seton found cardiovascular and neurologic problems to be the most common cause of postoperative morbidity in their series.[42] Data on the morbidity and mortality of mastectomy in the elderly are summarized in Table 24.2. Although mastectomy is an excellent method for obtaining local control of breast cancer with a minimum number of outpatient visits and elderly woman can undergo the procedure safely, these results are obtained at the expense of cosmesis.

TABLE 24.2. Morbidity and Mortality of Mastectomy in the Elderly

| Study | Age (years) | No. | Operative mortality (%) | Complications (%) |
|---|---|---|---|---|
| Hunt[41] | >65 | 94 | 1.0 | 20 |
| Schottenfield[43] | >65 | 437 | 0.2 | NS |
| Singletary[39] | >69 | 157 | 1.9 | 24 |
| Kessler[42] | >70 | 82 | 1.2 | 11 |
| Berg[44] | >70 | 242 | 2.0 | NS |
| Kraft[45] | >75 | 75 | 4.5 | NS |
| SEER 1967–1973[38] | >75 | NS | 0.9 | NS |
| Davis[40] | >80 | 96 | 3.0 | 7 |

NS, not stated.

## Breast-Conserving Surgery

Since 1970, six prospective randomized trials using modern radiation techniques, have compared survival after breast conservation treatment to survival after mastectomy for stage I and II breast cancer. No survival advantage has been noted for mastectomy. Although most of these trials did not include women over age 70, the biologic rationale for breast preservation can be extrapolated to the elderly population. Several studies have suggested that elderly women may have a lower rate of breast recurrence after partial mastectomy and radiotherapy than their younger counterparts.[46–48] Fourquet et al. reported a 97% rate of control at 10 years for women over age 55 compared to 85% for women aged 33–45 and 71% for women age 32 or younger in a series of 518 patients.[46] Veronesi et al.[47] and Clark et al.[48] have also reported a decreasing frequency of breast recurrence with increasing age. Some of these differences in local failure rates may be due to a higher incidence of adverse pathologic features, such as an extensive intraductal component or lymphatic invasion in young women, but old women appear to have lower local failure rates even after correction for pathologic features.

In addition, local recurrence rates can be affected by a number of treatment factors, such as the extent of surgical resection, the status of the surgical margin, and the use of adjuvant tamoxifen. In the National Surgical Adjuvant Breast Project (NSABP) B-14 trial, 2644 axillary node-negative patients, 38% of whom underwent breast-conserving therapy, were randomized to receive tamoxifen or placebo. After a median follow-up of 3 years, the rate of recurrence in the breast was 3.5% in the placebo arm compared to 1.9% in the tamoxifen group.[49] Thus in elderly women treated with breast-conserving therapy including breast irradiation and tamoxifen, the incidence of local failure is low and the small risk of a second surgery is not an appropriate reason to recommend that elderly women routinely undergo mastectomy. The standard contraindications to breast-conserving therapy (Table 24.3) used to determine the suitability of young women for breast-conserving therapy should be used in old women as well.

Despite the low rates of local recurrence seen in the elderly after lumpectomy and irradiation, radiation therapy is often omitted in this population. Kantorowitz et al. found that 82% of women under 60 years of age with stage I and II breast cancer were referred for irradiation, whereas only 40% of women over age 60 received radiation; moreover, the likelihood of referral decreased further with increasing age.[50] Wanebo et al. reported that 26.6% of women age 65 and older with stage IA and IB cancer were treated with lumpectomy alone compared to 9.4% of younger patients, and a decrease in 5-year survival was observed in these women when compared to those treated with lumpectomy, axillary dissection, and breast irradiation.[51] Four prospective randomized trials[52–55] have compared conservative surgery alone to conservative surgery with breast irradiation. Although these trials vary with regard to patient selection criteria and the techniques of surgery and irradiation (RT) employed, all of these studies demonstrate dramatic reductions in the incidence of local failure when RT is used, with an average crude rate of reduction of 85%. In the Milan trial,[55] some variation in the degree of benefit obtained from RT was observed related to age. At a follow-up of 39 months, the 3-year local recurrence rate after quadrantectomy alone was 17.5% in patients aged 55 and younger but only 3.8% in patients older than 55 years. Other studies demonstrate substantially higher rates of local recurrence in older women treated with more limited surgical resections. Reed and Morrison reported a 35% local failure rate 4 years after excision alone in 96 patients with a mean age of 76.[56] In another study, a 9% local failure rate was seen in 47 women treated with segmental mastectomy followed by RT compared with a 25% local failure rate in 20 women treated with segmental mastectomy and tamoxifen without RT.[57] The Joint Center for Radiation Therapy has reported the results of a prospective, single-arm trial of excision alone in a group of 87 patients with a median age of 67 years.[58] Entry criteria were a tumor size less than 2 cm, histologically negative axillary nodes, the absence of lymphatic invasion, an extensive intraductal component, and no cancer cells within 1 cm of the surgical margins. The average annual local recurrence rate was 3.6%, and the 3-year crude rate of local recurrence was 8.0%, resulting in early closure of the trial. In comparison, in a group of 45 patients with similar characteristics treated with breast irradiation at the same institution, the 3-year crude rate of local recurrence was 0%.

Breast irradiation has been shown to be well tolerated in the elderly population. A tolerance study by Wyckoff and colleagues demonstrated that radiation dose, duration of therapy, number of treatment interruptions, and toxicities were no different in women over the age of 65 compared to women younger than 65.[59] Even patients over 80 years of age tolerate breast irradiation. A patient's inability to travel to the hospital is often cited as a reason for omitting radiation therapy in the elderly. Morrow et al.[60] found that 80% of their elderly patients selected

TABLE 24.3. Contraindications to Breast-Conserving Therapy with Irradiation

| |
|---|
| Two or more primary tumors in separate quadrants of the breast |
| Diffuse malignant-appearing microcalcifications |
| Prior therapeutic irradiation to the breast region that requires retreatment to an excessively high total radiation dose |
| Persistent positive margins after reasonable surgical attempts |

breast conservation with irradiation when given the option, a finding similar to that reported by Stewart and Foster.[61]

It is likely that inability to travel to receive daily irradiation is a factor in the omission of this modality for some elderly patients, and alternative methods of delivering radiation are being studied. Maher et al. treated 70 patients with a median age of 81 years with tamoxifen and high-dose-per-fraction once-weekly radiotherapy consisting of seven exposures of 6.5Gy given over 60 weeks. At a median follow-up of 36 months, the local control rate was 86%.[62] Bolton et al.[63] have reported use of a high-dose implant to the tumor bed with in-hospital irradiation given for 72 hours after lumpectomy and no external beam treatment. Results in a pilot study demonstrated good local control rates and satisfactory cosmesis, but large studies are needed to define the appropriate role of this alternate form of irradiation.

When considering whether to omit breast irradiation after limited surgery, it is important to remember that most local failures occur within 6 years of surgery, leaving many elderly women at risk of this occurrence. Irradiation is well tolerated in the elderly population, and chronologic age alone is not an indication for its omission from breast-conserving therapy. In patients who do not undergo breast irradiation, a wider surgical resection (quadrantectomy) appears to decrease the risk of local recurrence.

## Axillary Dissection

Lymph node metastases remains the single best predictor of survival for patients with operable invasive breast cancer. For decades, knowledge of axillary node status has played a critical role in determining the need for adjuvant systemic therapy, and accurate staging has been considered an integral part of the management of invasive cancer. In addition, axillary dissection is an effective method for maintaining local control in the axilla with isolated axillary failures seen in only 1–2% of patients after the procedure.[64,65]

Major complications of axillary dissection, including injury or thrombosis of the axillary vein and injury to the motor nerves of the axilla, are uncommon, although, significant short- and long-term morbidity is associated with the procedure (Table 24.4). Of the potential sequelae of the procedure, lymphedema of the arm is potentially associated with the greatest disability. The incidence of lymphedema following axillary dissection ranges from 1.5% to 62.5%,[66–69] depending on the definition used, the length of follow-up, the method of detection employed, and the population studied. Several studies have suggested that older age is a risk factor for the development of lymphedema. Pezner et al.[69] noted lymphedema following breast-conserving treatment (including RT) in 25% of women age 60 or older compared to 3 of 46 younger women (7%) ($p = 0.02$). Other studies have failed to identify an association between age and lymphedema.[66,68] Axillary dissection has also been shown to cause pain and decreased upper arm mobility,[70] factors that can cause significant functional impairment in women with preexisting limitations due to neurologic disease or arthritis.

TABLE 24.4. Morbidity of Axillary Dissection

| Morbidity | Incidence (%) |
|---|---|
| Pain | 15–33 |
| Numbness | 70–80 |
| Reduced strength/ decreased ROM | 10–20 |
| Lymphedema | 2–30 |
| Breast edema | 15–50 |
| surgery using General anesthesia | 100 |

ROM, range of motion.

In the past, knowledge of nodal status was critical, as only patients with axillary metastases received systemic therapy. Today, most women have systemic therapy regardless of nodal status; tamoxifen is often the therapy of choice for women age 70 and older, regardless of nodal status.[71] This raises the question of whether axillary dissection is necessary solely to maintain local control. For patients with a clinically negative axilla, RT to the axilla is as effective as axillary dissection in maintaining local control.[64] A substantial portion of the lower axilla is often included in the standard breast radiation ports, so local control may be achieved without addition of a separate axillary field. This represents a viable alternative to dissection when the morbidity of the procedure is thought to be excessive. In the presence of palpable adenopathy, surgical dissection remains the treatment of choice because failure rates seen after irradiation alone are significantly higher than those reported after surgical dissection.

Although there has been a trend toward eliminating axillary dissection, particularly in the elderly population, knowledge of the status of the axilla is still the most important predictor of breast cancer outcome; and patients of all ages often desire this prognostic information. The emergence of the sentinel lymph node biopsy is an alternative therapeutic option that is particularly attractive for the elderly patient: It eliminates the need for an axillary dissection in patients found to have a negative sentinel node while identifying node-positive patients who may benefit from further surgical intervention.

## Sentinel Lymph Node Biopsy

The concept of lymphatic mapping and sentinel lymphadenectomy was popularized by Morton et al. in their

TABLE 24.5. Results of Sentinel Node Biopsy

| Study | No. of patients | Technique | Identification rate (%) | False-negative rate (%) |
|---|---|---|---|---|
| Giuliano[73] | 174 | Blue dye | 66 | 4.4 |
| Giuliano[74] | 107 | Blue dye | 94 | 0 |
| Krag[75] | 443 | Radioactive | 91 | 11 |
| Albertini[76] | 62 | Radioactive and blue dye | 92 | 0 |
| Veronesi[77] | 163 | Radioactive | 98 | 2.5 |
| Shons[78] | 243 | Radioactive and blue dye | 92 | 0.5 |
| Galimberto[79] | 213 | Radioactive | 99 | 2.9 |

work with melanoma patients.[72] The sentinel node is defined as the first draining lymph node of a particular cancer and, if correctly identified, accurately predicts the histologic status of the lymphatic basin. The sentinel node is identified by injecting the breast tissue around the primary tumor site with a blue dye or a radioactive tracer, which is picked up by the lymphatics. Several groups have reported their experience with sentinel lymphadenectomy for breast cancer and have shown promising results (Table 24.5). The success rate for identification of the sentinel node ranges from 66% to 99% and improves with experience.[72–79] The sentinel node is an accurate predictor of the status of the remaining nodes in the axilla in 97–100% of cases.[72–79] Giuliano and coworkers[80] demonstrated an increased incidence of nodal metastases in the sentinel node with the addition of immunohistochemical staining using anti-cytokeratin antibodies to identify occult metastases. This increase was specific to the sentinel node as demonstrated by a study by Turner and coworkers.[81] In that study, all nonsentinel nodes were examined using the same immunohistochemical staining techniques as for the sentinel node. Only 1 of 1087 nonsentinel nodes was found to have a metastasis, whereas 42% of sentinel nodes contained metastases, a statistically significant difference.

Many elderly patients are not offered axillary staging because the complications of such staging outweigh the potential benefits of the procedure. The sentinel node biopsy is a promising alternative and may allow all patients to undergo axillary staging, thereby providing the patient and the physician with accurate prognostic information with minimal morbidity.

## Tamoxifen as an Alternative Local Therapy

Because of concerns regarding the morbidity and mortality of conventional surgical therapy for breast cancer in elderly women with co-morbid conditions, considerable attention has been given to the use of tamoxifen as a primary treatment. In 1982, Preece and coauthors[82] reported a pilot study in which 67 consecutive women over age 75 received tamoxifen, 20–40 mg daily, as primary therapy for localized breast cancer. A 73% response rate was noted, although 18% of patients took more than 12 months to achieve the maximum response. At the same time, Helleberg et al.[83] reported remission in 21 of 27 women treated with tamoxifen, 40 mg daily. In 15 cases, remission was complete by both clinical and radiographic criteria, and the mean time to complete response was 14 months.

Several subsequent reports[84] of tamoxifen as primary therapy describe complete response rates ranging from 10%[85] to 50%[86] and failure of response or progression of disease in 23%[87] to 58%[88] of cases. These data are summarized in Table 24.6. A median duration of response of 19 months was noted by Allan et al.[84] in a study of 100 patients. Of 14 deaths occurring in this study, only 5 were due to carcinoma. Auclerc and coauthors[91] reported a median duration of response of 35 months in their group of tamoxifen-treated women, and more than 50% of the deaths occurring in this study were due to causes other than breast cancer. Conflicting evidence exists regarding the value of hormone receptors for predicting response to primary tamoxifen therapy. Foudraine et al.[88] did not find a relation between estrogen or progesterone receptor status and tumor response in the 19 patients in whom these data were available. In contrast, Gaskell et al.[85] observed a 26% response rate and no tumor progression in 31 women whose tumors showed more than 25% of cells staining for the estrogen receptor by immunocytochemistry, compared with no responses and a 100% progression rate in nine women in whom no staining was observed. Further study on larger numbers of women is needed to clarify this point.

The value of tamoxifen as a sole therapy has been further addressed in three randomized trials comparing tamoxifen alone with some form of surgical therapy. Gazet et al.[92] randomized 116 women aged 70 and over who were believed to have technically operable breast cancer to treatment with tamoxifen, 20 mg daily,

TABLE 24.6. Response Rates to Tamoxifen as Primary Breast Cancer Therapy

| Study | Number | Complete response (%) | Partial response (%) | Nonresponse or progression (%) |
|---|---|---|---|---|
| Allan et al.[84] | 100 | 39 | 29 | 32 |
| Robertson et al.[86] | 68 | 50 | 17 | 33 |
| Falk et al.[87] | 43 | 32 | 44 | 23 |
| Foudraine et al.[88] | 40 | 43 | | 58 |
| Bates et al.[89] | 183 | 33 | 15 | 53 |
| Margolese et al.[90] | 30 | 17 | 47 | 37 |
| Auclerc et al.[91] | 78 | 23 | 29 | 28 |

or surgical resection. Of the 56 women in the surgery arm, 37 (66%) were treated by local excision of the tumor only. At 3 years, no difference in the incidence of local failure or distant relapse was noted between groups, leading the authors to conclude that the treatments were equivalent. However, the surgical arm of this study does not represent the best available conventional therapy because irradiation was not employed in the lumpectomy group and no systemic therapy was given.

Bates and coauthors[89] randomized 381 women aged 70 and older to tamoxifen, 40 mg daily, or "optimal surgery" plus tamoxifen. Patients were selected for wide excision or mastectomy at the discretion of the surgeon. At a median follow-up of 34 months, 64 local failures (35%) were seen in the tamoxifen group compared with 21 (13%) in the surgery group. Of the 21 local failures among the surgical patients, only one occurred following mastectomy. No difference in mortality was observed between the two treatment groups. This study also assessed quality of life at a mean 12 months after diagnosis. The surgery and tamoxifen groups were well matched for demographic characteristics, and approximately half the women in each group lived alone. No differences were observed between treatment groups when physical malaise, anxiety, social dysfunction, and depression were assessed.

The third randomized trial of tamoxifen[86] versus surgery assigned 135 women aged 70 or older to 40 mg of tamoxifen daily or "wedge mastectomy," defined as removal of the pendulous portion of the breast at its base, without creating skin flaps. At a mean follow-up of 65 months, no differences in survival were noted between groups. Sixty-seven percent of the tamoxifen-treated women achieved a response, but at 5 years 40 women (59%) had locoregional progression of disease, primarily in the breast. Only 20 locoregional failures were seen in the surgery group, and half of them occurred in untreated axillary nodes ($p < 0.001$ vs. tamoxifen). The high local failure rate in the tamoxifen-treated women led the authors to conclude that in elderly women able to tolerate surgery, mastectomy should be done to maintain local control.

Three randomized trials comparing the treatment of operable breast cancer with tamoxifen alone to surgery or surgery plus tamoxifen, failed to demonstrate a survival advantage in favor of the surgical procedure. Despite the fact that the surgical procedures utilized do not represent the best available therapy, significant improvements in local control were observed in the surgically treated women. Response rates to primary tamoxifen treatment are high, but often 12 months or more are needed to achieve the best response; and with long-term follow-up the likelihood of disease progression is significant. Because mastectomy or lumpectomy and radiotherapy are well tolerated by most elderly women, there is no reason to substitute tamoxifen as a routine treatment. However, for the elderly woman with a limited life-span and a high risk of operative mortality due to co-morbid conditions, tamoxifen represents a viable alternative as a primary therapy.

## Systemic Therapy

Adjuvant therapy has come to play an increasingly large role in breast cancer management. Tamoxifen is well established as an effective therapy for postmenopausal, estrogen receptor-positive women with node-positive or node-negative breast cancer. An overview analysis[93] of 37,000 women treated with adjuvant tamoxifen demonstrated a 47% reduction in the risk of breast cancer recurrence and a 26% reduction the odds of breast cancer death in treated women. With tamoxifen treatment for longer than 2 years, even greater benefits are observed. For the subgroup of women aged 70 and older, the reductions in the odds of recurrence and death were 54% and 34%, respectively.

A study specifically designed to evaluate the benefits of tamoxifen in elderly postmenopausal women has been done by the Eastern Cooperative Oncology Group (ECOG).[94,95] The effect of 2 years of adjuvant tamoxifen in 170 women over age 65 with stage II breast cancer, was studied in this prospective, double-blind study. Women were stratified on the basis of their estrogen receptor status and number of positive axillary nodes. One-third of the patients in the study were age 71–75, and 21% were older than 75. The median time to treatment failure was 4.4 years for the placebo group versus 7.4 years for the tamoxifen group ($p = 0.001$). A reduction in contralateral breast cancers (one vs. five) was also noted in the tamoxifen-treated women. Overall, 61% of the deaths in this study were due to breast cancer, indicating significant benefit for adjuvant tamoxifen even in the elderly. In a similar study, Castiglione et al.[96] examined the effect of tamoxifen, 20 mg daily plus low-dose prednisone given for 1 year, on survival in a group of patients with node-positive breast cancer aged 66–80 years. With a median follow-up of 96 months, 9.1% of patients had died of other causes and 1.9% had developed a second malignant neoplasm. The 8-year disease-free survival for the tamoxifen group was 36 ± 4% compared to 22% for the untreated controls ($p = 0.004$).

There is considerably more controversy regarding the use of adjuvant chemotherapy in elderly women. Although combination chemotherapy was clearly shown to improve both relapse-free and overall survival in postmenopausal women in the overview analysis, the magnitude of benefit was not as large as that observed in premenopausal women.[93] In women younger than age 50, chemotherapy reduced mortality by 27% compared to an 18% reduction in women age 60–69. In women over 70, no significant survival benefit was noted. One potential explanation for these results is the use of lower doses of chemotherapy in an effort to reduce toxicity in the elderly. Bonnadonna and Valagussa[97] noted that most patients age 65 and older in an adjuvant breast cancer trial were treated with a reduced dose of chemotherapy. A definite dose-response relation was observed, with patients treated at lower doses having lower rates of 5-year disease-free survival and shorter durations of overall survival. Begg et al.[98] found that 4.5% of breast cancer patients age 60 and older treated in randomized trials from the ECOG were underdosed compared to 2.1% of their younger counterparts. Increased toxicity of cancer chemotherapy in the elderly is a potential explanation for underdosing, although studies that examined the relation between chronologic age and toxicity failed to demonstrate a relation. ECOG[98] reviewed data on 298 patients treated on six protocols to determine the effect of age on toxicity due to chemotherapy. Patients over age 60 were considered "elderly" in the breast cancer studies (owing to an upper age limit for study entry of 65), and patients aged 70 or more in other studies were classified as elderly. No significant differences in any type of toxicity (hematologic, mucosal, vomiting, infection, neurologic, cardiac) were noted on the basis of age. The authors concluded that, although it is conventional to treat the elderly cancer patient in a more conservative fashion, no clear biologic rationale exists for this approach. Further support for this conclusion comes from the Piedmont Oncology Association experience with combination chemotherapy in women over age 70 with metastatic breast cancer.[99] A comparison of toxic effects, dose delivery, and dose delay for women over age 70, those aged 50–69, and those younger than 50 demonstrated no differences between groups. Time to disease progression and survival were also not influenced by age.

Ganz et al.[100] studied the psychosocial morbidity of chemotherapy in elderly patients and found that the frequency of anxiety related to chemotherapy, before and after chemotherapy nausea, and problems with daily living resulting from treatment did not differ for young and old patients. In addition, the severity of these problems seemed to be greater in the young patients. Nerenz et al.[101] also found that elderly patients interviewed during chemotherapy seemed to have lower levels of emotional distress or interruption of daily activities than younger patients. These studies suggest that chemotherapy can be delivered with acceptable toxicity in the elderly. Decisions regarding the use of chemotherapy should be made on the basis of the patient's risk of breast cancer recurrence, overall health status, and current and future quality of life. At present, tamoxifen remains the mainstay of adjuvant therapy for women over age 70. In patients at high risk of relapse, such as those with multiple positive lymph nodes and negative estrogen receptor status, the use of chemotherapy should be considered.

## Patterns of Care in the Elderly

A number of studies suggest that age at breast cancer diagnosis is a major determinant of the type of therapy received. Busch et al.[102] examined patterns of care for women age 75 and older treated in 1983 ($n$ = 3496) and 1990 ($n$ = 5643). A total of 17,128 patients from 1983 and 24,115 from 1990 were studied. Only minor differences in the use of mastectomy and breast-conserving therapy were reported between age groups. However, the older women were significantly less likely than their younger counterparts to receive breast irradiation for both time periods, with 72% of older women treated in 1983 and 49% treated in 1990 receiving no radiation. Axillary dissection was omitted in 20.6% of the older women compared to 10.0% of the younger women in 1990. Similar findings were reported by Wanebo et al.,[51] using data from the Rhode Island Tumor Registry, with omission of axillary dissection and breast irradiation, the most common differences in the local therapy of old and young women.

Greenfield and coauthors[103] reviewed the charts of 374 women aged 50 and older treated at seven hospitals between 1980 and 1982, to determine the effect of age and co-morbidity on treatment. Only 67.4% of women age 70 and older received treatment deemed appropriate, compared with 83.4% of women age 50–69 ($p$ = 0.0001). These differences persisted after controlling for co-morbidity and were particularly pronounced in women with stage III and IV disease. Allen et al.[104] noted major age-related differences in the use of adjuvant systemic therapy in a study of 1795 women, including 405 age 65 and older treated at Duke University Medical Center. Among women age 65 and older with regional node metastases, 67% received no adjuvant chemotherapy or hormonal therapy compared to 37% of women under age 55. In addition, although the 1990 SEER data indicated that 47.7% of breast cancers occurred in women age 65 and older, only 17.3% of women treated in National Cancer Institute (NCI)-sponsored breast cancer clinical trials fell into this age group.[4] The lack of representation of older women in these trials makes it difficult to generalize their results to the elderly population. Overall, the pattern of less aggressive local therapy in the elderly and the decreased utilization of adjuvant systemic therapy suggest that inadequate treatment may be responsible for some of the breast cancer-related mortality observed in this age group.

## References


1. Landis SM, Murray T, Bolden S, Wingo PA. Cancer statistics 1998. CA Cancer J Clin 1998;48:6–29.
2. Bergman I, Kekker G, Van Leeuwen F, et al. The effect of age on treatment choice and survival in elderly breast cancer patients. Cancer 1991;67:2227–2234.

3. Goodwin J, Hunt W, Humble C, et al. Cancer protocols: who gets chosen? Arch Intern Med 1988;148:2258–2261.
4. Trimble El, Carter CL, Cain D, et al. Representation of older patients in cancer treatment trials. Cancer 1994;74:2208–2212.
5. MacMahon B, Cole P, Brown J. Etiology of human breast cancer: a review. J Natl Cancer Inst 1973;50:21–42.
6. Waterhouse J, Muis C, Correa P, et al. (eds). Cancer Incidence in Five Continents, vol 3. AIRC Scientific Publications 15. Lyon International Agency for Research on Cancer: Lyon, 1976.
7. Miller BA, Feur EJ, Hankey BF. The significance of the rising incidence of breast cancer in the United States. In: Devita V, Hellman S, Rosenberg S (eds) Important Advances in Oncology 1994. Lippincott: Philadelphia, 1994:193–207.
8. Yancik R, Ries LG, Yates JW. Breast cancer in aging women: a population based study of contrasts in stage, surgery, and survival. Cancer 1989;63:876–981.
9. Chu KC, Tarone RE, Kessler LG, et al. Recent trends in U.S. breast cancer, incidence, survival and mortality rates. J Natl Cancer Inst 1996;88:1571–1579.
10. Bernardo G, Plastina B, Strada M, et al. Breast cancer in elderly patients: our experience about some features. Ann Oncol 1994;5:59–63.
11. Rosen P, Lesser M, Kinne D. Breast carcinoma at the extremes of age: a comparison of patients younger than 35 years and older than 75 years. J Surg Oncol 1995:28:90–95.
12. Swanson R, Sawicka J, Wood W. Treatment of carcinoma of the breast in the older geriatric patient. Surg Gynecol Obstet 1991;173:465–469.
13. Von Rosen A, Gardelin A, Auer G. Assessment of malignancy potential in mammary carcinoma in elderly patients. Am J Clin Oncol 1987;10:61–67.
14. Schottenfeld D, Robbins G. Breast cancer in elderly women. Geriatrics 1971;3:121–126.
15. Schaefer G, Rosen P, Lesser M, et al. Breast carcinoma in elderly women: pathology, prognosis, survival. Pathol Ann 1984:195–219.
16. McCarty KS, Silva JS, Cox EB, et al. Relationship of age and menopausal status to estrogen receptor content in primary carcinomas of the breast. Ann Surg 1983;197:123–127.
17. Meyer JS, Hixon B. Advanced stage and early relapse of breast carcinomas associated with high thymidine labeling indices. Cancer Res 1979;39:4942–4047.
18. Van Dijck JAAM, Holland R, Verbeek ALM, Hendriks JHCL, Mravanuc M. Efficacy of mammographic screening of the elderly: a case referent study in the Nijmegen program in The Netherlands. J Natl Cancer Inst 1994;86: 934–938.
19. Fletcher S, Black W, Harris R, et al. Report of the International Workshop on Screening for Breast Cancer. J Natl Cancer Inst 1993;85:1644–1649.
20. Kerlikowske K, Grady D, Rubin S, et al. Efficacy of screening mammography: a meta-analysis. JAMA 1995;273: 49–52.
21. Andersson I, Aspergren K, Janzon L, et al. Effect of mammographic screening on breast cancer mortality in an urban population in Sweden: results from the randomized mammographic screening trial. Br Med J 1988;297:943–948.
22. Shapiro S, Venet W, Strax P, et al. Periodic screening for breast cancer: The Health Insurance Plan Project and Its Sequelae, 1963–1986. Johns Hopkins University Press: Baltimore, 1988.
23. Tabar L, Fagerberg G, Duffy S, et al. The Swedish two country trial of mammographic screening for breast cancer: recent results and calculation of benefit. J Epidemiol Commun Health 1989;42:197–214.
24. Van Dijck JAAM, Verbeek ALM, Beer LVAM, et al. Breast cancer mortality in a non-randomized trial on mammographic screening in women over age 65. Int J Cancer 1997;70:165–168.
25. Faulk R, Sickles E, Sollitto R, et al. Clinical efficacy of mammographic screening in the elderly. Radiology 1995;194: 193–298.
26. Wilson T, Helvie M, August D. Breast cancer in the elderly patient: early detection with mammography. Radiology 1994;190:203–209.
27. Mandelblatt J, Wheat M, Monane M, et al. Breast cancer screening for elderly women with and without co-morbid conditions. Ann Intern Med 1992;116:722–730.
28. Moskowitz M. Breast cancer: age specific growth rates and screening strategies. Radiology 1986;161:37–41.
29. Boer R, deKoning JH, van Oortmarssen GJ, Vander Maaas PJ. In search of the best upper age limit for breast cancer screening. Eur J Cancer 1995;31A:2040–2043.
30. Guide to Clinical Preventive Services: An Assessment of the Effectiveness of 169 Interventions. Report of the US Preventive Services Task Force. Williams & Wilkins: Baltimore, 1989.
31. Brown JT, Hulka BS. Screening mammography in the elderly: a case control study. J Gen Intern Med 1988;3: 126–131.
32. NCI Breast Cancer Screening Consortium. Screening mammography: a missed clinical opportunity. JAMA 1990;264: 54–58.
33. Hayward R, Shapiro M, Freeman H. Who gets screened for breast and cervical cancer? Arch Intern Med 1988;148: 1177–1181.
34. Harris R, Fletcher S, Gonzalez J, et al. Mammography and age: are we targeting the wrong women? Cancer 1991;67: 2010–2014.
35. Weinberger M, Saunders A, Samsa G, et al. Breast cancer screening in older women: practices and barriers reported by primary care physicians. J Am Geriatr Soc 1991;39: 22–29.
36. Leather DS, Roberts MM. Older women's attitudes towards breast disease, self-examination, and screening facilities. Br Med J 1985;290:668–670.
37. Fox SA, Siu Al, Stein JA. The importance of physician communication on breast cancer screening of older women. Arch Intern Med 1994;154:2059–2068.
38. Schneiderman M, Axtell L. Deaths among female patients with carcinoma of the breast treated by surgical procedure alone. Surg Gynecol Obstet 1979;148:193–196.
39. Singletary SE, Shallenberger R, Guinee VF. Breast cancer in the elderly. Ann Surg 1993;218:667–671.
40. Davis S, Karrer F, Moor B, et al. Characteristics of breast cancer in women over 80 years of age. Am J Surg 1985;150: 655–658.

41. Hunt K, Fry D, Bland K. Breast carcinoma in the elderly patient: an assessment of operative risk, morbidity and mortality. Am J Surg 1980;140:339–342.
42. Kessler H, Seton J. The treatment of operable breast cancer in the elderly female. Am J Surg 1978;135:664–666.
43. Schottenfeld D, Robbins G. Breast cancer in elderly women. Geriatrics 1971;26:121–131.
44. Berg J, Robbins G. Modified mastectomy for older, poor risk patients. Surg Gynecol Obstet 1961;113:631–634.
45. Kraft R, Block G. Mammary carcinoma in the aged patient. Ann Surg 1962;156:981–985.
46. Fourquet A, Campana F, Zafrani B, et al. Prognostic factors of breast recurrence in the conservative management of early breast cancer: a 25 year follow up. Int J Radiat Oncol Biol Phys 1989;17:719–725.
47. Veronesi U, Salvadori B, Luini A, et al. Conservative treatment of early breast cancer: long term results of 1232 cases treated with quadrantectomy, axillary dissection and radiation. Ann Surg 1990;211:250–259.
48. Clark R, Wilkinson R, Miceli P, et al. Breast cancer: experiences with conservative therapy. Am J Clin Oncol 1987;10: 461–468.
49. Margolese R. Surgical considerations in selecting local therapy. J Natl Cancer Inst Monogr 1992;11:41–46.
50. Kantorowitz D, Poulter C, Sischy B, et al. Treatment of breast cancer among elderly women with segmental mastectomy or segmental mastectomy plus postoperative radiotherapy. Int J Radiat Oncol Biol Phys 1988;15: 263–270.
51. Wanebo MJ, Cole B, Chung M, et al. Is surgical management compromised in elderly patients with breast cancer? Ann Surg 1997;225:579–589.
52. Fisher B, Redmond C, Poisson R, et al. Eight year results of a randomized clinical trial comparing total mastectomy and lumpectomy with or without irradiation in the treatment of breast cancer. N Engl J Med 1989;320:822–828.
53. Liljegren G, Holmberg L, Adani MO, et al. Sector resection with and without postoperative radiotherapy for stage I breast cancer: five year results of a randomized trial. J Natl Cancer Inst 1994;86:717–722.
54. Clark R, McCulloch P, Levine M, et al. Randomized clinical trial to assess the effectiveness of breast irradiation following lumpectomy and axillary dissection for node-negative breast cancer. J Natl Cancer Inst 1992;84:683–689.
55. Veronesi U, Luini A, Del Vecchio M, et al. Radiotherapy after breast preserving surgery in women with localized cancer of the breast. N Engl J Med 1993;328:1587–1591.
56. Reed M, Morrison J. Wide local excision as the sole primary treatment in elderly patients with carcinoma of the breast. Br J Surg 1989;76:898–900.
57. Plowman P, Gilmore O, George S. Tamoxifen versus surgery in elderly patients with breast cancer. Lancet 1988;2: 891–892.
58. Schnitt SJ, Hayman J, Gelman R, et al. A prospective study of conservative surgery alone in the treatment of selected patients with stage I breast cancer. Cancer 1996;77: 1094–1100.
59. Wyckoff J, Greenberg H, Sanderson R, et al. Breast irradiation in the older woman: a toxicity study. J Am Geriatr Soc 1994;42:150–154.
60. Morrow M, Bucci C, Rademaker A. Medical contraindications are not a major factor in the underutilization of breast conserving therapy. J Am Coll Surg 1998;186:269–274.
61. Stewart J, Foster R. Breast cancer and aging. Semin Oncol 1989;16:677–681.
62. Maher M, Campanor F, Mosseri V, et al. Breast cancer in elderly women: a retrospective analysis of combined treatment with tamoxifen and once-weekly irradiation. Int J Radiat Oncol Biol 1995;31:783–789.
63. Bolton J, Kuske R, McKinnon W, et al. Phase 1/11 trial of wide field brachytherapy as the sole method of breast irradiation in TIS 1,2 No-1 breast cancer. In: Proceedings of the 47th Cancer Symposium of the Society of Surgical Oncology, 1992:7.
64. Fisher B, Redmond C, Fisher E. Ten year results of a randomized trial comparing radical mastectomy and total mastectomy with or without radiation. N Engl J Med 1985;312:674–681.
65. Halverson K, Taylor M, Perez C, et al. Regional nodal management and patterns of failure following conservative surgery and radiation therapy for stage I and II breast cancer. Int J Radiat Oncol Biol Phys 1993;26:593–597.
66. Britton R, Nelson P. Causes and treatment of post mastectomy lymphedema of the arm: report of 114 cases. JAMA 1962;180:95–98.
67. Budd D, Cochran R, Sturetz D, et al. Surgical morbidity after mastectomy operations. Am J Surg 1978;135:218–220.
68. Larson D, Weinstein M, Goldberg I. Edema of the arm as a function of the extent of axillary surgery in patients with stage I–II carcinoma of the breast treated with primary radiotherapy. Int J Radiat Oncol Biol Phys 1986;12: 1575–1582.
69. Pezner R, Patterson M, Hill L, et al. Arm lymphedema in patients treated conservatively for breast cancer: relationship to patient age and axillary node dissection technique. Int J Radiat Oncol Biol Phys 1986;12:2079–2083.
70. Hladiuk M, Huchcroft S, Temple W, et al. Arm function after axillary dissection for breast cancer: a pilot study to provide parameter estimates. J Surg Oncol 1992; 50:47–50.
71. Glick J, Gelber R, Goldhirsch A, Senn HJ. Meeting highlights adjuvant therapy for primary breast cancer. J Natl Cancer Inst 1992;84:1479–1485.
72. Morton D, Wen D-R, Wong J, et al. Technical details of intraoperative lymphatic mapping for early stage melanoma. Arch Surg 1992;127:392–399.
73. Giuliano AE, Kirgan DM, Guenther JM, et al. Lymphatic mapping and sentinel lymphadenectomy for breast cancer. Ann Surg 1994;220:391–401.
74. Giuliano AE, Jones RC, Brennan M, et al. Sentinel lymphadenectomy in breast cancer. J Clin Oncol 1997;15: 2345–2350.
75. Krag DN, Weaver DL, Ashikaga T, et al. The sentinel node in breast cancer. A multicenter validation study. N Engl J Med 1998;337:941–946.
76. Albertini JJ, Lyman GH, Cox C, et al. Lymphatic mapping and sentinel node biopsy in the patient with breast cancer. JAMA 1996;276:1818–1823.
77. Veronesi U, Paganelli G, Galimberto V, et al. Sentinel node biopsy to avoid axillary dissection in breast cancer with

clinically negative lymph nodes. Lancet 1997;349:1864–1869.
78. Shons A, Joseph E, Cox CE, et al. Predictors of sentinel lymph node metastases in the lymphatic mapping of breast cancer patients. Breast Cancer Res Treat 1997;46:24.
79. Galimberto V, Zurrida S, Veronesi U, et al. Can sentinel node biopsy and axillary dissection in no breast cancer patients? Breast Cancer Res Treat 1997;46:24.
80. Giuliano AE, Dale PS, Turner RR, et al. Improved axillary staging of breast cancer with sentinel lymphadenectomy. Ann Surg 1995;222:394–401.
81. Turner RR, Ollila DW, Krasne PL, Giuliano AE. Histopathologic validation of the sentinel lymph node hypothesis for breast cancer. Ann Surg 1997;226:271–278.
82. Preece P, Wood R, Mackie C, et al. Tamoxifen as initial sole treatment of localized breast cancer in elderly women: a pilot study. Br Med J 1982;284:869–870.
83. Helleberg A, Lundgren B, Norin T, et al. Treatment of early localized breast cancer in elderly patients by tamoxifen. Br J Radiol 1982;55:511–515.
84. Allan S, Rodger A, Smyth J, et al. Tamoxifen as primary treatment of breast cancer in elderly or frail patients: a practical management. Br Med J 1985;290:358.
85. Gaskell D, Hawkins R, Sangsterl K, et al. Relation between immunocytochemical estimation of estrogen receptor in elderly patients with breast cancer and response to tamoxifen. Lancet 1989;1:1044–1046.
86. Robertson J, Ellis I, Elston C, et al. Mastectomy or tamoxifen as initial therapy for operative breast cancer in elderly patients: 5 year follow-up. Eur J Cancer Clin Oncol 1992; 28A:908–910.
87. Falk G, Gywnne-Jones D, Gray J. Efficacy of tamoxifen as the primary treatment of operable breast cancer in the high risk patient. Aust NZ J Surg 1989;59:543–545.
88. Foudraine N, Verhoef L, Burghouts J. Tamoxifen as sole therapy for primary breast cancer in the elderly patient. Eur J Cancer Clin Oncol 1992;14:900–903.
89. Bates T, Riley D, Houghton J, et al. Breast cancer in elderly women: a Cancer Research Campaign trial comparing treatment with tamoxifen and optimal surgery with tamoxifen alone. Br J Surg 1991;78:591–594.
90. Margolese R, Foster R. Tamoxifen as an alternative to surgical resection for selected geriatric with primary breast cancer. Arch Surg 1989;124:548–551.
91. Auclerc C, Khayat D, Borel C, et al. Tamoxifen as sole treatment in patients aged 65 and over with primary breast cancer. Proc Am Soc Clin Oncol 1990;9:A173.
92. Gazet J, Markopoulos C, Ford H. Prospective randomized trial of tamoxifen versus surgery in elderly patients with breast cancer. Lancet 1988;1:679–681.
93. Early Breast Cancer Trialists' Collaborative Group. Tamoxifen for early breast cancer: an overview of the randomized trials. Lancet 1998;351:1451–1460.
94. Cummings F, Gray R, Davis T, et al. Adjuvant tamoxifen treatment of elderly women with stage II breast cancer. Ann Intern Med 1989;103:324–329.
95. Cummings F, Gray R, Tormey D, et al. Adjuvant tamoxifen versus placebo in elderly women with node positive breast cancer: long-term follow-up and causes of death. J Clin Oncol 1993;11:29–35.
96. Castiglione M, Gelber RD, Goldhirsch A. Adjuvant systemic therapy for breast cancer in the elderly: competing causes of mortality. J Clin Oncol 1990;8:519–526.
97. Bonnadonna G, Valagussa P. Dose-response effect of adjuvant chemotherapy in breast cancer. N Engl J Med 1981; 304:10–15.
98. Begg C, Cohen J, Ellerton J. Are the elderly predisposed to toxicity from chemotherapy? Cancer Clin Trials 1980;3: 369–374.
99. Christman K, Muss H, Case L, et al. Chemotherapy of metastatic breast cancer in the elderly: the Piedmont Oncology Association experience. JAMA 1992;268: 57–62.
100. Ganz PA, Schag CC, Heinrich RL. The psychosocial impact of cancer on the elderly: a comparison with younger patients. J Am Geriatr Soc 1985;33:429–435.
101. Nerenz DR, Love RR, Leventhal H, et al. Psychosocial consequences of cancer chemotherapy for elderly patients. Health Serv Res 1986;20:961–976.
102. Busch E, Kemeny M, Fremgen A, et al. Patterns of breast cancer care in the elderly. Cancer 1996;78:101–111.
103. Greenfield S, Bianco D, Elashoff RM, Ganz PA. Patterns of care related to age of breast cancer patients. JAMA 1987; 257:2766–2770.
104. Allen C, Cox EB, Manton KG, Cohen JH. Breast cancer in the elderly: current patterns of care. J Am Geriatr Soc 1986;34:637–642.

# *Part II*
# *Specific Issues in Geriatric Surgery*

## Section 3
## Eyes, Ears, Nose, and Throat

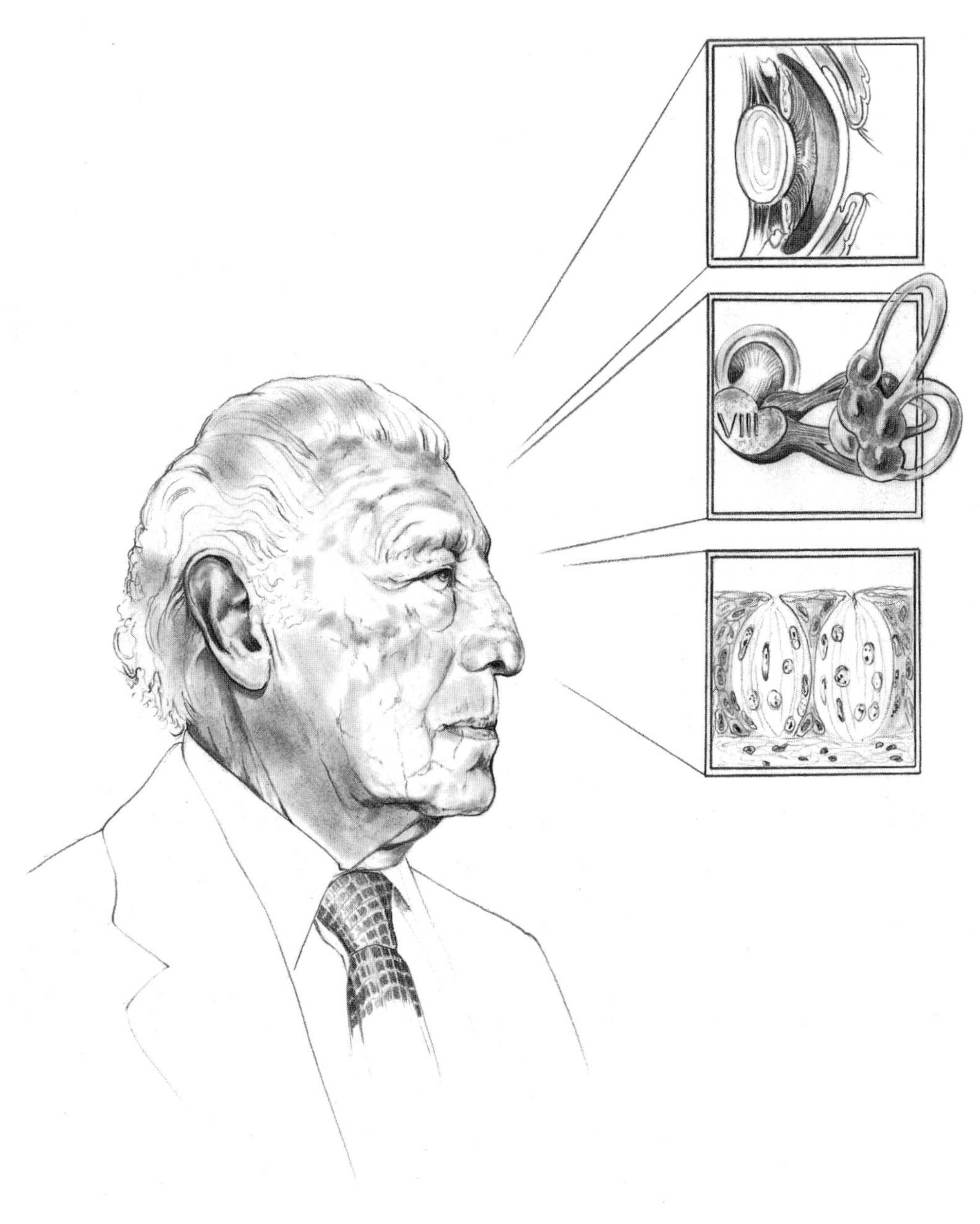

# Invited Commentary

Charles W. Cummings

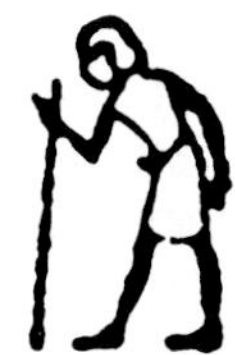

I am most appreciative for the opportunity to write a chapter denoting the highlights and substantial milestones of the evolution of otolaryngology as it exists today from the past quarter of a century. As with all other medical disciplines, technologic advancement has transformed the configuration of the specialty. My good fortune has been to be an interested passenger on this rather meteoric ride toward the amelioration of substantial disease processes and rehabilitation of the compromised patient. My intention is to review briefly the traditional areas of concern for the larynx, ear, nose, and oral cavity, as well as the oncologic advances that have occurred as they apply to head and neck cancer.

Certainly laryngeal disorders, both benign and malignant, have been brought into far sharper focus literally, through the use of the operating microscope and figuratively, through the marshaling of the interest of talented basic and clinical researchers. Miniaturization and understanding of laser technology began during the 1960s to affect the way laryngologists viewed and treated benign and malignant diseases. Papillomatous diseases of the larynx, as well as small benign, even malignant, true vocal cord pathologies were found to be suitably treated by the $CO_2$ laser with few side effects. Success with this modality has allowed further development, so now the indications for laser surgery include even laryngeal cancers, the claim being that the treatment is less invasive than more traditional surgical approaches. Conservation laryngeal surgery has remained an integral component of the management of laryngeal cancer. Through better understanding of laryngeal embryology and lymphatic outflow patterns, substantial components of the laryngeal skeleton may be removed, providing a long-term cancer-free status in a patient who remains able to communicate in a quasinormal fashion. One of the most effective contributions to the surgical management of laryngeal cancer has been the development of the tracheoesophageal fistula, a valved prostheses that is now used commonly in patients who are totally laryngectomized. This one-way conduit allows the patient to eat normally and, by diverting air into the upper cervical esophagus and hypopharynx, phonate with an effective, if not normal, voice. The mainstreaming of a laryngectomized patient is no longer an insurmountable task.

The operating microscope has fostered miniaturization of instruments and the development of a totally new concept of vocal cord surgery. Today small, yet functionally debilitating polyps or nodules affecting the mucosal or submucosal space, may be removed with substantially less scarring and postoperative morbidity than heretofore possible. These procedures, in concert with effective, aggressive speech therapy, have contributed substantially to an improved state of laryngeal function.

The laryngeal dystonias, originally thought to be functional disorders, are now recognized to be organic neurologic entities. Furthermore, using the neuroparalytic qualities of botulinusm toxin, the adductor and abductor dystonias can be treated successfully, lifting the often crushing burden of phonatory incompetence from the patient's back. This treatment is a truly remarkable intervention. One of the most innovative and satisfying advancements with respect to laryngeal dysfunction has been the development of a family of procedures that focus on vocal rehabilitation of patients afflicted with adductor paralysis (which has a profoundly negative effect on the ability to phonate). The effect of augmenting the paralyzed and atrophic vocal cord so its mucosal surface effectively interfaces with the opposite vocal cord was initially achieved by injecting Teflon paste into the endolaryngeal tissue lateral to the cricoarytenoid muscle. This technique was neither tunable nor reversible, but it was quite effective for the most part. Subsequently, a series of procedures were developed that allow introduction of variously sized prostheses so the voice can be tuned at the operating table and reversed should the need arise.

The advancements made by the audiologic and otologic community are far-reaching and have an extraordinary impact. Aural rehabilitation has been transformed during the past quarter-century, again through the wonders of miniaturization and electronic advancement. Hearing aids have become frequency selective and inordinately tunable. Amplification of sound through air conduction has been finely tuned and in some cases supplanted by transforming the ossicles or bony capsule of the cochlea. Furthermore, in the presence of the totally deafened ear where the auditory nerve is still intact, cochlear prostheses have bypassed the external and middle ear entirely to allow totally deafened patients to become mainstreamed into society. Cochlear prosthesis technology has allowed schoolchildren to receive an education and to communicate and compete effectively in society. Again, through microscope visualization, procedures have been developed that allow tumors to be dissected free of the auditory nerve at the brain stem with preservation of hearing. If the tumors are small, facial nerve function is preserved as well. Reconstitution of the ossicular chain damaged by trauma or infection and reconstruction of the tympanic membrane to re-create an air-containing middle ear cleft are the end-products of this surgical revolution.

The most common otologic affliction—secretory otitis media—affects hundreds of thousands of children and, if allowed to persist, has a substantially detrimental effect on the ability to learn in the classroom. Myringotomy with an indwelling ventilation tube, despite its simplicity, probably has had more impact on childhood growth and development than any other surgical or medical maneuver.

Until the past decade, vestibular disease, manifested by vertigo and unsteadiness, were poorly understood and even less enthusiastically addressed by the physician. This complex mechanism has now been unraveled to the point where objective vestibular testing can be done in a reproducible, understandable fashion; and further treatments have been developed to treat those individuals afflicted with benign positional vertigo. This therapy, in the form of vestibular positioning exercises, has been most effective. In this arena, as in no other associated with the head and neck, diagnostic imaging has contributed extraordinarily through enhanced computed tomography and magnetic resonance scans. Small abnormalities such as acoustic neuromas are now diagnosed and treated before irreversible sequelae ensue.

Without question, the nose and paranasal sinuses are the source of more symptoms of illness than any other segment of the body. The olfactory sense remains the least understood of the senses, yet one whose absence may have a devastating effect. Scientific advancement of olfactory physiology has only recently been modestly successful. Observations such that alterations in smell (and trace metal abnormalities) are symptoms of early Alzheimer's disease are recent. A biopsy of the olfactory sensory epithelium may allow diagnosis of Alzheimer's disease to become apparent though the nuclear clumping that occurs. During the mid-1970s, paranasal sinus surgery involved destructive procedures that removed substantial segments of the normal anatomy in the quest to provide drainage for sequestered areas of trapped mucous purulent debris. Minimally invasive endoscopic sinus surgery has essentially supplanted the methods of the past, so that now preservation of normal anatomy and thus normal nasal function, while at the same time evacuating the focus of disease is the norm. Similarly, orbital decompression for exophthalmos is done endoscopically rather than openly. Transsphenoidal pituitary resection and excision of early-stage inverted papillomas or in some cases, malignant tumors, are being accomplished endoscopically as well. With these techniques the postoperative morbidity is substantially reduced. Surgical repair for spinal fluid leak starting in the fovea ethmoidalis can be accomplished transnasally rather than cranially. When dealing with malignant tumors that involve the ethmoid region, removal of the anterior cranial base while preserving the dura has become the procedure of choice. The neuroradiologist, through collaboration with the otorhinolaryngologist, has transformed procedures with high morbidity (e.g., removal of juvenile angiofibromas) to a scenario where tumors may be removed subsequent to embolization with minimal blood loss and marked reduction in operating room anxiety.

No single development with respect to nasal function remotely competes with the contributions of pharmacology through topically administered nasal steroids. The treatment of vasoreactive nasal mucositis, allergically or nonallergically based, with long-term nasal steroids has substantially reduced the incidence of nasal surgery for chronic sinusitis.

Although not specific to the head and neck, medical and surgical advances and diagnosis and treatment for oncologic conditions have advanced profoundly. Through the wonders of molecular biology, genetic abnormalities at *p53*, *p9*, and *p16* of overexpression or underexpression have been observed to have an intimate relation with head and neck cancers. Molecular biologic assessment of surgical margins has been successfully prognostic. It has been shown that although the histology may appear to be normal at the margin, there may in fact be genetic abnormalities (*p53*) that affect the long-term prognosis of the patient and thus, in turn, direct a more aggressive adjunctive approach to the tumor site. The early stages of gene therapy are now upon us, so those predisposed to head and neck malignancies may be identified and undergo genetic manipulation as a means to alleviate the susceptibility. Protocols for advanced head and neck disease, predominantly oropharyngeal and laryngeal, have evolved utilizing chemotherapy and radiation therapy in an attempt to preserve laryngeal or oral function. Organ preservation protocols, unheard of two decades ago, have assumed a role of respectability and hope. Surgery remains the modality of choice in most instances, and it is here that the menu of options has shifted rather profoundly such that now it is commonplace for a patient to undergo an extensive resection with immediate reconstruction. For a high-grade malignant parotid tumor involving resection of the facial nerve and the lateral base of the skull, primary reconstruction at the same surgery using free tissue transfer, dynamic muscular slings, and implantation of a gold weight in the upper lid provides optimal care in facial reanimation/rehabilitation. Immediate reconstruction has become the norm as well with respect to mandibular reconstruction. Surgical management of cervical nodal metastases using radical neck dissection (removal of the jugular vein and strap muscles as well as the spinal accessory nerve) has been transformed to a selective neck dissection where almost invariably the accessory nerve is preserved unless it is intimately involved by the tumor. Sternocleidomastoid muscle and jugular vein preservation is the norm rather than the exception. An awareness that reconstruction and rehabilitation are as important as extirpation is a concept that has finally matured to the patient's benefit.

The anatomic region of the head and neck, including the ears, nose, and throat, has benefited extraordinarily by technologic and procedural advances. Much has evolved since the 1970s. The chapters in this section support this statement.

# 25
# Pathogenesis and Surgical Management of Common Geriatric Ophthalmic Disorders

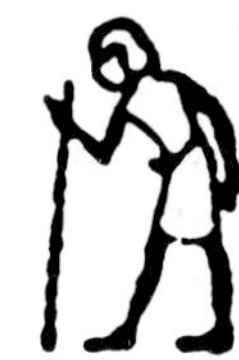

Ray F. Gariano, Jayne N. Ge, and Kathleen M. Stoessel

Visual loss is a leading cause of morbidity in elderly patients in industrialized and developing countries. Decreased visual acuity interferes with activities such as reading, driving, walking without assistance, and numerous daily tasks that allow employment and independent living. It has been estimated that in the United States 10% of persons over the age of 75 years have a visual disability, and 2.2% over age 65 years are legally blind (defined as acuity of 20/200 or worse in the better eye or visual field constriction to less than 20 degrees).[1–4] Many cases of legal blindness are preventable with early detection and treatment.[5,6]

Table 25.1 is a partial compendium of ophthalmic diseases that are more prevalent in the geriatric population, arranged according to anatomic location from the front to the back of the eye. This chapter describes pathogenesis and laser and surgical treatment for several of these disorders, with an emphasis on more common intraocular conditions. References are provided for readers interested in more detailed coverage of topics.

## Clinical Ocular Anatomy

A brief review of ocular anatomy can clarify later discussion of surgical approaches (Fig. 25.1). The eye is supported within the bony orbit by fat deposits. Six extraocular muscles control eye movements and arise from the posterior orbit and insert onto the anterior third of the globe (the superior oblique tendon and inferior oblique muscle arise from the anteromedial orbital wall and insert onto the posterior sclera). Eyelids consist of anterior (muscle fibers and skin) and posterior (tarsal plate and palpebral conjunctiva) lamellae. Conjunctiva lines the back of the lids and extends onto the sclera.

The cornea is the transparent curved anterior aspect of the eye, and provides approximately two-thirds of the eye's optical dioptric power. Clarity is achieved in part by an anhydrous state maintained by ion-pumping mechanisms in the posterior endothelial layer. The cornea is lubricated by tears secreted by glands within the palpebral conjunctiva and by the lacrimal gland in the anterior superotemporal orbit. The cornea is continuous with the tough white outer scleral coat of the eye, which in turn invests the optic nerve behind the globe and is continuous with dura mater of the central nervous system.

Just posterior to the cornea and anterior to the pigmented iris is the anterior chamber, filled with clear aqueous humor produced by the ciliary body located behind the iris root. Aqueous humor enters the anterior chamber mostly through the pupil and exits the eye mostly via channels in the trabecular meshwork, located in the "angle" between the peripheral iris and the cornea. The balance between aqueous humor production and outflow yields the intraocular pressure. In addition to its role in intraocular pressure, aqueous humor, along with oxygen in the external air, provides nourishment to the avascular cornea. Pupil size is adjusted by iris sphincter and dilator muscles, which are controlled by parasympathetic and sympathetic innervation, respectively.

The lens provides about one-third of the dioptric power of the eye and is suspended just posterior to the pupil by thin fibers (zonules) arising from the ciliary body. Parasympathetic innervation to the ciliary muscle relaxes zonular tension and increases lens power (accommodation). The lens is an avascular tissue without direct neural innervation. A layer of epithelial cells lines the anterior surface, and the lens cortex and nucleus are comprised of concentrically arranged cellular fibers.

The vitreous cavity is the largest cavity of the eye and is filled with approximately 4 ml of viscous vitreous humor that adheres to the posterior lens capsule anteriorly and to the neurosensory retina posteriorly. Rod and cone photoreceptors and vertically and horizontally oriented neural circuits within the retina initiate processing for functions of visual perception, including contrast, color, and motion. The retinal "output" neuron is the ganglion cell, and more than one million retinal ganglion cell axons collect to form the optic nerve, which projects via the optic chiasm to thalamic sensory nuclei. A significant proportion of optic nerve fibers projects to brain stem nuclei involved in pupillary reactions and coordinated eye movements.

TABLE 25.1. Selected Ophthalmic Disorders Associated with Aging

Eyelids
- Ptosis
- Dermatochalasis
- Entropion
- Ectropion
- Blepharospasm
- Malignancies[a]
- Herpes zoster ophthalmicus
- Trichiasis

Cornea, conjunctiva, sclera
- Keratitis sicca (dry eye)
- Epiphora (tearing)
- Infectious corneal ulceration
- Inflammatory corneal and scleral ulceration[b]
- Bullous keratopathy
- Inherited corneal dystrophies
- Benign and malignant growths[c]

Lens
- Presbyopia
- Cataract

Glaucoma
- Primary open-angle glaucoma
- Angle-closure glaucoma
- Neovascular glaucoma

Retina and vitreous
- Macular degeneration
- Retinal vascular occlusions
- Diabetic retinopathy
- Epiretinal membrane
- Retinal break
- Retinal detachment
- Endophthalmitis
- Macular hole
- Drug toxicity (e.g., Plaquenil)

Intraocular tumors
- Uveal malignant melanoma[d]
- Uveal metastasis[d]
- B cell lymphoma

Neuroophthalmic disorders
- Cranial nerve III, IV, and VI palsies
- Bell's palsy
- Ischemic optic neuropathy
- Giant cell (temporal) arteritis
- Myasthenia gravis
- Stroke

Ocular trauma
- Hyphema
- Corneoscleral laceration
- Lens dislocation/subluxation
- Vitreous hemorrhage
- Choroidal rupture

[a] Basal, squamous, and sebaceous cell carcinomas, for example.
[b] May be associated with vasculitides such as polyarteritis nodosa and rheumatoid arthritis.
[c] Pterygium and conjunctival intraepithelial neoplasia, for example.
[d] Most commonly in the choroid.

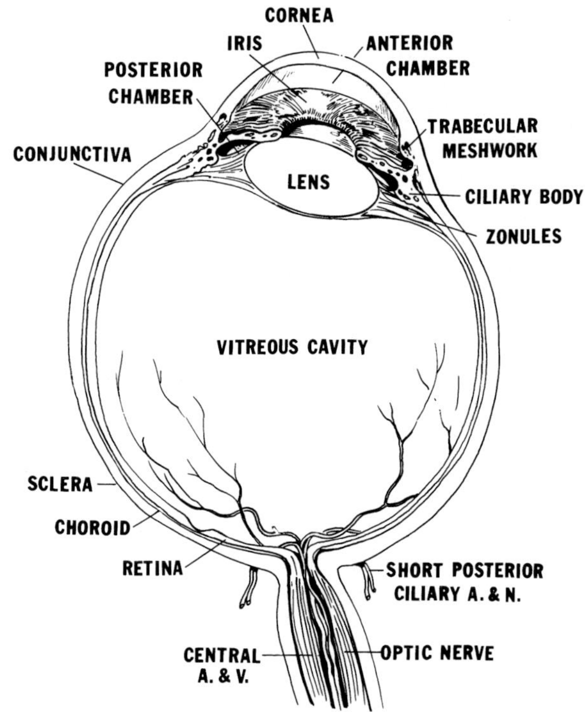


FIGURE 25.1. Eye removed from the orbit and disconnected from extraocular muscles, nerves, and vessels.

The retina; optic nerve, chiasm, tract, and radiations; lateral geniculate nuclei; and visual cortex are visuotopically arranged. Thus, the central portion of the retina, or macula, and the centermost region, the fovea, are specialized for fine acuity, whereas more peripheral portions of the retina subserve the peripheral visual field. Intraretinal arterioles and venules enter and exit the eye at the optic nerve head. Between the retina and the outer scleral eyewall are interposed pigment epithelial and vascular choroidal laminae that, among other functions, supply nutrients to and remove waste products from the highly metabolically active photoreceptors.

## Ocular Examination

Examination of anterior ocular structures is facilitated by the slit-lamp. Because this binocular microscope projects a thin beam of light tangentially, structures such as the cornea, chamber, and lens are viewed in cross section. Pathology can thus be localized within a tissue (e.g., in the lens nucleus or cortex) and even to a single cellular layer (e.g., in the corneal endothelium).

The direct ophthalmoscope is familiar to all clinicians and is valuable to examine the optic nerve head and macula, especially after pupillary dilation. The head-mounted indirect binocular ophthalmoscope, however, is essential to obtain stereoscopic views of the fundus and to view more anterior retina. For these reasons, ocular disease may be difficult to exclude without use of a slit-lamp and indirect ophthalmoscopy.

Ancillary testing in ophthalmology includes formal visual field testing (e.g., to detect glaucomatous or neurologic field loss), fluorescein angiography (e.g., to diagnose retinal and choroidal vascular diseases), ultrasonography (e.g., to detect intraocular tumors when the ophthalmoscopic view is obscured), radiographic studies (e.g., to detect foreign bodies and orbital tumors), and visual electrophysiology (visual evoked potentials, electroretinogram, electrooculogram) to assess the functional status of visual pathways.

## Perioperative Considerations

The most feared risk of ocular and periocular surgery is blindness. Inadvertent administration into the eye of medications, such as a local anesthetic, have rarely occurred and may cause total loss of vision.[7] Postoperative intraocular infection can also result in blindness.[8] Other complications such as anterior chamber or vitreous hemorrhage, persistent or severe intraocular inflammation (uveitis), elevated intraocular pressure, and retinal detachment are more successfully managed, although loss of vision may occur.

General anesthesia is employed in children and patients unable to lie still because of physical or mental impairment. General anesthesia is also desirable for long procedures, in cases of ocular trauma with corneal or scleral lacerations, and for procedures involving manipulation deep within the orbit (e.g., enucleation), for which local anesthetic blocks may be inadequate. A common anesthetic scenario for eye surgery combines mild intravenous sedation with local anesthetic blocks.[9] Certain minor procedures are performed using only local or topical anesthetic drops.

Special considerations by the anesthesiologist for eye surgery include (1) the oculocardiac reflex mediated by the trigeminal (afferent) and vagal (efferent) nerves, by which manipulation of extraocular muscles induces bradycardia; (2) avoidance of succinylcholine in patients taking echothiophate for glaucoma; (3) discontinuation of nitrous oxide 10–15 minutes prior to intravitreal infusion of gas to be left in the eye, so diffusion of anesthetic gas into the eye and increased intraocular pressure do not occur; (4) avoidance of intraoperative bucking or movements that may cause extrusion of intraocular contents; and (5) unusual positioning requirements upon awakening (e.g., face-down after certain retinal procedures).[9]

Periocular anesthesia has four objectives. First, pain relief is achieved by blocking branches of the ophthalmic division of the fifth (trigeminal) cranial nerve. Second, ocular movement is minimized by reducing activity of the oculomoter and abducens nerves (the third and sixth cranial nerves, respectively). Third, visual perception is inhibited with a block of the optic nerve. Retrobulbar and peribulbar blocks accomplish these three objectives by their effects on crainial nerves II, III, V, and VI; the trochlear nerve is spared. The fourth objective, suppression of lid closure, is achieved with a facial (seventh) nerve block.

Sites of administration for ocular anesthesia are depicted in Figure 25.2. The anesthetic mixture generally includes a faster-acting agent such as 1% or 2% lidocaine and a longer-acting agent such as 0.75% bupivacaine. Complications of retrobulbar and peribulbar anesthetic injections are rare but serious; they include retrobulbar hemorrhage, globe or optic nerve perforation, and intradural anesthetic injection.[7,9] Subconjunctival and subcutaneous eyelid injections generally include epinephrine 1:1000 to minimize bleeding.

Most intraocular surgeries are performed with the patient supine, the lids held apart with a speculum, and with an operating microscope positioned over the eye. Microscope controls include X and Y movement, focus, magnification, and lighting adjustments; they are manipulated by foot with a control panel. Many oculoplastic surgeries and extraocular procedures, such as scleral buckling and enucleation, are performed using overhead operating room lighting and surgical loupes if desired.

The unique and delicate nature of ocular tissues requires needles, sutures, and instruments of commensurate specialization. The reader is referred to other

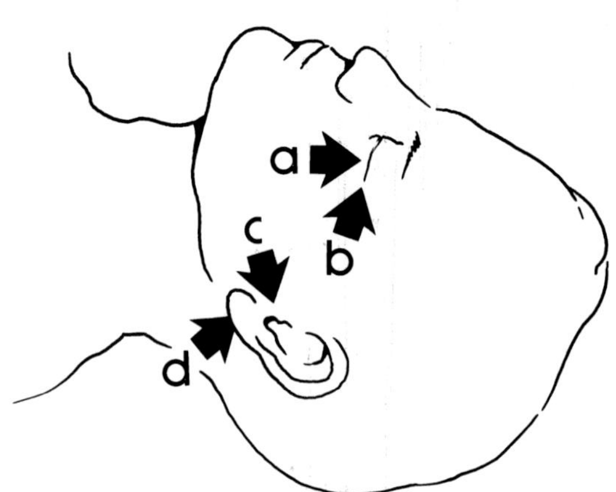


FIGURE 25.2. Sites of administration for commonly used anesthetic blocks. Retrobulbar (a) and peribulbar injections inhibit vision, pain fibers, and ocular motility (cranial nerves II, III, V, VI). The facial nerve can be blocked at the terminal branches (Van Lint) (b), the temporomandibular joint (O'Brien) (c), or the stylomastoid foramen (Nadbath) (d).

sources for details regarding ophthalmic surgical instrumentation.[10,11]

Wound care is of paramount concern during the postoperative period, as relatively fine sutures are employed in ocular surgery, and dehiscence may entail reoperation. Patients are usually instructed to avoid straining and heavy lifting for at least 2 weeks. An eye shield is often used for several weeks during sleep or activities in which injury may occur. Absorbable vicryl and plain gut sutures are used to close external wounds when possible to obviate suture removal. Medical therapy after eye surgery may include cycloplegic, antibiotic, and antiinflammatory eyedrops. Perioperative systemic antibiotics are indicated for certain orbital or nasolacrimal procedures, and in the setting of ocular trauma.

## Eyelid Lesions

Age-induced atrophy of eyelid tissues manifests as loss of skin elasticity and muscle tone. It predisposes the elderly to a number of functional and cosmetic conditions.

Dermatochalasis, or redundancy of the skin of the eyelids, is frequently associated with orbital fat herniation through the orbital septum into the anterior lid. Blepharoplasty[12] of the upper or lower lids (or both) corrects both conditions and is considered for superior visual field compromise or for cosmesis (Fig. 25.3).

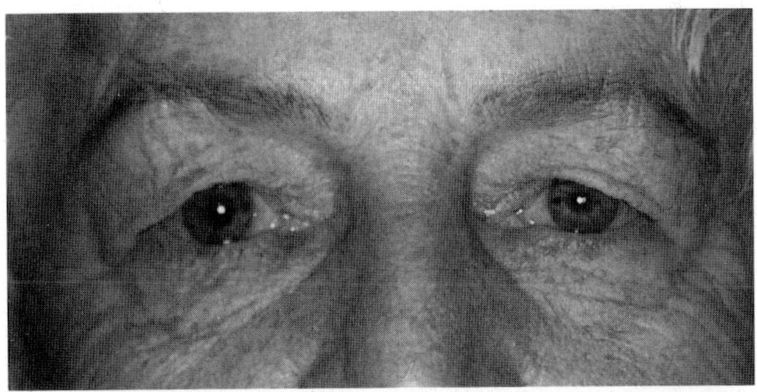

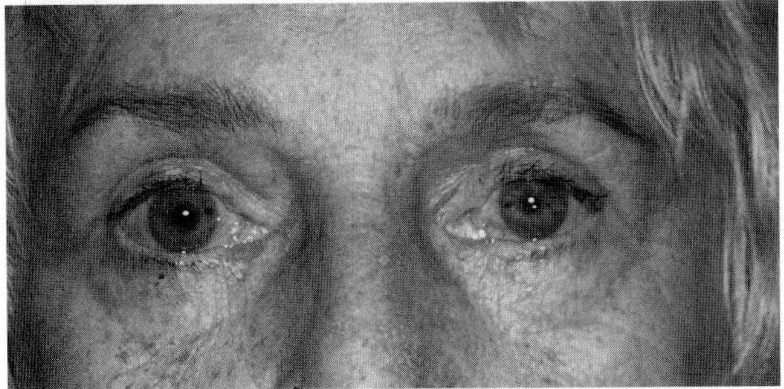

FIGURE 25.3. (Top) Dermatochalasis, or drooping eyelids due to excessive lax skin, may obstruct the superior or even the central visual field. (Bottom) Same patient, after bilateral blepharoplasty. (Courtesy of Jane Olsen, MD)

Senile ptosis is due to attenuation of the levator muscle or disinsertion of its aponeurosis from the tarsal plate in the upper lid. Ptosis repair is indicated for visual field obstruction or symptoms such as brow fatigue.[13] Brow ptosis is due to inferior displacement of the eyebrow below the supraorbital bony rim. Brow ptosis should be corrected by browplasty before lid ptosis and dermatochalasis can be properly evaluated.[14]

Entropion, or inward turning of the eyelid margins, is due in elderly patients to horizontal laxity to the eyelid, overriding of the preseptal orbicularis, and involutional enophthalmos. Foreign body sensation, redness, and tearing result as the lashes rub the cornea and conjunctiva. Surgical correction aims to rotate the lid outward by tissue resection, tightening lid retractors, or shortening the lower lid.[15]

Ectropion, or outward turning of the eyelid margin, occurs frequently in elderly patients owing to lower eyelid margin laxity. Poor apposition of the lid to the globe may cause tearing if the drainage puncta in the lids are not in contact with the tear film. Ectropion may also exacerbate dry eye symptoms and in severe cases may lead to corneal ulceration. Common procedures for senile ectropion are horizontal eyelid shortening and lateral tarsal strip.[16]

Blepharospasm is an involuntary, tonic spasmodic, bilateral contraction of the orbicularis oculi muscles lasting several seconds to several hours. Essential blepharospasm is poorly understood; in some patients basal ganglia dysfunction is implicated.[17] It occurs mainly in individuals over 45 years of age, may include other facial muscles, and if severe, causes both cosmetic deformity and visual impairment. Initial evaluation addresses irritative factors that may trigger spasm (e.g., dry eye, trichiasis, and stress). Periodic injection of botulinum toxin into the affected muscle is successful in 90% of patients.[17,18] In refractory cases, orbicularis oculi extirpation, oral tranquilizers, or neuroleptics are considered.

Eyelid tumors seen in elderly persons include benign lesions such as seborrheic keratosis, actinic keratosis, keratoacanthoma, xanthelasma, and papilloma; and malignant lesions such as basal cell carcinoma, sebaceous cell carcinoma, squamous cell carcinoma, and melanoma. The clinical history and examination of the lesion usually differentiate these lesions,[19,20] but definitive diagnosis requires histologic study of a biopsy specimen. If a tumor is malignant, complete excision is necessary. Moh's micrographic surgery, with stepwise excision and microscopic monitoring of surgical margins, has been reported to reduce recurrence and minimize damage to adjacent tissue for selected malignancies.[21] Oculoplastic reconstruction of the resulting defect is accomplished via primary closure if possible or with a mucocutaneous flap or graft.

## Lacrimal System Lesions

Dry eye symptoms associated with decreased tear production or poor apposition of the lid to the cornea due to lid laxity are the most common cause of red and irritated eyes in people over 65 years of age.[22] Dry eye together with xerostomia suggests Sjögren syndrome, a chronic lymphocytic infiltration of the lacrimal and salivary glands often associated with rheumatoid arthritis. Sjögren syndrome may be present in up to 3% of women over the age of 55 years.[23]

Dry eye symptoms are usually relieved with instillation of lubricating drops or ointments. Procedures to improve eyelid malpositions may be indicated (see discussion of ectropion and entropion, above). In severe cases, occlusion with silicone or collagen plugs of eyelid puncta through which tears enter the nasolacrimal drainage system can be curative;[24] permanent occlusion is achieved with electrodesiccation or thermal cautery of the puncta and canaliculus.[24] Temporary tarsorrhaphy (closure of the lids with sutures) is performed if dry eye leads to progressive corneal deterioration.

Conversely, tearing (epiphora) is also common in older patients and results from increased production or decreased drainage of tears. Increased tear production frequently results from surface irritation, such as dry eye syndrome, trichiasis (in-turned lashes), and abnormal lid positions. Decreased tear drainage occurs with stenosis or obstruction within the nasolacrimal drainage system. Simple probing and flushing of the system may relieve blockage. In persistant cases, dacryocystorhinostomy bypasses the obstruction by creating an osteotomy in the lacrimal bone between the lacrimal sac and the nasal cavity.[25]

## Corneal Disorders

Elderly patients are predisposed to corneal diseases because of reduced tear production, exposure, and dryness due to involutional eyelid malpositions and Bell's palsy, loss of corneal endothelial ion-pumping function, enhanced risk for infections and malignant and benign tumors, greater cumulative lifetime exposure to ultraviolet radiation, and predilection for surgical and nonsurgical trauma.[26] Because the cornea is the major refractive surface of the eye, these factors may result in optical aberrations or loss of clarity.

The most common cause of corneal opacification in the elderly in industrialized nations is pseudophakic bullous keratopathy.[27] With this disease, prior cataract surgery accelerates corneal endothelial decompensation, which leads to corneal edema and opacification. If the opacity is visually disabling, corneal transplantation (penetrating keratoplasty) is considered (Fig. 25.4). The benefits of acquiring a clear donor cornea are weighed against the risks of rejection and recurrence of the initial disorder. Details of this procedure, which is performed more than 40,000 times annually in the United States, are found elsewhere.[28]

## Lens

Accomodation is the mechanism by which the lens alters its shape—and thereby its power—to focus from distant to near images. The lens is relatively malleable during early life. Upon contraction of the ciliary muscle, tension in the zonule fibers relaxes, the lens assumes a more spherical shape, and optical power increases.[29] Presbyopia is a reduced capacity for accommodation resulting from age-related hardening of the lens, loss of zonules, and atrophy of ciliary muscle.

Infants have an accommodative reserve of more than 20 diopters, which allows them to focus on objects as close as 5 cm from the eyes. At age 40, the accommodative power is approximately 6 diopters, and difficulties with near vision may appear. By age 70–75 years, essentially all accommodative power is lost.[30]

Treatment of presbyopia with spectacles provides additional dioptric power to establish a focal point comfortable for reading and other near-vision activities. The

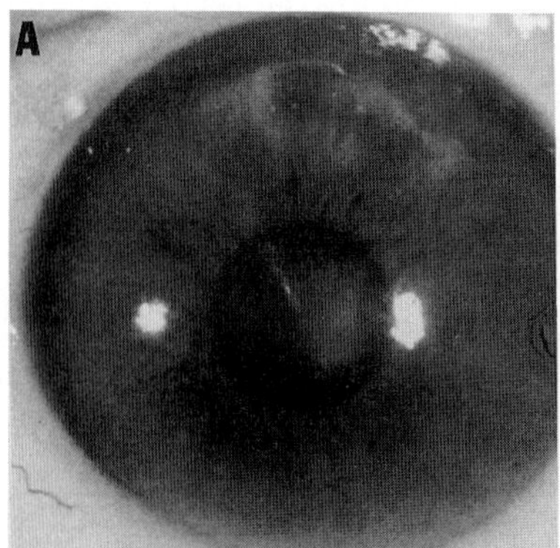


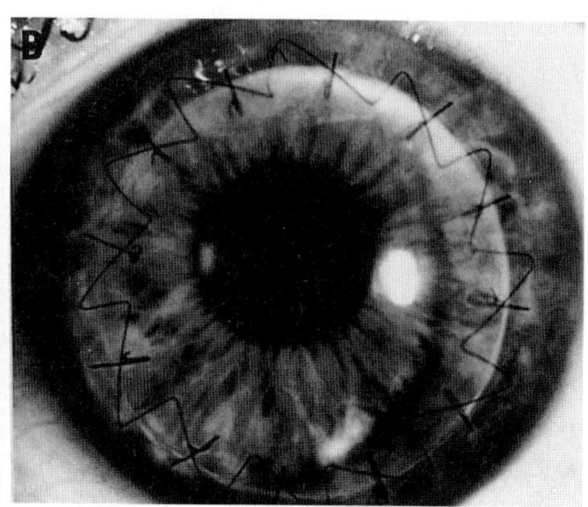


FIGURE 25.4. A. Corneal opacification in the right eye of a 71-year-old woman with prior cataract surgery. B. Clear donor cornea sutured in place with 12 interrupted radial sutures and a single continuous circumferential suture (10-0 nylon). Note the improved visualization of iris detail. Interrupted sutures may be cut selectively and removed postoperatively to reduce irregular corneal curvature and astigmatism. (Courtesy of Peter Gloor, MD)

power prescribed is a function of age and is provided either as separate reading glasses or as an "add" to the patient's distance-vision correction placed in the lower portion of glasses (e.g., bifocals). Contact lenses and prosthetic intraocular lenses have been developed to correct presbyopia, but their use is limited.[31]

## Cataract

Cataract, or loss of lens clarity, is the most common cause of decreased vision worldwide.[32] Although cataracts are associated with numerous factors, including trauma, inflammation, genetic predisposition, metabolic diseases, corticosteroid use, ultraviolet light exposure, and cigarette smoking, by far the most common association is aging.[33] Visually significant cataract has been found in more than 50% of persons 75 years of age or older.[32,34]

Senile cataracts are classified clinically according to their location within the lens capsule, cortex, or nucleus (Fig. 25.5). In many patients more than one type are present. The most common symptoms are blurring and glare.

Nuclear cataractogenesis, similar to other "molecular condensation diseases" such as sickle cell and Alzheimer's disease, includes loss of molecular solubility as a primary pathogenetic feature.[35] Mitotic divisions of the lens epithelium result in increasing concentric deposition of lens fibers and compression of the nucleus with advancing age. Breakdown of intercellular membranes within the lens nucleus, dehydration and accumulation of pigment, and slow conversion of soluble to insoluble proteins ensue. Biochemical modifications (e.g., disulfide cross-links, glycosylation, racemization, carbamoylation, oxidation) and other factors lead to lens protein aggregation and subsequently to increased light scattering and nuclear cataract.[35]

Nuclear cataracts are slowly progressive and bilateral though often asymmetric. Lens opacity causes blurring, and yellowing of the lens diminishes color discrimination. Nuclear thickening may induce myopia.

Cortical cataract is caused by changes in the ionic composition of the lens cortex and subsequent changes in hydration of the lens fibers. Early signs of cortical cataract are vacuoles and "spokes" that radiate from near the periphery of the lens toward the center. Later, wedge-shaped opacities may enlarge and coalesce. Patients with cortical cataract complain of decreased vision or partial obstruction of visual field, glare, and less often diplopia. Posterior subcapsular cataracts are accumulations of granular material between the posterior lens cortex and capsule. Glare is a prominent symptom, and visual function can be quite compromised despite relatively good visual acuity.

Indications for cataract surgery are tailored to individual visual disabilities and needs. Generally, the discrepancy between visual requirement and visual function depends on the visual acuity, severity of the cataract, glare symptoms, and visual needs for driving, reading,

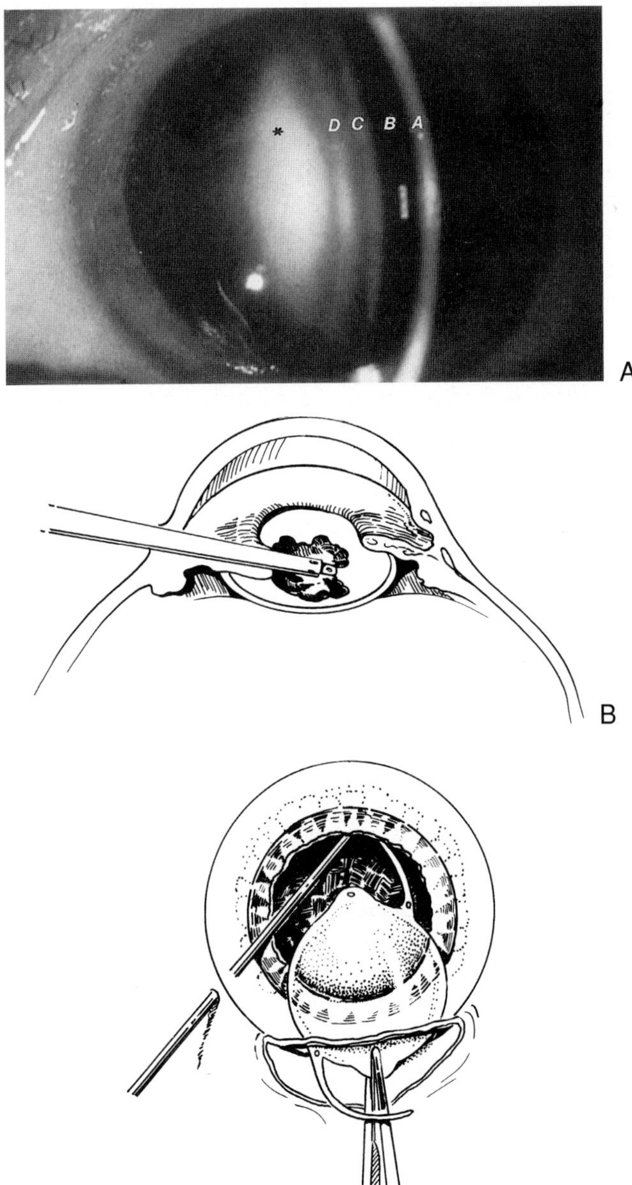


FIGURE 25.5. A. Opacities commonly occur in the lens cortex, nucleus, and posterior subcapsular regions. After cataract surgery, opacification may recur in the posterior capsule. A, cornea, B, anterior chamber, C, lens capsule, D, lens cortex, *, lens nucleus. B. Phacoemulsification tip with ultrasonic energy delivery, irrigation, and aspiration is introduced into the eye through a corneal limbal incision. An anterior lens capsule opening enables placement of the instrument within the lens nucleus, where the cataract is emulsified and removed. The posterior capsule is left intact to support the prosthetic lens. C. Placement of a prosthetic lens in the posterior capsular "bag." If insufficient posterior capsule remains, a lens implant can be placed in the anterior chamber on the iris surface or sewn to the internal eye wall.

self-care, hobbies, and employment. Systemic and ophthalmic conditions that pose additional risks for cataract surgery (e.g., diabetes mellitus, congestive heart failure, glaucoma, severe myopia, blepharitis, corneal edema), life expectancy, amblyopia, status of the fellow eye, and response of the fellow eye to prior cataract surgery, are also considered.[36] Thus although visual acuity is an important factor in cataract evaluation, arbitrary acuity levels (e.g., 20/50) are not absolute indications for cataract surgery.

Visual acuity is not accurately predicted by the clinical appearance of the cataract, and alternative explanations of decreased vision must be excluded prior to surgery. In elderly patients, three especially common causes of visual loss—macular degeneration, glaucoma, diabetic retinopathy—often coexist with cataract and must be evaluated to assess their relative contribution to the visual disability. Diabetic retinopathy is of particular concern in the setting of cataract extraction, as retinopathy may progress rapidly following surgery.[37] If the cataract is too dense to allow visualization of the fundus, ophthalmic ultrasonography is indicated; and visual potential is estimated by pupillary responses, color perception, entoptic imagery, and light projection. Finally, because cataracts can alter the lens power, new spectacle correction may improve acuity sufficiently to allow deferral of cataract removal. Tinted lenses may relieve some glare symptoms.

Thick, aphakic spectacles can compensate for loss of lens power after cataract extraction, but these are associated with marked optical aberrations. Postoperative visual function is greatly enhanced if the cataractous lens is replaced with a prosthetic intraocular lens (IOL). Numerous IOL materials and designs allow flexibility in the choice and anatomic placement of the lens (Fig. 25.5). The power of the IOL is calculated by a regression formula using variables of axial eye length and corneal curvature. The reader is referred elsewhere for a more complete discussion of issues related to cataract evaluation.[38,39]

The first known cataract removal in human history dates to 800 BC. Cataract extraction today is the most common surgical procedure in individuals 65 years of age and older in the United States,[40] with approximately half a million extractions performed each year. Technical refinements have made cataract surgery relatively safe and effective, and continued innovations may be expected. More than 95% of patients with otherwise normal eyes achieve reading and driving vision after cataract extraction.[41]

The most common techniques of cataract removal are phacoemulsification, extracapsular extraction, and intracapsular extraction. The choice of technique depends on surgeon preference and type of cataract. Today, most cataract extractions in the United States use phacoemulsification, and most of the rest are done via extracapsular technique. The visual results are similar with either technique. The intracapsular method is commonly employed in developing countries.

The phacoemulsification unit has several modes of operation, including irrigation, aspiration, and emulsification power controlled by the surgeon using a multifunction foot pedal. As shown in Figure 25.5, the phacoemulsification instrument tip is introduced into the anterior chamber through a small (usually 3 mm) corneoscleral opening, and the lens is emulsified and aspirated.[42,43] The posterior lens capsule is left intact to accommodate an IOL in the same location as the original lens. Use of smaller shelved incisions and foldable or injectable IOLs facilitates wound closure and obviates the need for sutures in some cases.

Dense or hard lens nuclei may be more easily removed with the extracapsular technique, in which the incision is made large enough (usually 11 mm) to allow expression of the entire lens nucleus from the eye. Residual cortical material is removed from the adherent posterior capsule by aspiration, an IOL is placed, and the incision is closed with interrupted or X-mattress sutures.

Complications of cataract surgery are numerous. Posterior capsular rupture may preclude IOL placement or may allow the cataract to pass into the vitreous cavity. Rarely, intraoperative ocular hypotony engenders massive choroidal hemorrhage. Postoperative complications include acute glaucoma, wound dehiscence, retinal detachment, macular edema, corneal edema, IOL dislocation, and endophthalmitis.[44,45] Opacification of the residual lens capsule occurs weeks to months after surgery in as many as one-fourth of patients. If visually significant, an opening can be created in the capsule (capsulotomy) in the office or clinic using a YAG laser.[46]

Despite these risks, modern cataract extraction is highly successful. More than 90% of otherwise healthy eyes achieve postoperative visual acuity of 20/40 or better (20/40 in at least one eye is the minimum vision required for a driver's license in most states), and fewer than 5% fail to improve.[41,44,47]

## Glaucoma

Glaucoma is the second most common cause of blindness in the United States and the leading cause among African Americans. More than two million Americans suffer from glaucoma, and 80,000 of them are blind from glaucoma.[48–50] The prevalence rises from a low level in young adults to as high as 10% in African Americans in their eighth decade and beyond; the prevalence in black persons is four- to fivefold greater than in whites[49] (Table 25.2).

TABLE 25.2. Prevalence of Definite Primary Open-angle Glaucoma by Age and Race in the Baltimore Eye Survery

| | Percent with glaucoma | |
|---|---|---|
| Age (years) | Whites | Blacks |
| 40–49 | 0.92 | 0.95 |
| 50–59 | 0.41 | 3.58 |
| 60–69 | 0.88 | 5.05 |
| 70–79 | 2.89 | 7.74 |
| 80+ | 2.16 | 10.88 |

Glaucoma is a progressive optic neuropathy with a characteristic appearance of the optic disc, nerve fiber layer, and visual field. Elevated intraocular pressure (IOP) is a significant risk factor in the development of glaucomatous optic nerve damage and visual field loss. Although acute glaucoma with extremely elevated IOP can present with painful loss of vision, most cases are chronic, painless, and progressive. Because irreversible visual field loss may be asymptomatic until the late stages when central acuity is affected, early detection and prevention are critical. It has been estimated that fewer than 50% of patients with glaucoma in developed countries are aware of their disease, and even fewer cases are detected in the developing world.[50]

Glaucoma can be classified into open-angle or closed-angle types, both of which increase in incidence with age. With closed-angle glaucomas access of aqueous humor to the trabecular meshwork in the "angle" is mechanically obstructed; with the open-angle types, aqueous humor reaches the angle unobstructed, yet egress of fluid is insufficient. The most common type in the United States is primary open angle glaucoma (POAG).

Age-related structural changes in the ciliary body, trabecular meshwork, and optic nerve head are believed to be responsible for the increased incidence of POAG during old age.[51,52] The ciliary body thickens with accumulation of connective tissue, and the epithelium of the ciliary process becomes attenuated. Trabecular meshwork fibers undergo sclerosis and thickening and compromise aqueous humor drainage from the eye, thereby elevating the IOP. The IOP increases with age,[53] and the optic nerve of elderly persons is more susceptible to pressure-induced damage, possibly due to a vascular etiology. Genetic factors are implicated in the pathogenesis of glaucoma.[54]

Diagnosis is based on a characteristic optic nerve head appearance, retinal nerve fiber layer loss, and visual field changes (Fig. 25.6). Elevated IOP is generally

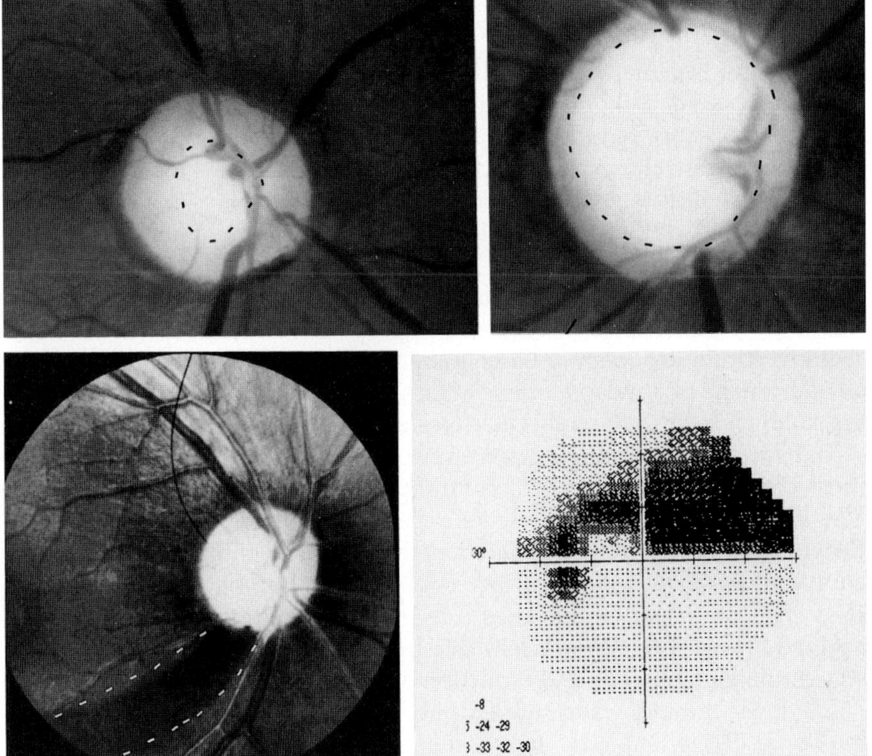


FIGURE 25.6. A. Optic nerve head with normal central depression (cup, dashes) occupying approximately one-third of the total disc area. B. Advanced glaucomatous optic nerve damage with extensive loss of central nerve; only a thin rim of normal nerve remains at the edges of the enlarged cup (dashes). The cup/disc ratio is approximately 0.85. C. Inferotemporal defect in the right retinal nerve fiber layer (between white dashed curves) indicates focal glaucomatous optic nerve damage with retrograde atrophy of the affected retinal ganglion cell axons. D. Automated 30-degree visual field of the left eye. An arcuate scotoma arching superiorly from the physiologic blind spot and a nasal defect that respects the horizontal midline are typical of glaucoma. (Courtesy of Bruce Shields, MD)

present. However, a subset of patients with glaucoma have normal IOP (10–22 mmHg), presumably because of a special susceptibility of the optic nerve to pressure-induced damage. Ophthalmoscopically detectable damage typical of glaucoma includes generalized enlargement of the central cup within the optic nerve head, focal notching of the cup, asymmetry of cupping between the two eyes, and loss of the retinal nerve fiber layer (Fig. 25.6). Typical visual field defects are paracentral and arcuate scotomas, nasal step, temporal wedge, and generalized constriction. As glaucoma progresses, visual field defects enlarge or coalesce, and the patient experiences dramatic loss of vision if the defect reaches central fixation.

Despite recognition that multiple factors contribute to glaucomatous optic nerve damage, current treatments, whether pharmacologic, laser, or operative procedures, are directed only at IOP reduction by reducing production or increasing outflow of aqueous humor.[55] Therapies for glaucoma rarely improve visual acuity but aim to prevent further loss of visual field. This, combined with a lack of symptoms early in the disease and the chronicity of the condition and its treatment, underscore the difficulty and importance of screening, careful follow-up, and compliance with drug therapies.

The variety of agents in common use for glaucoma (topical β-adrenergic receptor antagonists, adrenergic agonists, parasympathomimetics, prostaglandin analogues, and topical, oral, or intravenous carbonic anhydrase inhibitors) attest to the surprisingly complex physiologic and neurohormonal regulation of fluid flow within the eye.[56] Oral or intravenous hyperosmotic agents reduce the IOP by decreasing the vitreous volume. β-Blockers decrease aqueous production and may cause significant cardiovascular effects after topical administration; parasympathetic drugs enhance the aqueous outflow.[57] The reader is referred to reviews for discussions of the systemic side effects of glaucoma medications.[56,57]

Laser trabeculoplasty significantly lowers the IOP in many patients, but half of them require additional therapy within 2–5 years.[58] Laser trabeculoplasty facilitates drainage of aqueous humor after application of an argon green laser to the trabecular meshwork.

Trabeculectomy, or filtering procedure, is the operation most commonly performed to control IOP in POAG.[59] The surgical objective is to create a permanent fistula through the sclera from the anterior chamber into the subconjunctival space, to allow egress of aqueous humor (Fig. 25.7). With partial-thickness filtering, the fistula is covered by a split-thickness scleral flap that lessens excessive outflow of aqueous and reduction of IOP.

The most common cause of failure of trabeculectomy is closure of the fistula by scar tissue arising from episcleral fibroblast proliferation. Measures undertaken to reduce postoperative scarring include treatment of preoperative and postoperative inflammation with topical and oral antiinflammatory agents and minimization of intraoperative tissue manipulation and trauma. In addition, mitomycin C can be briefly applied to the scleral flap intraoperatively, and multiple 5-fluorouracil subconjunctival injections can be given for several weeks after surgery.[60,61] These antimetabolite adjuncts have improved the success rate of trabeculectomy in selected patients.

For patients who have failed or who are at high risk to fail conventional filtering surgery, a prosthetic drainage reservoir can be sewn externally to the sclera underneath the conjunctiva and connected by tubing to the anterior chamber (Fig. 25.7). These implant devices may incorporate a valve feature to allow outflow of aqueous humor when the IOP surpasses a designated value. Long-term success rates of 55–79% are reported.[62]

Ciliodestructive techniques reduce aqueous production by controlled ablation of the ciliary body. External freezing or infrared laser burns are placed circumferentially 1.5 mm posterior to the cornea to ablate the ciliary body transclerally; internal laser ablation of the ciliary body is accomplished with an endolaser probe. Ciliodestructive procedures are not easily titrated to IOP reduction, and their use is limited to patients with advanced glaucoma and poor vision.[63]

## Retina and Vitreous

### Age-Related Macular Degeneration

Age-related macular degeneration (ARMD) is the most common cause of visual loss in individuals over 50 years of age in the United States and the United Kingdom. The prevalence of this condition increases with age; it is estimated to be approximately 11% for persons 65–74 years of age and 28% for persons 75–84 years old.[64] People with northern European ancestry are at higher risk to suffer from ARMD, as are persons with light iris color. In many cases the disease is familial, with an autosomal dominant inheritance pattern and variable expressivity and penetrance. ARMD is rarely a cause of visual loss in black persons.

ARMD affects the macula, or central region, of the retina and the underlying choroidal capillaries (choriocapillaris) and pigment epithelium, thus causing deterioration of vision in the central visual field. The much larger peripheral visual field is generally spared, so total blindness is rare.

Normal senescence results in alterations within the outer retina, retinal pigment epithelium and adjacent choroid that predispose to development of ARMD, but the precise cause is unknown. Aging changes thought to be relevant include an increased accumulation of lipofuscin granules in the cytoplasm of pigment epithelial cells that in part result from phagocytosis and

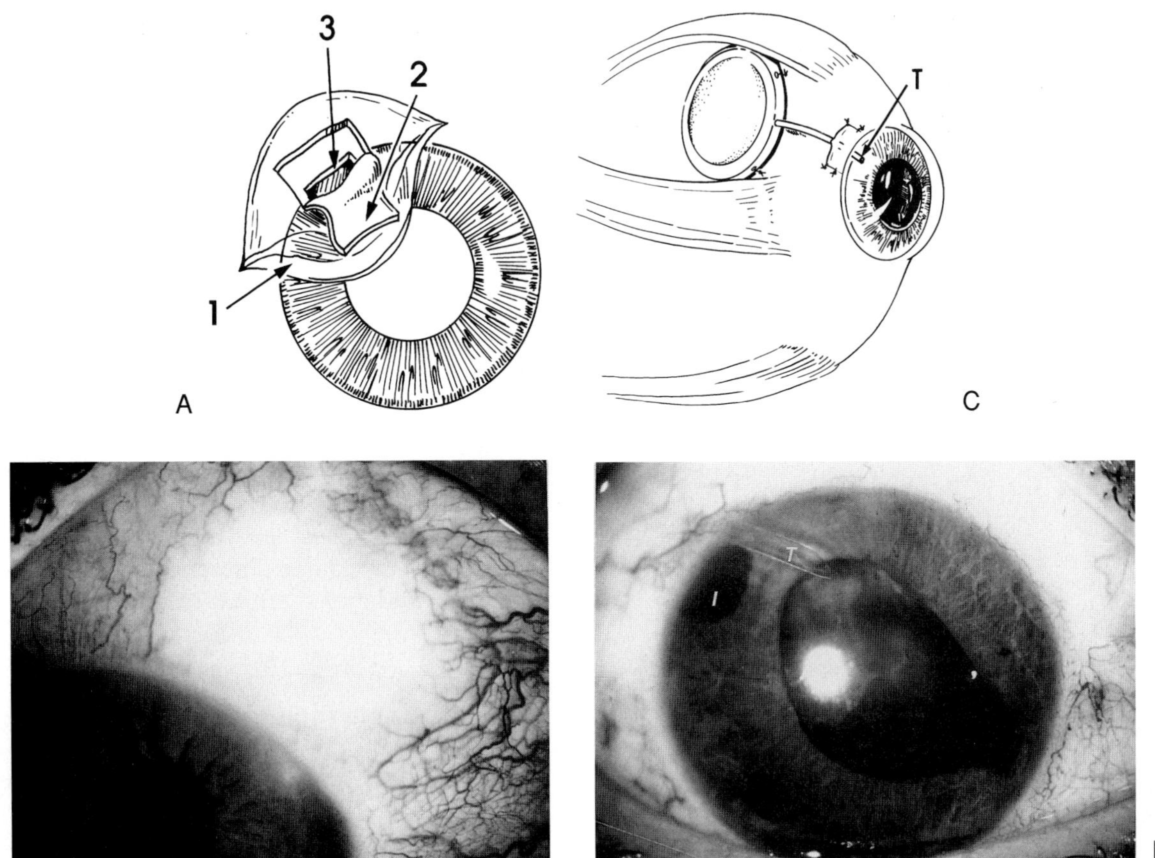


FIGURE 25.7. A. Trabeculectomy creates a surgical fistula between the anterior chamber and the subconjunctival space. The conjunctiva and a split-thickness scleral flap (1) are reflected to expose the fistula site (2) and iridectomy (3). B. Elevated conjunctiva (large white area) adjacent to a trabeculectomy site due to adequate aqueous humor outflow from fistula. C. Plate reservoir sutured to the sclera, with the connecting tube ending in the anterior chamber. D. Tubing tip (T) in the anterior chamber after reservoir and valve placement. Note also the peripheral iridectomy (I) that allows free flow of aqueous into the anterior chamber. (Courtesy of Marc Weizman, MD)

digestion of shed photoreceptor outer segments, reduced photoreceptor density, and thickening of Bruch's membrane between the pigment epithelium and choroid. Drusen are clinically detectable localized depositions of a hyaline-like material between the pigment epithelium and retina. They are an important feature of ARMD (Fig. 25.8A).[65]

Clinically, two forms of ARMD are recognized and may exist separately or together. The atrophic, or "dry," form is more common and often affects vision minimally, though it is occasionally severe. Ophthalmoscopically detectable yellow-white drusen may be present, as may pigment atrophy and pigment hypertrophy (Fig. 25.8A).

The exudative, or "wet," form afflicts only 10% of patients with ARMD but is responsible for 90% of blindness with this disorder. Possibly, ischemic and inflammatory stimuli of unknown origin lead to neovascular growth from the choriocapillaris into the potential spaces underneath the retina and retinal pigment epithelium. Neovascular complexes may leak fluid, lipoprotein, or frank blood underneath the retina, with resulting loss of central acuity (Fig. 25.8B). If left untreated, exudative lesions may progress to fibrosis with permanent destruction of the outer retina (Fig. 25.8C).

Antioxidant therapy has been proposed for ARMD, in part because (1) the macula is a region of high metabolic rate and blood flow; (2) cumulative blue light exposure throughout life may play a role in the development of ARMD; and (3) antioxidant pigments are present in the macula.[66]

Although a lifelong diet rich in leafy green vegetables is associated with a lower rate of ARMD, short-term clinical trials employing nutritional supplements have so far failed to support a major role for these vitamins in the treatment of dry ARMD.[67]

Argon laser photocoagulation of the choroidal neovascular complex is a proven effective treatment for the exudative form of ARMD. The multicenter Macular Photocoagulation Study clarified the role of laser therapy for

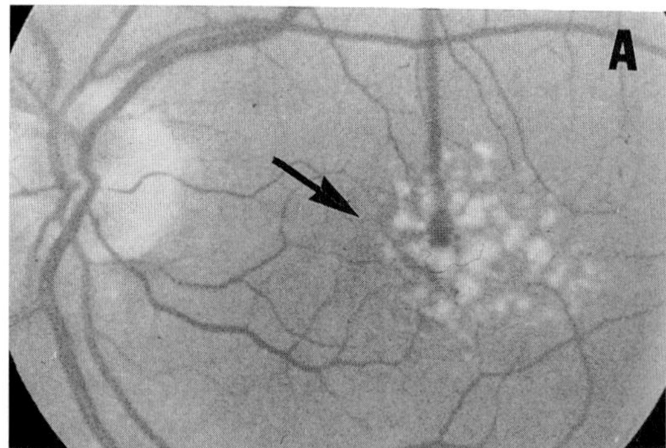


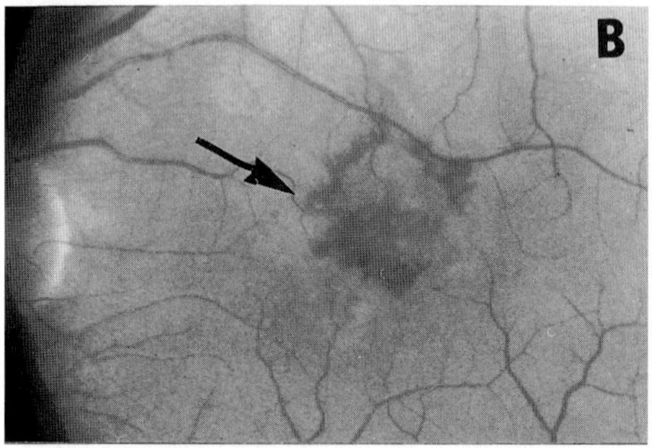


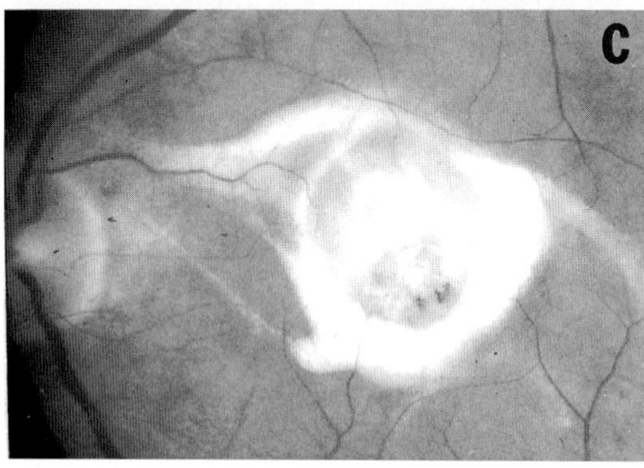


FIGURE 25.8. A. Dry or atrophic macular degeneration with numerous yellow-white deposits (drusen, arrow) underneath the macula. Visual acuity is 20/30. The vertical line in the upper half of the photograph is a fixation pointer. B. Wet or exudative macular degeneration, with hemorrhage (arrow) and fluid underneath the macula. Visual acuity is 20/100. C. Same patient as in B. 3 months later. The blood and exudation have organized into a subretinal scar; and vision has deteriorated to 5/200.

neovascular lesions of varying size, location, and fluorescein angiographic features.[68,69] A key requirement for effective treatment of a neovascular lesion is that its borders must be well defined, so the lesion is completely ablated with minimal laser-associated damage to healthy adjacent retina. A well-defined lesion is seen in Figure 25.9, before and after obliteration with laser. Unfortunately, only a minority of patients have neovascular lesions that meet criteria for laser treatment. Furthermore, although treatment is better than the long-term natural course, it often causes an immediate scotoma and reduction of vision, and recurrence is common.[70] Photodynamic therapy is a new approach to macular degeneration involving intravenous injection of a photosensitive drug that preferentially localizes within the choroidal neovascular complex. Illumination of the macula with a laser then activates the drug and results in a cytotoxic effect limited to the neovascular tissue. A beneficial effect of photodynamic therapy in selected patients has been demonstrated in clinical trials. Alternate means to prevent or treat exudative ARMD are under intense investigation, including external-beam irradiation of proliferating choroidal neovascular lesions.[71] Antiangiogenic drugs have inhibited the development of choroidal neovascularization in animal models.[72]

Surgical approaches have been developed to remove choroidal neovascular membranes and their associated subretinal exudation.[73] These techniques have not yet

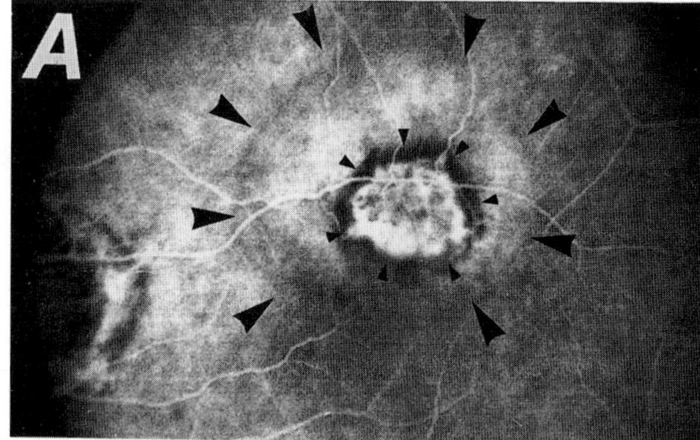


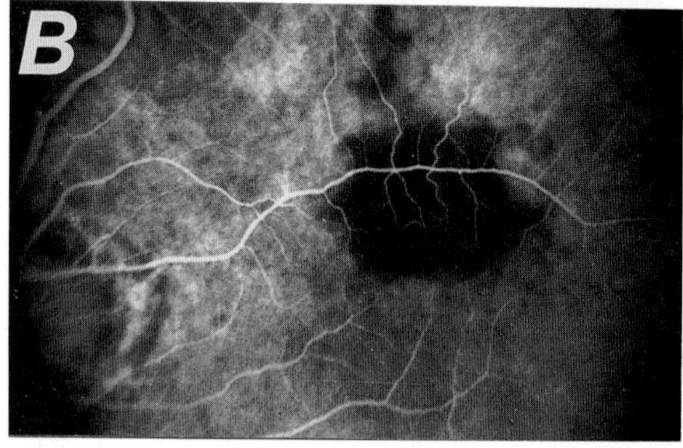


FIGURE 25.9. A. Patient with acute vision loss due to exudative macular degeneration. Angiography reveals a well-defined hyperfluorescent choroidal neovascular membrane (small arrowheads) whose inferior edge is just above the foveal center. Note also the elevated rim of edema surrounding the neovascular lesion (large arrowheads). Visual acuity is 20/80. B. Angiogram obtained 3 weeks after laser ablation of the neovascular complex. Exudation (hyperfluorescence) is absent. Visual acuity improved to 20/50, but a paracentral scotoma is present owing to the laser-induced damage to the overlying retina.

proven beneficial for most elderly patients, probably because abnormalities in the underlying pigment epithelium and choroid preclude full restoration of retinal function. Transplantation of pigment epithelium or of retina or retinal photoreceptors, is a technically feasible approach to macular degeneration but is unproven.[74]

## Retinal Detachment

With retinal detachment (RD), the retina separates from the underlying pigment epithelium and choroid, with resultant loss of photoreceptor function and vision. Three major etiologies for detachment are recognized. With exudative RD, inflammatory or rheologic factors cause accumulation of fluid underneath the retina. With traction RD, usually fibrovascular tissue (e.g., from prior trauma) lifts the retina off the eye wall. In rhegmatogenous RD, a full-thickness retinal break (a hole or flap tear) occurs in the retina and allows liquid vitreous humor to pass underneath, and detach, the retina.

Rhegmatogenous RD is the most common type in all age groups and occurs most often in persons over the age of 50 years.[75] The usual events leading to formation of retinal breaks and detachment, shown in Figure 25.10, are as follows: Biochemical alteration of collagen and hyaluronic acid macromolecules in vitreous humor occurs normally with aging and increases the vitreoretinal traction forces. The gel eventually separates from the retinal surface, a situation known as posterior vitreous detachment. By the age of 65 years, 25–65% of adults exhibit vitreous detachment; by age 75 it increases to more than 90%.[76] In 10–15% of cases of vitreous detachment, retinal breaks form as the vitreous pulls away from the retinal surface.[76] Breaks accompanied by symptoms such as light flashes (photopsia) and floaters progress to detachment in 28–35% of patients, whereas more common asymptomatic breaks found incidentally rarely progress.[77]

Severe myopia predisposes to retinal break formation, as do areas of retinal tissue structurally weakened by past trauma or congenital or acquired lesions. Of special relevance to the geriatric population is that prior eye surgery (particularly cataract surgery) accelerates vitreous syneresis and greatly increases the risk for retinal breaks and detachment. Approximately 30–40% of all patients with retinal detachment have had prior cataract surgery, whereas the risk of detachment after standard cataract surgery is about 1%.[75,78]

Retinal breaks without detachment are surrounded with laser- or cryotherapy-induced burns that enhance adhesion of the retina to underlying pigment epithelium. Laser and cryotherapy of retinal breaks is typically performed in an office or clinic setting and is highly successful in halting progression to detachment.[79]

Rhegmatogenous retinal detachment nearly always results in irreversible blindness if untreated. The goals of surgical treatment are to (1) relieve vitreoretinal traction and (2) seal retinal breaks with laser or cryotherapy.

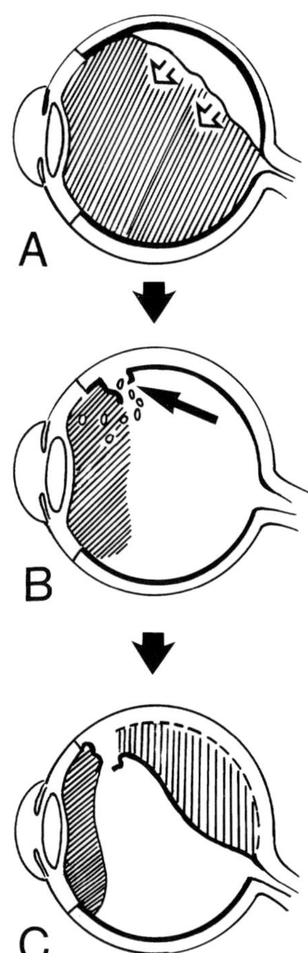


FIGURE 25.10. Critical role of the vitreous in the pathogenesis of retinal breaks and detachment. A. As vitreous gel within the eye shrinks, a centripetally directed (arrow) vitreoretinal traction develops. B. Further shrinkage and liquefaction of the gel may result in a peripheral retinal break. Cells gain access into the vitreous cavity if rupture of a retinal vessel or sloughing of pigment epithelium (arrow) occurs. Patients experience these cells as floaters. C. Passage of liquid vitreous through the break (arrow) and underneath the retina creates a detachment.

Vitreoretinal traction can be relieved by removing vitreous gel via pars plana vitrectomy and air–fluid exchange (Fig. 25.11). An inert gas, infused in the eye intraoperatively to provide internal tamponade of the retina, is replaced by aqueous fluid from the ciliary body over 2 weeks or more, during which time laser- or cryotherapy-induced adhesions around retinal tears become firm. Long-term internal tamponade is achieved with silicone oils and perfluorocarbon liquids.[80]

A more common means to relieve vitreoretinal traction is permanent placement of a silicone rubber element on the sclera (scleral buckling). Mattress sutures are used to indent the exoplant to reduce internal vitreoretinal trac-

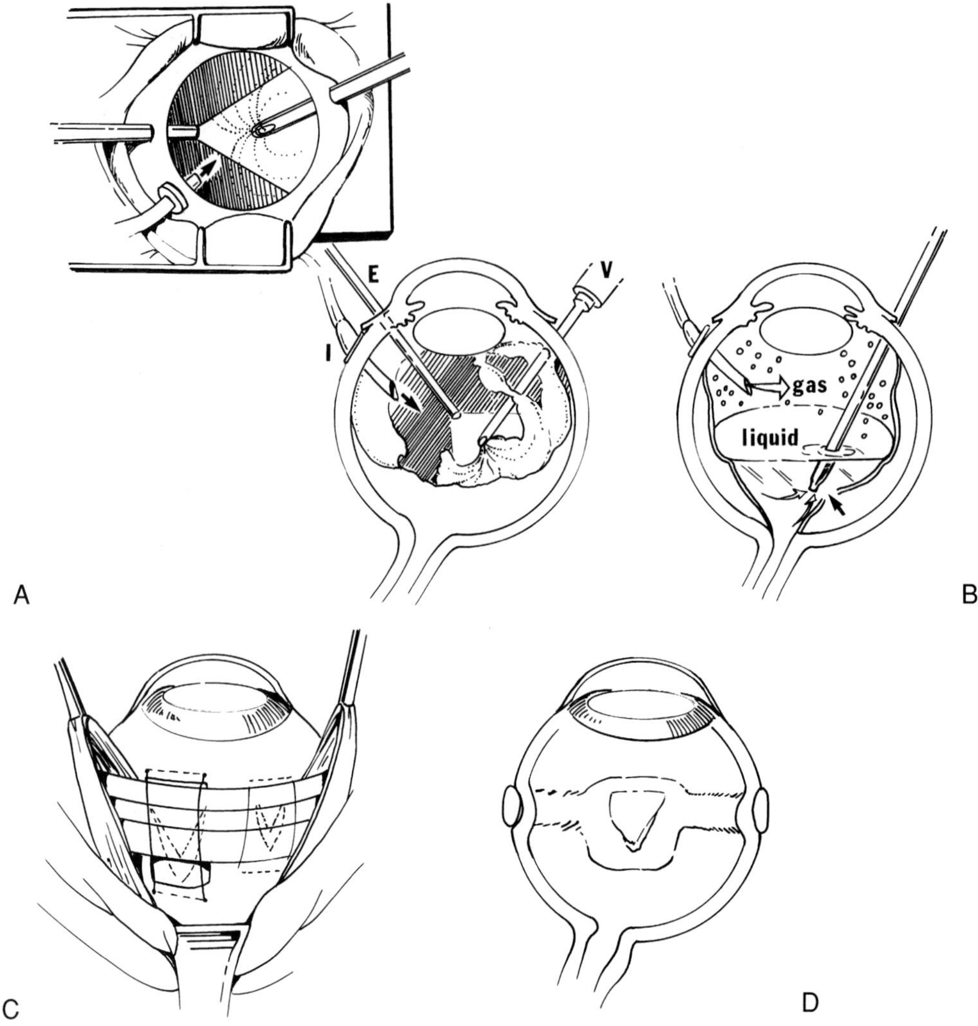


FIGURE 25.11. Retinal detachment repair aims to reduce vitreoretinal traction. A. Removal of the vitreous gel by pars plana vitrectomy. The vitrector has a cutting and aspirating tip. The infusion line (I) maintains eye volume during vitreous removal, and the endoscopic light pipe (E) provides illumination. Vitrectomy is performed also in the absence of detachment to remove vitreous opacity, such as diabetic hemorrhage. B. After removal of vitreous, the retina is repositioned against the eyewall by internal tamponade with air. Air–fluid exchange simultaneously infuses gas as vitreous and subretinal fluid is aspirated. C. A silicone buckling element secured to the eye. Mattress suture width is 2 mm wider than the exoplant width, so the element indents the sclera D. to relieve internal vitreoretinal traction and reappose the retina to the pigment epithelium.

tion and approximate the break(s) to underlying pigment epithelium (Fig. 25.11).

Pneumatic retinopexy is an alternative offered to selected patients in an office setting.[81] Briefly, an inert gas is injected into the vitreous cavity, and the patient is positioned for 3–5 days so the intraocular bubble covers the retinal break and repositions the retina. As with scleral buckling and vitrectomy, breaks are treated with laser or cryotherapy.

The choice of procedure is based on several factors. Pneumatic retinopexy requires that the retinal break be located in the upper fundus. Scleral buckling is superior for anterior breaks, where the buckling material can be easily placed. Vitrectomy techniques are valuable if intravitreal blood obscures retinal detail. All three procedures have excellent success rates: 70–95% for primary rhegmatogenous RD.[81–83]

Failure of retinal detachment surgery is usually due to growth on the retinal surface or fibrosis (proliferative vitreoretinopathy) that reestablishes retinal traction and elevation. Management of proliferative vitreoretinopathy is surgically challenging and often requires a combination of augmented scleral buckling, vitrectomy with excision and segmentation of fibrotic tissue, intraocular laser application, and long-acting gas or oil for internal tamponade; reported reattachment rates are 50–75%.[84]

Pharmacologic inhibition of postoperative intravitreal cellular proliferation may reduce the incidence of recurrent detachment.[85,86]

## Diabetic Retinopathy

Diabetes mellitus can affect the visual system in many ways, including increased risk for cataract, glaucoma, and microvascular infarcts of cranial nerves III, IV, and VI. Retinopathy is by far the most serious and common ocular consequence of diabetes and is the leading cause of blindness in adults in the United States. The risk of developing retinopathy and the severity of the retinopathy are related to the duration of diabetes: 50% of patients after 7 years and 90% after 17–25 years have retinopathy. Use of insulin, poor control of serum glucose, and systemic hypertension and carotid occlusive disease also relate to the development and progression of retinopathy.[87,88]

Diabetic retinopathy is a disease of the intraretinal vasculature. Several hypotheses have been suggested to explain how elevated serum glucose levels lead to retinal angiopathy, including nonspecific and enzymatic glycosylation of proteins, rheologic disturbances of white blood cells, increased platelet adhesion and erythrocyte aggregation, accumulation of sorbitol and galactitol, and growth hormone abnormalities associated with diabetes mellitus.[89]

Early pathologic changes during diabetic retinopathy are thickening of the capillary basement membrane and loss of capillary pericytes.[90] Loss of retinal blood flow autoregulation and breakdown of the blood–retina barrier ensue and result in intraretinal exudation of serum with lipid and proteins (hard exudates), hemorrhage, and edema (Fig. 25.12). Microaneurysms especially may be sites of extravasation. Capillary closure causes clinically detectable microinfarcts of the retinal nerve fiber layer, known as cotton-wool spots (Fig. 25.12);

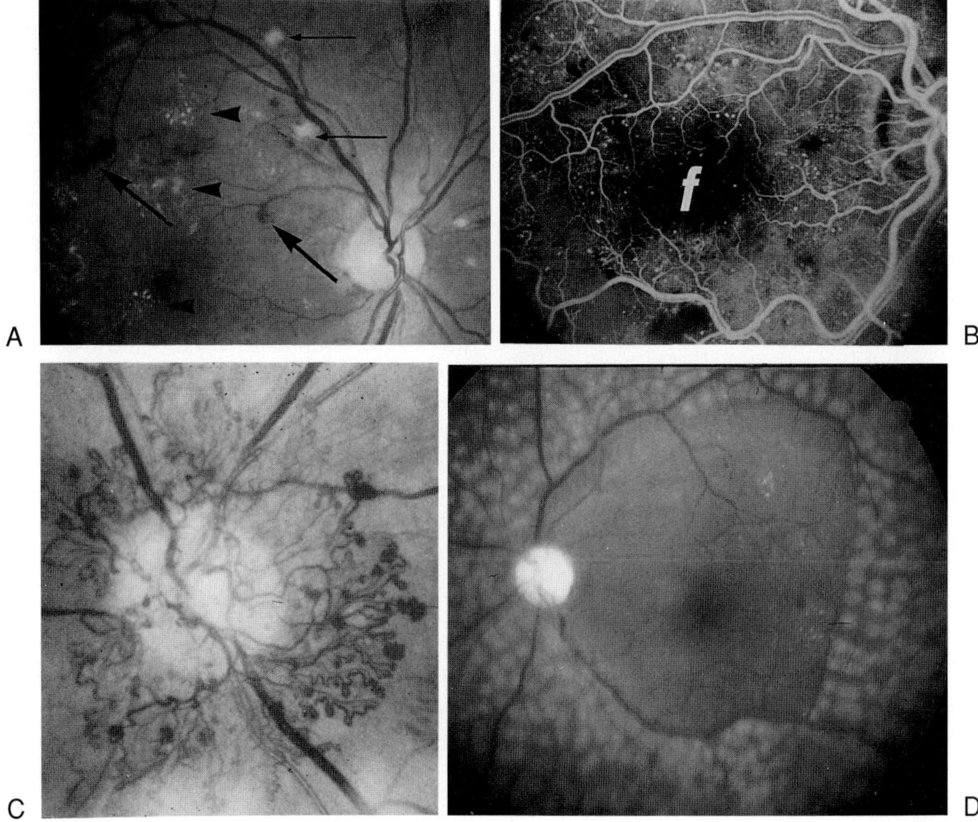


FIGURE 25.12. A. A 67-year-old man had diabetes mellitus for 15 years with typical signs of nonproliferative diabetic retinopathy: intraretinal blot hemorrhage (thick arrows); refractile yellow lipoprotein exudation (arrowheads), white nerve fiber layer microinfarcts ("cotton wool spots," thin arrows), and macular edema. B. Fluorescein angiogram from another patient with diabetic maculopathy. The macula and fovea (f) are demarcated by intraretinal arcade venules and arterioles that fluoresce owing to retained fluorescein. The pale, diffuse white background fluorescence reflects retinal and choroidal capillary filling. Abnormalities include microaneurysms that appear as numerous hyperfluorescent punctate lesions and abnormal dark regions (bottom and superotemporal to the fovea) due to capillary closure and nonperfusion. C. Proliferative diabetic retinopathy. Thin tortuous neovascular vessels extend from the optic nerve head into the vitreous. D. Panretinal laser photocoagulation covers the retina with dense, nearly confluent burns but spares the macula. Neovascularization has regressed.

closure of perifoveal capillaries may result in ischemic maculopathy. These changes fall under the rubric nonproliferative diabetic retinopathy (NPDR).

Visual loss in NPDR results usually from macular edema and less often from macular ischemia. When edema involves or threatens the center of the fovea, laser photocoagulation of the macula is indicated; it reduces the risk of moderate vision loss by 50%.[91] Macular laser therapy is directed at edematous areas in a grid pattern and focally to sites of leakage (e.g., microaneurysms) identified by fluorescein angiography (Fig. 25.12). Small laser spot size (50–100 μm) and low laser energy are employed to avoid creation of central scotomas.

Proliferative diabetic retinopathy (PDR) involves growth of neovascular tissue from retinal veins in regions of marked tissue ischemia. Neovascular growths tend to extend along the inner surface of the retina and into the vitreous cavity. Although retinal neovascularization may appear to be a desirable response to retinal ischemia, the new vessels do not alleviate hypoxia. Rather, these vessels can lead to two severe complications of PDR: vitreous hemorrhage and tractional retinal detachment. Vitreous hemorrhage may be partial (Fig. 25.13A), or it may completely obscure vision. Retinal detachment results from fibrosis of neovascular tissue, with resulting tractional elevation of the retina (Fig. 25.13B).

Laser therapy for PDR is aimed at the extramacular retina. Specifically, widespread areas are ablated (panretinal photocoagulation) using larger laser spots (500 μm) with high energies (Fig. 25.12). The rationale for this destruction of peripheral retina is that it lowers the metabolic demands of retinal tissue, thereby reducing ischemia and hypoxia and hence the angiogenic stimulus. Treatment causes regression of neovascular tissue in most patients and reduces severe visual loss (less than 5/200) by 60%.[91,92] Better understanding of the molecular basis of retinal angiogenesis may enable nondestructive novel pharmacologic therapies for PDR.[93]

The most common indication for surgery of diabetic retinopathy is a nonclearing vitreous hemorrhage arising from neovascular fronds. In many patients settling and clearing of the hemorrhage occurs spontaneously within weeks; it is facilitated by elevating the head of the bed during sleep. For patients in whom spontaneous clearing does not occur, the rationale for pars plana vitrectomy is threefold. First, removal of blood clears the visual axis and restores sight. Second, it allows placement of panretinal photocoagulation to reduce the likelihood of recurrent hemorrhage. Third, the vitreous is thought to provide a scaffold for growth of neovascular tissue, and its removal may facilitate regression of proliferative disease.

The timing of vitrectomy for diabetic vitreous depends on many factors, including visual potential, the presence of retinal detachment, anesthetic risk, and the status of the fellow eye. Guidelines provided by the multicenter Diabetic Retinopathy Vitrectomy Study recommend that vitrectomy be deferred up to 3 months after the onset of hemorrhage in type I diabetics and 6 months in type II diabetics.[94] Approximately 80% of patients achieve marked restoration of visual acuity.[95]

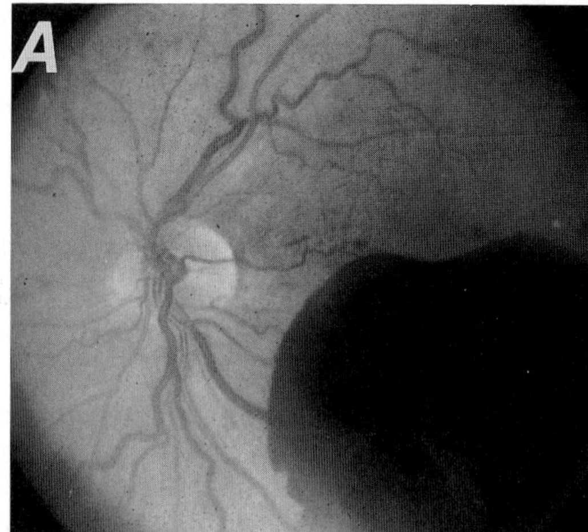


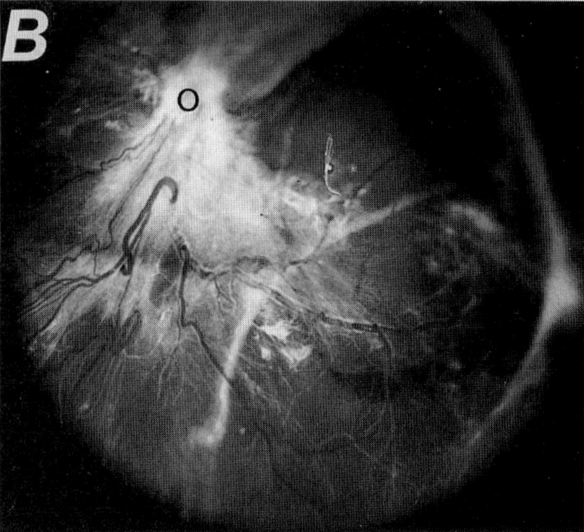


FIGURE 25.13. Complications of proliferative diabetic retinopathy. A. Vitreous hemorrhage obscures the inferior macula and extends into the inferotemporal periphery. B. Dense white fibrotic tissue arising from past hemorrhage and vascular leakage is seen in front of and underneath the retina, which is detached, and distorted into irregular folds. Much of the fibrosis appears to arise from the optic nerve head (O). Recurrent retinal detachment associated with proliferative vitreoretinopathy in nondiabetic patients may have a similar appearance.

The second indication for surgical intervention for diabetic retinopathy is traction retinal detachment. Contraction of preretinal fibrosis associated with neovascular growths can detach the retina, and severe loss of vision ensues if detachment involves the macula.

Surgical management of diabetic traction detachments is similar to that described above for recurrent rhegmatogenous retinal detachment. Reattachment rates are

60–85%, but improved visual acuity is seen in only 26–65% owing to advanced retinopathy and risks of iatrogenic retinal trauma.[95]

## Endophthalmitis

Endophthalmitis is a sight-threatening intraocular infection or inflammation involving the vitreous chamber. It is classified as endogenous (due to spread into the eye of a systemic process) or exogenous (e.g., introduced during surgery); infectious or inflammatory (e.g., from a foreign body, chemical toxicity, or condition such as Bechet's disease); and acute or chronic. In elderly patients the most common type of endophthalmitis is acute postoperative bacterial infection, which occurs with an incidence of approximately 0.07% following cataract surgery.[8]

Symptoms of acute endophthalmitis include pain, redness, and visual loss. Examination usually reveals severe intraocular inflammation. Vitreous and anterior chamber paracentesis is indicated to obtain samples for microbiologic testing. If visual acuity decreases to light perception, pars plana vitrectomy is performed to remove intravitreal purulent material and clear the visual axis. Initial antimicrobial therapy consists of intravitreal injection of broad-spectrum antibiotics; subsequent medication is tailored based on culture and sensitivity results from vitreous specimens. Corticosteroids may be administered to minimize inflammation. Prompt, aggressive management preserves useful vision in many patients.[96]

## Intraocular Tumors

The most common intraocular tumor in elderly patients is uveal metastasis, followed by uveal malignant melanoma and B-cell lymphoma. Uveal metastases most commonly arise from breast and lung cancer and less often from genitourinary, gastrointestinal, skin, and other malignancies.[97] Uveal metastes are far more common in the choroid than in the iris or ciliary body; and they typically appear as placoid masses, often with overlying effusion. Visual loss occurs if the macula is affected. Of note, 20% of patients presenting with uveal metastasis have not yet been diagnosed with the primary cancer.[97] Treatment is directed at the primary tumor if possible. Local therapy is indicated for visual loss or glaucoma. Uveal metastases generally respond to external beam or plaque irradiation, with return of vision.[98] Metastasis to the orbit also occurs and may present with proptosis, diplopia, limitation of eye movement, and pain.

Uveal melanomas also present most often in the choroid during the fifth to seventh decades. The incidence in the United States is six per million and is much lower among nonwhite populations.[99] Diagnosis is made by the typical funduscopic appearance of a mushroom-shaped choroidal mass, usually pigmented, with characteristic low internal reflectivity on A-scan ultrasonography, internal vasculature on fluorescein angiography, and documented growth at sequential examinations (Fig. 25.14). Small tumors may be followed or treated with laser photocoagulation or thermotherapy. Treatment options for medium and large tumors include

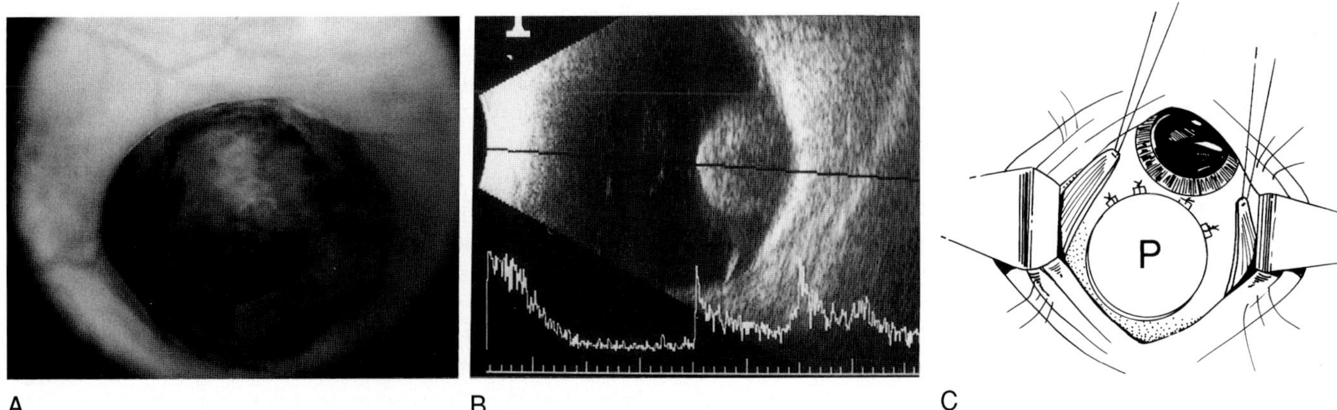


FIGURE 25.14. A. Choroidal malignant melanoma in the inferotemporal midperipheral fundus of a 73-year-old man. B. Cornea (anterior) is seen at the left and the orbit (posterior) at the right. B-mode ultrasonography shows a typical mushroom or collar button shape, associated retinal detachment at the tumor margins due to exudation, and decreased echoes toward the tumor base. An A-mode scan directed through the tumor apex (bottom tracing) shows characteristic low internal reflectivity between the apex and scleral spikes. C. Suturing of an $^{125}$I plaque (P) to the sclera is located above a melanoma. Measurements of the tumor diameter and thickness obtained by ultrasonography are used by the radiation oncologist to design a radioactive plaque specific to the tumor. The plaque is typically removed after 4 days.

surgical external placement of a radioactive plaque over the tumor (Fig. 25.14), external beam irradiation, and removal of the eye (enucleation). Selected tumors are excised along with adjacent choroid through a scleral incision.[100]

Intraocular non-Hodgkin's lymphoma is a rare disease with a mean age of onset of 60 years.[101] It may be associated with central nervous system or visceral disease and often presents with eye-related symptoms such as floaters and blurring. Funduscopy may reveal intravitreal and subretinal infiltrates and white blood cells floating in the vitreous cavity. The diagnosis is secured by cytologic analysis of a vitreous biopsy and by radiographic detection of brain or visceral lesions. Treatment, with chemotherapy and irradiation, is disappointing, and most patients die within 2 years.[102]

## Neuroophthalmic disorders

Vascular insufficiency of the eye, optic nerve, and visual areas of the central nervous system is more common in elderly patients owing to a higher prevalence of stroke, hypertension, and cardiac, carotid, atherosclerotic, and inflammatory vascular diseases in this population. Ocular ischemic syndrome, a rare condition of insufficient blood flow to the eye, can cause eye pain and decreased vision owing to retinal or anterior segment ischemia. Carotid occlusion is a frequent finding in these patients, and carotid endarterectomy may result in dramatic improvement if marked ophthalmic artery arteriosclerosis is not present as well.[103] Laser ablation of the peripheral retina, as described above for proliferative diabetic retinopathy, decreases retinal metabolic needs and hypoxia, and it can reverse retinal and iris neovascular complications of ocular ischemic syndrome.

Ischemic optic neuropathy, a nonembolic infarction of the optic nerve head, presents with sudden loss of vision and optic nerve head swelling. An idiopathic nonarteritic form is associated with systemic hypertension and usually affects one eye of patients over 50 years of age.

The arteritic form of ischemic optic neuropathy is an ocular manifestation of a generalized inflammatory disease of large and medium-sized arteries, termed giant cell or temporal arteritis. Blindness may result from involvement of posterior ciliary arteries supplying the anterior optic nerve. It is described almost exclusively in patients over 55 years of age; most patients are more than age 70. Clinical criteria most strongly suggestive of giant cell arteritis are jaw claudication, C-reactive protein level above 2.45 mg/dl, neck pain, and an erythrocyte sedimentation rate of 47 mm/hr or more.[104] Other associations are polymyalgia rheumatica, weight loss, fatigue, and scalp tenderness. Visual loss, seen in about 20% of patients, can be acute and severe; it is usually initially unilateral, with a high risk of spread to the other eye.[104–106]

Definitive diagnosis requires histologic identification of giant cell inflammation and disruption of the internal elastic lamina in an arterial biopsy specimen. The superficial temporal artery is chosen for biopsy because it is readily accessible and is frequently involved. A large specimen (3–5 cm) is removed to reduce false-negative results due to "skip" areas of pathology.

If giant cell arteritis is suspected, high-dose corticosteroid therapy is instituted immediately; the biopsy can be scheduled anytime within 2 weeks without loss of sensitivity. Treatment typically does not restore vision in the affected eye but protects the contralateral eye and thereby prevents bilateral blindness.[105]

Diplopia is the cardinal symptom in ocular muscle palsies. The most common causes are cranial nerve III, IV, and VI infarcts associated with microvascular diseases such as diabetes and hypertension, cerebrovascular accidents, tumors of the brain and orbit, intracranial aneurysms, trauma, thyroid orbitopathy, and myasthenia gravis.[107] Spontaneous recovery usually occurs within 3–6 months with a microvascular etiology. Prismatic power incorporated into eyeglasses achieves alignment in some patients with residual diplopia. Strabismus surgery is considered to realign the eyes and may involve resection, recession, myectomy, and transposition of extraocular muscles.

## Low Vision

Low vision exists when eyeglasses, contact lenses, medical treatment, and surgery cannot restore sight to the normal range. Low vision encompasses many types and etiologies of vision loss, such as central scotoma from macular degeneration or constricted visual field from stroke or glaucoma. Patients with low vision should be referred to low vision specialists for evaluation, counseling, and training.

The goal of low vision services is to ameliorate functional disability for specific tasks using optical or nonoptical devices.[108,109] Hand-held magnifiers or stand magnifiers may enable legally blind persons to read newspaper print and perform other near work. Telescopic devices improve distance vision (e.g., street signs); tinted lenses reduce glare; and mirrors and prisms enlarge visual fields. Closed-circuit television monitors can magnify reading materials, improve contrast sensitivity, and reduce glare; but they are expensive and not portable. Nonoptical aids include large-print reading materials, books-on-tape, and specially designed clocks, scales, and thermometers. Additional low vision services are mobility training, in-house assessment of the living environment, disability counseling, braille teaching, lists of local community resources, and guide-dogs.

## References


1. Friedenwald JS. The eye. In: Cowdry EV (ed) The Problems of Aging, 2nd ed. Williams & Wilkins: Baltimore, 1942:535.
2. Caird FI, Wiliamson J. The Eye and Its Disorders in the Elderly. Wright: Bristol, 1986.
3. US Department of Health and Human Services. Current Estimates from the National Health Interview Survey: United States. US Public Health Service Publ. No. 86–1582, Series 10, No. 154. OHHS: Hyattsville, MD, 1983.
4. Podgor MJ, Leske MC, Ederer F. Incidence estimates for lens changes, macular changes, open-angle glaucoma and diabetic retinopathy. Am J Epidemiol 1983;118:206–212.
5. Butler RN, Faye EE, Guazzo E, Kupfer C. Keeping an eye on vision: primary care of age-related ocular disease: part 1. Geriatrics 1997;52(8):30–41.
6. Rosenberg LF. Glaucoma: early detection and therapy for prevention of vision loss. Am Fam Physician 1995;52: 2289–2298.
7. Wong DH. Regional anesthesia for intraocular surgery. Can J Anaesth 1993;40:645–657.
8. Kattan HM, Flynn HW, Pflugfelder SC, Robertson C, Forster RK. Nosocomial endophthalmitis survey: current incidence of infection after intraocular surgery. Ophthalmology 1991;98:227–238.
9. Troll GF. Regional ophthalmic anesthesia: safe techniques and avoidance of complications. J Clin Anesth 1995; 7:163–172.
10. Lindquist TD, Lindstrom R. Ophthalmic Surgery. Looseleaf and Update Service. Mosby: St. Louis, 1990.
11. Buckley EG, Shields MB. Atlas of Ophthalmic Surgery, vol III: Strabismus and Glaucoma. Mosby-Year Book: St. Louis, 1995.
12. Pastorek N. Upper-lid blepharoplasty. Facial Plast Surg 1996;12:157–169.
13. Berlin AJ, Vestal KP. Levator aponeurosis surgery: a retrospective review. Ophthalmology 1989;96:1033–1036.
14. Koch RJ, Troell RF, Goode RL. Contemporary management of the aging brow and forehead. Laryngoscope 1997; 107:710–715.
15. Dresner SC, Karesh JW. Transconjunctival entropion repair. Arch Ophthalmol 1993;111:1144–1148.
16. Anderson RL, Gord DD. The tarsal strip procedure. Arch Ophthalmol 1979;97:2192–2196.
17. Mauriello JA Jr, Dhillon S, Leone T, Pakeman B, Mostafavi R, Yepez X. Treatment selections of 239 patients with blepharospasm and Meige syndrome over 11 years. Br J Ophthalmol 1996;80:1073–1076.
18. Cole H. Botulinum toxin may help blepharospasm sufferers. JAMA 1985;254:1688–1690.
19. Kass LG, Hornblass A. Sebaceous carcinoma of the ocular adnexa. Surv Ophthalmol 1989;33:477–490.
20. Margo CE, Waltz K. Basal cell carcinoma of the eyelid and periocular skin. Surv Ophthalmol 1993;38:169–192.
21. Leshin B, Yeatts P. Management of periocular basal cell carcinoma: Mohs' micrographic surgery versus radiotherapy. Surv Ophthalmol 1993;38:193–212.
22. Muenzier WS. The dry eye: a working outline of etiology, symptoms, diagnosis, and treatment. Geriatr Ophthalmol 1986;2:219–223.
23. Price EJ, Venables PJ. The etiopathogenesis of Sjogren's syndrome. Semin Arthritis Rheum 1995;25:117–133.
24. Anonymous. Punctal occlusion for the dry eye: three-year revision; American Academy of Ophthalmology. Ophthalmology 1997;104:1521–1524.
25. Tarbet KJ, Custer PL. External dacryocystorhinostomy: surgical success, patient satisfaction, and economic cost. Ophthalmology 1995;102:1065–1070.
26. Wigham CG, Hodson SA. Physiological changes in the cornea of the ageing eye. Eye 1987;1:190–196.
27. Morrison LK, Waltman SR. Management of pseudophakic bullous keratopathy. Ophthalmic Surg 1989;20:105–210.
28. Boruchoff SA. Penetrating keratoplasy. In: Albert DM, Jakobiec FA (eds) Principles and Practice of Ophthalmology, vol I. Saunders: Philadelphia, 1994:325–342.
29. Gillum W. Mechanisms of accommodation in vertebrates. Ophthalmic Semin 1976;1:253–286.
30. Duane A. Normal values of the accommodation at all ages. JAMA 1912;59:1010–1013.
31. Javitt JC, Wang F, Trentacost DJ, Rowe M, Tarantino N. Outcomes of cataract extraction with multifocal intraocular lens implantation: functional status and quality of life. Ophthalmology 1997;104:589–599.
32. Kupfer C, Underwood B, Gillen T. Leading causes of visual impairment worldwide. In: Albert DM, Jakobiec FA (eds) Principles and Practice of Ophthalmology: Basic Sciences. Saunders: Philadelphia, 1994:1249–1255.
33. Klein BE, Klein R, Moss SE. Incident cataract surgery: the Beaver Dam eye study. Ophthalmology 1997;104:573–580.
34. Kahn HA, Leibowitz HM, Ganley JP, et al. The Framingham eye study: outline and major prevalence findings. Am J Epidemiol 1977;106:117.
35. Benedek GB. Cataract as a protein condensation disease. Invest Ophthalmol Vis Sci 1997;38:1911–1922.
36. Lee PP, Hiborne L, McDonald L, et al. Documentation patterns before cataract surgery at ten academic centers. Ophthalmology 1996;103:1179–1183.
37. Jaffe GJ, Burton TC, Kuhn E, Prescott A, Hartz A. Progression of nonproliferative diabetic retinopathy and visual outcome after extracapsular cataract extraction and intraocular lens implantation. Am J Ophthalmol 1992;114: 448–456.
38. Steinberg EP, Javitt JC, Sharkey PD, et al. The content and cost of cataract surgery. Arch Ophthalmol 1993;111:1041–1049.
39. Curbow B, Legro MW, Brenner MH. The influence of patient-related variables in the timing of cataract extraction. Am J Ophthalmol 1993;115:614–622.
40. Rutkow IM. Surgical operations in the United States: then (1983) and now (1994). Arch Surg 1997;132:983–990.
41. Desai P. The National Cataract Surgery Survey. II. Clinical outcomes. Eye 1993;7:489–494.
42. Fine IH. The chip and flip phacoemulsification technique. J Cataract Refract Surg 1991;17:366–371.

43. Gimbel HV. Divide and conquer nucleofractis phacoemulsification: development and variations. J Cataract Refract Surg 1991;17:281–291.
44. Javitt JC, Vitale S, Canner JK, et al. National outcomes of cataract surgery: endophthalmitis following inpatient surgery. Arch Ophthalmol 1991;109:1085–1089.
45. Tezel G, Kolker AE, Kass MA, Wax MB. Comparative results of combined procedures for glaucoma and cataract. I. Extracapsular cataract extraction versus phacoemulsification and foldable versus rigid intraocular lenses. Ophthalmic Surg Laser 1997;28:539–550.
46. Apple DJ, Solomon KD, Tetz MR, et al. Posterior capsule opacification. Surv Ophthalmol 1992;37(2):73–116.
47. Steinberg EP, Tielsch JM, Schein OD, et al. National study of cataract surgery outcomes: variation in 4-month postoperative outcomes as reflected in multiple outcome measures. Ophthalmology 1994;101:1131–1140.
48. Kahn HA, Leibowitz HM, Ganley JB. Framingham eye study. I. Outline and major prevalence findings. Am J Epidemiol 1977;106:17.
49. Tielsch JM, Sommer A, Katz J, Royall RM, Quigley HA, Lavitt J. Racial variations in the prevalence of primary open-angle glaucoma. JAMA 1991;266:369–374.
50. Quigley HA. Number of people with glaucoma worldwide. Br J Ophthalmol 1996;80:389–393.
51. Millard CB, Tripathi BJ, Tripathi RC. Age-related changes in protein profiles of the normal human trabecular meshwork. Exp Eye Res 1987;45:623–631.
52. Albon J, Karwatowski WS, Avery N, Easty DL, Duance VC. Changes in the collagenous matrix of the aging human lamina cribrosa. Br J Ophthalmol 1995;79:368–375.
53. Colton T, Ederer F. The distribution of intraocular pressures in the population. Surv Ophthalmol 1980;25:123–129.
54. Butler RN, Faye EE, Guazzo E, Kupfer C. Keeping an eye on vision: new tools to preserve sight and quality of life; a roundtable discussion, part 2. Geriatrics 1997;52(9):48–50, 53–56.
55. Quigley HA. Reappraising the risk and benefits of aggressive glaucoma therapy. Ophthalmology 1997;104:1985–1986.
56. Roy H, Tindall R. An update on the use of drugs for common eye problems in older patients. Geriatrics 1991;46(11):51–54, 57–60.
57. Prakash UB, Rosenow EC III. Pulmonary complications from ophthalmic preparations. Mayo Clin Proc 1990;65:521–529.
58. Glaucoma Laser Trial Research Group: The glaucoma laser trial and glaucoma laser trial follow-up study. 7. Results. Am J Ophthalmol 1995;120:718–731.
59. Nouri-Mahdavi K, Brigatti L, Weitzman M, Caprioli J. Outcomes of trabeculectomy for primary open-angle glaucoma. Ophthalmology 1995;102:1760–1769.
60. Fluorouracil Filtering Surgery Study Group. Three-year follow-up of the Fluorouracil Filtering Surgery Study. Am J Ophthalmol 1993;115:82–92.
61. Palmer SS. Mitomycin as adjunct chemotherapy with trabeculectomy. Ophthalmology 1991;98:317–321.
62. Price FW Jr, Wellemeyer M. Long-term results of Molteno implants. Ophthalmic Surg 1995;26:130–135.
63. Mastrobattista JM, Luntz M. Ciliary body ablation: where are we and how did we get here? Surv Ophthalmol 1996;41:193–213.
64. Leibowitz HM, Krueger DE, Maunder LR, et al. Framingham eye study monograph. Surv Ophthalmol 1980;24(suppl):335–610.
65. Green WR, Key SN. Senile macular degeneration: a histopathological study. Trans Am Ophthalmol Soc 1977;75:180–254.
66. Mainster MA. Light and macular degeneration: a biophysical and clinical perspective. Eye 1987;1:304–310.
67. Mares-Perlman JA, Klein R, Klein BE, et al. Association of zinc and antioxidant nutrients with age-related maculopathy. Arch Ophthalmol 1996;114:991–997.
68. Macular Photocoagulation Study Group. Argon laser photocoagulation for neovascular maculopathy: three-year results from randomized trials. Arch Ophthalmol 1986;104:694–701.
69. Macular Photocoagulation Study Group. Argon laser photocoagulation for neovascular maculopathy: five-year results from randomized trials. Arch Ophthalmol 1991;109:1109–1114.
70. Moisseiev J, Alhalel A, Masuri R, Treister G. The impact of the macular photocoagulation study results on the treatment of exudative age-related macular degeneration. Arch Ophthalmol 1995;113:185–189.
71. Yonemoto LT, Slater JD, Friedrichsen EJ, et al. Phase I/II study of proton beam irradiation for the treatment of subfoveal choroidal neovascularization in age-related macular degeneration: treatment techniques and preliminary results. Int J Radiat Oncol Biol Phys 1996;36:867–871.
72. Sakamoto T, Soriano D, Nassaralla J, et al. Effect of intravitreal administration of indomethacin on experimental subretinal neovascularization in the subhuman primate. Arch Ophthalmol 1995;113:222–226.
73. Ibanez HE, Williams DF, Thomas MA, et al. Surgical management of submacular hemorrhage: a survey of 47 consecutive cases. Arch Ophthalmol 1995;113:62–69.
74. Kaplan HJ, Tezel TH, Berger AS, Wolf ML, Del Priore LV. Human photoreceptor transplantation in retinitis pigmentosa: a safety study. Arch Ophthalmol 1997;115:1168–1172.
75. Haimann MH, Burton TC, Brown CK. Epidemiology of retinal detachment. Arch Ophthalmol 1982;100:289.
76. Byer NE. Natural history of posterior vitreous detachment with early management as the premier line of defense against retinal detachment. Ophthalmology 1994;101:1503–1513; discussion 1513–1514.
77. Byer NE. The natural history of asymptomatic retinal breaks. Ophthalmology 1982;89:1033–1039.
78. Scheie HG, Morse PH, Aminlari A. Incidence of retinal detachment following cataract extraction. Arch Ophthalmol 1973;89:293.
79. Kramer SG, Benson WE. Prophylactic therapy of retinal breaks. Surv Ophthalmol 1977;22:41–47.
80. McCuen BW, Azen SP, Stern W, et al. Vitrectomy with silicone oil or perfluoropropane gas in eyes with severe proliferative vitreoretinopathy: silicone study report 3. Retina 1993;13:279–284.

81. Tornambe PE, Hilton GF. Pneumatic retinopexy: a multicenter randomized controlled clinical trial comparing pneumatic retinopexy with scleral buckling: the Retinal Detachment Study Group. Ophthalmology 1989;96: 772–783.
82. McAllister IL, Meyers SM, Zegarra H, Gutman FA, Zakov ZN, Beck GJ. Comparison of pneumatic retinopexy with alternative surgical techniques. Ophthalmology 1988;95: 877–883.
83. Escoffery RF, Olk RJ, Grand MG, Boniuk I. Vitrectomy without scleral buckling for primary rhegmatogenous retinal detachment. Am J Ophthalmol 1985;99:275–281.
84. Hanneken A, Michels RG. Vitrectomy and scleral buckling methods for proliferative vitreoretinopathy. Ophthalmology 1988;95:865–869.
85. Berger AS, Cheng CK, Pearson PA, et al. Intravitreal sustained release corticosteroid-5-fluorouracil conjugate in the treatment of experimental proliferative vitreoretinopathy. Invest Ophthalmol Vis Sci 1996;37:2318–2325.
86. Gariano RF, Assil KK, Wiley CA, Munguia D, Weinreb RN, Freeman WR. Retinal toxicity of the antimetabolite 5-fluorouridine 5′-monophosphate administered intravitreally using multivesicular liposomes. Retina 1994;14:75–80.
87. Palmberg P, Smith M, Waltman S, et al. The natural history of retinopathy in insulin-dependent juvenile-onset diabetes. Ophthalmology 1981;88:613–618.
88. Ohkubo Y, Kishikawa H, Araki E. Intensive insulin therapy prevents the progression of diabetic microvascular complications in Japanese patients with non-insulin-dependent diabetes mellitus: a randomized prospective 6-year study. Diabetes Res Clin Pract 1995;28:103–117.
89. Frank RN. On the pathogenesis of diabetic retinopathy: a 1990 update. Ophthalmology 1991;98:586–593.
90. Cogan DG, Toussaint D, Kuwabara T. Retinal vascular patterns. IV. Diabetic retinopathy. Arch Ophthalmol 1961; 66:366–378.
91. Anonymous. Early photocoagulation for diabetic retinopathy: ETDRS report number 9: Early Treatment Diabetic Retinopathy Study Research Group. Ophthalmology 1991; 98(suppl 5):766–785.
92. Anonymous. Treatment techniques and clinical guidelines for photocoagulation of diabetic macular edema: early treatment diabetic retinopathy study report number 2; Early Treatment Diabetic Retinopathy Study Research Group. Ophthalmology 1987;94:761–774.
93. Danis RP, Bingaman DP, Jirousek M, Yang Y. Inhibition of intraocular neovascularization caused by retinal ischemia in pigs by PKC beta inhibition with LY333531. Invest Ophthalmol Vis Sci 1998;39:171–179.
94. Anonymous. Early vitrectomy for severe vitreous hemorrhage in diabetic retinopathy: four-year results of a randomized trial: diabetic retinopathy vitrectomy; study report 5. Arch Ophthalmol 1990;108:958–964.
95. Ho T, Smiddy WE, Flynn HW. Vitrectomy in the management of diabetic eye disease. Surv Ophthalmol 1992;37: 190–202.
96. Anonymous. Results of the endophthalmitis vitrectomy study: a randomized trial of immediate vitrectomy and of intravenous antibiotics for the treatment of postoperative bacterial endophthalmitis; Endophthalmitis Vitrectomy Study Group. Arch Ophthalmol 1997;113:1479–1496.
97. Shields CL, Shields JA, Gross NE, Schwartz GP, Lally SE. Survey of 520 eyes with uveal metastases. Ophthalmology 1997;104:1265–1276.
98. Rudoler SB, Corn BW, Shields CL, et al. External beam irradiation for choroid metastases: identification of factors predisposing to long-term sequelae. Int J Rad Oncol, Biol, Physics 1997;38:251–256.
99. Scotto J, Fraumeni JF, Lee JAH. Melanomas of the eye and other noncutaneous sites: epidemiologic aspects. J Natl Cancer Inst 1976;56:489–491.
100. Shields JA, Shields CL. Current management of posterior uveal melanoma. Mayo Clin Proc 1993;68:1196–1200.
101. Freeman LN, Schachat AP, Knox DL, Michels RG, Green WR. Clinical features, laboratory investigations, and survival in ocular reticulum cell sarcoma. Ophthalmology 1987;94:1631–1639.
102. Margolis L, Fraser R, Lichter A, Char DH. The role of radiation therapy in the management of ocular reticulum cell sarcoma. Cancer 1980;45:688–692.
103. Neupert JR, Brubaker RF, Kearns TP, Sundt TM. Rapid resolution of venous stasis retinopathy after carotid endarterectomy. Am J Ophthalmol 1976;81:600–602.
104. Hunder GG, Bloch DA, Michel BA, et al. The American College of Rheumatology 1990 criteria for the classification of giant cell arteritis. Arthritis Rheum 1990;33: 1122–1128.
105. Hayreh SS. Giant cell arteritis: validity and reliability of various diagnostic criteria. Am J Ophthalmol 1997;123: 285–296.
106. Stevens RJ, Hughes R. The aetiopathogenesis of giant cell arteritis. Br J Rheumatol 1995;34:960–965.
107. Magram I, Schlossman A. Strabismus in patients over the age of 60 years. J Pediatr Ophthalmol Strabismus 1991;28:28–31.
108. Warren M. Providing low vision rehabilitation services with occupational therapy and ophthalmology: a program description. Am J Occup Ther 1995;49:877–883.
109. Swanson MW, Brock J, Houston R. Older Alabamians System of Information and Services (OASIS): a model title VII chapter 2 low vision rehabilitation program. J Am Optom Assoc 1995;66:357–361.

# 26
# Physiologic Changes in the Ears, Nose, and Throat

John F. Kveton and Ravi Goravalingappa

Aging, a phenomenon common to all multicellular organisms, results in multisystem dysfunction and ultimately death. The timing and rate of the aging process is species-dependent, which has led to the development of the concepts of chronologic age versus biologic age. The specific control mechanisms of the aging process are poorly understood, but aging has been theorized to be completely controlled by genetic and other biochemical changes that result from replication errors in RNA synthesis.[1]

The effects of aging in the head and neck region are extensive, ranging from the cosmetic effects on the integumentary system to functional disorders involving respiration, swallowing, the special senses, and changes in higher cortical function. Such changes not only alter the specific system-related functions, they have an impact on the patient as a whole and potentially how a patient responds to surgical alterations that occur in other body systems. This chapter describes the changes that occur in the special senses of hearing, balance, and chemosensation during aging and the potential impact of these changes on the patient.

## Presbyacusis

Hearing loss is a common disorder in the general population but affecting the elderly patient disproportionately. Most hearing loss in the elderly is caused by changes within the inner ear (sensorineural hearing loss) rather than the external or middle ears (conductive hearing loss). Hearing loss usually begins in the high frequency range, beyond the frequency characteristics of the human voice; so it is imperceptible to the patient. With advancing age, the hearing loss encroaches on the speech frequencies, with impairment now being recognized especially by the patient's family and friends. Hearing loss is first noted during conversation in noisy environments, in situations with multiple stimuli, and in interactions with persons with high-pitched voices. As hearing loss increases, speech recognition is increasingly impaired, often resulting in the unconscious development of lip reading. In such cases patients begin to recognize their impairment only when they are not capable of speaking face to face with the individual. If left untreated, such a progressive hearing deficit invariably leads to curtailment of socialization and to loneliness and depression.

Hearing loss in the elderly is often multifactorial, so presbyacusis may not be the sole cause of the hearing impairment. The plasticity of the auditory system, unlike many other organ systems, is mainly determined by genetics and multiple environmental factors, especially noise exposure.

Emphasis must be placed on the family history of hearing loss and other conditions that may affect the inner ear directly, such as neoplastic, infectious, inflammatory, or metabolic disorders. Auditory perception also requires intact central nervous system (CNS) pathways from the brain stem to the cerebral cortex. The recognized alteration of cortical function with age can be accelerated by metabolic or vascular changes in the CNS, which in turn have an additive effect on the patient's auditory impairment.

### Anatomy

Sensorineural hearing loss requires an understanding of the anatomy of the cochlea, auditory nerve, and CNS pathways of the auditory system.

#### *Cochlea*

The cochlea is the anterior portion of the inner ear (the bony labyrinth), which also contains the vestibule and the semicircular canals. This hollow bone contains the neuroepithelium for auditory perception (cochlea) and balance perception (vestibule and semicircular canals). The cochlea is a spiral canal with an axial length of about 5mm. This canal, in which lies the membranous canal

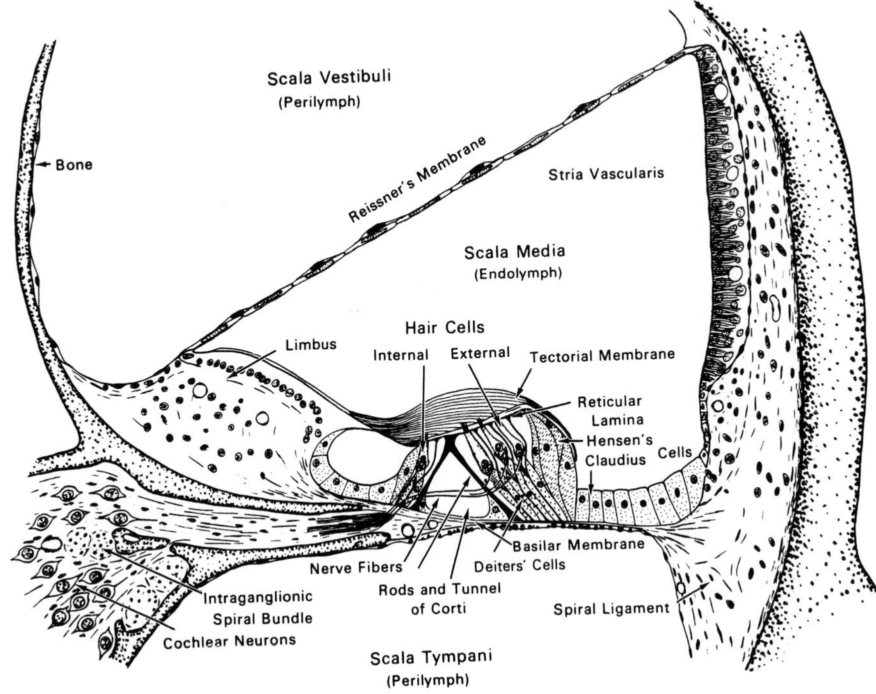


FIGURE 26.1. Anatomy of the organ of Corti. (From Schuknecht,[21] with permission.)

known as the cochlear duct, wraps around a central bony core, the modiolus, for two and a half to two and three-quarter turns through which the auditory nerve fibers penetrate. The cochlear duct is divided into three compartments: the scala tympani, scala media, and scala vestibuli. The scala media has a fluid composition (endolymph) different from that of the other two compartments (perilymph) and contains the organ of Corti (Fig. 26.1), which is the sensory organ of hearing. The organ of Corti rests on the basilar membrane, which separates the scala media from the scala tympani. The organ of Corti contains afferent nerve endings (3500 inner hair cells), afferent/efferent nerve endings (12,000 outer hair cells), and a variety of other supporting cells. The hair cells communicate with the dendritic terminals of the bipolar cochlear neurons whose cell bodies are located within the modiolus.

### *Auditory Nerve*

The auditory nerve consists of about 30,000 afferent and 1000 efferent bipolar neurons. Ninety-five percent of the spiral ganglion is composed of myelinated (type 1) fibers that innervate only inner hair cells, and nonmyelinated (type 2) fibers innervate outer hair cells. The spiral ganglion is the most dense at the mid and basal portions of the modiolus. The nerve fibers course in the nerve trunk in an orderly spatial arrangement (basal fibers located at the periphery and inferior portion of the nerve) through the temporal bone into the cerebellopontine angle into the pons to enter the cochlear nuclei.

### *Central Nervous System*

There are three morphologically distinct auditory nuclei within the pons. Upon entering the pons each fiber divides into an anterior branch, which terminates in the anterior part of the ventral cochlear nucleus, and a posterior branch, which again divides to terminate in the posterior part of the ventral cochlear nucleus and the dorsal cochlear nucleus. Cells from these nuclei send axons in a complex pattern from the contralateral superior and accessory olive areas to the lateral lemniscus, the inferior colliculus, and through the medial geniculate body to the auditory cortex in the temporal lobe.

## Physiology

Sound perception begins by the vibration of the ossicular chain produced when sound waves enter the external auditory canal to contact the tympanic membrane. The excursions of the stapes footplate within the vestibule set up a traveling wave within the perilymph of the scala tympani.

The mammalian cochlea is unique in the way the basilar membrane is supported to perceive forces and pressures from this traveling wave. Because of differences in the mechanical compliance along the length of the cochlear duct, specific regions of the organ of Corti are stimulated to produce a tonotopic map of the cochlear duct. For example, high frequency tones tend to produce maximal basilar membrane displacement in the basal turn, and low frequency tones produce maximal displacement near the apex.[2] The hair cells serves as mechanoreceptors, converting the mechanical energy of basilar membrane displacement into an action potential to stimulate the ganglion cells. The cochlea's capacity to analyze the periodicity, synchrony rate, phase, and spread of excitation of sound results in specific ganglion cell population stimulation and ultimately the perception of sound frequency patterns in the auditory cortex.[3]

## Pathologic Findings with Aging

### *Peripheral Nervous System*

Most agree that presbyacusis is caused by changes in the inner ear rather than in the tympanic membrane, ossicles, or ossicular ligaments. Crowe et al.[4] noted atrophy of the organ of Corti in the basal turn of the cochlear duct in association with high frequency sensorineural hearing loss and changes in the auditory nerve. These findings have been documented by various authors. The vascular effects of aging on the cochlea were recognized by Van Fiedant and Saxen,[5] who described atherosclerotic changes within the stria vascularis and collapse of the cochlear duct due to aging. These changes lead to eventual hair cell loss, producing marked degenerative changes in the neural fibers, decreasing the number of synapses at the base of the hair cells. Accumulation of cochlear debris in the spiral bundles, abnormalities of the dendritic fibers and their sheaths in the osseous spiral lamina, and degenerative changes in the spiral ganglion cells and axons follow.

### *Central Nervous System*

Changes within the CNS can be secondary to peripheral nervous system dysfunction or the result of primary neural loss. The primary physiologic changes in the CNS due to aging are a decrease in astrocytes in the frontal and parietal cortex, neuronal loss in the hippocampal cortex, and a decrease in Purkinje cells in the cerebellum after the fifth decade.[6] Wong Riley[7] studied the effects of peripheral dysfunction on central activity. Deafness led to diminished spontaneous neural activity with corresponding functional and morphologic changes in the central auditory system from the cochlear nucleus to the inferior colliculus. Loss of spiral ganglion cells leads to terminal degeneration within the cochlear nucleus and transneural degeneration to the level of the superior colliculus.

## Types of Presbyacusis

Four types of presbyacusis have been hypothesized to exist based on the auditory characteristics with which a patient presents and the histologic correlates. These types may occur alone or in combination. They present clinically as bilateral, symmetric, slowly progressive losses.

### *Sensory Presbyacusis*

Sensory presbyacusis presents clinically as a bilateral, symmetric, high frequency sensorineural hearing loss characterized by an abrupt, down-sloping threshold pattern. As the high frequency loss becomes more severe, speech discrimination deficits involving consonants became apparent. Morphologically, the basal turn of the cochlea demonstrates loss of both hair cells and supporting cells in the organ of Corti. The degeneration does not include the middle or apical turns of the cochlea. Speech discrimination is inversely related to the range of frequencies involved and usually remains within an acceptable range.

### *Neural Presbyacusis*

Neural presbyacusis can occur at any age and is due to loss of cochlear neurons. These degenerative changes appear to be controlled by genetic factors and vary in time of onset. Neural presbyacusis usually affects hearing late in life when the population of cochlear neurons falls below the number required for effective transmission of neural flow. The loss of speech discrimination is relatively more severe than pure tone hearing loss. Histologically, the organ of Corti is intact, but there is loss of spiral ganglion cells. Elderly patients with rapidly progressive neural presbyacusis usually demonstrate other CNS findings consistent with generalized neuronal loss, such as motor weakness, tremor, irritability, and memory loss.

### *Strial Presbyacusis*

Atrophy of the stria vascularis is common with aging and is usually associated with hair cell loss. The stria participates in the formation of endolymph and is probably the most important structure for maintaining its ionic composition. Patchy atrophy of strial cells predominantly in the middle and apical turns produces a characteristic flat, pure tone sensorineural hearing loss with excellent speech discrimination scores with a familial tendency. Such patients are excellent candidates for amplification.

### *Cochlear Conductive Presbyacusis*

Cochlear conductive presbyacusis produces a gradual, sloping high frequency loss rather than the abrupt loss seen with sensory presbyacusis. Ramdan and Schuknecht[8] postulated that such linear decrements of function are related to the physical anatomic gradients that determine the resonance characteristics of the cochlear duct. To support this concept, Nadol[9] demonstrated marked thickening of the basilar membrane due to an increase in the number of fibrillar layers.

## Summary

Although elderly patients experience progressive increases in the pure tone thresholds, only 8% have significant changes in the pure tone pattern. In the clinical setting, alterations due to aging of the other areas of the CNS are as important as hearing loss in diminished communication abilities.

The types of presbyacusis may be characterized as follows: (1) Sensory presbyacusis manifests clinically as high tone hearing loss with good speech discrimination. (2) Neural presbyacusis is seen as a severe loss of speech discrimination with minimal sensorineural hearing loss. (3) Strial presbyacusis manifests as a flat threshold pattern with excellent speech discrimination. (4) Cochlear conductive presbyacusis produces a gradual, sloping high tone loss with speech discrimination that is inversely related to the steepness of the slope.

# Presbyastasis

The vestibular system, like the auditory system, is not spared from the ravages of aging. The sense of head and body motion in space depends on the interaction of the inputs from virtually every sensory system of the body, with the vestibular, visual, and proprioceptive systems being primary. These interactions are necessary if one is to perform the complex tasks of retinal image stabilization, orientation, balance, and smooth, coordinated locomotion with speed and accuracy.

The symptoms of vestibular dysfunction vary on a continuum from severe vertigo to lightheadedness. The sudden onset of a sense of movement (vertigo) is generally a sign of acute vestibular dysfunction, whereas the more chronic symptoms of lightheadedness, imbalance, or vertigo on positional changes reflect either poor compensation due to an acute vestibular injury or chronic deterioration of the vestibular system. The latter symptoms are much more common in the elderly. Belal and Glorig[10] coined the term presbyastasis to describe these symptoms. By age 80, one in three of the elderly suffers from dysequilibrium, with women affected more than men. Such symptoms play a role in causing falls by the elderly, which is a significant health cost to society when considering the cumulative costs of hospitalization, rehabilitation services, and nursing home care. Although falls are often induced by cardiac arrhythmias, postural hypotension, Parkinson's disease, seizure disorders, cerebral ischemia, poor proprioception, and visual loss, dysequilibrium can be a contributing factor.

Deterioration or degeneration of the vestibular system changes can occur at peripheral or central sites. The inner ear and vestibular nerve comprise the peripheral vestibular system, and the central vestibular system involves the vestibular nuclei and the brain stem pathways to the visual and cerebellar nuclei and the spinal cord.

## Peripheral Vestibular System

### Vestibular Labyrinth

The vestibular system, located within the inner ear (bony labyrinth) along with the cochlea, is made up of the vestibule and the semicircular canals. The vestibule is a spherical structure about 4 mm in diameter that separates the cochlea from the semicircular canals. Three bony semicircular canals, each making two-thirds of a circle, join the posterior and medial portion of the vestibule. These semicircular canals are situated at right angles from each other and are named the horizontal, superior, and posterior semicircular canals. The horizontal canal is oriented 30 degrees from the horizontal head plane. At one end of each semicircular canal is the ampulla, a ballooning of the canal that houses the sensory neuroepithelium of each semicircular canal.

Within the bony labyrinth is the membranous labyrinth, which contains the sensory structures of the vestibular end-organ. The membranous labyrinth is suspended within the bony labyrinth by fluid (perilymph) and a web-like network containing blood vessels. The membranous labyrinth itself is filled with endolymph, which differs from perilymph in having high potassium/low sodium concentrations. The membranous labyrinth in the vestibule is divided into the saccule and the utricle, each demonstrating a defined thickening called macula. The three semicircular canals communicate with the utricle via openings. Three of these openings are enlarged to form the membranous ampullae. A crest-like septum, the crista, crosses the base of each ampulla and is covered with vestibular sensory epithelium. The sensory epithelium in both the vestibule and the semicircular canals is similar to that found within the cochlea. Type 1 hair cells are similar to inner hair cells, and type 2 hair cells are similar to outer hair cells. Type 1 hair cells appear to be more concentrated on the summit of the crista and in a central region of the macula. These hair cells project into a gelatinous matrix that fills the remaining space within the membranous ampulla and a gelatinous matrix in the utricle and macula that is covered with a layer of oblong crystals called otoconia.

### Vestibular Nerve

The vestibular ganglion contains bipolar neurons that project to the sensory neuroepithelium of the semicircular canals and vestibule and to the vestibular nuclei in the brain stem. A ganglion is located on both the superior and inferior divisions of the vestibular nerve within the internal auditory canal. The superior division supplies the cristae of the superior and horizontal semicircular canals and the macula of the utricle; and the inferior division supplies the crista of the posterior semicircular canal and the macula of the saccule.

### *Central Vestibular System*

The vestibular nuclei, located in the pons in proximity to the cochlear nuclei, include the superior, lateral, medial, and descending vestibular nuclei. All fibers from the vestibular ganglion bifurcate into ascending and descending branches once they enter the brain stem. Ascending fibers from the semicircular canals pass to the superior nucleus and ultimately to the cerebellum. Descending fibers mainly pass to the medial nucleus, with contributions to the lateral and descending nuclei. Fibers from the utricle and saccule terminate in the medial nuclei. Projections from the vestibular nuclei then extend to the cerebellum, extraocular nuclei, reticular formation, spinal cord, and cerebral cortex.

## Physiology

The sense of balance is elicited through depolarization of the vestibular hair cells located in the maculae of the utricle and saccule and the cristae of the semicircular canals. The utricle and saccule respond to linear acceleration. Linear acceleration causes the hair cells embedded in the macula to bend owing to the inertial effect of acceleration on the otoconia embedded in the gelatinous layer of the macula. Angular accelerations set in motion endolymph in the membranous portion of the semicircular canals. The flow patterns affect the hair cells of each ampulla differently, producing excitation in one and inhibition in the others. Working concurrently, both peripheral vestibular organs send excitatory and inhibitory information to the vestibular nuclei to control visual fixation and proprioception.

## Electron Microscopic Findings with Aging

### *Peripheral Vestibular System*

The degenerative changes in the otoconia have been well documented.[11] Pitting of the surface of the otoconia is followed by cavitation of the surfaces, demineralization, and finally fragmentation. There are also changes in the sensory epithelium in the maculae and cristae, including alterations in the hair cell length and number, accumulation of inclusion bodies (including lipofuscin), vacuoles, and the disappearance of some cells with replacement by scar tissue. There is a sequential pattern of loss of nerve fibers between the vestibule and Scarpa's ganglion. This loss is rather rapid after the fifth decade. A decrease in the number of ganglion cells in Scarpa's ganglion usually begins at about age 60, with recognizable decreases in the cell population apparent after age 70.[12,13] The appearance of increased amounts of lipofuscin in the receptors and neurons of the vestibular system during advanced age is thought to be caused by accumulation of protein due to intracellular transport.

### *Central Vestibular System*

Few data are available on changes in the vestibular nuclei with aging. Purkinje cells of the cerebellum are known to decrease after the fifth decade along with a reduction in astrocytes in the frontal and parietal cortex and neuronal loss in the hippocampus.[14]

## Types of Presbyastasis

There are four types of presbyastasis for which there are distinct clinical manifestations. Three of the conditions involve the peripheral vestibular system; they may occur alone or in combination.

### *Benign Paroxysmal Positional Vertigo*

Benign paroxysmal positional vertigo manifests as severe, brief episodes of vertigo predicated by certain head positions. It is usually self-limiting, lasting weeks to months; but if it develops insidiously in an aged person it may be permanent. Because of the sudden nature of the attacks, the episodes may induce falling. Pathologically, the disorder appears related to the accumulation of otoconial debris in the posterior semicircular canal. The accumulation of deposits in this area appear to alter the function of the posterior semicircular canal ampulla.

### *Ampullary Dysequilibrium*

Patients with ampullary dysequilibrium experience a sense of rotatory movement in their field of vision with angular head movements. They experience a sensation of movement. Unsteadiness may last several hours after a severe angular movement. Theoretically, these symptoms are due to the accumulation of lipofuscin granules in the hair cells of the cristae.

### *Macular Dysequilibrium*

With macular dysequilibrium, vertigo and severe dysequilibrium occur after a change in head position relative to the direction of gravitational force after the head has been maintained in a position for some time. Patients afflicted with this condition cannot rise from bed without progressing from the supine and sitting position in stages over several minutes. This condition can be differentiated from orthostatic hypotension by the absence of other signs of intracranial ischemia and visual blackout. Theoretically, this condition is caused by degenerative changes in the otolithic membranes or sensory epithelium of the saccule or utricle.

### *Vestibular Ataxia of Aging*

Patients with vestibular ataxia of aging manifest a constant unsteadiness on ambulation. Symptoms are absent when sitting or standing, but there is an inability to control the center of gravity when walking. It occurs predominantly during the seventh and eighth decades. The peripheral vestibular system appears intact, but the symptoms suggest loss of vestibular control over the lower extremities, implying a central vestibular system dysfunction.

### Summary

Vestibular dysfunction in the elderly is as prevalent as auditory dysfunction but more difficult to document. Although episodic vestibular disorders can occur in the elderly, the insidious onset of symptoms of dysequilibrium is the more common presentation, suggesting age-induced degeneration of the vestibular apparatus.

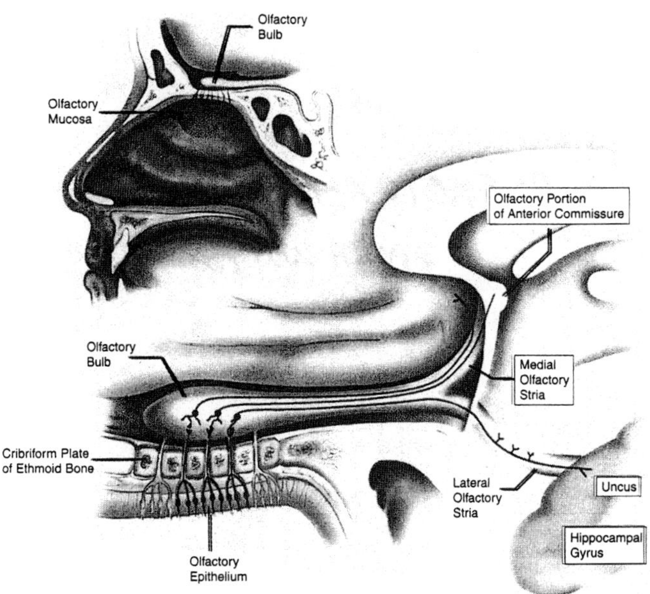


FIGURE 26.2. Olfactory nerve pathways.

## Chemosensation with Aging

A large proportion of the population, apart from age-related health issues, have significant age-related sensory loses involving olfaction and taste. These changes affect this vulnerable population by altering food choices, leading to impaired nutrition and immunity, weight loss, and possibly exacerbation of preexisting diseases. In addition, loss of an intact sensory system for smell and taste puts the individual at risk for food poisoning.

The chemosensory system includes olfactory and taste perception along with a contribution of the trigeminal system for pain and mechanoreception. This system is mediated by specialized receptors that lie in the nasal cavity, oral cavity, pharynx, and larynx. These receptors are mediated by the olfactory, trigeminal, facial, glossopharyngeal, and vagal nerves. Some chemicals are almost pure olfactory stimulants (e.g., phenyl ethyl alcohol), whereas others are sensed through trigeminal nerve stimulation.

### Olfaction

#### *Anatomy and Physiology*

Olfactory receptor cells are located in the olfactory neuroepithelium (olfactory cleft), which is in the roof of the nasal cavity, superior to the superior turbinate, and on the upper portion of the nasal septum (Fig. 26.2). The olfactory neuroepithelium contains Bowman's glands, which are ciliated for intrinsic mobility, and specialized bipolar neuron cells, which undergo constant renewal every 30 days. The olfactory receptor cells number about 6 million and contain unique protein (olfactory marker protein). Odorants bind to the olfactory receptor cells, which belong to the G-protein class.[15] Codes for the quality of the odor are compound-specific.

The axons of specific olfactory bipolar neurons cells (which are unmyelinated) traverse the cribriform plate of the ethmoid bone to synapse in the olfactory bulb, which is the first-order neuron. These intricate synapses are termed glomeruli and are located in single and double layers at the margin of the olfactory bulb. The mitral cells are the secondary neurons and are the largest cells in the bulb. The axons of the mitral cells project through the internal plexiform layer and proceed caudally within the granular layer. Tufted cells are located between the glomeruli and the mitral cell layer. Arising from the olfactory bulb, the olfactory tract projects caudally to the olfactory nucleus to the olfactory tubercle, the prepiriform cortex, and the amygdala. Olfactory information is ultimately relayed to the hypothalamus.

Once inhaled, odorant molecules are absorbed in the nasal mucus and reversibly bind to the protein receptor sites. This action induces intracellular biochemical changes in the receptor proteins, producing action potentials in the primary receptor neurons. Intensity appears to be related to the rate of production of the potentials, but odor perception quality is poorly understood. The quality of the odor perception may be related to the spatial distribution of the receptor cells within the neuroepithelium.

#### *Changes with Aging*

Anatomic and physiologic changes occur in both the peripheral end-organ and central pathways during aging.

The olfactory glomeruli atrophy along with the changes in the upper respiratory tract epithelium. As these fibers degenerate, the olfactory bulb takes on a moth-eaten appearance. The reduction in the number of the cells in the olfactory bulb is due to diminished levels of neurotransmitters. These changes are more exaggerated in individuals with Alzheimer's disease and other neurodegenerative process in the brain.[16]

Smell perception in the elderly is synergistically impaired, with losses occurring at both threshold and superthreshold concentrations.[17] Many psychophysical studies of smell indicate that age-related losses occur at the threshold concentration.[18] The degree of olfactory loss tends to be more uniform for volatile compounds, with different stimuli from those for taste. Interestingly, many patients with the diagnosis of failure to thrive have anosmia. Elderly populations have reduced capacity to differentiate the degree of odors compared to the younger population, but these differences are profoundly increased in those with Alzheimer's disease and other neurodegenerative brain diseases.

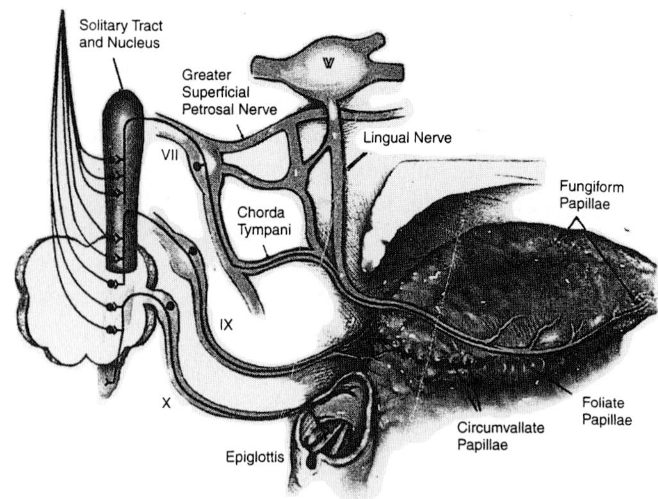


FIGURE 26.3. Peripheral taste pathways.

## Taste

### Anatomy and Physiology

The taste receptor cells are spherical cells located in the taste buds. On the surface of each taste bud is a pore from which microvilli of the receptor cells project. The taste buds are concentrated heavily on the tongue in three areas: in the foliate papillae on the lateral margin of the tongue, in the fungiform papillae on the dorsum of the tongue, and in the circumvallate papillae at the junction of the anterior two-thirds and posterior one-third of the tongue. A much lower concentration of taste buds can be found on the palate and epiglottis. The receptor cells of the taste buds have a limited life-span (measured in days) and are continually replaced by basal cells.

Cranial nerves VII, IX, and X provide afferent input from the taste buds to the CNS (Fig. 26.3). The facial nerve subserves taste along the anterior two-thirds of the tongue via the chorda tympani nerve and along the palate via the greater superficial petrosal nerve. The circumvallate papillae receive innervation from the pharyngeal branches of the glossopharyngeal nerve; and the vagus nerve, through the internal branch of the superior laryngeal nerve, carries afferent input from the epiglottis.

The taste afferents arise from unipolar cell bodies. The cell bodies in the facial nerve are located in the geniculate ganglion within the temporal bone. Cell bodies from the glossopharyngeal nerve are located in the superior petrosal ganglion, and those in the vagus nerve are located in the nodose ganglion. The rostral half of the tractus solitarius nucleus in the brain stem is the termination site of the second-order neuron afferent tract. Taste projections from the medulla terminate in the most medial thalamic ventroposteromedial nucleus adjacent to neurons that respond to somatosensory stimulation of the tongue and the nasal cavity. Clinical and electrophysiologic studies support projections from the thalamus to the ipsilateral circular sulcus that separates the frontal operculum from the insula.

There are four primary qualities of taste: sweet, sour, salty, and bitter. Salt and acids (which are ionic stimuli) interact with ionic channels in the membrane, and bitter and sweet substances (which are organic) interact with receptors in the membrane. The response patterns of gustatory afferent fibers can be grouped into classes based on the stimulus chemicals that produced the greatest response.

### Changes with Aging

Aging appears to be less of a determinant of gustatory sensitivity than it is for olfactory sensitivity. Taste buds have the capacity to regenerate after various direct injuries due to inflammation, infection, radiation injury, medications, and degenerative diseases of the oral cavity. The taste bud degenerates if the gustatory afferents have been transected. Interestingly, transection does not necessarily lead to taste loss, as a release of inhibition phenomenon appears to increase activity in unaffected areas.

Age-related decrements in taste sensitivity, as measured by detection or recognition threshold tests have been noted for standard sweet, sour, bitter, and salty tastants. However, loss of taste as a result of advancing age seems to have less effect than loss of smell. It is a general consensus that elderly individuals are less sensitive to salt than the young.[19] Studies of anatomic losses in the structures of the taste system in the elderly have been equivocal. Taste losses from natural aging are due to changes in the taste cell membrane rather than loss of taste buds.[20] Medications and preexisting medical conditions appear to play a key role in dysgeusia and taste loss.

## Summary

A significant proportion of the elderly population bitterly complain of loss of taste, and it is referable to age-related deficits observed in olfaction rather than loss of taste. Evaluation of aging patients with chemosensory dysfunction should be ascertained with a thorough history, physical examination, and psychophysical testing. Quantifying the loss of smell or taste by psychophysical testing provides an objective measure for correlating patients' complaints. Imaging studies may play a role in excluding neoplasm or fracture.

Sensory olfactory losses are caused by viral infection, head injury (cribriform plate fracture), neurologic surgical procedures, and other demyelinating disorders. Disturbances in taste are classified as (1) transport causes—the condition interferes with the access of tastant molecules to the receptor cells (e.g., xerostomia, heavy metal intoxication, fungus and bacterial colonization); and (2) neural causes—temporal bone fracture, surgical injury, neoplasia. These common causes should be considered before attributing the loss to age-related disease.

## References

1. Rossman I. Clinical Geriatrics. Lippincott: Philadelphia, 1971.
2. Clopton B. Micromechanics of the cochlea. Semin Hearing 1986;7(1):15–26.
3. Pfingst B. Encoding of frequency and level information in the auditory nerve. Semin Hearing 1986;7(1):5–63.
4. Crowe SJ, Guild ST, Plovogt LM. Observations on the pathology of high tonal deafness. Bull Johns Hopkins Hosp 1934;54:315.
5. Von Fiedant H, Saxen A. Pathologie and Klinikder Alterschwerhorigkeit. Acta Otolaryngol (Stockh) 1937;23(suppl).
6. Brody H. The nervous system and aging. In: Behnke JA, Finch CE, Moment GB (eds) The Biology of Aging. Menium Press: New York, 1978.
7. Wong Riley M. Maintenance of neuronal activity by electrical stimulation of unilaterally deafened cats demonstrable with cytochrome oxidase technique. Ann Otol Rhinol Laryngol 1981;90(suppl 90):30–32.
8. Ramdan H, Schuknecht HF. Is there a conductive type of presbyacusis? Otolaryngol Head Neck Surg 1986;101:520–525.
9. Nadol JB Jr. Electron microscopic findings in the presbyacusis degeneration of the basal turn of the human cochlea. Otolaryngol Head Neck Surg 1979;87:818–836.
10. Belal A Jr, Glorig A. Dysequilibrium of ageing (presbyastasis). J Laryngol Otol 1986;81:1037–1041.
11. Ross MD, Johnsson L-G, Peacor D, Allard LF. Observations on normal and degenerating human otoconia. Ann Otol Rhinol Laryngol 1976;85:310–326.
12. Richter E. Quantitative study of human Scarpa's ganglion and vestibular sensory epithelia. Acta Otolaryngol (Stockh) 1980;90:199–208.
13. Rosenhaall U, Rubin W. Degenerative changes in the human vestibular sensory epitihelia. Acta Otolaryngol (Stockh) 1975;79:67–80.
14. Brody H. The nervous system and aging. In: Behnke JA, Finch CE, Moment GB (eds) The Biology of Aging. Menium Press: New York, 1978.
15. Breer H. Odour recognition and second messenger signaling in olfactory receptor neurons. Semin Cell Biol 1994;5:25–32.
16. Leopold DA, Bartoshuk L, Doty RL, et al. Aging of the upper airway and senses of taste and smell. Asch Otolaryngol Head Neck Surg 1995;121:630–635.
17. Doty RL, Shaman P, Applebaum SL, Giberson R, Sikorskil, Rosenberg L. Smell identification ability: changes with age. Science 1984;226:1441–1443.
18. Murphy C. Age-related effects on the threshold, psychophysical function and pleasantness of mental. J Gerontol 1983;38:217–222.
19. Grzegorczyk PB, Jones SW, Mistretta CM. Age-related differences in salt taste acuity. J Gerontol 1979;34:834.
20. Mistretta CM. Aging effects on anatomy and neurophysiology of taste and smell. Gerontology 1984;3:131–136.
21. Schuknecht HF. *Pathology of the Ear.* Howard University Press: Cambridge, MA, 1974.

# 27
# Head and Neck Cancer in the Elderly

Michael Coomaraswamy and Loren Kroetsch

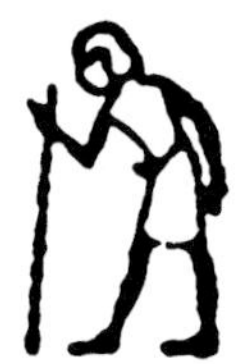

A large variety of malignant neoplasms occur in the region of the head and neck. They include cutaneous lesions such as melanomas, basal and squamous cell carcinomas, tumors arising from the mucosal lining of the upper aerodigestive tract, and metastatic lesions from thoracic or even abdominal primaries.

In this chapter discussion is limited to the pathophysiology, diagnosis, and treatment of squamous cell carcinomas of the head and neck (SCCHNs) arising from the mucosal lining of the upper aerodigestive tract. Approximately 90% of cancers in this region are of squamous cell origin.[1] The tumor biology and clinical behavior of SCCHNs are distinct from that of most other neoplasms arising in this anatomic region; nonetheless, many of the treatment principles reviewed are broadly applicable to the treatment of less common head and neck malignancies in the elderly population.

## Epidemiology

SCCHN is primarily a disease of the elderly. The age-adjusted incidence and mortality rates for SCCHNs in the oral and pharyngeal subsites are shown in Figure 27.1.[2–4] These data demonstrate a marked increase in the incidence of these cancers starting at approximately 60 years of age with the incidence continuing to increase into the oldest aged cohort of the population. SCCHN arising in other anatomic subsites (larynx, hypopharynx) show similar age distribution.[5,6] There is a marked male predominance in the incidence of these cancers at all subsites, although the relative proportion of women diagnosed with laryngeal cancer in particular is rising,[5] probably reflecting an increase in cigarette smoking in this group.

Demographic data from the U.S. Bureau of the Census and other sources indicate that there is an unprecedented shift in the age structure of the population taking place at this time.[7–9] This will result in a substantial increase in both the absolute number and the proportion of the population who are more than 65 years of age. In 1982 roughly 11% of the population (25.5 million people) were more than 65 years of age; by 1996 the proportion of elderly had risen to 13% (33.6 million persons). In 2030, the year in which the "baby boom" expansion is expected to peak, it is projected that one in five Americans (70 million persons) will be over the age of 65.

Further examination of the demographic data for the population over age 65 indicates that the aged population is itself becoming older. In 1950 only 3% of the population were more than 75 years of age; by 2030 this age group will represent 9% of the population.[7]

Based on these data it is clear that the incidence of SCCHNs is a reflection of the age structure of the population; and the anticipated expansion in the population at greatest risk is likely to result in a significant increase in the number of patients diagnosed with these cancers. The presence of serious co-morbidities, already a significant factor in treatment planning decisions in these patients, is also likely to assume even greater importance as the "oldest-old" cohort expands.

## Genetic Basis of SCCHNs

The current concepts regarding the genetic basis of SCCHNs have grown from the related clinical observations that synchronous squamous cell cancers are found in 4–10% of patients under evaluation for an index lesion,[10,11] and that among patients successfully treated for an index cancer new cancers develop at the rate of 4–6% per year.[12,13] Slaughter et al.[14] in 1953 first coined the term "field cancerization" to explain the often multicentric origins of squamous cell cancers arising in the mucosa of the upper aerodigestive tract. The authors conceptualized that the entire mucosa was more or less uniformly exposed to carcinogens in cigarette smoke and was thus condemned to an increased cancer risk.

A comprehensive review of the molecular pathogenesis of SCCHN was reported by Papadimi-

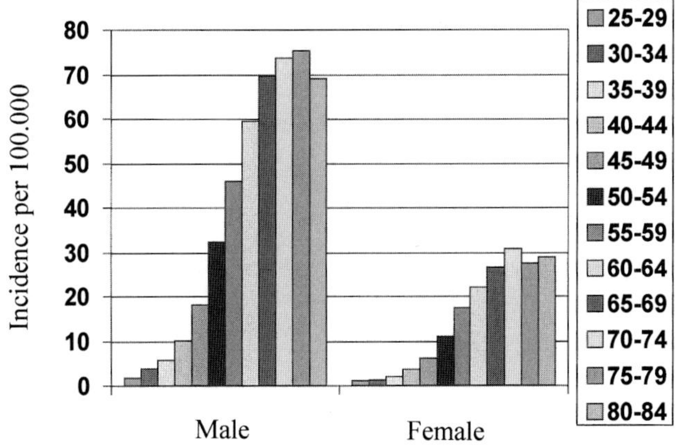


FIGURE 27.1. SEER data on the incidence of squamous cell cancer of the head and neck, by age. A similar trend is seen for mortality.

trakopoulou et al.[15] At a molecular level, it is believed that the progression from normal mucosa to dysplasia to preinvasive cancer and ultimately to invasive carcinoma is the result of a stepwise accumulation of mutations at multiple genetic loci. These mutations result in activation of proto-oncogenes and inactivation of tumor-suppressor genes, culminating in a malignant phenotype.

Most mutations in SCCHNs are somatic, that is, caused by exposure to environmental carcinogens. Cigarette smoking and alcohol consumption are the most widely recognize risk factors for these cancers. Polycyclic aromatic hydrocarbons present in cigarette smoke form DNA adducts that induce G to T transversions, producing point mutations in exposed cells. Ethanol has been shown to inhibit DNA repair processes in vitro,[16] which may explain the observation that smoking and alcohol act synergistically to promote these cancers.

Epstein-Barr virus (EBV) and human papilloma virus (HPV) have also been implicated in the development of SCCHN. Serologic evidence of EBV infection has been found in a high percentage of patients with the undifferentiated variant of nasopharyngeal cancer,[17] and evidence of incorporation of the viral genome has been demonstrated in tumor cell cultures. HPVs have been linked to the development of verrucous carcinomas of the oral cavity, tonsil, and larynx.[18]

Evidence for a multistep process of tumorigenesis in SCCHNs is compelling. Multiple nonrandom chromosomal changes involving rearrangements, deletions, translocations, and substitutions have been demonstrated in established and short-term cultures of head and neck cancers.[19,20] Investigators using polymerase chain reaction (PCR)-based techniques have shown frequent loss of heterozygosity at chromosomes 3p, 5q, 9p, 11q, 13q, and 17p in whole-tissue specimens of head and neck cancers, which implies that some or all of these areas of chromosomal loss contain important suppressor/recessive oncogenes.[21–23]

Correlating these frequently observed chromosomal abnormalities with activation of proto-oncogenes or inactivation of tumor-suppressor genes is an area of active research. Overexpression of certain gene products, such as epidermal growth factor receptor (EGFR), transforming growth factor-$\alpha$ (TGF-$\alpha$), and cyclin D1 has been demonstrated in dysplastic and malignant cell lines,[24,25] and the level of expression of these products has been correlated with phenotypic progression and the risk of recurrence after treatment. Mutations of the *p53* tumor-suppressor gene are frequent in SCCHNs. The *p53* gene encodes a nuclear protein that induces apoptosis during the replication of genetically damaged cells.[26] Loss of the *p53* gene product facilitates clonal expansion of genetically damaged cells, which is a key step in tumorigenesis. The importance of *p53* mutations in the genesis of SCCHNs can be inferred from experimental data in which an adenovirus vector was used to incorporate wild-type *p53* gene in SCCHN cell lines. Reestablishing a functional gene product led to marked inhibition of tumor cell growth in vitro and to a significant decrease in tumor cell mass in a nude mouse xenograph model.[27] It is likely that this and other gene-based therapies will be introduced into the therapeutic armamentarium in the not too distant future.

The emerging molecular model of tumorigenesis in SCCHNs helps explain the observed increase in the incidence of these cancers with age. The accumulation of genetic damage is, to some extent, a time-dependent phenomenon. Other changes associated with aging, such as a decline in T cell function[28,29] and decreased free radical scavenging capacity of older cells,[30] may also be relevant to the development of these cancers. An explanation for the observation that most elderly patients with long histories of smoking and alcohol use do not develop SCCHN is more difficult to derive from the model of tumorigenesis described above. Clearly, heritable and environmental factors help determine an individual's susceptibility to environmental carcinogens or the ability to repair mutations caused by these agents. Assays for sensitivity to bleomycin-induced chromosomal breaks in peripheral lymphocytes have been used to assess the risk of developing second primary cancers[31] and to select patients for chemoprevention protocols.[32]

## Tumor Biology/Clinical Behavior

SCCHNs arise from mucosal cells as the result of clonal expansion of a genetically altered cell population. Once an in situ carcinoma has become established, tumors with invasive potential elaborate a number of proteases and induce the production of related substances by local fibroblasts. These compounds, which include type I and type IV collagenases and stromelysins,[33] lead to destruction of the basement membrane underlying the tumor and facilitate tumor entry into the mesenchymal compartment. Once the epithelial compartment is breached, there is potential for regional and systemic metastatic spread.

Established tumors grow by local extension and metastasize to regional lymph nodes in a predictable, sequential pattern.[34] Distant metastases, although uncommon at initial presentation, eventually become clinically apparent in 10–30% of patients.[35,36] Distant metastases are most frequently noted in patients with uncontrolled locoregional disease[37] and in those with an advanced nodal stage on presentation.[38] Lung, bone, and liver are, in decreasing order, the most frequent sites of systemic metastases. Because most systemic metastases occur in the lung, chest radiography is an adaquate initial screening test for patients without bone pain or liver function abnormalities. Survival of patients with distant metastases is usually less than 1 year.[35] The prognosis of a patient with SCCHN is dependent on a number of factors, including clinical stage at presentation, tumor grade, and the anatomic subsite in the upper aerodigestive tract from which the tumor arises.

The upper aerodigestive tract is divided into a number of distinct anatomic subsites, which are discussed in detail below. There are marked differences in the clinical behaviors of SCCHNs depending on the anatomic subsite from which the tumor arises. Many of these differences are a function of the density of local lymphatic drainage, which varies widely throughout the mucosa of the upper aerodigestive tract. Carcinomas that arise from the epithelium of the true vocal cords, where lymphatics are sparse, rarely metastasize at an early stage. This behavior is in marked contrast to that of cancers arising in the hypopharynx, where there is a rich lymphatic network. Hypopharyngeal primaries, characterized by rapid regional and systemic spread, have the worst prognosis of all head and neck cancers.

The capacity of various subsites in the upper aerodigestive tract to accommodate a primary tumor before symptoms are apparent also varies widely. Nasopharyngeal cancers often present with regional metastases before the primary tumor is clinically apparent, whereas glottic lesions as small as 1–2 mm cause hoarseness by altering the vibratory characteristics of the vocal ligament. These factors influence the stage at diagnosis, which directly influences prognosis.

SCCHNs are staged according to a tumor/nodes/metastasis (TNM) system, as outlined in the *American Journal of the College of Cardiology* (AJCC) manual for staging cancer.[39] There are five T categories from Tis (in situ) to T4. The definition of the T stage is unique to each anatomic subsite (Table 27.1). N stage is determined on the basis of the size, number, and distribution (unilateral or bilateral) of metastatic lymph nodes. The absolute size of the largest node is recognized as the most prognostically significant feature of nodal stage (Table 27.2). Metastatic disease is simply defined as M0 or M1, that is, absent or present. Staging for head and neck cancer is delineated in Table 27.3. Crude 5-year survival estimates by stage are roughly 80% for stage I disease, declining to 20% or less for stage IV.

Although the AJCC staging system for SCCHNs has the advantage of being relatively easy to apply, there are a number of shortcomings that limit its usefulness.[40] Prognostically important tumor characteristics, such as tumor morphology and depth of invasion, are not incorporated; nor are performance status or patient comorbidities taken into account.

TABLE 27.1. TNM System for Head and Neck Cancer: T Definitions, by Site

| | |
|---|---|
| **Primary tumor (T)** | |
| TX | Primary tumor cannot be assessed |
| T0 | No evidence of primary tumor |
| Tis | Carcinoma in situ |
| **Oropharynx** | |
| T1 | Tumor ≤2 cm in greatest dimension |
| T2 | Tumor >2 cm but not >4 cm in greatest dimension |
| T3 | Tumor >4 cm in greatest dimension |
| T4 | Tumor invades adjacent structures [e.g., cortical bone, soft tissue of neck, deep (extrinsic) muscle of tongue] |
| **Nasopharynx** | |
| T1 | Tumor limited to one subsite or nasopharynx |
| T2 | Tumor invades more than one subsite or nasopharynx |
| T3 | Tumor invades nasal cavity or oropharynx |
| T4 | Tumor invades skull or cranial nerve(s) |
| **Hypopharynx** | |
| T1 | Tumor limited to one subsite of hypopharynx |
| T2 | Tumor invades more than one subsite of hypopharynx or an adjacent site, *without* fixation of hemilarynx |
| T3 | Tumor invades more than one subsite of hypopharynx or an adjacent site, *with* fixation of hemilarynx |
| T4 | Tumor invades adjacent structures (e.g., cartilage or soft tissues of neck) |
| **Supraglottis** | |
| T1 | Tumor limited to one subsite of supraglottis with normal vocal cord mobility |
| T2 | Tumor invades more than one subsite of supraglottis or glottis, with normal vocal cord mobility |
| T3 | Tumor limited to larynx with vocal cord fixation or invades postcricoid area, medial wall of piriform sinus, or preepiglottic tissues |
| T4 | Tumor invades thyroid cartilage, or extends to other tissues beyond the larynx (e.g., to oropharynx, soft tissues of neck) |
| **Glottis** | |
| T1 | Tumor limited to vocal cord(s) (may involve anterior or posterior commissures) with normal mobility |
| T1a | Tumor limited to one vocal cord |
| T1b | Tumor involves both vocal cords |
| T2 | Tumor extends to supraglottis or subglottis, or with impaired vocal cord mobility, or any combination of these |
| T3 | Tumor limited to the larynx with vocal cord fixation |
| T4 | Tumor invades thyroid cartilage or extends to other tissues beyond the larynx (e.g., oropharynx, soft tissues of neck) |

*Source:* American Joint Committee on Cancer,[39] with permission.

TABLE 27.2. TNM System for Head and Neck Cancer: N Definitions

| | |
|---|---|
| NX | Regional lymph nodes cannot be assessed |
| N0 | No regional lymph node metastasis |
| N1 | Metastasis in a single ipsilateral lymph node, ≤3 cm in greatest dimension |
| N2 | Metastasis in a single ipsilateral lymph node, >3 cm but not >6 cm in greatest dimension; or in multiple ipsilateral lymph nodes, none >6 cm in greatest dimension; or in bilateral or contralateral lymph nodes, none >6 cm in greatest dimension |
| N2a | Metastasis in a single ipsilateral lymph node >3 cm but not >6 cm in greatest dimension |
| N2b | Metastasis in multiple ipsilateral lymph nodes, none >6 cm in greatest dimension |
| N2c | Metastasis in bilateral or contralateral lymph nodes, none >6 cm in greatest dimension |
| N3 | Metastasis in a lymph node >6 cm in greatest dimension |

*Source:* American Joint Committee on Cancer,[39] with permission.

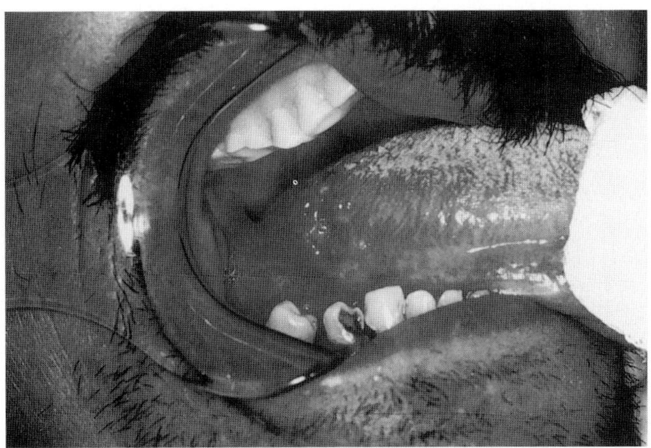

FIGURE 27.2. Squamous cell carcinoma arising from the lateral border of the tongue.

Functional status as measured by the Karnofsky Performance Status[41] and the presence and degree of co-morbidities as classified by the Kaplan-Feinstein Co-morbidity Index,[42] in particular, have a profound influence on prognosis independent of tumor stage.[43] A thorough appreciation of the influence of co-morbidity and functional status on prognosis of patients with SCCHN is vital and makes it easier to formulate appropriate treatment plans for elderly patients with head and neck cancer.[44,45]

## General Concepts of Diagnosis and Treatment

Most SCCHNs present as raised, ulcerated lesions with significant local induration (Fig. 27.2). Suspicious lesions in the oral cavity and nasopharynx can be biopsied under local or topical anesthesia in the cooperative patient. Cancers situated in the base of the tongue, hypopharynx, and larynx are usually biopsied at the time of staging examination (panendoscopy) under general anesthesia. Examination under anesthesia and triple endoscopy—laryngoscopy, rigid esophagoscopy, bronchoscopy—has traditionally been performed to assess the extent of the primary lesion accurately and to evaluate the entire mucosal surface of the upper aerodigestive tract for synchronous cancers.[46]

TABLE 27.3. TNM System for Head and Neck Cancer: Stage Grouping for All Head and Neck Sites

| | |
|---|---|
| Stage I | T1N0M0 |
| Stage II | T2N0M0 |
| Stage III | T3N0M0 |
| | T1 or T2 or T3N1M0 |
| Stage IV | T4N0 or N1M0 |
| | Any T N2 or N3M0 |
| | Any T any N M1 |

*Source:* Snow GB, Balm AJ, Arendse JE, et al. Prognostic factors in neck node metastasis. *In*: Larson DL, Ballantyne AJ, Guillamondegui OM (eds) Cancer in the Neck: Evaluation and Treatment. Macmillan, New York, 1986:53, with permission.

Neck masses suspicious for metastatic disease can be diagnosed with fine-needle aspiration biopsy (FNAB) for cytology. FNAB is a simple technique with almost no morbidity that is highly accurate for diagnosing metastatic SCCHNs in enlarged neck nodes.[47]

Chest radiography is routinely performed to exclude metastatic or primary lung cancer in patients with SCCHNs. Chest computed tomography (CT), although more sensitive, can probably be reserved for patients with abnormalities on chest radiography. Liver and bone scans should be performed only in patients with symptoms or laboratory abnormalities that suggest metastases to these organs.

Surgery and radiation therapy used alone or in combination are the mainstays of treatment for SCCHNs. Each modality offers certain advantages and should be viewed as complementary rather than competing forms of treatment.

The role of chemotherapy in the treatment of SCCHNs is still a matter of some debate. Improved survival has been achieved with cisplatin-based regimens and concomitant radiation therapy for treatment of nasopharyngeal cancer; and induction chemotherapy is part of the standard larynx-preservation protocol.[48,49] The use of chemotherapy for treatment of resectable SCCHNs outside of these settings has not been shown to improve survival.[50]

The basic concepts for surgical treatment of SCCHNs are wide excision of the primary tumor and involved structures and simultaneous neck dissection to remove potential or proven regional metastatic spread. These operations, when applied to primary cancers in the

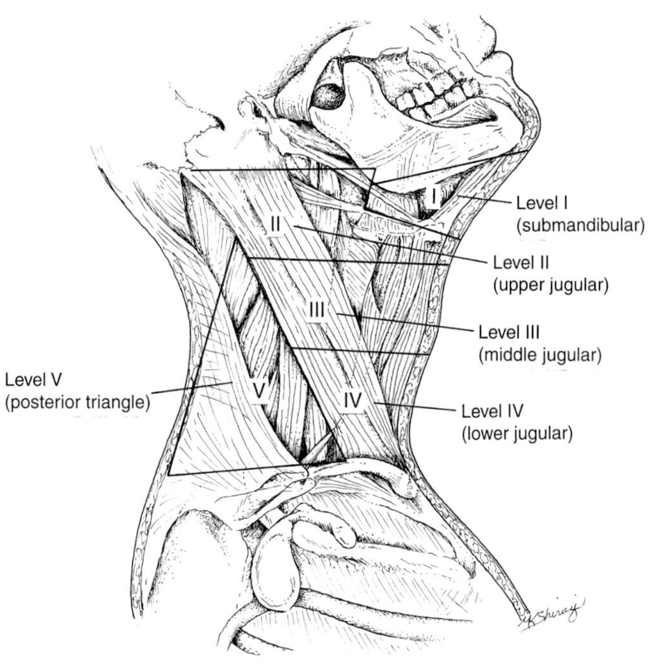


FIGURE 27.3. Anatomic drawing showing relevant neck anatomy for neck dissection. Level I, submandibular; level II, upper jugular; level III, middle jugular; level IV, lower jugular; level V, posterior triangle.

oropharynx, have been termed composite resections, commando procedures, or jaw-neck operations. The classic approach to treatment of SCCHNs in the neck has been radical neck dissection (RND). This operation involves en bloc removal of lymphatic structures from the submandibular area (level I), the upper, middle, and lower jugular chain (levels II, III, IV), and the posterior triangle (level V) in the neck as well as the internal jugular vein, sternocleidomastoid muscle, and spinal accessory nerve (Figs. 27.3, 27.4). The cosmetic and functional disability caused by RND are significant, and as a result most surgeons attempt preservation of an uninvolved spinal accessory nerve (functional radical neck dissection) or perform selective neck dissections in which only nodes in at-risk areas are excised. Despite a trend toward more selective management of the neck,[51] the overall approach to surgical ablation of SCCHNs has changed little during the nearly five decades these operations have been performed. There have, however, been significant advances in the reconstruction of soft tissue and bony defects left after radical surgical ablation of SCCHNs, including reliable regional flaps such as the pectoralis major myocutaneous flap,[52] advances in plating systems, and the widespread use of free tissue transfer such as radial forearm and free fibular grafts[53,54] (Figs. 27.5, 27.6). Thus the outlook for acceptable cosmetic and functional results after radical surgery has improved greatly.

Currently, external beam irradiation and brachytherapy are used extensively for treatment of SCCHN. Common sources of external radiation include photons in the 4- to 10-MV energy range and electrons in the 4- to 18-MV range. Iridium192 and cesium137 are common isotopes used for brachytherapy. X-irradiation works by causing breaks in a cell's DNA either by direct action on this molecule or by inducing local free radical formation. Cells that sustain sufficient damage to their DNA usually die during the next mitotic cycle.[55] Tumor cells are susceptible to irradiation because they are rapidly proliferating and the ability of cancer cells to repair sublethal genetic damage is less than that of nonneoplastic cells. Radiation oncologists strive to achieve a balance between the destruction of cancer cells and damage to surrounding tissue. This relation is conceptualized as the therapeutic ratio.[56] The relation between the tumor response and the dose of radiation is asymptotic at higher delivered doses; consequently, it is likely that normal tissue in the radiation field will be destroyed with little additional therapeutic benefit when doses of more than about 70 Gy are given. The therapeutic ratio is maximized by appropriately targeting the tumor volume to be irradiated via proper selection of radiation fields and types of radiation administered and by delivering the total dose of radiation in fractions.

Radiation is usually given in a series of equal daily doses of 180–200 cGy over several weeks. Fractionation

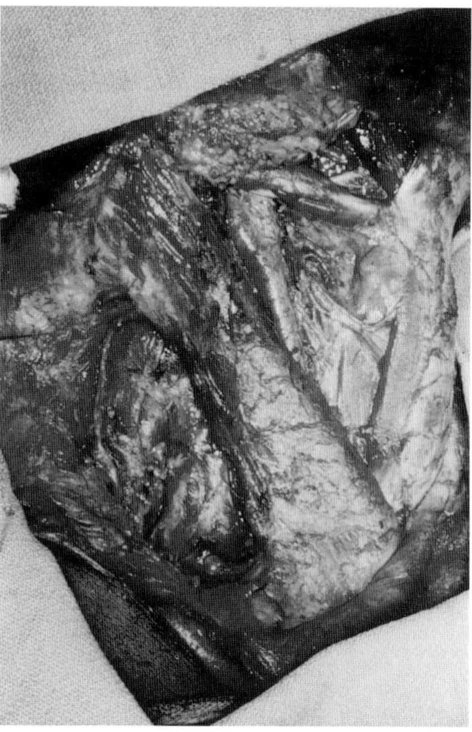

FIGURE 27.4. Appearance of the neck right after modified radical neck dissection. Node-bearing tissue has been excised from levels I–V with preservation of the sternocleidomastoid muscle and the spinal accessory nerve.

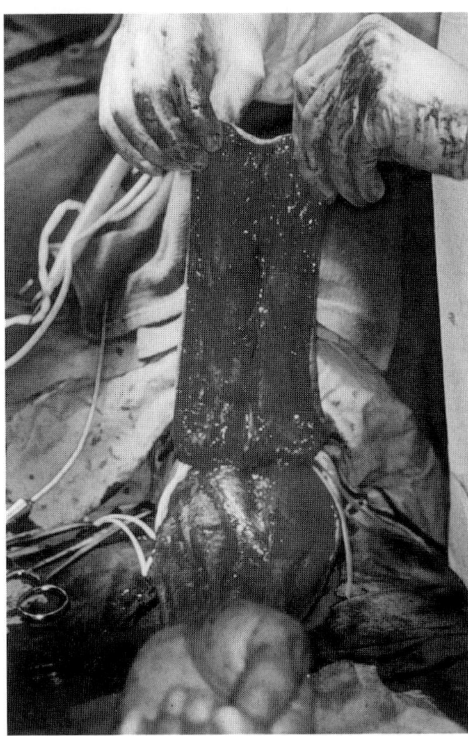

FIGURE 27.5. Radial forearm flap. The appearance of the donor site after elevation of a radial forearm flap. This tissue is transferred to the neck to reconstruct a large soft tissue defect on the floor of the mouth. Microvascular anastamoses to the radial artery and cephalic vein are than performed to restore inflow and venous drainage to the graft.

helps to increase the therapeutic ratio by exploiting a number of differences in the responses of normal and neoplastic cells to radiation. Because nonneoplastic cells in the radiation field are able to repair sublethal genetic damage more efficiently than the tumor cells, the time interval between radiation doses results in preferential sparing of normal cells. Repopulation of normal proliferating tissue occurs as stem cells replace those killed by radiation. This normal response to injury is also more pronounced in normal mucosa than in neoplastic cells.

Radiation is much more lethal to cells in certain phases of the mitotic cycle; as a result, the population of cells surviving after a fraction of radiation has been given are "synchronized" in a radioresistant phase of the cell cycle. The time interval between doses of radiation allows the surviving population of cells to redistribute within the mitotic cycle, resulting in a new subpopulation of radiosensitive cells. Although redistribution within the mitotic cycle is a feature of both cancerous and proliferative tissue (e.g., mucosa), this redistribution is not seen to the same degree in more static tissues such as bone and cartilage, which might otherwise show late effects from radiation. Finally, a feature of tumors that limits the efficacy of radiation as a single modality in the treatment of large tumor masses is the existence of underperfused and hence relatively hypoxic cells within the core of tumors. Hypoxic cancer cells are two to three times more radioresistant than are well-perfused cells located on the periphery of the tumor.

Neovascularization of the tumor core occurs as the normoxic peripheral cells are killed. Reperfusion of the tumor core is facilitated by fractionation.[55]

From the above discussion, the basis of the complementary roles of surgery and irradiation in the treatment of SCCHNs should be evident. Irradiation is most effective in eradicating small or subclinical tumor deposits, whereas surgery can be used to ablate large tumors or residual disease after radiation has been administered.

Patients who receive therapeutic doses of radiation for head and neck cancer often develop xerostomia owing to destruction of minor salivary glands in the submucosa of the upper tract. Mucositis, or painful ulceration of the oropharyngeal mucosa, also occurs frequently and can severely limit a patient's ability to maintain adequate caloric intake. Other complications associated with radiation include tissue fibrosis and well-recognized impairment of wound healing in the radiation field.[57]

There are theoretic concerns that because of a reduction in the number of mucosal stem cells with age, radiation therapy administered to patients at the extremes of age may cause greater therapeutic toxicity. There is, however,

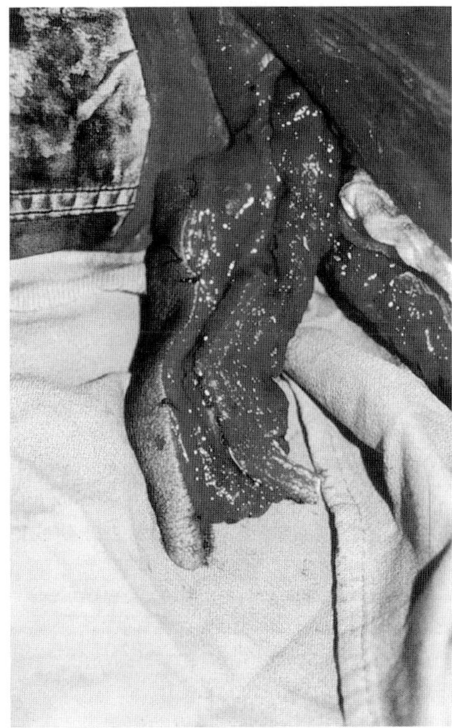

FIGURE 27.6. Free fibular graft. A neomandible has been fashioned from the patient's fibula. This tissue is transferred to the neck to reconstruct a soft tissue and bony defect after composite resection.

little clinical evidence that acute or late radiation toxicity is greater in elderly patients undergoing irradiation.[58]

## Comorbidities

Most patients presenting with SCCHNs in Western countries have long histories of alcohol abuse and smoking. As such, the incidence of significant co-morbidities in these patients is high. Although it is important to recognize the importance of functional status and comorbidities on the overall prognosis of patients with head and neck cancer, it is equally important to diagnose and treat these problems to optimize a patient's functional status and perhaps improve outcome. Concomitant pulmonary and cardiovascular dysfunction are common in elderly patients with SCCHNs, and dysfunction of these organ systems is associated with a known increased surgical risk.[59,60] Less well recognized are nutritional deficits in patients with head and neck cancer. Malnutrition is common in patients with SCCHNs because many of these tumors compromise a patient's ability to take in an adequate diet and because both irradiation and surgery commonly interfere with the function of deglutition. Roughly one-third of patients with SCCHNs are severely malnourished by standard nutritional assessment,[61] and another one-third have lesser degrees of malnutrition. Patients with severe malnutrition have a higher incidence of postoperative complications and decreased survival when compared with patients with lesser degrees of nutritional impairment.[62] A variety of nutritional parameters are used to assess nutritional status, but a weight loss of more than 10% has shown the highest correlation with poor outcome in these patients.[63] Nutritional therapy, using the enteral route whenever possible, should be initiated in all patients judged to be severely malnourished before surgery or radiation therapy is initiated. All patients in whom definitive therapy is likely to lead to impaired ability to swallow for an extended period of time should have secure enteral access placed in the form of a gastrostomy or feeding jejunostomy.

## Nasopharynx

The nasopharynx is a roughly cuboidal structure. The roof is formed from the undersurface of the sphenoid bone and the posterior wall by the anterior arch of the atlas and the body of C2. The superior surface of the soft palate forms the floor of this structure, and the lateral walls contain the pharyngeal ostium of the auditory tube. This ostium is surrounded by an incomplete cartilaginous ring, or crura, which forms an elevation in the mucosa. Medially this crura forms the torus tubarius and medial to this is a slit-like structure termed the fossa of Rosenmuller.

The mucosal lining of the nasopharynx contains abundant lymphoid tissue and a rich submucosal lymphoid plexus, which drains to the retropharyngeal and deep cervical nodal basins. There are three histologic variants of nasopharyngeal carcinoma according to the classification established by the World Health Organization (WHO).[64] WHO type 1 is keratinizing squamous carcinoma, type 2 is nonkeratinizing squamous cell carcinoma, and type 3 is undifferentiated carcinoma. The latter is characterized by an abundant nonneoplastic lymphoid infiltrate, which has led to the term "lymphoepithelioma" for this variant. WHO type 2 and 3 tumors are more radiosensitive and so are associated with a better prognosis.

Squamous cell cancer of the nasopharynx is an uncommon malignancy in Western countries, but these cancers are among the most common malignancies in southern China, where the incidence is as high as 50 per 100,000 in the province of Guangdong (Canton).[65] The disease is much more common in men, with a male/female incidence ratio of 3:1. As mentioned previously, there is a strong association with Epstein-Barr virus (EBV) infection and nasopharyngeal carcinoma (NPC), particularly the undifferentiated (WHO type 3) histologic variant. Elevated immunoglobulin A (IgA) antibody titers to EBV viral capsid antigen and early intracellular antigen have been used as a screening tool in high risk populations. In a large prospective study, Sham et al. found a 5.4% incidence of NPC in patients with elevated IgA anti-EBV antibody.[66] It is likely that other heritable, dietary, and environmental factors play a role in promoting these cancers as well.[67,68]

Most patients with NPC present with an ipsilateral enlarged upper jugular lymph node. FNAB is highly reliable and safe for diagnosing cervical metastatic disease.[47] Symptoms related to the primary tumor are rare on initial presentation but may include unilateral nasal obstruction, serosanguineous nasal discharge, serous otitis media due to obstruction of the eustacian tube orifice, or symptoms of cranial nerve involvement.

Endoscopic examination of the nasopharynx can be performed with either flexible or rigid instruments under topical anesthesia. The primary tumor may be visible as a submucosal bulge, most often in the fossa of Rosenmuller on the lateral wall of the nasopharynx. Deep biopsy specimens should be obtained to improve the yield.

Contrast-enhanced CT and MRI are both helpful for delineating the extent of disease in NPCs. The CT scan is superior to MRI for detecting bony erosion by the tumor and nodal involvement, particularly in the retropharyngeal nodal bed which is difficult to assess on examination. MRI provides excellent soft tissue detail and has multiplanar capabilities that are useful for determining the extent of the primary tumor.[69]

Radiation therapy is the mainstay of NPC treatment. Surgical approaches to the nasopharynx are hazardous, and en bloc resection of these tumors is difficult. Retropharyngeal lymph nodes are not routinely removed with even a radical neck dissection, and indeed the highest level retropharyngeal nodes are not approachable through the neck. Fortunately the most common histologic variants of NPC (WHO types 2 and 3) are radiosensitive. Standard irradiation protocols include radiation to the primary site and bilateral neck through opposed lateral portals to a dose of 45 Gy in 1.8- to 2.0-Gy daily fractions followed by an additional boost of 25 Gy to the primary site and upper neck such that the total dose to the primary lesion is 70 Gy, and the upper neck and lower neck are treated with 65 Gy and 50 Gy, respectively.[70] Careful treatment planning is necessary to minimize the risks of serious radiation side effects, such as panhypopituitarism and myelitis.

The prognosis of patients with NPC is related to the histology and disease stage, particularly the extent of nodal disease. With regard to histologic variants, keratinizing squamous cell tumors (WHO type 1) are the least radiosensitive and are associated with the worst prognosis. Undifferentiated squamous variants (WHO type 3) are highly radiosensitive, and the overall survival of patients with this histology is 60–70%.[71] Patients with advanced nodal disease at the time of diagnosis are at increased risk for systemic metastases and may benefit from adjuvant chemotherapy.[48]

## Oral Cavity

The boundaries of the oral cavity begin at the wet and dry lines of the vermilion border of the lips and extends posteriorly at its superior aspect to the junction of the hard and soft palates. Inferiorly, it extends to the junction of the anterior two-thirds of the tongue, with the posterior third at the circumvalate papilla. The oral cavity includes the anterior two-thirds of the tongue, floor of mouth, buccal mucosa of the cheeks, and gingival tissues including the retromolar trigone.

SCCHNs in this subsite are most commonly found in the anterior floor of the mouth and the lateral margin of the tongue.[72,73] These "high risk" areas are in a more dependent position within the oral cavity and as a result are subject to more prolonged and concentrated exposures to the carcinogens in tobacco and alcohol. Oral cavity cancers appear as raised, ulcerated lesions with indistinct borders (Fig. 27.7).

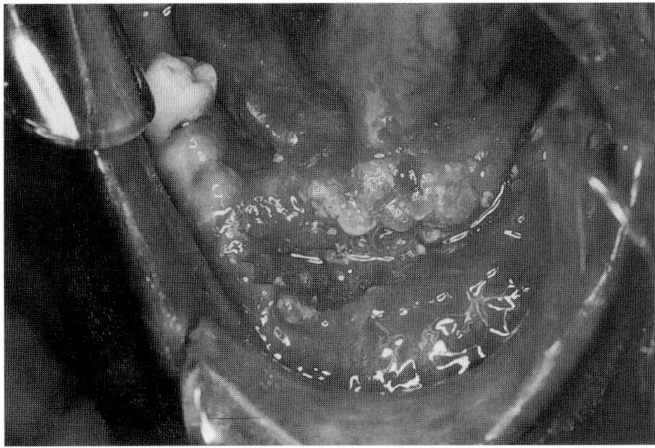

FIGURE 27.7. Squamous cell carcinoma arising in the anterior floor of the mouth.

A discussion of oral cancer should include a brief description of premalignant lesions. They are histologically benign mucosal abnormalities associated with an increased risk of malignant transformation within the lesion itself or elsewhere in the mucosa of the upper aerodigestive tract. Premalignant mucosal abnormalities of the oral cavity include white lesions, red lesions, and mixed white and red lesions. The term oral leukoplakia describes a white patch or plaque that cannot be removed by scraping (Fig. 27.8). On histologic examination areas of leukoplakia usually exhibit only hyperkeratosis. Overall rates of malignant transformation in oral leukoplakia range from 0.13% to 6.00%[74] with higher rates noted in studies with longer follow-ups. The presence of dysplasia on biopsy and the occurrence of this lesion in patients who do not have a history of tobacco use is associated with a markedly increased risk of malignant transformation.[75]

Erythroplasia describes a mucous membrane with erythematous papular projections, and erythroleukoplakia describes a lesion with mixed red and white components (Fig. 27.9). Both erythroplasia and erythroleukoplakia are associated with a risk of malignant transformation four to seven times greater than that of leukoplakia alone.[74,75] Early cancers of the oral cavity cause few symptoms, which underscores the importance of routine examina-

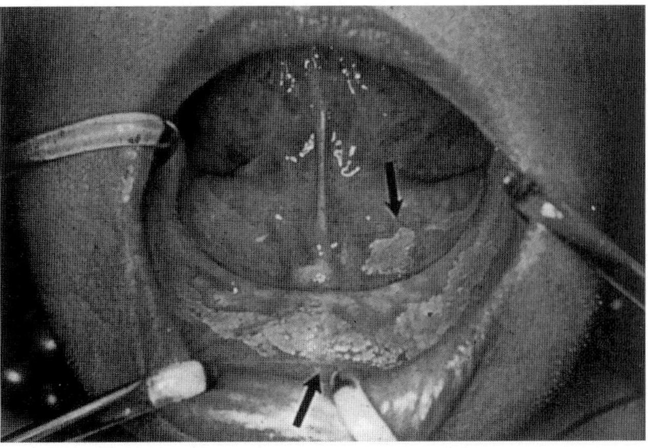

FIGURE 27.8. Oral leukoplakia (arrows).

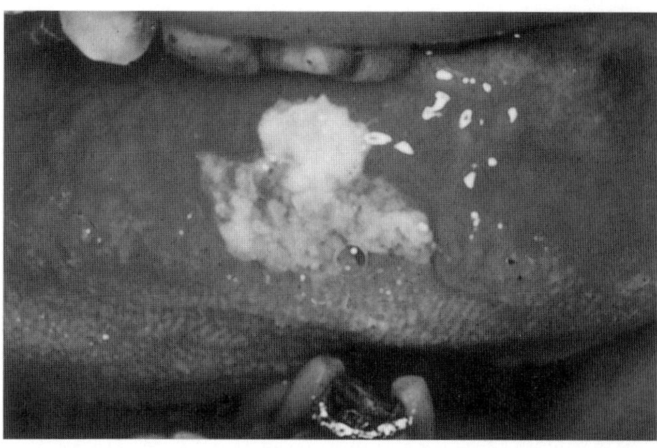

FIGURE 27.9. Erythroleukoplakia.

tion of the oral cavity in elderly patients at risk for these cancers. Patients presenting with more advanced cancers may complain of a change in denture fit or pain associated with a nonhealing ulcer. Numbness of the lower lip is diagnostic of involvement of the inferior alveolar nerve, implying spread of tumor to the mandibular bone. Cancers arising on the lateral border of the tongue often infiltrate deeply into the intrinsic musculature, which presents little barrier to spread. Difficulty swallowing and a change in speech is noted when tongue mobility is impaired.

Regional metastatic spread of SCCHNs arising in the oral cavity is to level I (submandibular area) and level II (upper jugular area) initially (Fig. 27.3). Lower jugular and posterior nodes are involved sequentially and later.[76] The risk of regional metastases is related to the absolute size of the cancer (T stage) and to the depth of invasion.[77] Suspicious lesions of the oral cavity are easily biopsied under local anesthesia in the outpatient setting. Enlarged neck nodes are sampled with FNAB for cytology. Contrast CT scanning is routinely employed to supplement the clinical examination of the oral cavity primary and to assess the neck for occult metastases. Mandibular involvement with tumor can be difficult to diagnose on clinical grounds but is an important determination to make because radiation therapy does not effectively eradicate cancer in bone. Panorex examination of the mandible is an excellent test for determining mandibular involvement with tumor and is not subject to dental artifact as is CT.

Premalignant lesions of the oral cavity should be biopsied, being mindful that areas of erythroplasia in mixed lesions are preferentially sampled. Mucosal lesions with dysplasia should be excised or ablated using the $CO_2$ laser. Patients with hyperkeratosis on biopsy should be encouraged to discontinue all mucosal irritants and must be followed closely. The role of chemoprevention with a variety of antioxidants and vitamin A analogues when treating these lesions is still not clear.[78]

In patients with oral cavity cancer the decision to employ surgery, irradiation, or a combination of these modalities must be based on a good knowledge of what is achievable with each technique and their likely side effects. Patients with mandibular involvement and advanced nodal stage disease require segmental mandibular resection and radical neck dissection if they are to have a reasonable chance of cure. Radiation therapy administered under these circumstances is likely to result in osteoradionecrosis and severe neck fibrosis apart from a poor therapeutic result.

## Oropharynx

The oropharynx is located immediately posterior to the oral cavity. It begins at the junction of the hard and soft palate and extends posteriorly toward the posterior pharyngeal wall. Inferiorly, the oropharynx begins at the junction of the anterior two-thirds and the posterior third of the tongue at the circumvalate papilla, extending to the epiglottis. Oropharyngeal structures include the base of tongue, tonsillar pillars and fossa, soft palate, and posterior pharyngeal walls. The mucosa of the oropharynx is surrounded by supporting musculature, including the pharyngeal constrictors. The parapharyngeal and retropharyngeal spaces lie lateral and posterior to this musculature. Tumor extension into these spaces is associated with a grim prognosis.

Squamous cell carcinomas of the oropharynx are less common than tumors arising from the oral cavity mucosa. Those arising in the oropharyngeal subsite cause few early symptoms, and as a result carcinomas arising in this anatomic area are rarely diagnosed at an early stage. In a study by Krause et al., 81% of patients with oropharyngeal primaries presented with stage III or stage IV disease.[79]

Nodal metastases from oropharyngeal cancer occur early owing to the rich lymphatic drainage in this area. Metastases occur most frequently at levels I and II, but lower jugular spread (level III, IV) and level V nodal spread is a common feature of more advanced lesions (Fig. 27.3). Primary lesions in the base of tongue, soft palate, and posterior pharyngeal walls show a high incidence of bilateral metastatic spread.[76]

The tonsillar fossa is the most common site of origin for cancers of the oropharynx.[80] Patients with tonsillar primaries may complain of mild local irritation, a foreign body sensation, or otalgia. More advanced tonsillar lesions cause difficult or painful swallowing and trismus if the deep musculature of the pharynx becomes infiltrated with tumor.[81] Roughly two-thirds of patients have palpable metastatic nodes on presentation; and in many an enlarged cervical node is the only manifestation.[79]

Cancers arising in the base of the tongue are notoriously difficult to diagnose at an early stage.[82] The tongue base is not open for easy inspection, and clinicians must therefore rely on digital palpation for initial assessment of this area. Panendoscopy and biopsy under anesthesia are usually required for accurate staging.

Radiation therapy is the cornerstone of treatment for small (T1 and T2) primary cancers in the base of the tongue and the tonsil. Rates of local control of early lesions achieved with irradiation are equivalent to those obtained with surgery, and the functional morbidity is often less.[83,84] Patients presenting with advanced locoregional disease are generally treated with surgery and postoperative radiation therapy.[79]

## Larynx

The larynx is a common site of SCCHNs. Primaries arising from this subsite are second in frequency only to cancers arising in the oral cavity.

The larynx is divided into three distinct anatomic regions: supraglottic, glottic, and subglottic. Cancers arising in each anatomic region of the larynx have marked differences in clinical presentation and patterns of both local and regional spread. Differences in clinical behavior are a function of variations in the density of lymphatic drainage, the "capacitance" of the site to contain a tumor, and local barriers to spread within the laryngeal framework. Knowledge of local patterns of spread is vital when selecting appropriate treatment for these lesions.

The supraglottic larynx is defined anatomically as that part of the larynx superior to a horizontal plane passing through the laryngeal ventricle. Structures included in the supraglottic larynx include the epiglottis, aryepiglottic folds, arytenoids, and false vocal cords. Cancers arising in the suprahyoid portion of the epiglottis are characterized by rapid, somewhat unpredictable local growth and early regional spread, which is often bilateral. Cancers arising in the infrahyoid area invade the preepiglottic space but tend not to cross the ventricle to involve the true vocal cords. The supraglottic larynx has a rich lymphatic system that drains through the thyrohyoid membrane to the jugular chain of nodes (levels 2, 3, and 4) sequentially.[85] Bilateral cervical metastases are a hallmark of supraglottic cancers.[34,86]

Patients with early supraglottic cancers generally have few symptoms but may complain of sore throat and dysphagia. Otalgia (referred ear pain) is a less common but more ominous complaint that should prompt an aggressive search for a malignancy in this area. Because supraglottic primaries can grow to a large size before causing overt symptoms of hoarseness or stridor, the first sign of disease in many patients is the appearance of a metastatic node in the neck.

Fiberoptic examination of the larynx is useful for confirming the presence of a mass and assessing its size and extension. Contrast-enhanced CT scans with thin (1.5–2.0 mm) cuts through the larynx parallel to the plane of the vocal cords provides excellent image quality and can provide details regarding framework invasion and lymph node status to complement the clinical evaluation.[87]

Early cancers of the supraglottic larynx can be approached surgically with supraglottic laryngectomy or irradiation alone. Vocal cord-sparing surgical approaches are feasible because of the barrier to spread represented by the laryngeal ventricle, allowing a close but safe margin in this area. Local control of early supraglottic cancers with supraglottic laryngectomy is on the order of 90–95%,[88] and most patients maintain an intelligible voice. Patients' ability to protect their airway after supraglottic laryngectomy is compromised, and consequently supraglottic laryngectomy is rarely the approach of choice in an elderly or extremely debilitated patient, especially if pulmonary reserve is poor. Radiation therapy with surgical salvage of treatment failures is an attractive alternative in this group and yields equivalent rates of local control; however, recurrent or persistent disease after definitive irradiation is difficult to detect, and most patients failing radiation require total laryngectomy.[89] As a practical matter the clinically N0 neck is usually treated with the same modality as the primary lesion, taking into account the frequent bilateral regional spread of supraglottic cancers.

Surgical treatment of advanced (T3 and T4) supraglottic cancers requires total laryngectomy in most patients. Irradiation protocols with surgical salvage produce equivalent rates of local control with the ability to preserve the larynx in some patients but at the cost of significant radiation side effects and increased surgical complications when salvage laryngectomy is performed in patients who have received a full course of radiation.

The most important prognostic factor for advanced supraglottic cancer is the extent of regional disease and the presence of extracapsular spread in metastatic nodes.[90] Bilateral selective neck dissections with preservation of one or both internal jugular veins are usually performed in the patient with a clinically positive neck in the setting of advanced supraglottic disease. Surgical treatment of both necks combined with irradiation has resulted in improved regional control but not a significant increase in overall survival.[85]

The glottic larynx includes the true vocal cords and the anterior and posterior commissures. Cancers arising from the epithelium in this region are, in their early stages, confined to the loose areolar tissue overlying the vocal ligament and bound inferiorly by the conus elasticus (Reinke's space). More advanced (T3) lesions usually cause vocal cord fixation by invasion of the thyroarytenoid muscle, as superior extension is blocked by the thyroglottic ligament. Framework invasion and extralaryngeal extension can occur as the tumor "outflanks" the thyroglottic ligament anteriorly or by invasion of the conus elasticus, which allows spread into the paraglottic space.[91]

Fortunately, most glottic cancers are symptomatic at an early stage, causing hoarseness long before vocal cord mobility is impaired. Lymphatic spread from an early glottic cancer is uncommon owing to the paucity of lymphatic channels in Reinke's space. These factors combine to make early glottic cancers the most treatable variety of SCCHN and emphasize the importance of performing a mirror examination or fiberoptic laryngoscopy in any patient with new onset of hoarseness.

Single-modality therapy with surgery or radiation therapy is effective treatment for early glottic cancer; the two modalities give equivalent rates of local control. A variety of open and endolaryngeal surgical techniques are effective in appropriately selected patients. In general, surgical treatment of early glottic cancer is probably most appropriate for early invasive lesions in which precise endolaryngeal excision is easily accomplished and can spare a patient the need for an extended course of radiation. Surgery is also appropriate for more advanced lesions, particularly T2 lesions with impaired vocal cord mobility where there is an increased risk of treatment failure with irradiation.[86,92] In contrast to supraglottic primaries, regional spread of early glottic cancer is rare. Routine dissection of the clinically negative neck is not required for early glottic cancers, but ipsilateral functional neck dissection should be considered in patients undergoing surgery for irradiation failure, as there may be an increased risk of regional failure in these patients.[93]

Treatment of advanced glottic cancers is an area of intense controversy. Laryngectomy, although effective therapy for these advanced lesions, obviously causes major functional and cosmetic disability. Consequently there has been increased emphasis on laryngeal preservation protocols. The crux of this dilemma is the concern that cure rates and overall survival may be compromised when aggressively pursuing laryngeal preservation in patients with resectable disease. In a large multiinstitutional study conducted by the Department of Veterans Affairs Laryngeal Cancer Study Group,[94] patients with advanced laryngeal cancer were given induction chemotherapy with cisplatin and 5-fluorouracil. Patients with a clinical response to this regimen after two cycles were treated with a third cycle of chemotherapy and then given definitive radiation therapy. Patients in whom a clinical response to chemotherapy was not achieved were treated with total laryngectomy followed by irradiation. Overall survival in the two study arms was not significantly different at 2 years, and laryngeal preservation was achieved in roughly two-thirds of the patients who responded to induction chemotherapy. Based on this study it appears that prioritizing laryngeal preservation need not necessarily compromise overall rates of cure and survival and that emphasis should be placed on identifying tumor or patient factors that predict a good response to irradiation.

Primary cancers arising in the subglottis are rare. This site is usually involved secondarily by subglottic extension of a glottic cancer. There is a high incidence of metastases to the thyroid and to paratracheal and upper mediastinal nodes, which usually mandates combined surgery and irradiation to treat these cancers.

## Hypopharynx

The hypopharynx is contiguous with the oropharynx and consists of the piriform sinuses, pharyngeal walls, and postcricoid area. SCCHNs arising in this subsite are highly lethal. Systemic metastases are frequent, and 5-year survivals are in the range of 11–27% for all stages,[95–97] which are among the worst rates for all head and neck subsites. Reasons for the poor prognosis associated with hypopharyngeal primaries include the fact that most areas of the hypopharynx can accommodate a large tumor mass before overt symptoms are evident. The lymphatic drainage of this area is extensive; there is a rich submucosal lymphatic plexus that drains to the retropharyngeal and jugular chain of nodes and contributes to extensive submucosal spread of the primary tumor. These factors combine to make locoregional control of these tumors difficult.

The piriform sinuses are two roughly pear-shaped mucosal pouches lying on either side of the larynx. Approximately 75% of hypopharyngeal cancers occur in this area. Symptoms of early cancer in this region include mild dysphagia and a foreign body sensation; referred ear pain can occur as a result of irritation of the internal branch of the superior laryngeal nerve, leading to reflex stimulation of the auricular nerve.[98] Large piriform sinus cancers can cause hoarseness, stridor, or airway obstruction due to laryngeal extension or mass effect. Most patients have clinically positive cervical lymph nodes at the time of diagnosis. Tumors arising in the pharyngeal walls and the postcricoid area are less common than piriform sinus cancers but have a similar clinical presentation and course.

Most hypopharyngeal cancers are visible on fiberoptic examination, although the extent of a lesion may be difficult to gauge. Instructing the patient to perform a Valsalva movement during fiberoptic examination may inflate the piriform sinuses and aid the visualization of small or more deeply situated cancers. Barium swallow is highly sensitive and can usually reveal the mucosal extent of a cancer; it is a poor study, however, to determine involvement of adjacent structures. Contrast CT is used routinely to determine invasion of adjacent structures such as the thyroid cartilage and tracheal wall and to help determine the extent of lymph node metastases.

CT is particularly useful for diagnosing suspicious nodes in the retropharyngeal position, an area difficult to assess clinically.[87]

Most patients with hypopharyngeal cancers present with stage III and IV disease. They require laryngectomy or pharyngolaryngectomy in addition to neck dissection and postoperative irradiation if surgery is chosen as the primary treatment modality. Although sometimes a noncircumferential pharyngeal defect can be closed primarily, the need for wide excision margins with SCCHNs at this subsite often results in pharyngeal defects that require reconstruction to reestablish oropharyngeal continuity. Noncircumferential pharyngeal defects can be reconstructed using a pectoralis major myocutaneous flap or a radial forearm free flap. The former, though bulky, is technically easier to perform and can provide muscle coverage of the carotid artery in patients in whom a radical neck dissection has been performed. The radial forearm flap is more pliable and hence more versatile but requires a microvascular anastomosis to maintain the viability of the graft. Large pharyngeal defects can be reconstructed with a gastric pull-up or a jejunal free graft.[99]

The use of radiation therapy or combined chemoradiation protocols as a primary modality for treatment of hypopharyngeal primaries generally results in inferior rates of local control,[97,100–102] though not necessarily in decreased overall survival. Although laryngeal preservation may be achieved in some patients, the ability to swallow and to protect the airway may be compromised. Surgery for radiation failures is associated with a greatly increased rate of postoperative complications usually related to poor wound healing in the postirradiated patient.[103]

In addition to tumor stage, treatment planning for patients with hypopharyngeal cancer must take into account such factors as patient functional status, co-morbidities, and nutritional status. It is likely that other tumor characteristics, such as the response to induction chemotherapy or molecular characteristics predicting the response to therapy, will assume greater importance in treatment decisions in the future.

## Conclusion

Squamous cell carcinoma of the head and neck is primarily a disease of the elderly. Ongoing changes in the age structure of American society make it likely that physicians in practice treating adult and elderly patients will care for increased numbers of patients with head and neck cancer.

Optimal care of patients with SCCHN is rendered in a multidisciplinary setting. Accurate assessment of tumor burden, functional status, co-morbidities, and nutritional status as well as an appreciation of a patient's social network and coping skills are required to arrive at an appropriate plan of treatment for each patient. It is hoped that the emerging understanding of the molecular pathogenesis of head and neck cancers will lead to gene-based and other highly directed therapies that will revolutionize the treatment of these tumors.

## References

1. Wolf G, Lippman SM, Laramore G, Hong WK. Head and neck cancer. In: Holland JF, Frei E, Bast RC, Kufe DW, Morton DL, Weichselbaum R (eds) Cancer Medicine, 3rd ed. Lea & Febiger: Philadelphia, 1993:1211–1275.
2. Parker SL, Tong T, Bolden S, Wingo PA. Cancer statistics, 1996. CA Cancer J Clin 1996;46:5–27.
3. Swango PA. Cancers of the oral cavity and pharynx in the United States: an epidemiologic overview. J Public Health Dent 1996;56:309–318.
4. Kosary CL, Ries LAG, Miller BA, Hankey BF, Harras A, Edwards BK (eds). SEER Cancer Statistics Review, 1973–1992. NIH Publ. No. 96-2789. National Cancer Institute: Bethesda, 1995.
5. Cancer: Rates and Risks, 4th ed. NIH Publ. No. 96-691. National Institutes of Health, National Cancer Institute: Bathesda, 1996:158–162.
6. Lampe HB, Lampe MK, Skillings J. Head and neck cancer in the elderly. J Otolaryngol 1986;15:235–238.
7. Yancik R. Cancer burden in the aged: an epidemiologic and demographic overview. Cancer 1997;80:1273–1283.
8. US Bureau of the Census. Current Population Reports: Special Studies: 65+ in the United States. Government Printing Office: Washington, DC, 1996:23–29.
9. Day JC. Projections of the population of the United States by age, sex, race and Hispanic origin:1993–2050; US Bureau of the Census, current population reports: P25-1104. Government Printing Office: Washington, DC, 1993.
10. Dhooge IJ, De Vos M, Albers FW, Van Cauwenberge PB. Panendoscopy as a screening procedure for simultaneous primary tumors in head and neck cancer. Eur Arch Otorhinolaryngol 1996;253:319–324.
11. Gluckman JL, Crissman JD, Donegan JO. Multicentric squamous cell carcinoma of the upper aerodigestive tract. Head Neck Surg 1980;3:90.
12. Cooper JS, Pajak TF, Ruben P, et al. Second malignancies in patients who have head and neck cancer: incidence, effect on survival and implications based on the RTOG experience. J Int Radiat Oncol Biol Phys 1989;17:449–456.
13. Lippman SM, Spitz M, Zoltan T, Benner SE, Waun KH. Epidemiology, biology and chemoprevention of aerodigestive cancer. Cancer 1994;74:2719–2725.
14. Slaughter DP, Southwick HW, Smejkal W. Field cancerization in oral stratified squamous epithelium: clinical implications of multicentric origin. Cancer 1953;6:963–968.
15. Papadimitrakopoulou VA, Shin DM, Hong WK. Molecular and cellular biomarkers for field cancerization and multistep process in head and neck tumorogenesis. Cancer Metast Rev 1996;15:53–76.
16. Hsu TC, Furlong C. The role of ethanol in oncogenesis of the upper aerodigestive tract, inhibition of DNA repair. Anticancer Res 1991;11:1995–1998.

17. Vasef MA, Ferlito A, Weiss LM. Nasopharyngeal carcinoma, with emphasis on its relation to Epstein-Barr virus. Ann Otol Rhinol Laryngol 1997;106:348–356.
18. Steinberg BM, DeLorenzo TP. A possible role for human papilloma viruses in head and neck cancer. Cancer Metast Rev 1996;15:91–112.
19. Van Dyke DL, Worsham MJ, Benninger MS, et al. Recurrent cytogenetic abnormalities in squamous cell carcinoma of the head and neck region. Genes Chromosomes Cancer 1994;9:192–206.
20. Carey TE, Van Dyke DL, Worsham MJ. Nonrandom chromosome aberrations and clonal populations in head and neck cancer. Anticancer Res 1993;13:2561–2568.
21. Ah-See KW, Cooke TG, Pickford IR, Soutar D, Balmain A. An allelotype of squamous cell carcinoma of the head and neck using microsatellite markers. Cancer Res 1994;54: 617–621.
22. El-Naggar AK, Lee MS, Wang G, Luna MA, Goepfert H, Batsakis JG. Polymerase chain reaction-based restriction fragment length polymorphism analysis of the short arm of chromosome 3 in primary head and neck squamous cell carcinoma. Cancer 1993;72:881–886.
23. Field JK. Genomic instability in squamous cell carcinoma of the head and neck. Anticancer Res 1996;15:2421–2432.
24. Grandis JR, Tweardy DJ. Elevated levels of transforming growth factor-alpha and epidermal growth factor receptor messenger RNA are early markers of carcinogenesis in head and neck cancer. Cancer Res 1993;53:3579–3584.
25. Michalides R, van Veelen N, Hart A, Loftus B, Wientjens E, Balm A. Overexpression of cyclin D1 correlates with recurrence in a group of forty-seven operable squamous cell carcinomas of the head and neck. Cancer Res 1995;55: 975–978.
26. Hartwell LH, Kastan MB. Cell cycle control and cancer. Science 1994;266:1821–1828.
27. Clayman GL, Ta-Jen L, Overholt SM, et al. Gene therapy for head and neck cancer: comparing the tumor suppressor gene p53 and a cell cycle regulator WA F1/CIP1(p21). Arch Otolaryngol Head Neck Surg 1996;122:489–493.
28. Gillis S, Kozak R, Durante M, Weksler ME. Decreased production and response to T-cell growth factor by lymphocytes from aged humans. J Clin Invest 1981;67:937–942.
29. Miller RA. The aging immune system: primer and prospectus. Science 1996;273:70–74.
30. Schal RS, Allen RG. Oxidative stress as a causal factor in differentiation and aging: a unifying hypothesis. Exp Gerontol 1990;25:499–522.
31. Spitz MR, Fueger JJ, Beddingfield NA, et al. Chromosomal sensitivity to bleomycin induced mutagenesis: an independent risk factor for upper aerodigestive tract cancer. Cancer Res 1989;49:4626–4628.
32. Spitz MR, Hoque A, Trizna Z, et al. Mutagen sensitivity as a risk factor for second malignant tumors following malignancies of the upper aerodigestive tract. J Natl Cancer Inst 1994;86:1681–1684.
33. Boyd D. Invasion and metastases. Cancer Metast Rev 1996;15:77–89.
34. Candela FC, Shah J, Jaques DP, et al. Patterns of cervical node metastases from squamous carcinoma of the larynx. Arch Otolaryngol Head Neck Surg 1990;116:432.
35. Calhoun KH, Fulmer P, Weiss R, Hokanson JA. Distant metastases from head and neck squamous cell carcinomas. Laryngoscope 1994;104:1199–1205.
36. Zbaren P, Lehmann W. Frequency and sites of distant metastases in head and neck squamous cell carcinomas: an analysis of 101 cases at autopsy. Arch Otolaryngol Head Neck Surg 1987;113:762.
37. Leibel SA, Scott CB, Mohiuddin M, et al. The effect of locoregional control on distant metastatic dissemination in carcinomas of the head and neck: results of an analysis from the RTOG database. Int J Radiat Oncol Biol Phys 1991;21: 549–556.
38. Shintani S, Matsuura H, Hasegawa Y, Nakayama B, Hasegawa H. Regional lymph node involvement affects the incidence of distant metastasis in tongue squamous cell carcinomas. Anticancer Res 1995;15:1573–1576.
39. American Joint Committee on Cancer. Manual for Staging of Cancer, 4th ed. Lippincott: Philadelphia, 1992.
40. Piccirillo JF, Pugliano FA. Evaluation, classification and staging. In: Myers EN, Suen JY (eds) Cancer of the Head and Neck, 3rd ed. Saunders: Philadelphia, 1996.
41. Karnofsky DA, Abelmann WH, Craver LF, et al. The use of nitrogen mustards in the palliative treatment of carcinoma. Cancer 1948;1:634.
42. Kaplan MH, Feinstein AR. The importance of classifying the initial co-morbidity in evaluating the outcome of diabetes mellitus. J Chronic Dis 1974;27:387.
43. Piccirillo JF, Wells CK, Sasaki CT, et al. New clinical severity staging system for cancer of the larynx: five-year survival rates. Ann Otol Rhinol Laryngol 1994;103:83.
44. List MA, D'Antonio LL, Cella DF, et al. The Performance Status Scale for head and neck cancer patients and the functional assessment of cancer therapy: head and neck scale; a study of utility and validity. Cancer 1996;77: 2294–2301.
45. Piccirillo JF. Inclusion of comorbidity in a staging system for head and neck cancer. Oncology (Huntingt) 1995;9: 831–836.
46. Dhooge IJ, DeVos M, Albers FW, Van Cauwenberge PB. Panendoscopy as a screening procedure for simultaneous primary tumors in head and neck cancers. Eur Arch Otorhinolaryngol 1996;253:319–324.
47. Layfield LJ. Fine needle aspiration of the head and neck. Pathology (Phila) 1996;4:409–438.
48. Pfister DG, Shaha AR, Harrison LB. The role of chemotherapy in the curative treatment of head and neck cancer. Surg Oncol Clin N Am 1997;6:749–768.
49. Vokes EE. Combined-modality therapy of head and neck cancer. Oncology (Huntingt) 1997;11(suppl 9):27–30.
50. Catimel G. Head and neck cancer: guidelines for chemotherapy. Drugs 1996;51:73–88.
51. Clayman GL, Frank DK. Selective neck dissection of anatomically appropriate levels is as efficacious as modified radical neck dissection for elective treatment of the clinically negative neck in patients with squamous cell carcinoma of the upper respiratory and digestive tracts. Arch Otolaryngol Head Neck Surg 1998;124:348– 353.
52. Ariyan S. Further experiences with the sternocleidomastoid myocutaneous flap: a clinical appraisal of 31 cases. Plast Reconstr Surg 1997;99:61–69.

53. Zenn MR, Hidalgo DA, Cordeiro PG, et al. Current role of the radial forearm free flap in mandibular reconstruction. Plast Reconstr Surg 1997;99:1012–1017.
54. Ferri J, Piot B, Rubin B, Mercier J. Advantages and limitations of the fibular free flap in mandibular reconstruction. J Oral Maxillofac Surg 1997;55:440–448.
55. Withers HR. Biological basis of radiation therapy for cancer. Lancet 1992;339:156–159.
56. Paterson R. The Treatment of Malignant Disease by Radiotherapy, 2nd ed. Williams & Wilkins: Baltimore, 1963.
57. Sassler AM, Esclamado RM, Wolf GT. Surgery after organ preservation therapy: analysis of wound complications. Arch Otolaryngol Head Neck Surg 1995;121:162–165.
58. Olmi P, Cefaro GA, Balzi M, Becciolini A, Geinitz H. Radiotherapy in the aged. Clin Geriatr Med 1997;13:143–167.
59. Ross AF, Tinker JH. Evaluation of the adult patient with cardiac problems. In: Rogers MC, Tinker JH, Covino BG, Longnecker DE (eds) Principles and Practice of Anesthesiology. Mosby: St. Louis, 1993.
60. Boyson PG. Evaluation of the patient with pulmonary disease. In: Rogers MC, Tinker JH, Covino BG, Longnecker DE (eds) Principles and Practice of Anesthesiology. Mosby: St. Louis, 1993.
61. Goodwin WJ, Byers PM. Nutritional management of the head and neck cancer patient. Med Clin North Am 1993; 77:597–610.
62. Lopez MJ, Robinson P, Madden T, Highbarger T. Nutritional support and prognosis in patients with head and neck cancer. J Surg Oncol 1994;55:33–36.
63. Van Bokhorst de van der Schueren MA, van Leeuwen PA, Sauerwein HP, et al. Assessment of nutritional parameters in head and neck cancer and their relation to postoperative complications. Head Neck 1997;19:419–425.
64. Shanmugaratnam K. Histopathology of nasopharyngeal carcinoma: correlation with epidemiology, survival rates and other biologic characteristics. Cancer 1979;44:1029–1044.
65. Yu MC. Nasopharyngeal carcinoma: epidemiology and dietary factors. IARC Sci Publ 1991;105:39–47.
66. Sham JST, Wei WI, Zong Y, et al. Detection of subclinical nasopharyngeal carcinoma by fiberoptic endoscopy and multiple biopsies. Lancet 1990;335:371–374.
67. Ho JHC. An epidemiologic and clinical study of nasopharyngeal carcinoma. Int J Radiat Oncol Biol Phys 1978;4: 183–197.
68. Vasef MA, Ferlito A, Weiss LM. Nasopharyngeal carcinoma with emphasis on its relationship to the Epstein-Barr virus. Ann Otol Rhinol Laryngol 1997;106:348–356.
69. Dillon WP, Harnsberger HR. The impact of radiologic imaging on staging of cancer in the head and neck. Semin Oncol 1991;18:64–79.
70. Wang CC. Radiation Therapy for Head and Neck Neoplasms, 3rd ed. Wiley-Liss: New York, 1997.
71. Hoppe RT, Williams J, Warnke R, Goffinet DR, Bagshaw MA. Carcinoma of the nasopharynx: the significance of histology. Int J Radiat Oncol Biol Phys 1978;4:199–205.
72. Oliver AJ, Helfrick JF, Gard D. Primary oral squamous cell carcinoma: a review of 92 cases. J Oral Maxillofac Surg 1996;54:949–954.
73. Mashberg A, Meyers H. Anatomical site and size of 222 early asymptomatic oral squamous cell carcinomas: a continuing prospective study of oral cancer II. Cancer 1976;37: 2149–2157.
74. Silverman S, Gorsky M, Losada F. Oral leukoplakia and malignant transformation: a follow-up study of 257 patients. Cancer 1984;53:563–568.
75. Silverman S. Precancerous lesions and oral cancer in the elderly. Clin Geriatr Med 1992;8:529–541.
76. Lindberg R. Distribution of cervical lymph node metastases from squamous cell carcinoma of the upper respiratory and digestive tracts. Cancer 1972;29:1446–1449.
77. Spiro RH, Huvos AG, Wong GY, Spiro JD, Gnecco CA, Strong EW. Predictive value of tumor thickness in squamous carcinoma confined to the tongue and floor of mouth. Am J Surg 1986;152:345–350.
78. Berwick M, Schantz S. Chemoprevention of aerodigestive cancer. Cancer Metast Rev 1997;16:329–347.
79. Kraus DH, Vastola P, Huvos AG. Surgical management of squamous cell carcinoma of the base of tongue. Am J Surg 1993;166:384–388.
80. Cancer Statistics 1993. CA Cancer J Clin 1993;43:18.
81. Civantos FJ, Goodwin WJ. Cancer of the oropharynx. In: Myers EN, Suen JY (eds) Cancer of the Head and Neck, 3rd ed. Saunders: Philadelphia, 1996:361–380.
82. Gluckman JL, Black RJ, Crissman JD. Cancer of the oropharynx. Otolaryngol Clin North Am 1985;18:451–459.
83. Weber RS, Gidley P, Morrison WH, et al. Treatment selection for carcinoma of the base of tongue. Am J Surg 1990;160:415–419.
84. Jaulerry C, Rodriguez J, Brunin F, et al. Results of radiation therapy in carcinoma of the base of tongue. Cancer 1991;67:1532–1538.
85. Myers EN, Alvi A. Management of carcinoma of the supraglottic larynx: evolution of current concepts and future trends. Laryngoscope, 1996;106:559–567.
86. Sinard RJ, Netterville JL, Gaelyn-Garret C, Ossof RH. Cancer of the larynx. In: Myers EN, Suen JY (eds) Cancer of the Head and Neck. Saunders: Philadelphia, 1996:381–421.
87. Mancuso AA. Evaluation and staging of laryngeal and hypopharyngeal cancer by computed tomography and magnetic resonance imaging. In: Silver CE (ed) Laryngeal Cancer. Thieme: New York, 1991.
88. Spriano G, Antognoni P, Piantanida R, et al. Conservative management of T1-T2 N0 supraglottic cancer: a retrospective study. Am J Otolaryngol 1997;18:299–305.
89. De Santo LW, Lillie JC, Devine KD. Surgical salvage after radiation for laryngeal cancer. Laryngoscope 1976;86: 649–657.
90. Moe K, Wolf GT, Fisher SG, Hong WK. Regional metastases in patients with advanced laryngeal cancer. Arch Otolaryngol Head Neck Surg 1996;122:644–648.
91. Kirchner JA. Spread and barriers to spread of cancer within the larynx. In: Silver CE (ed) Laryngeal Cancer. Thieme: New York, 1991.
92. Wiggenraad RG, Terhaard CH, Hordijk GJ, et al. The importance of vocal cord mobility in T2 laryngeal cancer. Radiother Oncol 1990;18:321.
93. Menderhall WM, Parsons JT, Brant TA, et al. Is elective neck treatment indicated for T2N0 squamous cell carcinoma of the glottic larynx? Radiother Oncol 1989;14:199.

94. Department of Veterans Affairs Laryngeal Cancer Study Group. Induction chemotherapy plus radiation compared with surgery plus radiation in patients with advanced laryngeal cancer. N Engl J Med 1991;324:1685–1690.
95. Thompson AC, Quraishi SM, Morgan DA, Bradley PJ. Carcinoma of the larynx and hypopharynx in the elderly. Eur J Surg Oncol 1996;22:65–68.
96. Grau JJ, Cuchi A, Traserra J, et al. Follow-up study in head and neck cancer: cure rate according to tumor location and stage. Oncology 1997;54:38–42.
97. Elias MM, Hilgers FJ, Keus RB, et al. Carcinoma of the piriform sinus: a retrospective analysis of treatment results over a 20-year period. Clin Otolaryngol 1995;20:249– 253.
98. Marshall JA, Mahanna GK. Cancer in the differential diagnosis of orofacial pain. Dental Clin North Am 1997;41: 355–365.
99. Urken ML, Cheney ML, Sullivan MJ, Biller HF. Atlas of Region and Free Flaps for Head and Neck Reconstruction. Raven: New York, 1995.
100. Zelefsky MJ, Kraus DH, Pfister DG, et al. Combined chemotherapy and radiation versus surgery and postoperative radiotherapy for advanced hypopharyngeal cancer. Head Neck 1996;18:405–411.
101. Clayman GL, Weber RS, Guillamondegui O, et al. Laryngeal preservation for advanced laryngeal and hypopharyngeal cancers. Arch Otolaryngol Head Neck Surg 1995; 121:219–223.
102. Kim KH, Sung MW, Rhee CS, et al. Neoadjuvant chemotherapy and radiotherapy for the treatment of advanced hypopharyngeal carcinoma. Am J Otolaryngol 1998;19:40–44.
103. Sassler AM, Esclamado RM, Wolf GT. Surgery after organ preservation therapy: analysis of wound complications. Arch Otolaryngol Head Neck Surg 1995;121:162–165.

# *Part II*
# *Specific Issues in Geriatric Surgery*

## Section 4
## Respiratory System

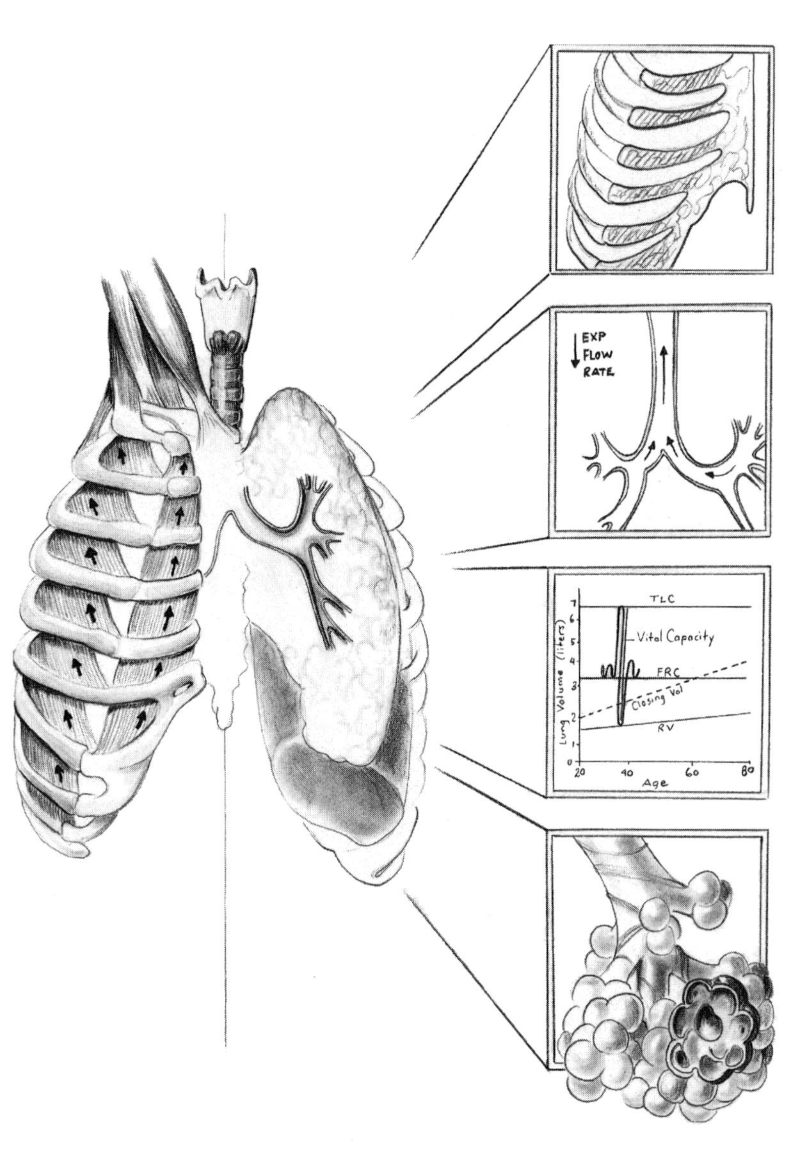

# Invited Commentary

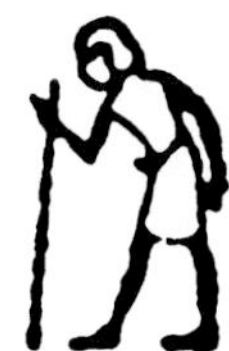

Earle W. Wilkins, Jr.

Preparing this invited commentary presents a unique challenge. Why unique? The commentary precedes two chapters on the respiratory system, *and* I have not seen the contents of those chapters. On the other hand, I am permitted freedom of perspective: "factual, philosophical, and/or personal." I choose, therefore, to do this as Past, Present, and Future, that is, the pioneering, modern and future as they related to my experience.

First, the **Pioneering Era**. My admission to medical school in 1941 and acceptance into a major teaching hospital residency program in 1944 allow me to think of the years before 1941 as the period when the foundations of modern pulmonary surgery evolved. In his Honored Speaker's Address before the fiftieth anniversary meeting of the American Association for Thoracic Surgery (AATS) in 1970 Leo Eloesser, distinguished scholarly surgeon of the pioneering era, discussed his nominations for milestones in the evolution of chest surgery.[1] Let me borrow his first three milestones (the fourth was Gibbon's development of the heart-lung machine). These three established the foundations on which all resectional surgery are based today.

1. *Intraoperative control of respiration*. Eloesser gave priority to Johann von Mikulicz, who wrote an early paper on the negative-pressure chamber in 1904. Sauerbruch was his pupil. Samuel Meltzer and John Auer of New York in 1909 proposed "continuous respiration without respiratory movements" via the intratracheal insufflation of a continuous stream of air and anesthetic vapor. It was another four decades before development of the inflatable cuffed endotracheal tube. (Its modifications with low-pressure cuffs to minimize damage to the tracheal wall and with double-lumen variants to permit operating on the quiet lung are still evolving.) It was essential, however, first to provide ventilation of the lungs in the open chest.

2. *Principles of one-stage lobectomy*. Early efforts at lobectomy for bronchiectasis included mass ligature of the pulmonary hilus and two-stage resections, often leading to horrendous double-digit surgical mortality. Harold Brunn of San Francisco carried out the first successful "modern" lobectomy with individual ligature of vessels and oversuture of the bronchial stump in a single-stage procedure in 1918. It is surprising in today's retrospective that it took another two decades before lobectomy utilizing hilar dissection and individual ligature became the norm.

3. *Pneumonectomy for bronchogenic carcinoma*. The most recognized name in early lung cancer surgery is that of Evarts Graham, who in 1933 carried out the first successful pneumonectomy for a squamous cell carcinoma of the left upper lobe bronchus. (The patient lived cancer-free for 30 years.) It is important to cite this early operation for bronchogenic carcinoma in order to identify the starting point from which modern resectional surgery for pulmonary neoplasms has evolved. In the interest of historical priority, it is intriguing to note that Batirel reports Graham acknowledged primacy of pneumonectomy to Rudolf Nissen (2000).[2]

Now, to the **Modern Era**. Allow me to present three areas of development in the refinement of the principles of pulmonary surgery as they have evolved over the second half of the twentieth century, the period of my active participation in general thoracic surgery.

1. *Extent of resection*. Graham's successful pneumonectomy had by 1950 established it as the standard operation for lung cancer. During the discussion of Churchill, Sweet, et al.'s paper[3] before the AATS that year, there was a huge outcry against lobectomy. Before 1948 in work at the Massachusetts General Hospital (MGH), 31 lobectomies and 87 pneumonectomies had been carried out with similar survivals. Graham: "We should distinguish between . . . the ideal operation for cancer and one which theoretically is not ideal but will sometimes work." Alton Ochsner: "Lobectomy should be limited to those cases in which pneumonectomy is contraindicated, not those in which lobectomy can be done." Eloesser then provided the historically approved commentary: "The attempt to

eradicate cancer by progressively increasing the anatomic limits of operation is not the right road to follow."

By the end of the 1950s the principle of lobectomy as the standard operation (where possible) had finally been accepted. Indeed, a later paper[4] from the MGH in 1978, comprising resectional experience from 1931 to 1971, reported that nine segmental resections were done as the definitive operation for bronchogenic carcinoma. It was from that institution that the classic work by Churchill and Belsey[5] defined the pulmonary segment as the basic anatomic unit of the lung (1939). When the extent of carcinoma is confined to a segment or segments of the lung, there is no contraindication to segmental resection as a procedure of choice.

The critical issue in any of these resections is lymphatic invasion. The situation is somewhat akin to the situation with breast carcinoma, where once traditional radical mastectomy has been replaced by lesser procedures *but* determination of lymphatic invasion is mandatory and easily accomplished by dissection or biopsy of the axilla. Similarly, lesser resections of lung parenchyma must be accompanied by dissection, or at least sampling, of mediastinal lymph nodes. This provides the information necessary for making decisions concerning adjuvant therapy.

2. *Staging*. An aspect of surgery for pulmonary carcinoma that became standard some two decades ago is staging, here primarily concerned with preoperative or evaluative staging. One technique, popularized by Pearson,[6] is mediastinoscopy. This procedure is routinely employed by many general thoracic surgeons but may have greater universal utility when biopsying enlarged mediastinal lymph nodes identified on computed tomographic (CT) study. Whether mediastinoscopy is necessary in the absence of adenopathy, as seen by CT, remains controversial. True mediastinoscopy is a procedure for the skilled thoracic surgeon who performs it more than occasionally. There are definite pitfalls in a too-aggressive technique. A reasonable approach is to rely on CT for preoperative staging. Finding unanticipated lymph node metastasis at the time of resection can be compensated by dissection and adjuvant therapy.

3. *Respiratory care*. The concept of specialized postoperative care for the patient undergoing pulmonary resection, especially pneumonectomy, was introduced during this era. The first respiratory intensive care unit (ICU) established at the MGH in 1958, evolved from the need for postthymectomy care in myasthenia gravis patients. Its role in the postoperative care of patients undergoing pulmonary resection soon became clear. Thoracic surgeons could tackle patients with borderline pulmonary reserve or complicating cardiovascular problems more confidently. Respiratory therapy became an integral component of pulmonary surgical care.

The development of endotracheal tubes with low-pressure cuffs evolved from studies conducted on patients requiring long-term intubation in the respiratory ICU. Prevention of the devastating complication of tracheal wall necrosis and ensuing stricture became essential in the everyday management of the complicated respiratory patient.

On to the **Future**, the post-1986 era for me. Happily, progress marches steadily onward. Here, once again, I note three areas of ongoing development.

1. *Video-assisted thoracoscopic surgery*. This technique, termed VATS, is certainly the most striking advance in the field of general thoracic surgery in recent decades. It is truly revolutionary. The surgeon utilizes mini-incisions, remarkable magnifying fiberoptic visualization, and an impressive armamentarium of dissecting and clipping instruments. Surgeons now look at a monitoring screen rather than at the patient. VATS has required acquisition of an entirely new and different skill for the surgeon. For the patient it means more comfortable and far shorter hospital stays.

The ultimate role of VATS is still developing. Its utilization in tissue diagnosis, staging of carcinoma, and excision of peripheral pulmonary nodules is firmly established. Whether it permits more limited pulmonary resections and lessens morbidity, especially in the elderly, remains to be seen. Similarly, the role of VATS in major pulmonary resections is not yet clear. Lobes, even entire lungs, can be removed by modifications of this technique, but it appears doubtful that this use will become routine.

2. *Adjuvant therapy*. Irradiation of the mediastinum seems to be standard postoperative therapy when mediastinal, or even bronchial, lymph nodes are involved in metastatic disease from carcinoma of the lung. The role of adjuvant chemotherapy is less well settled, in contradistinction to its use in patients with breast carcinoma with nodal metastasis. At the present time, chemotherapy in non-small-cell carcinoma is little utilized for overall postresection therapy. Extensive studies utilizing chemotherapy in association with irradiation are under way in stage III carcinoma patients. Where this modality will fit with resectional surgery, especially in the elderly patient, is certainly not clear.

3. *Extended resections*. Is there a place for surgical resections beyond the so-called routines of lobectomy and pneumonectomy with or without lymph node dissections? For years surgeons have been successfully resecting the chest wall when it is involved with bronchogenic carcinoma. Particular progress has been made in surgery for apical pulmonary carcinoma (the Pancoast tumor), especially with routes of access. The most remarkable progress has come from the pioneering efforts of Grillo[7] in carinal and tracheal resections when involved in stage III disease. Sleeve and parenchyma-sparing resections allow patients with limited pulmonary reserve to go

forward with surgery. It does seem, however, that we have reached the limits of surgical resection and what surgery per se can accomplish.

In the spirit of latitude provided me by the editors, permit me to "freewheel" about the status of surgery for bronchogenic carcinoma with special reference to the geriatric patient. It has long been evident that elderly patients with normal cardiovascular status and adequate pulmonary reserve readily tolerate pulmonary resection. With age 65 as a basic definition of the geriatric patient, 54 of 220 patients undergoing lobectomy or pneumonectomy *prior* to 1956 at the MGH were senior citizens.[8] The risk to life was no greater for this select number than for the entire group. Chronologic age in itself is not a contraindication to pulmonary resection in the geriatric patient. Physiologic age may be a determinant.

It is also clear to me, after a half century of involvement in the field of general thoracic surgery, that surgical resections per se have reached their limit of success in curing lung cancer. Looking back, I question whether the overall cure rate for lung cancer has really improved over the past quarter century. Selection of candidates for resection by accurate staging has refined surgical cure rates by eliminating from consideration for surgery those patients with disease out of surgical bounds. Improved methods of anesthesia and the availability of respiratory care have reduced morbidity and mortality, permitting increased survival. The possibility of more limited resections certainly adds to the candidacy lists for operation. The cure rates after surgical resection have indeed improved, but the 5-year survival rate for *all* patients diagnosed with lung cancer remains distressingly near 10% for this most common of all neoplasms. We have a long way to go in devising other forms of therapy in our efforts to cure the disease.

Surgical success in pathologic stage I patients is conclusively certain and can approach 100%. Stage II (perhaps) and stage III patients (certainly) merit consideration for combined therapy with the only other proved forms of therapy: irradiation and chemotherapy. Progress in this arena, with the possible exception of small-cell carcinoma, has been dismally slow. There is enormous room for innovation and progress but it will not likely come from us, the surgeons.

Finally, let me propose some recommendations for the geriatric patient with bronchogenic carcinoma.

1. Whenever possible, treat the geriatric lung cancer patient like any other lung cancer patient.
2. Stage the patient preoperatively with CT, reserving mediastinoscopy for positive radiographic findings.
3. Utilize as limited a pulmonary resection as can rid the patient of primary disease.
4. Do not give up conventional thoracotomy for VATS during segmentectomy, lobectomy, or pneumonectomy. Limited muscle-sparing incisions are still the order of the day.
5. Consider mediastinal irradiation for node metastases.
6. Withhold chemotherapy, as it is available today, in the resected patient.
7. Contraindications to pulmonary resection come from physiologic, not chronologic, age. Particular attention must be directed to cardiovascular status, pulmonary function, and the presence of metabolic or other malignant disease.

Remember: *The geriatric patient is, by his very survival, already self-selected* and becomes therefore a reasonable operative risk.

## References

1. Eloesser L. Milestones in chest surgery. J Thorac Cardiovasc Surg 1970;60:157–165.
2. Batirel HF, Yuksel M. Rudolf Nissen's years in Bosphorus and the pioneers of thoracic surgery in Turkey. Ann Thorac Surg 2000;69:651–654.
3. Churchill ED, Sweet RH, Soutter L, Scannell JG. The surgical management of carcinoma of the lung. J Thorac Surg 1950; 20:349–365.
4. Wilkins EW Jr, Scannell JG, Craver JG. Four decades of experience with resections for bronchogenic carcinoma at the Massachusetts General Hospital. J Thorac Cardiovasc Surg 1978;76:364–368.
5. Churchill ED, Belsey RHR. Segmental pneumonectomy in bronchiectasis; the lingular segment of left upper lobe. Ann Surg 1939;109:481–499.
6. Pearson FG. Mediastinoscopy: a method of biopsy in the superior mediastinum. J Thorac Cardiovasc Surg 1965;49: 11–21.
7. Grillo HC. Carinal resection. Ann Thorac Surg 1982;34: 356–373.
8. Churchill ED, Sweet RH, Scannell JG, Wilkins EW Jr. Further studies in the surgical management of carcinoma of the lung. J Thorac Surg 1958;36:301–308.

# 28
# Physiologic Changes in Respiratory Function

Edward J. Campbell

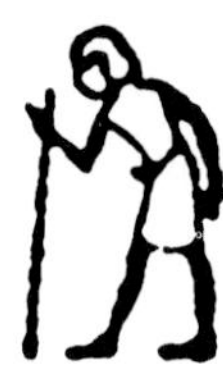

A substantial proportion of the excess operative risk among elderly patients is attributable to respiratory complications. The excess risk is explained in part by structural and functional changes in the respiratory system associated with aging. These changes are progressive even in individuals who enjoy apparently good health and are most marked beyond 60 years of age.

In youth, healthy individuals have a physiologic reserve (a marked excess of functional capacity over the amount needed to meet metabolic needs at rest or with stress). The respiratory system draws on this reserve as its function declines with age. Aged individuals thus become vulnerable to the stress, disease, and injuries that are weathered much more easily by the young.

The routine activities of healthy elderly persons are not limited by this decreasing respiratory system function. Thus the effects of age may not be apparent until they need to draw on their physiologic reserves during stress, such as postoperative recovery or complications. An awareness of the inevitable, but possibly hidden, age-related changes in the respiratory system help the surgeon anticipate and treat respiratory complications in elderly patients.

The purely age-related changes in the respiratory system are complicated by other accompaniments of aging. The lungs are exposed to a lifetime of environmental stresses, including tobacco smoke, respiratory infections, air pollutants, and occupational exposures to dusts and fumes. Elderly individuals also often have increasingly sedentary life styles and decreasing fitness.

As an introduction to the topics to be reviewed in this chapter, the various components of the respiratory system are shown in Table 28.1. Table 28.1 also contains introductory comments about structural and functional changes with age.

## Airways and Lung Parenchyma

### Lung Shape

The lungs are closely applied to the chest wall, and their overall shape is determined by of the chest wall shape. The increases in anteroposterior diameter of the lungs with age and the more rounded shape that results are presumably due to changes in the shape of the surrounding thoracic cage. These changes are not thought to have functional consequences.

### Conducting Airways

The conducting airways consist of the air passages from the mouth to the level of the respiratory bronchioles. The volume of the conducting airways determines the anatomic deadspace. Their size, shape, and branching pattern are the major determinants of airway resistance. The large cartilaginous airways show a modest increase in size with age, resulting in slight but probably functionally insignificant increases in anatomic deadspace.[1] Calcification of cartilage in the walls of the central airways and hypertrophy of bronchial mucous glands are seen during advanced age, but these and other changes in the extraparenchymal conducting airways appear to have little or no physiologic significance.

### Lung Parenchyma

The respiratory bronchioles and alveolar ducts undergo progressive enlargement with age, beginning as early as age 30 or 40 but observable most prominently after the age of 60 (Fig. 28.1). The proportion of the lung made up of alveolar ducts increases, and alveolar septa become

TABLE 28.1. Respiratory System and Changes with Aging

| Functional division | Components | Function | Change(s) with aging |
|---|---|---|---|
| Conducting airways | Airways not involved in gas exchange | Transport gas to and from lung parenchyma | Calcification and other minor changes |
| Lung parenchyma | Respiratory bronchioles through alveoli and supporting structures | Exchanges gas between alveoli and pulmonary capillaries | Enlarged alveolar ducts; ventilation-perfusion mismatching |
| Bellows apparatus | Chest wall and respiratory muscles | Provides support for lung structure and applies force to lung | Increased rigidity of chest wall; some decrease in respiratory muscle strength |
| Ventilatory control | Respiratory control center; carotid and aortic bodies | Alters ventilation to match metabolic needs | Markedly decreased responses to hypoxemia and hypercapnia |

shortened, leading to a flattened appearance of the alveoli. The proportion of alveolar air decreases as the volume of air in alveolar ducts increases.[2] The distance between alveolar walls (the mean linear intercept, or MLI) increases, whereas the surface/volume ratio of the lung decreases. As a result of these changes, the alveolar surface area decreases by approximately 15% by age 70.

Superficially, the morphologic changes in the lung with aging are similar to those observed with mild pulmonary emphysema. To be classified as emphysema, however, the anatomic changes must consist of airspace enlargement in the gas-exchanging zone of the lung (distal to the terminal bronchioles) and must show evidence that the airspace enlargement is due to alveolar wall destruction, with fusion of adjacent airspaces.[3] For a time there was considerable debate as to the cause and classification of the airspace enlargement seen with advanced age. Debate centered on whether the airspace enlargement was a "senile" form of emphysema.

Pump[4] and several early authors thought they could identify "emphysematous" lesions in aged lungs. However, Pump studied only two lungs (from 78- and 80-year-old men), one of whom had been a heavy smoker. Ryan and colleagues resisted the term "emphysema" and called the age-related structural changes "ductectasia" because of the prominent finding of enlarged alveolar ducts.[5] Significant alveolar wall destruction as a cause of emphysema appears to be unlikely, as Thurlbeck and Angus have shown that the number of alveoli per unit

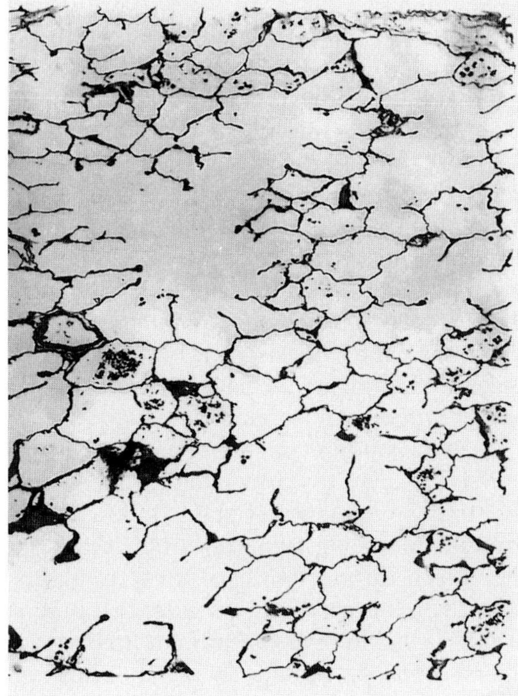

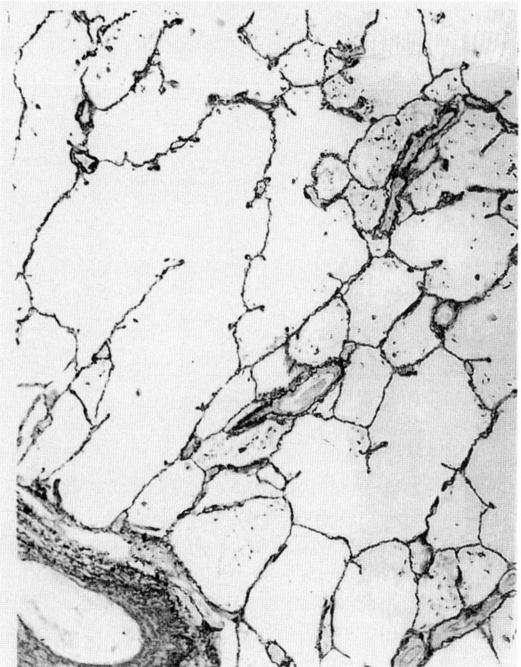

FIGURE 28.1. Histologic changes in the aging lung. (Left) Normal lung of a 36-year-old woman. (Right) Lung of a 93-year-old woman. Alveolar ducts are dilated, and shortening of interalveolar septa is observed. (Photomicrographs courtesy of Charles Kuhn III, MD, with permission of the Mayo Foundation.)

area remains constant in mature lungs.[2] The latter authors considered the changes to be a "rearrangement of the geometry of the lung." A National Heart, Lung, and Blood Institute Workshop on the definition of emphysema, weighed the available evidence and decided not to include age-related changes in the lung parenchyma under the definition of emphysema.[3] To avoid confusion and to simplify the nomenclature, they recommended use of the term "aging lung" to apply to the uniform airspace enlargement that develops with increasing age.

## Mechanical Properties of the Lungs

The lungs exert an inward force in the intact thoracic cage. The retractile force of the lungs, or "elastic recoil," can be measured during life by estimating the pleural pressure with an esophageal balloon. Measurements are taken at progressively decreasing lung volumes from total lung capacity to functional residual capacity, when the airways are open and there is no airflow. The negative pleural pressure is generated by the lungs' elastic recoil forces.

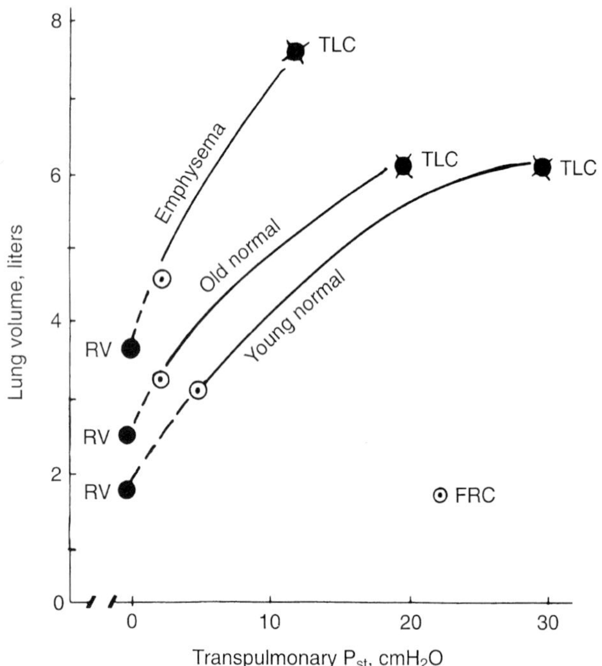


FIGURE 28.2. Static pressure–volume curves of the lungs illustrating elastic recoil forces and compliance. To generate these data, transpulmonary pressure (which reflects lung elastic recoil) is measured at various lung volumes with an esophageal balloon. At any lung volume, the recoil pressure is less in the aged than in the young individual. This results in a pressure–volume relation that is shifted upward and to the left. A curve for a patient with emphysema is shown for comparison. With emphysema, recoil pressures are much less than in normal elderly individuals, and lung compliance (the slope of the curve) is markedly abnormal. (From Pride,[6] with permission.)

Figure 28.2 compares the elastic recoil pressures of a young man, a normal elderly adult, and a patient with emphysema. The normal elderly individual and the patient with emphysema have a greater decrease in elastic recoil pressure than does a young person. This is reflected in the leftward shift of their pressure–volume curves.[7,8] Emphysema produces a much greater loss of elastic recoil than is caused by aging alone.

There has been some disagreement as to whether aging changes lung compliance (the slope of the curve in Fig. 28.2) or, alternatively, is accompanied by a parallel leftward shift of the pressure–volume curve with aging (no change in compliance). There is general agreement if small changes in lung compliance do occur, they are not physiologically significant.

### Changes in Lung Recoil Due to Surface Forces

The loss of surface area with age reduces the area of gas–liquid interface, resulting in a decrease in the surface tension forces. This ultimately causes a decrease in the lung elastic recoil. This change has important effects on lung function (especially on the function of small airways and expiratory flow).

### Changes in Structural Macromolecules

Elastic fibers consist in large part of an extremely hydrophobic, highly cross-linked, and highly elastic macromolecule (elastin). They form a continuous skeleton that follows the airways and pulmonary vessels and extends to a fine meshwork in the alveolar septa.[9] These fibers are thought to contribute substantially to lung elasticity. The amount of elastin in the lungs has been studied in an attempt to determine the cause of decreasing lung elastic recoil with age. Analysis of whole lungs has revealed that the elastin content actually increases (rather than decreases) with age.[10] More recent evidence indicates that the increase in lung elastin with age is accounted for by an increase in pleural elastin; parenchymal elastin does not change.[9]

Careful studies of the elastic fibers in the lung parenchyma by two independent methods have shown that they are remarkably stable following postnatal lung growth. Modeling of radiocarbon data[11] indicates that the "mean carbon residence time" in elastin is 74 years (Fig. 28.3). It is correct to consider that lung parenchymal elastin is stable over the human life-span. These elastic fibers probably provide a metabolically inert scaffold for the structure of the lung. Thus there are no age-related changes in lung elastin that provide an explanation for the decrease in elastic recoil forces observed in the elderly.

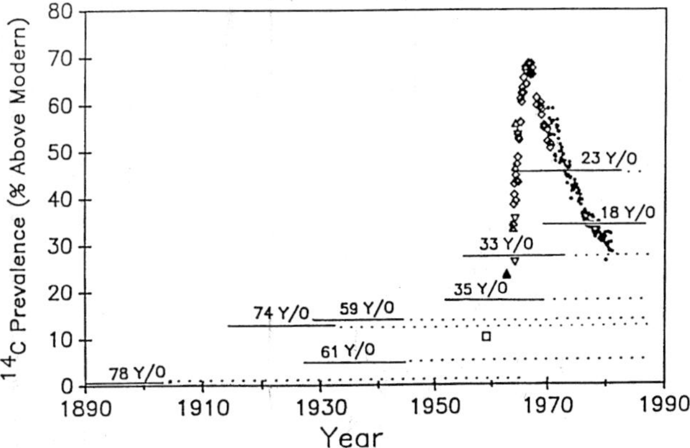


FIGURE 28.3. Turnover of elastic fibers in human lung parenchyma. Radiocarbon ($^{14}$C) prevalence in lung elastin is shown on the ordinate, with zero being the level before atmospheric nuclear weapons testing began. Levels above zero reflect protein synthesis that has occurred since the 1960s (% Above Modern). The symbols are data from human tissues that exhibit rapid turnover, sampled during the years shown.[11] Each horizontal line represents an analysis of human lung parenchymal elastin from a single individual. The age at time of death is shown for each subject. The lengths and positioning of the solid portions of the lines correspond to timing and duration of fetal and postnatal lung growth, and the interrupted portions of the lines represent the remainder of the individuals' life-spans. The vertical position of each line represents the $^{14}$C prevalence measured in that sample. Note that the $^{14}$C prevalence measured in the elastin samples reflects the $^{14}$C prevalence in the biosphere during the period of lung growth. Individuals whose lungs had ceased growing before the nuclear weapons age had little nuclear weapons-related $^{14}$C in their lung elastin, demonstrating that minimal lung elastin turnover occurred during adulthood. (From Shapiro et al.,[11] with permission.)

Although human studies have not been done, studies in rodents and birds suggest that lung collagen fibers, like elastic fibers, are long-lived. Finally, although some qualitative changes in collagen during aging have been described (decreases in solubility and increases in intermolecular cross-links), they appear to have no relation to changes in lung elastic recoil.

## Chest Wall

The chest wall becomes more rigid with advancing age.[8,12] As can be seen in Figure 28.4, the static pressure–volume curve of the chest wall is shifted to the right and is less steep (indicating decreased compliance) with increasing age.[13] It is known that the articulations of the ribs with the sternum and the spinal column may become calcified, and the compliance of the rib articulations decreases with age. The changes in rib articulations may be compounded by the development of kyphosis due to osteoporosis. The decreasing compliance of the chest wall demands more work from the respiratory muscles. For example, in a 70-year-old person approximately 70% of the total elastic work of breathing is expended on the chest wall, whereas this value is 40% in a 20-year-old.

## Muscles of Respiration

Age-related changes in nonrespiratory skeletal muscle include decreased work capacity owing to alterations in the efficiency of muscle energy metabolism, atrophy of motor units, and electromyographic abnormalities. Based on lessons learned with other skeletal muscles, it at first appeared likely that age-related abnormalities in respiratory muscles would also be found.

An early study by Black and Hyatt[14] appeared to confirm age-related decrements in respiratory muscle function by measuring maximal inspiratory pressure

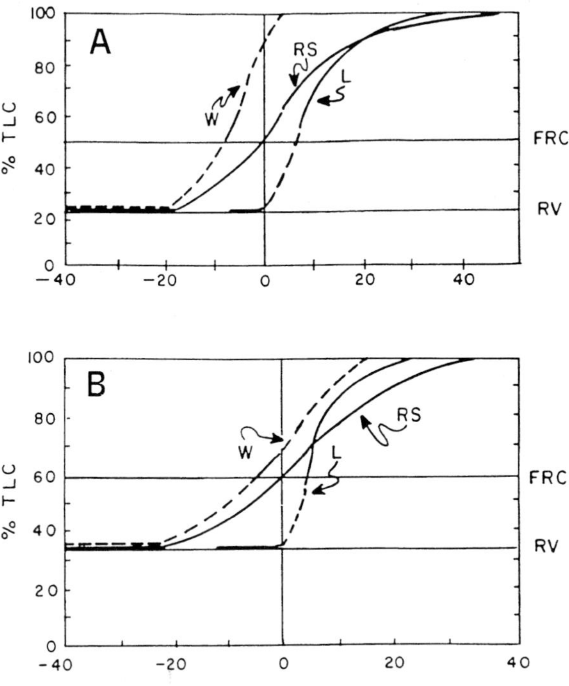


FIGURE 28.4. Static compliance relations of the components of the respiratory system. L, lungs; W, chest wall; RS, total respiratory system; TLC, total lung capacity; FRC, functional reserve capacity; RV, residual volume; P, pressure gradient, (A) A 20-year-old man; (B) A 60-year-old man. Note that the static compliance of the chest wall is substantially decreased (reduced slope) in the older individual, whereas functional residual capacity (resting volume of the respiratory system, or the point at which the pressure gradient across the respiratory system is zero) increases somewhat. Note again (compare with Fig. 28.2) that the static recoil pressure of the lungs is reduced in the older subject.

($PI_{max}$) and maximal expiratory pressure ($PE_{max}$) in 120 normal individuals (both smokers and nonsmokers) between the ages of 20 and 70. Maximal respiratory pressures in women were 65–70% of those in men. No significant age-related changes were observed in individuals under the age of 55. Trends toward reduced maximal respiratory pressure with age were seen for both sexes and with both $PI_{max}$ and $PE_{max}$. With the numbers of men studied, the change with age in $PI_{max}$ was not statistically significant for the male gender.

More recently, McElvaney and coworkers[15] came to a different conclusion in a similar study of 104 healthy individuals over the age of 55. They found large variation in maximal respiratory pressures from individual to individual (as had Black and Hyatt) but no significant correlation with age. In contrast, in a third population of 160 healthy individuals who ranged in age from 16 to 75 years, Chen and Kuo found significant gender differences in maximal respiratory pressures as well as trends toward decrements with age for both $PI_{max}$ and $PE_{max}$ in both genders.[16] The age-related change in $PE_{max}$ in the male subjects was not statistically significant with the sample size studied. When the 40 individuals of both genders in the youngest age group (16–30 years) were compared with the 40 individuals in the oldest group (61–75 years), the decrement in $PI_{max}$ was 32–36%, and the decrement in $PE_{max}$ was 13–23%. Representative findings for maximal respiratory pressures in women are illustrated in Figure 28.5.

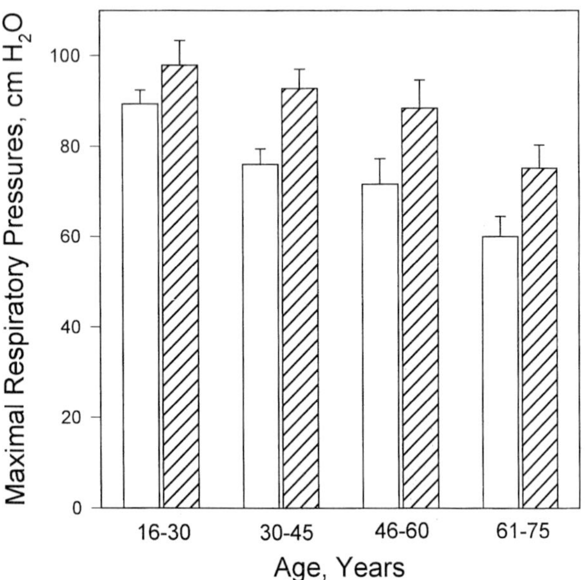


FIGURE 28.5. Representative variations in maximal respiratory pressure with age among women. Inspiratory and expiratory measurements were made at residual volume and total lung capacity, respectively. Open bars, maximal inspiratory pressure; hatched bars, maximal expiratory pressure. Error bars are standard errors of the mean. The variations with age were statistically significant but were small in magnitude. (From Chen and Kuo,[16] with permission.)

Chen and Kuo measured inspiratory muscle endurance against a resistive load and found significant decrements with age.[16] Physically active men had greater inspiratory muscle endurance than sedentary men.

In summary, it appears that when populations of healthy individuals of widely differing ages are studied, moderate age-related decrements in respiratory muscle strength and endurance can be found. These studies usually define "healthy" only by the absence of disease and do not control for physical activity. They are complicated by marked interindividual variability, and longitudinal studies have not been reported. Respiratory muscle function may be better preserved with age than that of other skeletal muscles because of a straining effect of the continuous respiratory muscle activity. Finally, physical activity may have an additional straining effect that enhances inspiratory muscle endurance in all age groups.

## Control of Breathing

Stanley and colleagues have found that elderly subjects (mean age 69 years) have a slower, more variable respiratory rate than a young control group.[17,18] It is doubtful that this isolated observation has any functional significance, but it did suggest that ventilatory control changes with aging.

More important is that ventilation becomes much less responsive to stress in elderly individuals. It is well known that in young individuals sensitive ventilatory control mechanisms match minute ventilation closely to metabolic demands. As a result, arterial blood–gas values remain stable throughout a wide range of activities from rest to strenuous exertion, whereas oxygen consumption and carbon dioxide production vary widely. Similarly, when the efficiency of gas exchange is diminished by a variety of lung problems (e.g., atelectasis and pneumonia) or congestive heart failure, appropriate increases in minute ventilation minimize the potential for resulting hypercapnia or hypoxemia in healthy young individuals.

To compare old and young individuals, ventilatory control mechanisms have typically been tested by inducing either hypoxemia or hypercapnia while monitoring ventilatory parameters. Such tests have shown striking differences between young and elderly individuals in ventilatory and cardiac responses.[19–22]

### Diminished Ventilatory Response to Hypercapnia

Kronenberg and Drage[21] compared the ventilatory responses to hypercapnia while $PaCO_2$ was allowed to rise to 65 mmHg. The elderly individuals had a significantly diminished ventilatory response to hypercapnia,

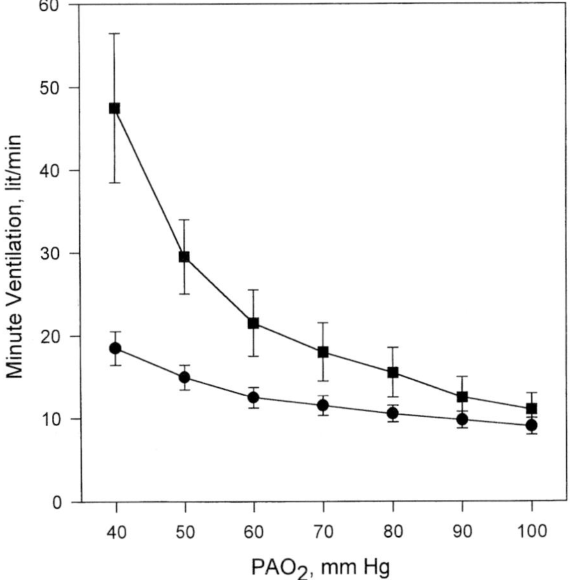


FIGURE 28.6. Variations in ventilatory responses to hypoxia, with age. Eight normal men aged 64–73 years (mean 69.6 years) (circles) were compared to young controls aged 22–30 years (mean 25.6 years) (squares). Ventilation was measured while the subjects were exposed to isocapnic progressive hypoxia by a rebreathing method. Values are means ± SEM. Note that the ventilatory responses were strikingly attenuated in the older individuals. (From Kronenberg and Drage,[21] with permission.)

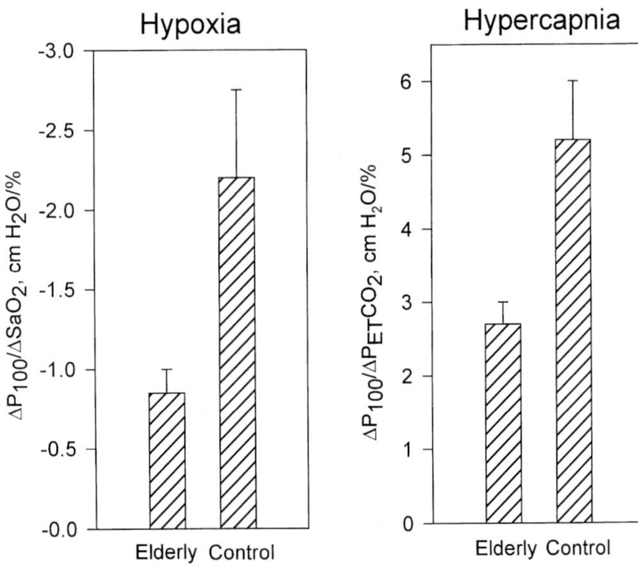


FIGURE 28.7. Variations in occlusion pressure responses to hypoxia and hypercapnia, with age. Data are slopes of the relations between occlusion pressure responses and either $SaO_2$ or end-tidal $PCO_2$; error bars are the SEM. Occlusion pressure responses are an indicator of ventilatory drive independent of chest wall compliance and respiratory muscle strength. The elderly individuals showed significantly and strikingly diminished ventilatory drives in response to both hypoxia and hypercapnia. (From Peterson and Fishman,[23] with permission.)

measured as the slope of the relation between ventilation and $P_ACO_2$.

## Diminished Ventilatory Response to Hypoxia

When these same authors[21] measured the ventilatory response to hypoxia, the contrasts between young and aged individuals were even more dramatic (Fig. 28.6). The ventilatory response to $P_AO_2$ 40 mmHg was uniformly smaller in the old subjects, and there was no overlap between the groups. The mean minute ventilation values at $P_AO_2$ 40 mmHg were 40.1 and 10.2 L/min in the young and old groups, respectively.

## Diminished Occlusion Pressure Responses

Peterson and Fishman[23] showed that the differences in responses of elderly subjects to both hypercapnia and hypoxia are due to a lesser increase in tidal volume during stress, whereas the ventilatory rate increases normally. These authors also measured airway occlusion pressures, which are valuable indices of respiratory drive that are not affected by either respiratory muscle strength or respiratory mechanics. The measurements, called $P_{100}$, are the negative pressures at the mouth when measured 100 ms after the start of inspiration against an occluded airway. The occlusion pressure responses to both hypoxia and hypercapnia (Fig. 28.7) were significantly reduced in 10 elderly subjects (mean age 73.3 years) when compared to those of 9 young control subjects (mean age 24.4 years).[22]

In summary, the compensatory change in tidal volume in response to either hypoxemia or hypercapnia is reduced (often strikingly) with age. The less-effective homeostasis is apparently due to reduced responsiveness of either the ventilatory drive or the neural output from the respiratory center. It has not been determined whether the diminished ventilatory drive results from altered chemoreceptor function or altered function of the respiratory center. Kronenberg and Drage favored altered receptor function based on their observation that elderly subjects responded to an alveolar oxygen tension of 40 mmHg with only an 11% increase in heart rate, whereas the young subjects responded with a 45% increase.[21]

## Respiratory Load Compensation and Dyspnea

Normally, when there is a change in the mechanical workload of the respiratory system (e.g., with lung disease, changes in posture, or mouth versus nose breathing), there is a reflex compensation that maintains the ventilation constant. To study the effects of aging, Akiyama and colleagues[24] measured responses to inspiratory flow-resistive loading in young and elderly individuals. In the young control group, inspiratory loading resulted in an increase in $P_{100}$ at each level of induced hypercapnia, such that inspiratory loading did not change the ventilatory response to hypercapnia. In marked contrast, the $P_{100}$ in the elderly group did not change when an inspiratory load was applied. Thus ventilatory responses to hypercapnia were reduced during inspiratory loading in the elderly group.

At each level of $PCO_2$, the intensity of perceived dyspnea in response to inspiratory loading was higher in the elderly than in the control group. Thus the sensation of dyspnea was intact or enhanced in the elderly subjects while their compensatory responses were reduced.

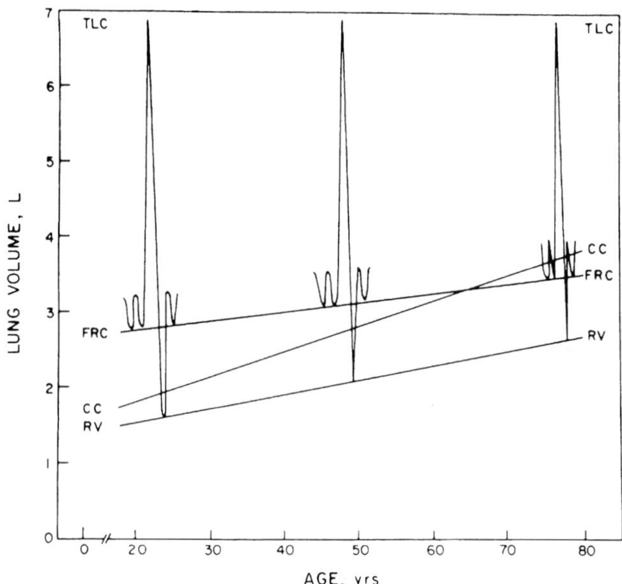


FIGURE 28.8. Lung volume changes with age. TLC, total lung capacity; CC, closing capacity; FRC, functional residual capacity; RV, residual volume. Although not labeled, the vital capacity is TLC minus RV. The most consistent age-related changes are an increase in RV and a decrease in ventilatory capacity. (From Peterson and Fishman,[23] with permission.)

## Pulmonary Circulation

Pulmonary artery catheterization studies have typically been biased in that only subsets of patients have been reported. The reported studies were performed on individuals who had signs and symptoms that led to referral for heart catheterization. These individuals are probably not representative of "healthy" young and old cohorts. Furthermore, age-related changes in the pulmonary circulation are difficult or impossible to distinguish from changes due to heart disease or age-related changes in cardiac function. Even if they are real, the minor increases in pulmonary vascular resistance and age-related increases in pulmonary artery wedge pressure are probably not physiologically significant.

## Pulmonary Function Tests

Several measurements of lung function and exercise capacity decline with age. However, descriptions of "normal" age-related changes are confounded by an increasing prevalence of disease, chronic illness, medication use, and an increasingly sedentary life style. The influences of all of these factors are difficult to distinguish from each other. Superficially, it appears that longitudinal studies would provide the optimal design for distinguishing the effects of age from other influences. Longitudinal studies, however, have methodologic problems and biases of their own, the most obvious being that the healthy elderly represent a healthy survival population. Regardless, it does seem that age alone has potentially important effects on lung function.

### Lung Volumes

Figure 28.8 illustrates typical lung volume changes with aging based on cross-sectional studies. Total lung capacity (TLC), the volume of air in the lungs at the end of a maximal inspiration, is marked by the point at which the recoil pressure exerted by the respiratory system is exactly counterbalanced by the maximal inspiratory pressure generated by the respiratory muscles. Cross-sectional studies of TLC summarized by the European Coal and Steel Community,[25,26] when combined, demonstrated no significant age coefficients for either men or women.[25,26]

Both slow and forced vital capacity (FVC) decline with age more rapidly in men than women. Average decrements in vital capacity per year vary considerably; in cross-sectional studies declines range from 21 to 33 ml/year in men and 18 to 29 ml/year in women. Ware and colleagues,[27] in a study containing both longitudinal and cross-sectional computations, found cross-sectional decreases in FVC for men and women to be −34 and −27.8 ml/year, respectively. Cross-sectional studies of residual volume (RV) and the RV/TLC ratio consistently show increases with age. In the young, RV (the volume of air in the lungs at the end of a maximal expiration) is the volume at which the outward static recoil pressure of the respiratory system is counterbalanced by the maximal pressure exerted by the expiratory muscles. In old subjects the expiratory flow never completely reaches zero, and RV is determined in part by the length of time an individual can maintain the expiratory effort. Other factors leading to an increased RV with aging include loss of lung recoil, decreased chest wall compliance, decreased expiratory muscle force, and increased small airway closure (air trapping) in dependent lung zones.[6]

Functional residual capacity (FRC) is also determined by the balance of the elastic recoil forces of the lung and chest wall, but in this instance the equilibrium occurs at the end of a quiet (unforced) exhalation. Because lung recoil decreases and the chest wall stiffens with age, one would expect the FRC to increase. Cross-sectional studies, however, show inconsistent results, with most showing no change in FRC with aging. Studies that do find an increase in FRC with aging show a small positive age coefficient on the order of 7–16 ml/year. McClaran et al.'s longitudinal study found the FRC to increase 40 ml/year, but again the change was not significant.[28] Despite the conflicting data, it is generally believed that FRC increases somewhat with aging.

Loss of lung recoil also changes the volume at which airway closure occurs. When adults exhale fully, small airways close in the region of the terminal bronchioles in dependent lung zones. The lung volume at which this closure begins is measured as the closing volume or, if it is added to the residual volume, closing capacity. Closing volume increases linearly with age from about 5–10% of TLC at age 20 to about 30% of TLC at age 70. The loss of lung elastic recoil, a possible decrease in the recoil of the intrapulmonary airways, and decreases in small airway diameter probably explain most of the change in closing volume.

On average, closing volume encroaches on tidal volume by about age 44 when subjects are supine and at about age 65 when they are seated (Fig. 28.8). Airway closure during tidal breathing explains part of the decrease in arterial oxygen tension observed with aging.

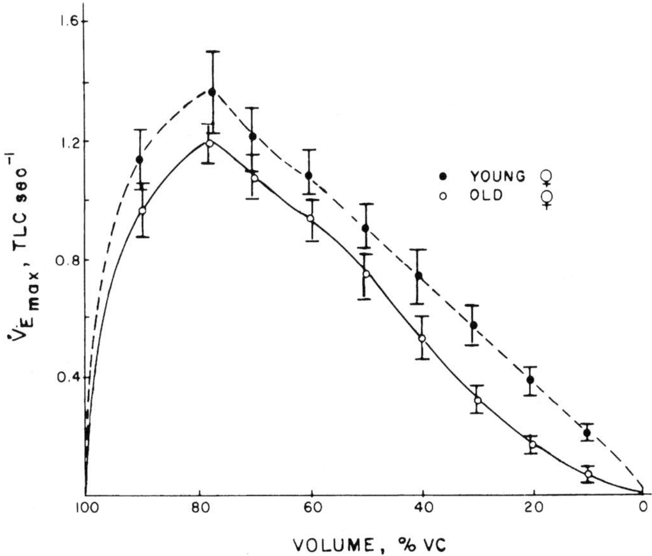


FIGURE 28.9. Maximal flow–volume curves, showing the changes in expiratory flow rates with age. Data are for elderly women (mean age 63 years) and control young women (mean age 25 years). Although all flows tend to be reduced with aging, the reduction in flow is most evident at lower lung volumes, where the flow–volume curve is concave in regard to the volume axis. (From Peterson and Fishman,[23] with permission.)

## Airflow

Although essentially all expiratory flows measured during a maximum expiratory maneuver decrease with age, the declines are most evident at low lung volumes (Fig. 28.9). Nunn and Dregg,[29] in a study of 225 male and 228 healthy female nonsmokers, reported a modest decrease in peak expiratory flow (PEF) with aging. The rate of decline in FVC and forced expiratory volume at 1 second ($FEV_1$) with age tends to be more in (1) men, (2) tall individuals; (3) individuals with large baseline values; and (4) individuals with increased airway reactivity. Total airways resistance, measured at FRC, does not change with aging.

## Gas Exchange

The carbon monoxide diffusing capacity ($DL_{CO}$) declines with age. Early cross-sectional studies reported a linear decline in $DL_{CO}$ of about −0.1 ml CO/min/mmHg per year for men and −0.15 ml/min/mmHg per year for women.[30,31] These declines are roughly 0.5% per year. In a large representative sample of U.S. adult men, Neas and Schwartz[32] found an almost identical linear fall in $DL_{CO}$. In women, however, they found a nonlinear, quadratic decline in $DL_{CO}$ with age. After age 47 the nonlinear component was not significant, and the decline in $DL_{CO}$ was identical to that in the earlier studies. The decline in $DL_{CO}$ with age did not vary with race.

The decline in $DL_{CO}$ with age is not explained by increased nonhomogeneity of gas distribution. Measured $DL_{CO}$ decreases as the alveolar $PO_2$ increases and the venous hemoglobin concentration falls. Neither alveolar $PO_2$ nor hemoglobin concentration varies enough with age to explain the aging-related decline in $DL_{CO}$. The magnitude of the decline in $DL_{CO}$ corresponds fairly well to the magnitude of the known aging-related decrease in the internal surface area of the lung.

Although alveolar oxygen pressure ($PAO_2$) remains constant with age, arterial $PO_2$ decreases and the alveolar-arterial oxygen tension gradient ($PA\text{-}aO_2$) increases with aging (Fig. 28.10). The decline in $PaO_2$ with aging is more pronounced when subjects are studied in a recumbent as contrasted with an upright position. The most likely explanation for the decline in $PaO_2$ with aging is increased mismatching of ventilation to blood flow ($\dot{V}/\dot{Q}$) as airway closure begins to occur during tidal breathing.

## Summary and Implications for Geriatric Surgery

Aging is accompanied by readily measurable changes in respiratory system mechanics, gas exchange, ventilatory control, and respiratory muscle strength. Despite these changes, the activities of normal elderly individuals are not limited because they have substantial functional

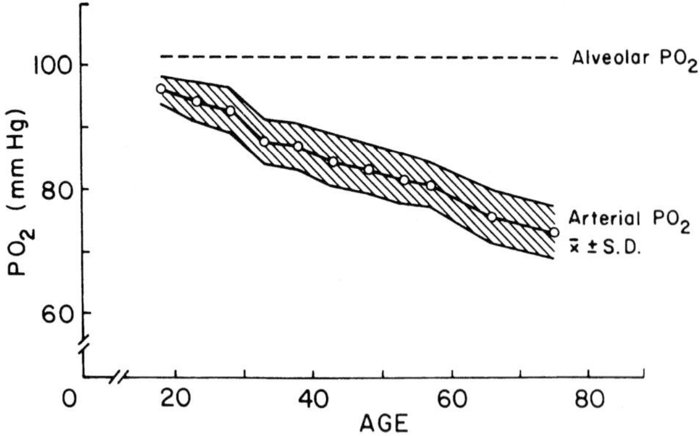


FIGURE 28.10. Decreasing arterial oxygen tension ($PO_2$) with age. The lack of change in alveolar oxygen tension is also shown for comparison with $PaO_2$. The widening alveolar–arterial partial pressure difference for oxygen results from the development of basilar areas of low ventilation/perfusion ratios due to airway closure in the elderly. (Modified from Sorbini et al.,[32] with permission.)

reserve of the respiratory system early in their lives. When anticipating operative morbidity and potential operative complications, however, the surgeon must be aware that elderly patients have lost much, or all, of their respiratory reserve. Operative stresses, pain, and bed rest are always less well tolerated by the respiratory system of elderly patients.

Changes in ventilatory control among geriatric patients deserve special attention. Because of changes in chemoreceptor function and respiratory center function, elderly individuals respond differently to hypoxemia and hypercapnia than their younger counterparts. Thus an elderly patient who is developing respiratory failure may appear comfortable and may not be tachypneic or tachycardiac. Vigilance and awareness on the part of the health care team allows detection of respiratory complications early, through measurement of oxygen saturation and arterial blood gases. Such vigilance allows appropriate *nonemergent* interventions.

## Acknowledgment

Supported in part by U.S. Public Health Service grant 46440.

## References

1. Gibellino F, Osmanliev DP, Watson A, Pride NB. Increase in tracheal size with age: implications for maximal expiratory flow. Am Rev Respir Dis 1985;132:784–787.
2. Thurlbeck WM, Angus GE. Growth and aging of the normal human lung. Chest 1975;67:3S–7S.
3. Snider GL, Kleinerman J, Thurlbeck WM, Bengali ZH. The definition of emphysema: report of a National Heart, Lung, and Blood Institute, Division of Lung Diseases workshop. Am Rev Respir Dis 1985;132:182–185.
4. Pump KK. The aged lung. Chest 1971;60:571–577.
5. Ryan SF, Vincent TN, Mitchell RS, Filley GF, Dart G. Ductectasia: an asymptomatic pulmonary change related to age. Med Thorac 1965;22:181–187.
6. Pride NB. Pulmonary distensibility in age and disease. Bull Eur Physiopathol Respir 1974;124:103–108.
7. Knudson RJ, Clark DF, Kennedy TC, Knudson DE. Effect of aging alone on mechanical properties of the normal adult human lung. J Appl Physiol 1977;43:1054–1062.
8. Turner JM, Mead J, Wohl ME. Elasticity of human lungs in relation to age. J Appl Physiol 1968;25:664–671.
9. Pierce JA, Ebert RV. Fibrous network of the lung and its change with age. Thorax 1965;20:469–476.
10. Pierce JA, Hocott JB, Ebert RV. The collagen and elastin content of the lung in emphysema. Ann Intern Med 1961;55:210–222.
11. Shapiro SD, Pierce JA, Endicott SK, Campbell EJ. Marked longevity of human lung parenchymal elastic fibers deduced from prevalence of D-aspartate and nuclear weapons-related radiocarbon. J Clin Invest 1991;87:1828–1834.
12. Mittman C, Edelman NH, Norris AH, Shock NW. Relationship between chest wall and pulmonary compliance and age. J Appl Physiol 1965;20:1211–1216.
13. Crapo RO, Campbell EJ. Aging of the respiratory system. In: Fishman AP, Elias JA, Fishman JA, Grippi MA, Kaiser LR, Senior RM (eds) Fishman's Pulmonary Diseases and Disorders. McGraw-Hill: New York, 1998:251–264.
14. Black LF, Hyatt RE. Maximal respiratory pressures: normal values and relationship to age and sex. Am Rev Respir Dis 1969;99:696–702.
15. McElvaney GL, Blackie S, Morrison NJ, Wilcox PG, Fairbarn MS, Pardy RL. Maximal static respiratory pressures in the normal elderly. Am Rev Respir Dis 1995;139:277–281.
16. Chen H-S, Kuo C-S. Relationship between respiratory muscle function and age, sex, and other factors. J Appl Physiol 1989;56:1143–1150.
17. Stanley G, Verotta D, Craft N, Siegel RA, Schwartz JB. Age and autonomic effects on interrelationships between lung volume and heart rate. Am J Physiol 1996;270:H1833–H1840.
18. Stanley G, Verotta D, Craft N, Siegel RA, Schwartz JB. Age effects on interrelationships between lung volume and heart rate during standing. Am J Physiol 1997;273:H2128–H2134.
19. Brichetto MJ, Millman RP, Peterson DD, Silage DA, Pack AI. Effect of aging on ventilatory response to exercise and $CO_2$. J Appl Physiol 1984;56:1143–1150.
20. Chapman KR, Cherniack NS. Aging effects on the interaction of hypercapnia and hypoxia as ventilatory stimuli. J Gerontol 1987;42:202–209.
21. Kronenberg RS, Drage CW. Attenutation of the ventilatory and heart rate responses to hypoxia and hypercapnia with aging in normal men. J Clin Invest 1973;53:1812–1819.
22. Peterson DD, Pack AI, Silage DA, Fishman AP. Effects of aging on the ventilatory and occlusion pressure responses to hypoxia and hypercapnia. Am Rev Respir Dis 1981;124:387–391.

23. Peterson DD, Fishman AP. Aging of the respiratory system. In: Fishman AP (ed) Update: Pulmonary Diseases and Disorders. McGraw-Hill: New York, 1992:1–17.
24. Akiyama Y, Nishimura M, Kobayashi S, Yamamoto M, Miyamoto K, Kawakami Y. Effects of aging on respiratory load compensation and dyspnea sensation. Am Rev Respir Dis 1993;148:1586–1591.
25. Quanjer PH. Standardized lung function. Bull Eur Physiopathol Res 1983;19:45–51.
26. Quanjer PH. Standardized lung function. Bull Eur Physiopathol Res 1983;19:66–92.
27. Ware JH, Dockery DW, Louis TA, et al. Longitudinal and cross-sectional estimates of pulmonary function decline in never-smoking adults. Am J Epidemiol 1990;131:685–700.
28. McClaran SR, Babcock MA, Pegelow DF, Reddan WG, Dempsey JA. Longitudinal effects of aging on lung function at rest and exercise in healthy active fit elderly adults. J Appl Physiol 1995;78:1957–1958.
29. Nunn AJ, Gregg I. New regression equations for predicting peak expiratory flow in adults. Br Med J 1989;298:1068–1070.
30. Crapo RO, Gardner RM. Single breath carbon monoxide diffusing capacity (transfer factor): recommendations for a standard technique. Am Rev Respir Dis 1987;136:1299–1307.
31. Stam H, Hrachovina V, Stijnen T, Versprille A. Diffusing capacity dependent on lung volume and age in normal subjects. J Appl Physiol 1994;76:2356–2363.
32. Neas LM, Schwartz J. The determinants of pulmonary diffusing capacity in a national sample of U.S. adults. Am J Respir Crit Care Med 1966;153:656–664.
33. Sorbini CA, Grassi V, Solinas E, Muiesan G. Arterial oxygen tension in relation to age in healthy subjects. Respiration 1968;25:3–13.

# 29
# Pulmonary Malignancies: Pathophysiology and Treatment

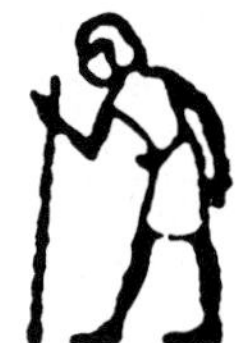

David S. Schrump

Lung cancer is a highly lethal neoplasm, with the worldwide incidence expected to have exceeded one million cases annually by the start of this millennium. Presently, it is the most frequent cause of cancer-related death in both men and women in the United States. Approximately 178,100 new lung cancer cases were diagnosed in 1997, and 160,400 deaths will be attributed to this disease.[1] Metastatic disease involving the lungs is observed in a vast number of additional malignancies, including those of gastrointestinal, genitourinary, breast, and mesenchymal origin; in some cases (particularly soft tissue sarcomas), pulmonary disease represents the sole site of distant metastases. This chapter focuses on current aspects of the pathophysiology and treatment of primary and metastatic tumors involving the lungs.

## Histology, Epidemiology, and Molecular Biology

Most primary lung cancers can be classified on the basis of light microscopy, immunohistochemistry, and cytology criteria into two major groups: non-small-cell lung cancer (NSCLC), for which surgery remains a major component of therapy, and small-cell lung cancer (SCLC), which is primarily a nonsurgical disease. NSCLCs constitute 75% of primary lung cancers and are comprised of epidermoid carcinomas, large-cell undifferentiated carcinomas, and adenocarcinomas including bronchoalveolar lung cancers. Nearly 65% of NSCLCs exhibit significant heterogeneity, with 45% of these specimens containing both adeno and squamous features[2]; minor heterogeneities (i.e., subtypes of adenocarcinomas) are observed in the remaining 20%. SCLCs account for nearly 20% of primary lung malignancies; the remaining 5% are carcinoids, sarcomatous malignancies, and unclassified neoplasms.[3]

Squamous cell carcinomas represent nearly 30% of all primary lung cancers and typically arise in lobar or segmental bronchi, often as cavitary tumor masses with intravascular invasion. The predominant histologic features include intracellular bridging, pearl formation, and keratinization. Believed to arise via progression from squamous metaplasia, to dysplasia, carcinoma in situ, and ultimately invasive neoplasms, squamous cell carcinomas occasionally arise de novo in apparently normal mucosa.[4,5]

Adenocarcinomas account for more than 30% of primary lung cancers and are typically subclassified into acinar, papillary, mucinous, and bronchoalveolar neoplasms.[3] Arising from Clara cells or type 2 pneumocytes, these tumors most often present as peripheral masses, occasionally associated with dense fibrotic scars.[6] Bronchoalveolar carcinomas are unique adenocarcinomas that grow in a lepidic manner along alveolar septa[7]; features of bronchoalveolar cancer often are observed at the periphery of more common forms of adenocarcinomas. Pure bronchoalveolar carcinomas exhibit uniform histologies with preservation of alveolar architecture. Nearly 50% of bronchoalveolar carcinomas are mucin-producing and multicentric; in contrast, nonmucinous variants tend to present as solitary lesions.[8,9] In general, nonmucinous bronchoalveolar carcinomas are slightly less aggressive than multicentric mucinous neoplasms.[8,9]

Large-cell carcinomas are poorly differentiated neoplasms lacking typical features of squamous cell carcinomas, adenocarcinomas, or small-cell lung cancers. These tumors, which account for approximately 10% of primary lung cancers, present as central or peripheral masses with extensive necrosis. Histologically, these tumors contain large pleomorphic cells with abundant cytoplasm, vesiculated nuclei, and prominent nucleoli.[7,10] Occasionally the tumors exhibit features of neuroendocrine differentiation (frequently in patients with extensive tobacco exposure) and display unusually aggressive metastatic potential.[11,12]

Small-cell lung cancers are highly lethal neoplasms that represent approximately 20% of primary lung cancers and exhibit unique molecular genetic, biochemical, and clinical characteristics that distinguish them from NSCLCs.[13] Most SCLCs present as hilar masses, often with extensive submucosal infiltration, and distant metastatic disease. SCLCs are further divided into oat cell type, mixed small-cell/large-cell lung cancer, and combined small-cell lung cancers containing adeno or squamous cell components.[14] Histologically, SCLCs are composed of cells of relatively small size with large nuclei with granular chromatin and scant cytoplasm; these neoplasms often exhibit "crush artifact," with brisk mitotic activity and extensive necrosis on pathologic examination.[14]

Small-cell lung cancers are believed to represent part of a spectrum of pulmonary neuroendocrine tumors that include typical and atypical carcinoids and large-cell neuroendocrine cancers.[11] Carcinoids most often present as central fleshy endobronchial masses, frequently causing hemoptysis, dyspnea, or postobstructive pneumonitis. Believed to arise from neuroendocrine (Kulshitsky) cells, these neoplasms demonstrate relatively uniform features of organoid growth patterns with cells containing moderate eosinophilia and nuclei with granular chromatin.[11] Atypical carcinoids are distinguished from typical carcinoids on the basis of increased mitotic activity, abnormal nuclear/cytoplasm ratios, bizarre chromatin patterns, and architectural distortion and necrosis.[15] In general, carcinoid tumors are relatively low grade neoplasms even in the presence of mediastinal nodal metastases. Surgical resection is the treatment of choice irrespective of lymph node involvement; patient survival depends on a variety of factors including stage, size of the primary lesion, lymph node metastases, atypical histology, and vascular invasion.[15–18] Although operable in the absence of gross mediastinal metastases, large-cell undifferentiated carcinomas with neuroendocrine features are nearly as aggressive as highly lethal SCLCs, which typically are not resected owing to extensive mediastinal and visceral metastases associated with them.[12]

Following the initial Surgeon General's report implicating tobacco abuse in the pathogenesis of lung cancers,[19] substantial data have confirmed that the extent and type of tobacco exposure significantly influence the incidence and the histology of these neoplasms. The relative risk of lung cancer ranges between 10 and 20 for smokers compared to nonsmokers.[20] Following smoking cessation, relative risk remains approximately 15 for 5 years, decreases to 7 between 5 and 9 years, and plateaus thereafter between 2 and 5, signifying that lung cancer risk in former smokers never returns to baseline.[21–23] Currently, 50% of all lung cancers occur in former smokers.[24] These clinical observations may be explained by recent studies demonstrating that molecular genetic changes induced by tobacco in bronchial epithelia persist despite regression of histologic abnormalities following smoking cessation[25]; clearly, many patients with preneoplastic lesions progress to lung cancer despite abstinence from tobacco.

Cigarette smoke contains 300 chemicals of which more than 40 are potential carcinogens, including polyaromatic hydrocarbons (PAH), aromatic amines, *N*-nitrosamines, benzo-a-pyrene, arsenic, acetaldehyde, and polonium 210. Most of these compounds are produced by pyrolysis immediately adjacent to the burning tip.[26] The size and depth of inhalation of particulate matter in smoke determine the sites of deposition in central or peripheral airways. Low tar (low yield) cigarettes deliver approximately 1 mg nicotine and 13 mg tar in contrast to approximately 2.7 mg nicotine and 38 mg tar delivered by cigarettes of the 1950s; reduced nicotine and tar content in current products is related to filters as well as tobacco blends.[27] Filters may reduce lifetime lung cancer risk by 20–40%.[28,29] Interestingly, smokers of low yield cigarettes often compensate by smoking more intensely and inhaling deeper, thus exposing the distal airways to more carcinogens. The newer tobacco blends have higher nitrate contents, resulting in a two- to threefold increase in nitrogen oxides and *N*-nitrosamines in smoke; one of these nitrosamines [*NNK*-(4-methylnitrosamino)—(1,3-pyridyl)—(1-butanone)] is known to be a potent initiator of pulmonary adenocarcinomas in laboratory animals.[30] In all likelihood the more intense smoking, deeper inhalation, and increased yield of nitrosamines have contributed to the increasing incidence of pulmonary adenocarcinomas noted during recent years.[31]

Environmental smoke (released from the burning tip and exhaled by the smoker) contains a variety of carcinogens, including nitrosamines, 4-amino-biphenyl, and benzo-a-pyrene, with higher levels than in mainstream smoke. Involuntary ("passive") smokers are exposed to the equivalent of one-half a cigarette per day.[32] A 25–30% increase in lung cancer risk has been reported among nonsmoking female spouses of heavy smokers relative to nonsmoking spouses of nonsmokers.[33] Environmental smoke may account for 2–3% of lung cases annually in the United States.

Epidemiologic studies have demonstrated a familial risk of lung cancer and suggest that the development of this disease at an early age (less than 50 years) may be related to inheritance of a rare autosomal co-dominant allele.[34] No clear inheritance patterns have been associated with most lung cancers typically presenting in patients more than 50 years of age. Although tobacco consumption has been implicated in the pathogenesis of lung cancer, only 10% of smokers develop these neoplasms, suggesting that complex genetic factors determine lung cancer susceptibility. At least 20 genes influence lung cancer development in mice, one of which is the k-*ras* proto-oncogene.[35] Increased transcriptional activity induced by a polymorphism within this gene renders it more accessible to mutagens in tobacco smoke.[36,37] Additional genes involved in bioactivation of chemical carcinogens also appear to contribute to lung cancer susceptibility in laboratory animals. Similar mechanisms may be relevant during human lung carcinogenesis.

The incidence of lung cancer in men is slowly plateauing due primarily to a gradual decline in smoking prevalence among men; in contrast, the incidence of lung cancer continues to rise among women, a phenomenon that cannot be accounted for solely on the basis of changing trends in tobacco consumption.[31,38] In general, women with lung cancer have less tobacco exposure than men owing to the fact that men start smoking earlier, inhale deeper, and smoke more cigarettes than women. In a large case–control study, Zang and Wynder[38] noted that the incidence of squamous cell lung cancer was much higher in men, whereas adenocarcinoma and bronchoalveolar carcinoma were more common in women. Although the mean tar yields and total number of cigarettes per day were higher among men, the odds ratios for lung cancer at each level of tobacco exposure were consistently higher for women than men (odds ratio 1.2–1.7) for epidermoid, small-cell, and adenocarcinoma histologies. Among individuals who never smoked (particularly if more than 55 years of age), adenocarcinoma was the most frequent histology; most of the patients in this category were women. McDuffee et al.[39] have observed that women with lung cancer are two to three times more likely than men to never have smoked. Furthermore, Begg et al.[40] reported increased susceptibility to second primary aerodigestive tract cancers in women.

Differences in lung cancer susceptibility associated with gender or racial characteristics may be related to genetic factors regulating tobacco metabolism. White women and black individuals have lower plasma clearance of nicotine than white men. A variety of P450 isozymes are involved in either bioactivation or detoxification of carcinogens such as PAHs, nitrosamines, and aromatic anines. Several studies have suggested that polymorphisms involving P450 isozymes 1A1, 1A2, 2E1, and 2A6, which are associated with differences in enzyme activities, may correlate with lung cancer susceptibility. The fact that some components of the P450 system pathways are regulated by androgens suggests a mechanism by which these biochemical pathways may influence gender-related lung cancer susceptibility.[38]

## Molecular Mechanisms of Pulmonary Carcinogenesis

Carcinomas of the aerodigestive tract arise via multistep mechanisms in cancerization fields. The concept of "field cancerization" was initially proposed by Slaughter et al.[41] to explain an unusually high incidence of second primary aerodigestive tract tumors in patients with oropharyngeal carcinomas; subsequent studies revealed similar risks for patients with primary lung or esophageal cancers. In 1961 Auerbach et al.[42] used conventional histology techniques to document precancerous lesions throughout the lungs of smokers, the frequency and severity of which correlated with extent of tobacco exposure. Utilizing molecular biology techniques, Smith et al.[43] and Thiberville et al.[44] observed widespread genetic defects throughout the respiratory tract of smokers; similar changes were not detected in normal individuals (never smokers). Collectively, these data demonstrate that premalignant lesions occur extensively throughout the aerodigestive tract in smokers, and that malignant transformation is a relatively rare event. Although histologic regression of preneoplastic lesions may occur following smoking cessation, molecular genetic defects remain, some of which facilitate malignant transformation several years later,[45,46] accounting for the fact that nearly 50% of lung carcinomas occur in former smokers.

Lung cancers arise via stochastic events that disrupt cell cycle regulation in respiratory epithelia. In normal cells proliferation is governed by complex interactions between stimulatory and inhibitory signals mediated by proto-oncogenes and tumor suppressor genes, respectively. Growth factor stimulation resulting from epithelial injury induces movement of quiescent ($G_0$) cells into the $G_1$ phase of the cell cycle (Fig. 29.1). Progression through $G_1$ is dependent on external mitogenic stimuli until the restriction point is traversed, when the cell becomes committed to divide independent of exogenous growth factor support.[47] Following $G_1$ phase, cells progress to S phase, where DNA replication occurs, and then proceed through $G_2$ and undergo mitosis during M phase. Checkpoints at the $G_1$–S and $G_2$–M transitions normally prevent abnormal DNA replication and improper chromosomal segregation, respectively.[48]

Movement through individual phases of the cell cycle is governed via orchestrated expression of proteins referred to as cyclins, which associate with their respective cyclin-dependent kinases (cdks) to form enzyme complexes that activate multiple regulatory proteins involved in cell proliferation. Cyclins A and B regulate progression through the S and $G_2$ phases of the cell cycle. During early to mid-$G_1$, signal transduction from a variety of mitogenic pathways is mediated via cyclin $D_1$, whereas $G_1$–S transition is regulated by cyclin E; thus D- and E-type cyclins appear to be critical regulators of $G_1$ progression in normal cells.[49,50] Perturbation of cell cycle integrity via alterations in cyclin levels or disruption of physiologic checkpoints by oncogene or tumor supressor gene mutations results in genomic instability, DNA amplification, and malignant transformation.

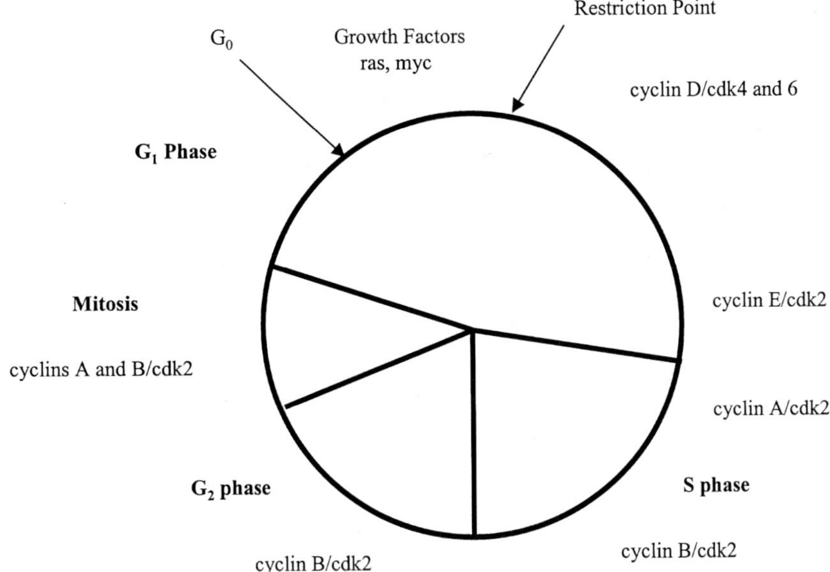


FIGURE 29.1. Eukaryotic cell cycle.

Loss of $G_1$ restriction point integrity is a common theme of multistep carcinogenesis; and a variety of oncogene and tumor suppressor gene mutations observed in lung cancers and their precursor lesions influence this aspect of cell cycle control (Table 29.1). The restriction point is regulated via the retinoblastoma (Rb) protein, which in its hypophosphorylated state sequesters $E_2F$ transcription factors (Fig. 29.2). During mid-$G_1$, Rb is phosphorylated by cyclin D/cdk4 or cyclin D/cdk6 complexes, thereby liberating $E_2F$ and enabling transcription of genes required for S phase. The *p16* tumor suppressor gene product regulates the restriction point by inhibiting association of cdk4 with cyclin D. Enhanced expression of k-*ras* by mutations directly involving this oncogene or overexpression of upstream growth factor receptors, induces expression of *cyclin* $D_1$.[51,52] The *p53* gene controls cell cycle progression in part by regulating the expression of *p21* (*waf1*), which sequesters cdk4 and cdk6, preventing their interaction with cyclin D.[53] From this simplified model it is apparent that $G_1$ restriction point control can be abrogated by loss of *Rb*, *p16*, or *p53* tumor-suppressor gene expression or by overexpression of the *cyclin* $D_1$ proto-oncogene; all of these events result in promiscuous $E_2F$ liberation. Data from cell lines and tumor specimens suggest that an inverse relation exists whereby cells that lack Rb expression tend to have normal cyclin $D_1$ and p16 expression.[54,55] In contrast, cells that retain Rb expression circumvent $G_1$ restriction point control via overexpression of cyclin $D_1$ with or without *p16* inactivation.[56] Although highly simplified, this model provides a useful framework for understanding mechanisms of pulmonary carcinogenesis and for designing strategies for molecular intervention in this disease.

## Growth Factor Receptors and Protooncogenes

A variety of growth factors and growth factor receptors are aberrantly expressed in lung cancers, some of which may be relevant to the biology and treatment of these neoplasms. Gastrin-releasing peptide (GRP) is a 27-amino-acid homologue of an amphibian hormone referred to as bombesin, which has been found in neural, bronchial, endocrine, and fetal lung tissues.[57] High affin-

TABLE 29.1. Oncogene and Tumor Suppressor Gene Mutations in Lung Cancers

| Growth factor | Oncogene | Tumor suppressors |
|---|---|---|
| Gastrin-releasing peptide (GRP) | *myc* | 3p (FHIT) |
| Transforming growth factor-α (TGF-α) | *ras* | Rb |
| Platelet-derived growth factor (PDGF) | *EGFr* | p53 |
| Insulin growth factor (IGF) | *ErbB2* | APC/MCC |
| | *cyclin D* | DCC |
| | | p16 |

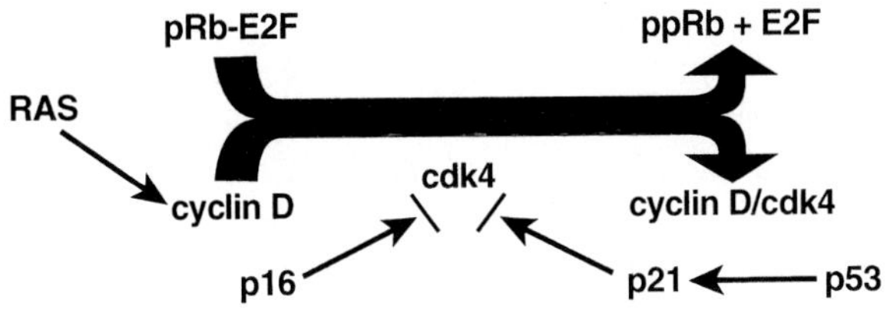


FIGURE 29.2. Regulation of the $G_1$ restriction point.

ity GRP receptors are present on SCLCs and, to a lesser extent, NSCLCs.[58] SCLCs secrete GRP, which functions as an autocrine growth factor for these neoplasms.[59] In vitro proliferation and tumorigenicity of SCLCs can be inhibited by bombesin antagonists, thus demonstrating the relevance of GRP in autocrine-mediated growth of these neoplasms.[60]

The epidermal growth factor receptor (EGFR) is a tyrosine kinase glycoprotein that is aberrantly expressed via gene amplification or overexpression of a normal or mutated receptor gene product.[61] Approximately 45% of lung cancers overexpress EGFR; nearly 60% of these tumors express transforming growth factor-$\alpha$ (TGF-$\alpha$), which functions as a ligand for EGFR-mediated autocrine stimulation of lung cancer cells.[62–64] EGFR overexpression has been observed in adenocarcinomas and squamous cell cancers; and proliferation of these cells can be inhibited by EGFR agonists. Several studies suggest a statistically significant association between EGFR overexpression and diminished survival in NSCLC patients.[65]

The *erbB2/NEU* gene encodes a 185-kilodalton (kDa) tyrosine kinase receptor molecule that is structurally related to EGFR and is present on normal ciliated epithelium, mucous cells, and type 2 pneumocytes of the adult lung.[66] Overexpression of *erbB2* has been observed in approximately 40% of pulmonary adenocarcinomas or squamous cell cancers.[67] Multivariate analysis has revealed that *p185* expression may be associated with reduced survival independent of tumor stage in patients with pulmonary adenocarcinomas.[68] Additional studies suggest that *erbB2* expression may correlate with in vitro drug resistance, substantiating the clinical relevance of *erbB2* overexpression in NSCLCs.[69]

Overexpression of platelet-derived growth factor (PDGF), PDGF receptor (PDGFR), or both have been observed in lung cancer cells; and significantly elevated levels of PDGF have been detected in metastatic pleural effusions associated with pulmonary adenocarcinomas.[70,71] Normal pulmonary epithelia do not express PDGF ligand or receptor transcripts, whereas lung cancer cells express PDGF and PDGFRs.[72] Interestingly, PDGF and PDGFR expression can be induced in epithelial tissues by trauma[73]; conceivably these molecules mediate autocrine stimulation of preneoplastic lung tissues.

Stimulation of PDGFRs induces quantitative and qualitative alterations in insulin-like growth factor-1 (IGF-1) receptors, activation of which is critical for initiating cell cycle progression in quiescent cells.[74,75] Enhanced expression of IGF ligands and receptors have been observed in lung cancers relative to normal lung tissues.[76,77] In all likelihood, mitogenic stimulation induced by epithelial injury facilitates malignant transformation by recruiting cells into the cell cycle, rendering them more susceptible to chemical carcinogens.

The *cyclin* $D_1$ proto-oncogene maps to 11q13 and is amplified in approximately 10% of large-cell and squamous cell lung cancers. Overexpression without gene amplification has been observed by immunohistochemistry techniques in approximately 50% of resected NSCLCs irrespective of histology.[78] Cyclin $D_1$ expression can be induced by *ras* mutations or by aberrant mitogenic stimuli transduced via EGFR, PDGFR, and IGFR pathways.[51,52] Several recent publications suggest that cyclin $D_1$ overexpression correlates with a high proliferation rate and poor cytoplasmic differentiation of NSCLCs, as well as diminished survival of patients with these neoplasms.[78,79] Additional studies are required to elucidate fully the mechanisms and implications of cyclin $D_1$ overexpression during pulmonary carcinogenesis.

The h-*ras*, k-*ras*, and n-*ras* genes are members of an evolutionarily conserved supergene family encoding 21-kDa proteins localized to the inner plasma membrane and that function as intermediates in a variety of signal transduction pathways.[80] Essentially all mutations in *ras* genes occur in codons 12, 13, or 61 and serve to stabilize *ras* in an activated conformation, resulting in unabated growth stimulation in part via cyclin $D_1$ overexpression.[51] Although not observed in SCLCs, k-*ras* mutations occur in approximately 40% of pulmonary adenocarcinomas, particularly those from patients with extensive tobacco exposure; only 5% of pulmonary adenocarcinomas from nonsmokers exhibit k-*ras* mutations.[81] Activation of k-*ras* is the earliest molecular event detected in mouse lung cancers induced by tobacco carcinogens; mutations involving this oncogene are observed in atypical adenomatous hyperplasias—putative precursor lesions for pulmonary adenocarcinomas in humans.[82,83] Lung cancer patients with k-*ras* mutations have significantly reduced survival relative to that of similarly staged patients with normal k-*ras* expression in their tumors.[81,84]

The *myc* gene family consists of three closely related genes (C, L, N) that encode DNA transcription factors containing helix loop helix and lucine zipper motifs.[85] Heterodimerization with another protein designated max is essential for transcriptional regulation by myc proteins, which are critical for initiating movement of quiesent cells ($G_0$) into and through the $G_1$ phase of the cell cycle.[86] Although infrequently detected in NSCLCs, aberrant *myc* expression is commonly observed in SCLCs particularly following chemotherapy exposure.[87] Individuals with c-*myc* amplification have significantly reduced survival relative to patients without c-*myc* amplification. In contrast to k-*ras* mutations, c-*myc* amplification occurs as a relatively late event during pulmonary carcinogenesis, enhancing tumor progression and metastases. Multiple mechanisms exist whereby mutations involving oncogenes or tumor-suppressor genes may deregulate *myc* expression, thus enhancing the malignant phenotype of lung cancer cells.

## Tumor Suppressor Genes

Cytogenetic analyses have revealed that lung cancers contain multiple genetic alterations. Most of these neoplasms are aneuploid with complex karyotypes; however, nonrandom chromosomal abnormalities are frequently observed in primary cancer specimens and irradiated bronchial epithelial cells, suggesting that these events may be causally related to pulmonary carcinogenesis. In addition to trisomy 7, commonly detected abnormalities include 1p, 3p, 5q, 7q, 9p, 11q, 11p, 13q, and 17p.[88,89] Using fractional allelic loss analysis,* Field et al.[90] observed that lung cancers with high fractions of allelic loss contain a preponderance of mutations involving chromosomes 3p, 9p, and 17p. Loss of heterozygosity at these three loci occurs less frequently in tumors exhibiting low frequency of allelic loss; these cancers tend to exhibit mutations involving 5p, 5q, 8p, 13q, 16q, and 19q, suggesting that different sets of tumor-suppressor genes can be sequentially inactivated during pulmonary carcinogenesis.

Deletions involving 3p have been detected in nearly 100% of SCLCs and most NSCLCs. Mutations involving 3p identified by polymerase chain reaction/loss of heterozygosity (PCR/LOH) techniques have been detected in preneoplastic epithelia; in some studies 3p allelic loss is the earliest molecular event associated with pulmonary carcinogenesis.[91] Whereas the region of 3p deletion in NSCLCs appears to cluster around 3p21, deletions in SCLCs have been observed at 3p14, 3p21, and 3p25.[92,93] The tumor suppressor genes targeted by mutations in these fragile chromosome regions have not been identified conclusively. Interestingly, a DNA repair gene that excises oxidatively damaged guanine residues is localized to the 3p25 region commonly deleted in lung cancers.[94] Recently the *FHIT* gene, involved in hydrolyzing dinucleotide triphosphates, has been mapped to 3p14.2; mutations involving this gene have been detected in a significant number of lung cancers and preneoplastic lung lesions.[95] Additional studies suggest that mutations involving *FHIT* correlate with tobacco exposure, and that loss of *FHIT* expression is associated with diminished survival of lung cancer patients.[96,97] Restoration of *FHIT* activity inhibits in vitro proliferation and tumorigenicity of cancer cells, confirming that *FHIT* functions as a tumor-suppressor gene.[98]

The retinoblastoma (*Rb*) gene is located on 13q14 and encodes a 105-kDa nuclear phosphoprotein intimately involved in regulation of the $G_1$–S checkpoint.[99] As previously discussed, the Rb protein has complex interactions with a variety of regulatory proteins including cyclin-dependent kinases, transcription factors, and viral oncoproteins.[100] Loss of Rb expression as the result of sequestration by viral oncoproteins or gene mutation disrupts restriction point control and facilitates malignant transformation.

The mechanisms of *Rb* gene inactivation in lung cancers are complex and often involve subtle point mutations that disrupt RNA splicing, resulting in an inability of the cell to express an intact Rb protein.[101] Rb expression is absent in approximately 20%, 40%, and 60% of adeno, squamous, and large-cell lung cancers, respectively, and virtually all SCLCs.[102,103]

The *p16* tumor suppressor gene product encoded on 9p21 acts to sequester cdk4, thereby inhibiting formation of the cyclin $D_1$–cdk4 complex required for Rb phosphorylation and cell cycle progression.[50] *p16* mutations detected by loss of heterozygosity or point mutations are observed in nearly 40% of NSCLCs.[104] A second mechanism of *p16* inactivation involving promoter methylation accounts for *p16* silencing in an additional 30% of NSCLCs.[105] In contrast to allelic deletions and point mutations, which are irreversible events, *p16* methylation can be reversed by agents such as 5-azacytidine, resulting in suppression of lung cancer cell growth.[106]

As previously discussed, there appears to be an inverse correlation between Rb expression, cyclin $D_1$ overexpression, and *p16* inactivation in lung cancer cells.[54,55] Typically, cyclin $D_1$ expression is normal, whereas p16 expression is either normal or slightly increased in SCLCs that do not express Rb protein. In contrast, overexpression of cyclin $D_1$ and loss of p16 expression are commonly observed in NSCLCs, in which Rb protein expression is less frequently disrupted. The relative oncogenic effects of mutations involving *Rb*, cyclin $D_1$, and *p16* during pulmonary carcinogenesis have not been fully defined. Cyclin $D_1$ overexpression, *p16* mutations, or both have no apparent effect on cell cycle kinetics in *Rb*-deficient cells, although they can be additive in cells that retain Rb expression.[56] These relations may have relevance with respect to future pharmacologic or gene therapy approaches to lung cancer treatment.

The *p53* gene located on 17p13 encodes a 53-kDa polypeptide that regulates cell cycle progression in normal and malignant cells via complex mechanisms involving sequence-specific DNA binding, transcriptional activation and repression, and protein interactions, some of which affect expression and function of other oncoproteins.[107] DNA damage from a variety of physical or chemical agents induces p53 expression. A nonspecific DNA binding domain in the carboxy-terminal region of p53 protein recognizes mutated DNA; depending on the extent of DNA damage, a sequence-specific DNA binding site in the central region of p53 mediates either $G_1$ cell cycle arrest and DNA repair, or programmed cell death (apoptosis).[108] *p53* mediates

* Fractional allelic loss equals the number of chromosome arms showing loss of heterozygosity per number of informative chromosome arms.

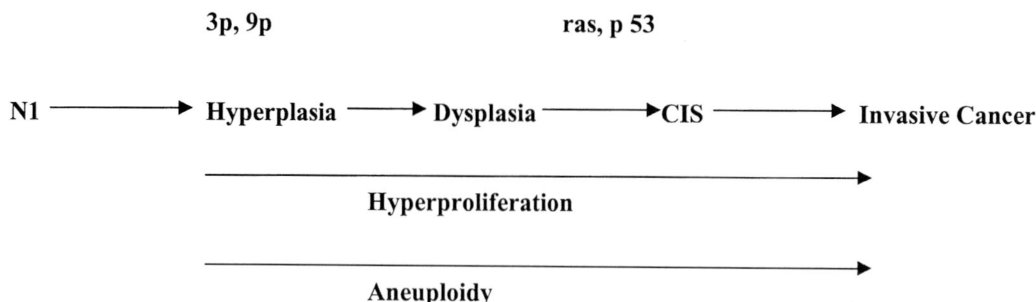


FIGURE 29.3. Multistep pulmonary carcinogenesis. Although *ras* mutations appear to occur late during squamous cell carcinogenesis, these mutations may occur much earlier during pulmonary adenocarcinogenesis.

cell cycle arrest in part by inducing expression of p21, which sequesters a variety of cyclin-dependent kinases thereby inhibiting Rb phosphorylation.[109] *p53* mediates apoptosis via induction of BAX (a proapoptic protein), which competes with BCL-2 (a cell survival protein) to activate irreversibly the enzyme pathways involved in programmed cell death.[107]

Although the *p53* gene contains 10 exons spanning an open reading frame of approximately 20 kilobases (kb), most *p53* mutations tend to occur in evolutionarily conserved residues within exons 5–8, disrupting the sequence-specific DNA binding domain.[110] Benzo-a-pyrene (a potent tobacco carcinogen) preferentially forms DNA adducts at "hotspots" within the *p53* gene, implicating tobacco exposure with *p53* mutations.[111] Molecular biology or immunohistochemical analyses* have revealed that nearly 70% of SCLCs and 50–60% of NSCLCs contain *p53* mutations. Several studies suggest that *p53* mutations correlate with metastases and reduced survival in lung cancer patients irrespective of pathologic stage.[112,113] Restoration of *p53* expression by gene therapy techniques induces cell cycle arrest and apoptosis in lung cancer cells.[114,115]

Examination of preneoplastic lesions adjacent to established cancers has provided considerable insight into sequential genetic events during pulmonary carcinogenesis. Histologic abnormalities are observed in 97% of bronchoscopic biopsies from current smokers in contrast to 25% of biopsies from former smokers; histologic abnormalities are exceedingly uncommon in biopsy specimens from never-smokers. More than 80% of biopsy specimens from smokers exhibit allelic loss at one or more tumor suppressor gene loci; multiple mutations are commonly observed in smokers less than 45 years old. Interestingly, nearly 25% of smokers exhibit loss of heterozygosity at one or more tumor suppressor gene loci in every bronchoscopic biopsy specimen. In contrast to *p16* and *p53* tumor suppressor gene loci, the frequency of allelic loss at 3p is higher in smokers than in former smokers.[45,46] The frequency of allelic loss involving 3p is greater than that for *p16*, which in turn is greater than that for *p53* or *Rb*. In general, no genetic abnormalities are identified in bronchoscopic biopsy specimens from normal individuals (never-smokers). Collectively, these data confirm that multiple genetic abnormalities are evident in smokers, some of which persist for extended periods of time despite smoking cessation. Fifty percent of histologically normal biopsies from smokers exhibit allelic loss. The sequence of genetic events correlating with histologic progression to malignancy in pulmonary epithelium is depicted in Figure 29.3.

* Mutations stabilize p53 protein expression, thereby enhancing detection by immunohistochemistry methods.

## Staging and Preoperative Assessment of Lung Cancer Patients

Histology and stage at presentation are the two most significant factors affecting survival in lung cancer patients. The major question regarding histology is whether a newly identified primary neoplasm represents an NSCLC (for which surgery may be considered) or an SCLC (for which surgery is rarely indicated). Histology may determine the extent of staging studies. Presently, NSCLCs are staged according to the modified system presented by Mountain.[116] Based on T, N, and M classifications, this staging system has been shown to correlate well with patient survival (Table 29.2). The tumor descriptor (T) is determined by the size, location, and extent of invasion of local structures by the primary carcinoma. The N factor defines regional nodal involvement, where N0 signifies absence of nodal metastases, N1 refers to disease lateral to the hilum, and N2 depicts mediasti-

TABLE 29.2. TNM Staging System for Lung Cancer

| | |
|---|---|
| Primary tumor | |
| TX | Positive malignant cells; no lesion seen |
| T1 | <3 cm diameter |
| T2 | >3 cm diameter; distal atelectasis |
| T3 | Extension to pleura, chest wall, diaphragm, or pericardium, <2 cm from carina or total atelectasis |
| T4 | Invasion of mediastinal organs; malignant pleural effusion |
| Regional lymph node involvement | |
| N0 | No involvement |
| N1 | Ipsilateral bronchopulmonary or hilar |
| N2 | Ipsilateral or subcarinal mediastinal; ipsilateral supraclavicular nodes |
| N3 | Contralateral mediastinal hilum or supraclavicular |
| Metastatic involvement | |
| M0 | None |
| M1 | Metastases present |

nal nodal invasion; N3 describes contralateral mediastinal involvement, implying systemic disease. The M factor designates metastatic disease: M0 and M1 refer to the absence or presence of distant metastases, respectively. Clinical staging often underestimates the pathologic extent of disease, particularly with regard to mediastinal nodal disease. In general, however, survival diminishes with increasing T and increasing N status within and between stages, correlating with the extent of disease.

Initial staging of suspected primary lung cancers should include posteroanterior and lateral chest roentgenograms as well as computed tomography (CT) scans of the chest and upper abdomen including liver and adrenals. In general, brain CT and bone scans are not cost-effective for NSCLC patients, as the incidence of occult metastases in these individuals is less than 5%. However, bone and brain scans should be obtained during evaluation of patients with SCLCs, as metastases to these organs occur frequently. Magnetic resonance imaging (MRI) scans typically are not indicated for staging early lung cancers, although they may be of considerable benefit during evaluation of central neoplasms invading great vessels, or vertebral bodies; they are particularly useful for staging superior sulcus (pancoast) tumors invading apical ribs, subclavian vessels, and brachial plexus.

Although it has not yet replaced CT scans for noninvasive staging of lung cancers, fluorodeoxyglucose positron-emission tomography (FDG-PET) appears superior with regard to predicting malignancy in solitary pulmonary nodules and for detecting microscopic mediastinal lymph node metastases. Dewan et al.[117] reported that the likelihood ratio for malignancy in a pulmonary nodule detected by FDG-PET was 7.1 in contrast to 0.06 when the PET scan was negative. In additional studies, Guhlmann et al.[118] retrospectively compared the efficacy of FDG-PET and CT scanning techniques in 46 individuals undergoing resection of solitary lung lesions (32 patients with NSCLCs and 14 with benign nodules). All patients with NSCLCs had complete mediastinal lymph node dissections. The sensitivity, specificity, and accuracy were 80%, 100%, and 88%, respectively, for PET, in contrast to 50%, 75%, and 60%, respectively, for CT. The absence of lymph nodes metastases was established by PET in all 12 NSCLC patients with N0 disease; metastases were correctly identified in three of five patients with N1 disease, nine of eleven patients with N2 disease, and all four patients with N3 disease. These results were superior to those obtained by CT. Similar data have been reported by Scott et al.[119] who prospectively observed that FDG-PET correctly staged the mediastinum in all 27 patients undergoing resection for NSCLC. The sensitivity, specificity, and positive predictive values of FDG-PET for evaluating mediastinal lymph nodes were 100%, 98%, and 91%, respectively, in comparison with 60%, 93%, and 60%, respectively, for CT. More recently, Steinert et al.[120] prospectively evaluated 47 patients undergoing resection of NSCLCs. The sensitivity, specificity, positive predictive value, negative predictive value, and accuracy of FDG-PET were 89%, 99%, 96%, 97%, and 96%, respectively, in contrast to 57%, 94%, 76%, 87%, and 85%, respectively, for CT. Nodal status was correctly predicted in 96% of cases by PET but in only 79% of cases by CT. Collectively, these data suggest that although false-positives occasionally occur, FDG-PET is superior to CT for predicting malignancy in a pulmonary nodule and for determining the likelihood of mediastinal lymph node metastases. Further evaluation of FDG-PET is required before this technique replaces more traditional invasive methods for accurately staging mediastinal lymph nodes in lung cancer patients.

Bronchoscopy remains the most important procedure for analysis of endobronchial extent of disease and confirmation of histology. About 25–50% of all lung cancers can be visualized by fiberoptic bronchoscopy; centrally located epidermoid, large-cell, or small-cell cancers are more accessible than peripheral adenocarcinomas, which occasionally can be biopsied via fluoroscopic brushing techniques. Frequently, fine-needle aspiration (FNA), with or without CT guidance, is the preferred technique for evaluating peripheral lesions, although nodules less than 1 cm may be difficult to biopsy.

Recent data indicate that FNA is a safe and highly effective method for histopathologic evaluation of newly diagnosed lung lesions, particularly when combined with CT guidance and immediate assessment of the aspirate. Diagnostic accuracy using optimal techniques approaches 100%, with complication rates ranging between 10% and 20%. The most frequent complication is pneumothorax.[121,122] Although this procedure may not be necessary in patients with lesions that regardless of histology will be resected, FNA should be performed in patients who are either medically unfit or refuse to undergo resection of a presumed primary neoplasm or in individuals for whom significant changes regarding management would be anticipated (i.e., SCLC vs. centrally located NSCLC). Patients with indeterminate peripheral nodules should undergo complete staging followed by excisional biopsy and definitive resection if indicated via video-assisted thoracoscopic techniques or thoracotomy depending on the expertise of the surgeon and the location of the lesions.

Nearly 70% of all lung cancers are inoperable because of extensive mediastinal nodal or distant metastatic disease. The prevalence of microscopic lymph node metastases is approximately 15% in patients with clinical stage I NSCLC.[123] In 1959 Carlens introduced cervical mediastinoscopy as a technique for accurately evaluating paratracheal and subcarinal lymph nodes.[124] Disease identified in these locations indicates stage III lung cancer for which survival may be expected to be 10–30%.[125] As such, mediastinoscopy is extremely useful for distinguishing patients who may benefit from immediate surgical resection from those who should be considered for more aggressive multimodality protocols.[126]

Because only 70% of mediastinal nodes larger than 1 cm contain metastases and because 15–20% of lymph nodes less than 1 cm contain micrometastases, mediastinoscopy should be considered during comprehensive staging of all lung cancers that are potentially resectable. The morbidity of mediastinoscopy ranges between 1% and 4%, and mortality is less than 1%; the accuracy of cervical mediastinoscopy is 80–90%. Subcarinal (level 7) nodes are the most difficult to assess accurately. Furthermore, levels 5 and 6 (aortopulmonary window and ascending aorta) cannot be evaluated by standard mediastinoscopy; these stations may be reached by extended cervical mediastinoscopy techniques (in which the mediastinoscope passes anterior to the innominate artery)[127] or by anterior mediastinotomy (Chamberlain procedure), which provides direct visual access to the aortopulmonary window via a small parasternal incision through the second, third, or fourth intercostal space.[128] Scalene nodes can be biopsied directly during cervical mediastinoscopy; biopsy of these nodes should be considered in patients with extensive ipsilateral mediastinal lymph node metastases in whom surgical resection is contemplated, as the incidence of metastases in this patient population may be as high as 20%.[129] Typically, metastases to scalene nodes represent N3 disease, for which surgery is not indicated.

Thoracoscopy was originally introduced by Jacobsen in 1910 as a means to induce pneumothorax in patients with pulmonary tuberculosis. Presently, video-assisted thoracoscopic techniques are useful for evaluating mediastinal lymph nodes, resecting peripheral lesions, and assessing chest wall or direct mediastinal invasion.[130,131] Essentially all mediastinal lymph node stations are accessible via thoracoscopy, and this technique offers a minimally invasive alternative modality for evaluating stations 5, 6, and 7 which as previously stated may be difficult to biopsy by cervical mediastinoscopy techniques.[132]

The operative staging of lymph nodes remains the gold standard against which all other staging modalities must be compared. Thoracotomy enables complete mediastinal lymph node dissection, thereby allowing precise pathologic staging of a resected cancer. Most controversies arise regarding level 10, which is classified in the Japanese staging system as a hilar (N1) station, in contrast to representing mediastinal (N2) lymph node disease in the staging system proposed by the American Society of Thoracic Surgeons. In general, metastases to station 10 behave like mediastinal, rather than hilar, nodal metastases (particularly on the right, where the mainstem bronchus is short). Ipsilateral stations 2, 3, 4, 7, 8, and 9 should be dissected for all resected lung cancers; for left-sided lesions, stations 5 and 6 should be evaluated as well. On the left side, lower paratracheal nodes (level 4) may be difficult to resect completely without mobilization of the aortic arch. This technique requires significant technical expertise to avoid morbidity from recurrent laryngeal nerve injury and bleeding from the aortic arch or intercostal arteries.

Overall, the present staging system has proved useful for stratifying patients relative to extent of disease and prognosis. However, survival rates vary considerably among individuals within given stages due to heterogeneity regarding histology, size of lesions, and nodal status. For instance, stage IIIA includes patients with chest wall lesions and negative lymph nodes (T3N0) whose expected postsurgical survival may be as high as 40–50%, as well as individuals with small lesions and positive mediastinal nodes (T1N2 or T2N2) in whom survival may be less than 10%.[133] Patients with carcinomas involving multiple nodal stations, extracapsular disease, or metastases within the highest resected nodes have significantly worse prognoses relative to individuals with less extensive nodal metastases. Furthermore, patients with stage IIIB also represent a heterogeneous group of individuals having tumors associated with malignant effusion or involvement of the aorta, pulmonary artery, superior vena cava (SVC), atrium, carina, or esophagus (T4 lesions) as well as contralateral (N3) nodal disease. Lung cancers associated with documented malignant effusions or contralateral nodal metastases are inoperable, and median survival for patients with these neoplasms is approximately 12 months. However, resection in properly selected patients with T4 lesions (i.e., those with SVC or atrial involvement or with carinal neoplasms without mediastinal lymph node metastases) results in 5-year survivals approximating 30%.[134,135] Survival of patients with early-stage lung cancer varies considerably in relation to T and N status as well as histology. As such, a more refined staging system has been proposed to accommodate these prognostic factors (Table 29.3).

TABLE 29.3. Current and Proposed Staging Systems for Lung Cancer

| Stage | Descriptors | 5-Year survival rate (%) |
|---|---|---|
| Current system | | |
| I | T1-2, N0, M0 | 60–80 |
| II | T1-2, N1, M0 | 25–50 |
| IIIA | T3, N0-1, M0 | 25–40 |
| | T1-3, N2, M0 | 10–30 |
| IIIB | Any T4 or any N3, M0 | <5 |
| IV | Any M1 | <5 |
| Proposed staging system | | |
| Ia | T1, N0, M0 | 75 |
| Ib | T2, N0, M0 | 60 |
| IIa | T1, N1, M0 | 50 |
| IIb | T2, N1, M0 | 40 |
| | T3, N0-1, M0 | 40 |
| IIIa | T1-3, N2, M0 | 10–30 |
| IIIb | Any T4, any N3, M0 | <10 |
| IV | Any M1 | <2 |

Because of field carcinogenesis, metachronous lung cancers develop in more than 10% of patients surviving more than 3 years following treatment of their primary cancer. Survival depends on the stage of the second lesion and the interval between the first and second cancers. Staging of the metachronous lesion should follow criteria outlined above for primary cancers.

The modified staging system can be utilized for staging SCLCs, although most often the Veterans' Administration Lung Cancer (VALG) system is utilized.[13] With this staging system tumors are classified as limited or extensive. Limited disease refers to neoplasms confined to a single hemithorax, with metastases to ipsilateral or contralateral mediastinal node groups that can be encompassed in a single radiation therapy port. If pericardial effusion or distant metastases are present (as is the case in nearly 90% of all SCLCs) the disease is classified as extensive. Infrequently, SCLCs present as solitary pulmonary nodules, in which case the TNM staging classification is appropriate; survival following resection of these limited-stage SCLCs is comparable to that following resection of similarly staged NSCLCs. Staging of primary lung cancers has been comprehensively reviewed by Nesbitt and Moores.[136]

Most lung carcinomas arise in individuals of advanced age, many of whom have significant additional illnesses such as obesity, diabetes mellitus, atherosclerosis, chronic obstructive pulmonary disease (COPD), and interstitial lung disease from tobacco or industrial exposure. These co-morbid conditions may affect the ability of an individual to tolerate optimal therapy. In general, surgery is the treatment of choice for stage I and stage II NSCLCs; in addition, surgery remains the best modality for local control and potential cure for stage IIIA NSCLCs, although the extent of ipsilateral disease may influence survival, and the results of irradiation and chemotherapy approximate those obtained by surgery alone in these patients.[125] Because many individuals have at least stage IIIA disease based on clinical staging criteria, every effort should be made to rule out contralateral nodal (stage IIIB) or distant metastatic (stage IV) disease for which surgery is typically contraindicated. Individuals with lung cancers and isolated brain or adrenal metastases are unique stage IV patients who should be considered for resection of the primary and metastatic lesions, systemic chemotherapy, and radiation therapy; 25% of these patients may be salvaged with aggressive multimodality treatment.[137,138]

Because postoperative pulmonary complications represent the leading causes of morbidity and mortality after lung resection, pulmonary function tests including spirometry, carbon monoxide diffusion in the lung (DLCO), and arterial blood gas should be evaluated in all lung cancer patients for whom resection is contemplated. Although there are no absolute criteria for excluding patients from curative resection, relative risks depend on the percent predicted postoperative pulmonary reserve, predicted postoperative spirometry and DLCO values have been shown to correlate significantly with morbidity and mortality following lung cancer resection. In general, patients tolerate lung resection, including pneumonectomy, provided the postoperative percent predicted forced expiratory volume in 1 second ($FEV_1$) and DLCO exceed 40%. Both should be evaluated, as individuals may have relatively normal mechanics but extremely low DLCO values resulting from interstitial lung disease.[139] Because significant V/Q mismatch or shunt may be associated with lung cancers superimposed on chronic lung disease, any patient with $FEV_1$ less than 2 liters (or <80% predicted) in whom pneumonectomy may be required, should undergo split-function ventilation perfusion (V/Q) scanning to quantitate the amount of ventilation and perfusion to each pulmonary segment and to predict accurately the postoperative pulmonary reserve. Split-function V/Q scans should also be obtained in individuals with severe pulmonary dysfunction for whom lesser procedures are contemplated because of the significant asymmetry of lobar ventilation and perfusion that occurs with COPD. Individuals with severe obstructive airways disease should undergo echocardiography and possibly right heart catheterization with exercise and sequential arterial blood gases to determine the presence and severity of pulmonary hypertension.

Patients with borderline pulmonary reserve evidenced by spirometry or DLCO indices should undergo oxygen consumption studies, which represent the most comprehensive means of evaluating cardiopulmonary reserve.[140] In general, individuals with oxygen consumption values ($\dot{V}O_2$) less than 10 ml/kg/min have a significant risk of postoperative pulmonary dysfunction (including 30% risk of death), whereas individuals with oxygen

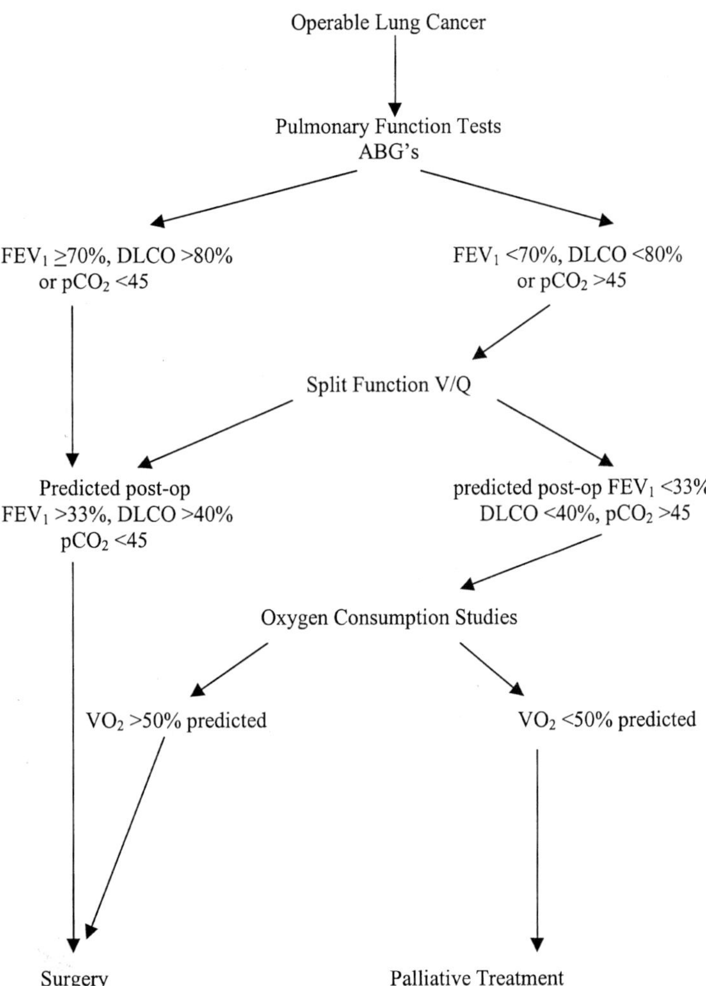


FIGURE 29.4. Algorithm for preoperative assessment of pulmonary risk. ABGs, arterial blood gases; FEV1, forced expiratory volume in 1 second; DLCO, carbon monoxide diffusion in lung; V/Q, ventilation/perfusion; $VO_2$, volume of oxygen utilization.

consumption values higher than 15 ml/kg/min have minimal risk of pulmonary complications and death. Patients with an oxygen consumption of 10 to 15 ml/kg/min have intermediate risks, and treatment should be tailored based on the likelihood of complete resection, the expertise of the surgical team, and the extent of co-morbid factors.[141]

Walsh et al. prospectively evaluated the role of exercise oxygen consumption in a group of high risk individuals with resectable NSCLCs.[142] Criteria for entry into the study included preoperative $FEV_1$ <40% predicted, postoperative $FEV_1$ <33% predicted, $PCO_2$ ≥45 mmHg, recent myocardial infarction (MI), class III angina, estimated left ventricular election fraction (LVEF) <50%, significant valvular heart disease, atrial fibrillation, or a history of cerebrovascular accident (CVA) or transient ischemic attack (TIA). No deaths occurred in 20 surgically treated patients whose $\dot{V}O_2$ was >15 ml/kg/min, whereas one of five patients whose $\dot{V}O_2$ was <15 ml/kg/min died postoperatively. The median survival was 48 months for the surgical patients whose $\dot{V}O_2$ exceeded 15 ml/kg/min; in contrast, the median survival of 45 similarly staged patients with $\dot{V}O_2$ less than 15/ml/kg treated with radiation therapy (41 patients) or surgery (4 patients) was only 17 months. These data indicate that exercise oxygen consumption studies can identify a subgroup of "high risk" patients for whom surgery can be safely performed and improved survival anticipated. The role of surgery in patients with $\dot{V}O_2$ less than 15 ml/kg/min remains to be determined by large scale prospective randomized studies. An algorithm for evaluating potentially resectable lung cancer patients is depicted in Figure 29.4.

## Surgical Management of Lung Cancer

Surgical resection is the preferred treatment modality for stages I, II, and IIIA NSCLCs. Nonsurgical management of stage I or II NSCLC using radiation therapy results in survival rates less than 25%[143,144]; as such, radiation therapy alone is rarely indicated in patients who can tolerate pulmonary resection. In general, stage III patients have limited survival (less than 14 months) following radiation therapy with or without chemotherapy. Because most SCLC patients have extensive (inoperable) disease at presentation, these individuals are currently treated with combined chemotherapy and irradiation. Although nearly 80% of SCLC patients respond initially to treatment, these individuals typically succumb to metastatic disease within 2 years of diagnosis. Comprehensive treatment of SCLCs, which is beyond the scope of this chapter, has been summarized in several publications.[13,145]

Survival of patients undergoing surgery for stage I or II NSCLC depends on the size and histology of the lesions and the extent of lymph node metastases. A comprehensive analysis revealed that survival ranged between 55% and 72% for nearly 4000 patients undergoing lobectomy for stage I lung cancer. Further analysis demonstrated that the 5-year survival for patients with T1N0 tumors was approximately 75%, in contrast to 60% for patients with T2N0 lesions. Furthermore, patients with T1N0 squamous cell cancers had postoperative survival rates of 83% in contrast to 69% for patients with T1N0 adenocarcinomas. No consistent correlation between differentiation status of the tumors and survival was observed.[146]

Similar trends have been observed for stage II NSCLCs. In general, 5-year postsurgical survival rates for patients with T1N1 tumors ranged between 40% and 63% compared to 38–45% for T2N1 tumors. Survival of stage II patients also depended on histology, with 58% survival noted for individuals with squamous cell cancers in contrast to 35% for patients with adenocarcinomas. Furthermore, survival of stage II patients was influenced by the number of diseased nodes; Martini et al. observed that patients with single N1 nodal involvement had a 45% survival rate compared to a 31% survival rate for individuals with multiple N1 nodal metastases.[147] A survival rate of 12.5% highlights the prognostic significance of satellite lesions in stage II patients; these dismal survival rates approximate those observed for individuals with stage III lung cancer. Collectively, these data indicate that postoperative survival of patients with stage I and II NSCLCs correlates with the size and histology of their cancers and the presence and extent of lymph node metastases. For reasons that are not clear, survival in these stages appears better for women than men, which is intriguing given the data suggesting increased lung cancer susceptibility in women.[38,39] Survival of patients with stage III or IV NSCLC depends primarily on the extent of nodal metastases and the size and location of the primary lesion.

The principles of operative management of NSCLC involve complete extirpation of the primary neoplasm with histologically negative margins, en bloc removal of regional (N1) lymph nodes, and thorough mediastinal (N2) lymph node dissection for staging purposes. Complete evaluation of mediastinal nodes should be performed for all lung cancers including clinical stage I lesions, as 15–20% of these cancers have micrometastases involving mediastinal (N2) nodes.[123]

As previously discussed, lung cancers often arise in elderly patients with limited pulmonary reserve and significant co-morbid conditions. Several series have evaluated the efficacy of limited pulmonary resections [anatomic segmentectomy or nonanatomic wedge excision via thoracotomy or video-assisted thoracic surgery (VATS)] relative to lobectomy in patients with stage I NSCLCs. A randomized trial performed by the Lung Cancer Study Group (LCSG) revealed that individuals undergoing segmentectomy had a 20% local recurrence rate, but overall survival rates comparable to those of lobectomy patients.[148] Warren and Faber[149] analyzed results of segmental pulmonary resection in 68 patients relative to lobectomy in 105 patients with stage I NSCLC. Although the local recurrence rate was nearly fivefold higher for the segmentectomy group, no difference in survival was noted for patients with T1 tumors treated by segmentectomy and those treated by lobectomy. Patients with T2 tumors had local recurrence rates of 22% following segmentectomy compared to 5% following lobectomy; survival at 5 years was significantly inferior in patients with T2 lesions treated by segmentectomy. More recently, Landreneau and colleagues[150] evaluated survival in 42 patients undergoing open wedge resection relative to 60 patients undergoing VATS resection and 117 patients receiving lobectomy for T1N0 NSCLCs. One-year survival and local recurrence rates were comparable for the groups. Five-year survival was decreased in the wedge resection patients primarily due to markedly inferior pulmonary reserve, which contributed to noncancer deaths in these individuals. Collectively, these studies have demonstrated that generous wedge resection (or preferably anatomic segmentectomy) may be acceptable alternatives to lobectomy in T1N0 stage I lung cancer patients with marginal pulmonary reserve. Lobectomy is still the procedure of choice for T2N0 stage I and stage II NSCLCs.

Numerous surgeons have advocated anatomic resections via video-assisted thoracoscopic methods for early-stage lung cancers.[151] Yim and Liu[152] reported their experience with 71 lobectomies, 1 segmentectomy, and 6 pneumonectomies performed for lung cancer using VATS techniques. Selection criteria included tumor size <5 cm, peripheral location without chest wall invasion, clinical stage I, and complete or near-complete fissures. One perioperative death and five nonfatal complications occurred in these patients. Kawahara et al.[153] described their experience with VATS resections noting that 3 of 11 patients in the VATS group required thoracotomy owing to anatomic considerations. Kaseda et al.[154] compared results of 36 VATS lobectomies with 32 conventional lobectomies performed during the same period, noting that the number of mediastinal lymph nodes obtained, complication rates, and short-term survival rates were comparable for the two groups. Iwasaki et al.[155] also demonstrated that mediastinal lymphadenectomy performed using VATS techniques is comparable to that achieved by thoracotomy.

Collectively, these data suggest that VATS lobectomy with mediastinal lymph node dissection may be an alternative to conventional lobectomy for stage I NSCLC. In experienced hands, complication rates including bleeding, prolonged air leak, and chest tube drainage, are similar to those recorded for conventional lobectomy. However, port site recurrence and long-term survival data for VATS procedures are not available. Although postoperative pain may be diminished in patients undergoing a VATS resection, routine use of optimal analgesic modalities [i.e., thoracic epidural analgesia or intravenous patient-controlled analgesia (PCA)] tend to negate the relevance of this issue. Furthermore, VATS procedures cannot be advocated for resection of large or central neoplasms (most lung cancers), which tend to be technically challenging during thoracotomy because of involvement of the chest wall, pulmonary vessels, or obliteration of fissures. Anatomic resection by VATS does not improve resectability in patients with marginal pulmonary reserve; in contrast, resectability of central lesions may be increased by thoracotomy, which enables utilization of bronchoplasty or arterioplasty techniques that preserve lung parenchyma without compromising patient survival. Thus the role of VATS in lung cancer resection has yet to be defined.

The treatment of stage III lung cancer has undergone considerable evolution during recent years. Comprehensive analysis of data from more than 1000 patients undergoing surgery for stage IIIA NSCLC reveals survival rates of 14–30%, with most series reporting rates of 10–15%.[125,133,156] Median survival for patients with clinically evident nodes (IIIA or IIIB) is approximately 12–14 months. Adjuvant chemotherapy has no proven benefit in patients with completely resected stage III lung cancer; and although adjuvant radiation therapy enhances local control, it does not improve long-term survival in these individuals.

During the 1980s considerable efforts were made to improve survival of stage IIIA patients by administering preoperative chemotherapy. The rationale for the use of induction (neoadjuvant) therapy was derived from the Goldie–Coldman hypothesis, which states that chemoresistance due to spontaneous mutations in cancer cells increases with tumor burden.[157] Additional factors supporting the use of induction therapy include improved drug delivery to the mediastinum via the microvasculature (which had not yet been disrupted by surgery) and a potential decrease in the number and viability of cancer cells shed from a tumor during resection. Initial nonrandomized phase II studies involving more than 450 patients revealed response rates of 50–75%, resectability rates of 65–90%, median survival of 13–22 months, and survival rates ranging between 17% and 40%.[158–160]

In 1994 Rosell et al.[133] reported results of a randomized trial comparing preoperative chemotherapy and surgery with surgery alone in 60 patients with stage IIIA NSCLC. Patients were randomly allocated to receive three cycles of mitomycin, ifosfamide, and cisplatin followed by surgery, or to surgery alone. Patients in the two groups were comparable in terms of histology and TNM status. Response to chemotherapy was 60%; median survival was 26 months for patients receiving induction chemotherapy compared to 8 months for patients treated with surgery alone. Disease-free survival was 20 months in the induction chemotherapy group versus 5 months in the surgery-alone group. The trial was terminated prematurely on the basis of ethical considerations due to the large survival difference between the two groups. Subsequent analysis revealed that significantly more cancers in the surgery-alone group contained k-*ras* mutations, which could account in part for the extremely poor survival noted in the noninduction therapy patients.[81,161]

In a subsequent study, Roth et al.[156] reported results of a randomized trial comparing perioperative chemotherapy (cyclophosphamide/etoposide/cisplatin: two cycles preoperatively and one cycle postoperatively) and surgery versus surgery alone in 60 stage IIIA NSCLC patients. Major response to chemotherapy was 35%. Patients treated with perioperative chemotherapy and surgery had an estimated median survival of 64 months compared to 11 months for patients treated with surgery alone. The estimated 3-year survival rates were 56% for the chemosurgery group and 15% for the surgery-alone group. This trial was also terminated early on ethical grounds because of the statistical significance of the data. Collectively, these two randomized trials support the use of perioperative chemotherapy in patients with resectable stage IIIA NSCLCs. Long-term follow-up is necessary to verify the provocative early results of these two trials.

Based on data from nonrandomized trials conducted during the 1980s, several more recent studies have evaluated the efficacy of combined induction chemotherapy and radiation therapy in patients with stage III NSCLCs. Favaretto et al.[162] treated 24 stage IIIA patients and 15 stage IIIB patients with two cycles of cisplatin/etoposide with concurrent radiation therapy (2560 cGy per cycle). Significant hematologic toxicity was observed, and 50% of the patients required delay between the first and second cycles of therapy. The overall response was 67%, with a 16% complete response rate. Fourteen stage IIIA and six stage IIIB patients underwent resection following induction therapy. Pathologic complete response (CR) was observed in 3 patients (14%), microscopic disease was noted in 8 patients (38%), and macroscopic disease was detected in 10 patients (48%). Of the 23 individuals achieving CR by multimodality treatment, 5 experienced subsequent local recurrence and 11 relapsed at distant sites. The overall median survival was 16 months, and the 5-year survival was 15%. Patients with resection had a median survival of 21 months compared to 10 months for those without resection. No survival difference between stage IIIA and IIIB patients was observed in this trial.

In an additional study, Choi et al.[163] evaluated the impact of induction chemotherapy with concurrent radiation therapy in 42 patients with Stage IIIA NSCLCs. Patients received two cycles of cisplatin, vinblastine, 5-fluorouracil (5-FU) with concurrent radiation therapy (total dose 4200 cGy), and an additional cycle of chemotherapy without irradiation postoperatively. Significant toxicities included esophagitis, myelosuppression, and neutropenic sepsis; however, overall treatment-related mortality was only 7%. Ninety-three percent of patients underwent resection. The 3- and 5-year survival rates were 67% and 37%, respectively. Downstaging from N2 to N1 disease was observed in 33% of patients, whereas downstaging from N2 to N0 was seen in 24% of individuals. The impact of downstaging with respect to survival was significant, with survival rates of 79%, 42%, and 18% observed for patients with posttreatment pathologic N0, N1, or N2 disease, respectively.

Collectively, data for stage III (N2) NSCLC demonstrate that 5-year survival following surgery alone ranges between 10% and 30% (most studies report survivals closer to 15%). Survival for stage III patients receiving radiation with or without chemotherapy yields comparable results. Recent studies suggest improved survival of these individuals following aggressive multimodality treatment including chemotherapy, irradiation, and surgery.[164] Additional prospective studies will be required to fully ascertain the importance of each of these modalities in achieving long-term survival of patients with locally advanced lung cancer.

Because available data support multimodality treatment for stage III lung cancers, it is logical to think that induction chemotherapy may be efficacious in patients undergoing resection of T2N0 stage I or stage II NSCLCs.[165] As previously discussed, survival of patients with early lung cancers may be as low as 40% depending on specific prognostic factors. Cote et al.[166] observed occult bone marrow metastases in 29% of patients with stage I or II NSCLCs and 46% of patients with stage III disease. Stage I and II patients with occult bone marrow metastases had significantly diminished disease-free intervals and overall survival rates relative to similarly staged individuals without marrow metastases. These data clearly explain why complete resection of early lung cancers cannot guarantee cure. As such, although it cannot be advocated as standard care, induction therapy should be considered for patients with high risk stage I (T2, adeno) and stage II lung cancers. Multicenter trials are currently under way to examine this issue.

In summary, lung cancer is the leading cause of cancer-related deaths in men and women in the United States. It will constitute a major health problem well into the new millenium. Most lung cancers are incurable at presentation owing to ineffective agents for systemic therapy. Surgery remains the primary treatment modality for patients with stage I, II, and IIIA NSCLCs. The roles of chemotherapy and irradiation as induction or adjuvant modalities for stages I to III NSCLCs have yet to be fully defined.

Most lung cancers are preventable, as they are caused by cigarette smoking. Although the genetic basis of lung cancer susceptibility may ultimately be elucidated, considerable emphasis must be placed on tobacco abstinence, particularly in adolescents, who are targeted by tobacco companies.

Continued analysis of multistep lung carcinogenesis may reveal novel genetic defects that can be targeted using pharmacologic agents or gene therapy techniques. Recent trials involving retroviral or adenoviral delivery of *p53*[167,168] demonstrate the potential of gene replacement in lung cancer. Ongoing analysis of immune recognition in lung cancer patients may facilitate immunologic approaches to the treatment and prevention of lung cancer.[169]

## Pulmonary Metastases

Pulmonary metastases occur in 20–54% of patients dying from extrathoracic malignancies, and approximately 15–25% of all such patients have metastases confined to the lungs.[170,171] Primary tumors metastasize via hematogenous or lymphatic routes to the right heart, where they embolize into the pulmonary arterial circulation. Typically, tumor emboli are 100–200 μm in size and become lodged in spaces between bronchovascular bundles of the secondary pulmonary lobules and the perilobular structures. Preferential growth of cancer cells in distant organs correlates with distinct patterns of adhesion molecule expression and the ability of these cells to induce neovascularization.[172,173] Primary and secondary lung neoplasms derive significant nutrient support from the bronchial arterial circulation.[174,175]

In 1930 Torek resected a right lower lobe metastasis from a patient 2 years after she had undergone a hysterectomy for a uterine adenocarcinoma.[176] In 1947 Alexander and Haight[177] reported 24 pulmonary resections for metastatic disease; eight patients had sarcomas, and 16 had carcinomas. Six of eight sarcoma patients, and 6 of 16 carcinoma patients were rendered free of disease by surgery alone. One patient was a 22-year-old woman who initially underwent several resections of a locally recurrent upper extremity sarcoma. Two years later she developed a pulmonary metastasis treated by right lower lobectomy, and approximately 1 year later she underwent a left upper lobectomy for a second solitary pulmonary recurrence; she remained free of disease thereafter. On the basis of their experience, Alexander and Haight defined criteria for pulmonary metastasectomy that included control of the primary tumor, no extrapulmonary metastases, and the ability of the patient to tolerate the proposed resection. These criteria remain valid today for selecting patients with metastatic disease who might benefit from surgical resection.

In 1953 Mannix[178] performed a basilar segmentectomy and a lingular wedge resection to remove six metastases from a patient with a history of tibial osteochondroma, rendering the individual free of disease. Shortly thereafter, Gliedman et al.[179] reported their experience with wedge resection in 29 patients (11 with sarcomas and 18 with carcinomas). Of the 29 patients, 6 had incomplete resections. Overall, the 3-year survival was 20% in this study.

In 1965 Thomford et al.[180] reported their results of a 21-year experience with pulmonary metastasectomy at the Mayo Clinic. A total of 221 operations were performed in 201 patients; 80% had carcinomas, and 20% had sarcomas. Of 185 patients for whom follow-up could be documented, survivals were 77%, 39%, and 30% at 1, 3, and 5 years, respectively. Survival of patients with multiple metastases was approximately equal to that for patients undergoing resection of solitary metastases. These data confirmed a favorable outcome for patients after complete metastasectomy with parenchyma-sparing techniques. Collectively, these initial reports demonstrated the potential efficacy of pulmonary metastasectomy in patients with a variety of primary malignancies.

Although sarcoma metastases are rarely associated with mediastinal lymph node involvement, nodal metastases are often observed in association with metastases from colon, breast, renal, and thyroid malignancies. Furthermore, recurrence of sarcomas following pulmonary metastasectomy is most often in the lungs, whereas recurrence of other malignancies (e.g., carcinomas and melanomas) often involves extrapulmonary sites.

Because the deposition of tumor emboli is dependent on blood flow characteristics, most pulmonary metastases are located in peripheral regions of the lower lobes. As such, most pulmonary metastases are asymptomatic. If present, symptoms usually are due to advanced disease with pleural or endobronchial involvement or cardiopulmonary insufficiency due to compression or diffuse metastatic disease.

Currently, the surgical approach to pulmonary metastases depends on the size, number, and location of these lesions.[181] In general, posterolateral muscle-sparing thoracotomy provides excellent exposure to all aspects of the hemithorax and enables palpation of lesions 1–2 mm in diameter, which are not detected by conventional CT scanning techniques; sequential thoracotomies are required to treat bilateral disease. Median sternotomy allows access to both lung fields and is particularly good for resection of lesions in anterior aspects of the upper lung fields; left lower lobe and central regions are difficult to assess well using this approach. The clam-shell incision (bilateral anterior thoracotomies with lateral sternotomy) allows access to both hemithoraces and is well tolerated. Because survival following metastasectomy depends on complete resection, the role of VATS for treating pulmonary metastases may be limited because it is difficult to resect deep lesions and does not allow palpation of the lungs for identifying subclinical metastases.[182] Although there is no proof that survival of patients with occult metastases is inferior to those without undetected disease, it is likely that resection of all disease not detected by CT scans, prolongs the disease-free interval and decreases the likelihood of recurrent metastatic disease. Gundry et al.[183] observed microscopic foci of tumor cells adjacent to resected pulmonary nodules, noting recurrent disease in 92% of patients with microscopic residual disease, in contrast to only 40% of patients who had no obvious microscopic disease adjacent to their nodules. Furthermore, pulmonary parenchymal and port-site recurrences have been reported following VATS resection of pulmonary malignancies,[184,185] possibly due to manipulation of tissue during application of stapling devices. With current modalities for pain management during thoracic surgery, including PCA narcotics and epidural analgesia, the surgical approach to pulmonary metastases should be dictated by the anatomy of the metastatic process and the goal of complete resection.

Prior to the era of chemotherapy, nearly 80% of patients undergoing amputation for osteogenic sarcoma eventually developed bilateral pulmonary metastases, many of whom succumbed to isolated pulmonary disease, suggesting that pulmonary micrometastases are present in most patients with localized sarcomas. The utilization of pulmonary metastasectomy as an integral component of the multimodality treatment of sarcoma patients was stimulated by the observation by Martini et al.[186] that osteogenic sarcoma patients rendered free of disease following pulmonary metastasectomy had a 45% three-year survival if the primary site was controlled. These observations have been confirmed by Putnam et al.,[187] who evaluated 80 patients entered onto prospective trials at the National Cancer Institute. Thirty-nine patients underwent pulmonary resection with an actuarial 5-year survival of 40%. Similar data were reported by Goorin et al.,[188] who noted an 82% disease-free survival in patients with complete resections compared to only 13% disease-free survival in those with incomplete resections at a median follow-up of 42 months; a 32% five-year survival following complete metastasectomy was observed in the study. Comparable results have been observed following pulmonary metastasectomy in patients with primary soft tissue sarcomas.

Although chemotherapy may conceivably reduce the number of micrometastases, response to chemotherapy does not necessarily correlate with prolongation of survival following complete resection of isolated pulmonary metastases. In a retrospective study, Lanza et al.[189] evaluated 24 sarcoma patients undergoing chemotherapy followed by pulmonary metastasectomy. Time from initiation of treatment to surgery ranged from 1 to 57 months. Five patients had a radiographic complete response, but their disease recurred 5–57 months later. Seven patients had partial responses, and 12 patients had either no response or disease progression. Patients with resections had a median survival of 30 months and an actuarial 5-year survival of 25%; survival could not be predicted on the basis of the chemotherapy response. Despite these data, sarcoma patients with resectable lesions should be evaluated in the context of multidisciplinary protocols involving administration of chemotherapeutic agents intended to control micrometastatic disease, which in all likelihood contributes to the failure of metastasectomy in most patients with soft tissue sarcomas. In the absence of a documented benefit of salvage chemotherapy in these individuals, reoperative pulmonary resections should be considered for all patients with recurrent sarcomatous pulmonary metastases, provided the resection criteria previously outlined are fulfilled. Pogrebniak et al.[190] evaluated 43 patients undergoing repeat resections for sarcomatous metastases. Of the 43 patients, 72% were rendered free of disease following a second thoracotomy, with a median survival of 25 months compared to 10 months for those with unresectable lesions. Operative mortality was 0%. Complete resection and disease-free interval of more than 1.5 years between thoracotomies appeared to correlate with prolonged survival.

Extensive experience in large centers confirms the role of pulmonary resection for the treatment of sarcomatous pulmonary metastases. Overall, the age, gender, histology, disease-free interval, and number of metastases have not correlated consistently with survival duration in these patients. Because 60–80% of patients with pulmonary metastases ultimately fail therapy, evaluation of new systemic chemotherapeutic regimens should continue in an attempt to enhance long-term survival of these individuals.

Approximately 20% of patients undergoing potentially curative resection for colorectal cancers develop distant metastases in the absence of local recurrences; yet only 2% of these patients have isolated pulmonary metastases. Thus the results of pulmonary resection in patients with colorectal metastases are derived from a cohort of highly selected individuals. In a large retrospective review, McCormack et al.[191] reported their experience involving 287 patients undergoing pulmonary resection for colorectal metastases during a 30-year period at Memorial Sloan-Kettering Cancer Center. Altogether, 230 patients had unilateral metastases, of whom 165 had solitary lesions; 57 patients had bilateral disease, 10 of whom had single metastases in each lung. Patients undergoing complete metastasectomy had 40% five-year survival; no obvious correlations between initial stage of the primary tumor, disease-free interval, or synchronous versus metachronous lesions and survival were noted in this study. Interestingly, 36 of 80 patients undergoing mediastinal lymph node dissection had evidence of nodal metastases, a situation much different from that seen in sarcoma patients, in whom the frequency of nodal metastases is considerably lower.

In additional studies, Okimura et al.[192] analyzed 159 patients with colorectal metastases. The overall 5-year survival was 40%. They identified three prognostic factors that correlated with survival: lung as the first site of metastatic disease, solitary metastasis, and no hilar or mediastinal lymph node metastases. The 5-year survival for patients fulfilling all criteria was 62% compared to 22% for those failing to meet one or more criteria. Girard et al.[193] evaluated results of pulmonary metastasectomy in 86 patients with colorectal cancer. The overall 5-year survival was 25%; site of the primary tumor, disease-free interval, and previous resection of hepatic metastases did not correlate with survival. Multivariate analyses revealed that complete resection and a normal preoperative carcinoembryonic antigen (CEA) level were associated with prolonged survival. McAfee et al.[194] evaluated 139 consecutive patients undergoing resection at the Mayo Clinic, noting a 5-year overall survival of 30%. Lymph node metastases were observed in 10% of patients. Survival of individuals undergoing repeat thoracotomy for recurrent disease or having pulmonary metastasectomy following resection of liver metastases was 30% as well. Collectively, these studies demonstrate the efficacy of pulmonary metastasectomy in patients with colorectal cancer provided extrapulmonary sites of disease are controlled. Because there is no documented role of chemotherapy in metastatic colorectal cancer, all patients with potentially resectable pulmonary metastases should be considered for surgical intervention.

A number of studies have addressed the role of pulmonary resections in patients with metastatic renal cell carcinoma, and data indicate that 5-year survival rates of 35–60% can be achieved in properly selected individuals. Pogrebniak et al.[195] evaluated the results of 23 patients undergoing 28 pulmonary resections for metastatic renal cell carcinoma, 18 of whom had received prior interleukin-2 (IL-2)-based immunotherapy. Survival following resection was in excess of 49 months (median survival was not reached at the time of the report), in contrast to 16 months for patients not rendered free of disease following surgical resection. Survival of individuals with complete resection did not depend on synchronous versus metachronous presentation of metastases, number of nodules resected, or previous immunotherapy. More recently, Kavolius et al.[196] retrospectively reviewed the results of pulmonary metastasectomy for renal carcinoma performed during a 13-year period at Memorial Sloan-Kettering Cancer Center. The 5-year survival of 141 patients having complete resection was 44%, compared to 14% and 11%, respectively, for 70 patients undergoing incomplete resection or medical therapy alone. Survival rates of 110 patients undergoing second and third metastasectomies were approximately 45%. Multivariate analysis revealed that favorable predictors of survival were single sites of first recurrence, complete metastasectomy, and metachronous presentation of pulmonary metastases. Interestingly, renal cell carcinoma patients often have mediastinal lymph node metastases similar to what has been observed in patients with metastatic colorectal carcinomas. Nevertheless, these data and those by Jett et al.,[197] and Cerfolio et al.,[198] indicate that similar to patients with sarcomas and colorectal carcinomas, properly selected individuals with metastatic renal cell carcinoma can experience significant prolongation of survival after pulmonary metastasectomies.

Pulmonary metastases occur in a significant number of patients with disseminated breast cancer, and data indicate that survival rates of 35–55% can be achieved following complete pulmonary metastasectomy in these individuals. In a retrospective study, Lanza et al.[199] reviewed the results of pulmonary metastasectomy for breast carcinoma performed in 44 women during a 10-year period at M.D. Anderson Cancer Center. A total of 47 thoracotomies were performed without operative mortality. The median survival of 37 individuals with complete resection was 47 months, with an actuarial 5-year survival of 49.5%. In an additional single institution study, Staren et al.[200] evaluated the results of pulmonary metastasectomy in a large cohort of breast cancer patients at Rush Presbyterian Hospital. During an 18-year period ending in 1990, a series of 5143 breast cancer patients were evaluated, of whom 284 had pulmonary metastases; 63 of these individuals had isolated pulmonary metastases, 33 of whom underwent surgical resection (criteria for resection were not clearly delineated); 30 women received medical treatment only. The mean survival of patients undergoing resection was 55 months compared to 33 months for the nonsurgical patients. An overall 5-year survival rate of 36% was noted in the surgical patients compared to 11% for patients in the medical group. In this study and that by Lanza et al.,[199] survival was not correlated with hormone receptor status or number of pulmonary nodules resected. Although Lanza et al.[201] noted that the disease-free interval appeared to correlate with prolonged survival following pulmonary resection, no consistent correlation has been observed in other studies. However, studies by Friedel et al.[201] and Vogt-Moykopf et al.[202] suggested that the number of pulmonary nodules adversely affects survival in breast cancer patients. Whereas Lanza et al.[199] noted that a disease-free interval of 12 months or more was associated with prolonged survival following pulmonary resection, no consistent correlation has been observed in other studies. Overall, these data indicate that complete pulmonary metastasectomy improves survival of properly selected patients with breast carcinoma.

A number of studies have evaluated the role of pulmonary metastasectomy in melanoma patients. Gorenstein et al.[203] analyzed 56 individuals undergoing pulmonary resections for histologically proven malignant melanoma at M.D. Anderson Cancer Center. Fifty percent of patients undergoing thoracotomy had pulmonary metastases as the initial site of tumor recurrence. Survival was not dependent on the location of the primary tumor, Clark's level or Breslow thickness, histology, or type of resection performed; but it was statistically associated in an adverse manner with the presence of regional nodal disease. Patients undergoing resection of pulmonary metastases as the initial site of tumor recurrence had a median survival of 30 months compared to 17 months for patients undergoing pulmonary metastasectomy in the presence of locoregional recurrence. Interestingly, approximately 15% of patients in this study had occult primary malignant melanoma metastatic to the lungs. Survival in this subset of patients was similar to individuals with known primary melanomas following pulmonary metastasectomy.

In a large retrospective analysis, Harpole et al.[204] analyzed their experience with the treatment of 945 melanoma cases with pulmonary metastases. During a 20-year period ending in 1990, a series of 7564 melanoma patients were evaluated at Duke University Medical Center, of whom 945 developed pulmonary metastases, with 1-, 3-, and 5-year survival rates of 30%, 9%, and 4%, respectively. Altogether 543 of these patients had evidence of advanced bilateral pulmonary disease; 109 individuals underwent pulmonary metastasectomy. The median survival of patients undergoing complete resection was approximately 18 months compared to 6 months for patients having no resection or incomplete resection. Multivariate analysis revealed that complete resection, disease-free interval, chemotherapy, number of nodules, and absence of lymph node metastases correlated significantly with prolonged survival. The 5-year survival rate for patients undergoing pulmonary metastasectomy was 20% compared to 4% of patients treated medically. These data are consistent with those reported by Tafra and colleagues,[205] who observed a median survival of approximately 25 months and a 5-year survival of 33% in patients undergoing complete metastasectomy compared to a median survival of less than 12 months in patients having incomplete resections or medical treatment alone. Further analysis revealed patients with resection of one to four lung metastases experienced a 30% five-year survival; in contrast, no patient with more than five lung metastases survived longer than 3 years following resection. Patients with a solitary pulmonary metastasis treated by surgical resection had a 5-year survival rate of 40%. Multivariate analysis revealed that complete surgical resection and immunotherapy correlated independently with prolonged survival. Collectively, these data indicate that approximately one-third of all melanoma patients with isolated pulmonary metastases can be salvaged by metastasectomy.

Aggressive resection of metastatic lesions for purposes of local control, palliation of symptoms, or potential cure is justified based on data reported by Putnam et al.[206] pertaining to 38 patients undergoing extended resection (primarily pneumonectomy or lesser pulmonary resection with en bloc resection of the chest wall, cava, or pericardium) for a variety of metastatic cancers. These authors noted 5% operative mortality, a median survival of 28 months, and an actuarial 5-year survival of 25%. These data and those reported by Schrump,[207] suggest that extended resections can be performed in properly selected metastatic disease individuals with acceptable mortality and reasonable salvage rates. As such, all patients with potentially resectable metastases should be referred to thoracic surgeons experienced in the treatment of locally invasive intrathoracic malignancies.

Because patients undergoing pulmonary metastasectomies represent relatively small cohorts of individuals with metastatic cancers, much of the experience regarding the treatment of these individuals has accumulated at large referral centers in the United States and Europe. In 1991 an international registry of lung metastases was established to assess collectively the long-term results of pulmonary metastasectomy performed at 18 institutions in North America and Europe. Recent analysis[208] revealed that 2260 patients (47%) had carcinomas, and 2173 (45%) had sarcomas; 328 patients (8%) had germ cell tumors or melanomas. Clinical staging was accurate in only 37% of patients with bilateral disease; the extent of disease was underestimated in 39% and overestimated in 25% of these individuals. Operative mortality was less than 1% for all patients entered into the registry. Subset analysis revealed that following complete resection sarcomas and melanomas had a 64% likelihood of relapse compared to a 46% recurrence rate for epithelial primaries and a 25% recurrence rate for germ cell tumors. Furthermore, most primary sarcomas relapsed in the chest, whereas most melanomas relapsed at extrathoracic sites. Epithelial and germ cell tumors were intermediate with regard to patterns of relapse. A 5-year actuarial survival rate of 68% was observed for patients with metastatic germ cell tumors; in contrast, a 5-year actuarial survival rate of 21% was noted for melanoma patients undergoing pulmonary metastasectomy. Actuarial 5-year survivals of patients with epithelial malignancies and sarcomas were 37% and 31%, respectively. Using three criteria (resectability, disease-free interval ≥36 months, solitary metastasis), four prognostic groups could be defined which correlated with median and actuarial 5-year survival rates (Table 29.4). Collectively, data analysis performed by the International Registry of Lung Metastases, confirmed the results of pulmonary metastasectomy reported in single-institution studies, providing guidelines for the treatment of patients with metastatic disease involving the lungs.

TABLE 29.4. Survival Following Pulmonary Metastasectomy

| Prognostic group | Actuarial 5-year survival (%) | Median survival (months) |
|---|---|---|
| Resectable, no risk factors | 50 | 61 |
| Resectable, one risk factor | 37 | 34 |
| Resectable, two risk factors | 25 | 24 |
| Unresectable | 12 | 14 |

*Source:* Adapted from data summarized by Pastorino et al.[208]

Despite impressive data demonstrating that some patients with pulmonary metastases can be salvaged by metastasectomy alone, it is clear that most individuals either present with or eventually develop multiple metastases that are inoperable. Although the efficacy of systemic chemotherapy for the treatment of pulmonary metastases is debatable,[209] it is conceivable that delivery of high doses of cytotoxic agents via isolated lung perfusion (ILuP) techniques may reduce the number of micro- and macrometastases while minimizing systemic toxicity, thereby enabling prolongation of survival in cancer patients.

A number of preclinical studies involving rodents and large animals have demonstrated the safety and potential efficacy of a variety of chemotherapeutic agents administered via ILuP. Methods for delivery of chemotherapeutic agents by selective lung perfusion were originally described by Jacobs et al.[210] and Pierpont and Blades.[211] Johnson et al.[212] evaluated lung perfusion using escalating doses of doxorubicin (Adriamycin) (1–10 μg/ml perfusate) in six patients with unresectable pulmonary metastases or bronchoalveolar lung cancers. Three patients underwent isolated single-lung perfusion, whereas three patients had bilateral simultaneous lung perfusions. Isolated perfusion circuits provided excellent separation of pulmonary and systemic circulations, and drug levels in pulmonary tissues increased with escalating drug doses. Doxorubicin could be detected in mediastinal lymph nodes following lung perfusion. Reversible pulmonary toxicity (pneumonia) was observed in one patient. No objective responses were noted in this pilot study in which a maximum tolerated dose was not determined.

In a phase I study at Memorial Sloan-Kettering Cancer Center,[213] five patients were treated with doxorubicin

40 mg/m$^2$ administered via single-pass isolated lung perfusion. Following ILuP, the FEV1, DLCO, and ventilation/perfusion ratio in the treated lung decreased relative to pretreatment values; pulmonary tissue levels of doxorubicin exceeded 20 μg/g tissue compared to no detectable doxorubicin in the systemic circulation. Two patients had partial responses, two had stable disease, and one patient experienced disease progression in this trial.

In another phase I study conducted at M.D. Anderson Cancer Center, Putnam et al.[214] treated 12 patients with sarcomatous pulmonary metastases using escalating doses of doxorubicin administered via single-pass isolated lung perfusion technique. Eight patients received 200 mg/ml (60 mg/m$^2$), and four patients received 250 mg/ml (75 mg/m$^2$) doxorubicin in 1 liter of crystalloid solution administered over 20 minutes. One patient experienced a major response, and four individuals had stabilization of their disease. Acute irreversible pulmonary toxicity (interstitial pneumonitis) occurred in one individual, and a second patient experienced reversible pulmonary toxicity, both of whom were in the higher dose cohort. Late pulmonary toxicity evidenced by diminution of ventilation and perfusion consistent with interstitial fibrosis was observed in several patients in this study (J. Putnam, personal communication). Extensive pharmacokinetic data have not yet been reported, although no doxorubicin was detected in the systemic circulation of any patient following lung perfusion. In this trial and those performed by Johnson et al.[212] and Mürdter et al.,[215] doxorubicin levels in normal tissues exceeded those in tumor nodules, which may account for the short- and long-term pulmonary toxicities observed following ILuP with doxorubicin.

Pass et al.[216] used isolated lung perfusion with tumor necrosis factor (TNF) and moderate hyperthermia in 15 patients with pulmonary metastases from a variety of malignancies. There were no operative deaths, and reduction of disease (not meeting criteria for a partial response) was observed in three patients in this study. One patient experienced reversible pulmonary toxicity (interstitial pneumonitis) requiring mechanical ventilation.

In a more recent study, Ratto et al.[217] delivered cisplatin (200 mg/m$^2$) to six patients with sarcomatous pulmonary metastases via 60-minute normothermic ILuP. Two patients developed reversible interstitial pneumonitis, one of whom required mechanical ventilatory support. No systemic toxicity was observed. Total platinum concentrations in pulmonary and systemic plasma were 12.8 ± 5.6 and 0.3 ± 0.2 mg/ml, respectively. Cisplatin levels in normal lung and metastatic lesions were comparable, ranging between 60 and 70 μg/g tissue. In all likelihood, the low protein content of the perfusate (approximately one-seventh that of normal serum) enhanced drug delivery via ILuP. Indices of interstitial injury (notably DLCO, PO2, and PCO2 assessed at 10, 30, and 90 days postoperatively) were essentially unchanged. (DLCO was slightly reduced commensurate with pulmonary metastasectomy, which was performed subsequent to the ILuP.) Response to therapy was not evaluated in this trial.

The aforementioned studies confirm the potential benefits of isolated lung perfusion, including intensification of drug delivery to the lungs with minimal systemic toxicity and optimization of subsequent therapy on the basis of drug levels and biochemical endpoints in perfused lung tissues. However, a major limitation of ILuP presently relates to the apparent lack of specificity with regard to uptake and cytotoxicity of drugs in normal lung tissues relative to metastatic lesions. This phenomenon has been well substantiated for doxorubicin[215,218]; additional agents such as melphalan or TNF may be expected to have limited use in isolated lung perfusion owing to their potential for significant interstitial pneumonitis. Attempts must be made in the future to reduce pulmonary toxicity via evaluation of pharmaceuticals with improved therapeutic profiles, including proactive drugs selectively activated in tumor tissues,[215] and identification of medicines specifically intended to protect the normal pulmonary parenchyma without inhibiting the tumoricidal activity of chemotherapeutic agents.[219] Furthermore, conventional techniques in which perfusate is administered antegrade via the pulmonary artery may not be optimal with respect to delivery of drug to primary or secondary lung neoplasms, which often derive their blood supply primarily from the bronchial artery (systemic) circulation[174,175]; selective bronchial artery infusion of chemotherapeutic agents can significantly reduce the size of lung neoplasms.[220] Conceivably, administration of a drug in a retrograde manner under steady perfusion pressure may enhance delivery of the drug to tumor masses via collaterals between the pulmonary and bronchial veins and overcome interstitial pressures within solid tumor masses that impede uptake of the drug.[221] These issues must be kept in mind as ILuP trials are commenced to ensure maximum therapeutic benefit of limited but intense exposure of the lungs to cytotoxic agents.

Based on pharmacokinetic and toxicity data derived using a large animal model,[222] an ILuP protocol utilizing retrograde perfusion of escalating doses of paclitaxel has been initiated at the National Cancer Institute (D.S.S., Principal Investigator). Paclitaxel is an attractive agent for use in ILuP given its ability to induce $G_2$–M arrest and apoptosis in a variety of epithelial malignancies, sarcomas, and melanomas and its apparent lack of toxicity in normal cells. Matsuoka et al.[223] evaluated in vitro proliferation and cell cycle kinetics of gastric carcinoma cells and normal fibroblasts following taxol exposure. Paclitaxel mediated dose-dependent growth inhibition as well as $G_2$–M arrest in gastric cancer cells; however, no significant growth inhibition or cell cycle perturbations were observed in normal fibroblasts exposed to similar taxol doses. Donaldson et al.[224] noted a 150-fold decrease in the sensitivity of normal lung fibroblasts to taxol relative to cancer cells.

Continuous taxol exposure induces $G_2$–M block in proliferating cells and inhibits $G_0$–$G_1$ transit in quiescent cells[224,225]; 1 hour of treatment also may be cytotoxic by mechanisms that have not yet been fully elucidated.[227] Donaldson et al.[224] demonstrated that synchronized cells emerging from quiescence were highly sensitive to taxol during early $G_1$ and $G_2$–M phases. In contrast, actively cycling cells were relatively resistant to taxol during $G_1$ but thereafter exhibited increasing sensitivity as they progressed through S phase into $G_2$–M. In addition to forming asters during mitosis, taxol facilitates tubulin bundling throughout the cell cycle, the extent of which correlates with cytotoxicity.[228] Induction of taxol-mediated apoptosis coincides with phosphorylation of BCL-2.[229] Additional studies suggest that paclitaxel sensitivity correlates with intrinsic levels of apoptosis in untreated cancer cells[230] and that cells containing *p53* mutations are more likely to undergo $G_2$–M arrest and apoptosis following taxol exposure than cells expressing wild-type *p53*.[231] Thus far, however, clinical studies have not demonstrated any correlation between *p53* expression and the response to taxol.[232]

In vitro data have demonstrated a steep dose–response curve with respect to taxol-mediated growth arrest and apoptosis in cancer cells; a dose response has also been observed in several clinical trials. As a result, efforts are under way to maximize the intensity of systemic taxol exposure in patients with advanced malignancies. Maier-Lenz et al.[233] evaluated the toxicity and pharmacokinetics of intravenous paclitaxel administered over 1 hour in 34 patients with incurable malignancies. The paclitaxel dose was escalated from 150 mg/m$^2$ to 250 mg/m$^2$; dose-limiting neurotoxicity was observed in two of three patients treated with 250 mg/m$^2$. No pulmonary toxicity was observed at any dose level. In patients receiving 250 mg/m$^2$, peak serum paclitaxel levels were approximately 19.2 µg/ml (approximately 23 µM). One-hour paclitaxel infusions can mediate tumor regression comparable to more traditional dose regimens but with less toxicity in patients who have a variety of solid tumors.[233–235] *Collectively, these data demonstrate that high levels of paclitaxel can be administered systemically without risk of pulmonary toxicity in patients without underlying interstitial lung disease, and suggest that this drug may have significant therapeutic potential as a chemotherapeutic agent delivered via isolated lung perfusion.*

Although paclitaxel can induce P-glycoprotein expression and multidrug resistance in tumor cells,[236] the high concentrations of Cremophor EL in which paclitaxel is solubilized may act to negate this activity. Clinical studies have demonstrated that Cremophor concentrations over 1 µl/ml have been shown to reverse drug resistance *in vitro*. Plasma concentrations of Cremophor following 3-, 6-, and 24-hour infusions of paclitaxel 175 mg/m$^2$ were reported at 1.47, 1.24, and 0.65 µl/ml, respectively.[237] Although this concentration may not be enough to inhibit drug efflux mediated by high levels of P-glycoprotein, it may be sufficient to reverse resistance mediated by the lower levels of P-glycoprotein typically found in clinical samples. Conceivably, paclitaxel administered alone or in conjunction with other drugs currently being evaluated in animal perfusion models at the National Cancer Institute, will prove efficacious in ILuP of patients with pulmonary metastases or unresectable primary lung cancers.

In summary, pulmonary metastases constitute a significant cause of morbidity and mortality in cancer patients. Pulmonary metastasectomy can salvage 25–40% of properly selected individuals. Investigation must continue to identify novel chemotherapeutic agents delivered systemically or by isolated lung perfusion techniques that can ablate the micrometastases responsible for disease recurrence and death in these patients.

## References


1. Parker SL, Tong T, Bolden S, Wingo PA. Cancer statistics, 1996. CA Cancer J Clin 1996;46:5–27.
2. Roggli VL, Vollmer RT, Greenberg SD, McGavrin MH, Spjut HJ, Yesner R. Lung cancer heterogeneity: a blinded and randomized study of 100 consecutive cases. Hum Pathol 1985;16:569–579.
3. Travis WD, T.L.D.S. Lung cancer. Cancer 1995:191–192.
4. Carter D. Squamous cell carcinoma of the lung: an update. Semin Diagn Pathol 1985;2:226–234.
5. Melamed MR, Zaman MB, Flahinger BJ, Martini N. Radiologically occult in situ and incipient invasive epidermoid lung cancer: detection by sputum cytology in a survey of asymptomatic cigarette smokers. Am J Surg Pathol 1977;1:5–16.
6. Kung IT, Lui IO, Loke SL. Pulmonary scar cancer: a pathologic reappraisal. Am J Surg Pathol 1985;9:391–400.
7. World Health Organization. Histological typing of lung tumors. In: International Histologic Classification of Tumors. World Health Organization: Geneva, 1981:1–1.
8. Daly RC, Trastek VF, Pairolero PC. Bronchoalveolar carcinoma: factors affecting survival. Ann Thorac Surg 1991:51:368–377.
9. Manning JT Jr, Spjut HJ, Tschen JA. Broncholoalveolar carcinoma: the significance of two histopathologic types. Cancer 1984;54:525–534.
10. Colby TV, Koss MN, Travis WD. Tumors of the lower respiratory tract. 3. Armed Forces Institute of Pathology: Washington, DC, 1995.
11. Travis WD, Linnoila RI, Tsokos MG. Neuroendocrine tumors of the lung with proposed criteria for large-cell neuroendocrine carcinoma: an ultrastructural, immunohistochemical, and flow cytometric study of 35 cases. Am J Surg Pathol 1991;15:529.
12. Rush W, Zeren H, Griffin JL, et al. Histologic subtypes of pulmonary neuroendocrine carcinomas: prognostic correlations [abstract]. Mod Pathol 1995;8:10.

13. Ihde DC, Pass HI, Glatstein E. Small cell lung cancer. In: DeVita VT Jr, Hellman S, Rosenberg SA (eds) Cancer: Principles and Practice of Oncology. Lippincott-Raven: Philadelphia, 1997:911–949.
14. Hirsch FR, Matthews JM, Aisner S. Histopathologic classification of small cell lung cancer: changing concepts and terminology. Cancer 1988;62:973–977.
15. Arrigoni MG, Woolner LB, Bernatz PE. Atypical carcinoid tumors of the lung. J Thorac Cardiovasc Surg 1972;64: 413–421.
16. McCaughan BC, Martini N, Bains MS. Bronchial carcinoids: review of 124 cases. J Thorac Cardiovasc Surg 1985; 89:8–17.
17. Paladugu RR, Benfield JR, Pak HY, Ross RK, Teplitz RL. Bronchopulmonary Kulchitzky cell carcinomas: a new classification scheme for typical and atypical carcinoids. Cancer 1985;55:1303–1311.
18. Bonato M, Cerati M, Pagani A. Differential diagnostic patterns of lung neuroendocrine tumours: a clinicopathological and immunohistochemical study of 122 cases. Virchows Arch 1992;420:201–211.
19. Advisory Committee to the Surgeon General of the US Public Health Service. Smoking and health. Government Printing Office: Washington, DC, 1964:1103.
20. Osann KE, Anton-Culver LT, Korosak T, Taylor T. Sex differences in lung cancer risk associated with cigarette smoking. Int J Cancer 1993;54:44–48.
21. Doll R, Peto R. Cigarette smoking and bronchial carcinoma: dose and time relationships among regular smokers and life-long nonsmokers. J Epidemiol Community Health 1978;32:303–313.
22. Freedman DA, Navidi WC. Ex-smokers and the multistage model for lung cancer. Epidemiology 1990;1:21–29.
23. Halpern MT, Gillespie BW, Warner KE. Patterns of absolute risk of lung cancer mortality in former smokers. J Natl Cancer Inst 1993;85:457–464.
24. Tong L, Spitz MR, Fueger JJ, Amos CA. Lung carcinoma in former smokers. Cancer 1996;78:1004–1010.
25. Wistuba II, Lam S, Behrens C, et al. Molecular damage in the bronchial epithelium of current and former smokers. J Natl Cancer Inst 1997;89:1366–1373.
26. International Agency for Research on Cancer (IARC). Tobacco smoking: IARC monographs on the evaluation of carcinogenic risk of chemicals to humans. IARC 1986:38.
27. Wynder EL, Muscat JE. The changing epidemiology of smoking and lung cancer histology. Environ Health Perspect 1995;103:143–148.
28. Lubin JH, Blot WJ, Berrino F. Patterns of lung cancer risk according to type of cigarette smoked. Int J Cancer 1984;33:569–576.
29. Wilcox H, Schoenberg J, Mason T. Smoking and lung cancer: risk as a function of cigarette tar content. Prev Med 1988;17:263–272.
30. Malkinson AM. Primary lung tumors in mice: an experimentally manipulable model of human adenocarcinoma. Cancer Res 1992;52:2670s–2676s.
31. Thun MJ, Lally CA, Flannery JT, Calle EE, Flanders WD, Heath CW Jr. Cigarette smoking and chages in the histopathology of lung cancer. J Natl Cancer Inst 1997;89: 1580–1586.
32. US Surgeon General. The Health Consequences of Involuntary Smoking. US Department of Health and Human Services, Centers for Disease Control: Washington, DC, 1986.
33. Schottenfeld D. Epidemiology of lung cancer. In: Pass HI, Mitchell JB, Johnson DH, Turrisi AT (eds) Lung Cancer: Principles and Practice. Lippincott-Raven: Philadelphia, 1996:305–321.
34. Ooi WL, Elston RC, Chen VW, Bailey-Wilson JE, Rothschild H. Increased familial risk for lung cancer. J Natl Cancer Inst 1986;76:217–222.
35. Malkinson AM. The genetic basis of susceptibility to lung tumors in mice. Toxicology 1989;54:241–271.
36. Chen B, Johanson L, Wiest JS, et al. The second intron of the K-ras gene contains regulatory elements associated with mouse lung tumor susceptibility. Proc Natl Acad Sci USA 1994;91:1589–1593.
37. Sithanandam G, Ramakrishna G, Diwan BA, Anderson LM. Selective mutation of K-ras by N-ethylnitrosourea shifts from codon 12 to codon 61 during fetal mouse lung maturation. Oncogene 1998;17:493–502.
38. Zang EA, Wynder EL. Differences in lung cancer risk between men and women: examination of the evidence. J Natl Cancer Inst 1996;88:183–192.
39. McDuffie HH, Klassen DJ, Dosman JA. Men, women and primary lung cancer—a Saskatchewan personal interview study. J Clin Epidemiol 1991;44:537–544.
40. Begg CB, Zhang ZF, Sun M, Herr HW, Schantz SP. Methodology for evaluating incidence of second primary cancers with application to smoking-related cancers from S.E.E.R. Am J Epidemiol 1995;142:653–665.
41. Slaughter DP, Southwick HW, Smejkal W. "Field cancerization" in oral stratified squamous epithelium. Cancer 1953;6:963–968.
42. Auerbach O, Stout AP, Hammond EC, Garfinkel L. Changes in bronchial epithelium in relation to cigarette smoking and in relation to lung cancer. N Engl J Med 1961;265:253–267.
43. Smith AL, Hung J, Walker L, et al. Extensive areas of aneuploidy are present in the respiratory epithelium of lung cancer patients. Br J Cancer 1996;73:203–209.
44. Thiberville L, Payne P, Vielkinds J, et al. Evidence of cumulative gene losses with progression of premalignant epithelial lesions to carcinoma of the bronchus. Cancer Res 1995;55:5133–5139.
45. Mao L, Lee JS, Kurie JM, et al. Clonal genetic alterations in the lungs of current and former smokers. J Natl Cancer Inst 1997;89:857–862.
46. Wistuba II, Lam S, Behrens C, et al. Molecular damage in the bronchial epithelium of current and former smokers. J Natl Cancer Inst 1997;89:1366–1373.
47. Hunter T, Pines J. Cyclins and cancer. II. Cyclin D and CDK inhibitors come of age. Cell 1994;79:573–582.
48. Sherr CJ. Cancer cell cycles. Science 1996;274:1672–1677.
49. Martín-Castellanos C, Moreno S. Recent advances on cyclins, CDKs and CDK inhibitors. Trends Cell Biol 1997;7:95–98.
50. Grana X, Reddy EP. Cell cycle control in mammalian cells: role of cyclins, cyclin dependent kinases (CDKs), growth suppressor genes and cyclin-dependent kinase inhibitors (CKIs). Oncogene 1995;11:211–219.

51. Filmus J, Robles AI, Shi W, Wong MJ, Colombo LL, Conti CJ. Induction of cyclin $D_1$ overexpression by activated *ras*. Oncogene 1994;9:3627–3633.
52. Lukas J, Bartkova J, Bartek J. Convergence of mitogenic signalling cascades from diverse classes of receptors at the cyclin D-cyclin-dependent kinase-pRb-controlled $G_1$ checkpoint. Mol Cell Biol 1996;16:17–25.
53. El-Deiry WS, Tokino T, Velculescu VE, et al. WAF1, a potential mediator of p53 tumor suppression. Cell 1993; 75:817–825.
54. Schauer IE, Siriwardana S, Langan TA, Sclafani RA. Cyclin D1 overexpression vs retinoblastoma inactivation: implications for growth control evasion in non-small cell and small cell lung cancer. Proc Natl Acad Sci USA 1994;91:7827–7831.
55. Sreekantaiah C, Ladanyi M, Rodriguez E, Chaganti R. Chromosomal aberrations in soft tissue tumors. Am J Clin Pathol 1994;111:121–134.
56. Lukas J, Aagaard L, Strauss M, Bartek J. Oncogenic aberrations of $p16^{INK4/CDKN2}$ and cyclin D1 cooperate to deregulate $G_1$ control. Cancer Res 1995;55:4818–4823.
57. Wharton J, Polak JM, Bloom SR, et al. Bombesin-like immunoreactivity in the lung. Nature 1978;273:769–770.
58. Moody TW, Carney DN, Cuttitta F, Quattrocchi K, Minna JD. High affinity receptors for bombesin/GRP-like peptides on human small-cell lung cancer. Life Sci 1985;37:105–113.
59. Carney DN, Cuttitta F, Moody TW, Minna JD. Selective stimulation of small-cell lung cancer clonal growth by bombesin and gastrin-releasing peptide. Cancer Res 1987; 47:821–825.
60. Layton JE, Scanlon DB, Soveny C, Morstyn G. Effects of bombesin antagonists on the growth of small cell lung cancer cells in vitro. Cancer Res 1988;48:4783–4789.
61. Hunter T. The epidermal growth factor gene and its product. Nature 1984;311:414–416.
62. Veale D, Kerr N, Gibson GJ, Harris AL. Characterization of epidermal growth factor receptor in primary human non-small cell lung cancer. Cancer Res 1989;49:1313–1317.
63. Rusch V, Baselga J, Cordon-Cardo C, et al. Differential expression of the epidermal growth factor receptor and its ligands in primary non-small cell lung cancers and adjacent benign lung tissue. Cancer Res 1993;53:2379–2385.
64. Wong ST, Winchell LF, McCune BK, et al. The TGF-$\alpha$ precursor expressed on the cell surface binds to the EGF receptor on adjacent cells leading to signal transduction. Cell 1989;56:495–506.
65. Veale D, Kerr N, Gibson GJ, Kelly PJ, Harris AJ. The relationship of quantitative epidermal growth factor receptor expression in non-small cell lung cancer to long term survival. Br J Cancer 1993;68:162–165.
66. Bargmann CI, Hung M-C, Weinberg RA. The neu oncogene encodes on epidermal frowth factor receptor-related protein. Nature 1986;319:226–230.
67. Shi D, He G, Cao S, et al. Overexpression of the c-erbB-2/neu-encoded p185 protein in primary lung cancer. Carcinogenesis 1992;5:213–218.
68. Kern JA, Schwartz DA, Nordberg JE, et al. p185neu expression in human lung adenocarcinomas predicts shortened survival. Cancer Res 1990;50:5184–5191.
69. Tsai C-M, Chang K-T, Perng R-P, et al. Correlation of intrinsic chemoresistance of non-small cell lung cancer cell lines with HER-2/neu gene expression but not with ras gene mutations. J Natl Cancer Inst 1993;85:897–901.
70. Heldin C-H, Westermark B. Platelet-derived growth factor: mechanism of action and possible *in vivo* function. Cell Regul 1990;1:555–556.
71. Safi A, Sadmi M, Martinet N, et al. Presence of elevated levels of platelet-derived growth factor (PDGF) in lung adenocarcinoma pleural effusions. Chest 1992;102: 204–207.
72. Antoniades HN, Galanopoulos T, Neville-Golden J, O'Hara CJ. Malignant epithelial cells in primary human lung carcinomas coexpress *in vivo* platelet-derived growth factor (PDGF) and PDGF receptor mRNAs and their protein products. Proc Natl Acad Sci USA 1992;89: 3942–3946.
73. Antoniades HR, Galanopoulos T, Neville-Golden J, Kiristy CP, Lynch SE. Injury induces *in vivo* expression of platelet derived growth factor (PDGF) and PDGF receptor mRNAs in skin epithelial cells and PDGF mRNA in connective tissue fibroblasts. Proc Natl Acad Sci USA 1991;84:565–569.
74. Rechler MM, Nissley SP. The nature and regulation of the receptors for insulin-like growth factors. Annu Rev Physiol 1985;47:425–442.
75. Pietrzkowski Z, Lammers R, Carpenter G, et al. Constitutive expression of insulin-like growth factor 1 and insulin-like growth factor 1 receptor abrogates all requirements for exogenous growth factors. Cell Growth Differ 1992;3:199.
76. Macaulay VM, Everard MJ, Teale JD, et al. Autocrine function for insulin-like growth factor I in human small cell lung cancer cell lines and fresh tumor cells. Cancer Res 1990;50:2511–2517.
77. Kaiser U, Schardt C, Brandscheidt D, Wollmer E, Havemann K. Expression of insulin-like growth factor receptors I and II in normal human lung and in lung cancer. J Cancer Res Clin Oncol 1993;119:665–668.
78. Caputi M, DeLuca L, Papaccio G, et al. Prognostic role of cyclin $D_1$ in non-small cell lung cancer: an immunohistochemical analysis. Eur J Histochem 1997;41:133–138.
79. Mate JL, Ariza A, Aracil C, et al. Cyclin $D_1$ overexpression in non-small cell lung carcinoma: correlation with Ki67 labelling index and poor cytoplasmic differentiation. J Pathol 1996;180:395–399.
80. Feig LA. The many roads that lead to ras. Science 1993; 260:767–768.
81. Rodenhuis S, Slebos RJC. Clinical significance of *ras* oncogene activation in human lung cancer. Cancer Res 1992;52:2665s–2669s.
82. Horio Y, Chen A, Rice P, Roth JA, Malkinson AM, Schrump DS. Ki-ras and p53 mutations are early and late events, respectively, in urethane-induced pulmonary carcinogenesis in A/J mice. Mol Carcinog 1996;17:217–223.
83. Westra WH, Baas IO, Hruban RH, et al. K-*ras* oncogene activation in atypical alveolar hyperplasias of the human lung. Cancer Res 1996;56:2224–2228.
84. Harada M, Dosaka-Akita H, Miyamoto H, Kuzumaki N, Kawakami Y. Prognostic significance of the expression of ras oncogene product in non-small cell lung cancer. Cancer 1992;69:72–77.

85. Koskinen PJ, Alitalo K. Role of myc amplification and overexpression in cell growth, differentiation and death. Cancer Biol 1993;4:3–12.
86. Amati B, Brooks MW, Levy N, Littlewood TD, Evan GI, Land H. Oncogene activity of the C-myc protein requires dimerization with max. Cell 1993;72:233–245.
87. Brennan J, O'Connor T, Makuch RW, et al. Myc family DNA amplification in 107 tumors and tumor cell lines from patients with small cell lung cancer treated with different combination chemotherapy regimens. Cancer Res 1998; 51:1708–1712.
88. Testa EH, Siegfried JM. Chromosome abnormalities in human non-small cell lung cancer. Cancer Res 1992;52: 2702–2706.
89. Whang-Peng J, Knutsen T, Gazdar A, et al. Nonrandom structural and numerical chromosome changes in non-small-cell lung cancer. Genes Chromosomes Cancer 1991;3:168–188.
90. Field JK, Neville EM, Stewart MP, et al. Fractional allele loss data indicate distinct genetic populations in the development of non-small-cell lung cancer. Br J Cancer 1996;74:1968–1974.
91. Hung J, Kishimoto Y, Sugio K, et al. Allele-specific chromosome 3p deletions occur at an early stage in the pathogenesis of lung carcinoma. JAMA 1995;273:558–563. Erratum. JAMA 1995;273:1908.
92. Hibi K, Takahashi T, Yamakawa K, et al. Three distinct regions involved in 3p deletion in human lung cancer. Oncogene 1992;7:445–449.
93. Whang-Peng J, Knutsen T, Gazdar A, et al. Nonrandom structural and numerical chromosome changes in non-small-cell lung cancer. Genes Chromosom Cancer 1991; 3:168–188.
94. Lu R, Nash HM, Verdine GL. A mammalian DNA repair enzyme that excises oxidatively damaged guanines maps to a locus frequently lost in lung cancer. Curr Biol 1997; 7:397–407.
95. Fong KM, Biesterveld EJ, Virmani A, et al. FHIT and FRA3B 3p14.2 allele loss are common in lung cancer and preneoplastic bronchial lesions and are associated with cancer related FHIT cDNA splicing aberrations. Cancer Res 1997;57:2256–2267.
96. Nelson HH, Wiencke JK, Gunn L, Wain JC, Christiani DC, Kelsey KT. Chromosome 3p14 alterations in lung cancer: evidence that FHIT exon deletion is a target of tobacco carcinogens and asbestos. Cancer Res 1998;58:1804–1807.
97. Burke L, Khan MA, Freedman AN, et al. Allelic deletion analysis of the FHIT gene predicts poor survival in non-small cell lung cancer. Cancer Res 1998;58:2533–2536.
98. Siprashvili Z, Sozzi G, Barnes LD, et al. Replacement of FHIT in cancer cells suppresses tumorigenicity. Proc Natl Acad Sci USA 1997;94:13771–13776.
99. Chen PL, Riley DJ, Lee WH. The retinoblastoma protein as a fundamental mediator of growth and differentiation signals. Crit Rev Eukaryot Gene Expr 1995;1:79–95.
100. Ewen ME. The cell cycle and the retinoblastoma protein family. Cancer Metastasis Rev 1994;13:45–66.
101. Harbour JW, Lai S-L, Whang-Peng J, Gazdar AF, Minna JD, Kaye FJ. Abnormalities in structure and expression of the human retinoblastoma gene in SCLC. Science 1988; 241:353–357.
102. Reissman PT, Koga H, Takahashi R, et al. Inactivation of the retinoblastoma susceptibility gene in non-small-cell lung cancer. Oncogene 1993;8:1913–1919.
103. Horowitz JM, Park SH, Bogenmann E, et al. Frequent inactivation of the retinoblastoma anti-oncogene is restricted to a subset of human tumor cells. Proc Natl Acad Sci USA 1990;87:2775–2779.
104. Okamoto A, Hussain SP, Hagiwara K, et al. Mutations in the p16$^{INK4}$/MTS1/CDKN2,P15$^{INK4B}$/MTS2, and p18 genes in primary and metastatic lung cancer. Cancer Res 1995; 55:1448–1451.
105. Merlo A, Herman JG, Mao L, et al. 5'CpG island methylation is associated with transcriptional silencing of the tumour suppressor p16/CDKN2/MTS1 in human cancers. Nat Med 1995;1:686–692.
106. Otterson GA, Khleif SN, Chen W, Coxon AB, Kaye FJ. CDKN2 gene silencing in lung cancer by DNA hypermethylation and kinetics of p16$^{INK4}$ protein induction by 5-aza 2'deoxycytidine. Oncogene 1995;11:1211–1216.
107. Kastan MB, Canman CE, Leonard CJ. p53, cell cycle control and apoptosis: implications for cancer. Cancer Metastasis Rev 1995;14:3–15.
108. Kastan MB, Onyekwere O, Sidransky D, Vogelstein B, Craig R. Participation of p53 protein in the cellular response to DNA damage. Cancer Res 1991;51:6304–6311.
109. El-Deiry WS, Harper JW, O'Connor PM, et al. WAF1/CIP1 is induced in p53-mediated $G_1$ arrest and apoptosis. Cancer Res 1994;54:1169–1174.
110. Hollstein M, Sidransky D, Vogelstein B, Harris CC. *p53* mutations in human cancers. Science 1991;253:49–53.
111. Denissenko MF, Pao A, Tang M, Pfeifer GP. Preferential formation of benzo[a]pyrene adducts at lung cancer mutational hotspots in p53. Science 1996;274:430–432.
112. Marchetti A, Buttitta F, Merlo G, et al. p53 Alterations in non-small cell lung cancers correlate with metastatic involvement of hilar and mediastinal lymph nodes. Cancer Res 1993;53:2846–2851.
113. Horio Y, Takahashi T, Kuroishi T, et al. Prognostic significance of p53 mutations and 3p deletions in primary resected non-small cell lung cancer. Cancer Res 1993; 53:1–4.
114. Zhang WW, Fang X, Mazur W, French BA, Georges RN, Roth JA. High-efficiency gene transfer and high-level expression of wild-type p53 in human lung cancer cells mediated by recombinant adenovirus. Cancer Gene Ther 1994;1:5–13.
115. Roth JA, Nguyen D, Lawrence DD, et al. Retrovirus-mediated wild-type p53 gene transfer to tumors of patients with lung cancer. Nat Med 1996;2:985–991.
116. Mountain CF. A new international staging system for lung cancer. Chest 1986;89:225S–233S.
117. Dewan NA, Shehan CJ, Reeb SD, Gobar LS, Scott WJ, Ryschon K. Likelihood of malignancy in a solitary pulmonary nodule: comparison of bayesian analysis and results of FDG-PET scan. Chest 1997;112:416–422.
118. Guhlmann A, Storck M, Kotzerke J, Moog F, Sunder-Plassmann L, Reske SN. Lymph node staging in non-small cell lung cancer: evaluation by [$^{18}$F]FDG positron emission tomography (PET). Thorax 1997;52:438–441.
119. Scott WJ, Gobar LS, Terry JD, Dewan NA, Sunderland JJ. Mediastinal lymph node staging of non-small-cell lung

cancer: a prospective comparison of computed tomography and positron emission tomography. J Thorac Cardiovasc Surg 1996;111:642–648.
120. Steinert HC, Hauser M, Allemann F, et al. Non-small cell lung cancer: nodal staging with FDG PET versus CT with correlative lymph node mapping and sampling. Radiology 1997;202:441–446.
121. Santambrogio L, Nosotti M, Bellaviti N, Pavoni G, Radice F, Caputo V. CT-guided needle aspiration cytology of solitary pulmonary nodules: a prospective, randomized study of immediate cytologic evaluation. Chest 1997;112: 423–425.
122. Stewart CJ, Stewart IS. Immediate assessment of fine needle aspiration cytology of lung. J Clin Pathol 1996;49: 839–843.
123. Takizawa T, Masanori T, Koike T, Akamatsu H, Kurita Y, Yokoyama A. Mediastinal lymph node metastasis in patients with clinical stage I peripheral non-small-cell lung cancer. J Thorac Cardiovasc Surg 1997;113:248–252.
124. Carlens E. Mediastinoscopy: a method for inspection and tissue biopsy in the superior mediastinum. Chest 1959; 36:343–348.
125. Lee JD, Ginsberg RJ. The multimodality treatment of stage III A/B non-small cell lung cancer: the role of surgery, radiation, and chemotherapy. Hematol Oncol Clin North Am 1997;11:279–301.
126. Pearson FG, Delarue NC, Ilves R, Tood TRJ, Cooper JD. Significance of positive superior mediastinal nodes identified at mediastinoscopy in patients with resectable cancer of the lung. J Thorac Cardiovasc Surg 1982;83:1–11.
127. Ginsberg RJ. Extended cervical mediastinoscopy. Chest Surg Clin North Am 1996;6:21–30.
128. McNeill TM, Chamberlain JM. Diagnostic anterior mediastinotomy. Ann Thorac Surg 1996;2:532–535.
129. Lee JD, Ginsberg RJ. Lung cancer staging: the value of ipsilateral scalene lymph node biopsy performed at mediastinoscopy. Ann Thorac Surg 1996;62:338–341.
130. Mack MJ, Aronoff RJ, Acuff TE, et al. Present role of thoracoscopy in the diagnosis and treatment of diseases of the chest. Ann Thorac Surg 1992;54:403–409.
131. Rusch VW, Bains MS, Burt ME, McCormack PM, Ginsberg RJ. Contribution of videothoracoscopy to the management of the cancer patient. Ann Surg Oncol 1994;1:94–98.
132. Landreneau RJ, Hazelrigg SR, Mack MJ, et al. Thoracoscopic mediastinal lymph node sampling: useful for mediastinal lymph node stations inaccessible by cervical mediastinoscopy. J Thorac Cardiovasc Surg 1993;106: 554–558.
133. Rosell R, Gómez-Condina J, Camps C, et al. A randomized trial comparing preoperative chemotherapy plus surgery with surgery alone in patients with non-small-cell lung cancer. N Engl J Med 1994;330:153–158.
134. Dartevelle PG. Extended operations for the treatment of lung cancer. Ann Thorac Surg 1997;63:12–19.
135. Mathisen DJaGHC. Carinal resection for bronchogenic carcinoma. J Thorac Cardiovasc Surg 1991;102:16–23.
136. Nesbitt JC, Moores DWO. Staging of lung cancer. In: Roth JA, Ruckdeschel JC, Weisenburger TH (eds) Thoracic Oncology. Saunders: Philadelphia, 1995:84–103.
137. Burt M, Wronski M, Arbit E, Galicich JH, Martini N, Ginsberg RJ. Resection of brain metastases from non-small-cell lung carcinoma: results of therapy. J Thorac Cardiovasc Surg 1992;103:399–411.
138. Luketich JD, Burt ME. Does resection of adrenal metastases from non-small cell lung cancer improve survival? Ann Thorac Surg 1996;62:1614–1616.
139. Ferguson MK, Little L, Rizzo L, et al. Diffusing capacity predicts morbidity and mortality after pulmonary resection. J Thorac Cardiovasc Surg 1988;96:894–900.
140. Morice RC, Peters EJ, Ryan MB, Putnam JB Jr, Ali MK, Roth JA. Exercise testing in the evaluation of patients at high risk for complications from lung resection. Chest 1992; 101:356–361.
141. Morice RC. Preoperative evaluation of the patient with lung cancer. In: Roth JA, Cox JD, Hong WK (eds) Lung Cancer. Blackwell Science: Malden, MA, 1998:73–86.
142. Walsh GL, Morice RC, Putnam JB, et al. Resection of lung cancer is justified in high-risk patients selected by exercise oxygen consumption. Ann Thorac Surg 1994; 58:704–711.
143. Smart J, Hilton G. Radiotherapy of cancer of the lung: results in a selective group of cases. Lancet 1956;1:880.
144. Morrison R, Deeley TJ, Cleland W. The treatment of carcinoma of the bronchus: a clinical trial to compare surgery and super-voltage radiotherapy. Lancet 1963;1:683.
145. Dombernowsky P, Hansen HH. Small cell lung cancer: clinical presentation and natural history of small cell lung cancer. In: Roth JA, Ruckdeschel JC, Weisenburger TH (eds) Thoracic Oncology. Saunders: Philadelphia, 1995: 188–200.
146. Nesbitt JC, Putnam JB, Walsh GL, Roth JA, Mountain CF. Survival in early-stage non-small cell lung cancer. Ann Thorac Surg 1995;60:466–472.
147. Martini N, Burt ME, Bains MS, et al. Survival after resection of stage II non-small cell lung cancer. Ann Thorac Surg 1992;54:460–466.
148. Ginsberg RJ, Rubenstein LA. A randomized comparative trial of lobectomy versus limited resection for patients with T1N0 non-small cell lung cancer. Lung Cancer 1991;7: 83–88.
149. Warren WH, Faber LP. Segmentectomy versus lobectomy in patients with stage I pulmonary carcinoma. J Thorac Cardiovasc Surg 1994;107:1087–1094.
150. Landreneau RJ, Sugarbaker DJ, Mack MJ, et al. Wedge resection versus lobectomy for stage I (T1 N0 M0) non-small cell lung cancer. J Thorac Cardiovasc Surg 1997; 113:691–700.
151. Landreneau RJ, Mack MJ, Dowling RD, et al. The role of thoracoscopy in lung cancer management. Chest 1998;113: 6S–12S.
152. Yim AP, Liu HP. Thoracoscopic major lung resection—indications, technique, and early results: experience from two centers in Asia. Surg Laparosc Endosc 1997;7:241–244.
153. Kawahara K, Iwasaki A, Shiraishi T, Okabayashi K, Shirakusa T. Video-assisted thoracoscopic lobectomy for treating lung cancer. Surg Laparosc Endosc 1997;7:219–222.
154. Kaseda S, Hangai N, Yamamoto S, Kitano M. Lobectomy with extended lymph node dissection by video-assisted thoracic surgery for lung cancer. Surg Endosc 1997;11: 703–706.
155. Iwasaki A, Shirakusa T, Kawahara K, Yoshinaga Y, Okabayashi K, Shiraishi T. Is video-assisted thoracoscopic

surgery suitable for resection of primary lung cancer? Thorac Cardiovasc Surg 1997;45:13–15.
156. Roth JA, Fossella F, Komaki R, et al. A randomized trial comparing perioperative chemotherapy and surgery with surgery alone in resectable stage III non-small cell lung cancer. J Natl Cancer Inst 1994;86:673–680.
157. Goldie JH, Coldman AJ. The genetic origin of drug resistance in neoplasms: implications for systemic therapy. Cancer Res 1984;44:3643–3653.
158. Strauss GM, Herndon JE, Sherman DD, et al. Neoadjuvant chemotherapy and radiotherapy followed by surgery in stage IIIA non-small-cell carcinoma of the lung: report of a cancer and leukemia group B phase II study. J Clin Oncol 1992;10:1237–1244.
159. Martini N, Kris MG, Flehinger BJ, et al. Preoperative chemotherapy for stage IIIa (N2) lung cancer: the Sloan-Kettering experience with 136 patients. Ann Thorac Surg 1993;55:1365–1374.
160. Weiden PL, Piantadosi S. Preoperative chemotherapy (cisplatin and fluorouracil) and radiation therapy in stage III non-small-cell lung cancer: a phase II study of the lung cancer study group. J Natl Cancer Inst 1991;83:266–273.
161. Silini EM, Bosi F, Pellegata NS, et al. K-ras gene mutations: an unfavorable prognostic marker in stage I lung adenocarcinoma. Virchows Arch 1994;424:367–373.
162. Favaretto A, Paccagnella A, Tomio L, et al. Pre-operative chemoradiotherapy in non-small cell lung cancer stage III patients: feasibility, toxicity and long-term results of a phase II study. Eur J Cancer 1996;31A:2064–2069.
163. Choi N, Mathisen D, Carey R, et al. Assessment of preoperative accelerated radiotherapy (RT) and chemotherapy (CT) in stage IIIA non-small cell lung cancer (NSCLC) [abstract]. Proc Am Soc Clin Oncol 1994;13:a1097–a1097.
164. Lee JD, Ginsberg RJ. The multimodality treatment of stage III A/B non-small lung cancer: the role of surgery, radiation, and chemotherapy. Hematol Oncol Clin North Am 1997;11:279–301.
165. Martini N, Kris MG, Ginsberg RJ. The role of multimodality therapy in locoregional non-small cell lung cancer. Surg Oncol Clin North Am 1997;6:769–791.
166. Cote RJ, Beattie EJ, Benjaporn C, et al. Detection of occult bone marrow micrometastases in patients with operable lung carcinoma. Ann Surg 1995;222:415–425.
167. Roth JA. A clinical trial of retroviral gene transfer of wild-type p53 in lung cancer patients with mutant p53 tumor. Nat Med 1996;2:985–991.
168. Swisher SG, Roth JA, Lawrence DD, et al. Adenoviral mediated p53 gene transfer in patients with advanced non-small cell lung cancer (NSCLC) [abstract]. Proc Am Soc Clin Oncol 1997;16:437a.
169. Carbone DP. Immunologic and biologic approaches to lung cancer therapy. In: Roth JA, Cox JD, Hong WK (eds) Lung Cancer. Blackwell Science: Malden, MA, 1998: 343–368.
170. Abrams HL, Spiro R, Goldstein N. Metastases in carcinoma: analysis of 1000 autopsied cases. Cancer 1950;3:74.
171. Farrell JT Jr. Pulmonary metastasis: a pathologic, clinical, roentgenologic study based on 78 cases seen at necropsy. Radiology 1935;24:444.
172. Fidler IJ. Special lecture: critical factors in the biology of human cancer metastasis: twenty-eight GHA; Clowes memorial award lecture. Cancer Res 1990;50:6130–6138.
173. Fidler IJ, Balch CM. The biology of cancer metastasis and implications for therapy. Curr Probl Surg 1987;24:137–209.
174. Miller BJ, Rosenbaum AS. The vascular supply to metastatic tumors of the lung. Surg Gynecol Obstet 1967;125: 1009–1012.
175. Neyazaki T, Ikeda M, Mitusi K, Kimura S, Suzuki M, Suzuki C. Angioarchitecture of pulmonary malignancies in humans. Cancer 1970;26:1246–1255.
176. Torek F. Removal of metastatic carcinoma of the lung and mediastinum: suggestions as to technic. Arch Surg 1930; 21:1416–1421.
177. Alexander J, Haight C. Pulmonary resection for solitary metastatic sarcoma and carcinoma. Surg Gynecol Obstet 1947;85:129–146.
178. Mannix EP Jr. Resection of multiple pulmonary metastases fourteen years after amputation for osteochondrogenic sarcoma of tibia: apparent freedom from recurrence two years later. J Thorac Surg 1953;26:544–549.
179. Gliedman ML, Horowitz S, Lewis FJ. Lung resection for metastatic cancer: 29 cases from the University of Minnesota and a collected review of 264 cases. Surgery 1957;42:521–532.
180. Thomford NR, Woolner LB, Clagett OT. The surgical treatment of metastatic tumors in the lungs. J Thorac Cardiovasc Surg 1965;49:357–363.
181. Lanza LA, Putnam JB. Resection of pulmonary metastases. In: Roth JA, Ruckdeschel JR, Weisenburger TH (eds) Thoracic Oncology. Saunders: Philadelphia, 1996:569–589.
182. McCormack PM, Bains MS, Begg DB, et al. Role of video-assisted thoracic surgery in the treatment of pulmonary metastases: results of a prospective trial. Ann Thorac Surg 1996;62:213–216.
183. Gundry SR, Coran AG, Lemmer J. The influence of tumor microfoci on recurrence and survival following pulmonary resection of metastatic osteogenic sarcoma. Ann Thorac Surg 1984;38:473–478.
184. Buhr J, Hurtgen M, Heinrichs CM, Weimar B, Morr H, Schwemmle K. Tumor dissemination after thoracoscopic resection of malignant pulmonary coin lesions. Chirurg 1996;67:81–85.
185. Johnstone PA, Rohde DC, Swartz SE, Fetter JE, Wexner SD. Port site recurrences after laparoscopic and thoracoscopic procedures in malignancy. J Clin Oncol 1996;14:1950–1956.
186. Martini N, Huvos AG, Mike V, Marcove RC, Beattie EJ. Multiple pulmonary resections in the treatment of osteogenic sarcoma. Ann Thorac Surg 1971;12:271–280.
187. Putnam J, Roth JA, Wesley MN, Johnston MR, Rosenberg SA. Survival following aggressive resection of pulmonary metastases from osteogenic sarcoma: analysis of prognostic factors. Ann Thorac Surg 1983;38:516–523.
188. Goorin AM, Delorey MJ, Lack EE. Prognostic significance of complete surgical resection of pulmonary metastases in patients with osteogenic sarcoma: analysis of 32 patients. J Clin Oncol 1984;2:425–431.
189. Lanza LA, Putnam JB, Benjamin RS, Roth JA. Response to chemotherapy does not predict survival after resection of sarcomatous pulmonary metastases. Soc Thorac Surg 1991;51:219–224.

190. Pogrebniak HW, Roth JA, Steinberg SM, Rosenberg SA, Pass HI. Reoperative pulmonary resection in patients with metastatic soft tissue sarcoma. Ann Thorac Surg 1991;52: 197–203.
191. McCormack PM, Burt ME, Bains MS, Martini N, Rusch VW, Ginsberg RJ. Lung resection for colorectal metastases: 10-year results. Arch Surg 1992;127:1403–1406.
192. Okimura S, Kondo H, Tsubai M. Pulmonary resection for metastatic colorectal cancer: experience with 159 patients. J Thorac Cardiovasc Surg 1996;112:867–874.
193. Girard P, Ducreux M, Baldeyrou P. Surgery for lung metastases from colorectal cancer: analysis of prognostic factors. J Clin Oncol 1996;14:2047.
194. McAfee MK, Allen MS, Trastek VF, Ilstrup DM, Deschamps C, Pairolero PC. Colorectal lung metastases: results of surgical excision. Ann Thorac Surg 1992;53: 780–786.
195. Pogrebniak HW, Haas G, Linehan WM, Rosenberg SA, Pass HI. Renal cell carcinoma: resection of solitary and multiple metastases. Ann Thorac Surg 1992;54:33–38.
196. Kavolius JP, Mastorakos DP, Pavlovich C, Russo P, Burt ME, Brady MS. Resection of metastatic renal cell carcinoma. J Clin Oncol 1998;16:2261–2266.
197. Jett JR, Hollinger CG, Zinsmeister AR, Pairolero PC. Pulmonary resection of metastatic renal cell carcinoma. Chest 1983;84:442–445.
198. Cerfolio RJ, Allen MS, Deschamps C, et al. Pulmonary resection of metastatic renal cell carcinoma. Ann Thorac Surg 1994;57:339–344.
199. Lanza LA, Natarajan G, Roth JA, Putnam JB Jr. Long-term survival after resection of pulmonary metastases from carcinoma of the breast. Ann Thorac Surg 1992;54: 244–248.
200. Staren ED, Salerno C, Rongione A, Witt TR, Faber LP. Pulmonary resection for metastatic breast cancer. Arch Surg 1992;127:1282–1284.
201. Friedel G, Linder A, Toomes H. The significance of prognostic factors for the resection of pulmonary metastases of breast cancer. Thorac Cardiovasc Surg 1994;42:71–75.
202. Vogt-Moykopf I, Krysa S, Bulzebruck H. Surgery for pulmonary metastases: the Heidelberg experience. Chest Surg Clin North Am 1994;4:85–112.
203. Gorenstein LA, Putnam JB Jr, Natarajan G, Balch CA, Roth JA. Improved survival after resection of pulmonary metastases from malignant melanoma. Ann Thorac Surg 1991;52:204–210.
204. Harpole DH Jr, Johnson CM, Wolfe WG, George SL, Seigler HF. Analysis of 945 cases of pulmonary metastatic melanoma. J Thorac Cardiovasc Surg 1992;103:743–750.
205. Tafra L, Dale PS, Wanek LA, Ramming KP, Morton DL. Resection and adjuvant immunotherapy for melanoma metastatic to the lung and thorax. J Thorac Cardiovasc Surg 1995;110:119–129.
206. Putnam JB Jr, Suell DM, Natarajan G, Roth JA. Extended resection of pulmonary metastases: is the risk justified. Ann Thorac Surg 1993;55:1440–1446.
207. Schrump DS. Cardiopulmonary Bypass for Extended Resection of Thoracic Malignancies. In: Franco KL, Putnam JB (eds) Advanced Therapy in Thoracic Surgery. B.C. Decker, Inc.: London, 1998:238–243.
208. Pastorino U, Buyse M, Friedel G, et al. Long-term results of lung metastasectomy: prognostic analyses based on 5206 cases. J Thorac Cardiovasc Surg 1997;113:49.
209. Roth J. Treatment of the patient with lung metastases. Curr Probl Surg 1996;33:892–952.
210. Jacobs JK, Flexner JM, Scott HW Jr. Selective isolated perfusion of the right lung. J Thorac Cardiovasc Surg 1961;42:546–552.
211. Pierpont H, Blades B. Lung perfusion with chemotherapeutic agents. Cardiovasc Surg 1960;39:159–165.
212. Johnson MR, Minchen RF, Dawson CA. Lung perfusion with chemotherapy in patients with unresectable metastatic sarcoma to the lung or diffuse branchioloalveolar carcinoma. J Thorac Cardiovasc Surg 1995; 110:368–373.
213. Weksler B, Burt M. Isolated lung perfusion with antineoplastic agents for pulmonary metastases. Chest Surg Clin N Am 1998;8:157–182.
214. Putnam JB, Madden T, Tran HT, Benjamin RS. Isolated single lung perfusion (ISLP) with Adriamycin® for unresectable sarcomatous metastases [abstract]. Proc ASCO 1997;16:500a.
215. Mürdter TE, Sperker B, Kivistö KT, et al. Enhanced uptake of doxorubicin into bronchial carcinoma: β-glucuronidase mediates release of doxorubicin from a glucuronide prodrug (HMR 1826) at the tumor site. Cancer Res 1997;57:2440–2445.
216. Pass HI, Mew DJY, Kranda KC, Temeck BK, Donington JS, Rosenberg SA. Isolated lung perfusion with tumor necrosis factor for pulmonary metastases. Ann Thorac Surg 1996;61:1609–1617.
217. Ratto GB, Toma S, Civalleri D, et al. Isolated lung perfusion with platinum in the treatment of pulmonary metastases from soft tissue sarcomas. J Thorac Cardiovasc Surg 1996;112:614–622.
218. Benjamin RS, Putnam JB, Tran HT, Hager HK, Madden T. High levels of doxorubicin in human lung and pulmonary metastases following single-pass isolated-single-lung perfusion [abstract]. 88th Annual Meeting. Am Assoc Cancer Res 1997;38:609.
219. Taylor CW, Wang LM, List AF, et al. Amifostine protects normal tissues from paclitaxel toxicity while cytotoxicity against tumour cells is maintained. Eur J Cancer 1997;33:1693–1698.
220. Neyazaki T, Ikeda M, Seki Y, Egawa N, Suzuki C. Bronchial artery infusion therapy for lung cancer. Cancer 1969;24: 912–922.
221. Nicholson KM, Bibby MC, Phillips RM. Influence of drug exposure parameters on the activity of paclitaxel in multicellular spheroids. Eur J Cancer 1997;33:1291–1298.
222. Schrump DS, Zhai S, Nguyen DM, Weiser TS, et al. Pharmacolcinetics and Acute Toxicity of Paclitaxel Administered via Hyperthermic Retrograde Isolated Lung Perfusion. 2000, Submitted for publication.
223. Matsuoka H, Furusawa M, Tomoda H, Seo Y. Difference in cytotoxicity of paclitaxel against neoplastic and normal cells. Anticancer Res 1994;14:163–168.
224. Donaldson KL, Goolsby GL, Wahl AF. Cytotoxicity of the anticancer agents cisplatin and taxol during cell proliferation and the cell cycle. Int J Cancer 1994;57:847–855.

225. Crossin KL, Carney DH. Microtubule stabilization by taxol inhibits initiation of DNA synthesis by thrombin and epidermal growth factor. Cell 1981;27:341–350.
226. Schiff PB, Horowitz SB. Taxol stabilizes microtubules in mouse fibroblast cells. Proc Natl Acad Sci USA 1980;77:1561–1565.
227. Hennequin C, Giocanti N, Favaudon V. S-phase specificity of cell killing by docetaxel (Taxotere) in synchronized HeLa cells. Br J Cancer 1995;71:1194–1198.
228. Rowinsky EK, Donehower RC, Jones RJ, Tucker RW. Microtubule changes and cytotoxicity in leukemic cell lines treated with taxol. Cancer Res 1988;48:4093–4100.
229. Blagasklonny MV, Schulte T, Nguyen P, Trepel J, Kneckers LM. Taxol-induced apoptosis and phosphorylation of Bcl-2 protein involves c-Raf-1 and represents a novel c-Raf-1 signal transduction pathway. Cancer Res 1996;56: 1851–1854.
230. Milross CG, Mason KA, Hunter NR, Chung WK, Peters LJ, Milas L. Relationship of mitotic arrest and apoptosis to antitumor effect of paclitaxel. J Natl Cancer Inst 1996; 88:1308–1314.
231. Wahl AF, Donaldson KL, Fairchild C, et al. Loss of normal p53 function confers sensitization to taxol by increasing G2/M arrest and apoptosis. Nat Med 1996; 2:72–79.
232. Safran H, King T, Choy H, et al. p53 mutations do not predict response to paclitaxel/radiation for nonsmall cell lung carcinoma. Cancer 1996;78:1203–1210.
233. Maier-Lenz H, Hauns B, Haering B, et al. Phase I study of paclitaxel administered as a 1-hour infusion: toxicity and pharmacokinetics. Semin Oncol 1997;24:S19-16–S19-19.
234. Hainsworth JD, Raefsky EL, Greco FA. Paclitaxel administered by a 1-hour infusion: a phase I–II trial comparing two schedules. Cancer J Sci Am 1995;1:281–287.
235. Hainsworth JD, Thompson DS, Greco FA. Paclitaxel by 1-hour infusion: an active drug in metastatic non-small-cell lung cancer. J Clin Oncol 1995;13:1609–1614.
236. Greenberger LM, Williams SS, Horowitz SB. Biosynthesis of heterogeneous forms of multidrug resistance-associated glycoproteins. J Biol Chem 1987;262:13685–13689.
237. Rischin D, Webster LK, Millward MJ, et al. Cremophor pharmacokinetics in patients receiving 3-, 6-, and 24-hour infusions of paclitaxel. J Natl Cancer Inst 1996;88: 1297–1301.

# *Part II*
# *Specific Issues in Geriatric Surgery*

## Section 5
## Cardiovascular System

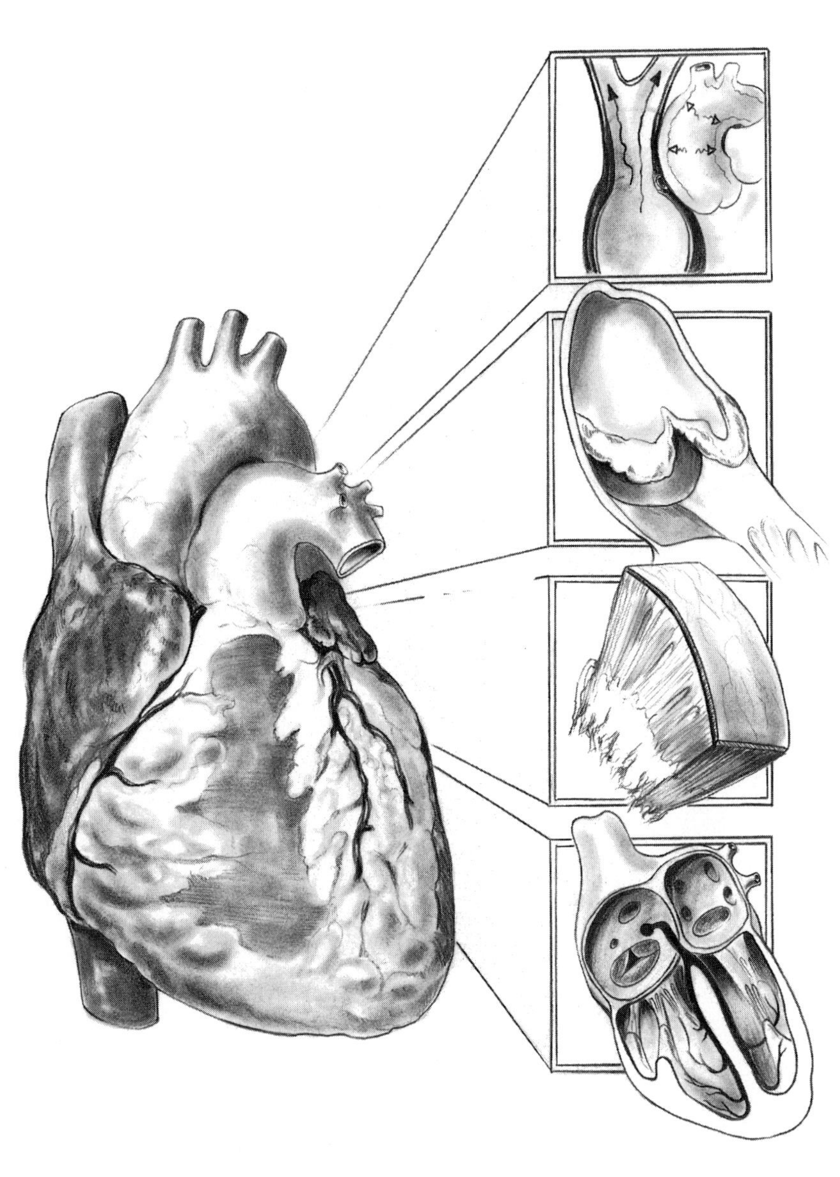

# Invited Commentary

Timothy J. Gardner

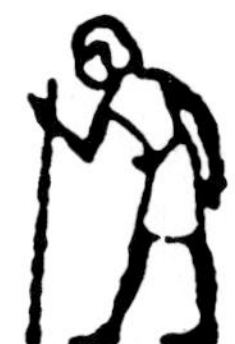

Cardiovascular illnesses in the elderly are, in many respects, a natural consequence of aging. The aging process is associated with degeneration of organs and their functions, including the brain, heart, musculoskeletal system, and vascular system. Cardiovascular illnesses, such as ischemic heart disease, peripheral vascular disease, and congestive heart failure can be expected to occur in some form or other as we age; and nearly everyone who survives into their eighties has evidence of cardiovascular pathology. It is interesting that when questioned about their preferred mode of demise, many older people indicate that they would choose to sustain a sudden fatal cardiac event over such unpleasant terminal illnesses as cancer, stroke, dementia, or other afflictions of the elderly.

Many of the dramatic advances in the management of cardiovascular diseases during the past 30 years have been directed toward premature or "unnatural" cardiovascular conditions such as ischemic heart disease in young people, cardiomyopathies causing heart failure in young adults, valvular heart conditions creating disability in middle-aged people, and the like. Coronary bypass grafting and percutaneous coronary angioplasty were offered initially only to young patients with disabling angina. Heart transplantation was undertaken initially only in patients 50 years or younger. Even today, cardiac transplantation is considered inappropriate for people in their late fifties and older.

Along with the survival improvement and increased longevity for young people with heart disease that has occurred over the past two to three decades, the general population, especially in prosperous and developed countries, has been blessed with increasing longevity, as many preventable causes of early deaths are being dealt with successfully. With the enhanced life expectancy has come changing expectations among our aging fellow citizens. Retirement is no longer viewed as the end of one's useful lifetime but, rather, as a period of enrichment during which the rewards of a productive life can be realized and enjoyed. One's ability to function successfully as an elderly member of society—that is, being able to remain independent and to participate in a variety of important social, physical, and intellectual activities—ends up defining one's quality of life. If an elderly individual develops a cancer that is unfavorable for successful treatment, that patient and his or her family usually accept the inevitability of death and attempt to deal with the pain and suffering associated with the disease and the need to prepare for dying. The prevailing attitude toward many cardiovascular conditions in the elderly, however, is often different. We often do not accept as readily the inevitability of continued deterioration and death from cardiovascular illnesses, even when such problems occur in older individuals.

What, then, should be the proper approach to cardiovascular disease in the elderly? Because heart and vascular diseases are a natural consequence of aging, should we develop limits indicating at what age one should cease and desist from treating the cardiovascular condition invasively and let "nature takes its course"? Should a patient's age of 75 or 80 become the cutoff for such advanced cardiovascular therapies as angioplasty, coronary bypass grafting, or placement of internal cardiac defibrillators? On the other hand, in view of our observation that most elderly people want to live as long as possible with a suitable quality of life, should we offer aortic valve replacement to the octogenarian who is functionally intact except for heart-related episodes of syncope from isolated critical aortic valve stenosis? Should we broaden the criteria for eligibility for heart transplantation to old patients who may, in fact, have an extended life expectancy if the current disabling heart failure is adequately managed by cardiac transplantation? There are no easy answers to these and similar questions. They involve a host of considerations beyond the scope of whether an operation can be done safely on a given patient or if there are identifiable preoperative patient characteristics that allow accurate risk factor analysis.

What must be acknowledged by all who are concerned with health care for the elderly is that there will be a continuing and dramatic increase in the percent of elderly in the population and a notable increase in the number of those surviving beyond 80 years of age. Because of the nature of cardiovascular illnesses, it is likely that such conditions will predominate among our aging population, and that illnesses such as unstable angina in an 80-year-old woman who is living alone successfully will mandate interventional treatment even though the risk of death or complications with angioplasty or surgery is increased. Likewise, the 85-year-old man who is living comfortably in a retirement home but develops an acute myocardial infarction should be given the opportunity to receive intravenous thrombolytic therapy despite his age and despite the increased risk of adverse bleeding events.

The challenge that must be faced when considering the expanded application of advanced or invasive therapies for cardiovascular disease in the elderly is that of defining and predicting the expected outcomes of various treatments in terms of immediate and long-term survival along with complications, morbidities, and the restoration of one's quality of life. Epidemiologic methods and techniques should be used in an attempt to account for survival differences among elderly patients with specific cardiovascular conditions. Using such information, risk profiles that are based on the individual's health characteristics and are predictive of treatment success or failure can be developed and discussed before undertaking advanced treatments.

In addition, it is mandatory to recognize differences between elderly patients and younger individuals with cardiovascular illnesses. Even such simple concepts as variations in pharmacokinetics in an old patient compared to that in the young, "general population" in whom most clinical trials have been performed becomes an important challenge. For example, despite the fact that there may be statistically validated efficacy associated with the use of a β-blocker for certain cardiovascular conditions, such a medication when used in an elderly patient may result in disabling complications, such as syncope or heart block. Percutaneous coronary angioplasty or intraarterial stenting from the usual femoral artery approach may be precluded in the elderly patient with severe peripheral vascular disease. Coronary artery bypass grafting, which has negligible mortality risks in otherwise healthy young patients, is much riskier even in the "healthy" elderly patient, with a substantially higher likelihood of death or disabling stroke.

Treatments for cardiovascular illness that, when successful, prolong life and enhance the quality of that life should not be withheld from an elderly patient simply based on that individual's age. On the other hand, we must recognize that invasive therapies, including catheter interventions and especially major surgical procedures, are likely to be less successful and more often associated with complications because of age-related comorbidities and other degenerative conditions. To determine accurately the risk–benefit relation of a suggested treatment, we must be able to stratify the risks according to the patient's individual characteristics including his or her advanced age. Successful treatment of the elderly individual with cardiovascular disease requires also the committed interest and attention of specialists who are willing and able to view their elderly patients with the same discrimination that pediatric specialists are called upon to utilize when caring for young children.

Finally, a commitment to preserve and sustain the useful life of our elderly patients must be supported by a societal commitment to support advanced medical therapies for these individuals. In virtually every developed country of the world, health care for the elderly is provided through government support for medical care. Each society must continuously renew its commitment to supporting and caring in the most appropriate way for its elderly citizens. The challenge and responsibility for those in medicine is to provide advanced medical care to elderly patients only when it is appropriate, that is, when it can be expected to sustain useful life for that patient. The challenges of the aging society, which we will face for the foreseeable future, are immense. It is predictable that much of the focus in medical care will remain on management of cardiovascular illnesses in the elderly.

# 30 Physiologic Changes in Cardiac Function with Aging

Wilbert S. Aronow and William H. Frishman

Age-related changes in the cardiovascular system, overt and occult cardiovascular disease, and decreased physical activity affect cardiovascular function in older persons. With aging, there is a loss of myocytes in both the left and right ventricles with a progressive increase in myocyte cell volume per nucleus in both ventricles.[1] There is also a progressive decrease in the number of pacemaker cells in the sinus node, with only 10% of the number of cells present at age 20 remaining at age 75.[2]

## Afterload

Resistance to the ejection of blood by the left ventricle is termed afterload. There are two components to afterload: peripheral vascular resistance and characteristic aortic impedance. Peripheral vascular resistance is the steady-state component and provides opposition to steady blood flow. Characteristic aortic impedance is the dynamic component and opposes pulsatile blood flow. Peripheral vascular resistance is calculated by dividing the mean arterial pressure by the cardiac output; it is inversely proportional to the cross-sectional area of the peripheral vascular beds. Characteristic aortic impedance is measured as the time variation in mean arterial pressure/flow through the aorta; it is inversely proportional to the arterial compliance (the distensibility of the arterial wall). An indirect measurement of afterload is the pulse wave velocity, which measures the propagation speed of pressure waves traveling from proximal to distal arterial segments; it increases as arteries become less compliant.

With aging, the large elastic arteries become dilated with a decrease in compliance.[3] Progessive thickening of the aortic media and intima are associated with aortic enlargement.[4] There is an age-associated increase in arterial stiffness resulting from changes in the arterial media, such as thickening of the smooth muscle layers, increased fragmentation of elastin, an increase in the amount and characteristics of collagen, and increased calcification.[5] These structural changes are associated with a decrease in aortic distensibility due to increased aortic stiffness with an increase in pulse wave velocity.[6] The structural changes in the arterial wall are independent of coexisting atherosclerosis. Avolio et al.[6] showed an increase in pulse wave velocity with age in farmers from Guanzhou Province in southern China despite a low prevalence of atherosclerosis in this population. The age-associated increase in stiffness and decrease in distensibility of large elastic arteries is not found in distal arteries.[7]

Impedance spectral patterns have demonstrated an age-related increase in characteristic aortic impedance and peripheral vascular resistance.[8] The decrease in arterial compliance contributes more to the age-related increase in afterload than does the loss of peripheral vascular beds.[8] Peripheral vascular resistance was not age-related in healthy persons screened for occult coronary artery disease in the Baltimore Longitudinal Study of Aging,[9] but increased with age in persons not screened for occult coronary artery disease.[10] Arterial stiffening appearing as an increase in pulse wave velocity is associated with degeneration of the vascular media independent of atherosclerosis. Arterial stiffening causes earlier occurrence of wave reflection from peripheral sites to the ascending aorta during left ventricular ejection. Therefore aortic and carotid phasic pressures increase to a greater magnitude at a later time during left ventricular ejection, causing an increase in systolic and pulse pressures and a delayed peak in the aortic pressure pulse contour.

Circulating levels of catecholamines increase with age, especially with stress, although β-adrenergic vasodilation of vascular smooth muscle decreases.[11] α-Adrenergic vasoconstriction of vascular smooth muscle does not change with age.[12] The impaired vasodilator response to β-adrenergic stimulation with age is most important during exercise and contributes to the increased afterload associated with aging.

Increased afterload results in an increase in blood pressure. With aging, there is an increase in systolic blood pressure and a widened pulse pressure. A slight reduction in diastolic blood pressure occurs after the sixth decade.[13] The increase in systolic blood pressure is due to interactions of aging, cardiovascular disease, and life style factors, such as dietary sodium intake, body weight, and level of physical activity. An age-associated increase in the index of aortic stiffening was not found in normotensive persons on a low sodium chloride diet.[14] The increase in carotid augmentation index (an index of aortic stiffening) in highly trained elderly men was half of that expected on the basis of age alone.[15]

As aortic compliance decreases with aging, the transfer of kinetic energy from the blood ejected during left ventricular systole to potential energy stored in the elasticity of the aortic wall is reduced. Consequently, return of the potential energy stored in the elasticity of the aortic wall back to the kinetic energy of blood flow during diastole also is reduced. Therefore the left ventricle must eject its stroke volume into a less compliant aorta with greater pressure and force to achieve adequate cardiac output. The increased pulse wave velocity also causes the pressure in the aorta to increase and peak later during systole, contributing to the increased systolic blood pressure and widened pulse pressure.

Posterior left ventricular wall thickness increased with increasing age in normotensive men and women screened for occult coronary artery disease in the Baltimore Longitudinal Study of Aging.[3] Data from persons in this study suggested that the increase in left ventricular wall thickness associated with aging is mediated by an increase in systolic blood pressure.[16] Aging is also associated with an increase in the prevalence of hypertension and cardiovascular disease and, therefore, with the left ventricular hypertrophy seen by echocardiography.

Age-associated left ventricular hypertrophy is caused by an increase in the volume but not in the number of cardiac myocytes. Fibroblasts undergo hyperplasia, and collagen is deposited in the myocardial interstitium. Increased afterload results in an increase in left ventricular systolic stress and the addition of sarcomeres, in parallel, which causes increased left ventricular wall thickness with a normal or reduced left ventricular chamber size and an increased relative wall thickness.

In the Framingham Heart Study, echocardiographic left ventricular hypertrophy was observed in 33% of men and 49% of women older than 70 years.[17] In our elderly population, echocardiographic left ventricular hypertrophy was found in 226 of 554 men (41%) with a mean age of 80 years and in 539 of 1243 women (43%) with a mean age of 82 years.[18]

In our elderly population systolic or diastolic hypertension was present in 255 of 664 men (38%) with a mean age of 80 years and in 651 of 1488 women (44%) with a mean age of 82 years.[19] In another study of our elderly population, systolic or diastolic hypertension occurred in 108 of 215 Blacks (50%) with a mean age of 81 years, in 411 of 1140 Whites (36%) with a mean age of 82 years, and in 19 of 54 Hispanics (35%) with a mean age 81 years.[20] Echocardiographically diagnosed left ventricular hypertrophy occurred in 66 of 92 hypertensive Blacks (72%), in 194 of 346 hypertensive Whites (56%), and in 8 of 15 hypertensive Hispanics (53%).[20] However, it was observed in only 2 of our 88 elderly persons (2%) without hypertension or overt cardiac disease.[21]

## Preload

Preload is the filling volume of the left ventricle. Preload is determined by many factors that influence blood return to the heart and by the mechanical properties of the heart during diastolic filling of the left ventricle.

Resting left ventricular end-diastolic volume, measured by radionuclide ventriculography using multiple gated pool acquisition imaging or by echocardiography, is not age-related in healthy persons, indicating that the resting preload does not change with age.[3,9,22] Although resting preload does not change with age, left ventricular early diastolic filling decreases with age.

Passive filling of the left ventricle occurs during the rapid filling and diastasis phases of early diastole. With age, left ventricular stiffness is increased, left ventricular compliance reduced, left ventricular wall thickness increased, left ventricular relaxation impaired, and left ventricular early diastolic filling reduced. This may result in hypotension if preload is reduced. An age-related increase in systolic blood pressure also decreases left ventricular early diastolic filling, leading to hypotension if preload is decreased. Left ventricular filling during early diastole is reduced 50% from age 20 to age 80.[3,23,24]

Despite the decrease in early diastolic filling of the left ventricle with age, preload is maintained because left atrial contraction becomes more vigorous to increase late diastolic filling of the left ventricle.[3,22–28] Augmentation of late diastolic filling of the left ventricle prevents a reduction in left ventricular end-diastolic volume. The ratio of late diastolic Doppler peak transmitral velocity (peak atrial, or A wave, velocity) to early diastolic Doppler peak transmitral velocity (peak rapid filling, or E wave, velocity) increases from approximately 0.6 at 30 years of age to 1.2 at 70 years of age.[29] A reduction in the E/A wave ratio with age reflects a decrease in left ventricular compliance. An age-related increase in left atrial size resulting from increased wall stress due to increased left atrial pressure counteracts the effects of reduced left ventricular compliance with age. In our older population, 619 of 1797 older persons (34%) had echocardiographic left atrial enlargement.[18]

Age was the most powerful independent variable for left ventricular filling in healthy persons in the Framingham Heart Study.[30] Age was inversely associated with the E wave (peak early diastolic filling velocity) and was directly associated with the A wave (peak late diastolic filling velocity). Other independent variables that contribute to a lesser degree to left ventricular filling were heart rate, PR interval measured from the electrocardiogram (ECG), gender, left ventricular systolic function, and systolic blood pressure. Increasing the heart rate decreases peak early diastolic filling and increases peak late diastolic filling velocity. The PR interval on the ECG is inversely associated with peak early diastolic filling velocity. Women have slightly higher peak early diastolic filling velocities than men. Left ventricular systolic function is directly associated with peak early diastolic filling velocity. Increasing the systolic blood pressure increases the peak late diastolic filling velocity.[30,31]

A decrease in preload is not well tolerated in older persons. Decreased intravascular volume, reduced venous return to the heart, vasodilation by drugs or disease states, and use of drugs such as nitrates or diuretics decrease preload and may cause reduced cardiac output and hypotension in older persons. Reduced compliance of the left ventricle and decreased cardiac and vascular responsiveness to β-adrenergic stimulation[32] cause elderly persons to be highly dependent on the Frank-Starling mechanism to increase cardiac output. Older persons are more susceptible to developing orthostatic hypotension.[33–35] Impaired baroreceptor reflex sensitivity,[36] reduced cardiac responsiveness to β-adrenergic stimulation,[32] loss of arterial compliance, reduced venous return due to increased venous distensibility, impaired compensatory mechanisms for maintenance of fluid volume and electrolyte balance, increased incidence of common precipitating diseases and disorders, and the use of multiple drugs contribute to orthostatic hypotension. Older persons are also more susceptible to developing postprandial hypotension.[37–39]

Marked decreases in postprandial systolic blood pressure in the elderly may predispose them to symptomatic hypotension and to falls, syncope, angina pectoris, and transient cerebral ischemic attacks.[37–41] At 29-month follow-up, a marked reduction in postprandial systolic blood pressure in older persons was associated with an increased incidence of falls, syncope, new coronary events, new stroke, and total mortality.[41] Whether therapeutic interventions to prevent a marked decrease in postprandial systolic blood pressure in elderly persons can reduce the incidence of falls, syncope, new coronary events, new stroke, and total mortality at long-term follow-up must be investigated.

Because left atrial contraction can contribute up to 50% of left ventricular filling in a poorly compliant left ventricle, the development of atrial fibrillation may result in a marked decrease in cardiac output because of loss of the left atrial contribution to left ventricular late diastolic filling. A rapid ventricular rate associated with atrial fibrillation also decreases the time for diastolic filling of the left ventricle, resulting in a marked reduction in cardiac output.

The incidence of chronic atrial fibrillation also is increased with age.[42,43] In 2101 elderly persons in a nursing home, the prevalence of chronic atrial fibrillation was 5% in persons aged 60–70 years, 13–14% in persons aged 71–90 years, and 22% in persons 91 years and older.[43] Atrial fibrillation in old persons is associated with an increased incidence of new thromboembolic stroke[42,43] and new coronary events.[44,45]

Cardiac output increases during exercise in healthy old persons owing to an increase in venous return to the heart, increasing the diastolic filling of the left ventricle and allowing an increased stroke volume to be ejected during exercise.[46] This is the Frank-Starling mechanism. The maximal heart rate response to exercise decreased with age in healthy persons in the Baltimore Longitudinal Study of Aging,[9] whereas exercise stroke volume increased with age to maintain the exercise cardiac output.[9] The increase in exercise stroke volume resulted from an increase in left ventricular end-diastolic volume (preload) via the Frank-Starling mechanism. In contrast, healthy nonelderly persons achieved an increase in exercise cardiac output primarily by an increase in heart rate. Exercise stroke volume increased in nonelderly healthy persons owing to a slight increase in the left ventricular end-diastolic volume and a large reduction in the left ventricular end-systolic volume. The exercise-induced increase in heart rate and decrease in left ventricular end-systolic volume in nonelderly persons is probably mediated by β-adrenergic stimulation. The increase in left ventricular end-diastolic volume during exercise in healthy older persons suggests that the age-associated decrease in resting early diastolic filling of the left ventricle does not persist during exercise.

## Contractility

The intrinsic ability of the heart to generate force does not change with age in healthy persons, although the duration of contraction and relaxation is prolonged in senescent animals.[47,48] Prolongation of the left ventricular ejection time[49] and the preejection period[50] with age in healthy persons indicates that prolongation of contraction occurs with age. Prolongation of the duration of contraction in senescent animals is associated with increased muscle stiffness and prolongation of the action potential duration.[51] These age-related changes are associated with cellular changes in the excitation-contraction coupling mechanism[52] and are an adaptive response to preserve contractile function in response to an age-induced increase in afterload.

There is no decrease in resting left ventricular ejection fraction (LVEF) or circumferential fiber shortening in old persons with no evidence of heart disease.[3,9,22,53,54] However, systolic function with exercise decreases with age. In the Baltimore Longitudinal Study of Aging, old persons showed less exercise-induced increase in LVEF than did younger persons because of an age-related increase in left ventricular end-systolic volume.[9] However, the absolute values of LVEF at maximal exercise in healthy old persons rarely decrease from basal values.[9] Age-associated decreases in maximal heart rate and left ventricular contractility during maximal exercise, are manifestations of reduced β-adrenergic responsiveness, with aging partially offset by exercise-induced dilation of the left ventricle.[55]

TABLE 30.1. Prevalence of Normal Left Ventricular Ejection Fraction in Old Persons with Congestive Heart Failure

| Study | Results for patients with CHF and normal LVEF |
|---|---|
| Wong[69] | 41% of 54 persons, mean age 80 years |
| Aronow[70] | 47% of 247 persons, mean age 82 years |
| Cardiovascular Health Study[71] | 47% of old persons, mean age 73 years |
| Framingham Heart Study[72] | 52% of 72 persons, mean age 73 years |
| Pernenkil[73] | 34% of 501 persons, mean age 81 years |
| Aronow[68] | 50% of 572 persons, mean age 82 years |

LVEF, left ventricular ejection fraction; CHF, congestive heart failure.

## Diastolic Function

Aging is associated with prolongation of the isovolumic relaxation time, decreased early diastolic filling of the left ventricle, and augmented late diastolic filling of the left ventricle.[23,26,29] Normal aging changes that affect the left ventricular diastolic function include increased systolic blood pressure, increased left ventricular wall thickness, reduced left ventricular early diastolic filling, prolonged left ventricular diastolic relaxation, increased left atrial size, and increased left ventricular late diastolic filling.[56]

With age occurs slowing of the rate at which calcium is sequestered by the sarcoplasmic reticulum following myocardial excitation, which causes decreased relaxation of the left ventricle.[52,57,58] Accumulation of calcium at the onset of diastole may decrease left ventricular diastolic relaxation and early diastolic filling.[57] Decreased oxidative phosphorylation and cumulative mitochondrial peroxidation occurring with age may also decrease the left ventricular diastolic function.[59,60]

Increased left ventricular stiffness with age due to increased interstitial fibrosis and cross-linking of collagen in the heart impairs left ventricular diastolic relaxation and filling.[1,61–63] Myocardial ischemia in the absence of coronary artery disease caused by decreases in capillary density and coronary reserve with age may further reduce left ventricular diastolic function in old persons.[1,64]

In addition to a decrease in left ventricular diastolic relaxation and early diastolic filling caused by age, old persons are more likely to have left ventricular diastolic dysfunction because they have an increased prevalence of hypertension, myocardial ischemia due to coronary artery disease, and left ventricular hypertrophy due to hypertension, coronary artery disease, valvular aortic stenosis, hypertrophic cardiomyopathy, and other cardiac disorders. The increased stiffness of the left ventricle and prolonged left ventricular relaxation time reduce left ventricular early diastolic filling and cause higher left ventricular end-diastolic pressures at rest and during exercise in old persons.[65,66]

In patients with congestive heart failure (CHF) associated with left ventricular systolic dysfunction, the LVEF is less than 50%. There is a reduced amount of myocardial fiber shortening, the stroke volume is decreased, the left ventricle is dilated, and the patient is symptomatic.

With CHF due to left ventricular diastolic dysfunction with normal left ventricular systolic function, the LVEF is normal. Kitzman et al.[67] showed that during exercise persons with CHF and normal left ventricular systolic function but abnormal left ventricular diastolic function were unable to increase stroke volume normally, even in the presence of increased left ventricular filling pressure. Myocardial hypertrophy, ischemia, or fibrosis causes slow or incomplete left ventricular filling at normal left atrial pressures. The left atrial pressure increases to augment left ventricular filling, resulting in pulmonary and systemic venous congestion. The development of atrial fibrillation may also cause a decrease in cardiac output and the development of pulmonary and systemic venous congestion because of loss of the left atrial contribution to left ventricular late diastolic filling and reduced diastolic filling time due to a rapid ventricular rate.

In a prospective study of 2535 persons older than 60 years (mean 82 years), CHF developed in 677 (27%).[68] Elderly persons are more likely than nonelderly persons to develop CHF because of abnormal left ventricular diastolic dysfunction with normal left ventricular systolic function. Table 30.1 shows that the prevalence of normal LVEF in older persons with CHF ranges from 34% to 52%.[68–73] The prevalence of normal LVEF with CHF is also higher in old women than in old men.[68,70,72,73]

## Cardiovascular Response to Exercise

The maximal oxygen consumption ($VO_2$max) is the best overall measurement of cardiovascular fitness.[74] $VO_2$max is the product of cardiac output and systemic arteriovenous oxygen difference at peak exercise. Maximal cardiac output—the heart rate multiplied by the stroke volume at peak exercise—is a more direct measurement of car-

TABLE 30.2. Cardiovascular Responses to Exercise in Healthy Old Persons

---

Maximal heart rate is reduced with age.
Exercise stroke volume is increased with age to maintain cardiac output.
Increased exercise stroke volume with age results primarily from increase in left ventricular end-diastolic volume by Frank-Starling mechanism.
Reduction in muscle mass with age plays role in age-associated decreases in systemic arteriovenous oxygen difference and in $VO_2$max at peak exercise.
Left ventricular end-diastolic and end-systolic volumes are increased during peak exercise with age.
Peak exercise left ventricular ejection fraction is reduced with age.
Exercise-induced decrease in the left ventricular end-systolic volume index and increases in the cardiac index, stroke volume index, and left ventricular ejection fraction from rest are greater in old men than in old women.

---

diovascular reserve than is $VO_2$max.[74] $VO_2$max is reduced with age.[75,76] The degree of reduction of $VO_2$max with age is affected by physical conditioning, subclinical coronary artery disease, smoking, and body weight. Table 30.2 lists the cardiovascular responses to exercise in healthy old persons.

In the Baltimore Longitudinal Study of Aging, older male athletes had a higher peak exercise $VO_2$max than older sedentary men.[77] The greater peak exercise $VO_2$max in older male athletes than in older sedentary men was achieved by a higher cardiac index and a greater systemic arteriovenous oxygen difference. The higher peak exercise cardiac index in older male athletes than in older sedentary men was due to a higher stroke volume index with similar maximal heart rates. Long-term endurance training also is associated with enhanced ventricular diastolic filling indices.[78]

A reduction in maximal systemic arteriovenous oxygen difference occurs with age.[79] The decrease in muscle mass with age may play a major role in the decrease in systemic arteriovenous oxygen difference at peak exercise and in $VO_2$max.[80]

Fleg et al.[81] also investigated the effect of age on peak upright cycle exercise in healthy sedentary men and women aged 22–86 years in the Baltimore Longitudinal Study of Aging. Peak cycle work rate was reduced with age in both men and women but was greater in men than in women at any age. Both men and women had peak exercise reductions in heart rate, cardiac index, and LVEF and increases in the left ventricular end-diastolic volume index and end-systolic volume index with age. Peak exercise stroke volume index did not vary with age in men or women. The exercise-induced decrease in left ventricular end-systolic volume index and the increases in cardiac index, stroke volume index, and LVEF from rest were greater in older men than in older women.

## Age-Related Changes in Cardiovascular Function

Table 30.3 lists some age-related changes in cardiovascular function in healthy old persons. Contractility at rest does not change with age, but the duration of left ventricular contraction and relaxation is prolonged. Age-associated reductions in maximal heart rate and in left ventricular contractility during maximal exercise are manifestations of reduced β-adrenergic responsiveness with age partially offset by exercise-induced dilation of the left ventricle.

Reduced arterial compliance contributes more to the age-related increase in afterload than does the loss of peripheral vascular beds. The impaired vasodilator response to β-adrenergic stimulation with age is most important during exercise and contributes to the increased afterload associated with age. Resting preload does not change with age. Left ventricular early diastolic filling is reduced with age. Augmentation of late diastolic filling of the left ventricle prevents a reduction in left ventricular end-diastolic volume with age. The maximal heart rate response to exercise is reduced with age. Exercise stroke volume is increased with age to maintain the exercise cardiac output, resulting from an increase in preload by the Frank-Starling mechanism. $VO_2$max and the systemic arteriovenous oxygen difference at peak exercise are reduced with age. Aging also selectively impairs endothelium-dependent function.[82]

In addition to age-related changes in cardiovascular function and deconditioning due to a sedentary life style, old persons also have a higher prevalence and incidence of cardiovascular disorders that impair cardiovascular performance than do nonelderly persons. Old persons are more likely than nonelderly persons to develop CHF secondary to abnormal left ventricular diastolic dysfunction with normal left ventricular systolic function.

TABLE 30.3. Some Age-Related Changes in Cardiovascular Function in Healthy Old Persons

---

Contractility at rest does not change with age.
Duration of left ventricular contraction and relaxation is prolonged with age.
Reduction in arterial compliance contributes more to age-related increase in afterload than does loss of peripheral vascular beds.
Resting preload does not change with age.
Left ventricular early diastolic filling is reduced with age.
Augmentation of late diastolic filling of the left ventricle prevents a reduction in left ventricular end-diastolic volume with age.
Cardiovascular responses to exercise with age are noted in Table 30.2.
Age-associated reductions in maximal heart rate and left ventricular contractility during maximal exercise are manifestations of reduced β-adrenergic responsiveness with age partially offset by exercise-induced dilation of the left ventricle.
Aging selectively impairs endothelium-dependent function.

---

## Treatment of Congestive Heart Failure

The LVEF should be measured in all persons with CHF so appropriate therapy may be given.[83,84] For example, digoxin should not be used to treat persons with CHF and normal LVEF if a sinus rhythm is present.[56,85] By augmenting contractility through increasing the intracellular calcium ion concentration, digoxin may increase left ventricular stiffness, increasing left ventricular filling pressure and adversely affecting CHF due to left ventricular diastolic dysfunction. Persons with CHF due to abnormal LVEF tolerate higher doses of diuretics than do persons with CHF and normal LVEF. Persons with CHF as a result of left ventricular diastolic dysfunction with normal LVEF need high left ventricular filling pressures to maintain an adequate stroke volume and cardiac output; they cannot tolerate intravascular depletion. These persons should be treated with a low salt diet and cautious use of diuretics rather than with large doses of diuretics. Nitrates should also be used cautiously in these persons.

Calcium channel blockers such as diltiazem, nifedipine, and verapamil exacerbate CHF in persons with CHF associated with abnormal LVEF.[86] Diltiazem increased mortality in patients with pulmonary congestion associated with abnormal LVEF after myocardial infarction.[87] The Multicenter Diltiazem Postinfarction Trial showed, in persons with an LVEF less than 40%, that late CHF at follow-up was increased in patients randomized to diltiazem (21%) versus those randomized to placebo (12%).[88] Recent prospective studies have found that the vasoselective calcium channel blockers amlodipine[89] and felodipine[90] did not significantly affect survival compared with placebo in patients with CHF associated with abnormal LVEF. There was a significantly higher incidence of pulmonary edema in the persons treated with amlodipine (15%) than in persons treated with placebo (10%).[89] On the basis of these data, calcium channel blockers should not be given to persons with CHF associated with abnormal LVEF.

However, calcium channel blockers may be used for therapy of persons with CHF associated with normal LVEF.[91] In a study of persons with CHF associated with normal LVEF and impaired left ventricular diastolic filling that compared verapamil to placebo, Setaro et al.[91] found that verapamil improved exercise capacity, peak left ventricular filling rate, and a clinicoradiographic heart failure score.

### Abnormal Left Ventricular Ejection Fraction

Old persons with CHF associated with abnormal LVEF should be treated with a low sodium diet and with diuretics plus an angiotensin-converting enzyme (ACE) inhibitor.[92,93] Losartan should be given if the persons cannot tolerate treatment with ACE inhibitors because of adverse effects such as cough, rash, or altered taste sensation.[94] If CHF persists despite diuretics with ACE inhibitors, digoxin should be added.[95] If CHF still persists, isosorbide dinitrate and hydralazine[96] or a β-blocker[97] is added to the regimen.

### Normal Left Ventricular Ejection Fraction

Old persons with CHF associated with normal LVEF should be treated with a low sodium diet and diuretics plus an ACE inhibitor.[98] Losartan is given if the person cannot tolerate ACE inhibitors because of adverse effects such as cough, rash, or altered taste sensation. If CHF persists, a β-blocker,[99] isosorbide dinitrate plus hydralazine,[100] or a calcium channel blocker[91] is added to the regimen.

In old persons with CHF associated with normal LVEF, pulmonary congestion is reduced by a low sodium diet, diuretics, and nitrates. Sinus rhythm is maintained to increase the left ventricular filling time. The ventricular rate is slowed below 90 beats per minute by a β-blocker to increase left ventricular filling time. Myocardial ischemia should be decreased and is best achieved by giving a β-blocker. Elevated systolic blood pressure is decreased by diuretics and an ACE inhibitor. The left ventricular mass is reduced by an ACE inhibitor. Left ventricular relaxation should be improved by ACE inhibitors, β-blockers, or calcium channel blockers.

## Cardiovascular disease

In addition to age-related changes in cardiovascular function and deconditioning due to a sedentary life style, old persons also have a higher prevalence and incidence of cardiovascular disorders, which impair cardiovascular performance, than nonelderly persons. Table 30.4 lists the prevalence of some cardiovascular disorders in an elderly population in a long-term health care facility.[18,19,43,68,101–104]

## Aortic Valve Disease

Valvular aortic stenosis in old persons is usually due to stiffening, scarring, and calcification of aortic valve leaflets. Calcific deposits in the aortic valve are common and may lead to valvular aortic stenosis.[18,105–107] Calcific deposits in the aortic valve were present in 22 of 40 necropsied patients (55%) aged 90–103 years.[106] Echocardiography demonstrated calcific deposits in the aortic valve in 95 of 473 old persons (20%) (mean age 82 years).[107]

Calcific valvular aortic stenosis was present at autopsy in 18% of 366 octogenarians.[108] Valvular aortic stenosis was diagnosed by continuous-wave Doppler echocardi-

TABLE 30.4. Prevalence of Cardiovascular Disorders in Old Persons in a Long-Term Health Care Facility

| Cardiovascular disorder | Mean age (years) | Prevalence No. | % |
|---|---|---|---|
| Coronary artery disease[19] | 81 | 895 / 2152 | 42 |
| Atherothrombotic brain infarction[101] | 81 | 551 / 2152 | 26 |
| Peripheral arterial disease[102] | 81 | 449 / 1834 | 24 |
| 40–100% Extracranial carotid arterial disease[103] | 82 | 239 / 1482 | 16 |
| Congestive heart failure[68] | 82 | 677 / 2535 | 27 |
| Hypertension[19] | 81 | 906 / 2152 | 42 |
| Aortic stenosis[18] | 81 | 301 / 1797 | 17 |
| Mitral annular calcium[18] | 81 | 859 / 1797 | 48 |
| ≥1+ Mitral regurgitation[18] | 81 | 591 / 1797 | 33 |
| ≥1+ Aortic regurgitation[18] | 81 | 526 / 1797 | 29 |
| Rheumatic mitral stenosis[18] | 81 | 22 / 1797 | 1 |
| Hypertrophic cardiomyopathy[18] | 81 | 62 / 1797 | 3 |
| Idiopathic dilated cardiomyopathy[18] | 81 | 16 / 1797 | 1 |
| Atrial fibrillation[43] | 81 | 283 / 2101 | 13 |
| Pacemaker rhythm[104] | 82 | 50 / 1153 | 4 |
| Abnormal left ventricular ejection fraction[18] | 81 | 422 / 1797 | 23 |
| Left ventricular hypertrophy[18] | 81 | 765 / 1797 | 43 |
| Left atrial enlargement[18] | 81 | 619 / 1797 | 34 |

ography in 301 of 1797 old persons (17%) with a mean age 81 years.[18] Severe aortic stenosis was present in 40 of these 1797 old persons (2%).[18] Severe aortic stenosis was also diagnosed in 3% of 501 persons aged 75–86 years in the Helsinki Ageing Study.[109]

The prevalence of aortic regurgitation also increases with age.[18,110,111] Aortic regurgitation was diagnosed by pulsed Doppler recordings of the aortic valve in 526 of 1797 old persons (29%) with a mean age of 81 years.[18] Severe or moderate aortic regurgitation was diagnosed by pulsed Doppler recordings of the aortic valve in 74 of 450 old patients with a mean age of 82 years.[112] Margonato et al.[110] linked the increased prevalence of aortic regurgitation with age to aortic valve thickening.

## Mitral Valvular Disease

Two degenerative aging processes—mitral annular calcification and mucoid (or myxomatous) degeneration of the mitral valve leaflets and chordae tendineae—can cause significant mitral valvular dysfunction.[113–115] Mitral annular calcification was diagnosed by two-dimensional echocardiography in 194 of 554 old men (35%) (mean age 80 years), and in 665 of 1243 old women (53%) (mean age 82 years).[18] Mitral annular calcium was present in 11 of 57 persons (19%) 62–70 years of age, in 53 of 158 persons (34%) 71–80 years of age, in 190 of 301 persons (63%) 81–90 years of age, in 75 of 85 persons (88%) 91–100 years of age, and in 3 of 3 persons (100%) 101–103 years of age.[116]

TABLE 30.5. Prevalence of Conduction Defects in 1153 Old Persons

| Defect | Prevalence (%) |
|---|---|
| First-degree atrioventricular block | 6 |
| Left anterior fascicular block | 8 |
| Right bundle branch block | 10 |
| Left bundle branch block | 4 |
| Intraventricular conduction defect | 3 |
| Second-degree atrioventricular block | 1 |
| Pacemaker rhythm | 4 |

*Source:* Adapted from Aronow.[104]

Mitral annular calcification and aortic cuspal calcium may coexist.[107,115,117] Breakdown of lipid deposits on the ventricular surface of the posterior mitral leaflet at or below the mitral annulus and on the aortic surfaces of the aortic valve cusps is probably responsible for the calcification.[118]

## Conduction Defects

The increased prevalence of conduction defects in old persons is due to age-related degeneration of the conduction system and to the development of cardiovascular disease. Table 30.5 lists the prevalence of conduction defects in 1153 old persons (mean age 82 years).[104] At a 45-month follow-up, old persons with second-degree atrioventricular block, left bundle branch block, intraventricular conduction defect, and pacer rhythm had an increased incidence of new coronary events.[104] At the 45-month follow-up, old persons with first-degree atrioventricular block, left anterior fascicular block, or right bundle branch block did not have an increased incidence of new coronary events.[104]

## Conclusions

Cardiovascular function in elderly persons is significantly affected by the aging process itself and by those acquired diseases of the cardiovascular system that are more prevalent with age. These physiologic and pathologic changes of the aging cardiovascular system must be taken into consideration during the clinical assessment and management of elderly patients who need to undergo surgical procedures and general anesthesia.

## References

1. Olivetti G, Melissari M, Capasso JM, et al. Cardiomyopathy of the aging human heart: myocyte loss and reactive cellular hypertrophy. Circ Res 1991;68:1560–1568.

2. Davies MJ. The pathological basis of arrhythmias. Geriatr Cardiovasc Med 1988;1:181–183.
3. Gerstenblith G, Fredericksen J, Yin FCP, et al. Echocardiographic assessment of a normal adult aging population. Circulation 1977;56:273–278.
4. Safar M. Aging and its effects on the cardiovascular system. Drugs 1990;39(suppl 1):1–8.
5. Yin FCP. The aging vasculature and its effects on the heart. In: Weisfeldt ML (ed) The Aging Heart: Its Function and Response to Stress. Raven: New York, 1980:137–214.
6. Avolio AP, Fa-Quan D, Wei-Qiang L, et al. Effects of aging on arterial distensibility in populations with high and low prevalence of hypertension: comparison between urban and rural communities in China. Circulation 1985;71: 202–210.
7. Boutouyrie P, Laurent S, Benetos A, et al. Opposing effects of ageing on distal and proximal large arteries in hypertensives. J Hypertens 1992;10:587–591.
8. Nichols WW, O'Rourke MF, Avolio AP, et al. Effects of age on ventricular-vascular coupling. Am J Cardiol 1985;55: 1179–1184.
9. Rodeheffer RJ, Gerstenblith G, Becker LC, et al. Exercise cardiac output is maintained with advancing age in healthy human subjects: cardiac dilatation and increased stroke volume compensate for a diminished heart rate. Circulation 1984;69:203–213.
10. Brandfonbrener M, Landowne M, Shock NW. Changes in cardiac output with age. Circulation 1955;12:557–566.
11. Pan HY, Hoffman BB, Pershe RA, et al. Decline in beta-adrenergic receptor-mediated vascular relaxation with aging in man. J Pharmacol Exp Ther 1986;239:802–807.
12. Buhler F, Kowski W, Van Brumeler P. Plasma catecholamines and cardiac, renal and peripheral vascular adrenoceptor mediated response in different age groups in normal and hypertensive subjects. Clin Exp Hypertens 1980;2:409–426.
13. Landahl S, Bengtsson C, Sigurdsson JA, et al. Age-related change in blood pressure. Hypertension 1986;8:1044–1049.
14. Avolio AP, Clyde KM, Beard TC, et al. Improved arterial distensibility in normotensive subjects on a low salt diet. Arteriosclerosis 1986;6:166–169.
15. Vaitkevicius PV, Fleg JL, Engel JH, et al. Effects of age and aerobic capacity on arterial stiffness in healthy adults. Circulation 1993;88:1456–1462.
16. Lima JAC, Gerstenblith G, Weiss JL, et al. Systolic blood pressure, not age mediates the age-related increase in left ventricular wall thickness within a normotensive population [abstract]. J Am Coll Cardiol 1988;11:81A.
17. Levy D, Anderson KM, Savage DD, et al. Echocardiographically detected left ventricular hypertrophy: prevalence and risk factors: the Framingham heart study. Ann Intern Med 1988;108:7–13.
18. Aronow WS, Ahn C, Kronzon I. Prevalence of echocardiographic findings in 554 men and in 1243 women aged >60 years in a long-term health care facility. Am J Cardiol 1997;79:379–380.
19. Aronow WS, Ahn C. Risk factors for new coronary events in a large cohort of very elderly patients with and without coronary artery disease. Am J Cardiol 1996;77:864–866.
20. Aronow WS, Kronzon I. Prevalence of coronary risk factors in elderly Blacks and Whites. J Am Geriatr Soc 1991;39: 567–570.
21. Aronow WS, Koenigsberg M, Schwartz KS. Usefulness of echocardiographic left ventricular hypertrophy in predicting new coronary events and atherothrombotic brain infarction in patients over 62 years of age. Am J Cardiol 1988;61:1130–1132.
22. Gardin JM, Henry WL, Savage DD, et al. Echocardiographic measurements in normal subjects: evaluation of an adult population without clinically apparent heart disease. J Clin Ultrasound 1979;7:439–447.
23. Bryg RJ, Williams GA, Labovitz AJ. Effect of aging on left ventricular diastolic filling in normal subjects. Am J Cardiol 1987;59:971–974.
24. Iskandrian AS, Aakki A. Age related changes in left ventricular diastolic performance. Am Heart J 1986;112: 75–78.
25. Spirito P, Maron BJ. Influence of aging on doppler echocardiographic indices of left ventricular diastolic function. Br Heart J 1988;59:672–679.
26. Miyatake K, Okamoto J, Kinoshita N, et al. Augmentation of atrial contribution to left ventricular flow with aging as assessed by intracardiac Doppler flowmetry. Am J Cardiol 1984;53:587–589.
27. Sartori MP, Quinones MA, Kuo LC. Relation of Doppler-derived left ventricular filling parameters to age and radius/thickness ratio in normal and pathologic states. Am J Cardiol 1987;59:1179–1182.
28. Fleg JL, Shapiro EP, O'Connor F, et al. Left ventricular diastolic filling performance in older male athletes. JAMA 1995;273:1371–1375.
29. Gardin JM, Rohan MK, Davidson DM, et al. Doppler transmitral flow velocity parameters: relationship between age, body surface area, blood pressure and gender in normal subjects. Am J Noninvas Cardiol 1987;1: 3–10.
30. Benjamin EG, Levy D, Anderson KM, et al. Determination of Doppler indexes of left ventricular diastolic function in normal subjects (the Framingham heart study). Am J Cardiol 1992;70:508–515.
31. Villari B, Hess OM, Kaufmann P, et al. Effect of aortic valve stenosis (pressure overload) and regurgitation (volume overload) on left ventricular systolic and diastolic function. Am J Cardiol 1992;69:927–934.
32. Lakatta EG. Age-related alterations in the cardiovascular response to adrenergic mediated stress. Fed Proc 1980;39: 3173–3177.
33. Robbins AS, Rubenstein LZ. Postural hypotension in the elderly. J Am Geriatr Soc 1984;32:769–774.
34. Aronow WS, Lee NH, Sales FF, et al. Prevalence of postural hypotension in elderly patients in a long-term health care facility. Am J Cardiol 1988;62:336.
35. Lipsitz LA, Jonsson PV, Marks BL, et al. Reduced supine cardiac volumes and diastolic filling rates in elderly patients with chronic medical conditions: implications for postural blood pressure homeostasis. J Am Geriatric Soc 1990;38:103–107.
36. Gribbin B, Pickering TG, Sleight P, et al. Effect of age and high blood pressure on baroreflex sensitivity in man. Circ Res 1971;29:424–431.

37. Lipsitz LA, Nyquist RP Jr, Wei JY, et al. Postprandial reduction in blood pressure in the elderly. N Engl J Med 1983;309:81–83.
38. Vaitkevicius PV, Esserwein DM, Maynard AK, et al. Frequency and importance of postprandial blood pressure reduction of elderly nursing-home patients. Ann Intern Med 1991;115:865–870.
39. Aronow WS, Ahn C. Postprandial hypotension in 499 elderly persons in a long-term health care facility. J Am Geriatr Soc 1994;42:930–932.
40. Kamata T, Yokota T, Furukawa T, et al. Cerebral ischemic attack caused by postprandial hypotension. Stroke 1994;25: 511–513.
41. Aronow WS, Ahn C. Association of postprandial hypotension with incidence of falls, syncope, coronary events, stroke, and total mortality at 29-month follow-up in 499 older nursing home residents. J Am Geriatr Soc 1997;45: 1051–1053.
42. Wolf PA, Abbott RD, Kannel WB. Atrial fibrillation as an independent risk factor for stroke: the Framingham study. Stroke 1991;22:983–988.
43. Aronow WS, Ahn C, Gutstein H. Prevalence of atrial fibrillation and association of atrial fibrillation with prior and new thromboembolic stroke in elderly patients. J Am Geriatr Soc 1996;44:521–523.
44. Kannel WB, Abbott RD, Savage DD, et al. Epidemiologic features of chronic atrial fibrillation: the Framingham study. N Engl J Med 1982;306:1018–1022.
45. Aronow WS, Ahn C, Mercando AD, et al. Correlation of atrial fibrillation, paroxysmal supraventricular tachycardia, and sinus rhythm with incidences of new coronary events in 1359 patients, mean age 81 years, with heart disease. Am J Cardiol 1995;75:182–184.
46. Poliner LR, Dehmer GJ, Lewis SE, et al. Left ventricular performance in normal subjects: a comparison of the responses to exercise in the upright and supine positions. Circulation 1980;62:528–534.
47. Fraticelli A, Josephson R, Danziger R, et al. Morphological and contractile characteristics of rat cardiac myocytes from maturation to senescence. Am J Physiol 1989;257:H259–H265.
48. Capasso JM, Malhotra A, Remly RM. Effects of age on mechanical and electrical performance of rat myocardium. Am J Physiol 1983;245:H72–H81.
49. Willems JL, Roelandt H, DeGeest H, et al. The left ventricular ejection time in elderly subjects. Circulation 1970;42: 37–42.
50. Shaw DJ, Rothbaum DA, Angell CS, et al. The effect of age and blood pressure upon the systolic time intervals in males aged 20–89 years. J Gerontol 1973;28:133–139.
51. Lakatta EG. Do hypertension and aging have similar effects on the myocardium? Circulation 1987;75(suppl I):69–77.
52. Lakatta EG, Yin FCP. Myocardial aging: functional alterations and related cellular mechanisms. Am J Physiol 1982;242:H927–H941.
53. Port S, Cobb FR, Coleman RE, et al. Effect of age on the response of the left ventricular ejection fraction to exercise. N Engl J Med 1980;303:1133–1137.
54. Aronow WS, Stein PD, Sabbah HN, et al. Resting left ventricular ejection fraction in elderly patients without evidence of heart disease. Am J Cardiol 1989;63:368–369.
55. Fleg JL, Schulman S, O'Connor F, et al. Effect of acute β-adrenergic receptor blockade on age-associated changes in cardiovascular performance during dynamic exercise. Circulation 1994;90:2333–2341.
56. Tresch DD, McGough MF. Heart failure with normal systolic function: a common disorder in older people. J Am Geriatr Soc 1995;43:1035–1042.
57. Wei JY, Spurgeon HA, Lakatta EG. Excitation-contraction in rat myocardium: alterations with adult aging. Am J Physiol 1984;246:H784–H791.
58. Morgan JP, Morgan KG. Calcium and cardiovascular function: intracellular calcium levels during contraction and relaxation of mammalian cardiac and vascular smooth muscle as detected with aequorin. Am J Med 1984;77(suppl 5A):33–46.
59. Bandy B, Davison AJ. Mitochondrial mutations may increase oxidative stress: implications for carcinogenesis and aging? Free Radic Biol Med 1990;8:523–539.
60. Corral-Debrinski M, Stepien G, Shoffner JM, et al. Hypoxemia is associated with mitochondrial DNA damage and gene induction: implications for cardiac disease. JAMA 1991;266:1812–1816.
61. Lie JT, Hammond PI. Pathology of the senescent heart: anatomic observations on 237 autopsy studies of patients 90 to 105 years old. Mayo Clin Proc 1988;63:552–564.
62. Schaub MC. The aging of collagen in the heart muscle. Gerontologia 1964;10:38–41.
63. Verzar F. The stages and consequences of aging collagen. Gerontologia 1969;15:233–239.
64. Hachamovitch R, Wicker P, Capasso JM, et al. Alterations of coronary blood flow and reserve with aging in Fischer 344 rats. Am J Physiol 1989;256:H66–H73.
65. Ogawa T, Spina R, Martin WH III, et al. Effects of aging, sex and physical training on cardiovascular responses to exercise. Circulation 1992;86:494–503.
66. Manning WJ, Shannon RP, Santinga JA, et al. Reversal of changes in left ventricular diastolic filling associated with normal aging using diltiazem. Am J Cardiol 1989;67: 894–896.
67. Kitzman DW, Higginbotham MB, Cobb FR, et al. Exercise intolerance in patients with heart failure and preserved left ventricular systolic function: failure of the Frank-Starling mechanism. J Am Coll Cardiol 1991;17:1065–1072.
68. Aronow WS, Ahn C, Kronzon I. Normal left ventricular ejection fraction in older persons with congestive heart failure. Chest 1998;113:867–869.
69. Wong WF, Gold S, Fukuyama O, et al. Diastolic dysfunction in elderly patients with congestive heart failure. Am J Cardiol 1989;63:1526–1528.
70. Aronow WS, Ahn C, Kronzon I. Prognosis of congestive heart failure in elderly patients with normal versus abnormal left ventricular systolic function associated with coronary artery disease. Am J Cardiol 1990;66: 1257–1259.
71. Gardin JM, Arnold A, Kitzman D, et al. Congestive heart failure with preserved systolic function in a large community-dwelling elderly cohort: the Cardiovascular Health Study [abstract]. J Am Coll Cardiol 1995;25: 423A.

72. Vasan RS, Benjamin EJ, Evans JC, et al. Prevalence and clinical correlates of diastolic heart failure: Framingham heart study [abstract]. Circulation 1995;92(suppl I):666.
73. Pernenkil R, Vinson JM, Shah AS, et al. Course and prognosis in patients ≥70 years of age with congestive heart failure and normal versus abnormal left ventricular ejection fraction. Am J Cardiol 1997;79:216–219.
74. Fleg JL. Alterations in cardiovascular structure and function with advancing age. Am J Cardiol 1986;57: 33C–44C.
75. Dehn MM, Bruce RA. Longitudinal variations in maximal oxygen intake with age and activity. J Appl Physiol 1972;33:805–807.
76. Heath GW, Hagberg JM, Ehsani AA. A physiological comparison of young and older endurance athletes. J Appl Physiol 1981;51:634–640.
77. Fleg JL, Schulman SP, O'Connor FC, et al. Cardiovascular responses to exhaustive upright cycle exercise in highly trained older men. J Appl Physiol 1994;77:1500–1506.
78. Forman DE, Manning WJ, Hauser R, et al. Enhanced left ventricular diastolic filling associated with long-term endurance training. J Gerontol 1992;47:M56–M58.
79. Julius S, Amery A, Whitlock LS, et al. Influence of age on the hemodynamic response to exercise. Circulation 1967; 36:222–230.
80. Fleg JL, Lakatta EG. Role of muscle loss in the age-associated reduction in $VO_{2max}$. J Appl Physiol 1988;65: 1147–1151.
81. Fleg JL, O'Connor F, Gerstenblith G, et al. Impact of age on the cardiovascular response to dynamic upright exercise in healthy men and women. J Appl Physiol 1995;78:890–900.
82. Chauhan A, More RS, Mullins PA, et al. Aging-associated endothelial dysfunction in humans is reversed by L-arginine. J Am Coll Cardiol 1996;28:1796–1804.
83. Aronow WS. Echocardiography should be performed in all elderly patients with congestive heart failure. J Am Geriatr Soc 1994;42:1300–1302.
84. Konstam MA, Dracup K, Baker DW, et al. Heart Failure: Evaluation and Care of Patients with Left-Ventricular Systolic Dysfunction. No. 11 AHCPR Publ. No. 94-0612. Agency for Health Care Policy and Research, Public Health Service, US Department of Health and Human Services: Rockville, MD, 1994:37–40.
85. Aronow WS. Digoxin or angiotensin converting enzyme inhibitors for congestive heart failure in geriatric patients: which is the preferred treatment? Drugs Aging 1991; 1:98–103.
86. Elkayam U, Amin J, Mehra A, et al. A prospective, randomized, double-blind, crossover study to compare the efficacy and safety of chronic nifedipine therapy with that of isosorbide dinitrate and their combination in the treatment of chronic congestive heart failure. Circulation 1990;82:1954–1961.
87. Multicenter Diltiazem Postinfarction Trial Research Group. The effect of diltiazem on mortality and reinfarction after myocardial infarction. N Engl J Med 1988; 319:385–392.
88. Goldstein RE, Boccuzzi SJ, Cruess D, et al. Diltiazem increases late-onset congestive heart failure in postinfarction patients with early reduction in ejection fraction. Circulation 1991;83:52–60.
89. Packer M, O'Connor CM, Ghali JK, et al. Effect of amlodipine on morbidity and mortality in severe chronic heart failure. N Engl J Med 1996;335:1107–1114.
90. Cohn JN, Ziesche SM, Loss LE, et al. Effect of the calcium antagonist felodipine as supplementary vasodilator therapy in patients with chronic heart failure treated with enalapril. V-HeFT III. Circulation 1997;96:856–863.
91. Setaro JF, Zaret BL, Schulman DS, et al. Usefulness of verapamil for congestive heart failure associated with abnormal left ventricular diastolic filling and normal left ventricular systolic performance. Am J Cardiol 1990;66: 981–986.
92. Cohn JN, Johnson G, Ziesche S, et al. A comparison of enalapril with hydralazine-isosorbide dinitrate in the treatment of chronic congestive heart failure. N Engl J Med 1991;325:303–310.
93. Garg R, Yusuf S, Collaborative Group on ACE Inhibitor Trials. Overview of randomized trials of angiotensin-converting enzyme inhibitory on mortality and morbidity in patients with heart failure. JAMA 1995;273:1450–1456.
94 Pitt B, Segal R, Martinez FA, et al. Randomised trial of losartan versus captopril in patients over 65 with heart failure (Evaluation of Losartan in the Elderly Study, ELITE). Lancet 1997;349:747–752.
95. Digitalis Investigation Group. The effect of digoxin on mortality and morbidity in patients with heart failure. N Engl J Med 1997;336:525–533.
96. Cohn JN, Archibald DG, Ziesche S, et al. Effect of vasodilator therapy on mortality in chronic congestive heart failure: results of a Veterans Administration cooperative study. N Engl J Med 1986;314:1547–1552.
97. Packer M, Bristow MR, Cohn JN, et al. The effect of carvedilol on morbidity and mortality in patients with chronic heart failure. N Engl J Med 1996;334:1349–1355.
98. Aronow WS, Kronzon I. Effect of enalapril on congestive heart failure treated with diuretics in elderly patients with prior myocardial infarction and normal left ventricular ejection fraction. Am J Cardiol 1993;71:602–604.
99. Aronow WS, Ahn C, Kronzon I. Effect of propranolol versus no propranolol on total mortality plus nonfatal myocardial infarction in older patients with prior myocardial infarction, congestive heart failure, and left ventricular ejection fraction ≥40% treated with diuretics plus angiotensin-converting-enzyme inhibitors. Am J Cardiol 1997;80:207–209.
100. Cohn JN, Johnson G, Veterans Administration Cooperative Study Group. Heart failure with normal ejection fraction: the V-HeFT Study. Circulation 1990;81(suppl III): 48–53.
101. Aronow WS, Ahn C, Gutstein H. Risk factors for new atherothrombotic brain infarction in 664 older men and 1488 older women. Am J Cardiol 1996;77:1381–1383.
102. Aronow WS, Ahn C. Correlation of serum lipids with the presence or absence of atherothrombotic brain infarction and peripheral arterial disease in 1834 men and women aged ≥62 years. Am J Cardiol 1994;73:995–997.
103. Aronow WS, Ahn C, Kronzon I, et al. Association of extracranial carotid arterial disease, prior atherothrombotic brain infarction, systemic hypertension, and left

ventricular hypertrophy with the incidence of new atherothrombotic brain infarction at 45-month follow-up in 1482 older patients. Am J Cardiol 1997;79:991–993.
104. Aronow WS. Correlation of arrhythmias and conduction defects on the resting electrocardiogram with new cardiac events in 1153 elderly patients. Am J Noninvas Cardiol 1991;5:88–90.
105. Roberts WC, Perloff JK, Costantino T. Severe valvular aortic stenosis in patients over 65 years of age. Am J Cardiol 1971;27:497–506.
106. Waller BF, Roberts WC. Cardiovascular disease in the very elderly: an analysis of 40 necropsy patients aged 90 years or over. Am J Cardiol 1983;51:403–421.
107. Aronow WS, Schwartz KS, Koenigsberg M, Correlation of serum lipids, calcium, and phosphorus, diabetes mellitus and history of systemic hypertension with presence or absence of calcified or thickened aortic cusps or root in elderly patients. Am J Cardiol 1987;59:998–999.
108. Shirani J, Yousefi J, Roberts WC. Major cardiac findings at necropsy in 366 American octogenarians. Am J Cardiol 1995;75:151–156.
109. Lindroos M, Kupari M, Heikkila J, et al. Prevalence of aortic valve abnormalities in the elderly: an echocardiographic study of a random population sample. J Am Coll Cardiol 1993;21:1220–1225.
110. Margonato A, Cianflone D, Carlino M, et al. Frequence and significance of aortic valve thickening in older asymptomatic patients and its relation to aortic regurgitation. Am J Cardiol 1989;64:1061–1062.
111. Akasaka T, Yoshikawa J, Yoshida K, et al. Age-related valvular regurgitation: a study by pulsed Doppler echocardiography. Circulation 1987;76:262–265.
112. Aronow WS, Kronzon I. Correlation of prevalence and severity of aortic regurgitation detected by pulsed Doppler echocardiography with the murmur of aortic regurgitation in elderly patients in a long-term health care facility. Am J Cardiol 1989;63:128–129.
113. Sell S, Scully RE. Aging changes in the aortic and mitral valves. Am J Pathol 1965;46:345–365.
114. Pomerance A, Darby AJ, Hodkinson HM. Valvular calcification in the elderly: possible pathogenic factors. J Gerontol 1978;33:672–676.
115. Roberts WC. The senile cardiac calcification syndrome. Am J Cardiol 1986;58:572–574.
116. Aronow WS, Schwartz KS, Koenigsberg M. Correlation of atrial fibrillation with presence of absence of mitral annular calcium in 604 persons older than 60 years. Am J Cardiol 1987;59:1213–1214.
117. Aronow WS, Schwartz KS, Koenigsberg M. Correlation of serum lipids, calcium and phosphorus, diabetes mellitus, aortic valve stenosis and history of systemic hypertension with presence or absence of mitral annular calcium in persons older than 62 years in a long-term health care facility. Am J Cardiol 1987;59:381–382.
118. Roberts WC, Perloff JK. Mitral valvular disease: a clinicopathologic survey of the conditions causing the mitral valve to function abnormally. Ann Intern Med 1972;77: 939–975.

# 31 Risk Factors for Atherosclerosis in the Elderly

Wilbert S. Aronow and William H. Frishman

Coronary artery disease (CAD) is the leading cause of death in elderly persons. CAD, peripheral arterial disease (PAD), atherothrombotic brain infarction (ABI), and extracranial carotid arterial disease (ECAD) are more common in old individuals than in middle-aged ones. CAD is the leading cause of death in old persons with PAD, ABI, or ECAD. This chapter discusses risk factors for CAD, PAD, ABI, and ECAD in old persons.

## Cigarette Smoking

### Coronary Artery Disease

The Chicago Stroke Study demonstrated that current cigarette smokers, ages 65–74, had a 52% higher mortality from CAD than nonsmokers, ex-smokers, and pipe and cigar smokers.[1] Ex-smokers who had stopped smoking for 1–5 years had similar mortality from CAD as nonsmokers. The Systolic Hypertension in the Elderly Program pilot project found that smoking was a predictor of a first cardiovascular event and myocardial infarction (MI)/sudden death.[2] During a 30-year follow-up of subjects 65 years of age and older in the Framingham Heart Study, cigarette smoking was not associated with the incidence of CAD but was associated with mortality from CAD.[3]

During a 12-year follow-up of men ages 65–74 in the Honolulu Heart Program, cigarette smoking was an independent risk factor for nonfatal MI and fatal CAD.[4] The absolute excess risk associated with cigarette smoking was 1.9 times higher in old men than in middle-aged men. At 5-year follow-up of old subjects (age 65 and older) in three communities, cigarette smokers were shown to have a higher incidence of cardiovascular mortality than nonsmokers.[5] The relative risk for cardiovascular mortality was 2.0 in male smokers and 1.6 in female smokers. The incidence of cardiovascular death in former smokers was similar to that for those who had never smoked.[5]

At 40-month follow-up of 664 old men (mean age 80 years) and 48-month follow-up of 1488 old women (mean age 82 years), cigarette smoking was demonstrated by multivariate analysis to increase the relative risk of new coronary events 2.2 and 2.0 times, respectively (Table 31.1).[6] During a 42-month mean follow-up of 410 old Blacks and Whites with hypertension (mean age 81), the odds ratio for developing new coronary events was 2.0 in cigarette smokers.[9] It has also been observed that cigarette smoking aggravates angina pectoris and precipitates silent myocardial ischemia in old persons with CAD.

In the Coronary Artery Surgery Study Registry, subjects over the age of 65 who continued smoking had an increased risk of developing MI or sudden death compared to those who stopped smoking during the year before enrolling in the study.[10] Furthermore, increasing age did not decrease the beneficial effects of smoking cessation.

In the Bronx Longitudinal Aging Study (BAS), whose cohort consisted of subjects 75 to 85 years of age at study onset, 10% of the cohort were smoking at study onset, and 46% reported having smoked in the past.[11] In the various BAS multivariate analyses, cigarette smoking history was shown to be an independent predictor of both cardiovascular morbidity and mortality and the development of MI.

### Peripheral Arterial Disease

Numerous studies have shown that cigarette smoking is a risk factor for PAD in men and women.[7,12–19] In a study of 869 old subjects (mean age 82 years), current cigarette smoking was shown to increase the prevalence of PAD 2.5 and 2.9 times in old men and women, respectively (Table 31.1).[7] At 43-month follow-up of 291 old subjects (mean age 82 years) with PAD, multivariate analysis demonstrated that cigarette smoking was an independent predictor of new coronary events, with a relative risk of 1.6.[20]

TABLE 31.1. Association of Cigarette Smoking with New Coronary Events, Peripheral Arterial Disease, and New Atherothrombotic Brain Infarction in Elderly Men and Women

| Study | Elderly men | | | Elderly women | | |
|---|---|---|---|---|---|---|
| | No. of pts. | Mean follow-up (months) | Relative risk | No. of pts. | Mean follow-up (months) | Relative risk |
| Incidence of new coronary events[6] | 664 | 40 | 2.2 | 1488 | 48 | 2.0 |
| Prevalence of PAD[7] | 244 | — | 2.4 | 625 | — | 2.9 |
| Incidence of new ABI[8] | 664 | 42 | 1.5* | 1488 | 48 | 1.9 |

PAD, peripheral arterial disease; ABI, atherothrombotic brain infarction.
* $p = 0.065$.

### Atherothrombotic Brain Infarction

A meta-analysis of 32 studies showed that cigarette smoking is a risk factor for ABI in men and women and carries a relative risk of 1.9.[21] In the Medical Research Council Trial, the incidence of strokes was 2.3 times higher in smokers than in nonsmokers.[22] Moreover, nonsmokers who received propranolol as antihypertensive therapy, had a reduction in the incidence of stroke that cigarette smokers did not have. In the Framingham Heart Study, during a 26-year follow-up, cigarette smoking increased the incidence of new ABI 1.6 and 1.9 times in men and women, respectively.[23] Furthermore, the incidence of stroke in smokers who used more than 40 cigarettes daily was twice as high as in those who used fewer than 10 cigarettes daily. The impact of cigarette smoking did not diminish with increasing age. The risk of stroke was substantially decreased within 2 years of quitting smoking, with the incidence of stroke returning to the level of nonsmokers 5 years after smoking cessation. Although elderly individuals who quit smoking have higher cerebral perfusion levels than old persons who continue to smoke, their cerebral perfusion levels are lower than those who have never smoked.[24]

At 42-month follow-up of 664 old men (mean age 80) and 48-month follow-up of 1488 old women (mean age 82), cigarette smoking was demonstrated by multivariate analysis to increase the relative risk for ABI 1.5 and 1.9 times in men and women, respectively (Table 31.1).[8]

### Extracranial Carotid Arterial Disease

Numerous studies have demonstrated that cigarette smoking is a strong risk factor for ECAD.[25–32] In a study of 1063 old subjects (mean age 81 years), cigarette smoking was found by multivariate analysis to increase the prevalence of 40–100% ECAD 4.2 times.[31]

On the basis of the available data, old men and women who smoke should be strongly encouraged to stop. In these individuals, cigarette smoking is a risk factor for CAD, PAD, ABI, and ECAD, as well as for other disorders including pulmonary disease and lung cancer. Smoking cessation should reduce mortality due to CAD, stroke, and other cardiovascular diseases and all-cause mortality in elderly persons.

## Hypertension

### Coronary Artery Disease

Increased peripheral vascular resistance is the cause of systolic and diastolic hypertension in old persons. *Systolic hypertension* is diagnosed if the systolic blood pressure is 140 mmHg or higher on three occasions, and *diastolic hypertension* is diagnosed if the diastolic blood pressure is 90 mmHg or higher on three occasions.[9] *Isolated systolic hypertension* is diagnosed when the systolic blood pressure is 140 mmHg or higher on three occasions but diastolic blood pressure is normal.[9]

In a study of 499 old individuals with hypertension, isolated systolic hypertension occurred in two-thirds of the persons. In 1414 old subjects (mean age 82 years), the prevalence of systolic or diastolic hypertension was higher in Blacks (50%) than in Hispanics (35%) or Whites (36%).[33] Although both diastolic and isolated systolic hypertension are associated with increased cardiovascular morbidity and mortality in old individuals, increased systolic blood pressure is the greater risk factor.[34]

The higher the systolic or diastolic blood pressure, the greater the morbidity/mortality from CAD in old men and women. During a 30-year follow-up of subjects 65 years and older in the Framingham Heart Study, systolic hypertension correlated with the incidence of CAD in men and women.[3] Diastolic hypertension correlated with CAD in old men but not in old women.[3] At 40-month follow-up of 664 old men and 48-month follow-up of 1488 old women, systolic or diastolic hypertension was demonstrated by multivariate analysis to increase the relative risk of new coronary events 2.0 and 1.6 times, respectively (Table 31.2).[6]

In the BAS[11] no relation was found between hypertension and the development of fatal MI, but a relation did exist for the development of clinically unrecognized MI, especially among hypertensives not on medication. Antihypertensive drugs have been shown to reduce new coro-

TABLE 31.2. Association of Systolic or Diastolic Hypertension with New Coronary Events, Peripheral Arterial Disease, and New Atherothrombotic Brain Infarction in Elderly Men and Women

| | Elderly men | | | Elderly women | | |
|---|---|---|---|---|---|---|
| Study | No. of pts. | Mean follow-up (months) | Relative risk | No. of pts. | Mean follow-up (months) | Relative risk |
| Incidence of new coronary events[6] | 664 | 40 | 2.0 | 1488 | 48 | 1.6 |
| Prevalence of PAD[7] | 244 | — | 1.7 | 625 | — | 1.5 |
| Incidence of new ABI[8] | 664 | 42 | 2.2 | 1488 | 48 | 2.4 |

nary events in the elderly hypertensive population.[35–38] The Joint National Committee on Detection, Evaluation and Treatment of High Blood Pressure recommends diuretics or β-blockers as initial drug therapy because these drugs have been demonstrated to reduce cardiovascular morbidity and mortality in controlled clinical trials.[39] The particular antihypertensive selected as monotherapy should depend on the associated medical conditions. For example, old individuals with hypertension who have had an MI or who have angina pectoris, myocardial ischemia or complex ventricular arrhythmias, should be treated initially with a β-blocker.[40] Old hypertensive persons with congestive heart failure associated with abnormal or normal left ventricular ejection fraction, should receive both a diuretic and an angiotensin-converting enzyme (ACE) inhibitor.[41] Old persons with hypertension who have diabetes mellitus or left ventricular hypertrophy should initially be treated with an ACE inhibitor.

## Peripheral Arterial Disease

Numerous studies have demonstrated that hypertension is a risk factor for PAD.[7,12,13,15–17,19] In a study of 869 old subjects, systolic or diastolic hypertension was observed to increase the prevalence of PAD 1.7 times in men and 1.5 times in women (Table 31.2).[7] At 43-month follow-up of 291 old subjects with PAD (mean age 82), new coronary events developed in 165 patients (57%).[20]

## Atherothrombotic Brain Infarction

Numerous studies have documented that both systolic and diastolic hypertension increase the incidence of stroke in old persons.[8,12,35–38,42–45] Indeed, the higher the systolic or diastolic blood pressure, the greater the incidence of stroke. During a 30-year follow-up of men and women ages 65–94 years in the Framingham Heart Study, systolic blood pressure was the single risk factor most strongly correlated with ABI or transient cerebral ischemic attack.[12] At 42-month follow-up of 664 old men and 48-month follow-up of 1488 old women, systolic or diastolic hypertension was demonstrated by multivariate analysis to increase the relative risk of ABI 2.2 times in men and 2.4 times in women (Table 31.2).[8]

In the BAS, subjects with measured hypertension had a significantly increased incidence of stroke (1.9/100 person-years) compared to that in controls (0.6/100 person-years).[11] Previous studies have used a definition of hypertension as systolic blood pressure >160 mmHg, diastolic blood pressure >95 mmHg, or both to show an increased risk of stroke.[46] The findings in the BAS extended the risk of stroke to this oldest-old age group; and considering the strict study values used, it suggested that the risk exists even at levels of blood pressure not previously uniformly considered to be elevated by others.

Antihypertensive drug therapy has been shown to reduce the incidence of new ABI in old individuals.[35–38,43] A systolic blood pressure of 140–160 mmHg causes an increased risk for cardiovascular disease that is equivalent to a diastolic blood pressure of 95–105 mmHg.[34,47] Consequently, the clinician should consider treatment of old persons with systolic blood pressures in this range. Although nonpharmacologic interventions are indicated,[48] there are currently no data showing that drug therapy for systolic blood pressures of 140–160 mmHg reduces the incidence of stroke in old persons. Nevertheless, the presence of left ventricular hypertrophy, target organ damage, and other risk factors for stroke would cause the authors to treat these individuals with antihypertensive drug therapy.

## Extracranial Carotid Arterial Disease

Numerous studies have demonstrated by univariate analysis that hypertension is a risk factor for ECAD.[25,27,29,31,49] According to multivariate analysis, however, hypertension is a risk factor in some studies[27,49] but not in others.[25,31] In a study of 1283 old subjects (mean age 81), left ventricular hypertrophy was more prevalent in those with systolic or diastolic hypertension and ECAD than in those with systolic or diastolic hypertension alone.[50]

## Left Ventricular Hypertrophy

### Coronary Events

Left ventricular hypertrophy caused by hypertension or other cardiovascular disease is not only a marker of but also a contributor to cardiovascular morbidity and mortality in the elderly population. Indeed, old persons with electrocardiographic (ECG)[9,51–53] and echocardiographic[9,52,54–58] evidence of left ventricular hypertrophy have an increased risk of developing new coronary events.

During a 4-year follow-up of 406 old men and 735 old women in the Framingham Heart Study, echocardiographic left ventricular hypertrophy was 15.3 times more sensitive for predicting new coronary events in men and 4.3 times more sensitive in women than ECG left ventricular hypertrophy.[54] The relative risk for new coronary events per 50g/m increases in left ventricular mass/height was 1.67 and 1.60 for old men and women, respectively.[54]

At a 37-month follow-up of 360 old subjects (mean age 82 years) with hypertension or CAD, echocardiographic left ventricular hypertrophy was 4.3 times more sensitive for predicting new coronary events than was ECG left ventricular hypertrophy.[52] Multivariate analysis of 472 old hypertensive subjects followed for 45 months showed that echocardiographic left ventricular hypertrophy was an independent risk factor for new coronary events, with a relative risk of 3.2.[58]

In the BAS a multivariate analysis showed that baseline ECG left ventricular hypertrophy is an independent predictor of MI and overall mortality. Those subjects who developed new left ventricular hypertrophy on ECG during follow-up had a 3.4 times higher total death rate and a 6.6-fold greater relative risk of cardiovascular death.[11]

### Atherothrombotic Brain Infarction

Elderly persons with ECG[9,51–53] and echocardiographic[9,52,55,58–60] left ventricular hypertrophy have an increased risk of developing a new ABI. During an 8-year follow-up of 447 old men and 783 old women in the Framingham Heart Study, the hazard ratio for new cerebrovascular events was 1.45 for each quartile increase in the left ventricular mass/height ratio after adjustments were made for age, sex, and cardiovascular disease.[59] At the 37-month follow-up of 360 old persons with hypertension and CAD, echocardiographic left ventricular hypertrophy was 4.0 times more sensitive for predicting a new ABI than ECG left ventricular hypertrophy.[52] Multivariate analysis of 472 old subjects with hypertension followed for 45 months revealed that echocardiographic left ventricular hypertrophy was an independent risk factor for a new ABI, with a relative risk of 2.9.[58] Among 1482 old persons (mean age 82 years) followed for 45 months, multivariate analysis also showed that echocardiographic left ventricular hypertrophy was an independent risk factor for a new ABI, with a risk ratio of 2.3.[60]

Physicians should try to prevent left ventricular hypertrophy from developing or progressing in persons with hypertension or other cardiovascular disease. The effect of various antihypertensive drugs on reducing left ventricular mass is discussed elsewhere.[61,62] A meta-analysis of 109 treatment studies showed that ACE inhibitors are more effective than other antihypertensive drugs in decreasing left ventricular mass.[62]

Reduction of left ventricular mass with antihypertensives does not cause deterioration of left ventricular systolic function and may improve left ventricular diastolic function. Data from the Framingham Heart Study have shown a decrease of cardiovascular events in patients with regression of left ventricular hypertrophy.[63] In patients with uncomplicated hypertension followed for 10.2 years, the Cornell group found that the development of left ventricular hypertrophy increases and the regression of left ventricular hypertrophy probably decreases the incidence of new cardiovascular events.[64] In addition, the BAS demonstrated that old subjects who developed new ECG left ventricular hypertrophy had a higher incidence of cardiovascular morbidity and mortality than old persons without ECG left ventricular hypertrophy[53] based on a 10-year follow-up. Old persons in whom the ECG pattern of left ventricular hypertrophy disappeared over time had a lower incidence of cardiovascular morbidity and mortality than old persons with persistent left ventricular hypertrophy.[53]

## Dyslipidemia

### Serum Total Cholesterol and Coronary Artery Disease

Serum total cholesterol was an independent risk factor for CAD in old men and women in the Framingham Heart Study.[65] Among subjects with prior MI in this study, serum total cholesterol was most strongly related to death from CAD and to all-cause mortality in persons age 65 years and older.[66] Many other studies have demonstrated that a higher serum total cholesterol level is a risk factor for new coronary events in old men and women.[2,6,67–69]

During a 9-year follow-up of 350 men and women with a mean age of 79 years, the BAS demonstrated that a consistently elevated low density lipoprotein (LDL) cholesterol was associated with the development of MI in women.[70] In the Established Populations for Epidemiologic Studies of the Elderly study, serum total cholesterol was a risk factor for CAD-associated mortality in old women but not in old men.[71] At 40-month follow-up of 664 old men and 48-month follow-up of 1488 old women, there was a 1.12 times higher probability of developing new coronary events in men and women for each 10mg/dl increase in serum total cholesterol (Table 31.3).[6]

During a 5.4-year median follow-up of 4444 men and women with CAD and hypercholesterolemia in the Scan-

TABLE 31.3. Association of Abnormal Serum Lipids with New Coronary Events in 664 Old Men and 1488 Old Women

| | Relative risk | |
|---|---|---|
| Parameter | Men | Women |
| Serum total cholesterol | 1.12* | 1.12* |
| Serum HDL-cholesterol | 1.70** | 1.95** |
| Serum triglycerides | NS | 1.02*** |

*Source:* Adapted from Aronow and Ahn.[6]
HDL, high density lipoprotein; NS, not significant.
* For an increment of 10 mg/dl of serum total cholesterol; ** for a decrement of 10 mg/dl of serum HDL-cholesterol; *** for an increment of 10 mg/dl of serum triglycerides.

dinavian Simvastatin Survival Study, patients treated with simvastatin had a 34% reduction in major coronary events, 42% reduction in coronary death, and 30% reduction in overall mortality.[72] The decreases in coronary events and total mortality were similar in men and women 60–70 years of age at study entry and those who were younger.[72]

In the Cholesterol and Recurrent Events (CARE) trial, 4159 men and women with MI, serum total cholesterol levels <240 mg/dl, and serum LDL-cholesterol ≥115 mg/dl were followed over a 5-year period.[73] The trial showed a 27% reduction in major coronary events in subjects 60–75 years of age who were randomized to pravastatin at study event; a 20% reduction in major coronary events was observed in subjects younger than 60 years of age who were randomized to pravastatin. Furthermore, the reduction in coronary events was greater in women (46%) than in men (20%). On the basis of these data, old men and women with CAD and elevated total or LDL-cholesterol should be treated with a statin drug.

## Serum HDL-Cholesterol and Coronary Artery Disease

A low level of serum high density lipoprotein (HDL) cholesterol is a risk factor for new coronary events in old men and women.[2,6,65,70,71,74,75] In the Framingham Heart Study[65] and in the Establshed Populations for Epidemiologic Studies of the Elderly study,[71] a low serum HDL was a more powerful predictor of new coronary events than was the total cholesterol.

During a 9-year follow-up of 350 men and women in the BAS, a consistently low HDL-cholesterol level was independently associated with the development of MI, cardiovascular disease, or death in men.[70] At a 40-month follow-up of 664 old men and 48-month follow-up of 1488 old women, multivariate analysis showed there was a 1.7 times higher probability of developing new coronary events in men and 1.95 times higher probability in women for each 10 mg/dl decrement in serum HDL-cholesterol (Table 31.3).[6]

## Serum Triglycerides and Coronary Artery Disease

High serum triglycerides have been reported to be a risk factor for new coronary events in old women but not in old men.[6,65] At a 40-month follow-up of 664 old men and 48-month follow-up of 1488 old women, multivariate analysis showed that serum triglyceride levels were not a risk factor for new coronary events in the men and were a weak risk factor in the women (Table 31.3).[6]

## Serum Lipids and Peripheral Arterial Disease

Some studies have shown an association between increased serum total cholesterol and PAD,[12,14,76,77] but other studies have not.[16,78,79] A low serum HDL-cholesterol level, however, has been shown to be associated with PAD.[14,76,77,79] In a study of 559 old men and 1275 old women (mean age 81 years), an inverse association was found between serum HDL-cholesterol and PAD.[79] Multivariate analysis demonstrated a 1.24 times higher probability of having PAD for each 10 mg/dl decrement of serum HDL-cholesterol.

Increased serum triglycerides have been associated with PAD in some studies[14,16,77] but not in others.[7,76,79] In a study of 559 old men and 1275 old women, serum triglycerides were associated with PAD in both men and women according to univariate analysis but not according to multivariate analysis.[79]

## Serum Lipids and Atherothrombotic Brain Infarction

The Framingham Study found that serum total and HDL-cholesterol levels were not associated with new ABIs in old men or women.[44] However, the serum total cholesterol HDL-cholesterol ratio was associated with new ABIs in the women but not the men. Very low density lipoprotein (VLDL) levels were not associated with new ABIs in older men or women.[44]

The Multiple Risk Factor Intervention Trial revealed an association between serum total cholesterol and death from nonhemorrhagic stroke in men.[80] Bihari-Varga et al.[81] demonstrated an inverse relation between serum HDL-cholesterol and ABIs in men and women. At 42-month follow-up of 664 old men and 48-month follow-up of 1488 older women, multivariate analysis showed no association between serum lipids and new ABIs in the men. There was an association between serum total cholesterol and an inverse association between HDL-cholesterol and new ABIs in the women (Table 31.4).[24] In this population there was a 1.06 times higher probability of developing a new ABI for each 10 mg/dl increment in serum total cholesterol. Likewise, there was a 1.14 times higher probability of developing a new ABI for each 10 mg/dl decrement in serum HDL-cholesterol.

TABLE 31.4. Association of Abnormal Serum Lipids with New Atherothrombotic Brain Infarction in 664 Old Men and 1488 Old Women

| Parameter | Relative risk | |
|---|---|---|
| | Men | Women |
| Serum total cholesterol | NS | 1.06* |
| Serum HDL-cholesterol | NS | 1.14** |
| Serum triglycerides | NS | NS |

*Source:* Adapted from Aronow et al.[24]
HDL, high density lipoprotein; NS, not significant.
* for an increment of 10 mg/dl of serum total cholesterol; ** for a decrement of 10 mg/dl of serum HDL-cholesterol.

In the Scandinavian Simvastatin Survival Study, patients treated with simvastatin had a 27% reduction in new ABIs.[72] In the Cholesterol and Recurrent Events trial, patients treated with pravastatin had a 31% reduction in new ABIs.[73] A meta-analysis of four primary prevention trials and eight secondary prevention trials of CAD that used simvastatin, pravastatin, or lovastatin to reduce serum total cholesterol levels, demonstrated a 27% reduction in new ABIs.[82] These data support the use of statins to reduce elevated serum total and LDL-cholesterol levels in old men and women to prevent new ABIs and new coronary events.

## Serum Lipids and Extracranial Carotid Arterial Disease

Elevated serum total cholesterol[26,31,83,84] and decreased serum HDL-cholesterol[26,27,29–31,48,83,84] are risk factors for ECAD. In 1189 persons age 66–93 years in the Framingham study, there was a strong association between the severity of ECAD and the serum total cholesterol, as measured 8 years before the carotid studies.[83] In women, but not in men, there was a strong inverse association between the severity of ECAD and the serum HDL-cholesterol level measured 8 years before the carotid studies and concurrently.[83]

In a study of 1063 old persons, increased total cholesterol and decreased HDL-cholesterol, but not serum triglycerides, were found to be risk factors for ECAD.[31] There was a 1.17 times higher probability of having 40–100% ECAD for each 10 mg/dl increment of serum total cholesterol and a 1.66 times higher probability of having 40–100% ECAD for each 10 mg/dl decrement of serum HDL-cholesterol. Many studies have demonstrated the beneficial effects of lipid-lowering drug therapy on carotid atherosclerosis and on coronary events.[85–87]

# Diabetes Mellitus

## Coronary Artery Disease

Diabetes mellitus is a risk factor for new coronary events in old men and women.[6,88] At a 40-month follow-up of 664 old men and 48-month follow-up of 1488 old women, diabetes mellitus was shown by multivariate analysis to increase the relative risk of new coronary events 1.9 and 1.8 times in men and women, respectively (Table 31.5).[6]

In the BAS diabetes mellitus, by history or a fasting blood glucose level >140 mg/dl was associated with an increased incidence risk of all-cause mortality and cardiovascular disease.[11]

Diabetic patients are more often obese and have higher serum LDL- and VLDL-cholesterol levels and lower serum HDL-cholesterol levels than do nondiabetics. Diabetics also have a higher prevalence of hypertension and left ventricular hypertrophy. These risk factors contribute to their higher incidence of new coronary events and new ABIs and the higher prevalence of PAD and ECAD. The drug of choice for treating hypertension in diabetics is an ACE inhibitor.

## Peripheral Arterial Disease

Diabetes mellitus is a risk factor for PAD in men and women.[7,12–15,18,19] In a study of 244 old men and 625 old women, diabetes mellitus was found to increase the prevalence of PAD 2.4 times in men and 3.0 times in women (Table 31.5).[19]

## Atherothrombotic Brain Infarction

Diabetes mellitus is a risk factor for new ABIs in old men and women.[24,44,89] At a 42-month follow-up of 664 old men and a 48-month follow-up of 1488 old women, diabetes was found by multivariate analysis to increase the rela-

TABLE 31.5. Association of Diabetes Mellitus with New Coronary Events, Peripheral Arterial Disease, and New Atherothrombotic Brain Infarction in Old Men and Women

| Study | Older men | | | Older women | | |
|---|---|---|---|---|---|---|
| | No. of pts. | Mean follow-up (months) | Relative risk | No. of pts. | Mean follow-up (months) | Relative risk |
| Incidence of new coronary events[6] | 664 | 40 | 1.9 | 1488 | 48 | 1.8 |
| Prevalence of PAD[7] | 244 | — | 2.4 | 625 | — | 3.0 |
| Incidence of new ABI[8] | 664 | 42 | 1.5 | 1488 | 48 | 1.5 |

tive risk for new ABIs 1.5 times in both men and women (Table 31.5).[24]

### Extracranial Carotid Arterial Disease

Some studies[31,90] have shown an association between diabetes mellitus and ECAD, whereas other studies[27,30] have not. In a study of 1063 old men and women, diabetes mellitus was demonstrated by multivariate analysis to increase the prevalence of 40–100% ECAD 1.7 times.[31]

## Obesity

In the Framingham Heart Study, obesity was demonstrated to be a risk factor for new coronary events in old men and women.[88] A disproportionate distribution of fat to the abdomen, as assessed by the waist/hip circumference ratio, has also been shown to be a risk factor for cardiovascular disease, mortality due to CAD, and total mortality.[91,92] At a 40-month follow-up of 664 old men and a 48-month follow-up of 1488 old women, obesity was shown to be a risk factor for new coronary events in both men and women by univariate but not multivariate analysis.[6]

In the BAS, body surface area was also not predictive. There were no subjects with major obesity problems.[11] In elderly subjects, maintenance of weight and appetite is a sign of health. Indeed, when old subjects lose weight and have reductions in their cholesterol, it may signify starvation, an occult malignancy, or a major cognitive problem.

The Framingham Heart Study showed that relative weight, according to Metropolitan Life Insurance criteria, was not associated with intermittent claudication in women but was inversely associated with intermittent claudication in men.[12] In a study of 244 old men and 625 old women, obesity did not significantly increase the prevalence of PAD in the men, but it did increase the prevalence of PAD 1.8 times in the women.[7]

The Framingham Heart Study showed that relative weight was not a risk factor for new ABIs in old men but was a weak risk factor in old women.[44] Barrett-Connor and Khaw[89] observed no association between body mass index and new ABIs in old men and women. At a 42-month follow-up of 664 old men, obesity was not a risk factor for new ABIs.[24] At a 48-month follow-up of 1488 old women, obesity was a risk factor for new ABIs by univariate analysis but not multivariate analysis.[24] Obesity is not a risk factor for ECAD.[27,31]

## Physical Inactivity

Physical inactivity is associated with obesity, hypertension, dyslipidemia, and hyperglycemia. Paffenbarger et al.[93] found that individuals age 65–79 with a physical activity index of more than 2000 kcal/week have a better survival rate than those with an index less than 2000 kcal/week. Wenger[94] discussed physiologic bases for the decrease in habitual physical activity with age and noted studies suggesting that physical activity is beneficial in preventing CAD. The relation of physical inactivity to ABI is unclear.[44,95,96]

Moderate exercise programs suitable for old persons include walking, climbing stairs, swimming, and bicycling. Exercise training programs are not only beneficial for preventing CAD[94] but have also been demonstrated to improve endurance and functional capacity in old men with CAD.[97]

## Age

The incidence of new coronary events increases with age in old men and women.[6,88] In the Framingham Heart Study, the incidence of PAD[13] and ABI[44] also increased with age.

In the BAS, age was the strongest independent predictor of total mortality, cardiovascular mortality, MI, stroke, and dementia.[11]

## Gender

At a 40-month follow-up of 664 old men (mean age 80) and a 48-month follow-up of 1488 old women (mean age 82), the incidence of new coronary events was not significantly different in the men (45%) and the women (43%) (Table 31.6).[6] The prevalence of PAD in 244 old men (34%) (mean age of 82) was higher than in 625 old women (23%) of the same mean age (Table 31.6).[19] At a 42-month follow-up of 664 old men and a 48-month follow-up of 1488 old women, the incidence of new ABIs was higher in the men (21%) than in the women (17%) (Table 31.6).[24] The prevalence of 40–100% ECAD was not significantly different for 435 old men (18%) and 1057 old women (15%) with a mean age of 82 years (Table 31.6).[60] In the BAS, the incidence of MI was higher in women than in men.[11]

## Race

Black men are 2.5 times more likely to die of stroke than white men, and black women are 2.4 times more likely to die of stroke than white women.[98] Table 31.7 shows the prevalence of CAD, PAD, and ABI in 268 elderly Blacks (mean age 81), 71 elderly Hispanics (mean age 81), and 1310 elderly Whites (mean age 82).[99] The prevalence of CAD was not significantly different among the Blacks, Hispanics, and Whites. However, the prevalence of PAD was significantly higher in the Blacks than

TABLE 31.6. Association of Gender with Incidence of New Coronary Events, Prevalence of Peripheral Arterial Disease, Incidence of New Atherothrombotic Brain Infarction, and Prevalence of 40–100% Extracranial Carotid Arterial Disease in Old Men and Women

| Study | Old men | | | Old women | | |
|---|---|---|---|---|---|---|
| | No. of pts. | Mean follow-up (months) | Incidence or prevalence (%) | No. of pts. | Mean follow-up (months) | Incidence or prevalence (%) |
| Incidence of new coronary events[6] | 664 | 40 | 45 | 1488 | 48 | 43 |
| Prevalence of PAD[7] | 244 | — | 34* | 625 | — | 23 |
| Incidence of new ABI[8] | 644 | 42 | 21** | 1488 | 48 | 17 |
| Prevalence of 40–100% ECAD[60] | 435 | — | 18 | 1057 | — | 15 |

ECAD, extracranial carotid arterial disease.
* $p < 0.05$; ** $p = 0.043$.

in Whites. Likewise, the prevalence of ABI was significantly higher in the Blacks than in either Hispanics or Whites.

## Prior Coronary Artery Disease, Peripheral Arterial Disease, and Atherothrombotic Brain Infarction

At a 40-month follow-up of 664 old men and a 48-month follow-up of 1488 old women, prior CAD was shown by multivariate analysis to increase the relative risk of new coronary events 1.7 times in men and 1.9 times in women.[6] At a 43-month follow-up of 291 old persons (mean age 82) with PAD, prior CAD was shown to be an independent risk factor for new coronary events, with a relative risk of 2.7.[20]

In the BAS, over an average range of 5–8 years of follow-up, the incidence of cardiovascular disease and mortality in subjects with evidence of infarct at baseline were 8.8 and 5.9 per 100 person-years versus 4.7 and 3.9 per 100 person-years in controls, respectively. The rates of development of unrecognized MI (Q-wave) were 2.4 and 3.2 per 100 person-years, respectively, for recognized MI. The rate of development of either a recognized or unrecognized MI was three times more likely in those with a history of a prior infarct.[11]

Old persons with prior ABI or transient cerebral ischemic attacks have a higher incidence of ABI.[9,24,44,100] At a 42-month follow-up of 664 old men and a 48-month follow-up of 1488 old women, multivariate analysis showed that a prior ABI increased the relative risk of a new ABI 2.6 times in men and 2.9 times in women.[24]

TABLE 31.7. Prevalence of Coronary Artery Disease, Peripheral Arterial Disease, and Atherothrombotic Brain Infarction in Elderly Blacks, Hispanics, and Whites

| Disorder | Prevalence (%) | | |
|---|---|---|---|
| | Blacks ($n = 268$) | Hispanics ($n = 71$) | Whites ($n = 1310$) |
| CAD | 46 | 34 | 41 |
| PAD | 29* | 24 | 23 |
| ABI | 47** | 31 | 22 |

*Source:* Adapted from Aronow.[99]
* $p < 0.05$ comparing Blacks with Whites; ** $p < 0.001$ comparing Blacks with Whites and <0.02 comparing Blacks with Hispanics.

## Coexistence of Coronary Artery Disease, Peripheral Arterial Disease, and Atherothrombotic Brain Infarction

Persons with PAD[20,101,102] or cerebrovascular disease[103–106] are at increased risk for developing new coronary events. The Framingham Heart Study demonstrated that the age-adjusted incidence of stroke was more than doubled in patients with CAD.[44] In a study of 110 old persons (mean age 82) with chronic atrial fibrillation, logistic regression analysis revealed that a prior MI was an independent predictor of thromboembolic stroke, with an odds ratio of 4.8.[57] Table 31.8 shows the prevalence of coexistence of CAD, PAD, and ABI in a study of 1886 old persons (580 men, 1306 women) whose mean age was 81 years.[107]

TABLE 31.8. Prevalence of Coexistence of Coronary Artery Disease, Peripheral Arterial Disease, and Atherothrombotic Brain Infarction in 1886 Elderly Persons

| Condition | Prevalence (%) | | |
|---|---|---|---|
| | CAD | PAD | ABI |
| ABI present | 53 | 33 | — |
| PAD present | 58 | — | 34 |
| CAD present | — | 33 | 32 |

*Source:* Adapted from Aronow and Ahn.[107]

Table 31.9. Factors Associated with Increased Independent Risk of Incident Morbidity or Cardiovascular Disease in the Oldest Old[a]: Bronx Longitudinal Aging Study

| |
|---|
| Age |
| Smoking history |
| Diabetes mellitus |
| History of past myocardial infarction (MI) (clinically apparent or silent) documented on electrocardiography (ECG) |
| Left ventricular hypertrophy by ECG (including new onset) |
| Cardiomegaly by chest radiography (including new onset) |
| Nonsustained ventricular tachycardia on 24-hour Holter ECG |
| Persistent HDL-cholesterol ≤30 mg/dl in men; persistent LDL-cholesterol ≥171 mg/dl in women |
| Hypertension, both combined systolic and diastolic and isolated systolic |
| Prolongation of the RR interval on resting ECG |
| Nonspecific ST and T wave abnormalities on resting ECG (unrelated to left ventricular hypertrophy or past MI) |
| Digoxin use |
| Unfavorable baseline self-rated health assessment |
| Development of dementia |
| High vitamin $B_{12}$ level |

*Source:* Frishman et al.,[11] with permission.
[a] Age 75–85 years.

## Conclusion

Many of the risk factors and markers for atherosclerosis complicated by CAD, cerebrovascular disease, and PAD seen during middle age continue to be operative in the elderly (Table 31.9).

## References


1. Jajich CL, Ostfield AM, Freeman DH Jr. Smoking and coronary heart disease mortality in the elderly. JAMA 1984;252:2831–2834.
2. Siegel D, Kuller L, Lazarus NB, et al. Predictors of cardiovascular events and mortality in the systolic hypertension in the elderly program pilot project. Am J Epidemiol 1987; 126:385–399.
3. Kannel WB, Vokonas PS. Primary risk factors for coronary heart disease in the elderly: the Framingham study. In: Wenger NK, Furberg CD, Pitt B (eds) Coronary Heart Disease in the Elderly. New York: Elsevier, 1986:60–92.
4. Benfante R, Reed D, Frank J. Does cigarette smoking have an independent effect on coronary heart disease incidence in the elderly? Am J Public Health 1991;81:897–899.
5. LaCroix AZ, Lang J, Scherr P, et al. Smoking and mortality among older men and women in three communities. N Engl J Med 1991;324:1619–1625.
6. Aronow WS, Ahn C. Risk factors for coronary events in a large cohort of very elderly patients with and without coronary artery disease. Am J Cardiol 1996;77:864–866.
7. Aronow WS, Sales FF, Etienne F, et al. Prevalence of peripheral arterial disease and its correlation with risk factors for peripheral arterial disease in elderly patients in a long-term health care facility. Am J Cardiol 1988;62:644–646.
8. Aronow WS, Ahn C, Gutstein H. Risk factors for new atherothrombotic brain infarction in 664 older men and 1488 older women. Am J Cardiol 1996;77:1380–1383.
9. Aronow WS, Ahn C, Kronzon I, et al. Congestive heart failure, coronary events and atherothrombotic brain infarction in elderly blacks and whites with systemic hypertension and with and without echocardiographic and electrocardiographic evidence of left ventricular hypertrophy. Am J Cardiol 1991;67:295–299.
10. Hermanson B, Omenn GS, Kronmal RA, et al. Beneficial six-year outcome of smoking cessation in older men and women with coronary artery disease: results from the CASS registry. N Engl J Med 1988;319:1365–1369.
11. Frishman WH, Sokol S, Aronson M, Wassertheil-Smoller S, Katzman R. Risk factors for cardiovascular and cerebrovascular diseases and dementia in the elderly: findings from the Bronx Longitudinal Aging Study. Curr Probl Cardiol 1998;23:1–68.
12. Stokes J III, Kannel WB, Wolf PA, et al. The relative importance of selected risk factors for various manifestations of cardiovascular disease among men and women from 35 to 64 years old: 30 years of follow-up in the Framingham study. Circulation 1987;75(suppl V):V65–V73.
13. Kannel WB, McGee DL. Update on some epidemiologic features of intermittent claudication: the Framingham study. J Am Geriatr Soc 1985;33:13–18.
14. Pomrehn P, Duncan B, Weissfeld L, et al. The association of dyslipoproteinemia with symptoms and signs of peripheral arterial disease: the Lipid Research Clinics Program Prevalence Study. Circulation 1986;73(suppl I): 100–107.
15. Juergens JL, Barker NW, Hines EA Jr. Arteriosclerosis obliterans: review of 520 cases with special reference to pathogenic and prognostic factors. Circulation 1960;21:188–195.
16. Hughson WG, Mann JI, Garrod A. Intermittent claudication: prevalence and risk factors. Br Med J 1978;1:1379–1381.
17. Schroll M, Munck O. Estimation of peripheral arteriosclerotic disease by ankle blood pressure measurements in a population study of 60 year old men and women. J Chronic Dis 1981;34:261–269.
18. Beach KW, Brunzell JD, Strandness DE Jr. Prevalence of severe arteriosclerosis obliterans in patients with diabetes mellitus: relation to smoking and form of therapy. Arteriosclerosis 1982;2:275–280.
19. Reunanen A, Takkunen H, Aromaa A. Prevalence of intermittent claudication and its effect on mortality. Acta Med Scand 1982;211:249–256.
20. Aronow WS, Ahn C, Mercando AD, et al. Prognostic significance of silent ischemia in elderly patients with peripheral arterial disease with and without previous myocardial infarction. Am J Cardiol 1992;69:137–139.
21. Shinton R, Beevers G. Meta-analysis of relation between cigarette smoking and stroke. Br Med J 1989;298:789–794.
22. Medical Research Council Working Party. MRC trial of treatment of mild hypertension: principal results. Br Med J Clin Res 1985;291:97–104.
23. Wolf PA, D'Agostino PS, Kannel WB, et al. Cigarette smoking as a risk factor for stroke: the Framingham study. JAMA 1988;259:1025–1029.

24. Rodgers RL, Meyer JS, Judd BW, et al. Abstention from cigarette smoking improves cerebral perfusion among elderly chronic smokers. JAMA 1985;253:2970–2974.
25. Candelise L, Bianchi F, Galligoni F, et al. Italian multicenter study on reversible cerebral ischemic attacks. III. Influence of age and risk factors on cerebrovascular atherosclerosis. Stroke 1984;15:379–382.
26. Ford CS, Crouse JR III, Howard G, et al. The role of plasma lipids in carotid bifurcation atherosclerosis. Ann Neurol 1985;17:301–303.
27. Crouse JR III, Toole JF, McKinney WM. Risk factors for extracranial carotid artery atherosclerosis. Stroke 1987;18: 990–996.
28. Tell GS, Howard G, McKinney WM, et al. Cigarette smoking cessation and extracranial carotid atherosclerosis. JAMA 1989;261:1178–1180.
29. Bots ML, Breslau BJ, Briet E, et al. Cardiovascular determinants of carotid artery disease: the Rotterdam Elderly Study. Hypertension 1992;19:717–720.
30. Prati P, Vanuzzo D, Casaroli M, et al. Prevalence and determinants of carotid atherosclerosis in a general population. Stroke 1992;23:1705–1711.
31. Aronow WS, Ahn C, Schoenfeld MR. Risk factors for extracranial internal or common carotid arterial disease in elderly patients. Am J Cardiol 1993;71:1479–1481.
32. Tell GS, Polak JF, Ward BJ, et al. Relation of smoking with carotid artery wall thickness and stenosis in older adults: the Cardiovascular Health Study. Circulation 1994;90: 2905–2908.
33. Aronow WS, Kronzon I. Prevalence of coronary risk factors in elderly blacks and whites. J Am Geriatr Soc 1991;39:567–570.
34. Applegate WB, Rutan GH. Advances in management of hypertension in older persons. J Am Geriatr Soc 1992;40: 1164–1174.
35. Amery A, Birkenhager W, Brixko P, et al. Mortality and morbidity results from the European Working Party on Hypertension in Elderly Trial. Lancet 1985;1:1349–1354.
36. Dahlof B, Lindholm LH, Hansson L, et al. Morbidity and mortality in the Swedish Trial in Old Patients with Hypertension (STOP Hypertension). Lancet 1991;338:1281–1285.
37. SHEP Cooperative Research Group. Prevention of stroke by antihypertensive drug treatment in older persons with isolated systolic hypertension: final results of the Systolic Hypertension in the Elderly Program (SHEP). JAMA 1991;265:3255–3264.
38. MRC Working Party. Medical Research Council Trial on treatment of hypertension in older adults: principal results. Br Med J 1992;304:405–412.
39. Joint National Committee on Detection, Evaluation and Treatment of High Blood Pressure. The Sixth Report of the Joint National Committee on Detection, Evaluation and Treatment of High Blood Pressure (JNC VI). Arch Intern Med 1997;157:2413–2444.
40. Aronow WS, Ahn C, Mercando AD, et al. Effect of propranolol versus no antiarrhythmic drug on sudden cardiac death, total cardiac death, and total death in patients ≥62 years of age with heart disease, complex ventricular arrhythmias, and left ventricular ejection fraction ≥40%. Am J Cardiol 1994;74:267–270.
41. Aronow WS, Kronzon I. Effect of enalapril on congestive heart failure treated with diuretics in elderly patients with prior myocardial infarction and normal left ventricular ejection fraction. Am J Cardiol 1993;71:602–604.
42. Garland C, Barrett-Connor E, Suarez L, et al. Isolated systolic hypertension and mortality after age 60 years: a prospective population-based study. Am J Epidemiol 1983;118:365–376.
43. Coope J, Warrender TS. Randomised trial of treatment of hypertension in elderly patients in primary care. Br Med J 1986;293:1145–1151.
44. Wolf PA. Cerebrovascular disease in the elderly. In: Tresch DD, Aronow WS (eds) Cardiovascular Disease in the Elderly Patient. New York: Marcel Dekker, 1999:125–147.
45. Shekelle RB, Ostfeld AM, Klawans HL. Hypertension and risk of stroke in an elderly population. Stroke 1974;5:71–75.
46. Lavie CJ, Ventura HO, Messerli FH. Left ventricular hypertrophy in the elderly. Cardiol Elderly 1994;2:362–369.
47. Stamler J, Neaton JD, Wentworth DN. Blood pressure (systolic and diastolic) and risk of fatal coronary heart disease. Hypertension 1989;13(suppl I):2–2.
48. Applegate WB, Miller ST, Elam JT, et al. Nonpharmacologic intervention to reduce blood pressure in older patients with mild hypertension. Arch Intern Med 1992; 152:1162–1166.
49. Ruben S, Espeland MA, Ryu J, et al. Individual variation in susceptibility to extracranial carotid atherosclerosis. Arteriosclerosis 1988;8:389–397.
50. Aronow WS, Kronzon I, Schoenfeld MR. Left ventricular hypertrophy is more prevalent in patients with systemic hypertension with extracranial carotid arterial disease than in patients with systemic hypertension without extracranial carotid arterial disease. Am J Cardiol 1995;76: 192–193.
51. Kannel WB, Dannenberg AL, Levy D. Population implications of electrocardiographic left ventricular hypertrophy. Am J Cardiol 1987;60:85I–93I.
52. Aronow WS, Koenigsberg M, Schwartz KS. Usefulness of echocardiographic and electrocardiographic left ventricular hypertrophy in predicting new cardiac events and atherothrombotic brain infarction in elderly patients with systemic hypertension or coronary artery disease. Am J Noninvas Cardiol 1989;3:367–370.
53. Kahn S, Frishman WH, Weissman S, et al. Left ventricular hypertrophy on electrocardiogram: prognostic implications from a 10 year cohort study of older subjects: a report from the Bronx Longitudinal Aging Study. J Am Geriatr Soc 1996;44:524–529.
54. Levy D, Garrison RJ, Savage DD, et al. Left ventricular mass and incidence of coronary heart disease in an elderly cohort: the Framingham Heart Study. Ann Intern Med 1989;110:101–107.
55. Aronow WS, Koenigsberg M, Schwartz KS. Usefulness of echocardiographic left ventricular hypertrophy in predicting new coronary events and atherothrombotic brain infarction in patients over 62 years of age. Am J Cardiol 1988;61:1130–1132.
56. Aronow WS, Epstein S, Koenigsberg M, et al. Usefulness of echocardiographic left ventricular hypertrophy, ventricular tachycardia, and complex ventricular arrhythmias in predicting ventricular fibrillation or sudden

cardiac death in elderly patients. Am J Cardiol 1988;62: 1124–1125.
57. Aronow WS, Gutstein H, Hsieh FY. Risk factors for thromboembolic stroke in elderly patients with chronic atrial fibrillation. Am J Cardiol 1989;63:366–367.
58. Aronow WS, Ahn C, Kronzon I, et al. Association of plasma renin activity and echocardiographic left ventricular hypertrophy with frequency of new coronary events and new atherothrombotic brain infarction in older persons with systemic hypertension. Am J Cardiol 1997;79:1543–1545.
59. Bikkina M, Levy D, Evans JC, et al. Left ventricular mass and risk of stroke in an elderly cohort: the Framingham Heart Study. JAMA 1994;272:33–36.
60. Aronow WS, Ahn C, Kronzon I, et al. Association of extracranial carotid arterial disease, prior atherothrombotic brain infarction, systemic hypertension, and left ventricular hypertrophy with the incidence of new atherothrombotic brain infarction at 45 month follow-up of 1482 older patients. Am J Cardiol 1997;79:991–993.
61. Aronow WS. Left ventricular hypertrophy. J Am Geriatr Soc 1992;40:71–80.
62. Dahlof B, Pennert K, Hansson L. Reversal of left ventricular hypertrophy in hypertensive patients: a meta-analysis of 109 treatment studies. Am J Hypertens 1992;5: 95–110.
63. Kannel WB, D'Agostino RB, Levy D, et al. Prognostic significance of regression of left ventricular hypertrophy [abstract]. Circulation 1988;78(suppl II):89.
64. Koren MJ, Savage DD, Casale PN, et al. Changes in left ventricular mass predict risk in essential hypertension [abstract]. Circulation 1990;82(suppl III):29.
65. Castelli SP, Wilson PWF, Levy D, et al. Cardiovascular risk factors in the elderly. Am J Cardiol 1989;63:12H–19H.
66. Wong ND, Wilson PWF, Kannel WB. Serum cholesterol as a prognostic factor after myocardial infarction: the Framingham study. Ann Intern Med 1991;115:687–693.
67. Benfante R, Reed D. Is elevated serum cholesterol level a factor for coronary heart disease in the elderly? JAMA 1990;263:393–396.
68. Barrett-Connor E, Suarez L, Khaw K-T, et al. Ischemic heart disease risk factors after age 50. J Chronic Dis 1984;37:903–908.
69. Rubin SM, Sidney S, Black DM, et al. High blood cholesterol in elderly men and the excess risk for coronary heart disease. Ann Intern Med 1990;113:916–920.
70. Zimetbaum P, Frishman WH, Ooi WL, et al. Plasma lipids and lipoproteins and the incidence of cardiovascular disease in the very elderly: the Bronx Aging Study. Arterioscler Thromb 1992;12:416–423.
71. Corti M-C, Guralnik JM, Salive ME, et al. HDL cholesterol predicts coronary heart disease mortality in older persons. JAMA 1995;274:539–544.
72. Scandinavian Simvastatin Survival Study Group. Randomised trial of cholesterol lowering in 4444 patients with coronary heart disease: the Scandinavian Simvastatin Survival Study (4S). Lancet 1994;344:1383–1389.
73. Sacks FM, Pfefer MA, Moye LA, et al. The effect of pravastatin on coronary events after myocardial infarction in patients with average cholesterol levels. N Engl J Med 1996;335:1001–1009.
74. Aronow WS, Ahn C. Correlation of serum lipids with the presence or absence of coronary artery disease in 1793 men and women aged ≥62 years. Am J Cardiol 1994;73:702–703.
75. Lavie CJ, Milani RV. National Cholesterol Education Program's recommendations and implications of "missing" high-density lipoprotein cholesterol in cardiac rehabilitation programs. Am J Cardiol 1991;68:1087–1088.
76. Fowkes FGR, Housley E, Riemersma RA, et al. Smoking, lipids, glucose intolerance, and blood pressure as risk factors for peripheral atherosclerosis compared with ischemic heart disease in the Edinburgh Artery Study. Am J Epidemiol 1992;135:331–340.
77. Beach KW, Brunzell JD, Conquest JD, et al. The correlation of arteriosclerosis obliterans with lipoproteins in insulin-dependent and non-insulin-dependent diabetes. Diabetes 1979;28:836–840.
78. Criqui MH, Browner D, Fronek A, et al. Peripheral arterial disease in large vessels is epidemiologically distinct from small vessel disease: an analysis of risk factors. Am J Epidemiol 1989;129:1110–1119.
79. Aronow WS, Ahn C. Correlation of serum lipids with the presence or absence of atherothrombotic brain infarction and peripheral arterial disease in 1834 men and women aged ≥62 years. Am J Cardiol 1994;73:995–997.
80. Iso H, Jacobs DR Jr, Wentworth D, et al. Serum cholesterol levels and six year mortality from stroke in 350,977 men screened for the Multiple Risk Factor Intervention trial. N Engl J Med 1989;320:904–910.
81. Bihari-Varga M, Szekely J, Gruber E. Plasma high density lipoproteins in coronary, cerebral and peripheral vascular disease: the influence of various risk factors. Atherosclerosis 1981;40:337–345.
82. Crouse JR III, Byington RP, Hoen HM, et al. Reductase inhibitor monotherapy and stroke prevention. Arch Intern Med 1997;157:1305–1310.
83. O'Leary DH, Anderson KM, Wolf PA, et al. Cholesterol and carotid atherosclerosis in older persons: the Framingham study. Ann Epidemiol 1992;2:147–153.
84. Salonen R, Seppanen K, Raurmaa R, et al. Prevalence of carotid atherosclerosis and serum cholesterol levels in eastern Finland. Arteriosclerosis 1988;8:788–792.
85. Blankenhorn DH, Selzer RH, Crawford DW, et al. Beneficial effects of colestipol-niacin therapy on the common carotid artery: two and four year reduction of intima-media thickness measured by ultrasound. Circulation 1993;88:20–28.
86. Furberg CD, Adams HP, Applegate WB, et al. Effect of lovastatin on early carotid atherosclerosis and cardiovascular events. Circulation 1994;90:1679–1687.
87. Crouse JR III, Byington RP, Bond MG, et al. Pravastatin, lipids and atherosclerosis in the carotid arteries (PLAC-II). Am J Cardiol 1995;75:455–459.
88. Vokonas PS, Kannel WB. Epidemiology of coronary heart disease in the elderly. In: Tresch DD, Aronow WS (eds) Cardiovascular Disease in the Elderly Patient. New York: Marcel Dekker, 1999:139–164.
89. Barrett-Connor E, Khaw K-T. Diabetes mellitus: an independent risk factor for stroke. Am J Epidemiol 1988;128: 116–123.
90. Bogousslavsky J, Regli F, Van Melle G. Risk factors and concomtants of internal carotid arterial occlusion or steno-

sis: a controlled study of 159 cases. Arch Neurol 1985; 42:864–867.
91. Kannel WB, Cupples LA, Ramaswami R, et al. Regional obesity and risk of cardiovascular disease. J Clin Epidemiol 1991;44:183–190.
92. Folsom AR, Kaye SA, Sellers TA, et al. Body fat distribution and 5 year risk of death in older women. JAMA 1993;269:483–487.
93. Paffenbarger RS Jr, Hyde RT, Wing AL, et al. Physical activity, all-cause mortality, and longevity of college alumni. N Engl J Med 1986;314:605–613.
94. Wenger NK. Physical inactivity as a risk factor for coronary heart disease in the elderly. Cardiol Elderly 1994;2: 375–379.
95. Paffenbarger RS Jr, Wing AL. Characteristics in youth predisposing to fatal stroke in later years. Lancet 1967;1:753–754.
96. Paffenbarger RS Jr. Factors predisposing to fatal stroke in longshoremen. Prevent Med 1972;1:522–527.
97. Williams MA, Maresh CM, Aronow WS, et al. The value of early outpatient cardiac exercise programs for the elderly in comparison with other selected age groups. Eur Heart J 1984;5(suppl E):113–115.
98. Gillum RF. Stroke in blacks. Stroke 1988;19:1–9.
99. Aronow WS. Prevalence of atherothrombotic brain infarction, coronary artery disease and peripheral arterial disease in elderly blacks, Hispanics and whites. Am J Cardiol 1992;70:1212–1213.
100. Aronow WS, Ahn C, Schoenfeld M, et al. Extracranial carotid arterial disease: a prognostic factor for atherothrombotic brain infarction and cerebral transient ischemic attack. NY State J Med 1992;92:424–425.
101. Hertzer NR, Beven EG, Young JR, et al. Coronary artery disease in peripheral vascular patients: a classification of 1000 coronary angiograms and results of surgical management. Ann Surg 1984;199:223–233.
102. Smith GD, Shipley MJ, Rose G. Intermittent claudication, heart disease risk factors and mortality: the Whitehall study. Circulation 1990;82:1925–1931.
103. Hertzer NR, Young JR, Beven EG, et al. Coronary angiography in 506 patients with extracranial cerebrovascular disease. Arch Intern Med 1985;145:849–852.
104. Chimowitz MI, Mancini GBJ. Asymptomatic coronary artery disease in patients with stroke: prevalence, prognosis, diagnosis and treatment. Stroke 1992;23:433–436.
105. Aronow WS, Ahn C, Schoenfeld MR, et al. Prognostic significance of silent myocardial ischemia in patients >61 years of age with extracranial internal or common carotid arterial disease with and without previous myocardial infarction. Am J Cardiol 1993;71:115–117.
106. Aronow WS, Schoenfeld MR. Forty-five month follow-up of extracranial carotid arterial disease for new coronary events in elderly patients. Coron Artery Dis 1992;3:249–251.
107. Aronow WS, Ahn C. Prevalence of coexistence of coronary artery disease, peripheral arterial disease, and atherothrombotic brain infarction in men and women ≥62 years of age. Am J Cardiol 1994;74:64–65.

# 32
# Cardiac Surgery in the Elderly

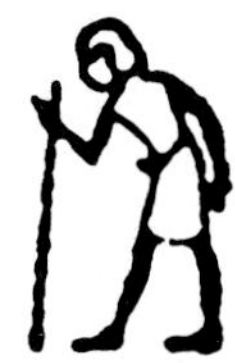

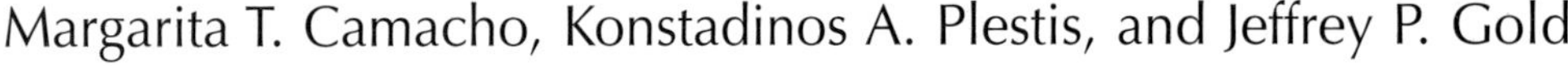
Margarita T. Camacho, Konstadinos A. Plestis, and Jeffrey P. Gold

As the elderly population steadily rises each year, so does the number of patients referred for cardiac surgical procedures. The U.S. Census Bureau predicted that at least 6.2% of the United States population would be more than 80 years of age by the year 2000.[1] Recent statistical actuarial data demonstrate that an individual aged 80 can expect to live an additional 8.1 years.[2] A formidable challenge facing cardiologists and cardiac surgeons is the appropriate treatment of the 40% of a growing elderly population that suffers from symptomatic cardiovascular disease.[3] The morbidity and mortality associated with cardiac surgical procedures in the elderly has substantially decreased since the late 1980s,[4] although it is still somewhat higher than that of younger counterparts less than 75 years of age.[5,6] Reports of acceptable mortality rates and improved long-term quality of life justify cardiac operations in most symptomatic elderly patients. Only recently have large studies focused on risk analyses and outcomes in an effort to provide the clinician with as much evidence-based literature as possible to make the most appropriate decisions for many of these complex elderly patients.

## Characteristics of the Elderly Cardiac Surgery Population

Despite the lack of consensus regarding the definition of "elderly," the perioperative cardiac surgery mortality rates rise significantly in patients older than 75 years of age.[5,6] An individual older than age 80 has more than three times the risk of death after coronary artery bypass than does a similar 50-year-old patient.[7] The increased risks of death and major complications are due not only to the natural processes of aging that result in associated co-morbidities but also to the fact that cardiovascular disease, the major cause of death and disability among elderly patients, is diagnosed at a more advanced state in this old population.

The aging process is influenced by a variety of genetic and environmental factors and occurs at somewhat different rates in every individual. The older the patient, the more likely is the presence of multiple chronic noncardiac diseases, increased tissue fragility, and limited organ reserves for stressful events.[7] Postoperative complications such as pneumonia, renal failure, stroke, and dementia are more prevalent and contribute significantly to perioperative morbidity and mortality. More than 50% of elderly individuals have at least one or more chronic medical conditions.[8] In addition to the routine preoperative assessment, other issues that must be evaluated include the degree of cognitive, neurologic, renal, respiratory, and immune impairment and the presence of other noncoronary atherosclerosis. Approximately one in three patients older than age 80 has some degree of cognitive dysfunction,[9] and it is important to establish a baseline level of performance prior to surgical intervention.[10] Such tests as the Folstein Mini-Mental Status Examination (MMSE) evaluates orientation, memory, attention span, concentration, and language capabilities.[11] Patients with previously compromised cognitive function are at highest risk for such postoperative complications as delirium and progressive cognitive dysfunction. Depression is a common problem in patients of all ages and has been reported to follow cardiac surgery. It is clearly more pronounced in the elderly patient who may live alone and have few social support systems.

By age 80 there is a 25% decrease in kidney mass and 40% reduction in glomerular filtration rate (GFR).[10] Due to the decrease in lean muscle mass, a decrease in GFR may not be reflected by an increase in serum creatinine concentration, and therefore a "normal" creatinine level in an octogenarian may be misleading. A more useful assessment of renal function in the elderly patient is the age-related creatinine clearance (Ccr)

$$\text{Ccr(ml/min)} = \frac{(140 - \text{age}) \times \text{(ideal body weight in kilograms)}}{72 \times \text{serum creatinine}}$$

where normal is 75–125 ml/min. Renal function should be evaluated both before and after cardiac catheterization, and the amount of renally excreted dye used during angiography should be kept to an absolute minimum, employing nonionic contrast materials. The transient episodes of hypotension that inevitably occur during cardiopulmonary bypass may worsen any preexisting renal dysfunction; in this age group, perioperative renal insufficiency is a strong positive predictor of postoperative mortality.[12–14]

Old patients have declining cellular immunity and are therefore more predisposed to developing invasive bacterial and viral infections.[10] In addition to the bacterial colonization of the respiratory, urinary, and gastrointestinal tracts, there is a risk of infection from other monitoring lines and catheters used during cardiac surgery, such as central lines, Swan-Ganz catheters, and mediastinal drainage tubes. Leukocytosis is frequently absent or depressed in an elderly patient, who otherwise commonly exhibits atypical signs of infection such as hypothermia or confusion. Although most cardiac surgery patients are not cachexic or nutritionally depleted owing to their cardiac disease, it is important to assess the preoperative nutritional status of an elderly individual whose other organ reserves are already limited. Adequate nutrition is vital for wound healing and for avoiding infection and ventilatory dependence. Ideally, the serum albumin concentration should be >3.5 mg/dl, and there should be no history of recent significant (>5%) weight loss.

Numerous physiologic changes affect the cardiovascular system with advancing age. There is a decrease in vascular elasticity: The aorta and large arteries become much less compliant, resulting in an increase in peripheral vascular resistance. Left ventricular stiffness is increased,[15] as is the ventricular septal thickness,[16] and may require higher filling pressures to maintain adequate forward flow. During exercise there is a decrease in peak heart rate and ejection fraction, likely due to reduced responsiveness to circulating catecholamines.[17–19] Autopsy studies of octogenarians revealed that atherosclerotic heart disease with more than 75% narrowing in at least one major coronary vessel was the most common abnormality (present in 60% of patients). In fact, coronary disease was the most common single cause of death, with the most frequent manifestation being acute myocardial infarction.[16] Finally, compared to younger age groups, the heart of the elderly individual has smaller ventricular cavities and tortuous coronary arteries.[20–22] In light of these morphologic findings, it is not surprising that by age 80 at least 20% of this population have an established clinical diagnosis of coronary artery disease, and that eventually 67% of elderly patients die from this disease.

Elderly patients tend to have more advanced coronary artery disease than their younger counterparts by the time they are referred for cardiac surgery. Compared to the Coronary Artery Surgery Study (CASS) with a patient population of mean age 68 years,[23] octogenarians were found to have a higher incidence of three-vessel coronary disease (87% vs. 61%; $p < 0.05$), left main or left main-equivalent disease (50% vs. 3%, $p < 0.0001$), and significant left ventricular dysfunction (19% vs. 4% had an ejection fraction <35%, $p < 0.01$).[24] Older patients are more symptomatic on presentation; many series report that more than 90% of octogenarians are New York Heart Association (NYHA) functional class III–IV preoperatively.[13,25–31] When compared to younger patients, a significantly higher percentage of elderly patients are referred for more urgent or emergent procedures, which carry substantially increased risks of major morbidity and mortality.[7,13,24,29,31–34] This underscores the need to prevent emergent and urgent surgical interventions.

A common finding in elderly patients is calcification and intimal disease of the aorta, which can crack and embolize when the ascending aorta is clamped or manipulated during cardiac operations. Such embolization to cerebral vessels is the principal cause of perioperative stroke in this age group.[35] Other causes of surgery-related neurologic deficits include transient episodes of systemic hypotension during cardiopulmonary bypass and air embolism from procedures that necessitate opening cardiac chambers or great vessels, such as aortic or mitral valve operations. Although aortic valve calcification is present in more than 55% of patients over the age of 90, only 5% eventually develop significant hemodynamic valvular stenosis.[36] One important difference between aortic and mitral valve disorders in the elderly is that aortic valve disease is usually associated with preserved left ventricular function, whereas mitral valve disease in the elderly is often ischemic in nature and is associated with significant ventricular dysfunction. Davis and coworkers[37] noted that only 29% of elderly patients with significant aortic valve disease had concomitant disease of two or more coronary vessels, compared with 46% of patients with significant mitral valve disease.

## Predictors of Perioperative Morbidity and Mortality

As experience with the surgical treatment of cardiac disease in septuagenarians has grown, the literature has focused on the surgical outcome in octogenarians (Table 32.1). Many of these studies have reported predictors of perioperative morbidity and mortality based on extensive univariate and multivariate analyses. This information has proved vital in identifying specific factors that may be optimized preoperatively and has provided physicians and patients with the ability to make timely treatment decisions based on expected short-term and long-term outcomes.

TABLE 32.1. Cardiac Surgical Procedures in the Octogenarian: Results and Average Length of Hospital Stay

| Study | Year | No. | Procedure | Mortality (%) | Complication rate (%) | Mean postop. LOS | % Survival (years) |
|---|---|---|---|---|---|---|---|
| Deiwick[34] | 1997 | 101 | Mixed | 8 | 73 | | 88 (1)<br>73 (5) |
| Gehlot[38] | 1996 | 322 | AVR mixed | 14 | 53 | 11.0 | 83 (1)<br>60 (5) |
| Sahar[39] | 1996 | 42 | Mixed | 7 | 24 | | |
| Logeais[40] | 1995 | 200 | Mixed | 12 | 35 | 12.7 | 82 (1)<br>75 (2)<br>57 (5) |
| Cane[12] | 1995 | 121 | Mixed | 9 | 49 | | |
| Klima[41] | 1994 | 75 | Mixed | 8 | 21 | | |
| Yashar[42] | 1993 | 43 | Mixed | 9 | 38 | | |
| Glower[26] | 1992 | 86 | CABG | 14 | 29 | 10.0 | 64 (3) |
| Freeman[31] | 1991 | 191 | Mixed | 20 | 30 | 16.4 | 92 (1)<br>87 (2)<br>82 (3)<br>78 (4) |
| Tsai[43] | 1991 | 157 | CABG | 7 | 20 | | 85 (1)<br>62 (5) |
| Ko[28] | 1991 | 100 | CABG | 12 | 24 | | |
| Mullany[44] | 1990 | 159 | CABG | 11 | 73 | | 84 (1)<br>71 (5) |
| Naunheim[33] | 1990 | 103 | Mixed | 17 | 71 | | 90 (1) |
| Kowalchuk[45] | 1990 | 53 | Mixed | 11 | 38 | | 81 (2) |
| Fiore[46] | 1989 | 25 | Mixed<br>Valve | 20 | 72 | 18.0 | 79 (1)<br>69 (2) |
| Naunheim[24] | 1987 | 23 | Mixed | 22 | 67 | 14.3 | 94 (1)<br>82 (2) |
| Rich[47] | 1985 | 25 | Mixed | 4 | 92 | 19.5 | 84 (2) |

Mixed, series includes valve and coronary bypass procedures and/or valve + coronary bypass procedures; AVR, aortic valve replacement; CABG, coronary artery bypass grafting; LOS, length of stay in hospital.

Several studies have shown that a decreased ejection fraction is a significant predictor of hospital mortality following cardiac surgery. This is even more predictive of an adverse outcome in octogenarians. A number of series have reported hospital mortality rates of 3–6%, 5–13%, and 24–43% in patients with normal, moderately impaired, and severely impaired (ejection fraction < 0.30) left ventricular function, respectively.[48–50] In a multivariate analysis of factors involving 159 octogenarians who underwent isolated coronary artery bypass, Mullaney and coworkers[44] found that an ejection fraction less than 0.50% was the most important predictor of adverse survival ($p < 0.01$). Ko and coworkers, who analyzed 100 consecutive octogenarians undergoing isolated coronary artery bypass, also found a decreased ejection fraction to be the most significant predictor of perioperative mortality ($p < 0.002$). In fact, an ejection fraction less than 30% was associated with a mortality rate of 43%.[28]

High NYHA functional cardiac class was highly predictive of hospital mortality in numerous studies.[3,6,13,16,19,22,25,26,31,45] In their series of 76 octogenarians undergoing a variety of cardiac surgery procedures, Tsai and coworkers[48] found that 94% of the hospital deaths were in patients who presented in NYHA functional class IV. In a study of 24,461 patients 80 years and older who underwent isolated coronary artery bypass, measures of more acute coronary disease, such as acute myocardial infarction (MI) before bypass surgery, predicted higher procedural and long-term mortality rates.[49] This relation with acute coronary artery disease has been borne out by numerous other authors.[6,24,26,28]

Combined coronary surgery procedures and mitral valve replacement have been shown to carry significantly higher hospital mortality rates in the elderly population.[19,27,32,36,37,39,42,45] Davis and coworkers reported operative mortality rates of 5.3% for aortic valve replacement, 20.4% for mitral valve replacement, and 5.8% for isolated coronary artery bypass[37]; and Naunheim et al. reported even higher hospital mortality rates of 50% for mitral valve replacement, 9% for aortic valve replacement, and 67% for double valve replacement combined with coronary revascularization.[33] The outcome after valve replacement in elderly patients is primarily a function of the myocardial performance, which decreases as the severity of any associated coronary artery disease increases. Old patients undergoing aortic valve replacement tend to have a well-functioning ventricle; the degree of coronary artery disease tends to be less than that in

TABLE 32.2. Comparison of Mortality Rates by Procedure Status (Elective vs. Urgent vs. Emergent)

| Study | Year | No. | Procedure | Mortality (%) | | | |
|---|---|---|---|---|---|---|---|
| | | | | Overall | Elective | Urgent | Emergency |
| Diewick[34] | 1997 | 101 | Mixed | 7.9 | 4.7 | | 23.5 |
| Williams[13] | 1995 | 300 | CABG | 11.0 | 9.6 | 11.0 | 33.3 |
| Diegeler[29] | 1995 | 54 | Mixed | 9.2 | 6.1 | | 40.0 |
| Freeman[31] | 1991 | 191 | Mixed | 18.8 | | | 35.9 |
| Ko[28] | 1991 | 100 | CABG | 12.0 | 2.8 | 13.5 | 33.3 |
| Naunheim[32] | 1990 | 103 | Mixed | 16.5 | | 10.0 | 29.0 |
| Naunheim[24] | 1987 | 23 | Mixed | 22.0 | 11.0 | | 75.0 |

See Table 32.1 for explanation of abbreviations.

patients undergoing mitral valve replacement. Patients requiring mitral valve surgery tend to have more serious ischemic disease, which irreversibly damages the myocardium and results in higher perioperative mortality.[20–22,27] Furthermore, combined procedures require longer cardiopulmonary bypass times and longer ischemic cross-clamp times, two factors that were found to be predictors of operative mortality as well.[19,24,26,28]

In addition to presenting with more advanced disease than their younger counterparts, a higher percentage of octogenarians are referred for urgent or emergent surgical intervention. As noted in Table 32.2, urgent and emergent operations are associated with extremely high mortality rates, particularly if a mitral valve procedure is performed independently or in combination with other procedures. A recent multicenter randomized study evaluating the benefit of emergency revascularization in cardiogenic shock patients has shown much higher mortality in elderly patients than in their younger counterparts (Dr. Judith F. Hochman, personal communication). These increased mortality rates reflect the progression and severity of the cardiac disease and the lack of functional reserve for stressful events in this older population. Another related factor, preoperative hemodynamic instability, was described by several authors as the need for an intraaortic balloon pump,[15,19,24,25,33,39] preoperative admission to the coronary care unit,[34,38,44] and preoperative use of inotropes and vasoactive medications.[33,50] Each was found to be a significant predictor of hospital mortality. Multivariate analyses by Williams and coworkers, who studied a group of 300 octogenarians who underwent isolated coronary artery bypass, revealed that preoperative renal dysfunction (creatinine >2.0 mg/dl), pulmonary insufficiency, and postoperative sternal wound infection were strong predictors of hospital mortality.[13] Tsai and coworkers found that 67% of the elderly patients with postoperative mediastinal bleeding necessitating reoperation ultimately died.[48]

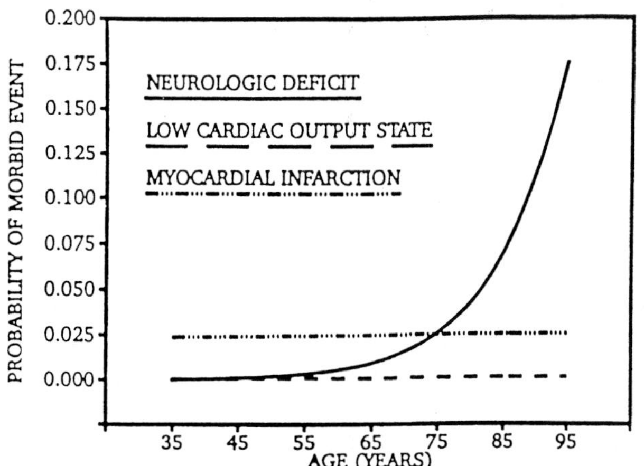


FIGURE 32.1. Effect of advanced age on the predicted probability of neurologic and cardiac morbidity. (From Tuman et al.,[51] with permission.)

In a prospective study of 2000 patients undergoing coronary artery bypass, Tuman and coworkers[51] studied the effect of age on neurologic outcome. The rate of neurologic complications rose significantly with age; patients <65 years old had a 0.9% stroke rate, whereas those aged 65–74 and >75 had rates of 3.6% and 8.9% respectively ($p$ = 0.0005). Suspected causes of serious neurologic events (in patients unresponsive for more than 10 days) include atheromatous emboli from the ascending aorta, hypotension or low-flow state during cardiopulmonary bypass, and preexisting critical extracranial or intracranial cerebrovascular disease. The mortality rate in this group of patients who sustained significant strokes was 74% (Fig. 32.1).[51] Perioperative mortality associated with perioperative stroke in younger patients, although still formidable, was less than half of this frequency (24–26%).

## Quality of Life

Although the short-term and intermediate-term survival for elderly patients undergoing cardiac surgery is somewhat less than their younger cohorts, the long-term survival for octogenarians after open heart surgery compares favorably with survival for the general

United States population of similar age. In a series of 600 consecutive patients 80 years or older undergoing various open heart procedures, the 5-year actuarial survival, including hospital mortality, was 63 ± 2%. Survival in this group was identical to that for the simultaneous general U.S. octogenarian population.[14] Excellent long-term results have been achieved by several groups in octogenarians after mitral valve surgery, aortic valve surgery, and coronary artery bypass surgery.[40,52,53]

Of as great importance to the elderly as survival is the associated quality of life. Several authors have shown that most (81–93%) of the octogenarians who survive open heart surgery "feel" as good and frequently better than before their operations.[14,29,40,53] An equally high percentage (75–84%) of octogenarians believed in retrospect that having decided to have a cardiac surgical procedure after age 80 had been a good choice.[14,54] The precise and objective measurements of quality of life may be difficult to quantify. Based on well-studied populations, it has been possible to construct instruments that reliably assess the various domains of daily living, thereby producing a meaningful reproducible measurement of quality of life.[55–57]

The NYHA angina functional class and cardiac failure functional class reflect symptom-free living in regard to chest pain and dyspnea. Octogenarians have consistently demonstrated substantial improvement in their NYHA angina functional class and cardiac failure functional class after open heart surgery. In several reports, most (68–92%) of the octogenarians who survived open heart surgery were in NYHA functional class I or II during long-term follow-up. This improvement was seen after isolated coronary artery bypass operations, valve operations, and combined operations (Table 32.3). When a well-validated health care index, the SF-36, was employed to study prospectively a cohort of elderly and nonelderly patients, those over 75 years of age enjoyed an identical long-term improvement in each of the seven domains of the SF-36. Indeed, as many of the elderly patients had low quality of life SF-36 scores preoperatively as their younger cohorts, their improvements were even greater, as both populations ended up with statistically identical SF-36 scores 6 months following surgery. Any neurologic injury associated with the diagnostic and surgical process dramatically affected their quality of life adversely when compared to those old patients who did not suffer any neurologic injury.

Many octogenarian patients live alone and consequently have impaired ability to carry out activities of daily living, which places them at a significant disadvantage. Karnofsky dependency category (KDC) and social support index (SSI) reflect the degree of help needed by patients. Glower and coworkers, using the KDC, showed that the median performance status in a group of octogenarians undergoing isolated coronary artery bypass grafting improved from 20% preoperatively to 70% at hospital discharge, with 89% of survivors being discharged home.[26] Kumar et al. showed that when there was a significant decrease in the level of social support needed by octogenarians after open heart surgery the mean KDC and mean SSI decreased significantly at the short-term follow-up (less than 2 years).[54] These improvements were also present but significantly less evident at the long-term follow-up (more than 5 years). It is likely that significant co-morbid conditions limit the ability of octogenarians to live independently long term, although they remain symptom-free from a cardiac point of view and do well in the short term.

TABLE 32.3. Change in Functional Class after Cardiac Surgical Procedures

| Study | Year | No. | Procedure | Functional class change (%) | |
|---|---|---|---|---|---|
| | | | | Preoperative FC III–IV | Postoperative FC I–II |
| Deiwick[34] | 1997 | 101 | Mixed | 88 | 83 |
| Morris[25] | 1996 | 474 | CABG | 93 | 92 |
| Gehlot[38] | 1996 | 322 | Mixed | 86 | 82 |
| Sahar[39] | 1996 | 42 | Mixed | 87 | 90 |
| Williams[13] | 1995 | 300 | CABG | 98 | 98 |
| Logeais[40] | 1995 | 200 | Mixed | 74 | 99 |
| Cane[12] | 1995 | 121 | Mixed | 69 | 84 |
| Diegeler[29] | 1995 | 54 | Mixed | 100 | 92 |
| Adkins[58] | 1995 | 42 | Mixed | 64 | 97 |
| Tsai[27] | 1994 | 528 | Mixed | 99 | 70 |
| Yashar[42] | 1993 | 43 | Mixed | 98 | 79 |
| Tsai[43] | 1991 | 157 | CABG | 96 | 73 |
| Ko[28] | 1991 | 100 | CABG | 100 | 94 |
| McGrath[30] | 1991 | 54 | Mixed | 96 | 94 |
| Mullaney[44] | 1990 | 159 | CABG | 97 | 89 |
| Merrill[59] | 1990 | 40 | Mixed | 100 | 100 |
| Edmunds[60] | 1988 | 100 | Mixed | 90 | 98 |
| Naunheim[24] | 1987 | 23 | Mixed | 94 | 83 |

FC, functional class.

As mentioned above, the subjective indicators of quality of life for octogenarians after open heart surgery are complex and involve a number of modalities relating to various domains of life. In the study by Kumar et al., indices for satisfaction with marriage, children, and overall life, feelings about the present life, and general affect were assessed. In the short term, the indices for satisfaction with overall life and eight bipolar items assessing general affect showed significant improvements, although all these improvements became less evident at long-term follow-up.[54] Perhaps the symptomatic benefits and the value of cardiac surgery as seen subjectively by the patients lie in the question, "Would you choose to undergo cardiac surgery again?" Virtually all the current studies in the literature have shown that most octogenarians would have made the same decision to undergo open heart surgery retrospectively.

## Possible Strategies to Decrease Operative Risk

Improvements in surgical techniques and anesthesia have increased the confidence of cardiac surgeons performing operations on an elderly population with increased perioperative risk. Awareness of the problems unique to this growing population of elderly patients, along with recent statistical data highlighting the impact of these problems on morbidity and mortality, can help the medical team recommend the most appropriate treatment choice and timing of intervention in each individual case.

The two principal causes of perioperative cerebrovascular accidents (CVAs) in elderly patients undergoing cardiac surgery are embolization (air, atheroma, calcific debris) and hypotension resulting in inadequate perfusion of the central nervous system. Preoperative evaluation of the ascending aorta and carotid arteries and intraoperative assessment of the proximal aorta using transesophageal or epiaortic echocardiography may alter the conduct of the procedure, minimize intraoperative manipulation, and thereby significantly reduce the incidence of stroke.[34,39,51,61,62] Such information enables the surgeon to avoid cannulation or direct manipulation of heavily diseased portions of the aorta where atheromas may dislodge or where plaque disruption may cause aortic dissection. The presence of extensive atheromatous or calcific disease, which precludes safe manipulation of the ascending aorta in patients with advanced coronary disease, leaves the surgeon with several choices.

1. Abandon the surgical procedure and consider nonoperative or nonbypass revascularization, such as angioplasty, transmyocardial revascularization, or angiogenesis.

2. Perform surgical revascularization on a beating heart, using one or both internal thoracic arteries or nonaortic-based grafts.

3. Establish cardiopulmonary bypass via the femoral, axillary, or other systemic nondiseased artery and perform graft replacement or endarterectomy of the ascending aorta.[34,62] The latter alternative is an aggressive, complex procedure and in the elderly population should be reserved for the very good risk patient with no significant co-morbidities.

Diffuse systemic atherosclerosis is more prevalent in the elderly than in younger patients; as such, special precautions should be taken to ensure adequate cerebral and renal perfusion perioperatively. Maintaining high perfusion pressures while on cardiopulmonary bypass can help decrease the incidence of ischemic stroke.[63–64] Control of atrial arrhythmias and avoidance of episodes of sustained arterial hypotension due to hypovolemia or medications are important during the immediate postoperative period. Although there is still controversy regarding the management of asymptomatic carotid disease, it is believed that known carotid disease in the elderly population is a risk factor for postoperative CVA.[14,34,44,51] Morris and coworkers[25] recommended routine preoperative assessment of carotid artery disease in octogenarians and advocated carotid endarterectomy if significant disease is found. If symptomatic carotid artery disease is diagnosed prior to cardiac surgical intervention, consideration should be given to performing a staged or a combined procedure. If asymptomatic significant carotid disease is discovered by Doppler preoperatively (>75% stenosis bilaterally or lesser degrees of unilateral stenosis in the presence of an occluded contralateral artery), concomitant carotid endarterectomy may decrease the risk of perioperative stroke.[61]

Because of the significant increase in mortality associated with urgent or emergent operative procedures (Table 32.2), all possible measures must be taken to optimize the elderly patient preoperatively and possibly convert an urgent or emergent situation to a more elective one. Careful selection of elderly patients in this setting is critical, and one must evaluate the patient's mental status and existing co-morbidities when determining the potential for meaningful survival before recommending operation. Aggressive preoperative medical management includes the use, when necessary, of intravenous nitroglycerin or heparin (or both), inotropic and ventilatory support, and if absolutely necessary, the intraaortic balloon pump (IABP). Although numerous studies have reported that preoperative use of the IABP is a significant predictor of perioperative mortality,[12,14,33,50] it likely reflects the severity of the elderly patient's underlying cardiac disease, rather than any inherent risk in using the device. Sisto and coworkers[65] reported that in 25 consecutive octogenarians requiring IABP insertion, there were no significant complications related to device insertion; and of 20 patients who eventually underwent surgery after IABP, only 2 patients (10%) died in hospital. This operative mortality rate is significantly better than that reported by others for urgent/emergent cases (Table 32.2).

There is a strong association between early postoperative death and prolonged ventilatory dependence,[60] which can develop quickly in the elderly patient. As soon as the patient awakens from general anesthesia, respiratory muscles must be exercised. Pulmonary hygiene and physiotherapy must be aggressive with early and progressive ambulation. Unlike their younger counterparts, elderly patients have much less functional reserve, and therefore a successful first attempt at extubation and mobilization ensures the best outcome. Intraoperatively, exquisite care must be taken to avoid injury to the phrenic nerve during harvesting of the internal thoracic artery, and use of bilateral internal thoracic arteries should generally be avoided.[66]

Nephrotoxic drugs should be avoided; or, if necessary, doses should be adjusted in light of the decreased renal function in elderly patients. Intravenous renal dosage dopamine hydrochloride (1–2 µg/kg/min) may have benefit when used for any patient with preexisting renal insufficiency. Because of the high mortality associated with perioperative renal failure in this population,[13,38,43,67,68] an aggressive approach to optimize preoperative renal function is essential. Although rigorous studies demonstrating the benefit of "renal dopamine" are inconclusive, many centers use this drug to enhance urine flow during and immediately after cardiac surgery.

Cognitive function is one of the most important factors affecting overall outcome and is one of the most difficult neurologic outcome parameters to measure and assess. Delirium and confusion are common in the postoperative elderly individual and can hinder important initial attempts to extubate and mobilize a patient. Encephalopathy changes are seen in as many as 30% of all bypass patients and 50% of elderly patients. Sensory deficits such as those due to hearing or vision impairments can be addressed as soon as the patient awakens by providing hearing aids and eyeglasses. Invasive lines and monitoring equipment should be removed as soon as is medically possible to facilitate mobilization. Transfer out of an intensive care unit (ICU) setting, when possible, helps restore the sleep–wake cycle. Family members should stay with confused patients to offer reassurance and encouragement. Long-acting benzodiazepines should be avoided or other sedative/hypnotic medications altered to prevent excessive sedation, confusion, and respiratory depression. Haloperidol is a more appropriate drug for management of delirium in this patient population because of its short-acting effect and safety margin in the postoperative cardiothoracic patient. Small doses are usually effective, and the patient can be rapidly weaned in conjunction with professional and family encouragement.

Octogenarians are more likely to develop sternal dehiscence due to osteoporosis of the sternum. For this reason, Utley and Leyland routinely use 12 wires to close the sternum.[69] The use of bilateral internal thoracic arteries should be avoided. Sternal wound infection has been shown to be a positive predictor of mortality in this group of patients.[13]

Aggressive management is essential and includes early institution of intravenous antibiotics, timely débridement and primary reconstruction, and adequate nutrition and pulmonary physiotherapy. Staged closures are to be avoided in this population, other than for the most advanced infections, which should then undergo coverage and secondary closure as rapidly as possible.

Utley and Leyland described a highly selected group of 25 patients over the age of 80 who underwent coronary artery bypass with no hospital deaths.[69] Patients were selected on the basis of their ability to achieve acceptable functional recovery after operation. All patients were living at home alone or with relatives preoperatively, and they were ambulatory and capable of caring for their own personal needs. They were counseled preoperatively regarding the importance of early ambulation and self-care postoperatively. Four patients were rejected for surgery based on mental or physical senility, previous debilitating strokes, or a history of long-term institutional care. Anesthetic management included the use of short-acting agents and minimal use of postoperative sedation. Patients were extubated within 9–48 hours postoperatively, and many were ambulatory and eating on the first postoperative day. Although this restrictive degree of patient selection is not appropriate in most cases, it illustrates how outcome can be strongly influenced by preexisting functional status and meticulous perioperative care.

## Nonsurgical Alternatives

During the current era of health care reform, there is considerable interest in providing the most appropriate care for patients more than 80 years of age at an "acceptable" cost.[70] As coronary bypass surgery is the most common major operation performed in the United States (more than 300,000 done annually), the use of coronary bypass in the very elderly is an important issue in the present cost-conscious environment. Medicare data from 1987 to 1990 indicated that the use of this operation in patients more than 80 years of age increased by 67% during that time period.[49] The projected rise in the number of coronary bypass procedures to be done in these patients and associated costs is impressive (Fig. 32.2).[49] Numerous studies have shown a considerable increase in length of stay (3–4 days longer) and hospital costs ($3000–$6000 more) in patients over 80 years old versus their younger

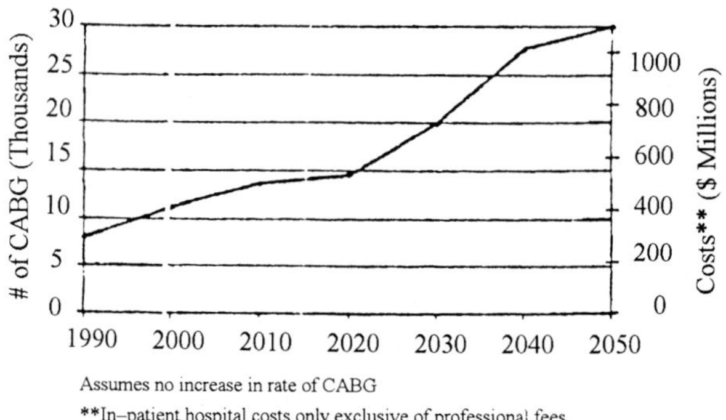


FIGURE 32.2. Projected number of bypass surgery (CABG) procedures performed per year in octogenarians (left axis) and the corresponding projected costs for these procedures (in 1990 dollars) (right axis). (From Peterson et al.,[49] with permission.)

counterparts. Failure to provide this service, however, often results in repeated and prolonged hospitalization, the need for multidrug therapy, and poorer quality of life, not to mention the emotional impact on patients and their families.[7,49]

In one series of octogenarians, when coronary surgery was compared to medical therapy, the overall cost, annual reinterventions, coronary disease-associated readmissions, and mortality were favored in the surgical group. Several studies have attempted to compare the treatment results of less expensive alternatives to coronary bypass surgery. In elderly patients, percutaneous transluminal coronary angioplasty (PTCA) has the advantages of shorter hospital stay, less immobilization, and lower cost compared to coronary artery bypass; however, coronary bypass confers greater and more durable freedom from angina, less need for future repeat interventional measures, and overall improved quality of life.[36,71,72] Whereas Mick and coworkers[73] reported that the procedural complication rates in matched groups of patients undergoing coronary bypass versus PTCA were similar, Braunstein et al.[71] observed that PTCA in the setting of unstable angina was associated with high initial morbidity but long-term survival roughly equivalent to that after coronary bypass surgery. As mentioned above, compared to medical noninterventional therapy, coronary artery bypass provides a significant survival advantage and improved quality of life. Ko and coworkers[72] compared 36 octogenarians who underwent coronary artery bypass to 29 octogenarians who continued medical noninterventional therapy and found that the functional class did not change in the latter group but improved significantly in the former group (NYHA functional class decreased from 3.4 to 1.2, $p < 0.01$). The 3-year survival rate of 77% for the surgical group was similar to the survival of octogenarians in the general U.S. population and was significantly better than that of 55% for the medical group. In summary, coronary bypass surgery provided improved long-term survival and functional benefit compared to medical therapy and improved the quality of life compared to PTCA.

## Guidelines for Therapy in the Elderly Cardiac Surgery Patient

During the process of deciding whether to offer cardiac surgical intervention to elderly patients, the relief of symptoms and improvement in quality of life should assume more importance than the issue of increased life expectancy. When surgical revascularization is considered in this patient population, numerous social, ethical, and clinical issues arise. Co-morbidities, quality of life, and concerns raised by the patient's family should be acknowledged and factored into the decision-making process. It is important to integrate the patient's and family's wishes, but one must focus the therapeutic decisions on the patient's advance directives. Emergency cases in these patients may be associated with more than 70% mortality risk, and therefore nonoperative treatment must be strongly considered. Asymptomatic patients should continue medical treatment unless there is critical (>70%) left main coronary artery stenosis, which is associated with significantly reduced life expectancy. Numerous groups (Table 32.2) have observed significant increased mortality when combined procedures were performed. One study, comparing the operative mortalities for isolated aortic valve replacement (AVR) and isolated coronary artery bypass to combined AVR + coronary bypass, demonstrated five- to sixfold increased operative mortality in the combined-procedure group.[48] In situations where two or three disease processes exist, the surgical plan should be modified to avoid such increased risks. For example, in an elderly patient with angina, severe coronary artery disease, and noncritical aortic stenosis, coronary revascularization alone may be the best option. Such patients are usually not at risk for a serious morbid event due to their aortic stenosis.[36] Conversely, in a patient with critical aortic stenosis, congestive heart failure, preserved or mildly impaired left ventricular function, and noncritical coronary lesions (<70–80% stenosis), valve replacement alone may be the best alternative. Fiore and coworkers[46] noted that of the early deaths of patients undergoing combined AVR + coronary bypass, 60% were due to low cardiac output; the patients who had died had little or no angina preoperatively, but each had considerable congestive heart failure and may have been better served by valve replacement alone.

Definitive treatment of isolated aortic stenosis is surgical replacement of the valve, preferably with a bioprosthesis that prevents a lifelong requirement for anticoagulation. The tissue valves have demonstrated impressive freedom from structural deterioration and reoperation at 10 or even 15 years in patients older than 65 years of age. Stentless bioprostheses may have some advantage in elderly small aortic root patients, but long-term benefit and durability remain unproven. Percutaneous balloon valvuloplasty may offer effective initial palliation, but medium- and long-term durability results have been disappointing. Symptoms recurred within 1 year in most patients and necessitated subsequent surgery.[74,75]

Chronic aortic regurgitation may be well tolerated for several decades before congestive heart failure occurs. Once symptoms appear and ventricular dilatation begins, aortic valve replacement should be offered before chronic volume overload results in symptomatic irreversible myocardial and pulmonary damage. The most appropriate time to replace the valve is soon after left ventricular dilatation begins.

Surgery is usually recommended for mitral stenosis patients with NYHA functional class II–III heart failure and a calculated mitral valve area less than 1.0 $cm^2$. Percutaneous balloon mitral valvuloplasty, unlike the similar treatment for stenotic aortic valves, may be useful when only the mitral valve leaflets are impaired and there is no significant calification or regurgitation. The subvalvular apparatus should be functional and not destroyed, as can happen with advanced rheumatic valve disease.[76] Mitral valve balloon valvuloplasty usually provides relatively long-term relief of dyspnea but is frequently not possible in elderly patients with advanced disease and heavily calcified mitral valves. Mitral valve replacement (MVR), although the definitive treatment for mitral valve stenosis, carries significantly increased procedural mortality either alone or combined with other procedures in the elderly. Naunheim et al.[33] observed operative risks of 42% for either MVR alone or MVR + coronary bypass. Combined MVR + AVR was associated with a 67% risk of surgical mortality, further suggesting a limited role for MVR in this elderly population. These procedures require prolonged periods of cardiopulmonary bypass and global cardiac ischemia, both of which are poorly tolerated by such patients with limited cardiac and other organ reserve. For these reasons, Fiore and coworkers[46] recommended that every effort be made to keep such operations simple and expeditious.

In patients with advanced coronary artery disease who may be at high risk for complications arising from cardiopulmonary bypass, such as those with severe calcific disease of the ascending aorta (precluding safe insertion of cannulas), a history of stroke, or end-stage pulmonary or renal failure, an alternate option is surgical revascularization on a beating heart. Technologic advances in pericardial retraction systems and stabilization devices has enabled the surgeon to perform anastomoses on a beating heart with the use of newer surgical techniques. However, there is a significant learning curve, as the surgical field is not nearly as optimal as that produced by cardiopulmonary bypass and ischemic arrest. Recent reports have observed a failure rate of 10% even in experienced hands. Although a reasonable alternative for patients who would otherwise have no interventional options, the increased risk of technical failure must be kept in mind and discussed with the patient and family.

## Conclusions

As the elderly population has grown, so have the number of elderly patients being referred for cardiac surgery and their disease complexity. For the most part, these patients can be offered conventional surgical procedures with acceptable mortality, morbidity, and long-term quality of life expectations. Indeed, the perioperative complications are somewhat more numerous than for younger patients even when they are compared procedure for procedure and matched for other risk factors.

This incremental morbidity and mortality is seen across the entire population but is most pronounced in emergently operated patients. With the availability of new and different techniques to accomplish myocardial revascularization and valvular repair and replacement, the range of procedures available for elderly patients with hemodynamically important heart disease is increasing at a rate almost faster than the population itself has grown. The use of minimally invasive techniques and off-pump techniques are but two of these promising alterations of standard cardiac surgical procedures. It is therefore critical that the health care professionals caring for these older patients are aware of ongoing developments in these areas and carefully stratify the preoperative risk factors to best select the least morbid and most effective procedure that is currently available.

## References


1. Specer G. US Bureau of the Census: Projections of the Population of the United States, by Age, Sex and Race: 1988 to 2080. Current Population Reports, Series P-25, No. 1018. Government Printing Office: Washington, DC, 1989.
2. National Center for Health Statistics. Vital Statistics of the United States, 1989. Vital Health Statistics, vol 2. Government Printing Office: Washington, DC, 1992:11.
3. National Center for Health Statistics. Current Estimates From the National Health Interview Survey, 1989. Vital and Health Statistics, Series 10. Government Printing Office: Washington, DC, 1990:No. 176.
4. Peterson ED, Jollis JG, Bebchuk JD, et al. Changes in mortality after myocardial revascularization in the elderly. Ann Intern Med 1994;121:919–927.
5. Horvath KA, DiSesa VJ, Peigh PS, et al. Favorable results of coronary artery bypass grafting in patients older than 75 years. J Thorac Cardiovasc Surg 1990;99:92–96.
6. Salomon NW, Page US, Bigelow JC, et al. Coronary artery bypass grafting in elderly patients: comparative results in consecutive series of 469 patients older than 75 years. J Thorac Cardiovasc Surg 1991;101:209–218.
7. Alexander KP, Peterson ED. Coronary artery bypass grafting in the elderly. Am Heart J 1997;134:856–864.
8. Kern LS. The elderly heart surgery patient. Crit Care Nurs Clin North Am 1991;3:749–756.
9. Mezey MD, Rauckhorst LH, Stokes SA. Health Assessment of the Older Individual, 2nd ed. Springer: New York, 1993.
10. Smith Rossi M. The octogenarian cardiac surgery patient. J Cardiovasc Nurs 1995;9(4):75–95.
11. Folstein MF, Folstein SE, McHugh PR. Mini-Mental State: a practical method for grading the cognitive state of patients for the clinician. J Psychiatr Res 1975;12:189–198.
12. Cane ME, Chen C, Bailey BM, et al. CABG in octogenarians: early and late events and actuarial survival in comparison with a matched population. Ann Thorac Surg 1995;60: 1033–1037.

13. Williams DB, Carrillo RG, Traad EA, et al. Determinants of operative mortality in octogenarians undergoing coronary bypass. Ann Thorac Surg 1995;60:1038–1043.
14. Akins CW, Daggett WM, Vlahakes GJ, et al. Cardiac operations in patients 80 years old and older. Ann Thorac Surg 1997;64:606–615.
15. Iskandrian AS, Segal BL. Should cardiac surgery be performed in octogenarians? J Am Coll Cardiol 1991;18:36–37.
16. Shirani J, Yousefi J, Roberts WC. Major cardiac findings at necropsy in 366 American octogenarians. Am J Cardiol 1995;75:151–156.
17. Iskandrian AS, Hakki AH. The effects of aging after coronary artery bypass grafting on the regulation of cardiac output during upright exercise. Int J Cardiol 1985;7:347–360.
18. Hakki AH, DePace NL, Iskandrian AS. Effect of age on left ventricular function during exercise in patients with coronary artery disease. J Am Coll Cardiol 1983:645–651.
19. Iskandrian AS, Hakki AH. Age-related changes in left ventricular diastolic performance. Am Heart J 1986;112:75–78.
20. Roberts WC. Ninety three hearts ≥90 years of age. Am J Cardiol 1993;71:599–602.
21. Waller BF, Roberts WC. Cardiovascular disease in the very elderly: analysis of 40 necropsy patients aged 90 years or older. Am J Cardiol 1983;51:403–421.
22. Roberts WC. The aging heart. Mayo Clin Proc 1988;63: 205–206.
23. Gersh BJ, Kronmal RA, Schaff HV, et al. Long-term (5 year) results of coronary bypass surgery in patients 65 years or older: a report from the Coronary Artery Surgery Study. Circulation 1983;66(suppl II):190–199.
24. Naunheim KS, Kern MJ, McBride LR, et al. Coronary artery bypass surgery in patients aged 80 years or older. Am J Cardiol 1987;59:804–807.
25. Morris RJ, Strong MD, Grunewald KE, et al. Internal thoracic artery for coronary artery grafting in octogenarians. Ann Thorac Surg 1996;62:16–22.
26. Glower DD, Christopher TD, Milano CA, et al. Performance status and outcome after coronary artery bypass grafting in persons aged 80 to 93 years. Am J Cardiol 1992;70:567–571.
27. Tsai T, Chaux A, Matloff JM, et al. Ten-year experience of cardiac surgery in patients aged 80 years and over. Ann Thorac Surg 1994;58:445–451.
28. Ko W, Krieger KH, Lazenby WD, et al. Isolated coronary artery bypass grafting in one hundred consecutive octogenarian patients. J Thorac Cardiovasc Surg 1991;102:532–538.
29. Diegeler A, Autschbach R, Falk V, et al. Open heart surgery in the octogenarians: a study on long-term survival and quality of life. Thorac Cardiovasc Surg 1995;43:265–270.
30. McGrath LB, Adkins MS, Chen C, et al. Actuarial survival and other events following valve surgery in octogenarians: comparison with age-, sex-, and race-matched population. Eur J Cardiothorac Surg 1991;5:319–325.
31. Freeman WK, Schaff HV, O'Brien PC, et al. Cardiac surgery in the octogenarian: perioperative outcome and clinical follow-up. J Am Coll Cardiol 1991;18:29–35.
32. Bashour TT, Hanna ES, Myler RK, et al. Cardiac surgery in patients over the age of 80 years. Clin Cardiol 1990;13: 267–270.
33. Naunheim KS, Dean PA, Fiore AC, et al. Cardiac surgery in the octogenarian. Eur J Cardiothorac Surg 1990;4:130–135.
34. Deiwick M, Tandler R, Mollhoff TH, et al. Heart surgery in patients aged eight years and above: determinants of morbidity and mortality. Thorac Cardiovasc Surg 1997;45: 119–126.
35. Wareing TH, Davila-Roman VG, Barzilai B, et al. Management of the severely atherosclerotic ascending aorta during cardiac operations. J Thorac Cardiovasc Surg 1992;103: 453–462.
36. Cannon LA, Marshall JM. Cardiac disease in the elderly population. Clin Geriatr Med 1993;9:499–525.
37. Davis EA, Gardner TJ, Gillinov AM, et al. Valvular disease in the elderly: influence on surgical results. Ann Thorac Surg 1993;55:333–338.
38. Gehlot A, Mullany CJ, Ilstrup D, et al. Aortic valve replacement in patients aged eighty years and older: early and long-term results. J Thorac Cardiovasc Surg 1996;111: 1026–1036.
39. Sahar G, Raanani E, Sagie A, et al. Surgical results in cardiac patients over the age of 80 years. Isr J Med Sci 1996;32: 1322–1325.
40. Logeais Y, Roussin R, Langanay T, et al. Aortic valve replacement for aortic stenosis in 200 consecutive octogenarians. J Heart Valve Dis 1995;4(suppl 1):S64–S71.
41. Klima U, Wimmer-Greinecker G, Mair R, et al. The octogenarians: a new challenge in cardiac surgery? Thorac Cardiovasc Surg 1994;42:212–217.
42. Yashar JJ, Yashar AG, Torres D, Hittner K. Favorable results of coronary artery bypass and/or valve replacement in octogenarians. Cardiovasc Surg 1993;1:68–71.
43. Tsai T, Nessim S, Kass RM, et al. Morbidity and mortality after coronary artery bypass in octogenarians. Ann Thorac Surg 1991;51:983–986.
44. Mullany CJ, Darling GE, Pluth JR, et al. Early and late results after isolated coronary artery bypass surgery in 159 patients aged 80 years and older. Circulation 1990;82 (suppl IV):229–236.
45. Kowalchuk GJ, Siu SC, McAuliffe LS, et al. Coronary artery bypass in octogenarians: early and late results. J Am Coll Cardiol 1990;15:35A.
46. Fiore AC, Naunheim KS, Barner HB, et al. Valve replacement in the octogenarian. Ann Thorac Surg 1989;48:104–108.
47. Rich MW, Sandza JG, Kleiger RE, et al. Cardiac operations in patients over 80 years of age. J Thorac Cardiovasc Surg 1985;90:56–60.
48. Tsai TP, Matloff JM, Gray RJ, et al. Cardiac surgery in the octogenarian. J Thorac Cardiovasc Surg 1986;91:924–928.
49. Peterson ED, Cowper PA, Jollis JG, et al. Outcomes of coronary artery bypass graft surgery in 24,461 patients aged 80 years or older. Circulation 1995;92(suppl II):85–91.
50. Curtis JJ, Walls JT, Boley TM, et al. Coronary revascularization in the elderly: determinants of operative mortality. Ann Thorac Surg 1994;58:1069–1072.
51. Tuman KJ, McCarthy RJ, Najafi H, et al. Differential effects of advanced age on neurologic and cardiac risks of coronary artery operations. J Thorac Cardiovasc Surg 1992;104: 1510–1517.
52. Lee EM, Porter JN, Shapiro LM, et al. Mitral valve surgery in the elderly. Heart Valve Dis 1997;6:22–31.
53. Culliford AT, Galloway AC, Colvin SB, et al. Aortic valve replacement for aortic stenosis in persons aged 80 years and over. Am J Cardiol 1991;67:1256–1260.

54. Kumar P, Zehr KJ, Cameron DE, et al. Quality of life in octogenarians after open heart surgery. Chest 1995;108:919–926.
55. Remington M, Tyrer PJ, Newson-Smith J, et al. Comparative reliability of categorical and analogue rating scales in the assessment of psychiatric symptomatology. Psychol Med 1979;9:765–770.
56. Campbell A, Converse PE, Ridgers WL. The Quality of American Life. Russell Sage: New York, 1976:1–583.
57. Bradburn NM. The structure of psychological well-being. Aldine: Chicago, 1969:214–215.
58. Adkins M, Amalfitano D, Harnum NA, et al. Efficacy of combined coronary revascularization and valve procedures in octogenarians. Chest 1995;108:927–931.
59. Merrill WH, Steward JR, Frist WH, et al. Cardiac surgery in patients age 80 years or older. Ann Surg 1990;211:772–776.
60. Edmunds LH, Stephenson LW, Edie RN, et al. Open-heart surgery in octogenarians. N Engl J Med 1988;319:131–136.
61. Berens ES, Kouchoukos NT, Murphy SF, et al. Preoperative carotid artery screening in elderly patients undergoing cardiac surgery. J Vasc Surg 1992;15:313–323.
62. Wareing TH, Davila-Roman VG, Barzilai B, et al. Management of the severely atherosclerotic ascending aorta during cardiac operations: a strategy for detection and treatment. J Thorac Cardiovasc Surg 1992;103:453–462.
63. Grawlee GP, Cordell AR, Graham JE, et al. Coronary revascularization in patients with bilateral internal carotid occlusion. J Thorac Cardiovasc Surg 1985;90:921–925.
64. Brener BJ, Bried DK, Alpert J, et al. The risk of stroke in patients with asymptomatic carotid stenosis undergoing cardiac surgery: a follow-up study. J Vasc Surg 1987;5:269–279.
65. Sisto DA, Hoffman DM, Fernandes S, Frater RWM. Is use of the intraaortic balloon pump in octogenarians justified? Ann Thorac Surg 1992;54:507–511.
66. He GW, Acuff TE, Ryan WH, et al. Determinants of operative mortality in elderly patients undergoing coronary artery bypass grafting. J Thorac Cardiovasc Surg 1994;108:73–81.
67. Ennabli K, Pelletier LC. Morbidity and mortality of coronary artery surgery after the age of 70 years. Ann Thorac Surg 1986;42:197–200.
68. Higgins TL, Estafanous FG, Loop FD, et al. Stratification of morbidity and mortality outcome by pre-operative risk factors in coronary artery bypass patients: a clinical severity score. JAMA 1992;267:2344–2348.
69. Utley JR, Leyland SA. Coronary artery bypass grafting in the octogenarian. J Thorac Cardiovasc Surg 1991;101:866–870.
70. Weintraub WS. Coronary operations in octogenarians: can we select the patients? Ann Thorac Surg 1995;60:875–876.
71. Braunstein EM, Bajwa TK, Andrei L, et al. Early and late outcome of revascularization for unstable angina in octogenarians. J Am Coll Cardiol 1991;17:2:151A.
72. Ko W, Gold JP, Lazzaro R, et al. Survival analysis of octogenarian patients with coronary artery disease managed by elective coronary artery bypass surgery versus conventional medical treatment. Circulation 1992;86(suppl II):191–197.
73. Mick MJ, Simpfendorfer C, Arnold AZ, et al. Early and late results of coronary angioplasty and bypass in octogenarians. Am J Cardiol 1991;68:1316–1320.
74. Dancy M, Dawkins, Ward D. Balloon dilatation of the aortic valve; limited success and early restenosis. Br Heart J 1989;60:236–239.
75. Litvack F, Jakubowski AT, Buchbinder NA, et al. Lack of sustained clinical improvement in an elderly population after percutaneous aortic valvuloplasty. Am J Cardiol 1988;62:270–275.
76. Palacios I, Block PC, Brandi S, et al. Percutaneous balloon valvotomy for patients with severe mitral stenosis. Circulation 1987;75:778–786.

# Invited Commentary: Vascular System

John A. Mannick

Modern vascular surgery is principally focused on the surgery of arteries and is therefore in large part surgery of the elderly because of the slowly progressive nature of the arteriosclerotic process that underlies the pathology requiring the attention of vascular surgeons. In contrast, arterial surgery is itself a relatively young field with a history of approximately 50 years. Before 1950 the term vascular surgery referred to the treatment of venous disease of the lower extremities, amputations for the complications of arterioscleroisis, and in some centers sympathectomy.

Although there had been isolated reports of direct surgical repair of injured arteries and even the use of vein grafts for such purposes, it was not until the report of Kunlin and associates in 1948 on the use of autogenous reversed saphenous vein grafts for the repair of occlusive disease in the legs and that of DosSantos at about the same time describing the use of endarterectomy for the same purpose that modern arterial surgery began. At nearly the same time Dubost described successful replacement of an abdominal aortic aneurysm with an arterial homograft. Only 3 years later Eastcott, Pickering, and Rob described the first successful repair of occlusive disease of the internal carotid artery. Thus in a period of approximately 5 years the technical feasibility of arterial surgery was demonstrated in the areas discussed in the three subsequent chapters in this volume.

## Occlusive Disease of the Extremities

The history of the surgery of arterial occlusive disease of the lower extremities over the past 50 years has been one of repeated cycles of disillusionment with alternative operative procedures and return to the use of autogenous saphenous vein bypass grafts, as originally proposed by Kunlin, as the most successful method of reconstruction for femoral-popliteal-tibial arteriosclerotic disease. The use of endarterectomy originally championed by Wiley and Barker in the United States was ultimately largely abandoned for infrainguinal arterial reconstruction because of its relatively high rate of recurrent stenosis and disappointing long-term results and because of technical problems with the closed or semiclosed techniques of endarterectomy popular at that time.

Many surgeons during the early 1950s who attempted to perform autogenous saphenous vein reconstructions for lower extremity occlusive disease, found that anastomoses between the vein and relatively noncompliant arteries presented annoying technical difficulties. It was partly a reflection of thc inexperience of most surgeons with arterial anastomoses and reliance on techniques suitable for intestinal suturing during early attempts at arterial reconstruction. The saphenous vein grafts simply puckered and became distorted when sutured to arteries in many of these early attempts. Therefore surgeons turned with some relief to the use of cryopreserved arterial homografts, which were much easier to handle, and then, upon failure of these conduits because of degeneration of the wall and aneurysm formation, to fabric arterial prostheses. The demonstration during the early 1950s by Voorhees of the feasibility of fabric arterial grafts proved to be an enormous step forward in the surgery of larger arteries; but in the leg, nylon, Teflon, and Dacron fabric prostheses, though rather easy to insert, were ultimately shown to have a high failure rate and poor long-term results.

A great step forward in surgery of occlusive disease in the extremities and elsewhere during the 1950s was the popularization by DeBakey of the fact that arteriosclerosis tended to be a segmental disease in most patients and thus could often by treated by the bypass principle of reconstruction, which left occluded arteries in place and did not interrupt collateral circulation. Early attempts in the United States at femoropopliteal reconstruction, for example, had often consisted of complete resection of the diseased arterial segment and in situ replacement with a homograft or vein graft.

By the early 1960s, most surgeons had become disillusioned with the fabric arterial prostheses then available because it was apparent that these prostheses failed quickly when implanted in patients with poor runoff, that is, those with diseased distal arteries providing outflow below the distal anastomosis of the prosthesis. Thus the patients who needed the reconstruction most to prevent ischemic limb loss were those in whom the operation was most likely to fail. It also became apparent that even in patients with relatively good outflow prostheses implanted below the level of the knee joint had a poor patency rate.

At this time of general disillusionment, a report by Linton and Darling of their long-term experience with autogenous vein grafts in the femoropopliteal position with more than 70% five-year patency, was a true revelation. Linton had himself visited Kunlin shortly after his first reports of the success of vein grafts in the leg and had learned from Kunlin the technique of a broad spatulated end-to-side anastomosis between vein graft and artery. Utilizing and perfecting this technique of anastomosis on his service, Linton had continued to perform successful femoropopliteal vein grafts during the 1950s when others had abandoned the technique. After Linton's landmark report, vascular surgeons gradually accepted autogenous saphenous vein grafts as the preferred method for infrainguinal arterial reconstruction and quickly mastered the essentials necessary for technical success. Early converts to vein grafting included Szilagyi, Dale and DeWeese, Hume and the present author. During these years, it was also gradually realized that vein grafts could be carried down to the tibial arteries with reasonable success.

Because of the unavailability of the greater saphenous vein in a number of patients and the operative time necessary to place a vein graft meticulously, new arterial prostheses for use in infrainguinal arterial reconstruction were introduced during the late 1960s and 1970s. The most durable of these prostheses in terms of surgeon acceptance has been the expanded polytetrafluoroethylene (PTFE) prosthesis. However, after more than two decades of experience with this prosthesis it has again become obvious that it, like the Dacron prostheses of the 1950s and the 1960s, yields satisfactory results in the hands of most surgeons only when the lower anastomosis of the prosthesis is kept above the level of the knee joint and when there is good outflow. Thus in many patients with severe occlusive disease the PTFE prosthesis can be expected to yield disappointing long-term results.

With these facts in mind, many surgeons have abandoned the routine use of PTFE prostheses and have exerted every effort to find appropriate autogenous vein grafts even in patients whose greater saphenous veins are diseased or surgically absent. Other possible grafts include arm veins and lesser saphenous veins, whose long-term results are in general slightly inferior to those of greater saphenous vein grafts but clearly superior to prostheses. It has been estimated by several groups with wide experience in infrainguinal reconstruction, that the percentage of patients with severe infrainguinal occlusive disease in whom an autogenous vein graft cannot be performed, is as low as 4–5%.

Fortunately, there is now convincing evidence that the success of autogenous vein grafts can be significantly improved if they are subjected to careful surveillance by duplex ultrasonography during the first postoperative year. Any vein graft stenoses encountered can be treated prior to occlusion of the graft with anticipated long-term success equal to that of grafts in which no stenotic lesions are detected. Autogenous vein grafting in the infrainguinal region can now be performed with the expectation of approximately 80% long-term graft patency and an equally high percentage of long-term limb salvage in patients operated on for this indication. Operative mortality in most modern series is 2% or less.

Balloon angioplasty of femoropopliteal occlusive disease has in general proved disappointing in contrast to the relatively high rate of success for this technique in the iliac arteries. Reasonable results in most series are obtained only when balloon angioplasty is applied to short stenotic lesions of the superficial femoral artery. Patients with such lesions ordinarily have symptoms only of mild claudication and are not in urgent need of intervention for limb salvage.

Dacron prostheses, in contrast to their record in infrainguinal reconstruction, have proved highly satisfactory for treatment of aortoiliac occlusive disease with excellent long-term results. The use of such prostheses for this indication however, has recently begun to decline because of the success achieved by percutaneous balloon angioplasty of iliac lesions with or without intraluminal stenting. Whether intraluminal grafts inserted through the femoral route will prove superior to balloon angioplasty and stenting for treatment of aortoiliac or femoropopliteal occlusive disease has yet to be determined.

## Aneurysms

Once the principle of graft replacement of aortic aneurysms was demonstrated during the early 1950s, subsequent efforts in this area of vascular surgery have been mainly directed at improving the safety of the operation and expanding its application to more proximal aneurysms in the aorta and in the peripheral arteries. The decades of the 1950s and 1960s showed a gradual reduction in mortality due to elective abdominal aortic aneurysm repair, from approximately 20% to approximately 5%. Among the factors responsible for this improvement were changes in operative technique to diminish the operating time and blood loss. Whereas most aneurysms during the 1950s were excised in toto, the graft inclusion technique, first described by Creech, was gradually adopted during the 1960s. Using this technique, only enough dissection is done to expose the neck of the aneurysm below the renal arteries and the iliac arteries below the aneurysm. After clamping these vessels, the entire operation is performed from inside the aneurysm, suturing the prosthesis to the normal arteries above and below the aneurysm from within the aneurysm cavity.

Other improvements included the realization that the common occurrence of renal failure in patients after abdominal aneurysm surgery could be avoided by administering sizable amounts of electrolyte solution during surgery and not clamping a debris-filled aorta immediately below the renal artery orifice. Respiratory and cardiac complications of aneurysm surgery were gradually reduced by improvements in postoperative care and the advent of modern intensive care units. With further refinements in intra- and postoperative patient management, the mortality rate due to elective abdominal aortic aneurysm repair in experienced hands is now often reported at 2% or less. Replacement of autogenous blood lost during the operative procedure through cell-saver techniques has also significantly reduced the number of transfusions of banked blood required and has increased the long-term safety of the operative procedure.

The safety of thoracoabdominal aneurysm surgery was also greatly enhanced during the 1970s and 1980s through application of the graft inclusion technique to such aneurysms, as described by Crawford. Again, surgery is carried out principally from within the aneurysm cavity, suturing buttons of aortic wall containing the origins of important branches to the side of the prosthesis.

The aortic aneurysm size that mandates surgical repair remains a subject of debate. Although some surgeons are convinced that surgery is indicated for most aneurysms more than 4.0 cm in diameter, available evidence from population-based studies and aneurysm screening protocols, suggests that 5.0 or 5.5 cm may be the diameter at which the danger of rupture exceeds the operative mortality.

At present, there is great interest in the use of endovascular techniques for repair of abdominal aortic aneurysms. With these still experimental procedures, repair of the aneurysm is carried out through femoral arterotomies in the groin with insertion of prostheses anchored in place with vascular stents or other devices. Initial experience with these techniques has shown that endografting may be applicable to some fraction of patients with abdominal aneurysms, perhaps as many as 50% in the more optimistic estimates. In the short run in a number of small series, the endografting techniques have effectively excluded the aneurysm from the arterial circulation. At present, however, the mortality from such procedures has not been demonstrated to be lower than that associated with conventional aneurysm repair, and the long-term durability of endografting is not yet known.

Among the disturbing features of early series has been an incidence of aneurysm rupture several months after endograft insertion in individuals in whom arterial blood flow had leaked around graft insertion points back into the aneurysm cavity. Nevertheless, it seems likely that because of its potential to diminish postoperative hospitalization and morbidity, endovascular repair will be refined sufficiently in the future to be the technique of choice for repair of some abdominal aortic aneurysms and for some less common aneurysms in peripheral arteries in areas difficult to expose surgically.

## Extracranial Vascular Disease

It had been convincingly demonstrated through careful autopsy studies during the late 1940s and early 1950s, that occlusive disease of the internal carotid artery was associated with ipsilateral ischemic brain infarcts, almost certainly establishing a causal relation between these two pathologic conditions. Although the first repair of internal carotid artery occlusive disease was not endarterectomy, the feasibility of localized endarterectomy for removing internal carotid artery disease was probably first established by DeBakey during the mid-1950s. It is therefore somewhat surprising how long it has taken for carotid endarterectomy to be accepted as an appropriate procedure for the prevention of strokes. This lack of acceptance was perhaps caused by the essential conservatism of the neurologic community and the fact that in the hands of surgeons unfamiliar with the technical requirements of the procedure, carotid endarterectomy could be associated with unacceptably high rates of perioperative stroke or death from stroke. Nevertheless, the operation clearly removed the most likely cause of stroke in many patients; and it gradually became evident that once the internal carotid had thrombosed, attempts to reopen the vessel were unlikely to be successful. It also became clear from prospective and retrospective analyses that patients with internal carotid occlusion were at markedly increased risk for stroke in the ipsilateral hemisphere at the time of carotid occlusion and for many years thereafter. It also became evident by the early 1960s that surgeons with a large experience of carotid endarterectomies and who had come to understand the technical demands of the procedure, could perform it with low perioperative stroke and mortality rates. Their patients in long-term follow-up also appeared to have, in most cases, long-term freedom from ipsilateral stroke.

Critics of the procedure accused these experienced surgeons, unfairly as it now seems, of bias in their reporting and maintained a barrage of criticism in the medical and lay press. The issue was further clouded by a prospective multiinstitutional study conducted during the late 1960s in which the clear benefits of successful carotid endarterectomy for patients having transient ischemic attacks (TIAs) and appropriate ipsilateral carotid stenosis was negated in the entire study population by high complication and death rates at the hands of several surgical groups participating in the study. However, the principal investigator of the study, a neurologist, concluded that if surgical groups could perform carotid endarterectomy with low morbidity and mortality, surgery appeared to be the appropriate therapy for patients with TIAs and significant ipsilateral carotid stenosis. There was little consensus in the neurologic community on this issue, however, and many reports during the 1970s suggested that treatment with antiplatelet agents, usually aspirin, was far more likely to produce beneficial results than surgery even in patients with TIAs.

By the 1970s, with widespread use of computed tomography (CT), it was becoming apparent that symptoms in patients with carotid disease did not always match their pathology. In fact, asymptomatic patients with high grade carotid stenoses were found not infrequently to have silent infarcts by CT imaging. By the late 1970s Thompson, a pioneer in carotid surgery, reported experience with prophylactic carotid endarterectomy in asymptomatic patients with high grade stenoses. These patients were compared with an unoperated control group and were found to do much better during follow-up with respect to ipsilateral strokes and death from stroke. Because this study was not prospective or randomized it was greeted with derision by critics in the neurologic community; but it altered the thinking of many vascular surgeons who had become increasingly aware of the sometimes devastating consequences of allowing patients to proceed to carotid occlusion even if they had no prior symptoms.

Fortunately, the controlled prospective randomized studies of the early 1990s, in which the surgical groups participating were prescreened with respect to mortality and morbidity, have convincingly demonstrated that what had seemed logical during the mid-1950s was in fact true: that removal of a hemodynamically significant internal carotid stenosis would prevent stroke if the operation could be performed safely. This is now known to be the case for both symptomatic and asymptomatic patients.

As might be anticipated, not all issues surrounding the treatment of carotid artery occlusive disease have been settled. Surgeons remain divided on the choice of anesthesia (local vs. general), the appropriate intraoperative monitoring techniques to detect and correct hypoperfusion of the ipsilateral hemisphere, and those used to detect the occurrence of cerebral emboli during the surgical procedure. Arguments for and against the routine use of indwelling shunts to continue perfusion of the ipsilateral hemisphere during surgery are still heard, and there remains a difference of opinion about the desirability of routine versus selective patching of the carotid arterotomy wound. Fortunately for the patients involved, experienced surgeons on both sides of the above-mentioned debates are producing excellent long- and short-term outcomes for the individuals under their care.

Perhaps of greater potential hazard is the current interest in the treatment of internal carotid occlusive disease by angioplasty and stenting techniques. If such techniques are ever to become clinically accepted, they must demonstrate equal safety and long-term symptom-free patency when compared to conventional carotid endarterectomy. Preliminary uncontrolled studies so far appear to demonstrate an unacceptably high incidence of procedure-related embolic stroke, which does not seem surprising to anyone who has looked at the inside of a stenotic carotid bulb at the time of endarterectomy.

Other operations for cerebrovascular occlusive disease are performed much less frequently than carotid endarterectomy. In appropriate patients with vertebrobasilar symptoms and bilateral vertebral artery stenoses, vertebral artery reimplantation or, in some instances, vertebral orificial endarterectomy or bypass grafting can be performed with safety and the expectation of a high rate of success. Treatment of stenoses or occlusions of the origins of the great vessels arising from the aortic arch has also been reasonably well standardized and can be performed directly or indirectly with expectation of low morbidity and mortality and a high rate of hemodynamic and symptomatic success.

All in all, the story of surgical treatment of arterial occlusive disease in the elderly during the past 50 years has been one of continuing technical refinement and an increase in the appreciation of the natural history of the disease in areas where arteriosclerosis most commonly produces clinically important effects. In most instances these advances have yielded gradual reduction in mortality and improved success of the operative procedures employed. As the field of vascular surgery reaches middle age, it appears to have matured as a clinical discipline.

# 33
# Surgical Treatment of Occlusive Vascular Disease in the Elderly

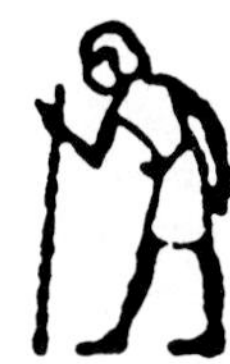

William D. Suggs, Frank J. Veith, and Luis A. Sanchez

Severe arterial occlusive disease can manifest as incapacitating claudication or limb-threatening ischemia of the lower extremities. Male cigarette smokers under the age of 65 have been considered in the past as the group with the highest prevalence of aortoiliac occlusive disease. Over the past 20 years it has been noted that there are increasing numbers of women affected with occlusive disease of the aortoiliac segment.[1] In addition, with the "graying" of the population and the increased life expectancy of individuals, the number of elderly patients presenting with significant aortoiliac occlusive disease is continuously increasing and becoming a significant and increasing percentage of the patients who require intervention for this disease.[2] During the 1990s, the average age of patients requiring aortoiliac reconstructions at our institution increased from 63 years to 68 years. The options for treatment of aortoiliac occlusive disease have evolved since the 1950s, when the initial aortoiliac reconstructions were performed using an arterial prosthesis. Multiple options for arterial reconstructions have been developed to accommodate varied patient arterial anatomy and risks of intervention. Advances in catheter-based techniques, vascular imaging, and other noninvasive tests have paralleled the development of new surgical techniques and procedures. Further advances in the treatment of aortoiliac occlusive disease are based on the combination of percutaneous techniques and surgical skills used to develop and perform endoluminal bypass.

Enormous advances have also occurred in the treatment of lower limb ischemia with management strategies developed to treat virtually all patterns of atherosclerosis underlying limb-threatening ischemia. Bypasses to the infrainguinal arteries utilizing autologous vein have become routine for limb salvage. As this technique has evolved, the distal limits of revascularization have been extended to arteries near the ankle or in the foot for patients who have no patent arteries for a bypass to more proximal arteries. In addition, some patients present with patent popliteal arteries but have three-vessel distal occlusive disease and forefoot gangrene that requires a bypass to a distal tibial or tarsal vessel.[3]

## Patient Assessment

The initial evaluation of elderly patients with arterial occlusive disease is critical. Atherosclerotic disease of the aortoiliac segment is often asymptomatic in many elderly patients secondary to their sedentary life style. Few elderly patients present with lower extremity or buttock claudication secondary to either isolated infrainguinal or aortoiliac disease. Instead, they more commonly present with limb-threatening lower extremity ischemia (rest pain, ischemic ulceration, gangrene) secondary to multilevel arterial occlusive disease. The combined aortoiliac and infrainguinal arterial occlusive disease can be more difficult to assess and treat in this patient population. After a complete physical examination that includes a careful pulse examination, noninvasive studies are helpful for evaluating the patient's arterial disease. The vascular laboratory may aid in the evaluation and selection of patients for single or multilevel revascularization.[4] If an intervention is indicated, further necessary invasive studies are performed to define the best intervention for the individual patient.

### Ankle-Brachial Indices, Segmental Pressures, and Pulse Volume Recordings

The ankle-brachial index (ABI) is determined by dividing the ankle pressure in each lower limb by the higher of the two brachial pressures. Patients with normal circulation have ABIs of 1.0–1.2, those with claudication have ABIs of 0.40–0.95, and those with limb-threatening ischemia have ABIs of 0–0.5. An important limitation of measuring lower extremity pressure occurs in patients with heavily calcified vessels, mostly diabetics and patients with end-stage renal disease. In these patients the ABIs are falsely elevated owing to the higher pressure required to occlude calcified vessels, and in some cases the vessels are not occluded even with pressures higher than 300 mmHg.

Pulse volume recordings (PVRs) are obtained using a calibrated air plethysmograph. A PVR waveform is generated for different levels of the lower extremity using standard blood pressure cuffs. The increase in pressure within the cuff resulting from the volume increase during systole is recorded as a pulse wave. The tracings are characterized as normal when there is a brisk rise during systole and a dicrotic notch, as moderately abnormal when there is loss of the notch and a more prolonged downslope, and as severely abnormal when there is a flattened wave. The absolute amplitudes are not comparable from patient to patient, but serial PVRs have been shown to be highly reproducible, making them useful for following the course of patients with severe peripheral vascular disease.[5] In addition, this test cannot differentiate proximal femoral disease from iliac occlusive disease.

## Duplex Scanning

Duplex scanning can be a useful noninvasive technique for assessing the aortoiliac and infrainguinal arterial system. A variety of studies have evaluated the ability of this technique to predict iliac artery stenoses. Kohler et al. initially suggested that duplex scanning had excellent sensitivity (89%) and specificity (90%) when used to predict an iliac stenosis of 50% or more.[6] Three subsequent studies by Langsfeld et al.,[7] Moneta et al.,[8] and Legemate et al.[9] corroborated these findings with sensitivities ranging from 81% to 89% and specificities ranging from 88% to 99%. These noninvasive evaluations may be useful for evaluating the elderly prior to invasive procedures such as angiography and angioplasty.

## Spiral CT Scanning and Magnetic Resonance Angiography

Conventional computed tomography (CT) has limited use in the evaluation of aortoiliac occlusive disease, but it can be helpful for identifying severely calcified arteries or lesions and may alter treatment plans. In addition, faster, new spiral CT scanners that have the capability of three-dimensional reconstructions may provide better images, but these studies are not used routinely for evaluating patients with aortoiliac occlusive disease.

Magnetic resonance angiography (MRA) is noninvasive, does not require contrast agents, and allows good arterial imaging. Owens et al.[10] and Carpenter et al.[11] showed that MRA may be more sensitive than arteriography when imaging distal lower extremity runoff vessels. Carpenter et al.[12] also reported that MRA had a 100% positive predicted value (PPV) and a 98.6% negative predicted value (NPV) when compared to contrast angiography for evaluating patients with aortoiliac occlusive disease. These findings have not been widely reproduced, but this noninvasive modality has the potential to replace contrast arteriography in the evaluation of these patients. Current images are generally inadequate for therapeutic planning in most centers; but as the associated hardware and software improve, the role of MRA in the assessment of occlusive disease of the aortoiliac segments will increase.[13]

## Angiography

Intraarterial contrast angiography is considered the gold standard for evaluating patients with arterial occlusive disease. This modality provides the diagnostic information necessary to plan the treatment of most vascular patients with arterial occlusive disease. Complete evaluation of the existing arterial disease from the aorta to the pedal vessels is necessary for elderly patients because they commonly have multilevel occlusive disease. The addition of intraarterial pressure measurements at the time of arteriography improves the accuracy of detecting clinically significant stenosis. Pressure measurements after intraarterial injection of a vasodilatory drug such as papaverine, are used to evaluate the significance of aortoiliac stenoses under conditions of stress that require increased blood flow through these vessels. A systolic pressure gradient across the lesion of more than 15 mmHg is considered hemodynamically significant.[14]

The complication rate of arteriography in the general population is only 1.7–3.3%.[15] Elderly patients with severe aortoiliac or infrainguinal disease must be carefully evaluated before the procedure, as local and systemic complications are more likely than in the general population. The transfemoral approach is the safest, but other options (e.g., translumbar, transbrachial, or transaxillary approach) may have to be used for patients with weak or nonpalpable femoral pulses. These alternative approaches have higher local complication rates. Complications include hematomas, pseudoaneurysms, dissections, thrombosis, and embolization.

Renal insufficiency is an important complication of angiography. Renal impairment associated with contrast agents occurs in 6.5–8.2% of patients who undergo arteriography.[16,17] Patients with preexisting azotemia and a baseline serum creatinine level >2.0 mg/dl are at the highest risk of renal complications after angiography. Elderly patients have a low creatinine clearance rate for a given serum creatinine level, so they should always be considered at high risk for nephrotoxicity. All possible precautions must be taken to limit the renal insult. The use of low osmolar contrast agents has been shown by some to decrease the incidence of renal impairment,[18,19] but these findings are not universal.[20] Adequate hydration prior to arteriography is an effective maneuver to diminish the risk of contrast nephropathy. Mannitol is used for its osmotic diuretic effect to help prevent contrast toxicity. Vasodilators such as dopamine have also been used because the nephrotoxic effect of contrast agents is considered to be partly due to intrarenal vasoconstriction. Dopamine has been shown to be better than mannitol for preventing contrast-related renal insufficiency.[21] Unfortunately, many elderly patients have moderate to severe cardiac disease, and aggressive hydration may lead to congestive heart failure, cardiac ischemia, and arrhythmias. In addition, the use of dopamine may lead to cardiac complications. Careful hydration and judicious use of mannitol, dopamine, and contrast agents can decrease the incidence of renal impairment associated with arteriography.

## Therapeutic Options

Elderly patients with mainly aortoiliac occlusive disease rarely require an intervention. Patients with claudication should be treated initially by maximizing the management of the known risk factors for the development of atherosclerosis, an exercise or walking program, and the use of potentially helpful oral agents such as pentoxifylline. The small group of patients with severe, debilitating claudication that has failed the initial treatment protocol generally request an intervention. In addition, patients who present with limb-threatening ischemia secondary to multilevel occlusive disease should be considered for intervention.

### Percutaneous Transluminal Angioplasty and Stents

The use of percutaneous balloon angioplasty for the treatment of aortoiliac occlusive disease and superficial femoral arterial disease, with or without the use of intravascular stents, has flourished over the past decade. The location of the lesion must be considered before therapy is determined. Isolated aortic stenoses are uncommon, though several small series of aortic angioplasties for stenotic disease have been reported. The initial success ranges from 90% to 100%,[22–26] with 5-year patency rates of 70%.[22,24]

Stenotic lesions of the iliac arteries have been treated successfully with balloon angioplasty. The 5-year patency rate of iliac angioplasty in a large literature review by Becker et al. was 72%.[27] Multiple series in the literature have described a variety of factors that can affect the long-term results of iliac angioplasty. Predictors of a long-term successful outcome after balloon angioplasty include the location of the lesion (common iliac lesions respond better than external iliac artery lesions), indication for therapy (patients with claudication respond better than those with limb-threatening ischemia), severity of the lesion (arterial stenoses respond better than arterial occlusions), and arterial runoff distal to the lesion (lesions with good runoff respond better than those with poor runoff). Johnston et al. reported a 60% five-year patency rate for common iliac artery angioplasty compared to a 48% five-year patency rate for external iliac artery lesions.[22] Series containing predominantly claudicants have 5-year secondary patency rates of up to 83%.[28] An early series by Spence et al. reported 2-year patency rates of 79% for patients with claudication and 50% for those treated for limb salvage.[29] A more recent study on diabetics reported 5-year patency rates of 70% for claudicants and only 29% for patients with limb-threatening ischemia.[30] Johnston et al. found that common iliac artery stenoses with good runoff had a 65% five-year patency rate versus a 52% rate for arteries with poor runoff.[22] In diabetics the 5-year patency rate for lesions with good runoff has been reported at 76%, whereas it was only 20% for those lesions with poor runoff.[30]

In 1990 Palmaz et al. reported on 171 procedures in 154 patients in whom stents were placed in the iliac arteries to treat occlusive disease.[31] The indications at that time were for unsatisfactory angioplasty, restenosis of previous angioplasry, or complete occlusion. At an average 6-month follow-up, 113 of 154 patients remained asymptomatic. A randomized German trial of iliac stent placement versus angioplasty alone implied that stenting was superior to angioplasty. The 5-year patency for stenting was 92% versus 64% for angioplasty.[32] Other studies have supported the use of stents in the iliac arteries particularly for total occlusions, dissection, and restenosis[33–36] (Fig. 33.1). Vorwerk and Gunther reported a 90% initial success rate in their last series of 50 patients with total occlusions.[37] The use of stents for treatment of angioplasty failures, dissections, or more complex lesions has improved the results of iliac artery interventions, but the long-term durablity of treatment of complex lesions has yet to be confirmed.

The results of infrainguinal percutaneous transluminal angioplasty (PTA) are reported to have patencies ranging from 12% to 100% with lower patencies reported for series when the indication for treatment was limb salvage; superior results were seen in series with large numbers of patients being treated for intermittent claudication.[38–41] Hunink et al.[42] reported a meta-analysis of patency results of percutaneous and surgical revascularization for femoropopliteal arterial disease. A 5-year patency of 68% was demonstrated when angioplasty of a stenotic femoropopliteal lesion was performed for claudication, whereas it was 12% when angioplasty of occlusions was performed for critical ischemia. Treiman et al. reported on the results of below-knee popliteal and tibial artery angioplasty for limb salvage in 25 patients and found a high rate of lesion and symptom recurrence that required subsequent surgical revascularization. In addition, an analysis of cost did not demonstrate a

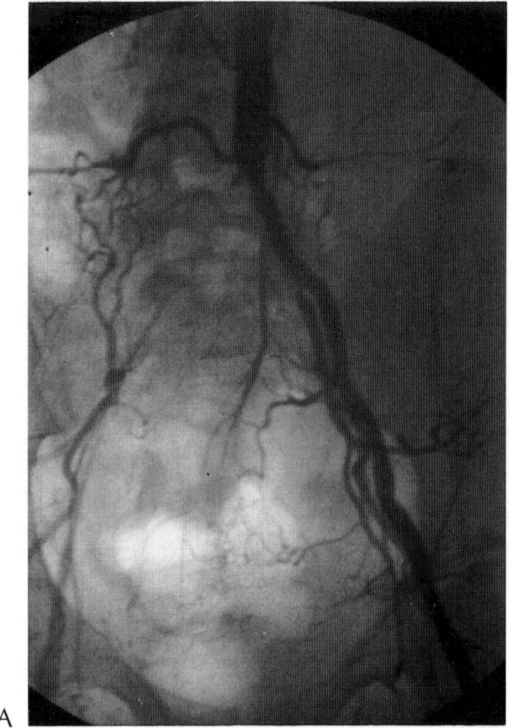

A

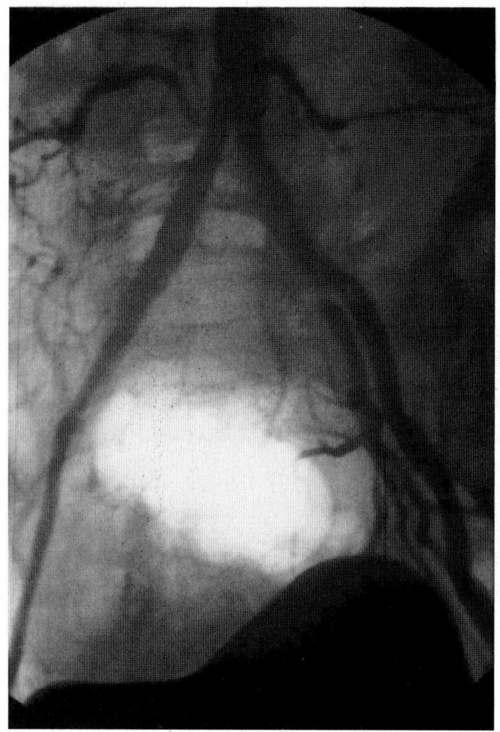

B

FIGURE 33.1. A 65-year-old woman was admitted with one half block right leg claudication with a history of two failed femorofemoral artery bypasses. A. Pelvic angiogram shows total occlusion of the right common iliac artery. B. Iliac artery occlusion was corrected by balloon angioplasty and wall stent placement. (Reprinted from Sanchez LA, Suggs WD, and Veith FJ, Vascular Disease in the Elderly, Futura Publishing Company, New York 1997, with permission.)

savings with PTA when compared to bypass surgery.[43] London et al. treated 54 patients with limb-threatening ischemia using angioplasty alone, with apparently better results; they reported a 2-year symptomatic improvement rate of 77%. These patients represented 23% of the total number of patients treated (232 limbs) by this group for limb-threatening ischemia.[44]

Currie and colleagues noted that 22 of 23 femoropopliteal angioplasties of lesions longer than 5 cm failed within 6 months in patients with critical ischemia; lesions less than 5 cm tended to perform better, with 10 of 15 open at 6 months.[45] A report by Stanley et al. on 176 patients treated by angioplasty of superior femoral artery (SFA) and popliteal artery lesions showed a 2-year cumulative patency of 46%. However, 74% of these patients were treated for claudication.[46] These discrepant results after PTA make the various reports difficult to interpret. Moreover, many studies continue to report technical or symptomatic success as an endpoint.

## Aortofemoral Bypass

Aortofemoral bypass remains the standard to which other procedures must be compared for treatment of aortoiliac occlusive disease. Operative morbidity and mortality are low, with 5-year patency rates of 80–90%.[47–50] Ten-year patency rates of 70–80% have been achieved in patients who have ceased smoking after operation[47,48] (Fig. 33.2). A significant portion of patients requiring iliac reconstruction also have significant femoropopliteal disease. Most of these patients are best served by correcting their inflow disease prior to infrainguinal reconstruction. Patients with severe rest pain or those with gangrene or nonhealing ulcerations may need simultaneous aortoiliac and infrainguinal bypass to achieve limb salvage.

## Femoral-to-Femoral Bypass

Crossover bypass for unilateral iliac artery occlusion has been traditionally reserved for high-risk patients but have been used more recently in good risk patients. This procedure can be performed easily under regional or local anesthesia if required. Patency rates have ranged from 60% to 90% at 5 years.[49–53] When concurrently performed femorofemoral bypasses were compared to aortobifemoral bypass in low-risk patients, femorofemoral bypass was inferior in terms of patency and hemodynamic performance to aortobifemoral bypass (primary patency 61% vs. 87% at 3 years). Interestingly, in this series limb salvage rates were similar for the two procedures in patients initially admitted with limb-threatening ischemia.[50] Femorofemoral graft is also useful

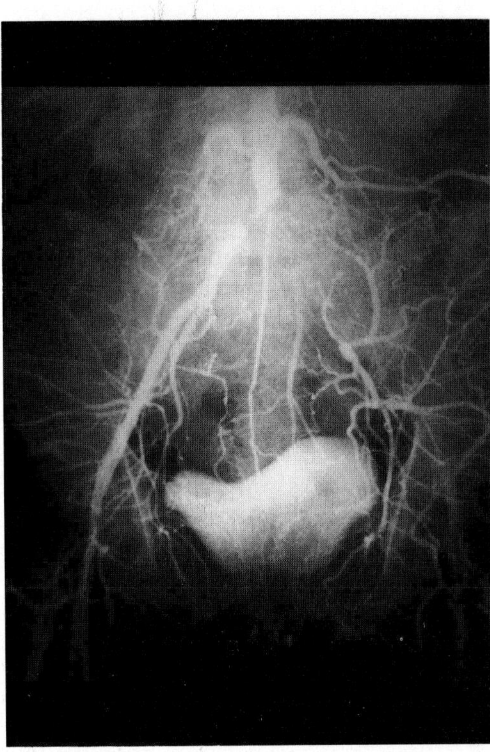

FIGURE 33.2. Aortogram of a 72-year-old woman with left leg rest pain. She underwent reconstruction with an aortobifemoral bypass.

to treat a unilateral occlusion of a limb of a bifurcated aortic graft.[54]

Direct iliofemoral bypass is another option for unilateral iliac artery occlusion. In a randomized study in France, aortofemoral and iliofemoral bypasses were compared with femorofemoral or iliofemoral crossover bypass. Primary patency rates for direct reconstruction were better at 4 years (89%) than for crossover grafts (52%), with no difference in morbidity.[51] Five-year secondary patency rates for iliofemoral versus femorofemoral bypass were 69% versus 65%, respectively, in a report by Harrington et al.[52]

## Axillofemoral Bypass

Traditionally, high risk patients with aortoiliac occlusive disease have been treated with axillofemoral bypass. Axillofemoral grafts were considered inferior to aortobifemoral grafts in terms of long-term patency. However, after the introduction of externally supported prostheses by Sauvage's group,[55] patency rates of axillofemoral grafts dramatically improved. Recent papers have demonstrated patency rates for axillary grafts that approach those from historic series for aortobifemoral grafts.[56,57] Passman et al.[50] found that axillofemoral grafts compared favorably with aortic graft in terms of limb salvage. In their comparative series of concurrently performed procedures, the aortic grafts had better long-term patency but equivalent results in terms of limb salvage. In this report the group of patients undergoing axillofemoral artery bypasses were an older and sicker group of patients with a significantly decreased survival when compared to the patients undergoing aortic procedures. Therefore, one can conclude that patients with limited life expectancy can achieve results from axillary bypass that should be equivalent to those of aortic reconstruction, but one would continue to use direct aortic reconstruction for the younger, better risk patients.[58]

## Endoluminal Grafts

An alternative method for treating long-segment aortoiliac disease employs endovascular stented grafts placed across the area of occlusion or stenoses. These devices may be inserted under local or regional anesthesia, require less operative dissection, and can be done with minimal blood loss. They can be applied to long or multiple lesions for which balloon angioplasty and stents have not proven to be durable.[59–61] Preliminary reports of aortoiliac reconstruction utilizing stented grafts in 43 high risk patients demonstrated primary and secondary patency rates at 18 months of 77% and 95%, respectively.[26] In addition, these endoluminal grafts can be combined with conventional infrainguinal bypass techniques to achieve limb salvage. Seventeen such cases have been successfully performed with a 1-year patency rate of 94% and a limb rate of 93%.[62] These methods will undoubtedly have increased application in the management of multilevel aortoiliac and infrainguinal occlusive disease as technology improves.

## Femoropopliteal Bypass

Patients whose limbs are threatened should undergo femoropopliteal bypass when the superficial femoral or popliteal artery is occluded and the patent popliteal artery segment distal to the occlusion has luminal continuity with any of its three terminal branches on arteriographic examination. This is true even if one or more of these branches ends in an occlusion anywhere in the leg. Even if the popliteal artery segment into which the graft is to be inserted is occluded distally, femoropopliteal bypass to this isolated segment can be considered when the segment is more than 7 cm in length.[63–65] If the isolated popliteal segment is less than 7 cm in length or there is extensive gangrene or infection in the foot, a femoral-to-distal artery bypass or sequential bypass is sometimes performed in one or two stages.[63,65] Femoropopliteal bypasses performed with greater saphenous vein have 4-year primary patency rates that range from 68% to 80%, with limb salvage rates of 75–80% (Fig. 33.3). Femoropopliteal bypasses done with polytetrafluoroethylene (PTFE)

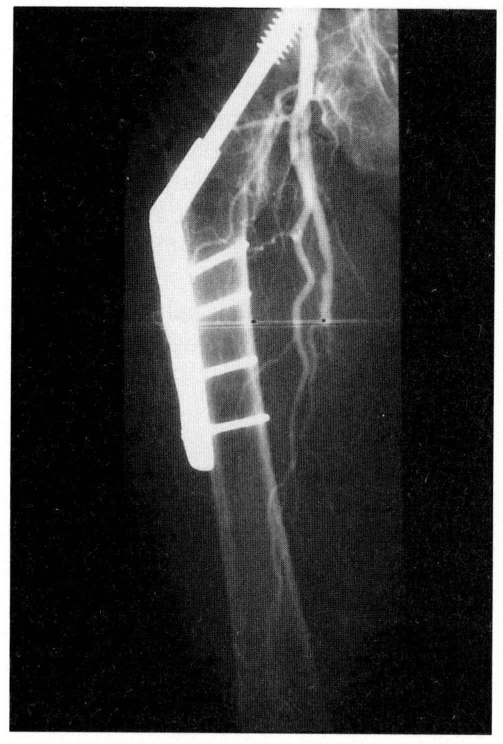


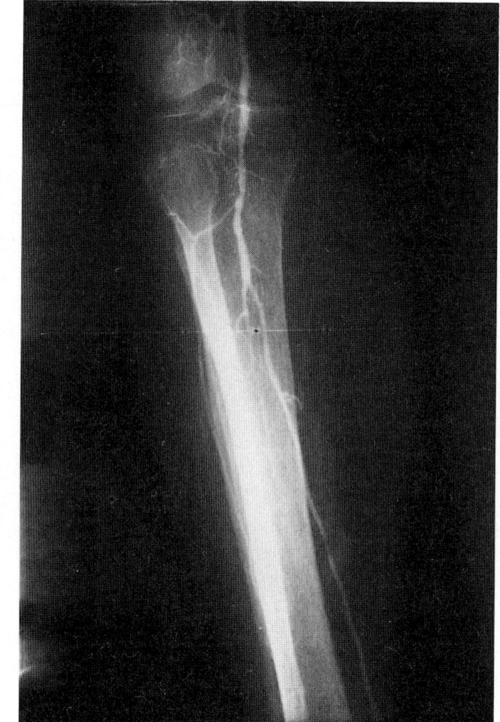


FIGURE 33.3. An 89-year-old ambulatory man who presented with a nonhealing right leg ulcer. A. Angiogram revealed occlusion of the right superficial femoral artery. B. Angiogram shows reconstitution of the right popliteal artery with posterior tibial runoff. This patient had a right femoropopliteal bypass.

have patency rates similar to that with vein if the bypass is to the above-knee popliteal artery; bypasses constructed with PTFE to the below-knee politeal artery do not perform as well.

## Infrapopliteal Bypass

Bypasses to arteries beyond the popliteal (small-vessel bypasses) are performed only when femoropopliteal bypass is not deemed possible, according to the foregoing criteria. These small-vessel bypasses are performed to the posterior tibial, anterior tibial, or peroneal artery, in that order of preference. A tibial artery is generally used only if its lumen runs without obstruction into the foot, although vein bypasses to isolated tibial artery segments and other disadvantaged outflow tracts have been performed and have remained patent more than 4 years.[66,67] A peroneal artery is usually used only if it is continuous with one or two of its terminal branches, which communicate with foot arteries. Absence of a plantar arch and vascular calcification are not considered contraindications to reconstruction.[66] Some patients require a bypass to an artery or an arterial branch in the foot.[2,66,67] Few patients fail to have an artery that meets these requirements in their leg or foot, so fewer than 1% of our patients are now considered not to be candidates for reconstruction on the basis of angiographic findings.[2]

With both femoropopliteal and small-vessel bypasses, stenosis of less than 50% of the diameter of the vessel is acceptable at or distal to the site chosen for the distal anastomosis. Although an effort is made to find the most disease-free segment of artery to use for the distal anastomosis, this may be tempered by the advisability of using the most proximal patent segment possible to shorten the length of the bypass. Bypasses to tibial arteries should be performed with autogenous vein by the reversed technique or the in situ technique. These bypasses should have 5-year primary patency rates that range from 60% to 67%, with limb salvage rates of 70–75%. The secondary patency of all of these grafts is improved with close patient follow-up and graft surveillance.

## Bypass to an Ankle or Foot Artery

Some patients present who have no patent or usable artery above the level of the ankle, and they require bypass to the distal perimalleolar and inframalleollar arteries. Visualization of these distal arteries requires excellent preoperative angiography. Bypass to a dorsalis pedis artery has yielded results comparable to those performed to more proximal tibial vessels, with 3-year primary patency rates of 58–60% and limb salvage rates of 75–95% (see Fig. 33.4). With careful follow-up, the assisted primary patency rates for these grafts have

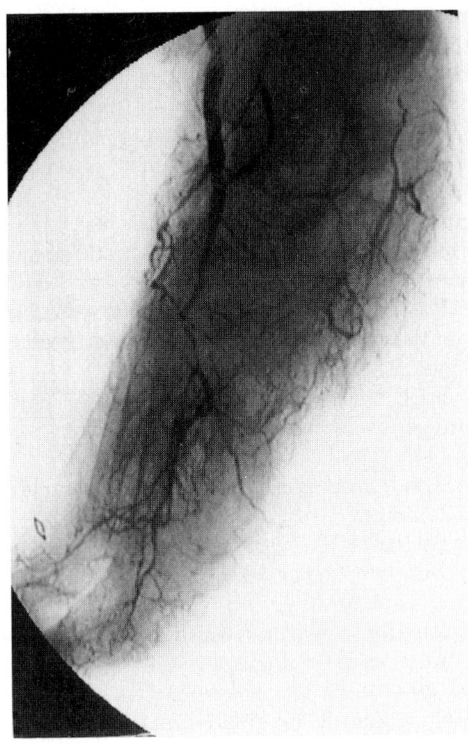

FIGURE 33.4. Completed angiogram of an 86-year-old woman with a nonhealing toe amputation site. This patient had a popliteal-to-dorsalis pedis bypass with saphenous vein.

substantially improved.[68,69] In addition, bypasses to the plantar and tarsal arteries have provided limb salvage when the dorsalis pedis and posterior tibial arteries were unsuitable for bypass. Visualization of the dorsalis pedis and posterior tibial arteries and their branches, and our use of them for bypass insertion, have been major factors in reducing the proportion of patients whose arterial disease was so distal that they were "unsuitable for an attempt at limb salvage" or inoperable.[66,67] The effectiveness of these bypasses to pedal arteries and their main branches has been documented, and these procedures are now more widely being performed and advocated.

## Failing Graft Concept

Intimal hyperplasia, progression of proximal or distal disease, or lesions within the graft itself can produce signs and symptoms of hemodynamic deterioration in patients with a prior arterial reconstruction without producing concomitant thrombosis of the bypass graft.[70–72] We have referred to this condition as a "failing graft" because if the lesion is not corrected, graft thrombosis will almost certainly occur.[71] The importance of this failing graft concept lies in the fact that many difficult lower extremity revascularizations can be salvaged for protracted periods by relatively simple interventions if the lesion responsible for the circulatory deterioration and diminished graft blood flow can be detected before graft thrombosis occurs.

Since the early 1990s, we have detected approximately 190 failing grafts and have corrected the lesions before graft thrombosis has occurred.[71–73] Invariably, the corrective procedure is simpler than the secondary operation that would be required if the bypass went on to thrombose. Vein grafts tend to fail as the result of hyperplastic lesions associated with the body or anastomotic areas of the graft. In contrast, PTFE grafts tend to fail as the result of proximal or distal progression of atherosclerotic disease. Solitary vein graft lesions 15 mm or less in length can be treated by PTA. Longer or multiple-vein graft lesions should be treated by an interposition graft or a proximal or distal graft extension depending on the lesion location. Some of the PTAs of these lesions have failed and required a second reintervention; others have remained effective in correcting the responsible lesion, as documented by arteriography, more than 2–5 years later. If the failing graft is a vein bypass, detection of the failing state permits accurate localization and definition of the responsible lesion by arteriography as well as salvage of any undiseased vein. In contrast, if the graft is allowed to thrombose, the responsible lesion may be difficult to identify, the vein may be difficult or impossible to thrombectomize, and the patient's best graft, the ipsilateral greater saphenous vein, may have to be sacrificed, rendering the secondary operation even more difficult and more likely to fail with associated limb loss. Most importantly, the results of reinterventions for failing grafts, in terms of both continued cumulative patency and limb salvage rates, have been far superior to the results of reinterventions for grafts that have thrombosed and failed.[71–75] The inflow and outflow arterial lesions responsible for the failing state of PTFE grafts can be treated with PTA when they are short occlusions (3–5 cm) or stenoses. Longer or more complex lesions require a graft extension to above or below the responsible lesion.

The improved results associated with reintervention for failing grafts mandate that surgeons performing bypass operations follow their patients closely during the postoperative period and indefinitely thereafter. Ideally, noninvasive laboratory tests, including duplex studies, should be performed with similar frequency.[72–74] If the patient has any recurrence of symptoms or if the surgeon detects any change in peripheral pulse examination or other manifestations of ischemia, the circulatory deterioration must be confirmed by noninvasive parameters and urgent arteriography.

## Conclusions

Functional status is maintained by performing lower extremity bypass in elderly patients with threatened limbs. In a study from Oregon, approximately 95% of patients maintained their preoperative life style after an arterial bypass was performed for limb salvage.[75] Elderly patients are not good candidates for extensive rehabilitation; therefore, following a major amputation they do not ambulate well and often lose their independence.

The dollar cost of an aggressive approach to salvage limbs is high, with a mean cost of $19,000 for femoropopliteal bypass and $29,000 for small-vessel bypass. These figures include all physician, hospital, and rehabilitation costs, including reoperations. On the other hand, the mean total cost of below-knee amputation, which in 26% of our patients resulted in failed rehabilitation with a need for chronic institutional care or professional assistance at home, was $27,000. Thus limb salvage surgery is expensive but no more so than the less attractive alternative of amputation.[76,77]

With the increasing age of our population the number of elderly individuals who present with significant aortoiliac or infrainguinal occlusive disease will also increase. The types of interventions employed to treat these elderly patients' disease process should be tailored to their age and medical condition. The increasing utilization of interventional techniques such as angioplasty with stents and endoluminal stented grafts should allow treatment of the elderly patient while minimizing interventional morbibity and mortality.

## References


1. Cronenwett JL, Davis JR Jr, Gooch JB, et al. Aortoiliac occlusive disease in women. Surgery 1980;88:775–784.
2. Veith FJ, Gupta SK, Wengerter KR, et al. Changing atherosclerotic disease patterns and management strategies in lower-limb threatening ischemia. Ann Surg 1990;212: 402–414.
3. Ascer E, Veith FJ, Gupta SK. Bypasses to plantar arteries and other tibial branches. J Vasc Surg 1988;8:434–441.
4. Moneta GL, Yeager RA, Taylor LM Jr, et al. Hemodynamic assessment of combined aortoiliac/femoropopliteal occlusive disease and selection of single or multilevel revascularization. Semin Vasc Surg 1994;7:3–10.
5. Baker JD, Dix D. Variability of Doppler ankle pressures with arterial occlusive disease: an evaluation of ankle index and brachial-ankle pressure gradient. Surgery 1976;79:134–137.
6. Kohler TR, Nance DR, Cramer MM, et al. Duplex scanning for diagnosis of aortoiliac and femoropopliteal disease: a prospective study. Circulation 1987;76:1074–1080.
7. Langsfeld M, Nupute J, Hershey FB, et al. The use of deep duplex scanning to predict hemodynamically significant aortoiliac stenoses. J Vasc Surg 1988;7:395–399.
8. Moneta GL, Yeager RA, Antonovic R, et al. Accuracy of lower extremity arterial duplex mapping. J Vasc Surg 1992; 15:275–284.
9. Legemate DA, Teeuwen C, Hoenveld H, et al. Value of duplex scanning compared with angiography and pressure measurement in the assessment of aortoiliac lesions. Br J Surg 1991;78:1003–1008.
10. Owens RS, Carpenter JP, Baum RA, et al. Magnetic resonance imaging of angiographically occult runoff vessels in peripheral arterial occlusive disease. N Engl J Med 1992; 326:1577–1581.
11. Carpenter JP, Owens RS, Baum RA, et al. Magnetic resonance angiography of peripheral runoff vessels. J Vasc Surg 1992;16:807–815.
12. Carpenter JP, Owens RS, Holland GA, et al. Magnetic resonance angiography of the aorta, iliac, and femoral arteries. Surgery 1994;116:17–23.
13. Arlart IP, Guhl L, Edleman RR. Magnetic resonance angiography of the abdominal aorta. Cardiovasc Intervent Radiol 1992;15:43.
14. Brewster DC, Waltman AC, O'Hara PJ, et al. Femoral artery pressure measurement during aortography. Circulation 60:120–124.
15. Hessel SJ, Adams DF, Abrams HL. Complications of angiography. Radiology 1981;138:273–281.
16. Gomes AS, Baker JD, Martin-Paredero V, et al. Acute renal dysfunction after major arteriography. AJR 1985;145:1249–1253.
17. Martin-Paredero V, Dixon SM, Baker JD, et al. Risk of renal failure after major angiography. Arch Surg 1983;118:1417–1420.
18. Nikonoff T, Skau T, Berglund J, et al. Effects of femoral arteriography and low osmolar contrast agents on renal function. Acta Radiol 1993;34:88–91.
19. Katholi RE, Taylor GJ, Woods WT, et al. Nephrotoxicity of nonionic low-osmolality versus ionic high-osmolality contrast media: a prospective double-blind randomized comparison in human beings. Radiology 1993;186:183–187.
20. Lautin EM, Freeman NJ, Schoenfeld AH, et al. Radiocontrast-associated renal dysfunction: a comparison of lower-osmolality and conventional high-osmolality contrast media. AJR 1991;157:59–65.
21. Hall KA, Wong RW, Hunger GC, et al. Contrast-induced nephrotoxicity: the effects of vasodilator therapy. J Surg Res 1992;53:317–320.
22. Johnston KW, Rae M, Hogg-Johnston SA, et al. 5-Year results of a prospective study of percutaneous transluminal angioplasty. Ann Surg 1987;206:403.
23. Ravimandalam K, Rao VRK, Kumar S, et al. Obstruction of the infrarenal portion of the abdominal aorta: results of treatment with balloon angioplasty. AJR 1991;156:1257–1262.
24. Odunry A, Colapinto RF, Sniderman KW, et al. Percutaneous transluminal angioplasty of abdominal aortic stenoses. Cardiovasc Intervent Radiol 1989;12:1–6.
25. Yakes WF, Kumpe DA, Brown SB, et al. Percutaneous transluminal aortic angioplasty: techniques and results. Radiology 1989;172:965–970.
26. Marin ML, Veith FJ, Cynamon J, et al. Transfemoral endovascular stented graft treatment of aortoiliac and femoropopliteal occlusive disease for limb salvage. Am J Surg 1994;168:156–162.
27. Becker GJ, Katzen BT, Dake MD. Noncoronary angioplasty. Radiology 1989;170:403–412.
28. Gallino A, Mahler F, Probst P, et al. Percutaneous transluminal angioplasty of the arteries of the lower limbs: a 5-year follow-up. Circulation 1984;70:619–623.

29. Spence RK, Freiman DB, Gatenby R, et al. Long-term results of transluminal angioplasty of the iliac and femoral arteries. Arch Surg 1981;116:1377–1386.
30. Stokes KR, Strunk HM, Campbell DR, et al. Five-year results of iliac and femoropopliteal angioplasty in diabetic patients. Radiology 1990;174:977–982.
31. Palmaz JC, Garcia OJ, Schatz RA, et al. Placement of balloon-expandable intraluminal stents in iliac arteries: first 171 procedures. Radiology 1990;174:969–975.
32. Richter GM, Roeren T, Brado M, et al. Further update of the randomized trial: iliac stent placement versus PTA-morphology, clinical success rates, and failure analysis. J Vasc Interv Radiol 1993;4:30.
33. Liermann D, Strecker EP, Peters J. The Strecker stent: indications and results in iliac and femoropopliteal arteries. Cardiovasc Intervent Radiol 1992;15:298.
34. Palmaz JC, Laborde JC, Rivera FJ, et al. Stenting of the iliac arteries with the Palmaz stent: experience from a multicenter trial. Cardiovasc Intervent Radiol 1992;15:291–297.
35. Hausegger KA, Cragg AH, Lammer J, et al. Iliac artery stent placement: clinical experience with a Nitinol stent. Radiology 1994;190:199–202.
36. Vorwerk D, Gunther RW. Stent placement in iliac arterial lesions: three years of clinical experience with the Wallstent. Cardiovasc Intervent Radiol 1992;15:285–290.
37. Vorwerk D, Gunther RW. Chronic iliac artery occlusion. Presented at the International Congress, University of Heidelberg, Zermatt, April 1993.
38. Blair JM, Gewertz BL, Mossa H, et al. Percutaneous transluminal angioplasty versus surgery for limb-threatening ischemia. J Vasc Surg 1989;9:698–703.
39. Becker GJ, Katzen BT, Dake MK. Noncoronary angioplasty. Radiology 1989;170:921–940.
40. Wilson SE, Wolf GL, Cross AP. Percutaneous transluminal angioplasty versus operation for peripheral arteriosclerosis. J Vasc Surg 1989;9:1–9.
41. Murray RR, Hewes RC, White RI, et al. Long-segment femoropopliteal stenosis: is angioplasty a boon or a bust? Radiology 1987;162:473–476.
42. Hunink MM, Wong JB, Donaldson MC, et al. Patency results of percutaneous and surgical revascularization for femoropoplitealerial arterial disease. Med Decis Making 1994;14: 17–81.
43. Treiman GS, Treiman RL, Ichikawa L, et al. Should percutaneous transluminal angioplasty be recommended for treatment of infrageniculate popliteal artery or tibioperoneal trunk stenosis? J Vasc Surg 1995;22:457–465.
44. London NJ, Varty K, Sayers RD, et al. Percutaneous transluminal angioplasty for lower-limb critical ischaemia. Br J Surg 1995;82:1232–1235.
45. Currie IC, Wakeley CJ, Cole SEA, et al. Femoropopliteal angioplasty for severe limb ischaemia. Br J Surg 1994;81: 191–193.
46. Stanley B, Teague B, Raptis S, et al. Efficacy of balloon angioplasty of the superficial femoral artery and popliteal artery in the relief of leg ischemia. J Vasc Surg 1994;23:679–685.
47. Brewster DC, Darling RC. Optimal methods of aortoiliac reconstruction. Surgery 1978;84:739–748.
48. Piotrowski JJ, Pearce WH, Jones DN, et al. Aortobifemoral bypass: the operation of choice for unilateral iliac occlusion? J Vasc Surg 1988;8:211–218.
49. Schneider JR, Besso SR, Walsh DB, et al. Femorofemoral versus aortobifemoral bypass: outcome and hemodynamic results. J Vasc Surg 1994;19:43–57.
50. Passman MA, Taylor LM Jr, Moneta GL, et al. Comparison of axillofemoral and aortofemoral bypass for aortoiliac occlusive disease. J Vasc Surg 1996;23:263–271.
51. Hanafy M, McLoughlin GA. Comparison of iliofemoral and femorofemoral crossover bypass in the treatment of unilateral iliac arterial occlusive disease. Br J Surg 1991;78:1001–1002.
52. Harrington ME, Harrington EB, Haimov M, et al. Iliofemoral versus femorofemoral bypass: the case for an individualized approach. J Vasc Surg 1992;16:841–842.
53. Farber MA, Hollier LH, Eubanks R, et al. Femorofemoral bypass: a profile of graft failure. South Med J 1990;83: 1437–1443.
54. Nolan KD, Benjamin ME, Murphy TJ, et al. Femorofemoral bypass for aortofemoral graft limb occlusion: a ten-year experience. J Vasc Surg 1994;19:851–857.
55. Kenney DA, Sauvage LR, Wood SJ, et al. Comparison of noncrimped, externally supported (EXS) and crimped, nonsupported Dacron prostheses for axillofemoral and above-knee femoropopliteal bypass. Surgery 1982;92:931–946.
56. El-Massry S, Saad E, Sauvage LR, et al. Axillofemoral bypass with externally supported, knitted Dacron grafts: a follow-up through twelve years. J Vasc Surg 1993;17:107–115.
57. Taylor LM Jr, Moneta GL, McConnell DB, et al. Axillofemoral grafting with externally supported polytetrafluoroethylene. Arch Surg 1994;129:588–595.
58. Harrington ME, Harrington, EB, Haimov M, et al. Axillofemoral bypass: compromised bypass for compromised patients. J Vasc Surg 1994;20:195–201.
59. Martin EC. Percutaneous therapy in the management of aortoiliac disease. Semin Vasc Surg 1994;7:17.
60. Tegtmeyer CJ, Hartwell GD, Selby JB, et al. Results and complications of angioplasty in aortoiliac disease. Circulation 1991;83(suppl I):53–60.
61. Johnston KW. Iliac arteries: reanalysis of results of balloon angioplasty. Radiology 1993;186:207–212.
62. Marin ML, Veith FJ, Sanchez LA, et al. Endovascular aortoiliac grafts in combination with standard infrainguinal arterial bypasses in the management of limb-threatening ischemia: preliminary report. J Vasc Surg 1995;22:316–325.
63. Veith FJ, Gupta SK, Daly V. Femoropopliteal bypass to the isolated popliteal segment: is polytetrafluoroethylene graft acceptable? Surgery 1981;89:296.
64. Kram HB, Gupta SK, Veith FJ, et al. Late results of 217 femoropopliteal bypasses to isolated popliteal segments. J Vasc Surg 1991;14:386.
65. Flinn WR, Flanigan DP, Verta MJ, et al. Sequential femoroal-tibial bypass for severe limb ischemia. Surgery 1980;88: 357.
66. Veith FJ, Ascer E, Gupta SK. Tibiotibial vein bypass grafts: a new operation for limb salvage. J Vasc Surg 1995;2: 552.
67. Ascer E, Veith FJ, Gupta SK. Bypasses to plantar arteries and other tibial branches: an extended approach to limb salvage. J Surg 1988;8:434.

68. Harrington EB, Harrington ME, Schanzer H, et al. The dorsalis pedis bypass: moderate success in difficult situations. J Vasc Surg 1992;15:409.
69. Schneider JR, Walsh DB, McDaniel MD, et al. Pedal bypass versus tibial bypass with autogenous vein: a comparison of outcome and hemodynamic results. J Vasc Surg 1993;17: 1029.
70. O'Mara CS, Flinn WR, Johnson ND, et al. Recognition and surgical management of patent but hemodynamically failed arterial grafts. Ann Surg 1981;193:467.
71. Veith FJ, Weiser RK, Gupta SK, et al. Diagnosis and management of failing lower extremity arterial reconstructions. J Cardiovasc Surg 1984;25:381.
72. Sanchez L, Gupta SK, Veith FJ, et al. A ten-year experience with one hundred fifty failing or threatened vein and polytetrafluoroethylene arterial bypass grafts. J Surg 1991; 14:729.
73. Sanchez LA, Suggs WD, Veith FJ, et al. Is surveillance to detect failing polytetrafluoroethylene bypasses worthwhile? Twelve-year experience with ninety-one grafts. J Vasc Surg 1993;18:981.
74. Bandyk DF, Bergamini TM, Towne JB, et al. Durability of vein graft revision: the outcome of secondary procedures. J Vasc Surg 1991;13:200.
75. Abou-Zamzam AM Jr, Lee RW, Moneta GL, Taylor LM, Porter JM. Functional outcome after infrainguinal bypass for limb salvage. J Vasc Surg 1997;25:287–297.
76. Gupta SK, Veith FJ, Ascer E, et al. Cost factors in limb-threatening ischemia due to infraingual arteriosclerosis. Eur J Vasc Surg 1988;2:151.
77. Gupta SK, Veith FJ. Inadequacy of diagnosis related group (DRG) reimbursements for limb salvage lower extremity arterial reconstructions. J Vasc Surg 1990;11: 348.

# 34
# Natural History and Treatment of Aneurysms

Jeffrey M. Reilly and Gregorio A. Sicard

Abdominal aortic aneurysms (AAAs) are principally a disease of the elderly. Until the middle of the twentieth century, AAAs were lethal unless some other disease process killed the patient first. Their anatomic location and the physiologic and technical challenges aortic surgery presented to both surgeon and patient, prevented their direct repair. However, several ingenious but uniformly unsuccessful indirect methods of preventing aneurysm rupture were tried including intraluminal thrombosis, wrapping the aneurysm with cellophane, or injecting sclerosants around the aneurysm wall.[1] In 1951 in France, Dubost et al. successfully repaired an AAA via a left retroperitoneal approach with excision of the aneurysm and homograft replacement of the infrarenal aorta.[2] Subsequent refinements of the endoaneurysmorrhaphy technique by Creech and DeBakey, coupled with the development of durable prosthetic grafts, ushered in the modern era of aneurysm surgery.[3] During this early period elective aneurysm repair was accompanied by significant morbidity and mortality, but evolutionary improvements in preoperative evaluation, surgical and anesthetic techniques, and perioperative management have changed this situation, with major centers reporting an operative mortality of 5% or less for elective AAA repair, despite the high incidence of medical comorbidities in this elderly patient population.[4]

## Incidence and Epidemiology

Aneurysms can occur anywhere along the length of the aorta, but approximately 80% involve only the infrarenal aorta.[5] AAAs are a relatively common disease of the elderly, with a reported incidence of 1.8–6.6% in several autopsy series.[6–8] The incidence increases after the age of 55 in men and after the age of 70 in women.[8] There is also an increasing incidence of AAAs with reports from the United States, Great Britain, and Australia all documenting an increasing incidence of AAAs over the past several decades.[8–12] A portion of this increase has been attributed to improved detection of AAAs secondary to the widespread use of B-mode ultrasonography, computed tomography (CT), and magnetic resonance imaging (MRI) for general diagnostic purposes and to the general aging of the population. However, age-specific mortality rates and age-specific aneurysm rupture rates have increased, indicating a true increase in the incidence.[11–14] Curiously, this increase has occurred simultaneously with a steadily decreasing mortality rate from stroke and cardiac disease in the same population.[15]

The epidemiology of AAA is characterized by a large male preponderance of patients in both clinical and autopsy series with a male/female ratio between 3:1 and 8:1.[6,7,14,16–22] The most recent series show that the incidence in women begins to approach that of men after the seventh decade of life.[8,23] The male preponderance is due principally to a preponderance of white men, with the incidence of AAAs in black men, black women, and white women all being approximately one-third the incidence in white men.[24,25]

Traditional teaching states that AAAs are a manifestation of atherosclerosis. Those who develop AAAs tend to have many risk factors for atherosclerosis and to have clinically significant atherosclerosis in other arterial beds.[26] The atherogenic risk factors of hypertension, cigarette smoking, and hypercholesterolemia are widely prevalent in patients with AAAs.[26–29] Despite this fact, only a small fraction of patients with aortic atherosclerosis develop aneurysms.[30] This dichotomy has yet to be explained and is currently an area of active research.

Aside from being an elderly Caucasian man, the strongest risk factors for the development of AAAs, are smoking and hypertension. In a large prospective, longitudinal study begun during the 1950s, the development of AAAs was strongly correlated with smoking, hypertension, or both.[29] In a later study, the same conclusions were drawn by Cronenwett and colleagues.[26] In autopsy series, the reported incidence of hypertension in the AAA population ranges between 38% and 50%.[6,7] One series of unruptured aneurysms reported a 60% incidence of hypertension.[26] In another series, patients with both hypertension and smoking incurred a cumulative rupture rate of 72%,[31] and a separate large autopsy study strongly correlated the risk of rupture with hypertension ($p < 0.001$).[32] Smoking is widely prevalent among patients with AAAs. In a recent large surgical series, the incidence of smoking in patients undergoing elective AAA repair was about 85%.[20] More recently, the Aneurysm Detection and Management (ADAM) study group documented that smoking was the risk factor most strongly associated with the development of AAAs (odds ratio 5.57), and smoking was calculated to account for 78% of all AAAs larger than 4.0 cm.[33] There are, however, patients who neither smoke nor have hypertension who develop aneurysms. Additionally, there is well-documented familial clustering of AAAs.[34] These data illustrate the multifactorial nature and possible heterogeneity of the etiology of AAAs.

Atherosclerosis is widely prevalent in patients with AAA, which is not unexpected given the relatively advanced age of this patient population. Clinically significant coronary artery disease is present in 33–68% of patents,[26,28] and cerebrovascular disease is present in 20%.[26] A full one-fourth of patients with AAAs have symptomatic lower extremity occlusive disease,[20] and ultrasound screening studies have documented an increased incidence of AAAs in patients with lower-extremity atherosclerotic occlusive disease.[35,36] An objective review of the data suggests that AAAs are strongly associated with atherosclerosis; and that if atherosclerosis is not the etiologic factor, it is at least a permissive factor in the development of AAAs.[37]

## Pathophysiology

Although AAAs are traditionally thought to be a manifestation of atherosclerosis, their etiology is unclear. The risk factors for atherosclerosis are highly prevalent in patients who develop AAAs,[26–29] but it has become clear that this disease entity has its own specific genetic environmental and biochemical determinants.[38] The hallmark pathophysiologic feature of AAA disease is destruction of the elastin matrix of the media of the aorta,[39,40] resulting in vessel dilatation and elongation. Microscopic examination of aneurysmal aortic tissue reveals complete fragmentation of the medial elastic lamellae. Biochemical analysis confirms the same finding; that is, there is a depletion of normal aortic elastin,[41] in contradistinction to what is normally found in occlusive atherosclerotic lesions. With occlusive disease the media is largely preserved, although there are sometimes penetrating ulcers, which result in focal disruption of the elastic matrix of the media. The finding of depleted elastin within aneurysms is a global finding. Currently, the central question driving aneurysm research is the cause of this elastin destruction and medial thinning.

Another characteristic feature of AAAs is an intense inflammatory infiltrate associated with the aortic wall. Unlike the inflammation associated with atherosclerotic plaques within the intima, this inflammatory infiltrate originates from the adventitial side of the artery, not the luminal side.[40] It has the characteristics of a chronic inflammatory infiltrate with mononuclear cells, consisting principally of T and B lymphocytes, plasma cells, and macrophages.[42] It is widely believed by investigators in the field that this inflammatory process is involved in the destruction of the media, although the inciting factor for this inflammatory response is not known.

Among the inflammatory cells, the macrophage is thought to play a pivotal role in AAA pathogenesis. Macrophages are capable of elaborating a variety of enzymes that are involved in normal tissue remodeling, as well as in pathologic states. Studies have demonstrated that macrophages associated with AAAs produce a variety of matrix metalloproteases capable of degrading the aortic wall[43–46] and urokinase-type plasminogen activator,[47] which synergistically enhances the ability of macrophages to destroy extracellular matrix.[48] It is becoming more widely accepted that the macrophages are driving the destruction of the aortic wall in aneurysm disease.

As previously stated, the inciting cause of the inflammation is unknown. It is most likely perpetuated by the inflammatory response, which generates a positive feedback cycle. Elastin degradation products are known to be chemotactic for other inflammatory cells.[49] Therefore once the elastin destruction has begun, it creates a positive feedback loop leading to more inflammation and more elastin destruction. Currently the inciting event leading to this inflammatory response is not known. It may be an immunologic phenotype that results in a specific patterned response to an injury to the aortic wall. It is unclear whether this is an injury caused by atherosclerosis or perhaps another injury related to hypertension or cigarette smoking, both of which are widely prevalent in the patient population with AAAs. This is obviously an area of ongoing research.

## Natural History

Estes reported in 1950 that the 1-year mortality in patients with large AAAs was high (33%), and that approximately two-thirds of the deaths were secondary to aortic rupture.[50] Other studies from this period noted a similar natural history with extremely poor 5-year survival in patients with AAA.[51,52] The inclusion of a significant number of patients with large or symptomatic aneurysms and a significant number of patients unfit for surgery biased these studies, and as a result they likely overestimated the true mortality associated with all AAAs: small and asymptomatic aneurysms were mostly excluded. Despite these facts, DeBakey and colleagues reported a 58% five-year survival in patients undergoing AAA repair (including a 9% perioperative mortality rate), suggesting that operative management was a means of improving survival of patients with AAAs.[53] The landmark study of Szilagyi and associates in 1966, clearly established the efficacy of AAA repair in terms of improving long-term patient survival.[54] This retrospective study compared the survival of patients who were not unfit for surgery but did not undergo AAA repair to those patients with similar characteristics who underwent aneurysm repair. It documented that the risk of rupture and long-term survival were directly correlated to aneurysm diameter. AAAs were categorized as being large (>6 cm diameter) or small (<6 cm diameter). The 5-year survival of untreated patients with small AAAs was 47.8% compared to 6% for patients with large AAAs. The cumulative 5-year risk of rupture was 20% for small AAAs and 43% for large AAAs. AAA rupture accounted for 33% of all deaths in patients not undergoing aneurysm repair, with coronary artery disease being the next most common cause. More importantly, patients who had a successful AAA repair appeared to have a long-term survival comparable to that of age-matched controls. A contemporary report of a small series of patients with AAAs by Foster and colleagues, essentially confirmed these findings.[31] Although these studies were imperfect because they lacked precise methods to determine aneurysm size and were retrospectively performed, their general conclusions have proven accurate except for the effect of successful repair on long-term survival. A more recent study once again documented the poor outcome of patients who do not have their aneurysms repaired. Englund and associates reported on 101 patients who were considered to have prohibitive surgical risks. In this group the 5-year survival of patients with AAAs ≤ 5.0 cm was 42% compared to 25% in patients with AAAs > 5 cm; 30% of deaths were secondary to ruptured AAAs.[55]

Although successful aneurysmorrhaphy clearly prolongs the survival of patients with AAAs, their long-term survival is still not as good as that of age-matched controls. Their 5- and 10-year survival is significantly less than that of an age-matched cohort. The 5-year survival was 60% for those with AAAs compared to 79% for those without an AAA[56]; similarly, their 10-year survival was 38% compared to 52% for the controls.[57] The principal cause of this late excess mortality in patients with AAAs is cardiac disease.[55–57]

It is now clear that aneurysm size correlates with the risk of aneurysm rupture. This has been borne out in the above-mentioned clinical series and in autopsy studies. Darling and colleagues reported that at the time of autopsy 10% of aneurysms <4.0 cm were ruptured and were the cause of death compared to 46% of aneurysms 7.1–10.1 cm.[30] Rupture rates of 5% for AAAs <5 cm in diameter, 39% for AAAs 5.1–6.9 cm, and 65% for those ≥7 cm were reported in an autopsy series involving 297 patients.[58]

The conclusions of these two studies are correct: that aneurysm size correlates with risk of rupture. However, each of these studies has been criticized for overestimating the risk of small aneurysm rupture for two reasons. The first is that the aortic diameters were determined postmortem and not under physiologic blood pressure; and accordingly, the measurements reported are likely too small. The second reason is that patients who die suddenly from rupture of an unsusupected aneurysm are more likely to come to autopsy than those who die of known causes. Therefore ruptured aneurysms are disproportionately represented in autopsy series. Determining the risk of rupture is of critical importance because the decision to recommend surgical repair is based on a risk/benefit ratio. If the risk of rupture of a small AAA is lower than the predicted mortality from surgery, it would be safest to manage it expectantly. Conversely, if the risk of rupture is high, surgical repair is warranted.

Two population-based studies have supported the contention that the risk of small aneurysm rupture is overestimated by the above-mentioned autopsy series. Both Nevitt and colleagues[59] at the Mayo Clinic and Gilmaker and colleagues[56] reported low rupture rates for aneurysms <5.0 cm. However, just as the autopsy studies were flawed, these too have been criticized as underestimating the risk of small aneurysm rupture. The conclusions based on the Mayo Clinic study have been questioned because 24% of the patients underwent elective AAA repair (i.e., their risk of rupture was eliminated).[55,59] Additionally, one would assume that the AAAs that were repaired were done so for a reason (i.e., the risk of rupture must have been perceived as increasing). The net result is that nearly one-fourth of the patients in the study were removed from analysis; and once again, one assumes that this group comprised the patients at highest risk for rupture. Similar criticisms apply to the study of Gilmaker and colleagues.[56] The true incidence of rupture of small aneurysms has been difficult to ascertain but is probably better estimated by the study of Gjuirguis and Barker.[57] In this series only 6% of 300 patients with small aneurysms underwent elective surgical repair, and the incidence of rupture of small (<5.0 cm) AAAs was 2% over the course of the study.

Several studies have attempted to manage small aneurysms selectively. In general, these studies have included a large proportion of patients who were considered high surgical risks; therefore their mortality related to their other co-morbidities is higher than in the general patient population with AAAs. These studies utilized a threshold value of 5 or 6 cm for recommending elective surgical repair. During an average follow-up of 42 months, approximately 40% of patients required elective intervention, and 2% required urgent or emergent intervention; 28% of patients survived without surgery, and the remainder died from other causes. Overall, the mortality was not significantly different from that for patients who were operated on the basis of aneurysm size alone.[60–64] A recent, prospective study of 142 patients with small (<4.0 cm) aneurysms was reported from the United Kingdom. Over the 9-year study period, 23 patients underwent elective repair, and only one patient (who had refused surgery) died of a ruptured aneurysm.[60] It is noteworthy that in the series of Cronenwett et al.[64] and Littoy et al.[61] the risk of rupture or need for surgical intervention correlated with the size of the aneurysm and the age of the patient at the time of initial presentation, with large AAAs and young patients being much more likely to require surgery.

Despite the data supporting the concept of "watchful waiting," the management of patients with small aneurysms remains controversial. One study that utilized a computer model to evaluate various clinical scenarios concluded that early intervention is better than expectant management.[65] Support for this position is provided by a prospective study reported by Brown et al.[63] A series of 492 patients with AAAs < 5.0 cm were followed prospectively. For patients who were deemed good surgical risks, elective repair was recommended when the AAA exceeded 5.0 cm. If the patient was a poor risk, the AAA was managed expectantly. In this study, AAAs of 4.5–4.9 cm expanded the most rapidly with an average rate of 0.7 cm/year. Additionally, in unfit patients with AAAs > 5.0 cm ($n$ = 176), 10 ruptures occurred, with 6 of them in patients with AAAs 5.0–5.6 cm in diameter. On the strength of these data the authors strongly advocated elective repair of AAAs > 4.5 cm, citing both the relatively rapid expansion rate of AAAs in the 4.5–4.9 cm range and the significant risk of rupture of AAAs 5.0–5.6 cm in diameter.[63] Presently, the management of small aneurysms remains unresolved. Sound arguments supported by numerous studies can be made for early surgery or for expectant management. Obviously, the decision to repair an aneurysm must be individualized, taking into account the size of the AAA, the risk factors for rupture, the medical co-morbidities of the patient, and the predicted operative mortality for elective repair.

The optimal management of patients with AAAs would require that one be able to identify those aneurysms at risk for rupture. An oversimplification, and what passes for common knowledge, is that the natural history of aneurysms is one of continued expansion until rupture. The only way for the unfortunate patient with an AAA to avoid this fate is to die of something else first or to undergo a successful aneurysm repair.[30] A review of the available data does not support this position. Reported aneurysm expansion rates range on average from 0.2 to 0.8 cm/year,[32,61,63,66,67] and the generally accepted rate of expansion is approximately 0.4 cm/year.

TABLE 34.1. Actuarial Risk of Rupture of AAAs Based on Their Size

| Aneurysm size (cm) | 5-Year risk of rupture (%) |
|---|---|
| <5.0 | 2[a] |
| 5.0–5.9 | 25 |
| 6.0–6.9 | 35 |
| ≥7.0 | 75 |

*Source:* Data from Darling et al.,[30] Foster et al.,[31] Brown et al.,[63] and Collin et al.[66]

[a] As mentioned in the text, the natural history of small aneurysms is not well defined.

In some, but not all, series two risk factors associated with accelerated expansion and rupture are hypertension and severe chronic obstructive pulmonary disease.[26,32,64–69] Chang and colleagues used multivariate analysis to evaluate the risk factors associated with rapid growth of small AAAs.[70] Risk factors that were statistically significant included advanced age, severe cardiac disease, previous stroke, and a history of cigarette smoking. The incidence of rapid expansion was also noted to be higher in young patients who presented with AAAs > 4.0 cm in diameter.[70] Unfortunately, the expansion of an AAA is neither constant nor predictable. AAAs can expand irregularly, with long periods of stability followed by periods of rapid expansion. Large aneurysms can remain stable for extended periods, and small aneurysms can rupture. Despite the numerous studies that have attempted to define the determinants of aneurysm rupture, aneurysm size at the time of presentation remains the single best predictor of the risk of rupture. The risk of rupture is depicted in Table 34.1.

## Clinical Presentation

The most common presentation of an AAA is as an incidental finding by the patient or by the physician on physical examination, diagnostic imaging study, or in the operating room at time of laparotomy for another reason. The most feared and dramatic presentation of an AAA is rupture. Free rupture into the peritoneal cavity is almost uniformly fatal, with patients presenting with sudden hemodynamic collapse and death within minutes from exsanguinating hemorrhage. Fortunately, AAAs more commonly rupture into the retroperitoneum, and the rupture is usually contained initially. This situation represents the "leaking" aneurysm. Patients present with symptoms related to impingement of the hematoma on adjacent retroperitoneal structures. These symptoms may include abdominal, back, or flank pain. The abdominal pain is often diffuse and cannot be well localized by the patient; but on physical examination, the aneurysm itself is often tender. Back pain is most often related to the pressure of the contained hematoma or occasionally to erosion of the aneurysm into an adjacent lumbar vertebral body.[71] Similarly, flank pain is secondary to pressure from the hematoma, and it often also radiates to the left groin, most likely secondary to pressure on the left ureter. It must be emphasized that an aneurysm can be ruptured without signs of hemodynamic instability. This fact is sometimes overlooked, and the patient who presents to the emergency room with back or flank pain is discharged with a diagnosis of a musculoskeletal problem only to return in hemorrhagic shock secondary to a ruptured AAA. A leaking aneurysm must always be a part of the differential diagnosis of back pain and should be excluded by physical examination or an appropriate diagnostic test before the patient is discharged with a diagnosis of muscloskeletal pain.

Aneurysms may also be symptomatic without being ruptured. AAAs may present as vague abdominal pain, and on physical examination there is tenderness over the aneurysm. In this setting a CT scan shows an intact aneurysm but may also show signs of recent expansion as well. In particular, the crescent sign, which is enhancement within the mural thrombus representing fresh blood, is thought to represent recent expansion and is considered an indicator of impending aneurysm rupture.[72] Any patient with a symptomatic aneurysm should undergo urgent repair (i.e., within 24 hours of presentation).

Aneurysms do not necessarily rupture into the peritoneum or retroperitoneum; they can also rupture into the vena cava or the duodenum. An aortocaval fistula results from erosion of the aneurysm into the adjacent vena cava with secondary rupture. The typical presentation is high-output (forward) congestive heart failure in association with venous hypertension, lower extremity swelling, a widened pulse pressure, and a continuous (machine-like) abdominal bruit. Erosion of the anterior wall of the aneurysm into the third portion of the duodenum followed by aneurysm rupture results in an aortoduodenal fistula. The usual presentation of a primary aortoduodenal fistula is a small, or sentinel, episode of upper gastrointestinal (GI) bleeding followed by massive, exsanguinating GI hemorrhage. The initial bleed is secondary to the mucosal injury caused by erosion of the aneurysm into the duodenum, and the exsanguinating hemorrhage occurs when the aneurysm ruptures. It is imperative that this diagnosis be confirmed or excluded in any patient with an AAA who presents with GI bleeding. Misdiagnosis is uniformly fatal. The appropriate treatment is emergent aneurysm repair with vigorous volume resuscitation.

Aneurysms can produce symptoms not due to rupture or impending rupture. Large aneurysms can cause partial obstruction of the third portion of the duodenum. Patients present with symptoms of a high partial small bowel obstruction. This presentation is distinctly unusual. The diagnosis can be made by an upper GI series, which demonstrates extrinsic compression of the third portion of the duodenum by the aneurysm. Similarly, CT scanning with oral contrast can provide the same information and has the additional benefit of defining the extent of the aneurysm.

Inflammatory aneurysms, which are a well-recognized variant of AAAs, also produce symptoms in approximately two-thirds of patients. These aneurysms are characterized by an intense desmoplastic reaction around the infrarenal aorta that involves adjacent structures. These aneurysms produce both local and systemic symptoms.[73] The most frequent presenting symptom is vague abdominal or back pain. Additional symptoms may include weight loss, malaise, and anorexia. The erythrocyte sedimentation rate (ESR) is elevated in nearly three-fourths of patients with this entity. The occurrence of weight loss and abdominal or back pain in a patient with an AAA suggests that an inflammatory aneurysm is present, and evaluation of the patient should proceed accordingly. Additionally, the desmoplastic reaction associated with an inflammatory AAA usually involves adjacent retroperitoneal structures including, in order of frequency, the duodenum (90%), inferior vena cava and left renal vein (50%), and ureters (25%). Ureteral involvement can result in ureteral colic.[73]

Although rupture is the most feared presentation, AAAs can also present with thromboembolic symptoms. Most AAAs are lined with laminated mural thrombus, which can embolize distally, resulting in lower extremity embolization. For this reason, AAA is always included in the differential diagnosis of emboli to the lower extremities. Thrombosis is more often associated with peripheral aneurysms, but AAAs can also thrombose, although they rarely do so.

## Preoperative Evaluation

Because cardiac complications are the most common cause of postoperative mortality, ideally patients at risk are identified preoperatively. Any potentially reversible or correctable cardiac problems are then addressed. Some of the best data on preoperative cardiac evaluation of patients undergoing abdominal aortic aneurysm repair comes from the Cleveland Clinic. Hertzer et al. reported on coronary angiography in 1000 consecutive patients undergoing vascular surgical procedures, including 263 patients with AAAs.[73] Findings in the patients with AAAs were that 6% of the patients had normal coronary arteries, 29% had mild to moderate coronary artery disease, 29% had advanced but compensated coronary artery disease, 31% had severe uncorrectable coronary artery disease, and 5% had inoperable coronary artery disease. The goal of their study was to identify patients with severe but correctable coronary artery disease, and fully

35% of patients with suspected coronary artery disease had severe but correctable disease. Surprisingly, another 12–15% of patients with no clinical suggestion of coronary artery disease had angiographically demonstrable severe correctable coronary artery lesions. Other risk factors such as age, hypertension, and diabetes, did not influence the incidence of severe correctable coronary artery disease. In their study a significant number of patients without clinical evidence of cardiac disease by history and physical examination, electrocardiography, and standard preoperative evaluation had significant, correctable, coronary artery disease that potentially threatened their perioperative survival. It was also suggested by the study that even if the patients survived AAA repair without cardiac complications their long-term survival was reduced. For this reason, coronary revascularization prior to AAA repair is recommended. At follow-up the actuarial 5-year survival for patients who underwent coronary revascularization demonstrated a significant improvement in the long-term survival [86.2% coronary artery bypass graft (CABG) patients vs. 63.5% without CABG, $p < 0.0001$]. Although this study is more than a decade old, the findings of this report are still important. Specifically, there is a high incidence of subclinical coronary artery disease in patients with AAAs, and its appropriate management significantly affects the long-term survival of patients with AAA disease.

Despite the recognition that coronary artery disease has a significant effect on perioperative and long-term mortality in patients with AAA disease, the ideal method for identifying these patients has not been clearly established. Although cardiac catherization provides excellent anatomic detail, it cannot be advocated in all patients undergoing AAA repair. Not only is it associated with specific risks, it is expensive. Currently, the standard of practice in most medical centers is that patients with ischemic changes on their electrocardiogram (ECG) or those with significant coronary artery disease, are screened using noninvasive cardiac stress tests (e.g., adenosine/dipyridamole thallium imaging or dobutamine stress echocardiography). It is believed that using these noninvasive screening tests can effectively identify patients at risk for perioperative myocardial ischemic events.[74]

Langen and colleagues used dobutamine stress echocardiography to risk-stratify 81 patients undergoing aortic surgery. They were able to identify three groups: (1) normal; (2) resting abnormalities but no inducible ischemia (fixed defects); and (3) dobutamine-induced ischemia. The first two groups of patients underwent aortic surgery without cardiac complications or death. Of the 25 patients in group three, 5 refused surgery, 4 underwent CABG, and 16 underwent AAA repair. There were no deaths, but three (19%) had myocardial infarctions.

Long-term survival of patients following AAA surgery is clearly related to cardiac evaluation and management of inducible myocardial ischemia at the time of the repair.[74] Roger et al.[75] reported a marked reduction in long-term survival in 131 patients who underwent elective aneurysm repair if they had symptomatic or demonstrable myocardial ischemia. They had a 34% survival rate at 8 years, compared to those without coronary artery disease who had a 59% survival at 8 years.[75] It is noteworthy that the presence of uncorrected coronary artery disease also increased the risk of nonfatal cardiac events by a factor of four.

Our current practice at Washington University Medical Center is based on the fact that there is a high incidence of coronary artery disease in this patient population and that appropriate identification of patients with coronary artery disease undergoing elective AAA repair can improve their long-term survival. To optimize the patients' survival, patients who have a history of coronary artery disease, symptoms suggestive of active cardiac disease, or an abnormal ECG are subjected to dobutamine stress echocardiography or adenosine/dipyridamole thallium imaging. Only those patients who have no cardiac complaints and have normal ECGs undergo surgery without further evaluation.

Aside from coronary disease, there is a high prevalence of cigarette smoking within the patient population. Therefore pulmonary function tests are often necessary. It is important to document the severity of pulmonary impairment and identify any reversible component due to bronchospastic disease. Often a preoperative pulmonary medicine consultation and a preoperative course of bronchodilators and pulmonary therapy is beneficial.

There is a high incidence of cerebral vascular disease in this patient population as well. If there is a history of transient ischemic attacks (TIAs) or stroke referable to the carotid arteries, or if a carotid bruit is identified on physical examination, the patient should undergo a preoperative duplex scan. If a high grade stenosis is identified or the patient has symptomatic stenosis, staged carotid endarterectomy is usually recommended prior to undergoing abdominal aortic aneurysmorrhaphy. Additional evaluation of other organ systems such as the kidneys depends on the patient's medical history and any evidence of symptoms referable to these systems.

In terms of imaging studies, the most useful study is abdominal and pelvic CT scanning. CT scans accurately determine the size of the aneurysm and more importantly, determine the extent of the aneurysm. For surgical decision-making, it is critical to determine the location of the neck of the aneurysm and plan therapy appropriately. In many ways repair of an infrarenal aneurysm is a different operation from repairing a juxtarenal or suprarenal AAA. Additionally, the CT scan gives information about the iliac arteries and determines whether they are aneurysmal, and it provides information on the venous anatomy. Arteriography demonstrates only the luminal diameter and because of a mural thrombus, often underestimates the true size of the aneurysm. For the same reason, it also may not accurately define the neck of the aneurysm.

Although some centers routinely perform arteriography on patients with an AAA, it is not necessary if a high quality CT scan has been performed. There are specific indications for performing arteriography: (1) In patients with hypertension or chronic renal insufficiency where renovascular disease is a possibility, arteriography should be performed to evaluate for renal artery stenosis. (2) In patients who have a history of claudication, it is important to perform arteriography to identify occlusive lesions, particularly in the iliac arteries, which may harbor coexisting infrarenal AAA disease. (3) Arteriography is done in patients in whom mesenteric ischemia is suspected. (4) In patients suspected to have a juxtarenal aneurysm, it is important to identify the location of the major branches of the aorta. Once preoperative evaluation and testing are completed, the patient can be subjected to AAA repair.

## Surgical Technique

The techniques for repair of infrarenal abdominal aortic aneurysms are well described elsewhere.[76–78] Briefly, there are two standard approaches to the infrarenal AAA. The most commonly employed approach is transabdominal, which can be done through a midline or a transverse abdominal incision. When aneurysm surgery is performed transabdominally, the aneurysm is approached by incising the peritoneum just lateral to the ligament of Treitz and mobilizing the third and fourth portions of the duodenum. The neck of the aneurysm is then exposed by dissecting up to the level of the left renal vein. If necessary, the left renal vein can be circumferentially mobilized, including ligation of its principal branches (adrenal, gonadal, posterior lumbar). Once the neck is exposed, the dissection proceeds distally so control can be obtained of the iliac arteries. After this dissection has been completed, vascular isolation is obtained with clamps, and the aneurysm is repaired using the endoaneurysmorrhaphy technique as described by Creech.[3] With this technique the aneurysm is repaired by opening the aneurysm and sewing a prosthetic graft within the sac of the aneurysm to the healthy proximal neck and distally to the distal aorta, the common iliac arteries, or the external iliac or femoral arteries, as dictated by the patient's anatomy. Following this step, the aneurysm sac is closed over the prosthetic graft. The peritoneum is closed taking care to make sure that the duodenum or any other viscera do not come in contact with the prosthetic graft.

Alternatively, the retroperitoneal approach can be used. The retroperitonel approach has proven to be advantageous in certain situations. Specifically it is useful in patients who have a hostile abdomen (history of multiple previous surgeries or extensive peritonitis), ostomies, and where it may be necessary for whatever reason to clamp above the level of the renal arteries. With this approach, an incision is made typically from the tip of the twelfth rib to the border of the rectus muscle midway between the umbilicus and the symphisis pubis. If necessary, the incision can be extended in either direction for better exposure. The retroperitoneal space is entered, and the peritoneal envelope is swept medially. The ureter is identified and circumferentially dissected free to avoid a traction injury. The dissection plane is developed between Gerota's fascia and the peritoneal envelope so the left kidney can be left to lie posteriorly. The gonadal vein is then identified and ligated at its origin from the left renal vein. At this point the neck of the aneurysm can be isolated at the level of the left renal vein. The left common iliac artery is then circumferentially dissected free so a clamp can be applied. It is our custom to not isolate the right common iliac artery, as it is technically difficult through this approach, but to occlude it from within the aneurysm after the sac is open using a Pruitt catheter. Once the aorta and the left common iliac artery are clamped, the aneurysm sac is opened and the Pruitt catheter is placed within the lumen of the left common iliac artery. A standard aortic aneurysm repair is then carried out. In the case of the left retroperitoneal approach, if it is necessary to carry the bypass down to the level of the right external iliac artery, a counterincision is made in the right lower quadrant. Alternatively, an incision can be made in the right groin and a graft placed down to this level. Once the aneurysm is repaired, the aneurysm sac is once again closed over the prosthetic graft.

Once the aneurysm repair is completed, the wound is closed in standard fashion. The patients are typically taken to the surgical intensive care unit. In uncomplicated cases, the patient is discharged to a step-down unit on postoperative day 1 and to the regular floor on postoperative day 2. Once GI function returns and the patient is ambulatory and taking a regular diet he or she is discharged to home, typically between postoperative days 5 and 8.

## Postoperative Complications

Repair of an AAA is a major surgical procedure, and as such it carries with it the risk of significant complications. There is often significant blood loss associated with opening the aneurysm sac. There is a period where the lumbar arteries and the inferior mesenteric artery are back-bleeding. Once these vessels are oversewn, the hemorrhage is controlled. The use of a blood scavenging suction system (Cell Saver) allows this blood to be scavenged and returned to the patient. Other bleeding, however, typically results from technical misadventure. The most common error is to injure one of the major veins. During infrarenal AAA repair, the left renal vein is at the superior extent of the dissection and courses over the anterior surface of the aorta. To the medial side of the aorta is the vena cava, and the iliac veins are in close juxtaposition to the iliac arteries. Any of these structures may be injured intraoperatively. An uncommon but well-recognized cause of catastrophic intraoperative hemorrhage results from injury to an unrecognized retroaortic renal vein. On occasion the left renal vein is not identified in its normal position. If the surgeon assumes that it is present but just not in the field of dissection and cross-clamps the aorta, the aberrant left renal vein, which tends to course more caudad than a normal left renal vein, is torn, resulting in massive hemorrhage from the renal vein posterior to the aorta. Fortunately, the aberrant left renal vein is easily identified by CT scanning, and the widespread use of this imaging modality has greatly reduced the incidence of this complication. Management of these problems intraoperatively consists of careful repair of the venous injury and rapid, appropriate volume resuscitation for the patient if there has been massive blood loss.

During the early postoperative period, continued bleeding can result from persistent bleeding from suture holes, bleeding along the anastomotic sites, or unrecognized bleeders in the retroperitoneal space. Persistent blood loss during the early postoperative period mandates an emergent return to the operating room.

The incidence of cardiac complications is discussed in the section on preoperative evaluation. There is a high incidence of tobacco abuse among patients undergoing AAA repair, and a corresponding high incidence of chronic obstructive pulmonary disease (COPD). As mentioned previously, there must be an attempt to identify these patients during the preoperative period and to optimize their pulmonary function. The risk factors that predict pulmonary complications after elective aortic surgery include American Society of Anesthesiologists (ASA) class IV, age more than 70 years, weight more than 150% of ideal body weight, a forced vital capacity (FVC) less than 80% of predicted, crystalloid infusion intraoperatively of more than 6 liters, and an operation duration of more than 5 hours.[79] In an attempt to limit pulmonary complications, epidural anesthesia is used as an intraoperative adjuvant and a primary means of postoperative pain control. Its advantage is that intraoperatively, the combined epidural plus general anesthesia blunts the hemodynamic changes associated with aortic cross-clamping and decreases the need for postoperative ventilatory support.[80] Compared to the traditional parenteral narcotic analgesia, epidural analgesia reduces the incidence of postoperative pulmonary complications. It also appears that epidural analgesia helps reduce postoperative cardiac complications, presumably by reducing nociceptive stimuli and their associated tachycardic response.[81]

Pulmonary complications after AAA repair are treated in standard fashion. Patients with ventilatory insufficiency are supported on a ventilator until they can be extubated. If prolonged ventilatory dependence develops, tracheostomy can be performed for improving pulmonary toilet and patient comfort. Respiratory tract infections, either pneumonia or bronchitis, are treated with antibiotics targeted at the specific organisms as determined by culture and sensitivity tests. Atelectasis is treated with pulmonary physiotherapy, which includes frequent use of incentive spirometry and systematic clearing of secretions with endotracheal suctioning as needed. Additionally, mobilizing the patients, including getting out of bed to chair and ambulating, during the early postoperative period, helps limit pulmonary complications.

Renal dysfunction occurs in 1–8% of patients following elective AAA repair,[82] but profound renal dysfunction with the need for dialysis is extremely unusual, with only 0.6% of all patients requiring it during the postoperative period.[83] Renal dysfunction occurs much more commonly in the setting of emergent AAA repair, with an incidence of 8–46% and an associated mortality of 57–95%.[84] Several factors contribute to perioperative renal dysfunction. During the preoperative period, the use of contrast agents for arteriography or CT scanning can result in renal dysfunction, although it is usually transient. In patients who do suffer significant deterioration of renal function following an imaging study, the surgery should be postponed until renal function returns to its baseline value. It is important that patients be adequately hydrated prior to arriving in the operating room. The combination of preoperative fasting and contrast loads with their attendant osmotic diuresis, as well as bowel preparation, can result in relative dehydration. Therefore, patients should receive intravenous fluids beginning the night before surgery. More unusual causes of nephrotoxicity include side effects of the perioperative antibiotics or anesthetic agents. If a suprarenal cross-clamp is required intraoperatively, the resulting warm renal ischemia time can result in the development of acute tubular necrosis. If the ischemic time is limited to less than 30 minutes, usually no permanent renal dysfunction results. Occasionally, clamping the infrarenal aorta results in plaque or thrombus adjacent to the renal arteries being dislodged, with embolization to the kidneys.[85] Similarly, prolonged ischemia of the lower extremities can result in myonecrosis with myoglobin release. This complication of elective aneurysm repair is unusual, as the aorta cross-clamp times must exceed 6 hours for it to occur. Should it occur, it is treated by maintaining a high urine flow via intravenous hydration with isotonic solutions and alkalization of the urine. Intraoperatively, division of the left renal

TABLE 34.2. Operative Mortality Rates

| Study | Year | Mortality (%) |
|---|---|---|
| Bernstein[94] | 1988 | 0.8 |
| Sicard[95] | 1987 | 1.4 |
| Johnson[96] | 1988 | 4.5 |
| Branchereau[97] | 1990 | 2.5 |
| Clark[98] | 1990 | 2.0 |
| Olsen[99] | 1991 | 4.8 |
| Sicard[100] | 1995 | 1.8 |
| Feinglass[101] | 1995 | 2.9 |
| Lloyd[102] | 1996 | 2.4 |

vein to facilitate exposure is associated with an increased risk of postoperative renal dysfunction.[86] Finally, placement of an infrarenal aortic cross-clamp stimulates the renin–angiotensin system, which creates a renal cortical vasospasm.[87] Sometimes this problem can be avoided by administration of mannitol.[88] If acute tubular necrosis (ATN) occurs, treatment is basically supportive, with particular attention paid to avoiding ongoing renal or new renal injury. It is important to optimize the patient's volume status and to monitor the electrolytes, blood urea nitrogen, and creatinine to avoid hyperkalemia and uremic symptoms. If the ATN is profound, dialysis is required; but as mentioned previously, this requirement is unusual after elective AAA repair.

## Results of Surgical Intervention

Despite the advances made in operative management of AAAs, the mortality rate for repair of ruptured aneurysms remains high and has not improved significantly over the past 40 years. Several series reported during the early 1990s documented an approximately 50% operative mortality rate.[89–92] This underestimates the true mortality associated with ruptured AAAs, as many patients die before they can reach the hospital. The patients who do survive experience a high complication rate. During the early era of AAA repair, elective surgical intervention was a risky proposition, with early surgical series reporting perioperative mortality rates as high as 21%.[53,54,93] Currently, elective AAA repair is a much safer endeavor. The recently reported surgical series almost uniformly report operative mortality rates of 5% or less (Table 34.2). In summary, elective AAA repair, although a major surgical procedure, has proved to be an effective treatment with low, acceptable rates of surgical morbidity and mortality.

## References


1. Mitchell MB, Rutherford RB, Krupski C. Infrarenal aortic aneurysms. In: Rutherford RB (ed) Vascular Surgery. Saunders: Philadelphia, 1995:1032–1059.
2. Dubost C, Allary M, Oecomomos N. A propos detraitement des aneurysms de l'aorte ablation de l'aneurysm: retablissment dela continuite par graffe d'aorte humaine conservee. Mem Acad Chir (Paris) 1951;77:281.
3. Creech O Jr. Endo-aneurysmorrhaphy and treatment of aortic aneurysm. Ann Surg 1966;164:935.
4. Nehler MR, Taylor LM, Moneta GL, Porter JM. Indications for operation for infrarenal abdominal aortic aneurysms: current guidelines. Semin Vasc Surg 1995;8:108–114.
5. Crawford ES, DeBakey ME, Cooley DA, et al. Surgical correlations of aneurysms and atherosclerotic occlusive lesions of the aorta and major arteries. Postgrad Med 1961; 29:151.
6. Carlsson J, Sternby N. Aortic aneurysms. Acta Chir Scand 1964;127:466–473.
7. Turk K. Post-mortem incidence of abdominal aortic aneurysms. Proc R Soc Med 1965;58:869–870.
8. Bengtsson H, Bergqvist D, Sternby NJ. Increasing prevalence of abdominal aortic aneurysm: a necropsy study. Eur J Surg 1992;158:19.
9. Melton L, Bickerstaff L, Hollier L, et al. Changing incidence of abdominal aortic aneurysms: a population based study. Am J Epidemiol 1984;120:379–386.
10. Fowkes FGR, Macintyre CCA, Ruckley CV. Increasing incidence of aortic aneurysms in England and Wales. Br Med J 1989;298:33–35.
11. Mealy K, Salman. The true incidence of ruptured abdominal aortic aneurysms. Eur J Vasc Surg 1988;2:405–408.
12. Castleden W, Merecer J. Abdominal aortic aneurysms in western Australia: descriptive epidemiology and patterns of rupture. Br J Surg 1985;72:109–112.
13. Lillienfeld D, Gunderson P, Sprafka J, et al. The epidemiology of abdominal aortic aneurysms: mortality trends in the United States 1951–1980. Arteriosclerosis 1987;7:637–643.
14. Bickerstaff LK, Hollier LH, Ban Peenan HJ, et al. Abdominal aortic aneurysms: the changing natural history. J Vasc Surg 1984;1:6–12.
15. Garaway WM, Whisnant JP, Burlan AJ. The declining incidence of stroke. N Engl J Med 1979;300:449–452.
16. Morris T, Bouhoutos J. ABO blood groups in occlusive and ectatic arterial disease. Br J Surg 1973;60:892–893.
17. Tilson MD, Stansel H. Differences in results for aneurysm vs. occlusive disease after bifurcation grafts. Arch Surg 1981;115:1173–1175.
18. Donaldson MC, Rosenberg JM, Bucknam CA. Factors affecting survival after ruptured abdominal aortic aneurysm. J Vasc Surg 1985;2:564–570.
19. Reigel MM, Hollier LH, Kazmier FJ, et al. Late survival in abdominal aortic aneurysm patients: the role of selective myocardial revascularization on the basis of clinical symptoms. J Vasc Surg 1987;5:222–227.
20. Johnston KW, Scobie TK. Multicenter prospective study of nonruptured abdominal aortic aneurysms. I. Population and operative management. J Vasc Surg 1988;7:69–81.
21. Leather RP, Shah DM, Kaufman JL, et al. Comparative analysis of retroperitoneal aortic replacement for aneurysm. Surg Gynecol Obstet 1989;168:387–393.
22. Sicard GA, Allen BT, Munn JS, Anderson CB. Retroperitoneal versus transperitoneal approach for repair of

abdominal aortic aneurysms. Surg Clin North Am 1989;69: 795–806.

23. McFarlane MJ. The epidemiologic necropsy for abdominal aortic aneurysm. JAMA 1991;265:2085–2088.
24. Johnson JG, Avery A, McDougal G, et al. Aneurysms of the abdominal aorta: incidence in Blacks and Whites in North Carolina. Arch Surg 1985;120:1138–1140.
25. Kitchen ND. Racial distribution of aneurysms in Zimbabwe. J R Soc Med 1989;82:136–138.
26. Cronenwett JL, Murphy TE, Zelenock GB, et al. Actuarial analysis of variables associated with rupture of small abdominal aortic aneurysms. Surgery 1985;98:472.
27. Reed D, Reed C, Stemmermann G, et al. Are aortic aneurysms caused by atherosclerosis? Circulation 1992;85: 205–211.
28. Norrgard O, Anguist KA, Dahlen G. High concentrations of Lp(a) lipoproten in serum are common among patients with abdominal aortic aneurysms. Int Angiol 1987;7:46–49.
29. Hammond JE, Garfinkel L. Coronary heart disease, stroke, and aortic aneurysm. Arch Environ Health 1969;19: 167.
30. Darling RC, Messina CR, Brewster DC, et al. Autopsy study of unoperated abdominal aortic aneurysms. Circulation 1977;56 (suppl II):161.
31. Foster JH, Bolasny BL, Govvel WG, et al. Comparative study of elective resection and expectant treatment of abdominal aortic aneurysm. Surg Gynecol Obstet 1969; 129:1.
32. Sterpetti AV, Cavallaro A, Cavallari N, et al. Factors influencing the rupture of abdominal aortic aneurysm. Surg Obstet Gynecol 1991;173:175.
33. Lederle FA, Johnson GR, Wilson SE, et al. Prevalence and associations of abdominal aortic aneurysms detected through screening: Aneurysm Detection and Management (ADAM) Veterans Affairs Cooperative Study Group. Ann Intern Med 1997;126:441–449.
34. Darling RC III, Brewster DC, Darling RC, et al. Are familial abdominal aortic aneurysms different? J Vasc Surg 1989; 10:39–43.
35. Berridge DC, Griffifth CDM, Amar SS, et al. Screening for clinically unsuspected abdominal aortic aneurysms in patients with peripheral vascular disease. Eur J Vasc Surg 1989;3:421–422.
36. Shapira OM, Pasik S, Wassermann JP, et al. Ultrasound screening of abdominal aortic aneurysms in patients with atherosclerotic peripheral vascular disease. J Cardiovasc Surg 1990;31:172–179.
37. Grange JJ, Davis V, Baxter BT. Pathogenesis of abdominal aortic aneurysm: update and look toward the future. J Cardiovasc Surg 1997;5:256–265.
38. Reilly JM. Abdominal aortic aneurysms: incidence, etiology and pathogenesis. In: Callow AD, Ernst CB (eds) Vascular Surgery: Theory and Practice. Appleton & Lange: Norwalk, CT, 1995:859–872.
39. Tilson CD. Histochemistry of aortic elastin in patients with nonspecific AAA disease. Arch Surg 1988;123:503–505.
40. Brophy CM, Reilley JM, Smith GJW, et al. The role of inflammation in nonspecific aneurysm disease. Ann Vasc Surg 1991;5:229–233.
41. Sumner DS, Hokanson DE, Standress DE. Stress-stained characteristics and collagen-elastin content of AAA's. Surg Gynecol Obstet 1970;130:459–466.
42. Koch AE, Haines GK, Rizzo RJ, et al. Human abdominal aortic aneurysms: immunophenotypic analysis suggesting an immune-mediated response. Am J Pathol 1990;137: 1199–1213.
43. Newman KM, Malon AM, Shin RD, et al. Matrix metalloproteinases in old aortic aneurysms, characterization, purification and their possible sources. Connect Tissue Res 1994;30:265–276.
44. Thompson RW, Holmes D, Merten RA, et al. Production and localization of 92-kilodalton gelatinase in abdominal aortic aneurysms: an elastolytic metalloproteinase expressed by aneurysm infiltrating macrophages. J Clin Invest 1995;96:318.
45. Reilly JM, Brophy CM, Tilson CD. Characterization of an elastase from aneurysmal aorta which degrades intact aortic elastin. Ann Vasc Surg 1992;6:499–502.
46. Curci JA, Liao S, Huffman MD, et al. Expression and localization of macrophage elastase (matrix metalloprotease 12 in abdominal aortic aneurysms. J Clin Invest 1998;102: 1900–1910.
47. Reilly JM, Sicard GA, Lucore CL. Differential expression of plasminogen activators in abdominal aortic aneurysm and occlusive disease. J Vasc Surg 1994;19:865–872.
48. Werb Z, Banda MJ, Jones PA. Degradation of connective tissue matrices by macrophages. J Exp Med 1980;152: 1340–1356.
49. Senior RM, Griffin GL, Mecham RP. Chemotactic activity of elastin derived peptides. J Clin Invest 1980;66:859–862.
50. Estes E. Abdominal aortic aneurysm: a study of 102 cases. Circulation 1950;2:258.
51. Wright IS, Urdenata E, Wright B. Re-opening the case of the abdominal aortic aneurysm. Circulation 1956;13:754.
52. Schatz IJ, Fairbairn JF, Jugens JL. Abdominal aortic aneurysms: a reappraisal. Circulation 1962;26:200.
53. DeBakey ME, Crawford ES, Cooley DA, et al. Aneurysm of abdominal aorta: analysis of results of graft replacement therapy one to eleven years after operation. Ann Surg 1964; 160:622.
54. Szilagyi DE, Smith RF, DeRusso FJ, et al. Contribution of abdominal aortic aneurysmectomy to prolongation of life. Ann Surg 1966;164:678.
55. Englund R, Perera D, Hanel KC. Outcome for patients with abdominal aortic aneurysms that are treated nonsurgically. Aust NZ J Surg 1997;67:260–263.
56. Gillmaker H, Holmberg L, Elvin A, et al. Natural history of patients with abdominal aortic aneurysm. Eur J Vasc Surg 1991;5:125.
57. Gjuirguis EM, Barber GG. The natural history of abdominal aortic aneurysms. Am J Surg 1991;162:481.
58. Sterpetti AV, Cavallaro A, Cavallari N, et al. Factors influencing the rupture of abdominal aortic aneurysm. Surg Obstet Gynecol 1991;173:175.
59. Nevitt MP, Ballard DJ, Hallett JW. Prognosis of abdominal aortic aneurysms: a population based study. N Engl J Med 1989;321:1009.
60. Brown PM, Pattenden R, Butlius JR. The selective management of small abdominal aortic aneurysms: the Kingston study. J Vasc Surg 1992;15:21.

61. Littoy FN, Steffan G, Greisler HP, et al. Use of sequential B-mode ultrasonography to manage abdominal aortic aneurysms. Arch Surg 1989;124:419.
62. Katz DA, Littenberg B, Cronenwett JL. Management of small abdominal aortic aneurysms: early surgery vs. watchful waiting. JAMA 1992;268:2678.
63. Brown PM, Pattenden R, Vernooy C, et al. Selective management of abdominal aortic aneurysms in a prospective measurement program. J Vasc Surg 1996;23:213–221.
64. Cronenwett JL, Sargent SK, Wall MH, et al. Variables that affect the expansion rate and outcome of small abdominal aortic aneurysms. J Vasc Surg 1990;11:260.
65. Michaels JA. The management of small abdominal aortic aneurysms: a computer simulation using Monte Carlo methods. Eur J Vasc Surg 1992;6:551.
66. Collin J, Aerugo L, Walton J. How fast do very small aneurysms grow? Eur J Vasc Surg 1989;3:15.
67. Krupski WC, Bass A, Thurston JDW, et al. Utility of computed tomography for surveillance of small abdominal aortic aneurysms. Arch Surg 1990;125:1345.
68. Bernstein EF, Eilley RB, Goldberger LE, et al. Growth rates small abdominal aortic aneurysms. Surgery 1976;80:765.
69. Chang JB, Stein TA, Liu JP, Dunn ME. Risk factors associated with rapid growth of small abdominal aortic aneurysms. Surgery 1998;121:117–122.
70. Johnson G, McDevitt NB, Procter HJ, et al. Emergent or elective operation for symptomatic abdominal aortic aneurysm. Arch Surg 1980;115:51.
71. Mehard WB, Heiken JP, Sicard GA. High-attenuating crescent in abdominal aortic aneurysm wall at CT: a sign of acute or impending rupture. Radiology 1994;192:359–362.
72. Pennell RC, Holiew LH, Lie JT, et al. Inflammatory abdominal aortic aneurysms: a 30-year review. J Vasc Surg 1985;2:859.
73. Hertzer NR, Young JR, Kramer RJ, et al. Routine coronary angiography prior to elective aortic reconstruction. Arch Surg 1979;114:1336.
74. Langan EM, Youkey JR, Franklin DP, et al. Dobutamine stress echocardiography for cardiac risk assessment before aortic surgery. J Vasc Surg 1993;18:905–913.
75. Roger VL, Ballard DJ, Hallet JW, et al. Influence of coronary artery disease on morbidity and mortality after abdominal aortic aneurysmectomy: a population-based study, 1971–1987. J Am Coll Cardiol 1989;14:1245–1252.
76. Reilly JM, Sicard GA. Left retroperitoneal approach to the aorta and its branches. Part I. Ann Vasc Surg 1994;8: 212–291.
77. Reilly JM, Sicard GA. Right retroperitoneal approach to the aorta and its branches. Part II. Ann Vasc Surg 1994;8: 318–323.
78. Mitchell MB, Rutherford RB, Krupski WC. Infrarenal aortic aneurysms. In Rutherford RB (ed) Vascular Surgery. Saunders: Philadelphia, 1995:1032–1059.
79. Caligaro KD, Azurin DG, Dougherty MJ, Dandora R, et al. Pulmonary risk factors for elective abdominal aortic surgery. J Vasc Surg 1993;18:914–921.
80. Her C, Kizelshteyn G, Walker V, et al. Combined epidural and general anesthesia for abdominal aortic surgery. J Cardiothorac Anesth 1990;4:552–557.
81. Major CP Jr, Greer MS, Russell WL, Roe SM. Postoperative pulmonary complications and morbidity after abdominal aneurysmectomy: a comparison of postoperative epidural versus parenteral intravenous analgesia. Am Surg 1995; 62:45–51.
82. Castronova JJ, Flanigan DP. Renal failure complicating vascular surgery. In: Bernhard VM, Towne JB (eds) Complications in Vascular Surgery. Grune & Stratton: Orlando, 1985:258–274.
83. Diehl JT, Cali RF, Hertzer NR, et al. Complications of abdominal aortic reconstruction: an analysis of perioperative risk factors in 557 patients. Ann Surg 1983;197: 49–56.
84. Abbott WM, Able RM, Beck CH, et al. Renal failure after ruptured aneurysm. Arch Surg 1975;110:11110.
85. Iliopoulos JI, Zdon MJ, Crawford BG, et al. Renal microembolization syndrome: a cause for renal dysfunction after abdominal aortic reconstruction. Am J Surg 1983;146:779–783.
86. Huber D, Harris HP, Walker PG, May J, Tyre RP. Does division of the left renal vein during aortic surgery adversely affect renal function? Ann Vasc Surg 1991;5:77–79.
87. Berkowitz HD, Shetty S. Renin release and renal cortical ischemia following aortic crossclamping. Arch Surg 1974; 109:612–618.
88. Abbott WM, Austen WG. The reversal of renal cortical ischemia during aortic occlusion by mannitol. J Surg Res 1974;16:482–489.
89. Ouriel K, Geary K, Green RM, et al. Factors determining survival after ruptured aortic aneurysm: the hospital, the surgeon, and the patient. J Vasc Surg 1990;11:493.
90. Cohen JR, Birnbaum E, Dassan M, Wise L. Experience in managing 70 patients with rutpured abdominal aortic aneurysms. NY State J Med 1991;91:97.
91. Harris LM, Gaggioli GL, Fielder R, et al. Ruptured abdominal aortic aneurysms: factors affecting mortality rates. J Vasc Surg 1991;14:812.
92. Gloviczki P, Pairolero PC, Mucha P Jr, et al. Ruptured abdominal aortic aneurysms: repair should not be denied. J Vasc Surg 1992;15:851.
93. Thompson JE, Hollier LH, Patman RD, et al. Surgical management of abdominal aortic aneurysms: factors influencing mortality and morbidity; a 20 year experience. Ann Surg 1975;181:654.
94. Bernstein EF, Diley RB, Randolph HF. The improving outlook for patients over seventy years of age with abdominal aortic aneurysms. Ann Surg 1988;207:318.
95. Sicard GA, Freeman MB, VanderWoude JC, et al. Comparison between the transabdominal and retroperitoneal approach for reconstruction of the infrarenal abdominal aorta. J Vasc Surg 1987;5:19.
96. Johnson KW, Scobie TK. Multicenter prospective study of nonruptured abdominal aortic aneurysms. I. Population and operative management. J Vasc Surg 1988;7:69.
97. Branchereau A, Nazet J, Colavolpe JC, et al. Combined morbidity and mortality of direct surgical treatment of abdominal aortic aneurysms. Ann Surg 1988;207:318.
98. Clark ET, Gewertz BL, Bassiouny HS, et al. Current results: elective aortic reconstruction for aneurysmal and occlusive disease. J Cardiovasc Surg (Torino) 1990;31:438.
99. Olsen PS, Schroeder T, Agerskov K, et al. Surgery for abdominal aortic aneurysms: a survey of 656 patients. J Cardiovasc Surg 1991;32:636.

100. Sicard GA, Reilly JM, Rubin GB, et al. Transabdominal versus retroperitoneal incision for abdominal aortic surgery: report of a prospective randomized trial. J Vasc Surg 1995;21:174–183.
101. Feinglass J, Cowper D, Dunlop D, et al. Late survival risk factors for abdominal aortic aneurysm repair: experience from 14 Department of Veterans Affairs hospitals. Surgery 1995;118:16–24.
102. Lloyd WE, Paty PS, Darling RC III, et al. Results of 1000 consecutive elective abdominal aortic aneurysm repairs. Cardiovasc Surg 1996;4:724–726.

# 35
# Natural History and Treatment of Extracranial Cerebrovascular Disease in the Elderly

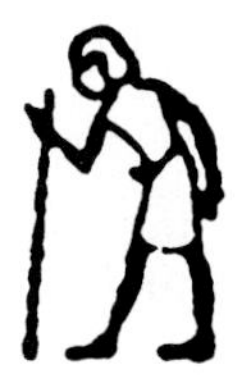

George H. Meier

Cerebrovascular disease, specifically stroke, continues to increase despite improvements in the treatment and outcomes of cardiovascular disease in general. Many believe that the development of cerebrovascular atherosclerosis is simply a normal consequence of aging, as the incidence of stroke increases with age, rising almost sevenfold between the ages of 55 and 85.[1] Despite a nearly 20% reduction in the death rate from stroke over the past 20 years, cerebrovascular disease remains the third leading cause of death in the United States.[2] It is therefore not surprising that carotid endarterectomy remains the most common peripheral vascular operation done in the United States.[3] Current estimates suggest that the population over the age of 65 will increase more than threefold over the next 25 years,[4] during which time the increase in cerebrovascular disease will result in a marked impact on medical care. The correct and cost-effective management of cerebrovascular disease is therefore increasingly important as the population ages.

Cerebral infarction can be caused by intracerebral hemorrhage or embolic disorders. Although hemodynamic flow limitations can occur, flow-related cerebral ischemia is rare. Previous studies have suggested that about 60% of cerebrovascular events originate with atherosclerotic disease outside the heart.[5] Thus most embolic strokes should be preventable if the extracranial vascular disease can be diagnosed and treated prior to an irreversible cerebrovascular event. This intervention may be as simple as limiting plaque growth once carotid disease is discovered, or it may require complex reopening of the arterial supply with surgical or endovascular techniques. Stroke prevention requires not only modification of risk factors for atherosclerosis but also effective selection of patients for intervention prior to the occurrence of a limiting cerebrovascular event.

Risk factor modification in those with atherosclerosis is an area of intense, ongoing investigation and review. Traditional risk factors for atherosclerotic disease such as smoking,[6] hypertension,[7] and diabetes[8] remain significant for patients with extracranial atherosclerosis. Research suggests that other risk factors such as homocysteine[9] and low density lipoprotein (LDL) cholesterol[10–12] may be important in lowering the ultimate risk of stroke. Elevated homocysteine levels in the bloodstream have been implicated in numerous atherosclerotic disease processes.[13,14] Whereas homozygous individuals with a deficiency in enzymes to metabolize homocysteine often die at a young age secondary to coronary disease,[15] heterozygous individuals maintain function but appear to have an increased tendency to develop atherosclerosis. The management of these elevations is relatively simple, as three inducible enzyme systems allow breakdown of homocysteine to safer metabolites. These inducible systems increase their activity in response to folate, vitamin $B_6$, and vitamin $B_{12}$, respectively. Therefore, trials have been initiated to evaluate stroke risk reduction using high doses of these vitamins.

The cholesterol saga has been a fundamental issue with respect to coronary disease for years. Cholesterol has traditionally been linked to coronary atherosclerosis[16] but has also been implicated strongly in cerebrovascular disease.[17] Whereas atherosclerotic plaque initiation is little influenced by cholesterol levels, progression of plaque already in place is clearly accelerated by elevated cholesterol levels. Presumably, the cholesterol becomes deposited in plaques, influenced directly by the cholesterol gradient from the bloodstream to the surrounding tissues. The permeability of the abnormal tissue in the plaque appears to be increased, so cholesterol can migrate into the plaque, leading to plaque progression. Evidence suggests that the reduction of cholesterol using 3-hydroxy-3-methylglutaryl coenzyme A (HMG-CoA) reductase inhibitors, even in individuals with normal levels, may lower the risk of subsequent cardiac events.[18] Extension of these studies to stroke populations is in progress, with early results suggesting a benefit in stroke reduction as well.

## Pathophysiology

Atherosclerotic disease begins early in life as plaque initiation starts in areas at risk for atherosclerotic degeneration.[19,20] Most atherosclerosis is well explained by this mechanism, although some fundamental contradictions remain. If atherosclerosis is a progressive degenerative disease, it would be reasonably expected that its incidence would continue to increase with increasing age. Indeed, this appears to be true for cerebrovascular disease, but it is distinctly contrary to existing data relative to both coronary[21] and iliac[22] disease. In those distributions, a plateau occurs in the incidence of atherosclerosis, with decreasing incidence of disease once a certain age is reached. The explanation for this discrepancy is complex, and whether there is a real plateau in disease progression in these anatomic areas or a selection bias exists remains unclear. What data are available suggest that no such plateau exists for cerebrovascular disease, with the incidence of disease increasing with increasing age.[23,24] Additionally, the increased incidence of cerebrovascular disease further explains the resultant increased incidence of stroke with increasing age.[25]

The atherosclerotic plaque of cerebrovascular disease is no different from that associated with coronary or peripheral vascular disease. The initiating event appears to be the development of a lesion on the intimal surface of the artery, particularly in areas of low shear stress.[26] The carotid bifurcation has been studied extensively, as plaque formation in this distribution is more anatomically consistent than that seen in other locations. Essentially, the bifurcation of the carotid artery generates an area of high velocity (and therefore high shear stress) at the septum between the external and internal carotid arteries and an area of low shear stress at the bulb of the internal carotid artery opposite the bifurcation. In fact, with the advent of color flow duplex ultrasonography, this area of flow separation and reversal can be easily defined in normal individuals. The flow phantom models of shear-related atherosclerosis have been best defined in this anatomic location. These models clearly demonstrate the areas of flow separation and resultant flow reversal opposite the bifurcation, where atherosclerosis is found consistently. Therefore flow patterns at the carotid bifurcation appear to be important in the initiation and progression of atherosclerotic plaque in the cerebrovascular system.

A second issue associated with atherosclerotic plaque progression is the concept of intraplaque hemorrhage. With coronary artery disease, intraplaque hemorrhage is a well-accepted mechanism of sudden plaque progression associated with an acute myocardial event. Similarly, carotid atherosclerosis has been studied extensively relative to plaque morphology and intraplaque hemorrhage. The small blood vessels that traverse the complex intimal plaque of mature atherosclerosis are subject to significant hemodynamic effects, resulting in an increased risk of vessel rupture, with attendant intraplaque hemorrhage. The association of intraplaque hemorrhage with increasing stenosis has been well documented.[27] Additionally, there has been a significant association of intraplaque hemorrhage with symptomatic carotid stenosis.[28–31] In this instance, the presence of subintimal hemorrhage results in intimal ulceration and embolization of residual intraplaque clot and debris, producing the characteristic microemboli associated with transient ischemic attacks (TIAs).[32] Thus intraplaque hemorrhage is associated with the severity of stenosis as well as the symptoms, suggesting that intraplaque hemorrhage may be the link between degree of stenosis and the incidence of symptoms.

The origin of symptoms related to carotid atherosclerosis has not always been well defined. According to the hemodynamic theory, the symptoms associated with carotid stenosis were related to flow limitations and resultant cortical ischemia. In contrast, the embolic theory held that degeneration of the atherosclerotic plaque resulted in microemboli, and clot formation caused macroemboli and stroke. The stumbling block for the embolic theory was the recurrent nature of similar symptoms with repeated episodes of transient ischemia. If a second TIA occurred, it was often with the same symptoms as seen during the previous attacks. How embolic debris could produce such repetitive symptoms was unclear. Two landmark studies served to resolve the conflict. First, the hemodynamics were evaluated by Kendall and Marshall.[33] In this study, patients with TIAs were subjected to pharmacologically induced hypotension. As the blood pressure was decreased, the patients were monitored for neurologic changes. None of these patients developed symptoms when their mean blood pressure was decreased significantly. Therefore hemodynamic causes of transient ischemia seemed less likely.[34]

The second study that ended the hemodynamic-embolic controversy was performed by Millikin at the Mayo Clinic.[35] In this study, baboons were anesthetized, and needles were inserted into the carotid flow. Small metallic beads were injected via these needles, and the brains were evaluated for the ultimate location of the beads. In a classic illustration from that study, the brain of one of the baboons was seen to have six beads lined up in the middle cerebral artery. The insertion of the beads at a specific point in the flow resulted in emboli at a specific destination determined by the laminar flow patterns in the artery. In other words, the origin of the embolus determined its ultimate resting point. Thus in one clear demonstration, the issue of recurrent symptoms resulting from multiple embolic events was resolved, confirming the embolic theory to be the best explanation for both TIAs and strokes.[36,37]

Given this evolution, the issue of hemodynamics has become a secondary issue in symptomatic cerebrovascular disease. Nonetheless, although certain patients clearly have flow compromise as an etiology for symptoms, the definition of them remains difficult. Anatomic studies have demonstrated that the circle of Willis, the traditional anatomic structure responsible for flow redistribution at the base of the brain, is incomplete in at least 25% of patients.[38,39] With an incomplete circle of Willis, blood flow may be limited in its redistribution, resulting in areas of potential underperfusion. With additional atherosclerotic obstruction of the cerebral vessels, collateral flow may be compromised because of one of these congenital abnormalities in the circle of Willis. With a complete circle of Willis, normal anterior (carotid) circulation equates with normal posterior perfusion, even in the absence of native vertebral flow. In contrast, if one or both posterior communicating arteries are absent, vertebral or basilar artery disease may result in posterior circulation symptoms with completely normal anterior circulation. Given the frequency of abnormalities in the circle of Willis, maldistribution of flow is certainly possible in the setting of severe carotid or vertebral artery stenosis or occlusion.

Hemodynamic issues remain important when discussing watershed ischemia. Watershed ischemia occurs when perfusion to a segment of the brain is limited hemodynamically to a level below the blood flow necessary to maintain cell integrity. Infarctions then occur at the junction between two blood supplies, the so-called watershed zones. Watershed ischemia remains a topic of some controversy, but its occurrence remains ill-defined and sporadic. The classic scenario for watershed infarction due to underlying hemodynamic compromise occurs most commonly with open heart surgery using cardiopulmonary bypass. If a critical stenosis or occlusion is present, the diminished perfusion associated with the nonpulsatile, limited pressure flow of the heart–lung machine can produce watershed infarction in an area at risk. Carotid endarterectomy prior to or simultaneous with coronary artery bypass surgery is done in an attempt to prevent these watershed infarctions.[40–42]

The possibility of hemodynamic flow disturbance is reinforced by the occurrence of reperfusion syndromes after surgical correction of severe carotid stenoses. In this scenario the severe upstream stenosis results in loss of autoregulation in the downstream cerebrovascular bed, with localized brain edema and risk of intracerebral hemorrhage resulting from reperfusion.[43,44] Clearly, this loss of autoregulation represents a flow-limited response to a hemodynamically significant stenosis.[45] The difficulty is that flow-related ischemia is diffuse rather than focal, and evaluation of flow limitation is difficult with conventional intracranial imaging. Nonetheless, positron emission tomography has provided a window into overall brain blood flow and metabolism[46] and provides experimental insights into the frequency of flow limitation in the clinical setting. For the present, however, the basis for diagnosis and treatment of cerebrovascular disease focuses on the presence of a potential embolic focus, rather than on any potential for cerebrovascular flow limitation.

## Diagnosis

Diagnostic testing in patients with cerebrovascular disease is essentially limited to two major areas: extracranial arterial imaging and intracranial arterial imaging. Each plays a fundamental role in the assessment of patients for carotid intervention. Because cerebral revascularization is focused on the extracranial carotid and vertebral arteries, arterial imaging is most important in these locations. Intracranial arterial imaging remains important, but its role continues to evolve as new modalities and technologies become available.

Anatomic definition in extracranial cerebrovascular disease is limited to two fundamental testing modalities: color duplex ultrasonography and arteriography. Each of these modalities has significant advantages and disadvantages, requiring more complete definition of their utility. Color duplex ultrasonography is a noninvasive technique for evaluating blood flow in any location accessible to an ultrasound beam. The carotid and vertebral circulations were the initial focus of vascular ultrasonography development and remain the test bed for ongoing research in ultrasonographic diagnosis. Consistent visualization can be achieved in this location, resulting in reproducible diagnostic assessment of the severity and pattern of stenosis. Estimation of the degree of stenosis is based on several criteria, including peak systolic velocity, internal carotid/common carotid velocity ratios, and end-diastolic velocity. The most widely used criteria are those of Strandness.[47] These criteria were developed to define percentage narrowing of the carotid bulb and have been verified in studies involving both angiographic and pathologic correlates.[48] Nonetheless, these criteria were developed to assess the degree of stenosis based on carotid bulb diameter reduction, rather than the more recent North American Symptomatic Carotid Endarterectomy Trial (NASCET) criteria. The true minimum arterial diameter occurs in the outflow vessel, away from the carotid bulb. For this reason, under NASCET guidelines the residual lumen in the bulb is compared to the minimum native internal carotid diameter distal to the bulb where the arterial walls become parallel once again. This system of measurement makes a given degree of bulb stenosis less impressive, requiring an adjustment in the percentage stenosis necessary for intervention. Nonetheless, all major studies on the carotid system now use the NASCET criteria rather than bulb diameter reduction.

The arteriographic assessment of cerebrovascular disease has remained essentially unchanged since the first cerebral angiogram by Moniz in 1927.[49] Angiography results from injection of a radiopaque tracer intraluminally followed by exposure of an x-ray film. The choice of tracer includes conventional iodine-containing high-osmolar contrast dye or newer low-osmolar contrast. Similarly, both conventional cut-film radiographs or digital subtraction images may be used for the permanent copy. No specific combination of techniques dominates the arteriographic diagnosis of cerebrovascular disease, and institutional experience is more important than perceived advantages of one technique over another.

The diagnosis of atherosclerosis by arteriography requires documentation of intraluminal narrowing of the involved artery viewed in two planes. Because angiography is fundamentally a two-dimensional technique and atherosclerosis is three-dimensional, the assessment of luminal narrowing requires perpendicular perspectives to state the degree of narrowing accurately. Measurement of internal carotid narrowing has traditionally been a calculation of the minimum residual lumen relative to an estimated arterial diameter in the carotid bulb. This estimation of the carotid bulb diameter is subject to interpretation and often results in overestimation of the degree of luminal narrowing. Fundamentally, the significance of any carotid stenosis resides in the degree of luminal encroachment relative to the outflow arterial diameter. As stated above, this approach was first applied to the assessment of arteriographic diameter reduction in the NASCET trial[50] and subsequently was used for the Asymptomatic Carotid Atherosclerosis Study (ACAS)[51] as well. This method has become the standard for measuring the arteriographic degree of carotid stenosis and should be the standard for reporting results.

With recent advances in magnetic resonance techniques, the possibility of a noninvasive technique for arterial imaging becomes more likely.[52] The difficulty with magnetic resonance angiography (MRA) lies in differentiating stenosis from occlusion. Any significant stenosis results in downstream turbulence. As a result, turbulence mixes once-aligned magnetic dipoles, resulting in signal dropout. Similarly, an absence of magnetic dipoles as is seen with arterial occlusion can also lead to signal dropout. Therefore conventional time-of-flight MRA techniques overestimate arterial stenoses, making diagnosis of stenosis versus occlusion reliant on other imaging techniques. Nonetheless, the combination of arterial imaging with intracranial parenchymal imaging makes MRA attractive in symptomatic patients. If surgery is contemplated, however, carotid evaluation with duplex ultrasonography or angiography in addition is necessary.

## Treatment

### Management of the Symptomatic Patient

Over the past few years, management of symptomatic carotid disease has progressed from an algorithm based on anecdotal reports to one based on significant scientific data owing primarily to publication of the NASCET study.[53] Thus with few exceptions, the prognosis of surgical versus medical management is clearly defined for the symptomatic population. Despite the data that exist, numerous questions arise specific to an elderly population.

The NASCET trial for patients with symptomatic carotid disease enrolled only patients less than 80 years of age for a randomized study of surgery versus medical therapy. Therefore although the conclusions remain important, the results of necessity must be extrapolated to the elderly population over 79 years of age. The NASCET trial was terminated early in the high-grade stenosis group because of the significant benefit of surgery relative to medical therapy in patients with more than 70% stenosis by NASCET criteria. Recently, these results have been extended to the patient population with 49–70% stenosis demonstrating similar (though more limited) benefits to surgical management.[54] Although these data remain the cornerstone of treatment decisions for symptomatic patients, many assumptions are necessary for applying these data to the elderly population.

In the NASCET severe stenosis (> 70%) group, a statistically beneficial result from surgical treatment was seen at the 3-month follow-up. Therefore patients with symptomatic carotid disease would be expected to benefit from surgery if their operative risk was acceptable and their life expectancy was at least 3 months. Obviously, most patients treated surgically would be expected to have a life expectancy of at least 3 months. Therefore the main issue of the decision to treat elderly symptomatic patients rests in the estimation of operative risk.

The operative risk associated with carotid disease centers on two factors: stroke risk and cardiac risk. Either factor may result in morbidity or mortality, but most studies report their results as a combined risk of stroke or death after endarterectomy. American Heart Association (AHA) guidelines[55] suggest that the upper limits for an acceptable stroke/death rate after carotid endarterectomy for TIAs should be 5%. In the NASCET trial, it was in fact 5.8% overall. Monitoring surgeon-specific and institution-specific stroke/death rates after carotid endarterectomy are a basic requirement for recommending surgical revascularization. Many investigators have studied the stroke/death rates after carotid endarterectomy in elderly patients.[56–73] There does not appear to be dramatically increased operative risks due to age alone, as most studies support the use of surgical endarterectomy in the elderly. Nonetheless, all surgical series suffer from an inherent selection bias: Patients at too high risk or who are too ill may simply never be offered the procedure, skewing the results further in favor of operative intervention. In the NASCET trial this bias was applied equally to both groups, as the randomization occurred between medical and surgical therapy only after patient entry. Therefore all candidates in this study were appropriate for surgical management. In retrospective studies concerning the safety of carotid endarterectomy in the elderly, these controls do not exist, resulting in potential selection bias. These data demonstrate that the stroke/death rate after carotid endarterectomy in the elderly is not significantly increased over that of a more traditional patient population.

The risk of anesthesia for carotid endarterectomy has been a topic of debate for many years. Although general anesthesia is a safe, effective technique for operations on the carotid artery, proponents of local or regional anesthesia argue that the intensive care unit (ICU) stay[74] and overall length of stay[75] are both reduced, thus decreasing cost. The basic philosophy is inextricably bound to that of shunt usage: Surgeons who routinely shunt intraoperatively are more likely to use general anesthesia, as neurologic monitoring is optional. If selective shunting is employed, the decision to shunt rests on the detection of neurologic changes suggestive of cerebral ischemia. In the patient under general anesthesia, this can be provided by continuous electroencephalographic (EEG) monitoring using either a formal 16-lead EEG or compressed spectral array EEG. In the patient under regional anesthesia, neurologic monitoring is more direct, resulting from changes in the patient's neurologic examination while undergoing surgery. No evidence exists to support one anesthetic or shunting technique over another in the elderly patient undergoing carotid endarterectomy.

In summary, any patient who is symptomatic because of extracranial carotid atherosclerosis and is an acceptable operative risk should be offered surgical intervention. The benefits of surgical revascularization are clear-cut, with improved outcome at both short-term and long-term follow-up. The anesthetic and shunt techniques used for carotid surgery are equally applicable in this population and remain safe.

Despite the data supporting carotid endarterectomy as a safe, effective technique for managing extracranial carotid disease, some studies[76] have proposed that operative intervention is too great a risk for some patients and therefore percutaneous intraluminal treatment should be offered using balloon angioplasty and placement of carotid stents. If a role exists for this modality, it is likely in the high risk symptomatic patient, in whom the risk of any anesthesia or operative intervention is prohibitive. Many authors are at a loss to define such a high risk group, and it is likely that the National Institutes of Health (NIH) will fund a prospective trial of carotid endarterectomy versus carotid angioplasty and stent for the patient with carotid atherosclerosis in the near future. Carotid angioplasty and stenting remains an experimental technique and should be reserved for use in centers participating in its evaluation and study. The safety and efficacy of carotid endarterectomy under regional anesthesia is so well established it can be utilized in most patients in need of intervention, including the high risk patient with a high bifurcation of the carotid artery or even reoperative carotid intervention.[77,78] Therefore the ultimate role of carotid angioplasty and stent placement remains to be defined.[79–81]

## Management of the Asymptomatic Patient

With publication of the ACAS trial,[82] many questions related to the management of asymptomatic extracranial vascular disease were answered, but many more were raised. Although a statistically significant decrease in stroke rate was achieved in patients with at least 60% stenosis of the internal carotid artery, this protocol was limited to a population less than 79 years old. Therefore extrapolation is necessary to apply these data to the very elderly population. In the ACAS trial, the patient group who most significantly benefited from prophylactic carotid endarterectomy were men, with a 79% risk reduction at the 5-year follow-up. Nonetheless, in this group the absolute risk reduction at 5 years was only 8%, yielding a yearly risk reduction of only 1.6%. Given this modest risk reduction, the procedure-related stroke/death rate of 2.3% becomes an important determinant of the overall benefit. If the operative morbidity and mortality of carotid endarterectomy are excessive, the benefit is reduced further and the overall efficacy reduced. Once again, the surgeon-specific and institution-specific risks must be accurately defined prior to recommending intervention. Similarly, the risk of operation in any given patient must be considered carefully, as any increase in operative stroke or death risk tempers the benefits seen. The stroke/death risk of cerebral angiography in the ACAS trial was surprisingly high at 1.2%. Therefore the routine use of angiography further elevates the morbidity and mortality, potentially compromising the benefit of endarterectomy. Currently, many centers have adopted new strategies to lower the risk of carotid intervention in asymptomatic individuals. Foremost in this strategy is the elimination of routine arteriography prior to carotid surgery. Angiography is reserved for patients in whom unexplained findings are present on preoperative duplex ultrasonography. Using this strategy of selective angiography, preoperative arteriograms can be avoided in up to 85% of the patients, lowering the risk of angiography (by extrapolation of ACAS data) to less than 0.2%. The loss of routine preoperative angiography in carotid surgery has two risks: failure to diagnose tandem intracranial or proximal lesions and failure to diagnose the high carotid bifurcation preoperatively. The risk of tandem lesions resides in the limitations to flow imposed across a fresh endarterectomy by a proximal or downstream lesion. Nonetheless, the risk of stroke following endarterectomy has not been documented to be higher in patients with tandem lesions.[83,84] Similarly, tandem lesions do not seem to impose an increased stroke risk after successful extracranial carotid endarterectomy.[85,86] Therefore the risk of surgery and the risk of subsequent stroke are not significantly increased by the presence of tandem lesions. It appears that tandem carotid and intracranial stenosis occurs in fewer than 10–15% of patients with carotid stenosis,[87] implying that angiography contributes little to the management of most of these patients.[88,89]

The relative risk imposed by a high carotid bifurcation is much more difficult to define. Although numerous strategies have been developed to assist the surgical approach to the high carotid lesion, none has been without complications. The incremental benefit of knowing preoperatively that the bifurcation is higher than usual resides in the ability to change the surgical approach to compensate for the anatomic variation and improve the ease of operation. Because there does not appear to be a widely accepted alternative to the conventional approach, the preoperative diagnosis of a high carotid bifurcation serves only to provide a psychological advantage to the surgeon rather than a physical one. No data exist to justify the use of preoperative angiography to define the high carotid bifurcation.

Although operation for asymptomatic carotid stenosis is an accepted technique, particularly in the male patient, there clearly are questions about who should undergo this treatment option. Foremost in this regard is the estimation of the patient's life expectancy. If an annual benefit of 1.2% stroke reduction is to be realized with surgery compared to medical management, the longer the patient survives after endarterectomy the greater the benefit of operation. Similarly, as discussed above, if the patient is at high risk during surgery (for any reason), the annual benefit of surgery decreases. Therefore patient selection for asymptomatic carotid endarterectomy requires consideration of the patient's risk during operation and the patient's overall health and life expectancy. If for any reason the patient's risk during operation is increased, medical management should be considered. Likewise, if the patient's health is so fragile that reliable long-term life expectancy cannot be assumed, medical management may be the best option.

In an in-depth cost analysis of carotid endarterectomy for asymptomatic disease, Cronenwett and colleagues estimated the cost-effectiveness of carotid endarterectomy with advancing age.[90] Although the cost-effectiveness of carotid endarterectomy under age 72 seemed conclusive, the costs increased exponentially to age 79 where the cost-effectiveness was marginal. By this algorithm, carotid endarterectomy for asymptomatic disease would not be considered cost-effective at age 80 or above. This is a theoretic issue related to an "average" elderly population. Obviously, some elderly patients have sufficient long-term survival to warrant carotid endarterectomy. Others just as obviously are medical candidates only. The difficulty remains in those in-between cases where selection criteria and operative risk are not clear-cut. In these situations, an in-depth analysis of risk and benefit is probably secondary to a truly informed consent discussion with the patient and family. In this way, the ultimate decision is left to the individual most directly involved, with the surgeon providing guidance where appropriate.

## Special Issues Related to Aging

Although carotid disease in general increases with increasing age, certain issues arise with aging that require further discussion. All of these problems can occur at any age, but the increased incidence in the elderly population requires explanation and elaboration.

### Tortuosity of the Carotid Arteries

The coiling and kinking of the carotid arteries can be severe, resulting in stenosis or even complete vascular loops. The first references to carotid artery tortuosity appeared in relation to tonsillectomy, where the tortuous artery proved to be at risk for inadvertent injury.[91] The first recognition of neurologic symptoms referable to carotid artery tortuosity was during the early 1950s, with recommendations for arteriopexy of the artery to the sternocleidomastoid muscle.[92] During the late 1950s, cases of cortical stroke associated with carotid kinks were reported, with successful treatment in all cases by arterial resection.[93] From this point forward, the standard treatment of carotid coils was resection of the redundant artery, which continues to be the treatment of choice today.

For a number of reasons, the exact incidence of extreme tortuosity of the extracranial carotid arteries is difficult to determine. Many patients are asymptomatic and may never come to medical attention. This situation is further confused by the lack of standard definitions as to what constitutes a kink, a coil, or a tortuosity. Tortuosity has been defined as excessive length of an artery. This is a relative judgment, and the lengthening of the arterial tree is limited by fixation at branch points. Therefore elongation often results in tortuosity moving away from bifurcations. If the elongation occurs between two points of fixation, kinks or coils can occur. Kinks are defined as an abrupt change in the direction of the artery, reducing the diameter of the arterial lumen. Coils are redundant loops of artery without luminal encroachment, lacking the acute change in direction. Both kinks and coils are subsets of the vessels exhibiting tortuosity, all of which can lead to boundary layer separation with an associated increased risk of cerebrovascular events.

Angiographic studies suggest that tortuosity is common in the carotid circulation, occurring in 31% of 1438 consecutive carotid arteriograms in one study.[94] In the same series, coils were seen in 7% and kinks in 5%. An additional study of 1000 consecutive arteriograms suggested a 16% incidence of kinks.[95] The incidence of kinks has been associated with female sex, advanced age, hypertension, kyphosis, and obesity.[17,18,96] Estimates have suggested that fewer than 5% of patients with carotid atherosclerosis who come to operative intervention have clinically significant associated carotid tortuosity.

As previously outlined, the main therapy for carotid tortuosity or kinking is resection of the redundant segment. A detailed discussion of the techniques of resection and reanastomosis is beyond the scope of this chapter, but segmental resection of either the internal or common carotid artery, with or without carotid endarterectomy, is the standard treatment. Using this technique, successful outcomes with low stroke rates are the norm.[97]

## "Dizziness" and Other Global Symptoms

The incidence of dizziness, vertigo, and syncope in the elderly population is epidemic, affecting an estimated 50% of the population over 65 years of age.[98] The causes of these symptoms are myriad, including inner ear problems, vision problems, loss of sympathetic tone, and cerebrovascular disease. Of all the symptoms related to cerebrovascular disease, this one remains unlikely to be related to cerebral blood flow. Because dizziness is a global rather than cortical symptom, the extent of cerebrovascular disease must be extreme if the symptoms are to arise from atherosclerotic disease.

Typical "drop" attacks associated with posterior circulation disease relates to loss of motor function due to cerebellar ischemia, often without loss of consciousness (cortical perfusion). These episodes are rare in the absence of combined system disease; if posterior circulation vascular disease is the only atherosclerosis present, no symptoms occur. Only when posterior disease is combined with circle of Willis or carotid disease do symptoms typically occur. If only 15% of the population over age 65 have carotid disease, a substantially smaller population of these individuals would be expected to have significant posterior circulation disease in addition. No matter how the calculations are derived, most dizziness cannot be accounted for by atherosclerotic obstruction.

## Postmenopausal Hormone Replacement and Carotid Disease

Perhaps the major risk factor for atherosclerosis is being of the male sex, presumably because of the effects of estrogen on the arterial wall. Therefore changes in the hormonal milieu after menopause may predispose to the development of atherosclerosis in women. Hormone replacement therapy (HRT) seems to be associated with a significant decrement in cardiovascular risk.[99,100] Because of its ready accessibility, the cerebrovascular circulation is an area of intense investigation regarding the mechanisms of atherosclerosis reduction associated with HRT. At least three changes associated with HRT in postmenopausal women have been noted in the carotid circulation: intimal thickness and the predisposition to atherosclerosis, changes in plasma fibrinolytic activity, and changes in cerebral blood flow with hormonal therapy.

The most readily accessible site for assessment of early atherosclerosis remains the carotid bifurcation.[101] The presence of significant vascular disease can be predicted with reasonable accuracy using duplex ultrasonography to measure wall thickness. Therefore as a screening tool for atherosclerosis, carotid duplex ultrasonography may play an increasing role in the future.

## Conclusions

Carotid disease is a continuing issue in the care of the elderly. The incidence of cerebrovascular disease is increasing as the population ages, resulting in an ever-greater focus on the appropriateness of vascular care in this population. Although future studies may refine the overall management of cerebrovascular disease in the elderly, the need for endarterectomy in symptomatic and asymptomatic patients with significant carotid disease has been better defined than vascular disease in virtually any other distribution. No other area of vascular disease has been subjected to two large, prospective, randomized trials as has been done with carotid disease. Therefore the utility of carotid endarterectomy has been uniquely studied, unlike any other surgical procedure.

The future direction of carotid intervention clearly includes trials of carotid angioplasty and stent placement. Nonetheless, current standards of carotid endarterectomy allow accurate comparisons with any future results from trials of these therapies. These data are critical to making effective therapeutic decisions for this increasingly common disease.

## References

1. Robins M, Baum HM. National survey of stroke incidence. Stroke 1981;12(suppl 1):45–57.

2. Matsumoto N, Whisnant JP, Kurland LT, et al. Natural history of stroke in Rochester, Minnesota, 1955 through 1969: an extension of a previous study, 1945 through 1954. Stroke 1973;4:20–29.
3. Pokras R, Dyken ML. Dramatic changes in the performance of endarterectomy for diseases of the extracranial arteries in the head. Stroke 1988;19:1289–1296.
4. Day JC. Population Projections of the United States by Age, Sex, Race, and Hispanic Origin: 1995 to 2050. U.S. Bureau of the Census, Current Population Reports, P25–1130. Government Printing Office: Washington, DC, 1996.
5. Wolf PA, Kannel WB, Dawber TR. Prospective investigation: the Framingham study and the epidemiology of stroke. Adv Neurol 1978;19:107–120.
6. Tell GS, Polak JF, Ward BJ, et al. Relation of smoking with carotid artery wall thickness and stenosis in older adults: the Cardiovascular Health Study; the Cardiovascular Health Study (CHS) Collaborative Research Group. Circulation 1994;90:2905–2908.
7. Glagov S, Rowley DA, Kohut R. Atherosclerosis of human aorta and its coronary and renal arteries. Arch Pathol Lab Med 1961;72:558–562.
8. Bell ET. Atherosclerotic gangrene of the lower extremities in diabetic and nondiabetic persons. Am J Clin Pathol 1957;28:27–35.
9. Selhub J, Jacques PF, Bostom AG, et al. Association between plasma homocysteine concentrations and extracranial carotid-artery stenosis. N Engl J Med 1995;332: 286–291.
10. Kannel WB, Castelli WP, Gordon T, et al. Serum cholesterol, lipoprotein, and the risk of coronary heart disease: the Framingham study. Ann Intern Med 1971;74:1–12.
11. Lipids Research Clinics Program. The Lipids Research Clinics Primary Prevention Trials results. II. The relationship of reduction and incidence of coronary heart disease to cholesterol lowering. JAMA 1984;251:365–374.
12. Multiple Risk Factor Intervention Trial Research Group. Multiple Risk Factor Intervention Trial: risk factor changes and mortality rates. JAMA 1982;248:1465–1477.
13. Kang SS, Wong PW, Malinow MR. Hyperhomocyst(e)inemia as a risk factor for occlusive vascular disease. Annu Rev Nutr 1992;12:279–298.
14. Ueland PM, Refsum H, Brattström L. Plasma homocysteine and cardiac disease. In: Francis RB (ed) Atherosclerotic Cardiovascular Disease, Hemostasis, and Endothelial Function. New York: Marcel Dekker, 1992:183–236.
15. Nygärd O, Nordrehaug JE, Refsum H, et al. Plasma homocysteine levels and mortality in patients with coronary artery disease. N Engl J Med 1997;337:230–236.
16. Cornfeld J. Joint dependence of risk of coronary heart disease on serum cholesterol and systolic blood pressure. Fed Proc 1962;21(suppl 2):58.
17. O'Leary DH, Anderson KM, Wolf PA, et al. Cholesterol and carotid atherosclerosis in older persons: the Framingham study. Ann Epidemiol 1992;2:147–153.
18. Sacks FM, Pfeffer MA, Moye LA, et al. The effect of pravastatin on coronary events after myocardial infarction in patients with average cholesterol levels. N Engl J Med 1996;335:1001–1009.
19. Ross R. The pathogenesis of atherosclerosis: an update. N Engl J Med 1986;14:488–500.
20. Ross R. Atherosclerosis: an inflammatory disease. N Engl J Med 1999;340:115–126.
21. Bild DE, Fitzpatrick A, Fried LP, et al. Age-related trends in cardiovascular morbidity and physical functioning in the elderly: the cardiovascular health study. J Am Geriatr Soc 1993;41:1047–1056.
22. Weber G, Bianciardi G, Bussani MD, et al. Atherosclerosis and aging: a morphometric study on arterial lesions of elderly and very elderly necropsy subjects. Arch Pathol Lab Med 1988;112:1066–1070.
23. Homma S, Ishida H, Hasegawa H, et al. Carotid intima-medial thickness and the occurrence of plaque in centenarians: data from the Tokyo Centenarian Study. Jpn J Geriatr 1997;34:139–146.
24. Weber G, Bianciardi G, Bussani R, et al. Atherosclerosis and aging: a morphometric study on arterial lesions of elderly and very elderly necropsy subjects. Arch Pathol Lab Med 1988;112:1066–1070.
25. Shuaib A, Boyle C. Stroke in the elderly. Curr Opin Neurol 1994;7:41–47.
26. Zarins CK, Giddens DP, Bharadvaj BK, et al. Carotid bifurcation atherosclerosis: quantitative correlation of plaque localization with flow velocity profiles and wall shear stress. Circ Res 1983;53:502–514.
27. Theile BL, Strandness DE. Distribution of intracranial and extracranial arterial lesions in patients with symptomatic cerebrovascular disease. In: Bernstein EF (ed) Vascular Diagnosis, 4th ed. Mosby: St. Louis, 1993:302–307.
28. Imparato AM, Riles TS, Mintzer R, et al. The importance of hemorrhage in the relationship between gross morphologic characteristics and cerebral symptoms in 376 carotid artery plaques. Ann Surg 1983;197:195–203.
29. Lusby RJ, Ferrell LD, Ehrenfeld WK, et al. Carotid plaque hemorrhage: its role in production of cerebral ischemia. Arch Surg 1982;117:1479–1488.
30. Fryer JA, Myers PC, Appleberg M. Carotid intraplaque hemorrhage: the significance of neovascularity. J Vasc Surg 1987;6:341–349.
31. Persson AV, Robichaux WT, Silverman M. The natural history of carotid plaque development. Arch Surg 1983;118:1048–1052.
32. Polak JF, O'Leary DH, Kronmal RA, et al. Sonographic evaluation of carotid artery atherosclerosis in the elderly: relationship of disease severity to stroke and transient ischemic attack. Radiology 1993;188:363–370.
33. Kendall RE, Marshall J. Role of hypotension in the genesis of transient focal cerebral ischemic attacks. Br Med J 1963; 2:344–248.
34. Fazekas JF, Alman RW. The role of hypotension in transitory focal cerebral ischemia. Am J Med Sci 1964;248: 567–570.
35. Millikin CH. The pathogenesis of transient focal cerebral ischemia. Circulation 1965;32:438–448.
36. Brass LM, Fayad PB, Levine SR. Transient ischemic attacks in the elderly: diagnosis and treatment. Geriatrics 1992; 47:36–53.
37. Perez-Burkhardt JL, Gonzalez-Fajardo JA, Rodriguez E, Mateo AM. Amaurosis fugax as a symptom of carotid artery stenosis: its relationship with ulcerated plaque. J Cardiovasc Surg (Torino) 1994;35:15–18.

38. Alpers BJ, Berry RG, Paddison RM. Anatomical studies of the circle of Willis in normal brain. Arch Neurol Psychiatry 1959;81:409–422.
39. Powers WJ, Press GW, Grubb RL, et al. The effect of hemodynamically significant carotid artery disease on the hemodynamic status of the cerebral circulation. Ann Intern Med 1987;106:27–35.
40. Berens ES, Kouchoukos NT, Murphy SF, Wareing TH. Preoperative carotid artery screening in elderly patients undergoing cardiac surgery. J Vasc Surg 1992;15:313–321.
41. Halpin DP, Riggins S, Carmichael JD, et al. Management of coexistent carotid and coronary artery disease. South Med J 1994;87:187–189.
42. Sayers RD, Thompson MM, Underwood MJ, et al. Early results of combined carotid endarterectomy and coronary artery bypass grafting in patients with severe coronary and carotid artery disease. J R Coll Surg Edinb 1993;38:340–343.
43. Reigel MM, Hollier LH, Sundt TM, et al. Cerebral hyperperfusion syndrome: a cause of neurologic dysfunction after carotid endarterectomy. J Vasc Surg 1987;5:628–634.
44. Powers AD, Smith RR. Hyperperfusion syndrome after carotid endarterectomy: a transcranial Doppler evaluation. Neurosurgery 1990;26:56–60.
45. Naylor AR, Merrick MV, Gillespie I, et al. Prevalence of impaired cerebrovascular reserve in patients with symptomatic carotid artery disease. Br J Surg 1994;81:45–48.
46. Syrota A, Castaing M, Rougemont D, et al. Tissue acid-base balance and oxygen metabolism in human cerebral infarction studied with positron emission tomography. Ann Neurol 1983;14:419–428.
47. Zierler RE, Phillips DJ, Beach KW, et al. Noninvasive assessment of normal carotid bifurcation hemodynamics with color-flow ultrasound imaging. Ultrasound Med Biol 1987;13:471–476.
48. Zierler RE, Kohler TR, Strandness DE. Duplex scanning of normal or minimally diseased carotid arteries: correlation with arteriography and clinical outcome. J Vasc Surg 1990;12:447–454.
49. Moniz E. L'encéphalographie artérielle, son importance dans la localisation des tumeurs cérébrales. Rev Neurol 1927;2:72.
50. Eliasziw M, Smith RF, Singh N, et al. Further comments on the measurement of carotid stenosis from angiograms. Stroke 1994;25:2445–2449.
51. Executive Committee for the Asymptomatic Carotid Atherosclerosis Study. Endarterectomy for asymptomatic carotid artery stenosis. JAMA 1995;273:1421–1428.
52. Mittl RL Jr, Broderick M, Carpenter JP, et al. Blinded-reader comparison of magnetic resonance angiography and duplex ultrasonography for carotid artery bifurcation stenosis. Stroke 1994;25:4–10.
53. North American Symptomatic Carotid Endarterectomy Trial Collaborators. Beneficial effects of carotid endarterectomy in symptomatic patients with high-grade carotid stenosis. N Engl J Med 1991;325:445–453.
54. Barnett HJM, Taylor DW, Eliasziw M, et al. Benefit of carotid endarterectomy in patients with symptomatic moderate or severe stenosis. N Engl J Med 1998;339: 1415–1425.
55. Moore WS, Barnett HJ, Beebe HG, et al. Guidelines for carotid endarterectomy: a multidisciplinary consensus statement from the Ad Hoc Committee, American Heart Association. Circulation 1995;91:566–579.
56. Treiman RL, Wagner WH, Foran RF, et al. Carotid endarterectomy in the elderly. Ann Vasc Surg 1992;6: 321–324.
57. Nunnelee JD, Kurgan A, Auer AI. Carotid endarterectomy in elderly vascular patients: experience in a community hospital. Geriatr Nurs 1995;16:121–123.
58. Perler BA, Dardik A, Burleyson GP, et al. Influence of age and hospital volume on the results of carotid endarterectomy: a statewide analysis of 9918 cases. J Vasc Surg 1998; 27:25–33.
59. Fisher ES, Malenka DJ, Solomon NA, et al. Risk of carotid endarterectomy in the elderly. Am J Public Health 1989;79:1617–1620.
60. Schultz RD, Feldhaus RJ. Carotid endarterectomy in octogenarians and nonagenarians. Surg Gynecol Obstet 1988;166:245–251.
61. Wong DT, Ballard JL, Killeen JD. Carotid endarterectomy and abdominal aortic aneurysm repair: are these reasonable treatments for patients over age 80? Am Surg 1998;64:998–1001.
62. Kerdiles Y, Lucas A, Podeur L, et al. Results of carotid surgery in elderly patients. J Cardiovasc Surg (Torino) 1997;38:327–334.
63. Van Damme H, Lacroix H, Desiron Q, et al. Carotid surgery in octogenarians: is it worthwhile? Acta Chir Belg 1996;96:71–77.
64. Thomas PC, Grigg M. Carotid artery surgery in the octogenarian. Aust NZ J Surg 1996;66:231–234.
65. Favre JP, Guy JM, Frering V, et al. Carotid surgery in the octogenarian. Ann Vasc Surg 1994;8:421–426.
66. Coyle KA, Smith RB, Salam AA, et al. Carotid endarterectomy in the octogenarian. Ann Vasc Surg 1994;8:417–420.
67. Perler BA, Williams GM. Carotid endarterectomy in the very elderly: is it worthwhile? Surgery 1994;116:479–483.
68. Meyer FB, Meissner I, Fode NC, et al. Carotid endarterectomy in elderly patients. Mayo Clin Proc 1991;66:464–469.
69. Brooks RH, Park RE, Chassin MR, et al. Carotid endarterectomy for elderly patients: predicting complications. Ann Intern Med 1990;113:747–753.
70. Pinkerton JA, Gholkar VR. Should patient age be a consideration in carotid endarterectomy? J Vasc Surg 1990;11:650–658.
71. Ouriel K, Penn TE, Ricotta JJ, et al. Carotid endarterectomy in the elderly patient. Surg Gynecol Obstet 1986;162: 334–336.
72. Perler BA. Vascular disease in the elderly patient. Surg Clin North Am 1994;74:199–216.
73. Roques XF, Baudet EM, Clerc F. Results of carotid endarterectomy in patients 75 years of age and older. J Cardiovasc Surg (Torino) 1991;32:726–731.
74. Back MR, Harward TR, Huber TS, et al. Improving the cost-effectiveness of carotid endarterectomy. J Vasc Surg 1997;26:456–462.
75. Allen BT, Anderson CB, Rubin BG, et al. The influence of anesthetic technique on perioperative complications after carotid endarterectomy. J Vasc Surg 1994;19:834–843.
76. Yadav JS, Roubin GS, Iyer S, et al. Elective stenting of the extracranial carotid arteries. Circulation 1997;95: 376–381.

77. Imparato AM, Ramirez A, Riles T, et al. Cerebral protection in carotid surgery. Arch Surg 1982;117:1703–1708.
78. Hafner CD, Evans WE. Carotid endarterectomy with local anesthesia. J Vasc Surg 1988;7:231–239.
79. Stanley JC, Abbott WM, Towne JB, et al. Statement regarding carotid angioplasty and stenting. J Vasc Surg 1996;24: 900.
80. Beebe HG, Archie JP, Baker WH, et al. Concern about the safety of carotid angioplasty. Stroke 1996;27:197–198.
81. Bergeon P, Rudondy P, Benichou H, et al. Transluminal angioplasty for recurrent stenosis after carotid endarterectomy: prognostic factors and indications. Int Angiol 1993;12:256–259.
82. Executive Committee for the Asymptomatic Carotid Atherosclerosis Study. Endarterectomy for asymptomatic carotid artery stenosis. JAMA 1995;273:1421–1428.
83. Moore WS. Does tandem lesion mean tandem risk in patients with carotid artery disease? J Vasc Surg 1988;7: 454–455.
84. Lord RS, Raj TB, Graham AR. Carotid endarterectomy, siphon stenosis, collateral hemispheric pressure and perioperative cerebral infarction. J Vasc Surg 1987;6:391–397.
85. Schuler JJ, Flanigan DP, Lim LT, et al. The effect of carotid siphon stenosis on stroke rate, death, and relief of symptoms following elective carotid endarterectomy. Surgery 1982;92:1058–1067.
86. Borozean PG, Schuler JJ, LaRosa MP, et al. The natural history of isolated carotid siphon stenosis. J Vasc Surg 1984;1:744–749.
87. Akers DL, Bell WH, Kerstein MD. Does intracranial dye study contribute to evaluation of carotid disease? Am J Surg 1988;156:87–90.
88. Ricotta JJ, Holen J, Schenk E, et al. Is routine angiography necessary prior to carotid endarterectomy? J Vasc Surg 1984;1:96–102.
89. Moore WS, Ziomek S, Quiñones-Baldrich WJ, et al. Can clinical evaluation and noninvasive testing substitute for arteriography in the evaluation of carotid artery disease? Ann Surg 1988;298:91–94.
90. Cronenwett JL, Birkmeyer JD, Nackman GB, et al. Cost-effectiveness of carotid endarterectomy in asymptomatic patients. J Vasc Surg 1997;25:298–311.
91. Kelly AB. Pulsating vessels in the pharynx. Glasgow Med J 1891;49:28–30.
92. Riser MM, Geraud J, Ducoudray J, et al. Dolicho-carotide interne avec syndrome vertigneux. Rev Neurol 1951;85: 10–12.
93. Quattlebaum JK, Upson ET, Neville RL. Stroke associated with elongation and kinking of the internal carotid artery. Ann Surg 1959;150:824–832.
94. Weibel J, Fields WS. Tortuosity, coiling and kinking of the internal carotid artery. I. Etiology and radiographic anatomy. Neurology 1965;15:7–11.
95. Metz H, Murray-Leslie RM, Bannister RG, et al. Kinking of the internal carotid artery. Lancet 1961;1:424–426.
96. Bauer R, Sheehan S, Meyer JS. Arteriographic study of cerebrovascular disease. II. Cerebral symptoms due to kinking, tortuosity, and compression of carotid and vertebral arteries in the neck. Arch Neurol 1961;4:119.
97. Mascoli F, Mari C, Liboni A, et al. The elongation of the internal carotid artery: diagnosis and surgical treatment. J Cardiovasc Surg 1987;28:9–11.
98. Yardley L, Owen N, Nazareth I, Luxon L. Prevalence and presentation of dizziness in a general practice community sample of working age people. Br J Gen Pract 1998;48: 1131–1135.
99. Jonas HA, Kronmal RA, Psaty BM, et al. Current estrogen-progestin and estrogen replacement therapy in elderly women: association with carotid atherosclerosis: CHS Collaborative Research Group Cardiovascular Health Study. Ann Epidemiol 1996;6:314–323.
100. Manolio TA, Furberg CD, Shemanski L, et al. Associations of postmenopausal estrogen use with cardiovascular disease and its risk factors in older women: the CHS Collaborative Research Group. Circulation 1993;88:2163–2171.
101. Niskanen L, Rauramaa R, Miettinen H, et al. Carotid artery intima-media thickness in elderly patients with NIDDM and in nondiabetic subjects. Stroke 1996;27:1986–1992.

# *Part II*
# *Specific Issues in Geriatric Surgery*

## Section 6
## Gastrointestinal System

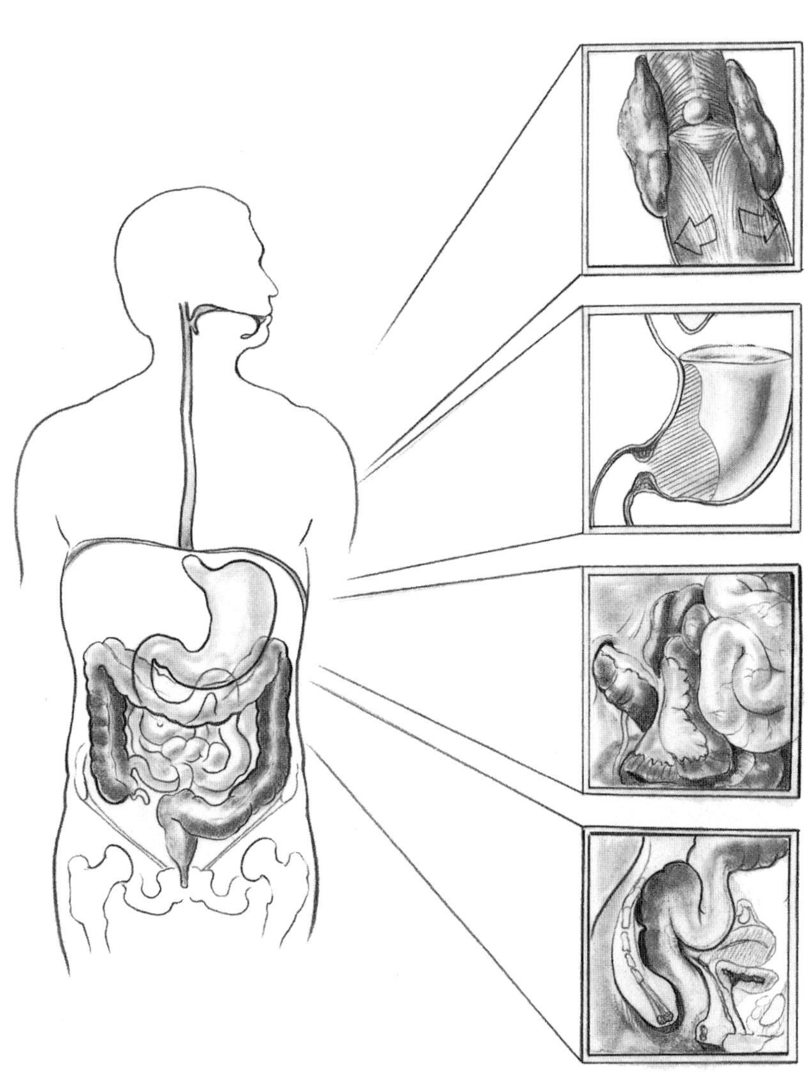

# Invited Commentary: Gastrointestinal System

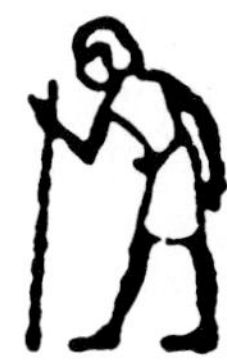

William Silen

There are two basic tenets of gerontology: (1) do not harm the aged with large numbers or amounts of poisonous drugs; and (2) excessive and traumatic manipulations are to be scrupulously avoided. When consideration is given to surgical procedures in the aged, physiologic and functional status are far more important than chronologic age. To assess these factors, an exquisitely detailed history and physical examination are in order so the surgeon is prepared to manage the octogenarian more readily pre- and postoperatively. Unfortunately, the advent of superspecialization and managed care has seriously eroded the ability and inclination of the surgeon to engage in such activities, to the detriment of both the patient and the surgeon. Excellent surgeons are eclectic physicians with one additional therapeutic tool not available to other specialists. Whether such eclecticism will become extinct in the current milieu remains to be seen.

The aged usually require only small doses of drugs and should be given narcotics sparingly. This is not a cruel practice but, rather, recognizes that pain is often of a much lesser magnitude than in younger persons. The most catastrophic of intraabdominal events (e.g., an embolus to the superior mesenteric artery) may be accompanied by surprisingly mild pain, especially during the first 24 hours. Confusion and disorientation are common and are most often caused by doses of narcotics usually well tolerated by younger individuals. Confinement to bed and somnolence induced by relatively small doses of narcotics often result in pulmonary atelectasis and pneumonia.

Well-conditioned octogenarians tolerate operations and the accompanying perturbations much more readily than do those who have been sedentary and whose functional reserve is small. Nevertheless, multiple investigations and manipulations such as colonoscopy followed by an encounter on the same or succeeding day with a computed tomography (CT) scanner are extremely debilitating for even the well-conditioned, older person. The need for repeated tests and procedures should be carefully considered and kept to an absolute minimum when possible. Maneuvers that tie the patient to a bed, such as nasogastric tubes attached to suction, should be avoided. Parenthetically, the routine use of nasogastric tubes during the postoperative period for patients undergoing extensive gastrointestinal surgery has been shown conclusively in several excellent studies to be adverse.[1] Yet their reflexive use on many services continues to plague patients, especially the elderly, despite the demonstration that not only do these tubes cause more complications (e.g., sinusitis otitis, sore throat, pulmonary atelectasis and infections, gastroesophageal reflux), but, amazingly enough, recovery from ileus is less rapid than when such tubes are omitted completely. It is a serious reflection on our profession that solid evidence-based data are ignored because of anecdotal experience or preconceived notions.

Abdominal incisions are solely a means of access and as such should be as free of morbidity as possible. The two currently most commonly employed incisions, the midline and the unilateral or bilateral subcostal incisions, have been shown conclusively to be associated with far more morbidity than other, safer approaches such as a paramedian incision.[2] The midline incision is heir to the development of incisional hernia in about 15% of cases by 2–3 years, the permanent repair of which is no insignificant task, whereas incisional hernia occurs in only 0.33% of paramedian incisions at 1 year. Dehiscence, which develops in less than 0.05% of paramedian incisions, occurs in about 2–3% of midline incisions. Are a few minutes saved while opening and closing midline incisions worth these complications? Has anyone compared the savings in time of execution of a midline incision (15–20 minutes in most studies) with the lost time and morbidity of the dehiscences and hernias these incisions generate? Dehiscence in an octogenarian is a complication of major proportion and in some instances, begins the all too common cascade of adverse events leading ultimately in death.

Subcostal incisions result in irreparable damage to intercostal nerves, causing atrophy and weakness of the rectus muscles of varying degree, depending on how far laterally the incisions are carried. Many of these patients suffer significant difficulty when arising from the supine position, especially after the bilateral procedure. This is a serious handicap to the elderly, sedentary patient. We must examine in a most critical way the continued employment of such morbid procedures in all patients and especially in the aged. The advent of laparoscopic techniques has reduced some of these problems, but because open operations are still required in many instances, rigid adherence to the use of morbid incisions is to be denounced.

Complications are tolerated far more poorly in the aged than in younger, fitter individuals. Thus every effort must be made to plan operative procedures that are associated with the lowest possible morbidity. Less radical and more conservative operations should always be given the most serious consideration in the aged patient.

Surgery has come a long way during the past 10–15 years, but we still have a long road to travel. Only evidence-based practice can help us along this journey. We must imbue the next generation of surgeons with the knowledge and will to exercise the most careful evaluation of what we do and how we practice. We must vigorously oppose external influences, such as managed-care moguls, from causing us to use techniques that produce short-term financial gains.

## References

1. Cheadle WG, Vitale GC, Mackie CR, Cushieri A. Prophylactic postoperative nasogastric decompression: a prospective study of its requirement and the influence of cimetidine in 200 patients. Ann Surg 1985;202:361–366.
2. Cahalane MJ, Shapiro ME, Silen W. Abdominal incision: decision of indecision. Lancet 1989;8630:146–148.

# 36
# Age-Related Physiologic Changes in the Gastrointestinal Tract

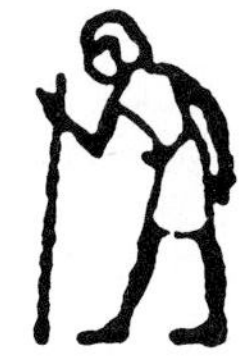

Joshua L. Levine and Michael E. Zenilman

The multitude of changes that take place in the gastrointestinal tract throughout the life of a human have various clinical and surgical repercussions. Although our knowledge of age-related changes is growing, their consequences are still the subject of much debate and controversy. One problem when assessing the effects of aging on humans is the extreme physiologic variability seen among elderly individuals. As individuals age, differences among them increase, such as those relating to their genetic distinctions, exposure to toxins, and environmental, psychological, and physical factors. Additionally, it becomes increasingly difficult to isolate control groups of healthy subjects because the elderly commonly have multiple medical problems. Many of these illnesses, such as diabetes, tend to confound study outcomes by adversely affecting the organs studied. Another obstacle to studying age-related changes involves the vast reserve capacity with which the human body is endowed. Some areas of the gastrointestinal tract and liver are capable of handling many times the quantitative functional capacity required during normal life and compensate well for normal physiologic loss with aging, which makes it difficult to detect age-related changes in function even though they may be apparent on a microscopic level.

## Esophagus

In the upper third of the human esophagus the longitudinal and the circular muscles are striated. The second third is composed of both striated and smooth muscle fibers, and the lower third is entirely smooth muscle. Normal esophageal motor function is characterized by a peristaltic wave, which begins at the upper esophageal sphincter (UES) and propagates through the striated and smooth muscle layers to terminate in closure of the lower sphincter (LES). This peristaltic wave is initiated by swallowing, which is controlled centrally, or by a bolus within the upper esophageal lumen (primary and secondary peristalsis, respectively). Activation of intrinsic peripheral control, which can function independently of the central control mechanism, helps propel the peristaltic wave forward. The function of the LES, which is controlled both locally and centrally, depends on various factors, including myogenic specialization, excitatory and inhibitory neural elements, and circulating hormones.

Swallowing impairment is more prevalent in the elderly.[1] Problems with swallowing are related to a variety of physiologic parameters including oral, pharyngeal, and esophageal. Ekberg and Feinberg found 84% of 56 healthy elderly subjects (mean age 83 years) to have abnormal deglutition compared to that considered normal in young persons.[1] Evaluation of videofluoroscopy and radiographs with the subjects erect and recumbent found problems at each phase of swallowing. Altogether, 63% of the swallowing problems were due to oral abnormalities (difficulty ingesting, controlling, and delivering the bolus relative to swallowing initiation), 25% were due to pharyngeal dysfunction (bolus retention and lingual propulsion or pharyngeal constrictor paresis), 39% were due to pharyngoesophageal abnormalities (mostly cricopharyngeal muscle dysfunction), and 36% were due to intrinsic esophageal abnormalities (mostly motor in nature).

Various UES abnormalities have been shown to be related to advanced age. Mean resting UES pressure has been shown to be decreased in elderly subjects, and UES relaxation is delayed.[2] This and the fact that the sensitivity of the cough reflex appears to be significantly reduced in elderly subjects[3] may increase the risk of aspiration leading to pneumonia. Both increased age and aspiration are risk factors for nosocomial pneumonia, which is three time more prevalent in older age groups than in the general population.[4] Older subjects also tend to have markedly elevated pharyngeal contraction pressures with a reduction in duration of upper esophageal contraction.[5] These findings help explain dysphagia in some patients.

Presbyesophagus, or degenerating motor function in the esophagus, has long been associated with advanced age. Whether old age in and of itself is the cause, however, remains controversial. Early studies by Zboralske et al.[6] and Soergel et al.[7] found that a reduced rate of peristalsis following swallowing in the elderly is accompanied by an increase in nonpropulsive contractions. This results in discoordination of muscular activity in the esophagus. Other age-related changes found were a defect in initiation of LES relaxation and of primary peristalsis shown by cineradiography, intraluminal manometry, and balloon kymography in nonagenarians. These studies found esophageal motor function to be disorganized and inefficient, with various abnormalities, including reduced or absent peristalsis, frequent and prominent tertiary contractions, delayed esophageal emptying, and dilation of the esophagus.[7] Radiographic evaluations on nonagenarians have also shown a higher incidence of intrathoracic LES (which normally straddles the diaphragmatic hiatus).[6] These studies have been criticized for having included patients with diabetes and senile dementia, diseases that can contribute to esophageal dysmotility.

A later study that controlled for these diseases but used younger subjects (70–87 years old), found decreased amplitude of esophageal peristalsis in the elderly but no increase in abnormal motility.[8] More recently Adamek et al. confirmed that age is of little significance in esophageal motility. This study also showed, however, a tendency among the older subjects toward an increase in the following parameters: distal pressure amplitudes, quotient of distal and proximal pressure amplitudes, distal duration, and percentage of simultaneous waves. The percentage of propulsive waves and proximal pressure amplitude and duration tended to decrease in these subjects.[9] It should also be pointed out that the "older" subjects' median age in this study was just 62.4 years.

The contribution of aging to presbyesophagus remains to be fully elucidated. Some evidence suggests that dysphagia and aperistalsis can be attributed to aging alone in a distinct, small group of patients. Meshkinpour et al. performed esophageal manometry in 562 patients and found that in 29 aperistaltic patients no secondary explanation was detected. Of these patients, 26 were 65 years or older and only 3 were 40 years or younger. They concluded that aging remains a possible explanation.[10]

Another recent study used only healthy volunteers to evaluate secondary esophageal peristalsis, which is believed to play an important role in the volume clearance of the esophagus of ingested material left behind after a swallow. This investigation found that in healthy elderly volunteers secondary peristalsis is either absent or its stimulation is inconsistent and significantly less frequent compared to that in younger volunteers. The frequency of stimulation of LES relaxation in response to intraesophageal air distension in the elderly was also significantly lower than that of the young. These elderly subjects demonstrated normal primary peristalsis, indicating an intact central, preganglionic, ganglionic, and postganglionic control mechanism. This finding suggests an intrinsic defect in the afferent neural pathway, reduced concentration (or absence) of tension-sensitive receptors within the esophageal wall, or both.[11]

Degenerative esophageal neurologic changes in the elderly have also been suggested by studies of other esophageal functions. Graded intraesophageal balloon distension was used to evaluate the visceral pain threshold in patients older than 65 compared to those in the young age group. Investigators found that upon inflation of the balloon 10cm above the LES the mean pain threshold balloon volumes in the young subjects was $17.0 \pm 0.8$ ml of air, and for the elderly subjects it was $27.0 \pm 1.4$ ml ($p < 0.01$). In the elderly group, five patients felt no pain even at the maximum inflatable volume of the balloon (30ml). These data suggest an age-related decrease in visceral pain threshold.[12]

Some data have suggested neurologic loss as a possible mechanism to explain defects in both motility and sensory thresholds. Filho et al. showed that patients over 70 years of age had a decreased number of neurons along the esophagus compared to subjects aged 20–40 years of age. This decrease in number was accompanied by an increase in the size of the neurons, suggesting that compensatory growth may be an attempt to maintain neuronal density.[13] Despite the abundance of data indicating that there are neurologic and functional changes in the esophagus with age, it has been difficult to show a significant correlation between these changes and clinical dysfunction. As more studies are done with a growing population of healthy elderly subjects, this potential mechanism will be further elucidated.

## Stomach

Many of the various functions of the stomach have been studied in the aging population. A brief overview of normal stomach physiology follows.

The epithelial lining of the stomach lumen is characterized by thick folds called rugae, which contain microscopic gastric pits. The mucosal surface of the stomach and the linings of the gastric pits are composed of mucin-secreting columnar cells. The gastric glands are contained within the gastric pits and are responsible for secreting hydrochloric acid (HCl), pepsinogen, gastrin, intrinsic factor, mucus, and various gastrointestinal hormones. The capacity of the stomach to produce HCl is directly proportional to the parietal cell mass in the glands of the body and fundus. The parietal cells secrete HCl by a process involving oxidative phosphorylation, the final step of which is accomplished by a sodium-potassium "proton pump" located in the apical membrane. Regulation of gastric acid secretion is controlled by histamine, gastrin, and postganglionic vagal fibers via muscarinic cholinergic receptors.[14]

The motor activity of the stomach is essential to digestion in both the fasting and fed states. Between meals, contractile patterns clear the stomach of undigested material, and the stomach then relaxes and expands to receive a food bolus. The meal is ground and delivered to the small intestine for further digestion. This delivery is accomplished by a complex series of muscular contractions in the proximal and distal stomach.[14] These distinct physiologic regions of the stomach must coordinate contractile function to deliver the stomach contents to the duodenum. Gastric emptying has been found to depend on the type of food it contains: liquid, solid, or fat.[14]

The cumulative effect of stress and exposure to various ingested substances over one's lifetime, such as ethanol, aspirin, and toxins, may damage the stomach mucosa and lead to atrophic gastritis, gastric atrophy, achlorhydria, and intrinsic factor deficiency. These changes are difficult to distinguish from those resulting from age alone.

## Acid Production

It is generally agreed that gastroduodenal secretory function changes with increased age, but the extent and the direction of the change remains controversial. Historically, it has been accepted that acid secretion declines as a consequence of normal aging. This observation, however, was based on studies that often included subjects with medical problems rather than healthy volunteers. These studies also predated understanding of the role of the bacterium *Helicobacter pylori* in acid production. *H. pylori*, found in more than 75% of individuals over the age of 60,[15] may cause transient hypochlorhydria in acutely infected patients. Although long-term studies have not been conclusive, epidemiologic data suggest that long-standing *H. pylori* infection may result in reduced acid secretion secondary to atrophic changes in the gastric mucosa.[16]

A large ($n = 437$) computer-selected family sample of the Finnish population aged 15 years or over was extensively studied in 1982 with pentagastrin stimulation and mucosal biopsies. Gastric acid output, expressed as millimoles per hour (mmol/hr), mmol/hr/kg of total body weight (TBW), mmol/hr/kg of lean body mass (LBM), and mmol/hr/kg of fat-free body weight (FFB), correlated with the changes in the body mucosa but not with those of the antrum. This investigation also found that gastric acid secretion declines with age but did not attribute this change to aging alone. Reduced acid production did, however, correlate with atrophic gastritis (Table 36.1). Male patients with normal mucosa had no significant change in acid output, and female patients with normal mucosa actually demonstrated an increase in acid production when expressed in FFB (Table 36.2).[17]

Goldschmiedt et al. in 1991 undertook a prospective, multivariate analysis to investigate basal and stimulated gastric acid output with aging. This study, which included 41 healthy volunteers, showed that aging is associated with an increase in gastric acid production (basal, meal-stimulated and gastrin-stimulated), and that infection with *H. pylori* is independently associated with decreased acid secretion rates.[18] This finding has since been confirmed by other studies that compared gastric

TABLE 36.1. Relation of Acid Output to Age, Sex, and Morphology of the Body Mucosa

| | Acid output | | | | | | | | |
|---|---|---|---|---|---|---|---|---|---|
| | Men (ages ≤30 to >70) | | | | Women (ages ≤30 to >70) | | | | |
| Parameter | ≤30 | 31–50 | 51–70 | >70 | ≤30 | 31–50 | 51–70 | >70 | Units |
| **Acid output per:** | | | | | | | | | |
| Total body weight | 0.47 ± 0.19 | 0.45 ± 0.19 | 0.33 ± 0.22 | 0.20 ± 0.20 | 0.39 ± 0.13 | 0.37 ± 0.16 | 0.24 ± 0.18 | 0.21 ± 0.18 | mmol/hr/kg TBW |
| Fat-free body weight | 0.60 ± 0.23 | 0.59 ± 0.25 | 0.46 ± 0.31 | 0.29 ± 0.29 | 0.54 ± 0.18 | 0.58 ± 0.24 | 0.40 ± 0.28 | 0.34 ± 0.29 | mmol/hr/kg FFBW |
| Lean body mass | 0.62 ± 0.23 | 0.62 ± 0.27 | 0.46 ± 0.31 | 0.28 ± 0.28 | 0.52 ± 0.17 | 0.55 ± 0.23 | 0.37 ± 0.27 | 0.32 ± 0.28 | mmol/hr/kg LBW |
| Prevalence of atrophic gastritis[a] (%) | 9 | 11 | 25 | 53 | 3 | 8 | 31 | 43 | |

*Source:* Adapted from Kekki et al.[17]
[a] Body gastritis.

TABLE 36.2. Acid Output in Relation to Morphologic State of the Body Mucosa

| Mucosal status | Acid output (mmol/hr) | | Acid output (mmol/hr/FFB) | |
|---|---|---|---|---|
| | Men | Women | Men | Women |
| Normal | 36.5 ± 13.2[a] | 24.2 ± 13.3[b] | 0.63 ± 0.20[c] | 0.60 ± 0.20[d] |
| Superficial gastritis | 31.5 ± 15.1[e] | 21.1 ± 17.9[f] | 0.57 ± 0.26[g] | 0.51 ± 0.22[h] |
| Slight atrophic gastritis | 15.2 ± 13.8[i] | 10.33 ± 18.4[j] | 0.31 ± 0.26[k] | 0.25 ± 0.28[l] |
| Moderate and severe atrophic gastritis | 2.2 ± 4.4[m] | 1.38 ± 4.0[n] | 0.04 ± 0.10[o] | 0.03 ± 0.09[q] |

*Source:* Adapted from Kekki et al.[17]
*a* vs. *b*, $p < 0.001$; *c* vs. *d*, NS; *e* vs. *f*, $p < 0.001$; *g* vs. *h*, NS; *i* vs. *j*, NS; *k* vs. *l*, NS; *m* vs. *n*, NS; *o* vs. *q*, NS; *a* vs. *e*, $p < 0.05$; *c* vs. *g*, NS; *e* vs. *i*, $p < 0.001$; *g* vs. *k*, $p < 0.001$; *b* vs. *f*, NS; *d* vs. *h*, $p < 0.01$; *f* vs. *j*, $p < 0.001$; *h* vs. *l*, $p < 0.001$; *j* vs. *n*, $p < 0.001$; *l* vs. *q*, $p < 0.001$.

acid secretion and *H. pylori* infection in young and old patients. These investigators concluded that gastric acid secretion does not decline as a result of healthy aging.[16,19] Only gastritis had a negative effect on acid secretion,[16] and *H. pylori* is commonly the causative agent.

Studies finding a correlation between atrophic gastritis and reduced gastric acid secretion during old age are supported by knowledge of the pathophysiology of pernicious anemia. Pernicious anemia is a disease of the elderly, the average patient presenting near age 60. With this condition atrophy of the gastric mucosa results in decreased intrinsic factor secretion (also a product of the parietal cells), leading to reduced cobalamin uptake.

## Gastric Emptying

Many studies have documented that gastric emptying slows with aging. The importance of this finding extends beyond the obvious morbidity it causes in affected patients. For example, the rate of gastric emptying can influence the rate and extent of absorption of orally administered drugs, thereby influencing the rate and duration of their pharmacologic effect.

Various radioisotope methods have been employed to evaluate gastric emptying in the elderly (Table 36.3). Horowitz et al. used a double isotope technique on healthy young ($n = 22$; age 21–62 years, mean age 34) and elderly ($n = 13$; age 70–84 years, mean age 77 years) subjects to evaluate gastric emptying of both liquids and solids. The data showed a statistically significant delay in both among the elderly subjects.[22] A similar study, performed more recently on healthy Chinese subjects, found that gastric emptying of solid foods did not change with age, but a delay in liquid phase emptying was observed.[23] In a similar study Moore et al. also demonstrated a delay in gastric emptying of liquids in the elderly.[21] Evans et al. used modified sequential scintiscanning after administration of the nonabsorbable chelated radiopharmaceutical technetium 99m-diethylenetriaminepentaacetic acid ($^{99m}$Tc-DTPA) to show that the rate of emptying was significantly longer in elderly subjects. The investigators concluded that it could explain a delay in absorption of drugs with aging. This study, however, did not control for the presence of concomitant chronic diseases such as parkinsonism, hypothyroidism, transient ischemic attacks, and strokes.[20]

Clarkston et al.[24] used two isotopes to evaluate the gastric emptying of solid and liquid foods. The patients were healthy young ($n = 19$, age 23–50 years) and old ($n = 14$, age 70–84 years) volunteers who were evaluated sitting at a 45-degree angle. Gastric emptying of both solids and liquids was found to be delayed in the elderly patients. This investigation also found that the elderly had reduced hunger and desire to eat after a meal, which was thought to be an effect of delayed gastric emptying.

An investigation of paracetamol, a drug that is rapidly absorbed from the small bowel but not from the stomach, found no significant difference in gastric emptying between young and elderly healthy subjects. This study was well controlled for health and other potentially confounding factors.[25]

Gastric emptying is regulated in part by stomach myoelectric activity, which occurs at the membrane level

TABLE 36.3. Gastric Emptying Studies Using Radiolabeled Foods

| Study | Year | Method | Mean age | | Elimination $T_{1/2}$[a] (minutes) | | |
|---|---|---|---|---|---|---|---|
| | | | Elderly | Young | Elderly (solids) | Young (solids) | Elderly (liquids) |
| Evans[20] | 1981 | $^{99m}$Tc-DTPA | 77 ($n = 11$) | 26 ($n = 7$) | — | — | 123 ± 23 |
| Moore[21] | 1982 | Dual isotope | 76.4 ($n = 10$) | 31 ($n = 10$) | 105 ± 17 | 104 ± 10 | 94 ± 13 |
| Horowitz[22] | 1984 | Dual isotope | 77 ($n = 13$) | 34 ($n = 22$) | 103 ± 8 | 78 ± 4 | 25 ± 3 |
| Koa[23] | 1993 | $^{99m}$Tc-phytate | 67 ($n = 39$) | 34 ($n = 37$) | 89.0 ± 17.8 | 88.0 ± 18.2 | 46.2 ± 11 |
| Clarkston[24] | 1997 | Dual isotope | 76 ($n = 14$) | 30 ($n = 19$) | 182 ± 26 | 127 ± 13 | 47 ± 4 |

[a] Half-life of elimination of radiolabeled foods from the stomach.

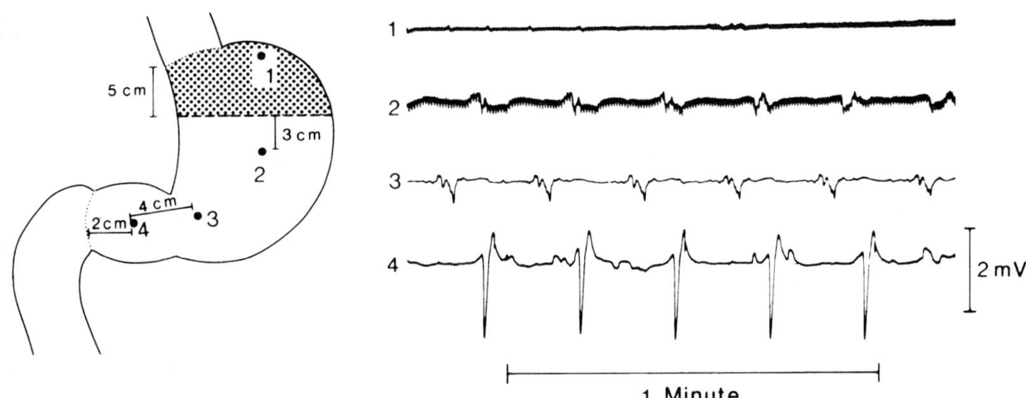


FIGURE 36.1. Myoelectric activity from the human stomach. Electrodes 1–4 were placed in the fundus, corpus, and proximal antrum and at the antral-pyloric juncture, respectively. The fundus is myoelectrically quiet. The basal electrical rhythm is seen in tracings 2 and 3 and are associated with cyclic membrane depolarization. No contractions are associated with the basal electrical rhythm (BER). Rapid depolarizations of the proximal corpus drive the myoelectric activity of the distal stomach. The pacemaker rests on the greater curvature of the stomach at the fundocorpal border. Spike potentials are seen in tracing 4 in the region of the antrum and pylorus. They are associated with contractions and, therefore, emptying of the stomach. (From Hinder and Kelly,[28] with permission.)

of the gastric smooth muscle. The electrical membrane potentials of each region of the stomach differ as measured by electrogastrography (EGG). EGG abnormalities occur in various pathologic states of the stomach. For example, gastric dysrhythmias have been reported in patients with gastroparesis, idiopathic or diabetic peptic ulcer disease,[14] functional dyspepsia (associated with tachygastria),[26] gastroesophageal reflux disease (associated with gastric dysrhythmias),[27] and chronic intestinal pseudoobstruction (associated with various gastric dysrhythmias). Despite these findings, abnormal EGG tracings alone do not necessarily correlate with symptoms.

The basal electrical rhythm (BER), or the slow wave, is a cyclic change in membrane potential, which varies in different regions of the stomach (Fig. 36.1). The membrane potential is generated by the membrane sodium-potassium pump. The BER is associated with minimal contractile activity and does not result in detectable gastric peristalsis. The BER in the stomach, which originates in a pacemaker located in the mid-corpus along the greater curve, is propagated through gap junctions between adjacent smooth muscle cells. Vagotomy in humans has been shown to have no effect on the amplitude, rhythm, frequency, direction, or velocity of propagation of the electrical potentials, implying that initiation of the current is a myogenic phenomenon.[28] This finding, along with an equally ineffectual denervation of non-vagal extrinsic stomach fibers, was recently confirmed in dogs.[29]

In the distal stomach and duodenum, a cyclic contractile pattern called the interdigestive migrating motor complex (MMC) exists and is characterized by four phases. The contractions are associated with myoelectric spike potentials superimposed on the basal electrical rhythm. The spikes are associated with rapid calcium influx into the cells. Phase I is characterized by a period of quiescence, phase II is irregular motor activity, phase III is regular contractions that sweep the gastrointestinal tract in a peristaltic manner, and phase IV represents a brief period of irregular activity.[14]

Abnormalities in gastric myoelectric activity have been associated with various gastric maladies, although patients with EGG disturbances alone do not necessarily have symptoms. There is recent evidence that the normal postprandial EGG frequency increase is less pronounced in elderly men.[30]

Some studies have shown delayed gastric emptying in the elderly, but it has been difficult to show that it is associated with any clinical deficit. Other studies have found that there is no difference in gastric emptying between young and elderly subjects. Studies that evaluated only neuromuscular changes similarly were inconclusive about clinical relevance. If aging alone results in any gastric motility impairment, it is probably not clinically relevant.

## Gastric Cancer

Because the peak incidence of gastric cancer is among patients older than 50 years, it is considered a disease primarily of the middle-aged and elderly. Gastric cancer is also of interest to those studying the elderly because although its incidence in young patients has remained consistent, that in elderly patients has increased. Also, despite similarities in young and elderly patients in terms of tumor biology [characterized, for example, by the magnitude of overexpression of the tumor supressor gene *p53*

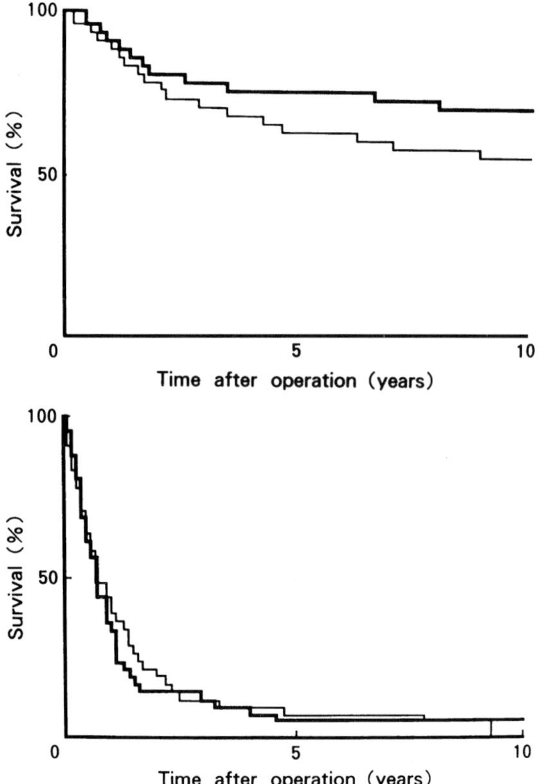


FIGURE 36.2. Survival time for patients undergoing curative resection for gastric cancer (top panel) or noncurative resection (bottom panel) in a Japanese study. The patients were stratified to young (<40 years, $n = 175$, thin line) and old groups (>70 years, $n = 356$, heavy line). Survival was no different for young patients if the tumor was unresectable, but survival was significantly better in young patients undergoing curative resection. (From Maehara Y, Emi Y, Tomisaki S, Oshiro T, Kakeji Y, Ichiyoshi Y, Sugimachi K. Age-related characteristics of gastric carcinoma in young and elderly patients. Cancer 1996;77:1774–1780, with permission.)

and increased levels of other cellular markers, such as proliferating cell nuclear antigen (PCNA)], the survival rate after curative resection has been shown to be decreased in the elderly (Fig. 36.2). Kitamura et al. also noted that elderly patients with gastric cancer have poorer survival than younger patients despite a similar rate of tumor extension. The reason for this difference is unclear. Kitamura et al. suggested it may be due to weakened defense status in the elderly, or it may reflect a reluctance on the part of the surgeon to undertake aggressive treatments such as extended resection, extensive lymph node dissection, and strong chemotherapy.[31] Others have postulated that the tumor is physiologically different in the aged from that in younger patients.

Loss of gastric acidity is related to an increased risk of developing gastric cancer. It is manifested in the elderly by achlorhydria, atrophic gastritis, or pernicious anemia. It can also be the result of previous gastric resection for ulcer disease. The loss of gastric acidity may permit bacterial growth of the pathogen *H. pylori*, adding another independent risk factor for gastric cancer.[32] The risk of gastric cancer has been shown to be increased fourfold in *H. pylori*-positive persons. Although this may not reflect a causative relation, infection by *H. pylori* creates an environment of chronic gastritis and intestinal metaplasia suitable for neoplastic change.[33]

Mucosa-associated lymphoid tissue (MALT), which progresses to MALT lymphomas, has also been found to be the result of *H. pylori* infection. Eradication of the *H. pylori* infection by oral antibiotic therapy has been shown not to eliminate MALT and may even result in remission of low-grade gastric MALT lymphomas.[34]

## Small Intestine

Over the course of an individual's life, enormous quantities of nutrients are processed through the small intestine. This makes the small intestine a likely place for potential changes with advancing age secondary to prolonged functioning and exposure to multitudes of potential carcinogens over time. Additionally, the small intestine is an organ of epithelial regeneration, turning over its cellular population often. This unique characteristic may be involved in the physiologic changes that occur with aging.

### Motility

Advanced age is associated with a decrease in body weight, reduced caloric intake, and frequent gastrointestinal complaints. In fact, as many as 15% of adults have functional bowel complaints.[35] The effect of advanced age on the motility of the small intestine, however, is still unknown.[36] One way to evaluate small bowel motility is by studying the migrating motor complex (MMC), the ordered array of myoelectric activity and muscular contractions that travel down the small intestine in an aboral direction during fasting. The four phases of the MMC can be monitored by electrical activity, muscular contractions, intraluminal pressure, and intestinal transit times.

Husebye and Engedal[36] prospectively studied 15 healthy elderly subjects (age 81–91) and 19 young healthy controls with ambulatory intraluminal manometry performed at home. This study found all subjects to have recurrent MMCs during fasting with similar periodicity in old and young adults ($p = 0.4$) (Fig. 36.3). Duration of postprandial motility, amplitude, and frequency of contractions during phase III and the postprandial state were also preserved in the elderly subjects. Interestingly, the propagation velocity was slower ($6.5 \pm 0.8$ vs. $10.8 \pm 1.2$ cm/min) and intermittent propagated clustered contractions were more frequent in the older subjects (Fig. 36.4). However, these minor to moderate changes were also within the range of healthy younger adults and are

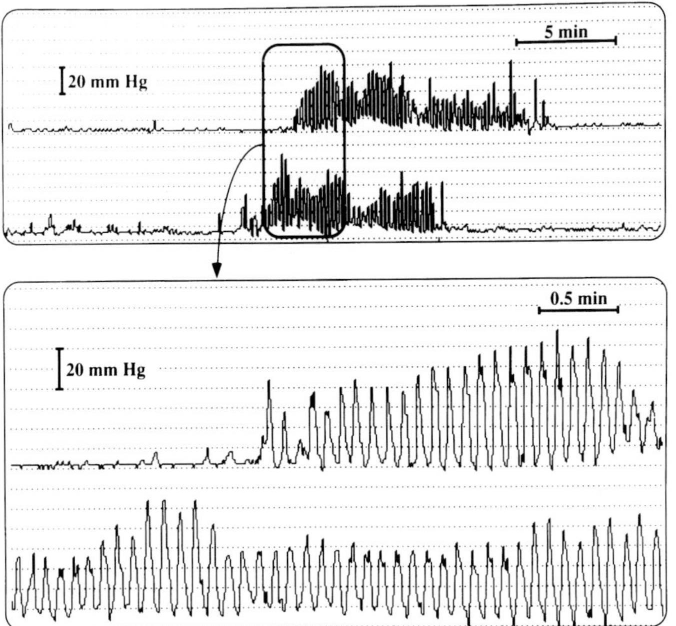


FIGURE 36.3. Fasting phase III of the migrating motor complex recorded in a healthy old individual. Intraluminal manometric sensors were located in the duodenum (bottom tracing) and the proximal jejunum (top tracing). Propagation of the waveform is seen. A slight decrease in propagation velocity is noted in the aged, but no difference is found between the periodicity of the fasting or fed pattern of the migrating myoelectric complex (MMC). (From Husebye and Engedal,[36] with permission.)

unlikely to be of clinical relevance. The investigators concluded that small intestinal motility, for the most part, is preserved in the healthy elderly subject. Intestinal disorders such as maldigestion, malabsorption, and bacterial overgrowth should not be attributed to age-related hypomotility.[36]

Madsen confirmed this concept with a more clinically practical study. He evaluated small-intestine transit time using radionuclide tracers in healthy elderly subjects and compared it to that of young healthy subjects. The 17 healthy young subjects and 16 healthy older subjects were fed a meal containing $^{99m}$Tc-labeled cellulose fiber and 2- to 3-mm $^{111}$In-labeled plastic particles. No difference was noted in mean small intestinal transit time between the groups.[37] Argeny et al. similarly evaluated transit times in 10 young and 9 elderly healthy volunteers (using $^{99m}$Tc-sulfur colloid-labeled eggs). They also found no difference between young and elderly subjects. There was, however, a wide normal range of transit times in normal subjects and significant intrasubject biologic variability.[38] This finding is not uncommon in motility studies and is an important point to consider when trying to understand the clinical significance of small bowel transit times.

## Morphology

There are few data concerning structural changes with increasing age on the human small bowel. In a study done in 1975, the jejunal mucosa from necropsies of 32 patients under the age of 60 (mean age 43 years) and 39 patients aged 67–90 years (mean age 80) were evaluated microscopically. Only minor differences were noted in the villous morphology between the young control group and the old subjects. Specifically, broader, shorter villi were found to be more common in the elderly. This led the authors to postulate that this minor difference in total villous surface explains some absorption problems in the elderly.[39]

Warren et al. compared the small intestine histology of 10 well-nourished elderly patients aged 60–73 to that of 10 similar patients in the age range 16–30. A highly significant reduction in the mucosal surface area was

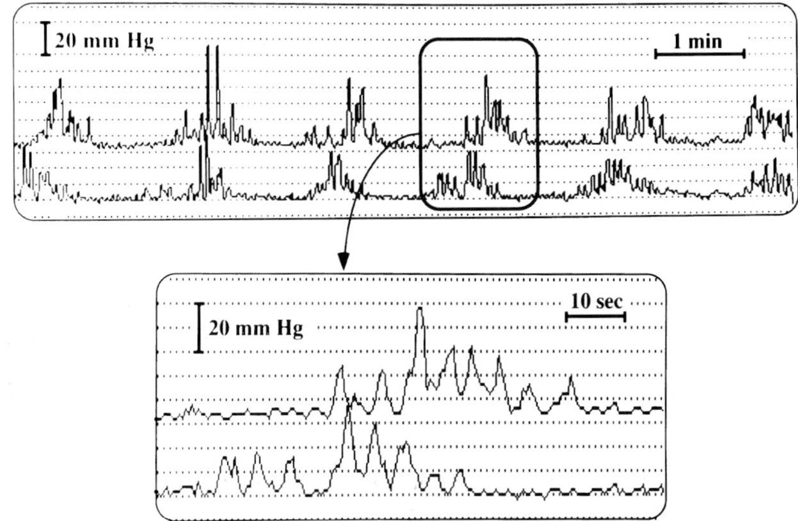


FIGURE 36.4. Propagated cluster contractions (PCCs) in the small intestine during the postprandial state in an old adult. A typical sequence of repeated PCCs at intervals of 1–2 minutes is shown. The bottom tracings in both boxes correspond to the duodenal sensor, and the top tracings show the recording from the proximal jejunum. These contractions are seen in increased frequency in the old person when compared to young controls. (From Husebye and Engedal,[36] with permission.)

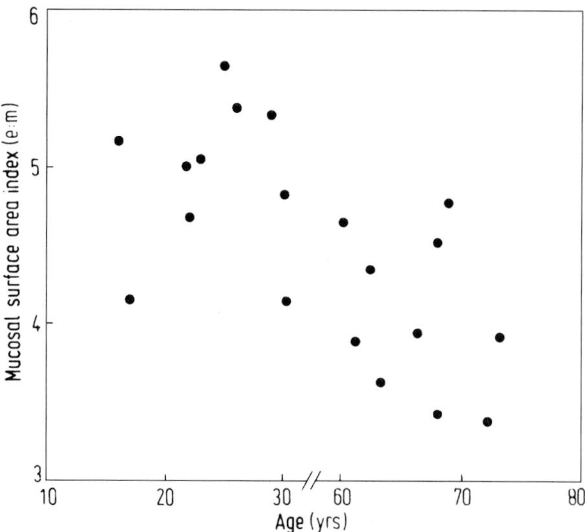


FIGURE 36.5. Relation of the intestinal mucosal surface area to the age of the patient. An indirect, statistically significant correlation is noted. (From Warren et al.,[40] with permission.)

found in the older age group (Fig. 36.5). The mean villous height was also slightly reduced and the breadth slightly increased, but these differences were not significant.[40]

Corazza et al. evaluated the small bowel mucosa of 16 elderly patients and 22 younger controls to determine the surface area/volume ratio of jejunal mucosa using microscopic point-counting techniques. This technique is performed by counting the number of times the standardized lines of a reticule intersects the jejunal mucosal surface under a set magnification. The surface area/volume ratio, which is an index of the extent of the mucosal surface area, was determined. Mean enterocyte height was also measured. No significant difference was found between the two groups for either parameter.[41] One noteworthy aspect in this study is the use of patients with "abdominal symptoms" rather than healthy volunteers.

Clarke found that the pattern of reduced villous height noted in aging humans was mirrored in the aging rat, but it was not associated with decreased nutrient absorption.[42] Atillasoy and Holt, on the other hand, found aged rats to have hyperproliferation of intestinal epithelial cells. These investigators found that the number of villous absorbing cells in the duodenum and the jejunum as well as the protein and DNA content per unit length of intestine did not differ in 4- to 5-month-old animals and 25- to 27-month-old-animals, but ileal cell numbers were increased. The older animals also had greater crypt cell numbers, and crypt cells of the older rats had 20–30% more proliferating cell DNA when labeled with [$^3$H]thymidine. These findings were confirmed with the metaphase arrest technique, which is a direct calculation of the crypt cell production rate. They postulated that there is a release in the normally tight control of proliferation seen in young animals.[43]

Brush border enzymes have been shown to increase in the senescent rat, which tends to support the finding of hyperproliferation of enterocytes. Raul et al. found hyperproliferation in older rat intestine, but they also found that in some segments (proximal intestine) there was a significant reduction in villous height.[44]

The integrity of the small intestinal mucosa may age along with the host. The lactulose/mannitol test has been used to evaluate intestinal permeability in humans. The test is based on comparing the absorption of a monosaccharide (mannitol), which is absorbed transcellularly, to a disaccharide (lactulose), which is absorbed paracellularly. The urinary lactulose/mannitol ratio after oral administration is a reproducible measure of small intestine mucosal integrity. This ratio is increased when the mucosal integrity is disrupted. In a prospective cohort study using healthy volunteers, Saltzman et al. found small intestinal permeability, or "leakiness," not to be significantly altered with age.[45] Riordan et al., using the same test, found that although intestinal permeability increases with small intestine bacterial overgrowth with colonic-type bacteria, this effect is independent of age.[46] Similarly, the thickness of the small bowel was found by de Souza et al. to be unchanged in the elderly. The latter investigation also found that the density of nerve cells in the myenteric plexus of the small bowel is decreased in the aged small intestine.[47] This implies that the intrinsic innervation of the human intestine is reduced during old age.

## Absorption

Malnutrition in the elderly has been theoretically attributed to malabsorption at the level of the intestinal epithelium.[48] However there is evidence that age alone does not adversely effect brush border enzymes. Wallis et al. collected 38 duodenal biopsy specimens from patients 55–91 years in age. Tissue was evaluated for the activity of the brush border enzymes maltase, sucrase, lactase, alkaline phosphatase, leucine aminopeptidase, and α-glucosidase. The study demonstrated no significant effect of age on the specific activities of these enzymes. It also found that glucose transport was not changed in the more elderly subjects.[49]

Using probe molecules that are absorbed by active and passive intestinal transport and then easily recovered in the urine, Beaumont et al. found no significant age-related decline in passive absorption of carbohydrate in either healthy nonhospitalized individuals or in elderly long-stay hospital residents.[50] In another study, Arora et al. investigated three aspects of intestinal absorption in the elderly and found no significant change. A series of

114 healthy adult volunteers (age 19–91) were started on a 100g of fat per day diet 1 day prior to testing. The subjects remained on the diet for the following 72 hours as their stools were collected and tested for fecal fat. There was no change with advancing age. In another arm of the study, 25g of D-xylose was given orally to 54 fasting volunteers (56–86 years of age; 20 men, 34 women). Serum and urinary xylose levels were measured. There was no significant difference in D-xylose serum levels between young and elderly volunteers. Although urinary excretion of D-xylose in the elderly was found to be significantly decreased ($p < 0.02$), there was a concomitant decrease in creatinine clearance with advancing age ($p < 0.01$). This suggests a decrease in renal function rather than a problem with absorption as the reason for the decreased urinary D-xylose levels in the elderly. In the third part of the study [$^{14}$C]glycocholate breath tests were performed in 60 healthy adult volunteers [30 were age ≥30 years (15 men, 15 women) 30 were age ≥60 years (15 men, 15 women)]. This test is used to assess increased deconjugation of bile salts, which suggests bacterial overgrowth of the small intestine. There was no evidence of an age-associated increase in bile salt deconjugation by intestinal bacteria.[51]

Malabsorption in the elderly has been shown to be often related to bacterial overgrowth. McEvoy et al. studied 490 patients over age 65 and found that 71% of the malnourished patients (those in whom poor diet alone was not a factor) had bacterial overgrowth of the small intestines.[52] MacMahon et al. evaluated 30 elderly patients between 68 and 90 years of age for small intestinal bacterial overgrowth (SIBO). Advancing age correlated significantly with rising counts of strict anaerobes in the small bowel. The investigators thought that malabsorption in these patients was not related to bacterial overgrowth because metabolic or nutritional abnormalities could be attributed to alternative causes.[53]

Because fat is a major source of caloric intake, its absorption is an important area of investigation in the healthy and ill elderly. Fat absorption is a complex process involving four major phases: (1) intraluminal processes (digestion and solubilization); (2) mucosal uptake; (3) intracellular reesterification and lipoprotein synthesis; and (4) export from the enterocyte into the lymph. Although disruption of any of these phases can lead to fat malabsorption, this too is rarely observed in elderly patients. In a study of 114 healthy, free-living subjects, aged 19–91 years, Arora et al. found that on a diet that included 100g of fat per day, fecal fat in a 72-hour collection did not increase with advancing age.[51] Lipid digestion and absorption are well preserved in aging individuals.[43]

## Liver and Biliary Function

The liver is responsible for the synthesis of clotting factors and the metabolism of toxins, including anesthetics, analgesics, and sedatives, all of which are important in the elderly surgical patients. The liver in adult man has been found to increase in size only marginally, from a median weight of 1820g at age 25 years to a median weight of 1840g at 55 years of age. It then decreases by 20% to a median weight of 1480g by age 75. The median weight of the female liver similarly changes, from 1430–1460g during the age range 20–60 years to 1180g by 75 years of age (Fig. 36.6).[54] Sherlock et al. used the Bromsulphalein technique to estimate hepatic blood flow in 29 men and found a decrease in flow with increasing age of about 1.5% per year. At age 65 hepatic blood flow would be expected to be reduced about 40–45% compared to that

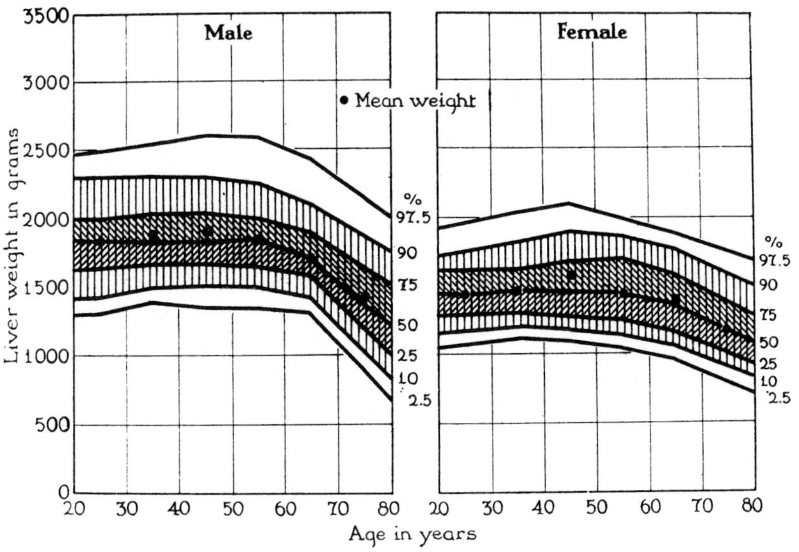


FIGURE 36.6. Pattern of change in human liver weight with respect to age. At age 55–60 the mean weight begins to decline in both men and women. (From Boyd,[54] with permission.)

of a 25-year-old.[55] There is some controversy as to whether a reduction in liver function with age is attributable to these physical changes, or there is some intrinsic age-related cellular change.[56]

In another branch of their study of 60 healthy, adult volunteers, Arora et al. performed [$^{14}$C]aminopyrine breath tests, which measures the rate of demethylation by the hepatic microsomes, thereby estimating the capacity of hepatic microsomal phase I monooxygenases. This study was unable to show a statistically significant difference between young and elderly subjects and concluded that hepatic functions are generally well preserved during the normal human aging process.[51]

Many pharmacokinetic studies in human subjects have suggested that the clearance of drugs metabolized by oxidation–reduction is reduced in the elderly by 10–50%.[56] One way to evaluate liver function in aging is to study the liver's store of cytochrome P450 and its functional capacity. Sotaniemi et al. investigated liver biopsy samples from 226 patients (102 women, 124 men) with equal histopathologic conditions. This was ensured by dividing the liver biopsies into three groups using standard histopathologic conditions: (1) apparently normal liver histologic diagnosis; (2) subjects with slight to moderate changes in liver parenchyma (fatty liver, fatty liver with fibrosis, degree of fibrosis 1–3, and reactive changes such as granulomas or portal infiltrates); and (3) subjects with severe changes (cirrhosis and hepatitis). They evaluated the cytochrome P450 contents in liver biopsy samples and the plasma antipyrine (phenzone) clearance rates, which tests for hepatic drug-metabolizing capacity. The study found that cytochrome P450 content in subjects 20–29 years of age was 7.2 ± 2.6 mmol/g; it increased during the fourth decade to 7.6 ± 2.5 (+7.2%, $p$ = NS) and declined after age 40 to 6.1 ± 2.2 (–16%, $p < 0.01$), a level that remained relatively constant until age 69. It declined further to 4.8 ± 1.1 after age 70 (–32%, $p < 0.001$). The antipyrine clearance rate in young subjects was 46.4 ± 18.5 ml/min, remained unaltered during the fourth decade, and declined after age 40 by a rate of 0.34 ml/min per year toward old age (–29%, $p < 0.001$). The antipyrine half-life also changed during old age, increasing linearly from 9.6 ± 2.0 hours in young subjects (20–29 years) to 12.1 ± 3.1 hours in the elderly (>70 years) (+26%, $p < 0.001$). There was also a decline in the apparent volume of distribution of the drug: 0.46 ± 0.12 L/kg in young subjects (20–29 years) and after a linear decline with aging to 0.40 ± 0.07 L/kg in middle-aged subjects (60–69 years) and to 0.41 ± 0.09 L/kg in the elderly (70 years) (–11%). This reduction of liver drug metabolism with age, along with a decline in cytochrome P450 content in livers of the elderly, suggests primary hepatic aging. The authors concluded that caution is advisable when using drugs metabolized by the liver in the elderly, and that elderly patients should be closely monitored for high blood levels caused by reduced drug metabolism, drug interactions, or both.[57] Aging of the liver may not be readily apparent in the healthy individual; and it is often unmasked only by stress, illness, or infection.

In addition to any changes due solely to aging, the liver is particularly susceptible to the toxic effect of environmental agents such as cigarettes and ethanol. Its decline in function secondary to decreased size and blood flow can be attributed to nonhepatic factors, such as reduced cardiac output and age-related reduction of trophic factors from the pancreas via the portal system such as insulin and glucagon.[56] Here again it is difficult to determine how much functional decline can be attributed solely to age, but there is at least some clear evidence of physical change.

Like other gastrointestinal organs, the liver has a large reserve capacity. This is illustrated by the successful transplant of an 86-year-old donated liver into a 65-year-old recipient performed by Wall et al. Immediate function of the graft was excellent. Aside from an elevation in serum transaminases and bilirubin, the development of ascites, and infection by cytomegalovirus (all of which cleared with appropriate therapy), the patient was reported well 6 months after the transplantation with normal liver function.[58]

Increasing age is known to be associated with a high incidence of gallstones in both men and women. This was recently confirmed by a large ($n$ = 1000) study in which multiple logistic regression was used to show that age was the most important variable associated with cholelithiasis.[59] Another study that supported this finding was the Multicenter Italian Study on Epidemiology of Cholelithiasis (MICOL). In this study, data from 29,584 individuals (15,910 men, 13,674 women) examined in 14 cohorts (with a participation rate above 50%) were collected. Increasing age was again found to be associated with an increased incidence of gallstone disease by both univariate and multivariate analysis in men and women. Interestingly, gallstone disease was also associated with decreased serum cholesterol,[60] which may be related to a high proportion of biliary cholesterol and the lithogenic index, which have been shown to be elevated in elderly women. Valdivieso et al. reported that 41.7% of elderly women had supersaturated bile compared to 8.3% of younger women.[61]

Liver regeneration is known to occur after resection, and this effect has been studied in the elderly. The livers of aged rats have been found to have decreased regenerative capacity by proliferating cell nuclear antigen (PCNA)[62] and [$^{3}$H]thymidine incorporation.[63] This finding, however, has not been supported in human studies, and in fact quite the opposite has been found. Increased age in humans is associated with no difference in[64] or even increased regenerative capacity following resection.[65]

## Pancreas

Like the liver, the pancreas progressively atrophies with old age. Similar to other areas of the gastrointestinal tract, the pancreas has enormous reserve capacity, so again it is difficult to attribute pancreatic changes solely to old age.[15]

Because acinar cells make up 80% of the pancreas, an effective way to evaluate pancreatic function is to test for exocrine output in response to infusion of secretin and cerulein. When this test was performed on 25 subjects over the age of 60, no statistically significant decrease in pancreatic output was observed compared with a group of 30 young controls.[66] The same group subsequently confirmed their findings with an updated, elegant method of evaluating pancreatic function, the fluorescein dilaurate (pancreolauryl) test. For this test subjects are administered the synthetic, poorly water-soluble ester fluorescein dilaurate orally. In the duodenum this compound is hydrolyzed by pancreatic arylesterases into lauric acid and free water-soluble fluorescein. The fluorescein is absorbed in the small intestine, conjugated in the liver, and excreted in the urine. Fluorescent activity in the urine output correlates with pancreatic function and digestive capacity. Sixty healthy elderly subjects (aged 66–88 years, mean 78 years) were compared to 36 healthy younger subjects (aged 21–57 years, mean 36 years). No significant differences in pancreatic function could be shown between the elderly under age 80 and those over age 80.[67]

Another way to evaluate pancreatic exocrine function is to determine serum levels of pancreatic enzymes. Carrere et al. compared immunoreactive trypsinogen and lipase in healthy elderly adults and younger adult controls. This investigation found that the pancreatic enzymes were similar in young and elderly adults, with no significant differences between the groups.[68]

It is well known that humans become more glucose-intolerant with age. It is still somewhat controversial, though, whether this change is due to beta cell failure, peripheral insulin resistance, or a combination of the two. Here again, discerning the effects of age only versus the effects of age-related changes, such as increased adiposity, decreased physical activity, and changes in diet is difficult. The glucose clamp study, in which a hyperglycemic state is induced, can differentiate the intrinsic function of beta cells from peripheral insulin resistance. In a study of 230 hyperglycemic clamps done on 85 young (24–39 years), 47 middle-aged (40–59 years), and 98 old (60–90 years) subjects (the latter group was further divided into old-normal and old-impaired, based on the results of oral glucose tolerance tests), Elahi et al. found that although oral glucose tolerance tests (OGTTs) were worse in the elderly group, insulin responses during the clamp were not statistically different for this group as a whole. Additionally, insulin-dependent glucose uptake, a measure of tissue sensitivity to insulin, was decreased in the old-impaired group at each hyperglycemic plateau except the highest. This finding supports the view that glucose intolerance is due to insulin resistance.[69]

In a study of 20 nonobese, nondiabetic men divided into young [$n$ = 10; 18–36 years old (mean ± SD, 27 ± 6 years)] and old ($n$ = 10; 57–82 years old (mean 69 ± 6 years)] groups, Chen et al. used the minimal model approach to evaluate age-related glucose intolerance. This method is based on the use of mathematic models to account for the dynamic relations between glucose and insulin by measuring insulin sensitivity and islet cell function during the frequently sampled intravenous glucose tolerance test (FSIGT). The older men were found to be glucose-intolerant (glucose disappearance rate 1.32%/min) compared with the younger men (glucose disappearance rate 2.21%/min; $p < 0.01$). This was found to be the result of both a beta cell defect and insulin resistance. There was no significant change in insulin clearance or insulin-independent glucose disappearance, however, so these factors are probably not involved in the decreased insulin levels.[70]

Alteration in beta cell function in the elderly has also been shown. In an experiment that involved the administration of OGTTs to nonobese middle-aged normal controls [control (CNT) group: $n = 38$; 40–64 years old], nonobese non-insulin-dependent diabetes mellitus (NIDDM) subjects ($n = 28$, 40–64 years old), and nonobese elderly subjects (OL group; $n$ = 17; 65–92 years old), Shimizu et al. found age-related alterations of beta cell function. The OL and NIDDM groups had hyperproinsulinemia compared to the CNT group, and the proinsulin/insulin or proinsulin/C-peptide ratios were significantly higher in the OL and NIDDM groups. These increases are likely the result of a dysfunction of the beta cell in processing proinsulin to insulin, as there was no evidence of beta cell hypersecretion or altered clearance of insulin and C-peptide.[71] A study that confirmd these results looked at 12 young controls [27 ± 1 (SE) years] and 12 elderly men (69 ± 2 years), all with normal OGTTs and normal insulin sensitivity. In a FSIGT, basal C-peptide was found to be lower in the old subjects: 0.43 ± 0.06 versus 0.70 ± 0.11 ng/ml ($p < 0.025$), suggesting reduced insulin secretion. Beta cell secretion was found to be lower in the elderly (total amount released in 240 minutes was 4.8 ± 0.6 nM in the elderly group vs. 7.5 ± 0.9 in the young group; $p < 0.025$). Hepatic extraction of insulin was also impaired in the elderly, such that virtually the same amount of insulin reached the periphery in both groups (2.7 ± 0.2 nM in the elderly and, 2.9 ± 0.3 in the young;

$p > 0.3$).[72] Here again beta cell function was found to be altered in the elderly. The similar serum levels of insulin can be explained by decreased hepatic extraction.

## Colon

Ample data suggest that there is no difference in colonic motility in the elderly when compared to that in the young. Loening-Baucke and Anuras studied sigmoid, rectosigmoid, and rectal transit times using intraluminal pressure transducers during fasting, during eating, and after consumption of a meal in 18 healthy young subjects (age 21–40 years, mean 29 years) and 18 healthy elderly subjects (age 65–82 years, mean 72 years). There was no difference in the percentage activity and the surface area under the curve between the two groups.[73] In a comparison of colonic transit times of a meal containing radiolabeled food particles in young versus elderly subjects, Madsen also reported no significant difference.[37] Using a "simplified assessment" in which subjects' total colonic and segmental transit times are estimated based on a single abdominal film obtained on the fourth day after ingestion of radiopaque markers of colonic transit, Metcalf et al. found no significant difference between young and old subjects.[74] In a study by Melkersson et al. a radioisotope was followed through the gut in 16 elderly subjects with constipation, 16 age-matched subjects without constipation, and 10 healthy younger subjects. Although constipated patients had slower transit times through the rectosigmoid, there was no difference in transit times between young and old with normal bowel habits.[75]

Despite the abundance of data suggesting that colonic transit time is not decreased in the elderly, constipation, defined as fewer than three bowel movements per week,[76] continues to be one of the most common chronic digestive complaints in this population.[77] About 9–34% of men and women over age 65 suffer from constipation compared to 4% of a younger population and 19% of a middle-aged population. The cause of constipation is usually attributed to a low-fiber diet, sedentary life style, and colonic motility disturbances[15] (Table 36.4). Of course, routine screening for colon cancer, including serial stool guiaic tests, flexible endoscopy, or barium enema, is mandatory for the workup of new constipation.

There is a high rate of laxative use in the elderly (reported in 32% of nursing home patients). Constipation in the elderly may produce serious complications, such as acute mental confusion, urinary retention, urinary incontinence, fecal impaction and stercoral ulceration. The primary symptom older people use to describe their constipation is the feeling of having to strain excessively to defecate. This may be due to outlet delay caused by pelvic dyssynergia, which is a paradoxical increase in anal canal pressure with attempts to defecate. This was found to be the predominant mechanism for constipation in 10 of 10 otherwise healthy patients over 65 in a study by Cheskin et al. Colonic inertia, or total gut transit time over 67 hours, was found in two of these patients, and rectosigmoid irritability, or multiple rectosigmoid contractions in response to balloon distension, was seen in only one subject.[78]

The explanation for constipation in the elderly is probably multifactorial, resulting from decreased muscle tone and motor function of the colon. One possible explanation is a decrease in neuron density in the myenteric plexus in the elderly. Gomez et al. found that there was a 37% decrease in the number of neurons in the myenteric plexus in six colon specimens from elderly patients (average age 77.7 ± 7.6 years) with no previous digestive pathology.[77] Similarly, Koch et al. found a significant decrease in inhibitory junction potentials in human colon with age, an association noted with other functional obstructions, as in Hirschsprung's disease.[79]

For many people, defecation is part of a morning routine beginning upon arising, which can initiate contraction in the distal colon.[80] Bed rest at any age is known to cause constipation, and many elderly people have a low activity level or are disabled. A nursing home study, which implemented a bowel management program, found that participating subjects had a significant decrease in their need for laxatives and an increase in their number of bowel movements. This program included increased fluid and fiber intake, daily ambulation, and exercise.[81]

Constipation is a side effect of many drugs commonly used in the elderly. In a study of 800 nursing home residents (age 65–105 years, mean 84.7 years) who were receiving psychoactive medication, Monane et al. evaluated the relation of these drugs to constipation. Consti-

TABLE 36.4. Causes of Constipation in the Elderly

| |
|---|
| Tumor, anatomic stricture |
| Low fiber diet |
| Dehydration, electrolyte imbalance |
| Sedentary life style, recent injury |
| Colonic motility problems |
| Colonic inertia |
| Rectosigmoid irritability |
| Anorectal functional problems |
| Outlet obstruction |
| Anismus |
| Rectal prolapse |
| Systemic disease |
| Diabetes mellitus |
| Acute illness |
| Medications |
| Antidepressants, antipsychotics |
| Opioids |
| Anticholinergics |

pation was assessed by measuring the frequency of laxative use. Altogether, 74% of residents were found to be taking laxatives daily, and 45% received more than one per day. Logical regression modeling was used to adjust for potential confounding. The investigators found that laxative use was significantly higher in residents taking highly anticholinergic antidepressants such as amitriptyline (odds ratio 3.12), diphenhydramine (odds ratio 2.18), or highly anticholinergic neuroleptics such as thioridazine (odds ratio 2.01); it was also high in the very old (≥85 years) (odds ratio 2.23). Among the factors that did not show a correlation with increased laxative use were gender, decreased functional status, impaired cognitive function, and the use of benzodiazepines or antiparkinsonian agents.[82]

## Anorectum

Anorectal physiology plays a major role in the function of large bowel and pelvic disorders.[83] The increase in fecal incontinence and constipation seen during old age is sometimes caused by mechanical changes in the rectum known as pelvic outlet obstruction.[84] Anal incontinence is seen predominantly in women, increases with advancing age, and is due to insufficient anal sphincter function. In a study of 49 healthy women with a mean age of 51 years (range 20–79 years), the anal pressure was recorded. Closing pressure (the difference between maximum resting anal pressure and rectal pressure), an important determinant of anal continence, was reduced with age. Age-related changes were also found for the length of the anal canal.[85]

Another study that set out to find a relation between age and anorectal function had similar results. Jameson et al. prospectively evaluated 91 healthy subjects (51 women age 19–70 years, mean 40 years; and 40 men age 16–85 years, mean 52 years) to determine the effect of age, sex, and parity on anorectal function.[83] Maximum resting pressures, voluntary contraction pressure, rectal sensation to distension, rectal and mid-anal electrosensitivity, perineal descent, pudendal nerve terminal motor latency, and fiber density of the external anal sphincter were all measured. Age was found to influence resting pressure, mid-anal electrosensitivity and rectal electrosensitivity. Increased age was also found to lead to perineal descent at rest, slowed pudendal nerve conduction, a fall in resting anal pressure, and decreased anorectal sensory function. Laurberg and Swash also found elderly subjects (women in the fifth decade) to have increased pudendal nerve terminal motor latency (indicating chronic damage to this nerve), but it was associated with a reduction in rectal "squeeze" pressure and not to a reduction in resting anal pressure. This study, which evaluated 102 women and 19 men without colorectal or pelvic floor disease, found these women to have increased perineal descent in the resting and straining positions. The investigators were reluctant to attribute these changes solely to aging, noting that menopausal effect and parity may be relevant.[86] Parity could not be shown to have any effect on rectoanal function in another evaluation of 68 normal subjects. This study used graded isobaric distension in combination with anal manometry and found that increasing age correlated with a decrease in rectal volume, resting anal pressure, and maximal squeezing pressure. An age-dependent increase was observed for the pressure threshold to produce an initial sensation of rectal filling and the rectoanal reflex.[87] This may be due to chronic damage resulting from constipation and passages of large fecal boluses.

Parity may, however, be associated with rectal prolapse, which has a higher incidence in women and the elderly and is thought to be related to pelvic floor disease. In this condition the rectum bulges into the perineum, tightening the puborectalis and increasing the anorectal angulation. Here again the pudendal nerve is stretched. The rectum herniates through the weakened anal sphincter.[80]

Anorectal physiology can be evaluated in terms of recovery of function following an operative procedure. Young and elderly patients who have undergone an ileoanal reservoir procedure following a colectomy for ulcerative colitis or familial polyposis have been compared.[88] These patients were evaluated pre- and postoperatively with manometry for anorectal pressures and clinical outcomes by a questionnaire. No difference in preoperative anorectal pressures or in clinical outcome was found between the two groups. Also, despite the transient impairment of internal anal sphincter function seen in these patients, there is complete recovery after ileostomy closure.

## Colorectal Cancer

The incidence of many types of neoplasia is increased as humans age. The proliferative potential of the gastrointestinal tract, which turns over its entire epithelium every 24–72 hours, makes it particularly susceptible to neoplasia.[35] The mean age of presentation of colon cancer is 71, and two-thirds of the 150,000 new cases of colon cancer each year occur in patients over age 65.[89]

A lifetime of repeated insults from environmental factors, such as chemicals and radiation, are important external influences affecting genetic stability. Yet aging itself may eventually become enough of a pathogenic influence for carcinogenesis. Colon cancer is associated with genetic abnormalities such as mutations and, more commonly, deletions of tumor-suppressor genes. Genomic entropy has been shown to increase with time, making genetic instability (and therefore the malfunction of genetic mechanisms such as DNA repair) more common in the elderly.[90]

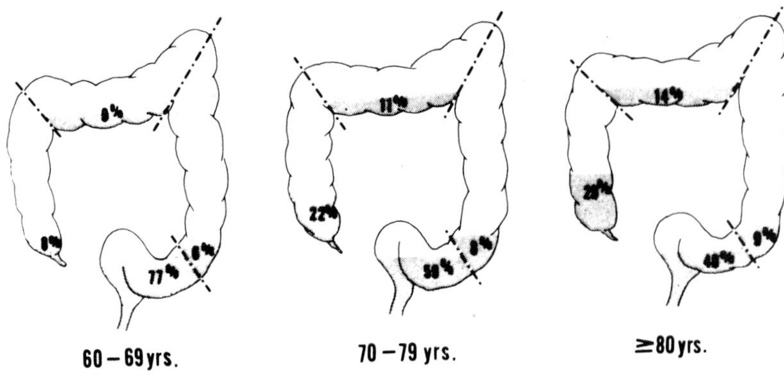


FIGURE 36.7. Location of colon cancers in 222 patients grouped by age. The authors found an increased incidence of right-sided colon cancer with age, associated with a concomitant fall in the number of rectosigmoid lesions. Interestingly, a more favorable staging pattern was noted with each. (From Schub and Steinheber,[92] with permission.)

Colorectal carcinomas appear to arise from adenomas, and the idea that carcinogenesis evolves in a multistage process is generally accepted.[90] It is described as a series of genetic alterations resulting in progressive derangement of the genetic factors that control normal growth. Vogelstein et al. looked at four genetic alterations in 172 colorectal tumor specimens representing various stages of neoplastic development: *ras* gene mutations and allelic deletions of chromosomes 5, 17, and 18. Specimens consisted of 40 predominantly early-stage adenomas from 7 patients with familial adenomatous polyposis, 40 adenomas (19 without associated foci of carcinoma and 21 with such foci) from 33 patients without familial polyposis, and 92 carcinomas resected from 89 patients. The *ras* gene mutations were found to have occurred in a significantly higher proportion of adenomas >1 cm and in carcinomas (58% and 47%, respectively) than in adenomas <1 cm in size (9%). Sequences on chromosome 5 that are linked to the gene for familial adenomatous polyposis were present in adenomas from patients with polyposis but were lost in 29% and 35% of adenomas and carcinomas, respectively, from other patients. Carcinomas and advanced adenomas showed a higher rate of deletion of a specific region of chromosome 18 (73% and 47%, respectively) than in earlier-stage adenomas (11–13%). Chromosome 17p sequences were usually lost only in carcinomas (75%). The clinical progression of the tumors developed synchronously with these four genetic alterations. These findings are consistent with the model of tumorigenesis in which the development of cancer occurs in a stepwise fashion, involving the mutational activation of an oncogene together with the loss of genes responsible for tumor suppression.[91]

In addition to a higher incidence in the elderly, colon cancer also has been shown to have characteristically different locations of occurrence. In a review of 222 patients with colon cancer over age 60, Schub and Steinheber found that there was a higher incidence of right-sided lesions and a decreased incidence of rectosigmoid lesions as the population aged. For patients in their sixth decade, 8% of the tumors were located in the right colon, 9% in the transverse colon, 6% percent in the descending colon, and 77% in the rectosigmoid. During the seventh decade, 22% were located in the right colon, 11% in the transverse colon, and 58% in the rectosigmoid area. In the oldest group (those 80 years of age and above) 29% were in the right colon, 14% in the transverse colon, 9% in the descending colon, and 49% in the rectosigmoid area. This trend was found to be statistically significant by chi-square analysis ($p < 0.05$). This "rightward shift" was also associated with a trend toward more favorable staging. The investigators believed that it reflects an increase in the proportion of elderly patients with cancer and a predilection toward right-sided lesions with aging[92] (Fig. 36.7).

Similarly, in a review of 1205 Japanese patients with colorectal cancer, Ikeda et al. found an increased incidence of proximal colon cancer in the elderly. In this study, though, it was true only for female patients ($p < 0.01$). The authors suggested a difference in the biologic mechanism in tumor development between the proximal and distal colon.[93]

## Conclusions

The aging of the gastrointestinal tract is associated with many somatic complaints, ranging from dyspepsia to constipation. The scientific explanation for these events has eluded us, as for the most part there are no real differences in histology, motility, or mucosal structure. The molecular aging of the gastrointestinal epithelial cell, however, is being studied and has yielded some explanations for the incidence of gastrointestinal malignancies. Diagnosis and treatment of ailments in specific organ systems are addressed in the chapters that follow.

## References

1. Ekberg O, Feinberg MJ. Altered swallowing function in elderly patients without dysphagia: radiologic findings in 56 cases. Am J Radiol 1998;156:1181–1184.
2. Fulp SR, Dalton CB, Castell JA, Castell DO. Aging-related alterations in human upper esophageal sphincter function. Am J Gastroenterol 1990;85:1569–1572.

3. Newnham DM, Hamilton SJC. Sensitivity of the cough reflex in young and elderly subjects. Age Ageing 1997; 26:185–188.
4. Harkness GA, Bently DW, Roghmann KJ. Risk factors for nosocomial pneumonia in the elderly. Am J Med 1990;89: 457–463.
5. Wilson JA, Pryde A, Macintyre CCA, Maran AGD, Heasing RC. The effects of age, sex, and smoking on normal pharyngoesophageal motility. Am J Gastroenterol 1990;85:686–691.
6. Zboralske FF, Amberg JR, Soergel KH. Presbyesophagus: cineradiographic manifestations. Radiology 1964;82:463–467.
7. Soergel KH, Zboralske FF, Amberg JR. Presbyesophagus: esophageal motility in nonagenarians. J Clin Invest 1964; 43:1472–1479.
8. Hollis JB, Castell DO. Esophageal function in elderly men; a new look at "presbyesophagus." Ann Intern Med 1974;80: 371–374.
9. Adamek JR, Wegener M, Weinbeck M, Gielen B. Long-term esophageal manometry in healthy subjects; evaluation of normal values and influence of age. Dig Dis Sci 1994; 39:2069–2073.
10. Meshkinpour H, Haghighat P, Dutton C. Clinical spectrum of esophageal aperistalsis in the elderly. Am J Gastroenterol 1994;89:1480–1483.
11. Ren J, Shaker R, Kusano M, et al. Effect of aging on the secondary esophageal peristalsis: presbyesophagus revisited. Am J Physiol 1995;268:G772–G779.
12. Lasch HC, Castell DO, Castell JA. Evidence for diminished visceral pain with aging: studies using graded intraesophageal balloon distension. Am J Physiol 1997;272:G1–G3.
13. Filho JM, Carvalho VC, deSouza RR. Nerve cell loss in the myenteric plexus of the human esophagus in relation to age: a preliminary investigation. Gerontology 1995;41:18–21.
14. DelValle J, Lucey MR, Yamada T. Gastric secretion. In: Yamada Y, Alpers DH, Powell DW, Owyang C, Silverstein FE (eds) Textbook on Gastroenterology. Philadelphia: Lippincott, 1995:295–326.
15. Shamburek RD, Scott RB, Farrar JT. Gastrointestinal and liver changes in the elderly. In: Katlic MR (ed) Geriatric Surgery: Comprehensive Care of the Elderly Patient. 1990: 97–113.
16. Katelaris PH, Seow F, Lin BPC, Napoli J, Ngu MC, Jones DB. Effect of age, Helicobacter pylori infection, and gastritis with atrophy on serum gastrin and gastric acid secretion in healthy men. Gut 1993;34:1032–1037.
17. Kekki M, Samloff IM, Ihamaki T, Varis K, Siuala M. Age- and sex-related behaviour of gastric acid secretion at the population level. Scand J Gastroenterol 1982;17:737–743.
18. Goldschmiedt M, Barnett CC, Schwartz BE, Karnes WE, Redfern JS, Feldman M. Effect of age on gastric acid secretion and serum gastrin concentrations in healthy men and women. Gastroenterology 1991;101:990–997.
19. Feldman M, Cryer B, Huet BA, Lee E. Effects of aging and gastritis on gastric acid and pepsin secretion in humans: a prospective study. Gastroenterology 1996;110:1043–1052.
20. Evans MA, Triggs JE, Broe GA, Creasey H. Gastric emptying rate in the elderly: implications for drug therapy. J Am Geriatr Soc 1981;29:201–205.
21. Moore JG, Tweedy C, Datz FL. Effect of age on gastric emptying of liquid-solid meals in man. Dig Dis Sci 1983; 28:340–344.
22. Horowitz M, Maddern GJ, Collins JP, Harding PE, Shearman DJ. Changes in gastric emptying rates with age. Clin Sci 1984;67:213–218.
23. Kao CH, Lai TL, Chen GH, Yeh SH. Influence of age on gastric emptying in healthy Chinese. Clin Nucl Med 1997; 19:401–404.
24. Clarkston WK, Pantano MM, Horowitz M, Littlefield JM, Burton FR. Evidence for the anorexia of aging: gastrointestinal transit and hunger in the healthy elderly vs. young adults. Am J Physiol 1997;272:R243–R248.
25. Gainsborough N, Maskrey VL, Keating J, Sherwood RA, Jackson SHD, Swift CG. The association of age with gastric emptying. Age Ageing 1993;22:37–40.
26. Pfaffenbach B. Adamek RJ, Bartholomaus C. Gastric dysrhythmias and delayed gastric emptying in patients with functional dyspepsia. Dig Dis Sci 1997;42:2094–2099.
27. Cucchiara S, Salvia G, Borrelli O, et al. Gastric electrical dysrhythmias and delayed gastric emptying in gastroesophageal reflux disease. Am J Gastroenterol 1997;92: 1103–1108.
28. Hinder RA, Kelly KA. Human gastric pacesetter potential: site of origin, spread, and response to gastric transection and proximal gastric vagotomy. Am J Surg 1977;133:29–33.
29. Spencer MP, Sarr MG, Hakim NS, Soper NJ. Interdigestive gastric motility patterns: the role of vagal and nonvagal extrinsic innervation. Surgery 1989;106:185–193.
30. Parkman HP, Harris AD, Fisher RS. Influence of age, gender, and menstrual cylcle on the normal electrogastrogram. Am J Gastroenterol 1996;91:127–133.
31. Kitamura K, Yamaguchi H, Taniguchi H, et al. Clinicopathologic characteristics of gastric cancer in the elderly. Br J Cancer 1996;73:798–802.
32. Mayer RJ. Gastrointestinal tract cancer. In: Fauci AS, Braunwald E, Isselbacher KJ, et al. (eds) Harrison's Principles of Internal Medicine. New York: McGraw-Hill, 1998:568–577.
33. Asaka M, Takeda H, Sugiyama T, Kato M. What role does Helicobacter pylori play in gastric cancer? Gastroenterology 1997;113:S56–S60.
34. Thiede C, Morgner A, Alpen B, et al. What role does Helicobacter pylori eradication play in gastric MALT and gastric MALT lymphoma? Gastroenterology 1997;113:S61–S64.
35. Isselbacher KJ, Podolsky DK. Approach to the patient with gastrointestinal disease. In: Fauci AS, Braunwald E, Isselbacher KJ, et al. (eds) Harrison's Principles of Internal Medicine. New York: McGraw-Hill, 1998:1579–1583.
36. Husebye E, Engedal K. The patterns of motility are maintained in the human small intestine throughout the process of aging. Scand J Gastroenterol 1992;27:397–404.
37. Madsen JL. Effects of gender, age, and body mass index on gastrointestinal transit times. Dig Dis Sci 1992;37:1548–1553.
38. Argeny EE, Soffer EE, Madsen MT, Bernbaum KS, Walkner WO. Scintigraphic evaluatioin of small bowel transit in healthy subjects: inter- and intrasubject variability. Am J Gastroenterol 1995;90:938–942.
39. Webster SGP, Leeming JT. The appearance of the small bowel mucosa in old age. Age Ageing 1975;4:168–174.

40. Warren PM, Pepperman MA, Montgomery RD. Age changes in small-intestinal mucosa. Lancet 1978;2:849–850.
41. Corazza GR, Frazzoni M, Gatto MRA, Gasbarrini G. Ageing and small-bowel mucosa: a morphometric study. Gerontology 1986;32:60–65.
42. Clarke RM. The effects of age on mucosal morphology and epithelial cell production in rat small intestine. J Anat 1977;123:805–811.
43. Atillasoy E, Holt PR. Gastrointestinal proliferation and aging. J Gerontol 1993;48:B43–B49.
44. Raul F, Gosse F, Doffoel M, Darmenton P, Wessely JY. Age related increase of brush border enzyme activities along the small intestine. Gut 1988;29:1557–1563.
45. Saltzman JR, Kowdley KV, Russell RM. Changes in small-intestine permeability with ageing. J Am Geriatr Soc 1995;-43:160–164.
46. Riordan SM, McIver CJ, Thomas DH, Duncombe VM, Bolin TD, Thomas MC. Luminal bacterial and small-intestinal permeability. Scand J Gastroenterol 1997;32:556–563.
47. De Souza RR, Moratelli HB, Borges N, Liberti EA. Age-induced nerve cell loss in the myenteric plexus of the small intestine in man. Gerontology 1993;39:183–188.
48. Holt PR. The small intestine. Clin Gastroenterol 1985;14: 689–723.
49. Wallis JL, Lipski PS, James OFW, Hirst BH. Duodenal brush-border mucosal glucose transport and enzyme activities in aging man and effect of bacterial contamination of the small intestine. Dig Dis Sci 1993;38:403–409.
50. Beaumont DM, Cobden I, Sheldon WL. Passive and active carbohydrate absorption by the ageing gut. Age Ageing 1987;16:294–300.
51. Arora S, Kassarjian Z, Krasinski SD, Croffey B, Kaplan MM, Russell RM. Effect of age on test of intestinal and hepatic function on healthy humans. Gastroenterology 1989;96: 1560–1565.
52. McEvoy S, Dutton J, James OFW. Bacterial contamination of the small intestine is an important cause of occult malabsorption in the elderly. BMJ 1983;287:789–793.
53. MacMahon M, Lynch M, Mullins E, et al. Small intestinal bacterial overgrowth—an incidental finding. J Am Geriatr Soc 1994;42:146–149.
54. Boyd E. Normal variability in weight of the adult human liver and spleen. Arch Pathol 1933;16:350–372.
55. Sherloch S, Bearn AG, Billing BH, Paterson JCS. Splanchnic blood flow in man by the bromsulfalein method: the relation of peripheral plasma bromsulfalein level to the calculated flow. J Lab Clin Med 1950;35:923–932.
56. MacMahon MM, James OFW, Holt PR. Liver disease in the elderly. J Clin Gastroenterol 1994;18:330–334.
57. Sotaniemi EA, Arranto AJ, Pelkonen O. Age and cytochrome P450-linked drug metabolism in humans: an analysis of 226 subjects with equal histopathologic conditions. Clin Pharmacol Ther 1997;61:331–339.
58. Wall W, Grant D, Roy A, Asfar S, Block M. Elderly liver donor. Lancet 1993;341(8837):121.
59. De Pancorbo CM, Carballo F, Horcajo P, et al. Prevalence and associated factors for gallstone disease: results of a population survey in Spain. J Clin Epidemiol 1997;50:1347–1355.
60. Attili AF, Capocaccia R, Carulli N, et al. Factors associated with gallstone disease in the MICOL experience. Hepatology 1997;26:809–818.
61. Valdivieso V, Palma R, Wunkaus R, Antezana C, Severin C, Contreras A. Effect of aging on biliary lipid composition and bile acid metabolism in normal Chilean women. Gastroenterology 1978;74:871–874.
62. Tanno M, Ogihara M, Taguchi T. Age-related changes in proliferating cell nuclear antigen levels. Mech Ageing Dev 1996;92:53–66.
63. Fry M, Silber J, Loeb LA, Martin GM. Delayed and reduced cell replication and diminishing levels of DNA polymerase-α in regenerating liver of aging mice. J Cell Physiol 1984; 118:225–232.
64. Yamamoto K, Takenada K, Matsumata T, et al. Right hepatic lobectomy in elderly patients with hepatocellular carcinoma. Hepatogastroenterology 1997;44:514–518.
65. Shimada M, Matsumata T, Maeda T, Itasaka H, Suehiro T, Sugimachi K. Hepatic regeneration following right lobectomy: estimation of regenerative capacity. Jpn J Surg 1994; 24:44–48.
66. Gullo L, Priori P, Daniele C, Ventrucci M, Gasbarrini GL. Exocrine pancreatic function in the elderly. Gerontology 1983;29:407–411.
67. Gullo L, Ventrucci M, Naldoni P, Pezzilli R. Aging and exocrine pancreatic function. J Am Geriatr Soc 1986;34: 790–792.
68. Carrere J, Serre G, Vincent C, et al. Human serum pancreatic lipase and trypsin 1 in aging: enzymatic and immunoenzymatic assays. J Gerontol 1987;42:315–317.
69. Elahi D, Muller DC, McAloon-Dyke M, Tobin JD, Andres R. The effect of age in insulin response and glucose utilization during four hyperglycemic plateaus. Exp Gerontol 1993;28: 393–409.
70. Chen M, Bergman RN, Pacini G, Porte D. Pathogenesis of age-related glucose intolerance in man: insulin resistance and decreased beta-cell function. J Clin Endocrinol Metab 1985;60:13–20.
71. Shimizu M, Kawazu S, Tomono S, et al. Age-related alteration of pancreatic beta-cell function. Diabetes Care 1996;19: 8–11.
72. Pacini G, Beccaro F, Valerio A, Nosadini R, Crepaldi G. Reduced beta-cell secretion and insulin hepatic extraction in healthy elderly subjects. J Am Geriatr Soc 1990;38: 1283–1289.
73. Loening-Baucke V, Anuras S. Sigmoidal and rectal motility in healthy elderly. J Am Geriatr Soc 1984;32:887–891.
74. Metcalf AM, Phillip SF, Zinsmeister AR, MacCarty RL, Beart RW, Wolff BG. Simplified assessment of segmental colonic transit. Gastroenterology 1987;92:40–47.
75. Melkersson M, Andersson H, Bosaeus I, Falkheden T. Intestinal transit time in constipated and non-constipated geriatric patients. Scand J Gastroenterol 1982;18:593–597.
76. Isselbacher KJ, Friedman L. Diarrhea and constipation. In: Fauci AS, Braunwald E, Isselbacher KJ, et al. (eds) Harrison's Principles of Internal Medicine. New York: McGraw-Hill, 1998:236–244.
77. Gomez OA, de Souza RR, Liberti EA. A preliminary investigation of the effects of aging on the nerve cell number in the myenteric ganglia of the human colon. Gastroenterology 1997;43:210–217.
78. Cheskin LJ, Kamal N, Crowell MD, Schuster MM, Whitehead WE. Mechanisms of constipation in older persons and effect of fiber compared with placebo. J Am Geriatr Soc 1995;43:666–669.

79. Koch TR, Go VLW, Szurszewski JH. Changes in some electrophysiological properties of circular muscle from normal sigmoid colon of the aging patient [abstract]. Gastroenterology 1986;90:1497.
80. Read NW, Celik AF, Katsinelos P. Constipation and incontinence in the elderly. J Clin Gastroenterol 1995;20:61–70.
81. Karam SE, Neis DM. Student/staff collaboration: a pilot bowel management program. J Gastroenterol Nurs 1994;20: 32–40.
82. Monane M, Avorn J, Beers MH, Everitt DE. Anticholinergic drug use and bowel function in nursing home patients. Arch Intern Med 1993;153:633–638.
83. Jameson JS, Chia YW, Kamm MA, Speakman CTM, Chye YH, Henrey MM. Effect of age, sex, and parity on anorectal function. Br J Surg 1994;81:1689–1692.
84. Lovat LB. Age related status changes in gut physiology and nutritional status. Gut 1996;38:306–309.
85. Haadem K. Dahlstrom JA, Ling E. Anal sphincter competence in healthy women: clinical implications of age and other factors. Obstet Gynecol 1991;78:823–827.
86. Laurberg S, Swash M. Effects of aging on the anorectal sphincters and their innervation. Dis Colon Rectum 1989; 32:737–742.
87. Arkervall S, Nordgren S, Fasth S, Oresland T, Pettersson K, Hulten L. The effects of age, gender and parity on rectoanal functions in adults. Scand J Gastroenterol 1990;25:1247–1256.
88. Jorges JMN, Wexner SD, James K, Nogueras JJ, Jagelman GD. Recovery of anal sphincer function after the ileoanal reservoir procedure in patients over the age of fifty. Dis Colon Rectum 1994;37:1002–1005.
89. McGinnis LS. Surgical treatment options for colorectal cancer. Cancer 1994;74:2147–2150.
90. Riggs JE. Aging, genomic entropy and carcinogenesis: implications derived from longitudinal age-specific colon cancer mortality rate dynamics. Mech Ageing Dev 1993;72: 165–181.
91. Vogelstein B, Fearon ER, Hamilton SR, et al. Genetic alterations during colorectal-tumor development. N Engl J Med 1988;3119:525–532.
92. Schub R, Steinheber FU. Rightward shift of colon cancer: a feature of the aging gut. J Clin Gastroenterol 1986;8:630–634.
93. Ikeda Y, Koyagani N, Mori M, et al. Increased incidence of proximal colon cancer in the elderly. J Clin Gastroenterol 1996;23:105–108.

# 37
# Benign Esophageal Disease in the Elderly

Seth A. Spector and Neal E. Seymour

Pathologic conditions of the esophagus that affect the elderly, exclusive of carcinoma, are similar to diseases that occur in the younger population, although the incidence of selected disorders may be either greater or smaller in older patients. Special consideration must be given to elderly patients' limited tolerance of symptoms and to the physiologic impact of treatments and treatment complications in this vulnerable population. Advances in minimally invasive surgery have made the surgical treatment of some esophageal diseases less traumatic than had previously been the case. Despite these and other improvements in therapy, benign esophageal disorders continue to present great challenges to practitioners treating the geriatric population.

## Gastroesophageal Reflux Disease

Gastroesophageal reflux disease (GERD) is the pathologic form of gastroesophageal reflux associated with symptoms and abnormalities of the esophagus. The full spectrum of GERD and its complications are observed in the elderly and present special management considerations compared to its treatment in the younger population. Although GERD does not itself present a significant risk for mortality in the elderly, it may impair quality of life and lead to considerable complication-related morbidity. Patient tolerance of severe symptoms is often poor, and complications such as peptic stricture, Barrett's esophagus, and chronic upper aerodigestive problems may be particularly difficult to manage in the elderly.

Although the prevalence of GERD and esophagitis increases with age, the precise prevalence after the seventh decade is uncertain. Current data suggest that patients more than 60 years of age present with more advanced esophagitis than do younger patients, and that a large percentage of less severe cases do not come to medical attention.[1,2] Zhu et al. reported that 21% of patients 65–76 years of age with symptomatic GERD present with endoscopically severe esophagitis, but that only 3.4% of those less than 64 years old have esophagitis of similar severity.[3] It has been suggested that elderly patients may as a group be less symptomatic of reflux as a result of either decreased refluxate acid concentration or blunted pain perception, but no firm data support this supposition. Some limited data suggest that Barrett's esophagus is also more common in the elderly with GERD.[4]

Few data address mechanical esophagogastric junction changes leading to GERD that may be specific to elderly patients. Some factors predisposing to GERD may be more active with advancing age. Major esophageal protective mechanisms are degraded through expected aging-related physiologic events, such as loss of primary esophageal peristalsis,[5] and diminished salivary secretion. These mechanisms may become relatively more important in the pathophysiology of GERD after the seventh decade. Although the concept that gastric acid secretion decreases with age has been challenged, it is unlikely that hyperacidity contributes significantly to GERD in the elderly. Increased esophageal acid exposure with age is probably due to commonly recognized mechanical factors (Table 37.1) in conjunction with a loss in mucosal barriers.[1–3,5] Translocation of the esophagogastric junction and lower esophageal sphincter (LES) into the mediastinum through the esophageal hiatus (type 1, sliding hiatal hernia) occurs more frequently after age 60 and is thought to contribute to pathologic reflux by exposing the LES to ambient extraluminal pressure in the chest that is lower than that in the abdomen (Fig. 37.1). This diminished extraluminal pressure permits LES tone to be more easily overcome by increased intragastric pressure, leading to reflux.

The tendency for elderly patients to present with more severe mucosal injury may be explained on the basis of altered patient perception of pain and regurgitation symptoms.[1,3] Mold et al. performed ambulatory 24-hour esophageal pH monitoring in 54 elderly patients with an average age of 72 years (range 62–96 years).[6] It was found that the prevalence of measurable gastroesophageal

TABLE 37.1. Pathophysiologic Factors Contributing to GERD

| |
|---|
| Mechanical deficiency of lower esophageal sphincter |
| Increased frequency and duration of transient lower esophageal sphincter relaxations |
| Hiatal hernia (loss of intraabdominal segment of esophagus) |
| Increased intragastric pressure |
| Loss of esophageal peristalsis |
| Loss of esophageal mucosal barrier function |

GERD, gastroesophageal reflux disease.

acid reflux was approximately 20% in this population. However, only 54% of those with pathologic reflux complained of significant GERD symptoms. Furthermore, 11% of those without pathologic gastroesophageal reflux complained of weekly heartburn. It was also unexpectedly found that 31% of patients had significant esophageal alkalinity. Of these patients, there was a smaller incidence of heartburn (29%) but a greater incidence of pulmonary symptoms (24% vs. 0%). Pellegrini et al. found that individuals with alkaline reflux may have less heartburn, regurgitation, and dysphagia but at least as much esophagitis and stricture risk as those with acid reflux. They also showed that the alkaline refluxers had a much higher frequency of pulmonary symptoms.[7]

Barrett's esophagus has been reported to occur in up to 10–15% of patients with GERD[8,9] and is a marker of more severe esophageal injury. Although its incidence is uncertain, some data suggest that Barrett's esophagus, or columnar metaplasia, is more frequent in the elderly.[4] Long-term follow-up of patients with dysplasia-free Barrett's esophagus has indicated that the incidence of dysplasia and cancer in patients treated medically were 19.7% and 1.3%, respectively, whereas those treated by fundoplication had 3.4% dysplasia and 0% cancer incidences.[10] Progression to dysplasia appears to be a time-dependent process, the impact of which remains to be elucidated in the elderly, where residual life expectancy may be significantly limited by co-morbid conditions. It is not clear that the same forceful arguments can be made in favor of operative treatment in elderly patients as can be made for the larger pool of patients with Barrett's esophagus.

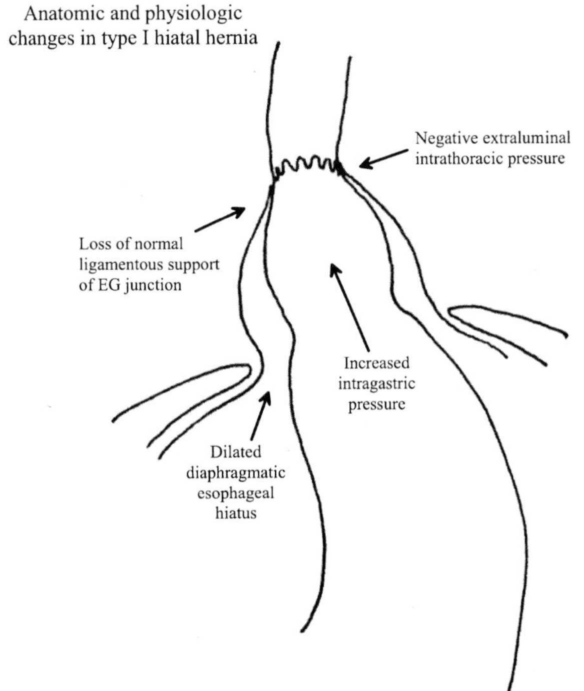


FIGURE 37.1. Hiatal hernia and gastroesophageal reflux disease (GERD).

## Diagnostic Studies

Several investigations are available to establish the diagnosis of GERD or to clarify selected aspects of a patient's GERD complaints (Table 37.2). These tests are generally reserved for patients with moderate to severe disease or are used in uncertain diagnostic situations. Upper endoscopy should be performed in any elderly patient with symptoms severe enough to require chronic medical treatment. It is currently the only reliable method to rule out Barrett's esophagus and determine the severity of the esophagitis. In those with dysphagia or suspected peptic stricture, carcinoma can usually be excluded. Although barium esophagography is not necessary in all patients, it can provide important additional information in those with dysphagia and suspected luminal narrowing. In addition, dynamic information regarding esophageal emptying and reflux can be obtained. Esophageal manometry is useful for clarifying potential motility disturbances in patients with dysphagia or chest pain. This study can also provide vital information regarding esophageal peristalsis and the possible risk of postoperative dysphagia after fundoplication.

Ambulatory esophageal pH monitoring is the most definitive diagnostic modality for GERD. This method directly tracks the spontaneous reflux events and

TABLE 37.2. Diagnostic Studies for GERD

| Test | Purpose of study |
|---|---|
| Barium esophogram | Presence of hiatal hernia, esophageal stricture, web, ring; reflux of contrast |
| Endoscopy | Presence of esophagitis, Barrett's, ulcer, tumor, gastroduodenal pathology; documentation of healing esophagitis |
| Esophageal manometry | Ascertain lower esophageal sphincter (LES) function, rule out esophageal dysmotility |
| 24-Hour pH probe study | Definitive diagnosis of GERD |

measures the degree of acid exposure experienced by the esophagus. Esophageal 24-hour pH monitoring is probably most useful for establishing the diagnosis of GERD in patients with significant symptoms but without esophagitis on endoscopy. It is advisable in (1) those who have failed a trial of medical therapy (particularly proton pump inhibitor treatment); (2) patients with atypical symptoms, chest pain of uncertain origin, or pulmonary symptoms; and patients who are under consideration for antireflux surgery. Furthermore, pH monitoring can be used to study the efficacy of GERD treatment.

As in the general population, the presence of the classic symptoms of GERD in the elderly does not necessitate a full diagnostic workup prior to a trial of medical therapy. Although the cardinal symptoms of GERD, heartburn and regurgitation, are neither entirely sensitive nor specific for the diagnosis,[11,12] a combination of the symptoms, response to pharmacologic treatment, and results of selective testing can accurately lead to the diagnosis of GERD. The investigative methods available to demonstrate pathologic reflux should be used selectively in elderly patients who have a poor response to medical therapy, dysphagia, repeated episodes of chest pain, or a complication associated with GERD. Chest pain symptoms in the elderly deserve special mention. The most obvious concern when dealing with chest pain in this population is to identify correctly any patients whose symptoms are cardiac in origin and then institute the proper treatment. Most patients with GERD-induced chest pain give a classic history of reflux symptoms in addition to their chest discomfort. In patients whose pain does not resolve promptly with medical treatment for GERD, studies of cardiac perfusion (radionuclide scans, cardiac catheterization) are required before the symptoms can be presumed to be noncardiac.

DeMeester et al. performed 24-hour pH probe studies in patients with typical angina pectoris symptoms and normal cardiac catheterizations and demonstrated reflux to be present in 46%.[13] In this group of 23 patients, 13 had chest pain during the pH probe study. These symptoms coincided with an episode of reflux in 12 of the 13 patients. Schofield et al. reported similar results and added that exercise testing was often needed to produce these chest pain-associated reflux episodes.[14] A positive correlation between chest pain episodes and acid reflux during the pH probe study can be demonstrated in up to 50% of patients with noncardiac chest pain.[15]

## Treatment

The goal of GERD therapy is to alleviate reflux-related symptoms and concurrently heal and prevent the relapse of esophagitis. The "step-up" approach to medical management of GERD, where patient symptom severity determines method of treatment, is most frequently used in the United States. Treatment begins with life style changes, including changes in diet and sleeping position. Assuming at least moderate reflux symptoms, first-line pharmacologic therapy consists of $H_2$-receptor antagonists, which can reduce heartburn and heal esophagitis in 60% of patients after 12 weeks of therapy.[16] If symptoms persist, omeprazole or lansoprazole, long-acting inhibitors the $H^+/K^+$-ATPase in the parietal cell are given. These agents induce healing of even the most severe esophagitis after 8–12 weeks of treatment.[17,18] This algorithm limits the number of patients on the most expensive medication. However, it is based on the assumption that patients' symptoms parallel the severity of their disease, which may be incorrect, particularly in elderly patients. In "step-down" treatment, patients begin therapy with a proton-pump inhibitor and then are subsequently switched to $H_2$-blocker treatment. This approach leads to faster healing of esophagitis and may be more appropriate in elderly patients, who as a group may present with more severe esophagitis for a given level of symptomatology. If necessary, patients may be maintained at the level of medical treatment that is determined to be required for adequate symptom relief or prevention of esophagitis. The response to a specific therapy determines the next appropriate treatment, and treatment algorithms can be constructed which lead ultimately to a surgical approach to GERD (Fig. 37.2).

The only prokinetic agent currently in common use in GERD therapy is cisapride, which promotes the release of acetylcholine at the esophageal myenteric plexus, increases LES tone, improves peristalsis, and accelerates gastric emptying. Despite data showing its effectiveness,[19] cisapride is rarely used for single-agent maintenance therapy. Specific benefits of prokinetic agents in the elderly have not been demonstrated.

With the rapid development since 1990 of laparoscopic techniques to deal with GERD, there has been a resurgence in the use of antireflux surgery in the United States. The procedures that have become most widely accepted are virtually identical to well-described open operations. The goals of surgical treatment are to establish a segment of the esophagus below the diaphragm and to wrap the proximal stomach around the distal esophagus to enhance LES function.[20] Data also suggest that restoration of LES function by fundoplication may preserve esophageal body motility.[21]

Virtually all laparoscopic antireflux surgery involves the construction of either a Nissen or a Toupet fundoplication (Fig. 37.3). The former is a complete (360 degree) wrap of gastric fundus around the distal esophagus, while the latter consists of a similarly constructed partial (270 degree) wrap. The Nissen fundoplication is much more frequently performed, and most worldwide experience with both open and laparoscopic antireflux surgery pertains to this procedure.

Acceptable indications for antireflux surgery are somewhat controversial (Table 37.3), but the major goals of any

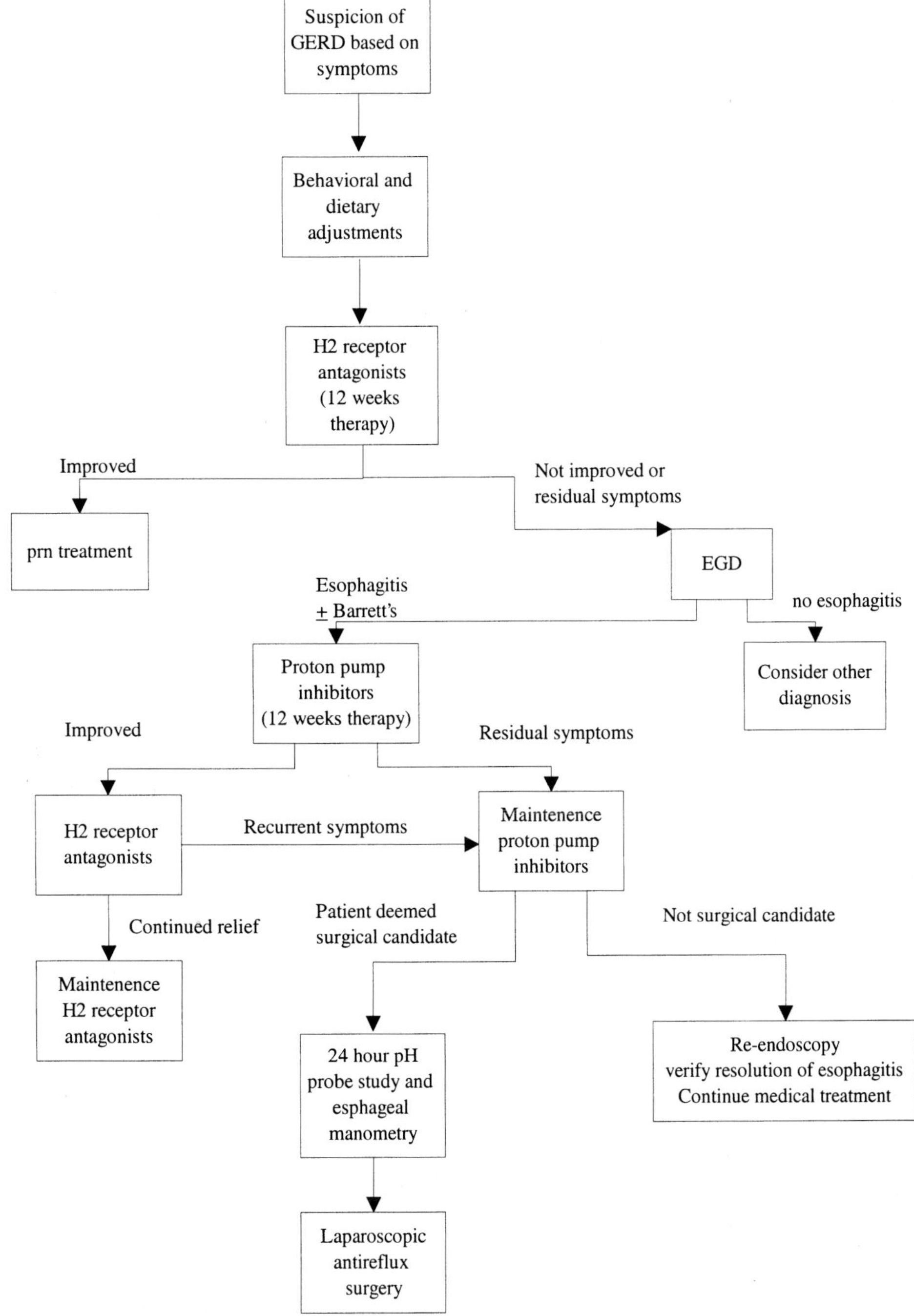


FIGURE 37.2. Algorithm for workup and treatment of GERD in the elderly.

operative intervention are to (1) relieve GERD symptoms, (2) heal esophagitis, and (3) eliminate the need for chronic medical therapy. The decision to proceed with surgical treatment most often is driven by the patient's unwillingness to deal with residual symptoms or to accept chronic medical treatment, the cost of which is not necessarily borne by medical insurance. Arguments in favor of surgical treatment based on economic considerations or possible health risks of prolonged proton pump inhibitor use cannot hold the same weight when considering elderly patients that they might when considering the general pool of GERD patients.

The only reports that have specifically examined surgical indications and results in elderly patients pertain to open procedures. Allen et al.[22] reviewed 103 surgically treated patients with GERD categorized as age >60 (average age 70.6 years, $n$ = 43) and <60 (average age 43.7 years). Altogether, 28 patients >60 were referred for surgery for complications of GERD (stricture, bleeding, aspiration, Barrett's esophagus) compared to only 4 in

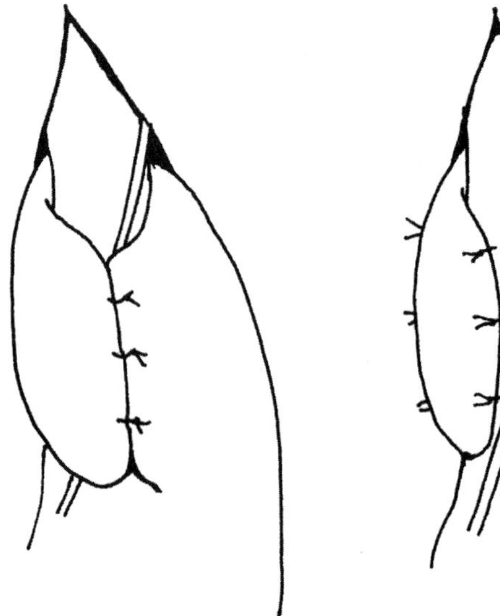


FIGURE 37.3. Laparoscopic antireflux procedures. Laparoscopic Nissen (left) and Toupet (right) fundoplications.

the younger group. The length of time between onset of symptoms and surgical treatment was significantly longer in the older patients (14 vs. 4 years) and may account for the greater incidence of GERD-related complications. Rates of intraoperative and postoperative complications were comparable in the two groups, and 86% of the older patients reported improvement in symptoms compared to 93% of the younger patients.

The laparoscopic method currently represents the standard surgical approach to esophagogastric junction. Current data indicate that laparoscopic approaches to GERD are at least as effective if not better than open procedures.[23] Minimally invasive antireflux procedures are associated with shortened hospitalization and recovery times, and are generally more acceptable to patients than open procedures. Although no data have examined specific benefits to elderly patients, earlier resumption of normal activity after laparoscopic antireflux surgery may avoid significant postoperative morbidity in this vulnerable population. In addition to other benefits of minimally invasive surgery, the use of angled-view magnifying telescopes and current video technology provides visualization of the area of the fundoplication that is superior to the direct exposure that is achieved in open surgery (Fig. 37.4).

TABLE 37.3. Indications for Surgical Treatment of GERD

| Indications |
|---|
| Residual symptoms despite medical treatment |
| Continued esophagitis despite medical treatment |
| Avoidance of long-term medication use |
| Medication intolerance or noncompliance |
| Recurrent peptic stricture |
| Barrett's esophagus |

Large series of laparoscopic Nissen fundoplications indicate that relief of heartburn is possible in more than 95% of patients, with overall morbidity less than 5% in combined populations of young and old patients. Increased complication rates in old patients have not been reported.[24,25]

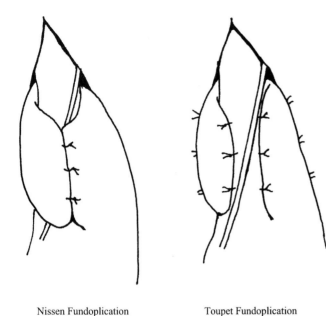

The authors make routine use of manometry for the workup of GERD prior to surgery, primarily to identify patients with impaired esophageal peristalsis. The mean LES pressure is measured but is not used as a diagnostic tool or to guide surgical decision-making. Although no clear guidelines have been established, we currently use a cutoff peristaltic amplitude of 30 mmHg to determine which patients undergo a partial fundoplication. Frequent nonphasic or nonpropagated contractions and preoperative dysphagia complaints influence this decision. Although specific data favoring this widely used approach are lacking, no effort to avoid postoperative dysphagia in elderly patients can be spared. Comparison of laparoscopic Nissen and Toupet fundoplications in combined populations, using abnormal esophageal motility as the indication for use of the partial wrap demonstrated that the two procedures were equally effective in relieving GERD symptoms (98% vs. 97%).[26] At the 6-month follow-up there was a slightly higher rate of dysphagia in the Nissen group, but by the 15-month follow-up there was no difference between the groups.

Immediate operative complications of laparoscopic antireflux surgery are infrequent. Esophageal perforations are rare and may result from dissection or bougie injuries. Bleeding and infection are likewise uncommon. Whereas splenic injury necessitating splenectomy was a not uncommon complication of open fundoplication, this

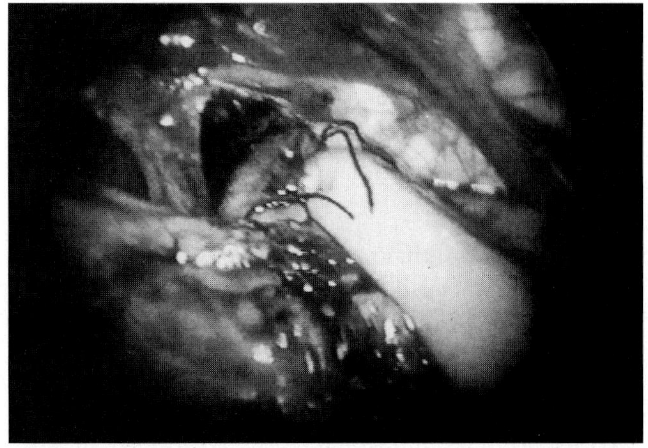

FIGURE 37.4. Laparoscopic Nissen fundoplication. Laparoscopic camera view of complete (360 degree) wrap of gastric fundus around the esophagogastric junction and distal esophagus.

TABLE 37.4. Postoperative Complications of Laparoscopic Antireflux Surgery

| Complication | Incidence (%) |
|---|---|
| Dysphagia | 5–30 |
| Early | 5–30 |
| Late | 0–10 |
| Gas bloat | 0–15 |
| Wrap failure | <5 |

event has all but vanished with laparoscopic antireflux procedures. Pneumothorax occurs in 1–5% of cases and is usually due to extensive dissection at the gastroesophageal (GE) junction and into the mediastinum. Chest tube placement is rarely required due to the rapid uptake of $CO_2$.

Postoperative chest radiography is reserved for cases of respiratory difficulty. Subcutaneous and mediastinal emphysema occurs occasionally and requires no specific treatment. Most concerns focus on postwrap complications, of which dysphagia is the most frequent (Table 37.4). These problems may occur to varying degrees and are generally related to wrap tightness. Technical considerations that minimize the likelihood of postoperative dysphagia include routine division of the gastrosplenic ligament and short gastric vessels and adequate fundic mobilization for a loose wrap. In most patients dysphagia is mild and limited to the early postoperative period. Gas-bloat symptoms and an inability to belch also generally resolve over time but can be distressing during the early postoperative period.

## Other Inflammatory Disorders

Infectious esophagitis secondary to fungal, bacterial, or viral illness occurs in the setting of impaired host immune defenses. Although there may be aging-related immune system degradation, esophageal infections have no special predilection for the elderly except in the setting of corticosteroid use, organ transplantation, chemotherapy, or human immunodeficiency virus (HIV) infection. Advancing age has been cited as a risk factor for *Candida*-related esophagitis,[27] but this remains an unusual condition in the absence of the above factors.

## Achalasia

The motility of the gastrointestinal tract is an early victim to aging. Esophageal motility studies have demonstrated a diminished amplitude of postdeglutitive pressure waves in elderly patients, with an associated incomplete relaxation of the LES.[28] These senile changes are similar to those seen with achalasia.

Achalasia is characterized by impaired LES relaxation during swallowing and evolving esophageal aperistalsis. Although achalasia may occur between the ages of 25 and 90, it is more a disease of the elderly than is GERD. Although the peak incidence is probably around the fifth decade, Sonnenberg et al. reported an average age of 78 years for patients with achalasia based on primary and secondary diagnosis codes for hospital admission, with a steady increase in hospitalization rates between the ages of 65 and 94 years.[29] Although occasional familial clustering of achalasia cases has been reported, most are sporadic and of uncertain etiology.[30] Viral infection has been proposed as a predisposing factor,[31,32] and information linking toxic agents, esophageal trauma, and ischemic esophageal damage to this disease are limited.

The most striking gross feature of achalasia is the often massive esophageal dilation (sigmoid esophagus) that accompanies a prolonged course of disease. It is a late finding, and minimal gross change may be observed in patients with early disease. The histologic characteristics of achalasia have been determined by evaluating resected esophageal specimens in advanced cases[33] or those obtained at autopsy. Early histologic changes are less well described. Wallerian-type degenerative changes, loss of myenteric ganglion cells, and hypertrophy of the muscularis propria of the distal esophagus may be observed. Extraesophageal changes include microscopic degeneration of the vagus nerve.[33] In studies of the muscle from achalasia patients, there is a selective loss of nitric oxide- and vasoactive intestinal peptide (VIP)-containing postganglionic inhibitory (LES-relaxing) neurons in the myenteric plexus, which may play a causative role in tonic cholinergic stimulation and impaired LES relaxation.[34–36] The presence of Lewey bodies in the myenteric plexus and loss of neurons in the dorsal motor nucleus of the vagus in both achalasia and Parkinson's disease suggests an as-yet unidentified link between these two diseases, which appear with high prevalence in the elderly.

The most common symptoms of achalasia are dysphagia to solid food (which may be progressive and interfere with ingestion of liquids in severe cases), regurgitation of esophageal contents, weight loss, and chest pain. Dysphagia due to impaired LES relaxation is exacerbated by impaired peristalsis in the dilated esophagus. The net result is profoundly diminished esophageal emptying and stasis of undigested food proximal to the LES. Patients develop techniques to allow them to eat, including slow, purposeful swallowing, avoidance of firm foods, postural changes (twisting, stretching), and ingestion of warm liquids with meals. Approximately 40% of patients have chest pain in the xiphoid or substernal areas, which often prompts evaluation for myocardial disease. This pain may be increased by exercise and relieved by rest.[37] Achalasia patients also commonly describe "heartburn," which is related to stasis of ingested material in the esophagus.[38]

TABLE 37.5. Diagnostic Studies in Achalasia

| Test | Information sought |
|---|---|
| Chest radiograph | Esophageal dilation (widened mediastinum, esophageal air-fluid level), lung pathology (abscess, pneumonia) |
| Esophagoscopy | Rule out malignant stricture |
| Barium esophagram | Esophageal dilation, impaired contrast clearance, "bird's beak" deformity, esophageal diverticuli |
| Esophageal manometry | Nonrelaxation of LES, impaired esophageal peristalsis |

Clouse et al. examined specific differences in clinical presentations of achalasia in patients more than 70 years of age and those younger than 70. In general, the symptoms at presentation were similar, with the notable exception that fewer of the older patients complained of chest pain. Basal LES pressures and esophageal peristalsis were similar in the two groups, although the residual LES pressure was significantly lower in the older patients; there was a weak inverse association between age and residual LES pressure.[39] These findings suggest that in elderly patients significant dysphagia can be experienced at lower-threshhold LES pressures.

The workup of clinically suspected achalasia is fairly standard irrespective of patient age (Table 37.5).[40] Radiologic techniques can be valuable for demonstrating advancd disease. A plain chest radiograph may demonstrate an air-fluid level in the posterior mediastinum and a widened mediastinum due to esophageal dilation. A barium esophogram effectively demonstrates the gross esophageal changes, which can include dilation, tortuosity, retention of food and barium, and a symmetric smooth tapering of the esophagus resembling a bird's beak (Fig. 37.5).

Upper endoscopy should be considered a mandatory study to exclude peptic stricture and malignancy. The latter condition may be associated with clinical changes similar to those of achalasia, particulary in patients over 60 years of age.[41,42] A diagnosis of pseudoachalasia can be firmly established only by biopsy and histologic demonstration of carcinoma.

Of all currently available studies, esophageal manometry establishes the diagnosis of achalasia most effectively. Although the resting LES pressure is normal in 40% of patients, up to 80% have absent or incomplete LES relaxation with wet swallows. It must be emphasized that the presence of LES relaxation does not exclude achalasia. Postdeglutitive relaxations may appear complete but usually are of short duration.[43,44] Loss of normal esophageal body peristalsis is manifested by simultaneous contractions following wet swallows. Contractile amplitudes are low (10–40 mmHg), with frequent prolonged and repetitive waves. Vigorous achalasia is characterized by normal- or high-amplitude but nonphasic contractions, which may be associated with intense chest pain.[45] This form of achalasia may be less frequent in elderly patients. Other clinical complaints associated with this disease include cervical-level dysphagia and difficulty belching. It has been suggested some symptoms are related to impaired upper esophageal sphincter relaxation.[46,47]

Numerous conditions may closely mimic achalasia. Although many of them occur in the elderly, most are exceedingly rare and do not have a marked predilection for this patient population. In addition to malignancy-associated pseudoachalasia, Chagas' disease, which is endemic in South America, can be observed in elderly patients and deserves special mention.

Patients with achalasia are at risk for developing chronic inflammation, ulceration, perforation, and fistulas as a result of chronic stasis and retention. It has been shown that there is a 33-fold increased risk of esophageal carcinoma in these patients, with a yearly incidence of 3.4/1000. The patients at highest risk are elderly patients with a long history of dysphagia and a markedly dilated esophagus.[48]

Treatment of achalasia in the elderly is geared toward adequate relief of symptoms. A variety of options are available (Fig. 37.6). Although LES pressure can be decreased by a variety of agents, calcium channel blockers and nitrates are the most commonly used pharmcologic therapies. Clinical improvement with both sublingual isosorbide dinitrite and nifedipine treatment has been reported.[49–52] These agents must be

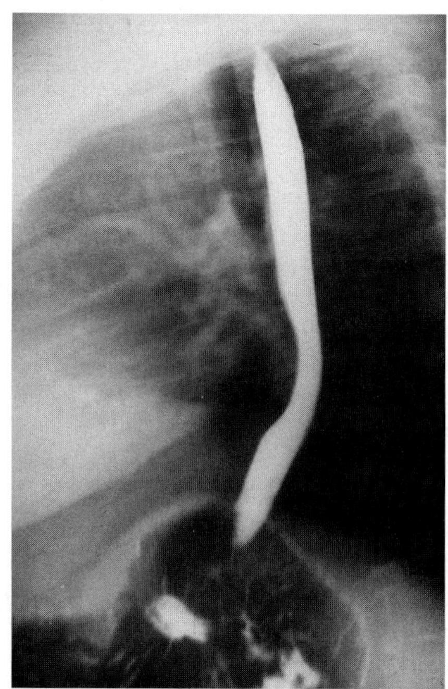

FIGURE 37.5. Bird's beak deformity of the distal esophagus in a patient with achalasia seen on a barium esophagram.

| Pneumatic Balloon Dilatation | | Botulinum Toxin Injection | | Laparoscopic Heller Myotomy | |
|---|---|---|---|---|---|
| **Advantages** | **Disadvantages** | **Advantages** | **Disadvantages** | **Advantages** | **Disadvantages** |
| -Effective | -Risk of perforation | -Safe | -Poor long-term reults | -Effective | -GERD risk without antireflux procedure |
| -Often definitive | -Multiple procedures often required | | -Need for repeated injections | -Lower relapse rate than other procedures | -Operative and anesthetic morbidity |

FIGURE 37.6. Treatment options for achalasia.

taken sublingually immediately prior to meals to achieve the desired result, and their long-term efficacy is uncertain. In elderly patients who are not good candidates for dilation treatment or myotomy, trials of pharmacotherapy are appropriate. The major potential side effects that might limit this treatment are headache and tachyphylaxis.

Intrasphincteric injection of botulinum toxin type A has been demonstrated to be effective in reducing both LES pressure and esophageal retention as well as relieving achalasia-associated dysphagia. A double-blind placebo-controlled study showed that botulinum toxin was significantly more effective than placebo, with 70% of patients having a symptomatic and objective improvement; only 40% of the patients required more than one injection.[53] Despite impressive early results, the long-term efficacy of this treatment has been questioned based on high 1-year relapse rates and less successful repeat injection.[54]

Pneumatic balloon dilatation has wide acceptance and is the mainstay of treatment for achalasia. This technique employs a rapidly inflated balloon in the distal esophagus to dilate and disrupt the circular smooth muscle fibers of the LES. Irrespective of the size of the initial balloon used, 15–48% of patients require repeat procedures.[55–57] The principal risk of pneumatic dilation is esophageal perforation, which in skilled hands is less than 2% with a significantly lower mortality rate. The initial results with pneumatic dilatation are excellent, with 70% of patients experiencing early relief of their dysphagia. When patients are followed over 5 years, the response rate drops to 40%. The success of pneumatic dilatation may not be as substantial in elderly patients, who require more dilation procedures, with each procedure yielding less improvement. The inevitable question of how many dilatation attempts can reasonably be made to achieve symptom relief in elderly patients is difficult to answer. The alternative is operative esophagomyotomy, which carries its own risks and expected results. There has been one randomized, controlled trial comparing surgery and dilatation; it suggested that surgical treatment is associated with a better long-term outcome.[58] This view is supported by a large series from the Mayo Clinic.[59]

Surgical treatment of achalasia consists of dividing the LES. Esophagomyotomy lowers the LES pressure 55–75% and also lowers the esophageal intraluminal pressure. Like pneumatic dilatation, esophagomyotomy does not alter LES relaxation; and 90% of achalasia patients have had good to excellent results after a follow-up of 1–36 years. Follow-up studies have demonstrated an improvement in esophageal emptying, increased LES diameter, and decreased esophageal diameter.[60–63]

The first thoracoscopically performed minimally invasive esophagomyotomy was reported in 1992.[64] Despite the excellent results achieved with this procedure, the transthoracic minimally invasive approach was quickly abandoned in favor of laparoscopic esophagomyotomy. The latter procedure offers a more technically straightforward approach to the LES, more favorable instrument placement for the myotomy, and decreased postoperative pain and length of hospitalization compared to the transthoracic procedure. It also greatly facilitates construction of a fundoplication. The overall complication rate for esophagomyotomy is 10%, with GERD being the most common postoperative problem if no antireflux procedure is performed at the time of myotomy. Toupet fundoplication in conjunction with esophagomyotomy is preferred by the authors not only for its effectiveness in preventing reflux but for the tendency of the wrap components to hold the myotomy open (Fig. 37.7).

Although no specific data are available, examining laparoscopic esophagomyotomy results in elderly patients or the need for concomitant antireflux procedure in this patient group, overall results of these procedures are impressive. Hunter et al. reported the results of laparoscopic myotomy in 40 patients up to age 84 years, 75% of whom had undergone previous repetitive treatments for achalasia.[65] All patients were scored pre- and postoperatively for dysphagia, heartburn, chest pain, and regurgitation. At a mean follow-up of 12.5 months, dysphagia was greatly alleviated or resolved in 90% of patients. Regurgitation, heartburn, and chest pain were also greatly reduced; 93% of the patients were discharged

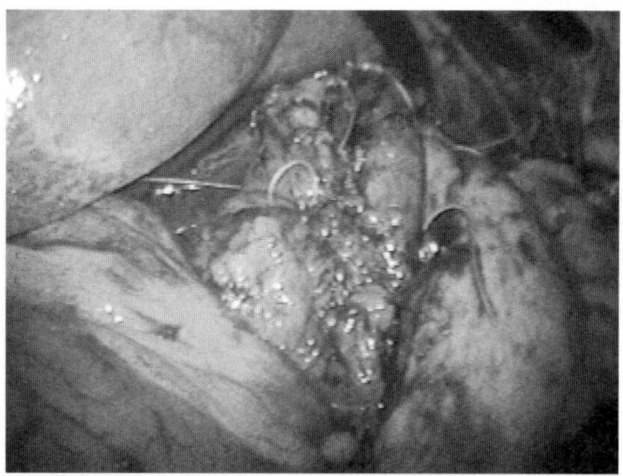

FIGURE 37.7. Completed laparoscopic esophagomyotomy (Heller myotomy) with Toupet fundoplication. The myotomy extends 5 cm proximal to the esophagogastric junction and 1 cm onto the anterior gastric wall.

within 72 hours of surgery. Routine antireflux procedures were performed in this series, which probably accounts for the small incidence of postoperative GERD symptoms. As larger numbers of patients undergo laparoscopic procedures for achalasia and longer-term data become available, surgical treatment may become a more attractive option for the elderly in whom safe, definitive therapy may offer significant advantages.

## Other Hypermotility Disorders

Several disorder of esophageal body motility have been described that, like achalasia, are associated with disordered peristalsis and possibly increased intramural muscular tone. These diseases are mentioned here because they may occur in elderly patients but for the most part appear prior to the sixth decade.

Diffuse esophageal spasm (DES) is a poorly understood motor disorder characterized clinically by dysphagia and episodic substernal chest pain as a result of a primary disorder of esophageal body motility. It is a rare condition, the etiology of which is unknown. Because the symptom that most often brings DES patients to medical attention is angina-like chest pain, formal workup for a cardiac etiology is almost always undertaken. DES is characterized manometrically by the frequent occurrence of simultaneous and repetitive contractions of abnormally high amplitude or long duration. The finding of 20% or more simultaneous contractions per 10 wet swallows is considered diagnostic of the disorder.[66] LES resting pressures and relaxation with swallows are usually normal. Because DES activity is intermittent, an episode must be precipitated during manometric assessment or else the study may be entirely normal. Ambulatory 24-hour manometry allows patients to go about their daily activities and receive whatever typical stimuli are necessary to precipitate esophageal spasm.[67] Many patients with DES have an underlying psychiatric history with diagnoses that include depression, psychosomatic complaints, and anxiety. These diagnoses have been reported in 80% of patients with manometric contraction abnormalities.[68]

A barium esophogram can help in the characterization of DES. Occasionally, a "corkscrew" esophagus caused by segmental contractions of circular muscle is identified. The finding of an esophageal pulsion diverticulum in a patient with characteristic chest pain is virtually diagnostic of DES. Esophagoscopy should be performed in all patients to exclude the possibility of a tumor, fibrosis, or esophagitis, which might cause esophageal narrowing that may be associated with proximal tertiary esophageal contractions.

Treatment of this condition may be difficult. As with achalasia, some patients respond to sublingual nitrates or calcium channel blockers before meals.[69,70] Esophageal dilation may alleviate symptoms of dysphagia for days to months and can be repeated for continued relief.[71] However, there is an increased risk of perforation with multiple dilations of a hypertrophic, spastic esophagus.

Surgical treatment, which helps selected patients, consists of a long myotomy aimed at reducing the simultaneous contractions and improving compliance, at the cost of abolishing peristalsis and reducing contraction amplitude.[72] It can be accomplished thoracoscopically,[73] with an 80% rate of diminished symptoms during the early postoperative period. As with achalasia treatment, a fundoplication is necessary to avoid reflux. After lengthy periods of followup (5.0–10.7 years), it appears that patients remain free of chest pain and dysphagia.[74]

### Paraesophageal Hernia

In contrast to type I (sliding) hiatal hernia, type II hernia or paraesophageal hernia is characterized by herniation of a peritoneal sac and intraabdominal viscera into the mediastinum through a true defect in the esophageal hiatus adjacent to the esophagogastric junction (Fig. 37.8). Type III hiatal hernia, a combined paraesophageal and sliding hernia, is the most common paraesophageal hernia variant. By far, the most commonly herniated structure in paraesophageal hernias is the gastric fundus, although the entire stomach and other viscera such as the transverse colon and greater omentum may also be involved.[75] Paraesophageal hernia is primarily a disease of the elderly with an average age at diagnosis of 60–70 years.[76] Although these hernias are far less common than sliding hiatal hernias, their actual incidence is unknown, as many are presumed to be asymptomatic. Symptoms at presentation include chest pain (or chest fullness) sometimes relieved by vomiting, ineffective vomiting, early satiety, and dysphagia. Patients also report classic reflux symptoms, which may not be directly related to the paraesophageal hernia. In 5–10% of patients, parae-

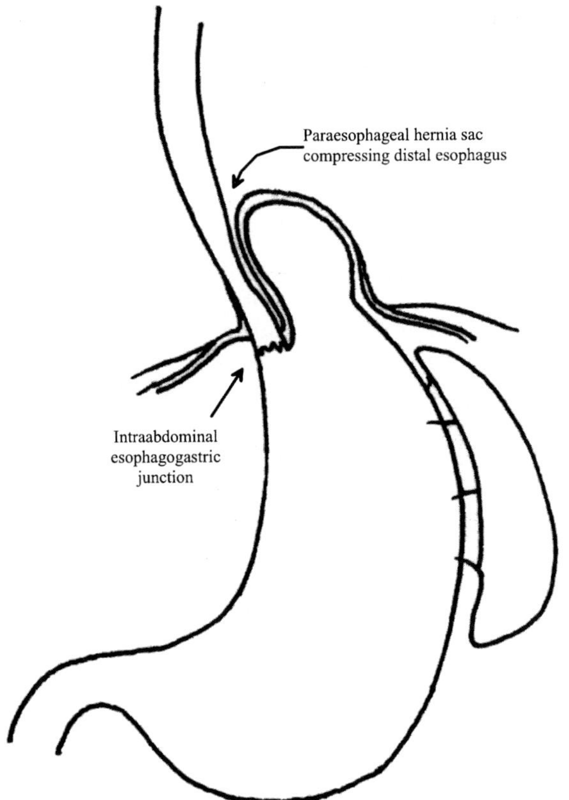


FIGURE 37.8. Paraesophageal hernia. Type II hiatal hernia with herniated proximal gastric fundus within a peritoneal sac adjacent to the intraabdominal esophagogastric junction.

may increase with time, expectant management of paraesophageal hernias is not generally recommended.

Surgical treatment of paraesophageal hernia can be accomplished safely and effectively in elderly patients using the same minimally invasive techniques employed for treatment of GERD.[77–80] In one recent series of 30 patients with a median age of 68 years, 86% of patients were reported to have resumed normal activities within 6 days of surgery; the remaining 14% reached this stage of recovery by 12 days after surgery.[80] The cardinal technical points of laparoscopic paraesophageal hernia repair include reduction and excision of the sac to reduce the risk of recurrence and effective hiatal closure. Although some authors describe hiatal closure anterior to the esophagus, this method effectively maneuvers the LES into the posterior mediastinum, causing functional shortening of the esophagus. With excision of the sac and mobilization of the esophagus and gastric fundus, a posterior reconstruction of the hiatus can be readily performed. Posterior closure transposes the esophagus forward, functionally increasing its intraabdominal length.[81] Prosthetic mesh may be used to close large defects, either alone or in conjunction with a separate posterior hiatal closure.[82]

Although the need for fundoplication at the time of paraesophageal hernia repair remains controversial, most surgeons support adding this procedure. As many as 60% of patients with type III hernias have diminished LES pressures and abnormal esophageal pH monitoring

sophageal hernias may be discovered during a workup for anemia attributed to ulcers in a herniated stomach.[77]

A chest radiograph may demonstrate an air-fluid level with a mass in the left chest. The diagnosis is most comonly made on an upper gastrointestinal (GI) contrast study that demonstrates the involved portion of stomach and the position of the esophagogastric junction (Fig. 37.9). Upper endoscopy can also aid in the diagnosis and is frequently the first study obtained for workup of the aforementioned symptoms.

Up to one-third of patients present in an emergent setting with gastric volvulus, incarceration, and obstruction or strangulation. Gastric volvulus in a paraesophageal hernia is referred to as organoaxial rotation (left to right and caudad to cephalad). Strangulation complicating either gastric volvulus or a simply herniated segment of stomach can lead to infarction and perforation, with a high attendant patient mortality. Surgical treatment is recommended for all symptomatic paraesophageal hernias. Whether small, asymptomatic paraesophageal hernias should be similarly managed remains controversial. Risk of catastrophic complication or of symptom progression cannot be accurately assessed in any given case. In old patients when the operative risk

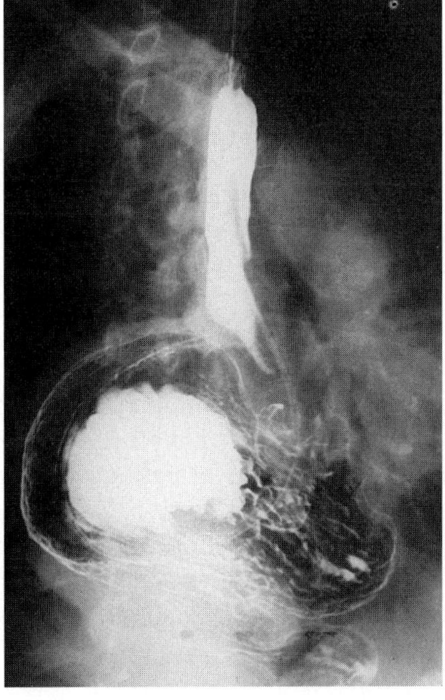

FIGURE 37.9. Barium esophagram of a large type III hiatal hernia with gastric volvulus and herniation of most of the stomach into the mediastinum and left chest, and an esophagogastric junction above the diaphragm.

studies.[83] However, others have reported that antireflux procedures are required in only 15% of patients with paraesophageal hernia and preoperative reflux-like symptoms, as detailed by preoperative endoscopy, pH testing, and manometry. Of the remaining patients with these symptoms, 98% had total resolution of heartburn with reduction of the hernia and closure of the hiatus.[84] Willekes et al. based the need for fundoplication on several factors: (1) 30% of patients report preoperative reflux symptoms; (2) some patients develop postoperative reflux despite the absence of preoperative reflux symptoms; and (3) the esophagogastric junction and LES physiology cannot be predicted once it has been surgically disturbed and all phrenoesophageal supporting attachments are divided.[80] Furthermore, the complication rate of fundoplication at the time of other esophageal surgery is predictably less in elderly patients than if the need for a second procedure arises. Despite a paucity of prospective data supporting the benefits of fundoplication in conjunction with paraesophageal hernia repair, it seems to be favored in most reports.[85,86] In addition to addressing the issue of potential postoperative GERD, the fundoplication may facilitate fixation of the LES below the diaphragm. However, among oldest-old often critically ill patients who present with bleeding, gangrene, or perforation as complications of a paraesophageal hernia, the decision to perform fundoplication must be weighed against the added time of the procedure and the absence of clear-cut, objective data demonstrating its advantages.

## Benign Tumors of the Esophagus

Benign tumors of the esophagus often go unreported and undiagnosed. Their exact incidence is not known, and those found at autopsy are directly dependent on the diligence of the pathologist. In two large autopsy series, the reported incidences of these tumors were 0.45% and 0.59%. Most benign esophageal tumors are intramural and of muscular origin.

### Leiomyoma

Leiomyomas are the most common benign tumor of the esophagus. They are observed in all age groups up to the ninth decade, although 92% of patients present between the ages of 20 and 59.[87] In a review of 838 cases, 56% were found in the lower third of the esophagus, 33% in the middle third, and 11% in the upper third.[88] Most are solitary, well-circumscribed ovoid masses that range in size from 3 to 10 cm.

Esophageal leiomyomas grow slowly and are usually not symptomatic until they reach about 5 cm. Smaller lesions are usually discovered incidentally. Symptoms are slowly progressive and consist of intermittent dysphagia, pain, a sense of fullness, aching or pressure, regurgitation, anorexia, belching, nausea, and vomiting. Severe complications such as obstruction, bleeding, or respiratory symptoms can occur with progression in size.[89] The submucosal mass is usually first observed as a luminal filling defect on the barium esophogram. Computed tomography demonstrates a well-demarcated submucosal mass that is diagnostic of leiomyoma in most cases.[90] Endoscopic ultrasonography is a sensitive method for diagnosing smooth muscle tumors of the esophagus. Leiomyomas appear as characteristic well-circumscribed hypoechoic masses.[91,92] Upper endoscopy demonstrates tumor bulging into the lumen with normal overlying mucosa. Endoscopic biopsy rarely yields diagnostic information owing to the submucosal location of the tumor.

Leiomyomas are surgically excised for relief of symptoms and pathologic confirmation of the diagnosis and to avoid future symptoms related to enlargement. Most lesions can be enucleated via thoracotomy, thoracoscopy, or the transabdominal approach for distal lesions.[93,94] On rare occasions, esophagogastrectomy is necessary for large, ulcerated, or firmly adherent lesions at the esophagogastric junction.[90]

### Fibrovascular Polyps of the Esophagus

Fibrovascular esophageal polyps are intraluminal polyploid lesions that appear most commonly in the upper esophagus near the cricopharyngeus muscle. These lesions occur predominantly in men during the sixth and seventh decades; and as a group they include fibromas, fibrolipomas, myomas, myxofibromas, pedunculated lipomas, and fibroepithelial polyps.[95,96] Early lesions consist of nodular submucosal tissue that may over time elongate into a pedunculated polyp. The geometric forces of peristalsis eventually cause the tip of the polyp to reach the distal esophagus. Fibrovascular polyps come to medical attention when large enough to cause intermittent dysphagia, substernal fullness, or regurgitation of recently ingested material. The presentation may be more acute if a pedunculated polyp obstructs the esophagogastric junction or becomes ulcerated and bleeds. Although rare, regurgitation of the tumor and asphyxiation secondary to acute glottic obstruction is an additional concern.[97] A barium esophogram demonstrates the smooth polyploid intraluminal filling defect. Under fluoroscopy barium flow is generally unimpeded, and the up and down movement of the tumor is seen with swallows.[98] Upper endoscopy can also be used to visualize the polyp and permits the stalk to be traced to its level of attachment. Endoscopic ultrasonography generally shows an intraluminal echo-dense mass and can be used to determine if a large vessel is present in the stalk.[98]

Fibrovascular polyps are resected to relieve symptoms and prevent aspiration and asphyxiation. Small polyps may be removed endoscopically. The surgical approach is through a cervical incision on the side of the neck opposite the stalk attachment. An esophagomyotomy is performed below the cricopharyngeal muscle, and the polyp is delivered into the wound and amputated at the base of the stalk. Polyps with bases a significant distance below the cricopharyngeal muscle may require a right-sided transthoracic approach.

## References


1. Collen MJ, Abdulian JD, Chen YK. Gastroesophageal reflux disease in the elderly: more severe disease that requires aggressive therapy. Am J Gastroenterol 1995;90:1053–1057.
2. Zhu H, Pace F, Sangaletti O, Bianchi-Porro G. Gastric acid secretion and pattern of gastroesophageal reflux in patients with esophagitis and concomitant duodenal ulcer. Scand J Gastroenterol 1993;28:387–392.
3. Zhu H, Pace F, Sangaletti O, et al. Features of symptomatic gastroesophageal reflux in elderly patients. Scand J Gastroenterol 1993;28:235–238.
4. Cameron AJ, Lomboy CT. Barrett's esophagus: age prevalence and extent of columnar epithelium. Gastroenterology 1992;103:1241–1245.
5. Hollis JB, Castell DO. Esophageal function in elderly men: a new look at "presbyesophagus." Ann Intern Med 1974; 80:371–374.
6. Mold JW, Reed LE, Davis AB, et al. Prevalence of gastroesophageal reflux in elderly patients in a primary care setting. Am J Gastroenterol 1991;86:965–970.
7. Pellegrini CA, DeMeester TR, Wernly JA, et al. Alkaline gastroesophageal reflux. Am J Surg 1978;135:177–183.
8. Winters CJ, Spurling TJ, Chobanian SJ, et al. Barrett's esophagus: a prevalent occult complication of gastroesophageal reflux disease. Gastroenterology 1987;92:118–124.
9. Mann NS, Tsai MF, Nair PK. Barrett's esophagus in patients with symptomatic reflux esophagitis. Am J Gastroenterol 1989;8:1494–1496.
10. Katz D, Rothstein R, Schned A, et al. The development of dysplasia and adenocarcinoma during endoscopic surveillance of Barrett's esophagus. Am J Gastroenterol 1998;93: 536–541.
11. Klauser AG, Schlindebeck NE, Muller-Lissner SA. Symptoms in gastrooesophageal reflux disease. Lancet 1990;335: 205–208.
12. Costantini M, Crookes PF, Bremner RM, et al. Value of physiologic assessment of foregut symptoms in surgical practice. Surgery 1993;114:780–787.
13. DeMeester TR, O'Sullivan GC, Bermudez G, et al. Esophageal function in patients with anginal-like chest pain and normal coronary arteriograms. Ann Surg 1982;196:488–498.
14. Schofield PM, Brooks NH, Colgan S, et al. Left ventricular function and oesophageal function in patients with angina pectoris and normal coronary angiograms. Br Heart J 1987;58:218–224.
15. Hewson EG, Sinclair JW, Dalton CB, et al. 24 Hour esophageal pH monitoring: the most useful test for evaluating non-cardiac chest pain. Am J Med 1991;90:576–583.
16. Sontag SJ. The medical management of reflux esophagitis: role of antacids and acid inhibition. Gastroenterol Clin North Am 1990;19:683–712.
17. Hetzel DJ, Dent J, Reed D, et al. Healing and relapse of severe peptic esophagitis after treatment with omeprazole. Gastroenterology 1988;95:903–912.
18. Feldman M, Harford WB, Fisher RS, et al. Treatment of reflux esophagitis resistance to $H_2$ receptor antagonists with lansoprazole, a new $H^+/K^+$-ATPase inhibitor: a controlled, double blind study. Am J Gastroenterol 1993;88:1212–1217.
19. Ramirez B, Richter JE. Promotility drugs in the treatment of gastroesophageal reflux disease. Aliment Pharmacol Ther 1993;7:5–20.
20. Sataloff DM, Pursnani K, Hoyo S, et al. An objective assessment of laparoscopic antireflux surgery. Am J Surg 1997; 174:63–67.
21. Rakic S, Stein HJ, Hinder RN. Role of esophageal body function in gastroesophageal reflux disease: implications for surgical management. J Am Coll Surg 1997;185:380–387.
22. Allen R, Rappaport W, Hixson L, et al. Referral patterns and the results of antireflux operations in patients more than sixty years of age. Surg Gynecol Obstet 1991;173: 359–362.
23. Richards KF, Fisher KS, Flores JH, Christensen BJ. Laparoscopic Nissen fundoplication: cost, morbidity, and outcome compared to open surgery. Surg Laparosc Endosc 1996;6:140–143.
24. Hinder RA, Filipi CJ, Wetscher G, et al. Laparoscopic Nissen fundoplication is an effective treatment for gastroesophageal reflux disease. Ann Surg 1994;220:472–481.
25. Richardson WS, Trus TL, Hunter JG. Laparoscopic antireflux surgery. Surg Clin North Am 1996;76:437–450.
26. Karim SS, Panton ON, Finley RJ, et al. Comparison of total versus partial laparoscopic fundoplication in the management of gastroesophageal reflux disease. Am J Surg 1997; 173:375–378.
27. Baehr PH, McDonald GB. Esophageal infections: risk factors, presentation, diagnosis and treatment. Gastroenterology 1994;106:509–532.
28. Szurszewski JH, Holt PR, Schuster MM. Proceedings of a workshop entitled "Neuromuscular function and dysfunction of the gastrointestinal tract in aging." Dig Dis Sci 1989; 34:1135–1146.
29. Sonnenberg A, Massey BT, McCarty DJ, Jacobsen JT. Epidemiology of hospitalization for achalasia in the United States. Dig Dis Sci 1993;38:233–244.
30. Bosher L, Shaw A. Achalasia in siblings: clinical and genetic aspects. Am J Dis Child 1981;84:1329–1330.
31. Robertson C, Martin B, Atkinson M. Varicella zoster virus DNA in the oesophageal myenteric plexus in achalasia. Gut 1993;34:299–302.
32. Jones D, Mayberry F, Rhodes J, Munro J. Preliminary report of an association between measles virus and achalasia. J Clin Pathol 1983;36:655–657.
33. Goldblum JR, Whyte RI, Orringer MB, Appelman HD. Achalasia: a morphologic study of 42 resected specimens. Am J Surg Pathol 1994;18:327–337.
34. Aggestrup S, Uddman R, Sundler F, et al. Lack of vasoactive intestinal peptide nerves in esophageal achalasia. Gastroenterology 1983;84:924–927.

35. Mearin F, Mourelle M, Guarner F, et al. Patients with achalasia lack nitrous oxide synthase in the gastro-esophageal junction. Eur J Clin Invest 1993;23:724–728.
36. Holloway RH, Dodds WJ, Helm JF, et al. Integrity of cholinergic stimulation to the lower esophageal sphincter in achalasia. Gastroenterology 1986;90:924–929.
37. Howard PJ, Maher L, Pryde A, et al. Five year prospective study of the incidence, clinical features, and diagnosis of achalasia in Edinburgh. Gut 1992;33:1011–1015.
38. Smart HL, Foster PN, Evans DF, et al. Twenty-four hour oesophageal acidity in achalasia before and after pneumatic dilatation. Gut 1987;28:883–887.
39. Clouse RE, Abramson BK, Todorczuk JR. Achalasia in the elderly: effects of aging on clinical presentation and outcome. Dig Dis Sci 1991;36:225–228.
40. Hewson EG, Ott DG, Dalton CB, et al. Manometry and radiology: complementary studies in the assessment of esophageal motility disorders. Gastroenerology 1990; 98:626–632.
41. Kahrilas PJ, Kishk SM, Helm JF, et al. Comparison of pseudoachalasia and achalasia. Am J Med 1987;82:439–446.
42. Rozman RW Jr, Achkar E. Features distinguising secondary achalasia from primary achalasia. Am J Gastroenterol 1990;85:1327–1330.
43. Cohen S, Lipshutz W. Lower esophageal sphincter dysfunction in achalasia. Gastroenterology 1971;61:814–820.
44. Katz PO, Richter JE, Cowan R, Castell DO. Apparent complete lower esophageal sphincter relaxation in achalasia. Gastroenterology 1986;90:978–983.
45. Goldenberg SP, Burrell M, Fette GG, et al. Classic and vigorous achalasia: a comparison of manometric, radiographic and clinical findings. Gastroenterology 1991;101:743–748.
46. Massey BT, Hogan WJ, Dodds WJ, Dantas RO. Alteration of the upper esophageal sphincter belch reflex in patients with achalasia. Gastroenterology 1992;103:1574–1579.
47. Dudnick RS, Castell JA, Castell DO. Abnormal upper esophageal sphincter function in achalasia. Am J Gastroenterol 1992;87:1712–1715.
48. Meijssen MAC, Tilanus HW, van Blankenstein M, et al. Achalasia complicated by oesophageal squamous cell carcinoma: a prospective study in 195 patients. Gut 1992; 33:155–158.
49. Berger K, McCallum RW. Nifedipine in the treatment of achalasia. Ann Intern Med 1982;96:61–62.
50. Bortolotti M, Labo G. Clinical and manometric effects of nifedipine in patients with esophageal achalasia. Gastroenterology 1981;80:39–44.
51. Gelfond M, Rozen P, Gilat T. Isosorbide dinitrite and nifedipine treatment of achalasia: a clinical, manometric and radionuclide evaluation. Gastroenterology 1982;83: 963–969.
52. Traube M, Dubovik S, Lange RC, McCallum RW. The role of nifedipine therapy in achalasia: results of a randomized, double-blind placebo-controlled study. Am J Gastroenterol 1989;84:1259–1262.
53. Pasricha PJ, Ravich WJ, Hendrix TR, et al. Intrasphincteric botulinum toxin for the treatment of achalasia. N Engl J Med 1995;322:774–778.
54. Pasricha PJ, Rai R, Ravich J, et al. Botulinum toxin for achalasia: long-term outcome and predictors of response. Gastroenterology 1996;110:1410–1415.
55. Barkin JS, Guelrud M, Reiner DK, et al. Forceful ballon dilation: an outpatient procedure for achalasia. Gastrointest Endosc 1990;36:123–126.
56. Kadakia SC, Wong RKH. Graded pneumatic dilation using Rigiflex achalasia dilators in patients with primary esophageal achalasia. Am J Gastroenterol 1993;88:34–38.
57. Wehrmann T, Jacobi V, Jung M, et al. Pneumatic dilation in achalasia with a low compliance balloon: results of a 5 year prospective evaluation. Gastrointest Endosc 1995;42: 31–36.
58. Csendes A, Braghetto I, Henriquez A, et al. Late results of a prospective randomized study comparing forceful dilatation and oesophagomyotomy in patients with achalasia. Gut 1089;30:299–304.
59. Okike N, Payne WS. Esophagomyotomy versus forceful dilatation for achalasia of the esophagus: results in 899 patients. Ann Thorac Surg 1979;28:119–125.
60. Ellis FH Jr. Oesophagomyotomy for achalasia: a 22 year experience. Br J Surg 1993;80:882–885.
61. Malthaner RA, Todd TR, Miller L, Pearson FG. Long term results in surgically managed esophageal achalasia. Ann Thorac Surg 1994;58:1343–1347.
62. Csendes A, Braghetto I, Mascaro J, Henriquez A. Late subjective and objective evaluation of the results of esophagomyotomy in 100 patients with achalasia of the esophagus. Surgery 1988;104:469–475.
63. Little AG, Soriano A, Ferguson MK, et al. Surgical treatment of achalasia: results with esophagomyotomy and Belsey repair. Ann Thorac Surg 1988;45:489–494.
64. Pellegrini CA, Leichter R, Patti M. Thoracoscopic esophageal myotomy in the treatment of achalasia. Ann Thorac Surg 1993;56:680–682.
65. Hunter JG, Trus TL, Branum GD, Waring JP. Laparoscopic Heller myotomy and fundoplication for achalasia. Ann Surg 1997;225:655–665.
66. Dent J, Holloway RH. Esophageal motility and reflux testing. Gastroenterology Clin North Am 1996;25:50–73.
67. Barham CP, Gotley DC, Fowler A, et al. Diffuse oesophageal spasm: diagnosis by ambulatory 24 hour manometry. Gut 1997;41:151–155.
68. Clouse RE, Lustman PJ. Psychiatric illness and contraction abnormalities of the esophagus. N Engl J Med 1983;309: 1337–1342.
69. Kikendall JW, Mellow MH. Effect of sublingual nitroglycerin and long acting nitrate preparations on esophageal motility. Gastroenterology 1980;79:703–706.
70. Drenth JP, Bos LP, Engels LG. Efficacy of diltiazem in the treatment of diffuse esophageal spasm. Aliment Pharmacol Ther 1990;4:411–416.
71. Irving D, Owen WJ, Linsell J, et al. Management of diffuse esophageal spasm with balloon dilatation. Gastrointest Radiol 1992;17:189.
72. Eypasch EP, DeMeester TR, Klingman RR, et al. Physiologic assessment and surgical management of diffuse esophageal spasm. J Thorac Cardiovasc Surg 1992;104:859–869.
73. Patti MG, Pellegrini CA, Arcerito M, et al. Comparison of medical and minimally invasive surgical therapy for primary esophageal motility disorders. Arch Surg 1995;130: 609–616.

74. Henderson RD, Ryder D, Marryatt G. Extended esophageal myotomy and short total fundoplication hernia repair in diffuse esophageal spasm: five year review in 34 patients. Ann Thorac Surg 1987;43:25–31.
75. Wichterman K, Geha AS, Cahow CE, Baue AE. Giant paraesophageal hiatus hernia with intrathoracic stomach and colon: the case for early repair. Surgery 1979;86:497–506.
76. Landrenau RJ, Johnson JA, Marshall JB, et al. Clinical spectrum of paraesophageal herniation. Dig Dis Sci 1992;37: 537–544.
77. Perdikis G, Hinder RA, Filipi CJ, et al. Laparoscopic paraesophageal hernia repair. Arch Surg 1997;132:586–589.
78. Kuster GGR, Gilroy S. Laparoscopic repair of hiatal hernias. Surg Endosc 1993;7:362–363.
79. Oddsdottir M, Franco AL, Laycock WS, et al. Laparoscopic repair of paraesophageal hernia. Surg Endosc 1995;9: 164–168.
80. Willekes CL, Edoga JK, Frezza EE. Laparoscopic repair of the paraesophageal hernia. Ann Surg 1997;225:31–38.
81. Skinner DB, Belsey RHR. Surgical management of esophageal reflux and hiatus hernia. J Thorac Cardiovasc Surg 1967;53:33–54.
82. Huntington TR. Laparoscopic mesh repair of the esophageal hiatus. J Am Coll Surg 1997;184:399–400.
83. Walther B, DeMeester TR, Lafontaine E, et al. Effect of paraesophageal hernia on sphincter function and its implication on surgical therapy. Am J Surg 1984;147:111–116.
84. Williamson WA, Ellis FH, Streitz JM, Shanian DM. Paraesophageal hiatal hernia: is an antireflux procedure necessary? Ann Thorac Surg 1993;56:447–452.
85. Fuller CB, Hagen JA, DeMeester TR, et al. The role of fundoplication in the treatment of type II paraesophageal hernia. J Thorac Cardiovasc Surg 1996;111:655–661.
86. Casabella F, Sinanan M, Horgan S, Pellegrini CA. Systematic use of gastric fundoplication in laparoscopic repair of paraesophageal hernias. Am J Surg 1996;171:485–489.
87. Skinner DB, Belsey RHR. Benign tumors of the esophagus. In: Management of Esophageal Disease. Philadelphia: Saunders, 1988:717.
88. Seremetis MG, Lyons WS, DeGuzman VC, et al. Leiomyomata of the esophagus: an analysis of 838 cases. Cancer 1976;38:2166.
89. Kramer M, Gibb P, Ellis H. Giant leiomyoma of the esophagus. J Surg Oncol 1986;33:166–169.
90. Rendeina EA, Venuta F, Pescarmona ED, et al. Leiomyoma of the esophagus. Scand J Thorac Cardiovasc Surg 1990;24: 79.
91. Tio TL, Tygat GNJ, denHartog Jager FCA. Endoscopic ultrasonography for the evaluation of smooth muscle tumors in the upper gastrointestinal tract: an experience with 42 cases. Gastrointest Endosc 1990;36:342.
92. Rosch T, Lorenz R, Dancygier H, et al. Endosonographic diagnosis of submucosal upper gastrointestinal tract tumor. Scand J Gastroenterol 1992;27:1–8.
93. Bardini R, Segalin A, Ruol A, et al. Video-thoracoscopic enucleation of esophageal leiomyoma. Ann Thorac Surg 1992;54:576–577.
94. Gossot D, Fourquier P, El Meteini M, Celerier M. Technical aspects of endoscopic removal of benign tumors of the esophagus. Surg Endosc 1993;7:102–103.
95. Rendeina EA, Venuta F, Pescarmona ED, et al. Leiomyoma of the esophagus. Scand J Thorac Cardiovasc Surg 1990;24: 79.
96. Avezzano EA, Fleischer DE, Merida MA, et al. Giant fibrovascular polyps of the esophagus. Am J Gastroenterol 1990;85:299.
97. Patel J, Kieffer RN, Martin M, et al. Giant fibrovascular polyp of the esophagus. Gastroenterology 1984;87:953.
98. Cochet B, Hohl P, Sans M, et al. Asphyxia caused by laryngeal impaction of an esophageal polyp. Arch Otolaryngol Head Neck Surg 1980;106:176.
99. Vrabec DP, Colley AT. Giant intraluminal polyps of the esophagus. Ann Otol Rhinol Laryngol 1983;92:344.

# 38
# Esophageal Cancer in the Elderly

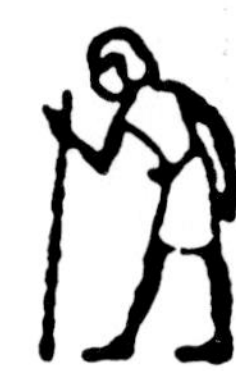

Richard F. Heitmiller and Arlene A. Forastiere

Esophageal cancers are aggressive tumors that tend to present in an advanced stage and that historically have been associated with poor survival despite therapy. There are two reasons a chapter on esophageal cancer is pertinent in this text on geriatric surgery. The first is that esophageal cancer is primarily a disease of the elderly. Thomas and Sobin,[1] reporting the Surveillance, Epidemiology, and End Results (SEER) data from the National Cancer Institute, demonstrated that the peak incidence for presentation of esophageal cancer occurred in patients over age 65 regardless of histologic cell type or gender (Fig. 38.1). The second reason is that esophageal cancer most frequently presents with dysphagia, weight loss, and fatigue, all of which threaten an elderly patient's personal and financial independence. Despite the fact that historically the outlook has been bleak for many patients with esophageal tumors, advancements in the identification of premalignant pathology, diagnosis and staging of tumors, therapeutic options, treatment safety, and survival have introduced a note of optimism into the management of this disease.

## Classification

Several classification schemes for esophageal tumors have been proposed. A detailed description of them and their respective attributes is beyond the scope of this chapter but may be found in the pathology literature. The classification with the greatest clinical application is based on tumor histology and cell type of origin and is shown in Table 38.1. Esophageal tumors are classified as epithelial, metastatic, lymphoma, or sarcoma. Epithelial tumors, including squamous cell, adenocarcinoma, small-cell, melanoma, and choriocarcinoma, are the most prevalent. In this chapter the focus is diagnosis and management of esophageal squamous cell carcinomas and adenocarcinomas.

## Location

The distribution of esophageal cancers along the esophagus is different and somewhat characteristic. Squamous cell cancer occurs most commonly in the middle third of the esophagus. Postlethwaite,[2] in a collective review of more than 28,000 patients with squamous tumors, reported these tumors to be in the upper, middle, and lower esophagus in 15%, 50%, and 35% of patients, respectively. Adenocarcinomas, on the other hand, tend to involve the lower esophagus. Ming,[3] reviewing a series of 4783 patients with adenocarcinoma, showed the tumor to be in the lower third in 67%. Ellis,[4] in a review of 310 patients with adenocarcinoma in 190, squamous cell cancers in 108, and miscellaneous cancers in 12, showed a distribution of tumors in the cervical esophagus, upper thoracic, lower thoracic, and esophagogastric junction (including cardia) in 2%, 23%, 27%, and 48%, respectively. Small-cell cancers occur with equal frequency in the middle and lower thirds, with the upper third involved in fewer than 5% of cases.[5] Esophageal melanoma and choriocarcinoma, though rare, seem to be most prevalent in the lower third. No specific pattern of distribution has been noted for esophageal sarcomas, lymphomas, or metastases.

## Incidence and Cell Type

Tumors of the esophagus other than squamous cell cancer and adenocarcinoma are rare. The reported incidence of these tumors are melanoma 0.1%,[6] small cell cancer 0.5–7.6%,[7–9] sarcomas 0.5%,[10] and metastases 3%. There is no evidence to suggest there is an increase in the frequency of these tumors. This section therefore focuses on the more common squamous cell cancer and adenocarcinoma. Esophageal cancer comprises 1.5% of all gastrointestinal cancers; it exceeds only small bowel tumors in frequency. Within the United States the incidence of esophageal cancer in patients under age 80 years is 3.2

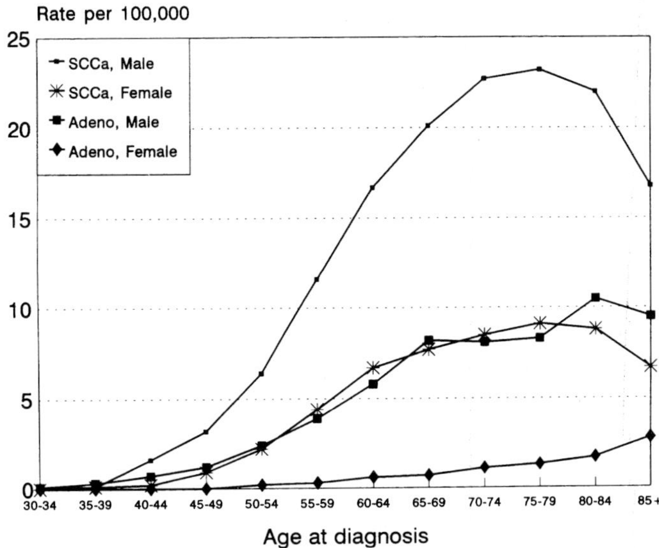


FIGURE 38.1. Incidence of esophageal cancer by age, gender, and cell type. (From Thomas and Sobin,[1] with permission.)

per 100,000 persons.[1] Overall, the incidence is only slowly increasing. On the other hand, the prevalence of esophageal cancer by cell type has shown dramatic changes. In a review of the Johns Hopkins Hospital pathology records from 1959 to 1994, Heitmiller and Sharma[11] demonstrated that squamous cell cancers have historically been most common but have been decreasing in frequency since 1992. Adenocarcinoma, uncommon before 1978, has been increasing in prevalence at a rapid pace since that time; and since 1992 it has become the most commonly diagnosed esophageal cancer (Fig. 38.2). Many authors from different institutions and geographic regions in the United States have demonstrated similar trends in cell type prevalence, noting an abrupt rise in the frequency of adenocarcinoma with a concurrent stable or decreasing frequency of squamous cell cancer.[12–15] Similar

TABLE 38.1. Classification of Esophageal Tumors

| |
|---|
| Epithelial |
| Squamous cell |
| Adenocarcinoma |
| Small cell |
| Melanoma |
| Choriocarcinoma |
| Metastatic tumors |
| Lymphoma |
| Sarcoma |

findings have been reported from the United Kingdom and western Europe.[16,17]

There are several consequences of this trend toward a prevalence of adenocarcinoma. Patients with adenocarcinoma are more likely to be treated surgically than nonsurgically, as shown in Figure 38.3. Therefore the predominance of adenocarcinoma in many U.S. surgical series results from two factors: an overall increase in the prevalence of adenocarcinoma since 1978 and an increase in the likelihood of resection for patients with these tumors. Adenocarcinoma invariably involves the lower third of the esophagus near the esophagogastric junction, which means that both the tumor and the regional lymph nodes are accessible through an abdominal approach. As a result, there has been growing interest and success using laparoscopy to stage esophageal cancers, as discussed later in this chapter. Finally, lower third tumors, which may be visualized through the hiatus and with which the regional lymph nodes are in the upper abdomen, are suitable for resection using the transhiatal esophagectomy (THE) technique. With the option of avoiding thoracotomy (using the THE approach), many elderly patients can now be offered esophagectomy who otherwise may not have been a candidate for surgical therapy.

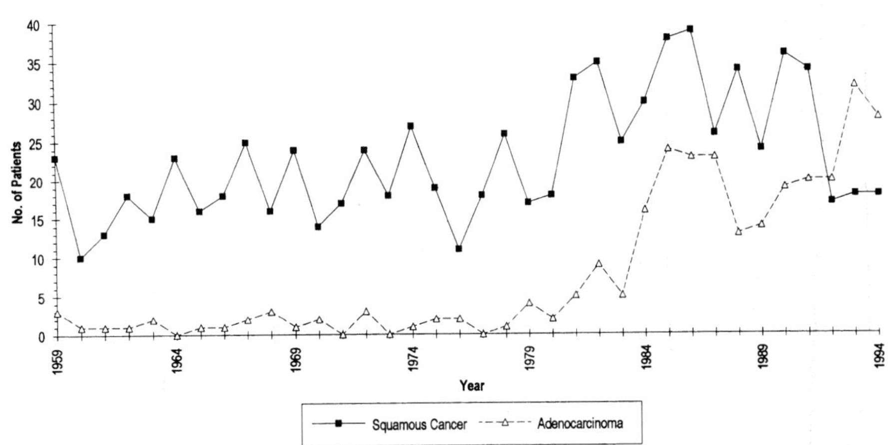


FIGURE 38.2. Prevalence of esophageal cancer at the Johns Hopkins Hospital by cell type for the years 1959–1994. (From Heitmiller and Sharma,[11] with permission.)

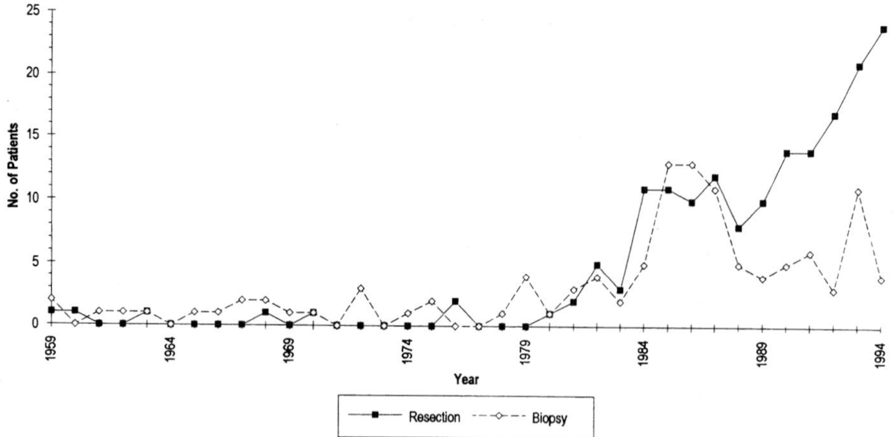


FIGURE 38.3. Comparison of surgical and nonsurgical (biopsy only) therapy for patients with adenocarcinoma. (From Heitmiller and Sharma,[11] with permission.)

## Pathogenesis

The exact etiology of esophageal cancer is unknown. The data support the hypothesis that the more common epithelial tumors arise as a result of chronic irritation of the esophagus from a wide range of behavioral, nutritional, and environmental sources, and that the likelihood of developing cancer may be increased in immunocompromised patients.

The relation between smoking and the development of squamous cell cancers is well documented for both men and women.[18–22] Choi and Kahyo[19] have shown a dose-dependent relation between the amount of smoking and the risk of developing cancer, and they have shown that this risk decreases with smoking cessation. Smokeless tobacco products have also been shown to increase the risk of cancer of the oropharynx, larynx, and esophagus.[23] Numerous studies have documented the relation between alcohol consumption and squamous cell cancer.[19–22,24,25] As with smoking, the risk appears to be dose-dependent. These risk factors, alcohol consumption and smoking, are additive.

Other factors implicated in the development of squamous cell cancer are diet, including meal composition, consistency, temperature, and rate of consumption, achalasia, lye ingestion, radiation therapy, Plummer-Vinson syndrome, and prior head and neck squamous cell cancer.

The development of adenocarcinoma has been most closely associated with gastroesophageal reflux disease and Barrett esophagus (BE) in particular. BE is a condition in which the normal stratified squamous mucosa is replaced by columnar epithelium, which is distally continuous with gastric mucosa. It is generally accepted to be a metaplastic change in which the normal squamous mucosa is injured, usually from reflux, then heals in the setting of continued reflux, and is replaced with columnar lined mucosa. BE presents in a characteristic demographic pattern. It is more common in men than women and in whites more than African-Americans. The frequency of BE increases with age. Whether the overall incidence of BE is increasing, or it is being diagnosed more frequently, is unclear. Many patients with BE are asymptomatic and evade clinical detection. Cameron et al.[26] demonstrated a clinical prevalence rate of 22.6 cases per 100,000 persons. Review of concurrent autopsy data revealed a prevalence rate considerably higher, at 376 cases per 100,000 persons. Of concern, 71% of cases found at autopsy had no other documentation of BE.

The association of BE and esophageal adenocarcinoma is well documented. Patients with BE have a risk of developing adenocarcinoma that is 30–40 times that of those without BE. Both BE and esophageal adenocarcinoma occur almost exclusively in white men. When followed prospectively, only 7–20% of cases progress to adenocarcinoma.[27–30] On the other hand, 63% of patients with adenocarcinoma who undergo resection are found to have BE in the resected specimen.[31] Some investigators believe that all esophageal adenocarcinoma is derived from BE.

Dysplasia in BE refers to histologic epithelial changes that are considered neoplastic. It is not a term used to describe inflammatory or reactive, atypical epithelium The dysplastic epithelium is subclassified into low, intermediate, and high grade dysplasia on the basis of mucosal architecture, epithelial morphology, and cytologic findings. Tygat and Hameeteman[32] have provided graphic evidence that dysplasia in Barrett mucosa is a prerequisite to adenocarcinoma, that low grade dysplasia is potentially reversible, and that once dysplasia reaches the threshold of high grade, it always progresses to invasive adenocarcinoma (Fig. 38.4). Furthermore, other have documented occult, invasive adenocarcinoma in 40–50% of patients who undergo esophagectomy for high grade dysplasia alone.[33–35] These two facts have led some to advocate aggressive surgical therapy (esophagectomy) for patients with high grade dysplasia. These same authors, however, specified that aggressive therapy should be recommended only in cases where the pathol-

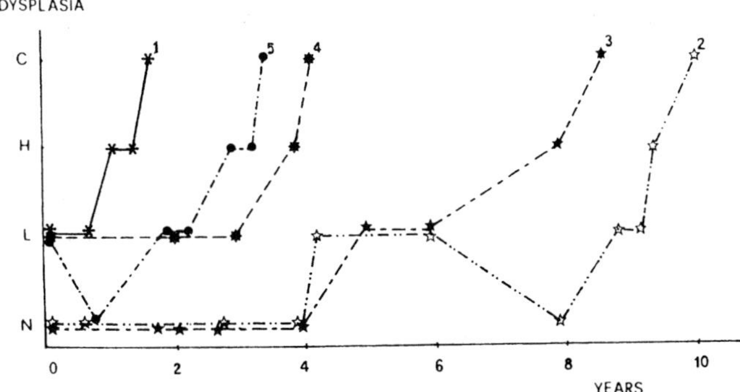


FIGURE 38.4. Progression of five patients from distinctive Barrett mucosa (N), to dysplasia (L, low grade; H, high grade), to invasive adenocarcinoma (C). (From Tygat and Hameeteman,[32] with permission.)

ogy has been confirmed by a pathologist experienced in making the diagnosis of high grade dysplasia, in patients who are suitable operative candidates, and be performed by surgeons experienced in esophagectomy. These caveats must be weighed carefully when assessing the elderly patient with dysplasia in BE. The principles of surgical therapy include resecting the esophagus as for malignant disease but reconstructing the esophagus as for benign disease. The authors' preferred approach is to use a transhiatal technique, described later in the chapter.

A great deal of progress has been made in understanding BE since the entity was first described by Barrett in 1950[36] and esophageal adenocarcinoma. However, many questions remain including why BE involves primarily white men, why only some of these patients progress to dysplasia and adenocarcinoma, and how long this process takes.

## Staging Classification System

Prior to 1987 preoperative clinical staging was based on tumor length (T1 < 5 cm; T2 > 5 cm; T3, evidence of extra-esophageal spread) and whether the tumor was circumferential or obstructing. Therefore, reports prior to 1988 often characterized patients at diagnosis by their "clinical" stage. Tumor length and degree of esophageal obstruction have proven to correlate poorly with operative findings and outcome. In 1987 the TNM staging system developed by the American Joint Cancer Committee (AJCC) was revised to consist of pathologic staging to more accurately reflect prognosis.[37] Tumor (T) stage is determined by the depth of esophageal wall penetration, nodal (N) stage by the presence or absence of regional lymph node metastases, and distant metastases as being present (M1) or not (M0). The current AJCC staging system is shown in Tables 38.2 and 38.3.

TABLE 38.2. TNM Classification

Primary tumor (T)
- Tx Primary tumor stage cannot be assessed
- T0 No evidence of primary tumor
- T1 Tumor invades lamina propria or submucosa
- T2 Tumor invades muscularis propria
- T3 Tumor invades adventitia
- T4 Tumor invades adjacent structures

Regional lymph nodes (N)
- Cervical esophagus
  - Nx Regional lymph nodes cannot be assessed
  - N0 No regional nodal metastases
  - N1 Regional nodal metastases
- Thoracic esophagus
  - N0 No regional nodal metastases
  - N1 Regional nodal metastases

Distant metastases (M)
- Mx Distant metastases cannot be assessed
- M0 No metastatic disease
- M1 Metastatic disease present

## Diagnosis

The process of diagnosis and staging frequently occur together as an overlapping process, the first to prove the presence of cancer, determine cell type, and identify associated conditions (e.g., Barrett mucosa) and the second to determine therapeutic options and prognosis.

### Clinical Characteristics

The typical presentation of the patient with esophageal cancer is a man in the sixth or seventh decade who presents with a 3- to 6-month history of progressive solid food dysphagia and weight loss. Often the amount of weight loss exceeds what would be expected for the degree of reported dysphagia. Cigarette and alcohol abuse are found in the social history of approximately 90% of patients with squamous cell tumors but in only about half of patients with adenocarcinoma. Patients with adenocarcinoma have a strong history of gastroesophageal reflux, chronic antacid use, and Barrett esophagus. Their characteristic demographics, invariably white men, reflects this strong association with Barrett

TABLE 38.3. Stage by TNM Grouping

| Stage | T | N | M |
|---|---|---|---|
| 0 | T(in situ) | N0 | M0 |
| I | T1 | N0 | M0 |
| IIA | T2 | N0 | M0 |
| IIB | T3 | N0 | M0 |
| III | T3 | N1 | M0 |
| | T4 | Any N | M0 |
| IV | Any T | Any N | M1 |

mucosa. A few patients with adenocarcinoma present with nonobstructive polypoid lesions that result in upper gastrointestinal bleeding.

Pain with swallowing is common, with obstructing tumors reflecting swallow-induced esophageal dilatation proximal to the obstruction. Persistent mid-back or epigastric pain unrelated to swallowing is suggestive of mediastinal invasion. Concurrent respiratory symptoms of persistent cough and hemoptysis in patients with upper-half esophageal tumors are suggestive of airway invasion. The presence of Horner syndrome, hoarseness from recurrent laryngeal nerve invasion (usually in the aorticopulmonary window), supraclavicular adenopathy, or symptoms of esophagorespiratory fistula are indicative of advanced, unresectable disease.

Symptoms of metastatic disease vary depending on the metastatic site. The most common sites and associated symptoms include celiac lymph nodes or liver with epigastric or right upper quadrant pain, pulmonary or pleural space metastases with shortness of breath and chest pain, and bone metastases with localized, severe, pain.

### Contrast Esophagography

In patients with dysphagia suspected of having an esophageal tumor, contrast esophagography should be undertaken. A localized, concentric, "apple-core" narrowing of the esophagus is highly suggestive of a carcinoma. Some benign disease, such as a peptic stricture and achalasia, may mimic cancer, and therefore endoscopy and biopsy are required to confirm the diagnosis.

### Upper Gastrointestinal Endoscopy

Esophagoscopy is performed to visualize the tumor for endoscopic biopsy or brushings for cytology, which can confirm the diagnosis. Additional endoscopic information that should be recorded at the same time includes the proximal and distal extent of the tumor and the presence and location of concurrent esophageal or gastric pathology (e.g., Barrett mucosa).

### Bronchoscopy

Any patient with a middle or proximal third esophageal tumor, especially if the patient reports a new cough with or without hemoptysis, should be staged with bronchoscopy. Flexible bronchoscopy is an outpatient procedure, is well tolerated, and is the single best method to determine if there is airway invasion by contiguous esophageal tumor. A patient who presents in such a fashion occasionally is first diagnosed as having esophageal cancer by bronchoscopic biopsy.

## Staging

Preresection staging has historically had limited utility in clinical practice. The correlation between preoperative staging and actual pathologic staging has been poor, and the choice of therapy was not affected by stage except for the detection of metastatic disease. Surgery evolved as the single best therapy for esophageal cancer. Preoperative staging required screening only for metastatic disease. All other stages in patients who were surgical candidates were eligible for resection. Postsurgical pathology became the gold standard means of staging these cancers and still is. The prospect of successful neoadjuvant chemoradiation, which administers chemoradiation therapy to patients with AJCC stage II and III tumors *before* surgery, has refocused the need to develop accurate, preresection staging. Today accurate pretherapy staging is essential to triage patients to appropriate therapy and to assess the presurgical results of neoadjuvant chemoradiation therapy. This topic is currently an area of active clinical research.

Computed tomography (CT) scanning of the chest and abdomen is the best initial staging test for patients with esophageal cancer. It is quick, well tolerated, and inexpensive relative to other staging options; and it has the specific advantages of screening for T4 disease (by imaging the tumor–mediastinal interface) and metastatic disease (M1) (by imaging the celiac lymph nodes, liver, and lungs, which are the most common sites of metastatic disease). The disadvantages of CT scanning are that it does not provide pathologic staging, it requires nodal enlargement to demonstrate nodal metastases, and it has demonstrated poor correlation between the CT scan staging and postresection pathologic staging.[38,39]

Magnetic resonance imaging (MRI) does not require contrast agent administration, can routinely display the findings in multiple planes (e.g., sagittal, coronal), and its ability to evaluate the tumor–vascular and tumor–vertebral interface is superior to that of CT scanning. On the other hand, MRI of the chest and abdomen takes longer than a CT scan of the same area and costs more. Furthermore, many claustrophobic patients are unable to tolerate the test altogether. Despite the advantages of MRI scanning listed above, the literature does not show any overall advantage of MRI over CT scanning for staging esophageal cancers. Quint et al.[40] compared MRI and postsurgical staging in 10 patients with esophageal cancer. Preresection staging was correct in only 40% of patients. Both of the patients with metastatic disease were correctly identified. In five patients (50%) the disease was overstaged, and in one patient (10%) it was understaged. Therefore it appears that MRI offers no documented overall advantage over CT scanning for staging esophageal cancer.

Transesophageal ultrasonography (TUS) is designed to determine size and depth of esophageal wall penetration by tumor. It is an outpatient procedure in which the endoscopic ultrasound probe is passed through the tumor site. The anatomic structures of the esophageal wall are represented by five bands on TUS, and the relation of the tumor to these layers can be directly imaged. The accuracy of T staging by TUS is well documented.[41,42] Enlarged paraesophageal lymph nodes, suggestive of regional nodal metastasis (N1 disease), may also be identified. In their series, Kallimanis et al.[43] were able to pass the endoscopic ultrasound probe directly in 62%, after dilatation in 22%, and not at all in 16% of patients. They reported no complications with or without dilatation as a consequence of this procedure. Chandawarkar et al.[44] reported overall accuracy, specificity, and sensitivity of 87%, 90%, and 37%, respectively. Holscher et al.[45] have made the point that TUS and CT scanning are complementary, not competing, staging modalities. The limitations of TUS include the inability to pass the endoscope through a tumor stenosis, distinguishing between benign and malignant lymph nodes, and distinguishing between mucosal and submucosal tumors.[46] High frequency TUS, in which the endoscope does not need to traverse the tumor stenosis to determine the size and depth of tumor invasion, and in which real-time TUS biopsy of paraesophageal lymph nodes is possible, may increase the accuracy of TUS staging.

One of the consequences of the observed increase in the prevalence of adenocarcinoma is that these tumors invariably involve the distal esophagus near the esophagogastric junction. Therefore the regional lymph nodes are located in the abdomen (in the lesser curvature region) and are visible laparoscopically. Standard laparoscopic equipment and techniques are employed. The abdomen is explored and the liver inspected to look for occult metastases. A jejunostomy may be placed during the same staging procedure. Krasna et al.[47] reported that laparoscopy accurately detected regional lymph node metastases in 94% of patients. Talamini et al.[48] demonstrated an unexpectedly high frequency of regional nodal metastases in nonenlarged lesser curvature nodes that were thought to be benign by other staging methods. In their series, laparoscopic staging kept 10 of 34 patients (29%) from receiving neoadjuvant chemoradiation therapy inappropriately. Finally, O'Brien et al.[49] reported that laparoscopic staging of esophageal cancer is superior to combined imaging (CT scanning and TUS).

Thoracoscopy has been used to sample and stage intrathoracic paraesophageal lymph nodes. General anesthesia, single-lung ventilation, and standard thoracoscopic techniques are employed. Thoracoscopy has a reported accuracy for nodal staging of up to 93%. In 7% of patients the nodal disease may be understaged, and in 7% the procedure could not be performed because of adhesions.[47] Despite these good results, the introduction of high frequency TUS and transesophageal biopsy techniques, which can provide similar information on an outpatient basis without general anesthesia, has significantly challenged the role of thoracoscopy in staging esophageal tumors.

Positron emission tomography (PET scan) with $^{18}$F-fluorodeoxyglucose is the most recent staging modality.[50] The proposed advantages of this test is that it provides one-step TNM staging as it scans for tumor activity at the primary site, in regional lymph nodes, and systemically to rule out metastatic disease. The disadvantages include cost, availability, and a scanner resolution that requires the tumor to be approximately 1 cm to be detected. Initial reports have shown it to be more sensitive than CT scanning for detecting regional and distant metastatic disease.

## Therapy

The goal of any therapy designed to manage patients with esophageal cancer is to relieve symptoms and treat the underlying cancer. The purpose of this chapter is not to present an exhaustive review of all treatment modalities but to cover those most commonly used and that may be applicable in the elderly patient. It is important for elderly patients and their families to be aware of their treatment options so the choice of therapy fits the patient's desires, life style, and personal and family support systems.

### Surgery

Surgery has emerged as the best single-modality therapy for patients with esophageal cancer in terms of durable control of dysphagia and survival. Historically, though, surgery has often been associated with significant morbidity, mortality, and lengthy hospital stays. Increased surgical experience, improved techniques, nutritional support, anesthesia, intensive care, and clinical care pathway strategies have dramatically lowered the risks and costs of surgical therapy, It is now the standard against which other potentially curative therapies are measured.

Standard esophagectomy for cancer involves subtotal esophageal resection and resection of the esophagogastric junction, gastric cardia, and regional lymph nodes. Technically, the procedure is termed a partial esophagogastrectomy,[51] as illustrated in Figure 38.5. A number of incisional approaches[52] are used to perform a partial esophagogastrectomy, including transhiatal, Ivor-Lewis, left thoracoabdominal, and three incision techniques (Fig. 38.6). In the past, proponents have argued that one operative technique was superior to others in terms of morbidity, mortality, and survival. Despite using different incisions, all of the techniques are partial esophagogastrectomies with similar reported results in terms of morbidity and mortality. Muller et al.[53] reviewed overall

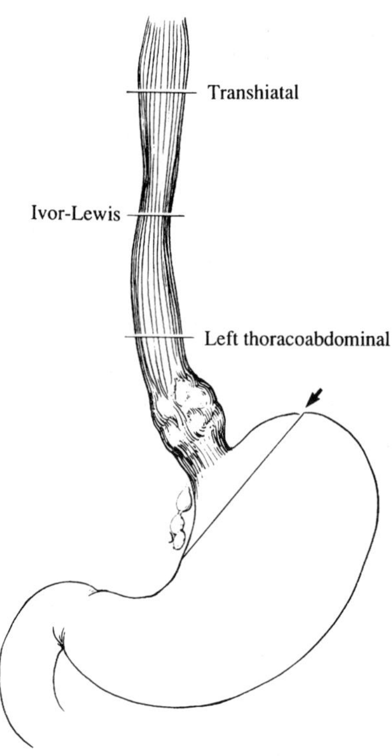


FIGURE 38.5. Standard esophagectomy for cancer involves subtotal esophagogastric resection along with removal of the regional lymph nodes. It is termed a partial esophagogastrectomy. Different incisional approaches result in variations in the amount of resected esophagus and the level of the esophageal anastomosis. (From Heitmiller,[51] with permission.)

postsurgical survival in 1000 patients from multiple institutions and found no statistical difference in survival based on operative techniques. Selection of the surgical technique is therefore based on tumor location, options for esophageal reconstruction, the patient's body habitus and past medical and surgical history, and the surgeon's experience. Only the most common surgical techniques are covered in this chapter.

Transhiatal esophagectomy does not use a thoracotomy. By doing so, esophagectomy may now be cautiously offered to some elderly and high risk patients who otherwise would not be candidates for surgery. Indications for THE include benign or malignant esophageal pathology usually involving the distal half of the intrathoracic esophagus in which there are options for long-segment esophageal replacement. The technique uses a midline laparotomy and left cervical incision. The intrathoracic esophagus is mobilized through the hiatus and transcervically. The resected portion of esophagus is reconstructed using stomach (also known as a gastric pull-up) or long-segment colon, which is passed up into the neck and anastomosed to the remaining cervical esophagus. Technical aids in performing THE were largely established by Orringer.[54] Additionally, Stone and Heitmiller[55] have described a technique to optimize exposure for the cervical anastomosis during THE. Advantages of the THE approach are that (1) it avoids thoracotomy, which results in less short-term incisional pain, reduced pain medication requirement, and greater mobility and independence; (2) it uses a cervical esophageal anastomosis, which minimizes the adverse consequences of anastomotic leakage; and (3) gastric pull-up with cervical esophagogastric anastomosis results in good, reliable, durable quality of swallowing. Disadvantages are that (1) it requires long-segment esophageal replacement; (2) it is associated with a risk of ipsilateral recurrent laryngeal nerve injury; (3) there is a chance of intrathoracic injury from the "blunt" transhiatal dissection; and (4) complete intrathoracic nodal dissection is not possible. Results include operative mortality of 0–11%, anastomotic leak in 0–13%, hoarseness in 4–9%, pneumonia in 3–21%, and anastomotic stricture in 14–42% of patients.[54,56–58] Length of hospital stay is generally 10–14 days. Orringer[56] has reported the quality of swallowing to be good to excellent in 78% of patients.

Partial esophagogastrectomy using a midline abdominal and right thoracotomy incisions, also known as the Ivor-Lewis[59] technique, is designed to optimize exposure of the intrathoracic esophagus, which passes through the upper two-thirds of the chest along the right posterior mediastinum. The involved portion of esophagus is freed from the mediastinum and resected along with the esophagogastric junction, proximal cardia, and regional lymph nodes. The resected esophageal segment is replaced by stomach, colon, or less frequently jejunum, which is passed into the chest along the esophageal bed and anastomosed to the proximal esophagus at or above the level of the carina. The advantage of this technique is the excel-

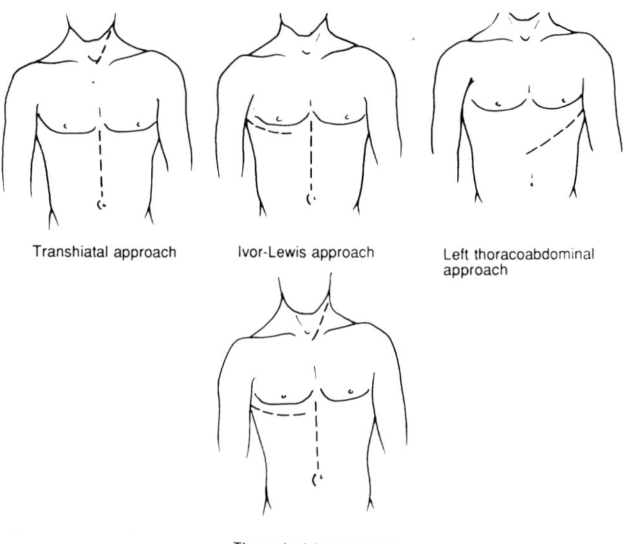


FIGURE 38.6. Incisions used for the more common esophagectomy techniques. (From Reichle et al.,[52] with permission.)

lent exposure of the mid- to upper intrathoracic esophagus and lymph nodes. The disadvantages are post-thoracotomy pain and the potential for intrathoracic esophageal anastomotic leak. Respiratory complications are reported in 11%, anastomotic leak in 3–7%, and wound infection in 5% of patients. Operative mortality ranges from 0% to 4%, with a reported length of hospital stay as low as 11.1 days.[60–64]

The left thoracoabdominal approach uses a single incision that extends from the left chest onto the left upper abdomen. It provides excellent exposure of the lower third of the esophagus and abdominal left upper quadrant. This technique is ideal for patients with tumors near the esophagogastric junction, especially when the extent of gastric invasion is uncertain, because it yields superb operative exposure and maximizes options for replacement of the lower third of the esophagus. Heitmiller[65] summarized the history, indications, technical aids, and options for using the left thoracoabdominal incision. Once the esophagogastric pathology is resected, the esophagus is replaced by stomach, isoperistaltic jejunum, or short-segment isoperistaltic colon. Advantages of this incision are its superb exposure of the lower third of esophagus and left upper abdomen and the fact that options for short-segment esophageal replacement are maximized. Disadvantages are incisional pain, healing complications especially at the divided costal margin, limited exposure of the upper esophagus, and a low intrathoracic anastomosis. Postoperative respiratory complications are common. At least some degree of lower lobe atelectasis, especially left-sided, occurs in most patients. Pneumonia is reported to occur in 0–24%, anastomotic leak in 0–12%, atrial fibrillation in 10%, and wound infection in 1.5–5.2% of patients. Operative mortality is 0–6.2%, and reported length of hospital stay is 11-21 days.[65–67]

Multiple-incision surgical approaches seek to combine the advantages of open thoracotomy and transhiatal techniques. The term "multiple incision" comes from the fact that cervical, abdominal, and thoracotomy incisions are utilized. The rationale for the thoracotomy incision is to permit direct surgical exposure of the intrathoracic esophagus and lymphatics, but a gastric pull-up with cervical anastomosis is used for esophageal replacement. The most common multiincision approach uses cervical, right thoracotomy, and midline laparotomy incisions as described by McKeown.[68] Although there have been reports detailing the technical details of these incisions, no large cumulative series have been reported. There is, however, no reason to assume that the morbidity, mortality, and length of hospital stay are significantly different from those of other thoracotomy techniques.

Some have attempted to improve postsurgical survival results by increasing the scope of the surgical resection by adding formal lymphadenectomy.[69–73] Esophageal lymphatic drainage has been categorized into cervical, thoracic, and abdominal regions. Standard esophagectomy involves one-field lymphadenectomy. Adding two- or three-field lymphadenectomy is known as extended, radical, or en bloc esophagectomy. These procedures are technically more challenging, take longer, and are associated with more morbidity and mortality than standard esophagectomy. Despite the fact that operative mortality has fallen to 2–10%, there are still no prospective randomized data to support routine use of this approach.

Postsurgical survival is discussed separate from specific surgical techniques to underscore the fact that survival is based on tumor biology and stage, not on the operative approach use. Cumulative 5-year survival rates of 5.0–39.8% have been reported. Ellis[4] reported a cumulative 5-year survival of 20.8% and the following survivals by stage: stage I and II, 38.4%; stage III, 13.3%; and stage IV, 0%. King et al.[60] reported similar figures from the Mayo Clinic. Their overall postsurgical survival was 22.8%, with the following results by stage: stage I, 85.7%; stage II, 34.1%; and stage III, 15.2%. A more recent review of postesophagectomy survival by stage and cell type by the authors (unpublished data) did not demonstrate improved survival overall or by stage. There was also no difference in survival between those patients with squamous cell carcinoma or adenocarcinoma.

The results listed include surgical treatment of patients of all ages. As stated in the introduction, most patients with esophageal cancer who undergo surgery are elderly. In most series the mean patient age ranges from 60 to 65 years. Table 38.4 summarizes the results of esophagectomy specifically in the elderly population. In most series morbidity and mortality rates for the elderly are higher than those for younger patients, documenting increased morbidity and mortality with increasing age. Thomas et al.[74] however, noted no difference in the complication rate, mortality, or 5-year survival in patients less than 70 years compared to those over 70 years of age. Naunheim et al.,[75] Muehrcke et al.,[76] and Adam et al.[77] clearly demonstrated that emergent indications for surgery in patients over 70 and 80 years, respectively, markedly increased operative mortality. Kuwano et al.[78]

TABLE 38.4. Esophagectomy in the Elderly

| Study | Age (years) | No. | Morbidity (%) | Mortality (%) | LOS (days) | 5-year survival (%) |
|---|---|---|---|---|---|---|
| Naunheim[75] | >70 | 38 | 68 | 18.0 | | 15–20 |
| Muehrcke[76] | >70 | 46 | 13 | 13.0 | 13.6 | 15.3 |
| Adam[77] | >80 | 31 | 39 | 10.7–16.0 | | 17 |
| Kuwano[78] | >80 | 8 | 25 | 12.5 | | |
| Thomas[74] | >70 | 56 | 13.6 (leak)<br>20.6 (resp.) | 11.2 | | 17 |

LOS, length of stay in hospital.

has shown that surgical complications and deaths decrease with time, although the reasons for this trend are not specifically addressed. In patients who have an uncomplicated course, length of hospital stay is comparable to that in young patients. All series have reported 5-year survival figures of 15–20%, which compares favorably with the collective results for all patients.

## Chemoradiation Followed by Surgery

Neoadjuvant chemoradiation (NAC) therapy followed by esophagectomy is designed to improve survival of patients with stage II or III esophageal cancer. It is not intended for use in stage I patients, for whom postsurgical survival is excellent, or in patients with metastatic disease (stage IV), where the goal is palliation, not cure. There is no age limit for entry into this therapy protocol, but the minimum requirements in terms of performance status, renal, and bone marrow function, and the lengthy and aggressive nature of this combination therapy, keeps many elderly patients from being eligible for it. The treatment plan calls for concomitant preoperative chemoradiation therapy over a 3- to 4-week period, followed by a break to allow recovery, followed by standard esophagectomy. Forastiere et al. reported pathologic complete response rates of 40% in their pilot NAC study.[79] There was a highly significant difference in survival between patients achieving a pathologic complete recovery and those who did not, as shown in Figure 38.7. These results are consistent with those in earlier pilot series using NAC from the University of Michigan.[80] Data from prospective randomized trials to determine the effectiveness of NAC therapy are becoming available. The results are somewhat conflicting, but some data suggest improved survival with NAC in trials with predominantly or exclusively adenocarcinoma.[81]

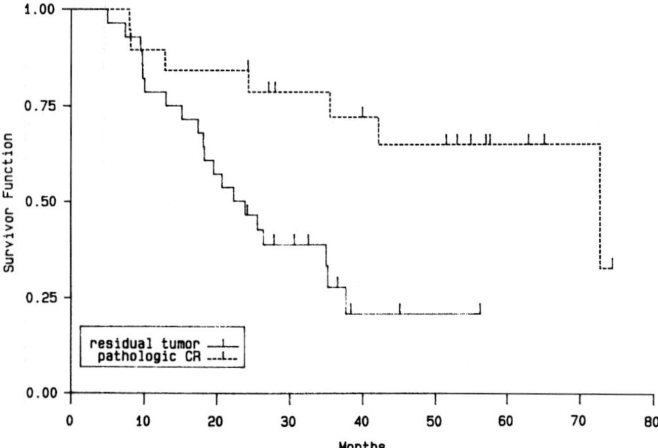


FIGURE 38.7. Kaplan-Meier survival curves following neoadjuvant chemoradiation therapy followed by surgery according to the pathologic response. Pathologic CR, complete histologic response. (From Forastiere et al.,[79] with permission.)

## Radiotherapy

The advantage of radiation therapy is that it is a generally well-tolerated, outpatient treatment. Tumor response to therapy relieves esophageal obstruction and associated dysphagic symptoms. The effectiveness of radiotherapy is highly dependent on tumor size. Small tumors (<5 cm) that are nonobstructing and noncircumferential can be treated with good local control and an estimated 5-year survival as high as 15–20%.[82–84] Most patients, however, present with larger, more extensive tumors and associated dysphagia and weight loss, which adversely affect treatment outcome. Radiation therapy for these patients results in a transient tumor response and therefore relief of symptoms (for an average 6–8 months in 75% of patients) but rarely results in cure.[85] Therefore, radiotherapy may be considered as primary curative therapy in two patient groups: (1) those with small (<5 cm), localized tumors as an alternative to surgery; and (2) those who have resectable localized disease and who refuse or are at high risk for surgery. No randomized trials comparing surgery to radiotherapy have been completed. In the absence of such data, surgery remains the preferred treatment for patients with localized disease. Radiation therapy continues to play an important role in the palliation of symptoms in patients with metastatic disease.

Chemotherapy has been used in combination with radiation therapy with the goal of increasing response rates, lengthening the disease-free interval, and improving survival. The Radiation Therapy Oncology Group (RTOG) compared four cycles of cisplatinum +5-fluorouracil (5-FU) + 50 Gy to radiotherapy alone with 64 Gy.[86] The trial was stopped early because the interim results demonstrated a significant survival advantage in the chemotherapy group: median survivals of 12.5 and 8.9 months and 2-year survivals of 50% and 38% for the chemoradiation and radiotherapy groups, respectively. Therefore patients with locally advanced disease who are not considered surgical candidates as a result of unresectable tumors or medical risks should now be considered for chemoradiation therapy rather than irradiation alone. For patients with resectable disease, surgery remains the standard of care until randomized trials demonstrate otherwise.

## Endoscopic Palliation

Endoscopic techniques to restore luminal patency are palliative procedures that may be used in patients who are not candidates for primary surgical therapy, in an adjuvant setting for patients receiving combination therapy, or in the setting of locally recurrent cancer. Endoscopic techniques include dilatation, thermal ablation with laser or coagulation probes, intubation with plastic or metal expandable stents, photodynamic therapy, or brachytherapy. The variables that must be considered when selecting the specific method are cost, tumor location and length, whether the tumor is circumferential, and the presence or absence of an esophagorespiratory fistula.

Esophageal dilatation may provide symptomatic relief of dysphagia in as many as 90% of patients, but the relief is transient.[87,88] Rigid, wire-guided dilators are preferred by most therapists. Because of the short-term relief of symptoms, dilatation is most often used in conjunction with some other means of endoscopic palliation.

Thermal ablation, using laser or coagulation probes, may be used to open an esophageal lumen narrowed by tumor. Laser techniques use an endoscopically directed neodymium: yttrium-aluminum-garnet (Nd: YAG) laser that emits a light wavelength in the infrared spectrum to ablate the obstructing tumor. To be a candidate for this therapy, the endoscope must be able to traverse the tumor. This determines the correct path through the tumor into the distal lumen and minimizes the risk of treatment-related perforation. Although shorter-length lesions may be opened in one session, most lesions require more than one session to achieve the desired result. Repeat treatments are usually needed to treat recurrent symptoms. Relief of dysphagia is reported in 69–100%[88] of patients. Individual success rates are related to the length of esophagus involved with circumferential tumor. For tumors longer than 4cm, the number of endoscopic sessions increases, and the chance of success decreases. Contraindications for laser therapy include completely obstructing cancers and esophagorespiratory fistulas. The effectiveness of therapy seems to be reduced with cervical lesions. Complications are reported in 4.1% of patients and include fever, perforation, aspiration pneumonia, and stricture formation. Treatment-related mortality occurs in 0–5% of patients.[88,89]

Electrocautery techniques use either a monopolar or bipolar (BICAP) coagulating probe to open the esophageal lumen narrowed by tumor. As with laser, it must be possible to traverse the tumor at least with a guidewire to prevent perforation. The monopolar probe directly coagulates the tumor under endoscopic guidance. The BICAP probe is passed through the narrowed lumen under guidewire control, coagulating the tumor blindly and circumferentially. Comparison of electrocoagulation and laser techniques have shown similar results in terms of morbidity, mortality, and ability to relieve dysphagia.[90,91] Contraindications for electrocoagulation techniques include completely obstructing tumors and esophagorespiratory fistulas. BICAP, as it coagulates circumferentially, is indicated for circumferential tumors only.

The practice of using a prosthetic funnel-shaped tube or wire coil to stent open a malignant esophageal stricture is not new. Historically, two techniques evolved to place these stents. The first involved transoral, endoscopic insertion ("push-through"), and the second added laparotomy and gastrotomy to pull a stent into place by means of a long "tail" ("pull-through"). Comparison of the two techniques has demonstrated the "push-through" endoscopic approach to be the safer approach.[92] Numerous endoscopic stents have been developed. The tubes differ in their shape, length, and flexibility; but there is no evidence that one is superior to any other. The technique involves esophagoscopy, dilatation, guidewire placement, and tube placement. The tube is positioned so its upper flange sits just at the proximal shelf of tumor, and its tip exits beyond the tumor into the distal lumen. Marked luminal angulation, inability to dilate a tumor, or complete obstruction are contraindications for stent insertion. Palliation of symptoms from an esophagorespiratory fistula is an acceptable indication. Reed,[88] in a review of 17 series on esophageal intubation, reported rates of failure of 0–15% (average 5.4%), perforation 0–14% (6.1%), hemorrhage 0–8.5% (3.5%), displacement 0–41.8% (13.2%), obstruction 0.4–28% (9.5%), and mortality 0–16.8% (6.8%). Obstruction and displacement were cited as late complications. Length of hospital stay was 3–5 days. In a large series reported by Cusumano et al.[93] using Celestin tubes, 20% of patients had no dysphagia, 60% could eat semisoft foods, and 20% were confined to a liquid diet. For patients with an esophagorespiratory fistula who were similarly treated, 73.5% of patients were able to resume oral feedings.

Expandable metal stents are designed to reduce the incidence of the esophageal perforation that may result from rigid tube placement while maintaining the favorable relief of dysphagia demonstrated by their rigid tube predecessors. These new stents achieve this goal by having a small insertion diameter, thereby requiring less rigid dilatation for successful insertion. Early uncovered expandable stents initially worked favorably but were plagued by tumor ingrowth, reobstruction, and return of dysphagia. This problem seems to have been largely solved by enclosing the expandable metal stent in a polyethelene sheath. These covered expandable stents are now largely favored by gastroenterologists because of studies demonstrating symptom palliation similar to that achieved with rigid stents but with reduced morbidity and mortality. Cook and Dehn[94] cited four major benefits of covered expandable stent use: (1) shorter hospital stay compared with rigid tube insertion; (2) use of a single hospital stay; (3) lack of readmission for recurrent obstruction from tumor ingrowth or food impaction; and (4) no procedure-related morbidity or mortality. The authors further stated that these benefits collectively make expandable stents more cost-effective than rigid tube use. The safety and early favorable results using these stents have resulted in rapid acceptance and increasing use of this palliative technique.

Photodynamic therapy (PDT) is a technique in which a chemical sensitizer is administered intravenously, which then accumulates in esophageal tumor tissue in preference to normal esophageal mucosa. About 40–50 hours later, the area of esophageal cancer is treated with an endoscopically directed laser light of a specific wavelength that activates the accumulated chemical sensitizer, resulting in tumor necrosis by means of a photochemical, not thermal, process. After 2–3 days patients are reendoscoped to débride necrotic tumor and to determine if additional treatments are needed. A maximum of three courses per month are permitted. Numerous studies have demonstrated the effectiveness of PDT. Additional studies show comparable effectiveness of PDT and laser ablation therapy. The advantages of PDT are low cost, technical ease, reduced incidence of perforation, and reduced treatment-related morbidity. The disadvantages include late stricture formation at the treatment site and prolonged skin photosensitivity. Clinical trials comparing PDT with stent insertion techniques are in progress.

Intracavitary brachytherapy uses and endoscopically placed afterloading catheter to deliver radiation seeds directly to the region of the tumor. The reported complication rate is low, and the procedure is well tolerated. The data do not clearly show an advantage of using brachytherapy over other palliative techniques.

## References


1. Thomas RM, Sobin LH. Gastrointestinal cancer. Cancer 1995;75 (suppl):154–170.
2. Postlethwaite RW. Squamous cell carcinoma of the esophagus. In: Surgery of the Esophagus, 2nd ed. Norwalk, CT: Appleton & Lange, 1986:369–342.
3. Ming S. Adenocarcinoma and other epithelial tumors of the esophagus. In: Ming S, Goldman H (eds) Pathology of the Gastrointestinal Tract. Philadelphia: Saunders, 1992: 459–477.
4. Ellis FH Jr. Treatment of carcinoma of the esophagus or cardia. Mayo Clin Proc 1989;64:945–955.
5. Ibrahim NB, Briggs JC, Corbishley CM. Extrapulmonary oat cell carcinoma. Cancer 1984;54:1645–1661.
6. Chalkiadakas G, Wihlm JR, Morand G, Weill-Boussan M, Witz JP. Primary malignant melanoma of the esophagus. Ann Thorac Surg 1985;39:472–475.
7. Briggs JC, Ibrahim NBM. Oat cell carcinoma of the oesophagus: a clinico-pathologic study of 23 cases. Histopathology 1983;7:261–277.
8. Doherty MA, McIntyre M, Arnott SJ. Oat cell carcinoma of the esophagus: a report of six British patients with a review of the literature. Int J Radiat Oncol Biol Phys 1984; 10:147–152.
9. Nichols GL, Kelson DP. Small cell carcinoma of the esophagus: the Memorial Hospital experience 1970–1987. Cancer 1989;64:1531–1533.
10. Partyka EK, Sanowski RA, Kozarek RA. Endoscopic diagnosis of a giant esophageal leiomyosarcoma. Am J Gastroenterol 1981;75:132–134.
11. Heitmiller RF, Sharma R. Comparison of incidence and resection rates in patients with esophageal squamous cell and adenocarcinoma. J Thorac Cardiovasc Surg 1996;112: 130–136.
12. Yang PC, Davis S. Incidence of cancer of the esophagus in the U.S. by histologic type. Cancer 1988;61:612–617.
13. Hesketh PJ, Clapp RW, Doos WG, Spechler SJ. The increasing frequency of adenocarcinoma of the esophagus. Cancer 1989;64:526–530.
14. Pera M, Cameron AJ, Trastek VF, Carpenter HA, Zinmeister AR. Increasing incidence of adenocarcinoma of the esophagus and esophagogastric junction. Gastroenterology 1993;104:510–513.
15. Blot J, Devesa SS, Kneller RW, Fraumeni JF. Increasing incidence of adenocarcinoma of the esophagus and gastric cardia. JAMA 1991;265:1287–1289.
16. Powell J, McConkey CC. Increasing incidence of adenocarcinoma of the gastric cardia and adjacent sites. Br J Cancer 1990;62:440–443.
17. Reed PI. Changing pattern of oesophageal cancer. Lancet 1991;338:178.
18. Newcomb PA, Carbone PP. The health consequences of smoking. Med Clin North Am 1992;76:305–331.
19. Choi SY, Kahyo H. Effect of cigarette smoking and alcohol consumption in the etiology of cancers of the digestive tract. Int J Cancer 1991;49:381–386.
20. Franceschi S, Talamini R, Barra S, et al. Smoking and drinking in relation to cancers of the oral cavity, pharynx, and esophagus in northern Italy. Cancer Res 1990;50:6502–6507.
21. DeStefani E, Munoz N, Esteve J, Vasallo A, Victora CG, Teuchmann S. Mate drinking, alcohol, tobacco, diet, and esophageal cancer in Uruguay. Cancer Res 1990;50:426–431.
22. Gray JR, Coldman AJ, MacDonald WC. Cigarette and alcohol use in patients with adenocarcinoma of the gastric cardia or lower esophagus. Cancer 1992;69:2227–2231.
23. Christen AG, McDonald JL Jr, Olsen BL, Christen JA. Smokeless tobacco addiction: a threat to the oral and systemic health of the child and adolescent. Pediatrician 1989;16:170–177.
24. Adami HO, McLaughlin JK, Hsing AW, et al. Alcoholism and cancer risk: a population-based cohort study. Cancer Causes Control 1992;3:419–425.
25. Kato I, Nomura AM, Stemmermenn GN, Chyon PH. Prospective study of the association of alcohol with cancer of the upper aerodigestive tract and other sites. Cancer Causes Control 1992;3:145–151.
26. Cameron AJ, Zinmeister AR, Ballard DJ, Carney JA. Prevalence of columnar-lined (Barrett's) esophagus: comparison of population-based clinical and autopsy findings. Gastroenterology 1990;99:918–922.
27. Sarr MG, Hamilton SR, Marrone GC, Cameron JL. Barrett's esophagus: its prevalence and association with adenocarcinoma in patients with symptoms of gastroesophageal reflux. Am J Surg 1985;149:1878–1892.
28. Hamilton SR, Smith RL. The relationship between columnar epithelial dysplasia and invasive adenocarcinoma arising in Barrett's esophagus. Am J Clin Pathol 1987;87: 301–312.

29. Naef AP, Savary M, Ozello L. Columnar-lined lower esophagus: an acquired lesion with malignant predisposition; report on 140 cases of Barrett's esophagus with 12 adenocarcinomas. J Thorac Cardiovasc Surg 1975;70:826–834.
30. Saubier EC, Gouillat C, Samaniego C, Guillard M, Moulinier B. Adenocarcinoma in columnar-lined Barrett's esophagus: analysis of 13 esophagectomies. Am J Surg 1985;150: 365–369.
31. Heitmiller RF. Esophageal tumors. In: Cameron JL (ed) Current Surgical Therapy, 5th ed. St. Louis: Mosby, 1995:45–49.
32. Tygat GNJ, Hameeteman W. The neoplastic potential of columnar-lined (Barrett) esophagus. World J Surg 1992;16: 302–312.
33. Heitmiller RF, Redmond M, Hamilton SR. Barrett's esophagus with high-grade dysplasia: an indication for prophylactic esophagectomy. Ann Surg 1996;224:66–71.
34. Pera M, Trastek VF, Carpenter HA, et al. Barrett's esophagus with high grade dysplasia: an indication for esophagectomy? Ann Thorac Surg 1992;54:199–204.
35. Altorki NK, Sunaagawa M, Little AG, Skinner DB. High-grade dysplasia in the columnar-lined esophagus. Am J Surg 1991;161:97–100.
36. Barrett NR. Chronic peptic ulcer of the oesophagus and "oesophagitis." Br J Surg 1950;38:175–182.
37. American Joint Committee on Cancer: Manual for Staging of Cancer, 3rd ed. Philadelphia: Lippincott, 1988.
38. Inculet RI, Keller SM, Dwyer A, Roth JA. Evaluation of non-invasive tests for the preoperative staging of carcinoma of the esophagus: a prospective study. Ann Thorac Surg 1985;40:561–565.
39. Greenberg J, Durkin M, Van Drunen M, Aranha GV. Computed tomography or endoscopic ultrasonography in preoperative staging of gastric and esophageal tumors. Surgery 1994;116:696–702.
40. Quint LE, Glazer GM, Orringer MB. Esophageal imaging by MR and CT: study of normal anatomy and neoplasms. Radiology 1985;156:727–731.
41. Lightdale CJ, Botet JF. Staging of esophageal cancer. Endoscopy 1993;25:655–659.
42. Lightdale CJ. Staging of esophageal cancer. I. Endoscopic ultrasonography. Semin Oncol 1994;21:438–446.
43. Kallimanis GE, Gupta PK, al-Kawas FH, et al. Endoscopic ultrasound for staging esophageal cancer, with or without dilatation, is clinically important and safe. Gastrointest Endosc 1995;41:540–546.
44. Chandawarkar RY, Kakegawa T, Fujita H, Yamana H, Toh Y, Fujitoh H. Endosonography for preoperative staging of specific nodal groups associated with esophageal cancer. World J Surg 1996;20:700–702.
45. Holscher AH, Dittler HJ, Siewert JR. Staging of squamous esophageal cancer: accuracy and value. World J Surg 1994;18:312–320.
46. Souquet JC, Napoleon B, Pujol B, et al. Endoscopic ultrasonography in the preoperative staging of esophageal cancer. Endoscopy 1994;26:764–766.
47. Krasna MJ, Flowers JL, Attar S, McLaughlin J. Combined thoracoscopy/laparoscopic staging of esophageal cancer. J Thorac Cardiovasc Surg 1996;111:800–806.
48. Talamini M, Kutka M, Heitmiller RF. Laparoscopic staging of esophageal cancer alters neoadjuvant therapy. Presented at the Society of the Alimentary Tract, May 1997.
49. O'Brien MG, Fitzgerald EF, Lee G, Crowley M, Shanahan F, O'Sullivan GC. A prospective comparison of laparoscopy and imaging in the staging of esophagogastric cancer before surgery. Am J Gastroenterol 1995;90:2191–2194.
50. Flanagan FL, Dehdashti F, Siegel BA, et al. Staging of esophageal cancer with $^{18}$F-fluorodeoxyglucose positron emission tomography. AJR 1997;168:417–424.
51. Heitmiller RF. Cancer of the Esophagus. In: Bayless TM (ed) Current Therapy in Gastroenterology and Liver Disease, 4th ed. St. Louis: Mosby, 1994:81–85.
52. Reichle R, Nixon M, Heitmiller RF, Fishman E. Post surgical evaluation of the esophagus: normal radiographic appearance and complications. Invest Radiol 1993;28:247–257.
53. Muller JM, Erasmi H, Stelzner M, et al. Surgical therapy of oesophageal carcinoma. Br J Surg 1990;77:845–857.
54. Orringer MB. Technical aids in performing transhiatal esophagectomy without thoracotomy. Ann Thorac Surg 1984;38:128–132.
55. Stone CD, Heitmiller RF. Simplified standardized technique for cervical esophagogastric anastomosis. Ann Thorac Surg 1994;58:259–261.
56. Orringer MB. Surgical options for esophageal reconstruction with stomach. In: Baue AE, Geha AS, Hammond GL, Laks H, Naunheim KS (eds) Glenn's Thoracic and Cardiovascular Surgery, 6th ed. Norwalk, CT: Appleton & Lange, 1996:899–922.
57. Shriver CD, Burt M. Transhiatal esophagectomy. Semin Thorac Cardiovasc Surg 1992;4:307–313.
58. Orringer MB, Marshall B, Stirling MC. Transhiatal esophagectomy for benign and malignant esophageal disease. J Thorac Cardiovasc Surg 1993;105:265–277.
59. Lewis I. The surgical treatment of carcinoma of the oesophagus with special reference to a new operation for growths of the middle third. Br J Surg 1946;34:18–31.
60. King MR, Pairolero PC, Trastek VF, Payne WS, Bernatz PE. Ivor Lewis esophagogastrectomy for carcinoma of the esophagus: early and late functional results. Ann Thorac Surg 1987;44:119–122.
61. Mathisen DJ, Grillo HC, Wilkins EW, Moncure AC, Hilgenberg AD. Transthoracic esophagectomy: a safe approach to carcinoma of the esophagus. Ann Thorac Surg 1988;45:137–143.
62. Barbier PA, Becker CD, Wagner HE. Esophageal carcinoma: patient selection for transhiatal esophagectomy; a prospective analysis of 50 cases. World J Surg 1988;12:263–269.
63. Mitchell RL. Abdominal and right thoracotomy approach as a standard procedure for esophagogastrectomy with low morbidity. J Thorac Cardiovasc Surg 1987;93:205–211.
64. Allen MS. Ivor Lewis esophagectomy. Semin Thorac Cardiovasc Surg 1992;4:320–323.
65. Heitmiller RF. The left thoracoabdominal incision. Ann Thorac Surg 1988;46:250–253.
66. Shahian DM, Neptune WB, Ellis FH Jr. Transthoracic versus extrathoracic esophagectomy: mortality, morbidity, and long-term survival. Ann Thorac Surg 1986;41:237–246.

67. Heitmiller RF. Results of standard left thoracoabdominal esophagogastrectomy. Semin Thorac Cardiovasc Surg 1992; 4:314–319.
68. McKeown KC. Total three-stage esophagectomy for cancer of the oesophagus. Br J Surg 1976;63:259–262.
69. DeMeester TR, Zaninolto G, Johansson KE. Selective therapeutic approach to cancer of the lower esophagus and cardia. J Thorac Cardiovasc Surg 1988;95:42–54.
70. Skinner DB. En bloc resection for neoplasms of the esophagus and cardia. J Thorac Cardiovasc Surg 1983;85:59–69.
71. Altorki NK, Skinner DB. En bloc esophagectomy: the first 100 patients. Hepatogastroenterology 1990;37:360–363.
72. Kato H, Watanabe H, Tachimori Y, Iizuka T. Evaluation of neck lymph node dissection for thoracic esophageal carcinoma. Ann Thorac Surg 1991;51:931–936.
73. Lerut T, DeLeyn P, Coosemans W, et al. Surgical strategies in esophageal carcinoma with emphasis on radical lymphadenectomy. Ann Surg 1992;216:583–590.
74. Thomas P, Doddoli C, Neville P, et al. Esophageal cancer resection in the elderly. Eur J Cardiothorac Surg 1996; 10:941–946.
75. Naunheim KS, Hanosh J, Zwischenberger J, et al. Esophagectomy in the septagenarian. Ann Thorac Surg 1993;56:880–884.
76. Muehrcke DD, Kaplan DK, Donnelly RJ. Oesophagectomy in patients over 70. Thorax 1989;44:141–145.
77. Adam DJ, Craig SR, Sang CT, Cameron EW, Walker WS. Esophagectomy for carcinoma in the octogenarian. Ann Thorac Surg 1996;61:190–194.
78. Kuwano H, Morita M, Baba K, et al. Surgical treatment of esophageal carcinoma in patients eighty years of age and older. J Surg Oncol 1993;52:36–39.
79. Forastiere AA, Heitmiller RF, Lee DJ, et al. Intensive chemoradiation followed by esophagectomy for squamous cell and adenocarcinoma of the esophagus. Cancer J Sci Am 1997;3:144–152.
80. Urba S, Orringer MB, Turrisi A, et al. A randomized trial comparing transhiatal esophagectomy to preoperative chemoradiation followed by esophagectomy in locoregional esophageal carcinoma. Proce ASCO 1995;14: 119.
81. Walsh TN, Noonan N, Hollywood D, et al. A comparison of multimodal therapy and surgery for esophageal adenocarcinoma. N Engl J Med 1996;335:462–467.
82. Langer M, Choi N, Orlow E. Radiation therapy alone or in combination with surgery in the treatment of carcinoma of the esophagus. Cancer 1986;58:1208–1213.
83. Okawa T, Kita M, Tanka M, Ikeda M. Results of radiotherapy for inoperable locally advanced esophageal cancer. Int J Radiat Oncol Biol Phys 1989;17:49–54.
84. Earlam R, Johnson L. 101 Oesophageal cancers: a surgeon uses radiotherapy. Ann R Coll Surg Engl 1990;72:32–40.
85. Caspers R, Welvaart K, Verkes R. The effect of radiotherapy on dysphagia and survival in patients with esophageal cancer. J Radiat Ther Oncol 1988;12:15–23.
86. Herskovic A, Martz, Al-Sarraf M, et al. Combined chemotherapy and radiotherapy compared with radiotherapy alone in patients with cancer of the esophagus. N Engl J Med 1992;326:1593–1598.
87. Shemesh E, Czerniak A. Comparison between Savary-Gillard and balloon dilatation of benign esophageal strictures. World J Surg 1990;14:518–521.
88. Reed CE. Endoscopic palliation of esophageal carcinoma. Chest Surg Clin North Am 1994;4:155–172.
89. Ell C, Demling L. Laser therapy of tumor stenosis in the upper gastrointestinal tract: an international inquiry. Lasers Surg Med 1987;4:491–[illegible].
90. Nava HR, Schuh ME, [illegible]mbisan R, Clark JL, Douglass HO Jr. Endoscopic ablation of esophageal malignancies with the neodymium-YAG laser and electrofulguration. Arch Surg 1989;124:225–228.
91. Jensen DM, Machicado G, Randall G, Tung LA, English-Zych S. Comparison of low-power YAG laser and BICAP tumor probe for palliation of esophageal cancer strictures. Gastroenterology 1988;94:1267–1270.
92. Lishman AH, Dellipiani AW, Devlin HB. The insertion of oesophagogastric tubes in malignant esophageal strictures: endoscopy or surgery? Br J Surg 1980;67:257–259.
93. Cusumano A, Ruol A, Seglin A, et al. Push-through intubation: effective palliation in 409 patients with cancer of the esophagus and cardia. Ann Thorac Surg 1992;53:1010–1014.
94. Cook TA, Dehn CB. Use of covered expandable metal stents in the treatment of oesophageal carcinoma and tracheo-oesophageal fistula. Br J Surg 1996;83:1417–1418.

# 39 Pathophysiology and Treatment of Benign Diseases of the Stomach and Duodenum

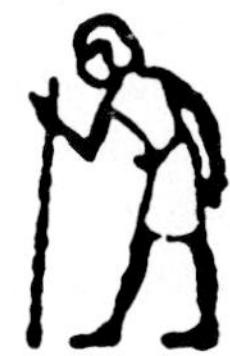

Robert R. Cima and David I. Soybel

Evaluation of the elderly patient with complaints of upper abdominal discomfort is often difficult and frustrating for both the patient and the physician. A multitude of processes may have similar presentations, including cardiac, respiratory, renal, and gastrointestinal processes. A malignant process must also be considered more frequently in the elderly patient than in the young or middle-aged patient. In the elderly patient, the presentation of a true pathologic process is often obscured by functional disorders of the upper digestive tract, which accounts for nearly 30% of all office visits.[1] Also confounding the evaluation of the elderly patient are the multiple co-morbid disease processes frequently encountered and the polypharmacy treatment regimens administered by different specialists.

The purpose of this chapter is to address some of the major benign disease processes of the stomach and duodenum that occur frequently in or are unique to the elderly patient. Gastritis and peptic ulcer disease are by far the most important benign processes in the upper digestive tract in the elderly patient and are responsible for significant morbidity and mortality in this population. The physiologic and functional issues of age-related changes in the gastrointestinal mucosa are discussed, as are the epidemiologic issues relevant to these diseases and the elderly population. An overview of the medical and surgical treatment of these processes is provided, and some of the major complications of these treatments in the elderly are evaluated. Rare occurrences, such as gastric and duodenal diverticula, duplications, and gastric volvulus, which have no specific age-related manifestations, are not discussed.

## Physiologic Changes with Age

Histologic and functional changes in the stomach and duodenum have been observed with increasing age in both humans and laboratory models. Age-related atrophic changes were once thought to represent a natural progression of changes related to the aging process itself. Until relatively recently the atrophic changes in the upper gastrointestinal tract were thought to be related to years of exposure to the intraluminal contents and gastric secretions. Most age-related atrophic changes were noted in the mucosa and parietal cell mass. However, Bird et al. showed that one-third of patients over age 80 and one-half of those over age 90 had normal gastric mucosa.[2] Similar biopsy findings were reported by Palmer.[3] Khanna et al. reported that in mice there was no evidence of superficial or atrophic gastritis with increasing age; and although they noted a decrease in parietal cell volume, it was only significant in extremely elderly mice.[4] Functionally, the loss of parietal cell mass in the elderly was thought to contribute to the higher rate of hypochlorhydria and achlorhydria in the elderly. However, there is now considerable evidence in the clinical and experimental literature that, in fact, histologic and functional changes previously attributed to the aging process may represent pathologic processes rather than physiologic changes.

Unlike the solid organs of the alimentary tract, in which growth ceases during adolescence, the gastrointestinal mucosa is maintained by constant cell turnover. Studies of gastric mucosal turnover in young rats have clearly shown a dramatic decrease in gastric mucosal proliferation.[5] Age-related changes in mucosal proliferation rates have not been clearly demonstrated. Majumdar et al.[6] showed that there is an increase in thymidine kinase activity (a reflection of proliferative activity) in the gastric mucosa of rats as they aged from 4 months to 16 months. Although there was evidence of increased proliferation, there was no evidence of increased DNA or protein content in the mucosa. These observations suggest that aging leads to increased cell turnover without an overall change in cell density. Subsequent studies in rats that carefully evaluated proliferative activity and histologic changes have shown that there was marked atrophy of the mucosal glandular height in rats as they aged from 4 months to 24 months.[7] There was also a decrease in the gland density, which resulted in a reduction of all epithelial cell types. Although there was a decrease in the gastric epithelial cells, there was a relative increase in the amount of connective tissue components of the lamina propria and extensive collagen deposition. This marked mucosal atrophy was accompanied by a significant increase in mucosal proliferative activity. Overall, the data from these studies indicate that aging leads to both a decrease in the epithelial cells of the gastric mucosa and an increase in the proportion of the remaining cellular components of the gastric mucosa. This age-related change of the gastric epithelial cell population in the apparently healthy aged rat may contribute to some of the functional changes reported in the aged gastric mucosa.

Whereas there is considerable evidence to indicate that there is a decrease in the gastric epithelial cellular component of the mucosa, there are conflicting observations on the functional consequences of these changes. Khalil et al. showed that both basal and gastrin-stimulated gastric acid secretion are decreased in 32-month-old rats compared to that in 3-month-old rats.[8] A subsequent study by the same investigators showed that gastrin release in response to bombesin or low dose carbachol is well preserved in aged rats.[9] It is of interest that in this same study they showed that the basal release of somatostatin from the gastric antrum decreases with age, which may indicate that changes in the relative balance of these two hormones could contribute to the altered secretory capacity of the stomach with age. These findings are of interest because morphometric studies have shown that the density of antral G-cells (gastrin-secreting cells) decreases by 40% as rats age from 4 months to 16 months, whereas the antral D-cell density (somatostatin-secreting cells) is unchanged.[6] Majumdar et al. also showed that, although the serum gastrin levels decreased significantly with age, the antral gastrin levels rose sharply. The decline in serum gastrin with age parallels a decline in gastric mucosal sensitivity to the trophic action of gastrin.[6] Similar age-related changes in mucosal prostaglandin levels have been reported in rats. Lee and Feldman showed that gastric mucosal prostaglandin formation, but not leukotriene formation, decreases by 70% from age 3 months to 21 months.[10] The decline in prostaglandins, which are known to have beneficial properties for gastric mucosal integrity, was shown to have an inverse correlation to the extent of gastric mucosal injury induced by aspirin.[10] Together the change in gastrin and prostaglandin levels with age may contribute to the increasing incidence of mucosal injuries that occur with age.

The data regarding age-related gastric mucosal changes in the rat are convincing, but studies in humans have not provided consistent observations. Many studies have found that acid secretion is decreased,[11] unchanged,[12] or increased[13,14] with age. One explanation for the lack of consistency is that most of these studies failed to account for the presence of gastritis and its influence on histologic and functional properties of the epithelial cells and glands. Kekki and associates showed that gastric acid secretion is maintained in the normal range by 75% of elderly people so long as there was no evidence of gastritis.[15,16] In their study, there was an age-related decrease in acid secretion that paralleled an increase in the severity of atrophic changes in the mucosa of the body. However, even when controlling for gastritis in asymptomatic healthy patients, the data are conflicting in regard to acid secretion. In the most recent evaluations of this process, Feldman has reported that advancing age has no independent effect on gastric acid secretion but is associated with reduced pepsin output independent of atrophic gastritis or *Helicobacter pylori* infection.[19] Similar results relating to acid secretion were reported by Katelaris,[17] who also reported that there was no change in serum gastrin with aging. Although the level of acid secretion in the healthy elderly person is unclear, all of the recent studies have shown a decrease in gastric acid secretion with chronic antral gastritis, *H. pylori* infection, and smoking, which were independent of age. Recently, however, Husebye et al. showed that in otherwise healthy patients over the age of 80 with no evidence of gastritis, approximately 80% had fasting hypochlorhydria.[18]

With regard to concentrations of prostaglandins in human gastric mucosa, there is a marked decrease in the prostaglandin concentration in the gastric and duodenal mucosa with increasing age and cigarette use.[14,19] There was no association between mucosal prostaglandin levels and *H. pylori* infection, ethanol use, or the presence of gastritis.

Another consideration in the elderly patient is the alteration in gastric emptying that may occur with age. If there is a delay in emptying, gastric acid or agents injurious to the mucosa, such as nonsteroidal antiinflammatory drugs (NSAIDs), may have prolonged contact with the mucosa, leading to injury. Similar to the effect of aging on the acid secretory capacity of the stomach, there are conflicting data regarding the influence of age on gastric motility. The most commonly used methods for measuring gastric emptying is to follow the transit of radiolabeled particles into the duodenum or the absorption of a nonmetabolized marker. Using variations of these methodologies, various teams of investigators have shown an increase,[20] no change,[21] or a decrease[22,23] in the rate of gastric emptying of solids or liquids with aging. In some studies there was a difference with aging between solids and liquids in which only the emptying of liquids was delayed with aging.[24] One consistent finding in studies of gastric emptying is a gender difference in which elderly women taking estrogen replacement have a decreased rate of gastric emptying compared to that of elderly men.[25]

From this brief review of the literature, it is clear that the functional consequences of aging on the stomach mucosa are not well understood. How these changes may contribute to disease processes of the stomach in the elderly patient are similarly unclear. For example, the role of acid secretion, which may or may not change with aging, in peptic ulcer disease has been significantly modified by recognition of the pathologic conditions of antral and NSAIDs gastritis and *H. pylori* infection, each of which plays a major role in ulcer formation in the elderly population. As is discussed later, both of these conditions occur with increasing prevalence in the elderly population and likely contribute to the high incidence of peptic ulcer disease and complications in this population.

## Epidemiology of Ulcer Disease

According to most epidemiologic studies, the incidence of ulcer disease in the United States has declined steadily since the early 1960s.[26] Although the morbidity related to peptic ulcer disease has also declined, it remains a significant health problem. In the United States, approximately 10% of all people suffer from peptic ulcer disease during their lifetime. The cost related to the medical care for ulcer disease is estimated to be more than $3 billion annually in the United States.[27] The decline in ulcer disease preceded the introduction of the antisecretory agents (e.g., cimetidine), but their introduction in 1977 had a profound impact on the treatment of ulcer disease. By the end of the 1970s, there was a nearly 50% reduction in the number of hospital discharges listing peptic ulcer disease as the cause of admission.[28] Although introduction of the antisecretory agents has reduced hospitalizations for uncomplicated ulcer disease, the number of hospitalizations for complications of ulcer disease seems to have remained unchanged.[29]

The apparent decline in the prevalence of peptic ulcer disease is due predominantly to a decreasing incidence in young and middle-aged patients. In the population over 65 years of age, there has been an increase in ulcer disease.[30] The explanation for the declining incidence in young people and increasing incidence of ulcer disease in the elderly is unclear. Though age-related changes in the upper gastrointestinal tract mucosal physiologic function may contribute modestly to ulcer disease in the elderly, many believe that the higher incidence of *H. pylori* infection, the more prevalent use of NSAIDs, and the greater prevalence of cigarette use among the elderly may explain the age-related differences. It is also interesting to note that this increase has a definite sex difference, with elderly women being disproportionately affected compared to elderly men.[31]

Ulcer disease has a significant impact on the health of the elderly population in the United States. Cryer and Feldman estimated that in 1994 approximately 700,000 people in the United States over the age of 65 would have experienced symptoms or complications of peptic ulcer disease.[32] It must also be noted that elderly patients have much higher morbidity and mortality rates from the complications of ulcer disease. Thus 80% of ulcer-related deaths in the United States in 1984 occurred in people over the age of 65.[33]

## Gastritis

Gastritis is one of the most commonly used terms for upper abdominal complaints of the elderly. It is also one of the most common endoscopic diagnoses.[34] Although the term is used widely, *gastritis* should be limited to a histologically proven inflammatory process of the stomach mucosa. Gastritis is classified as type A or type B. Type A gastritis predominantly involves the mucosa of the fundus, although the antrum may be involved to a lesser degree. In Finland, it occurs in approximately 8% of the population.[35] Type A gastritis is considered to be an autoimmune disorder, with most patients having antibodies to parietal cells and intrinsic factors. The loss of parietal cell mass is thought to result from immune-mediated destruction.

Histologically, type A gastritis is divided into superficial and atrophic gastritis. With superficial gastritis, the inflammatory process is limited to the outer mucosal layers, whereas with atrophic gastritis, the inflammatory process extends into the deeper layers of the mucosa. This deeper inflammation results in a decrease in the number of parietal and chief cells. In the atrophic gastric glands, there is metaplasia toward cell types found either in the antral region or small intestine. Type A gastritis is considered to evolve from a superficial form to an atrophic form over an approximately 20-year period.[36] During this period there is a reduction in the parietal and chief cell mass, which leads to decreased acid, pepsin, and intrinsic factor secretion.

Although many patients remain asymptomatic from the gastrointestinal changes associated with type A gastritis, the decrease in intrinsic factor leads to clinically significant pernicious anemia in approximately 10% of these patients.[34] Pernicious anemia is usually diagnosed 6–18 years after the first tissue diagnosis of gastritis. Treatment for pernicious anemia is directed at treatment of the anemia by vitamin $B_{12}$ replacement, which has no effect on the gastritis or its course. Of the patients who develop overt pernicious anemia, approximately 10% develop gastric carcinoma.[37]

Type B gastritis, also known as antral gastritis, is predominantly restricted to the antral mucosa. It is the more common form of chronic gastritis, than type A by 4:1.[28] Like type A gastritis, type B gastritis increases in prevalence with increasing age. It is not associated with any autoantibodies or predictable change in acid or pepsinogen production. In fact, there is preservation of the gastric glands. Until recently, the cause of type B gastritis was unknown. Circumstantial evidence indicates that most type B or chronic antral gastritis is caused by *H. pylori* infection of the gastric antral mucosa.[39] In a large series of elderly dyspeptic patients, Safe et al. reported that 81% of the patients with antral gastritis and 63% with gastric ulcers were *H. pylori*-positive.[40] It is notable that all the patients with *H. pylori*-negative antral gastritis were chronic users of NSAIDs. The users of NSAIDs had severe active gastritis that correlated with the presence of *H. pylori* but not with the number of NSAIDs used. In a similar study by Gillanders et al., *H. pylori*-positive elderly patients had a significantly higher association with features of severe active chronic antral gastritis than *H. pylori*-negative patients.[41] A more detailed discussion of the role of *H. pylori* infection and the elderly patient is presented below.

Although there may be relatively few changes in the physiology of the gastrointestinal tract related to aging, gastrointestinal dysfunction has a significant impact on the health of the aged. According to Levitan, approximately 18% of all patients in geriatric clinics have significant gastrointestinal problems and 20% of all geriatric deaths are caused by gastrointestinal diseases.[42] Peptic ulcer disease accounts for approximately 16% of gastrointestinal disorders in those older than 65 years, which is second only to functional disorders of the gastrointestinal tract.[43] As is discussed in more detail later in the chapter, the typical symptoms of peptic ulcer disease are often attenuated or even absent in the elderly. Often the initial presentation of ulcer disease in the elderly involves a life-threatening complication. Initial symptoms are often vague, and the description of pain, if there is any, is usually diffuse in nature. Other prominent symptoms related to ulcer disease are weight loss, anorexia, nausea, and constipation.[43]

## *Helicobacter pylori* and Ulcer Disease

With the discovery of *Helicobacter pylori* in the stomach, a considerable amount of evidence has indicated that this pathogen plays a causal role in chronic antral gastritis in the elderly and in the progression and continuation of gastric and duodenal ulcer disease in both the young and old. *H. pylori*, formerly *Campylobacter pylori*, is one of the most common bacterial pathogens in the world. It has been identified in all countries and affects all ages from children to the aged. *H. pylori* has been shown to be the major cause of chronic active type B gastritis peptic ulcer disease.[44] It has also been shown that *H. pylori*-associated gastritis is the most common histopathologic finding in the elderly dyspeptic patient.[43] Epidemiologic studies have suggested a possible role for *H. pylori* in gastric carcinoma[45] and mucosa-associated lymphoid tissue (MALT) gastric lymphoma.[46]

Humans are the only recognized host for *H. pylori*. Epidemiologic studies performed in developing countries, indicate that *H. pylori* infections are most likely to occur during childhood, with approximately 70% of children and teenagers infected.[47] In developed countries there is a lower childhood infection rate, which results in 40–50% *H. pylori* seropositivity in the population 20–60 years of age.[48] There is an approximately 1% per year infection rate in developed nations, which is about the same as the rate for newly diagnosed gastritis and dyspepsia.[48,49] There are two views regarding the increased prevalence of *H. pylori* in old people in developed nations. One is that individuals can acquire *H. pylori* at any time during their lives. If this is true, the reason for the increased prevalence in old people is that this population has had a longer time to acquire the infection. Another view is that *H. pylori* infections were more common during the past in developed countries, which has led to a cohort of people infected with *H. pylori*. The cohort hypothesis is strongly supported by the work reported by Cullen et al., in which *H. pylori* antibody titers in serum samples from a cohort of people obtained in 1969, 1978, and 1990 were analyzed.[50] The prevalence of *H. pylori* was 39.0%, 40.9%, and 34.8% for each of the years, respectively. Only 7% of the seronegative subjects in 1969 had seroconverted by 1990. This "cohort effect" is consistent with the overall decline in duodenal ulcer disease that started early in the twentieth century and the relatively higher frequency of duodenal ulcers in older people. This cohort phenomenon is also consistent with the epidemiologic data of *H. pylori* infections, which show a decrease in prevalence with increasing socioeconomic status.[48,51] This inverse relation most likely reflects better hygiene practices and environmental factors. The association is strongest with respect to the socioeconomic status of individuals during their childhood compared to their status as adults.[52]

Until recently the mode of acquisition and transmission of *H. pylori* was unclear, but it now appears that *H. pylori* is most likely transmitted via an oral-oral route rather than a fecal-oral route.[53] The infection appears to be lifelong unless specific eradication treatments are undertaken. *H. pylori* colonization and infection is localized to gastric-type surface cells.[53] Thus *H. pylori* is found predominantly in the stomach, primarily the antrum, and in areas of gastric metaplasia such as the diseased duodenum. The acute infection has been shown to cause dyspepsia-type symptoms and biopsy-proven gastritis.[54] The symptoms of dyspepsia are of variable duration and eventually resolve completely, but the gastritis may be present as long as *H. pylori* is present. It is believed that chronic *H. pylori* infection is the cause of the most common form of chronic gastritis, type B gastritis. Nearly 100% of patients with type B gastritis are infected with *H. pylori*.[44] More important is the fact that the eradication of *H. pylori* infection results in either marked improvement or complete resolution of the chronic gastritis.[39]

It is accepted that *H. pylori* plays a significant role in chronic gastritis and gastric ulcers and probably a causal role in the development of duodenal ulcers. This hypothesis is based on the nearly 100% association of *H. pylori* infection in the stomach and duodenum of patients suffering from duodenal ulcers.[39,55] The association of *H. pylori* with gastric ulcers in patients not taking NSAIDs is approximately 80%.[56] The putative relation between *H. pylori* infection and ulcer disease is strengthened by the greatly diminished recurrence rate (approximately 2–5% per year) of duodenal ulcer disease after effective treatment of *H. pylori* infection compared with standard antisecretory therapy, which has a 1-year recurrence rate of approximately 60–90%.[57] Because epidemiologic data indicate that *H. pylori* infection is chronic in nature, with most persons infected early in life, eradication of the infection in patients with duodenal ulcer disease should lead to long-term cure of the ulcer disease. Forbes et al. found that 7 years after effective *H. pylori* eradication treatment only 1 of 38 (3%) patients had endoscopic evidence of duodenal ulceration compared to 5 of 25 (20%) of *H. pylori*-infected control patients.[58]

Although most agree that *H. pylori* eradication treatment reduces the recurrence rate of duodenal and gastric ulcers, often the first-line therapy for ulcer disease in the elderly is the antisecretory or mucosal protective medications. These medicines are often preferred because of their relative ease of use and side effect profile. There are two problems with *H. pylori* eradication protocols as they relate to the elderly patient. One problem is ensuring compliance with the complex multiple-drug regimens used for effective *H. pylori* eradication. The second problem is the severe side effect profile associated with these regimens, which include severe nausea, vomiting, diarrhea, and abdominal pain. If treatment for *H. pylori* is required in the elderly patient, one might consider two-drug therapy rather than the standard triple-drug therapy because of the relatively higher levels of compliance and decreased side effects. The details of *H. pylori* eradication therapies are discussed below.

The mechanisms by which *H. pylori* infection contributes to ulcer formation and prevents ulcer healing are unclear. It should be emphasized that *H. pylori* infection does not inevitably mean development of an ulcer. However, it seems clear that *H. pylori* infection results in alterations in the gastric and duodenal mucosa that aggravate mucosal injury and prevent healing of ulcers after they occur.

## NSAIDs and Ulcer Disease

When discussing ulcer disease in the elderly, particular attention must be paid to the role of NSAIDs. These drugs contribute to gastric and duodenal injury by interfering with mucosal production of prostaglandins, which are an essential component of the normal mucosal defense mechanisms. The worldwide market for such medicines approaches $2 billion per year. On average, approximately 1% of the U.S. population uses NSAIDs on a daily basis, with nearly 70 million prescriptions written annually.[59] It is estimated that the use of NSAIDs by the elderly is three times greater than by younger age groups.[60] Henry and Robertson showed that during the 1980s, NSAIDs use increased in all age groups, but the greatest increase occurred in the over-65 age group.[61] This increased use was most pronounced in elderly women, whose use rose from 11.9% in 1979 to 22.5% in 1988.[61] This rise parallels the increase in ulcer but does not completely account for the increased prevalence.

With the increasing use of NSAIDs, the importance of the side effects of this class of drugs has also increased. NSAIDs have well-known gastrointestinal side effects, with NSAIDs-induced gastropathy being the most frequent drug side effect reported in the United States. Serious gastrointestinal (GI) side effects, including ulceration, perforation, and hemorrhage, are estimated at 2–4% annually.[62] Endoscopic evaluations of chronic NSAIDs users revealed that 20% have an ulcer crater.[63] Bellary et al. reported that there is a significant sex difference in endoscopically proven gastric ulcers related to NSAIDs use, with 25% of elderly women having ulcers compared to 8% of elderly men.[64] Overall, it is estimated that treatment of the upper GI side effects in arthritis patients in the United States using NSAIDs costs $3.9 billion annually.[65]

As mentioned previously, elderly patients are much less likely than young patients to report symptoms of ulcer disease. Unfortunately, NSAIDs-related ulcers in elderly patients often first present with complications from the ulcer disease.[66] Epidemiologic studies of patients more than 65 years of age, revealed a relative risk of developing peptic ulcer disease in NSAIDs users compared to nonusers of 4.1, with 34% of users requiring hospitalization compared to 13% of control patients.[67] In the same study, NSAIDs users had a relative risk of 4.9 (compared to nonusers) for complications of peptic ulcer disease. In a similar study of elderly patients, users of prescription NSAIDs were four times more likely to die from peptic ulcer disease or upper GI bleeding than nonusers.[68] In a study of patients with rheumatoid arthritis, GI-related hospitalizations were six times more frequent among patients taking NSAIDs than in those not taking them.[62] In this group of patients there was a steady increase in upper GI-related hospitalizations by age. The odds ratio for GI-related hospitalization for patients over age 60 years was 2.6 compared to patients under 60 years of age; and patients more than age 60 years had an odds ratio three times that for those under 60 years for GI-related death. Meta-analysis of 16 studies examining the relation between NSAIDs use and

GI complications revealed a nearly a threefold increase in the relative risk for serious gastrointestinal events among elderly NSAIDs users when compared to nonelderly users.[69]

As previously discussed, elderly patients are at higher risks of morbidity and mortality from complications of peptic ulcer disease. The relatively high use of NSAIDs in this population further increases this risk. Armstrong and Blower, reporting a large series of patients who presented with life-threatening complications of peptic ulcer disease, noted that 60% were taking NSAIDs.[66] Almost 80% of all deaths occurred in patients using NSAIDs. The patients using NSAIDs who required operation for treatment were significantly older and had an operative mortality of 24% compared to 10% in nonusers. Similar findings were reported by Gabriel et al.[69]

Overall, the data indicate that there is a causal relation between NSAIDs use and ulcer disease. There is evidence that the elderly use NSAIDs at a significantly higher level than other age groups and are much more prone to complications from the use of these drugs. Therefore it is important for physicians who care for elderly patients to be aware of the extent of NSAIDs use and to counsel their patients to minimize their use.

## Oral Anticoagulants and Ulcer Disease

Another group of elderly patients at high risk of peptic ulcer disease complications are those using oral anticoagulants. Hemorrhagic complications of all types occurred in approximately 30% of elderly patients during the course of therapy.[70] This risk is increased dramatically in patients concurrently using NSAIDs. In a retrospective cohort study of Medicaid patients more than 65 years of age, the use of NSAIDs in patients on oral anticoagulants was found to be similar to patients not using oral anticoagulants, or approximately 14%.[71] In that study oral anticoagulant users had an increased relative risk of 2.2 times that of nonusers for hospitalization for ulcer disease primarily due to hemorrhagic ulcer disease. However, concurrent use of oral anticoagulants and NSAIDs increased the relative risk of developing hemorrhagic peptic ulcer disease to nearly 13 compared to nonusers of either drug.

## Medical Management of Ulcer Disease

The objectives of medical management of peptic ulcer disease for any age patient are to relieve the symptoms, promote healing, prevent complications, and prevent recurrence. In the elderly patient, these goals are often difficult to achieve because of the natural history of peptic ulcer disease in this group of patients. As discussed previously, elderly patients often have few if any symptoms related to peptic ulcer disease, which makes the diagnosis difficult. They often have multiple medical problems requiring multiple medications, which together may hinder ulcer healing or directly contribute to ulcer formation and progression. The elderly patient is much more likely than the younger patient to present initially with a life-threatening complication of ulcer disease. For all of these reasons, it is important to have a high index of suspicion for peptic ulcer disease in high risk elderly patients and to treat them aggressively to avoid the complications of ulcer disease.

Currently, several medications are used effectively to treat the symptoms and course of ulcer disease. Although most trials of the efficacy of various antiulcer agents are carried out in younger and healthier patients, there is no evidence to suggest differences in the relative efficacy of these agents or any change in the standard dosage because of increasing age.[72] Although all of these agents are effective in the elderly patient, there is some evidence that the elderly patient may require a longer course of therapy than a younger patient.[73] The main difference between the age groups relates to compliance with the treatment regimen and side effect profiles, which become a slightly greater problem in the elderly patient.

Antacids are effective for relief of acute dyspeptic symptoms. However, antacids are not useful in the elderly patient for treatment of presumed or known ulcer disease. The frequent dosing regimen and severe GI side effects, most commonly diarrhea, significantly limit the use of antacids as sole treatment of ulcer disease in the elderly. Another disadvantage of frequent high dose antacid use in the elderly, is the interaction with many other medications and the high sodium load that may occur and may exacerbate underlying medical conditions.[33] The $H_2$-receptor antagonists are by far the most commonly used antiulcer agents in the elderly. More than one-third of all ranitidine prescriptions in the United States are filled by people age 65 years or older.[74] These agents, as a class, are well tolerated by the elderly, and side effects are relatively rare, being less than 2% for all possible side effects.[75]

Of importance in the elderly are adverse drug interactions of $H_2$-blockers, particularly cimetidine, because of inhibition of the cytochrome P-450 mixed-function oxidase system. The often commented on neuropsychiatric effects of $H_2$-blockers in the elderly are perhaps overestimated. The most commonly reported side effect is delirium, which tends to occur in either the extremely sick elderly patient or the patient with significantly impaired renal or hepatic function. Postmarket surveys have shown no significant increase in neuropsychiatric side effects in the elderly compared to those in younger users of $H_2$-blockers.[74] The overall reported frequency of adverse central nervous system (CNS) effects for $H_2$-blockers is less than 0.21%.[76]

Sucralfate falls into the class of mucosa-protective agents. It has minimal systemic absorption, so possible adverse drug interactions are minimized. However, it may interfere with the bioavailability of certain agents commonly used by the elderly, such as digoxin.[77] The most common adverse reaction reported in the elderly is constipation, which occurs in approximately 2%.[76]

Another group of agents that has been extensively studied include the prostaglandin analogues. Misoprostol is the most commonly prescribed agent in this class. These drugs have both antisecretory and cytoprotective properties. The antisecretory effects occur at higher doses than the cytoprotective effects. Unfortunately, at high doses there is a high rate of GI side effects. Diarrhea was reported in up to 39% of patients taking antisecretory doses and resulted in withdrawal of the agent in up to 8% of patients in the trial.[78] The reported GI side effects are minimal at the cytoprotective doses. Although the side effects of these agents may limit their broad usefulness in the elderly, one group of patients who may benefit are those elderly patients taking NSAIDs. In a study by Graham et al., patients taking NSAIDs and misoprostol decreased their incidence of gastric ulceration from 21% to 6% using low-dose misoprostol (100 µg qid) and as low as 1% using higher doses (200 µg qid).[78] Similar protective benefits of misoprostol in this high risk group of patients was recently reported by McKenna, who noted a two- to threefold decrease in gastroduodenal ulcerations in the group of patients using a combination regimen of misoprostol and diclofenac.[79]

The most recent addition to the antiulcer arsenal is the proton-pump inhibitor class of drugs, typified by omeprazole. The active agent binds irreversibly to the $H^+/K^+$-ATPase of the parietal cell, which prevents acid secretion. Omeprazole has been shown to result in more rapid relief of symptoms of peptic ulcer disease and higher healing rates than the $H_2$-blockers.[80] In many trials comparing omeprazole and $H_2$-blockers, omeprazole had more rapid healing than the $H_2$-blockers, but the longer treatment is continued, the smaller the difference between treatment results, with each agent achieving 80–90% healing rates.[80] Omeprazole has been shown to have a side effect profile similar to that of $H_2$-blockers. It may have interactions with medicines commonly used in the elderly because it is metabolized by the liver cytochrome P-450 oxidase system. Even though omeprazole has slightly better healing rates than $H_2$-blockers, there is no evidence that it prevents relapse after a normal course of, and then cessation of therapy.[81]

The high incidence of *H. pylori* infection in duodenal and gastric ulcer patients and the low recurrence of ulcer disease after eradication of *H. pylori* infection, has led to intense investigation into the most effective eradication protocols. By far, the most effective *H. pylori* eradication protocol is a triple-drug therapy consisting of bismuth and two antibiotics.[82] There are multiple reports of triple-drug regimens that have reported similar eradication rates, but meta-analysis of the bismuth/antibiotic treatments of *H. pylori* eradication showed the most successful to be bismuth (8 tablets/day), metronidazole (750 mg/day), and tetracycline (2 g/day) for 2 weeks.[83] This regimen resulted in a 93% eradication rate. Using this form of *H. pylori* eradication therapy, the recurrent infection rate is reported to be 3.4%.[84] Long-term follow-up of triple-drug therapy eradication protocols have shown them to be effective in lowering ulcer recurrence. Forbes et al. reported a 3% duodenal ulcer recurrence after effective triple therapy during a 7-year follow-up compared to a 20% recurrence in those patients who were *H. pylori*-positive.[58]

Because of the complexity and side effects of triple-drug therapy, the efficacy of double- and single-drug therapy has been evaluated. The most successful of these regimens has been the dual therapy of omeprazole (20 mg bid) and an antibiotic (usually metronidazole or amoxicillin). The reported eradication rate for dual therapy using omeprazole and an antibiotic is approximately 70–80%.[85,86] Although no studies have investigated the effectiveness of *H. pylori* eradication therapy solely in elderly patients, there is no evidence to suggest that the elderly have a different *H. pylori* clearance rate for the different therapies. Often the limiting factor when treating the elderly *H. pylori*-positive patients is their ability to tolerate the treatment regimen.

## Surgical Treatment of Ulcer Disease

Surgical treatment for peptic ulcer disease has changed dramatically over the past 30 years. Corresponding to the improved medical treatment for peptic ulcer disease, there has been a significant decline in the number of elective procedures performed for peptic ulcer disease, although the number of emergency operations for complications of peptic ulcer disease seems to have remained relatively constant at 10 per 100,000.[87,88] In a retrospective study of more than 1000 patients during a 12-year span (1974–1986) conducted at the Massachusetts General Hospital, the annual incidence of surgical admissions for peptic ulcer disease declined by 39%.[89] In the same study, the number of ulcer operations per year declined by 16%, but the number of operations for massive hemorrhage and acute perforation remained nearly constant.

Most of the reported series for ulcer surgery include both elective and emergent surgeries in the reported mortality figures. As expected, elective or semiurgent surgery for the complications of ulcer disease (i.e., intractable pain, obstruction, or continuing low level bleeding) are associated with a mortality rate of less than 4%.[89,90] On the other hand, emergency surgery for ulcer complications is always accompanied by much higher mortality rates, which vary from 6% to 100%.[89–98] Subgroup analysis reveals that the elderly are more likely to have postoperative complications and a higher mortality after emergency ulcer surgery.[66,89,90,98,99] Armstrong and Blower found, in a series of 235 patients operated on emergently for acute complications of ulcer disease, an overall mortality rate of 18%; by age, however, patients over 70 years of age had an operative mortality of 34.9%, whereas those under age 70 had a mortality of 7.9%.[66] This high mortality rate after emergent ulcer surgery is similar to that seen with other emergent gastrointestinal surgeries in elderly patients. In a large retrospective series, emergency gastrointestinal surgery in patients over age 75 resulted in a 33% mortality rate compared to 12.8% for elective procedures.[100]

The presentation of an elderly patient with an acute complication from peptic ulcer disease can often be subtle, leading to a delay in diagnosis. The stereotypical presentation of an intraabdominal catastrophe typical in young patients is frequently absent. Kane et al. reported that among 32 elderly patients with acute perforations of peptic ulcers, 27 [84%] reported minimal pain.[97] In that series, the diagnosis of a perforated ulcer was finally made in three patients only at the time of autopsy. Permutt and Cello found similar differences in the clinical presentation of the elderly with duodenal ulcer disease, with melena being the most common initial presentation.[101] In another study, 62% of patients who presented with pain-free bleeding were over the age of 70 years compared to 37% for those less than 70 years.[102] Because of the often atypical presentation of the elderly patient with a complication from peptic ulcer disease, these patients often wait longer before definitive treatment is undertaken.

The complications of ulcer disease that most frequently require urgent or emergent operative treatment are acute bleeding and perforation. Acute bleeding is the most common complication of ulcer disease in the elderly and accounts for 50–70% of peptic ulcer deaths.[103] In the case of acute bleeding, there should be an immediate attempt at endoscopic visualization and control of the bleeding after the initial resuscitation of the patient. The older belief that immediate operation after resuscitation in the elderly patient was indicated to prevent rebleeding was modified with the advent of excellent techniques for resuscitation and endoscopic management.[104] The proper initial management of the elderly patient with a bleeding ulcer is critical to minimize complications. The patient must be adequately volume-resuscitated, ideally in an intensive care unit. Hypotension is one of the most important prognostic factors for predicting outcomes in the elderly patient with a bleeding ulcer. Branicki et al. found a fourfold increase in mortality if the patient presented in shock at the time of admission.[105] In the same study, logistic regression analysis revealed that the major predictors of death were age over 60 years, preexisting medical illness, and ulcer size >1 cm. Acute perforation is the second most common complication of ulcer disease in the elderly. Similar to bleeding ulcers, outcomes analyses of perforated ulcers have shown that increasing age, concomitant medical illness, shock at the time of admission, and delay in diagnosis are predictors of complications or death.[92,93]

Although aggressive nonoperative management of a bleeding ulcer in the elderly patient is acceptable first-line treatment, early surgical intervention is indicated for massive or persistent hemorrhage. Likewise, nearly all ulcer perforations require operative management. It is commonly believed that in the elderly patient presenting with a complication of ulcer disease, the simplest operation is the best operation. However, some authors suggest that when choosing an operative approach to the management of an acute ulcer complication in the elderly, a more definitive procedure may be performed with comparable morbidity and mortality relative to the minimal required operation. In the setting of perforation, simple closure of the ulcer, which is advocated by many in the elderly patient, can result in a recurrence rate of up to 60% if the patient receives no further therapy.[106,107] In the series reported by Hamby and associates, it was concluded that patient outcome for perforated ulcer is dependent on preoperative conditions and is independent of the surgical procedure performed.[93] Although they reported that increasing age is one of three risk factors that predicted the likelihood of complications or death, these poor outcomes in elderly patients occurred independent of the operation performed. The other two predictors were hospitalization at the time of perforation and concomitant medical illness. They also found that the recurrent ulcer rate was significantly higher following simple closure with no further therapy than after definitive surgery. It was their conclusion that simple ulcer closure had no benefit compared to a definitive procedure unless there was persistent hemodynamic instability. Similarly, Boey and associates found in a large prospective series of perforated duodenal ulcers that definitive surgery resulted in fewer complications and comparable mortality relative to simple closure in patients without risk factors.[92] They identified three independent risk factors for the higher levels of mortality: severe medical illness, preoperative shock, and long-standing (>48 hours) perforation. Mortality increased with increasing number of risk factors, approaching 100% when all three are present regardless of the procedure performed. Age, however, was not found to be a risk factor that precluded treatment with a definitive operation. Perhaps the most persuasive reason for attempting definitive surgery is to reduce the high rate of recurrence after simple closure. In the setting of perforated gastric ulcer, Hodnett and associates suggested that nondefinitive surgery results in a significantly higher mortality rate (29%) than definitive surgery (11.3%).[96] It must be acknowledged that no studies to date have yet addressed the impact of a closely

TABLE 39.1. Surgical Treatment of Peptic Ulcer Disease in the Elderly

| Ulcer type | Bleeding | Perforation | Obstruction | Intractability |
|---|---|---|---|---|
| Duodenal | Oversew; V&P | Patch ± HSV or V&P | V&A (V&G-J for difficult duodenum) | HSV or V&A |
| Gastric | | | | |
| Type 1 | Excise ulcer; V&P | Excise ulcer ± HSV or V&P | Distal gastrectomy | Distal gastrectomy |
| Type 2/type 3 | Oversew; V&P | Patch ± V&P | V&A (V&G-J for difficult duodenum) | V&A |

*Source:* Adapted from McFadden and Zinner,[103] with permission.
HSV, highly selective (or parietal cell) vagotomy; V&P, vagotomy and pyloroplasty; V&G-J, vagotomy and gastrojejunostomy, use to avoid dissection and devascularization of a badly scarred duodenum; V&A, vagotomy and gastrectomy.

monitored program of medical management as a follow-up to less definitive operative treatment compared to definitive operative management.

Massive hemorrhage from an ulcer presents a special problem in the elderly. Elderly patients poorly tolerate blood loss and hypotension. In this setting, operative management is directed at minimizing further blood loss. Although aggressive resuscitation and endoscopic hemostasis should be attempted initially in nearly all cases, operative intervention should not be delayed if there is persistent hemodynamic instability. There also is a significant risk to postponing operative intervention if the patient initially presented in shock but was subsequently stabilized. Hunt reported that shock on admission was the most important risk factor for rebleeding regardless of age.[108] However, age is an important risk factor in those patients brought to the operating room for bleeding duodenal ulcers. Age over 60 years was found to be a significant risk factor for rebleeding postoperatively regardless of the procedure performed.[105] However, even in the setting of hemorrhage a case can be made for a more definitive initial operation. In the study by Welch et al. at the Massachusetts General Hospital, it appeared that, regardless of the location, a bleeding ulcer was best treated in patients less than 70 years of age with gastric resection, vagotomy, and ligation of the bleeding vessel. Those patients more than 70 years were treated with pyloroplasty, vagotomy, and arterial ligation.[89] Only in the most extreme cases was simple ligation of the bleeding vessel a viable operative choice.

In summary, taking an elderly patient to the operating room for acute complications of peptic ulcer disease is a serious matter. Aggressive resuscitation and optimizing preexisting medical problems are essential to improve outcomes. Although the choice of operation must be individualized, it is important to realize that in most cases the age of the patient alone should not dictate the choice of operation. The literature strongly suggests that in the healthy elderly patient without risk factors who presents with a complication from peptic ulcer disease, a definitive operation can be performed safely.

The other complications of ulcer disease, obstruction and intractable pain, are now rarely encountered in any age group and are not discussed here. McFadden and Zinner summarized the suggested operations for the various complications of peptic ulcer disease in the elderly patient (Table 39.1).[103]

## Complications of Gastric Surgery

Numerous complications can occur after gastric and duodenal operations for both benign and malignant disease. They can be divided into early and late complications. The early complications of gastric surgery include, but are not limited to, suture line leaks, intragastric bleeding, intraperitoneal bleeding, and ischemic necrosis. Although these early complications may be considered in part the result of technical errors, there are no indications that age alone contributes to the occurrence of these complications. However, as previously discussed, the elderly patient who experiences any operative complication is at higher risk for significant morbidity and mortality.

There are numerous late complications of gastric surgery, but the most important in the elderly patient relate to disturbances in gastric and intestinal motility and transit time: the dumping syndrome and diarrhea, respectively. The decrease in gastric motility after gastric surgery is known as gastric atony, which contributes to many of the late complications of gastric surgery. The most common and troublesome late complication is the dumping syndrome, which occurs in 15–50% of patients who have had gastric surgery,[109] although fewer than 1–5% of patients have debilitating symptoms.[110] The occurrence of the dumping syndrome and postoperative diarrhea, which may be seen after any gastric or duodenal operation, appears to be dependent on the type of surgery performed, with procedures that preserve the pylorus (i.e., highly selective vagotomy) being least likely to cause these complications.[111,112] Although none of these studies specifically showed that these complications occurred more frequently in elderly patients, in general, the elderly are less tolerant of the symptoms related to these complications. In one study that specifically addressed age and a dumping provocation test prior to and after gastric surgery for ulcer disease, age did not correlate with the occurrence of dumping symptoms induced by the test.[113]

Many of the symptoms related to the disturbances in intestinal motility after gastric surgery abate shortly afterward, but for those patients with persistent symptoms, medical management is required. Such management initially is based on dietary modifications, which include avoiding concentrated carbohydrates, increased frequency and decreased volume of meals, and taking solids at least 30 minutes prior to liquids. If these interventions fail, use of the long-acting somatostatin analogue octreotide has been used to treat dumping syndrome with reasonable success.[114] The long-term effects of octreotide use and in particular its use in the elderly has not been addressed. If medical management fails, numerous surgical interventions have been used to treat both the dumping syndrome and diarrhea. The details of these surgical procedures are beyond the scope of this chapter, but the most commonly used procedures are (1) stomal revisions, (2) pyloric reconstruction, (3) conversion of Billroth II to Billroth I anastomisis, (4) jejunal interpositions, and (5) Roux-en-Y conversion. Approximately 75–95% of patients who undergo these corrective operations report improvement in their symptoms. However, there is as yet no way to identify the subgroup of patients who will benefit from surgery.

Similar to the dumping syndrome and postvagotomy diarrhea, studies of the "Roux stasis syndrome," which is a postsurgical complication related to a motility dysfunction in the Roux limb in patients who undergo Roux-en-Y gastrojejunostomy, have not addressed specifically the impact of age on the frequency of this complication. However, 30% of patients who undergo this procedure, develop symptoms of decreased gastric emptying.[115] Unlike dumping syndrome and diarrhea, the Roux stasis syndrome does not respond well to medical management. Nearly all patients come to reconstructive surgery, with near-total gastrectomy and revision of the Roux limb being the most commonly used procedure. Unfortunately, a significant portion of patients do not experience alleviation of their symptoms.

## Gastric Bezoars

Gastric bezoars are concretions of material or foreign objects that are unable to pass through the pylorus. Some bezoars form in normal stomachs, but most occur as a complication of previous gastric surgery in which there is a loss of normal pyloric function and gastric atony. The symptoms of gastric bezoars commonly are nonspecific, such as epigastric fullness, regurgitation, nausea, and vomiting. The most common presentation of gastric bezoars, however, is small bowel obstruction due to a dislodged portion of the bezoar passing into the small intestine and causing an obstruction.[116,117] Although bezoars have been reported as early as 1 year after gastric surgery, most form years later. Therefore, the development of nonspecific abdominal complaints in an elderly patient who has had previous gastric surgery should raise the possibility of a bezoar. If the patient fails to respond to standard medical therapy for presumed gastritis or benign ulcer disease, endoscopic or radiologic evaluation should be undertaken to rule out malignant disease or the presence of a bezoar.

The treatment options vary depending on the type of bezoar. In the case of phytobezoars, endoscopic retrieval, segmentation, or chemical dissolution may be used.[118,119] In the case of bezoars that cannot be removed by endoscopic or chemical means, early surgical intervention is recommended.[117,120,121]

## Benign Tumors of the Stomach

Benign tumors of the stomach are relatively uncommon, comprising 1–5% of all tumors of the stomach.[122] The most common lesion is the hyperplastic polyp. In a review of the largest series of benign tumors of the stomach, Lanza reported that hyperplastic polyps accounted for 38% of all benign neoplasms. The most frequent intramural tumor was the leiomyoma, which represented 24% of all neoplasms. Leiomyomas account for approximately 3% of all gastric tumors.[122] Although leiomyomas occur most frequently in the fundus, they can be found anywhere in the stomach. In a large series of benign smooth muscle tumors of the gastrointestinal tract from the Massachusetts General Hospital, 131 patients were treated over 24 years.[123] The median age at diagnosis was 62 years, with a range of 19–89 years. Sixty-one percent of all the smooth muscle tumors in the gastrointestinal tract in their series occurred in the stomach. The presentation of the gastric lesions varied, with 31% asymptomatic, 38% presenting with occult or frank bleeding, and 37% presenting with either pain or dyspepsia. These tumors were treated by local excision with less than 1-cm margins in most cases; no patient received adjuvant therapy. At the long-term follow-up of 103 patients, there was only one recurrence of tumor in the stomach. Considering the relatively benign natural history of histologically diagnosed leiomyomas, some surgeons are now reporting the use of laparoscopic excision of these intramural tumors because of the small surgical margins required.[124] Laparoscopic excision of small (<4 cm) tumors may be the ideal treatment of symptomatic intramural tumors in the elderly patient because of the small amount of morbidity associated with these procedures. To date, however, there have been no large series to show that laparoscopic excision will have the similar low recurrence rate that open excision does with these tumors.

## Conclusions

Upper abdominal complaints in the elderly patient are frequently of unclear etiology. The classic history, signs, and symptoms of common disease processes are often attenuated or even absent in the elderly patient, making diagnosis and effective treatment difficult. The increased frequency of co-morbid diseases and polypharmacy in the elderly, add another layer of complexity. However, gastritis and peptic ulcer disease continues to be an important medical and surgical problem for the elderly patient. The higher prevalence of *Helicobacter pylori* infection, NSAIDs use, atypical presentations of ulcer disease, and co-morbid conditions contribute to a higher incidence of morbidity and mortality from ulcer disease in the elderly. It is important to consider seriously the diagnosis of ulcer disease in the elderly patient when confronted with vague abdominal or systemic complaints. Ulcer disease should be treated aggressively in the elderly to prevent complications because of the significantly increased risk of death in this population.

## References

1. Levitan R. GI problems in the elderly. Part II. Prevalent disease and disorders. Geriatrics 1989;44:80–86.
2. Bird T, Hall MR, Schade RO. Gastric histology and its relation to anemia in the elderly. Gerontology 1977;23:309–321.
3. Palmer E. Gastritis: a reevaluation. Medicine 1954;35: 199–210.
4. Khanna PB, Davies I, Faragher EB. Age-related changes in the stomach of laboratory mouse: a quantitative morphological study. Age Ageing 1988;17:257–264.
5. Majumdar APN, Johnson LR. Gastric mucosal cell proliferation during development in rats and effect of pentagastrin. Am J Physiol 1982;242:G135–G139.
6. Majumdar APN, Edgerton EA, Dayal Y, et al. Gastrin: levels and trophic action during advancing age. Am J Physiol 1988;254:G538–G542.
7. Majumdar APN, Jasti S, Hatfiels JS, et al. Morphological and biochemical changes in gastric mucosa of aging rats. Dig Dis Sci 1990;35:1364–1370.
8. Khaliil T, Fujimura SP, Townsend CM Jr, et al. Effect of aging on gastric acid secretion, serum gastrin, and antral gastrin content in rats. Dig Dis Sci 1988;33:1544–1548.
9. Kogire M, Ishizuka J, Parekh D, et al. Effects of aging on gastrin and somatostatin secretion from isolated perfused rat stomach. Dig Dis Sci 1993;38:303–308.
10. Lee M, Feldman M. Age-related reductions in gastric mucosal prostaglandin levels increase susceptibility to aspirin-induced injury in rats. Gastroenterology 1994;107: 1746–1750.
11. Blackman AH, Lambert DL, Thayer WR, et al. Computed normal values for peak acid output based on age, sex, and body weight. Am J Dig Dis 1970;15:783–789.
12. Cleator IGM, Stoller JL, Nunn PN, et al. Discriminant analysis of data in ulcer and nonulcer populations. Dig Dis Sci 1973;18:301–310.
13. Goldschmiedt M, Barnett CC, Schwarz BE, et al. Effect of age on gastric acid secretion and serum gastrin concentrations in healthy men and women. Gastroenterology 1991; 101:977–990.
14. Cryer B, Redfern JS, Goldschmiedt M, et al. Effects of aging on gastric and duodenal mucosal prostaglandin concentrations in humans. Gastroenterology 1992;102:1118–1123.
15. Kekki M, Sipponen P, Siurala M. Age behavior of gastric acid secretion in males and females with a normal antral and body mucosa. Scand J Gastroenterol 1983;18:1009–1016.
16. Kekki M, Samloff IM, Ihamaki T, Varis K, Siurala M. Age- and sex-related behavior of gastric acid secretion at the population level. Scand J Gastroenterol 1982;17:737–743.
17. Katelaris PH. Effects of age, Helicobacter pylori infection, and gastritis with atrophy on serum gastrin and gastric acid secretion in healthy men. Gut 1993;34:1032–1037.
18. Husebye E, Skar V, Hoverstad T, Melby K. Fasting hypochlorhydria with gram positive gastric flora is highly prevalent in healthy old people. Gut 1992;33:1331–1337.
19. Cryer B, Lee E, Feldman M. Factors influencing gastroduodenal mucosal prostaglandin concentrations: roles of smoking and aging. Ann Intern Med 1992;116:636–640.
20. Kupfer RM, Heppell M, Haggith JW, et al. Gastric emptying and small-bowel transit rate in the elderly. J Am Geriatr Scoc 1985;33:340–343.
21. Madsen JL. Effect of gender, age, and body mass index on gastrointestinal transit times. Dig Dis Sci 1992;37:1548–1553.
22. Horowitz M, Maddern GJ, Chatterton BE, et al. Changes in gastric emptying rates with age. Clin Sci 1984;67:213–218.
23. Moore JG, Tweedy C, Christian PE, et al. Effect of age on gastric emptying of liquid-solid meals in man. Dig Dis Sci 1983;28:340–344.
24. Kao CH, Lai TL, Wang SJ, et al. Influence of age on gastric emptying in healthy Chinese. Clin Nucl Med 1994;19: 401–404.
25. Wedmann B, Schmidt G, Wegener M, et al. Effects of age and gender on fat-induced gallbladder contraction and gastric emptying of a caloric liquid meal: a sonographic study. Am J Gastroenterol 1991;86:1765–1770.
26. Kurata, JH. Ulcer epidemiology: an overview and proposed research framework. Gastroenterology 1989;96: 569–580.
27. Kurata JH, Haile BM. Epidemiology of peptic ulcer disease. Clin Gastroenterol 1984;13:289–307.
28. Elashoff J, Grossman MI. Trends in hospital admissions and death rates for peptic ulcers in the United States from 1970 to 1978. Gastroenterology 1980;20:200–205.
29. Kurata JH, Corboy ED. Current peptic ulcer trends: an epidemiological profile. J Clin Gastroenterol 1988;10:259–268.
30. Bonnevie O. Changing demographics of peptic ulcer disease. Dig Dis Sci 1985;30(suppl):8S.
31. Kurata JH, Haile BM, Elashoff JD. Sex differences in peptic ulcer disease. Gastroenterology 1985;88:96–100.
32. Cryer B, Feldman M. Peptic ulcer disease in the elderly. Semin Gastrointest Dis 1994;5:166–178.
33. Gilinsky NH. Peptic ulcer disease in the elderly. Scand J Gastroenterol 1988;23(suppl 146):191–200.

34. Green L, Graham D. Gastritis in the elderly. Gastroenterol Clin North Am 1990;19:273–292.
35. Siurala M, Krohn K, Varis K. Parietal cell and intrinsic factor antibodies in a Finnish rural population sample. Scand J Gastroenterol 1969;4:521–527.
36. Siurala M, Salmi HJ. Long term follow-up of subjects with superficial gastritis or normal gastric mucosa. Scand J Gastroenterol 1971;6:459–463.
37. Siurala M, Lehtola J, Ihamaki T. Atrophic gastritis and its sequelae: results of 19–23 years of follow-up examinations. Scand J Gastroenterol 1974;9:441–446.
38. Cotran RS, Kumar V, Robbins SL (eds). Robbins' Pathologic Basis of Disease. Philadelphia: Saunders, 1989:844.
39. Rauws EA, Langenberg W, Houthoff HJ, Zanen HC, Tytgat GNJ. Campylobacter pyloris-associated chronic active antral gastritis: a prospective study of its prevalence and the effects of antibacterial and antiulcer treatment. Gastroenterology 1988;94:33–40.
40. Safe AF, Warren B, Corfield A, et al. Helicobacter pylori infection in elderly people: correlation between histology and serology. Age Ageing 1993;22:215–220.
41. Gillanders IA, Scott PJW, Smith GD. Helicobacter pylori and chronic antral gastritis in elderly patients. Age Ageing 1994;23:277–279.
42. Levitan R. GI problems in the elderly. Part I. Aging-related considerations. Geriatrics 1989;44(9):53–56.
43. Levitan R. GI problems in the elderly. Part II. Prevalent diseases and disorders. Geriatrics 1989;44(11):80–86.
44. Dooley CA, Cohen H, Fitzgibbons PL, et al. Prevalence of Helicobacter pylori infection and histologic gastritis in asymptomatic persons. N Engl J Med 1987;321:1562–1566.
45. Parsonnet J, Friedman GD, Vandersteen DP, et al. Helicobacter pylori infection and risk of gastric cancer. N Engl J Med 1991;325:1127–1131.
46. Wotherspoon AC, Ortiz-Hidalgo C, Falzon MR, Isaacson PG. Helicobacter pylori associated gastritis and primary B-cell gastric lymphoma. Lancet 1991;338:1175–1176.
47. Klein PD, Graham DY, Gaillour A, et al. Water source as risk factor for Helicobacter pylori infection in Peruvian children. Lancet 1991;337:1503–1506.
48. Graham DY, Malaty HM, Evans DG, Evans DJ Jr, Klein PD, Adam E. Epidemiology of Helicobacter pylori in an asymptomatic population in the United States: effect of age, race and socioeconomic status. Gastroenterology 1991; 100:1495–1501.
49. Perez-Perez GI, Dworkin BM, Chodos JE, Blaser MJ. Campylobacter pylori antibodies in humans. Ann Intern Med 1988;109:11–17.
50. Cullen DJ, Collins BJ, Christiansen KJ, et al. When is Helicobacter pylori infection acquired? Gut 1993;12:1681–1682.
51. Fiedorek SC, Evans DG, Evans DJ, et al. H. pylori infection epidemiology in children: importance of socioeconomic status, age, gender, and race. Gastroenterology 1990;98: A44.
52. Mendall MA, Goggin PM, Molineaux N, et al. Childhood living conditions and Helicobacter pylori seropositivity in adult life. Lancet 1992;85:944–948.
53. Lee A. The microbiology and epidemiology of Helicobacter pylori infection. Scand J Gastroenterol 1994;29(suppl 201):2–6.
54. Morris A, Nicholson G. Ingestion of Campylobacter pyloridis causes gastritis and raised fasting gastric pH. Am J Gastroenterol 1987;82:192–199.
55. Jiang SJ, Liu WZ, Zhang DZ, et al. Campylobacter-like organisms in chronic gastritis, peptic ulcer, and gastric carcinoma. Scand J Gastroenterol 1987;22:553–558.
56. Ateshkadi A, Lam NP, Johnson CA. Helicobacter pylori and peptic ulcer disease. Clin Pharmacokinet 1993;12: 34–48.
57. Tytgat GNJ. Peptic ulcer and Helicobacter pylori: eradication and relapse. Scand J Gastroenterol 1995;30(suppl 210):70–72.
58. Forbes GM, Glaser ME, Cullen DJ, et al. Duodenal ulcer treated with Helicobacter pylori eradication: seven-year follow-up. Lancet 1994;343:258–260.
59. Roth SH. Nonsteroidal anti-inflammatory drugs: gastropathy deaths and medical practice. Ann Intern Med 1988;109:353–354.
60. Beard K, Walker AM, Perera DR, Jicks H. Nonsteroidal anti-inflammatory drugs and hospitalization for gastroesophageal bleeding in the elderly. Arch Intern Med 1987; 47:1621–1623.
61. Henry D, Robertson J. Nonsteroidal anti-inflammatory drugs and peptic ulcer hospitalization rates in New South Wales. Gastroenterology 1993;104:1083–1091.
62. Fries JF, Miller SR, Spitz PW, Williams CA, Hubert HB, Bloch DA. Toward an epidemiology of gastropathy associated with nonsteroidal anti-inflammatory drug use. Gastroenterology 1989;96:647–655.
63. Roth SH, Bennett RE. Nonsteroidal anti-inflammatory drug gastropathy: recognition and response. Arch Intern Med 1987;147:2093–2100.
64. Bellary SV, Isaacs PE, Lee FI. Upper gastrointestinal lesions in elderly patients presenting for endoscopy: relevance of NSAID usage. Am J Gastroenterol 1991;86:961–964.
65. Hochberg MC. Association of nonsteroidal anti-inflammatory drugs with upper gastrointestinal disease: epidemiologic and economic considerations. J Rheumatol 1992;19(suppl 36):63–67.
66. Armstrong CP, Blower AL. Nonsteroidal anti-inflammatory drugs and life threatening complications of peptic ulceration. Gut 1987;28:527–532.
67. Griffen MR, Piper JM, Daugherty JR, Snowden M, Ray WA. Nonsteroidal antiinflammatory drug use and increased risk for peptic ulcer disease in elderly persons. Ann Intern Med 1991;114:257–263.
68. Griffen MR, Ray WA, Schaffner W. Nonsteroidal anti-inflammatory drug use and death from peptic ulcer in elderly persons. Ann Intern Med 1988;109:359–363.
69. Gabriel SE, Jaakkimainen L, Bombardier C. Risk for serious gastrointestinal complications related to use of nonsteroidal anti-inflammatory drugs. Ann Intern Med 1991; 115:787–796.
70. Levine MN, Raskob G, Hirsh J. Hemorrhagic complications of long-term anticoagulant therapy. Chest 1989;95: 26S–36S.
71. Shorr RI, Ray WA, Daugherty JR, Griffen MR. Concurrent use of nonsteroidal antiinflammatory drugs and oral anticoagulants place elderly persons at high risk for hemorrhagic peptic ulcer disease. Arch Intern Med 1993;153: 1665–1670.

72. Chiverton SG, Hunt RH. Pharmacokinetics and pharmacodynamics of treatments for peptic ulcer disease in the elderly. Am J Gastroenterol 1988;83:211–215.
73. Koop H, Arnold R, Classen M, Fischer M, Goebell H, Blum AL. Healing and relapse of duodenal ulcer during ranitidine therapy in the elderly: the Ruder Study Group. J Clin Gastroenterol 1992;15:291–295.
74. Sirgo MA, Mills R, Euler AR, Walker S. The safety of ranitidine in elderly versus nonelderly patients. J Clin Pharmacol 1993;33:79–83.
75. Humphries TJ, Myerson RM, Gifford LM, et al. A unique postmarket outpatient surveillance program of cimetidine: report on phase II and final summary. Am J Gastroenterol 1984;79:593–596.
76. Isenberg JI. Should safety concerns with available ulcer treatment influence drug selection. J Clin Gastroenterol 1990;12(suppl 2):S48–S53.
77. Lacz JP, Groschang AG, Giesing DH, Browne RK. The effect of sucralfate on drug absorption in dogs [abstract]. Gastroenterology 1982;82:1108.
78. Graham DY, Agrawal NM, Roth SH. Prevention of NSAID-induced gastric ulcer with misoprostol: multicentre, double blind, placebo-controlled trial. Lancet 1988;2: 1277–1280.
79. McKenna F. Efficacy and gastroduodenal safety of a fixed combination of diclofenac and misoprostol in the treatment of arthritis. Br J Rheumatol 1995;34(suppl 1):11–18.
80. Maton PN. Omeprazole. N Engl J Med 1991;324:965–975.
81. Graham DY, Colon-Pagan J, Morse RS, et al. Ulcer recurrence following duodenal ulcer healing with omeprazole, ranitidine, or placebo: a double-blind, multicenter, 6-month study. Gastroenterology 1992;102:1289–1294.
82. Hunt RH. Helicobacter pylori eradication: a critical appraisal and current concerns. Scand J Gastroenterol 1995;30(suppl 210):73–76.
83. Chiba N, Rao BV, Rademaker JW, et al. Meta-analysis of the efficacy of antibiotic therapy in eradicating H. pylori. Am J Gastroenterol 1992;87:1716–1722.
84. Cutler AF, Schubert TT. Long-term Helicobacter pylori recurrence after successful eradication with triple therapy. Am J Gastroenterol 1993;88:1359–1361.
85. Unge P, Ekstrom P. Effects of combination therapy with omeprazole and an antibiotic on Helicobacter pylori and duodenal ulcer disease. Scand J Gastroenterol 1993; 28(suppl 196):17–18.
86. Bayerdorffer E, Mannes GA, Sommer A, et al. Long-term follow-up after eradication of Helicobacter pylori with a combination of omeprazole and amoxicillin. Scand J Gastroenterol 1993;28(suppl 196):19–25.
87. Paimela H, Tuompo PK, Perakyla T, Saario I, Hockerstedt K, Kivilaakso E. Peptic ulcer surgery during the $H_2$-receptor antagonist era: a population-based epidemiological study of ulcer surgery in Helsinki from 1972–1987. Br J Surg 1991;78:28–31.
88. Gustavsson S, Kelly KA, Melton LJ III, Zinsmeister AR. Trends in peptic ulcer surgery: a population-based study in Rochester, Minnesota, 1956–1985. Gastroenterology 1988;94:688–694.
89. Welch CE, Rodkey GV, von Ryll Gryska P. A thousand operations for ulcer disease. Ann Surg 1986;204:454–467.
90. Walker LG Jr. Trends in the surgical management of duodenal ulcer: a fifteen year study. Am J Surg 1988;155:436–438.
91. McConnell DB, Baba GC, Deveney CW. Changes in surgical treatment of peptic ulcer disease within a veterans hospital in the 1970s and the 1980s. Arch Surg 1989;124: 1164–1167.
92. Boey J, Choi SKY, Alagaratnam TT. Risk stratification in perforated duodenal ulcers: a prospective validation of predictive factors. Ann Surg 1987;205:22–26.
93. Hamby LS, Zweng TN, Strodel WE. Perforated gastric and duodenal ulcer: an analysis of prognostic factors. Am Surg 1993;59:320–324.
94. Boey J, Wong J. Perforated duodenal ulcers. World J Surg 1987;11:319–324.
95. Feliciano DV, Bitondo CG, Burch JM, Mattox KL, Jordan GL Jr, DeBakey ME. Emergency management of perforated peptic ulcers in the elderly patient. Am J Surg 1984;148: 764–767.
96. Hodnett RM, Gonzalez F, Lee C, Nance FC, Deboisblanc R. The need for definitive therapy in the management of perforated gastric ulcers: review of 202 cases. Ann Surg 1989; 209:36–39.
97. Kane E, Fried G, McSherry CK. Perforated peptic ulcer in the elderly. J Am Geriatr Soc 1981;29:224–227.
98. Bliss DW, Stabile BE. The impact of ulcerogenic drugs on surgery for the treatment of peptic ulcer disease. Arch Surg 1991;126:609–612.
99. Svanes C, Salvesen H, Espehaug B, Soreide O, Svanes K. A multifactorial analysis of factors related to lethality after treatment of perforated gastroduodenal ulcer: 1935–1985. Ann Surg 1989;209:418–423.
100. Mendes da Costa PR, Lurquin P. Gastrointestinal surgery in the aged. Br J Surg 1993;80:329.
101. Permutt RP, Cello JP. Duodenal ulcer disease in the hospitalized elderly patient. Dig Dis Sci 1982;27:1–6.
102. Matthewson K, Pugh S, Northfield TC. Which peptic ulcer patients bleed? Gut 1988;29:70–74.
103. McFadden DW, Zinner MJ. Gastroduodenal disease in the elderly patient. Surg Clin North Am 1994;74:113–126.
104. Morris DL, Hawker PC, Brearly S, et al. Optimal timing of operation for bleeding peptic ulcer: prospective randomized trial. BMJ 1984;74:1277–1280.
105. Branicki FJ, Boey J, Fok PJ, et al. Bleeding duodenal ulcer: a prospective evaluation of risk factors for rebleeding and death. Ann Surg 1990;211:411–418.
106. McGuire HH, Horsley JS. Emergency operations for gastric and duodenal ulcers in high risk patients. Ann Surg 1986; 203:551–557.
107. Boey J, Lee NW, Koo J, Lam PHM, Wong J, Ong GB. Immediate definitive surgery for perforated duodenal ulcers: a prospective controlled trial. Ann Surg 1982;196: 338–344.
108. Hunt PS. Bleeding gastroduodenal ulcers: selection of patients for surgery. World J Surg 1987;11:289–294.
109. Lamers CB, Bijlstra AM, Haris AG. Octreotide, a long-acting somatostatin analog: in the management of postoperative dumping syndrome. Dig Dis Sci 1993;38: 359–364.
110. Sawyers JL. Management of postgastrectomy syndromes. Am J Surg 1990;159:8–14.

111. Hoffmann J, Jensen HE, Christiansen J, et al. Prospective controlled vagotomy trial for duodenal ulcer: results after 11–15 years. Ann Surg 1989;209:40–45.
112. Hoffmann J, Shokouh-Amiri MH, Klarskov P, et al. Gastrectomy for recurrent ulcer after vagotomy: five- to nineteen-year follow-up. 1986;99:517–522.
113. Kaushik SP, Ralphs DN, Hobsley M. Influences on the occurrences of dumping syndrome. Am J Gastroenterol 1983;78:155–158.
114. Geer RJ, Richards WO, O'Dorisio TM, et al. Efficacy of octreotide acetate in treatment of severe postgastrectomy dumping syndrome. Ann Surg 1990;212:678.
115. Herrington JL, Scott HW, Sawyers JL. Experience with vagotomy and antrectomy and Roux-en-Y gastrojejunostomy in the surgical treatment of duodenal, gastric and stomal ulcers. Ann Surg 1984;199:590–597.
116. Vellar DJ, Vellar ID, Pucius R, et al. Phytobezoars: an overlooked cause of small bowel obstruction following vagotomy and drainage operations for duodenal ulcer. Aust NZ J Surg 1986;56:635–638.
117. Robles R, Parrilla P, Escamilla C, et al. Gastrointestinal bezoars. Br J Surg 1994;81:1000–1001.
118. Rider JA, Foresti-Lorente RJ, Garrido J, et al. Gastric bezoars: treatment and prevention. Am J Gastroenterol 1984;79:357–359.
119. Klamer TW, Max MH. Recurrent gastric bezoars: a new approach to treatment and prevention. Am J Surg 1983;145: 417–419.
120. Krausz MM, Moriel EZ, Ayalon A, et al. Surgical aspects of gastrointestinal persimmon phytobezoar treatment. Am J Surg 1986;152:526–530.
121. Visvanathan R. Cement bezoars of the stomach. Br J Surg 1986;73:381–382.
122. Lanza FL. Benign and malignant tumors of the stomach other than carcinoma. In: Haubrich WS, Schaffner F, Bertk JE (eds) Bockus Gastroenterology, 5th ed. Philadelphia: Saunders, 1995:841–858.
123. Morgan BK, Compton C, Talbert M, et al. Benign smooth muscle tumors of the gastrointestinal tract: a 24-year experience. Ann Surg 1990;211:63–66.
124. Motson RW, Fisher PW, Dawson JW. Laparoscopic resection of a benign intragastric stromal tumor. Br J Surg 1995;82:1670.

# 40
# Small Bowel Obstruction in the Elderly

J. Chris Eagon

Small bowel obstruction (SBO) is a common surgical entity that can occur at any age. Although the general principles of diagnosis and treatment of SBO are similar across age groups, there are shifts in the incidence and etiology with age and important treatment considerations in the elderly population. The classic dilemmas associated with SBO management are true for the elderly and include (1) differentiating strangulated from nonstrangulated SBO; (2) differentiating ileus from SBO; and (3) determining optimal duration of conservative treatment for partial SBO. Resolution of these dilemmas is especially pertinent for the elderly because the risks of perioperative morbidity and mortality from an unnecessary laparotomy are greatest in the elderly.

There are few new data to suggest a recent change in the major etiologic causes of SBO, which remain adhesions, hernias, and neoplasms. However, several recent advances in medical technology will likely have a significant future impact on diagnosis and management of SBO in the elderly. Laparoscopic surgery is playing an increasing role in the etiology of SBO and potentially its treatment. The classic diagnostic modalities, including history, physical examination, and plain radiography, are today being augmented by other modalities including computed tomography (CT), contrast radiography, ultrasonography, and magnetic resonance imaging (MRI). Evaluation of the utility of these modalities is ongoing. With the increased emphasis on resource consumption and cost outcomes in the medical field, there have also been interesting studies measuring costs and long-term outcomes in patients with SBO.

Mechanical bowel obstruction can be defined as an abnormal decrease in the caliber of the large or small bowel such that the passage of liquid or solid intestinal content is impeded. As a result of the retroperitoneal nature of a large proportion of large bowel, the ileocecal valve, and the relatively short mesentery, the etiology and pathophysiology of large bowel obstruction are considerably different from those of SBO. Both types of obstruction are common in the elderly, but nearly 80% of all bowel obstructions are of the small bowel.

## Epidemiology

The incidence of SBO is difficult to determine precisely. Estimates can be obtained from population-based samples, such as state hospital discharge registries, although the clinical variables by which to classify patients may be limited by the granularity of classification schemes such as ICD-9 CM and the accuracy of the coding process. In Missouri in 1997, the overall age-adjusted rate of hospitalization for intestinal obstruction excluding hernia was 8.4 per 10,000.[1] Intestinal obstruction was the second most common gastrointestinal diagnosis after gastrointestinal bleeding. Figure 40.1 shows the age- and sex-specific rates of hospital discharge. There is a dramatic increase in the incidence of hospitalization for bowel obstruction with age. Although abdominal hernia and bowel obstruction are listed as the cause of death in only 1.5 per 100,000 population, age-specific rates from the Missouri data indicate that death is much more likely in the elderly (Fig. 40.2).

Another source of data regarding the incidence of SBO can be derived from surveys conducted by the National Center for Health Statistics. The National Hospital Ambulatory Medical Care Survey (NHAMCS) collects data on diagnosis and treatment of a probability sample of patients reporting to emergency rooms and other hospital-based ambulatory health care settings in the United States.[2] These data indicate that SBO (including ICD-9 CM diagnoses for unspecified SBO, specific types of SBO, ileus, fecal impaction, and SBO associated with abdominal wall hernias) was one of the three diagnoses listed for an estimated 408,000 emergency room (ER) visits in 1996. This represents an incidence of 15.4 per 10,000 population in the United States. These ER visits resulted in more than 276,000 hospital admissions for an incidence of hospitalization for SBO of 10.4 per

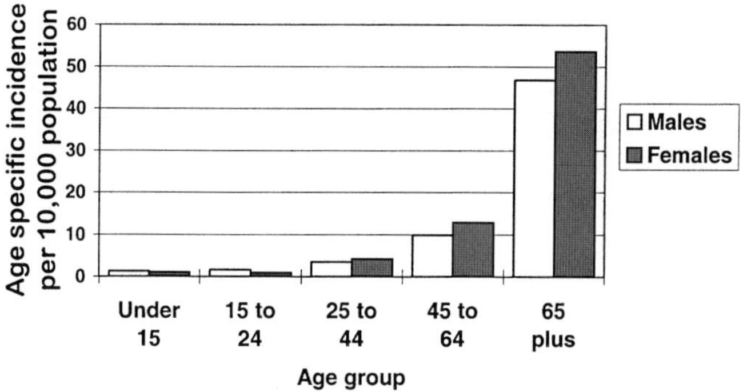


FIGURE 40.1. Age-specific rates of hospital discharge for the diagnoses "intestinal obstruction excluding hernia" for Missouri hospitals, 1997.

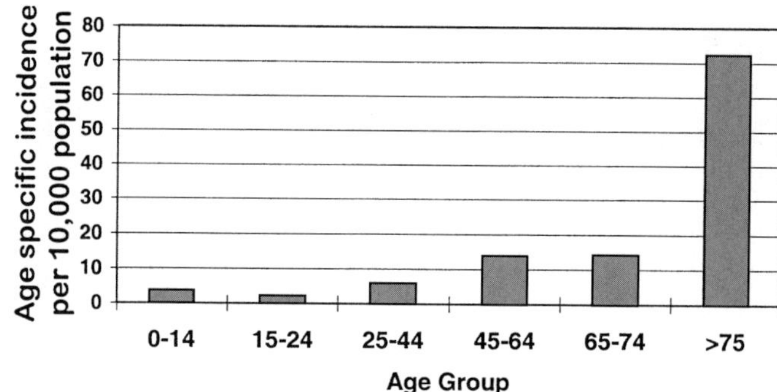


FIGURE 40.3. Age-specific incidence of hospital admission from U.S. hospital-based ambulatory health care settings for the diagnoses of intestinal obstruction without hernia (ICD-9 560*), inguinal hernia with obstruction (5501*), and other hernia of the abdominal cavity with obstruction (552*).

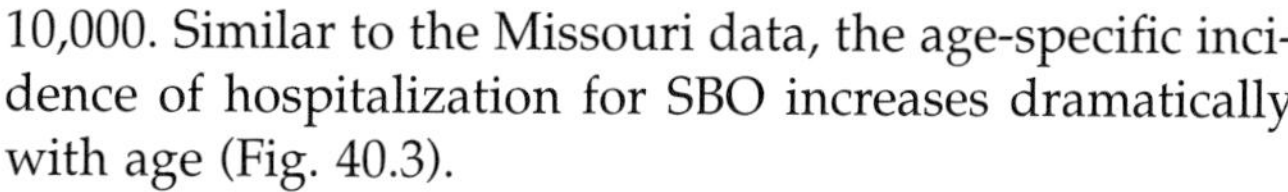
10,000. Similar to the Missouri data, the age-specific incidence of hospitalization for SBO increases dramatically with age (Fig. 40.3).

## Etiology

To predict the etiology of SBO and direct its treatment, it is useful to classify SBO using several characteristics. The degree of luminal obstruction may be partial or complete. The location of the obstruction along the axis of the small bowel can be categorized as proximal, mid-, or distal. A special category using this characteristic is the closed loop obstruction in which two areas of obstruction prevent flow of intestinal content from the loop in either the aborad or orad direction. The structure causing the obstruction can also be classified by its anatomic location perpendicular to the axis of the bowel. These structures may either be extrinsic to the bowel, intrinsic to the bowel wall itself,[3,4] or fill the lumen of the bowel segment in an obturation obstruction. In most cases, SBO starts out as a simple obstruction with adequate blood supply to the intestinal wall such that the bowel remains viable. SBO may progress to strangulation where local bowel ischemia occurs by direct compression of the affected segment by the obstructing lesion or by extreme dilation and increased pressure in the bowel just proximal to the obstruction, leading to diminished perfusion pressure.

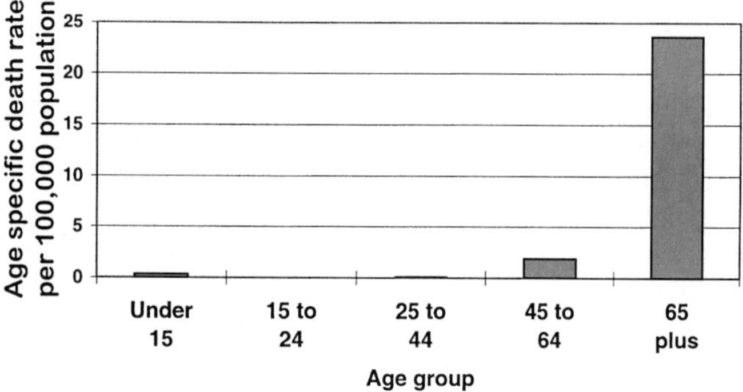


FIGURE 40.2. Age-specific mortality rates for "abdominal hernia and bowel obstruction" for Missouri, 1997.

Table 40.1 lists some of the common etiologies for SBO. Increasing age is a risk factor for many of the causes of SBO. Certain classes of etiology, such as the congenital atresias, webs, and malrotation, are much less likely to be seen in the elderly population. The three most common root causes of SBO—postoperative adhesions, hernias, and neoplasms—all have increasing prevalence in aged populations.

As minimally invasive techniques become a larger part of the medical diagnostic and treatment armamentarium, application of these techniques in the elderly is expanding because of reduced overall morbidity. With this change, new etiologic subclasses of iatrogenic causes of SBO have been reported with increasing frequency. Endoscopically placed foreign objects, such as percutaneous endoscopic gastrostomy tubes[5,6] and endoscopic retrograde cholangiopancreatography (ERCP) stents,[7,8] can become dislodged and lead to obturation obstruction. Numerous SBOs after laproscopic procedures have been reported.[9] Hernias can occur in trocar sites or through peritoneal defects created during the laparoscopic procedures.[10–14] Although postoperative adhesions are less likely, they do occur. Because of the different frequencies of causes of obstruction after laparoscopy, the general approach to the SBO after laparoscopy may differ from that after laparotomy. One recent report examining a series of patients with early postoperative SBO after laparoscopy found that all patients eventually required surgical intervention.[15]

TABLE 40.1. Etiologies of Small Bowel Obstruction in the Elderly

| |
|---|
| **Extrinsic lesions** |
| Postoperative adhesions |
| Abdominal wall hernias |
| Extrinsic neoplastic mass/carcinomatosis |
| Internal hernias |
| Volvulus |
| Inflammatory adhesions |
| Pseudocysts |
| Superior mesenteric artery (SMA) syndrome |
| **Intrinsic lesions** |
| Radiation stricture |
| Ischemic stricture |
| Crohn's disease |
| Small bowel neoplasms |
| Bowel hematoma |
| Duodenal/stomal/Meckel's ulcer |
| **Obturation obstruction** |
| Bezoars |
| Gallstones |
| Foreign bodies |
| Enteroliths |
| Intussusception |

## Pathophysiology and Clinical Features

Presenting symptoms of SBO, which are primarily determined by the anatomic level and degree of obstruction, include nausea and vomiting, abdominal distension, abdominal pain, and obstipation (lack of passage of stool or flatus). Proximal SBO is characterized by frequent vomiting of bilious material and dehydration early in the course of disease with relatively little abdominal distension. With distal SBO, swallowed air and gastrointestinal secretions lead first to small bowel and abdominal distension. Only later do patients develop vomiting, usually after bacterial overgrowth has resulted in a feculent character to the enteric content. Partial obstruction is accompanied by continued, though potentially diminished, passage of flatus or stool. Early complete obstruction may also be accompanied by seemingly normal bowel movements, but eventually obstipation occurs.

Strangulation is notoriously difficult to detect reliably. Classic signs of fever, tachycardia, hypotension, and severe pain or focal tenderness are especially unreliable in the elderly, where the inflammatory response may be muted. Similarly, an elevated white blood cell (WBC) count may be absent in the elderly patient. In a recent Mayo Clinic series,[16] strangulation was present in 13% of patients operated for SBO and was most commonly seen with the etiologies of hernia and small bowel volvulus. Only 52% of patients with strangulation had an elevated WBC count, and the mean WBC count for patients with strangulation was just 2000 cells/$mm^3$ higher than that for patients with simple obstruction.

## Diagnostic Considerations

Symptoms of SBO are common presenting complaints of elderly patients. The differential diagnosis for abdominal pain, nausea, and vomiting includes gastroenteritis, food poisoning, pancreatitis, biliary colic, porphyria, diabetic ketoacidosis, intestinal ischemia, constipation, paralytic ileus, and intestinal pseudoobstruction. Among these diagnoses, SBO is fairly common. In a review of ER visits to a regional trauma center by patients over 65 years of age, 12% of patients presenting with nontraumatic abdominal pain ultimately were found to have SBO.[17] Patients should be asked about any history of abdominal surgery or SBO; and during the physical examination evidence of abdominal wall hernias should be vigilantly elicited. Laboratory values that can help in the diagnosis and management of these patients include a complete blood count (CBC), basic metabolic profile, and serum amylase. Although the classic signs of strangulation are often absent in the elderly and a leukocytosis is not a reliable sign, elevated hematocrit and blood urea nitrogen (BUN) levels are often seen as a consequence of dehydration. Serum bicarbonate may be elevated because of loss of chloride-rich emesis and as part of a contraction alkalosis. These findings indicate significant fluid deficit, which should be aggressively corrected upon initial presentation.

Diagnostic imaging is an important part of the evaluation of every patient with suspected SBO. Supine and upright abdomen and upright PA chest films are often all that is required to confirm the diagnosis of complete SBO and to plan its treatment. Dilation of small bowel, paucity of colon and rectal gas, and air-fluid levels suggest complete SBO. In the Mayo Clinic series, 48% of patients with proven SBO had abdominal plain films that were consistent with SBO.[16] This, of course, means that almost half of patients with SBO have equivocal or even normal plain films, with residual colonic or rectal gas.

When these films are not diagnostic of complete SBO, the decision has traditionally been to rely on the clinical examination and serial plain films. CT scans may be useful in equivocal cases as an early diagnostic test[18] and alters management in up to 20% of patients.[19] Some centers have reported high accuracy of CT in identifying strangulation obstruction. A prospective evaluation of CT in 60 patients with high grade SBO (with 48% strangulation rate) showed that CT had 100% sensitivity and 61% specificity for detecting bowel ischemia.[20] The CT findings consistent with strangulation included bowel thickening and a high attenuation bowel wall on nonenhanced CT and abnormal bowel wall enhancement and mesenteric fluid on enhanced CT. A similar series of 100 patients from a different institution found a sensitivity of 83% and a specificity of 93%.[21] In contradistinction to these studies, several studies have compared CT with plain radiography and have found only modest differences in the overall accuracy of these tests when evaluating the grade of obstruction.[22,23] However, CT is much more likely to demonstrate the cause of SBO, particularly when the obstruction is not due to adhesions. CT also is helpful in patients with closed loop obstructions and patients who swallow little air and thus have a gasless proximal bowel, as these problems are difficult to detect on plain films.

Other diagnostic imaging modalities in the acute setting include ultrasonography[24–27] and MRI.[28] In the more subacute and chronic setting in patients with an intermittent or partial SBO, the CT scan can be useful, as can use of the enteroclysis (small bowel enema) and small bowel follow-through.[29,30] The passage of water-soluble oral contrast into the cecum within 4 hours after CT or small bowel follow-through, has been shown to be highly predictive of nonsurgical resolution of SBO.[31,32] Interestingly, there have also been two randomized controlled trials examining whether water-soluble contrast speeds the resolution of partial SBO. Assalia et al. found a therapeutic benefit in terms of a shorter hospital stay in those receiving the oral contrast in patients with SBO with a variety of etiologies,[33] whereas Feigin et al., looking specifically at patients with postoperative SBO, found no therapeutic benefit.[34]

A special case of the diagnostic dilemma between SBO and paralytic ileus occurs during the early postoperative period. At 1–6 weeks after abdominal surgery, inflammatory adhesion can be thick and highly vascular. For these reasons, the morbidity of reoperation can be considerable. Because these early adhesions are also in a somewhat fluid state of constant remodeling, there is also a good chance of resolution of even high grade partial obstructions without surgical intervention. It therefore becomes even more critical to define the degree of obstruction in these patients to avoid the higher morbidity of reoperation. CT scanning has been shown to be highly accurate for distinguishing ileus from complete SBO.[35] It is less precise for distinguishing partial SBO from ileus. In these cases where a persistent partial SBO is a problem, endoscopic placement of a long intestinal tube can be therapeutic and allow a high quality small bowel contrast study that more clearly characterizes the site of partial obstruction.

## Initial Treatment

Even the patient who clearly has a complete bowel obstruction benefits from initial nonsurgical measures including proximal decompression, aggressive fluid resuscitation, and correction of electrolyte abnormalities. A Foley catheter is critical in the elderly to assess organ perfusion and fluid status. Generally, a nasogastric tube is adequate to decompress the gastrointestinal (GI) tract; but in some patients in whom a prolonged course of nonoperative management is contemplated, as for early postoperative SBO or the patient with multiple previous laparotomies or known severe adhesions, a long nasointestinal tube should be considered strongly as the primary treatment.

Patients with complete SBO or with obvious signs of strangulation should be expeditiously resuscitated and then brought to the operating room. This strategy particularly applies to patients in whom the etiology is thought unlikely due to adhesions or neoplasm. The adage "do not let the sun rise or set on a small bowel obstruction" applies most aptly to these patients. However, most patients admitted for an SBO do not fall into this category. Two-thirds to three-fourths of patients with partial (primarily adhesive) SBO can be treated conservatively, with resolution of their acute episode.[36,37] In patients with a partial SBO, the duration of medical therapy continues to be a hotly debated issue. Recent series examining this question have consistently shown that partial SBOs that ultimately resolve generally do so within 24–72 hours. Delays beyond 48 hours have been associated with increased morbidity in some series,[38] whereas others have shown no increased morbidity with even longer delays.[39]

The potential arguments against maintaining a conservative approach are that the diagnosis of strangulation is inaccurate[40] and the duration of medical treatment may be proportional to the incidence of strangulation or need for bowel resection and the subsequent higher incidence of complications. These concerns are particularly relevant in elderly patients. Adhesive SBO requiring surgery in elderly patients ultimately requires bowel resection in up to 50% of cases,[41] whereas only 8% of patients of all ages required bowel resection in the Mayo Clinic series.[16] In that series, among patients in whom strangulation was found, delays of more than 4 hours from presentation to surgery were associated with higher morbidity rates. Mucha emphasized the importance of the underlying etiology when determining the mortality risk of delayed surgical intervention.[16] Data from the Mayo Clinic series showed that in the case of obstruction due to hernia, the time from presentation to operation was directly related to the mortality rate, but this relation with mortality did not exist for SBO caused by adhesions or malignancy.

We favor a selective approach in the elderly patient with SBO. The immediate strategy should be determined by consideration of (1) the evidence for current bowel ischemia and (2) the presumed etiology of the SBO and degree of obstruction. Patients with two or more signs of strangulation, radiographic signs of complete SBO, or both are operated on as soon as possible after adequate resuscitation is carried out. Nasogastric decompression and serial examinations are then planned for those in whom an adhesive SBO is likely. For those in whom the diagnosis of SBO is unclear or the etiology is in question,

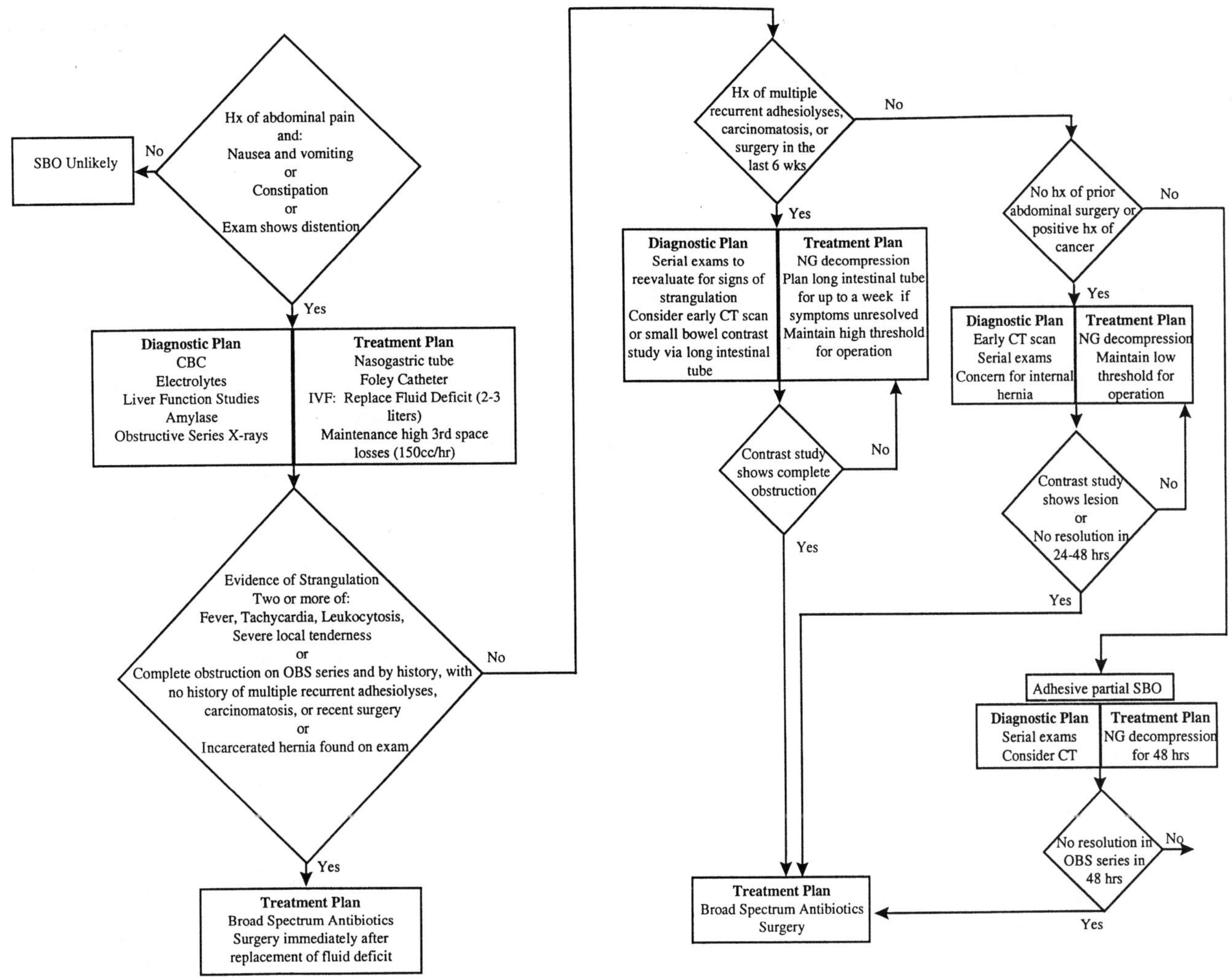


FIGURE 40.4. Diagnostic and treatment algorithm for small bowel obstruction. SBO, small bowel obstruction; Hx, history; CBC, complete blood count; IVF, intravenous fluid; CT, computed tomography; NG, nasogastric; OBS, obstructive series.

CT is performed. The longer-term strategy in patients initially treated nonoperatively should include both the above factors as well as (3) the likelihood of intraoperative and postoperative complications. These factors should be weighed against the likelihood of success using continued nonsurgical management. Figure 40.4 shows our diagnostic and treatment algorithm for patients with SBO.

## Surgical Treatment: General Principles

Preoperative antibiotic coverage to cover enteric organisms should be administered, as a number of cases involve bowel resection or inadvertent enterotomy. Although elderly patients are more likely to have underlying cardiovascular disease, increasing the risk of a perioperative cardiac event, invasive monitoring devices are rarely required. Hypotension upon induction of anesthesia should be avoided by attention to adequate preoperative fluid resuscitation often requiring 3–4 liters of intravenous isotonic crystalloid.

Laparotomy should be performed through a midline approach with at least part of the incision over virgin skin, if possible. Entry through the fascia is done with extreme care, avoiding the use of cautery, as transmitted heat can injure underlying bowel. Adhesions are usually stronger than the junctions between the small bowel muscle layers and the muscularis propria and submucosa, and this seems particularly true in the elderly patient. Sharp dissection with scissors or knife should therefore be performed to avoid seromuscular injuries. We generally lyse adhesions from the anterior abdominal wall first and then proceed to run the small bowel lysing adhesions as we progress from the terminal ileum to the ligament of Treitz.

While running the bowel, the etiology of the SBO and local bowel viability are assessed. The commonly available parameters include bowel color, peristalsis, and mesenteric pulsations. Although clearly viable and clearly dead extremes are easy to identify, many gradations of color are difficult to judge, and assessment of ultimate viability is prone to error. Adjuncts to these methods include Doppler flow probe assessment of mesenteric and antimesenteric blood flow,[42,43] intravenous fluorescein perfusion,[42,44] and electromyography (EMG). Although these methods have their advocates, none has consistently been shown to have higher accuracy than "clinical judgment" using visual and manual inspection. Our general strategy is to resect questionable bowel if possible. If resection would result in less than 4–5 feet of clearly viable intestine, questionable segments with the highest likelihood of viability should be left in situ with a planned reoperation within 24–48 hours.

To allow abdominal wall closure, frequently the bowel must be decompressed. This can be achieved with a long nasointestinal tube, but we favor gentle retrograde milking of the intestine toward the duodenum with fluid evacuation via a nasogastric tube. To minimize excessive distension and the risk of serosal tears, this process is first started in the mid-jejunum. The proximal jejunal segment is then evacuated of luminal content. The process is then repeated starting progressively more distally on the bowel. Prior to closing the abdomen, the bowel loops should be laid back in the abdomen in gentle folds. Some have advocated the use of long intestinal tubes to act as stents, particularly in the patient with recurrent SBO or pervasive adhesions.[45] Another option recently available is application of hyaluronidase-containing films to inhibit adhesion formation.[46,47] Although data show a dramatic decrease in the number and severity of adhesions with this technique,[48] it is not clear whether it will ultimately result in a decreased incidence of recurrent SBO.

## Laparoscopic Treatment of SBO

Laparoscopic surgery has theoretic advantages over open surgery including decreased postoperative pain, reduced wound complications, and decreased respiratory complications. These advantages are particularly attractive in elderly patients and have likely led to a decreased threshold for elderly patients seeking surgical management of biliary tract disease and gastroesophageal reflux disease. Thus far the laparoscopic approach to SBO has not been widely accepted, although several recent reports of SBO management using a laparoscopic approach have been documented.[49–53]

Several factors make laparoscopic treatment of SBO difficult and have prevented many laparoscopic surgeons from adopting this approach to SBO. Visualization can be difficult because of diffuse adhesions to the anterior abdominal wall and because distended bowel may have already increased the intraabdominal pressure and decreased the volume of pneumoperitoneum that can be achieved. It is generally best to use an open insertion technique and to select an initial insertion site remote from previous scars. Bowel distension should be minimized by preoperative nasogastric decompression, and some advocate use of long intestinal tubes prior to attempting laparoscopic treatment. Perhaps the most common reason for reluctance to use laparoscopy for SBO is concern that treatment may ultimately require an extensive adhesiolysis or resection that is impossible to achieve laparoscopically.

Despite these concerns, several selected and consecutive series of SBO treated with laparoscopy have reported favorable results.[51–53] About 70–86% of cases could be treated with a laparoscopic approach; and in some cases a laparoscopic assisted approach was used to minimize incisional morbidity. This approach is particularly attractive for adhesive SBOs where there is a single adhesive band. Conventional laparotomy is recommended for malignant SBOs and hernia-related SBOs, where there is a high rate of strangulation. The general principles of the laparoscopic approach are similar to those of the open approach. Adhesions are dissected sharply, and after adhesiolysis the bowel is inspected from the ileocecal valve to the ligament of Treitz.

Although one-half to two-thirds of patients may be treatable laparoscopically, one must anticipate a high conversion rate to open laparotomy; moreover, the mastery of laparoscopic skills is essential. A study by Bailey et al. compared SBOs treated in two surgical units, one with a special interest in laparoscopy.[54] The laparoscopy unit attempted laparoscopic treatment in 80% of SBOs, and among those cases, they completed treatment laparoscopically in 56%. The laparoscopically treated patients left the hospital 5 days earlier than the open procedure patients, but they also had a higher rate of unplanned reoperation (14% vs. 5%). It seems reasonable to attempt laparoscopic treatment in elderly patients with a likely adhesive SBO but to plan on converting to an open procedure if extensive adhesions or nonadhesive causes are identified.

## Outcomes of Treatment of SBO

Most studies of the outcomes of treatment of SBO have centered on traditional surgical outcomes, such as perioperative mortality, survival, and postoperative complications. Age is a risk factor for mortality from SBO (Fig. 40.2). In the Mayo Clinic series, 50% of the deaths occurred in patients over age 70.[16] Perioperative mortality is also related to the etiology. SBO with a malignant etiology had an in-hospital mortality of 21% and a median survival of 6 months compared to a 4–5% mortality risk for hernia and adhesive etiologies. Delay from symptom onset to presentation is not generally related to mortality risk except in the case of hernias, where there is also a higher risk of strangulation. Overall in-hospital morbidity is around 30%, but it is increased in patients with strangulation to 60%.

Attempts have been made to ascertain the longevity of treatment of SBO. Specifically, for patients treated nonsurgically, what is the likelihood and timing of recurrence, and how does this compare to patients treated surgically? Landercasper et al. retrospectively reviewed 309 consecutive patients with SBO and followed them for recurrence.[55] The SBOs recurred in 34% by 4 years and in 42% by 10 years. Those who were operated on had a lower recurrence rate (29%) than those who were treated nonoperatively (53%). Among those who had surgery, recurrences differed by etiology: malignant (56%), adhesive (28%), and hernia (0%). In this study, the number of prior obstructive episodes was not a risk factor for recurrence. Barkan et al. retrospectively studied 90 patients with SBO for up to 13 years for recurrence.[56] They found that an increased number of SBO episodes increased the risk of SBO in the future. SBO recurred after 53% of first episodes, but it recurred after 85% of second or later episodes. Recurrence appeared sooner and more frequently in patients treated nonoperatively and in patients with three or more prior episodes. Although patient selection may explain the differences in recurrence rates between surgically and nonsurgically treated patients, the likelihood of SBO recurrence is clearly high (30–50% in 10 years, with most recurring within 4 years) regardless of the treatment used.

In addition to recurrence risk, treatment choice affects the cost of care and utilization of health care resources. The costs of caring for patients with SBO are considerable. In a recent Swedish study, 60% of all bowel obstructions were due to adhesions; 65% of them required more than a 1-day hospital stay, and 45% of these required surgery. Calculating direct costs and extrapolating these data, $13 million are spent on adhesive SBO in Sweden (a country of 8.5 million population) annually.[57] In many cases, treatment choice is determined solely by the initial clinical presentation. Either the decision to undergo surgery occurs early or an initial short duration of medical management results in rapid clinical improvement and resolution of the SBO. However, in patients with high grade partial obstruction likely due to adhesions, an early decision to treat surgically is likely to have a favorable clinical outcome but may result in a longer hospital stay and higher cost of care compared to a nonsurgical approach. As one might expect, retrospective analysis of patients treated medically and surgically show that surgically treated patients have clinical outcomes similar to those treated medically but longer lengths of stay.[58] The additional costs of care in patients ultimately treated surgically may be as much as eight times higher than nonsurgically treated patients. This differential makes tests with improved diagnostic accuracy such as CT or ultrasonography potentially cost-effective for questionable partial SBO.[59]

## Etiology-Specific Considerations in the Elderly

### Adhesions

Adhesions account for 55–85% of SBOs, and more than 90% of adhesions occur after surgery. Other causes of inflammatory adhesions are pelvic inflammatory disease, diverticulitis, tuberculosis, and other forms of peritonitis. SBOs due to postoperative adhesions can occur from several days to 65 years after the initial operation, but most SBOs occur early during this interval. The reported median interval between operation and SBO varies among reports from 1.5 to 5.0 years.[16,58,60] The incidence rate of SBO after abdominal surgery thus appears to decrease over time, but the cumulative risk is high over the lifetime of the patient. Nieuwenhuijzen et al., reporting a series of 234 patients who underwent colectomy, found that 11% developed an SBO within the first postoperative year and 30% within the first 10 years.[61] A similar series from Norway showed a 9% cumulative incidence of SBO after colorectal resection over 5 years.[62]

Colorectal procedures, appendectomy, and multiple prior abdominal procedures (including adhesiolysis for SBO) each account for 20–25% of adhesive SBO, and gynecologic procedures account for an additional 10–15%.[60,63,64] Other operative procedures common in the elderly, such as vascular procedures, can also cause adhesive SBO.[65,66] Given these operative procedures, it is not surprising that more than half of all adhesions causing SBO involve the ileum and occur in the pelvis. In the Mayo Clinic series, 48% of adhesions consisted of only a single band, 40% were multiple bands, and only 10% were categorized as dense.[16] Band adhesions are more likely following appendectomy, colorectal, and gynecologic operations.[63] This finding argues for a greater role in laparoscopic management of adhesive SBO.

The overall incidence of strangulation in SBO is around 13%, and it is lower with adhesive SBO than for hernia-related SBO. Most adhesive partial SBOs resolve with nonsurgical management. The clinical indicators of strangulation are less reliable in the elderly. This fact, together with a high incidence of vascular insufficiency, high prevalence of co-morbid disease, and perhaps reluctance to undergo early surgery in the elderly, probably explains why the likelihood of strangulation and mortality is high in the elderly. There are no prospective studies that compare an aggressive surgical approach to a more conservative one to determine whether overall outcomes would improve with the more aggressive intervention in the elderly.

## Hernia

Hernias account for 15–20% of SBOs. The etiologic factors responsible for increased hernia incidence with age include benign prostatic hypertrophy, chronic obstructive pulmonary disease, constipation, and obesity. Around three-fourths of hernias involve the anterior abdominal wall, with 10–20% being incisional hernias. Internal hernias account for about 25% of hernia-associated SBOs and most of these are due to iatrogenic mesenteric defects created during prior surgery. They often occur through the mesentery at the site of a previous anastomosis and highlight the importance of closing such defects.

With SBOs due to a hernia, the overall mortality rate is around 4%. However, there are several factors that make this entity more worrisome in the elderly. The incidence of strangulated bowel in an SBO due to hernia is 28%, and delay in surgical treatment is associated with a higher mortality. The mortality and morbidity rates for elective hernia repair are 0% and 5%, respectively. With emergent repair, these same values are 8–14% mortality and >50% morbidity.[67] The underlying incidence of hernia in men over age 65 has been estimated at 13 per 1000.[68] Although the true risk of observation of hernias is not precisely known, a calculation based on the incidence of SBO (Fig. 40.3) and the percentage of SBO due to hernia indicates that roughly 10–15% of the incident cases of hernia occur in the setting of SBO. This is similar to other data showing that emergent hernia repairs account for 20% of all hernia repairs in the elderly compared with only 5% in the young.[69] This illustrates the reluctance of elderly patients to submit to surgery or the reluctance of physicians to appreciate the true risks of hernias. The low morbidity of elective repair and the high incidence of strangulation and considerably poorer outcome with emergent repair are strong reasons to advocate aggressive elective repair of hernias in elderly patients.

Of special interest in the elderly is the obturator hernia. Although this cause accounts for only 1–2% of all SBOs, this type of hernia is almost universally reported in elderly, thin women.[70–73] It is easily missed on physical examination. The obturator foramen is a rigid ring, and hernias in this location have a high incidence of strangulation (50%). For all these reasons, the mortality from obturator hernia-associated SBO is as high as 15–25%. Pressure and inflammation in the obturator foramen can lead to pain in the distribution of the femoral nerve; and the Howship Rhomberg sign (thigh pain on external rotation of the thigh) can be elicited in about one-third of patients. The key to diagnosis is acute suspicion for elderly women with no history of surgery and promptly obtaining a CT scan.[72,74]

## Neoplasms

Neoplasms account for 16% of SBOs. In the Mayo Clinic series, 92% of neoplasms originated in the abdomen, but only 2% were due to primary small bowel neoplasms.[16] Most are due to direct extension or metastases from colonic, pancreatic, and gastric tumors. The interval from cancer diagnosis to the onset of SBO ranges from 0 to 6 years, with the median time being 1–2 years for abdominal malignancies. Patients with SBO and a history of cancer still have a 55% chance of a benign cause for SBO; and even in patients with SBO and a known recurrence of colorectal cancer, SBO is due to benign causes in 10–30%.[75,76] The median interval between cancer diagnosis and SBO is longer (5 years) in patients who ultimately are found to have a benign cause for the SBO.[62]

For patients with malignant SBO, the outcome is grim. The 30-day mortality is 25–35%, and median survival is only 3–6 months. It is for this reason that many surgeons have a nihilistic view of patients with an SBO with known intraabdominal cancer. The combination of a partial SBO, short life expectancy due to known metastatic cancer, and poor operative risk should put operative management in question. However, given the significant incidence of benign causes in the face of recurrent cancer, an initial aggressive approach is warranted, including early surgical intervention. Once the malignant obstruction is diagnosed, heroic attempts at resection should be avoided in deference to palliative measures, including bypass of the obstructed segment and placement of a venting gastrostomy tube.

## Obturation Obstruction

A variety of objects can cause obturation obstruction, including bezoars, gallstones, enteroliths, ingested solid objects and medications, and parasites. Overall, obturation obstruction is relatively uncommon, but its incidence increases with age, particularly that due to bezoars and gallstones. Bezoars account for 2–3% of SBOs.[77–79] Risk factors for bezoar formation are increasing age and previous gastric surgery. It is likely that vagotomy reduces the contractile strength of the antrum and leads to increased gastric stasis. Treatment of bezoars should initially be medical, including treatment with digestive enzymes, prokinetic agents, and endoscopic morcellation. If this fails to resolve the problem, surgery should be undertaken. Gastric bezoars may spontaneously fragment or pieces may break off during morcellation and pass into the small bowel. Rarely, they can lead to obturation obstruction. At the time of surgery, bezoars are often fragmented, and they pass distally without the need of an enterotomy. The fragments should be passed into the colon. If this is not possible, the bezoar often can be milked into the more proximal small bowel that is less edematous for extraction via an enterotomy. Alternatively, small bowel resection is required. To prevent recurrence, patients should be advised to avoid high fiber foods, and consideration should be given to chronic use of a promotility agent.

Gallstone ileus is another obturation obstruction that is particularly prevalent in the elderly population. It accounts for 1–3% of SBOs, but is seen in up to 25% of the elderly with no history of surgery or detectable hernia.[80] The female/male ratio is 4:1, and 50–60% have symptomatic gallstones. The radiographic signs of gallstone ileus include ectopic gallstones and air in the biliary tree in addition to the findings of SBO. These patients require either enterotomy and stone extraction or segmental small bowel resection. In unstable patients or in the presence of a severe inflammatory reaction in the duodenum, lithotomy alone is recommended, leaving the cholecystoenteric fistula intact. In a review by Way, this was associated with only a 3.3% recurrence rate, and 8% of those patients die.[80] However, in a stable patient in whom a secure duodenal closure is thought possible, cholecystectomy and closure of the duodenum can be considered.[81] Enteroliths from duodenal,[82] jejunal,[83] and Meckel's[84,85] diverticula can also lead to obturation obstruction. Radiographic findings are similar to those seen with gallstone ileus, but there is no air in the biliary tree.

## Conclusions

Small bowel obstruction is a common disorder that primarily affects elderly patients. Postoperative adhesions, hernias, and intraabdominal cancer are the etiologies in most cases. The risks of strangulation, perioperative mortality, and morbidity are all higher in the elderly than in younger patients, which argues for aggressive early intervention in older patients. This must be tempered by the knowledge that unnecessary laparotomy also is associated with significant morbidity and mortality risk in the elderly population. Prompt resuscitation should be instituted while the history, physical examination, and selected radiologic studies are being performed to ascertain the likely cause of the SBO. CT scanning has shown promise with its ability to identify signs of bowel ischemia and particularly for identifying the etiology of SBO.

Early operative intervention is required in patients with signs of strangulation or complete SBO and in whom the etiology is thought to be a hernia. Conservative management of adhesive SBO seems safe for at least 48 hours and is likely to be successful in most cases. Conservative management is less costly than surgical management, although recurrence of SBO may appear sooner after conservative management than after surgical management. Population-based outcome studies of this problem are lacking in the current literature despite the high incidence of SBO. The increasing use of minimally invasive surgery will likely decrease the overall rate of adhesive complications, but port-site hernias comprise a new group of complications that must be identified. Minimally invasive surgery has made a seemingly small impact on the treatment of SBO in the elderly up to now, but its role in treating adhesive SBO should probably be expanded.

## References


1. Missouri Hospital Discharge Records. In: Missouri Information for Community Assessment. Missouri Department of Health, Jefferson City, 1997. (http://www.health.state.mo.us/BobHosp/allcod.html).
2. National Center for Health Statistics. National Hospital Ambulatory Medical Care Survey. Hyattsville: NCHS, 1996 (ftp://ftp.cdc.gov/pub/Health_Statistics/NCHS/Datasets/NHAMCS/ed1996.exe).
3. Neugut AI, Marvin MR, Rella VA, Chabot JA. An overview of adenocarcinoma of the small intestine. Oncology (Huntingt), 1997;11:529–536.
4. Gutstein DE, Rosenberg SJ. Nontraumatic intramural hematoma of the duodenum complicating warfarin therapy. Mt Sinai J Med 1997;64:339–341.
5. Waxman I, al-Kawas FH, Bass B, Glouderman M. PEG ileus: a new cause of small bowel obstruction. Dig Dis Sci 1991; 36:251–254.
6. Lambertz MM, Earnshaw PM, Short J, Cumming JG. Small bowel obstruction caused by a retained percutaneous endoscopic gastrostomy gastric flange. Br J Surg 1995;82: 951.
7. Lancaster JF, Strong RW, McIntyre A, Kerlin P. Gallstone ileus complicating endoscopic sphincterotomy. Aust NZ J Surg 1993;63:416–417.
8. Simpson D, Cunningham C, Paterson-Brown S. Small bowel obstruction caused by a dislodged biliary stent. J R Coll Surg Edinb 1998;43:203.
9. Tekin A. Mechanical small bowel obstruction secondary to spilled stones. J Laparoendosc Adv Surg Tech A 1998;8: 157–159.
10. Burney TL, Jacobs SC, Naslund MJ. Small bowel obstruction following laparoscopic lymphadenectomy. J Urol 1993; 150:1515–1517.
11. Hass BE, Schrager RE. Small bowel obstruction due to Richter's hernia after laparoscopic procedures. J Laparoendosc Surg 1993;3:421–423.
12. Spier LN, Lazzaro RS, Procaccino A, Geiss A. Entrapment of small bowel after laparoscopic herniorrhaphy. Surg Endosc 1993;7:535–536.
13. Vanclooster P, Meersman A, de Gheldere C. Small bowel obstruction after laparoscopic inguinal hernia repair: a case report. Acta Chir Belg 1995;95(suppl 4):199–200.
14. Bender E, Sell H. Small bowel obstruction after laparoscopic cholecystectomy as a result of a Maydl's herniation of the small bowel through a trocar site [letter]. Surgery 1996; 119:480.
15. Velasco JM, Vallina VL, Bonomo SR, Hieken TJ. Postlaparoscopic small bowel obstruction: rethinking its management. Surg Endosc 1998;12:1043–1045.

16. Mucha P. Small intestinal obstruction. Surg Clin North Am 1987;67:597–620.
17. Bugliosi TF, Meloy TD, Vukov LF. Acute abdominal pain in the elderly. Ann Emerg Med 1990;19:1383–1386.
18. Donckier V, Closset J, Van Gansbeke D, et al. Contribution of computed tomography to decision making in the management of adhesive small bowel obstruction. Br J Surg 1998;85:1071–1074.
19. Taourel PG, Fabre JM, Pradel JA, Seneterre EJ, Megibow AJ, Bruel JM. Value of CT in the diagnosis and management of patients with suspected acute small-bowel obstruction. AJR 1995;165:1187–1192.
20. Frager D, Baer JW, Medwid SW, Rothpearl A, Bossart P. Detection of intestinal ischemia in patients with acute small-bowel obstruction due to adhesions or hernia: efficacy of CT. AJR 1996;166:67–71.
21. Balthazar EJ, Liebeskind ME, Macari M. Intestinal ischemia in patients in whom small bowel obstruction is suspected: evaluation of accuracy, limitations, and clinical implications of CT in diagnosis. Radiology 1997;205:519–522.
22. Maglinte DD, Reyes BL, Harmon BH, et al. Reliability and role of plain film radiography and CT in the diagnosis of small-bowel obstruction. AJR 1996;167:1451–1455.
23. Fukuya T, Hawes DR, Lu CC, Chang PJ, Barloon TJ. CT diagnosis of small-bowel obstruction: efficacy in 60 patients. AJR 1992;158:765–769; discussion 771–772.
24. Ko YT, Lim JH, Lee DH, Lee HW, Lim JW. Small bowel obstruction: sonographic evaluation. Radiology 1993;188: 649–653.
25. Ogata M, Imai S, Hosotani R, Aoyama H, Hayashi M, Ishikawa T. Abdominal ultrasonography for the diagnosis of strangulation in small bowel obstruction. Br J Surg 1994;81:421–424.
26. Czechowski J. Conventional radiography and ultrasonography in the diagnosis of small bowel obstruction and strangulation. Acta Radiol 1996;37:186–189.
27. Schmutz GR, Benko A, Fournier L, Peron JM, Morel E, Chiche L. Small bowel obstruction: role and contribution of sonography. Eur Radiol 1997;7:1054–1058.
28. Regan F, Beall DP, Bohlman ME, Khazan R, Sufi A, Schaefer DC. Fast MR imaging and the detection of small-bowel obstruction. AJR 1998;170:1465–1469.
29. Makanjuola D. Computed tomography compared with small bowel enema in clinically equivocal intestinal obstruction. Clin Radiol 1998;53:203–208.
30. Maglinte DD, Nolan DJ, Herlinger H. Preoperative diagnosis by enteroclysis of unsuspected closed loop obstruction in medically managed patients. J Clin Gastroenterol 1991; 13:308–312.
31. Joyce WP, Delaney PV, Gorey TF, Fitzpatrick JM. The value of water-soluble contrast radiology in the management of acute small bowel obstruction. Ann R Coll Surg Engl 1992;74:422–425.
32. Chung CC, Meng WC, Yu SC, Leung KL, Lau WY, Li AK. A prospective study on the use of water-soluble contrast follow-through radiology in the management of small bowel obstruction. Aust NZ J Surg 1996;66:598–601.
33. Assalia A, Schein M, Kopelman D, Hirshberg A, Hashmonai M. Therapeutic effect of oral Gastrografin in adhesive, partial small-bowel obstruction: a prospective randomized trial. Surgery 1994;115:433–437.
34. Feigin E, Seror D, Szold A, et al. Water-soluble contrast material has no therapeutic effect on postoperative small-bowel obstruction: results of a prospective, randomized clinical trial. Am J Surg 1996;171:227–229.
35. Frager DH, Baer JW, Rothpearl A, Bossart PA. Distinction between postoperative ileus and mechanical small-bowel obstruction: value of CT compared with clinical and other radiographic findings. AJR 1995;164:891–894.
36. Brolin R. Partial small bowel obstruction. Surgery 1984; 95:145–149.
37. Peetz DJ, Gamelli RL, Pilcher DB. Intestinal intubation in acute, mechanical small-bowel obstruction. Arch Surg 1982;117:334–336.
38. Sosa J, Gardner B. Management of patients diagnosed as acute intestinal obstruction secondary to adhesions. Am Surg 1993;59:125–128.
39. Cox MR, Gunn IF, Eastman MC, Hunt RF, Heinz AW. The safety and duration of non-operative treatment for adhesive small bowel obstruction. Aust NZ J Surg 1993; 63:367–371.
40. Sarr MG, Bulkley GB, Zuidema GD. Preoperative recognition of intestinal strangulation obstruction: prospective evaluation of diagnostic capability. Am J Surg 1983;145: 176–182.
41. Zadeh BJ, Davis JM, Canizaro PC. Small bowel obstruction in the elderly. Am Surg 1985;51:470.
42. Mann A, Fazio VW, Lucas FV. A comparative study of the use of fluorescein and the Doppler device in the determination of intestinal viability. Surg Gynecol Obstet 1982; 154:53–55.
43. Cooperman M, Pace WG, Martin EW Jr, et al. Determination of viability of ischemic intestine by Doppler ultrasound. Surgery 1978;83:705–710.
44. Bulkley GB, Zuidema GD, Hamilton SR. Intraoperative determination of small intestinal viability following ischemic injury. Ann Surg 1981;193:628–637.
45. Rodriguez-Ruesga R, Meagher AP, Wolff BG. Twelve-year experience with the long intestinal tube. World J Surg 1995;19:627–630; discussion 630–631.
46. DeCherney AH, diZerega GS. Clinical problem of intraperitoneal postsurgical adhesion formation following general surgery and the use of adhesion prevention barriers. Surg Clin North Am 1997;77:671–688.
47. Diamond MP. Reduction of adhesions after uterine myomectomy by Seprafilm membrane (HAL-F): a blinded, prospective, randomized, multicenter clinical study: Seprafilm Adhesion Study Group. Fertil Steril 1996;66:904–910.
48. Beck DE. The role of Seprafilm bioresorbable membrane in adhesion prevention. Eur J Surg Suppl 1997;(577):49–55.
49. Keating J, Hill A, Schroeder D, Whittle D. Laparoscopy in the diagnosis and treatment of acute small bowel obstruction. J Laparoendosc Surg 1992;2:239–244.
50. Adams S, Wilson T, Brown AR. Laparoscopic management of acute small bowel obstruction. Aust NZ J Surg 1993; 63:39–41.
51. Franklin ME Jr, Dorman JP, Pharand D. Laparoscopic surgery in acute small bowel obstruction. Surg Laparosc Endosc 1994;4:289–296.
52. Ibrahim IM, Wolodiger F, Sussman B, Kahn M, Silvestri F, Sabar A. Laparoscopic management of acute small-bowel

obstruction. Surg Endosc 1996;10:1012–1014; discussion 1014–1015.
53. Parent S, Tortuyaux JM, Deneuville M, Bresler L, Boissel P. What are the small bowel obstructions to operate and how to do it? Acta Gastroenterol Belg 1996;59:150–151.
54. Bailey IS, Rhodes M, O'Rourke N, Nathanson L, Fielding G. Laparoscopic management of acute small bowel obstruction. Br J Surg 1998;85:84–87.
55. Landercasper J, Cogbill TH, Merry WH, Stolee RT, Strutt PJ. Long-term outcome after hospitalization for small-bowel obstruction. Arch Surg 1993;128:765–770; discussion 770–771.
56. Barkan H, Webster S, Ozeran S. Factors predicting the recurrence of adhesive small-bowel obstruction. Am J Surg 1995; 170:361–365.
57. Ivarsson ML, Holmdahl L, Franzen G, Risberg B. Cost of bowel obstruction resulting from adhesions. Eur J Surg 1997;163:679–684.
58. Wilson MS, Hawkswell J, McCloy RF. Natural history of adhesional small bowel obstruction: counting the cost. Br J Surg 1998;85:1294–1298.
59. Ogata M, Mateer JR, Condon RE. Prospective evaluation of abdominal sonography for the diagnosis of bowel obstruction. Ann Surg 1996;223:237–241.
60. Matter I, Khalemsky L, Abrahamson J, Nash E, Sabo E, Eldar S. Does the index operation influence the course and outcome of adhesive intestinal obstruction? Eur J Surg 1997; 163:767–772.
61. Nieuwenhuijzen M, Reijnen MM, Kuijpers JH, van Goor H. Small bowel obstruction after total or subtotal colectomy: a 10-year retrospective review. Br J Surg 1998;85:1242–1245.
62. Edna TH, Bjerkeset T. Small bowel obstruction in patients previously operated on for colorectal cancer. Eur J Surg 1998;164:587–592.
63. Cox MR, Gunn IF, Eastman MC, Hunt RF, Heinz AW. The operative aetiology and types of adhesions causing small bowel obstruction. Aust NZ J Surg 1993;63:848–852.
64. Meagher AP, Moller C, Hoffmann DC. Non-operative treatment of small bowel obstruction following appendicectomy or operation on the ovary or tube. Br J Surg 1993;80:1310–1311.
65. Franko E, Cohen JR. General surgical problems requiring operation in postoperative vascular surgery patients. Am J Surg 1991;162:247–250.
66. Siporin K, Hiatt JR, Treiman RL. Small bowel obstruction after abdominal aortic surgery. Am Surg 1993;59:846–849.
67. Rosenthal RA. Small-bowel disorders and abdominal wall hernia in the elderly patient. Surg Clin North Am 1994; 74:261–291.
68. Deysine M, Grimson R, Soroff HS. Herniorrhaphy in the elderly: benefits of a clinic for the treatment of external abdominal wall hernias. Am J Surg 1987;153:387.
69. Nehme AE. Groin hernias in elderly patients. Am J Surg 1983;146:257.
70. Yip AW, AhChong AK, Lam KH. Obturator hernia: a continuing diagnostic challenge. Surgery 1993;113:266–269.
71. Lo CY, Lorentz TG, Lau PW. Obturator hernia presenting as small bowel obstruction. Am J Surg 1994;167:396–398.
72. Ijiri R, et al. Obturator hernia: the usefulness of computed tomography in diagnosis. Surgery 1996;119:137–140.
73. Chung CC, Mok CO, Kwong KH, Ng EK, Lau WY, Li AK. Obturator hernia revisited: a review of 12 cases in 7 years. J R Coll Surg Edinb 1997;42:82–84.
74. O'Connell G, Cole A. Obturator hernia: diagnosis through medical imaging. Australas Radiol 1995;39:306–308.
75. Butler JA, Cameron BL, Morrow M, Kahng K, Tom J. Small bowel obstruction in patients with a prior history of cancer. Am J Surg 1991;162:624–628.
76. Ellis CN, Boggs HW Jr, Slagle GW, Cole PA. Small bowel obstruction after colon resection for benign and malignant diseases. Dis Colon Rectum 1991;34:367–371.
77. Ko S, Lee T, Ng S. Small bowel obstruction due to phytobezoar: CT diagnosis. Abdom Imaging 1997;22:471–473.
78. Chisholm EM, Leong HT, Chung SC, Li AK. Phytobezoar: an uncommon cause of small bowel obstruction. Ann R Coll Surg Engl 1992;74:342–344.
79. Lo CY, Lau PW. Small bowel phytobezoars: an uncommon cause of small bowel obstruction. Aust NZ J Surg 1994; 64:187–189.
80. Way LW. Gallstone ileus. In: Way LW, Pellegrini CA (eds) Surgery of the Gallbladder and Bile Ducts. Philadelphia: Saunders, 1987:275.
81. Day EA, Marks C. Gallstone ileus: review of literature and presentation of 34 new cases. Am J Surg 1975;129:552–558.
82. Yang HK, Fondacaro PF. Enterolith ileus: a rare complication of duodenal diverticula. Am J Gastroenterol 1992;87: 1846–1848.
83. Bowley D, Royle CA. Enterolith ileus as a complication of small bowel diverticulosis. J R Army Med Corps 1997; 143:169.
84. Lopez PV, Welch JP. Enterolith intestinal obstruction owing to acquired and congenital diverticulosis: report of two cases and review of the literature. Dis Colon Rectum 1991; 34:941–944.
85. Rudge FW. Meckel's stone ileus. Milit Med 1992;157:98–100.

# 41 Lower Gastrointestinal Bleeding in the Elderly

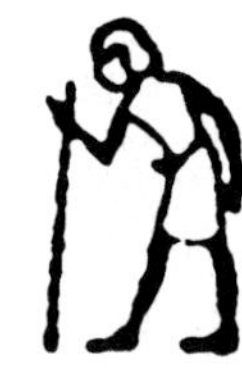

David McAneny and Craig L. Weinstein

Lower gastrointestinal (LGI) hemorrhages develop from sources distal to the ligament of Treitz and have a wide spectrum of presentations and acuities. This subject warrants special attention in the elderly. Bleeding from the upper gastrointestinal (UGI) tract occurs from practically the same causes in the elderly as in the young, albeit with differences among the prevalence of diagnoses. In contrast, a variety of degenerative changes develop over time in the LGI tract, so elderly patients are susceptible to bleeding from causes different from those in the young. Reinus and Brandt observed an interesting evolution of the explanations of LGI hemorrhage over the past 70 years.[1] Bleeding was commonly attributed to tumors and diverticulitis early in the twentieth century, but colonoscopy and arteriography have demonstrated that vascular ectasias and diverticular disease without acute inflammation actually comprise about two-thirds of cases.[2] Other problems to which the elderly are predisposed include ischemic colitis and neoplasms.

Elderly patients merit many considerations. They may suffer from co-morbid conditions and end-organ impairments. In addition, medications such as warfarin and nonsteroidal antiinflammatory drugs (NSAIDs) can contribute to bleeding. The mortality associated with acute UGI bleeding has been related to age in collected series,[3] although it is difficult to extrapolate the data to LGI hemorrhage and to distinguish the confounding issues. Series of colorectal cancer patients have suggested that age is not an independent risk factor for mortality after bowel resection.[4–7] Authors who have correlated age with increased mortality after colon surgery concede that systemic illnesses and emergency surgery are more critical factors than chronologic age.[8,9] Therefore, old patients certainly deserve and can tolerate treatment for LGI bleeding. In fact, the paradox is that the elderly might actually benefit from more aggressive care because they are less tolerant of repeated episodes of bleeding and shock.[10]

The goals of therapy for LGI bleeding are assessment of blood loss with commensurate volume resuscitation, identification of the source of hemorrhage, and correction of the bleeding if it persists or recurs.[3] The broad varieties of patients and bleeding intensities do not necessarily conform to rigid treatment algorithms. Furthermore, many evaluation and therapy options are available, so a team approach to the patient with LGI bleeding is essential among primary care physicians or geriatricians, gastroenterologists, intensivists, radiologists, and surgeons.

The intent of this chapter is to describe diagnostic studies, the culprits of LGI hemorrhage, their respective pathophysiologies, and treatment alternatives so clinicians caring for these challenging patients are well equipped. In general, the terms hemorrhage and bleeding refer to active blood loss. Occult or chronic oozing is examined separately.

## Effects of Aging on the Lower Gastrointestinal Tract

Distinct anatomic alterations develop in the gut with age.[11] The mucosa atrophies, and its glands change. Circular muscle wastes, and the longitudinal fibers become more pronounced. Anorectal sensory and effector mechanisms deteriorate. In addition, elastin deposition, arteriosclerosis, and decreased splanchnic blood flow contribute to the degenerative process. As a result, conditions affect the elderly that are rather unusual in younger patients.

Vascular ectasias of the colon, also known as angiodysplasias or arteriovenous malformations, are considered to be the consequence of aging on normal mural vessels.[12] In accordance with the law of Laplace, increased bowel wall tension occurs in the cecum and the proximal ascending colon, where most ectasias develop. This pressure produces repetitive partial occlusions of submucosal veins where they pierce the muscularis, eventually dilating the corresponding capillaries and arterioles, creating arteriovenous communications (Fig. 41.1). This acquired lesion is clearly related to age. About half of the individuals over

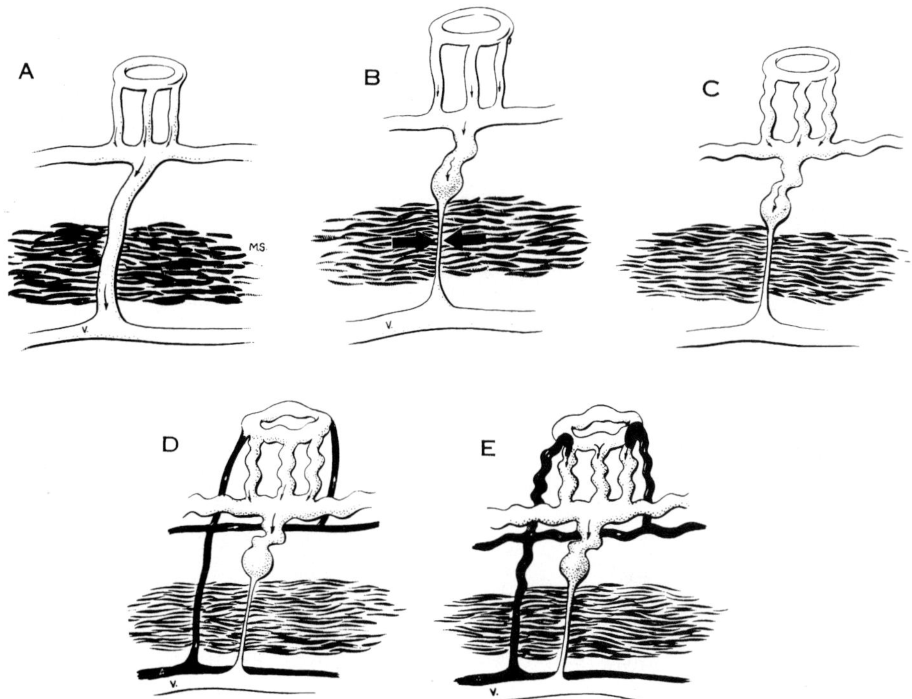


FIGURE 41.1. Proposed concept of the development of cecal vascular ectasias. (A) Normal state of vein perforating muscular layers. (B) With muscular contraction or increased intraluminal pressure, the vein is partially obstructed. (C) After repeated episodes over many years the submucosal vein becomes dilated and tortuous. (D) Later the veins and venules draining into the abnormal submucosal vein become similarly involved. (E) Ultimately the capillary ring becomes dilated, the precapillary sphincter becomes incompetent, and a small arteriovenous communication is present through the ectasia. (From Boley et al.,[12] with permission.)

60 years have either fully developed ectasias or histologic evidence of the formative stages.[12] Also, most patients diagnosed with this disorder are over age 50 years.[13] The pathophysiology of small bowel vascular ectasias is not as established as it is for those of the colon.[14]

Diverticulosis coli, another acquired lesion of the elderly, is characterized by pulsion pseudodiverticula, a condition unique to humans among herbivores.[13] Both the circular and longitudinal colon muscles become increasingly fibrotic with age, resulting in decreased complicance of the bowel wall and increased intraluminal pressure.[15] This environment promotes the protrusion of mucosa and muscularis mucosa through inherently weak sites where the vasa recta perforate the circular muscle between the teniae coli (Fig. 41.2).[13] A linear correlation exists between diverticular disease and age,[16] and the prevailing theory indicts the low fiber Western diet for diverticulosis.[17] A suggestion has been made that the increased intraluminal pressure responsible for this condition is due to the aversion of those in developed nations to pass flatus in public.[18] If that is the case, what an irony that, at a time of life when one may finally be less inhibited about this function, the die is already cast.

Although small bowel and colon neoplasms occur in the young, they are generally associated with older patients. The average age for small bowel tumors is 51 years,[19] and 90% of colorectal cancer patients are older than 55 years.[20] Fearon and Vogelstein proposed the sequence of gradual progression from colorectal epithelial hyperproliferative changes to adenocarcinomas.[21] The exponentially increasing disposition of cells to undergo malignant degeneration with age has also been calculated.[22]

Mesenteric ischemia may result from thromboembolic or hypoperfusion states. Ischemic colitis is usually multifactorial and occurs without a major vessel occlusion.[23] Although colonic ischemia presents in young patients in special circumstances, such as sickle cell anemia, long-distance running, and drug (illicit or prescribed)-induced reactions, most patients with colonic ischemia are over 60 years.[23]

To the extent that radiation therapy, the use of anticoagulants, constipation, and bowel instrumentation may be more common in elderly patients, other causes of LGI hemorrhage can be considered age-related as well.

## Initial Assessment and Resuscitation

As with any ailment, proper evaluation of the patient with LGI bleeding begins with obtaining a history and performing a physical examination. In the elderly patient, confusion or memory lapses can pose a problem, which

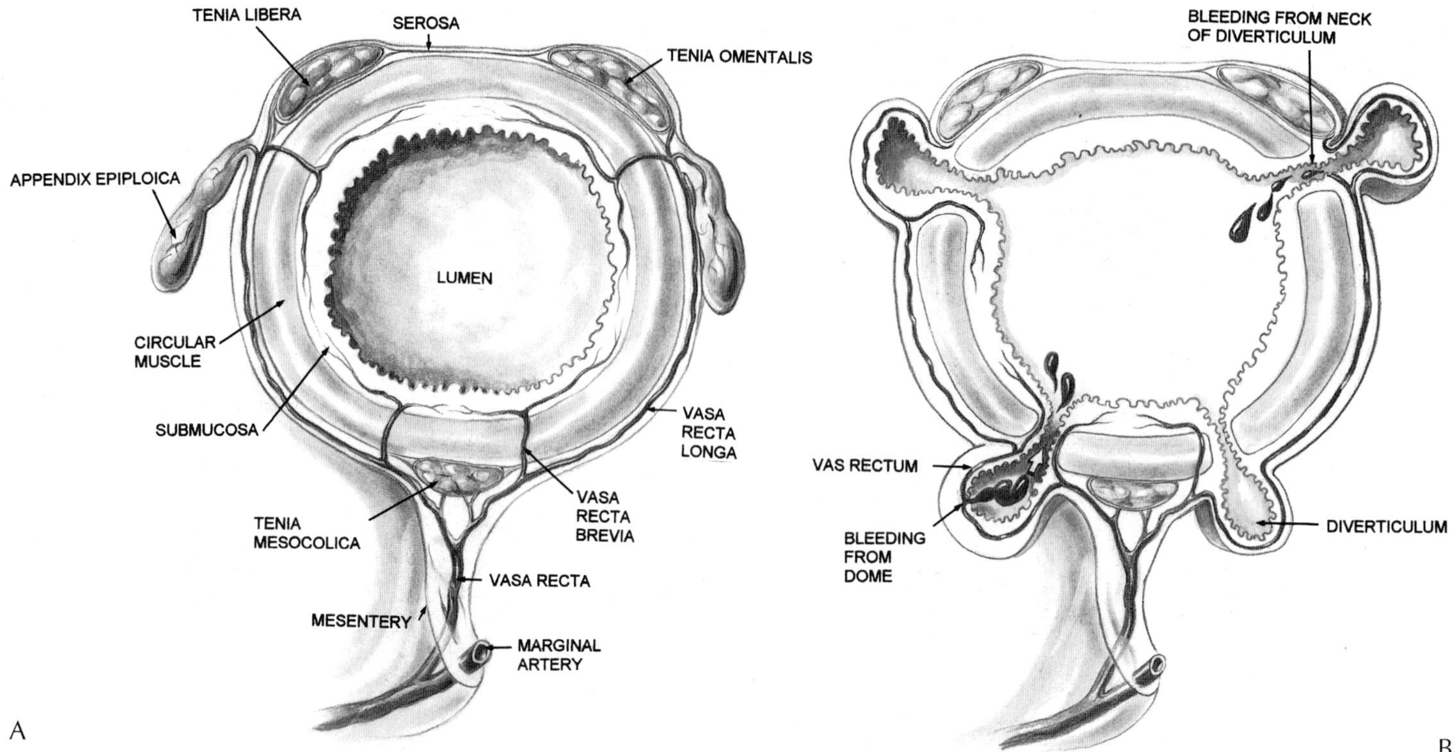


FIGURE 41.2. Acquired diverticulosis coli. Increased intraluminal pressure promotes the passage of mucosa and muscularis mucosa through inherently weak sites of the bowel wall where vasa recta pierce the circular muscle between teniae coli. Hemorrhage results when a vas rectum ruptures into either the dome or the neck of a diverticulum.

emphasizes the importance of cooperation with the patient's primary care physician or geriatrician, who may provide critical information. A severe hemorrhage abbreviates the initial evaluation to a perfunctory examination, so resuscitation is instituted immediately. When the situation settles, a more thorough history should be elicited.

Valuable information includes the acuity and volume of the bleeding, previous episodes of gastrointestinal hemorrhage and those evaluations, typical and recent bowel patterns, differentiation between melena and hematochezia, the presence of hematemesis, abdominal pain or cramps, anorectal symptoms, syncope or postural lightheadedness, medications, travel history or provocative meals, prior medical problems and operations, and chronic constitutional symptoms such as weight loss and fatigue. The passage of fresh clots or bright red blood generally indicates active LGI bleeding, although both can be seen with brisk UGI hemorrhage.[3] Melena is the product of the degradation of blood by coliform bacteria. Although more typical of UGI hemorrhage, melena can occur with LGI bleeding as well. The responses to the above inquiry may permit a reasonable estimation of the extent, location, and cause of the hemorrhage.

A physical examination incorporates the vital signs and a general assessment of the patient. The presence of wasting or peripheral adenopathy suggests a previously unrecognized malignancy. Stigmata of liver disease arouse suspicions of a UGI bleed or coagulopathy. During the abdominal examination, the physician should search for masses or tenderness. A digital rectal examination characterizes the blood and begins with gentle eversion of the buttocks and inspection rather than with abrupt, blind insertion of the digit. An inspection reveals anorectal pathology such as hemorrhoids, particularly thrombosed external or prolapsed internal complexes, fissures, abscesses, fistulas, or tumors.

Orifices must be scrutinized. Evaluation of the nasogastric tube aspirate is effective in discriminating between upper and lower gastrointestinal (GI) bleeding. When bile is present but no blood is discovered, the source is almost assuredly from the LGI tract. This simple maneuver is mandatory because about 10–15% of GI bleeding cases thought to be LGI in origin actually arise proximal to the ligament of Treitz.[24] It must be emphasized that a nonbloody and nonbilious aspirate is cautiously interpreted and does not preclude an endoscopic investigation of the UGI tract. Sigmoidoscopy should also be performed. This readily available study might determine an anorectal cause of the bleeding or identify mucosal changes representative of a more pervasive colorectal problem, such as proctocolitis from any number of causes. The procedure also allows one to procure a stool specimen when appropriate.

The laboratory assessment proceeds simultaneously with the history, physical examination, and resuscitation. A complete blood cell count (CBC) is essential for a baseline hematocrit and platelet count. Of course, a normal hematocrit may be registered despite significant bleeding if volume resuscitation and hemodilution have not yet begun. Prothrombin and partial thromboplastin times are important, particularly if the patient takes anticoagulants or has recently received antibiotics that alter gut flora and vitamin K absorption. The prothrombin time also reflects hepatic reserve. The determination of electrolytes, blood urea nitrogen (BUN), and creatinine are useful for assessing renal function. Furthermore, the BUN/creatinine ratio can help localize the bleeding.[25] About 95% of patients with LGI hemorrhage have a ratio less than 25:1 (allowing for the conversion from SI units to conventional units), whereas a higher ratio implies a more proximal source. An arterial blood gas assay is probably the most valuable laboratory determinant of hemodynamic instability and may be obtained at least during the initial evaluation of an acute GI bleed. Finally, the blood bank should receive a specimen for typing and cross-matching.

Early management includes the standard "ABCs" of resuscitation: control of the *a*irway and maintenance of *b*reathing and *c*irculation. Supplemental oxygen is administered to support the patient during the period of diminished oxygen-carrying capacity, whereas obtunded patients require intubation. An estimation of the acuity and amount of bleeding is crucial in the elderly patient, and the establishment of sufficient intravenous access and volume replacement with isotonic solutions ensue. Old patients with active hemorrhage and shock are well suited for the intensive care unit (ICU).

Blood component transfusion is dictated by hemodynamic instability, preceding and ongoing blood loss, coagulopathy, and platelet deficiency or dysfunction. The decreased perfusion and oxygen delivery associated with shock may compromise end-organs that are already impaired in the elderly. For example, angina pectoris or electrocardiogram (ECG) changes may be early manifestations of acute volume loss. Similarly, patients with chronic anemia due to a cecal cancer occasionally present with exertional chest pain or dyspnea. In addition, postural blood pressure changes may be especially sensitive to relatively mild blood loss as a result of weakened compensatory mechanisms (e.g., vasoconstriction) in older patients. This is particularly pronounced with certain medicines, including β-blockers. Central venous pressure monitoring and pulmonary artery catheterization are useful, although the initial volume expansion can be assessed on an empiric basis and guided by urine output. Pressors are not ordinarily indicated in the presence of hypovolemia and may actually contribute to end-organ ischemia. When anemia is identified by the baseline hematocrit during active bleeding, a chronic blood loss with a superimposed acute event is likely. Elderly patients are less tolerant of hemodynamic collapse than are the young, so resuscitation should be aggressive with a low threshhold for transfusions.

## Diagnostic Evaluation

Most cases of LGI hemorrhage among the elderly in the United States are due to vascular ectasias, diverticular disease, internal hemorrhoids, or neoplasms.[26] These lesions typically involve the colon and anorectum, but perhaps 3–5% of GI bleeding episodes originate in the small bowel.[14] Although LGI bleeding spontaneously resolves in 80% of patients, about 25% of cases recur.[27] The evaluation and management clearly depend on the acuity and severity of the hemorrhage. Therefore, active bleeding and occult blood loss are considered separately.

### Active Hemorrhage

The sequence of diagnostic assessment of the patient with active LGI bleeding has some variability, depending on personal expertise and philosophy and the institutional availability of tests and procedures. Clinical judgment is imperative to gauge the severity of bleeding and which diagnostic approach is favored. It should be emphasized that whereas barium enema is useful for evaluating chronic bleeding, it has no role in assessing active GI hemorrhage, as the barium interferes with both colonoscopy and arteriography. Once again, UGI endoscopy is indicated if the initial survey has failed to exclude the stomach and duodenum as potential sources.

#### *Nuclear Scintigraphy*

When active hemorrhage is determined to be from the LGI tract, accurate localization is a priority. If the blood loss is not massive, many investigators begin with technetium$^{99m}$ ($^{99m}$Tc)-labeled red blood cell (RBC) radionuclide scintigraphy.[10,13,28] This noninvasive scanning technique, which uses autologous RBCs labeled in vitro, is highly sensitive, detecting bleeding at rates of 0.1 ml/min.[29] Furthermore, the half-life of the radionuclide permits scans to be repeated for intermittent bleeding episodes up to 36 hours later.[30] In contrast, sulfur colloid scintigraphy is less sensitive, is dependent on an agent with a 3-minute half-life, and is difficult to interpret because of uptake of the sulfur colloid in the liver and spleen.[31] A 94% positive predictive value (PPV) of $^{99m}$Tc scintigraphy was cited in one study,[30] although these results are exceptional compared to the less impressive

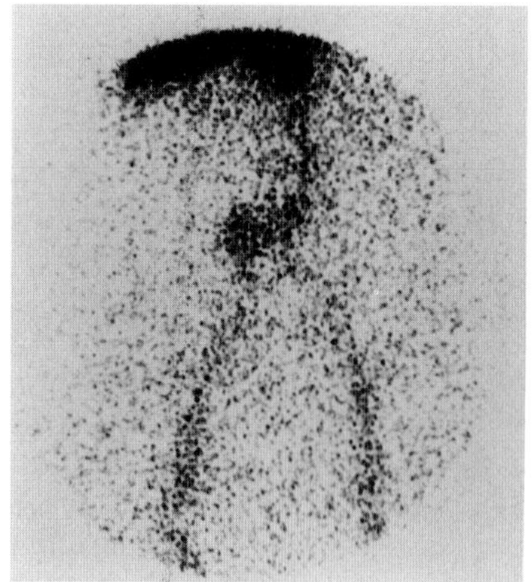

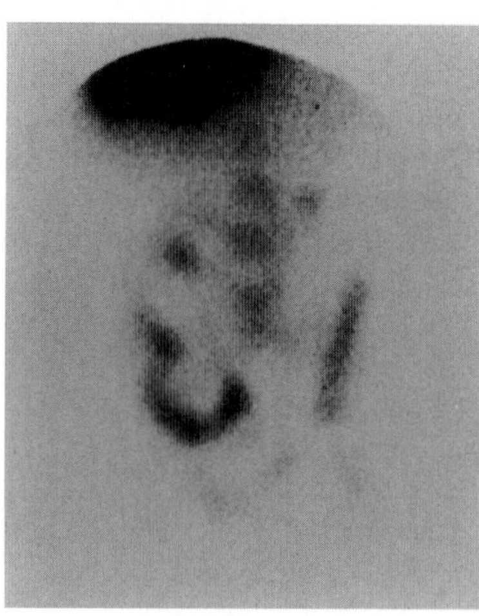

FIGURE 41.3. (Right) One-minute image from the flow phase of a $^{99m}$Tc-sulfur colloid bleeding scan showing extravasation of tracer above and to the right of the aortic bifurcation. (Left) Image at 45 minutes demonstrating the serpiginous course of tracer in the small bowel.

experiences typical of other series.[32,33] Few advocate scintigraphy alone to direct the extent of surgical resection.[28] Because LGI bleeding is so variable and intermittent, $^{99m}$Tc scintigraphy is most valuable for selecting patients in whom visceral arteriography would have the highest yield. Parenthetically, $^{99m}$Tc pertechnetate scintigraphy is possible for Meckel's diverticula containing heterotopic gastric mucosa. However, this is classically a source of LGI bleeding in young adults or children, not the elderly.

Nuclear scintigraphy suggests a small bowel source of bleeding when a serpiginous course of flow is apparent[14] (Fig. 41.3). Unfortunately, the radionuclide is more easily diluted in the small bowel than in the colon, and the precise site of bleeding is elusive among the multiple, overlapping loops of gut.

## *Arteriography*

Visceral arteriography is an invasive radiologic procedure with some morbidity, including thromboembolic complications and renal failure.[34,35] Less sensitive than $^{99m}$Tc scanning, arteriography cannot detect bleeding at a rate less than 0.5 ml/min.[36] Nevertheless, its accuracy in determining the site, and even the diagnosis, of the bleeding, is clearly superior to the radionuclide technique, and it offers therapeutic possibilities as well.[31] This procedure is performed when a nuclear scan suggests active blood loss. If bleeding is massive, one should forgo scintigraphy on the presumption that time is of the essence and a positive arteriogram is likely.

Arteriographic evidence of intraluminal extravasation precisely localizes the source of bleeding and is the sine qua non of active hemorrhage[31] (Fig. 41.4). This dramatic finding has been cited in as many as two-thirds of patients with diverticular hemorrhage and 10% of those with bleeding from vascular ectasias.[37] The accuracy of arteriography is about 50–72% with massive bleeding, although it declines to 25–50% when bleeding is intermittent or of a moderate degree.[38]

Arteriography is directed by scintigraphy results. It usually begins with injection of the superior mesenteric artery because most cases of diverticular hemorrhage and practically all bleeding from vascular ectasias occur in the right colon.[12,39] If that injection is nondiagnostic, studies of the inferior mesenteric artery and the celiac axis follow.

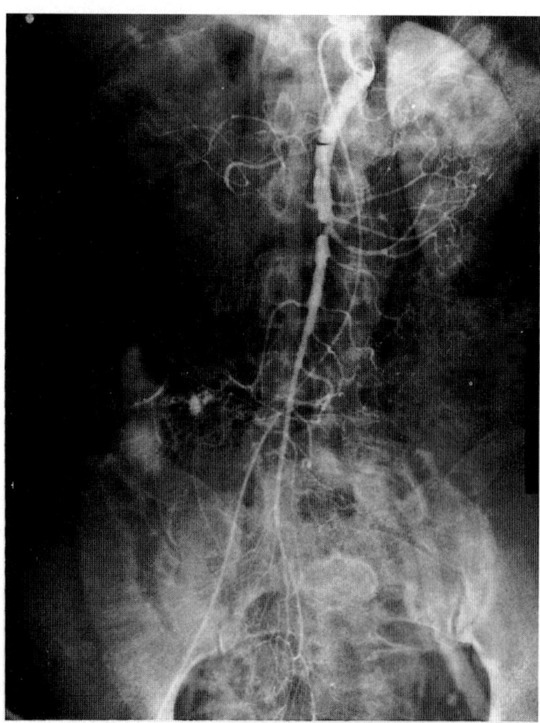

FIGURE 41.4. Superior mesenteric arteriogram demonstrating extravasation of contrast from an actively bleeding mid-ileal arteriovenous malformation.

In addition to defining bleeding sites, arteriographic findings may identify specific diagnoses. For example, vascular ectasias are characterized by a slowly emptying, densely opacified tortuous intramural vein, a vascular tuft, or an early-filling vein.[40] On the other hand, demonstration of contrast extravasating directly into a diverticulum during arteriography is uncommon.[1] Nevertheless, precise localization of the bleeding site in association with known diverticular disease is suggestive of this source. Finally, tumors often have characteristic neovascular changes.

Arteriographic techniques also permit therapeutic options.[31] Mesenteric arterial infusion of vasopressin or transcatheter embolization may be practiced in selected patients, as discussed below.

### Colonoscopy/Enteroscopy

Colonoscopy is probably most valuable for patients with intermittent bleeding or hemorrhage of relatively mild activity.[3] Blood itself is a cathartic, although most colonoscopists prefer to administer a purgative lavage.[34] Brisk hemorrhage may preclude a safe, adequate examination, but some investigators are comfortable performing colonoscopy in this situation.[34] An added benefit is the ability to control bleeding from vascular ectasias with laser, thermal, sclerosant, or electrocoagulation techniques.[34] Similar therapy for diverticular bleeding has been successful despite the seemingly increased risk of perforation through the thin-walled diverticulum.[41]

A perplexing situation occurs when arteriography or colonoscopy reveals common degenerative changes (e.g., diverticula or vascular ectasias) but fails to demonstrate active bleeding. Considering that most bleeding episodes from these sources cease spontaneously, it is prudent to reinstitute the evaluation if the bleeding recurs and not to empirically attribute blood loss to potential sites that were previously hemostatic.

When massive hemorrhage develops in the small intestine, nuclear scintigraphy or arteriography generally indicates this possibility.[14] A variety of enteroscopic methods are available, but an intraoperative examination is the most expeditious and thorough, particularly if massive bleeding prompts laparotomy.[14]

### Provocative Measures

Various agents have been employed to enhance the sensitivities of examinations that have failed to identify an intermittently bleeding source. Heparin infusion has been described with RBC scintigraphy.[42] Thrombolytic materials, heparin, and tolazoline have also been injected to precipitate bleeding during arteriography.[43] These measures may create an unwelcome degree of bleeding and are best reserved for particularly frustrating situations, such as nondiagnostic studies, despite persistent bleeding following bowel resection. Pentagastrin and cimetidine have enhanced the uptake of pertechnetate by parietal cells in Meckel's diverticula,[44,45] although these methods probably have little utility in the elderly. Finally, naloxone has a proven role in the colonoscopic identification of vascular ectasias that may be less obvious when narcotics have been administered during the procedure.

### Intraoperative Diagnosis

Unusual circumstances, especially massive bleeding, rarely demand laparotomy. A 31% yield from empiric laparotomies using transillumination and palpation was reported during the era before fiberoptic endoscopy.[46] However, it can be argued that, after adjusting for lesions that would now be discovered by endoscopy, the yield drops to 10%.[14]

Intraoperative arteriography is possible for small bowel bleeding, but it is cumbersome.[47] This technique identifies the lesion by referring to radiopaque clips placed on the bowel during surgery, palpating embolized metal coils, or injecting vital dyes.[47,48] Vascular ectasias have been located by Doppler ultrasonography or determination of mesenteric venous oxygen saturation.[49] Intraoperative scintigraphy has been utilized while sequentially clamping and scanning the bowel at limited intervals.[50]

Current surgical diagnostic options also include on-table lavage with colonoscopy[10] or enteroscopy[14] for localization of bleeding. The mortality rate of a "blind," empiric subtotal colectomy is particularly high for patients over age 70 years[51]; this operation is considered during desperate circumstances.[24]

## Occult Hemorrhage

Although occult GI blood loss does not have the dramatic urgency of active hemorrhage, the diagnostic dilemmas can be at least as perplexing. The vigor of the evaluation is a function of how the blood loss manifests, the presence of iron deficiency anemia, blood transfusion requirements, symptoms, and the patient's general condition.

### Fecal Occult Blood Tests

Normal, physiologic fecal blood loss is approximately 1 ml daily[52] and is rather constant with age.[53] Fecal occult blood tests (FOBTs) have been evaluated and refined for colorectal cancer screening, although their value for iron deficiency anemia is not established.[54] Despite many limitations, FOBTs have been associated with a 22–58% likelihood of predicting a colorectal neoplasm.[55] In the inpatient setting, this test has a less well-defined role in colorectal cancer detection,[55] and it frequently identifies peptic disease in elderly patients.[56,57]

The asymptomatic person with a positive FOBT should undergo colonoscopy or a combination of air-contrast barium enema and sigmoidoscopy.[53] It may be that the latter approach is more reasonable in some elderly patients, considering the natural history of diminutive polyps with respect to the individual's anticipated longevity. The UGI tract does not require a routine investigation because FOBTs are not especially sensitive to proximal gut blood loss. Moreover, stomach and duodenal tumors are not as common as colorectal malignancies and are less likely to be discovered at curative stages. Significant UGI pathology is uncommon in asymptomatic patients with positive FOBTs.[53]

### *Iron Deficiency Anemia*

In Western society, elderly patients with iron deficiency anemia generally have occult GI bleeding.[58,59] Therefore, aside from a digital anorectal examination, FOBTs are moot in the evaluation of these patients. Furthermore, a positive FOBT does not correlate with the discovery of GI pathology in this population.[60,61] An appropriate inquiry consists of colonoscopy (or air-contrast barium enema with sigmoidoscopy) and esophagogastroduodenoscopy. When those tests are unremarkable, some advocate empiric oral iron supplementation for the elderly without examining the small bowel.[62]

Patients who fail to respond to iron, particularly if they are transfusion-dependent, require a more thorough investigation. A barium small bowel series is reasonable, safe, and relatively inexpensive, although its yield is only 5%.[63] Enteroclysis is about twice as likely as a routine small bowel follow-through to indict a source of bleeding.[64] Several enteroscopic techniques are available. Standard push enteroscopy extends into only the most proximal 45–60 cm of jejunum,[65] but an overtube increases the distance to as far as 150 cm beyond the ligament of Treitz.[66] The yield of push enteroscopy is as high as 38%, and this technique also affords the opportunity to fulgurate lesions such as vascular ectasias or to perform biopsies.[65] Sonde enteroscopy relies on peristalsis to advance the tip of the instrument to the terminal ileum. Combined with push enteroscopy, the Sonde method has a diagnostic yield of 42%.[67] Although it extends the full length of the small intestine, the Sonde device is limited by an inability to maneuver its tip and by the lack of biopsy or therapy capabilities.

The next level of investigation includes arteriography and intraoperative video-enteroscopy. Because these studies are invasive, they should be invoked only if one is prepared to act on their findings and the patient is debilitated by the anemia. Arteriography can reveal small bowel vascular ectasias, although they are more difficult to distinguish than are corresponding lesions in the colon.[14] Intraoperative enteroscopy obviously requires laparotomy and can be associated with a prolonged ileus; but it provides a diagnosis in most patients.[68,69] The transilluminated bowel permits recognition of lesions from both the serosal aspect of the gut and the lumen.

When the patient with occult GI blood loss is symptomatic, the evaluation should be guided by the complaints. Contrast studies may be as rewarding as the more sophisticated examinations described above because the source is likely a gross lesion such as a tumor, Crohn's disease, or a peptic ulcer rather than an elusive vascular ectasia.

Finally, virtual colonoscopy is an emerging technology that involves software manipulation of computed tomography (CT) or magnetic resonance imaging (MRI) data to generate navigations through the colon, simulating conventional colonoscopy.[70] This technique may eventually provide a safe, noninvasive alternative to barium enema or diagnostic colonoscopy for evaluating chronic GI bleeding.

## Specific Diseases and Treatments

In the elderly, about two-thirds of cases of significant lower intestinal hemorrhage are from diverticular disease or vascular ectasias.[2] Even when these conditions are present, active bleeding is often not encountered during the evaluation due to the intermittent nature of LGI hemorrhage.[13] Furthermore, bleeding stops spontaneously in approximately 80% of episodes.[27] An appreciation of the various diseases and their natural histories contributes to the balance between judicious restraint and appropriate boldness in the care of these patients. There are numerous causes of LGI hemorrhage (Table 41.1), but this chapter addresses only the relatively common ones.

### Colorectal Lesions

#### *Diverticular Disease*

Despite the widespread prevalence of diverticula among the elderly, perhaps just 3–5% of patients with this problem exhibit bleeding.[71] Diverticular disease is usually concentrated in the sigmoid colon and only 10–15% of affected individuals have diverticula in the ascending colon.[72] Nevertheless, most diverticular hemorrhages emanate from the right colon.[39] This may be a function of the wider necks and domes of right colon diverticula, exposing more surface area of the thin mucosa and the underlying vasa recta to injury.[73]

Although bleeding into a diverticulum is normally not seen during arteriography,[1] it has been shown to result from rupture of a vas rectum in the dome or near the neck of the diverticulum[74] (Fig. 41.2). The mural architecture and attenuated media of the vasa recta promote bleeding into the lumen of the diverticulum rather than into the peritoneal cavity.[74] It must be emphasized that hemor-

TABLE 41.1 Causes of Lower Gastrointestinal Blood Loss

- Benign anorectal conditions
  - **Abscess**
  - **Fissure**
  - **Fistula-in-ano**
  - **Hemorrhoid**
  - Prolapse
- Diverticular diseases
  - Acquired: **diverticulosis coli**, jejunal diverticulosis
  - Congenital (e.g., Meckel's diverticulum)
- Enteritis/colitis/proctitis
  - **Antibiotic-associated colitis (e.g., *Clostridium difficile*)**
  - Crohn's disease
  - Diversion colitis
  - **Ischemic colitis** (see Table 41.2)
  - **Infectious enteritis or colitis**
    - **Bacteria** (e.g., *Campylobacter, Escherichia coli, Salmonella, Shigella*, typhoid fever, *Vibrio parahemolyticus, Yersinia*)
    - Parasite (e.g., *Ascaris, Entamoeba histolytica*, hookworm, *Strongyloides*)
    - Tuberculosis
  - Radiation-induced enteritis or colitis (acute or chronic)
  - Typhlitis
  - Ulcerative colitis
- Iatrogenic
  - **Instrumentation** (e.g., colonoscopy, sigmoidoscopy, biopsy)
  - **Medicines**
    - **Anticoagulation**
    - Chemotherapy (e.g., vincristine)
  - **Surgery** (e.g., anastomosis)
- Miscellaneous
  - Arsenic poisoning
  - Celiac sprue
  - **Coagulopathy**
  - Duplication cyst
  - Endometriosis
  - Eosinophilic gastroenteritis
  - Foreign body
  - Graft-versus-host disease
  - Impaction
  - Intussusception
  - Lymphangiectasia
  - Long-distance running
  - Physiologic blood loss
  - Pneumatosis cystoides intestinalis
  - Trauma
- Neoplasms
  - Primary anal
    - Epidermoid (squamous cell) carcinoma
    - Melanoma
    - Transitional-cloacogenic carcinoma
  - Primary colorectal or small bowel
    - **Adenoma**/polyposis syndromes
    - **Adenocarcinoma**
    - Carcinoid
    - Hamartoma (e.g., Peutz-Jeghers syndrome)
    - Lipoma
    - Lymphoma
    - Neurofibromatosis
    - Sarcoma (e.g., angiosarcoma, lymphosarcoma, Kaposi's)
    - Stromal tumor (e.g., leiomyoma/leiomyosarcoma)
  - Metastatic
    - Breast
    - Lung
    - Melanoma
    - Renal cell
    - Contiguous tumors (e.g., pelvic malignancies)
- Ulcers
  - Anastomotic ulcer
  - Idiopathic chronic ulcerative enteritis
  - **Medicine-induced** (e.g., NSAIDs, potassium tablets)
  - Solitary rectal ulcer syndrome (e.g., actinomycosis, cytomegalovirus, herpes, lymphogranuloma venerum, schistosomiasis, syphilis) (noninfectious causes: see Miller et al.[26])
  - Stercoral ulcer
  - Zollinger Ellison syndrome
- Vascular lesions
  - Aortoenteric fistula
  - Arteriovenous malformation
  - Dieulafoy's lesion (cirsoid aneurysm)
  - Hemangioma
  - Hereditary hemorrhagic telangiectasia
  - Phlebectasia
  - Portal hypertension colopathy
  - Varices
  - **Vascular ectasia**

Common causes of lower gastrointestinal blood loss are in boldface.

rhage occurs from noninflamed diverticula; diverticulitis rarely produces a significant amount of blood.[75] Moreover, although diverticula can be responsible for acute bleeding episodes, chronic anemia should not be ascribed to them.

Diverticular hemorrhage typically presents with spontaneous rectal bleeding, abdominal cramps with the urge to defecate, and signs and symptoms of hypovolemia. Medical management is sufficient for the 80% of patients in whom bleeding resolves spontaneously. However, one cannot predict when the bleeding will persist or recur, so the diagnostic evaluation must proceed as outlined above.

Therapeutic colonoscopic techniques have been applied to diverticular hemorrhage.[41] Because of the risk of bowel perforation from electrocoagulation,[76] these measures are safest when a mechanical bowel preparation and minimally active hemorrhage allow good visualization of the bleeding site. However, few clinicians possess the skill to locate and control diverticular bleeding consistently with the colonoscope.

When diverticular bleeding is recognized during arteriography, radiologic interventional techniques may provide hemostasis. The infusion of intraarterial vasopressin arrests hemorrhage in 80–90% of patients, although bleeding recurs in as many as 50% and the maneuver is not without significant morbidity.[38,77,78] It is also impossible to estimate how many patients might have stopped bleeding without this measure. Although it could be that vasopressin is as effective when given by peripheral vein as it is by intraarterial infusion for left colon diverticular bleeding,[13] the vasoconstrictive effects on the coronary vasculature from venous infusion can be undesirable in the elderly.[31] Of particular concern in older patients, mesenteric vessels with severe atherosclerosis do not respond well to vasopressin.[79] Selective arterial embolization is accomplished with a variety of agents and is an option if vasopressin fails, but it conveys a risk of bowel ischemia and infarction.[31] Mesenteric vasopressin and embolization are best reserved for patients who are not surgical candidates or as temporizing efforts while patients are prepared for an operation.

Surgical resection is likely necessary in the 20% of patients with diverticular bleeding that does not spontaneously subside. Segmental resections are highly preferable to "blind" subtotal colectomies. In one series of massive LGI hemorrhage, segmental resections guided by preoperative localization were associated with 7% mortality.[80] On the other hand, subtotal colectomies imparted a 30% death rate. The importance of localization is emphasized by the 42% incidence of recurrent bleeding for segmental resections with a negative arteriogram.[80] A prevalence of left colon diverticula should not influence surgery because most episodes of diverticular bleeding occur in the right colon. Subtotal colon resections are reserved as a last resort for massive bleeding that persists and cannot be localized. As stated earlier, the elderly are especially intolerant of protracted shock, so the determination to operate should not be delayed by efforts that are unlikely to succeed.[10]

### *Vascular Ectasias*

Vascular ectasias are typically degenerative lesions in the ascending colon, although they may also be congenital lesions, hereditary hemorrhagic telangiectasias, or findings related to systemic diseases.[81] Aortic stenosis has been implicated as an associated condition, but recent evidence seems to refute that notion.[82] The extent of hemorrhage is variable and is massive in about 15% of cases of bleeding vascular ectasias.[83] A similar number of individuals present with occult bleeding and iron deficiency anemia.[83] The signs and symptoms of vascular ectasias depend on the nature of the bleeding. Like diverticular hemorrhage, significant bleeding from vascular ectasias spontaneously resolves in 90% of cases.[83]

Although massive bleeding often precludes safe, thorough inspection, colonoscopy plays a greater role in the diagnosis and management of vascular ectasias than in diverticular bleeding. The various coagulation methods are similar to those applied in the UGI tract and include monopolar, bipolar, and multipolar electrocautery, the heater probe, and laser therapy.[84] Lasers such as argon and potassium-titanyl-phosphate 532 have limited depths of penetration and practically eliminate the risk of perforation.[84,85] However, these lasers are not widely or readily available. Colonoscopic coagulation therapy is valuable for minimally to moderately active bleeding, and its success rates range from 40% to 80%.[84] Parenthetically, incidentally discovered nonbleeding ectasias should be left undisturbed.[86] Conversely, nonbleeding ectasias encountered during evaluation of a chronic GI bleed should probably be coagulated.[87]

As with diverticular disease, vasopressin may be administered systemically or into the specific mesenteric artery that perfuses the vascular ectasia. Selective arteriographic embolization is also an option. The same risks of recurrent bleeding and ischemia for diverticular disease apply to vascular ectasias. Once again, the interventional arteriographic methods are best employed for patients who are poor operative risks or who refuse surgery or to allow stabilization of the patient until resection.

Surgery is indicated when significant bleeding persists or numerous vascular ectasias preclude coagulation therapy. The extent of resection is dictated by preoperative localization and normally involves a right colectomy as a result of the distribution of the lesions. Vascular ectasias can be elusive upon histologic examination of the specimen. Although clinical outcome determines the success of the resection, special preparation of the specimen with silicon rubber and methylsalicylate permits precise identification of ectasias, if necessary.[88]

Intermittent or chronic occult bleeding from vascular ectasias is especially vexing. Prophylactic estrogen therapy has been proposed for extensive ectasias or those that are not amenable to endoscopic techniques. However, a cohort study failed to find any efficacy for hormonal manipulation.[89]

### *Neoplasms*

Colon polyps and carcinomas do not ordinarily cause major hemorrhage. However, the passage of any blood per rectum by the elderly cannot be dismissed and must be regarded as a possible harbinger of malignancy, even in the presence of an obvious benign source such as a hemorrhoid. Left colon cancers classically present with obstructive symptoms. In contrast, right colon tumors commonly manifest as weakness, a right lower quadrant mass, and anemia. Rectal cancers often produce blood per rectum and may be palpated on digital examination.

Resection of colorectal tumors is usually advocated, even in palliative settings.[90] Furthermore, sphincter preservation is possible for most rectal cancers. In frail patients or those with extensive metastases, bleeding and obstruction are palliated with coagulative ablation techniques, stents, and radiation therapy.[84,90]

### Ischemic Colitis

Ischemic colitis is multifactorial and typically does not involve a major vascular occlusion.[23] The variety of etiologic factors are listed in Table 41.2. Patients present with crampy abdominal pain, diarrhea, hematochezia, and occasional abdominal distension and tenderness. The acute injury may be reversible or can result in a later stricture; peritonitis and shock become evident in the 15–20% of patients in whom the bowel insult is transmural. Ischemic colitis proximal to an obstructing lesion, such as a colon tumor, should be strongly considered in the elderly.

The expedient recognition of ischemic colitis requires clinical suspicion of this condition. Abdominal plain radiographs, barium enema, and CT scanning may be suggestive, but colonoscopy is generally the preferred diagnostic modality. Caution against overdistension of the colon must be exercised to avoid exacerbation of the colitis. Mesenteric arteriography is rarely necessary.

Supportive measures normally suffice and include gut rest and decompression, intravenous antibiotics, hydration, and maximization of the cardiopulmonary status. Reversible underlying conditions and the use of medications must also be addressed. Of course, patients with pneumoperitoneum or peritonitis should undergo immediate laparotomy without superfluous tests. Mortality in this situation is about 53–60%.[23] Chronic strictures require an evaluation to exclude a malignancy, and they are electively resected when symptoms are present.

### Other Colitides

Inflammatory bowel disease, such as ulcerative colitis and Crohn's disease, can initially present in the elderly[91] (see Chapter 43). Bloody diarrhea is a common manifestation of both conditions because Crohn's disease more often manifests as colitis than as ileitis in old patients.[91] Although there may be differences between the elderly and younger patients with respect to presenting symptoms and responses to certain therapies,[92] the principles of medical and surgical management are similar. Of course, it is crucial to consider ischemia and other causes of colitis in the elderly.

Infectious colitis results from numerous bacteria and parasites that produce fevers, bloody diarrhea, and

TABLE 41.2. Causes of Ischemic Colitis

| | |
|---|---|
| Idiopathic (spontaneous) | Hypovolemia |
| Major vascular occlusion | Sepsis |
| Trauma | Neurogenic insult |
| Thrombosis, embolization of mesenteric arteries | Anaphylaxis |
| Arterial embolus | Medications |
| Cholesterol embolus | Digitalis preparations |
| Aortography | Diuretics |
| Colectomy with inferior mesenteric artery ligation | Catecholamines |
| Midgut ischemia | Estrogens |
| Postabdominal aortic reconstruction | Danazol |
| Mesenteric venous thrombosis | Gold |
| Hypercoaguable states | Nonsteroidal antiinflammatory drugs |
| Portal hypertension | Neuroleptics |
| Pancreatitis | Colonic obstruction |
| Small-vessel disease | Colon carcinoma |
| Diabetes mellitus | Adhesions |
| Rheumatoid arthritis | Stricture |
| Amyloidosis | Diverticular disease |
| Radiation injury | Rectal prolapse |
| Systemic vasculitis disorders | Fecal impaction |
| Systemic lupus erythematosus | Volvulus |
| Polyarteritis nodosa | Strangulated hernia |
| Allergic granulomatosis | Pseudoobstruction |
| Scleroderma | Hematologic disorders |
| Behçet syndrome | Sickle cell disease |
| Takayasu's arteritis | Protein C deficiency |
| Thromboangiitis obliterans | Protein S deficiency |
| Buerger's disease | Antithrombin III deficiency |
| Shock | Cocaine abuse |
| Cardiac failure | Long-distance running |

*Source:* Gandhi et al.,[23] with permission.

abdominal cramps. The elderly are particularly susceptible to certain organisms. For example, *Salmonella* thrives in the presence of achlorhydria, disseminated carcinoma, lymphatic or hematologic malignancy, and immune-suppressed states.[24] *Escherichia coli* 0157:H7 has been associated with epidemics in nursing facilities and may foster a profound, even lethal hemorrhagic colitis.[93] *Clostridium difficile* infections are typically acquired in hospitals, but nosocomial outbreaks also occur in nursing homes and extended-care facilities.[94] Moreover, most patients with pseudomembranous colitis are over 60 years of age.[24] *C. difficile* is associated with a spectrum of presentations, including an asymptomatic carrier state, antibiotic-associated diarrhea, pseudomembranous colitis, and fulminant colitis. Occult bleeding may be detected, but gross LGI hemorrhage is rather unusual. Oral antibiotic therapy is successful for most patients; and meticulous hygiene among hospital staff, such as proper hand-washing, minimizes cross-infections. Emergency colectomy is infrequently necessary for fulminant infectious colitis.

Acute proctocolitis or enteritis develops transiently in as many as 50% of patients undergoing irradiation to pelvic viscera,[95] but only about 2% of patients suffer major acute gut complications. The radiation injury affects the rapidly proliferating GI mucosa, causing diarrhea, mucoid or bloody rectal discharge, tenesmus, constipation, nausea, vomiting, or abdominal cramps. These problems are managed with gut rest, supportive care, and cessation of the radiation therapy. Chronic radiation proctocolitis results in intramural vasculitis with chronic ischemia and fibrosis.[96] Patients experience fecal urgency, lower abdominal cramps, rectal pain, diarrhea, or bloody bowel movements. Management includes bulking agents for the stool and cholestyramine to reduce the intraluminal bile salts. Sodium pentosan polysulfate may be of value for more advanced proctitis, and intraluminal laser or electrocoagulation therapy is indicated for significant bleeding.

Diversion colitis results in patients with stomas and defunctionalized segments of colon or rectum.[97] It is postulated that the inflammation arises from the deprivation of short-chain fatty acid exposure to the colonic mucosa.[98] The condition is reversed with restoration of bowel continuity.

### *Anorectal Conditions*

Hemorrhoids and fissures occur in elderly patients and are typically associated with constipation. Management, which is the same as for the general population, includes hydration and efforts to soften and add bulk to stools. Internal hemorrhoid banding or ablation is reserved for refractory bleeding or other bothersome symptoms. Lateral internal sphincterotomy is an option for fissures, but preoperative sphincter tone should be particularly assessed in the elderly.

### *Miscellaneous Disorders*

Severe constipation can lead to stercoral ulcer formation, resulting in hemorrhage upon disimpaction.[24] Typhlitis develops in leukopenic patients and often responds to supportive care and antibiotics; its fulminant form requires resection and is devastating to the elderly. Intussusception can produce abdominal cramps and currant-jelly stools. Because tumors frequently act as lead points among elderly patients, intussuscepted bowel must be resected without attempting reduction. Finally, iatrogenic bleeding can arise after colonoscopy or bowel resection. Both situations are usually managed with supportive care, although persistent bleeding could prompt laparotomy or colonoscopy with coagulation.[99]

## Small Bowel Lesions

### *Vascular Ectasias*

Vascular ectasias account for 70–80% of cases of small intestine hemorrhage and can produce either brisk or occult bleeding.[14] Although the pathophysiology of the ectasias is not well established, they probably constitute a degenerative process, the average age of presentation being 69 years.[19]

Push enteroscopes afford the possibility of fulguration, but this is not an option with longer, more flexible devices. Arteriography is less helpful for small bowel ectasias than for those of the colon. A limited segment of small bowel with ectasias is certainly amenable to resection. Conversely, diffuse vascular ectasias present a complex situation and do not ordinarily prompt extensive bowel resection. Intraoperative laser therapy may be applied to diffuse disease, but it does not necessarily prevent recurrent bleeding.[69]

### *Neoplasms*

Tumors are responsible for 5–10% of cases of small bowel bleeding.[14] They include lipomas, hamartomas, adenomas and adenocarcinomas, benign and malignant stromal tumors, lymphomas, and carcinoid tumors.[100] Although most neoplasms are associated with occult blood loss, the stromal tumors are well known for brisk hemorrhage due to their propensity to undergo central necrosis. Melanoma, other metastatic malignancies from the breast, lung, or kidney, and Kaposi's sarcoma can also produce significant bleeding. Resection is indicated for these tumors.

### *Miscellaneous Disorders*

Crohn's disease commonly presents with abdominal pain, cramps, and altered bowel habits, but active bleeding infrequently occurs with terminal ileitis.[101] Hemorrhage typically abates spontaneously, and Crohn's disease is thereafter managed in accordance with standard practice. Tuberculosis is another granulomatous enteritis that can cause bleeding.

Medicines such as potassium chloride and NSAIDs are notorious for promoting bleeding from small intestine ulcers. The potassium tablets alter local mesenteric circulation, creating ischemic ulcers and eventually stenoses.[102]

Small bowel bleeding also arises from diverticula, aortoenteric fistulas, Dieulafoy lesions, vasculitides, various ulcerative lesions, Zollinger-Ellison syndrome, and a host of other relatively uncommon conditions.[26]

## Prevention of Lower Gastrointestinal Hemorrhage

Hospital admissions for GI bleeding among patients over 65 years of age is about five times more common than for middle-aged adults.[103] Therefore with a growing population of elders, emphasis must be placed on prevention of GI hemorrhage.

As stated earlier, dietary fiber has an influence on bowel habits and intraluminal pressure, potential factors in the development of diverticula, vascular ectasias, and other colonic disorders. Although correction of lifelong eating routines does not eliminate established lesions, it may reduce the progression of disease. Of course, dietary counseling benefits young patients who might not develop these problems in later years.

Some investigators have demonstrated that regular physical activity by the elderly conferred distinct benefits with regard to preventing GI bleeding.[104] Qualifying efforts included walking, gardening, or performing vigorous physical activity at least three times each week. The overall relative risk of a GI hemorrhage among active individuals was 0.7 [95% confidence interval (CI) 0.5–0.9] compared to sedentary members of the cohort. Multivariate analyses determined that this relation was independent of a variety of confounding factors including the usage of β-blockers, ibuprofen, other NSAIDs, aspirin, and coumarin derivatives. Interestingly, more vigorous efforts did not impart greater protective effects. The same group also determined that disabilities and curtailed activities of daily living independently predicted GI hemorrhage with a two- to threefold relative risk.[105] The authors proposed that the association between physical activity and the diminished risk of GI bleeding may be a function of more aerobic capacity, enhanced cardiac output and oxygen delivery, improved gut perfusion, attenuated sympathetic response to stress, decreased risk of atherosclerosis, and less constipation with its inherent risks of diverticular disease, stercoral ulcers, ischemic colitis, and vascular ectasias.

Several medications can provoke GI hemorrhage. For example, among elderly hypertensive patients, calcium channel blockers are associated with a twofold increased relative risk of GI hemorrhage compared to β-blockers.[106] Moreover, potassium supplements can cause small bowel ulcers and bleeding.[102] However, the shear prevalence of the usage of warfarin and NSAIDs poses a larger threat.

Based on several recent reports, an expanding elderly population will receive anticoagulants. One study found a 6-month regimen of oral anticoagulation better than a 6-week course for thromboembolic disease.[107] Furthermore, long-term or lifelong warfarin to maintain the international normalized ratio (INR) between 2.0 and 3.0 seems appropriate for patients with atrial fibrillation to ameliorate the risks of stroke and systemic embolization.[108,109] Because higher INR values are associated with an increased likelihood of hemorrhage,[110] physicians must closely monitor these levels and emphasize the importance of compliance. Although anticoagulated patients are clearly more likely to develop a GI hemorrhage, active or occult bleeding should not be lightly dismissed and left unexamined. A significant number of patients are found to harbor pathology, including a 25% incidence of neoplasms.[111]

An analysis was conducted of series of patients taking low-dose aspirin to prevent ischemic, thromboembolic, or cerebrovascular events.[112] Aspirin was related to an increased chance of GI bleeding [odds ratio (OR) 1.5; 95% CI 1.3–1.7]. Another meta-analysis demonstrated a similar association between NSAIDs and GI hemorrhage in the elderly (OR 5.5; 95% CI 4.6–6.6).[113] The association between aspirin or NSAID usage and UGI bleeding is well established, and adverse effects on the LGI tract have been described.[114] A comparison between adults with LGI complications and matched controls revealed a 2.6 relative risk (95% CI 1.4–4.8) of hemorrhage among those taking aspirin or NSAIDs.[115] A possible mechanism of NSAID-induced damage to the small intestine is nonspecific ulceration or inflammation.[116] A range of NSAID-induced enteropathies of the small and large bowel, including malabsorption, protein loss, and anemia, has also been proposed.[117] Finally, just as anticoagulants can unmask significant pathology, evaluations of overt bleeding or of positive FOBTs are warranted among patients taking NSAIDs. One series revealed GI neoplasms in one-third of patients with occult blood loss.[55]

Physicians must be particularly judicious about prescribing medications to the elderly. Certain drug interactions potentiate the effects of anticoagulants, aspirin, and

NSAIDs. In addition, hepatic and renal dysfunction and diminished lean body mass must be entertained with respect to drug metabolism.

## References


1. Reinus J, Brandt L. Upper and lower gastrointestinal bleeding in the elderly. Gastroenterol Clin North Am 1990;19:293–318.
2. Boley S, DiBiase A, Brandt L, et al. Lower intestinal bleeding in the elderly. Am J Surg 1979;137:57–64.
3. Lieberman D. Gastrointestinal bleeding: initial management. Gastroenterol Clin North Am 1993;22:723–736.
4. Arnaud J, Schloegel M, Ollier J, et al. Colorectal cancer in patients over 80 years of age. Dis Colon Rectum 1991; 34:896–898.
5. Hesterberg R, Schmidt W, Ohmann C, et al. Risk of elective surgery of colorectal carcinoma in the elderly. Dig Surg 1991;8:22–27.
6. Coburn M, Pricolo V, Soderberg C. Factors affecting prognosis and management of carcinoma of the colon and rectum in patients more than eighty years of age. J Am Coll Surg 1994;179:65–69.
7. Hobler K. Colon surgery for cancer in the very elderly. Ann Surg 1986;203:129–131.
8. Nwiloh J, Dardik H, Dardik M, et al. Changing patterns in the morbidity and mortality of colorectal surgery. Am J Surg 1991;162:83–85.
9. Bender J, Magnuson T, Zenilman M, et al. Outcome following colon surgery in the octogenarian. Am Surg 1996;62:276–279.
10. Shoji B, Becker J. Colorectal disease in the elderly patient. Surg Clin North Am 1994;74:293–316.
11. Geokas M, Conteas C, Majumdar A. The aging gastrointestinal tract, liver, and pancreas. Clin Geriatr Med 1985; 1:177–205.
12. Boley S, Sammartano R, Adams A, et al. On the nature and etiology of vascular ectasias of the colon: degenerative lesions of aging. Gastroenterology 1977;72:650–660.
13. Reinus J, Brandt L. Vascular ectasias and diverticulosis: common causes of lower intestinal bleeding. Gastroenterol Clin North Am 1994;23:1–20.
14. Lewis B. Small intestinal bleeding. Gastroenterol Clin North Am 1994;23:67–91.
15. Whiteway J, Morson B. Pathology of ageing: diverticular disease. Clin Gastroenterol 1985;75:829–846.
16. Morson B. Pathology of diverticular disease of the colon. Clin Gastroenterol 1975;4:37–52.
17. Burkitt D. A deficiency of dietary fiber may be one cause of certain colonic and venous disorders. Dig Dis Sci 1976;21:104–108.
18. Wynne-Jones G. Flatus retention is the major factor in diverticular disease. Lancet 1975;2:211–212.
19. Lewis B, Kornbluth A, Waye J. Small bowel tumours: yield of enteroscopy. Gut 1991;32:763–765.
20. Lieberman D. Endoscopic screening for colorectal cancer. Gastroenterol Clin North Am 1997;26:71–83.
21. Fearon E, Vogelstein B. A genetic model for colorectal tumorigenesis. Cell 1990;61:759–767.
22. Dix D. The role of aging in cancer incidence: an epidemiological study. J Gerontol 1989;44:10–18.
23. Gandhi S, Hanson M, Vernava A, et al. Ischemic colitis. Dis Colon Rectum 1996;39:88–100.
24. Reinus J, Brandt L. Lower intestinal bleeding in the elderly. Clin Geriatr Med 1991;7:301–319.
25. Snook J, Holdstock G, Bamforth J. Value of a simple biochemical ratio in distinguishing upper and lower sites of gastrointestinal haemorrhage. Lancet 1986;1:1064–1065.
26. Miller L, Barbarevech C, Friedman L. Less frequent causes of lower gastrointestinal bleeding. Gastroenterol Clin North Am 1994;23:21–52.
27. Nath R, Sequeira J, Weitzman A, et al. Lower gastrointestinal bleeding: diagnostic approach and management conclusions. Am J Surg 1981;141:478–481.
28. Ryan P, Styles C, Chmiel R. Identification of the site of severe colon bleeding by technetium-labeled red-cell scan. Dis Colon Rectum 1992;35:219–222.
29. Smith R, Copely D, Bolen F. $^{99m}$Tc RBC scintigraphy: correlation of gastrointestinal bleeding rates with scintigraphic findings. AJR 1987;148:869–874.
30. Nicholson M, Neoptolemos J, Sharp J, et al. Localization of lower gastrointestinal bleeding using in vivo technetium-99m-labeled red blood cell scintigraphy. Br J Surg 1989; 76:358–361.
31. Zuckerman D, Bocchini T, Birnbaum E. Massive hemorrhage in the lower gastrointestinal tract in adults: diagnostic imaging and intervention. AJR 1993;161:703–711.
32. Hunter J, Pezim M. Limited value of technetium 99m-labeled red cell scintigraphy in localization of lower gastrointestinal bleeding. Am J Surg 1990;159:504–506.
33. McKusick K, Froelich J, Callahan R, et al. $^{99m}$Tc red blood cells for detection of gastrointestinal bleeding: experience with 80 patients. AJR 1981;137:1113–1118.
34. Jensen D, Machicado G. Diagnosis and treatment of severe hematochezia: the role of urgent colonoscopy after purge. Gastroenterology 1988;95:1569–1574.
35. Schrock T. Colonoscopic diagnosis and treatment of lower gastrointestinal bleeding. Surg Clin North Am 1989;69: 1309–1325.
36. Nusbaum M, Baum S. Radiographic demonstration of unknown sites of gastrointestinal bleeding. Surg Forum 1963;14:374–375.
37. Jhangiani S, Pitchumoni C. Gastrointestinal bleeding in elderly patients. Compr Ther 1987;13:17–25.
38. Browder W, Cerise E, Litwin M. Impact of emergency angiography in massive lower gastrointestinal bleeding. Ann Surg 1986;204:530–536.
39. Casarella W, Kanter I, Seaman W. Right-sided colonic diverticula as a cause of acute rectal hemorrhage. N Engl J Med 1972;286:450–453.
40. Boley S, Sprayregen S, Sammartano R, et al. The pathophysiologic basis for the angiographic signs of vascular ectasias of the colon. Radiology 1977;125:615–621.
41. Johnston J, Sones J. Endoscopic heater probe coagulation of the bleeding colonic diverticulum. Gastrointest Endosc 1986;32:160.
42. Chaudhuri T, Brantly M. Heparin as a pharmacologic intervention to induce postive scintiscan in occult gastrointestinal bleeding. Clin Nucl Med 1984;9:187–188.

43. Koval G, Benner K, Rosch J, et al. Aggressive angiographic diagnosis in acute lower gastrointestinal hemorrhage. Dig Dis Sci 1987;32:248–253.
44. Baum S. Pertechnetate imaging following cimetidine administration in Meckel's diverticulum of the ileum. Am J Gastroenterol 1981;76:464–465.
45. Yeker D, Buyukunal C, Benli M, et al. Radionuclide imaging of Meckel's diverticulum: cimetidine versus pentagastrin plus glucagon. Eur J Nucl Med 1984;9:316–319.
46. Retzlaff J, Hagedorn A, Bartholomew L. Abdominal exploration for gastrointestinal bleeding of obscure origin. JAMA 1961;177:104–107.
47. Fazio V, Zelas P, Weakley F. Intraoperative angiography and the localization of bleeding from the small intestine. Surg Gynecol Obstet 1980;151:637–640.
48. Athanasoulis C, Moncure A, Greenfield A, et al. Intraoperative localization of small bowel bleeding sites with combined use of angiographic methods and methylene blue injection. Surgery 1980;87:77–84.
49. Cooperman M, Martin E, Evans W, et al. Use of Doppler ultrasound in intraoperative localization of intestinal arteriovenous malformation. Ann Surg 1979;190:24–26.
50. Biener A, Palestro C, Lewis B, et al. Intraoperative scintigraphy for active small intestinal bleeding. Surg Gynecol Obstet 1990;171:388–392.
51. Bender J, Wiencek R, Bouwman D. Morbidity and mortality following total abdominal colectomy for massive lower gastrointestinal bleeding. Am Surg 1991;57:536–541.
52. Ahlquist D, McGill D, Schwartz S. Fecal blood levels in health and disease: a study using HemoQuant. N Engl J Med 1985;312:1422–1428.
53. Richter J. Occult gastrointestinal bleeding. Gastroenterol Clin North Am 1994;23:53–66.
54. Moses P, Smith R. Endoscopic evaluation of iron deficiency anemia: a guide to diagnostic strategy in older patients. Postgrad Med 1995;98:213–226.
55. Pochapin M, Fine S, Eisorfer R, et al. Fecal occult blood testing in hospitalized patients. J Clin Gastroenterol 1994;19:274–277.
56. Mangla J, Pereira M, Murphy J. Diagnosis of occult gastrointestinal lesions by stool guaiac testing in a geriatric hospital. J Am Geriatr Soc 1981;29:473–475.
57. Wroblewski M, Ostberg H. Ulcer disease among geriatric inpatients with positive faecal occult blood test and/or iron deficiency anaemia: a prospective study. Scand J Gastroenterol 1990;25:489–495.
58. Cook I, Pavli P, Riley J, et al. Gastrointestinal investigation of iron deficiency anemia. BMJ 1986;292:1380–1382.
59. Hershko C, Vitells A, Braverman D. Causes of iron deficiency anemia in an adult inpatient population: effect of diagnostic workup on etiologic distribution. Blut 1984;49: 347–352.
60. Gordon S, Smith R, Power G. The role of endoscopy in the evaluation of iron deficiency anemia in patients over the age of 50. Am J Gastroenterol 1994;89:1963–1967.
61. Rockey D, Cello J. Evaluation of the gastrointestinal tract in patients with iron-deficiency anemia. N Engl J Med 1993;329:1691–1695.
62. Gordon S, Smith R. Long term follow-up of older patients with iron deficiency anemia after a negative gastrointestinal evalution. Gastroenterology 1994;106:A235.
63. Rabe F, Becker G, Besozzi M, et al. Efficacy study of the small-bowel examination. Radiology 1981;140:47–50.
64. Rex D, Lappas J, Maglinte D. Enteroclysis in the evaluation of suspected small intestinal bleeding. Gastroenterology 1989;97:58–60.
65. Foutch P, Sawyer R, Sanowski R. Push-enteroscopy for diagnosis of patients with gastrointestinal bleeding of obscure origin. Gastrointest Endosc 1990;36:337–341.
66. Barkin J, Lewis B, Reiner D, et al. Diagnostic and therapeutic jejunoscopy with a new, longer enteroscope. Gastrointest Endosc 1992;38:55–58.
67. Lewis B, Waye J. Small bowel enteroscopy for obscure GI bleeding. Gastrointest Endosc 1991;37:277.
68. Lewis B, Wenger J, Waye J. Small bowel enteroscopy and intraoperative enteroscopy for obscure gastrointestinal bleeding. Am J Gastroenterol 1991;86:171–174.
69. Lau W, Wong S, Yuen W, et al. Intraoperative enteroscopy for bleeding angiodysplasias of small intestine. Surg Gynecol Obstet 1989;168:341–344.
70. Fenlon H, Ferrucci J. Virtual colonoscopy: what will the issues be? AJR 1997;169:453–458.
71. McGuire H, Haynes B. Massive hemorrhage from diverticulosis of the colon: guidelines for therapy based on bleeding patterns observed in fifty cases. Ann Surg 1972;175:847–855.
72. Horner J. A study of diverticulitis of the colon in office practice. Gastroenterology 1952;21:223–229.
73. Lichtiger S, Kornbluth A, Salomon P, Waye J. Lower gastrointestinal bleeding. In: Taylor M, Gollan J, Peppercorn M, Steer M, Wolfe M (eds) Gastrointestinal Emergencies. Baltimore: Williams & Wilkins, 1992:358–373.
74. Meyers M, Alonso D, Gray G, et al. Pathogenesis of bleeding colonic diverticulosis. Gastroenterology 1976;71:577–583.
75. Heald R, Ray J. Bleeding from diverticula of the colon. Dis Colon Rectum 1971;14:420–427.
76. Wadas D, Sanowski R. Complications of the hot biopsy forceps technique. Gastrointest Endosc 1988;34:32–37.
77. Athanasoulis C, Baum S, Rosch J, et al. Mesenteric arterial infusions of vasopressin for hemorrhage from colonic diverticulosis. Am J Surg 1975;129:212–216.
78. Waltman A. Transcatheter embolization versus vasopressin infusion for the control of arteriocapillary gastrointestinal bleeding. Cardiovasc Intervent Radiol 1980; 3:289–297.
79. Rosch J, Dotter C, Antonovic R. Selective vasoconstrictor infusion in the management of arterio-capillary gastrointestinal hemorrhage. AJR 1972;116:279–288.
80. Parkes B, Obeid F, Sorensen V, et al. The management of massive lower gastrointestinal bleeding. Am Surg 1993; 59:676–678.
81. Richardson J. Vascular lesions of the intestines. Am J Surg 1991;161:284–293.
82. Imperiale T, Ransohoff D. Aortic stenosis, idiopathic gastrointestinal bleeding, and angiodysplasia: is there an association? A methodologic critique of the literature. Gastroenterology 1988;95:1670–1676.
83. Boley S, Brandt L. Vascular ectasias of the colon—1986. Dig Dis Sci 1986;31:26S–42S.
84. Forde K. Therapeutic colonoscopy. World J Surg 1992;16: 1048–1053.

85. Hunter J. Endoscopic laser applications in the gastrointestinal tract. Surg Clin North Am 1989;69:1147–1166.
86. Church J. Angiodysplasia. Semin Colon Rectal Surg 1994; 5:43:49.
87. Brandt L. A cecal angiodysplastic lesion is discovered during diagnostic colonoscopy performed for iron-deficiency anemia associated with stool positive for occult blood: what therapy would you recommend? Am J Gastroenterol 1988;83:710–711.
88. Aldabagh S, Trujillo Y, Taxy J. Utility of specimen angiography in angiodysplasia of the colon. Gastroenterology 1986;91:725–729.
89. Lewis B, Salomon P, Rivera-MacMurray S, et al. Does hormonal therapy have any benefit for bleeding angiodysplasia? J Clin Gastroenterol 1992;15:99–103.
90. Abel M, Rosen L, Kodner I, et al. Practice parameters for the treatment of rectal carcinoma: supporting documentation. Dis Colon Rectum 1993;36:991–1006.
91. Brandt L. Colitis in the elderly. Am J Gastroenterol 1992; 87:692–695.
92. Zimmerman J, Gavish D, Rachmilewitz D. Early and late onset ulcerative colitis: distinct clinical features. J Clin Gastroenterol 1985;7:492–498.
93. Griffin P, Ostroff S, Tauxe R, et al. Illnesses associated with Escherichia coli 0157:H7 infections: a broad clinical spectrum. Ann Intern Med 1988;109:705–712.
94. Kelly C, Pothoulakis C, LaMont J. Clostridium difficile colitis. N Engl J Med 1994;330:257–262.
95. Deitel M, Vasic V. Major intestinal complications of radiotherapy. Am J Gastroenterol 1979;72:65–70.
96. Coia L, Myerson R, Tepper J. Late effects of radiation therapy on the gastrointestinal tract. Int J Radiat Oncol Biol Phys 1995;31:1213–1236.
97. Glotzer D, Glick M, Goldman H. Proctitis and colitis following diversion of the fecal stream. Gastroenterology 1981;80:438–431.
98. Harig J, Soergel K, Komorowski R, et al. Treatment of diversion colitis with short-chain fatty acid irrigation. N Engl J Med 1989;320:23–28.
99. Rosen L, Bub D, Reed J, et al. Hemorrhage following colonoscopic polypectomy. Dis Colon Rectum 1993;36: 1126–1131.
100. Ashley S, Wells S. Tumors of the small intestine. Semin Oncol 1988;15:116–128.
101. Farmer R, Hawk W, Turnbull R. Clinical patterns in Crohn's disease: a statistical study of 615 cases. Gastroenterology 1975;68:627–635.
102. Boley S, Allen A, Schultz L, et al. Potassium-induced lesions of the small bowel. JAMA 1965;193:997–1000.
103. US Department of Health and Human Services. Vital and Health Statistics: Detailed Diagnoses and Procedures, National Hospital Discharge Survey, 1988. Hyattsville, MD: Public Health Service, Centers for Disease Control, 1991.
104. Pahor M, Guralnik J, Salive M, et al. Physical activity and risk of severe gastrointestinal hemorrhage in older persons. JAMA 1994;272:595–599.
105. Pahor M, Guralnik J, Salive M, et al. Disability and severe gastrointestinal hemorrhage: a prospective study of community-dwelling older persons. J Am Geriatr Soc 1994; 42:816–825.
106. Pahor M, Guralnik J, Furberg C, et al. Risk of gastrointestinal hemorrhage with calcium antagonists in hypertensive persons over 67 years old. Lancet 1996;347: 1061–1065.
107. Schulman S, Rhedin A, Lindmarker P, et al. A comparison of six weeks with six months of oral anticoagulant therapy after a first episode of venous thromboembolism. N Engl J Med 1995;332:1661–1665.
108. Stroke Prevention in Atrial Fibrillation Investigators. Adjusted-dose warfarin versus low-intensity, fixed-dose warfarin plus aspirin for high-risk patients with atrial fibrillation: Stroke Prevention in Atrial Fibrillation III randomized clinical trial. Lancet 1996;348:633–638.
109. Hylek E, Skates S, Sheehan M, et al. An analysis of the lowest effective intensity of prophylactic anticoagulation for patients with nonrheumatic atrial fibrillation. N Engl J Med 1996;335:540–546.
110. Fihn S, McDonell M, Martin D, et al. Risk factors for complications of chronic anticoagulation: a multicenter study. Ann Intern Med 1993;118:511–520.
111. Jaffin B, Bliss C, LaMont T. Significance of occult gastrointestinal bleeding during anticoagulation therapy. Am J Med 1987;83:269–272.
112. Stalnikowicz-Darvasi R. Gastrointestinal bleeding during low-dose aspirin administration for prevention of arterial occlusive events: a critical analysis. J Clin Gastroenterol 1995;21:13–16.
113. Gabriel S, Jaakkimainen L, Bombardier C. Risk for serious gastrointestinal complications related to use of nonsteroidal anti-inflammatory drugs: a meta-analysis. Ann Intern Med 1991;115:787–796.
114. Kessler W, Shires G, Fahey T. Surgical complications of nonsteroidal antiinflammatory drug-induced small bowel ulceration. J Am Coll Surg 1997;185:250–254.
115. Langman M, Morgan L, Worrall A. Use of anti-inflammatory drugs by patients admitted with small or large bowel perforations and haemorrhage. BMJ 1985; 290:347–349.
116. Allison M, Howatson A, Torrance C, et al. Gastrointestinal damage associated with the use of nonsteroidal antiinflammatory drugs. N Engl J Med 1992;327:749–754.
117. Bjarnason I, Hayllar J, MacPherson A, et al. Side effects of nonsteroidal anti-inflammatory drugs on the small and large intestine in humans. Gastroenterology 1993;104: 1832–1847.

# 42 Ischemic Disorders of the Large and Small Bowel

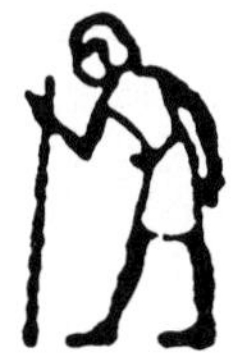

Jeffrey M. Reilly and Gregorio A. Sicard

Intestinal ischemia is usually a disease that affects the elderly. It is useful to categorize it as acute or chronic because of the different presentations of patients and the urgency of treatment. It can also be further subdivided by etiology; causes include arterial insufficiency secondary to thrombosis or embolus, venous thrombosis, and nonocclusive mesenteric ischemia.

To understand the etiology of mesenteric ischemia, it is helpful to review the basic vascular anatomy of the gastrointestinal (GI) tract. The gut is supplied basically by three arteries: celiac axis, superior mesenteric artery, and inferior mesenteric artery. The celiac axis branches almost immediately into the common hepatic, left gastric, and splenic arteries. The celiac axis communicates with the superior mesenteric artery recirculation via the gastroduodenal artery and the pancreaticoduodenal arcades. The superior mesenteric artery originates from the aorta usually approximately 1 cm below the celiac axis. This occurs at the level of the L1 vertebra. The superior mesenteric artery supplies the mid-gut, and its major branches are the inferior pancreaticoduodenal branches, middle colic artery, right colic artery, ileal branches, and ileocolic artery. The middle colic artery comes off the proximal superior mesenteric artery and supplies the transverse colon. It also communicates directly with branches of the inferior mesenteric artery. The ileocolic artery is the terminal branch of the superior mesenteric artery and supplies the terminal ileum, cecum, and ascending colon. The inferior mesenteric artery is the most distal and smallest of the mesenteric arteries and is also a ventral branch of the aorta. It arises approximately 6–7 cm below the superior mesenteric artery, which corresponds to the level of the L3 vertebra. It supplies the hind gut, which includes the distal transverse colon, descending colon, sigmoid colon, and rectum. The left colic artery communicates with the superior mesenteric artery via the marginal artery.

To understand the pathophysiology of mesenteric ischemia, it is important to understand the anatomic collateral pathways. For collateral circulation between the celiac axis and the superior mesenteric artery, the principal pathways are the gastroduodenal and pancreaticoduodenal arteries. Unusual anatomic variations can also provide collateral flow, such as a replaced right hepatic artery or a pancreatic or middle colic artery originating from the celiac axis. Additionally, there is an infrequent but well-recognized collateral pathway known as the arc of Buhler, which represents a direct collateral pathway between the celiac artery and the superior mesenteric artery. This is thought to be due to persistence of an embryonic ventral segment artery.

There are three major anastomotic pathways between the superior mesenteric artery and the inferior mesenteric artery, the most significant of which is the marginal artery of Drummond. This artery runs within the mesentery of the colon and gives rise to the vasa recta. It receives branches from the ileocolic, right colic, middle colic, and the left colic arteries. It usually runs close to the mesenteric border of the colon. Normally, this artery is not particularly large; but with occlusion of the superior mesenteric artery, it can enlarge significantly. The arc of Riolan also lies within the mesentery, but is much closer to its base. This collateral connects the middle and left colic arteries. The final potential collateral pathway between the superior and inferior mesenteric arteries is the meandering or wandering mesenteric artery. Occasionally this is a markedly hypertrophied arc of Riolan, and other times there is a distinct anastomotic pathway between the superior and mesenteric arteries. The inferior mesenteric artery can be collateralized not only by the superior mesenteric artery but also by branches from the lumbar branches of the aorta, as well as from the internal iliac artery and its branches.

The venous drainage of the gut is principally via the splenic vein for the foregut, the superior mesenteric vein for the midgut, and the inferior mesenteric vein for the hindgut. These vessels all drain into the portal vein and hence through the liver.

Mesenteric blood vessels are highly reactive; and, accordingly, mesenteric blood flow can fluctuate between

10% and 35% of cardiac output.[1] They react to a large variety of endogenous cytokines and exogenous medications. The teleologic reason given for the vasoreactivity is the widely varying metabolic needs of the gut based on the fasting and fed states. Absolute blood flow through the celiac axis and the superior mesenteric artery ranges from 300 to 1200 ml/min.[1–4] At rest (fasting state) the mesenteric flow is low due to high resistance with low diastolic flow with flow reversal, which is typical of high resistance beds. In the fed state there is both systolic and continuous diastolic flow.

Although the nutritional state of the individual is often the principal determinant of blood flow, there is also extensive extrinsic and intrinsic control of splanchnic blood flow. Sympathetic tone to the gut is supplied by preganglionic cholinergic fibers of the greater splanchnic nerves.[5] These synapse in the paired celiac ganglia next to the celiac axis. Postganglionic adrenergic fiber stimulation of the celiac axis ganglia results in vasoconstriction of the mesenteric arteries and arterioles.[6,7] The renin-angiotensin axis and vasopressin can both cause profound vasoconstriction. These substances are released in settings of hypovolemia.[7,8] The net effect of their secretion is to preserve cerebral and renal circulation at the expense of the mesenteric circulation.

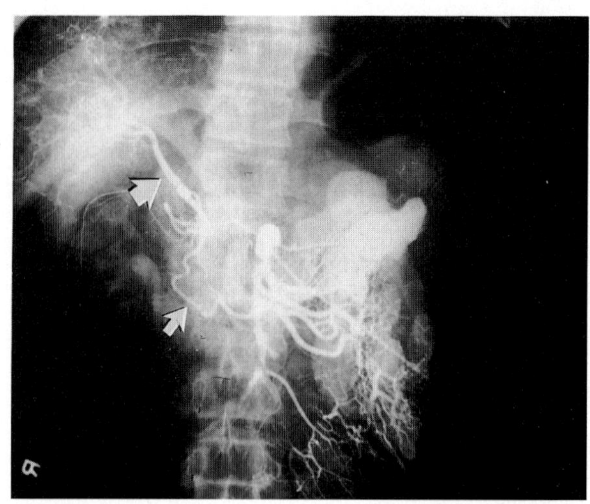

FIGURE 42.1. Selective superior mesenteric artery (SMA) arteriogram of patient with abdominal pain and a type B aortic dissection. Note the dissection of the SMA with incomplete filling of the branches. Note also filling of the right hepatic artery (large arrow) through the pancreatic duodenal arcade (small arrow) as a result of the dissection and obstruction of the celiac axis.

## Acute Mesenteric Ischemia

The most dramatic and feared form of mesenteric ischemia is *acute* mesenteric ischemia. Despite broad advances in diagnostic capabilities, surgical techniques, and perioperative management, the mortality associated with acute mesenteric ischemia is high ranging from 60% to 90% in most series.[9,10] The risk factors for acute mesenteric ischemia are essentially those associated with advancing age, including cardiac arrhythmias, low cardiac output states secondary to congestive heart failure, severe valvular cardiac disease or recent myocardial infarction, generalized atherosclerosis, and intraabdominal malignancy.

Acute arterial insufficiency to the small bowel results from occlusion of the superior mesenteric artery (SMA). Approximately 50% of acute SMA occlusions are due to emboli, and an additional 25% of cases are secondary to in situ thrombosis superimposed on preexisting atherosclerotic lesions.[11] Other, more unusual causes include dissection of the SMA occurring in isolation or as part of extensive aortic dissection (Fig. 42.1).[12–14]

Another cause of acute mesenteric ischemia is nonocclusive mesenteric ischemia (NOMI), which accounts for the remainder of cases of acute intestinal ischemia. The cause of NOMI is usually a low-flow state in the setting of preexisting atherosclerotic lesions, often coupled with the administration of vasoconstricting medications or digitalis.

Acute arterial embolization is the most common cause of acute mesenteric ischemia, and most of the emboli are cardiac in origin. They originate from left atrial or ventricular mural thrombi or from cardiac valvular lesions. They often occur in the setting of cardiac arrhythmias, particularly atrial fibrillation, or immediately following acute myocardial infarction. Although the emboli can lodge at the origin of the SMA, approximately 85% lodge more distally, usually 3–10 cm beyond the origin of the SMA where it begins to taper. The typical point of occlusion is just distal to the middle colic artery. It is important to realize that in approximately 20% of cases patients with SMA emboli also have emboli to other beds.[15] Often the intestinal ischemia caused by the embolus is exacerbated or compounded by reflexive mesenteric vasoconstriction. This compounds the ischemic insult to the bowel.

Acute mesenteric arterial thrombosis occurs in the setting where patients have acute thrombosis superimposed on preexisting high-grade atherosclerotic lesions. Although the SMA is most commonly affected, the celiac axis may be involved. Often even though these patients present acutely, on questioning they give a history consistent with chronic mesenteric ischemia. Anatomically, these lesions usually occur at the origin of the SMA and not distally, as with embolic disease. Substantial weight loss secondary to "food fear" is common. Food fear refers to the fact that patients do not eat because when they do they incur intestinal angina. Additionally, the patients may complain of diarrhea.

As mentioned previously, mesenteric ischemia does not necessarily occur in the setting of an occlusive lesion.

It can occur during periods of low mesenteric blood flow, which can be exacerbated in the setting of preexisting atherosclerotic occlusive lesions. The causes of these low-flow states were enumerated earlier but are most often seen in the setting of cardiac failure, sepsis, or with administration of digitalis or other vasoconstrictive drugs. The diagnosis of NOMI is based on a high index of clinical suspicion followed by arteriography. It requires an even higher index of suspicion than other causes of acute mesenteric ischemia because the presentation is sometimes more insidious. Mortality in the setting of NOMI is high and reflects not only the morbidity associated with mesenteric ischemia but probably more likely the underlying medical conditions that precipitated the episode of mesenteric ischemia.[16]

The first case of NOMI was described at autopsy when it was recognized that there were patients with a small intestinal infarction but without arterial or venous occlusive lesions.[17,18] It is estimated that NOMI is the underlying cause in approximately 25% of cases of acute mesenteric ischemia, and its mortality is approximately 70%.[19–21] The incidence of NOMI is decreasing despite the general aging of the population. The likely reasons are the widespread use of systemic vasodilators in coronary care units and the improved treatment of cardiogenic shock.[22] The best chance for avoiding poor clinical outcome with NOMI resides in making the correct diagnosis and treating the underlying precipitating cause of the NOMI. It has been postulated that low flow results in peripheral hypoxemia and a paradoxical splanchnic vasospasm, which precipitates intestinal ischemia. Laboratory studies have confirmed that mesenteric vasoconstriction, intestinal hypoxia, and ischemia/reperfusion injury may play a role in the pathogenesis of NOMI. In low-flow states the neurohormonal mediators of mesenteric vasoconstriction appear to be vasopressin and angiotensin.[22,23]

The precipitating event for NOMI is usually cardiogenic or hypovolemic shock. In an attempt to maintain homeostasis, there is peripheral and splanchnic vasoconstriction. The use of digoxin is common in patients with NOMI, and in in vitro and in vivo studies it has been shown to enhance mesenteric arterial vasoconstriction.[24,25] Once set in motion, mesenteric vasospasm can become persistent, even after correcting the underlying precipitating event. The persistence of prolonged vasoconstriction is responsible for the development of intestinal ischemia and subsequent infarction in NOMI.[26] The treatment of NOMI is complicated by the fact that correction of the vasospasm may result in a reperfusion injury to the bowel.[27]

As with other forms of mesenteric ischemia, the key to improved patient outcome is diagnosis in a timely fashion. It requires a high index of suspicion. This diagnosis should be entertained when *elderly patients* present with the risk factors previously mentioned, including acute myocardial infarction with cardiogenic shock, congestive heart failure, arrhythmias, hypovolemic shock from sepsis, or hemorrhage or in the setting of burns and pancreatitis. Additionally, the use of splanchnic vasoconstrictors including digitalis and α-agonists, are commonly seen in patients who develop NOMI. Although patients with SMA occlusion usually present with pain out of proportion to their physical findings, a significant portion of patients with NOMI (20–25%) may not have severe abdominal pain.[28] When present, the pain is often less severe or more variable in intensity, character, and location than it is in classic occlusive arterial mesenteric ischemia. Even in patients without pain, if there is unexplained abdominal distension, GI bleeding, fever, diarrhea, nausea, or vomiting, the diagnosis of NOMI should be entertained. As with other forms of mesenteric ischemia, once a patient develops abdominal tenderness or localized peritonitis, it indicates that the mesenteric ischemia has progressed to transmural bowel infarction.

Obviously, early diagnosis is of critical importance. Laboratory tests, although often abnormal, are nonspecific. Leukocytosis is common, as is hemoconcentration secondary to extracellular fluid loss.[29] As with other forms of intestinal ischemia, metabolic acidosis, with a rise in serum glutamic oxaloacetic transaminase (SGOT), lactate dehydrogenase (LDH), and creatinine phosphokinase (CPK), occurs late in the course of intestinal ischemia, as does a rise in serum amylase and hyperphosphatemia. These are usually indicative of irreversible ischemia with bowel infarction.[30]

Although plain films of the abdomen may be useful in helping to exclude other causes of abdominal pain, such as a small bowel obstruction or a perforated viscus, a normal radiographic study does not rule out intestinal ischemia. In the setting of abdominal pain with normal radiographs, a diagnosis of NOMI must be entertained. Plain films can be abnormal, but they are usually only suggestive of mesenteric ischemia. Nonspecific findings include ileus, bowel wall edema, thumbprinting; and late in the course of the disease process, once intestinal infarction has occurred, pneumatosis or portal venous air may be observed. With NOMI, plain films are suggestive of intestinal ischemia in only 20–60% of the cases.[31] As mentioned earlier, definitive diagnosis and treatment of nonocclusive mesenteric ischemia relies on mesenteric angiography prior to the onset of intestinal infarction and necrosis.[32]

Four diagnostic criteria were described by Sigelman et al. with the diagnosis of nonocclusive mesenteric ischemia[33]: (1) narrowing of the origins of multiple branches of the superior mesenteric artery; (2) alternative dilatation and narrowing of the intestinal branches ("string of sausages" sign); (3) spasm of the mesenteric arteries; and (4) delayed filling of intramural vessels. Once the diagnosis is made by angiography, intraarterial papaverine into the SMA is started with the usual dose

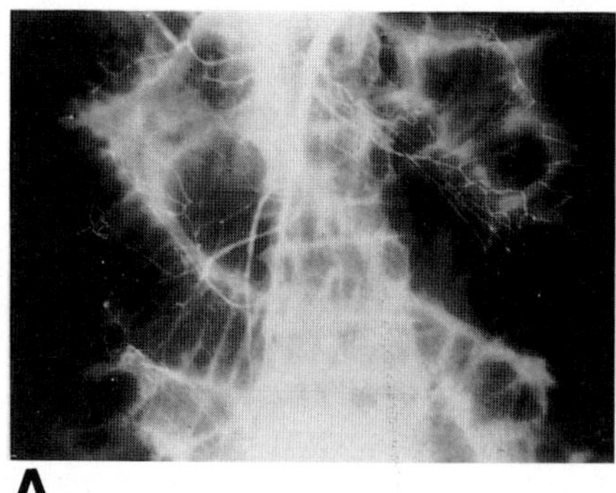


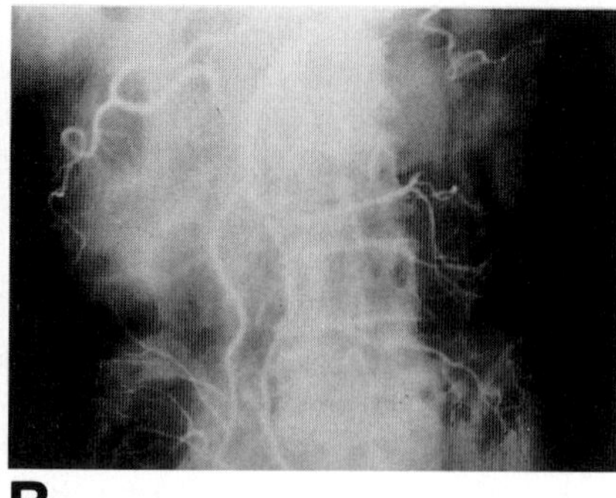


FIGURE 42.2. A. Selective superior mesenteric artery (SMA) arteriogram in a patient with nonocclusive mesenteric ischemia (NOMI). Note the significant vasoconstriction of all branches. B. Repeat SMA arteriogram (1 hour) after selective infusion of papaverine at 40 mg/hr. Note the vasodilatation of the mesenteric branches.

range of 30–60 mg/hr (Fig. 42.2). The patient's response to vasodilator therapy is monitored by clinical and angiographic criteria. Of importance is that there is resolution of abdominal pain. Arteriography should be repeated to document that the vasospasm has been broken. Once the vasospasm is broken, papaverine treatment should continue for another 24 hours. It is important to monitor carefully patients receiving intraarterial vasodilator therapy, as marked hypotension can result. These patients obviously must be cared for in an intensive care unit (ICU).

The indications for surgical intervention remain the same even in the setting of papaverine infusion. If there is an increasing leukocytosis, evidence of GI bleeding, free intraabdominal air, or the development of peritonitis, immediate exploratory laparotomy is warranted. At the time of surgery for nonocclusive mesenteric ischemia, the aims of the operation are the same as for any other cause of bowel ischemia. Simply, the goals are to (1) assess the amount of viable bowel left; (2) resect any necrotic bowel; and (3) decide whether a second-look laparotomy should be performed within 24 hours. If there is any question about the viability of the bowel, exteriorization of the bowel is recommended, as well as second-look laparotomy. Even in the setting of segmental infarction development, it is recommended that papaverine infusion continue. Unlike the setting of embolic mesenteric ischemia, systemic anticoagulation is not required for NOMI. This current treatment regimen is frequently successful, and often the underlying morbidity and mortality in these patients are not related to the nonocclusive mesenteric ischemia but to the disease states that precipitated it.

## Mesenteric Venous Thrombosis

Mesenteric venous thrombosis is the least common form of mesenteric ischemia. It currently accounts for only 5–15% of all cases of mesenteric ischemia.[34–36] As with arterial ischemia, mesenteric venous thrombosis can be divided into acute and chronic presentations. Acute mesenteric venous thrombosis is a process in which the patient presents with less than 4 weeks of symptoms. Patients who present with more than 4 weeks of symptoms without evidence of bowel infarction, or those who have a diagnosis of mesenteric venous thrombosis made incidentally and it is clinically insignificant, are classified as having chronic mesenteric venous thrombosis.[37]

The etiology of mesenteric venous thrombosis is classified into one of two categories: primary or secondary. Primary mesenteric venous thrombosis is a spontaneous, idiopathic event with thrombosis of the mesenteric veins that is not associated with any other disease process or a hypocoagulable state.[38] The frequency of this diagnosis has decreased with the improved ability to diagnose hypercoagulable states. The conditions associated with secondary mesenteric venous thrombosis are hypercoagulability, malignancy, cirrhosis, splenomegaly, intraabdominal infection, trauma, and pancreatitis. The hypercoagulable states are usually related to hematologic disorders and include protein C and S deficiency, antithrombin III deficiency, dysfibrinogenemia, abnormal plasminogen, polycythemia vera, thrombocytosis, sickle cell disease, and more recently, factor V Leiden mutation.[39–42]

Although patients with acute mesenteric venous thrombosis can present with a picture similar to that of acute arterial thrombosis, their presentation is usually not as dramatic and the symptoms not as severe. There is less incidence of bowel infarction. Because of this more protean presentation, there is often a delay in diagnosis. This delay is a major contributory factor to the relatively high mortality reported in the literature secondary to mesenteric venous thrombosis.[36,43–47] Patients usually present with a several-day to several-week history of diffuse, nonspecific, and often intermittent abdominal pain. Typically, these symptoms are gradually progressive. Aside from abdominal pain, other symptoms occur much less frequently. Physical findings are often vague, with abdominal distension being the most common, but is seen in only approximately 50% of patients. Peritonitis is present only in advanced cases that have progressed to bowel infarction.

As with nonocclusive mesenteric ischemia, laboratory tests are usually not helpful for diagnosing acute mesenteric venous ischemia. Leukocytosis is seen in some patients, as are elevated amylase and LDH levels; but once again this is in the setting of mesenteric infarction.

Mesenteric venous thrombosis is diagnosed by radiographic means. Plain abdominal films are usually nonspecific and help little with the diagnosis. The most common finding is a nonspecific ileus.[36] Computed tomography (CT) scanning has proved to be the most sensitive diagnostic test for mesenteric venous thrombosis. CT scanning accurately identified thrombus within the superior mesenteric vein and the portal vein.[48,49] Magnetic resonance imaging (MRI) has also proved to be sensitive.[50] Duplex scanning of the mesenteric veins can be performed as well but has a slightly lower sensitivity than CT scanning.[36] Unlike with other forms of mesenteric ischemia, mesenteric arteriography has proved not to be diagnostically sensitive. Evidence of venous thrombosis can be seen on the venous phase of a selective SMA injection. As with other forms of mesenteric ischemia, any patient who presents with evidence of peritonitis or other signs of bowel infarction, should undergo exploratory laparotomy. If mesenteric venous thrombosis is diagnosed prior to surgery, anticoagulation with intravenous heparin should be instituted immediately. If it is diagnosed at the time of laparotomy, heparin should be administered immediately.

The guidelines for bowel resection are the same as with any other form of mesenteric ischemia. Frankly necrotic segments are excised. If there are questionable areas, a second-look laparotomy is performed. In general, venous thrombectomy is not recommended, as it is almost uniformly unsuccessful; although it may be indicated in a few select circumstances, such as when it can be clearly documented that there is thrombus within the superior mesenteric vein within 1–3 days of the initial symptoms.[51] More recently, thrombolytic therapy has been used, but its efficacy is unclear, and its use remains controversial.[52,53] In patients who do not present with peritonitis or who have evidence of bowel necrosis, optimal management consists of anticoagulation and observation. Anticoagulation with intravenous heparin acutely is followed by chronic anticoagulation with warfarin (Coumadin). It is recommended that this regimen continue for the life of the patient.[44] Once again the mortality is usually related to a delay in diagnosis of mesenteric ischemia.

Treatment of mesenteric venous thrombosis is more successful than that of acute arterial thrombosis, but it still has a high mortality. This success is attributed to improved diagnosis and the recognition that lifelong anticoagulation is indicated. The outcome of these patients has recently improved. In the Mayo Clinic experience,[37] chronic anticoagulation was associated with improved survival compared to the survival of those who did not undergo anticoagulation. The underlying cause of the mesenteric venous thrombosis does not appear to affect the survival. Additionally, the recurrence rate tends to remain generally high, and recurrence is usually during the acute hospitalization or within 30 days of surgery.[37]

Chronic mesenteric venous thrombosis is different from acute mesenteric venous thrombosis. Patients usually present only with vague abdominal pain or slight distension. The most frequent presentation is asymptomatic, with the theombosis being an incidental finding on diagnostic imaging for another complaint. No specific therapy is generally indicated.

## Chronic Arterial Mesenteric Ischemia

Chronic mesenteric ischemia is a relatively rare diagnosis, and there is a paucity of surgical literature involving its treatment. This being said, it appears that the number of elective operations for chronic mesenteric ischemia is increasing; and given the general aging of the population, it is expected that it will continue to increase.[54] Chronic mesenteric ischemia is most common during late middle age, with the typical patient being approximately 58 years old at the time of presentation.[55] Most patients who present are smokers; and in contradistinction to vascular disease in other beds, most of the patients (60%) are female. Additionally, there is a high incidence of other factors for vascular disease including a high incidence of hypertension, coronary artery disease, and cerebrovascular disease.[56] It is interesting to note that, although clinically significant chronic mesenteric ischemia is uncommon, asymptomatic atherosclerosis of the mesenteric circulation is common, with autopsy series showing significant stenoses in approximately 50% of celiac axes, in 30% of the superior mesenteric arteries, and in 30% of inferior mesenteric arteries.[57,58] The prevalance of mesenteric atherosclerotic disease increases with age, with two-thirds of patients over 80 years of age having significant stenoses.

Councilman's report was the first to recognize the syndrome of chronic mesenteric ischemia with its pathognomonic symptom of postprandial pain.[59] He described three patients who presented with epigastric and midabdominal pain following eating. Typically, this pain occurs 1–2 hours after a meal. The degree of pain correlates well with the quantity and the fat content of the ingested meal. Although the pain is typically described as a dull, crampy pain, there is some variability in presentation, with symptoms ranging from vague pain to severe sharp pains that can penetrate to the back.[60] In advanced cases, patients may have persistent or continuous pain, and sometimes it progresses to acute mesenteric ischemia (in situ thrombosis of mesenteric vessels in the setting of advanced occlusive disease).[61] Because of the postprandial pain, the patients often experience what has been termed "food fear." Food fear results in the patient being unwilling to eat, which in turn results in the most common physical finding of chronic mesenteric ischemia: weight loss. The weight loss has been described as malignant cachexia without malignancy. Frequently these patients have been evaluated for a GI malignancy prior to making the correct diagnosis of mesenteric ischemia.[60] It is worthwhile to note, however, that a few patients present without weight loss. Presenting symptoms other than abdominal pain and weight loss that are also GI in nature, include nausea, vomiting, diarrhea, and constipation. It is thought that the symptoms may relate to the distribution of the vascular occlusive disease, with foregut ischemia (celiac distribution) leading to nausea and vomiting, midgut ischemia (superior mesenteric artery) leading to the common postprandial abdominal pain and subsequent weight loss, and hindgut ischemia leading to constipation (inferior mesenteric artery).[62]

On physical examination the most obvious finding in patients with chronic mesenteric ischemia is evidence of weight loss. Signs of peripheral vascular disease may also be noted and the presence of an abdominal bruit.

The diagnosis of chronic mesenteric ischemia is often delayed. Because of the nonspecific symptoms with which patients present, they are often evaluated for other diseases including cholecystitis, liver disease, peptic ulcer disease, and occult malignancy.[54,60] As with acute mesenteric ischemia, the diagnosis of chronic mesenteric ischemia requires a high index of clinical suspicion. Often these patients have undergone extensive evaluations prior to being referred to a vascular surgeon for evaluation. Due to the prolonged nature of their illnesses, nonspecific laboratory findings may include evidence of malnutrition, such as anemia, hypoalbumenemia, hypocholesterolemia, and evidence of impaired immune function. Patients have frequently undergone both plain and contrast radiologic studies of their abdomen and GI tract, but these tests are of little value. They have also often undergone both upper and lower GI endoscopy, which occasionally documents evidence of ischemia.[62] The key to making the diagnosis is documenting occlusive lesions involving the mesenteric vessels. Among the noninvasive studies available, duplex scanning has been used to assess the mesenteric circulation. However, this test is dependent on the expertise of the person performing the test, and it is often limited by overlying bowel gas or the presence of significant obesity. Findings on the duplex scan suggestive of significant stenoses include a peak systolic velocity of more than 275 cm/s in the SMA and 200 cm/s in the celiac artery. Additional findings include evidence of poststenotic turbulence as well as retrograde flow in the hepatic artery, which is suggestive of occlusion or high grade stenosis of the celiac artery.[63,64] At present it is only in centers of expertise that duplex scanning appears to be a fairly specific and sensitive test for screening patients for superior mesenteric and celiac artery stenoses.[64,65] Once a diagnosis is suspected and surgical intervention is being contemplated, contrast angiography is necessary.

Magnetic resonance imaging is also under investigation, but at present it does not have widespread applicability.[66] Therefore, arteriography with selective injection of the mesenteric vessels is the critical test for diagnosing mesenteric ischemia and for planning any revascularization. To document stenoses of the origins of the superior mesenteric artery and celiac axes, lateral views are best (Figs. 42.3, 42.4). Usually involvement of at least two mesenteric vessels is required to diagnose symptomatic chronic mesenteric ischemia. It is unusual for a patient to be symptomatic from occlusion of only one vessel. Additional evidence of chronic ischemia is evidenced by hypertrophy of collateral pathways including the marginal artery of Drummod and the arc of Rioland (Fig. 42.5).

Because the natural history of symptomatic mesenteric ischemia is one of progressive malnutrition, weight loss, and possible progression to visceral infarction, vascular reconstruction is generally indicated. If the patient is an acceptable operative risk, mesenteric revascularization is indicated.[67] Simply stated, the indication for mesenteric revascularization is the presence of symptomatic chronic mesenteric ischemia. The ultimate goal is to restore a normal mesenteric circulation, thereby allowing normalization of the nutritional status and alleviation of abdominal pain. Three basic techniques are available for revascularization: bypass grafting, transaortic endarterectomy, and more recently, angioplasty. The choice of therapy must be individualized not only to the patient's anatomic lesions but also to the patient's comorbidities. The ideal procedure for chronic mesenteric ischemia remains a subject of debate.[68] Preoperative evaluation of patients for mesenteric revascularization is no different from preparing for any other major vascular reconstruction. As indicated by the patient's general medical condition, he or she should be evaluated for coronary artery disease, cerebrovascular disease, or renal vascular disease.

It is important to realize also that these patients are often nutritionally debilitated and as a result are both volume-contracted and anemic. These conditions should be approached in an urgent, aggressive manner prior to surgery. Because of the high incidence of multisystem disease, invasive intraoperative monitoring with radial artery and pulmonary artery catheters is recommended. As part of this goal, it is hoped that the progression of mesenteric ischemia to visceral infarction is avoided as well. In unusual circumstances, prophylactic mesenteric revascularization is undertaken in patients undergoing major aortic reconstruction who have had incidentally identified significant mesenteric artery stenoses.[58] The rationale for doing this is that the patient may be at increased risk for perioperative visceral infarction due to

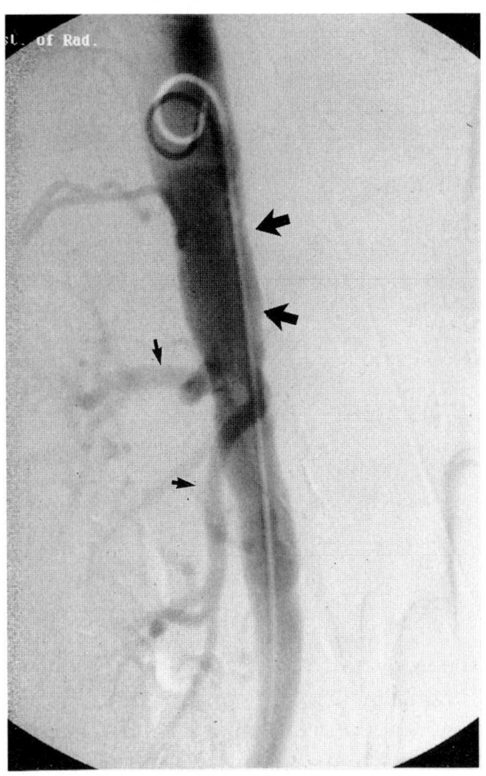


FIGURE 42.3. Lateral aortogram of a patient with acute mesenteric ischemia showing complete occlusion of the celiac axis and superior mesenteric artery (large arrows). Note the patent renal arteries (small arrows).

unexpected hypovolemia, hypotension, or disruption of the collateral circulation by the periaortic dissection. In the absence of performing aortic procedures, prophylactic mesenteric revascularization is not usually recommended. As previously noted, mesenteric artery occlusive disease is widely present in autopsy series, but most of it was asymptomatic.

Several techniques are available for performing mesenteric bypasses. Because mesenteric ischemia usually results from multiple-vessel disease, multiple-vessel reconstruction is usually recommended. Bypasses are generally categorized into two broad techniques: antegrade and retrograde. Antegrade bypass grafts generally originate from the supraceliac aorta, which is an excellent site for originating a bypass graft because it is usually spared significant atherosclerotic or aneurysmal disease. Autologous material or synthetic grafts can be used without any documented difference in efficacy. Polytetrafluoroethylene (PTFE) and Dacron grafts have been used (Fig. 42.6). If there is any question of contamination at the time of surgery (e.g., if bowel resection is necessary) an autologous conduit, usually the saphenous vein, should be used.

The supraceliac aorta is usually exposed transabdominally, which can be done through either a midline incision or bilateral subcostal incisions. After thorough exploration of the abdomen, the supraceliac aorta is exposed by first mobilizing the lateral segment of the left lobe of the liver, which is retracted inferiorly and to the right. The gastrohepatic omentum is divided and the lesser sac entered. Care is taken not to injure the esophagus, which is easily identified by palpating the

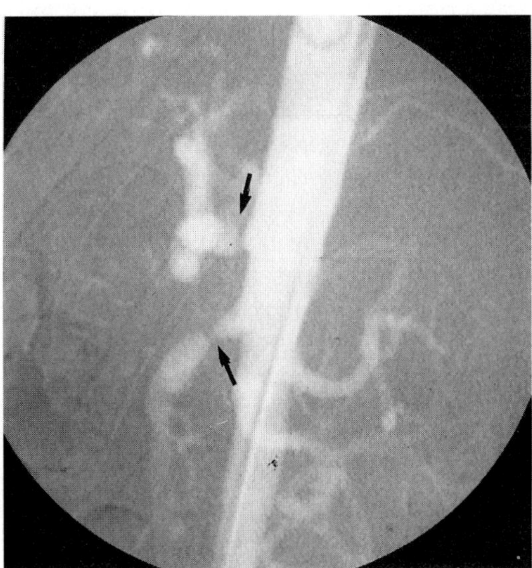

FIGURE 42.4. Lateral superior mesenteric arteriogram of a patient with chronic mesenteric ischemia. Note the high grade stenosis of the celiac axis and superior mesenteric artery (arrows).

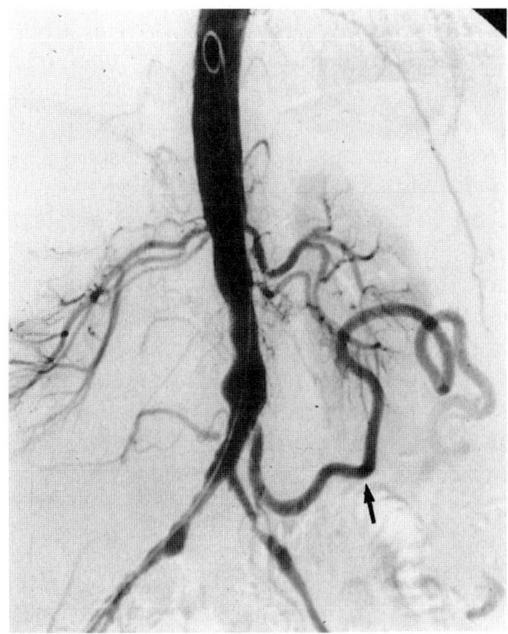

FIGURE 42.5. Anteroposterior aortogram showing a meandering artery (arrow) from the inferior mesenteric artery in patient with chronic mesenteric ischemia.

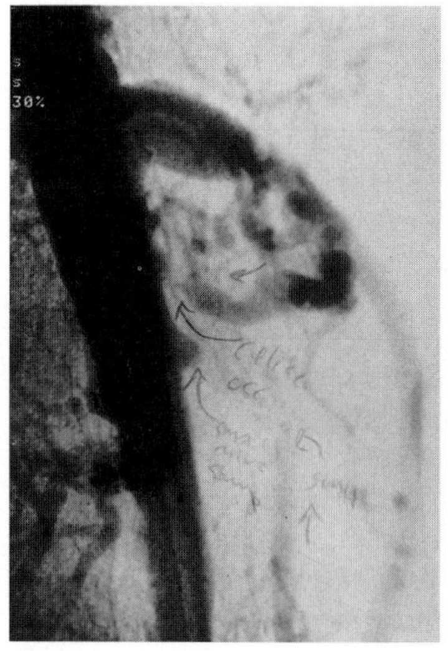

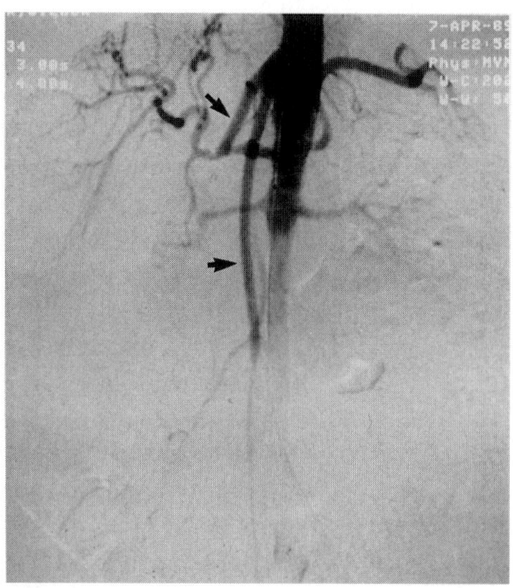

A B

FIGURE 42.6. A. Lateral arteriogram of patient with chronic mesenteric ischemia treated by a supraceliac aortohepatic superior mesenteric artery bypass. B. Anteroposterior view of the arteriogram in the same patient. Note the limbs of the bifurcated graft to the hepatic artery and superior mesenteric artery (arrows).

nasogastric tube within its lumen. The right crus of the diaphragm is divided with electrocautery. In this fashion, approximately 7–10 cm of distal thoracic and proximal abdominal supraceliac aorta can typically be isolated. The celiac axis is then easily exposed through this as well. The celiac axis and SMA are skeletonized. The rationale for doing multivessel revascularization is to maximize symptomatic relief and prevent symptomatic recurrence and visceral infarction, which may result from single-graft failure.[69,70] Supraceliac aortic control is obtained with a partially occluding clamp if possible. This step helps limit the large increase of afterload on the heart that can result from supraceliac cross-clamping, as well as renal and visceral ischemia. If a synthetic graft is used, a bifurcated graft of appropriate size is chosen. The proximal anastomosis is sewn in an end-to-side fashion to the aorta. One limb is then sewn in end-to-end into the celiac axis. In a similar fashion, an end-to-end anastomosis is preformed to the SMA. Sometimes if it is necessary to completely cross-clamp the supraceliac aorta, but the proximal anastomosis can usually be completed in 20 minutes or less, and this amount of visceral and renal ischemia time is well tolerated. A straight graft to the SMA is placed with reimplantation of the celiac axis onto that graft. Additionally, as mentioned, the SMA anastomosis can usually be performed to the proximal SMA anterior to the pancreas. If necessary, due to extensive disease within the proximal SMA, the graft can be tunneled behind the pancreas with construction of the distal anastomosis to the SMA distal to the point where the SMA has passed through the uncinate of the pancreas.

An alternative technique uses an autologous conduit. This is done in the setting of the contaminated or clean-contaminated case secondary to the need for bowel resection. One effective and simple technique is to perform an inline bypass using saphenous vein to the SMA, with the hood of the vein graft forming a patch angioplasty at the origin of the celiac axis. In this fashion, both the celiac axis and the superior mesenteric artery are revascularized. Once revascularization is completed, blood flow is restored to the viscera. This is done in coordination with the anesthesia team to avoid declamping hypotension. Following this step, the bowel is carefully inspected to ensure that adequate flow has been restored.

Occasionally, the supraceliac aorta is not suitable as the origin for antegrade bypass because of aneurysmal or atherosclerotic disease or secondary to previous surgery at the diaphragmatic hiatus. Also, some patients cannot tolerate supraceliac cross-clamping. In this situation, retrograde bypass from either the infrarenal aorta or the iliac vessels can be performed (Fig. 42.7). The infrarenal aorta is also often used as the inflow source if mesenteric revascularization is being performed at the time of concomitant infrarenal aortic reconstruction. The synthetic aortic prosthesis provides an excellent inflow vessel. Standard transperitoneal exposure of the iliac vessels or of the infrarenal aorta is performed. It is necessary to mobilize the ligament of Treitz fully, and then the proximal SMA is isolated below the inferior border of the pancreas at the base of the small bowel mesentery. Once again the choice of conduit can be saphenous vein or prosthetic graft (PTFE or Dacron). The proximal anastomosis is performed to either the distal infrarenal aorta or the proximal right common iliac artery in an end-to-side fashion. The conduit is left with a long, gentle curve around the base of the mesocolon, which not only facilitates the anastomosis to the SMA but helps avoid kinking, which tends to occur with short grafts, particularly saphenous vein grafts.[71,72] The anastomsis to the SMA can be performed in an end-to-end or end-to-side fashion. In the event that the celiac axis is to be revascularized at the same time, a bifurcated graft can be used, or a "piggyback" graft can be sewn onto

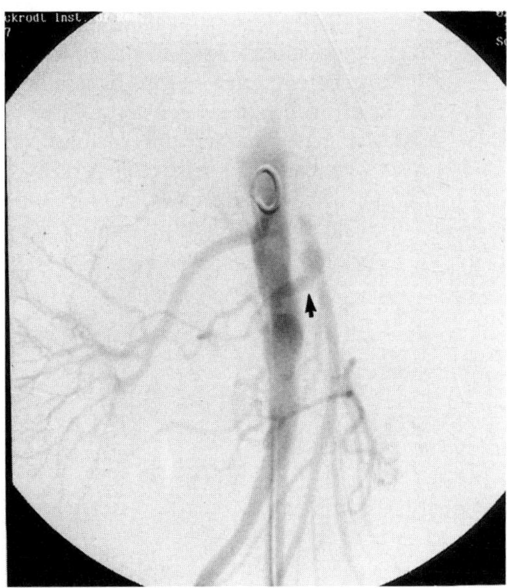

FIGURE 42.7. Postoperative arteriogram from a patient with chronic mesenteric ischemia treated with saphenous vein aortomesenteric bypass (arrow).

the SMA graft. The celiac axis is exposed as previously described. Once again the graft is tunneled to a retropancreatic tunnel and can be anastomosed to the celiac axis or the common hepatic artery.

These operations, as might be expected, are associated with significant perioperative mortality, which averages approximately 6% for patients undergoing revascularization for chronic mesenteric ischemia.[73] These patients, despite their significant co-morbidities, have an approximately 75–80% three-year survival following surgery.[70,73] Graft thrombosis with visceral infarction is a significant cause of both early and late mortality.[74,75] The rate of symptomatic graft failure has been documented to be 15% at an average follow-up of 38 months.[70] Another more recent series has shown that an objective primary patency rate of 89% at 72 months was obtained in a single series.[70] In that series, there was no difference between primary patency rates in patients undergoing retrograde or antegrade bypass. There were also no differences noted for the type of conduit used. Overall, given the extensive co-morbidities of these patients and their underlying atherosclerotic disease, visceral revascularization is a durable procedure, and the morbidity and mortality of the procedure are acceptable.

For occlusive disease limited to the origins of the visceral vessels, transaortic mesenteric endarterectomy is a well-described technique for mesenteric revascularization. The advantages of endarterectomy are that: (1) it eliminates the occlusive lesion; (2) it is an anatomic revascularization and is therefore not subject to turbulent flow or problems with graft compression or alignment; and (3) it provides an autogenous method for multiple-vessel reconstruction.[75] In addition to being able to address mesenteric ischemia, transaortic endarterectomy allows concomitant ostial renal artery disease to be addressed.

The patients are prepared for surgery in a fashion similar to that for other mesenteric revascularizations. The surgery is performed under general anesthesia with radial and pulmonary artery catheters. The visceral abdominal aorta can be exposed through a thoracoabdominal incision or a midline or extended left subcostal incision using medial visceral rotation. The advantage of medial visceral rotation is that it avoids entering the thoracic cavity. Exposure of the upper abdominal aorta is accomplished via left-sided medial visceral rotation. First the splenic flexure of the colon is mobilized by dividing its peritoneal attachments, and then the descending colon is mobilized along its lateral peritoneal reflection. In a similar fashion, the spleen is mobilized by dividing its lateral peritoneal attachments, and it is rotated medially. The dissection plane is established in the retroperitoneum and lies between Gerota's fascia and the peritoneal envelope and posterior to the tail of the pancreas. Once the spleen and pancreas are mobilized medially, the left renal vein is identified and is dissected free from the renal hilum to the vena cava. Division of the adrenal and lumbar branches of the renal vein allow the vein to be retracted inferiorly, thereby providing optimal exposure of the perirenal aorta. The left crus of the diaphragm is divided along the left anterior lateral aorta. Once it is divided, the distal thoracic aorta is exposed, which is the site of proximal aortic control. The site of distal control depends on the extent of the planned endarterectomy. Usually infrarenal aortic control is necessary because of the proximity of the SMA to the renal arteries. The origins of all the visceral vessels are circumferentially dissected free. When circumferentially dissecting the vessels, care is taken to palpate the vessels to make sure the dissection proceeds beyond the margins of the disease. If the disease goes well beyond the ostium, aortic endarterectomy is not possible.

Once vascular isolation is obtained, an aortotomy is performed. The extent of the aortotomy depends on whether endarterectomy of the renal vessels is planned. A standard endarterectomy is performed around the base of each vessel. Usually with ostial disease, gentle eversion endarterectomy suffices and good endpoints are obtained. Once the endarterectomy is completed, the aortotomy is closed using continuous Prolene sutures. On occasion it is not possible to complete the SMA endarterectomy through the transaortic incision. In this case, an arteriotomy can be made on the SMA, and a good endpoint can be obtained. If the more distal SMA is diseased, and it is thought that endarterectomy cannot suffice, a longitudinal arteriotomy can be performed and then closed with a patch angioplasty using saphenous vein.

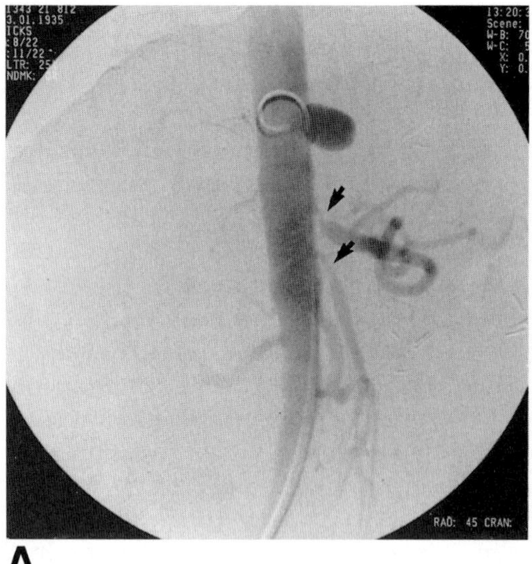

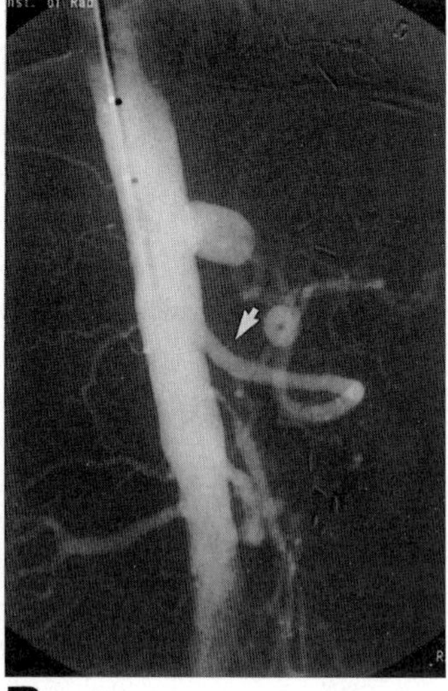

A B

FIGURE 42.8. A. Lateral aortogram 18 months after supraceliac aortohepatic superior mesenteric artery (SMA) bypass in a patient with recurrent symptoms of chronic mesenteric ischemia and poor medical condition. Note the severe celiac axis and SMA stenosis (arrows). B. Lateral aortogram after balloon dilatation and stent placement in the celiac axis.

This operation has proved to be durable. Its drawback is that the patient must be able to tolerate an extensive abdominal dissection as well as a supraceliac aorta cross-clamp. Additionally, there is the anatomic constraint that the occlusive disease must be limited to the ostia.

The final option for mesenteric revascularization is percutaneous transluminal mesenteric angioplasty. The application of angioplasty techniques to mesenteric ischemia is in its infancy. Currently, there are no standard guidelines for the application of angioplasty, and the literature suggests that it is being reserved for patients considered to be "extremely poor surgical candidates."[76] The improving technology for angioplasty including better cathethers, guidewires, balloons, and stent technology have made angioplasty more applicable to increasingly complex lesions.[77] Ideal lesions for angioplasty are short-segment ones that are not being caused by extrinsic constriction. It goes without saying that any patient who presents with acute mesenteric ischemia and evidence of intestinal infarction requires immediate laparotomy, not angioplasty. The technique for angioplasty of a mesenteric vessel is similar to that of any other lesion. The lesion must be able to be crossed with a guidewire. Following placement of the guidewire, a balloon must be passed over the wire across the lesion. Additionally, if necessary, a stent may be placed (Figs. 42.8, 42.9). The reports in the literature are still essentially anecdotal, and the procedure has been used in desperate situations. It is anticipated that in the future this technique will gain widespread applicability. Complications due to the angioplasty are related to occlusion or dissection of the SMA.[76,78,79]

To date, the published experience on mesenteric angioplasty of chronic intestinal ischemia is limited. The largest series comprises only 19 patients. It is also noteworthy that there are few large surgical series dealing with chronic mesenteric ischemia (because chronic mesenteric ischemia is relatively rare). Long-term follow-up is also

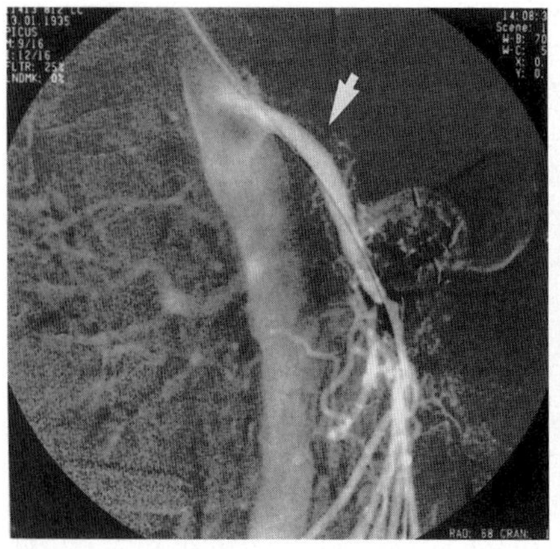

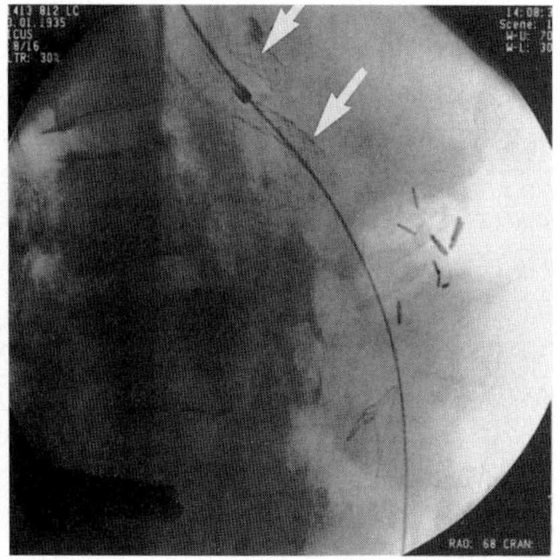

A B

FIGURE 42.9. A. Lateral aortogram of same patient as in Figure 42.8 one month after celiac axis balloon dilatation and stent placement. The patient developed worsening symptoms despite a patent celiac axis. Note the successful superior mesenteric artery balloon dilatation and stent placement (arrow) with resolution of symptoms. B. Note the stents in the celiac axis and superior mesenteric axis (arrows).

not available on these patients, and obviously the resolution of clinical symptoms and the durability of a bypass along with the periprocedural morbidity and mortality will determine the ultimate efficacy of percutaneous transluminal angioplasty. Review of the literature suggests that patients, after a relatively short follow-up, have had a 30–50% recurrence rate.

## Ischemic Colitis

The final category of mesenteric ischemia in the elderly to be considered here is ischemic colitis. As with other causes of mesenteric ischemia, ischemic colitis can be caused by occlusive or nonocclusive lesions. The colon is normally supplied on the right side by the SMA and on the left by the inferior mesenteric artery (IMA) and branches of the hypogastric arteries. The collateral pathways that exist between the SMA, the IMA, and the hypogastric arteries were described earlier in the chapter. Ischemic colitis results when there is obviously decreased flow in one of these vascular beds. Patients susceptible to this problem are those who have absent or poorly developed collateral pathways. It is important to know that previous colonic surgery can interfere with these pathways. The splenic flexure of the colon is in a watershed area between the IMA and the SMA. It is more susceptible than the rest of the colon to ischemic injury. In 5% of the population the marginal artery of Drummond is absent or diminutive, and it is also poorly developed in the right colon of nearly 50% of the population. This helps explain the relatively frequent occurrence of right-sided ischemic colitis.[80] Ischemic colitis results when the colon is rendered ischemic for any of the reasons presented previously.

Ischemic colitis tends to produce local and systemic symptoms. In particular, there is a release of inflammatory cytokines and other mediators of inflammation, which is thought to be secondary to endotoxemia and portal bacteremia. These situations result from the increased mucosal permeability caused by ischemia.[81,82] Also, if there is reperfusion of the ischemic areas, there can be release of oxygen-free radicals and other toxins, resulting in further systemic symptoms. Moreover, recent studies suggest that neutrophils activated during the ischemia/reperfusion process play an important role.[83,84] It is therefore not surprising that patients with ischemic colitis can be extremely ill, and that their mortality is often secondary to multisystem organ failure.

The typical patient who presents with ischemic colitis is an elderly man with co-morbid conditions, including cardiac disease, peripheral vascular disease, diabetes mellitus, or renal insufficiency. The presentation of ischemic colitis can be insidious, with patients complaining of abdominal pain, distension, and diarrhea. Progression to lower GI hemorrhage occurs at an advanced stage of ischemic injury. It usually results from sloughing of the mucosa.

Three degrees of severity of ischemic colitis have been described.[83] The mildest form involves only the colonic mucosa and submucosa. It is estimated that more than half of all patients with ischemic colitis have experienced this degree of the disease. These patients typically have abdominal pain and bloody diarrhea, but the symptoms typically resolve with conservative measures and surgery is not required.[85] The most severe form of ischemic colitis, which affects only 10–20% of patients, involves full-thickness necrosis of the colon, requiring immediate surgical resection. The intermediate form of ischemic colitis involves the mucosa, submucosa, and the muscularis layer of the colon. It can lead to chronic stricture due to scarring when the lesion heals or to persistent symptoms.[86] Often, in patients with the two milder forms of ischemic colitis, the initial presenting symptoms are vague and nonspecific. Once again, as with other forms of mesenteric ischemia, a high index of suspicion should be maintained in patients who present with GI symptoms.

As with other forms of mesenteric ischemia, blood tests, although providing collaborative evidence of colonic ischemia, are nonspecific.[87] As with mid-gut ischemia, the presence of metabolic acidosis and elevated CPK and LDH levels are indicative of advanced colonic ischemia. The most definitive way to diagnose ischemic colitis is by endoscopic evaluation. Acutely, pale mucosa with areas of petechial hemorrhage is seen with mild ischemia; more severe degrees of ischemia are indicated by a dark (blue to black) mucosa, which may be accompanied by mucosal sloughing and ulceration.[88–90] Because the findings at time of endoscopy can be confused with other colitides, biopsy and histologic examination may prove useful.[91] With ischemic colitis there is destruction of the crypts, sloughing of the epithelium, edema, thrombosis of capillaries, and a relative lack of inflammatory cells. Later findings include stricture and fibrosis; biopsy reveals extensive transmural fibrosis with mucosal atrophy.[91]

Unlike other forms of mesenteric ischemia due to arterial lesions, angiography is usually not helpful in this setting. This is because often the lesions leading to ischemic colitis are more peripheral and therefore more difficult to detect.[92] CT scans are often obtained owing to the unclear diagnosis in the patient presenting with abdominal pain; they are often normal in these patients, particularly those who present early in the course of their illness.[93] A late finding highly suggestive of ischemic colitis is pneumatosis.[94] The most frequent positive finding is circumferential thickening of the colonic wall, which is secondary to edema or hemorrhage, but it is nonspecific.[95] The use of other imaging studies remains experimental, and so far they have proved to be insensitive.[96,97] As with other forms of ischemia, findings on plain films are not often seen, are usually nonspecific, and when seen usually are due to advanced ischemia. Such findings include pneumatosis, portal venous air, and free intraabdominal air.[98] Contrast studies are infrequently used to evaluate patients with acute abdominal pain; if obtained, thumbprinting due to submucosal edema and hemorrhage is the classic finding of ischemic colitis.[99]

The management of patients with ischemic colitis is individualized and depends on the patient's presentation. Most patients who present with ischemic colitis do not have an acute abdomen, and therefore emergent surgery is usually not necessary.[86,92] These patients are managed supportively by vigorous rehydration with intravenous solutions, administration of broad-spectrum antibiotics, and stopping oral intake. The precipitating events for ischemic colitis, which are often low-flow states, should be corrected. Within 1 week most patients with a mild form of ischemic colitis respond well to treatment.[98,99] In the patient who presents with ischemic colitis with no clear cause, visceral angiography can be considered; but once again it has a relatively low yield.

Any patient who presents with an acute abdomen requires emergent surgery. Those who fail to respond to conservative measures and who have persistent bleeding or low-grade sepsis, require surgical intervention. Surgical treatment involves resecting the ischemic segments of colon. It is recommended that patients have a colostomy or an ileostomy, with a subsequent procedure to restore intestinal continuity.[100] Patients with ischemic colitis have a relatively high mortality, but it is usually due to the underlying condition that precipitated the ischemic colitis. In this sense it is similar to nonocclusive mesenteric ischemia. Obviously patients who require surgery have an even higher mortality rate.[101,102] Elective aortic reconstruction for aneurysm disease is associated with a 1–2% incidence of ischemic colitis.[103] In the emergent setting of a ruptured abdominal aortic aneurysm, the incidence of ischemic colitis has been reported to be as high as 60%.[104] Ischemic colitis following aortic surgery is associated with a high mortality rate, which has been reported to be in excess of 50%.[105] In the subgroup of patients who require emergent colectomy, mortality is nearly 90%. As with other forms of mesenteric ischemia, the key to a successful clinical outcome is a timely diagnosis, which requires a high index of clinical suspicion. Therefore, in any patient who has undergone aortic reconstruction and develops bloody or heme-positive diarrhea, has an unexplained high fluid resuscitation requirement, presents with fever and leukocytosis of unknown origin, or has an unexplained acidosis, the diagnosis of colitis should be suspected, and evaluation including endoscopy should be undertaken.

## References


1. McMillan WD, McCarthy WJ, Bresteker MR, et al. Mesenteric artery bypass: objective patency determination. J Vasc Surg 1995;21:729–741.
2. Buchardt-Hansen HJ. Abdominal angina: results of arterial reconstruction in 12 patients. Acta Chiurg Scand 1976;142:319–325.
3. Rapp JH, Reilly LM, Qvarfordt PG, et al. Durability of endarterectomy and antegrade grafts in the treatment of chronic visceral ischemia. J Vasc Surg 1986;3:799–806.
4. Schwartz LB, Puret CM, Craig DM, et al. Input impedance of revascularized skeletal muscle, renal, and mesenteric vascular beds. Vasc Surg (in press).
5. Ahlborg G, Weitzberg E, Lundberg JM. Circulating endothelin-1 reduces splanchnic and renal blood flow and splanchnic glucose production in humans. J App Physiol 1995;79:141–145.
6. VanHoutte PM. Heterogeneity in vascular smooth muscle cells. In: Caley G, Altura BM (eds). Microcirculation. Baltimore: University Park Press, 1978:181–308.
7. Reilly PM, Bulkley GB. Vasoactive mediators and splanchnic perfusion. Crit Care Med 1993;21:S55–S68.
8. Granger DN, Richardson PDI, Kvietys PR, Mortillaro NA. Intestinal blood flow. Gastroenterology 1980;78:837–863.
9. Heys SD, Brittenden J, Crofts TJ. Acute mesenteric ischemia: the continuing difficulty and early diagnosis. Postgrad Med J 1993;69:48–51.
10. Kaleya RN, Boley SJ. Acute mesenteric ischemia: an aggressive diagnostic and therapeutic approach: 1993 Roussel lecture. Can J Surg 1992;5:613–623.
11. Stoney RJ, Cunningham CG. Acute mesenteric ischemia. Surgery 1993;114:489–490.
12. Cambria RP, Brewster DC, Gertler J, et al. Vascular complications associated with spontaneous aortic dissection. J Vasc Surg 1988;7:199–209.
13. Cogbill TH, Gundersen AE, Travelli R. Mesenteric vascular insufficiency and claudication following acute dissecting thoracic aortic aneurysm. J Vasc Surg 1985;2:472–476.
14. Vignati PV, Welch JP, Ellison L, Cohen JL. Acute mesenteric ischemia caused by isolated superior mesenteric artery dissection. J Vasc Surg 1992;16:109–112.
15. Kaleya RN, Sammartano RJ, Boley SJ. Aggressive approach to acute mesenteric ischemia. Surg Clin North America 1992;72:157–182.
16. Deehan DJ, Heys SD, Brittenden J, Eremin O. Mesenteric ischaemia: prognostic factors and influence of delay upon outcome. J R Coll Surg Edinb 1995;40:112–115.
17. Case records of the Massachusetts General Hospital (case 35082). N Engl J Med 1949;240:308–310.
18. Haglund U, Lundgren O. Nonocclusive acute intestinal vascular failure. Br J Surg 1979;6:155–158.
19. Berger RL, Byrne JJ. Intestinal gangrene associated with heart disease. Surg Gynecol Obstet 1961;113:522–529.
20. Jenson CV, Smith GA. A clinical study of 51 cases of mesenteric infarction. Surgery 1956;40:930–937.
21. Wilson GSM, Block J. Mesenteric vascular occlusion. Arch Surg 1956;73:330–345.
22. Bassiouny HS. Nonocclusive mesenteric ischemia. Surg Clin North Am 1997;77:319–326.
23. McNeill JR, Stark RD, Greenway CV. Intestinal vasoconstriction after hemorrhage: roles of vasopressin angiotensin. Am J Physiol 1970;219:1342–1347.
24. Kim EH, Gewertz BL. Chronic digitalis administration alters mesenteric vascular reactivity. J Vasc Surg 1987; 5:382–389.

25. Mikkelsen E, Andersson DK, Pedersen OL. Effects of digoxin on isolated human mesenteric vessels. Acta Pharmacol Toxicol (Copenh) 1979;5:249–256.
26. Gewertz BL, Zarins CK. Postoperative vasospasm after antegrade mesenteric revascularization: a report of three cases. J Vasc Surg 1991;14:382–385.
27. Clark ET, Gewertz BL. Intermittent ischemia potentiates intestinal reperfusion injury. J Vasc Surg 1991;3:606.
28. Howard TJ, Plaskon LA, Wiebke EA, Wilcox MG. Nonocclusive mesenteric ischemia remains a diagnostic dilemma. Am J Surg 1996;171:405–408.
29. Boley SJ, Brandt LJ, Veith FJ. Ischemic disorders of the intestine. Curr Probl Surg 1978;15:1.
30. Jamieson WG, Lozon A, Durand D, Wall W. Changes in serum phosphate levels associated with intestinal infarction and necrosis. Surg Gynecol Obstet 1975;140:19–21.
31. Tomchek FS, Wittenberg J, Ottinger LW. The roentgenograph spectrum of bowel infarction. Radiology 1970; 96:249–260.
32. Boley SJ, Sprayregen SS, Veith FJ. An aggressive roentgenologic and surgical approach to acute mesenteric ischemia. In: Niehaus LM (ed). Surgery Annual. Norwalk, CT: Appleton-Century-Crofts, 1973:355.
33. Sigelman SS, Bragen S, Boley SJ. Angiographic diagnosis of mesenteric arterial vasoconstriction. Radiology 1974;22:533.
34. Kairaluoma MI, Karkola P, Heikkinene S, et al. Mesenteric infarction. Am J Surg 1977;133:188.
35. Ottinger LW, Austen WG. A study of 136 patients with mesenteric infarction. Surg Gynecol Obstet 1967;124:251.
36. Rhee RY, Gloviczki P, Mendonca CT, et al. Mesenteric venous thrombosis: still a lethal disease in the 1990s. J Vasc Surg 1994;20:688.
37. Rhee RY, Gloviczki P. Mesenteric venous thrombosis. Surg Clin North Am 1997;77:327.
38. Kitchens CS. Evolution of our understanding of the pathophysiology of primary mesenteric venous thrombosis. Am J Surg 1992;163:346.
39. Bontempo FA, Hassett AC, Faruki H, et al. The factor V Leiden mutation: spectrum of thrombotic events in laboratory evaluation. J Vasc Surg 1997;25:271–275.
40. Inagakia H, Sakakibara O, Miyaike H, et al. Mesenteric venous thrombosis and familiar-free protein S deficiency. Am J Gastroenterol 1993;88:134.
41. Tollefson DFJ, Friedman KD, Marlar RA, et al. Protein C deficiency; a cause of an unusual or unexplained thrombosis. Arch Surg 1988;123:881.
42. Wilson C, Walker ID, Davidson JF, et al. Mesenteric venous thrombosis and empty thrombin 3 deficiency. J Clin Pathol 1987;40:906.
43. Abdu R, Zakhour BJ, Dallis DJ. Mesenteric venous thrombosis 1911–1984. Surgery 1987;101:383.
44. Boley SJ, Kaleya RN, Brandt LJ. Mesenteric venous thrombosis. Surg Clin North Am 1992;72:183.
45. Carr N, Jamison MH. Superior mesenteric venous thrombosis. Br J Surg 1981;68:343.
46. Clavien PA, Harder F. Mesenteric venous thrombosis. Helv Chir Acta 1988;55:29.
47. Grieshop RJ, Dalsing MC, Ckrit DF, et al. Acute mesenteric venous thrombosis: revisited in time of diagnostic clarity. Am J Surg 1991;57:573.
48. Harward TRS, Green D, Bergan JJ, et al. Mesenteric venous thrombosis. J Vasc Surg 1989;9:328.
49. Rhmouni A, Mathieu D, Golli M, et al. Value of CT and sonography in the conservative management of acute splenoportal and superior mesenteric venous thrombosis. Gastrointest Radiol 1992;17:135.
50. Gehl HB, Bohndorf K, Klose KC, et al. Two-dimensional MR angiography in the evaluation of abdominal vein with gradient refocused sequences. J Comput Assist Tomogr 1990;14:619.
51. Inhara T. Acute superior mesenteric venous thrombosis: treatment by thrombectomy. Ann Surg 1971;74:956.
52. Bilbao JI, Rodriquez-Cabello J, Longo J, et al. Portal thrombosis: percutaneous transhepatic treatment with urokinase: a case report. Gastrointest Radiol 1989; 14:326.
53. Robin P, Gurel Y, Lang M, et al. Complete thrombolysis of mesenteric vein occlusion with recombinant tissue type plasminogen activator. Lancet 1988;1:1391.
54. Hallet JW, James ME, Ahlquist DA, et al. Recent trends in the diagnosis and management of chronic intestinal ischemia. Ann Vasc Surg 1990;4:126–132.
55. Moawad J, Gewertz BL. Chronic mesenteric ischemia: clinical presentation and diagnosis. Surg Clin North Am 1997;77:357–369.
56. Calderon M, Reul GJ, Gregoric ID, et al. Long-term results of the surgical management of symptomatic chronic intestinal ischemia. J Cardiovasc Surg 1992;33:723–728.
57. Derrick JR, Pollard HS, Moore RM. The pattern of atherosclerotic narrowing of the celiac and superior mesenteric arteries. Ann Surg 1959;149:684–689.
58. Reiner L, Himinez FA, Rodriquez FL. Atherosclerosis in the mesenteric circulation: observations and correlations with aortic and coronary atherosclerosis. Am Heart J 1963;66:200–209.
59. Councilman WT. Three cases of occlusion in the superior mesenteric artery. Boston Med Surg J 1894;130:410–411.
60. Gluecklich B, Deterling RA, Matsumoto GH, et al. Chronic mesenteric ischemia masquerading as cancer. Surg Gynecol Obstet 1979;148:49–56.
61. Lye CR. Chronic mesenteric ischemia. Can J Surg 1988; 31:159–161.
62. Watt JK. Arterial disease of the gut. Br Med J 1968;3:231–233.
63. Koslin DP, Mulligan SA, Burland LL. Duplex assessment of the splanchnic vasculature. Semin Ultrasound CT MR 1992;13:34–39.
64. Moneta GL, Lee RW, Yeager RA, et al. Mesenteric duplex scanning: a blinded perspective study. J Vasc Surg 1993;17:79–86.
65. McMillan WD, McCarthy WJ, Bresticker MR, et al. Mesenteric artery bypass: objective patency determination. J Vasc Surg 1995;21:729–741.
66. Li KC, Whitney WS, McDonnell CH, et al. Chronic mesenteric ischemia: evaluation with phase contrast-cine MR imaging. Radiology 1994;190:175–179.
67. Dunphy JE. Abdominal pain of vascular origin. Am J Med Sci 1936;192:109–113.
68. Shanley CJ, Ozaki KC, Zelenock GB. Bypass grafting for chronic mesenteric ischemia. Surg Clin North Am 1997; 7:381–395.

69. McAfee MK, Cherry KJ Jr, Nassens JM, et al. Influence of complete revascularization on chronic mesenteric ischemia. Am J Surg 1992;164:220–224.
70. McMillan WD, McCarthy WJ, Bresticker MR, et al. Mesenteric artery bypass: objective patency determination. J Vasc Surg 1995;21:729–740; discussion 740–741.
71. Baur GM, Millay DJ, Taylor LM, Porter JM. Treatment of chronic visceral ischemia. Am J Surg 1984;148:138–144.
72. Taylor LM Jr, Moneta GL. Intestinal ischemia. Ann Vasc Surg 1991;5:403–406.
73. Johnston KW, Lindsay TF, Walker PM, Kalman PG. Mesenteric arterial bypass grafts: early and late results on suggested surgical approach for chronic and acute mesenteric ischemia. Surgery 1995;118:1–7.
74. Cunningham CG, Reilly LM, Stoney R. Chronic visceral ischemia. Surg Clin North Am 1992;72:231–244.
75. Hansen KJ, Deitch S. Transaortic mesenteric endarterectomy. Surg Clin North Am 1997;77:397–407.
76. Allen R, Martin G, Rees C, et al. Mesenteric angioplasty in the treatment of chronic intestinal ischemia. J Vasc Surg 1996;24:415–423.
77. Bertran X, Muchart J, Planas R, et al. Occlusion of the superior mesenteric artery in a patient with polycythemia vera resolution with percutaneous transluminal angioplasty. Ann Hematol 1996;72:89–91.
78. Odurny A, Sniderman KW, Colapinto RF. Intestinal angina: percutaneous transluminal angioplasty of the celiac and superior mesenteric arteries. Radiology 1988; 167:59–62.
79. Rose SC, Quigley TM, Raker EJ. Revascularization for chronic mesenteric ischemia: comparison of operative arterial bypass grafting and percutaneous transluminal angioplasty. J Vasc Intervent Radio 1995;6:339–349.
80. Sonneland J, Anson LJ, Beaton LE. Surgical anatomy of the arterial supply of the colon from the superior mesenteric artery based upon a study of 60 specimens. Surg Gynecol Obstet 1958;106:385–397.
81. Bradley AW, Murie JA, Ruckley CV. Role of the leukocyte and the pathogenesis of vascular disease. Br J Surg 1993;80:1503–1512.
82. Turnage RH, Guice KS, Oldham KT. Endotoxemia and remote organ injury following intestinal reperfusion. J Surg Res 1994;56:571–578.
83. Bradbury AW, Brittenden J, McBride K, Ruckley CV. Mesenteric ischemia in multi-disciplinary approach. Br J Surg 1995;82:1446–1459.
84. Sisley AC, Desai T, Harig JM, Gewertz BL. Neutrophil depletion attenuates human intestinal reperfusion injury. J Surg Res 1994;57:192–196.
85. Boley SJ, Brandt LF, Veith SJ. Ischemic disorders of the intestines. Curr Probl Surg 1978;15:1–85.
86. Boley SJ. Colonic ischemia: 25 years later. Am J Gastroenterol 1990;85:931–934.
87. Thompson JS, Bragg LE, West WW. Serum enzyme levels during intestinal ischemia. Ann Surg 1990;211:369–373.
88. Andus CH. Endoscopic assessment of vascular disorders. Semin Colon Rectal Surg 1994;5:27–31.
89. Longo WE, Ballantyne GH, Gusberg BJ. Ischemic colitis: patterns and prognosis. Dis Colon Rectum 1992;35:726–730.
90. Scherpenisse J, VanHeese PAM. The endoscopic spectrum of colonic mucosal injury following aortic aneurysm resection. Endoscopy 1989;21:174–176.
91. Price AB. Ischemic colitis. Curr Top Pathol 1990;81:229–246.
92. Robert JH, Mentha G, Rohner A. Ischaemic colitis: two distinct patterns of severity. Gut 1993;34:4–6.
93. Alpern MB, Glazer PM, Francis IR. Ischemic or infarcted bowel: CT findings. Radiology 1988;66:149–152.
94. Philpotts LE, Heiken JP, Westcott MA, Gore RM. Colitis: use of CT findings and differential diagnosis. Radiology 1994;190:445–449.
95. Jacobs JE, Birnbaum BA. CT of inflammatory disease of the colon. Semin Ultrasound CT MR 1995;16:91–101.
96. Teefey SA, Roarke NC, Brink JA, et al. Bowel wall thickening: differentiation of inflammation from ischemia with color Doppler and duplex, ultrasound. Radiology 1996;198:547–551.
97. Wilkerson DK, Mezrich R, Drake C, et al. MR imaging of acute occlusive intestinal ischemia. J Vasc Surg 1990;11: 567–571.
98. Smerud MJ, Johnson CD, Stephens DH. Diagnosis of bowel infarction: a comparison of plain films and CT scans in 23 cases. Am J Radiol 1990;154:99–103.
99. Scholz FJ. Ischemic bowel disease. Radiol Clin North Am 1993;31:1197–1218.
100. Toursarkissian B, Thompson RW. Ischemic colitis. Surg Clin North Am 1997;77:461–470.
101. Guttormson N, Brubrick MP. Mortality from ischemic colitis. Dis Colon Rectum 1989;32:469–472.
102. Parrish KL, Chapman WC, Williams LF Jr. Ischemic colitis: a never changing spectrum? Am Surg 1991;57:118–121.
103. Ernst CB, Hagihara PF, Dougherty ME, et al. Ischemic colitis incidence following abdominal aortic reconstruction: a prospective study. Surgery 1976;80:417–421.
104. Hagihara PF, Ernst CB, Griffen WO Jr. Incidence of ischemic colitis following abdominal aortic reconstruction. Surg Gynecol Obstet 1979;149:571–573.
105. Longo WE, Lee TC, Barnett MG, et al. Ischemic colitis complicating abdominal aortic aneurysm surgery in the U.S. veteran. J Surg Res 1996; 60:351–354.

# 43 Inflammatory Bowel Disease in the Elderly

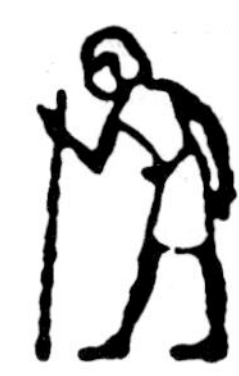

Tonia M. Young-Fadok and Bruce G. Wolff

Although inflammatory bowel disease is often considered an affliction of the young, significant proportions of those presenting with either Crohn's disease or Ulcerative Colitis are elderly. An understanding of the differences in disease presentation in the elderly compared to that in the young is important in making a timely diagnosis. In addition, operative approaches, when indicated, must be tailored to the needs of the aging patient.

## Epidemiology

### Incidence

Several factors influence the interpretation of data regarding the incidence of inflammatory bowel disease (IBD) in the elderly: the source of the data (population-based studies versus clinical series), the definition of elderly, the historic age of the series, and the criteria employed for disease definition.[1] More accurate data on the incidence of IBD in the elderly are derived from population-based studies because clinical series are typically retrospective descriptions of patients from a single institution, often a tertiary center where complicated cases may be overrepresented. Late-onset cases are variably defined in patients ranging from >40 years to those >65 years of age. Early reports may reflect changes in diagnosis and thoroughness of data collection, but they may not reveal true increases in the incidence of Crohn's disease.

#### *Crohn's Disease*

Crohn's disease (CD) has been called a disease of the twentieth century, having first been described by Crohn and his colleagues in 1932.[2] The incidence of the disease ranges from 2 to 5 per 100,000 population[3] and usually accounts for one-fourth to one-third of cases of IBD, although a multinational study of 3175 patients noted variations in the incidence ratio of Ulcerative Colitis (UC) to CD of 3.4 : 1.0 in favor of CD to 3.1 : 1.0 in favor of UC.[4] The proportion of elderly patients with CD varies in different population-based studies from 5.9% to 30.7%[1] with a mean of 16.0%,[5] the age of late-onset being variably defined as 50–60 years of age. More recent series suggest that older patients make up a larger proportion of Crohn's patients than originally reported. CD was diagnosed in only 4.2% of 600 patients seen over 37 years at the Mayo Clinic in a report in 1954,[6] whereas a recent population-based series from Stockholm, Sweden, noted an increase in the proportion of elderly patients (60 years and older) from 3.4% to 12.0% between 1955 and 1989.[7] The overall incidence of CD has also increased in most studies, with a tendency toward a plateau in recent years.[7]

#### *Ulcerative Colitis*

The incidence of UC shows interesting geographic differences. There has been a stable incidence in Stockholm,[8] Cardiff,[9] and Copenhagen,[10] compared with a marked increase in Iceland,[11] Faroe Islands,[12] Scotland,[13] and North Tees (UK)[14] since 1970. The greater incidence of both UC and CD in northern Europe was confirmed by the European Collaborative Study on IBD (EC-IBD).[15] Incidence data for UC are influenced by inclusion or exclusion of patients with ulcerative proctitis, as available data suggest this entity is more common in elderly individuals.[16] Population-based studies suggest that the proportion of patients with late-onset UC (defined variably as >50 years to >70 years) ranges from 8.1% to 43.9% with a mean of 12.0%. The EC-IBD study also found that the age-specific incidence of UC decreases in women with age but not in men, confirming reports by others.[13,16,17]

### Bimodality

Most epidemiologic studies have illustrated a bimodal distribution in the age at diagnosis of both UC[18–20] and CD.[19] The first peak (mode) occurs during the third decade, whereas the second varies between the ages of 50 and 80 years. This bimodal distribution has been noted to remain constant for CD in both Cardiff[21] and Scotland[13] over many years, despite a 2.6- to 5.0-fold increase in the incidence.

The reason for this striking age distribution pattern is not known, although several theories have been proposed. One suggestion has been that the two peaks represent two types of disease, or a differential effect of age on the underlying disease. The variation in the anatomic distribution of CD depending on the patient's age is an example of the latter. CD of the terminal ileum tends to present in young patients,[22] producing a unimodal age distribution for small bowel CD with a peak during the third and fourth decades.[23] Conversely, old patients tend to have purely colonic disease, and the second peak has been found to be comprised predominantly of elderly women with Crohn's colitis, often left-sided.[24,25]

An earlier theory that misdiagnosis was responsible for the second peak has gained less credence with time. As Crohn's colitis and UC came to be recognized as distinct clinical and pathologic entities during the middle part of the twentieth century, some authors ascribed the second peak to misclassification of such other conditions as ischemic and infectious colitis.[26] That may possibly have been so at one time, as was well shown in a retrospective review by Brandt et al.,[27] where of 81 patients older than 50 years with a diagnosis of colitis only 14% were thought to have UC and 5% to have CD after further consideration; ischemic colitis was the diagnosis assigned to three-fourths of the series. Even exclusion of ischemic colitis, however, has not abolished the second peak in UC; and the incidence of UC in the elderly has continued to increase, not decrease, in the face of improved diagnostic ability.

## Presentation and Natural History

### Presentation

The presentation of CD and UC in the elderly does not vary significantly from that in the young population. A review of the clinical features in patients more than 50 years of age with CD found abdominal pain (82%), diarrhea (70%), weight loss (56%), and rectal bleeding (26%) to be the most common presenting features.[28] Toxic dilatation at presentation was rare. The initial diagnosis is often incorrect (being correct in only 64% of patients older than 65 years versus 96% of younger patients[29]) or delayed (despite clinical characteristics similar to those in younger patients) because of confusion caused by a higher incidence of diverticular and cardiovascular disease.[30] A higher rate of complications has also been seen in old patients (36% vs. 16% in young patients) and a higher mortality rate, thought to be at least partly due to delay in diagnosis.[29]

### Natural History

There are conflicting reports on the natural history of CD and UC in the elderly. Gupta et al.[31] in a series of patients with both CD and UC found that few patients required operation. This concurred with the findings of Fabricius et al.,[32] who found that in elderly patients with CD the course of the disease was largely dependent on the site of the lesion. Most of those with distal ileal disease required laparotomy for obstruction, for peritonitis, or to rule out carcinoma; but thereafter the prognosis was good. In contrast, patients with colonic disease rarely required operation and were managed medically. This contrasted with findings from others[26,33,34] where 40–91% of those with colitis required surgery.

The natural history in UC is also the subject of controversy. Jones et al.[35] found that elderly patients were admitted more often with their first attack and were more likely to receive intravenous steroids than younger patients; but none required emergent surgery, and mortality on follow-up was no greater than that expected in the general population of the same age. The prognosis was found to be the same as in younger patients. This differs from Brandt et al.,[36] who noted that in a group of 11 patients with UC, 2 developed toxic dilatation, 3 underwent operation, and 3 died during the first admission, leading to the conclusion that the prognosis was worse than in younger patients.

## Differential Diagnosis

The diagnosis of IBD can be delayed by atypical presentation in the elderly or by classic symptoms such as weight loss, abdominal pain, or bleeding, prompting a workup for more common pathology such as colorectal carcinoma or diverticulitis. IBD should be considered during the evaluation of elderly patients with digestive complaints, particularly chronic diarrhea with or without bleeding. Symptoms in the elderly may not suggest IBD for reasons that include blunted response to pain, poor communication because of altered comprehension or hearing, fear of the medical system, and focus on cancer as the most likely cause of symptoms.[5] A delay in diagnosis is common in old patients with IBD and may result in inappropriate treatment and a higher rate of complications.[29]

The differential diagnosis of IBD in the elderly includes ischemic colitis, diverticular disease, infectious colitis, and of course, cancer. Less common entities that should be considered are collagenous colitis, lymphocytic colitis, radiation enterocolitis, lymphoma, carcinoid, vasculitis, and drug-induced colitis.[5] Diagnostic evaluation is generally unaffected by age. Prompt diagnostic evaluation may be particularly important in elderly patients, who may present with atypical symptoms. Two particularly common sources of diagnostic confusion are ischemic colitis and diverticulitis.

### Ischemic Colitis

A history of cardiovascular disease may suggest a diagnosis of ischemic colitis. Occasionally there is difficulty distinguishing ischemia from IBD. Brandt et al., in a study of 81 patients, found that half were originally diagnosed with CD, UC, or nonspecific colitis; but on retrospective review, ischemic colitis was diagnosed in 75% of the series.[36] The authors raised the question as to whether such incorrect diagnoses might explain why colitis is reported to behave differently in the elderly. That ischemic changes may mimic UC or CD has been reported by other authors.[37]

### Diverticulitis

Diagnosis may be difficult and confusing with segmental colitis in patients with diverticular disease.[38] Distinguishing segmental CD with diverticula from pure diverticulitis may be difficult, as each may have abdominal pain, diarrhea, fistula, and abdominal mass; blood in the stool, especially if in small amounts and frequent, suggests CD.[39] Peppercorn[40] described eight patients with segmental chronic active colitis associated with sigmoid diverticula. No patient less than 60 years of age with CD had these findings. Endoscopy reveals a characteristic appearance with patchy areas of hemorrhage in the sigmoid colon; biopsy demonstrates focal chronic active colitis without granulomas. It is important to consider this differential diagnosis, as major complications may follow surgery for suspected diverticulitis in elderly patients with unrecognized CD.[41]

## Surgical Therapy

Many aspects of the surgical therapy of Crohn's disease and ulcerative colitis are similar. This is particularly true with regard to indications (especially emergent ones), preoperative evaluation, and preoperative preparation. There are many excellent texts and atlases that deal with operative details.[42,43] Few describe adjustments that must be considered when operating on the elderly patient. This discussion concentrates on factors that may influence decision-making for the older patient.

### Crohn's Disease

Despite advances in the medical therapy of Crohn's disease, most patients undergo surgical intervention at some point during their lifetime. The National Cooperative Crohn's Disease Study reported operative rates of 78% at 20 years and 90% at 30 years from diagnosis.[44] The form of this intervention is determined by the operative indication, extent of disease, and site within the gastrointestinal tract.

#### *Indications for Elective Surgery*

##### Fistulas and Abscesses

Fistulas and abscesses, hallmark manifestations of Crohn's disease, are the most common indications for surgical intervention. The presence of fistulizing disease, with or without accompanying abscess, was the reason for operation in 35% of 482 patients in an early series reported by Farmer et al.[45] More recent series, including multicenter studies, have confirmed the prominence of this complication as an indication for operation.

The risk of developing fistulas is to some extent related to the site of the underlying Crohn's disease. Fistulas appear to arise more commonly from the ileocolic distribution; 44% occur in patients with ileocolitis, compared with 32% in patients with more proximal small bowel distribution, and 23% in those with colonic disease alone.

Fistulas may develop between diseased bowel and any structure or surface adjacent to the inflammatory process. They may be internal or external. Internal fistulas may, for example, be classified as enteroenteral or coloenteral, enterocolic, enterovesical, or enterovaginal. External fistulas are enterocutaneous, perianal, and perirectal. Accompanying abscesses may be within the peritoneal cavity (enteroparietal), interloop, intramesenteric, retroperitoneal, or perianal.

Symptomatic fistulas generally require operative intervention. Corticosteroids rarely result in fistula closure. Fistulas have been demonstrated to heal in 30–40% of patients given 6-mercaptopurine[46] but only in the absence of obstruction. Percutaneous drainage under antibiotic coverage is the first-line therapy for abscesses, followed by resection of the affected bowel.

##### Obstruction

Obstruction is the second most common indication for operation; in one report it occurred in 34% of patients undergoing surgical therapy of Crohn's disease.[45] It is seen in 55% of patients requiring operation for small bowel disease, 35% where there is ileocolic disease, and 12% in patients with Crohn's colitis. Early obstructive symptoms may improve with steroid therapy, but longer-standing symptoms generally indicate a fibrotic stricture that does not respond to medical therapy.

##### Refractory to Medical Therapy

In the absence of indications mandating prompt surgical therapy, patients with symptomatic Crohn's disease undergo medical therapy. The severity and extent of disease determine the role of sulfasalazine, 5-aminosalicylic acid (5-ASA) compounds, antibiotics, steroids, immunosuppressive drugs, or agents such as the recently Food and Drug Administration (FDA)-approved anti-tumor necrosis factor-α (TNF-α) medication infliximab. Operative intervention is indicated if the response to medical therapy is incomplete, side effects develop, or planned withdrawal of steroids, for example, is not possible once a response has been induced.

#### Carcinoma

There is an established association between Crohn's disease and carcinoma of the colon and the small bowel. The magnitude of this association is, however, controversial. Carcinoma complicating the inflammatory state can be difficult to recognize on preoperative radiologic studies and even macroscopically at operation. For this reason, it is advised that all sites of stricturing undergoing strictureplasty, rather than resection, should be biopsied to exclude underlying malignancy. Resection of malignancy that occurs in a background of Crohn's disease unfortunately has poor results, particularly in the small intestine.[47]

### *Indications for Emergency Surgery*

#### Toxic Colitis

A diagnosis of toxic colitis mandates emergent treatment. One of the most useful definitions includes a subjective and an objective component.[43,48] Toxic colitis is defined as an acute "flare" of Crohn's disease accompanied by two of the following: fever (>38.6°C); hypoalbuminemia (<3.0g/dl); leukocytosis ($>10.5 \times 10^9$ cells/L); tachycardia (>100 beats/min). Megacolon is additionally diagnosed by colonic dilatation of more than 5cm. A low threshold of suspicion is important in the elderly, where age alone can mask classic abdominal symptoms and signs, even in the absence of steroids or immunosuppressive agents, which may also conceal symptoms.

Therapy should be instituted as soon as the diagnosis is suspected. Emergent operative intervention is necessary in the presence of perforation, peritonitis, sepsis, and massive hemorrhage. In the absence of these findings, medical therapy is initiated with intravenous rehydration, high dose steroids or other immunosuppressive drugs, bowel rest, and broad-spectrum antibiotics. A vital component of treatment is frequent serial abdominal examinations and abdominal radiographs. Deterioration during therapy is a further indication for operation, as is failure to improve after 5–7 days of conservative treatment. Surgical management should be pursued aggressively in the elderly, who have little physiologic reserve and are less well able to survive the consequences of colonic perforation.

#### Perforation

Free perforation is unusual but may occur in the setting of acute disease or chronic disease. With acute toxic colitis, perforation occurs in the presence of a dilated, friable colon with transmural inflammation. Perforation in patients with chronic disease occurs in the presence of an acute exacerbation of small bowel disease often in association with obstruction. Perforation occurs in fewer than 2% of patients.[49] More commonly, the fistulizing nature of Crohn's disease results in adhesions to adjacent loops of bowel that contain the process and prevent free perforation; an abscess so formed may itself perforate and result in purulent peritonitis or fecal peritonitis if there is a free connection to the bowel lumen.

#### Hemorrhage

Hemorrhage, a relatively unusual complication of Crohn's disease,[50] should be treated in a fashion similar to that for significant gastrointestinal bleeding due to other causes. The patient's condition should be stabilized while investigations proceed to determine the site of bleeding. Emergent operative intervention is indicated for persistent hemodynamic instability after transfusion with 4–6 units of blood, recurrent bleeding, or an additional indication to resect the diseased bowel. The elderly, particularly those with coexisting cardiopulmonary disease, have little physiologic reserve, and early operative intervention should be considered in those who have demonstrated unstable vital signs.

### *Preoperative Preparation*

#### Completion of Workup

Initial studies are guided by the patient's symptoms. Once the primary site of Crohn's disease has been identified, the remainder of the gastrointestinal tract should be evaluated to identify the presence of coexistent sites of disease, which may determine the nature and extent of the operative approach. For example, the individual with obstructive-type symptoms may undergo a small bowel series that indicates ileocecal disease; the operative approach is different depending on whether the disease is localized or there is also coexistent extensive colitis demonstrated on colonoscopy. Such information is important when discussing the nature of the operative approach, the extent of resection, and the likely postoperative course.

#### Preoperative Discussion

Knowing the extent and severity of disease assists in preoperative discussions with the patient and family. Procedure-specific risks should be discussed and tailored to the patient and to the procedure contemplated. Such risks may include bleeding with the attendant risks of blood transfusion; wound infection; anastomotic leak and possible abscess, enterocutaneous fistula, or peritonitis; and the likelihood of the need for a temporary or permanent stoma. Co-morbidities, more prevalent in the elderly, also increase the risk of operation and anesthesia and should be discussed with the patient.

### Bowel Preparation

In the elective setting most patients tolerate some form of bowel preparation incorporating both a mechanical and an antibiotic component. Most commonly the mechanical bowel preparation is performed the day prior to operation with a clear liquid diet and 2–4 liters of polyethylene glycol. This regimen must be modified in the patient with obstructive symptoms and may include a longer period of clear liquids in addition to phospho-soda (90 ml) or magnesium citrate (60 ml). Enemas may also be helpful, particularly in the presence of obstructive symptoms. Despite the trend to perform bowel preparation in the outpatient setting, selected elderly patients, particularly those with cardiac disease such as aortic stenosis, may require hospitalization to prevent dehydration and hypotension.

Antibiotic preparation may be intravenous, oral, or a combination of the two. Oral antibiotics are given as part of the bowel preparation; one combination in use is neomycin 2 g and metronidazole 2 g given at 7 P.M. and 10 P.M. the night prior to operation. Intravenous antibiotics, usually a second- or third-generation cephalosporin and metronidazole, are administered within 2 hours prior to the skin incision and for two doses postoperatively.

### Steroid Preparation

Perioperative stress doses of corticosteroids are necessary if the patient has been treated with steroids within the preceding 6 months. Our preference is to administer methylprednisone 40 mg on call to the operating room, 30 mg every 12 hours for the next 24–48 hours, and then 30 mg daily. Continuation of the taper depends on the preoperative dose and duration of steroid therapy but generally occurs over a period of 6–8 weeks.

### Electrolyte and Nutritional Deficits

Appropriate preoperative testing may reveal abnormalities. Electrolyte derangements, anemia, dehydration, and coagulation deficits should be corrected in both elective and emergent settings. Correction of nutritional deficits, as evidenced by weight loss, hypoalbuminemia, and negative nitrogen balance, is controversial. The use of total parenteral nutrition (TPN) has been shown in some series to improve nutritional parameters but does not significantly reduce postoperative complications. One series[51] did show that the extent of small bowel resection was less in patients receiving preoperative TPN, but this finding is possibly of clinical value only in patients who would otherwise be at risk of short bowel syndrome.

### Enterostomal Therapy

Preoperative preparation of the patient for a stoma is invaluable, whether an ileostomy or colostomy is being considered and whether it is to be temporary or permanent. Preparation consists of marking the abdomen preoperatively and patient education. Such marking guides the correct siting of the stoma within the rectus muscle, away from bony prominences and skin creases and scars. Preoperative education and counseling, preferably from an enterostomal therapist, is valued by patients.

## *Operative Principles*

### Resection, Strictureplasty, or Bypass

Resection is generally the procedure of choice in patients whose symptoms are sufficient to merit operative intervention. In elderly patients the colon is the most common site of disease, and with rare exceptions symptomatic disease is resected. The surgery may take the form of segmental resection and anastomosis for limited colonic disease, or a subtotal colectomy with or without anastomosis, or proctocolectomy. With small bowel disease the ileocecal region is often affected most severely and merits resection.

Strictureplasty is generally employed in the small bowel to avoid resection. It is usually not necessary at a first operation but can be employed at subsequent procedures to widen the lumen of the bowel at short strictures. Although active Crohn's disease is left in situ by this method, it does not appear to increase the rate of subsequent reoperation and has proven invaluable for preserving small bowel length in patients who would otherwise be at risk of short bowel syndrome. Strictureplasty is less commonly used at anastomotic strictures but can be useful in this situation.

### Extent of Resection

The extent of resection is essentially based on the surgeon's judgment at operation and the ability to recognize diseased bowel. Typical small bowel disease is manifested by bowel wall thickening and induration; serositis and prominent vessels running on the surface of the serosa; "creeping fat" or encroachment of mesenteric fat over the bowel wall; and thickening along the mesenteric edge of the bowel. Correlating with these changes in the bowel are a characteristic thickening of the mesentery, with enlarged lymph nodes that may occur diffusely throughout the small bowel mesentery but are usually more prominent at sites of active disease. Establishing the extent of disease in the colon may be more problematic by inspection of the external appearance alone, and intraoperative colonoscopy may prove invaluable in such cases.

Adequate margins are obtained by resecting back to macroscopically normal bowel. Once a subject of controversy, radical margins of resection now are thought to sacrifice more functioning small bowel than is of benefit for reducing recurrence. Several retrospective series have demonstrated no relation between the presence of microscopic disease at resection margins and the rate of recurrence.[52,53] Hamilton et al.[54] compared patients undergoing frozen section evaluation of margins with a group whose margins were judged macroscopically free of disease; at 10 years the clinical recurrence rates were not significantly different (60% and 66%, respectively), nor were the reoperative rates (36% and 32%, respectively). More recently, a randomized prospective trial comparing macroscopically free margins of 2cm versus 12cm, revealed no difference in clinical or operative recurrence rates at 5 years.[55] The advent of postoperative medical prophylaxis with mesalamine, azathioprine, and other medications has made microscopic disease-free resection margins moot.[56]

### Anastomosis

Standard surgical principles apply to the creation of any anastomosis, ensuring good blood supply, lack of tension, and correct orientation. Use of suturing or stapling techniques depends on the surgeon's preference. As staples are not intended to be hemostatic, it is important to check the suture line for excessive oozing.

### Operative Approach: Laparoscopic versus Open

Laparoscopic techniques are being increasingly utilized for Crohn's disease, a disease that was once thought not to be compatible with the laparoscopic approach. Initial concerns centered on the inherent inflammatory nature of the disease, with its attendant thickened bowel and mesentery and frequent association with fistulas and abscesses, which can make even open surgery challenging. As experience with the technique has grown, however, the feasibility and benefits of this approach in selected patients are becoming more apparent. A large multicenter series[57] demonstrated that laparoscopic-assisted resection is possible for a range of procedures but particularly for isolated ileocecal and small bowel disease. The presence of fistulas and abscesses did not preclude a successful laparoscopic approach, this being possible in 75% of such patients. A similar success rate was demonstrated in patients who had undergone prior abdominal operations. The procedure results in statistically significant and clinically relevant benefits, with patients exhibiting less pain, more rapid resolution of ileus, and earlier discharge.[58]

Similar benefits have been demonstrated in elderly patients. A case–control series from the Mayo Clinic[59] of laparoscopic resection versus matched open resection, found in the former group that postoperative ileus resolved more rapidly, patients had fewer postoperative complications, and they were discharged sooner. In addition, a significantly larger percentage of patients in the laparoscopy group were discharged to their own homes and remained independent after operation, an important consideration in the elderly.

## *Management by Anatomic Site*

### Gastric and Duodenal Disease

Primary gastric disease is an unusual manifestation of CD.[45] Endoscopy may reveal gastric dilatation and superficial ulceration. The findings may be suggestive of peptic ulcer disease or may be difficult to distinguish from carcinoma. Biopsy may reveal characteristic granulomas. Patients may undergo gastrectomy if carcinoma cannot be excluded.

The duodenum may be the site of primary or secondary manifestations of CD. Primary CD is unusual; the early nonspecific symptoms are suggestive of peptic ulcer disease and may respond to antacids, hydrogen receptor blockers, and steroids. In the event of obstructing disease, highly selective vagotomy, and gastrojejunostomy has become the procedure of choice.[60] The addition of highly selective vagotomy prevents the marginal ulceration associated with bypass alone and avoids the postvagotomy diarrhea associated with truncal vagotomy. Duodenal strictureplasty is technically challenging and rarely performed, even in tertiary referral centers.

More commonly, the duodenum may be secondarily affected as a bystander adjacent to fistulizing disease in the ileum or colon, especially from a previous ileocolic anastomosis. This complication may be reduced by performing an ileoascending anastomosis, preserving as much of the right colon as possible at the time of ileocecal resection. The omentum should be used whenever possible to separate the anastomosis from the duodenum.

### Jejunoileal Disease

Manifestations of CD in the small bowel may be localized or diffuse. Most commonly, localized disease occurs distally and is generally amenable to resection, particularly at first operation. This also holds true for several segments of disease concentrated in one area, where a single resection and anastomosis is preferred rather than several anastomoses. Although sparing of the terminal ileum is relatively unusual with distal ileal disease, the ileocecal valve should be preserved if there is a distal disease-free area of more than 5cm allowing an anastomosis.

Surgical judgment faces stronger challenges in the event of diffuse small bowel disease. Occasionally, areas of small bowel dilatation serve as guides to points of significant stricturing; but often with diffuse disease, it is difficult to distinguish small bowel that is thickened secondary to CD, from bowel that is thickened from chronic obstruction proximal to a stricture. In such instances, it is helpful to make an enterotomy distally and insert a Baker tube (a long tube bearing an inflatable balloon near its tip) proximally as far as the ligament of Treitz. The balloon is then inflated to a diameter of 1.5–2.0 cm and withdrawn slowly. The balloon is held up at points of stricturing that can be marked with seromuscular sutures, and strictureplasties are performed at these sites.

### Ileocecal Disease

Ileocecal disease is the commonest indication for operative intervention in all patients but is less common in old than in young patients. Frequently, the right colon is affected only to the level of the ileocecal valve, and it is possible to perform an ileoascending anastomosis, preserving most of the right colon.

### Colonic Disease

The surgical approach to colonic disease is determined primarily by three factors: extent of disease (localized or diffuse); presence of rectal sparing; and function of the anal sphincter in preserving continence.

*Localized Colitis.* Among patients with disease limited to the colon, only 10%[61] exhibit limited or segmental disease of the colon. Unlike the situation with the small intestine, segmental resection of the colon has in the past been considered controversial because of the impression that recurrence rates were high and that an ileostomy would ultimately be required.[43] A series from the Mayo Clinic[62] of 49 patients undergoing limited colonic resection for segmental disease, showed that only 14% of patients over a mean follow-up period of 14 years ultimately required stoma construction. Those who ultimately required a stoma enjoyed a mean stoma-free interval of 23 months. Thus, a stoma was avoided in most of the patients. Even those in whom a stoma was eventually necessary benefited from an extended period of stoma avoidance. Social and body image arguably may be of more importance to young patients for avoiding a stoma. The elderly also benefit from this approach, particularly those in whom a previous small bowel resection has been performed and who potentially might be debilitated by profuse small bowel effluent through an ileorectal anastomosis or an ileostomy. The use of segmental colonic resection may increase with more widespread prescription of immunosuppressive drugs, such as azathioprine or 6-mercaptopurine for diffuse colitis; areas of most severe ulceration appear in some instances to heal with focal stricturing.

*Diffuse Colitis.* In the elective setting, the choice of procedure for treating pancolitis is determined in part by the presence or absence of rectal disease. In the patient with proctocolitis, the preferred option is proctocolectomy and Brooke ileostomy. Although some have suggested use of a low Hartmann closure of the rectum to allow perianal disease to regress, 40% of the patients (10/25) required a later perineal proctectomy, and three of these patients still exhibited wound problems.[63] The use of ileostomy alone improves general well-being in about two-thirds of patients but does not consistently avoid later proctocolectomy; and fewer than 10% ever experience restoration of intestinal continuity. Diversion alone may be a consideration in an elderly patient who refuses or who would not tolerate proctocolectomy.

The elderly patient with pancolitis but rectal sparing deserves careful evaluation. Measurement of anal canal pressures is not predictive of postoperative function, although Keighley et al.[64] found assessment of rectal compliance (by identifying those whose maximum tolerated rectal volume was >150 ml) to be helpful. The individual who remains continent despite loose stool during attacks of colitis has undergone the most rigorous physiologic test of continence and would be a candidate for total abdominal colectomy (subtotal colectomy) with ileosigmoid or ileorectal anastomosis. Those occasionally incontinent of loose stool probably have less than perfect control, but this situation may be preferable to having a stoma; it merits discussion with the patient. The individual who is frankly incontinent would be best served by a proctocolectomy or a subtotal colectomy, ileostomy, and retained rectal stump. Although some authors have suggested use of an ileal pouch to improve compliance if resection is necessary to the level of the mid-rectum,[43] this procedure is highly controversial, as known Crohn's disease is widely considered an absolute contraindication to use of a pouch, given the 45% risk of pouch failure secondary to complications.[65]

In the emergent setting, the guiding principle is to remove the site of disease as expeditiously as possible, avoid further complications, and perform a later staged procedure if necessary. In the setting of diffuse colonic involvement and megacolon, perforation, or hemorrhage, a subtotal colectomy with ileostomy is performed; and the rectum is either left long as a mucus fistula or short as an extraperitoneal stump. If hemorrhage is arising from the rectum in the face of diffuse disease, however, proctocolectomy cannot be avoided. Perforation resulting from localized disease in the colon is addressed with resection, proximal stoma, and mucus fistula or exclusion of the distal bowel. Perforation of localized rectal disease is approached by proximal colostomy and drainage of the pelvis, with proctectomy 3–6 months later.

### Perianal Disease

Crohn's disease manifestations in the perianal region include skin tags, fissures, ulcers, abscesses, fistulas, and anorectal stricture. These findings frequently occur after intestinal symptoms have resulted in a diagnosis of CD, but when perianal findings precede other symptoms, the diagnosis can present difficulties. Examination includes digital assessment, anoscopy, and rigid or flexible sigmoidoscopy. Discomfort may necessitate examination under anesthesia for full evaluation. Biopsy infrequently yields evidence of a granuloma, but other features are suggestive of CD: edematous, violaceous skin tags; fissures at sites other than the midline; indolent abscesses; complex fistulas; and stricturing without evidence of malignancy or prior anorectal surgery. A new diagnosis of CD should prompt evaluation of the entire gastrointestinal tract, although it is unclear whether disease activity more proximally affects perianal disease.[66,67]

Therapy must be individualized, bearing in mind treatment principles of relief of symptoms and avoidance of additional complications. Careful consideration should be given to appropriate medical and surgical approaches. Perianal skin tags and hemorrhoids are best approached conservatively, with control of diarrhea, sitz baths, and analgesia; surgical therapy of either is associated with a high rate of poor outcomes.[68] Symptomatic fissures should be evaluated to rule out underlying sepsis and then approached initially with medical therapy. In selected cases and when conservative therapy has failed, lateral internal sphincterotomy may be beneficial. Careful consideration must be given to issues of continence, however, particularly in the elderly. Abscesses should be treated with incision and drainage, making the incision into the abscess cavity as medial as possible to keep any subsequent fistula as short as possible.

Management of perianal fistulas is often challenging. As with other situations, therapy is aimed at relieving symptoms; hence, in the absence of associated sepsis, an asymptomatic fistula may require no specific therapy. Simple low fistulas without accompanying proctitis may be managed successfully with fistulotomy,[69,70] particularly when combined with therapy such as metronidazole or sulfasalazine.[71,72] When it is thought that sphincterotomy may result in fecal continence because the fistula is high or complex or because the elderly patient has borderline continence, other approaches are necessary. Noncutting setons achieve drainage without compromise of continence; despite the presence of a foreign body, most patients tolerate setons far better than undrained fistulas, particularly if the seton is of a soft material such as Silastic vessel loops.[43] If the rectal mucosa does not exhibit active disease the patient may be a candidate for a rectal mucosal advancement flap. An overall success rate of 60% has been reported for this approach to low fistulas,[73] but the success rate falls to approximately one-third in high, complex fistulas.[74] An alternative approach is the use of fibrin glue, which has a lower success rate than with non-Crohn's fistulas after a single application, but repeated applications may result in success and there is no risk of compromising the sphincter. A novel medication, anti-TNF (infliximab) is showing promise in therapy of perianal CD that would otherwise be considered an indication for proctectomy. Data in the elderly, however, are still limited or absent. Creation of a diverting ileostomy is occasionally a useful means for controlling severe perianal disease, but only one-third of patients ever achieve successful reversal.[43]

## Ulcerative Colitis

### *Indications for Elective Surgery*

#### Failure of Medical Therapy

Medical therapy may be considered to have failed when maximal therapy has not controlled symptoms or when symptoms are abolished only at the expense of side effects from the medications themselves. The inability to wean steroids completely or to an acceptable level is also an indication for operation. Inability or unwillingness to comply with a medical regimen may prompt surgical intervention.

#### Presence or Risk of Carcinoma

An increased risk of colorectal cancer has been documented in those with extensive long-standing ulcerative colitis.[75] The magnitude of this risk is controversial, with population-based studies suggesting that the risk is lower than previously thought.[76] It is best defined in patients whose disease onset occurred during childhood or the teenage years, those with extensive disease, and those whose duration of disease is more than 10 years; in these patients the risk of developing cancer is reported to be 2% per year.[77] The risk in patients with later age of onset is not well defined. Monitoring by screening colonoscopy for dysplasia has limitations, including patient compliance and the finding that carcinoma may not have evidence of preceding dysplasia.[78] At the time of colectomy for dyplasia, more than 50% already have invasive cancer.[79] In the absence of an absolute indication (i.e., stricture, evidence of dysplasia or a dysplasia-associated mass, existing cancer[80]) the role of surgery is less clear, despite results of a decision analysis that suggest prophylactic colectomy improves survival more than surveillance.[81] In the elderly, later onset of disease and shorter duration of remaining life compared with younger patients, probably results in surgery being used more for specific indications than for prophylaxis.

#### Extraintestinal Manifestations

Although up to 30% of all patients with inflammatory bowel disease present with at least one extraintestinal manifestation,[82] the incidence is not clear in the elderly. In addition, these presentations are rarely the primary indication for surgery.

### Indications for Emergency Surgery

#### Fulminant Colitis

The definition of fulminant colitis is identical to that described for CD. It is important to remember, particularly in the patient presenting with a fulminant first attack, that the differentiation between CD and UC may not be possible. The surgical approach is the same, whichever the underlying diagnosis. Although this diagnosis previously was associated with a high mortality rate, mortality is now less than 3%[83] due in part to aggressive surgical intervention and probably to changes in medical management; with the introduction of cyclosporine for severe colitis not responding to steroids, one series reported 70% of patients responding and being prepared for surgery on an elective basis.[84]

#### Toxic Megacolon, Perforation, Hemorrhage, Obstruction

In emergent settings, UC is often indistinguishable from CD. The principles of therapy outlined for CD, including the appropriate extent of resection in emergent settings, apply equally to either diagnosis.

### Preoperative Preparation

Many of the principles of preoperative preparation discussed for patients with CD apply equally to those with UC. They include correction of electrolyte abnormalities and severe anemia, bowel preparation, use of antibiotics, and stress doses of steroids. Possibly the most important aspect differentiating the patient with UC from one with CD, is consideration given to reconstructive surgery in the form of the ileal pouch–anal anastomosis (IPAA).

### Operative Procedure

Essentially, the choice of procedure depends on how much of the rectum is to be removed (all, part, or none), and if the anal sphincter is competent. If the patient is incontinent of stool due to an incompetent sphincter (and not to poor compliance in a diseased rectum) the decision is simple: proctocolectomy and Brooke ileostomy. In the individual without compromise of the sphincter, consideration may be given to proctocolectomy and ileostomy, subtotal colectomy and ileorectal anastomosis, or proctocolectomy and IPAA (or ileal pouch-distal rectal anastomosis) (Table 43.1).

Advanced age has generally been considered a contraindication to IPAA because of the high risk of fecal incontinence in the elderly. The clinical results in carefully selected patients over the age of 50, however, are equivalent to those of younger patients.[85] Anal sphincter strength does decline after the age of 70,[86] and almost no one beyond this age is a candidate for this operation.[42]

TABLE 43.1. Choice of Operation for Ulcerative Colitis in Elderly Patients

| Procedure | Contraindications | Comments |
|---|---|---|
| Proctocolectomy and Brooke ileostomy | None | Complete excision of disease |
| Subtotal colectomy and ileorectal anastomosis | Incompetent sphincter<br>Active rectal disease<br>Noncompliance with follow-up endoscopy of rectal remnant | Incomplete excision of disease<br>At risk for proctitis or development of rectal cancer |
| Proctocolectomy and ileal pouch–anal anastomosis | Incompetent sphincter<br>Age > 60 (relative)<br>Age > 70 (absolute) | Operation necessary to close temporary diverting ileostomy<br>Risk of pouchitis |
| Proctocolectomy and ileal pouch–distal rectal anastomosis | Incompetent sphincter<br>Age > 60 (relative)<br>Age > 70 (absolute)<br>Noncompliant | Easier operation to perform<br>Risk of pouchitis<br>Risk of cancer in retained rectal mucosa |
| Proctocolectomy, continent ileostomy | Most patients | Frequent reoperation<br>Rarely recommended, even in young patients |

## References


1. Grimm IS, Friedman LS. Inflammatory bowel disease in the elderly. Gastroenterol Clin North Am 1990;19:361–389.
2. Crohn BB, Ginzburg L, Oppenheimer GD. Regional ileitis: a pathologic and clinical entity. JAMA 1932;99:1323–1329.
3. Sandler RS, Golden AL. Epidemiology of Crohn's disease. J Clin Gastroenterol 1986;8:160–165.
4. Myren J, Bouchier IAD, Watkinson G, et al. The OMGE multinational inflammatory bowel disease survey 1976–1986: a further report on 3175 cases. Scand J Gastroenterol 1988;144(suppl):11–19.
5. Fleischer DE, Grimm IS, Friedman LS. Inflammatory bowel disease in older patients. Med Clin North Am 1994;78: 1303–1319.
6. Van Patter WN, Bargen JA, Dokerty MB, et al. Regional enteritis. Gastroenterology 1954;26:347.
7. Lapidus A, Bernell O, Hellers G, et al. Incidence of Crohn's disease in Stockholm County 1955–1989. Gut 1997;41: 480–486.
8. Nordenvall B, Brostrom O, Berglund M, et al. Incidence of ulcerative colitis in Stockholm County 1955–1979. Scand J Gastroenterol 1985;20:783.
9. Morris T, Rhodes J. Incidence of ulcerative colitis in the Cardiff region 1968–1977. Gut 1984;25:846.
10. Binder V, Both H, Hansen PK, et al. Incidence and prevalence of ulcerative colitis and Crohn's disease in the county of Copenhagen, 1962–1978. Gastroenterology 1982; 83:563.
11. Bjornsson S, Thorgeirsson T. Ulcerative colitis in Iceland: an epidemiologic study. Nord Med 1983;98:298–301.
12. Berner J, Kjaer T. Ulcerative colitis and Crohn's disease on the Faroe Islands 1964–1983. Scand J Gastroenterol 1986; 21:188–192.

13. Sinclair TS, Brunt PW, Mowat NAG. Nonspecific proctocolitis in northeastern Scotland: a community study. Gastroenterology 1983;85:1.
14. Devlin HB, Datta D, Dellipiani AW. The incidence and prevalence of inflammatory bowel disease in North Tees health district. World J Surg 1980;4:183–193.
15. Shivananda S, Pena AS, Nap M, et al. Epidemiology of Crohn's disease in Regio Leiden, The Netherlands. Gastroenterology 1987;93:966.
16. Softley A, Myren J, Clamp SE, et al. Inflammatory bowel disease in the elderly patient. Scand J Gastroenterol 1988;23(suppl 144):27–30.
17. Langholz E, Munkholm P, Haagen Nielsen O, et al. Incidence and prevalence of ulcerative colitis in Copenhagen County from 1962 to 1967. Scand J Gastroenterol 1991; 26:1247.
18. Evans JG, Acheson DE. An epidemiological study of ulcerative colitis and regional enteritis in the Oxford area. Gut 1965;6:311.
19. Garland CF, Lilienfeld AM, Mendeloff AI, et al. Incidence rates of ulcerative colitis and Crohn's disease in fifteen areas of the United States. Gastroenterology 1981;81:1115.
20. Sedlack RE, Nobrega FT, Kurland LT, et al. Inflammatory colon disease in Rochester, Minnesota 1935–1964. Gastroenterology 1972;62:935.
21. Rose JDR, Roberts GM, Williams G, et al. Cardiff Crohn's disease jubilee: the incidence over 50 years. Gut 1988;29:346.
22. Kyle J. Prognosis after ileal resection for Crohn's disease. Br J Surg 1971;58:735.
23. Lee FI, Costello T. Crohn's disease in Blackpool: incidence and prevalence 1968–1980. Gut 1985;26:274.
24. Lockhart-Mummery HE. Crohn's disease of the large bowel. Br J Surg 1972;59:823.
25. Walker MA, Pennington CR, Pringle R. Crohn's disease in the elderly. Br Med J Clin Res Educ 1985;291:1725–1726.
26. Shapiro PA, Peppercorn MA, Antonioli DA, et al. Crohn's disease in the elderly. Am J Gastroenterol 1981;76:132–137.
27. Brandt L, Boley S, Goldberg L, et al. Colitis in the elderly: a reappraisal. Am J Gastroenterol 1981;76:239–245.
28. Eisen GM, Schutz SM, Washington MK, et al. Atypical presentation of inflammatory bowel disease in the elderly. Am J Gastroenterol 1993;88:2098–2101.
29. Stalnikowicz R, Eliakim R, Diab R. Crohn's disease in the elderly. J Clin Gastroenterol 1989;11:411–415.
30. Harper PC, McAuliffe TL, Beeken WL. Crohn's disease in the elderly: a statistical comparison with younger patients matched for sex and duration of disease. Arch Intern Med 1986;146:753–755.
31. Gupta S, Saverymuttu SH, Keshavarzian A, et al. Is the pattern of inflammatory bowel disease different in the elderly? Age Ageing 1985;14:366–370.
32. Fabricius PJ, Gyde SN, Shouler P, et al. Crohn's disease in the elderly. Gut 1985;26:461–465.
33. Elliott PR, Ritchie JK, Lennard-Jones JE. Prognosis of colonic Crohn's disease. Br Med J 1985;291:178.
34. Serpell JW, Johnson CD. Complicated Crohn's disease in the over 70 age group. Aust NZ J Surg 1991;61:427–431.
35. Jones HW, Hoare AM. Does ulcerative colitis behave differently in the elderly? Age Ageing 1988;17:410–414.
36. Brandt LJ, Boley SJ, Mitsudo S. Clinical characteristics and natural history of colitis in the elderly. Am J Gastroenterol 1982;77:382–386.
37. Eisenberg RL, Montgomery CK, Margulis AR. Colitis in the elderly: ischemic colitis mimicking ulcerative and granulomatous colitis. Am J Radiol 1979;133:1113–1118.
38. Van Rosendaal G, Andersen MA. Segmental colitis complicating diverticular disease. Can J Gastroenterol 1996;10: 361–364.
39. Editorial. Crohn's disease in the elderly: a diagnostic problem. Br Med J 1973;873:188–189.
40. Peppercorn MA. Drug-responsive chronic segmental colitis associated with diverticula: a clinical syndrome in the elderly. Am J Gastroenterol 1992;87:609–612.
41. Tchirkow G, Lavery IC, Fazio VW. Crohn's disease in the elderly. Dis Colon Rectum 1983;26:177–181.
42. Heppell J, Kelly KA, Dozois RR. Surgery for ulcerative colitis. In: Nicholls RJ, Dozois RR (eds) Surgery of the Colon and Rectum. New York: Churchill Livingstone, 1997: 593–615.
43. Strong SA. Crohn's disease. In: Nicholls RJ, Dozois RR (eds) Surgery of the Colon and Rectum. New York: Churchill Livingstone, 1997:617–644.
44. Mekhijan HS, Sweitz DM, Watts HD, et al. National cooperative Crohn's disease study: factors determining recurrence of Crohn's disease after surgery. Gastroenterology 1979;77:907–913.
45. Farmer RG, Hawk WA, Turnbull RB Jr. Indications for surgery in Crohn's disease: analysis of 500 cases. Gastroenterology 1976;71:245–250.
46. O'Brien JJ, Bayless TM, Bayless JA. Use of azathioprine or 6-mercaptopurine in the treatment of Crohn's disease. Gastroenterology 1991;101:39–46.
47. Michelassi F, Testa G, Pomidor WJ, et al. Adenocarcinoma complicating Crohn's disease. Dis Colon Rectum 1993;36: 654–661.
48. Fazio VW. Toxic megacolon in ulcerative colitis and Crohn's colitis. Gastroenterology 1980;9:389–407.
49. Abscal J, Diaz-Rojas F, Jorge J, et al. Free perforation of the small bowel in Crohn's disease. World J Surg 1982;6: 216–220.
50. Homan WP, Tang CK, Thorbjarnason B. Acute massive hemorrhage from intestinal Crohn's disease. Arch Surg 1976;111:901–905.
51. Lashner BA, Evans AA, Hanauer SB. Preoperative total parenteral nutrition for bowel resection in Crohn's disease. Dig Dis Sci 1989;34:741–746.
52. Papaioannau N, Piris J, Lee ECG, Kettlewell MGW. The relationship between histological inflammation in the cut ends after resection of Crohn's disease and recurrence. Gut 1979;20:A916.
53. Kotanagi H, Kramer K, Fazio VW, Petras RE. Do microscopic abnormalities at resection margins correlate with increased anastomotic recurrence in Crohn's disease? Retrospective analysis of 100 cases. Dis Colon Rectum 1991;34: 909–916.
54. Hamilton SR, Reese J, Pennington L, et al. The role of resection margin frozen section in the surgical management of Crohn's disease. Surg Gynecol Obstet 1985;160:57–62.
55. Fazio VW, Marchetti F, Church JM, et al. Effect of resection margins on the recurrence of Crohn's disease in the small

bowel: a randomized controlled trial. Ann Surg 1996;224: 563–573.
56. McLeod RS, Wolff BG, Steinhart AH, et al. Prophylactic mesalamine treatment decreases postoperative recurrence of Crohn's disease. Gastroenterology 1995;109:404–413.
57. Young-Fadok TM, Nelson H, Fleshman J, et al. Laparoscopic resection of Crohn's disease. Poster presentation at Digestive Disease Week, New Orleans, May 1998.
58. Young-Fadok TM, Sgambati SA, Nelson H. Benefits of laparoscopic resection for Crohn's disease: a case-matched series. Presentation at Society of American Gastrointestinal and Endoscopic Surgeons, San Antonio, TX, March 1999.
59. Stocchi L, Nelson H, Young-Fadok TM, et al. Safety and advantages of laparoscopic versus open colectomy in the elderly: a matched-control study. Presentation at the American Society of Colon and Rectal Surgeons, Washington, DC, May 1999.
60. Nugent FW, Roy MA. Duodenal Crohn's disease: an analysis of 89 cases. Am J Gastroenterol 1989;84:249–254.
61. Goligher JC. The long-term results of excisional surgery for primary and recurrent Crohn's disease of the large bowel. Dis Colon Rectum 1985;28:51–55.
62. Prabhakar LP, Laramee C, Nelson H, et al. Avoiding a stoma: role for segmental or abdominal colectomy in Crohn's colitis. Dis Colon Rectum 1997;40:71–78.
63. Sher ME, Bauer JJ, Gorfine S, et al. Low Hartmann's procedure for severe anorectal Crohn's disease. Dis Colon Rectum 1992;35:975–980.
64. Keighley MRB, Buchmann P, Lee JR. Assessment of anorectal function in selection of patients for ileo-rectal anastomosis in Crohn's colitis. Gut 1982;23:102–107.
65. Sagar PM, Dozois RR, Wolff BG. Long-term results of ileal pouch-anal anastomosis in patients with Crohn's disease. Dis Colon Rectum 1996;39:893–898.
66. Wolff BG. Crohn's disease: the role of surgical treatment. Mayo Clin Proc 1986;61:292–295.
67. Buchmann P, Keighley MRB, Allan RN, et al. Natural history of perianal Crohn's disease: ten year follow-up: a plea for conservation. Am J Surg 1980;140:642–644.
68. Jeffrey PJ, Ritchie JK, Parks AG. Treatment of haemorrhoids in patients with inflammatory bowel disease. Lancet 1977;1:1084–1085.
69. Fry RD, Shemesh EI, Kodner IJ, Timmcke A. Techniques and results in the management of anal and perianal Crohn's disease. Surg Gynecol Obstet 1989;168:42–48.
70. Levien DH, Surrell J, Mazier W. Surgical treatment of anorectal fistulas in Crohn's disease. Surg Gynecol Obstet 1989;169:133–136.
71. Fuhrman GM, Larach SW. Experience with perirectal fistulas in patients with Crohn's disease. Dis Colon Rectum 1989;32:847–848.
72. Sohn N, Korelitz BI, Weinstein MA. Anorectal Crohn's disease: definitive surgery for fistulas and recurrent abscesses. Am J Surg 1980;139:394–397.
73. Makowiec F, Jehle EC, Becker HD, Starlinger M. Clinical course after transanal advancement flap repair of perianal fistula in patients with Crohn's disease. Br J Surg 1995;82: 603–606.
74. Crim RW, Fazio VW, Lavery IC. Rectal advancement flap repair in Crohn's patients—factors predictive of failure. Dis Colon Rectum 1990;33:P3.
75. Ekbom A, Helmick C, Zack M, et al. Ulcerative colitis and colorectal cancer: a population-based study. N Engl J Med 1990;323:1228–1233.
76. Hendriksen C, Kreiner S, Binder V. Long term prognosis in ulcerative colitis—based on results from a regional patient group from the county of Copenhagen. Gut 1985;26:158–163.
77. Devroede G. Risk of cancer in inflammatory bowel disease. In: Winawer SJ, Schottenfeld R, Sherlock R (eds) Colorectal Cancer: Prevention, Epidemiology, and Screening. Philadelphia: Lippincott-Raven, 1980.
78. Reiser JR, Waye JD, Janowitz HD, Harpaz N. Adenocarcinoma in strictures of ulcerative colitis without antecedent dysplasia by colonoscopy. Am J Gastroenterol 1994;89:119–122.
79. Blackstone MO, Riddle RH, Rogers BH, Levin B. Dysplasia-associated lesion or mass (DALM) detected by colonoscopy in long-standing ulcerative colitis: an indication for colectomy. Gastroenterology 1981;80:366–374.
80. Lennard-Jones JE. Colitic cancer: supervision, surveillance, or surgery? Gastroenterology 1995;109:1388–1391.
81. Provenzale D, Kowdley KV, Arora S, Wong JB. Prophylactic colectomy or surveillance for chronic ulcerative colitis? A decision analysis. Gastroenterology 1995;109:1188–1196.
82. Greenstein AJ, Janowitz HD, Sachar DB. The extraintestinal complications of Crohn's disease and ulcerative colitis: a study of 700 patients. Medicine 1976;55:401.
83. Hawley PR. Emergency surgery for ulcerative colitis. World J Surg 1988;12:169–173.
84. Hurst RD, Finco C, Rubin M, Michelassi F. Prospective analysis of perioperative morbidity in one hundred consecutive colectomies for ulcerative colitis. Surgery 1995;118: 748–755.
85. Lewis WG, Sagar PM, Holdsworth PJ, et al. Restorative proctocolectomy with end to end pouch-anal anastomosis in patients over the age of fifty. Gut 1993;34:948–952.
86. McHugh SM, Diamant NE. Effect of age, gender, and parity on anal canal pressures: contribution of impaired anal sphincter function to fecal incontinence. Dig Dis Sci 1987;32: 726–736.

# 44 Diverticulitis and Appendicitis in the Elderly

Scott C. Thornton

This chapter deals with diverticular disease and appendicitis in the elderly. Diverticular disease increases in incidence with age and also appears to present with diffuse peritonitis more frequently in old than in young patients. Acute appendicitis in the elderly accounts for 5–10% of all appendicitis, and old patients tend to present more frequently with advanced disease than do young groups. There is good evidence that the elderly present more frequently in an atypical fashion with both of these diseases compared with their younger counterparts. Abdominal pain may be absent or not greatly perceived in older patients. Furthermore, it is well known that emergency operations in the elderly are associated with significantly higher mortality and morbidity rates than similar operations on younger patients. Thus, old patients present atypically, often with more advanced disease and have higher complication and death rates than the young. This chapter attempts to explain these findings.

## Diverticular Disease

### Etiology

The cause of diverticulosis is unknown. Colonic diverticula are mucosal herniations through the muscle wall of the colon. The sigmoid colon is affected in 96% of patients, with this area being the only site of diverticulosis in two-thirds of patients.[1] Acute diverticulitis can occur anywhere in the colon and has been reported in the rectum.[2,3] Diverticula occur at the points of weakness where the blood supply to the mucosa penetrates the bowel wall. Most commonly, they occur between the mesenteric and antimesenteric teniae coli. Less commonly, they occur between the two antimesenteric teniae. Strong epidemiologic evidence suggests that a low fiber diet has a substantial etiologic role in the development of diverticulosis,[4,5] and low fiber intake has long been implicated as a cause of diverticulosis.[4,6] In the United States, diverticular disease has increased with decreasing fiber intake.[7] Vegetarians have been found to have a lower incidence of diverticular disease than nonvegetarians.[8] Other studies have confirmed these findings.[9–13]

The current speculation is that a diet low in fiber decreases stool bulk, causes narrowing of the colonic lumen, prolongs intestinal transit time, and increases intraluminal pressures. Painter et al.[14] combined manometry and cineradiography and found that the increased intraluminal pressure may be due to simultaneous contractions of circular muscular bands causing occlusion of short segments of bowel. Contraction rings are thus formed in the sigmoid colon, which produces segmentation of these short segments of bowel. Contraction of the muscle wall of these sections can result in intraluminal pressures of 90 mmHg or more. This pulsion pressure may lead to mucosal herniation along the weak points of the bowel wall, resulting in diverticula. Others have found that the contractile response to eating is exaggerated in people with diverticulosis.[15] Although consistent with the speculation that elevated pressures are particularly significant in combination with or potentiated by low fiber stools, experimentation with colomyotomy showed that decreased muscular activity did not affect intraluminal pressures.[16] Stool bulk may be related to intraluminal pressure only in that stool bulk increases the radius of the colon, thereby decreasing wall tension. Painter et al. suggested that a low fiber diet causes a narrower colonic lumen, which allows the colon to segment more efficiently, increasing the segmental intraluminal pressures.[14]

Colonic dysmotility may contribute to diverticular disease. Abnormally slow wave patterns have been found in patients with symptomatic diverticular disease.[17] Furthermore, patients with symptomatic diverticular disease return to normal motility patterns with ingestion of bran, whereas those with asymptomatic diverticulosis have no change in motility with bran intake.[18] Others have disputed these findings.[19] Colonic transit times can be decreased by adding bran to the diet,[20–22] and water-retaining fiber can decrease intraluminal pressure.[23]

One report[24] implicated localized ischemia as a causative factor for antimesenteric free perforation of the colon from diverticulitis. In patients with multiple bilateral pseudodiverticula arranged in a double row about the antimesenteric teniae, the vascular supply to the middle area of the antimesenteric wall is compromised. Careful histologic studies showed that free perforation associated with diverticulitis has the same histologic characteristics as ischemic bowel perforations. It is well known that microvascular changes predisposing to microvascular ischemia occur in the elderly. The more aggressive disease and higher perforation rates found in the elderly[25–28] may be related to this ischemic process.

Investigators have also touched on whether an intrinsic change in bowel wall composition is necessary for the development of diverticula. Young people with collagen vascular diseases such as Marfan syndrome,[29] have been reported with diverticular disease. Several authors have also documented an association of diverticular disease with degenerative disorders such as varicose veins,[30] hiatal hernias,[31] and arthritis.[32] The most important element with regard to strength of the colon wall is collagen.[33] Collagen fibrils in the left colon become more numerous but smaller in width with age, and this difference is greater with diverticular disease.[34] Similarly, elastin fibrils increase in number but decrease in quality with age.[35] Pace[35] found that colon wall thickness increases with age and is thickest in the distal colon. These factors combined to result in decreased tensile strength and decreased expandability of the aging colon wall.[36]

The distal sigmoid is the narrowest portion of the colon, and the distal sigmoid narrows with age.[37] The law of Laplace states that wall tension is directly proportional to the pressure times the diameter. Thus, as contractile pressures remain the same and the diameter is decreased, there is an increase in pressure delivered to the bowel wall. A simple example of Laplace's law is blowing up a balloon. It is most difficult when there is no air in the balloon and becomes easier as the diameter increases. Similarly, increased pressures are required in the narrower distal sigmoid to propel stool. As the lumen narrows with age, higher pressures are required. This increased stress further damages the colon, causing decreased elasticity and more loss of tensile strength.[36] Comparison studies show that populations with a low incidence of diverticular disease have stronger, more elastic distal colons than industrialized populations,[37] presumably due to years of more bulky stools keeping the lumen diameter large. Furthermore, with increasing wall tension pressures, there must be a concomitant decrease in microvascular perfusion,[38] possibly adding further weight to the vascular theory of free perforation of diverticulitis.[13] Combined with the following epidemiologic findings, evidence appears overwhelming that diets low in fiber produce diverticulosis.

## Epidemiology

Diverticulosis is an entity particular to the dietary patterns of Western society. There are linear increases in size, number, incidence, and symptoms of diverticula with age.[5,39] Diverticulosis in patients less than age 40 ranges from 2% to 5%, and one-third of people over age 45 and two-thirds over age 85 having radiographic or pathologic evidence of diverticulosis.[40] Deckman and Cheskin[41] cited a prevalence in the United States as high as 33%. In comparison, the prevalence may be as low as 1% in Korea,[31] with low incidences found in other, similar populations.[42–47]

Independent of age, prevalence is thought to be similar in men and women. However, in a large single institutional series by Rodkey and Welch,[48] when sex and age were examined jointly, women over the age of 70 predominated over men by more than 3:1. The reverse was found in patients under 50 years of age, with more than twice as many men affected as women. This ratio was also substantiated by Ouriel and Schwartz,[49] who found a predominance of men in the under-40 age group.

Nonsteroidal antiinflammatory drugs (NSAIDs) have also been linked to diverticular disease,[50] and others have implicated NSAIDs as a potential cause of acute diverticulitis.[51–53] Steroids have been linked to diverticulitis as well and may cause delays in diagnosis with resulting poor prognosis.[54–56]

## Pathogenesis

Diverticulitis is the inflammatory process that originates within colonic pseudodiverticula. The particular mechanisms of both the local and systemic infections have not been well characterized. It has been hypothesized that diverticulitis constitutes the same endpoint of localized luminal obstruction found with other intraabdominal visceral inflammatory processes such as appendicitis and cholecystitis.[57–59] Obstruction of the necks of the diverticula, presumably with inspissated stool, creates a closed microenvironment characterized by fluid sequestration, stasis, and bacterial overgrowth. Deitch[60] showed that even in the absence of perforation, obstruction alone is sufficient for bacterial translocation across the intestinal barrier. As the diameter of the diverticulum expands to accommodate the increased intraluminal pressure, venous and then arterial pressures are overcome. It results in congestion, ischemic necrosis, and perforation. Others cannot find supporting pathologic evidence and suggest that perforation is likely the result of increased intraluminal pressure.[41] Activation of local and systemic inflammatory mediators, in combination with microscopic or macroscopic perforation and soiling of the peritoneum, leads to the clinical manifestations of the disease. The role of localized ischemia was discussed earlier.[24]

Painful diverticular disease is an obscure clinical entity manifesting with lower abdominal pain, especially on the left side. Motility patterns may be abnormal in this subset of patients.[61] The pain is usually chronic, intermittent, and not associated with acute symptoms. Narrow stools and other changes in bowel habits may result. Attacks may come and go. Symptoms may be confused with irritable bowel syndrome. The diagnosis is difficult, with barium enema showing only diverticulosis and possibly spasm of the sigmoid colon. Endoscopic findings are generally nonspecific, although a tortuous colon may be found. Treatment is aimed at relieving symptoms. Bulk agents (psyllium seed) and a high fiber diet are usually helpful. Uncommonly, sigmoid resection is required to produce relief.

## Symptoms

The spectrum of disease produced by diverticula ranges from completely symptom-free to vascular collapse secondary to systemic sepsis from peritonitis. About 10–25% of patients with diverticulosis progress to diverticulitis.[62,63] Most of these patients never come to surgical attention.[62,63] A small number, estimated at fewer than 25% of those with diverticulitis, require inpatient management of their disease.[64] Complicated cases involving sepsis, obstruction, or peritonitis constitute approximately 40% of all those admitted. The elderly present with diffuse peritonitis up to twice as frequently as younger patients.[25,28]

Typically, patients with diverticulitis seek medical care owing to mild or moderate peritoneal irritation often accompanied by a change in bowel habits. Crampy left lower quadrant pain is also common. Approximately two-thirds of patients complain of constipation or diarrhea.[65] Other associated symptoms may include a palpable mass, abdominal distension, dysuria, excessive flatus, nausea, and vomiting. About 30–40% of patients have occult blood in their stool.[2] Fever and pain are the most consistent indicators of acute disease, occurring 45% of the time. Septic shock with diffuse peritonitis may be the presenting picture. With the presence of a redundant sigmoid colon, suprapubic or right lower quadrant pain may manifest. Occasionally, the diagnosis of appendicitis is the indication for surgical exploration when a redundant sigmoid colon and diverticulitis are found to be the culprit.

Considerable diagnostic overlap exists between diverticulitis and other acute abdominal processes. The spectrum of differential diagnoses range from relatively common urinary tract infections in the elderly to inflammatory bowel disease, colon cancer, closed loop obstruction, and ischemic bowel. These diagnoses and causes of abdominal pain must always be kept in mind during the initial evaluation.

Symptoms of diverticular fistulas may lead to an accurate preoperative diagnosis. Pneumaturia and fecaluria are diagnostic of an enteric–vesicular fistula and in the appropriate patients are highly suggestive of a diverticular origin. Similarly, flatus or stool via the vagina leads to common bowel sources. Thigh abscesses may originate from a diverticular abscess with tracking along the psoas muscle onto the skin.

Many investigators have found atypical presentations of diverticular disease in the elderly.[25,66–70] Wroblewski and Mikulowski[68] noted the absence of typical manifestation of peritonitis in the elderly to be associated with a poor outcome. They also found an absence of abdominal pain in half of their patients with peritonitis. Intraabdominal abscesses are the most common cause of fever of unknown origin in the elderly.[71] Others noted that elderly patients with intraabdominal infections have hypothermic temperatures more frequently than young patients. Similarly, old patients have less nausea, vomiting, diarrhea, and fever compared to the young.[66] Acute abdominal pain is more likely to require surgery in the elderly.[72,73] France et al.[67] examined 12 old patients who died of diverticulitis: 75% did not have symptoms typical of their disease, 3 of the 12 did not have abdominal symptoms, and another's symptoms did not warrant further investigation. Generalized peritonitis occurs in up to one-half of old patients.[25,26] Old patients require operations more frequently, have free perforation more commonly, and have higher mortality rates than young patients.[25,26,27,28,74] Watters et al.[25] attempted to explain this difference. They found that the mean time from the onset of symptoms to hospitalization for old and young patients with generalized diverticular peritonitis was the same. Thus, old patients have peritonitis and free perforation more frequently than the young do, and it is not due to a delay in seeking medical care. This finding suggests that the severity of disease in the elderly is determined early in its course and is independent of the passage of time or that symptoms begin later in the course of the disease. The former explanation further supports the theory that ischemia is the cause of the more frequent diffuse peritonitis found in the elderly.

## Diagnosis

Diverticulitis is usually diagnosed based completely on clinical grounds. This presents a unique problem in the elderly because, as previously shown, they often present atypically and abdominal pain is minimal or absent. A history of known diverticula seen by barium enema or endoscopy often aids the clinician. Useful serologic and hematologic tests include a complete blood count, serum electrolytes, urinalysis, and in the case of suspected ischemic bowel, arterial blood gas measurement.

Acute-phase reactants are also being evaluated as diagnostic agents. Physical examination reveals peritoneal irritation to some extent. Mild left lower quadrant tenderness to generalized peritonitis may be found. Rectal examination may reveal a pelvic abscess.

Several diagnostic modalities are helpful for establishing the diagnosis of diverticular disease and assessing the extent of inflammation. In preceding decades, contrast enema was the test of choice for diagnosis. The practice parameters of the American Society of Colon and Rectal Surgeons[75] cite a sensitivity of 94%, an accuracy of 77%, and a false-negative rate of 2–15% with water-soluble enemas. Radiographic findings include intramural or extramural sinus tracts, filling of the abscess cavity, or inferred extramural compression or spasm of the bowel lumen.

Ultrasonography may also provide useful information in the setting of suspected diverticular disease. Investigators have found it to be 84–98% sensitive.[76–78] Ultrasonography can detect abnormal segments of bowel, those with mural thickening, peridiverticular inflammation and abscess, and linear echogenic foci suggestive of fistulous tracts. Unfortunately, this technique is both operator-dependent and limited by the body habitus of the patient.

Computed tomography (CT) has emerged as the imaging modality of choice for evaluating suspected diverticulitis.[79–83] Though in some studies it is comparable to contrast enema, other investigators have found a clear advantage regarding diagnostic sensitivity and specificity. Hulnick et al.[83] found that CT not only stages the extent of the inflammatory process more accurately, it better differentiates the varying gradations of pericolic inflammation. Furthermore, CT has the distinct advantage over a contrast enema because of its ability to identify both the intraluminal and extraluminal components of diverticular disease. It is also the diagnostic modality of choice for identifying colovesicle and colovaginal fistulas. Findings suggestive of diverticulitis include inflammation of the pericolic fat, thickening of the sigmoid mesocolon, pericolic phlegmon, visualization of colonic diverticula themselves, and thickening of the colonic wall. CT is helpful for demonstrating the manifestations of intraabdominal abscess, particularly abscesses amenable to percutaneous drainage.[79–83] Despite these modalities, the diagnosis of diverticulitis can be obscure in the elderly.[68] Endoscopic evaluation is reserved until after the acute phase has resolved; it is used mainly to rule out carcinoma.

## Treatment

### *Uncomplicated Diverticulitis*

Most physicians suggest a high fiber diet with bulk-producing supplements (psyllium seed) for patients with asymptomatic diverticulosis.[84] Fiber has been shown to decrease intraluminal pressures and colonic transit time.[23,85–87] It also decreases symptoms attributed to diverticular disease.[84,86,88–91] A small number of physicians suggest restricted intake of nuts, popcorn, and foods with large seeds in an attempt to decrease the chance of obstructing the diverticula. Most acute diverticulitis is treated by primary physicians on an outpatient basis. Those with only mild tenderness, no clinical peritoneal signs, and the ability to achieve satisfactory pain control and tolerate adequate fluids orally may be treated empirically on an outpatient basis.[5] Treatment consists of oral antibiotics covering anaerobic and gram-negative bacteria for at least 7 days and liquid diet until resolution of symptoms. Significant systemic signs of infection including high fever and leukocytosis suggest the need for hospital treatment. Resolution is common. There is no place for outpatient management in the setting of significant concurrent medical disease or immune compromise or in patients on steroids, those with altered mental status, or patients without appropriate supervision.

Immune-compromised patients have a more aggressive lethal disease, are more likely to present with perforation, and have higher morbidity and mortality rates.[55,92] Perkins et al.[92] found a 100% failure rate with conservative treatment of immune-compromised patients. For this aggressive disease, some have suggested elective sigmoid resection in patients with a single prior attack when they are candidates for organ transplantation with its attendant long-term immune suppression.[93]

Patients who fail outpatient therapy or who present with significant systemic symptoms should be admitted to the hospital. Hospital treatment consists of complete bowel rest and parenteral broad-spectrum antibiotics to cover anaerobic and gram-negative bacteria. Triple-antibiotic or single-agent therapy are both effective. Nasogastric suction is required only with persistent vomiting or evidence of bowel obstruction. Laboratory evaluation includes a complete blood count and urinalysis. CT should be done to confirm the diagnosis and quantify the extent of inflammation. Conservative treatment of acute uncomplicated diverticulitis leads to resolution of symptoms in 70–100% of cases.[1,2,41,42,48,65,79,94] Oral intake is resumed with disappearance of symptoms. Following hospital discharge, oral antibiotics should be continued for 7–10 days. With complete resolution of the inflammation, patients should have endoscopic or radiographic evaluation of their colon to rule out carcinoma, and they should be started on long-term fiber supplementation. Psyllium seed or hydrophilic colloids have been shown to reduce recurrence by up to 70%.[90] One-fourth of patients have further attacks requiring hospitalization.[1,95]

Elective sigmoid resection is suggested after two or more attacks, after one attack with radiologic evidence of perforation, or abscess successfully managed medically, after one attack in patients requiring long-term immunosuppression, and if cancer cannot be ruled out.[57] Elective sigmoid resection after resolution of the acute inflammation should include adequate mobilization of the proximal bowel to provide a tension-free anastomosis. The proximal bowel need not be devoid of diverticulosis, but the bowel must be soft, supple, and free of diverticular thickening. Resection should include all thickened, diseased bowel. Splenic flexure mobilization is occasionally required to achieve these goals. Distal resection must include removal of the entire sigmoid to the rectum to significantly reduce recurrent attacks.[96] No diverticula should be left distal to the anastomosis. The site of distal transection should be at the point where the teniae coli are lost, signifying the beginning of the intraperitoneal rectum. Laparoscopic approaches can be used in the nonacute setting.

Up to one-third of all patients admitted to the hospital require urgent or emergent surgery.[1,40,41,51,94] Up to one-half of elderly patients present with generalized peritonitis requiring operative intervention.[25] Similarly, more old patients with diverticulitis require urgent or emergent operations.[26] Most patients requiring urgent or emergent surgery are undergoing their initial episode of diverticulitis.[2,95] Surgical treatment aims to relieve sepsis, remove the diseased bowel, minimize mortality and morbidity, and avoid stomas with their concomitant second operation to restore bowel continuity. Options include resection with primary anastomosis, resection with proximal colostomy and closure of the distal end (Hartmann's procedure), and diversion with drainage alone. The latter plays only a small role today, with only the most ill and unstable patients unable to tolerate removal of the infectious foci. Diversion alone leaves a column of undrained stool above the perforation that can further contribute to the septic process.[97,98] Resection with primary anastomosis for acute disease is occasionally possible with gentle preoperative bowel preparation and localized sepsis.[85,97] Mobilization of the colon should begin in an unaffected area to facilitate entrance into normal planes of dissection. The retroperitoneal structures (ureters and gonadal vessels) can be swept dorsally, elevating the sigmoid colon. Ureteral catheters can be helpful for acute inflammation and occasionally for elective resections.[99] It is not necessary to remove all proximal bowel containing diverticula. Soft, pliable proximal sigmoid or descending colon should be chosen for the proximal site of resection. Distal margins should provide soft, normal rectum free of diverticulosis and inflammation for anastomosis.[96] Hartmann's resection with diverting colostomy is recommended for unprepared bowel. Adequate diverticular resection requires removal of the distal sigmoid from the rectum when restoring bowel continuity after Hartmann's procedure. Removing the sigmoid from the rectum decreases recurrences of diverticular disease.[96] Furthermore, using the distal sigmoid instead of rectum for the anastomosis was found to be a risk factor in the development of postoperative colocutaneous fistulas.[100]

## *Complicated Diverticular Disease*

Complicating factors associated with diverticular disease include abscess formation, free perforation, fistula formation, obstruction, and bleeding. The presentation of complicated diverticular disease occurs in up to 32% of hospitalized patients[79] and more than 50% of the elderly.[25] Bleeding diverticular disease is discussed in Chapter 45. Complicated diverticulitis is associated with significant morbidity and mortality, and the need for operative intervention should be continually reassessed. Treatment of complicated diverticular disease requires accurate diagnosis and staging. The goal of treatment of complicated diverticular disease is to minimize morbidity and mortality and the number of subsequent operations. To achieve these goals, nonoperative techniques can convert complicated disease to medically manageable disease, thereby allowing elective resection with primary anastomosis. Hartmann's procedure is associated with high morbidity and mortality rates.[97,101,102] Retained colostomy rates after Hartmann's operation range from 5% to 58%.[97,103] Furthermore, colostomy closure is associated with significant complication and death rates, especially in the elderly.[104] Eisenstat et al.[105] recorded a lower mortality rate for complicated diverticular disease treated with elective resection than that treated with staged surgical procedures. Avoiding a stoma with its concomitant second operation is a major goal of operative treatment for complicated diverticular disease. Accurate preoperative diagnosis is helpful, as up to 25% of patients explored for abscess or fistula have a perforated cancer.[106]

Abscess formation is the most common complication of acute diverticulitis, occurring in 32–68% of complicated diverticular cases.[50,79–81,107] A wide spectrum of presentations may result: small occult abscesses; scrotal, buttock, or thigh abscess; and sepsis due to a large abscess. Diagnosis is best made with CT.[79,108] Treatment is aimed at relief of the sepsis and the diverticulitis. Small peri-colic abscesses or phlegmon may be managed conservatively with bowel rest and broad-spectrum intra- venous antibiotics. Elective, single-stage sigmoid resection with primary anastomosis can be done with resolution of symptoms. If symptoms worsen or are not alleviated, repeat CT scan with percutaneous drainage of the abscess should be considered. Exploration is reserved for patients whose abscesses are not amenable to percutaneous drainage or who fail conservative management. Primary anastomosis is possible if the proximal and distal bowel is healthy and the perforation is contained, and if a gentle preoperative mechanical preparation has been done.[81,103] The patient's underlying medical diseases and acute physiologic status must obviously be considered.

Large abscesses, including more distant pelvic abscesses, and smaller ones that do not respond to conservative treatment should be referred quickly for possible percutaneous drainage under CT guidance.[80,109] Percutaneous drainage of diverticular abscesses is associated with a success rate of 62–100%.[79,80,110–113] Following placement of a drainage catheter and aspiration of the pus, repeat radiologic evaluation should be undertaken to assess not only resolution of the abscess cavity but to identify potential fistulous communications to the small or large bowel. In the setting of appropriate drainage, treatment should progress as for uncomplicated diverticulitis. The catheter may be removed when the drainage stops or when complete collapse of the abscess cavity has been shown by sinography. At discharge, the catheter may also be left in place and removed during subsequent elective sigmoid resection.[80,99] The presence of a persistent colocutaneous fistula does not preclude elective resection with primary anastomosis.[79,80] Such a course of treatment allows complicated disease to be transformed nonoperatively to disease that responds to medical treatment, thereby avoiding emergent surgery with stoma formation. Subsequent elective sigmoid resection with primary anastomosis after resolution of inflammation (in about 6 weeks) becomes the only operative intervention required.[83] This has become the standard treatment for diverticulitis complicated by abscess formation.

Stabile et al.[80] followed three patients who refused surgery after catheter drainage for large abscesses. One required resection after a repeat diverticulitis attack 7 months later. The second required permanent catheter drainage for recurrent and persistent abscesses. The third died in hospital of sepsis. Ambrosetti et al.[81] followed one patient without operation after percutaneous drainage who required elective resection 11 months later owing to stenosis. The authors suggested that occasional small mesocolic abscesses can be managed without operation, but they stated that pelvic and abdominal abscesses behave aggressively and require surgical treatment. Thus, all patients, with the possible exception of those with small mesocolic abscesses, which are treated with percutaneous drainage, require elective sigmoid resection after resolution of inflammation to prevent future complications.

Pelvic abscesses can be drained transrectally and transvaginally in women as well. These techniques are being replaced by CT-guided drainage but should remain in the surgeon's arsenal. If large abscesses cannot be drained adequately or if sepsis does not resolve, operative exploration is required. Gentle preoperative mechanical bowel preparation can be performed in well-selected patients; and with normal proximal and distal bowel, resection and primary anastomosis can be performed safely.[103] The use of Hartmann's procedure is reserved for most other patients. One should remember that restoring bowel continuity after Hartmann's procedure has high morbidity and mortality rates, and a large percentage of "temporary" stomas become permanent.[97,103–105]

A few important technical aspects of resection must be emphasized. When possible, care should be taken in the face of peritonitis to avoid opening noninfected tissue planes such as the presacral space and the splenic flexure area. These areas are known to invite abscess formation and are best left intact and free from contamination by the infectious process. Ureteral catheters should be used generously, as the inflammatory process may obliterate the normal tissue planes and allow the ureters to be drawn into the inflammatory process.[114] The reader is referred to standard surgical textbooks for other technical aspects of sigmoid resection.

Free perforation of diverticulitis generally presents as acute sepsis or an acute abdominal crisis and some degree of shock. It occurs in approximately 10% of complicated cases.[79] More importantly, up to 50% of elderly patients present with diffuse peritonitis.[25,26] Rapid hydration with correction of electrolyte abnormalities is necessary. Broad-spectrum antibiotics are administered preoperatively. Immunocompromised patients may not exhibit classic abdominal findings. Physical examination and CT scans generally yield the diagnosis. A large number of old patients with peritonitis lack abdominal pain as a finding,[68] so a high index of suspicion is required when treating them. Emergent exploration with aspiration of pus, cleansing of fecal material, resection of the diseased bowel, and proximal end colostomy with oversewing of the distal stump (Hartmann's operation) are performed.[115,116] Only rarely are patients so sick that diversion and drainage without resection is appropriate.[115,117] In fact, one study[98] found higher mortality among patients treated with diversion only compared to those who underwent resection, despite more steroid use and fecal peritonitis in the resection group. The mortality rate associated with fecal peritonitis is as high as 35%.[98,115,118]

Fistula formation occurs in approximately 2% of diverticulitis cases but accounts for up to 22% of patients requiring surgery.[79,103,115,119,120] Multiple fistulas are uncommon.[119] Fistulas develop when inflammation or abscesses develop in close proximity to adjacent organs. The inflammatory process invades the adjacent normal organs and causes decompression, which spontaneously converts the acute complicated infectious process to controlled, drained, simple diverticulitis. It is diagnosed often on clinical grounds, and diagnostic tests are used to rule out cancer and other diagnoses. Expensive, complex testing is often unnecessary. In general, single-stage resection with primary anastomosis can be performed in a fashion similar to that used for complicated diverticulitis treated with percutaneous abscess drainage.

The bladder is affected most commonly.[119,121] Symptoms include pneumaturia and fecaluria. Sepsis can also occur. Diagnosis is made most commonly by the patient's history. CT scan is most accurate for diagnosis, showing air in the uninstrumentated bladder and inflammation of the sigmoid colon and dome of the bladder.[115] Contrast enema or endoscopic evaluation is required to rule out colon cancer. Cystoscopy may be performed to rule out a neoplastic process originating in the bladder. In some patients the fistula cannot be demonstrated. Elective sigmoid resection with primary anastomosis is curative.[97,122] The fistula is pinched off the bladder. A small bladder defect is best treated by Foley catheter drainage for 7–10 days. Large defects should be closed in two layers with absorbable suture and drained by Foley catheter for a similar length of time. Bladder resection should be reserved for malignant disease.[122]

Colovaginal fistulas occur most commonly in women who have had a hysterectomy. Diagnosis is simply made by the history, including flatus or stool per vagina. It is confirmed by transvaginal and transanal endoscopy. Air may be heard exiting from the vagina during sigmoidoscopy. Contrast enema or endoscopic evaluation of the colon is required to rule out neoplastic and inflammatory bowel disorders. Patients generally are not septic at the time of presentation and may undergo elective sigmoid resection with primary anastomosis. The vagina can be left open for drainage or may be closed with absorbable sutures and omentum interposed between the vagina and the anastomosis. Other organs, including the uterus, may be involved with the fistulous process. Hysterectomy may be required if the uterus is involved with the infectious process or if a neoplastic process is suspected.[123] Spontaneous colocutaneous fistulization is uncommon and can be treated with resection and primary anastomosis if sepsis is controlled.

Obstruction complicating diverticulitis occurs uncommonly.[79,124] Repeated episodes of edema, spasm, and inflammation cause a chronically strictured bowel lumen to become narrowed.[97] Acute inflammation can then complete the luminal obstruction. Gentle water-soluble enema or endoscopy by a skilled endoscopist with minimal air insufflation can confirm the diagnosis and exclude a neoplasm. With proper diagnosis and treatment, the inflammation usually resolves and the obstruction abates. This allows it to be treated as uncomplicated diverticulitis with preoperative bowel preparation followed by elective resection and primary anastomosis after complete resolution of inflammation. Emergency operation for obstruction due to diverticulitis generally requires removing the diseased bowel with creation of an end colostomy. The unprepared and dilated proximal bowel often precludes safe primary anastomosis. On-table lavage has been used more frequently in selected cases to allow primary anastomosis.[125]

## Appendicitis

Many investigators have tried to assign an immune function to the appendix, as it does secrete immunoglobins, but the appendix is an organ whose function is unknown. Certainly, normal life results after its removal. Inflammation and neoplastic transformation are by far the most common afflictions that affect the human appendix. Infectious diseases (typhoid and tuberculosis), regional enteritis, and congenital defects of the appendix are beyond the scope of this chapter. Similarly, neoplasms of the appendix are not addressed. Appendectomy is one of the most common operations performed, with more than 500,000 appendices removed annually in the United States; 5–10% of acute appendicitis occurs in the elderly. Old patients delay presentation, present atypically, and suffer delay in diagnosis and treatment more often than young patients. Perforation is found more frequently in the elderly. Higher mortality rates and prolonged hospital stays result. The following section attempts to explain these findings.

### Etiology

Obstruction of the lumen of the appendix is the predominant cause of appendicitis, and fecaliths are a common cause of obstruction. After the lumen is obstructed a closed microenvironment is produced, which allows fluid sequestration, stasis, distension, and bacterial overgrowth. Mucosal secretion and bacterial multiplication increase the distension and intraluminal pressure. As the diameter of the lumen expands to accommodate the increased pressure, venous and then arterial pressures are overcome. Ischemia, necrosis, bacterial translocation, and appendiceal perforation result. Interestingly, humans are one of the few animals able to secrete fluid into the lumen of the appendix at pressures high enough to produce necrosis and perforation.[126]

Perforation occurs owing to vascular compromise, causing necrosis, usually on an antimesenteric border. There are thought to be many differences in the elderly appendix that predispose it to obstruction and perforation. The appendiceal lumen is small or obliterated, and the blood supply is decreased, predisposing to necrosis; the mucosa is thinned, and there is fatty infiltration of the wall.[127] These changes may lead to increased rupture rates with decreased pressures, thus altering the natural history of appendicitis in the elderly. NSAIDs have been implicated in appendicitis as well. Campbell and DeBeaux[128] found that 37% of patients over the age of 50, with the diagnosis of acute appendicitis, were on NSAIDs compared with only 11% of a similar age group admitted with other emergencies.

## Epidemiology

Appendicitis is the most common acute surgical condition of the abdomen. Six to eight percent of the population will suffer from acute appendicitis in their lifetime.[129–131] Life-table analysis estimates that 12% of males and 23% of females have their appendixes surgically removed.[130] Acute appendicitis occurs at all ages but is most frequent during the teenage years.[130,132] This age peak is thought to result from the peak in lymph tissue in the appendix during these years. The extra lymph tissue presumably narrows the lumen, predisposing it to obstruction and the resulting appendicitis. Males are more commonly affected in young ages, but during later adult life the male/female ratio equals out.[132] There is a decrease in the incidence of acute appendicitis in the young over recent decades, and the reason is unknown.[127,130,132–134] Five to ten percent of all acute appendicitis occurs in the elderly,[129,131,134,135] and in fact the incidence of acute appendicitis in the elderly is increasing.[127,133,134] It may be due to longer life-spans, as Thorbjarnarson and Loehr[127] found that old patients accounted for only 1% of appendicitis between 1932 and 1937, whereas this percentage increased to 6–8% after 1957. Altogether, 1 of 35 women and 1 of 50 men over age 50 years develop acute appendicitis.[131] Furthermore, appendicitis accounted for 2.5–5.0% of all acute abdominal disease in patients over 60–70 years of age.[68,135]

Acute appendicitis is the third most common cause of abdominal pain in the elderly after gallbladder disease and small bowel obstruction.[136,137] It is the leading source of intraabdominal abscess, which in turn is the most common cause of fever of unknown origin in the elderly.[71] About 33–50% of the mortality due to acute appendicitis occurs in the elderly.[129,130,138] Whereas mortality from appendicitis in general has been decreasing, the percentage of deaths among the elderly is on the rise,[127] often due to delays in diagnosis and treatment. Also, lowered immune responses to foreign antigens and decreased production of lymphocytes with advancing age limits the older patients' ability to wall off peritoneal inflammation and fight overall infectious events.[139,140]

## Symptoms and Diagnosis

Abdominal pain, fever, and leukocytosis are the hallmarks of acute appendicitis. Distension of the obstructed appendix stimulates visceral afferent nerve fibers, producing vague, dull, mid-abdominal pain. Pain classically begins in the periumbilical area and migrates to the right lower quadrant within hours.[126,141] This pain is peritoneal in origin and as such is constant and increases with time. Anorexia is common. Vomiting occurs up to 75% of the time. Protracted vomiting and diarrhea should lead the clinician away from the diagnosis. There are many variations in presentation.

Physical examination reveals the site of peritoneal inflammation. Usually tenderness is found at McBurney's point. Rovsing's sign (pain referred to the right lower quadrant with palpation of the left side) indicates localized peritoneal irritation. The appendix may be found anywhere in the abdomen and thus can cause pain during psoas muscle stretch, obturator muscle stretch, rectal examination, or palpation of any abdominal site.[141] Continued irritation results in rebound and referred peritoneal irritation. Frank peritonitis can ultimately result with perforation. Elevated core temperature is usually not more than 39°C. The white blood cell (WBC) count is generally between 10,000 and 18,000/mm$^3$ with a left shift.[126] Higher or lower counts and extreme left shifts are indications of diffuse peritonitis. Acute-phase reactants are being examined in an attempt to increase the accuracy of the preoperative diagnosis. Urinalysis should be done but may be abnormal if the appendix is adjacent to the bladder or ureter.

The presentation and difficulty with diagnosis of acute appendicitis in the elderly deserves special consideration. An elderly patient with a perforated appendicitis who was incorrectly treated for alcohol withdrawal for 5 days prior to being accurately diagnosed has been reported.[142] Burns et al.[143] found that 20% of older patients with acute appendicitis had WBC counts less than 10,000/mm$^3$ and neutrophil counts less than 75%. Lau et al.[144] found only 43% of old patients with simple appendicitis to have elevated WBC counts. Thorbjarnarson and Loehr[127] recorded an average duration of symptoms prior to admission in patients over age 60 to be 2.5 days. Horattas et al.[145] found that one-third of patients over 60 years of age waited more than 48 hours from onset of symptoms before presenting to the hospital. Fewer than two-thirds had "typical" right lower quadrant pain, and one-half had a temperature <37.6°C. Similarly, Smithy et al.[146] found that only 55% of patients over age 80 had right lower quadrant pain, and 18% did not have abdominal pain. They also noted that only 1 of 13 patients had "typical" periumbilical pain localizing in the right lower quadrant. They hypothesized that because of the smaller lumen diameter of the elderly appendix, which requires less pressure to produce rupture, the old patient does not necessarily experience the prodromal phase of appendicitis with the generalized abdominal pain, anorexia, nausea, and vomiting thought to be caused by visceral distension. Nausea, vomiting, fever, and anorexia were found to be uncommon in old patients by others as well.[66,143] Burns et al.[143] compared the presentations of young and old patients. They found that twice as many young patients presented "classically," and old patients were more than two times more likely to delay presentation for more than 72 hours after onset of symptoms. Furthermore, in their study old patients were three times as likely to have operation delayed more than 24 hours after admission than were the young. Horattas et al.[145] found that 13% of patients had their operations delayed more than 48 hours after admission, further illustrating the difficulty of correctly diagnosing this age group. Samiy[147] described a blunted or absent pain response in the elderly and, perhaps more importantly, found that doctors often minimize the importance of the old patient's pain, attributing it to old age or concomitant diseases.[148–150] Clinicians must be more cognizant of the abdominal complaints in old patients if prompt diagnosis and treatment with resultant decreased morbidity and mortality are to be expected.

The confident diagnosis of acute appendicitis is difficult, and the experienced clinician is wrong 5–25% of the time.[132,151] Many books and articles have been written describing techniques for diagnosing acute appendicitis.[141,152–154] The combination of appropriate history, physical examination, and elevated WBC count is thought to be most important for diagnosing appendicitis correctly.[155] Unfortunately, these factors are not often present together.[154] Ultrasonography and focused CT have been used extensively for presurgical evaluation of patients.[152,153,156] Despite numerous advances in radiographic techniques, the rate of unnecessary explorations remains at 5–20%.[152,153,157]

C-reactive protein (CRP) has been studied as a tool to aid in the accurate diagnosis of appendicitis.[158] There is a decline in the production of inflammatory mediators and the immune system with aging.[139,140,159] CRP is preserved with age.[158] CRP has been found to be consistently elevated only in patients with perforation, perhaps because it first appears in the serum about 8 hours after the initial insult and takes 24–48 hours to reach peak blood levels.[158] Thus, elevated serum levels are often found only with prolonged symptoms, which corresponds to high perforation rates. Obviously, if symptoms progress rapidly, there is no time for serum CRP levels to rise. CRP is not specific for appendicitis: It also increases with any inflammation, surgical trauma, and acute myocardial infarcts.[158]

Exploratory laparotomy or laparoscopy remains the diagnostic test of choice in appropriately chosen patients. Despite the advances in preoperative modalities, an accurate diagnosis of acute appendicitis is made in only 30–77% of the elderly on admission and in only 70% preoperatively.[143,145,146,151,160] Between 14% and 33% of older patients have operations more than 24 hours after admission.[143–146,151]

## Treatment and Outcomes

Nonoperative care of acute appendicitis is appropriate only if emergent surgical expertise is unavailable. Recurrence within 18 months is seen in at least 35% of patients treated only with antibiotics.[161] Early, aggressive treatment is imperative to minimize mortality in the elderly. In fact, Burns et al.[143] suggested that "based on the lack of significant complications in those patients with a false-positive diagnosis and the 65% perforation rate in older patients, we feel an even earlier and more aggressive surgical approach is warranted." Operative treatment for acute appendicitis remains resection of the offending organ. Hydration and correction of electrolyte imbalances prior to urgent operation is prudent. Untoward delay before exploration may allow progression of the disease and ultimately free rupture of the organ with resultant peritonitis. Preoperative broad-spectrum antibiotics are administered intravenously and are continued postoperatively if necrosis or perforation is discovered. All pus should be evacuated, localized abscess cavities irrigated thoroughly, and appropriate closed-suction drains employed if abscess cavities are encountered.[143] The skin should be left open in complicated cases. When a normal appendix is discovered, the abdomen should be systematically examined to search for the origin of the symptoms; resection of the normal appendix is usually appropriate. Nonoperative management of abdominal abscesses is well known. CT-guided drainage of abscesses allows resolution of the acute septic process followed by elective, internal operative treatment, thereby avoiding emergency surgery with its attendant morbidity.[79,80,109,110,162] Acute appendicitis with a contained abscess responds well to drainage,[162] and most patients with appendicitis respond to antibiotics.[161,163] Interval appendectomy 6–12 weeks later, after resolution of the infectious process, is suggested because of the high recurrence rates. Some question the need for interval resection.[161–163] Recurrence rates in adult age groups approach 35%.[161] With the well-known delay in presentation, difficulty with accurate and timely diagnosis, and the increased morbidity and mortality seen in the elderly, interval appendectomy is suggested in all but the most frail. Neoplasm must be ruled out in those managed conservatively. Furthermore, elective interval appendectomy lends itself well to the laparoscopic approach, as stressed by Greig and Nixon.[164]

Ileocecal resection and primary anastomosis are reserved for the markedly inflamed cecum. Rarely, resection cannot be performed safely because of the inflammatory reaction. In these cases, irrigation and drainage are performed, and interval appendectomy is scheduled for 6–12 weeks later. The reader is referred to general surgical textbooks for the detailed operative technique.

More than 75% of young patients are found to have simple appendicitis at operation.[25,130,143,160] This is in contrast to 48–63% of patients over age 50 years having a ruptured appendicitis[160,165] and 49–92% of patients over age 70 years having perforation, an abscess, or both.[25,130,133,143,145,146,160] Luckmann[132] found an age-related increase in complex appendicular disease in a California population-based study. About 1.8–32.0% of the older patients succumb to their disease, mostly owing to sepsis.[127,130,132,135,144,146,151,160] In a countrywide population-based study, the mortality was 4.6% for patients over age 65 and only 0.2% for those less than 65.[130]

It is debated whether appendicitis in the elderly progresses more quickly than in younger patients, which may account for the higher perforation rates found in old patients. Children with symptoms for more than 48 hours have perforation rates up to 98%.[166] Franz et al.[160] studied a Veterans Administration hospital population and found that those with simple appendicitis had symptoms lasting a mean of 22 hours, perforated appendicitis patients a mean of 50 hours, and those with abscesses an average 66 hours prior to presentation. They concluded that the delay in seeking care accounts for the increased perforation and abscess rates in old patients. Watters et al.[25] agreed that prehospital delay accounted for the increased rate of perforation found in the elderly compared with the young. Paajanen et al.[167] agreed that duration of symptoms within an age group corresponds well with perforation rates for that group, thus dispelling the concept that in old patients appendicitis progresses more rapidly than in young patients. Others have found an increased rate of perforation in pregnant women, with symptoms lasting longer than 24 hours,[168] and in children, with symptoms more than 48 hours prior to operation.[166] Similarly, Temple et al.[169] examined 95 consecutive patients and found an average of 31 hours from onset of pain to operation for simple appendicitis, whereas patients with perforation had symptoms for 63 hours before operation. Interestingly, those with perforation spent less time in the hospital before operation. In contrast, Smithy et al.[146] observed a 92% perforation rate in patients more than 80 years of age, with an average time from admission to operation of 15 hours, bespeaking the difficulty of making the diagnosis in the elderly. Thus, the rate of evolution of appendicitis is not different in the elderly. Old patients more frequently delay seeking treatment, increasing the rate of perforation.

Lau et al.[144] found a 38% perforation rate in old patients operated on within 24 hours of the onset of symptoms, suggesting aggressive disease. Wolff and Hindman[170] agreed, finding a perforation rate of 41% in old patients with onset of symptoms within 24 hours of operation. However, Burns et al.[143] found that one-third of young and old patients operated within 24 hours had perforation. Von Tittle et al.[171] also found that roughly one-third of old patients with perforation had symptoms less than 24 hours. Thus, an equal number of their young and old patients progressed rapidly to advanced disease. They concluded that physicians are responsible for almost two-thirds of older patients' delays in diagnosis and treatment of appendicitis, with the patients themselves being responsible for the rest. Obviously, duration of symptoms correlates with perforation rates in all age groups. Luckmann[132] found that only 53% of patients over age 80 in California had their operation on the day of admission, compared to more than 80% of young patients. More impressively, in patients with abscesses, more than 85% of young patients had operations within 1 day of admission, compared to only 57% of those older than 80 years. This further attests to the difficulty accurately diagnosing and treating acute appendicitis in the elderly. One study revealed that 17% of elderly patients were treated without accurate diagnosis prior to being admitted with acute appendicitis.[143] Incorrect diagnosis rates in the elderly are as high as 25%.[172]

Most studies show that the progression of appendicular disease in the elderly is similar to that in younger groups. However, old patients frequently present with longer duration of symptoms and are more commonly misdiagnosed, resulting in delayed operation. This prolonged time from onset of symptoms to operation accounts for the increased perforation rates found in the elderly. Their concomitant medical problems most likely account for the high mortality rates reported. Incidental appendectomy should not be performed in patients over age 60 and probably not in those over 35 years of age.[130]

In-hospital observation has been shown to decrease negative operative rates safely without increasing the perforation rate.[172,173] This suggests that the out-of-hospital delay is most important for determining the aggressiveness of disease. Lau et al.[144] found a statistically significant increase in perforation rates in elderly patients when surgeons delayed operation for more than 25 hours. Klein et al.[151] also found increased perforation and abscess rates in old patients with increasing delays of operation. Because of the difficulty diagnosing old patients, attempting to decrease perforation rates through hospital observation in the elderly is unwise.

There has been an explosion of laparoscopic surgery in the United States. The laparoscopic approach compared with conventional surgery is touted to decrease pain, length of stay, costs, and rehabilitation time for many procedures. Most surgeons agree this is true for laparoscopic cholecystectomy. Appendicitis is a unique disease. The conventional operative intervention does not impart a significant physiologic insult to the patient, and early and late recovery appears to be more related to the severity of the disease and the underlying health of the patient than to the operative approach.

Many authors have examined laparoscopic versus open appendectomy.[174–178] One prospective randomized study found that patients used fewer analgesics and returned to full activities sooner compared to those exposed to conventional operative techniques.[177] Some have found fewer wound infections with laparoscopic techniques.[179–181] This good record is usually achieved with increased hospital costs. Others have found an increase in abdominal abscesses in laparoscopically treated patients.[182] One obvious advantage of laparoscopic appendectomy is the ability to view the entire abdomen and pelvis in cases where the diagnosis is in question. The reader is referred to a recent current status review for a more in-depth evaluation of laparoscopic appendectomy.[183]

## References


1. Parks TG. Natural history of diverticular disease of the colon: a review of 521 cases. Br Med J 1969;4:639–642.
2. Chiu TT, Bailey HR, Hernandez AJ Jr. Diverticulitis of the midrectum. Dis Colon Rectum 1983;26:59–60.
3. Hackford AW, Veidenheimer MC. Diverticular disease of the colon: current concepts and management. Surg Clin North Am 1985;65:347–363.
4. Painter NS, Burkitt DP. Diverticular disease of the colon: a deficiency disease of Western civilization. Br Med J 1971; 2:450–454.
5. Painter NS, Burkitt DP. Diverticular disease of the colon, a 20th century problem. Clin Gastroenterol 1975;4:3–21.
6. Burkitt DP. Related disease—related cause? Lancet 1969; 2:1229–1231.
7. Trowell H. Definition of dietary fiber and hypotheses that it is a protective factor in certain diseases. Am J Clin Nutr 1976;29:417–427.
8. Gear JSS, Fursdon P, Nolan DJ, et al. Symptomless diverticular disease and intake of dietary fiber. Lancet 1979; 1:511–514.
9. Segal I, Solomon A, Hunt JA. Emergence of diverticular disease in the urban South African Black. Gastroenterology 1977;72:215–219.
10. Aktan H, Ozden A, Kesim E, et al. Colonic function in rural and urban populations of Turkey. Dis Colon Rectum 1984;27:538–541.
11. Dabestani A, Aliabadi P, Shah-Rookh FD, et al. Prevalence of colonic diverticular disease in southern Iran. Dis Colon Rectum 1982;24:385–387.
12. Manousos O, Day NE, Tzonou A, et al. Diet and other factors in the aetiology of diverticulosis: an epidemiological study in Greece. Gut 1985;26:544–549.
13. Brodribb AJM, Humphreys DM. Diverticular disease: three studies. Part I. Relation to other disorders and fibre intake. Br Med J 1976;1:424–425.
14. Painter NS, Truelove SC, Ardran GM, et al. Segmentation and the localization of intraluminal pressures in the human colon, with special reference to the pathogenesis of colonic diverticula. Gastroenterology 1965;29:169–177.
15. Trotman IF, Misiewicz JJ. Sigmoid motility in diverticular disease and the irritable bowel syndrome. Gut 1988; 29:218–222.
16. Attisha RP, Smith A. Pressure activity of the colon and rectum in diverticular disease before and after sigmoid myotomy. Br J Surg 1696;56:891–894.
17. Snape WJ Jr, Carlson GM, Cohen S. Colonic myoelectric activity in the irritable bowel syndrome. Gastroenterology 1976;70:326–332.
18. Findlay JM, Smith AN, Mitchell WD, et al. Effects of unprocessed bran on colon function in normal subjects and in diverticular disease. Lancet 1974;1:146–149.
19. Painter NS. Diverticulosis of the colon: fact and speculation. Am J Dig Dis 1967;12:222–227.
20. Almy TP, Howel DA. Medical progress: diverticular disease of the colon. N Engl J Med 1980;302:324–330.
21. Muller-Lissner SA. Effect of wheat bran on weight of stool and gastrointestinal transit time: a meta analysis. Br Med J 1988;296:615–617.
22. Kirwan WO, Smith AN. Colonic propulsion in diverticular disease, idiopathic constipation, and the irritable colon syndrome. Scand J Gastroenterol 1977;12:331–335.
23. Smith AN, Drummond E, Eastwood MA. The effect of coarse and fine Canadian red spring wheat and French soft wheat bran on colonic motility in patients with diverticular disease. Am J Clin Nutr 1981;34:2460–2463.
24. Tagiacozzo S, Tocchi A. Antimesenteric perforation of the colon during diverticular disease. Dis Colon Rectum 1997;40:1358–1361.
25. Watters JM, Blakslee JM, March RJ, et al. The influence of age on the severity of peritonitis. Can J Surg 1996;39: 142–146.
26. Freischlag J, Bennion RS, Thompson JE Jr. Complications of diverticular disease of the colon in young people. Dis Colon Rectum 1986;29:639–643.
27. Ambrosetti P, Robert JH, Witzig JA, et al. Acute left colonic diverticulitis in young patients. J Am Coll Surg 1994; 179:156–160.
28. Ambrosetti P, Robert JH, Witzig JA, et al. Acute left colonic diverticulitis: a prospective analysis of 226 consecutive cases. Surgery 1994;115:546–550.
29. Mielke JE, Becker KL, Gross JB. Diverticulitis of the colon in a young man with Marfan's syndrome. Gastroenterology 1965;48:379–382.
30. Latto C. Diverticular disease and varicose veins. Am Heart J 1975;90:274–275.
31. Kim EH. Hiatus hernia and diverticulum of the colon: their low incidence in Korea. N Engl J Med 1964;271:764–768.
32. Klein S, Mayer L, Present DH, et al. Extraintestinal manifestations in patients with diverticulitis. Ann Intern Med 1988;108:700–702.
33. Fung YC. Biomechanics: Mechanical Properties of Living Tissues. New York: Springer, 1981.
34. Thomson HJ, Busuttil A, Eastwood MA, et al. Submucosa collagen changes in the normal colon and in diverticular disease. Int J Colon Dis 1987;2:208–213.
35. Pace JL. Cited by Watters DAK, Smith AN. Strength of the colon wall in diverticular disease. Br J Surg 1990;77: 257–259.
36. Iwasaki T. Cited by Yamada H. Strength of Biological Materials. Baltimore: Williams & Wilkins, 1970.
37. Watters DAK, Smith AN, Eastwood MA, et al. Mechanical properties of the colon: comparison of the features of the African and European colon in vitro. Gut 1985;26: 394– 397.
38. Watters DAK, Smith AN. Strength of the colon wall in the diverticular disease. Br J Surg 1990;77:257–259.
39. Sugihar K, Muto T, Morioka Y, et al. Diverticular disease of the colon: a review of 615 cases. Dis Colon Rectum 1984;27:531–537.
40. Welch CE, Allen AW, Donaldson GA. An appraisal of resection of the colon for diverticulitis of the sigmoid. Ann Surg 1953;138:332–343.
41. Deckman RC, Cheskin LJ. Diverticular disease in the elderly. J Am Geriatr Soc 1993;40:986–993.

42. Vajrabukka T, Saksornchai K, Jimakorn P. Diverticular disease of the colon in a Far-Eastern community. Dis Colon Rectum 1980;23:151–154.
43. Fatayer WT, Alkhalaf MM, Shalan KA, et al. Diverticular disease of the colon in Jordan. Dis Colon Rectum 1983;26:247–249.
44. Calder JF. Diverticular disease of the colon in Africans. Br Med J 1979;1:1465–1466.
45. Coode PE, Chan KW, Chan YT. Polyps and diverticula of the large intestine: a necropsy survey in Hong Kong. Gut 1985;26:1045–1048.
46. Chia JG, Chintana WC, Ngoi SS, et al. Trends of diverticular disease of the large bowel in a newly developed country. Dis Colon Rectum 1991;34:498–501.
47. Lee YS. Diverticular disease of the large bowel in Singapore: an autopsy survey. Dis Colon Rectum 1986;29: 330–335.
48. Rodkey GV, Welch CE. Changing patterns in the surgical treatment of diverticular disease. Ann Surg 1984;200: 466–478.
49. Ouriel K, Schwartz SI. Diverticular disease in the young patient. Surg Gynecol Obstet 1983;156:1–5.
50. Rampton DS. Non-steroidal anti-inflammatory drugs, and the lower gastrointestinal tract. Scand J Gastroenterol 1987;22:1–4.
51. Coutrot S, Roland D, Barbier J, et al. Acute perforation of colonic diverticula associated with short-term indomethacin. Lancet 1978;2:1055–1057.
52. Corder A. Steroids, non-steroidal anti-inflammatory drugs, and serious septic complications of diverticular disease. Br Med J 1987;295:1238.
53. Campbell K, Steele RJC. Non-steroidal anti-inflammatory drugs and complicated diverticular disease: a case-control study. Br J Surg 1991;78:190–191.
54. Warshaw AL, Welch JP, Ottinger LW. Acute perforation of colonic diverticula associated with chronic corticosteroid therapy. Am J Surg 1976;131:442–446.
55. Remine SG, McIlrath DC. Bowel perforation in steroid-treated patients. Ann Surg 1984;192:581–586.
56. Arsura EL. Corticosteroid-associated perforation of colonic diverticula. Arch Intern Med 1990;150:1337–1138.
57. Schoetz DJ Jr. Uncomplicated diverticulitis. Surg Clin North Am 1993;73:965–974.
58. Chappuis CW, Cohn I Jr. Acute colonic diverticulitis. Surg Clin North Am 1988;68:301–313.
59. Rege RV, Nahrwold DL. Diverticular disease. Curr Probl Surg 1989;26:133–189.
60. Deitch EA. Strength of the colon wall in diverticular disease. Br J Surg 1990;77:257–259.
61. Cortesini C, Pantalone D. Usefulness of colonic motility study in identifying patients at risk for complicated diverticular disease. Dis Colon Rectum 1991;34:339–342.
62. Cheskin LJ, Bohlman M, Schuster MM. Diverticular disease in the elderly. Gastroenterol Clin North Am 1990;19:391–403.
63. Parks TG. Natural history of diverticular disease of the colon. Clin Gastroenterol 1975;4:53–69.
64. Sarin S, Boulos PB. Long-term outcome of patients presenting with acute complications of diverticular disease. Ann R Coll Surg Engl 1994;76:117–120.
65. Zollinger RW. The prognosis in diverticulitis of the colon. Arch Surg 1968;97:418–422.
66. Cooper GS, Shlaes DM, Salata RA. Intraabdominal infection: differences in presentation and outcome between younger patients and the elderly. Clin Infect Dis 1994; 19:146–148.
67. France MJ, Vuletic JC, Koelmeyer TD. Does advancing age modify the presentation of disease. Am J Foresnsic Med Pathol 1992;13:120–123.
68. Wroblewski M, Mikulowski P. Peritonitis in geriatric inpatients. Age Ageing 1991;20:90–94.
69. Fenyo G. Acute abdominal disease in the elderly: experience from two series in Stockholm. Am J Surg 1982; 143:751–754.
70. Telfer S, Fenyo G, Holt PR, DeDombal FT. Acute abdominal pain in patients over 50 years of age. Scand J Gastroenterol Suppl 1988;23:47–50.
71. Esposito AL, Gleckman RA. Fever of unknown origin in the elderly. J Am Geriatr Soc 1978;26:498–505.
72. Brewer BJ, Golden GT, Hitch DC, et al. Abdominal pain: an analysis of 1000 consecutive cases in a university hospital emergency room. Am J Surg 1976;131:219–223.
73. Eisenberg RL, Montgomery CK, Margulis AR. Colitis in the elderly: ischemic colitis mimicking ulcerative and granulomatous colitis. Am J Radiol 1979;133:1113–1118.
74. Kahn AL, Heys SD, Ah-See AK, et al. Surgical management of the septic complications of diverticular disease. Ann R Coll Surg Engl 1995;77:16–20.
75. Roberts P, Abel M, Rosen L, et al. Practice parameters for sigmoid diverticulitis—supporting documentation. Dis Colon Rectum 1995;38:126–132.
76. Schwerk WB, Schwarz S, Rothmund M. Sonography in acute colonic diverticulitis: a prospective study. Dis Colon Rectum 1992;35:1077–1084.
77. Verbanck J, Lambrecht S, Rutgeerts L, et al. Can sonography diagnose acute colonic diverticulitis in patients with acute intestinal inflammation? A prospective study. J Clin Ultrasound 1989;17:661–666.
78. Taylor KJ, Wasson JF, de Graaff C, et al. Accuracy of grey scale ultrasound diagnosis of abdominal and pelvic abscesses in 220 patients. Lancet 1978;1:3–4.
79. Hachigian MP, Honickman S, Eisenstat TE, et al. Computed tomography in the initial management of acute left-sided diverticulitis. Dis Colon Rectum 1992;35:1123–1129.
80. Stabile BE, Puccio E, vanConnenberg E, Neff CC. Preoperative percutaneous drainage of diverticular abscesses. Am J Surg 1990;159:99–104.
81. Ambrosetti P, Robert J, Witzig JA, et al. Incidence, outcome, and proposed management of isolated abscesses complicating acute left-sided colonic diverticulitis. Dis Colon Rectum 1992;35:1072–1076.
82. Ambrosetti P, Robert J, Witzig JA, et al. Prognostic factors from computed tomography in acute left colonic diverticulitis. Br J Surg 1992;79:117–119.
83. Hulnick DH, Megibow AG, Balthazar EJ, et al. Computed tomography in the evaluation of diverticulitis. Radiology 1984;152:491–495.
84. Mendeloff AI. Thoughts on the epidemiology of diverticular disease. Clin Gastroenterol 1986;15:855–877.
85. Brodribb AJM, Humphries DM. Diverticular disease. Part II. Treatment with bran. Br Med J 1976;1:425–428.

86. Hodgson J. Effect of methycellulose on rectal and colonic pressures in the treatment of diverticular disease. Br Med J 1972;3:729–731.
87. Taylor I, Duthie HL. Bran tablets and diverticular disease. Br Med J 1976;1:988–990.
88. Andersson H, Bosaeus I, Falkheden T, et al. Transit time in constipated geriatric patients during treatment with a bulk laxative and bran: a comparison. Scand J Gastroenterol 1979;14:821–826.
89. Srivastava GS, Smith AN, Painter NS. Sterulica bulk-forming agent with smooth-muscle relaxant versus bran in diverticular disease. Br Med J 1976;1:315–318.
90. Hyland JMP, Taylor I. Does a high fibre diet prevent the complications of diverticular disease? Br J Surg 1980;76: 77–79.
91. Brodribb AJM. Treatment of symptomatic diverticular disease with a high-fibre diet. Lancet 1977;1:664–666.
92. Perkins JD, Shield CF III, Chang FC, et al. Acute diverticulitis: comparison of treatment in immunocompromised and nonimmunocompromised patients. Am J Surg 1984; 148:745–748.
93. Tyau ES, Prystowsky JB, Joehl RJ, et al. Acute diverticulitis: a complicated problem in the immunocompromised patient. Arch Surg 1991;126:855–589.
94. Parks TG, Connell AM. The outcome in 455 patients admitted for treatment of diverticular disease of the colon. Br J Surg 1970;57:775–778.
95. Kirson SM. Diverticulitis: management patterns in a community hospital. South Med J 1988;81:972–977.
96. Benn PL, Wolff BG, Ilstrup DM. Level of anastomosis and recurrent colonic diverticulitis. Am J Surg 1986;151:269–271.
97. Madoff RD. Complicated diverticular disease. Probl Gen Surg 1992;9:723–731.
98. Nagorney DM, Adson MA, Pemberton JH. Sigmoid diverticulitis with perforation and generalized peritonitis. Dis Colon Rectum 1985;28:71–75.
99. Krukowski ZH, Matheson NA. Emergency surgery for diverticular disease complicated by generalized and faecal peritonitis: a review. Br J Surg 1984;71:921–927.
100. Fazio VW, Church JM, Jagelman DG, et al. Colocutaneous fistulas complicating diverticulitis. Dis Colon Rectum 1987;30:89–94.
101. Finlay IG, Carter DC. A comparison of emergency resection and staged management in perforated diverticular disease. Dis Colon Rectum 1987;30:929–933.
102. Labow JM, Salvati EP, Rubin RJ. The Hartmann procedure in the treatment of diverticular disease. Dis Colon Rectum 1978;16:392–394.
103. Belmonte C, Klas JV, Perez JJ, et al. The Hartmann procedure: first choice or last resort in diverticular disease? Arch Surg 1996;131:612–615.
104. Berry AL, Turner WH, Mortensen NJM, Kettlewell MGW. Emergency surgery for complicated diverticular disease: a five-year experience. Dis Colon Rectum 1989;32:849–855.
105. Eisenstat TE, Rubin RJ, Salvati EP. Surgical management of diverticulitis: the role of the Hartmann procedure. Dis Colon Rectum 1983;26:429–432.
106. Colcock BP. Surgical management of complicated diverticulitis. N Engl J Med 1958;259:570–573.
107. Alexander J, Karl RC, Skinner DB. Results of changing trends in the surgical management of complications of diverticular disease. Surgery 1983;94:683–690.
108. Labs JD, Sarr MG, Fishman Ek, et al. Complications of acute diverticulitis of the colon: improved early diagnosis with computerized tomography. Am J Surg 1988;155: 331–336.
109. Schechter S, Eisenstat TE, Oliver GC, et al. Computerized tomographic scan-guided drainage of intra-abdominal abscesses. Dis Colon Rectum 1994;37:984–988.
110. Hemming A, Davis NL, Robins RE. Surgical versus percutaneous drainage of intraabdominal abscesses. Am J Surg 1991;161:593–595.
111. Mueller PR, Siani S, Wittenberg, et al. Sigmoid diverticular abscesses: percutaneous drainage as an adjunct to surgical resection in twenty-four cases. Radiology 1987;164: 321–325.
112. Neff CC, van Sonnengerb E, Casola G, et al. Diverticular abscesses: percutaneous drainage. Radiology 1987;163:15–18.
113. Saini S, Mueller PR, Wittenberg, et al. Percutaneous drainage of diverticular abscess. Arch Surg 1986;121:475–478.
114. Leff EI, Groff FW, Rubin RJ, et al. Use of ureteral catheters in colonic and rectal surgery. Dis Colon Rectum 1982; 25:457–460.
115. Rothenberger DA, Wiltz O. Surgery for complicated diverticulitis. Surg Clin North Am 1993;73:975–992.
116. Smirniotis V, Tsoutsos D, Totopoulos A, et al. Perforated diverticulitis: a surgical dilemma. Int Surg 1992;77:44–47.
117. Kronborg O. Treatment of perforated sigmoid diverticulitis: a prospective randomized trial. Br J Surg 1993;80:505–507.
118. Hackford AW, Schoetz DJ Jr, Coller JA, et al. Surgical management of complicated diverticulitis: the Lahey Clinic experience, 1967 to 1982. Dis Colon Rectum 1985;65:347–363.
119. Woods RJ, Lavery IC, Fazio VW, et al. Internal fistulas in diverticular disease. Dis Colon Rectum 1988;31:591–596.
120. Elliot TB, Yego S, Irvin TT. Five-year audit of the acute complications of diverticular disease. Br J Surg 1997; 84:535–539.
121. Pontari MA, McMillen MA, Garvey RH, et al. Diagnosis and treatment of entero-vesical fistulae. Am J Surg 1992;58:258–263.
122. Kirsh GM, Hampel N, Shuck JM, Resnick MI. Diagnosis and management of vesicoenteric fistulas. Surg Gynecol Obstet 1991;173:91–97.
123. Chaikof EL, Cambria RP, Warshaw AL. Colouterine fistula secondary to diverticulitis. Dis Colon Rectum 1985;28:358–360.
124. Greenlee HB, Pienkos FJ, Vanderbilt PC, et al. Proceedings: acute large bowel obstruction: comparison of county, Veterans' Administration and community hospital publications. Arch Surg 1974;108:470–476.
125. Dudley HA, Radcliffe AG, McGeehan D. Intra-operative irrigation of the colon to permit primary anastomosis. Br J Surg 1980;67:80–81.
126. Schwartz SI. Appendix. In: Schwartz SI (ed) Principles of Surgery, 5th ed. New York: McGraw-Hill, 1989.

127. Thorbjarnarson B, Loehr WJ. Acute appendicitis in patients over the age of sixty. Surg Gynecol Obstet 1967;125:1277–1280.
128. Campbell KL, DeBeaux AC. Non-steroidal anti-inflammatory drugs and appendicitis in patients over 50 years. Br J Surg 1992;79:967–968.
129. Norman DC, Yoshikawa TT. Intraabdominal infections in the elderly. J Am Geriatr Soc 1983;31:677–684.
130. Addis DG, Shaffer N, Fowler BS, Tauxe RV. The epidemiology of appendicitis and appendectomy in the United States. Am J Epidemiol 1990;132:910–925.
131. Peltokallio P, Jauhiainen K. Acute appendicitis in the aged patient. Arch Surg 1970;100:140–143.
132. Luckmann R. Incidence and case fatality rates for acute appendicitis in California. J Epidemiol 1989;129:905–918.
133. Nockerts SR, Detmer DE, Fryback DG. Incidental appendectomy in the elderly? Surgery 1980;88:301–306.
134. Peltokallio P, Tykka H. Evolution of the age distribution and mortality of acute appendicitis. Arch Surg 1981; 116:153–156.
135. Owens WB, Hamit HF. Appendicitis in the elderly. Ann Surg 1978;187:392–396.
136. Bott DE. Geriatric surgical emergency. BMJ 1960;1:832–836.
137. Williams JS, Hale HW Jr. Acute appendicitis in the elderly. Ann Surg 1965;162:208–212.
138. Hall A, Wright TM. Acute appendicitis in the geriatric patient. Am Surg 1976;42:147–150.
139. Weksler ME. Immune senescence. Ann Neurol 1994;35: S35–S37.
140. Roberts-Thomson IC, Whittingham S, Young-Chaiyud U, MacKay IR. Ageing, immune response and mortality. Lancet 1974;2:368.
141. Silen W (ed). Cope's Early Diagnosis of the Acute Abdomen, 19th ed. New York: Oxford University Press, 1996.
142. Agafonoff S, Hawke I, Khadra M, et al. The influence of age and gender on normal appendicectomy rates. Aust NZ J Surg 1987;57:843–846.
143. Burns RP, Cochran JL, Russell WL, Bard RM. Appendicitis in mature patients. Ann Surg 1985;201:695–702.
144. Lau WY, Fan ST, Yiu TF, et al. Acute appendicitis in the elderly. Surg Gynecol Obstet 1985;161:157–160.
145. Horattas MC, Guyton DP, Wu D. A reappraisal of appendicitis in the elderly. Am J Surg 1990;160:291–293.
146. Smithy WB, Wexner SD, Dailey TH. The diagnosis and treatment of acute appendicitis in the aged. Dis Colon Rectum 1986;29:170–173.
147. Samiy AH. Clinical manifestations of disease in the elderly. Med Clin North Am 1983;76:333–344.
148. Harkins SW, Chapman CR. Detection and decision factors in pain perception in young and elderly men. Pain 1976;2:253–264.
149. Hodgkinson HM. Common Symptoms of Disease in the Elderly, 2nd ed. Oxford: Blackwell Scientific, 1980.
150. Hunt TE. Management of chronic non-rheumatic pain in the elderly. J Am Geriatr Soc 1976;24:402–406.
151. Klein SR, Layden L, Wright JF, White RA. Appendicitis in the elderly. Postgrad Geriatr 1988;83:247–254.
152. Birnbaum BA, Balthazar EJ. CT of appendicitis and diverticulitis. Radiol Clin North Am 1994;32:885–898.
153. Yacoe ME, Jeffrey RB Jr. Sonography of appendicitis and diverticulitis. Radiol Clin North Am 1994;32:899–912.
154. Hale DA, Molloy M, Pearl RH, et al. Appendectomy: a contemporary appraisal. Ann Surg 1997;225:252–261.
155. Eskelinen M, Ikonen J, Lipponen P. The value of history-taking, physical examination, and computer assistance in the diagnosis of acute appendicitis in patients over 50 years old. Scand J Gastroenterol 1995;30:349–355.
156. Lane MJ, Katz DS, Ross BA, et al. Unenhanced helical CT for suspected acute appendicitis. Am J Radiol 1997;168: 405–409.
157. Andersson RE, Hugander A, Thulin AJG. Diagnostic accuracy and perforation rate in appendicitis: association with age and sex of the patient and with appendicectomy rate. Eur J Surg 1992;158:37–41.
158. Paajanen H, Maniskka A, Laato M, et al. Are serum inflammatory markers age dependent in acute appendicitis? J Am Coll Surg 1997;184:303–308.
159. Sansoni P, Cossarizza A, Brianti V, et al. Lymphocyte subsets and natural killer cell activity in healthy old people and centenarians. Blood 1993;82:2767–2773.
160. Franz MG, Norman J, Fabri PJ. Increased morbidity of appendicitis with advancing age. Am Surg 1995;61:40–44.
161. Erkisson S, Granstrom L. Randomized controlled trial of appendicectomy versus antibiotic therapy for acute appendicitis. Br J Surg 1995;82:166–169.
162. Hurme T, Nylamo E. Conservative versus operative treatment of appendicular abscess. Ann Chir Gynaecol 1995;84:33–36.
163. Ein SH, Shandling B. Is interval appendectomy necessary after rupture of an appendiceal mass? J Pediatr Surg 1996;31:849–850.
164. Greig JD, Nixon SJ. Correspondence: randomized controlled trial of appendicectomy versus antibiotic therapy for acute appendicitis. Br J Surg 1995;82:1000.
165. Ricci MA, Trevisani MF, Beck WC. Acute appendicitis: a 5 year review. Am Surg 1991;57:301–305.
166. Rappaport WD, Peterson M, Stanton C. Factors responsible for the high perforation rate seen in early childhood appendicitis. Am Surg 1989;55:602–605.
167. Paajanen H, Kettunen J, Kostianinen S. Emergency appendectomies in patients over 80 years. Am Surg 1994; 60:951–953.
168. Tamir LL, Bongard FS, Klein SR. Acute appendicitis in the pregnant patient. Am J Surg 1990;160:571–576.
169. Temple CL, Huchcroft SA, Temple WJ. The natural history of appendicitis in adults. Ann Surg 1995;221:278–281.
170. Wolff WI, Hindman R. Acute appendicitis in the aged. Surg Gynecol Obstet 1952;94:239–247.
171. Von Tittle SN, McCabe CJ, Ottinger LW. Delayed appendectomy for appendicitis: causes and consequences. Am J Emerg Med 1996;14:620–622.
172. Thomson HJ, Jones PF. Active observation in acute appendicitis. J R Coll Surg Edinb 1985;30:290–293.
173. White JJ, Santillana M, Haller JA. Intensive in-hospital observation: a safe way to decrease unnecessary appendectomy. Am Surg 1975;41:793–798.

174. Hale DA, Molloy M, Pearl RH, et al. Appendectomy: a contemporary appraisal. Ann Surg 1997;225:252–261.
175. Vallina VL, Velasco JM, McCulloch CS. Laparoscopic versus conventional appendectomy. Ann Surg 1993;218:685–692.
176. Attwood SE, Hill AD, Murphy PG, et al. A prospective randomized trial of laparoscopic versus open appendectomy. Surgery 1992;112:497–501.
177. Frazee RC, Roberts JW, Symmonds RE, et al. A prospective randomized trial comparing open versus laparoscopic appendectomy. Ann Surg 1994;219:725–731.
178. Minne L, Varner D, Burnell A, et al. Laparoscopic vs open appendectomy. Arch Surg 1997;132:708–712.
179. Hansen JB, Smithers BM, Schache D, et al. Laparoscopic vs. open appendectomy: prospective randomized trial. World J Surg 1996;20:17–21.
180. McAnena OJ, Austin O, O'Connell PR, et al. Laparoscopic versus open appendectomy: a prospective evaluation. Br J Surg 1992;79:818–819.
181. Tate JJT, Dawson JW, Chung SCS, et al. Laparoscopic versus open appendectomy: prospective randomized trial. Lancet 1993;342:633–637.
182. Ortega AE, Hunter JG, Peters JH, et al. A prospective randomized comparison of laparoscopic appendectomy with open appendectomy. Am J Surg 1995;169:208–213.
183. Slim K, Pezet D, Chipponi J. Laparoscopic or open appendectomy? Dis Colon Rectum 1998;41:398–403.

# 45
# Benign Colorectal Disease

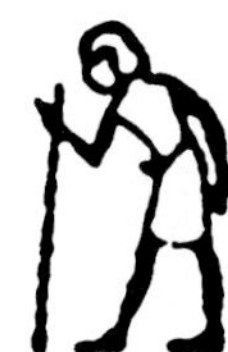

Elisa H. Birnbaum

The incidence of benign medical and surgical diseases of the colon and rectum increases with age. Although constipation, fecal incontinence, and several other associated benign conditions increase in frequency with aging, a paucity of information exists regarding the normal aging effect on gastrointestinal pathophysiology. Studies documenting anatomic, physiologic, and pathologic changes that occur in the aging colon have not been definitive; and many studies have reported conflicting results. Mucosal atrophy, atrophy of circular muscles, thickening of longitudinal muscles (taeniae coli), increased elastin deposition, and atherosclerosis are several of the changes seen in the aging bowel.[1] These changes may factor into the development of several disease states (i.e., diverticular disease and angiodysplasia). Myriad medications affect gastrointestinal function and many have constipation as a side effect. Preexisting diseases (cardiac, pulmonary, renal, neurologic, psychiatric) factor into the cause of several benign colorectal diseases, directly or secondarily, because of the medications used to treat the disease. In addition, these preexisting diseases affect the medical and surgical therapy, making geriatric operative risks higher. Early diagnosis and treatment is crucial even for seemingly benign diseases or symptoms. In this chapter, we address benign colorectal diseases frequently encountered in the elderly patient. Diseases common to both young and old persons, such as hemorrhoids and fissures, are not discussed.

## Constipation

Constipation is a frequent complaint in the United States and has been estimated to affect more than 4 million people. The complaint of constipation is reported to be more common in people more than 65 years old.[2] The overall prevalence of reported constipation in the elderly Western population is approximately 20–25%, but the prevalence differs according to the source of the sample.[3,4] The incidence of constipation is approximately 12% in the ambulatory geriatric population versus 41% in acute-care facilities and more than 80% in geriatric nursing homes and extended-care facilities. Elderly women are more likely to report symptoms of constipation than elderly men.[4] Although complaints of constipation increase in those over age 65, about 80–90% of subjects over age 60 report at least one bowel movement per day.[5,6] Further studies indicate large variation in bowel habits and frequent use of laxatives in as many as 30–50% of the elderly population.[5–7] Subjective complaints of constipation and laxative use increase with age, but true epidemiologic data suggest that clinical constipation does not.[8]

Several investigators have attempted to define "normal" bowel function in the elderly.[5,7] The normal range of bowel movements within the elderly population ranges from three per week to two or three per day and does not differ from that found among the young population. Total colonic transit times in healthy asymptomatic elderly subjects show no change with aging but are prolonged in healthy elderly subjects who report symptoms of constipation.[9,10] Although there may be normal physiologic aging of the colon and rectum, asymptomatic geriatric patients do not seem to differ significantly from their younger cohorts. Often symptoms do not correlate well with colonic and anorectal physiologic tests for constipation.[11] It is important to define constipation, as patients and their physicians frequently have different definitions.[12] It is generally accepted that patients with a reduced frequency in the number of bowel movements (fewer than three per week) are considered constipated.[13] However, many patients complain of constipation if they strain or have painful, hard stools. The distinction is important because the latter are more easily controlled with dietary manipulation.

Decreased motility or prolonged transit diffusely throughout the colon can be caused by several factors. Dietary factors (fluid and fiber) have frequently been implicated. Inadequate fluid intake may decrease the fecal bulk causing decreased intraluminal pressures in the colon, which in turn may decrease the number of propagating motor complexes generated.[8] The role fiber plays in the development and treatment of constipation is questionable. A meta-analysis showed that bran did not affect the stool output or transit time in constipated patients.[14] Many medications taken by the elderly are known to cause constipation.[15] Anticholinergics, tricyclic antidepressants, β-blockers, and calcium channel blockers are commonly implicated. Over-the-counter medications, such as aluminum and calcium antacids and laxatives, may also contribute to patients' symptoms. Chronic medical diseases such as hypothyroidism, diabetes, scleroderma, multiple sclerosis, and Parkinson's disease can result in decreased colonic motility. Psychiatric conditions (depression and dementia) have been associated with constipation, which may be behaviorally related.[2] Inability to ambulate to the bathroom because of arthritis, for example, or ignoring the call to defecate because of dementia may contribute to symptoms of fecal impaction, constipation, and the development of a megarectum.[2,6] Constipation is probably not a normal consequence of aging but is associated with and possibly caused by the immobility, chronic illnesses, and increased neuropsychiatric problems of the elderly population.

Generally, patients with constipation can be separated into four groups. The first are those who do not truly have significant constipation but complain of hard, dry stools that are difficult to evacuate. These patients can easily be treated with life style manipulation: increased fiber, increased fluid, and exercise. The second group comprises patients with colonic inertia. These patients have minimal to no motility of their colon and rarely have spontaneous bowel movements. Many of these patients report going for days and occasionally weeks without bowel function. This group of patients commonly report a long history of laxative use and abuse. Chronic laxative use, particularly with the anthracene laxatives, can cause degeneration of the myoneural chains and may impede motility irreversibly over time.[16] The third group are the patients with pelvic floor abnormalities. The pelvic floor abnormality or terminal reservoir syndrome has been identified with colonic transit marker studies and scintidefecography. These patients have normal transit to the sigmoid colon but are unable to evacuate their rectums easily despite having soft stool. This group is considered to have a terminal reservoir syndrome or rectal intussusception, and they give a history of straining often to the point of rectal and lower back pain. The fourth group are patients who are unable to evacuate their rectums owing to an anal outlet obstruction. The etiology of outlet obstruction is unclear, although dysfunction and discoordination of the pelvic floor muscles is the most common explanation. In patients with chronic fecal impaction, the rectal capacity increases over time and rectal sensation becomes blunted. These patients cannot feel the urge to defecate until a fecal bolus is too large to pass. These patients often report the need to use digital maneuvers, suppositories, or enemas to evacuate to their satisfaction.

Patients with complaints of severe constipation should be completely evaluated. Initially, a history and physical examination are performed. A detailed medication list, including all over-the-counter medications, is imperative. A diet and defecation diary is helpful to attempt to define the extent of the problem. Metabolic diseases such as diabetes and hypothyroidism should be ruled out. Carcinoma of the colon and rectum, inflammatory bowel disease, diverticulitis, and colonic volvulus may alter bowel patterns by causing partial or total obstruction. A digital rectal examination should be done to exclude low rectal carcinomas, anal strictures, and other anorectal abnormalities. Contrast studies or colonoscopy should be performed to rule out obstructing colonic lesions, particularly if the symptoms of constipation are recent or associated with bleeding, mucus, or altered stool caliber.

Several tests are available for assessment of constipation. Colonic transit times are measured to assess the bowel motility and can identify colonic inertia or possible outlet obstruction. Patients are placed on a high fiber diet and taken off all laxatives and enemas. A capsule with 20 radiopaque markers is given to the patient. A plain radiograph is obtained on the third and fifth days, and the markers are counted. The presence of more than 10% of the markers on the fifth day is considered to be an abnormal study. It is important to ensure that the patient took the capsule, did not take laxatives, and did not have abnormal bowel function (i.e., diarrhea) during the study period, as these possibilities may give a falsely normal examination. Patients with colonic inertia have markers scattered diffusely throughout the colon that remain through the fifth day. In patients with rectal intussusception or outlet obstruction, the markers move through the colon and are held up in the rectosigmoid region.

Scintidefecography may identify patients with severe rectal intussusception or rectal prolapse. This test is done by placing a thickened barium paste in the rectosigmoid to simulate a bowel movement. The patient is then placed on a commode and asked to evacuate the paste while radiographs are obtained. In a normal test the rectosigmoid remains stable along the presacral space, and the puborectalis is seen to relax as the patient passes the contrast bolus. With an abnormal test, the rectosigmoid falls away from its attachments to the presacral space, and the proximal rectum is seen to infold (intussuscept) (Fig. 45.1). Internal intussusception of the rectum can block the rectal outlet, resulting in incomplete evacuation of the rectal contrast. With severe straining, the intussusception may worsen, and occasionally the entire rectum is seen prolapsing through the anorectal ring. Intussusception is a common finding even in normal subjects, so it is important to obtain a clear bowel history from the patient.

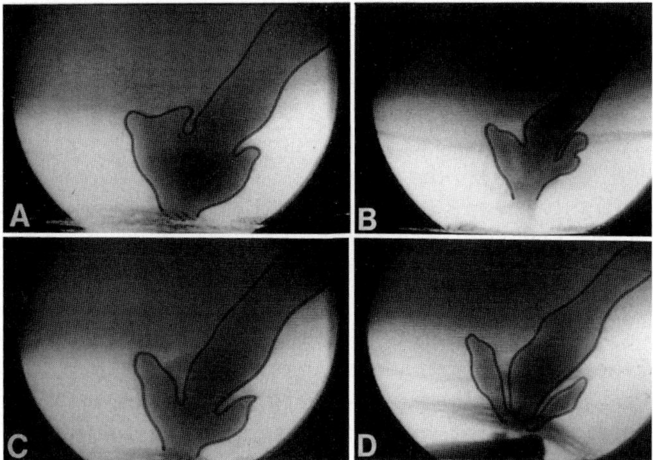


FIGURE 45.1. Scintidefecogram showing progressive outlet obstruction secondary to internal intussusception. (From Nyhus LM, ed. Surgery Annual, Vol. 24. New York: McGraw-Hill, 1992, with permission from the McGraw-Hill Companies.)

Anal manometry has limited value in the workup of constipation in the elderly. In select cases anal manometry, rectal anal inhibitory reflex, minimal sensory rectal volume, and balloon expulsion may identify adult Hirschsprung's disease, patients with megarectum, and patients with a nonrelaxing puborectalis. These tests require specialized manometric instruments and can be done utilizing a capillary perfusion system or microballoon system. The systems measure the pressures within the anal canal and test the function of the anal sphincter mechanism. Anal sensation is tested by inserting a rectal balloon just above the anal sphincter and insufflating increasing amounts of air until the patient notes sensation. Patients with megarectums require large amounts of distension before any sensation is noted. The rectoanal inhibitory reflex is absent in the setting of Hirschsprung's disease and may be absent in patients with megarectum who require large volumes to induce the inhibitory reflex. A rectal examination done on an "unprepped" patient distinguishes between Hirschsprung's disease and megarectum. Patients with Hirschsprung's disease have no stool in the rectal vault, whereas patients with megarectum have a rectum full of stool. It is rare that Hirschsprung's disease is diagnosed in a young adult and even rarer in the elderly. The inability to expel the rectal balloon is tested by asking the patient to evacuate a rectal balloon filled with 60cc of air in the privacy of the bathroom. If patients have an outlet obstruction and the puborectalis muscle does not relax properly they have difficulty doing this simple task. The inability to relax the puborectalis muscle and evacuate the contrast on scintidefecography helps confirm the diagnosis.

Treatment of constipation is generally medical, and treatment of the elderly constipated patient is no different. A trial of dietary fiber and increased fluid intake should be initially instituted once a malignancy has been ruled out (Fig. 45.2). A bowel evacuation routine is often helpful for those patients with outlet obstruction. The patient is instructed to take bulk-forming agents daily and to use a glycerine suppository or tap water enema at the same time daily. Biofeedback has had some success in the treatment of pelvic floor outlet obstruction but requires a motivated patient.[17] Surgical intervention is rarely necessary and is usually not indicated for treatment of pelvic floor abnormalities. A total colectomy with ileorectal anastomosis has been successful in the treatment of severe colonic inertia if there is no element of outlet obstruction. This operation should be reserved for

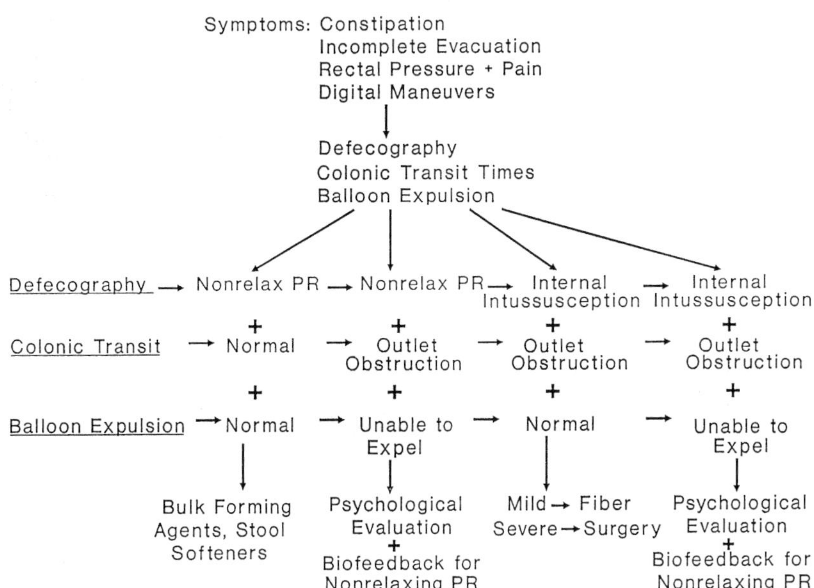


FIGURE 45.2. Management plan for the treatment of severe constipation. PR, puborectalis muscle. (From Schwartz SI, ed. Principles of Surgery, 6th Ed. New York: McGraw-Hill, 1998, with permission of The McGraw-Hill Companies.)

the young, medically stable patient. Other patients with colonic inertia are probably best treated by accepting the need for continuous laxative use.

## Rectal Intussusception

Rectal intussusception results from a loss of fixation of the rectum from the sacrum. The rectum folds in onto itself and acts as a valve that prevents normal emptying. Symptoms vary from mild constipation with rectal pressure to severe constipation with rectal pain and a "plugging" sensation. Incomplete evacuation and discharge of mucus and blood per rectum are frequent complaints. Other associated disease entities are colitis cystica profunda, solitary rectal ulcer syndrome, and mucosal prolapse.

On proctosigmoidoscopic examination, the typical patient with significant intussusception is found to have an erythematous anterior rectal wall approximately 5–8 cm from the mucocutaneous junction. Patients with solitary rectal ulcer syndrome frequently have more severe symptoms of straining, passage of bloody mucus per rectum, and incomplete evacuation. On examination, the solitary rectal ulcer appears as a heaped-up lesion in the anterior midline 5–8 cm from the mucocutaneous junction. This lesion can often be palpated and is frequently mistaken for a rectal tumor. Biopsy of the lesion reveals cystic proliferation of fibroblasts and muscle hypertrophy in the lamina propria, epithelial hyperplasia, colitis cystica profunda, or excess mucosal collagen.[18] Defecography may show profound intussusception.

Treatment of patients with intussusception is primarily medical. Surgery should be limited to patients who are incapacitated because of the pressure or who have a persistent solitary rectal ulcer after intensive medical therapy. Surgery involves low anterior resection or retrorectal sacral fixation of the mobile rectum. Many patients have persistent postoperative symptoms of constipation and difficulty emptying. Patients with symptoms of nonrelaxing puborectalis or colonic inertia must have these symptoms addressed and treated preoperatively to have a successful surgical result.[19]

## Rectal Prolapse

The most severe abnormality of the pelvic floor is rectal prolapse. Rectal prolapse can be partial (mucosal) or full (complete extrusion of the rectum through the anal canal). Circumferential rings are typical of a full rectal prolapse, whereas radial folds are more typical of mucosal prolapse or prolapsing hemorrhoids. Rectal prolapse is associated with chronic constipation and straining[20] and is more frequent in elderly women and institutionalized patients, who often have neurologic or psychiatric co-morbidities. In addition, many patients have other significant medical problems.[20,21]

Rectal pressure, mucous discharge, rectal bleeding, and fecal incontinence are frequent symptoms of rectal prolapse. Often the patient does not mention that the rectum extrudes through the anal canal, and it is not uncommon for the symptoms to be attributed to prolapsing hemorrhoids. Direct questioning may result in the history that the patient's rectum protrudes with bowel movements (especially with straining) and occasionally when assuming an upright position. Manual replacement by the patient or their caretakers is common. Incarceration or strangulation of the prolapsed rectum are rare presentations. A lax anal sphincter and prolapsing rectum are usually found on physical examination. An erythematous edematous circumferential region may be seen approximately 5–8 cm from the dentate line on proctosigmoidoscopic examination. Asking patients to strain to evacuate their rectum may allow visualization of the prolapse by the examiner. If the prolapse cannot be demonstrated in the office setting, defecography may be done to demonstrate the redundant prolapsing rectosigmoid. A complete evaluation with contrast studies or colonoscopy is necessary to rule out a tumor as a lead point of the rectal prolapse. Occasionally a solitary rectal ulcer is seen at the leading edge of the prolapsing rectum and may be confused with a rectal tumor. Biopsy of the ulcer should give a more definitive diagnosis. The anal sphincter may be assessed using anal manometry and electromyography. Unilateral or bilateral neurogenic injury may result from chronic stretching of the pudendal nerve. Stretch injury may also be a direct result of repeated trauma to the anal sphincter by the prolapsing rectum. Preoperative motility studies with colonic transit times should be done to identify a group of patients with colonic inertia and prolapse who may require more extensive resection.[22]

The surgical approach to rectal prolapse is transabdominal or perineal; more than 100 operations have been cited as forms of treatment for rectal prolapse. Surgical therapy must be tailored to the individual patient. Abdominal suture rectopexy with or without sigmoid resection can be done in patients who are good surgical risks.[22,23] Low anterior resection may improve the bowel habits of patients who complain of preoperative constipation in whom a markedly redundant distal colon is found[22,24] (Fig. 45.3A). Complete encirclement of the rectum with a band of mesh (Ripstein procedure) can be modified to leave the anterior bowel wall free[25,26] (Fig. 45.3B), which minimizes the stenosis by the foreign material and may decrease postoperative fecal impaction at the level of the mesh. Resection should not be done in the presence of foreign material. Modifications using the laparoscope to perform rectopexy have been described.[27]

Perineal procedures (anal encirclement or proctosigmoidectomy) can be done under regional anesthesia, minimizing the anesthetic risk in the high risk patient.

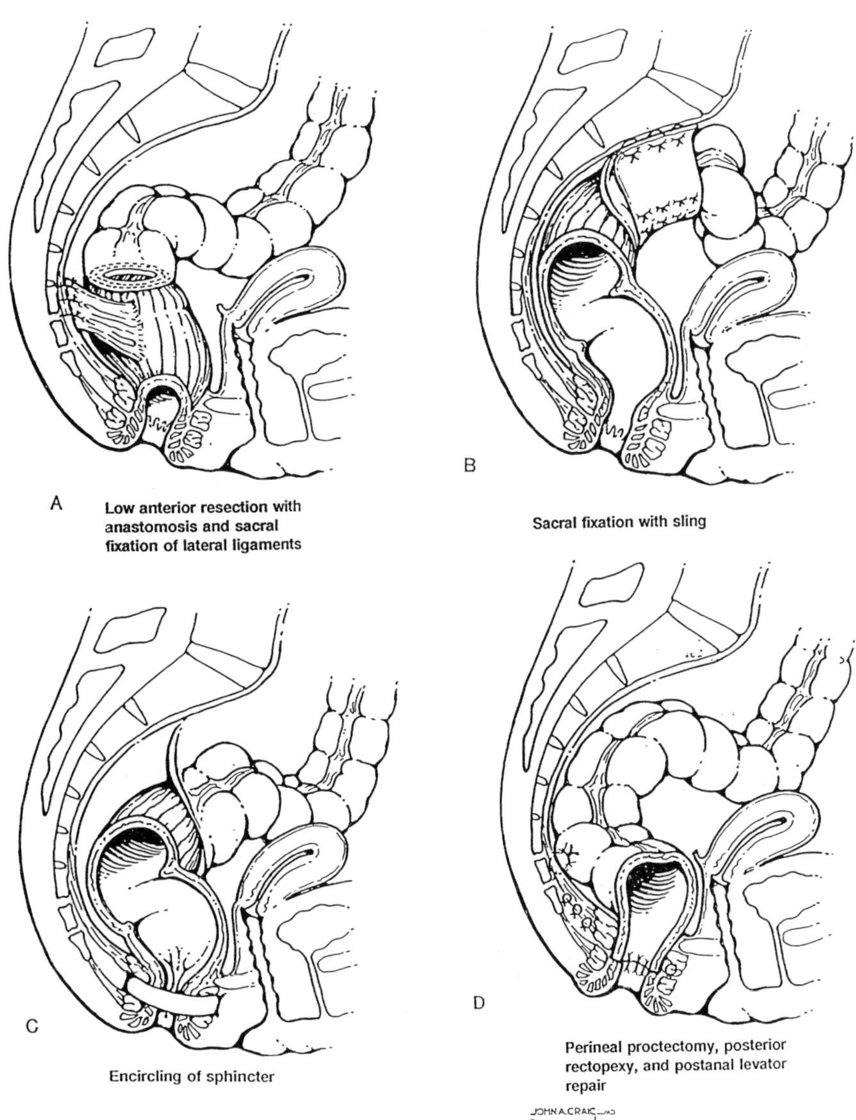


FIGURE 45.3. Surgical options for the treatment of rectal prolapse. (From Schwartz SI, ed. Principle of Surgery, 6th Ed. New York: McGraw-Hill, 1998 with permission of The McGraw-Hill Companies.)

Thiersch wire or other synthetic material may be used to encircle the anal canal to prevent rectal prolapse (Fig. 45.3C). The synthetic material acts as an obstruction to defecation and prevents the rectum from prolapsing through the anal canal. The anal encirclement procedures do not treat the underlying condition, and the symptoms of rectal intussusception persist in most patients. It is not uncommon for patients to require laxatives and enemas for fecal evacuation after anal encirclement, as the synthetic material acts as an obstruction to defecation. Because septic and mechanical complications are high, anal encirclement as a primary treatment for rectal prolapse is generally reserved for moribund patients with limited life expectancy.

Perineal proctosigmoidectomy, first described in 1889 by Mikulicz,[28] has been modified and popularized by others[20,29] (Fig. 45.3D). It can easily be performed under regional anesthesia in either prone jackknife or lithotomy position. The redundant rectum and portion of sigmoid colon can be easily removed via the anal incision. Addition of a posterior levator repair described by Prasad et al. re-creates the anatomic anorectal angle and may help patients gain fecal control postoperatively.[29] Minimal pain and little physiologic alteration are associated with this procedure, and most patients can be discharged from the hospital within 3–4 days. The recurrence rate of a perineal proctosigmoidectomy is related to the length of follow-up and ranges from 0% to 22%.[20,21,29] The morbidity is 3–12%, and mortality is less than 5%.[20,21,29]

## Stercoral Ulceration

Ischemic pressure necrosis by a stercoraceous mass causing fecal peritonitis is a rare cause of free perforation of the colon. Although considered a disease of the elderly, the average age of patients presenting with stercoral ulceration is in the fifties. Associated medical diseases occur in about one-third of patients, and almost all patients complain of chronic constipation requiring laxatives. The sigmoid and rectosigmoid are the most common sites of perforation, which almost always occurs along the antimesenteric border. The bowel wall adjacent to the perforation is usually thin and rarely inflamed, in contrast to the colonic findings of diverticulitis. The symptoms of abdominal pain and peritonitis start acutely. An upright chest radiograph shows free air under the diaphragm, and the clinical picture is usually one of sepsis. It is rarely diagnosed preoperatively. As in all cases of fecal peritonitis, broad-spectrum intravenous antibiotics are necessary. Irrigation of the abdominal cavity and distal rectal stump help to decrease the fecal load. Several surgical procedures are recommended for treatment in the literature, and they can be roughly grouped into three categories. Resection with end colostomy, with a mucous fistula or Hartmann's procedure has the lowest operative mortality rate (23%). A proximal colostomy with closure of the perforation is rarely done and carries a mortality of approximately 44%. Proximal loop colostomies and exteriorization of the perforation have the highest mortality rate (71%) and are probably not to be recommended.[30]

## Volvulus

Colonic volvulus occurs when an air-filled segment of colon twists about its elongated mesentery. In the United States, colonic volvulus is a rare cause of intestinal obstruction and accounts for approximately 3% of colonic obstructions.[31] In parts of Iran and Russia, colonic volvulus is one of the predominant causes of intestinal obstruction. The high incidence of sigmoid volvulus in other parts of the world has been attributed to the high fiber diets of those regions. Chagas' disease, which causes megacolon, may play a role in the development of sigmoid volvulus, particularly in countries where the disease is common.[32] In North America, the incidence increases over the age of 50. The disease is associated with chronic constipation, laxative use, psychiatric illness, and institutionalization.[31] A dilated, redundant colon with a narrow mesocolon is a prerequisite for a volvulus to occur, and therefore the intraabdominal portions of colon are at risk. Colonic volvulus most commonly occurs in the sigmoid colon; cecal volvulus and volvulus of the transverse colon occur less frequently (<10%) and are generally seen in young patients.

Patients with sigmoid volvulus usually present with abdominal distension, obstipation, and pain. Peritoneal irritation on physical examination, fever, or an elevated white blood cell (WBC) count indicates ischemic or gangrenous bowel. Plain abdominal radiographs may show an inverted, U-shaped, air-filled bowel loop ("bent inner tube"), with a dense line running toward the point of torsion. This radiologic finding is highly suggestive of a sigmoid volvulus. If peritonitis is not present, sigmoidoscopy should be performed to the point of obstruction. The volvulus can often be reduced by inserting a soft rectal tube past the point of obstruction. A release of gas and liquid stool follows successful detorsion. The rectal tube should be left in place for several days to assist with further decompression. The success rate with this technique is good, and reduction of the volvulus can be expected with approximately 75% of attempts. The colonoscope may be used to attempt reduction, but its use should be limited to patients in whom a rigid proctoscope has been unsuccessful in reaching the point of torsion. Contrast enemas may be necessary when plain radiographs are not diagnostic for volvulus but suggest a colonic obstruction. The column of contrast tapers at the point of torsion ("bird's beak" deformity) (Fig. 45.4). Occasionally, reduction occurs with contrast enemas, but detorsion occurs in fewer than 10% of attempts.[33] Evidence of mucosal ischemia, bloody discharge, or unsuccessful detorsion indicates strangulation and possibly gangrene. If the patient has signs of peritoneal irritation or if gangrene is suspected, contrast studies and tube decompression should not be attempted and the patient should undergo emergency exploration.

Nonoperative reduction is successful in approximately 90% of patients but does not constitute adequate treatment in good risk patients.[34] Recurrence rates following nonoperative reduction range from 20% to 60% but can be as high as 90%.[34,35] Once the volvulus is reduced,

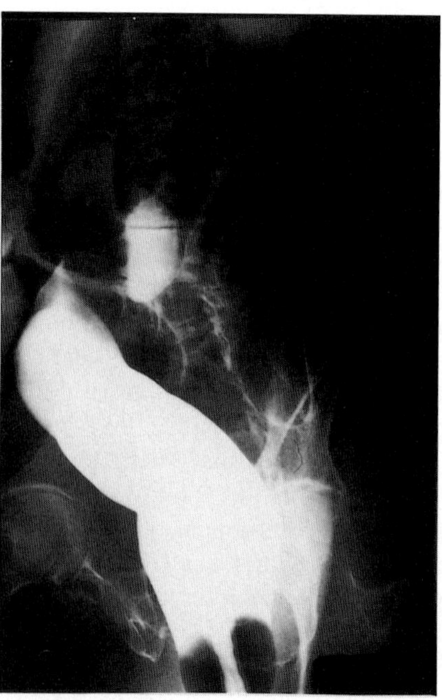

FIGURE 45.4. Hypaque enema showing sigmoid volvulus. Note the "bird's beak" deformity (arrow). (From Schwartz SI, ed. Principle of Surgery, with permission of The McGraw-Hill Companies.)

medically stable patients should undergo mechanical bowel preparation and elective resection. The choice of operation depends on the adequacy of the bowel preparation and the viability of the colon. A sigmoid resection with primary anastomosis can be done after bowel preparation and if the colon shows no signs of ischemia. The presence of ischemic or gangrenous bowel is an indication for resection and colostomy.

Mortality is related to the presence of gangrenous bowel and to delay in decompressing the ischemic bowel. The operative mortality following elective resection of a primary volvulus is approximately 6% versus 21% for recurrent volvulus.[34] Some investigators have found high mortality rates associated with elective resection and recommend elective resection only in good risk, young patients.[36] Patients who require emergency operation for sigmoid volvulus have a mortality rate of more than 30%.[34]

Cecal and transverse colonic volvulus are less common than sigmoid volvulus. Anomalous fixation of the cecum may be an important reason why cecal volvulus occurs in a young age group.[37] Other predisposing factors, such as prior abdominal surgery, pregnancy, and distal obstruction, have been implicated as causes of cecal volvulus. Ninety percent of patients with cecal volvulus have a full axial volvulus twisting the associated mesentery and blood vessels.[31] In the remaining patients, the cecum folds in an anterior cephalad direction (cecal bascule). Although a bascule is not a true volvulus around the mesentery, gangrene can result from tension on the bowel wall. Patients with cecal volvulus clinically appear to have a small bowel obstruction. Abdominal pain, nausea, vomiting, and obstipation are common symptoms. Many patients give a history of chronic intermittent symptoms of partial bowel obstruction.[31] Plain abdominal radiographs show the cecum as an air-filled, kidney-shaped structure pointing to the left upper quadrant. Multiple air-fluid levels are suggestive of a distal small bowel obstruction. Contrast enemas may show the "bird's beak" tapered edge of the contrast pointing toward the site of torsion (Fig. 45.5). Contrast studies are useful in difficult cases but should not be performed routinely if the diagnosis of cecal volvulus is clear. Contrast studies and colonoscopy have rarely been successful in reducting a cecal or transverse volvulus.

Once a cecal volvulus is diagnosed operative intervention should be undertaken. Operative detorsion alone has high recurrence and mortality rates and should not be performed as the sole procedure. Cecopexy, cecostomy, and resection have variable rates of recurrence and morbidity. The highest rates of postoperative complications, mortality, and recurrence are seen with cecostomy.[38] Cecostomy or appendicostomy allows decompression of the distended bowel and fixation of the cecum. Although the recurrence rate is similar to that for cecopexy, the intraabdominal and wound complications are more than 25%.[38] Cecopexy is done by anchoring the right colon to the parietal peritoneum by direct suture or by making a peritoneal flap. This technique eliminates the cecal hypermobility, but is technically challenging to perform if the cecum is dilated and thin-walled. The recurrence rate after cecopexy is variable, with some series reporting recurrence as high as 28%.[39] Patients who are medically stable should undergo a right hemicolectomy with primary anastomosis if there is no evidence of gangrenous bowel. Resection, ileostomy, and mucous fistula are indicated if

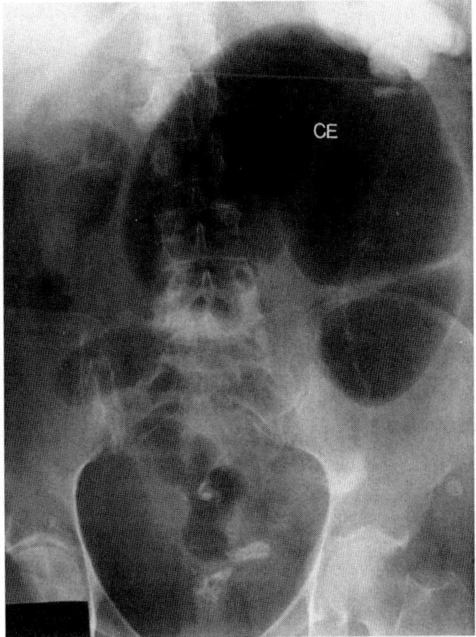


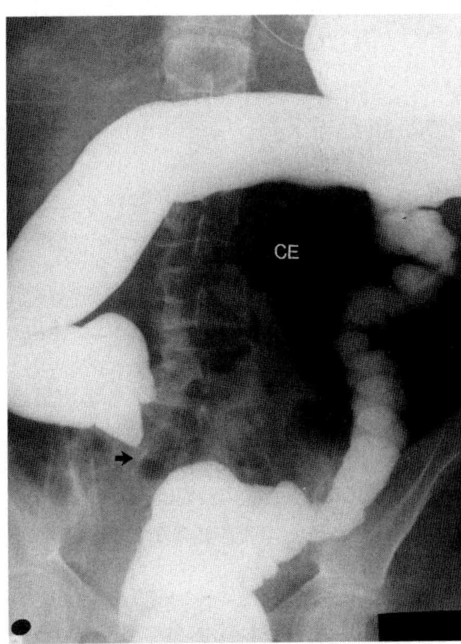


FIGURE 45.5. A. Cecal volvulus, plain radiograph. CE, cecum. B. Barium enema. Arrow indicates the point of obstruction. CE, cecum.

there is evidence of ischemia or gangrene. Mortality is increased in the presence of gangrenous bowel and is higher with cecal volvulus than with sigmoid volvulus (33% vs. 7%). This increased mortality rate with cecal volvulus is due to the increased presence of gangrenous bowel seen with cecal volvulus (21% vs. 7%).[31]

## Fecal Incontinence

Fecal incontinence is a disabling problem in the elderly. A community-based prevalence study estimated that fecal incontinence affects 2.2% of the general population.[40] The incidence of fecal incontinence is increased in persons over 65 years of age and in institutionalized patients.[41] More than 60% of patients who complain of fecal incontinence are women.[40] Certain physiologic factors have been shown to occur with aging: decreased rectal tone and weakening of the anal sphincter mechanism.[42,43] The anal sphincter may decrease in strength secondary to loss of muscle mass or neuropathy. These differences are more pronounced in elderly women. It may be due to weakening of connective tissues, possibly from decreased estrogen secretion. Physical limitations and poor general health are other predisposing factors that contribute to fecal incontinence.[40,41] The most common cause of fecal incontinence in the elderly, however, is fecal impaction with overflow incontinence.[41] Systemic diseases such as scleroderma, polymyositis, and multiple sclerosis can be associated with fecal incontinence. Colorectal carcinoma, colonic ischemia, and inflammatory bowel disease may cause symptoms of fecal urgency, and incontinence may be a result of the patient's inability to respond quickly.

Incontinence may be neurogenic, mechanical, mixed, or secondary to other medical conditions. Neurogenic incontinence may be due to central or peripheral denervation of the puborectalis muscle or external anal sphincter. Rectal prolapse or descending perineum syndrome may denervate the sphincter by a stretch injury to the pudendal nerve. Injury to the sphincter mechanism, traumatic or surgical, may lead to fecal incontinence immediately after the injury or during the ensuing years. Decreased anorectal sensation caused by radiotherapy or diabetes mellitus may lead to incontinence as well.

On initial evaluation, constipation with overflow incontinence must be ruled out by history and digital rectal examination. A complete colonic evaluation with colonoscopy or contrast enema should be done especially if the symptoms of fecal incontinence have a short history. The anal physiology laboratory can objectively evaluate the anal sphincter mechanism to determine the cause of fecal incontinence and direct treatment. Anal manometry, electromyography, and transrectal ultrasonography can help differentiate neurogenic from mechanical injury to the anal sphincter. Anal manometry assesses the resting and squeeze pressures generated by the anal sphincter. The sphincter length can be determined, and some systems can identify the specific quadrant involved in a sphincter defect. The minimal sensory rectal volume is useful for identifying patients with megarectum who do not sense the presence of a large bolus of fecal material in their rectum. Electromyography is used to evaluate the pudendal nerve terminal motor latency. The pudendal nerve innervates the external anal sphincter and the puborectalis muscle. Both muscles are involved in maintaining fecal continence; and denervation of these muscles, represented by prolonged pudendal nerve terminal motor latency, may cause neurogenic incontinence. Transrectal endoluminal ultrasonography has replaced needle electromyography as the preferred method for evaluating the anal sphincter for defects. Using this modality, the puborectalis muscle and the external and internal anal sphincters can be thoroughly evaluated for defects.

Initial treatment may be as simple as dietary alteration (avoidance of milk products and food with high fat content) and a bowel evacuation regimen (bulk-forming agents and glycerine suppositories). Biofeedback has had some success in patients, but requires the understanding and cooperation of the patient.[44] Anterior sphincter reconstructions with direct muscle repair has had success in the elderly population.[45] A Thiersch procedure obstructing defecation or a diverting colostomy is rarely necessary for control of the fecal stream in the elderly population. If the rectum is severely damaged by radiation injury, a diverting colostomy is probably the best treatment option for severely incontinent patients.

## References

1. Whiteway J, Morson B. Pathology of the aging: diverticular disease. Clin Gastroenterol 1985;14:829–846.
2. Everhart JE, Go VL, Johannes RS, et al. A longitudinal survey of self-reported bowel habits in the United States. Dig Dis Sci 1989;34:1153–1162.
3. Read NW, Celik AF, Katsinelos P. Constipation and incontinence in the elderly. J Clin Gastroenterol 1995;20:61–70.
4. Stewart RB, Moore MT, Marks RG, Hale WE. Correlates of constipation in an ambulatory elderly population. Am J Gastroenterol 1992;87:859–864.
5. Connell AM, Hilton C, Irvine G, et al. Variation of bowel habit in two population samples. Br Med J 1965;2:1095–1099.
6. Milne JS, Williamson J. Bowel habit in older people. Gerontol Clin 1972;14:56–60.
7. Donald IP, Smith RG, Cruikshank JG, et al. A study of constipation in the elderly living at home. Gerontology 1985;31:112–118.
8. Harari D, Gurwitz JH, Minaker KL. Constipation in the elderly. J Am Geriatr Soc 1993;41:1130–1140.
9. Metcalf A, Phillips S, Zinsmeister A, et al. Simplified assessment of segmental colonic transit. Gastroenterology 1987; 92:40–47.

10. Melkersson M, Andersson H, Bosaeus I, Falkheden T. Intestinal transit time in constipated and nonconstipated geriatric patients. Scand J Gastroenterol 1983;18:593–597.
11. Merkel IS, Locher J, Burgio K, et al. Physiologic and psychologic characteristics of an elderly population with chronic constipation. Am J Gastroenterol 1993;88:1854–1859.
12. Moore-Gillon V. Constipation: what does the patient mean? J R Soc Med 1984;77:108–110.
13. Johanson JF, Sonnenberg A, Koch TR. Clinical epidemiology of chronic constipation. J Clin Gastroenterol 1989;11: 525–536.
14. Muller-Lissner SA. Effect of wheat bran on weight of stool and gastrointestinal transit time: a meta-analysis. Br Med J 1988;296:615–617.
15. Campbell AJ, Busby WJ, Horwath CC. Factors associated with constipation in a community based sample of people aged 70 years and over. J Epidemiol Community Health 1993;47:23–26.
16. Smith B. Effect of irritant purgatives on the myenteric plexus in man and the mouse. Gut 1968;9:139–143.
17. Fleshman J, Dreznik Z, Meyer K, et al. Outpatient protocol for biofeedback therapy of pelvic floor outlet obstruction. Dis Colon Rectum 1992;35:1–7.
18. Tjandra JJ, Fazio VW, Church JM, et al. Clinical conundrum of solitary rectal ulcer. Dis Colon Rectum 1992;35:227–234.
19. Kuijpers HC, Schreve RH, ten Cate Hoedemakers H. Diagnosis of functional disorders of defecation causing the solitary rectal ulcer syndrome. Dis Colon Rectum 1986;29: 126–129.
20. Altemeier WA, Culbertson WR, Schowengerdt C, Hunt J. Nineteen years' experience with the one-stage perineal repair of rectal prolapse. Ann Surg 1971;173:993–1006.
21. Williams JG, Rothenberger DA, Madoff RD, Goldberg SM. Treatment of rectal prolapse in the elderly by perineal rectosigmoidectomy. Dis Colon Rectum 1992;35:830–834.
22. Watts JD, Rothenberger DA, Bulls JG, et al. The management of procidentia: 30 years' experience. Dis Colon Rectum 1985;28:96–102.
23. Kuijpers, HC. Treatment of complete rectal prolapse: to narrow, to wrap, to suspend, to fix, to encircle, to plicate or to resect? World J Surg 1992;16:826–830.
24. McKee RF, Lauder JC, Poon FW, et al. A prospective randomized study of abdominal rectopexy with and without sigmoidectomy in rectal prolapse. Surg Gynecol Obstet 1992;174:145–148.
25. Ripstein CB. Treatment of massive rectal prolapse. Am J Surg 1952;83:68–71.
26. Kuijpers JHC, DeMorree H. Toward a selection of the most appropriate procedure in the treatment of complete rectal prolapse. Dis Colon Rectum 1988;31:355–357.
27. Berman IR. Sutureless laparoscopic rectopexy for procidentia: technique and implications. Dis Colon Rectum 1992;35: 689–693.
28. Mikulicz J. Zur operativen behandlung des prolapsus recti et coli invaginati. Arch Klin Chir 1889;38:74–97.
29. Prasad ML, Pearl RK, Abcarian H, et al. Perineal proctectomy, posterior rectopexy, and postanal levator repair for the treatment of rectal prolapse. Dis Colon Rectum 1986; 29:547–552.
30. Guyton DP, Evans D, Schreiber H. Stercoral perforation of the colon: concepts of operative management. Am Surg 1985;51:520–522.
31. Ballantyne GH, Brandner MD, Beart RW, Ilstrup DM. Volvulus of the colon; incidence and mortality. Ann Surg 1985;202:83–92.
32. Habr Gama A, Haddad J, Simonsen O, Warde P, et al. Volvulus of the sigmoid colon in Brazil: a report of 230 cases. Dis Colon Rectum 1976;19:314–320.
33. Ballantyne GH. Review of sigmoid volvulus: history and results of treatments. Dis Colon Rectum 1982;25:494–501.
34. Bak MP, Boley SJ. Sigmoid volvulus in elderly patients. Am J Surg 1986;151:71–75.
35. Hines JR, Geurkink RE, Bass RT. Recurrence and mortality rates in sigmoid volvulus. Surg Gynecol Obstet 1967;124: 567–570.
36. Arnold GJ, Nance FC. Volvulus of the sigmoid colon. Ann Surg 1973;177:527–533.
37. Wolfer JA, Beaton LE, Anson BJ. Volvulus of the cecum: anatomical factors in its etiology; report of a case. Surg Gynecol Obstet 1942;74:882–894.
38. Rabinovici R, Simansky DA, Kaplan O, et al. Cecal volvulus. Dis Colon Rectum 1990;55:765–769.
39. Todd GJ, Forde KA. Volvulus of the cecum: choice of operation. Am J Surg 1979;138:632–634.
40. Nelson R, Norton N, Cautley E, Furner S. Community-based prevalence of anal incontinence. JAMA 1995;274: 559–561.
41. Barrett JA, Brocklehurst JC, Kiff ES, et al. Anal function in geriatric patients with faecal incontinence. Gut 1989;30: 1244–1251.
42. McHugh SM, Diamant NE. Effect of age, gender, and parity on anal canal pressures; contribution of impaired anal sphincter function to fecal incontinence. Dig Dis Sci 1987; 32:726–736.
43. Bannister JJ, Abouzekry I, Read NW. Effect of aging on anorectal function. Gut 1987;28:353–357.
44. Whitehead WE, Burgio KL, Engel BT. Biofeedback treatment of fecal incontinence in geriatric patients. J Am Geriatr Soc 1985;33:320–324.
45. Simmang C, Birnbaum EH, Kodner IJ, et al. Anal sphincter reconstruction in the elderly: does advancing age affect outcome? Dis Colon Rectum 1994;37:1065–1069.

# 46
# Neoplastic Diseases of the Colon and Rectum

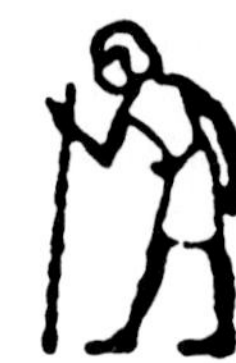

Jasleen Jasleen, Edward E. Whang, K. Robert Shen,
Elizabeth Breen, and Stanley W. Ashley

Colorectal cancer is primarily a disease of the elderly. The incidence of both colorectal carcinoma and its precursor lesions increase progressively with age. Although there is no evidence that the biologic aggressiveness of colorectal cancer increases with age, delays in diagnosis contribute to the presence of relatively advanced disease at presentation, and therefore a poorer prognosis, in the elderly. These delays in diagnosis also result in the development of complications of colorectal cancer, requiring emergent surgery. Recently reported series document excellent results for elderly patients undergoing elective operations for colorectal cancer. In contrast, the elderly, who are more likely to have co-morbid conditions, fare poorly with emergent procedures. It is ironic that the elderly population, which has the most to gain from early detection of colorectal neoplasms, is the least likely to undergo appropriate screening and diagnostic evaluation.

In this chapter, the epidemiology, pathology, diagnosis, and therapy of colorectal neoplasms are reviewed, with an emphasis on recent developments. Although the benefit of screening for colorectal cancer is universally accepted, the optimal strategies for doing so are controversial. Likewise, surveillance methods for detecting disease recurrence following curative resection are in evolution. The tools of modern biology have generated new insights into the pathogenesis of colorectal neoplasia and have identified specific genetic abnormalities in several inherited forms of colorectal cancer. Surgical techniques, particularly for rectal cancer, have also undergone recent evolution. There is an increasing emphasis on minimizing local recurrence rates and maintaining sphincter function. For rectal cancer, effective neoadjuvant therapies have altered the therapeutic approach to the disease. It is likely that these and other recent developments will dramatically improve the prognosis for patients with colorectal cancer.

## Epidemiology

Colorectal cancer is the third most frequently diagnosed cancer and the second leading cause of cancer-related mortality in the United States, where it accounts for 14% of cancer-related deaths. Altogether, 135,000 new cases and 55,000 deaths due to colorectal cancer were estimated to have occurred in the United States in 1997.[1] Epidemiologic studies have documented a broad variation in the incidence of colorectal cancer with geographic location, with the highest incidence in industrialized nations such as western Europe and North America (Fig. 46.1). This geographic variation is attributable, at least partially, to environmental factors, as populations migrating from regions associated with a low incidence of colorectal cancer to those with a high incidence experience an increased rate of acquiring the disease.[2]

The incidence of colorectal cancer in men is approximately equal to that in women. Its incidence progressively increases with advancing age, consistent with the hypothesis that colorectal cancer arises as the result of multiple genetic mutations accumulated over time. The median age at which patients in the United States are diagnosed with colorectal cancer is 70 years for men and 73 for women. Whereas the overall incidence of colon cancer in the United States is 17 per 100,000 population, in men and women over the age of 85, the incidence is 239 and 209 cases per 100,000 population, respectively. For rectal cancer the incidence in men and women over 85 years of age, is 142 and 226 cases per 100,000 population, respectively. The cumulative lifetime risk of developing colorectal cancer is approximately 5%.

Adenomatous polyps of the colon and rectum, which have the potential to undergo transformation into cancers, are found in approximately 25% of people by the age of 50 years, and their prevalence increases with advancing age. The prevalence of large (>1 cm in diame-

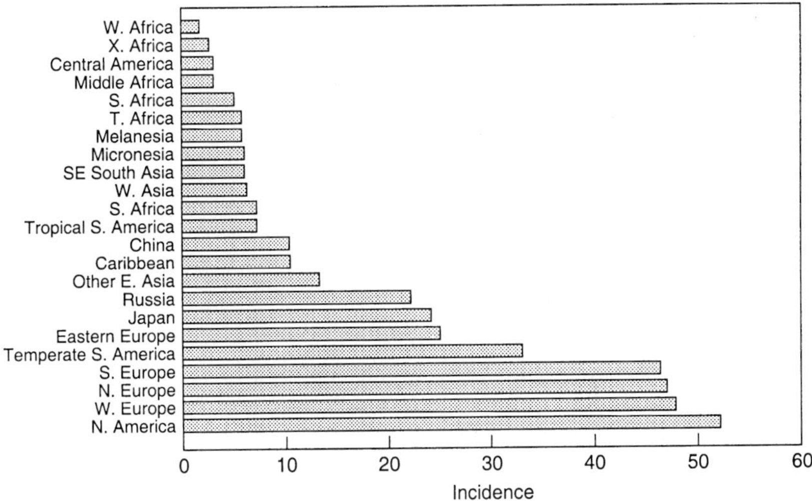


FIGURE 46.1. Incidence of colorectal cancer per 100,000 population in 23 geographic regions. (From Parkin et al.,[2] with permission.)

ter) polyps, which have the greatest probability of harboring cancer, also appears to be related to age. In one series, such large polyps were found in 4.6% of patients of age more than 54 years and in 15.6% of patients of age more than 75 years.[3]

Not only are the elderly at greater risk of developing colorectal cancer, they are also likely to have more advanced disease at the time of diagnosis. In one report, patients over 75 years of age were twice as likely to present with advanced, untreatable colorectal cancer as those under 65 years of age.[4] The relative contributions of physician bias, limited access to health care, poor social support, and impaired cognition to this observation are not clear.

## Risk Factors

Epidemiologic studies have suggested that an increase in the consumption of dietary fiber, fruits, and cruciferous vegetables and a reduction in the consumption of fat, is associated with a decrease in mortality from colorectal cancer. However, the efficacy of modifications in diet in preventing colorectal cancer has not yet been demonstrated in prospective trials. Epidemiologic studies have also suggested that aspirin use is associated with a reduction in the incidence of colorectal cancer, and that cigarette smoking is associated with an increased incidence of colorectal adenomas and cancers, with relative risk related to both dose and duration of smoke exposure. Again, the efficacy of modifying these risk factors in colorectal cancer prevention remains to be shown.

In addition to older age, factors clearly associated with an increased incidence of colorectal cancer include a history of colorectal cancer, either in oneself or in one's relatives. Patients with colorectal cancer are more likely to develop a subsequent (metachronous) lesion than is the general population to develop primary cancer. Patients who have a first-degree relative with colorectal cancer, but not one of the specific genetic syndromes discussed below, have approximately twice the probability of developing colorectal cancer as those without such a family history. This probability is higher if more than one first-degree relative is affected or if the age at diagnosis of the relative's cancer is less than 55 years. A similar increase in risk is found for patients with a first-degree relative found to have an adenomatous polyp prior to the age of 60.

In the United States, approximately 25% of cases of colorectal cancer occur in individuals with a family history of the disease or an underlying condition specifically associated with the development of colorectal cancer. Patients who have first-degree relatives with colorectal cancer, but not any of the defined genetic syndromes, account for most of these cases (15–20%). Hereditary nonpolyposis colon cancer (HNPCC) accounts for 4–7% of cases, and familial adenomatous polyposis (FAP) accounts for 1%. An additional 1% of cases is accounted for by a combination of patients with inflammatory bowel disease, Peutz-Jeghers syndrome, and familial juvenile polyposis (Table 46.1).

### Familial Adenomatous Polyposis

Affected individuals develop adenomatous polyps during the second and third decades of life, have hundreds to thousands of polyps throughout their colon by the third decade of life, and if they do not undergo prophylactic colectomy have almost a 100% probability of developing colorectal cancer by the fourth decade of life. Variants of FAP include Turcot syndrome (familial colorectal cancer and brain cancer) and Gardner syndrome (familial colorectal cancer, osteomas, and benign soft tissue tumors). These syndromes are inherited in an autosomal dominant manner and result from mutations in the adenomatous polyposis coli (*APC*) gene, located on the long arm of chromosome 5. Many distinct mutations of this gene have been identified in the kindreds studied.

TABLE 46.1. Risk Factors for Colorectal Cancer

| |
|---|
| General factors |
| Age > 40 years |
| Family history of colorectal cancer |
| Genetic factors |
| Co-morbid conditions |
| Crohn's disease |
| Ulcerative colitis |
| Prior colorectal malignancy |
| Neoplastic colorectal polyps |
| Pelvic irradiation |
| Breast or genital tract malignancy |
| Polyposis syndromes |
| Peutz-Jeghers syndrome (hamartomas) |
| Oldfield syndrome (sebaceous cysts) |
| Gardner syndrome |
| Turcot syndrome (CNS tumors) |
| Familial polyposis coli |
| Nonpolyposis syndromes |
| Lynch syndrome I |
| Lynch syndrome II |

Although genetic testing is useful for identifying the gene carriers within kindreds, such testing is not feasible as a screening measure in the general population.

## Hereditary Nonpolyposis Colon Cancer

There are two forms of HNPCC (also known as Lynch syndrome). With Lynch syndrome I, familial colorectal cancer occurs in isolation; with Lynch syndrome II, there is an increased familial occurrence of other cancers, especially ovarian and uterine cancer. The lifetime incidence of colon cancer in patients with HNPCC is 75–80%, and the cancers tend to become evident at an early age (typically during the fourth and fifth decades of life, although the range has been 15–75 years of age). Adenomatous polyps, although they do not occur in unusually large numbers, as in FAP, do occur with higher frequency and at a younger age in patients with HNPCC than in the general population. These polyps tend to be sessile and undergo more rapid transformation into invasive cancer. However, invasive cancers in these patients, which tend to be located proximal to the splenic flexure, are associated with a better prognosis than those in the general population.

In contrast to the polyposis syndromes, HNPCC lacks reliably distinctive clinical features. Therefore, an accurate family history is currently the most effective way of identifying the syndrome in a particular patient. The Amsterdam criteria for diagnosing HNPCC requires (1) the presence of three or more relatives with histologically documented colorectal cancer, one of whom is a first-degree relative of the other two; (2) one or more cases of colorectal cancer diagnosed prior to the age of 50 years; and (3) colorectal cancer involving at least two generations.[5] These criteria have been criticized as being too strict, and alternatives have been proposed, although the former remain the gold standard for diagnosis.[3] Mutations that have been identified in affected kindreds occur primarily on four genes on chromosomes 2, 3, and 7 (*MLH1*, *MSH2*, *PMS1*, *PMS2*). More mutations are likely to remain to be discovered, as the known mutations are found in only 70% of families with HNPCC, as defined by the Amsterdam criteria.

## Hamartomatous Polyposis Syndromes

The hamartomatous polyposis syndromes, in which hamartomas occur in the small and large intestine, are transmitted in an autosomal dominant fashion. With juvenile polyposis, these hamartomas develop during childhood. With Peutz-Jeghers syndrome, the hamartomas develop in conjuction with mucocutaneous pigmentation. Colonic adenomas can occur with both of these syndromes, and the risk of colorectal cancer is increased relative to that in the general population, although considerably less so than for HNPCC or FAP.

## Inflammatory Bowel Disease

The increased risk of developing colorectal cancer associated with ulcerative colitis is similar to that with Crohn's colitis when extent, duration, and age of onset of disease are taken into consideration. The strongest risk factor seems to be the anatomic extent of inflammation. The cumulative incidence of colorectal cancer in patients with pancolitis is 30% in 35 years. Disease duration is also a risk factor; cancer rarely arises prior to 8 years of disease activity. Earlier age at disease onset is also said to be a risk factor, although it is not clear whether this effect is independent of the duration and extent of disease. Because the level of activity of a patient's inflammatory bowel disease is not associated with an increased incidence of colorectal malignancy, it is important that even patients with quiescent disease undergo regular surveillance. Cancers arising in patients with inflammatory bowel disease tend to be flat and infiltrating and often arise from areas of epithelial dysplasia not associated with preexisting polyps. The probability of colorectal cancer being present in these patients in the setting of dysplasia is 30%.

# Pathology

## Polyps

Polyps are mucosal masses in the colon and rectum. There are several histologically distinct types of polyps of varying clinical significance (Table 46.2), including ade-

TABLE 46.2. Classification of Colorectal Polyps

| |
|---|
| Neoplastic epithelial polyps |
| Benign adenomas |
| Tubular |
| Tubulovillous |
| Villous |
| Malignant |
| Carcinoma in situ |
| Invasive carcinoma |
| Nonneoplastic epithelial polyps |
| Hyperplastic |
| Hamartomas |
| Juvenile |
| Peutz-Jeghers |
| Inflammatory |
| Mucosal |
| Inherited syndromes |
| Familial adenomatous polyposis (FAP) |
| Juvenile polyposis |
| Peutz-Jeghers |
| Submucosal polyps |
| Lymphoid |
| Lipomas |
| Carcinoids |
| Miscellaneous |

nomatous polyps (which are premalignant and represent 50–66% of all colorectal polyps), hyperplastic polyps (which are of no clinical importance and represent 10–30% of all polyps), mucosal tags (which are also of no clinical significance and represent 10–30% of polyps), and a variety of more unusual other histologic types, such as lipomas and hamartomas. Polyps in which the bulk of the lesion projects into the bowel lumen and is tethered to the mucosal surface through a narrow stalk of submucosa surrounded by mucosa, are characterized as pedunculated. Polyps that are flat and have a broad base are characterized as sessile.

Adenomatous polyps can be found throughout the colon and rectum, with approximately 30% occurring proximal to the splenic flexure. With advancing age, a larger percentage of adenomatous polyps are found in the proximal colon. Histologically, adenomatous polyps are subclassified as tubular, tubulovillous, and villous. Tubular and tubulovillous adenomas tend to be pedunculated, whereas villous adenomas tend to be sessile. The potential for malignant transformation is least for tubular adenomas and highest for villous adenomas.

The size of an adenomatous polyp is directly related to the probability that it is harboring high grade dysplasia, which is likely to be the direct precursor of preinvasive carcinoma, and that the patient will develop other adenomatous polyps and colorectal cancer (Fig. 46.2). In one report, 1.1% of adenomatous polyps <5 mm in diameter, 4.6% of those 5–9 mm in diameter, and 20.6% of those ≥1 cm, exhibited high-grade dysplasia.[6] Fewer than 1% of adenomatous polyps <1 cm in diameter harbor invasive carcinoma, whereas more than 10% of larger adenomatous polyps do so.

## Colorectal Cancer

Approximately 95% of all colorectal cancers are adenocarcinomas. Macroscopically, the lesions can have a polypoid, infiltrative, or ulcerated appearance. Histologically, they are characterized as being well differentiated, moderately differentiated, or poorly differentiated. Lesions that have an infiltrative or ulcerated appearance and are less well differentiated are associated with poorer prognosis. Cancers associated with increased production of mucin are typically characterized by the presence of signet ring cells. The prognostic implication of these signet ring cells is not clear-cut.

Extension of colorectal cancers occurs through three routes: (1) via the bloodstream to distant sites, particularly the liver; (2) via the lymphatics to regional lymph nodes and ultimately the systemic circulation; and (3) by direct extension into adjacent organs, such as the posterior vaginal wall, uterus, prostate, bladder, small intestine, stomach, and retroperitoneal structures.

The anatomic distribution of cancers is as follows: ascending colon 18%, transverse colon 9%, descending colon 5%, sigmoid colon 25%, and rectum 43%. Cancers are currently found with greater frequency in the proximal colon than they were earlier during the twentieth century. It is unknown whether the advent of colonoscopy (and its ability to detect more proximally located cancers) or a change in the biologic behavior of colorectal cancer explains this shift.

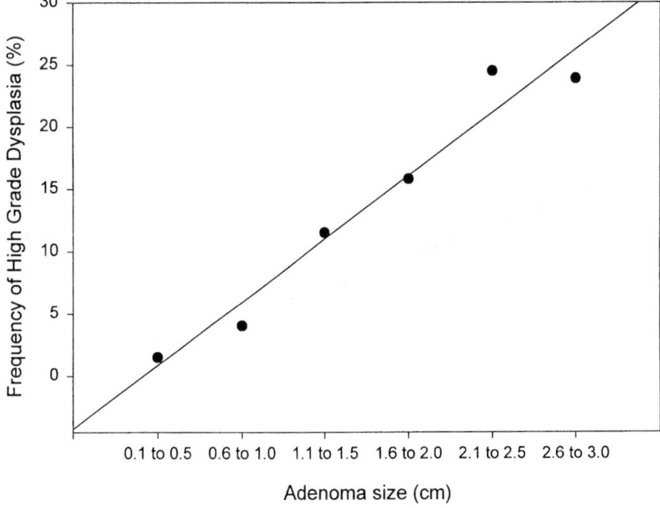


FIGURE 46.2. Frequency of high grade dysplasia versus adenoma size. (From O'Brien et al.,[6] with permission.)

## Staging

A variety of pathologic staging systems have been used. Dukes, a pathologist, in 1932 proposed a staging system for rectal cancer based on the depth of invasion of the bowel wall by the primary tumor. He described three stages: Stage A tumors involve the bowel wall without extension through the muscularis propria. Stage B lesions extend through the muscularis propria into the perirectal fat but are not associated with lymph node metastases. Stage C lesions are associated with regional lymph nodes metastases; the depth of penetration by the primary tumor may vary.

Several modifications of Dukes' original staging system have been described, but the Astler-Coller modification has seen the most widespread clinical application. Stage A lesions are limited to the mucosa. Stage B lesions are subclassified into B1, B2, and B3, depending on the depth of invasion and adjacent organ involvement. Stage C lesions are associated with regional lymph node metastases and are subclassified into C1, C2, and C3, based on the depth of invasion. Stage D lesions are associated with distant metastases.

With the TNM staging system, recommended by the American Joint Committee on Cancer (Table 46.3), staging is based on the depth of invasion of the primary tumor (T), status of regional lymph nodes (N), and the presence of distant metastasis (M). The advantage of the TNM staging system is its applicability to both presurgical clinical-diagnostic staging and postsurgical resection-pathologic staging.

TABLE 46.3. TNM Staging Classification of Colorectal Cancer

| Stage | Description |
|---|---|
| Primary tumor | |
| Tx | Primary tumor cannot be assessed |
| T0 | No evidence of tumor in resected specimen (prior polypectomy) or fulguration |
| Tis | Carcinoma in situ |
| T1 | Invades submucosa |
| T2 | Invades muscularis propria |
| T3/T4 | Depends on whether serosa is present |
| Serosa present | |
| T3 | Invades through muscularis propria into subserosa<br>Invades serosa (but not through)<br>Invades pericolic fat within the leaves of the mesentery |
| T4 | Invades serosa into free peritoneal cavity or through serosa into a contiguous organ |
| No serosa (distal two-thirds of rectum, posterior left or right colon) | |
| T3 | Invades muscularis propria |
| T4 | Invades other organs (vagina, prostate, ureter, kidney) |
| Regional lymph node involvement | |
| Nx | Nodes cannot be assessed |
| N0 | No regional node metastases |
| N1 | 1–3 Positive nodes |
| N2 | ≥4 Positive nodes |
| N3 | Central nodes positive |
| Distant metastasis | |
| Mx | Presence of distant metastases cannot be assessed |
| M0 | No distant metastases |
| M1 | Distant metastases present |

## Pathogenesis

Most colorectal cancers probably arise via transformation of preexisting adenomatous polyps. Several lines of circumstantial evidence support this assertion: (1) Cancers and adenomatous polyps occur with the same anatomic distribution; (2) cancers rarely arise in the absence of adenomatous polyps; (3) the average age of onset of adenomatous polyps precedes that of cancer by several years; (4) patients found to have large polyps are at increased risk for subsequently developing cancer, with most of these cancers arising at sites where these polyps are left in place; (5) patients with familial adenomatous polyposis are at markedly increased risk of developing cancer; and (6) the detection and removal of adenomatous polyps reduces the incidence of colorectal cancer.

The strongest evidence for the clinical relevance of the concept that most cancers arise from precursor adenomatous polyps is derived from the National Polyp Study. A group of 1418 patients was followed for an average of 5.9 years after removal of all identifiable colonic polyps. Only five subsequent malignant polyps (all being Dukes' stage A lesions) were found, and no deaths from colorectal cancer occurred during 8401 person-years of follow-up.[7] The incidence of malignant transformation of adenomatous polyps has been estimated to be 2.5 polyps per 1000 per year. The mean time required for an individual polyp to undergo such transformation has been estimated to be 10 years.[3]

The transformation of an adenomatous polyp to invasive cancer (and that of normal mucosa to adenomatous polyp) is associated with an accumulation of acquired genetic mutations. This model of tumorigenesis, proposed by Fearon and Vogelstein, is shown in Figure 46.3. Genetic changes include mutational activation of dominantly acting cellular oncogenes and mutational inactivation of recessive tumor-suppressor genes. Protooncogenes are present in normal cells; their protein products tend to be positive regulators of cell growth. When these genes undergo mutation, they can become oncogenes, whose protein products are produced in excessive quantities or act in an unregulated manner, thereby promoting tumor formation. The protein products of tumor-suppressor genes, on the other hand, tend to suppress cell growth, and their loss may promote tumor development.

Mutations characteristic of colorectal cancer have begun to be identified. Approximately 50% of colorectal cancers and adenomatous polyps >1 cm in diameter, have

FIGURE 46.3. Genetic model for colorectal tumorigenesis as proposed by Fearon and Vogelstein. (From Vogelstein et al.,[8] © Massachusetts Medical Society, with permission.)

| | | Chromosome | Alteration | Gene |
|---|---|---|---|---|
| Normal Epithelium | | | | |
| ⇓ | ⇐ | 5q | Mutation or Loss | FAP |
| Hyperproliferation Epithelium | | | | |
| ⇓ | | | | |
| Early Adenoma | ⇐ | DNA hypomethylation | | |
| ⇓ | ⇐ | 12p | Mutation | K-ras |
| Intermediate adenoma | | | | |
| ⇓ | ⇐ | 18q | Loss | DCC |
| Late Adenoma | | | | |
| ⇓ | ⇐ | 17p | Loss | p53 |
| Carcinoma | | | | |
| ⇓ | ⇐ | Other Alteration | | |
| Metastasis | | | | |

been found to harbor mutations in the *ras* oncogene,[8–10] whereas fewer than 10% of adenomas <1 cm in diameter are associated with such mutations. The highly conserved *ras* proto-oncogenes (N-*ras*, H-*ras*, K-*ras*) encode for the production of signal transduction G-proteins (guanosine triphosphate-binding proteins). Mutations in the *ras* gene result in the production of an abnormal G-protein that is associated with unregulated cell growth. In vitro and animal studies have suggested that mutations in the *ras* gene may also inhibit programmed cell death (apoptosis).

The development of colorectal cancer is also associated with the deletion of chromosomal fragments. This phenomenon is also known as *allelic loss* or *loss of heterozygosity*. This process primarily affects chromosomes 17 and 18 and to a lesser degree chromosome 5. The DNA lost in such deletions may contain tumor-suppressor genes. One such gene whose loss is associated with FAP, has been localized to chromosome 5q and is known as the adenomatous polyposis coli (*APC*) gene. The *APC* gene is thought to be a tumor-suppressor gene, although the function of its protein product is not yet known. Therefore, allelic loss of *APC* may promote neoplastic transformation. Allelic loss of chromosome 5q is present in approximately 20–50% of sporadic colorectal carcinomas and 30% of sporadic adenomatous polyps.

The loss of chromosome 17p, which contains the *p53* tumor-suppressor gene, is seen in 75% of sporadic colorectal cancers but rarely in adenomas of any size. Therefore loss of chromosome 17p may be particularly associated with progression of an adenoma to cancer. The allelic loss of chromosome 17p is also seen in a wide range of cancers, including those of the brain, breast, lung, and bladder. Evidence has indicated that reconstitution of wild-type *p53* expression in human and murine cell lines, inhibits growth through induction of cell cycle arrest, apoptosis, or both.

Approximately 70% of colorectal cancers and 50% of large adenomatous polyps, are associated with allelic deletions of chromosome 18q. *DCC* (deleted in colorectal carcinoma) is a candidate tumor-suppressor gene that has been mapped to chromosome 18q. The protein product of the *DCC* gene has significant homology to the neural cell adhesion molecule (N-CAM). It has been speculated that deletion of the *DCC* gene may modify cell–cell or cell–basement membrane interactions (or both), which are important for regulating cell growth and differentiation.

Several germ-line mutations (*MLH1*, *MSH2*, *PMS1*, *PMS2*) on chromosomes 2, 3, and 7, have been identified in patients with HNPCC. These genes are human homologues of the bacterial mutHLS complex, which is involved in genetic proofreading (the repair of mismatched basepairs in DNA). Loss of this function is thought to allow basepair mismatches to accumulate, resulting in a replication-error phenotype, which is seen in a high percentage of patients with HNPCC and approximately 15% of those with sporadic colorectal cancer.

It is likely that specific mutations, for sporadic and familial forms of colorectal cancer, will be identified at an increasingly rapid pace in the years to come. As the functions of the protein products of these abnormal genes are characterized, genetic interventions may become a reality.

## Screening

Screening for colorectal cancer has clearly been demonstrated to have efficacy in reducing cancer-related mortality. There has been controversy, however, related to which screening and surveillance methods are optimal, how frequently the tests should be done, who should undergo testing, and the cost-effectiveness of the various strategies. In addition, only a small number of the elderly population, who potentially have the most to gain from such testing, undergo screening of any kind for colorectal cancer. According to data from the National Health Interview Survey (NHIS), in 1992 only 17.3% of people aged 50 years or older, had undergone fecal occult blood testing (FOBT) during the previous year, and only 9.4% had undergone sigmoidoscopy during the previous 3 years.[11] Education (for both patients and physicians) and investigation related to screening would likely have a major impact on the overall management of colorectal cancer. In this section, the terminology related to screening is defined, tests used for screening strategies are discussed, and recommendations are outlined.

The terms screening, diagnosis, and surveillance have distinct clinical definitions. *Screening* identifies those patients who are at risk for having colorectal cancer or adenomatous polyps from among the population who are without signs or symptoms of the disease. *Diagnosis* classifies patients who, because of a positive screening test or symptoms, are suspected of having colorectal cancer or adenomatous polyps into those with and without the disease. *Surveillance* monitors patients with previously diagnosed colorectal disease (polyps, colorectal cancer, or inflammatory bowel disease, for example) for the development of adenomatous polyps or colorectal cancer.

Screening for a disease is justified when the following four criteria are met: (1) the disease is common and associated with serious morbidity and/or mortality; (2) screening tests are accurate for detecting early stage disease; (3) treatment after detection by screening improves prognosis relative to treatment after diagnosis in the absence of screening; and (4) potential benefits outweigh the potential harms and costs of screening. Screening for colorectal cancer fulfills all of these criteria.[3]

### Fecal Occult Blood Testing

The rationale for using FOBT to screen for colorectal cancer is based on the observation that colonic neoplasms have a greater tendency to bleed than does normal mucosa. This propensity increases with polyp size and cancer stage, although the bleeding is usually intermittent and unevenly distributed in the stool.

The most widely used test for fecal occult blood is the guaiac-based assay for peroxidase activity. Hemoglobin, which has pseudoperoxidase activity, in blood yields a positive test result. This test has considerable limitations. The test is not specific for cancer, as nonneoplastic processes, such as gum disease, gastritis, peptic ulcer disease, and hemorrhoids can also cause gastrointestinal hemorrhage. The test is also not specific for blood, as other substances with peroxidase or pseudoperoxidase activity, such as red meat, bacteria, and some fruits and vegetables can cause false-positive reactions. False-negative tests may result if the cancer did not bleed when the sampled stool was being formed or if the quantity of bleeding is below the limits of test detection. The antioxidant activity of vitamin C can interfere with the test reaction, causing a false-negative result. Iron supplements do not interfere with the reaction; but by making the stool dark they interfere with interpretation of the test results. The patient should therefore observe a diet restricted from these confounding substances for 2 days prior to stool sampling.

The sensitivity of FOBT is increased with the number of samples per stool and the number of stools sampled. Therefore it is recommended that patients provide several specimens from several consecutive stools and that each stool be sampled at two sites. A single specimen obtained by digital rectal examination has questionable value and should not be considered adequate when screening for colorectal cancer. Typically, several days elapse between stool collection and testing it for blood. The sensitivity of a guaiac-based test is increased if the test slide is rehydrated with a few drops of water before performing the test. The best available evidence that FOBT is effective in preventing death caused by colorectal cancer is from a study with rehydrated tests on two samples from each of three consecutive stools in patients who followed a restricted diet prior to testing.[12]

In a program of repeated screening (rather than a single test), the nonhydrated form of FOBT has a reported sensitivity for detecting cancer that ranges from 72% to 78%, a specificity of 98%, and a positive predictive value of 10–17%. Rehydrating the slides increases the sensitivity to 88–92% but decreases the specificity to 90–92%, and the positive predictive value to 2–6%.[3]

The FOBT for detecting colon cancer has been reported to be of lower specificity for patients over 60 years of age than for younger patients. This observation may be related to a higher prevalence of other etiologies for gastrointestinal hemorrhage with increasing age. On the other hand, there is no evidence that the value of FOBT is diminished in the very elderly. In fact, the positive predictive value of FOBT has been reported to increase with age from 1.6% for those under 60 years of age to 3.6% for those over 70 years of age.[13]

## Sigmoidoscopy

Although supporting data from randomized trials are lacking, several case–control studies support the efficacy of screening sigmoidoscopy for reducing mortality due to colorectal cancer. As a screening method, sigmoidoscopy has three advantages over FOBT: (1) the bowel is directly visualized; (2) lesions can be biopsied during the procedure; and (3) it has high sensitivity and specificity for detecting polyps in the bowel examined. Its primary limitation is that only the rectum and distal colon are examined.

Patients usually do not require sedation or full bowel preparation for screening sigmoidoscopy. Although lesions are biopsied, full polypectomies are not routinely done, as cautery used for polypectomies can result in explosions in colons subjected to less than full bowel preparation. Prophylactic antibiotics are given to patients at risk for developing endocarditis.

The performance of the flexible 60 cm sigmoidoscope is superior to that of the 25 cm rigid scope. With the flexible scope, a larger area of colon can be examined, the optics are better, and there is more comfort for both patient and examiner. Within the area of reach, nearly all cancers and all polyps >1 cm in diameter and 70–85% of smaller polyps are detected by flexible sigmoidoscopy. False-positive findings are rare, although many polyps identified prove to be nonadenomatous. The 60 cm scope, which reaches up to or beyond the proximal sigmoid colon in 80% of examinations, should be able to detect 40–60% of adenomatous polyps and cancers based on the known anatomic distribution of these lesions. The rigid scope would be able to detect only 20–30% of these lesions.

What constitutes a positive finding on screening sigmoidoscopy requiring full colonoscopy is somewhat controversial. Cancer or an adenomatous polyp >1 cm in diameter should be followed by colonoscopy. Polyps shown to be hyperplastic and normal mucosa do not require follow-up. It is not yet clear whether a small adenoma (<1 cm in diameter), especially if it is tubular and without high grade dysplasia, needs follow-up. When an adenomatous polyp is found in the rectosigmoid there is an approximately 33% probability that more proximally located adenomatous polyps are present. However, if the rectosigmoid adenoma is <1 cm in diameter, it is unlikely that adenomas >1 cm or with high grade dysplasia will be found more proximally.

## Barium Enema

Barium enema examination allows the entire colon and rectum to be evaluated, although there are no specific data that its use as a screening test is associated with a reduction in mortality from colorectal cancer. This test can be performed in two ways: as a single-contrast study using barium alone or as a double-contrast study, in which air is instilled into the colon after most of the barium is removed. With the single-contrast study lesions appear as filling defects, whereas with the double-contrast study lesions are outlined by the retained barium against a background of air. The double-contrast study has considerably more sensitivity and specificity than the single-contrast study and has generally replaced it, except in patients not able to tolerate the more complicated and uncomfortable study. The sensitivity of double-contrast barium enema has been reported as 50–80% for polyps <1 cm in diameter, 70–90% for polyps >1 cm in diameter, and 55–85% for Dukes' stage A and B cancers. False-negative results are related to inadequate visualization of segments of bowel, especially the sigmoid colon, and to errors in interpretation. False-positives are the result of stool in the bowel and of non-neoplastic mucosal irregularities. When a finding on double-contrast barium enema is interpreted as cancer, the false-positive rate is less than 1%; the rate ranges from 5% to 10% when the interpretation is a large polyp and 50% when it is a small polyp. Another limitation of the test is that 5–10% of studies are technically unsatisfactory, requiring another attempt at barium enema or colonoscopy.

## Colonoscopy

Colonoscopy is the only screening technique that offers the potential to both detect and remove premalignant lesions throughout the colon and rectum. With respect to technical difficulty and the risk to the patient, it is more formidable than either sigmoidoscopy or barium enema. Colonoscopy is poorly tolerated without intravenous sedation. Because there is potential for the development of cardiorespiratory complications, elderly patients, particularly those with significant co-morbidities, should undergo cardiorespiratory monitoring. As is the case for sigmoidoscopy, patients at risk for developing bacterial endocarditis should undergo appropriate antibiotic prophylaxis.

Sensitivity rates for colonoscopy are difficult to discern, as colonoscopy itself is often used as the gold standard for the presence or absence of lesions. However, studies in which colonoscopy is done prior to surgical resection for polyps and cancers, suggest that colonoscopy misses 3% of such lesions. In comparison to barium enema, colonoscopy has more sensitivity for detecting small polyps, but its ability to detect polyps >1 cm is equivalent. It is unclear which procedure causes less discomfort and is therefore associated with greater patient acceptability. Models of diagnostic strategies for patients with a positive screening FOBT have shown that barium enema and colonoscopy are associated with comparable cost-effectiveness.[14]

A limitation of colonoscopy is that in only 80–95% of procedures is the entire colon visualized. The probability of reaching the proximal colon depends primarily on the skill of the examiner and the adequacy of the bowel preparation. If the entire colon cannot be visualized, another examination is required: another attempt at colonoscopy or a barium enema.

## Digital Rectal Examination

A common practice is to screen for colorectal cancer by performing digital rectal examination, followed by a test for fecal occult blood if stool is present in the rectum. Based on the anatomic distribution of cancers, only 5–10% of lesions would be within reach of the examining finger. In addition, stool obtained from the digital rectal examination represents inadequate sampling and is associated with high false-negative rates. Digital rectal examination, by itself, is not an effective method of screening for colorectal cancer.

## Recommendations

Screening for colorectal cancer and adenomatous polyps should be offered to all men and women without special risk factors beginning at age 50. A positive screening test should be followed by a diagnostic evaluation. Five screening options have been proposed in guidelines defined by a multidisciplinary panel.[15,16] These guidelines have been endorsed by a wide range of organizations, including the American Cancer Society, the American Gastroenterological Association, and the American Society of Colon and Rectal Surgeons; and they represent the current standard of care.

1. *Yearly fecal occult blood screening*. Those with a positive test should undergo diagnostic evaluation with colonoscopy or double-contrast barium enema (with flexible sigmoidoscopy).
2. *Flexible sigmoidoscopy every 5 years*. If polyps >1 cm in diameter are found, colonoscopy should be done. Polyps <1 cm in diameter should be biopsied, and if adenomatous polyps or cancers are found, colonoscopy should be done. It is not clear whether patients with small tubular adenomas (<1 cm in diameter) should undergo colonoscopy.
3. *Combined fecal occult blood testing and flexible sigmoidoscopy*. The combination of these two methods theoretically compensates for some of the deficiencies of each. However, there are no good data proving that combining the two methods offers any advantage over either alone.
4. *Double-contrast barium enema every 5–10 years*. No data exist to support that this method reduces mortality due to colorectal cancer.
5. *Colonoscopy every 10 years*. No data exist to support that this method reduces mortality due to colorectal cancer.

## Patients with Particular Risk Factors

The guidelines published by the multidisciplinary panel also propose specific recommendations for patients at increased risk for developing colorectal cancer (Table 46.4).

### Family History

Patients with a first-degree relative who has had colorectal cancer or an adenomatous polyp should be offered the same options as average-risk patients but starting at age 40.

### Familial Adenomatous Polyposis

Patients with a family history of FAP should undergo genetic counseling and consider genetic testing to determine if they are gene carriers. A negative genetic test result eliminates the possibility of FAP only if an affected family member has an identified mutation. Gene carriers (or indeterminate cases) should be offered flexible sigmoidoscopy yearly, beginning at puberty to determine if they are expressing the gene. If polyposis is present, they should undergo proctocolectomy. Colonoscopy is unnecessary, as sigmoidoscopy alone is able to detect the

TABLE 46.4. Screening Guidelines for Colorectal Cancer

| Symptoms | Family history | Age to begin (years) | Evaluation |
|---|---|---|---|
| None | None | 50 | DRE; stool guiaic; colonoscopy: if negative repeat in 3–5 years, otherwise repeat in 1 year to ensure no new lesions |
| None | One or more FDR | 40 | As above |
| None | FAP | 10 | DRE; colonoscopy: repeat annually if polyps found or at 3 years if no polyps |
| None | HNPCC | Late teens | As for FAP |
| Present | None | 25 | DRE; stool guiaic; colonoscopy: if negative repeat in 3–5 years, otherwise repeat in 1 year to ensure no new lesions |

*Source:* Byers et al.,[16] with permission.
DRE, digital rectal examination; FDR, first-degree relative; FAP, familial adenomatous polyposis; HNPCC, hereditary nonpolyposis colorectal carcinoma.

adenomatous polyps, which occur throughout the bowel. Once the polyps occur, they are too numerous for colonoscopy to identify which ones harbor advanced pathology.

### *Hereditary Nonpolyposis Colorectal Carcinoma*

Patients with a family history of colorectal cancer in multiple close relatives and across generations should undergo genetic counseling and consider genetic testing for HNPCC. They should be offered examination of the entire colon every 1–2 years between the age of 20 and 30 and every year after age 40. Genetic tests are positive in only 80% of affected patients. Sigmoidoscopy is insufficient, as cancers tend to occur proximal to the splenic flexure in these patients.

### *Inflammatory Bowel Disease*

Patients with long-standing inflammatory bowel disease should undergo surveillance to detect dysplasia as a marker for an increased risk of cancer. The common practice is to perform colonoscopy every 1–2 years in patients who have had pancolitis for 8 years and left-sided colitis for 15 years.

## When to Stop Screening

There is no evidence to suggest that screening should stop at any given point.

## Cost-effectivencess of Screening for Colorectal Cancer

Cost-effectiveness analyses involve a number of assumptions and should therefore be interpreted with caution. In addition, current charges for the various screening tests vary greatly and may involve complex factors, some of which are difficult to measure. Nevertheless, recommended screening strategies are estimated to cost less than $20,000 per year of life saved. This figure is within an acceptable range by U.S. health standards and compares favorably with screening mammography in women for the detection of breast cancer.[17]

# Clinical Presentation

Symptoms of colorectal cancer are nonspecific and include abdominal pain, change in bowel movement patterns, and rectal bleeding (Table 46.5). In elderly patients particularly, the presentation may be varied and insidious, with vague symptoms such as apathy and weight loss sometimes being the only clue to the existence of cancer. Unfortunately, the incidence of benign colonic diseases associated with such nonspecific symptoms is increased in the elderly, and there is a tendency to procrastinate when proceeding with an appropriate diagnostic evaluation in this patient population.

TABLE 46.5. Signs and Symptoms of Colorectal Cancer

| |
|---|
| Right colon |
| Chronic anemia |
| Occult gastrointestinal bleeding |
| Fungating lesion |
| Left colon |
| Obstructing symptoms |
| Grossly bloody stool |
| Change in bowel habits |
| Circumferential lesion |
| Rectum |
| Tenesemus, perineal pain |
| Gross bleeding |
| Change in bowel habits |
| Palpable tumor |

There is some correlation between the location of the cancer and its resulting symptoms. Lesions in the right colon are frequently associated with such symptoms as a dull, aching pain in the right lower quadrant and fatigue and dizziness, which are related to the iron-deficiency anemia of chronic blood loss. Colonic obstruction is rare with cancers of the right colon. Transverse colon cancer frequently manifests as signs of obstruction or pain in the mid-epigastrium. Lesions of the left colon are often associated with an alteration in bowel habits and a decrease in stool caliber, with these changes being related to the narrower lumen and the presence of more solid stool in the left colon. Overt bleeding and colonic obstruction occur more frequently with rectosigmoid cancers than they do with more proximal lesions. Low rectal cancer tends to be associated with the presence of tenesmus, urgency, and perineal pain.

Signs of colorectal cancer include the presence of an abdominal or rectal mass or tenderness, anemia, and weight loss. Approximately 15% of colorectal cancers are first diagnosed in patients presenting with evidence of complete colonic obstruction. A smaller percentage of cancers present as colonic perforation, with most perforations occurring at the site of the tumor.

On occasion, signs and symptoms of metastatic disease are the first indication of the presence of colorectal cancer. Metastasis to the liver may manifest as jaundice and pruritus. Metastatic pulmonary disease may be seen on a chest radiograph in an otherwise asymptomatic patient. Signs of metastatic disease include the presence of ascites, hepatomegaly, and lymphadenopathy (in the supraclavicular and periumbilical areas, for example).

## Treatment

### Polyps

In general, sigmoidoscopy allows biopsy of polyps but not their complete removal. Full bowel preparation and colonoscopy are required for polypectomy. The current literature on the need for colonoscopy for small distal tubular adenomas found at sigmoidoscopy is controversial. Markowitz and Winawer,[18] in a review of the management of colorectal polyps, proposed the following guidelines. If a small polyp (<1 cm in diameter) biopsied on sigmoidoscopy is an adenoma, colonoscopic polypectomy with examination of the entire colon should be performed to look for synchronous neoplastic lesions. Read et al.,[19] in a prospective study of asymptomatic average risk individuals, reported that 31% of patients with benign adenomas on flexible sigmoidoscopy were found to have a synchronous neoplasm, and 8% with adenomas >1 cm in diameter had invasive cancers. If the polyp is >1 cm on sigmoidoscopy, however, rather than biopsy the lesion, colonoscopic polypectomy with examination of the proximal colon for synchronous lesions should be performed. Finding a nonneoplastic polyp at sigmoidoscopy requires no further evaluation. Radiographic detection of a polyp warrants full colonoscopy to resect the polyp and to examine the entire colon for the presence of synchronous lesions.

Polyps seen on colonoscopy should be excised endoscopically, unless they are sessile or too large to be removed endoscopically for technical reasons. For sessile polyps with invasive carcinoma, the incidence of lymph node metastasis is 15%, and the incidence of residual tumor after attempted endoscopic removal is 6%. A local recurrence rate of 21% can be anticipated if formal bowel resection is not done. For pedunculated lesions, polypectomy has the potential to be both diagnostic and therapeutic; although if invasive carcinoma is present in the polyp, further therapy may be indicated. Invasive carcinoma in a pedunculated polyp implies invasion of the cancer through the muscularis mucosa. The incidence of lymph node metastases in this circumstance ranges from 8% to 16%. Tumor features predictive of nodal metastasis are the presence of positive or close margins of resection, invasion of the neck or stalk of the polyp, poor differentiation status, and the presence of vascular and lymphatic invasion. In the absence of such adverse factors, complete polypectomy should be considered the definitive procedure. Formal colon resection should be performed if any of the high risk features are present.

Rectal polyps can be challenging. Although transanal sphincter-sparing excision is the procedure of choice, complete excision may require low anterior resection or abdominoperineal resection.

## Colorectal Cancer

### *Colorectal Surgery in the Elderly*

Most reported series of operations for colorectal cancer document a higher postoperative mortality rate in the elderly. This age-related increase in postoperative mortality rate is likely to be related to two factors: (1) the higher prevalence of coexisting illnesses in elderly patients; and (2) the higher incidence of emergency operations in elderly patients, as they are more likely to present with complications of colorectal cancer, such as intestinal obstruction and perforation. In one study, the subgroup of patients who were 70 years of age or older, who were without concomitant pulmonary, renal, hemopoietic, or cardiac disease, had a postoperative mortality rate of 4% following colon surgery; those younger than age 70 had a postoperative mortality rate of 3.2%.[20] In another review of 357 patients over the age of 50 undergoing colon resection, the postoperative mortality rate was directly correlated with the number of preexisting illnesses; age was not an independent risk factor for postoperative mortality. The postoperative mortality rate for all studied was 4.8%. For patients with no or one concomitant disease, the postoperative mortality rate for patients younger than age 70 was 0%, and it was 1.5% for those older than age 70.[21] In this study, for all age groups mortality for elective colon surgery was 3.4%, but it was 18% for emergency surgery. In another report of 101 colon resections in patients 70 years of age or older, the postoperative mortality rate was 5%, but no deaths occurred following elective procedures.[22]

It appears, as demonstrated in contemporary series, that elective colon resection can be performed safely in the elderly and that age is an independent risk factor for postoperative mortality following surgery for colorectal cancer. Existing data also suggest that early detection of colorectal cancer, allowing elective rather than emergent surgery, with careful preoperative assessment and optimization of organ system function, should be the goal in elderly patients.

When cancer stage is taken into account, the long-term survival rates following curative resection for colorectal cancer are comparable in elderly and younger patients. In one reported series, 3-year survival following surgery for colorectal cancer in patients older than 80 years was equivalent to that for patients under age 80, although increased age was associated with longer hospitalization and higher hospital costs.[23] Although there are few data regarding quality of life issues following surgery for colorectal cancer in the elderly, in one report of patients older than 80 years, 82% of those who were admitted to the hospital from home for colon surgery, were able to resume their normal level of activity postoperatively.[24]

### Preoperative Evaluation

Prior to surgery, elderly patients should undergo careful evaluation to diagnose and treat preexisting medical illnesses and to detect the presence of synchronous lesions and metastatic disease. The operative approach to be taken depends on the results of the preoperative evaluation.

Once a cancer in the colon or rectum has been diagnosed, the incidence of synchronous cancer is 5%, and the incidence of a synchronous adenomatous polyp is 28%. Preoperative colonoscopy or barium enema to detect such lesions is the standard of care. In general, colonoscopy is preferable; and if one has not already been performed, it is ideally performed the day prior to surgery, so only a single preparation is required. Barium enema is the test of choice if the cancer is nearly obstructing and prevents proximal passage of a colonoscope.

The hematocrit should be checked because of the possibility of anemia, which might require correction prior to surgery. Liver function tests should be checked, as they may indicate the presence of metastatic disease in the liver. Tumor markers such as carcinoembryonic antigen (CEA), CA 19-9, and CA-50 have been used for patients with colon cancer. Of these, CEA has had the most clinical application. Its preoperative concentration correlates well with tumor stage, as well as postoperative survival and recurrence rates. Elevated CEA concentrations are not specific for colorectal cancer, however. The CEA concentration in normal individuals ranges from 0 to 2.5ng/ml. Benign elevations in CEA concentration are usually less than 10ng/ml and are reversible. Known benign conditions associated with elevations in CEA concentration include biliary obstruction, hepatocellular dysfunction, cigarette smoking, bronchitis, gastric ulcer, gastritis, inflammatory bowel disease, diverticulitis, adenomatous polyps, renal disease, and benign prostatic hyperplasia. CEA concentration can also be elevated with noncolorectal cancers.

A preoperative chest radiograph is obtained to detect the presence of lung metastases and cardiopulmonary disease. For colon cancers, a preoperative computed tomography (CT) scan is not necessary, although in some practice settings it is obtained routinely. It would be indicated in patients with abnormal liver function tests or who have a palpable mass on physical examination.

Rectal cancers should undergo a somewhat different preoperative evaluation from cancers of the colon, to determine whether preoperative neoadjuvant therapies might be indicated or if a more conservative surgical approach can be used. A careful digital rectal examination should be done to evaluate tumor size, fixation, and ulceration and to evaluate possible extension of the cancer to pararectal lymph nodes or adjacent organs. A woman should have a complete pelvic examination to determine if the tumor has invaded the vagina or has spread to the ovaries. Rigid sigmoidoscopy is done to assess size, ulceration, and distance of the distal edge of the tumor to the anal verge. Flexible instruments are unreliable for assessing distance. CT scanning is indicated in patients with rectal cancer to evaluate pelvic extension and to look for distant metastases. Transrectal ultrasound examinations can accurately determine the depth of cancer invasion. Although lymph nodes can be visualized by ultrasonography, the presence of cancer within these nodes cannot be predicted accurately. Improved magnetic resonance imaging (MRI) techniques, positron emission tomography (PET) scanning, and monoclonal antibody scans might help in this aspect of staging in the future.

### Preoperative Bowel Preparation

The concentration of bacteria in the stool contained in the colon is approximately $10^9$/ml. As a result, operations performed on unprepared colon or rectum are associated with infectious complications in up to 70% of cases. A combined approach of mechanical washout and oral antibiotic administration decreases the infection rate to 10%. With the addition of parenteral antibiotic prophylaxis, infection rates are less than 5%.

In addition to reducing infection rates, evacuation of stool facilitates intraoperative bowel manipulation and minimizes the possibility of cautery-induced ignition of combustible gases found in the colon. Mechanical evacuation of stool is usually accomplished by administering polyethylene glycol (PEG), a nonabsorbable osmolar agent: 2–4 liters of PEG-containing solution are usually required to evacuate the colon. An alternative regimen is Fleet's Phospho-soda taken with 4 ounces of water followed by two 8-ounce glasses of water. This is then followed by two Dulcolax tablets taken orally. This method requires ingestion of lower volumes of fluid than PEG-based preparations and may be better tolerated by elderly patients, except those with renal or cardiac failure for whom the phosphate load and fluid shifts may be excessive.

A mixed flora exists in the colon, although the predominant organisms are obligate anaerobes. The most commonly used oral antibiotic regimen is the combination of neomycin and erythromycin base targeted to aerobes and anaerobes, respectively. Alternative oral antibiotic regimens include oral neomycin and metronidazole, oral neomycin alone, and oral metronidazole alone. Parenteral antibiotics are administered prior to skin incision and are selected to provide broad-spectrum coverage against both aerobes and anaerobes. Second-generation cephalosporins are used most often.

## Surgical Technique

### Colon Cancer

Operation with curative intent is possible in approximately 85% of patients diagnosed with colorectal cancer. The goal of curative resection is en bloc excision of the primary tumor along with its regional lymphatic system. Extensive central or retroperitoneal lymph node dissections are associated with increased operative morbidity but no survival advantage. Tumor-free margins proximal and distal to the lesion along the length of the intestine are easily achievable for colon cancer, as pathology studies have shown that longitudinal spread of the disease rarely exceeds 4 cm. Local extension into organs contiguous with the large intestine is found in approximately 10% of cases. Excision with tumor-free margins is still the goal in such cases, as 67% five-year survival has been reported for patients undergoing curative resection of B3 lesions.

Traditional resections for colon cancer are based on the pattern of lymphatic drainage. As the lymphatics course together with the major vascular supply of the colon, resection of lymphatic channels draining a particular colonic segment necessitates devascularization of that segment. This approach requires resection of large segments of colon beyond what longitudinal margins alone would require.

Cancers of the cecum and ascending colon are treated with a right hemicolectomy. The ileocolic artery, right colic artery, and right branch of the middle colic artery are ligated. This requires resection of the distal 5–8 cm of the ileum, cecum, ascending colon, and proximal transverse colon.

For cancers of the transverse colon, transverse colectomy with ligation of the middle colic artery and anastomosis between the ascending colon and the descending colon can be done, although there may be tension at the anastomosis, even after full mobilization of the colon. Cancers of the proximal and mid-transverse colon can be resected with an extended right hemicolectomy, with ligation of the ileocolic artery, right colic artery, and middle colic artery. The terminal ileum, cecum, ascending colon, hepatic flexure, transverse colon, and splenic flexure are resected; and an anastomosis between the ileum and the descending colon is performed.

Cancers of the splenic flexure and descending colon are treated by left hemicolectomy. The left colic artery is ligated, the splenic flexure and the descending colon are resected, and an anastomosis is created between the transverse colon and sigmoid colon.

A sigmoid colectomy is performed for sigmoid cancers. The inferior mesenteric artery is ligated distal to the origin of the left colic artery, and an anastomosis is created between the descending colon and the rectum.

### Rectal Cancer

Surgical options for curable rectal cancer are summarized in Table 46.6. The surgical approach to rectal cancer is different from that for colon cancer, largely because of anatomic factors. Wide excision of the cancer and surrounding structures, possible in colon cancer, is difficult for rectal cancer, as the rectum resides within the confines of the pelvis. The proximity of the anal sphincter mechanism, organs of the urogenital tract, and enervation of the urogenital system pose significant challenges.

The desired distal margin in rectal cancer excisions has been the focus of much interest. A 5 cm margin of normal tissue distal to the grossly visible lesion was once the standard of care. This concept was based on observations by Dukes, who failed to detect submucosal or lymphatic spread more than 4.5 cm distal to the tumor. Unfortunately, tumor differentiation status was not considered in his study. More recent pathology studies have shown that for well-differentiated and moderately well-differentiated rectal cancers a 2 cm distal margin is adequate. Poorly differentiated tumors probably still require a 5 cm distal margin. In recent years the importance of margins lateral to the rectum have received greater attention. These margins are often neglected during the pathology examination. Clearance of these margins is difficult to achieve, a factor that may account for the high local recurrence rates observed for rectal cancer.

Cancers of the upper rectum are treated by anterior resection, during which the proximal rectum is resected through an abdominal incision, and intestinal continuity is re-established by colorectal anastomosis. Resection of the rectosigmoid colon performed proximal to the pelvic peritoneal reflection is known as a high anterior resection, whereas an operation in which it is necessary to open the pelvic peritoneum is known as a low anterior resection. Typically, the sigmoid colon is resected in continuity with the rectum, as the inferior mesenteric artery has been

TABLE 46.6. Treatment Options for Curable Rectal Cancer

| |
|---|
| Mid and upper rectum (6–15 cm) |
| Anterior resection, stapled or hand-sutured |
| Lower rectum (0–5 cm) |
| Coloanal anastomosis, with or without a pouch |
| Transanal excision |
| Transsphincteric and parasacral approaches |
| Diathermy |
| Abdominal perineal resection |
| Primary radiation therapy |
| All sites |
| Adjuvant radiation therapy |

*Source:* DeCosse J, Tsioulias G, Jacobson J. Colorectal cancer: detection, treatment, and rehabilitation. CA Cancer J Clin 1994;44:27–42, with permission.

divided. The more generous collateral circulation to the descending colon provides a safer anastomosis.

Cancers of the lower rectum (less than 4 cm from the anorectal junction) have traditionally been treated by abdominoperineal resection (APR). Patients should understand that a permanent colostomy, which is integral to APR, does not signify a hopelessly advanced cancer. Other surgical options for low rectal cancers include a low anterior resection with coloanal anastomosis or local excision of the tumor, usually via a transanal approach. The option for these procedures is based on the preoperative stage.

Cancers of the middle third of the rectum require the most surgical judgment to determine whether a sphincter-sparing procedure should be done. Clearly, with the advent of stapling devices and an understanding that a distal margin of 2 cm is adequate, sphincter-sparing operations are more prevalent. Although the distance from the distal edge of the tumor to the anal verge is clinically the most often used criterion for determining whether a patient is a candidate for low anterior resection, other factors should play a role. These factors include body habitus, tumor size, mobility, histologic grade, the presence of metastatic disease, the preoperative continence status, the patient's willingness to accept a stoma and his or her ability to care for a stoma, and the general medical condition of the patient.

#### Total Mesorectal Excision

Given the probable contribution of inadequate lateral clearance of rectal cancers to high local recurrence rates, modifications of the traditional surgical techniques have been proposed. The technique of total mesorectal excision (TME) has been advocated initially by Heald.[25] With TME, the envelope of lymphovascular fatty tissue surrounding the rectum and mesorectum are completely excised under direct vision. The avascular plane between the mesorectum and the surrounding tissues is developed using sharp dissection. The excised specimen includes the whole posterior, distal, and lateral mesorectum; the inferior hypogastric plexuses are preserved. Anteriorly, Denonvilliers' fascia is included as part of the excised specimen.

Using TME, local recurrence rates of 4–8% have been reported.[25,26] These rates are significantly lower than those for historical controls, for whom recurrence rates range from 20% to 45%. However, TME has been associated with a high anastomotic leak rate (≥17%), leading some to advocate routine proximal colonic diversion following the procedure. TME also adds to the operating time. Although some have proposed TME as the standard of care, its overall role in the management of patients with rectal cancer is not yet clear, particularly given the improvements in neoadjuvant therapies.[27]

TABLE 46.7. Criteria for Local Management of Rectal Cancer

| |
|---|
| Diameter <3 cm |
| Mobile tumor |
| Exophytic |
| Confined to rectal wall (maximum T2) on transrectal ultrasonography |
| No evidence of extrarenal spread or distant metastases on computed tomography |
| Well-differentiated or moderately differentiated histology |

### *Local Therapies*

Although radical surgery is the treatment of choice for most patients, local treatment is a satisfactory alternative under defined conditions. Local resection should be considered with curative intent for early-stage rectal cancers that are too distal to allow a restorative resection and as a palliative measure in patients with metastatic disease or co-morbid medical conditions who may not be able to tolerate the stress of general anesthesia and a major abdominal operation.

Local techniques include excision, ablation, and irradiation. Local excision can be performed through transanal, transsacral, or transsphincteric approaches, with the transanal approach being used most frequently.[28] In patients who are particularly poor surgical candidates, transanal electrocoagulation, possibly in multiple stages, offers effective palliation.[29]

For curative resections, the success of local excision depends on stringent selection criteria, as described by Ogunbiyi[30] (Table 46.7). Transrectal ultrasonography should be performed to stage the lesions preoperatively. Candidate lesions should be small (<3 cm in diameter), mobile, confined to the rectal wall (T1 or T2), without evidence of regional or distant metastasis, exophytic, and well or moderately well differentiated. Graham et al. reported a 5-year cancer-specific survival of 89% in their series of local excisions for rectal cancer using such selection criteria.[31] The local recurrence in this series was 19%.

## Special Cases

### *Synchronous Lesions*

Total abdominal colectomy may be performed when synchronous lesions or multiple adenomatous polyps are present. This operation is also recommended for patients with HNPCC. Although this operation is associated with postoperative diarrhea, intestinal adaptation allows good long-term function. Total proctocolectomy with mucosal proctectomy and ileoanal anastomosis is done for younger patients with FAP; there is less experience with this operation in the elderly.

### *Colonic Obstruction*

Complete obstruction of the colon or rectum by an obstructing carcinoma is a surgical emergency. Obstructing cancer of the right or transverse colon can be treated by resection and anastomosis without proximal diversion, but treatment of left-sided obstruction is more controversial. The preferred approaches are resection without anastomosis, resection and anastomosis with a proximal diverting ileostomy, or subtotal colectomy with ileorectal anastomosis. In the presence of an extensively dilated proximal colon and unstable patient, a temporary proximal decompressing stoma may be appropriate. The preliminary experience with colonic stenting in patients with advanced tumors presenting with obstruction has been reported to be promising.[27] Such stents can be used for palliation or for recanalization to allow bowel preparation and safer elective surgery.

### *Perforated Colon Carcinoma*

The surgical approach is resection of the perforated segment of the bowel, together with involved adjacent structures. An anastomosis in a contaminated field should be protected by a proximal diverting stoma. Although the prognosis is poor, a curative operation should be attempted.

## Status of Laparoscopy for Colorectal Cancer

Laparoscopic technology has become widespread, especially because of its success in the treatment of biliary disease. For elderly patients, laparoscopy has the theoretic advantage of causing less physiologic derangement than open surgery. In one study of 18 patients over age 70 years and American Society of Anesthesiologists (ASA) class III–IV, there was no mortality when laparoscopic surgery was used to resect colorectal cancers electively.[32] Laparoscopy also offers the potential advantages of reduced pain, shorter hospital stay, and better cosmetic results.

Progress in laparoscopic surgery for colorectal cancer has been slow for several reasons. These procedures are considerably more technically difficult than laparoscopic cholecystectomy and require significant training time for surgeons not trained in advanced laparoscopic techniques.[33] There have also been numerous reports of cancer recurrences at laparoscopic port sites. Currently, a National Institutes of Health (NIH)-funded prospective randomized trial is under way to evaluate the risks and benefits of laparoscopic versus open surgery for colon cancer. The objectives of the study are threefold: (1) to examine whether disease-free and overall survival in patients undergoing laparoscopic surgery are comparable to those undergoing open procedures; (2) to compare the early and late morbidity and operative mortality for these two surgical approaches; and (3) to compare the cost-effectiveness of these two approaches. Until the results of this study are available, laparoscopic surgery for colon cancer should be confined to study protocols.

## Adjuvant Therapies

Adjuvant systemic therapies are designed to eradicate micrometastases present at the time of surgery, with the goal of reducing local recurrence rates and prolonging survival. Several chemotherapy regimens based on 5-fluorouracil (5-FU) have been shown to prolong survival in select groups of patients following curative resection for colon cancer. The American National Cancer Institute Intergroup Study reported a 41% reduction in tumor recurrence and a 33% reduction in cancer-related mortality during a 3-year observation period in node-positive patients treated with levamisole and 5-FU.[34]

Ongoing trials are designed to identify chemotherapeutic agents with more antitumor efficacy and to define which patients would benefit from such treatments. Although standard treatment for colon cancer includes adjuvant chemotherapy for patients with stage III disease but not for patients with stage II tumors (who have no lymph node metastases), 20% of patients with stage II tumors die of recurrent disease. The challenge is to identify the subset of patients with stage II disease who would benefit from adjuvant chemotherapy. In a recent report, 192 lymph nodes from 26 consecutive patients with stage II colorectal cancer were examined using a CEA-specific nested reverse-transcriptase polymerase chain reaction (RT-PCR) to detect the presence of micrometastases not otherwise identified by routine histologic methods. Micrometastases were detected by PCR in one or more lymph nodes from 14 of 26 patients (54%). The 5-year survival rate was 36% in this group, but it was 75% in the group without micrometastases. The groups were similar with respect to age, sex, tumor location, tumor differentiation, and tumor size.[35]

Adjuvant radiation therapy is rarely used following curative resection of colon cancers, as local recurrence rates are low and adjacent structures (e.g., small intestine) are sensitive to radiation-induced toxicity. For rectal cancer, however, the reported local recurrence rates are usually 30–35% for stage II disease and 40–60% for stage III disease. The use of adjuvant radiation therapy has clearly been shown to be associated with a reduction in local recurrence rates.[36–38] Postoperative adjuvant radiation therapy and chemotherapy for transmural and node-positive rectal cancer is the current standard of care. However, the optimal timing of adjuvant therapy for rectal cancer remains controversial.

The advantage of postoperative radiotherapy is that it allows patient selection based on surgical and histopathologic findings. Preoperative radiation therapy protocols may include patients who do not need such adjuvant treatments, given the limitations of currently available imaging studies. However, preoperative radiation therapy has the potential to downstage tumors and allow sphincter-sparing surgery in patients who otherwise might have required abdominoperoneal resection.

At least 10 modern randomized trials of preoperative radiation therapy for resectable rectal cancer have been reported. In five reports the authors found a significant reduction in the rate of local recurrence. In some studies, a significant improvement in survival, as determined in subgroup analyses, was reported. In only one trial was a significant survival advantage for the whole group of treated patients reported.[39] In this trial, done in Sweden, 1168 patients received either a short course (five fractions over one week) of radiation therapy preoperatively combined with surgery or surgery alone. Irradiation was not associated with an increase in postoperative mortality. The local recurrence rate was 11% in the group who underwent irradiation and 27% in the group who were subjected to surgery alone. The difference in local recurrence rate was statistically significant for lesions of all Dukes' stages. The overall 5-year survival rate was 58% in the group who received radiation and 48% in the surgery-alone group ($p = 0.004$).

The Swedish trial has been criticized, as more than 100 surgeons at 70 hospitals participated, with each surgeon, on average, performing fewer than four operations per year.[39] The local recurrence rate for Dukes' stage A cancers in the trial (4% after irradiation and 12% after surgery alone) was higher than is typically reported. This study also did not address the role of preoperative irradiation in combination with preoperative chemotherapy. Additional studies are required to define the optimal adjuvant therapy regimens for rectal cancer.

## Postoperative Surveillance

There are two goals of postoperative surveillance: (1) to increase the lead time in the detection of recurrent carcinoma to detect lesions at a potentially curable stage; and (2) to detect metachronous lesions. Recurrent disease following resection for colorectal cancer, even at distant sites, is potentially treatable. Hepatic resection for metastatic lesions is safe and appears to prolong survival in selected patients. In a report of 128 patients over the age of 70 undergoing major hepatic resections for colorectal metastasis, those over 80 years of age had perioperative outcomes and 5-year survival rates equivalent to those of younger patients. Hepatic resection for colorectal metastases with clear margins of resection is associated with a 5-year survival of 25–48% and mean survival of 20–40 months. The lung is the second most common site of metastases from colorectal cancers. In selected patients, complete resection of pulmonary metastases is associated with a 5-year survival of 20–44%.

The best surveillance strategies remain to be determined. Postoperative surveillance following surgery for colorectal cancer is highly variable in clinical practice. In one report, the number of office visits during the first 5 years ranged from 6 to 18, CEA measurements ranged from 0 to 44, liver ultrasound examinations ranged from 0 to 10, and sigmoidoscopy ranged from 0 to 13. Medicare charges per patient ranged from $910 to $26,717.[40]

Traditional surveillance protocols have included periodic history and physical examination, FOBT, complete blood count, liver function tests, tumor marker sampling, colonoscopy, and chest radiography. Surveillance tests are generally performed more frequently during the initial postoperative period, as 80–90% of all recurrences become evident during the first 2–3 years after surgery. One standard textbook of surgery has recommended that the history, physical examination, FOBT, and blood studies be obtained every 3 months during the first 3 years and every 6 months for an additional 2 years. Tumor markers are measured every 8 weeks by some investigators and monthly by others for 3 years and then every 3 months for another 2 years. Traditionally, colonoscopy has been done 6–12 months after resection, at yearly intervals for an additional 2 years, and at less frequent intervals thereafter.

Some studies have challenged these traditional approaches. Of 1356 Eastern Cooperative Oncology Group patients who had undergone surgical resection for Dukes' B2 and C colon carcinoma, 421 developed recurrent disease (mean follow-up 43.6 months). Ninety-six of these patients underwent resection of their recurrent disease with curative intent. Routine physical examination failed to identify a single resectable recurrence. The detection rate for CEA testing was 2.2% (cost per recurrence $5696). The detection rate by chest radiography was 0.9% (cost per recurrence $10,078). The detection rate of colonoscopy was 1% (cost per recurrence $45,810). The authors concluded that CEA measurements are the most cost-effective test for detecting potentially curable recurrent disease and that routine physical examination in the absence of specific symptoms is not helpful.[41]

In another recent report, the efficacy of a surveillance strategy using the history, physical examination, liver function tests, CEA assay, and colonoscopy 5 years postoperatively is as good as a more intensive strategy using yearly colonoscopy, CT, and chest radiography.[42] Survival rates were equivalent, regardless of the surveillance strategy used.

In guidelines recently published by a multidisciplinary panel, patients in whom large (>1 cm in diameter) or multiple adenomatous polyps have been removed, should have an examination of the entire colon 3 years after the initial examination. If the first follow-up is normal or if only a single, small, tubular adenoma is found, the next examination can be at 5 years.

Patients with a colorectal cancer that has been resected with curative intent (but who did not undergo complete adequate colonoscopic examination preoperatively) should have a complete examination of the colon within 1 year after resection. If this or a complete preoperative examination is normal, subsequent examination should be offered after 3 years and then, if normal, every 5 years.[43] As with original cancers, subsequent cancers are preceded by adenomatous polyps that occur with increased frequency. There is no evidence to suggest that these polyps progress to cancer at a different rate from those in average-risk people.

## References


1. Parker SL, Tong T, Boldern S, et al. Cancer statistics, 1997. CA Cancer J Clin 1997;47:5–27.
2. Parkin DM, Laara W, Muir CS. Estimates of the worldwide frequency of sixteen major cancers in 1980. Int J Cancer 1988;41:184–197.
3. Winawer SJ, Fletcher RH, Miller L, et al. Colorectal cancer screening: clinical guidelines and rationale. Gastroenterology 1997;112:594–642.
4. Kingston RD, Jeacock J, Walsh S, et al. The outcome of surgery for colorectal cancer in the elderly: a 12-year review from the Trafford databases. Eur J Surg Oncol 1995;21: 514–516.
5. Vasen HF, Mechlin JP, Khan PM, et al. The International Collaborative Group on Hereditary Non Polyposis Colorectal Cancer (ICG-HNPCC). Dis Colon Rectum 1991; 34:424–425.
6. O'Brien MJ, Winawer SJ, Zauber AG, et al. The National Polyp Study: patient and polyp characteristics associated with high-grade dysplasia in colorectal adenomas. Gastroenterology 1990;98:371–379.
7. Winawer SJ, Zauber AG, Ho MN, et al. Prevention of colorectal cancer by colonoscopic polypectomy. N Engl J Med 1993;329:1977–1981.
8. Vogelstein B, Fearon ER, Hamilton SR, et al. Genetic alterations during colorectal-tumor development. N Engl J Med 1988;319:525–532.
9. Bos JL, Fearon ER, Hamilton SR, et al. Prevalence of ras gene mutations in human colorectal cancers. Nature 1987;327: 293–297.
10. Forrester K, Almoguera X, Han K, et al. Detection of high incidence of K-ras oncogenes during human colon tumorigenesis. Nature 1987;327:298–303.
11. Anderson LM, May DS. Has the use of cervical, breast, and colorectal cancer screening increased in the United States? Am J Public Health 1995;85:840–842.
12. Mandel JS, Bond JH, Church TR, et al. Reducing mortality from colorectal cancer by screening for fecal occult blood: Minnesota Colon Cancer Control Study. N Engl J Med 1993;328:1365–1371.
13. Mandel JS, Bond JH, Bradley M, et al. Sensitivity, specificity, and positive predictivity of the hemoccult test in screening for colorectal cancers: the Minnesota Colon Cancer Control Study. Gastroenterology 1989;17:597–600.
14. Winawer SJ, Fletcher RH, Miller L, et al. Colorectal cancer screening: clinical guidelines and rationale. Gastroenterology 1997;112:594–642.
15. Winawer SJ, Fletcher RH, Miller L, et al. Colorectal cancer screening: clinical guidelines and rationale. Gastroenterology 1997;112:594–642.
16. Byers T, Levin B, Rothenberger D, et al. American Cancer Society guidelines for screening and surveillance for early detection of colorectal polyps and cancer: update 1997, American Cancer Society Detection and Treatment Advisory Group on Colorectal Cancer. CA Cancer J Clin 1997;47: 154–160.
17. Toribara MW, Sleisenger NH. Screening for colorectal cancer. N Engl J Med 1995;332:861–867.
18. Markowitz AJ, Winawer SJ. Management of colorectal polyps. CA Cancer J Clin 1997;47:93–113.
19. Read TE, Read JD, Butterfly LF. Importance of adenomas 5 mm or less in diameter that are detected by sigmoidoscopy. N Engl J Med 1997;336:8–12.
20. Greenberg AG, Salk RP, Pridhom D. Influence of age on mortality of colon surgery. Am J Surg 1985;150:65–70.
21. Boyd JB, Bradford B Jr, Watne AL. Operative risk factors of colon resection in the elderly. Ann Surg 1980;192:743–746.
22. Cohen H, Willis I, Wallack M. Surgical experience of colon resection in the extreme elderly. Ann Surg 1986;52: 214–217.
23. Hobler KE. Colon surgery for cancer in the very elderly: cost and 3 year survival. Ann Surg 1986;203:129–131.
24. Morel P, Egeli RA, Wachtl S, et al. Results of operative treatment of gastrointestinal tract tumors in patients over 80 years of age. Arch Surg 1989;124:662–664.
25. Heald RJ. Recurrence and survival after total mesorectal excision for rectal cancer. Lancet 1986;1:1479–1482.
26. MacFarlane JK, Ryall RD, Heald RJ. Mesorectal excision for rectal cancer. Lancet 1993;341:457–460.
27. Stamos MJ. Colon and rectal surgery. J Am Coll Surg 1998;186:134–140.
28. Bailey HR, Huval WV, Max E, et al. Local excision of carcinoma of the rectum for cure. Surgery 1992;111:555–561.
29. Madden JL, Kandalaft SI. Electrocoagulation as a primary curative method in the treatment of carcinoma of the rectum. Surg Gynecol Obstet 1983:157:164–179.
30. Ogunbiyi OA, Fleshman JW. Colorectal cancer and laparoscopic colorectal surgery in the elderly patient. Problems in General Surgery 1997;13:154–162.
31. Graham RA, Garnsey L, Jessup JM. Local excision of rectal carcinoma. Am J Surg 1990;160:306–312.
32. Vara-Thornbeck C, Garcia-Laballero M, Salvi M, et al. Indications and advantages of laparoscopy-assisted colon resection for carcinoma in elderly patients. Surg Laparosc Endosc 1994;4:110–118.
33. Senagore AJ, Luchtefeld MA, MacKeigan JM. What is the learning curve for laparoscopic colectomy? Am Surg 1995;61:681–685.
34. Moertel CG, Fleming TR, MacDonald JS, et al. Levamisole and fluorouracil for adjuvant therapy of resected colon carcinoma. N Engl J Med 1990;322:352–358.
35. Liefers GJ, Cleton-Jansen AM, van de Velde CJ, et al. Micrometastases and survival in stage II colorectal cancer. N Engl J Med 1998;339:223–228.

36. Kodner IJ, Shemesh EI, Fry RD, et al. Preoperative irradiation for rectal cancer: improved local control and long-term survival. Ann Surg 1989;209:194–199.
37. Mendenhall WM, Bland KI, Copeland EM, et al. Does preoperative radiation enhance the probability of local control and survival in high risk distal rectal cancer? Ann Surg 1992;215:696–706.
38. Roe JP, Kodner IJ, Walz BJ, et al. Preoperative radiation therapy for rectal carcinoma. Dis Colon Rectum 1982;25: 471–473.
39. Swedish Rectal Cancer Trial. Improved survival with preoperative radiotherapy in resectable rectal cancer. N Engl J Med 1997;336:980–988.
40. Lavery IC, Fazio VW, Lopez-Kostner R, et al. Correspondence. N Engl J Med 1997;337:346.
41. Virgo KS, Vernara AM, Longo WE. Cost of patient follow-up after potentially curative colorectal cancer treatment. JAMA 1995;273:1837–1841.
42. Graham RA, Wang S, Catalano PJ, et al. Post surgical surveillance of colon cancer; preliminary cost analysis of physician examination, carcinoembryonic antigen testing, chest x-ray, and colonoscopy. Ann Surg 1998;228:59–63.
43. Schoemaker D, Black R, Giles L. Yearly colonoscopy, liver CT, and chest rediography do not influence 5-year survival of colorectal cancer patients. Gastroenterology 1998;114: 7–14.

# 47 Abdominal Wall Hernia in the Elderly

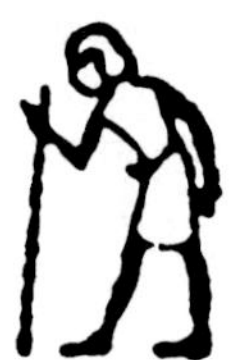

Seth A. Spector and Ronnie A. Rosenthal

Abdominal wall hernia repair is the most common surgical procedure in the United States. More than 500,000 herniorrhaphies are performed annually. The incidence of groin hernias, the most common type of abdominal wall hernia, in men over age 65 is approximately 13 per 1000 population.[1] The incidence in women is 12–25% that of men. In a British study of more than 30,000 inguinal hernia repairs, 27% were in an elderly population; 85.5% of these cases were elective repairs on patients age 65 or older, and the remaining 14.5% were classified as emergency procedures.[2]

All groin hernias arise from a common anatomic space, but they are named according to their location relative to specific inguinal structures. Hernias above the abdominocrural crease are termed inguinal, and those below are termed femoral. Inguinal hernias are divided into two types: direct and indirect. Indirect hernias pass through the deep inguinal ring, lie anterior and medial to the vas deferens within the spermatic cord, and descend through the inguinal canal to the scrotum. Direct hernias pass directly through the floor of the inguinal canal and point anteriorly. Femoral hernias are a variation of direct hernias in which the inguinal ligament prevents the sac from protruding through the inguinal floor. Instead, the sac passes through the femoral canal medial to the femoral vein (Fig. 47.1).[3]

Inguinal hernias in elderly persons are frequently long-standing. Many have been present for 10–20 years, although some may have occurred as long as 50–60 years prior to presentation for repair.[4–6] As a result of the chronic nature of these hernias, the surrounding normal anatomic architecture is disrupted and there is loss of the appropriate tissue planes to facilitate repair. Furthermore, with age comes the anticipated loss of muscle mass and tissue strength, making an anatomic repair more difficult. Increased co-morbidity in this age group can make elective repair challenging, but operative morbidity and mortality is still remarkably low. Prolonged neglect, however, results in a high incidence of preoperative complications, such as constipation and obstipation, bowel obstruction, incarceration, and strangulation. These conditions frequently necessitate emergency treatment. Incarcerated hernias are responsible for 33% of bowel obstructions in this age group.[7] Furthermore, incarceration and bowel obstruction account for 10–30% of all emergency abdominal operations in the elderly.[8,9]

## Etiology and Distribution

The etiology of abdominal wall hernias differs somewhat in the elderly population. Congenital hernias, although more common in young patients, do occur in the geriatric population as well. Acquired hernias, however, are more common with increasing age and are often associated with other physiologic changes or disease processes. In most cases the pathophysiologic mechanism of an acquired hernia is a structural inadequacy of the inguinal floor, which manifests as a direct inguinal hernia (hernia occurring medial to the inferior epigastric vessels through previously intact inguinal floor tissues). Previous studies of noninguinal floor tissues suggest that the basis for this defect is abnormal organization of connective tissue, the most important component of which is the structural protein collagen. Collagenous fibers are flexible and offer great resistance to pulling. Forces in excess of several hundred kilograms per square centimeter are necessary to disrupt the integrity of these fibers.[10]

Data indicate that direct inguinal hernias are associated with both biochemical and ultrastructural collagen abnormalities.[11–15] Electron microscopy demonstrates swelling of collagen fibrils and defective periodicity of banding, which represent an abnormal association of collagen chains.[16] The reasons for this are uncertain, but other studies of tissues from hernia patients demonstrate blunted fibroblast proliferation rates in tissue culture and decreased rates of incorporation of proline into skeletal muscle collagen.[11,15,16] There is evidence that a global connective tissue turnover defect occurs in cigarette smokers that may predispose to hernia formation. Cannon et al.

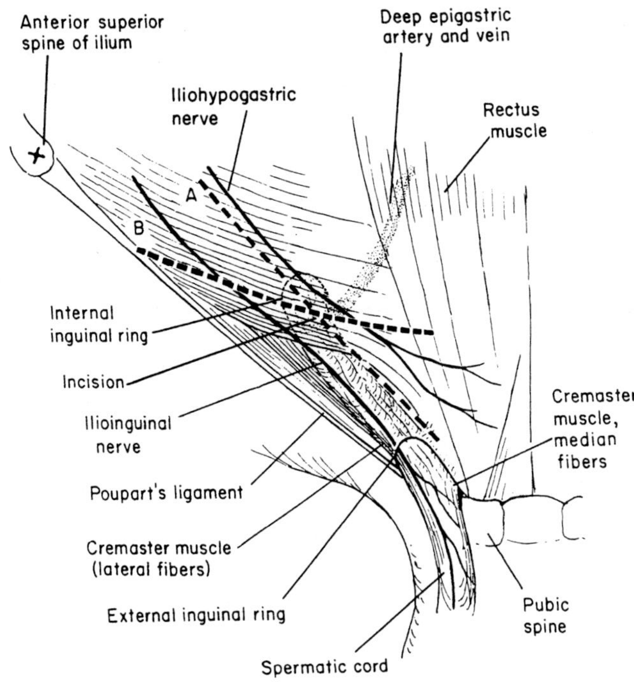


FIGURE 47.1. Anatomy of the inguinal canal. (From Zollinger and Zollinger,[3] with permission.)

reported that smokers with direct inguinal hernias had increased serum elastolase activity and decreased $\alpha_1$-antitrypsin activity, despite normal serum concentrations of these enzymes.[17] These are indications of a systemic process that could adversely affect vulnerable structural tissues.

Chronically increased intraabdominal pressure due to long-standing constipation and straining, bladder outlet obstruction, chronic cough, obesity, and kyphoscoliosis further predispose to the development of acquired hernias. In the elderly patient it is not uncommon for several of these factors to be present simultaneously. On occasion, this confluence of factors contributes to the development of a giant hernia or one with a large scrotal component. These hernias can become extremely large and may contain a significant portion of the abdominal viscera. When forced reduction of the viscera into the contracted abdominal cavity is attempted, severe respiratory compromise due to increased intraabdominal pressure and decreased diaphragmatic excursion may occur.

The relative frequency of the various types of abdominal wall hernia in the elderly reflects the differences in pathophysiologic mechanism. Indirect inguinal hernias, which comprise 90% of the hernias in young men, account for only 50–60% of hernias in older men. Direct hernias increase to 35% in men over age 65.[5] Furthermore, the incidence of sliding hernias also increases from 0.5% during the third decade of life to as much as 13% during the sixth to eighth decades.[19] Early studies reported a 3:1 predominance of femoral to indirect inguinal hernias in women, but it is now generally accepted that most hernias in both men and women are inguinal.[20] Femoral hernias are, however, more common in women. Umbilical and ventral hernias each account for 10% of abdominal wall hernias. In elderly women herniation of bowel through the obturator canal is a rare but insidious event. The obturator hernia is of special concern because it is associated with no external manifestations and therefore usually presents a diagnostic challenge (see Obturator Hernias, below).

Approximately 15–30% of all herniorrhaphies in the elderly are performed on an emergent basis as a result of incarceration: Overall, 50–60% are indirect and 17–25% are femoral. When separated by gender, 73% of incarcerated hernias in men are indirect and 15% are femoral, whereas femoral hernias account for 50% of incarcerations in women.[4,7,8] Once incarceration and strangulation have occurred, the hernia changes from a simple mechanical problem to a complex life-threatening systemic illness; and the repair changes from correction of a simple mechanical defect to reversal of a major abdominal catastrophe.

## Diagnosis

In most cases, the diagnosis of abdominal wall hernia in the elderly is clear. More than 70% of patients with groin hernias complain of a groin or scrotal mass and pain in the inguinal region. In many cases the patient has been aware of, or diagnosed with, a hernia for many years. Symptomatic control is often achieved at the expense of physical activity or with the encumberment of a truss.

The presence of a femoral hernia, however, is more difficult to recognize. Typically, poorly localized pain is present in the inguinal area without an obvious, visible bulge. Unfortunately, because of the subtle findings, femoral hernias are frequently not diagnosed until they incarcerate.[5]

Historic factors that contribute to the development of inguinal hernias should always be elicited. Respiratory symptoms with chronic cough, chronic constipation, and symptoms of bladder outlet obstruction, are most prevalent in an older population.

Examination for the presence of groin hernias should be part of the standard physical exam. Patients should be examined in the erect position, as a reducible hernia is sometimes more difficult to appreciate in the supine position. The only visible abnormality may be groin asymmetry. Indirect inguinal hernias appear as a small mass in the region of the deep ring, midway between the pubic tubercle and the anterior superior iliac spine. Direct hernias appear more medially, although this distinction is not always clear. Invaginating the skin of the scrotum and introducing the examining finger along the spermatic cord structures into the external inguinal ring is necessary for accurate diagnosis. Prolonged standing or increasing intraabdominal pressure by coughing or with Valsalva maneuver causes the sac and its contents to descend toward the examining finger, where it is felt as a mass or a transmitted impulse. A small hernia defect or a sac that is difficult to reduce presents the greatest risk for future incarceration. In women, inguinal hernias may be more difficult to diagnose until they become quite large.

It is important when examining the groin to include an examination of the upper thigh below the inguinal ligament as well. Most femoral hernias can be felt as a soft mass medial to the femoral vessels. Frequently, hernias in this location are mistaken for inguinal lymph nodes or lipomas. Increased intraabdominal pressure may transmit an impulse through the sac, but this too can be mistaken for normal transmission of the increased pressure in the femoral vein.

A rectal exam to assess prostate size, the presence of a rectal mass, and fecal occult blood, is an essential part of every physical exam for hernia, particularly in elderly patients. Although there is no association between inguinal hernia and colonic abnormalities, the high risk of colon neoplasm in these patients, in general, justifies a screening procedure, such as flexible sigmoidoscopy, for all patients over age 50 (see Elective Surgical Repair, below).

The diagnosis of an incarcerated hernia is usually not difficult to establish. Most often patients present with a previously recognized hernia that has recently become increasingly painful and "stuck out." In the case of a femoral hernia, a painful mass in the groin may be the first indication. Obstructive symptoms such as nausea, vomiting, and obstipation may not be present early in the course but develop if the incarceration goes untreated. Strangulation is indicated by increasing pain and signs of systemic sepsis. On physical examination, a tender, nonreducible mass is present in the groin. Erythema and edema of the overlying skin are suggestive of strangulation of bowel in a hernia sac, as is severe tenderness to palpation.

## Elective Surgical Repair

When an abdominal wall hernia is diagnosed, operative repair should always be considered. With increasing age, the consequences of incarceration or strangulation are magnified. In a 1983 study of patients over age 65 years, 26% of 1044 patients having elective hernia repairs, developed a complication and 1% died. Among the group of 235 patients who required emergency procedures, 56% had complications and 8% died.[4] It is evident that hernia surgery in the elderly is safe so long as the operations are performed under elective conditions. Once incarceration or strangulation occurs, the morbidity and mortality rise substantially.

Even when hernia defects are large and pose little risk of incarceration, surgical repair should always be considered. Occasionally, large hernias create mechanical problems with defecation particularly when most of the sigmoid colon has come to reside in the sac. Manual manipulation of the sac is sometimes necessary to enable defecation. Serious constipation and related disorders may develop. The elderly patient may also compensate for the discomfort of the hernia by avoiding activities, even those as simple as walking. This avoidance of physical activity leads to an overall functional decline and eventual loss of independence. The quality of life in these circumstances must be considered. Elective repair can be safely performed under local anesthesia in most cases, and patients can be restored to their preoperative functional status in just a few days. Hernia repair should be denied only to patients at extremely high risk and those for whom the overall life expectancy is because of other disease processes.

Prior to elective repair, conditions that may cause increased intraabdominal pressure should be investigated and corrected if possible. Increased intraabdominal pressure puts stress on the repair, interferes with normal wound healing, and predisposes to recurrence. Constipation, symptoms of prostatic hypertrophy, chronic cough, and obesity are common conditions associated with increased tension on the abdominal wall. Managing the first three conditions with medications sufficiently to proceed with operation can often be accomplished in several weeks. Obesity cannot, however, and should not be controlled rapidly. Therefore, significant weight loss should not be used as an absolute prerequisite for repair.

Although there is no direct association between inguinal hernia and colonic pathology, colonic screening procedures have been advocated in asymptomatic elderly patients undergoing elective hernia repair. Several studies have shown a 16–28% incidence of abnormal findings in patients over age 50, even when stool occult blood testing is negative.[21] Specifically, Ruben and colleagues performed flexible sigmoidoscopy on 110 patients (99% men) undergoing inguinal hernia repair and found that 36% had diverticulosis, 26% had colorectal polyps, and 3.6% had colorectal cancers. In their study, only 11% of patients had a positive stool occult blood test.[21] The high incidence of colonic abnormalities in the elderly justifies screening. For patients with primary care providers, this screening can be accomplished at any time. For those who enter the health care system primarily to have the hernia repaired, screening should be part of the preoperative assessment. Elective repair should not be extensively delayed, however, to perform a screening procedure.

## Anesthesia

The first step in elective hernia repair is the choice of anesthesia. Avoiding anesthetic techniques that place unnecessary stress on cardiac, pulmonary, and renal reserves may minimize the surgical morbidity and mortality. Both general and spinal anesthetic techniques are associated with perioperative complications. Guillen and Aldrete reported that in men over age 70 undergoing elective inguinal hernia repair the incidences of hypotension with spinal and inhaled anesthetic were 43% and 36%, respectively.[22] A significantly higher incidence of complications, particularly respiratory and urinary, has been reported in elderly patients receiving general and spinal anesthesia when compared to local block.[23] In a randomized trial of local versus general anesthesia, a significantly higher percentage of patients was able to ambulate and pass urine at 6 hours in the local anesthetic group.[24] These data support the concept that local field block is the ideal anesthesia method for elective hernia repair in the geriatric age group. There are, however, a few limitations to this method. Patients with dementia or those who for other reasons are unable to understand commands and lie still on the operative table, as well as those who are unusually anxious, are considered poor candidates for local blocks. The excessive use of sedation necessary to control these patients frequently worsens the confusion and results in respiratory complications, which defeat the whole purpose of the local anesthetic route. Further problems are encountered in obese patients for whom adequate local anesthesia may not be achievable because of limitations in dose and absorption.

With a detailed understanding of the neuroanatomy of the inguinal region, painless inguinal herniorrhaphy may be accomplished in the elderly patient.[25] The innervation of the inguinal region is complex (Fig. 47.2). A clear understanding of the intercostal nerve supply is paramount. Following the pattern of dermatome distribution, the tenth thoracic nerve innervates the umbilicus, the first lumbar nerve innervates the inguinal area, and the twelfth thoracic nerve innervates the area in between. The iliohypogastric and ilioinguinal nerves lie deep to the external oblique fascia, and lateral to the anterior superior iliac spine. The iliohypogastric originates at the first lumbar nerve and lies under the external oblique aponeurosis after penetrating the internal oblique muscle. This nerves supplies sensory fibers to the suprapubic region. The ilioinguinal nerve follows the same course as the iliohypogastric nerve but lies closer to the crest of the ileum and inguinal ligament. The ilioinguinal nerve penetrates the internal oblique muscle approximately 1.0–1.5 cm from the anterosuperior iliac spine and supplies sensory innervation to the base of the penis and part of the scrotum (and comparable areas in the female body). The penile skin and a small area of the scrotum are supplied by sensory fibers from the sacral plexus. When repairing a femoral hernia, more attention must be paid to the ilioinguinal nerve and the femoral branch of the genitofemoral nerve, which supply the upper thigh. The genitofemoral nerve originates from the first and second lumbar nerves to supply sensory fibers to the scrotum and upper thigh and motor fibers to the cremasteric muscle via the genital branch. The genital branch reaches the inguinal canal at the internal abdominal ring. When performing herniorrhaphy under local anesthesia, pain is also felt when traction is applied to the sac or the spermatic cord or when a finger is inserted into the peritoneal cavity.

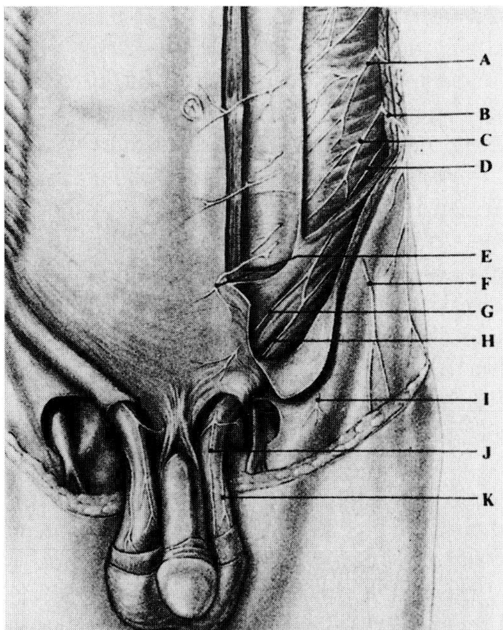


FIGURE 47.2. Innervation of the inguinal region. A, 11th thoracic nerve; B, lateral branch of 12th thoracic nerve; C, anterior branch of 12th thoracic nerve; D, iliohypogastric nerve; E, anterior branch of 12th thoracic nerve; F, lateral femoral cutaneous nerve; G, iliohypogastric nerve (anterior branch); H, ilioinguinal nerve; I, femoral branch of genitofemoral nerve; J, anterior scrotal nerve from the ilioinguinal nerve; K, genital branch of the genitofemoral nerve. (From Lichtenstein et al.,[18] with permission.)

To attain adequate anesthesia, Ponka described the following seven-step method (Fig. 47.3).[25] Step 1: The epidermal skin wheal is made by injecting 3–5 ml of anesthetic solution 2 cm above the anterosuperior iliac spine with a 25-gauge needle. Step 2: Through the skin wheal, a blunted 19-gauge needle is inserted and advanced until a small pop is felt as it passes under the external oblique fascia; 5–10 ml of anesthetic is injected at three different vertical levels to bathe the ilioinguinal and iliohypogastric nerves. Step 3: Through the skin wheal, intradermal injections are carried out in three directions: toward the umbilicus, above and parallel to the inguinal ligament, and vertically for a distance of 4 cm. Step 4: Once the skin incision is made, 3–5 ml of anesthetic is injected under the external oblique fascia at several points. Step 5: Once the external oblique fascia is incised, the ilioinguinal and iliohypogastric nerves are identified and retracted, and the cord is elevated out of the inguinal canal; the base of the cord is then injected with 3–5 ml of anesthetic solution. The goal is to block the sympathetic fibers to the cord and the genital branch of the genital femoral nerve and to infiltrate the peritoneum at the internal ring. Step 6: The local anesthetic is injected into the region of the pubic tubercle and Cooper's ligament. Step 7: Under direct vision, the peritoneum is injected at several points with 3–5 ml of anesthetic solution in a circumferential fashion.

The choice of anesthetic drugs is variable. One favored mixture contains 50 ml of 1% lidocaine with epinephrine (1:200,000) plus 50 ml 0.25% bupivacaine.[26] This is usually adequate and meets the tolerance limits of lidocaine (7 ml/kg) in a 75 kg patient. The duration of action of lidocaine is 1–2 hours, which is usually sufficient to complete the hernia repair. The addition of bupivacaine to the mixture, which has a duration of action of 5–7 hours, provides supplementary pain control during the early postoperative period and enables the patient to begin ambulating soon after the procedure. Regardless of the local anesthetic chosen, the addition of epinephrine to the mixture enhances surgical hemostasis and delays absorption of the local anesthetic, resulting in an increased duration of anesthesia and a decreased risk of systemic reactions.

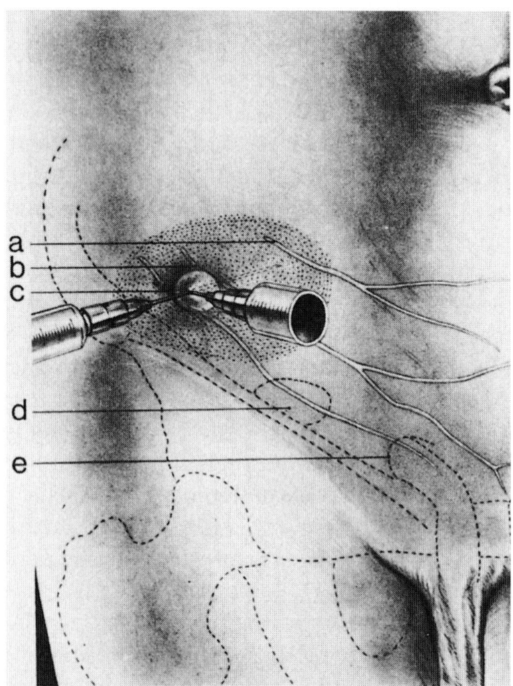


FIGURE 47.3. Ilioinguinal and iliohypogastric nerve block. a, 12th thoracic nerve; b, iliohypogastric nerve; c, ilioinguinal nerve; d, internal ring; e, external ring. (From Lichtenstein et al.,[18] with permission.)

In this era of cost analysis and health care economics, inguinal herniorrhaphy is becoming predominantly an outpatient procedure. Even though outpatient general anesthesia is possible, local block facilitates earlier ambulation and is associated with fewer immediate postoperative complications. Flanagan and Bascom reported that with the use of just a short-acting local anesthetic, pain control was not adequate to allow discharge in only 5% of patients. The addition of bupivacaine eliminates the need for oral analgesia for up to 24 hours postoperatively.[27]

## Tissue Repairs

Modern-day inguinal hernia repair has been dominated by an anterior, open approach that was first proposed by Bassini, who introduced the concept of repair of the inguinal floor in 1887. This basic tenet of hernia repair has undergone many modifications, with various combinations of suturing the transversalis fascia, conjoined tendon, internal oblique or transversus abdodinis to the inguinal or Cooper's ligament. The choice of herniorrhaphy technique must take into account the risk of recurrence and patient tolerance of the procedure. The actual rate of recurrence is difficult to establish. Questionnaires and telephone interviews are not an appropriate substitution for experienced examination, as 25% of recurrences are found on examination rather than by the patient. Furthermore, the duration of follow-up is critical, as only 22–50% of recurrences become apparent within the first 5 years of initial repair.[28,29] There are, however, no randomized, prospective studies comparing the various techniques with comparable lengths of follow-up in the world's literature. The best reported recurrence rates by conventional tissue repairs are generally less than 1.5% with 5–10 years of follow-up.[30,31] Many other series report recurrence rates as high as 15%. This may be a more accurate reflection of recurrences for repairs performed by the nonspecialized general surgeon. Prospective data on hernia repair in the elderly are even more difficult to interpret. There is no good evidence that the choice of technique significantly affects outcome. There is, however, a general move away from tissue repairs toward "tension-free" repairs using synthetic patches.

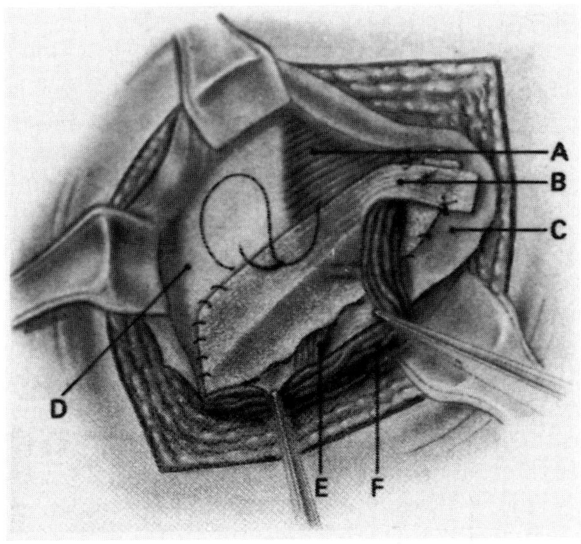


FIGURE 47.4. Tension-free inguinal herniorraphy. A, internal oblique muscle; B, mesh patch; C, external oblique muscle; D, rectus sheath; E, inferior cremasteric bundle containing the genitocrural nerve; F, spermatic cord. (From Lichtenstein et al.,[37] with permission.)

## Synthetic Repairs

In 1909, McGavin was the first to use a prosthetic material, a filigree of silver wire, to repair an inguinal hernia.[31] Throckmorton introduced tantalum gauze for use when there was insufficient tissue for adequate primary tissue repair. This material, however, did not prove to be durable. During the 1950s and 1960s, Usher et al. used polypropylene mesh to bolster primary tissue repairs of direct and indirect hernias.[32–34]

Collier and Griswold, in 1967, described the routine use of synthetic mesh for primary tension-free repairs.[35] The utility of the synthetic tension-free approach was further supported by Bellis, who reported a recurrence rate of less than 0.5% in more than 3000 repairs done with Dacron mesh. Patients in this study were also allowed to return to regular activity immediately after surgery.[36] It was not until 1986, with the published work of Lichtenstein and Shulman, that synthetic mesh became accepted for primary hernia repair without approximation of the underlying hernia margins (Figs. 47.4, 47.5).[38] A meta-analysis of more than 3000 cases from several subsequently published series showed a recurrence rate of 0.2% and an infection rate of 0.03% with no instance of mesh rejection.[39,40]

The excellent results of mesh repairs are also not confined to special centers or practitioners with special expertise. Janu et al. performed a retrospective review of patients undergoing primary inguinal hernia repair at a VA Medical Center over a 10-year period.[41] Patients were evaluated, operated on, and managed by surgical residents under staff supervision. There were 892 primary inguinal hernia repairs during the study period: 185 Bassini, 164 McVay, 101 Shouldice, 13 Marcy, 12 open preperitoneal, 26 laparoscopic, and 391 mesh (Lichtenstein type). Among the 391 mesh repairs, there was only one recurrence. This study confirms the durability and ease of the mesh repair across a wide range of operator skills.

The tension-free inguinal herniorraphy was further refined by Gilbert in 1992,[42] and Rutkow and Robbins in 1993,[43] to what is now known as the plug and patch repair. In addition to the onlay of mesh underneath or on top of the canal floor, a mesh plug is used to fill the hernia defect. Some believe this technique is superior to others because it requires less dissection and does not alter normal anatomy. The sphincter mechanism of the internal ring and the sling and shutter mechanism of the inguinal floor are also preserved.

## Laparoscopic Repairs

Shortly after the success of laparoscopic cholecystectomy became apparent, surgeons began to apply minimal access techniques to a wide variety of other surgical procedures. This approach has become generally accepted for some procedures, whereas for others there is still considerable disagreement. Hernia repair is one of the latter

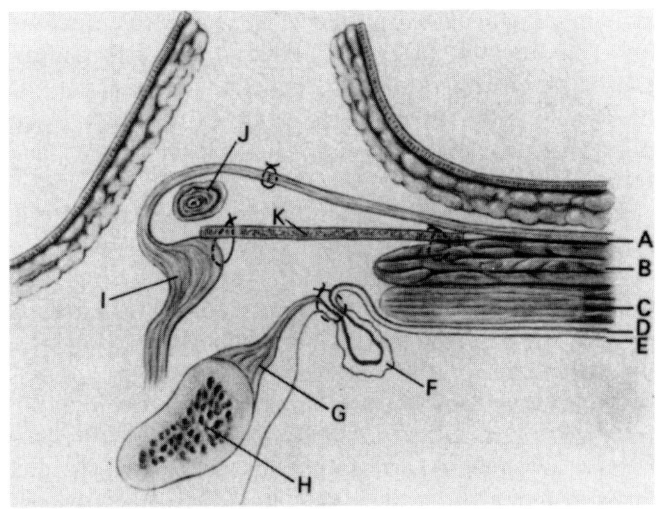


FIGURE 47.5. Sagittal view of tension-free inguinal herniorraphy. A, external oblique aponeurosis; B, internal oblique muscle; C, transversus aponeurosis; D, transversalis fascia; E, peritoneum; F, inverted direct sac; G, Cooper's ligament; H, pubis; I, inguinal ligament; J, spermatic cord; K, mesh patch bridging defect. (From Lichtenstein et al.,[37] with permission.)

group. Although some skilled laparoscopists prefer the approach for all inguinal hernias, many others believe the benefits do not outweigh the risks, particularly in the elderly.

The advantages of laparoscopic inguinal herniorrhaphy include less postoperative pain, reduced recovery time and earlier return to full activity, easier repair of recurrent hernia through unoperated tissues, the ability to treat bilateral inguinal hernias simultaneously through a single set of incisions, and improved cosmesis.[44–47]

The disadvantages, however, are not insignificant. Laparoscopic herniorrhaphy requires general anesthesia, is frequently performed by a transperitoneal route, is technically more difficult to understand and learn than mesh repairs, and in most hands, takes considerably longer. In comparisons of anesthetic techniques for open hernia repair, general anesthesia in the elderly is associated with far higher complication rates than local anesthesia. Therefore, the need for general anesthesia alone probably obviates most of the benefits of the laparoscopic approach in elderly patients. In addition, the transperitoneal route exposes the patient to the risk of inadvertent bowel injury, which in any age group could be devastating. Although the increased time to return to full activity may be an important consideration in a young person, the length of recovery may not be as important in old patients so long as mobility is not significantly compromised. Postoperative pain after the tension-free open approach is rarely severe enough to curtail activity.

The laparoscopic approach to the inguinal hernia may be performed by an extraperitoneal (TEP) rather than a transperitoneal (TAPP) approach. The TEP repair is possible in all patients except those who have had previous lower abdominal surgery or irradiation. This procedure can be performed under locoregional anesthesia, but at most centers the inability to tolerate general anesthesia is an absolute contraindication to laparoscopic hernia repair.

The difficulty when operating from either of these approaches is the ability to obtain adequate exposure of the inguinal anatomy. Most recurrences are due to incomplete dissection of the region and either a missed component or inadequate placement of mesh to cover the defect. The TAPP repair provides the largest operating space and the most unobstructed view of the inguinal region and is probably the procedure of choice to start with when learning to perform laparoscopic herniorrhaphy and master the elements of the preperitoneal space. However, because of the risk and consequences of possible visceral injury with the TAPP, TEP is preferred in the elderly patient. Given the experience required to master this approach, laparoscopic repair in the elderly should be performed only by the most skilled operators.

## Bilateral Hernias

The laparoscopic approach has been advocated for simultaneous repair of bilateral hernias. If a general anesthetic is needed to repair bilateral hernias, the laparoscopic route may be superior. In a series of 1000 bilateral Lichtenstein-type hernia repairs during 1994–1995 on patients between the ages of 25 and 76,[48] 98.3% were performed under local anesthesia. In this group of patients, postoperative pain was treated with oral pain medication for 1–5 days, with patients taking a total of 4–20 tablets over this period. The recurrence rate was 0.1% in 87% of the patients who had physician follow-up between 1 and 11 years (mean 5 years). Average time to return to work was 1 week for patients with sedentary jobs and 2 weeks for those who did heavy manual labor. It is evident from these studies that the postoperative pain and recovery period with a bilateral tension-free open mesh repair is comparable to that seen with laparoscopic repair. Furthermore, open repair avoids complications such as uncontrolled bleeding, intestinal or bladder perforation, postoperative small bowel obstruction, and trocar-site hernias associated with laparoscopic herniorraphy.[48]

## Emergency Repair

A presentative study reports incidence of incarcerated inguinal hernia as 16.8% in patients over age 65, compared to only 4.4% in younger patients.[49] Frequently in the elderly, the incarceration is chronic through a large hernia defect. Unfortunately, acute incarceration and the sequela, strangulation, are also more common in the elderly and less well tolerated. Strangulation occurs when the blood supply to the incarcerated organ becomes occluded at the neck of the hernia sac. Initially there is venous compression with subsequent edema, venous occlusion, and eventually arterial occlusion. Strangulation occurs in 1.3–3.0% of all groin hernias, most often in the elderly and children.[50] Indirect inguinal and femoral hernias are the most likely hernias to strangulate. The probability that an indirect inguinal hernia will strangulate is reported as 2.8% within 3 months of diagnosis and 4.5% after 2 years compared to 22% at 3 months and 45% at 21 months for femoral hernias.[51]

The approach to an incarcerated hernia in the elderly depends on the nature of the incarceration. Chronic incarcerations pose less of a threat of strangulation and can be treated on an elective basis (Fig. 47.6). Acute incarcerations, on the other hand, require immediate surgical treatment. Forceful attempts at nonoperative reduction may result in an en masse reduction of a compromised loop of intestine within the hernia sac. This ischemic bowel may not produce significant abdominal findings in the older patient until full-thickness necrosis and perforation occur.

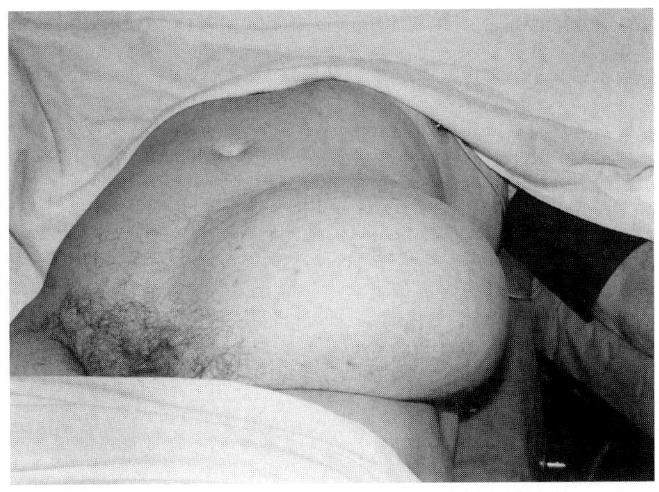

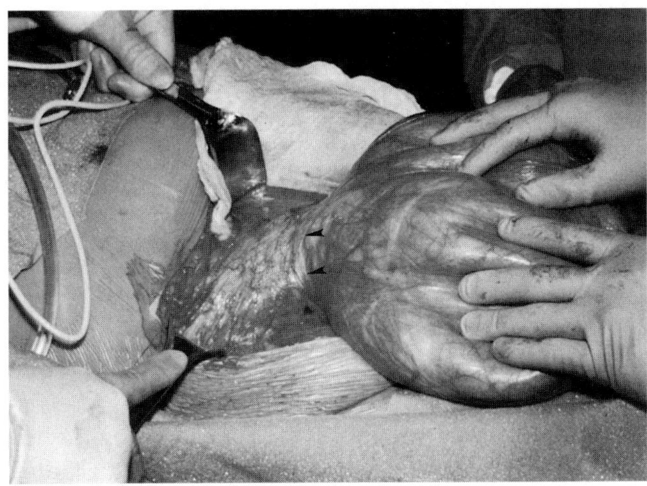

FIGURE 47.6. A. Large chronic incarcerated inguinal hernia. B. Arrowheads identify fibers of external oblique muscle through which the hernia presents.

The type of repair for incarcerated hernias depends to some extent on the viability of the contents of the hernia sac. A general or regional anesthetic is usually necessary. In the presence of inflammation, local anesthetic agents are usually not effective. In addition, the muscle relaxation provided by regional or general anesthesia may facilitate reduction of the incarcerated organ. If the incarceration is of short duration and there is no erythema or induration of the overlying skin suggesting strangulation, the choice of approach is less critical. Open anterior repair, which allows careful inspection of the sac contents outside the peritoneal cavity, is usually preferred. Frequently, a recently incarcerated hernia is reduced spontaneously or with minimal force when anesthesia is induced. In this setting, identifying the incarcerated loop of bowel through the hernia defect may be difficult but is usually not impossible. Skilled laparoscopists may prefer to inspect the bowel and repair the hernia laparoscopically through a transperitoneal approach.

If the incarceration is of longer duration or there are signs of local inflammation suggestive of strangulation, an open procedure is safest and most expeditious. The not infrequent need to use synthetic materials to repair the hernia defect in the presence of dead bowel creates a difficult clinical dilemma. Many surgeons prefer a direct anterior approach to the hernia. If ischemic bowel is found in the hernia sac, resection can generally be accomplished through the hernia defect. Every attempt is then made to repair the defect with tissue rather than synthetic material, accepting the higher risk of recurrence in exchange for a lower chance for infection. Others advise that if there is high suspicion for compromised bowel preoperatively, a small lower midline laparotomy should be performed for more careful inspection of the bowel and a more controlled resection. After the abdomen is closed, an open anterior repair of the hernia with mesh can be accomplished through a reprepared field.

## Recurrence

When performing hernia repairs, the primary focus of success is determined by the incidence of recurrence. There is a wide variation in the time frame over which recurrences are reported. There is, however, general agreement that follow-up should be at regular intervals and recurrence determined by direct examination rather than by patient report. Hernias recur for one or more reasons: tension on the tissues created by the repair, inherent abnormalities in collagen that predispose to the development of new hernias, an unrecognized second hernia component at the time of the initial repair (usually a small indirect component), and technical error.

Hernia recurrences can be classified as early or late. Most early recurrences are due to undue tension on the repair. For instance, when a hernia is due to a metabolic defect of the musculofascial abdominal wall, covering the defect with endogenous tissues results in suturing together tissues that are not normally juxtaposed. This then subjects these structures to undue tension.[53] Suture lines under tension exhibit an inadequate fibroblastic response for healing, which results in a weak scar and a subsequent recurrence of the hernia. Furthermore, these suture lines are subject to the same degenerative process that resulted in the initial herniation. Using a tension-free synthetic technique can minimize this type of recurrence.

Late recurrences are usually due to missed components or new hernias at the site of a previous repair or in a new location. This type of recurrence is more appropriately termed reherniation. Following a mesh repair, reherniation occurs because the mesh was not sutured in place or it was not of sufficient size to cover beyond the inguinal floor. Progression of tissue degeneration is of great concern and can be compensated for by placing a large sheet of mesh underneath the external oblique aponeurosis well beyond Hesselbach's triangle. This dissection is extensive but is necessary in some patients with severe tissue loss. According to Amid and Lichtenstein, recurrence rates can be reduced by a few simple methods. First, position the mesh so it overlaps the pubic bone by 1–2 cm and suture it down medial to and above the pubic tubercle. Second, use a large enough piece of mesh (6–8 cm wide) to create a substantial tissue–mesh interface. Third, allow adequate relaxation of the mesh by leaving small ripples. Fourth, create a new internal ring with a sling configuration by fixing both tails of the mesh to the inguinal ligament and suture the mesh in place to prevent displacement.[54]

Although tension and tissue factors are important determinants of recurrence, the experience of the operator is also significant. In a study of tissue repairs, Hay and colleagues compared the Shouldice repair to the Bassini and Cooper's ligament repair in 1247 patients with inguinal hernias.[55] With an average follow-up of 5.75 years, the Shouldice repair, which is a two-layer anatomic repair with the least tissue tension, had the lowest recurrence rate (6.1%). The Bassini repair, which approximates the medial edge of the transversalis fascia (conjoin tendon) and the inguinal ligament and is usually associated with an intermediate amount of tension, had a recurrence rate of 8.6%. The Cooper's ligament repair, which joins the medial edge of the conjoin tendon to Cooper's ligament, had the highest recurrence rate (11.2%). This is consistent with the fact that the Cooper's ligament repair frequently requires a medial relaxing incision to relieve the tension on the suture line. Although the influence of increasing tension on the recurrence rate is clear, the recurrence rate for Shouldice repairs in this group of unselected operators is many times higher than the recurrence rate for hernias repaired by this technique at the Shouldice Hernia Clinic. Because it is unrealistic to think that all hernia repairs can be performed by a hernia specialist, tension-free synthetic techniques that limit the other variables for recurrence and are easy to learn have become the most widely accepted.

## Other Hernias

Although groin hernias are by far the most common, there are several other types of hernia that are also of concern in the elderly: some because of the frequency and technical challenge they present, and others because they are relatively uncommon and are not discovered until they incarcerate.

### Incisional Hernias

Incisional hernias in the elderly are common and can often be challenging to repair. The incidence of hernias in patients with a midline surgical incision is 5–11%.[56] The etiology of these hernias is often multifactorial.[57] Wound infection, suture failure, malnutrition, increased age, obesity, excessive straining, ascites or peritoneal dialysis, chemotherapy or steroids, and tension on the wound closure are factors that have been implicated. The symptoms of incisional hernia often begin with the patient noticing a bulge in a previously healed incision. Although incarceration and subsequent strangulation can occur, the defects are frequently large enough to allow the contents to move in and out of the sac without difficulty. The size and discomfort caused by these hernias is often the most pressing consideration for repair.

Technically, these hernias may be challenging for several reasons. First, it is possible for most of the abdominal contents to become a fixed part of the hernia, which may result in a decrease in the intraabdominal compartment volume. This in turn complicates complete reduction of the contents at the time of repair. Second, the defects are usually multiple, reflecting failure of wound healing throughout the length of the incision. Identifying all the defects in the "Swiss cheese"-type abdominal wall and freeing all of the underlying adhesions may be tedious and time-consuming. Finally, extreme care must be exercised not to enter the bowel lumen during dissection because most incisional hernias are large and require synthetic materials for repair without tension.

### Umbilical Hernias

The umbilical hernia was first noted in 1 AD by the Hindu physician Charaka, who mistakenly believed it to be an abdominal tumor. The treatment of umbilical hernia has run the gamut from external compression devices to amputation. The modern repair is credited to William J. Mayo, who used a technique of overlapping abdominal wall fascia in a "vest-over-pants" manner. Jackson and Moglen, in a retrospective review of adult patients with umbilical hernias, reported that only 10.8% remembered the presence of the hernia during childhood. In adults, unlike in children, the hernia occurs through an umbilical canal that is bordered by the umbilical fascia, the linea alba, and the two rectus sheaths.[58] Because of the tight limitations of this canal, this type of hernia is apt to incarcerate and strangulate.

Umbilical hernias are common in cirrhotic patients and in those with ascites of other etiology because of the increased intraabdominal pressure against a thinned umbilical ring and fascia. An incidence as high as 24% has been reported in this patient population.[59] Umbilical hernia is also an important consideration in patients on peritoneal dialysis. Dialysis must be interrupted and

# *Part II*
# *Specific Issues in Geriatric Surgery*

## Section 7
## Hepatobiliary System

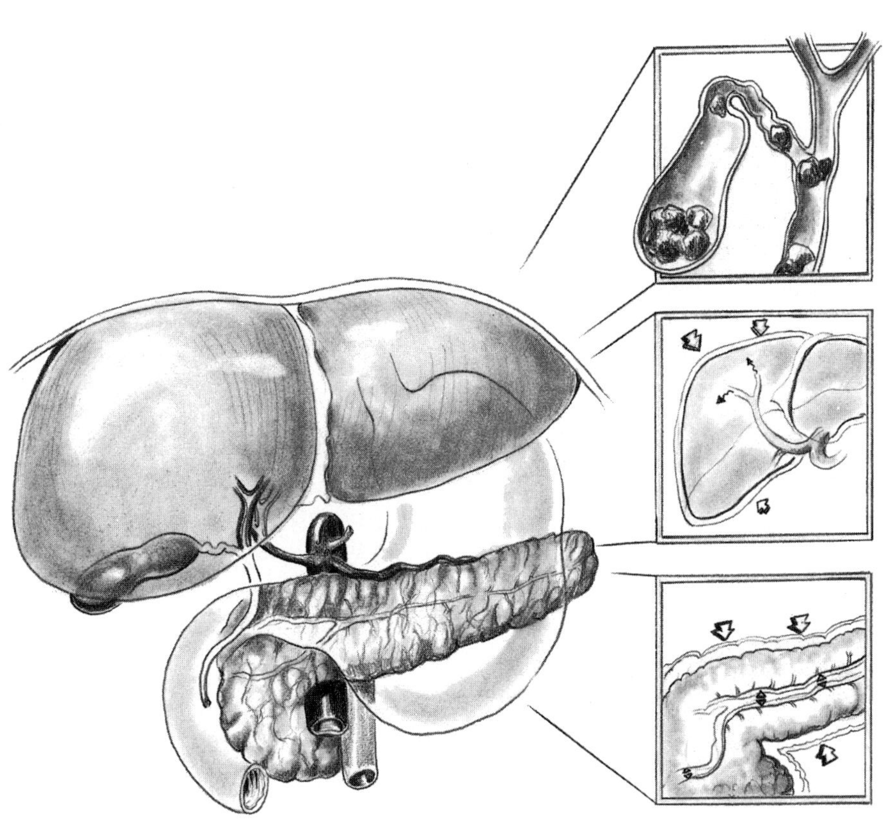

# Invited Commentary

Seymour Schwartz

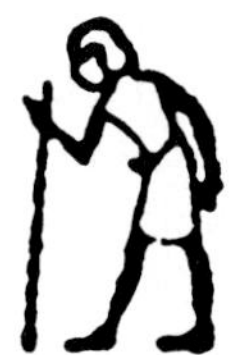

There has been a quantum change in the management of geriatric patients with hepatobiliary, pancreatic, and splenic disorders. The change is a consequence of two unrelated factors. The first factor is the disregard of the patient's chronologic age, replaced by an appreciation that it is the physiologic status of the patient that determines operative risk. The same major hepatic resections, pancreaticoduodenectomies, and complex biliary procedures that are applied with curative or palliative intentions for patients in their fifties and sixties can be performed in patients in their seventies and eighties with equivalent results. Improved intraoperative and perioperative care has been responsible for the change.

The second, unrelated factor is the introduction and rapid growth of minimally invasive surgery, which has been a by-product of the technologic age in which we live. Endoscopic equipment has been refined to extend the applicability of these procedures. Laparoscopic surgery, first applied to the gallbladder by general surgeons a little more than a decade ago, has been extended to the biliary tract, liver, pancreas, and spleen. Less invasive procedures have resulted in fewer adverse effects and more rapid recovery for patients. This is particularly meaningful for geriatric patients, who benefit by reducing the period of postoperative compromise and thereby maintaining quality of life.

In the realm of hepatic surgery, it has been shown that age precludes no resection, regardless of extent; and minor resections such as segmentectomies can be accomplished laparoscopically. Benign nonparasitic cysts are particularly amenable to laparoscopic unroofing and destruction of the epithelium adherent to the liver by endoscopic argon coagulation. The reduced risk of hepatic resections has liberalized the indications for operations to excise benign lesions. Enucleation of large symptomatic hemangiomas is usually accomplished without transfusion. Occasionally, resection is indicated for painful focal nodular hyperplasia. It is generally accepted that all adenomas should be removed because of the potential for malignant transformation. Age alone should not preclude resection of primary malignant lesions or metastatic tumors, particularly those of colonic, renal, or adrenal origin. The old nostrum that a portal systemic shunt in a patient older than 60 years is associated with a prohibitive risk of hepatic encephalopathy has been proved wrong.

Laparoscopic cholecystectomy is currently applicable to most patients with calculous disease of the gallbladder. This also pertains to the geriatric patient. The reduced length of hospitalization and the shortened recovery period is particularly advantageous for the elderly patient. The combination of laparoscopic cholecystectomy and endoscopic procedures on the common duct obviates more complex open procedures. The endoscopic approaches also address the critical problem of suppurative cholangitis, often a disease of the elderly. The necessary drainage and decompression (the basis of treatment) replaces the need for an urgent major operation.

The age limits for resection of carcinoma of the confluence of the bile ducts (Klatskin tumor) has been lifted, and concomitant hepatic resection to achieve a disease-free margin is tolerated by geriatric patients. In those patients in whom resection is not possible, endoscopic establishment of internal biliary drainage is indicated to provide palliation.

The most convincing evidence that elderly patients tolerate extensive operations relates to pancreaticoduodenectomy, for which there are data to indicate that patients over 70 years of age do as well as younger patients. There is also the suggestion that geriatric patients are better palliated by the Whipple procedure than by internal drainage. Pancreatic pseudocysts are readily drained by radiologic interventionalists, and laparoscopic pancreatic cystgastrostomy may facilitate the care of some old patients.

Laparoscopic surgery has been extended to the spleen, where there is increasing enthusiasm for removing the spleen in patients with idiopathic thrombocytopenic purpura by this approach. The spleen in these patients is characteristically small or of normal size, thereby lending itself to the procedure. Accessory spleens are identifiable and removable by this approach.

As the life-span is extended and the geriatric population consequently increases, attitudes about these patients are altered. With anticipated longer life ahead, a more aggressive attitude toward achieving cure or affording palliation is merited. The reduction in the risk of complex operative procedures and the possibility of achieving equivalent results by minimally invasive operations amplifies the applicability of surgical approaches. It is anticipated that the technology will continue to improve in an exponential fashion, particularly as related to operations on the liver, biliary tract, pancreas, and spleen. It is also anticipated that a better understanding of the physiologic consequences of the aging process will lead to more specific perioperative care of these patients. The result will be a reduction of risk and an extension of surgical horizons.

# 48
# Hepatobiliary and Pancreatic Function: Physiologic Changes

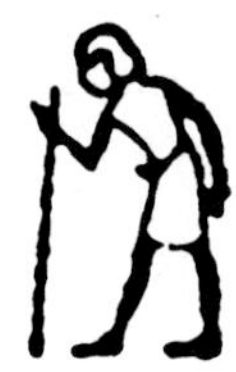

D. LaRon Mason and F. Charles Brunicardi

Normal variation in physiologic parameters of the hepatobiliary system and pancreas is increasingly recognized in the elderly. Appreciation of these alterations allows the surgeon to distinguish between expected physiologic variation and intercurrent pathophysiology in the clinical setting. It is with this goal in mind that we present this review of normal hepatobiliary and pancreatic physiology compared with recognized physiologic aging of these organ systems and select pathophysiology.

## Liver and Biliary System

### Liver Anatomy

The human liver is the largest intraabdominal organ, uniquely situated at the interface between the visceral and systemic circulation. Surgical anatomy of the liver divides its substance into lobes and segments important for performing anatomic resections (Fig. 48.1). Anatomic classification is based on intrahepatic branching of the bile ducts and vasculature, not on external topography. The interlobar line of Cantlie extending from the gallbladder fossa to the inferior vena cava divides the true right and left lobes of the liver. The portal vein, hepatic artery, and biliary ductal system generally run in parallel, each bifurcating just before entry into the hilum and sending major branches to each hepatic lobe. Further bifurcation of the left vasculature and ductal system divides the left lobe of the liver into medial and lateral segments; the right hepatic lobe is partitioned into anterior and posterior segments. In addition to this traditional classification of hepatic anatomy, Couinaud's classification divides the liver into eight segments according to the anatomic relation of portal vein and hepatic vein branches (Fig. 48.2).[1]

### Hepatic Physiology

In health, the liver provides a variety of functions necessary for metabolic homeostasis. The surplus or deficit of metabolic fuels at any given time directs the interplay of anabolic and catabolic processes within the hepatocytes. Anabolic functions of the liver include glycogenesis and synthesis of plasma proteins, such as albumin, transferrin, haptoglobin, and numerous coagulation factors. Catabolic functions include glycogenolysis, gluconeogenesis, and ketogenesis. Other vital functions include detoxification of exogenous and endogenous substances, filtration of pathogens that enter the hepatic reticuloendothelial system, and bile production.

The production of bile by the hepatocyte serves as a route of excretion for organic solutes, such as bilirubin, cholesterol, bile salts, and phospholipids. Additionally, bile facilitates the intestinal absorption of dietary lipids and fat-soluble vitamins. The liver secretes 500–1000 ml of bile per day, with secretion rates being enhanced by vagal stimulation, gastrin, secretin, and cholecystokinin (CCK).[1] Ultimately, bile salt synthesis by the liver is the most important regulator of the bile secretion rate, which in turn is regulated by the return of bile salts to the liver after absorption in the terminal ileum. This cycle of bile salt transport between the liver and intestines is aptly called the enterohepatic circulation.

The primary constituents of bile are bile salts, phospholipids, and cholesterol. The cholesterol secretion rate of the liver is dependent on the activity of two hepatocyte enzymes: 3-hydroxy-3-methylglutaryl coenzyme A (HMG-CoA) reductase, which catalyzes the rate-limiting step in the synthesis of cholesterol, and cholesterol 7-α-hydroxylase, which converts hepatic cholesterol to bile salts. Dietary intake and availability of lipoprotein carriers also affect cholesterol metabolism. Although insoluble in water, cholesterol remains soluble in bile if the relative concentrations of bile salts and phospholipids are maintained within certain limits. As first presented by Admirand and Small in 1968, the solubility characteristics of cholesterol are depicted by plotting the percentages of bile constituents on triangular coordinates[2] (Fig. 48.3). The area under the curve represents relative percentages of bile constituents that are required to main-

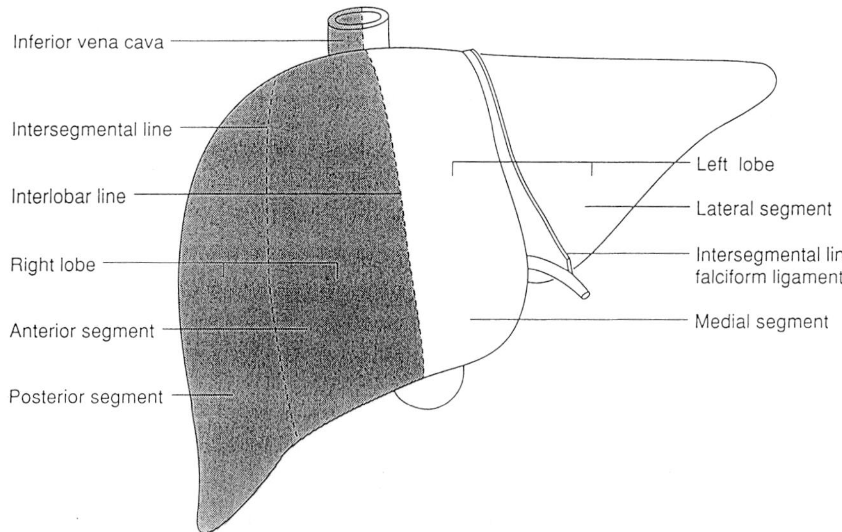


FIGURE 48.1. Anatomic division of the liver into right and left lobes by the interlobar line of Cantlie extending from the gallbladder fossa to the inferior vena cava. (From Greenfield LJ, ed. Surgery: Scientific Principles and Practice. Philadelphia: Lippincott, 1993, with permission.)

tain cholesterol in solution. If the relative percentages fall outside this area, supersaturation and crystallization of cholesterol can occur, which of course, can be a prelude to gallstone formation.

## Hepatic Function in the Elderly

The liver undergoes morphologic and physiologic changes with aging (Table 48.1), gradually decreasing in absolute and relative size, and conforming to the shape of adjoining structures. The characteristic gross change noted in the liver of the elderly has been called "brown atrophy." Histologically, it is associated with a decrease in the size of constituent lobules, although the absolute number of lobules remains constant. There is also a proliferation of bile ducts, particularly around portal tracts. The number of hepatocytes decreases, but there is a compensatory increase in mean cell volume, mitochondrial and lysosomal volume, endoplasmic reticulum, and DNA content. The incidence of binucleate or multinucleate hepatocytes is increased.[3] The cellular hypertrophy and hyperplasia seen in response to senescent cell loss is similar to the structural changes noted after surgical

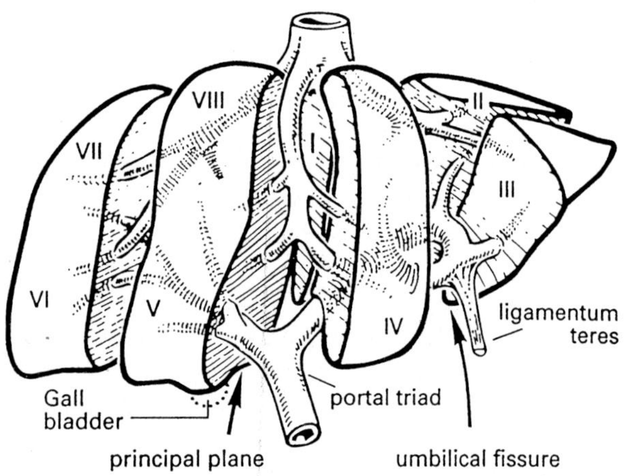

FIGURE 48.2. Hepatic segmental anatomy as defined by Couinaud, based on the anatomic relation of the portal vein and hepatic vein branches. (Blumgart LH, ed. Surgery of the liver and biliary tract. Edinburgh: Churchill Livingstone, 1994, with permission.)

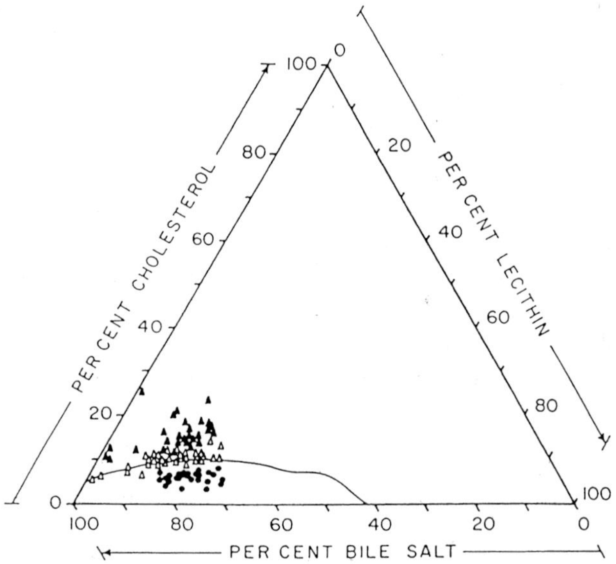


FIGURE 48.3. Triangular coordinates of the primary bile constituents for prediction of cholesterol solubility or crystallization. Any single point within the triangle represents a solution of bile with unique relative proportions of cholesterol, phospholipid (lecithin), and bile salt. Solutions represented by points under the curve are likely to maintain cholesterol in solution, whereas points above the curve are likely to represent solutions with cholesterol supersaturation and propensity to crystallization. (From Admirand and Small,[2] with permission.)

TABLE 48.1. Morphologic and Physiologic Changes Observed in the Liver of Elderly Persons

| Parameter | Change |
|---|---|
| Organ size (absolute and relative) | ↓ |
| Hepatocyte number | ↓ |
| Cell volume, ploidy, organelle constituents | ↑ |
| Hepatic blood flow | ↓ |
| Liver function tests | No change |
| Metabolic function | No significant change? |

↑, increased; ↓, decreased; ?, not proven or consistent.

resection or other traumatic injury to the hepatic parenchyma. The aforementioned brown coloration of the aged liver is caused by accumulation of pigmented lipofuscin granules in hepatocytes and Kupffer cells. These granules are thought to be the depository of residues, predominantly exogenous dietary contaminants, that the liver cannot metabolize.[3]

Hepatic blood flow, measured with dye clearance tests, shows a corresponding decrease with age at an estimated 0.3–1.5% decline per year, with obvious implications for drug metabolism dependent on hepatic clearance. Reduced blood flow is attributed to the diminution of hepatic parenchymal mass with aging. As a result of this decline, individuals aged 65 years have 40–45% less total hepatic blood flow than they had at age 25.[4]

Although the morphology of the liver may change with age, the great functional reserve of this organ allows little or no clinical impairment. Several studies have documented that standard liver function tests (LFTs) do not vary significantly with increasing age alone.[3,5,6] Abnormal liver chemistries in the elderly should be considered an indication of hepatobiliary disease. However, standard LFTs—including serum bilirubin, aminotransferases, and alkaline phosphatase—do not reflect the true dynamic function of the liver. Evaluation of dynamic hepatic function requires measuring clearance of anionic dyes, such as sodium sulfobromophthalein (Bromsulphthalein, or BSP) and $^{131}$I-rose bengal, or various drugs that require hepatic microsomal enzyme activity. Prior studies investigating hepatic clearance or retention in the elderly have been controversial and conflicting, requiring control for multiple co-morbid diseases, medications, and decreased hepatic blood flow.[5,7,8] To date, the most definitive study is that of Kampmann and associates, which demonstrated no significant variation in retention of anionic dyes in 43 carefully selected patients aged 50–88 years when compared with younger persons.[6] Patients who were obese, alcoholic, receiving potentially hepatotoxic medicines, or showing evidence of renal, hepatic, or bone disorders were excluded from this study. Additionally, liver biopsies were performed in all patients to rule out hepatic pathology that could secondarily elevate dye retention rates, such as fatty degeneration, cirrhosis, or chronic hepatitis.

In general, synthesis of most hepatic proteins remains intact with some impaired catabolism. This combination of metabolic alterations would partly explain the presence of excess proteinaceous material in some cells of the aging liver. Also, the activities of certain hepatic enzymes necessary for cholesterol metabolism are thought to be affected by the aging process. These age-related changes in hepatic enzyme activity may well be contributing factors in the pathogenesis of gallstone formation in the elderly.

## Biliary Anatomy

After being secreted by the hepatocyte, bile drains into progressively larger intrahepatic ducts that coalesce within each lobe to form the right and left lobar ducts. These lobar ducts exit the hilum and join to form the common hepatic duct (CHD). The gallbladder is a pear-shaped organ lying on the inferior surface of the liver that drains through the cystic duct. The cystic duct joins the CHD to form the common bile duct (CBD), extending distally to the ampulla of Vater within the duodenal wall. The sphincter of Oddi is a complex muscular structure surrounding the distal portions of the CBD, main pancreatic duct, and ampulla of Vater that is separate from the duodenal musculature. This sphincter coordinates appropriate release of biliary and pancreatic secretions during a meal while preventing harmful reflux of duodenal contents.

## Biliary Physiology

The electrolyte and water content of secreted bile are modified with passage from the liver to the extrahepatic biliary system by the secretory and absorptive capacities of biliary ductal epithelium. As described previously, gastrointestinal hormones, such as secretin, CCK, and gastrin, regulate this process. The main function of the gallbladder is to store and concentrate bile during the fasting state and allow coordinated release in response to a meal. The normal gallbladder volume is only 40–50 ml. Gallbladder mucosa has remarkable absorptive capacity, allowing it to accommodate the 500–1000 ml of bile produced by the liver each day.[1] However, the concentration of gallbladder bile allows more efficient mucosal absorption of sodium and water than cholesterol and calcium. This process may significantly affect the concentration and solubility of gallbladder cholesterol and calcium, both of which are important factors in gallstone pathogenesis.

Between meals, the gallbladder fills with bile in concert with tonic contraction of the ampullary sphincter. Every 60–120 minutes, the gallbladder empties about 10–30% of its concentrated bile while accepting dilute hepatic bile, analogous to the action of a set of "bellows." This process of partial emptying and filling seems to be coordinated with late phase II and phase III activity of the gastrointestinal migrating myoelectric complex (MMC), which is associated with increases in plasma concentrations of the hormone motilin.[9] The turnover of gallbladder bile during fasting may serve as a mechanism to prevent or expel cholesterol crystals prior to macroscopic stone formation.

In response to intraluminal fatty acids and certain amino acids, CCK is released from endocrine I cells of the duodenal and jejunal mucosa and serves as the main stimulus for simultaneous gallbladder contraction and relaxation of the sphincter of Oddi. This coordinated reflex allows flow of bile and pancreatic juice into the duodenum to aid in the digestive process. At physiologic levels, CCK seems to influence vagal cholinergic innervation of the gallbladder by means of CCK-A receptors on postganglionic neurons.[10] This neurohumoral interaction may provide control of basal gallbladder smooth muscle tone and coordination of postprandial gallbladder contraction.

### Biliary Function in the Elderly

There is little effect of aging on gallbladder size, contractility, or absorptive capacity (Table 48.2). Khalil and colleagues demonstrated that gallbladder sensitivity to CCK decreases with age, but fasting and fat-stimulated plasma levels of CCK are significantly higher in older individuals. These physiologic alterations appear to offset each other functionally, as the rate of gallbladder emptying in the elderly is similar to that of younger individuals.[11] An increase in serum concentration of pancreatic polypeptide with age is also speculated to slow gallbladder emptying, but further studies are needed to clarify the role of this hormone in hepatobiliary function in the elderly.

The common bile duct does undergo an age-related increase in luminal diameter similar to that of the main pancreatic duct. One study by Nagase and associates used intravenous cholangiography to measure the CBD size in 84 healthy Japanese persons and documented a mean diameter of 9.2mm at age 70 compared to 6.8mm at age 20.[12] The distal portion of the CBD and the sphincter of Oddi become progressively narrower with age, however.

TABLE 48.2. Morphologic and Physiologic Changes Observed in the Biliary System of Elderly Persons

| Parameter | Change |
|---|---|
| Bile duct size | ↑ |
| Gallbladder contractility | No change |
| Gallbladder absorptive capacity | No change |
| Cholecystokinin plasma levels | ↑ |
| Gallbladder cholecystokinin sensitivity | ↓ |
| Cholelithiasis incidence | ↑ |
| Bile cholesterol saturation | ↑ |

↑, increased; ↓, decreased; ?, not proven or consistent.

## Gallstone Pathogenesis

Gallstone disease is a significant health care problem in the United States, with an overall prevalence of 10–12%, translating to 25 million to 30 million people. Risk factors for gallstone development include female sex, obesity, and ethnicity.[13] The incidence of cholelithiasis is also known to increase with advancing age (Table 48.3).[14–18] In fact, the most common abdominal operation performed in the geriatric population is cholecystectomy, with the total number of cases performed annually for nonfederal inpatients 65 years of age and over approximating 161,000.[19] The elderly more commonly require urgent surgical intervention for biliary tract disease than the younger populace and usually suffer more complications, such as CBD obstruction, perforation, and gangrene.[20]

The formation of gallstones is a function of the relative concentrations of biliary solutes, primarily cholesterol and calcium salts. Gallstones are classified according to their cholesterol content as either cholesterol stones or pigment stones. Pigment stones are further classified as black or brown. In the United States, gallstones are most commonly composed of cholesterol (70–80%) with pigment stones accounting for the remaining 20–30%.[1] Biliary "sludge" is a pathologic precipitation of cholesterol crystals and calcium bilirubinate granules in a mucin gel matrix, not infrequently observed in states of prolonged bowel rest or with use of total parenteral nutrition (TPN).

### Cholesterol Gallstone Pathogenesis

Three independent but mutually inclusive processes appear to be necessary for gallstone formation: (1)

TABLE 48.3. Prevalence of Gallstones at Autopsy in Women in Various Countries

| Age | Prevalence of gallstones (%) | | | |
|---|---|---|---|---|
| (years) | UK[14] | USA[15] | Sweden[16] | Chile[17] |
| 10–19 | — | 0 | — | 7.2 |
| 20–29 | 6.8 | 4.2 | 14.3 | 25.1 |
| 30–39 | — | 8.6 | 16.7 | 26.4 |
| 40–49 | 9.7 | 12.1 | 15.0 | 46.5 |
| 50–59 | 28.0 | 23.3 | 27.6 | 55.6 |
| 60–69 | 31.5 | 27.5 | 40.0 | 65.3 |
| 70–79 | 33.6 | 30.6 | 52.7 | 63.7 |
| 80–89 | 42.6 | 34.9 | 51.9 | 77.1 |
| 90+ | 42.7 | 44.4 | 58.4 | — |

*Sources:* Data from Bateson,[14] Lieber,[15] Lindström,[16] and Marinovic et al.[17] The table illustrates the geographic variation of gallstone disease and increasing prevalence with advancing age.

cholesterol supersaturation; (2) nucleation; and (3) stone growth. As previously mentioned, cholesterol is a highly hydrophobic molecule requiring appropriate relative concentrations of bile salts and phospholipids to remain soluble in bile. These biliary solutes are arranged in cholesterol-phospholipid vesicles and mixed micelles when in solution. Excess biliary cholesterol can result from hypersecretion of cholesterol with a normal bile acid pool or with normal cholesterol secretion in conjunction with a diminished bile acid pool. Therefore, cholesterol supersaturation can be produced by decreased activity of cholesterol 7-α-hydroxylase (decreasing the conversion of hepatic cholesterol to bile acids), overactivity of HMG-CoA reductase (the rate-controlling enzyme in the synthesis of cholesterol), or terminal ileal disease or resection (interrupting the enterohepatic conservation of bile acids).

Although it is a necessary requirement, biliary cholesterol supersaturation alone appears insufficient to cause stone formation. In fact, cholesterol supersaturation of bile is a frequent finding in healthy individuals known to be free of biliary pathology.[21,22] Nucleation, or the precipitation of supersaturated bile cholesterol into solid cholesterol monohydrate crystals, is probably influenced by the interplay of multiple substances within the hepatobiliary system that can enhance or inhibit the process. Nucleation time, the rate at which cholesterol crystals form, is decreased from approximately 15 days in control patients free of biliary disease to 3 days in patients with gallstones.[22] Mucin glycoproteins secreted under prostaglandin control and immunoglobulins secreted by the gallbladder mucosa are thought to serve as pronucleating agents, perhaps using the mucous gel coating on the mucosa as a nucleation matrix. Other substances that have demonstrated pronucleating effects in vitro include phospholipase C, fibronectin, and a low density lipoprotein, whereas apolipoprotein A-I has been shown to inhibit nucleation.[23] Concentration of bile within the gallbladder causes the formation of large, cholesterol-rich multilamellar vesicles that can precipitate cholesterol crystals. Also, concentration of calcium salts within the gallbladder leading to saturation may serve as a nidus for nucleation.

Ultimately, for gallstones to be clinically significant, cholesterol crystals must attain sufficient size to cause mucosal injury or obstruction of the ductal system. Macroscopic stone formation from cholesterol crystals results from progressive enlargement of individual crystals with deposition of insoluble material onto its outer surface or by fusion of crystals into a larger conglomerate.

Although the pathogenesis of cholesterol gallstones is clearly multifactorial (Table 48.4), it has become increasingly clear that gallbladder mucosal function and contractility play key roles in this process. Gallbladder hypomotility with infrequent or incomplete emptying of the gallbladder contents may predispose to bile stasis and crystal formation. Patients with these conditions clearly are at increased risk for development of cholelithiasis. Conditions associated with impaired gallbladder emptying and an enhanced propensity to gallstone formation include administration of TPN, pregnancy, sickle cell anemia, administration of octreotide, or the presence of somatostatin-secreting tumors, spinal cord injuries, or truncal vagotomy.[24]

TABLE 48.4. Factors Contributing to Cholesterol Gallstone Formation

| |
|---|
| Cholesterol supersaturation |
| Cholesterol hypersecretion |
| Diminished bile acid pool |
| Ileal disease or resection |
| Nucleation |
| Mucin glycoproteins |
| Pronucleating substances: phospholipase C, fibronectin |
| Nucleation-inhibiting substances: apolipoprotein A1 |
| Calcium concentration |
| Gallbladder dysmotility |
| Altered cholecystokinin (CCK) plasma levels or receptors |
| Neurohumoral influences: CCK somatostatin, estrogen |
| Vagolysis, mechanical or functional |

Although gallstones are associated with abnormal gallbladder contractility, it is not known whether altered motility is the primary problem or a secondary consequence. The presence of cholesterol-supersaturated bile alone has been shown to impair gallbladder emptying before cholesterol crystals or gallstones are evident.[23] Mechanisms proposed to explain the apparent effect of cholesterol-rich bile or gallstones on gallbladder motility, include a possible myotoxic or neurotoxic effect of cholesterol or bile salts, the development of hypertrophic myopathy with chronic inflammation or inflammatory mediator release, and disordered regulation of hormonal influences, such as CCK, motilin, or somatostatin.[23,25]

As part of a series of studies evaluating the characteristics and regulation of gallbladder motility in patients with and without gallstones, Thompson and colleagues reported that most gallbladders containing gallstones contract like normal controls when evaluated by ultrasonography after a lipid meal.[26] These "contractors" exhibited a diminished release of endogenous CCK measured with plasma bioassay, but an increased sensitivity to the hormone was apparent relative to controls. A few patients with gallstones displayed depressed gallbladder contractility but with CCK output equivalent to that of the controls. Gallbladder muscle strips obtained from these "noncontractors" were subsequently shown to have significantly reduced in vitro responsiveness to CCK[27] and a decrease in the number of CCK receptors.[28] The cause-and-effect relation between gallstones, gallbladder dysmotility, and neurohumoral influences is an area of active investigation.

## Pigment Gallstone Pathogenesis

Calcium salts are now recognized as important components of most if not all gallstones, including those that are primarily cholesterol-containing. Factors that result in elevated concentrations of biliary calcium or the associated anions—unconjugated bilirubin, carbonate, phosphate, palmitate—predispose to pigment stone formation. The presence and physical characteristics of pigment gallstones are reflective of precipitating factors. Black pigment stones are more common in Western populations and are seen in states of hemolysis and cirrhosis. Excess unconjugated bilirubin combines with calcium, leading to stone formation. These stones are of solid consistency and most frequently found in the gallbladder. Brown pigment stones are more common in Asian populations and are associated with chronic biliary tract infections or bile stasis. The stones are much more fragile than cholesterol or black pigment stones, crumbling readily when manipulated. Brown pigment stones are usually found in the bile ducts where β-glucuronidase produced by bacteria hydrolyzes conjugated bilirubin to the free form, a hydrophobic solute that readily combines with calcium to produce a nidus for gallstone formation.

## Lithogenic Factors in the Elderly

The increased incidence of lithogenic bile and gallstones in the elderly is multifactorial, with several known contributing factors. Einarsson and associates demonstrated age-associated changes of biliary cholesterol saturation and bile acid kinetics in a group of nonobese, normolipidemic subjects known to be gallstone-free.[29] Specifically, this investigation was able to show a direct correlation between advancing age and increasing cholesterol saturation of bile, presumably due to an increased rate of hepatic cholesterol secretion (Fig. 48.4). Additionally, bile acid synthesis and pool sizes were noted to decrease with advancing age (Fig. 48.5). Each of these changes contributes to the enhanced lithogenicity of bile in the

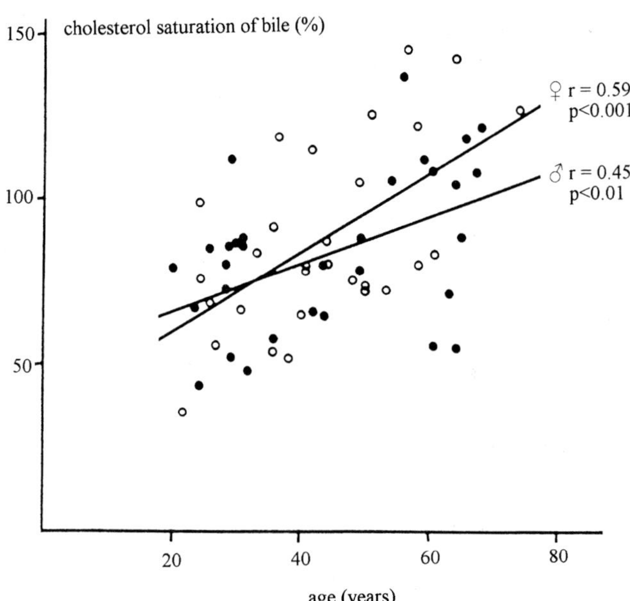


FIGURE 48.4. Relation between age and cholesterol saturation of bile. Open symbols denote women, and closed circles denote men. (From Einarsson et al.,[29] © Massachusetts Medical Society, with permission.)

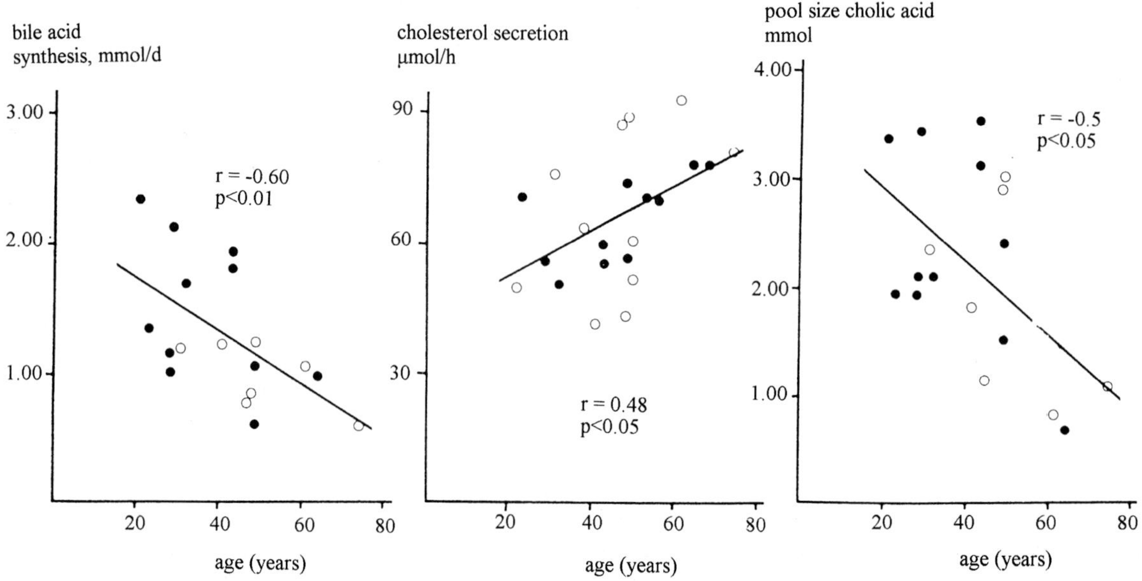


FIGURE 48.5. Relation between age and hepatic cholesterol secretion, total bile acid synthesis, and size of the cholic acid pool. Open circles denote women, and closed circles denote men. (From Einarsson et al.,[29] © Massachusetts Medical Society, with permission.)

elderly. The relation of these physiologic changes with possible age-related changes in hepatocyte enzyme activity for HMG-CoA reductase and 7-α-reductase has been investigated, with studies available that both support[30] and refute[31] this position.

Gallbladder stasis may also contribute to an increased incidence of gallstones in the elderly. Factors that may lead to gallbladder dysmotility in older patients include increasing saturation of bile with cholesterol and altered sensitivity of the gallbladder smooth muscle to CCK. Reviews of CCK receptor stimulants, motilin agonists, and procholinergic agents provide encouragement for emerging pharmacotherapy as treatment options for gallbladder hypomotility.[23,24]

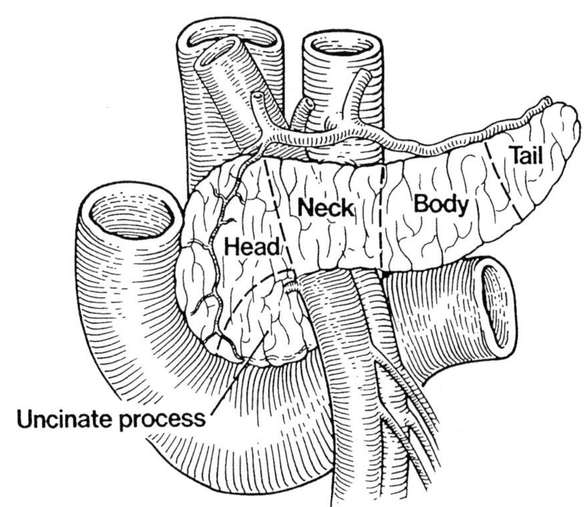


FIGURE 48.6. Anatomy of the mature pancreas, relative to surrounding structures. (Trede M, Carter DC, eds. Surgery of the Pancreas. Edinburgh: Churchill Livingstone, 1993, with permission.)

## Pancreas

### Pancreatic Development and Anatomy

The pancreas is a retroperitoneal organ of endodermal origin. Embryonic development is intimately associated with hepatobiliary organogenesis as the developing pancreas arises from ventral and dorsal buds of the primitive foregut. The ventral bud rotates 180 degrees clockwise around the duodenum and fuses with the dorsal pancreatic bud. The resulting mature organ consists of four portions, relative to surrounding structures: (1) the head, which fits snugly into the duodenal C loop; (2) the uncinate process, a ventral bud remnant off the pancreatic head extending posterior to the superior mesenteric vessels; (3) the neck, which lies over the superior mesenteric vessels; and (4) the body and tail, extending to the left of the superior mesenteric vessels into the splenic hilum (Fig. 48.6). The main pancreatic duct of Wirsung, formed by fusion of the ventral duct and the distal portion of the dorsal pancreatic duct, drains most of the pancreas into the duodenum at the ampulla of Vater. The diameter of the main pancreatic duct is 2.0–3.5 mm in healthy young adults.[32] The common bile duct joins with the main pancreatic duct at the ampulla of Vater and empties through the greater duodenal papilla. The proximal ductal system of the dorsal bud persists as the accessory pancreatic duct of Santorini, draining the superior portion of the pancreatic head via the lesser papilla into the duodenum proximal to the greater papilla.

### Pancreatic Physiology

The pancreas has many functions, including exocrine activity to facilitate digestion, neutralize gastric acid, and regulate luminal pH in the intestine. Pancreatic endocrine activity is necessary for glucose homeostasis. Because of the great functional reserve of this organ, 90% of pancreatic function can be lost before signs of insufficiency become clinically evident.[33]

#### *Exocrine Function*

The major components of the exocrine pancreas are the acinar cells and the ductal network. Acinar cells secrete enzymes responsible for digestion, and centroacinar cells and the ductal system direct the exocrine secretions to the duodenum, modifying the electrolyte concentration and water content of the pancreatic fluid as it passes.

Acinar cells synthesize enzymes necessary for digestion of carbohydrates, proteins, and fats. These enzymes include amylase (isoamylase type P), lipase, trypsinogen, chymotrypsinogen, procarboxypeptidases A and B, deoxyribonuclease, ribonuclease, proelastase, and trypsin inhibitor. The major proteolytic enzyme is trypsin, initially secreted within the pancreas in an inactive form but activated within the duodenum by increasing acidity and enterokinase, a hormone produced by duodenal mucosa. Only amylase is secreted directly from the acinus in an active form. The other enzymes are initially secreted as inactive proenzymes, requiring trypsin and the acidic environment of the duodenum for activation. Inappropriate early activation of enzymatic action can result in autodigestion of the pancreatic substance. Dietary alteration and specific nutrient stimulants alter the absolute amount and ratio of enzymes secreted. Regulation of enzyme secretion is primarily through the hormone CCK and acetylcholine. Secretin, vasoactive intestinal peptide (VIP), and pancreatic islet hormones weakly stimulate acinar secretion.[32]

Pancreatic fluid has a pH that varies from 7.6 to 9.0, depending on the rate of bicarbonate secretion from the ductal epithelium. An alkaline pH is necessary to carry inactive proteolytic enzymes to the appropriate acidic milieu of the duodenum for activation. The major stimulant for pancreatic electrolyte and water secretion is secretin, a hormone released from the mucosa of proximal small bowel in the presence of a local pH of less than 3.0. Cholecystokinin, gastrin, and acetylcholine also serve as weak stimulants. The anion content of pancreatic exocrine secretion varies according to the rate of secretion. As the rate of pancreatic fluid secretion increases, the bicarbonate concentration in the secreted fluid increases, with the chloride secretory rate varying inversely, such that the sum of these two anions remains constant and equal to that of plasma. Sodium and potassium concentrations remain constant and equivalent to that of plasma regardless of the pancreatic secretory rate.

### *Endocrine Function*

The endocrine functions of the pancreas are mediated by polypeptides produced in specialized nests of cells scattered throughout the pancreatic parenchyma. These nests are called islets of Langerhans and consist of four major cell types: alpha, beta, delta, and PP or F cells, which secrete glucagon, insulin, somatostatin, and pancreatic polypeptide, respectively.

Insulin is synthesized as a preprohormone in the beta cells of Langerhans islets. This 56-amino-acid polypeptide is broken down to its prohormone form and finally, with kallikrein as a catalyst, to insulin and C peptide. Insulin secretion is enhanced by elevated blood glucose levels and suppressed by hypoglycemia. Maximal secretion of insulin occurs at serum glucose concentrations of 400–500 mg/dl. Additional stimulants for insulin secretion include acetylcholine (parasympathetic stimulation), glucagon, CCK, sulfonylureas, and several amino acids (arginine, lysine, leucine). Norepinephrine (sympathetic stimulation) and somatostatin inhibit insulin secretion.[32]

Insulin binds to specific membrane-associated glycoprotein receptors that effect intracellular protein phosphorylation and a subsequent increase in membrane-bound glucose transporters (GLUT-1 to GLUT-5). The primary site for glucose disposal under hyperinsulinemic conditions is skeletal muscle, accounting for about 75% of whole-body glucose uptake.[34] In the liver, insulin facilitates glycogen deposition while inhibiting gluconeogenesis and glycogenolysis, resulting in a net increase in glucose uptake. Insulin also promotes lipogenesis and protein synthesis.

Like insulin, glucagon is synthesized as a precursor polypeptide but by histologically distinct alpha cells in the pancreatic islets. The actions of this counterregulatory hormone are generally antagonistic to those of insulin. Glucose, insulin, and somatostatin serve as negative regulators of glucagon secretion. Secretion is stimulated by hypoglycemia, acetylcholine, and generalized stressed states such as occur with infection, trauma, or inflammation. Glucagon promotes an elevation of blood glucose levels, with mobilization of intracellular fuels by glycogenolysis, gluconeogenesis, ketogenesis, and lipolysis. It is the provision of metabolic fuels during times of stress that resulted in glucagon being grouped with epinephrine, cortisol, and growth hormone as stress hormones.

Somatostatin is a 14-amino-acid polypeptide found in the delta cells of the pancreatic islets. It was originally isolated in 1973 as a hypothalamic extract that inhibited the release of growth hormone. The exact role of this hormone in the pancreas remains unclear, but it has been shown to inhibit the release of almost all peptide hormones and to inhibit gastric, pancreatic, and biliary secretion. Some researchers have suggested that somatostatin may regulate adjacent islet cell functions, but this has not been proven in vivo. The potent inhibitory effects of somatostatin and octreotide, a long-acting synthetic analogue, have been used to treat a variety of endocrine and exocrine disorders.

Pancreatic polypeptide (PP) is a 36-amino-acid polypeptide secreted exclusively by the F cells of the islet. Although they are distributed throughout the pancreas, the predominance of these cells is concentrated in the pancreatic head and uncinate process. The entire spectrum of normal physiologic activity remains unclear, but the peptide does serve as an important mediator of hepatic response to insulin. It has been demonstrated that abnormal glucose homeostasis associated with PP deficiency in patients with chronic pancreatitis is due to impaired suppression of hepatic glucose production by insulin.[35] This relative hepatic resistance to insulin is a consequence of diminished insulin receptor concentration, rather than altered receptor affinity, and can be ameliorated by administration of PP.[36] This mechanism of glucose metabolism has been further clarified by studies suggesting that hepatic insulin resistance in chronic pancreatitis is due to impaired transcription of the insulin receptor gene. Additionally, PP increases hepatic insulin-binding sites perhaps by upregulating insulin receptor gene expression.[37] PP is known to inhibit pancreatic exocrine secretion, choleresis, and motilin release.[38] PP release is augmented by cholinergic stimulation, with the normal postprandial rise in PP levels being ablated by vagotomy, antrectomy, or both.[32]

## Pancreatic Anatomy in the Elderly

Although the weight and size of the pancreas decrease moderately with age, postmortem and endoscopic retrograde cholangiopancreatography (ERCP) studies have documented age-associated changes in the ductal system manifested as an increase in the caliber of the main pancreatic duct and ectasia of branched ducts. One review by Kreel and Sandin[39] of in situ retrograde pancreatography

TABLE 48.5. Morphologic and Physiologic Changes Observed in the Aging Pancreas

| Parameter | Change |
|---|---|
| Organ size | ↓ |
| Ductal size | ↑ |
| Acinar glands | ↓ |
| Pancreatic lithiasis | ↑ |
| Exocrine function | No change |
| Glucose tolerance | ↓ |
| Glucagon levels | ↑ ? |
| Pancreatic polypeptide levels | ↑ |

↑, increased; ↓, decreased; ?, not proven or consistent.

at necropsy in 120 subjects older than 30 years revealed the main pancreatic duct width to increase with age at a rate of 8% per decade. The pancreatic duct widens proportionally along its entire length such that a uniform taper in caliber is maintained. This ductal anatomy can be distinguished from ductal dilatation associated with obstruction as seen with chronic pancreatitis and periampullary cancer. In some elderly patients, ductal ectasia becomes cystic as a variant of the aging pancreas. Acinar atrophy, an increased amount of intralobular fibrosis and fatty infiltration, and calcified pancreatic ductal calculi[40] seem to be common findings in the pancreas over the age of 70. Because of the increasing frequency of intercurrent disease states and degrees of malnutrition in the elderly, the proportion of these morphologic changes that are due to age alone versus pathology has yet to be determined. In summary, the morphologic changes of the aging pancreas can be considerable, requiring clinicians to take caution when interpreting ERCP and computed tomography (CT) findings in the elderly (Table 48.5).

## Aging of the Exocrine Pancreas

Pancreatic exocrine function seems to be altered minimally in the elderly. Although results of early studies looking at pancreatic exocrine function were inconclusive and at times contradictory, studies in patients over 65 years of age suggest significant decreases in the volume of pancreatic secretion and the concentrations of pancreatic protein and lipase with secretin and CCK stimulation.[41] However, the large functional reserve capacity of the pancreas ensures that these changes in secretion are clinically inconsequential. This principle was reinforced by the work of Gullo and associates, who tested the pancreatic exocrine function of 60 healthy subjects aged 66–88 years who exhibited no evidence of malnutrition.[42] This study used the fluorescein dilaurate test as an indicator of pancreatic function and found pancreatic exocrine function and digestive capacity to be unaffected by age.

## Aging of the Endocrine Pancreas

### *Insulin Resistance in the Elderly*

It has long been recognized that persons over 60 years of age more commonly exhibit dysfunction of glucose regulatory mechanisms in response to a glucose challenge.[43] Minimal morphologic alteration occurs in the aging endocrine pancreas, but a number of functional tests suggest progressive impairment of glucose tolerance in the elderly.[44–46] Clinical studies show an age-related increase in fasting blood glucose levels of about 1–2 mg/dl per decade, which may be less marked in lean, physically active individuals.[44,47]

Insulin resistance precedes and contributes to the development of the frank diabetic state, but its evolution is multifactorial with both genetic and environmental factors involved. Persons with insulin resistance maintain normoglycemia by compensatory hypersecretion of insulin, with progression to frank diabetes only after pancreatic beta cell secretion can no longer compensate for peripheral hormone resistance. In modern society, the clinical condition most commonly associated with insulin resistance is obesity, although other Western life style factors appear to be directly related, including diminished physical activity and consumption of diets high in fats and refined sugar. Studies of familial clustering and monozygotic twins suggest that insulin resistance is also conferred by genetic tendencies.[34]

Hypotheses to explain the loss of glucose tolerance with age are still subjects of considerable debate. Proposed mechanisms include altered insulin metabolism (depressed secretion, increased clearance, or diminished prohormone activation), increased resistance of peripheral tissues to insulin (receptor aberration, altered postreceptor pathways, or altered glucose transporter), and loss of hepatic sensitivity to insulin, causing reduced glycogenesis, increased glucagon levels, and an age-associated increase in adipose tissue.[48] The most accepted of these hypotheses is that aging is associated with a failure of insulin to facilitate appropriate peripheral glucose uptake. Most investigators agree that the number and affinity of insulin receptors are similar across the spectrum of age groups,[49] so the most recent area of interest has been at the postreceptor level with investigation of receptor-mediated phosphorylation/dephosphorylation events and generation of intracellular second messengers.[34]

### *Glucagon*

Little is known about glucagon metabolism and actions in the elderly. Berger and associates reported that fasting plasma glucagon levels are significantly higher after age 30 when compared to those of a younger cohort.[47] However, after age 30, plasma glucagon levels did not significantly increase with advancing age. These findings are compared with those from the more recent work of Simonson and DeFronzo,[50] who showed no correlation between advancing age and glucagon levels in 111 subjects aged 21–75 years. Additionally, this study demonstrated no difference in glucagon concentrations or clearance in young and old subjects receiving glucagon infusion, but hepatic sensitivity to the hormone appeared to be enhanced in the older age groups. Although the mechanism for this effect is not known, heightened hepatic sensitivity to glucagon in the elderly may be one of several factors contributing to progressive glucose intolerance of aging.

### Pancreatic Polypeptide

The physiologic capacity of PP remains unclear, but studies suggest that the peptide may serve as an important mediator of hepatic response to insulin.[35–37] Other possible functions include inhibition of pancreatic exocrine secretion, choleresis, and motilin.[38]

It has been previously noted that plasma levels of immunoreactive PP increase linearly with patient age.[47] The functional consequence of the age-related rise in PP levels is unknown. Studies using an isolated perfused human pancreas model reaffirmed this phenomenon and suggested that elevated PP levels in the elderly are due to enhancement of basal PP secretion, not reduced PP clearance.[38]

## References


1. Klein AS, Lillemoe KD, Yeo CJ, Pitt HA. Liver, biliary tract, and pancreas. In: O'Leary JP (ed) The Physiologic Basis of Surgery, 2nd ed. Baltimore: Williams & Wilkins, 1996:441–478.
2. Admirand WH, Small DM. The physicochemical basis of cholesterol gallstone formation in man. J Clin Invest 1968; 47:1043–1052.
3. Popper H. Aging and the liver. Prog Liver Dis 1986;8:659–683.
4. Mooney H, Roberts R, Cooksley WGE, et al. Alterations in the liver with aging. Clin Gastroenterol 1985;14:757–771.
5. Thompson EN, Williams R. Effect of age on liver function with particular reference to Bromsulphalein excretion. Gut 1965;6:266–269.
6. Kampmann JP, Sinding J, Møller-Jørgensen I. Effect of age on liver function. Geriatrics 1975;30:91–95.
7. Rafsky HA, Newman B. Liver function tests in the aged (the serum cholesterol partition, Bromsulphalein, cephalin-flocculation and oral and intravenous hippuric acid tests). Am J Dig Dis 1943;10:66–69.
8. Koff RS, Garvey AJ, Burney SW, et al. Absence of an age effect on sulfobromophthalein retention in healthy men. Gastroenterology 1973;65:300–302.
9. Qvist N. Motor activity of the gallbladder and gastrointestinal tract as determinants of enterohepatic circulation: a scintigraphic and manometric study. Dan Med Bull 1995;42:426–440.
10. Gadacz TR. Biliary anatomy and physiology. In: Greenfield LJ (ed) Surgery: Scientific Principles and Practice. Philadelphia: Lippincott, 1993:925–936.
11. Khalil T, Walker JP, Wiener I, et al. Effect of aging on gallbladder contraction and release of cholecystokinin-33 in humans. Surgery 1985;98:423–429.
12. Nagase M, Hikasa Y, Soloway RD, et al. Surgical significance of dilatation of the common bile duct: with special reference to choledocholithiasis. Jpn J Surg 1980;10:296–301.
13. Valdivieso V, Palma R, Wünkhaus R, et al. Effect of aging on biliary lipid composition and bile acid metabolism in normal Chilean women. Gastroenterology 1978;74:871–874.
14. Bateson MC. Gallbladder disease and cholecystectomy rate are independently variable. Lancet 1984;2:621–624.
15. Lieber MM. The incidence of gallstones and their correlation with other diseases. Ann Surg 1952;135:394–405.
16. Lindström CG. Frequency of gallstone disease in a well-defined Swedish population. Scand J Gastroenterol 1977; 12:341–346.
17. Marinovic I, Guerra C, Larach G. Incidencia de litiasis biliar en material de autopsias y analisis de composicion de los calculos. Rev Med Chil 1972;100:1320–1327.
18. Heaton KW. The epidemiology of gallstones and suggested aetiology. Clin Gastroenterol 1973;2:67–83.
19. National Center for Health Statistics. National Hospital Discharge Survey: Annual Summary, 1994. Series 13: Data from the National Health Care Survey, No. 128. DHHS Publ No. (PHS) 97-1789. Hyattsville, MD: National Center for Health Statistics, May 1997.
20. Reiss R, Deutsch AA. Emergency abdominal procedures in patients above 70. J Gerontol 1985;40:154–158.
21. Tang WH. Serum and bile lipid levels in patients with and without gallstones. J Gastroenterol 1996;31:823–827.
22. Holan KR, Holzbach RT, Hermann RE, et al. Nucleation time: a key factor in the pathogenesis of cholesterol gallstone disease. Gastroenterology 1979;77:611–617.
23. Portincasa P, Stolk MFJ, van Erpecum KJ, et al. Cholesterol gallstone formation in man and potential treatments of the gallbladder motility defect. Scand J Gastroenterol 1995;30(suppl 212):63–78.
24. Patankar R, Ozmen MM, Bailey IS, Johnson CD. Gallbladder motility, gallstones, and the surgeon. Dig Dis Sci 1995;40:2323–2335.
25. Schneider H, Sänger P, Hanisch E. In vitro effects of cholecystokinin fragments on human gallbladders: evidence for an altered CCK-receptor structure in a subgroup of patients with gallstones. J Hepatol 1997;26:1063–1068.
26. Thompson JC, Fried GM, Ogden WS, et al. Correlation between release of cholecystokinin and contraction of the gallbladder in patients with gallstones. Ann Surg 1982;195:670–676.
27. Zhu XG, Greely GH, Newman J, et al. Correlation of in vitro measurements of contractility of the gallbladder with in vivo ultrasonographic findings in patients with gallstones. Surg Gynecol Obstet 1985;161:470–472.
28. Upp JR, Nealon WH, Singh P, et al. Correlation of cholecystokinin receptors with gallbladder contractility in patients with gallstones. Ann Surg 1987;205:641–648.
29. Einarsson K, Nilsell K, Leijd B, Angelin B. Influence of age on secretion of cholesterol and synthesis of bile acids by the liver. N Engl J Med 1985;313:277–282.

30. Bowen JC, Brenner HI, Ferrante WA, Maule WF. Gallstone disease: pathophysiology, epidemiology, natural history, and treatment options. Med Clin North Am 1992;76:1143–1157.
31. Ahlberg J, Angelin B, Einarsson K. Hepatic 3-hydroxy-3-methylglutaryl coenzyme A reductase activity and biliary lipid composition in man: relation to cholesterol gallstone disease and effects of cholic acid and chenodeoxycholic acid treatment. J Lipid Res 1981;22:410–422.
32. Anderson DK, Brunicardi FC. Pancreatic anatomy and physiology. In: Greenfield LJ (ed) Surgery: Scientific Principles and Practice. Philadelphia: Lippincott, 1993:775–791.
33. DiMagno EP, Vay LWG, Summerskill WHJ. Relations between pancreatic enzyme outputs and malabsorption in severe pancreatic insufficiency. N Engl J Med 1973;288:813–815.
34. Youngren JF, Goldfine ID. The molecular basis of insulin resistance. Sci Med 1997;4(3):18–27.
35. Brunicardi FC, Chaiken RL, Ryan AS, et al. Pancreatic polypeptide administration improves abnormal glucose metabolism in patients with chronic pancreatitis. J Clin Endocrinol Metab 1996;81:3566–3572.
36. Seymour NE, Volpert AR, Lee EL, et al. Alterations in hepatocyte insulin binding in chronic pancreatitis: effects of pancreatic polypeptide. Am J Surg 1995;169:105–110.
37. Spector SA, Frattini JC, Zdankiewicz PD, et al. Insulin receptor gene expression in chronic pancreatitis: the effect of pancreatic polypeptide. In: Surgical Forum. Proceedings for the 52nd Annual Sessions of the Owen H. Wangensteen Surgical Forum; 1997 Oct 12–17; Chicago. Lawrence, KS: Allen Press, 1997:168–171.
38. Brunicardi FC, Druck P, Sun YS, et al. Regulation of pancreatic polypeptide secretion in the isolated perfused human pancreas. Am J Surg 1988;155:63–69.
39. Kreel L, Sandin B. Changes in pancreatic morphology associated with aging. Gut 1973;14:962–970.
40. Nagai H, Ohtsubo K. Pancreatic lithiasis in the aged. Gastroenterology 1984;86:331–338.
41. Laugier R, Sarles H. The pancreas. Clin Gastroenterol 1985;14:749–756.
42. Gullo L, Ventrucci M, Naldoni P, Pezzilli R. Aging and exocrine pancreatic function. J Am Geriatr Soc 1986;34:790–792.
43. Spence JC. Some observations on sugar tolerance, with special reference to variations found at different ages. Q J Med 1921;14:314–326.
44. Davidson MB. The effect of aging on carbohydrate metabolism: a review of the English literature and a practical approach to the diagnosis of diabetes mellitus in the elderly. Metabolism 1979;28:688–705.
45. Bennett PH. Diabetes in the elderly: diagnosis and epidemiology. Geriatrics 1984;39:37–41.
46. Taylor R, Agius L. The biochemistry of diabetes. Biochem J 1988;250:625–640.
47. Berger D, Crowther RC, Floyd JC Jr, et al. Effect of age on fasting plasma levels of pancreatic hormones in man. J Clin Endocrinol Metab 1978;47:1183–1189.
48. Timiras PS. The endocrine pancreas and carbohydrate metabolism. In: Timiras PS (ed) Physiological Basis of Aging and Geriatrics, 2nd ed. Boca Raton, FL: CRC Press, 1994:191–197.
49. Goldfine ID. The insulin receptor: molecular biology and transmembrane signaling. Endocr Rev 1987;8:235–255.
50. Simonson DC, DeFronzo RA. Glucagon physiology and aging: evidence for enhanced hepatic sensitivity. Diabetologia 1983;25:1–7.

# 49
# Gallstone Disease in the Elderly

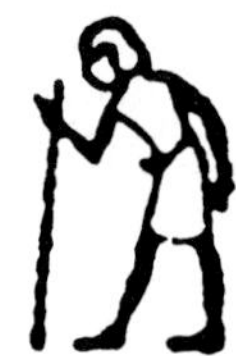

Kim U. Kahng and Jennifer A. Wargo

Disease of the biliary tract is common among adults in the United States: 10–15% of the adult population have gallstones, accounting for approximately 20 million people, and 1 million new cases are discovered annually. Gallstone disease is the most common and most costly digestive disease causing hospitalization, with an estimated annual cost exceeding $5 billion.[1] Among the elderly, biliary disease is the most common indication for abdominal surgery.[2] This is undoubtedly related to the progressive increase in the prevalence of cholelithiasis with advancing age, which in some reports exceeds 50% in those older than age 70.[3] In addition to being common, gallbladder disease in the elderly is more severe than in the young, as indicated by the higher proportion of elderly patients requiring cholecystectomy for acute rather than chronic cholecystitis.[4] Biliary tract disease in the elderly is further complicated by the greater incidence of choledocholithiasis. Common duct stones are found at the time of cholecystectomy in up to 30% of those in their sixties and in up to 50% of those in their seventies.[5]

Manifestations of biliary disease in the elderly differ significantly from those in the young, which may contribute to the higher morbidity and mortality in older patients.[6] The atypical presentation in elderly patients and the frequency of coincidental gastrointestinal complaints often lead to delays in diagnosis.[7] These delays contribute to the higher incidence of the known complications of cholelithiasis and the increased mortality of gallstone disease in the aged population.[8] Recognizing the frequency and understanding the clinical presentation of biliary disease in the elderly is thus imperative for the proper care and treatment of these patients.

## Cholelithiasis

### Incidence and Epidemiology

The prevalence of cholelithiasis varies widely among populations of the world. The considerable variation in the incidence of cholelithiasis among ethnic groups is perhaps best illustrated by the markedly increased rate of gallstone disease in Pima Indians. The prevalence of cholelithiasis in female Pima Indians exceeds 60% for those over 35 years of age.[9] To a lesser degree, an increased propensity for gallstone formation is also seen in the Scandinavian countries, Chile, and among Native Americans.[10] The prevalence of gallstones in Blacks, however, is roughly one-half that of Whites[5] and is as low as 3% in some African tribes.[11]

Regardless of geographic site or ethnicity, the two primary factors associated with the development of gallstones are gender and age. Female gender unquestionably contributes to an increased incidence of cholelithiasis, as women are twice as likely as men to develop gallstones.[10] Differences in the hormonal milieu have been implicated by studies showing that estrogen and progesterone increase the lithogenicity of bile and alter gallbladder motility.[11] Exogenous estrogen induces hypersecretion of cholesterol into bile in both men[12] and women[13] and affects the motility of the sphincter of Oddi in animal models.[14]

Advancing age is clearly associated with an increased prevalence of cholelithiasis (Fig. 49.1). This is true regardless of gender[4] or ethnicity. The effect of age may be magnified in the institutionalized elderly as indicated by a report that cholelithiasis was present in 60% of institutionalized women age 80–89 years and 80% of those older than 90 years.[15]

## Classification

Most gallstones in most Western countries, including the United States, are composed of a mixture of both cholesterol and pigment. Pure cholesterol stones account for only 10% and pure pigment stones for about 15% of gallstones in the United States.[16] Most mixed stones contain cholesterol as their principal constituent, with alternating layers of mucin glycoproteins.[10]

Pigment stones are composed mainly of bilirubin, usually in the form of calcium bilirubinate. These stones

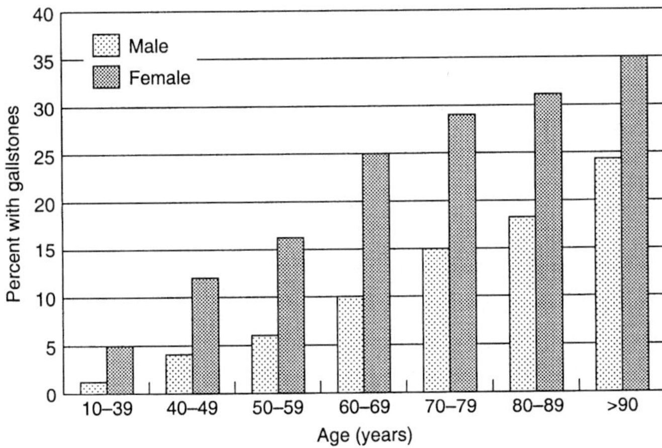


FIGURE 49.1. Incidence of gallbladder disease by age.

may be further categorized as either black or brown, with black stones seen more commonly in the presence of hemolytic disease or hepatic cirrhosis. Brown pigment stones are typically seen in Asian patients and are associated with biliary infection.[16] At the time of cholecystectomy, the percentage of stones that are pigmented increases with advancing age.[17] Whether the type of stone is related to the subsequent development of symptoms is debatable, but the differentiation between cholesterol and pigment stones is important when nonoperative management is considered, as black pigment stones are resistant to dissolution therapy.[18]

## Pathogenesis

### *Cholesterol Stones*

The pathogenesis of cholesterol stones involves a series of defects that ultimately lead to the formation of stones. These pathogenic factors include cholesterol hypersecretion with subsequent supersaturation of bile, gallbladder hypomotility leading to bile stasis, cholesterol crystallization in bile serving as a nidus for stone formation, hypersecretion of gallbladder mucus,[19] and increased concentration of biliary calcium.[20]

Hypersecretion of cholesterol is considered the primary requisite factor for the development of cholesterol gallstones in the Western world.[21] Cholesterol supersaturation of bile results mainly from increased secretion of cholesterol into bile by hepatocytes.[22] The increased hepatic secretion of cholesterol may result from a primary increase in hepatic synthesis of cholesterol[23] or secondary upregulation of cholesterol synthesis related to decreases in enzyme activity for hepatic bile salt and cholesterol ester synthesis.[24] This increased hepatic cholesterol secretion is associated with higher cytosolic cholesterol concentrations within hepatocytes.[25] Advancing age is associated with increased biliary secretion of cholesterol and decreased hepatic bile salt synthesis.[26] The increased biliary secretion of cholesterol may be related to changes in enzyme activity that occur with aging, namely a decrease in the activity of 7-α-hydroxylase and an increase in the activity of 3-hydroxy-3-methylglutaryl coenzyme A (HMG-CoA) reductase.[11] These changes in cholesterol secretion and bile salt synthesis may contribute to the increased prevalence of cholelithiasis in the elderly population.

Other factors may contribute to cholesterol supersaturation of bile in the elderly. One is the use of exogenous estrogens, which results in hypersecretion of cholesterol in both men and women.[12,13] Another is alteration in the serum lipid profile, although the relation between serum cholesterol and the formation of cholesterol gallstones is less clear. Increased risk of cholesterol stone formation does not correlate with total serum cholesterol levels but does seem to be related to diminished serum high density lipoprotein (HDL) and increased serum triglycerides.[27]

Although most patients with cholesterol gallstones have cholesterol hypersaturation of their bile,[28] increased biliary cholesterol is present in nearly half of normal individuals who do not have gallstone disease.[29] Thus the development of cholesterol stones is dependent on the presence of lithogenic factors in addition to increased cholesterol saturation of bile. This is further exemplified by considering nucleation time, which is defined as the number of days required for the formation of cholesterol monohydrate crystals in crystal-free bile incubated at 37°C in the dark. For any given level of cholesterol hypersaturation, the nucleation time is shorter in bile from patients with gallstone disease than in bile from gallstone-free individuals.[30] This may be related to the presence of promoters of nucleation, such as calcium bilirubinate,[31] or to the absence of inhibitors of nucleation, such as apolipoprotein A-I and A-II.[32]

One factor that may promote nucleation is the effect of cholesterol hypersecretion on gallbladder production of mucin. Normally, the gallbladder mucosa constantly secretes mucin glycoproteins, which are then expunged from the gallbladder and enter the duodenum.[33] Secretion of mucin glycoproteins by gallbladder epithelium is greatly increased during the formation of cholesterol gallstones.[24] Mucin gel has been identified as a potent agent promoting cholesterol crystallization in animal models[24] and humans.[34] Cholesterol supersaturation of bile is known to induce gallbladder production of mucin glycoproteins.[35] Production of mucin glycoproteins may also be induced by increased mucosal synthesis of prostanoids[33] or the toxicity of increased secondary bile salts in lithogenic bile.[36]

Increased concentrations of calcium in bile may also contribute to the formation of cholesterol gallstones.[37,38] Bile from patients with cholesterol cholelithiasis is typically supersaturated with calcium.[39] Calcium salts are frequently found in the center of both pigment and cholesterol gallstones, indicating their potential role in the development of these stones. A study of human gallstones from patients undergoing cholecystectomy demonstrated centrally located calcium salt precipitates in 88% of cholesterol stones and 100% of pigment stones.[40] Ionized calcium has been shown to reduce the solubility of biliary cholesterol[41] and accelerate cholesterol nucleation.[42] It has also been demonstrated to increase gallbladder production of mucin glycoproteins, thus indirectly promoting cholesterol crystallization.[43] In animal models of gallstone disease, there is a linear correlation between increased biliary calcium concentration and increased biliary protein, which may potentiate the pronucleating effects of both calcium and protein.[38] It is postulated that defects in gallbladder pH regulation may contribute to calcium supersaturation.[44] Increases in intracellular calcium may modify the absorptive and secretory capacity of the gallbladder mucosa, tipping the balance toward secretion and contributing to lithogenesis.[45]

In addition to factors related to bile composition, decreased gallbladder motility plays a significant role in gallstone formation. The risk of gallstone formation is significantly increased by conditions that impair normal gallbladder emptying, such as pregnancy,[46] treatment with total parenteral nutrition (TPN),[47] octreotide therapy for acromegaly,[48] diabetes mellitus,[49] sickle cell anemia,[50] and in patients who have suffered spinal cord injury[51] or who have undergone truncal vagotomy.[52]

Normally, there is a continuous flow of bile in and out of the gallbladder. The greatest flow of gallbladder bile is stimulated by food consumption,[53] which causes gallbladder contraction in a triphasic pattern of emptying, refilling, then emptying again.[4] Gallbladder emptying and refilling also occurs during fasting. Nearly 10% of gallbladder volume is ejected during fasting in association with migrating motor complexes (MMCs) in the duodenum.[54] This facilitates exchange of bile between the common duct and the gallbladder and may prevent stratification of bile within the gallbladder itself.[14] Gallbladder motility is influenced by several neurohumoral mechanisms. The entry of food into the duodenum stimulates the release of cholecystokinin (CCK) by intestinal endocrine cells. CCK has several effects, including increasing the flow of hepatic bile into the biliary tree and contracting the gallbladder with concomitant relaxation of the sphincter of Oddi.[14] Nearly three-fourths of the gallbladder volume is ejected in response to CCK,[55] with approximately 15% released prior to the onset of gastric emptying. The effect of CCK is modulated by several other peptide hormones as well. Secretin has no intrinsic effect on gallbladder motility, but it significantly potentiates the effects of CCK.[56] Somatostatin inhibits CCK-mediated gallbladder contraction and is thought to act as a physiologic "brake."[55] Other inhibitors of CCK-mediated gallbladder contraction include vasoactive intestinal polypetide (VIP),[57] pancreatic polypeptide,[58] and peptide YY.[59] In addition to CCK, several neurohumoral agents have prokinetic effects on gallbladder motility, including neuropeptide Y,[60] motilin,[61] substance P,[62] gastrin-releasing peptide,[63] and prostaglandins.[64] Parasympathetic (vagal) activity has a significant role in maintaining resting gallbladder tone,[53] and nitric oxide appears to play a role in gallbladder relaxation.[65]

In addition to neurohumoral control mechanisms, gallbladder motility may be influenced by the degree of cholesterol saturation of bile. Animal and human studies suggest that cholesterol hypersaturation of bile attenuates gallbladder motility. In animal models, 1 week of cholesterol feeding reduces the gallbladder ejection fraction from 76% to 26%.[66] Gallbladder contraction is considerably diminished in patients with cholesterolosis, or "strawberry gallbladder."[67] The ability to contract both spontaneously and in response to stimulation with CCK, acetylcholine, and potassium chloride is markedly reduced in gallbladders from patients with cholesterol cholelithiasis.[67] The presence of excess cholesterol within bile may lead to the esterification and storage of cholesterol within the mucosa and muscle cells of the gallbladder.[68] This may affect motility through cholesterol incorporation within cell membranes[24] or by altering intracellular stores of calcium secondary to changes in the membrane of the endoplasmic reticulum.[69] The decrease in gallbladder motility may also be mediated via an inositol triphosphate ($IP_3$)-related mechanism, as addition of $IP_3$ in vitro abrogates these effects.[70]

Several features surrounding gallbladder hypomotility contribute to the development of gallstones. Hypomotility promotes nucleation by allowing bile stasis to occur.[71] Hypomotility and bile stasis may divert a large fraction of hepatic bile into the duodenum, leading to contraction of the bile salt pool required to solubilize biliary cholesterol.[72] Additionally, an increase in the concentration of hydrophobic bile salts may directly damage muscle cells of the gallbladder,[73] further impairing gallbladder motility and worsening the degree of stasis. Chronic inflammatory changes within the gallbladder epithelium[20] may occur secondary to bile stasis with resultant bacterial overgrowth.[6]

Bile stasis may also lead to the formation of biliary sludge, a viscous aggregate composed of mucin glycoproteins, calcium bilirubinate, and cholesterol crystals.[14] The presence of sludge in the gallbladder can be detected by ultrasonography, and its formation is typically related to the presence of lithogenic bile and gallbladder hypomotility.[74] Biliary sludge has been found in 50% of patients receiving TPN for a period of 6 weeks and in nearly 100% of those receiving TPN for more than 6 weeks.[75] This is thought to be related to the lack of oral intake during therapy with TPN,[47] as enteral feeding may reverse the process of biliary sludge deposition.[75] The formation of both cholesterol and pigment stones is virtually always anteceded by the presence of biliary sludge.[6]

Investigation into the effects of aging on gallbladder motility have been confined primarily to changes in neurohumoral control mechanisms, particularly age-related changes in CCK sensitivity. In animal studies, aging is associated with a decrease in the gallbladder contractile reponse to CCK, which appears to be related to a decrease in the number of CCK receptors.[76] The increased incidence of gallstone formation seen in old animals can be prevented by the administration of exogenous CCK.[77] Human studies have also demonstrated markedly reduced gallbladder sensitivity to CCK with aging, but there appears to be a compensatory elevation in the level of serum CCK.[78] In addition to changes in CCK activity, aging is associated with increased levels of pancreatic polypeptide,[79] which may contribute to bile stasis because of decreased gallbladder contractility and increased sphincter of Oddi pressures.

### Pigmented Stones

Despite their relatively low incidence in the United States, pigment stones are the most common type of gallstone worldwide.[80] The etiology and pathogenesis differ between black and brown pigment stones. Black pigment stones form in the presence of increased secretion of bilirubin conjugates, which typically occurs with chronic hemolysis and to some degree with hepatic cirrhosis.[24] Normally, unconjugated bilirubin produced by the action of β-glucuronidase constitutes less than 1% of the total bile pigments.[81] In patients with hemolytic disease, the percent of unconjugated bilirubin may increase more than 10-fold,[82] thus exceeding its solubility in bile. The unconjugated bilirubin precipitates with calcium ions, leading to the formation of insoluble calcium salts.[83] Most pigment stones are composed primarily of calcium bilirubinate[79] and generally form in sterile bile.[84] The incidence of black pigment stones seems to be increased in the elderly population.[17]

Brown pigment stones form in the presence of chronic anaerobic infection of bile.[85] This particular type of pigment stone is endemic to Asia, probably owing to the high incidence of biliary infection in this area of the world.[86] The finding of significantly increased bacterial β-glucuronidase activity in the bile of patients with brown pigment stones is supporting evidence that biliary infection is an important etiologic factor.[87] The pathogenesis of brown pigment stones also involves biliary stasis, which predisposes to biliary infection.[81] The incidence of brown pigment stones in the common bile duct in the presence of preexisting cholelithiasis increases with age, probably owing to decreased biliary motility with subsequent stasis and infection of bile.[88]

## Natural History

### Asymptomatic Stones

Few studies have addressed the natural history of gallstone disease, particularly in the aged population. Understanding the natural history of cholelithiasis has become increasingly important with the widespread use of abdominal ultrasonography, as the incidental finding of gallstones occurs with significant frequency.[89] This is particularly pertinent in elderly patients in whom the prevalence of cholelithiasis is known to be much higher than in the general population.

Several studies have attempted to describe the natural history of asymptomatic gallstone disease, mainly focusing on the rate of symptom development and complications. Gallstone disease is considered symptomatic with the development of biliary pain or any of its associated complications such as acute cholecystitis, biliary obstruction, or biliary pancreatitis.[90]

An early report from the 1940s cited the development of symptoms in nearly 50% of patients with known gallstones when followed for 10–20 years. The complication rate in this study was roughly 19% over 15 years, accounting for an annual complication rate of approximately 1.4%.[91] In contrast, Gracie and Ransohoff reported much lower rates for the development of symptoms and associated complications.[92] The probability of symptom development in the presence of cholelithiasis in this study was estimated to be only 15% at 10 years and 18% at 15 and 20 years; the complication rate was approximately 20% in those who became symptomatic. Based on these findings, Gracie and Ransohoff introduced the concept of the "innocent gallstone." The population in their study, however, consisted of exclusively white, predominantly male subjects with a mean age of 54 years who had documented gallstone disease on oral cholecystography.[92] Atilli et al.[93] questioned the results of Gracie and Ransohoff[92] and reviewed the natural history of both asymptomatic and symptomatic gallstones in a much more representative population. The probability of symptom development in asymptomatic individuals in their study was nearly 12% at 2 years, 16.5% at 4 years, and close to 26% at 10 years. The complication rate in this study was approximately 3% after 10 years. The authors concluded that the natural history of gallstone disease is less benign than suggested by the studies of Gracie and Ransohoff.[92] A conservative annual rate of symptom development of approximately 2% with about 1.5% requiring cholecystectomy was reported by McSherry et al. in their study of 691 patients with gallstone disease enrolled in a large health maintenance organization.[94] Based on all of these studies it can be estimated that serious symptoms and complications of gallstone disease are likely to occur at an annual rate of about 2% in those with cholelithiasis, with roughly two-thirds of patients remaining asymptomatic over a period of 20 years.[95] In light of this information, prophylactic cholecystectomy for asymptomatic cholelithiasis in the general population is not recommended.[96]

The natural history of asymptomatic gallstones in the elderly is much less well defined. Studies that have included a significant number of older individuals have shown that elderly patients are more likely to present with complications of gallstone disease. In a study of 750 patients with gallstone disease, Wenckhert and Robertson demonstrated that nearly half of these patients developed severe complications within 11 years after the diagnosis of cholelithiasis.[97] Additionally, the complications of biliary disease are much less likely to be preceded by the typical symptoms ordinarily exhibited by younger individuals with biliary tract disease. In one study, nearly 80% of those who died from complications of gallbladder disease were previously classified as "asymptomatic."[98] Given the atypical presentation of gallstone disease and the relatively high rate of complicated gallstone disease in the elderly, the asymptomatic gallstone may never be truly "innocent" in this patient population.[6]

A related issue over the years has been the natural history of asymptomatic gallstone disease in the diabetic population. This has great significance when considering the risks of asymptomatic gallstones in the elderly, as the incidence of diabetes increases with age.

During the early 1950s, Liebner reported the incidence of cholelithiasis and its relation to associated disease conditions in his study of 29,779 autopsies of patients aged 20 to more than 90 years. The overall prevalence of gallstone disease in this study was 11.6%, but in diabetic patients the prevalence was 30.2%.[99] The prognosis of acute cholecystitis was also reported to be much less favorable in diabetic patients in a report by Mundth during the 1960s.[100] Both operative mortality and postoperative complications were significantly higher in diabetic patients undergoing cholecystectomy for acute cholecystitis in a series of 145 patients admitted to the Massachusetts General Hospital with a diagnosis of diabetes mellitus and either acute or chronic cholecystitis.[100] In a study by Turill et al.[101] of 481 patients admitted to Los Angeles County Hospital during 1953–1958, the mortality rate was nearly 20% in diabetic patients requiring surgery for complications of their gallstone disease. The authors concluded that prophylactic cholecystectomy should be considered in most diabetic patients before they attain old age.[101]

More recent studies have led to reexamination of this issue.[102,103] Ransohoff et al.[102] reported a significantly lower case-fatality rate in their study of 311 patients admitted to Cleveland Clinic Hospital between 1960 and 1981 for the management of acute cholecystitis. Their case-fatality rate of 7% for diabetic patients with acute cholecystitis is drastically lower than that reported by Mundth some 26 years earlier.[100] This difference in outcome was attributed to improvements in medical care, including the availability of antibiotics.[102] Other investigators[104] have corroborated the lower mortality rates reported by Ransohoff et al.[102]

The risk of elective surgery is an additional factor when considering the role of prophylactic cholecystectomy in diabetic patients. Sandler et al.[105] demonstrated that diabetic patients have higher complication rates following elective and emergent surgery when compared to patients without diabetes. Similar findings were reported by Hjortrup et al.[106] This increased morbidity in diabetic patients is most likely related to advanced age[105,107] and the presence of co-morbid conditions.[105]

Del Favero et al.[108] prospectively studied the natural history of gallstones in patients with non-insulin-dependent diabetes mellitus (NIDDM). In a study of 440 patients with NIDDM, they found similar rates of symptom development, complications, and cholecystectomy when compared to the general population.[108] Although a few may still disagree,[90] it is generally acknowledged that cholecystectomy should not be performed prophylactically in the diabetic population.[108]

Gallstones may be discovered when patients undergo laparotomy for other reasons. Incidental cholecystectomy is generally recommended in elderly patients undergoing abdominal surgery, provided the surgical incision affords adequate exposure and the patient's condition warrants the additional procedure.[109] Ouriel et al.[110] reported no significant increase in operative mortality, duration of operation, or length of hospital stay in their study of 18 patients who underwent concomitant abdominal aortic aneurysmectomy and cholecystectomy. Nine of eleven patients in the study with cholelithiasis who underwent aneurysmectomy without cholecystectomy developed acute cholecystitis during a 3-year follow-up period.[110] Other studies, however, have demonstrated a slightly higher rate of wound infection and increased length of hospital stay.[111]

### *Symptomatic Gallstones*

The natural history of symptomatic gallstones is understandably different from that of asymptomatic gallstones. Studies on the natural history of symptomatic cholelithiasis are somewhat sparse, as treatment is customarily recommended for patients within this population. Some studies are available, however. Annual rates of severe symptom development and cholecystectomy in patients with mildly symptomatic cholelithiasis were 44.0% and 3.2%, respectively, in the National Cooperative Gallstone Study.[112] Annual rates for cholecystectomy in patients with severe symptoms are typically 6–8%.[113] The rate of complications is not significantly different between patients with symptomatic and asymptomatic gallstone disease,[98] suggesting that the presence or absence of symptoms is not a reliable prognostic indicator for the development of complications in cholelithiasis.

## Symptomatic Cholelithiasis

The typical initial presentation of symptomatic gallstone disease is that of biliary colic or chronic cholecystitis.[114] Elderly patients are less likely to present with the "typical" symptoms of gallstone disease experienced by younger individuals.[2] Furthermore, elderly patients may present with complications of gallstone disease without any precursor symptoms of chronic cholecystitis.[115] Morrow et al.[116] reported minimal or absent prior symptoms in nearly 40% of elderly patients presenting with grave complications, such as gangrenous cholecystitis, gallbladder empyema, or gallbladder perforation. Because of atypical symptomatology and the predilection for presenting with complicated gallstone disease, clinicians must have a high index of suspicion for biliary tract disease when caring for elderly patients.

### *Chronic Cholecystitis*

The pain associated with chronic cholecystits, often referred to as biliary colic, is produced by a stone obstructing the cystic duct.[117] The term "colic" is deceiving, as the pain is abrupt in onset and constant in nature, unlike true "colicky" pain that is characterized by a waxing and waning course.[16] The pain is typically located in the right upper quadrant or epigastrium. Although radiation of pain is classically to the right shoulder or the inferior angle of the scapula, the pain may also radiate to other areas of the thorax or abdomen.[10] The pain usually occurs at night, often around midnight,[118] and lasts several hours. The frequency of recurrent pain varies among individuals, with intervals between attacks of pain ranging from days to weeks to occasionally months.[119]

Patients may also present with nonspecific symptoms, such as bloating, gassiness, indigestion, nausea, and fatty food intolerance.[121–122] Elderly patients are more likely to present with dyspepsia and vague epigastric discomfort.[123] The nonspecific nature of biliary symptoms commonly seen in aged patients, along with the multiplicity of coexisting gastrointestinal problems, clearly contribute to delays in diagnosis and treatment.[116]

Physical examination of the symptomatic patient may yield right upper quadrant tenderness but is likely to be normal when the patient is not experiencing symptoms. Laboratory values are usually normal with chronic cholecystitis.

Based primarily on the history, a diagnosis of chronic cholecystitis is confirmed by establishing the presence of gallstones. The use of ultrasonography to detect cholelithiasis is clearly established.[125] Gallstones are best visualized when the gallbladder is examined in both axial and sagittal planes after 8 hours of fasting.[125] Gallstones typically appear as echogenic foci that demonstrate acoustic shadowing and gravitational dependence. Ultrasonogrphy may detect stones as small as 1–2 mm in size, which when multiple, are often characterized as "gravel."[125] Gallbladder sludge, in contrast to gravel, appears as an echogenic layer that does not cast an acoustic shadow and is less gravitationally dependent.[126] The sensitivity and specificity of ultrasonography for cholelithiasis when chronic cholecystitis is suspected are 0.95 and 0.97, respectively.[127,128]

In addition to detecting the presence of gallstones, ultrasonography provides structural information about the gallbladder itself and the biliary ductal system. The ability to detect significant biliary ductal dilatation is particularly useful in the elderly because of the high incidence of common bile duct stones. Furthermore, information is provided about the liver, kidneys, and pancreas. For all these reasons, ultrasonography is the diagnostic study of choice for gallstone disease.

Several other radiologic studies can yield information about the biliary tree but have little role in the diagnosis of chronic cholecystitis. Plain roentgenography alone has limited usefulness in the diagnosis of cholelithiasis, as most of the stones are radiolucent.[129] Fewer than 20% of gallstones can be visualized on plain radiographs of the abdomen.[125] Abdominal CT is far less sensitive than ultrasonography for detecting gallstones,[130] as most stones are of the same attenuation as bile and therefore not well visualized. Cholescintigraphy has limited usefulness in the routine diagnosis of chronic cholecystitis, as it cannot provide anatomic information or identify gallstones.[131] In atypical cases of classic biliary symptomatology with no ultrasonographic abnormalities, the functional information provided by cholescintigraphy becomes important. In such cases, analyzing gallbladder motility in response to a prokinetic agent may be the only means of establishing gallbladder pathology.[14] It must be emphasized, however, that these atypical cases are rare.

When considering treatment for patients with symptomatic cholelithiasis, the natural history of the disease, the general life expectancy and medical condition of the individual, and the risks and benefits of the various treatment modalities are all factors that must be noted.[133] Expectant management of symptomatic gallstone disease is generally not advisable, as severe symptom development in patients with mildly symptomatic cholelithiasis is reported to be as high as 44% per year.[112] Particularly in the elderly, the risk of developing complicated biliary disease requiring emergent treatment with attendant high mortality, weighs strongly in favor of definitive treatment of symptomatic gallstones in an elective setting.

The definitive treatment for gallstone disease is cholecystectomy,[5] which is performed in patients with chronic cholecystitis to relieve symptoms and prevent potentially life-threatening complications.[134] Prior to the introduction of laparoscopic cholecystectomy, open cholecystectomy had been the gold standard for treating cholelithiasis for more than a century.[16] A comprehensive review by Roslyn et al.[135] of 42,474 open cholecystectomies performed at all non-Veterans Administration (VA) acute care hospitals in California and Maryland for a 12-month period, indicated that open cholecystectomy was a safe, effective treatment for gallstone disease. The study, which included patients undergoing emergent and elective cholecystectomy, reported an overall mortality rate of 0.17%.[135] This is significantly lower than the mortality rate of 1.77% reported by Glenn more than 15 years ago.[136] In this more contemporary study, however, advanced age (more than 65 years) was associated with significantly higher mortality (0.5% vs. 0.03%) and complication (25.7% vs. 10.1%) rates than for the less than 65-year-old group. Significant increases in length of stay and in-hospital charges were also noted in aged patients.[135] These results are consistent with those of other investigators.[137,138]

An extensive study by Escarce et al.[139] analyzed the outcomes of open cholecystectomy strictly in the elderly population before the era of laparoscopic procedures for gallstone disease. The postoperative mortality rate in this series, which included both emergency and elective surgery, was 2.1% at 60 days and 3.6% at 90 days. The 30-day postoperative mortality rate nearly doubled when common bile duct exploration was performed in addition to cholecystectomy. Postoperative complications occurred in almost 20% of patients and were most commonly secondary to cardiovascular events, pneumonia, urinary tract infections, and wound infections.[139]

Several factors contribute to the increased mortality and complication rates following open cholecystectomy in aged patients. A primary factor is the larger proportion of elderly patients compared to younger patients requiring emergency rather than elective cholecystectomy. Pigott and Williams[138] studied a group of 347 patients over 65 years of age who underwent open cholecystectomy for symptomatic gallstone disease. More than half of the patients in this study presented with an acute complication of gallstone disease, and they often required emergent surgical procedures. There may be multiple reasons for the greater tendency of the elderly to present with complicated gallstone disease. The early diagnosis of symptomatic gallstone disease at an uncomplicated stage (i.e., simple chronic cholecystitis) may not be made as readily, as elderly patients are more likely to present with atypical symptoms such as dyspepsia and vague epigastric discomfort.[123] Elderly patients are also more likely to present with complications of gallstone disease without antecedent symptoms of chronic cholecystitis.[115] Of those presenting with acute gallstone disease, a significant proportion of elderly patients have major complications (i.e., gangrenous cholecystitis, gallbladder empyema, free perforation) present with minimal or absent symptoms.[140] Finally, the increased incidence of choledocholithiasis adds to the complexity of biliary disease in the elderly.[141,142]

Laparoscopic cholecystectomy has changed the surgical management of symptomatic cholelithiasis dramatically since its advent during the late 1980s.[143] First performed in France by Dr. Phillipe Mouret in 1987,[144] and in the United States by McKernan and Saye in 1988 and Olsen and Reddick in 1989,[145] laparoscopic cholecystectomy is now established as the procedure of choice for symptomatic gallstone disease in the United States[146] and many other countries.[147] The laparoscopic approach offers many advantages when compared to open cholecystectomy, including reduced postoperative pain, shorter hospital stay and recovery, improved cosmetic results,[148] and lower cost.[149] The reduction of postoperative pain is a major benefit, resulting in decreased analgesic requirement and improved pulmonary function following surgery.[150]

Mortality rates for laparoscopic cholecystectomy are reportedly lower than those of open cholecystectomy in reviews of both European[147] and U.S. experiences,[151] averaging about 0.1%. One of the largest reported series is that of the Southern Surgeons Club, which included more than 1500 patients who underwent laparoscopic cholecystectomy for symptomatic cholelithiasis.[152] This study reported a 4.7% conversion rate to open cholecystectomy and a complication rate of 5.1%.[152] The most signficant complication of laparoscopic cholecystectomy is major bile duct injury, which is reported to occur in 5–10 per 1000 cases.[153] Bile duct injury tends to occur early in a surgeon's experience with laparoscopy.[154] A more recent study by the Southern Surgeons Club reported that 90% of bile duct injuries occurred during the first 30 cases performed by individual surgeons, clearly supporting the existence of a learning curve for laparoscopic cholecystectomy.[155] The overall complication rate for laparoscopic cholecystectomy is noted to be significantly lower than that of open cholecystectomy.[156]

Conversion to open cholecystectomy is generally required in approximately 5% of patients undergoing laparoscopic cholecystectomy,[157] most commonly because adhesions and chronic inflammation preclude the laparoscopic approach.[152] Advanced age, male gender, obesity, acute cholecystitis, and the presence of a thickened gallbladder wall on ultrasonography are factors associated with a significantly increased rate of conversion from laparoscopic to open cholecystectomy.[158] A study based on the Connecticut Laparoscopic Cholecystectomy Registry, reported a correlation between conversion rates and age among elderly patients. Conversion was necessary in roughly 8% of those aged 70–74 years, 12% of those aged 75–80 years, and more than 12% of those over 80 years of age.[146] Although conversion to an open procedure is not a complication of laparoscopic surgery and should never have a negative connotation, an appreciation for the likelihood of conversion is important when considering the risk of laparoscopic surgery in an elderly patient.

Laparoscopic cholecystectomy has significant implications in the treatment of elderly patients with gallstone disease. Several studies have reported favorable results in elderly individuals undergoing the laparoscopic procedure compared to those with the open approach.[159–162] A study of 233 patients by Massie et al.,[159] demonstrated a sevenfold reduction in postoperative morbidity following laparoscopic cholecystectomy compared to open cholecystectomy in elderly patients and younger patients with clinically significant associated illnesses. A more extensive study of 1677 patients at McGill University reported similar results.[160] As expected, elderly patients in this study were much more likely to present with evidence of complicated gallstone disease and were nearly twice as likely to require conversion to open cholecystectomy.[160] The mortality rate of 0.6% for elderly patients was roughly five times higher than that for patients under 65 years of age[160] but was markedly lower than rates reported for open cholecystectomy in the same age group.[5] Complication rates were also significantly lower after laparoscopic cholecystectomy in the elderly[160] compared to the complication rate following open cholecystectomy.[139] In particular, laparoscopic cholecystectomy in the older patients results in less postoperative impairment of pulmonary function compared to open cholecystectomy.[163]

There are few absolute contraindications to laparoscopic cholecystectomy. These include an uncorrected coagulopathy and the inability to tolerate general anesthesia.[16] Conditions that may increase a patient's risks for postoperative complications of laparoscopic cholecystectomy include cardiopulmonary disease, immunosuppression, and cirrhosis with portal hypertension.[164] These factors are particularly pertinent during the preoperative risk assessment of elderly patients, as their presence is associated with an increased frequency of complications.[162]

For those patients who are unwilling or unable to tolerate cholecystectomy, the nonoperative methods for treating chronic cholecystitis are primarily oral and contact dissolution as well as extracorporeal shock wave lithotripsy. These methods are limited by their variable efficacy, requiring careful patient selection. Furthermore, even when they successfully achieve clearance of gallstones, the rate of recurrent cholelithiasis approaches 50% over 5 years.[16] It must be noted that although these methods may find application in the treatment of uncomplicated symptomatic cholelithiasis, they should not be used to treat complicated gallstone disease.[165]

Oral dissolution therapy involves the use of litholytic bile acids. These substances act primarily by inhibiting the enzyme HMG-CoA reductase, thus decreasing the biosynthesis of cholesterol and the saturation of cholesterol in bile.[165] Chenodeoxycholic acid (CDCA) was the first of these agents to be used in the dissolution of gallstones.[166] CDCA had an unfavorable side effect profile and poor efficacy and in 1988 was replaced by ursodeoxycholic acid (UDCA).[167] Patients eligible for UDCA therapy include those with a history of biliary colic, radiolucent stones less than 1.5–2.0 cm in diameter, and a functional gallbladder. By these selection criteria, only 10–20% of those undergoing cholecystectomy would be eligible for UDCA therapy.[5] The dose is 8–10 mg/kg/day,[165] and the expense of therapy is approximately $2000 per year.[5] Although better than the results with CDCA, treatment with UDCA has limited efficacy, with complete dissolution occurring in 40% and partial dissolution in 20% after 2 years of therapy.[168]

For contact dissolution therapy, a catheter is placed transhepatically into the gallbladder, and organic solvents are infused to dissolve gallstones. This method of treatment was first used in 1891 by Walker,[169] 9 years after Langenbuch reported the use of cholecystectomy to treat symptomatic gallstone disease.[170] Its use was reevaluated in 1972 when Admirand and Way reported use of contact dissolution therapy to eradicate retained common duct stones.[171] The most commonly used solvent is methyl *tert*-butyl ether (MTBE). The efficacy of contact dissolution with MTBE is reported to be quite high, with complete dissolution of stones in more than 90% of patients.[172] Disadvantages of this technique, however, include a relatively high recurrence rate[173] and cost.

Extracorporeal shock wave lithotripsy (ESWL) for the treatment of gallstones was introduced in 1985.[174] It is used to fragment gallstones into particles small enough to be expelled by a functional gallbladder and often requires the use of general or epidural anesthesia.[175] Patients eligible for ESWL include those with a history of biliary colic who have one to three radiolucent stones with a combined diameter not exceeding 3 cm and a functional gallbladder.[5] The combination of ESWL and UDCA clears stone fragments in nearly 90% of patients after 1 year,[174] but 9% of patients are reported to have recurrent cholelithiasis 1 year after termination of therapy with UDCA.[176] The expense of therapy with ESWL is also noted to be quite high.[177]

In summary, laparoscopic cholecystectomy has found wide application for treatment of chronic cholecystitis, regardless of age, and has largely supplanted open cholecystectomy as the new gold standard, particularly in the young. The overall improvement in mortality rates and the clear demonstration of the benefits of laparoscopic compared to open cholecystectomy specifically in the elderly, makes it the preferred procedure for definitive treatment of chronic cholecystitis even in the elderly. The crux is diagnosing symptomatic gallstone disease at an early stage to allow elective rather than emergency cholecystectomy. Although it must be acknowledged that age increases the risk for cholecystectomy, it is crucial to understand how this risk is magnified when emergency surgery is required.

### Acute Cholecystitis

Acute cholecystitis is by far the most common complication of gallstone disease. It typically results from cystic duct obstruction due to impaction of a stone in the cystic duct itself or in Hartmann's pouch, with resultant bile stasis and distension of the gallbladder.[119] The consequent mucosal release of lysolecithin, prostaglandins, and phospholipase A result in local inflammation.[178] Bile becomes secondarily infected, resulting in positive bile cultures in nearly three-fourths of patients with acute cholecystitis.[16] The organisms most commonly isolated include *Escherichia coli*, *Klebsiella*, and *Enterococcus* species.[3]

The classic presentation of acute cholecystitis includes fever and localized right upper quadrant abdominal pain.[4] Initially the pain may resemble that of biliary colic, but it differs in its longer duration and greater propensity to localize to the right upper quadrant. Patients often have associated nausea and vomiting. Physical examination typically yields right upper quadrant tenderness and a positive Murphy's sign. Laboratory values usually reveal a mild to moderate polymorphonuclear leukocytosis and may demonstrate a mild rise in transaminases, bilirubin, and alkaline phosphatase,[3] but liver function studies are not universally elevated in those patients experiencing acute cholecystitis.[120]

Acute cholecystitis in the elderly can be a diagnostic challenge, as the presentation is commonly atypical[179] and may vary widely. Abdominal pain remains a common presenting symptom[117] but is often not accompanied by nausea, vomiting, fever,[6] or leukocytosis.[116] Symptoms, however, may be minimal and the presentation may be nonspecific mental and physical disability alone.[124] At the opposite end of the spectrum, nearly 12% of elderly patients with acute cholecystitis present in septic shock.[180] The physical examination may also be misleading. Morrow et al.[116] reported that nearly 40% of elderly patients presenting with acute cholecystitis were afebrile, and more than half did not have peritoneal signs on examination. The absence of these findings did not correlate with milder disease, as 40% of the patients studied had severe complications including gallbladder empyema, gangrenous cholecystitis, and gallbladder perforation.[116] Given the variability and atypical features of presentation, the initial diagnostic accuracy of acute abdominal pain in patients over age 80 is only 29%, which is significantly lower than in younger patients.[181]

When acute cholecystitis is suspected, the diagnosis may be established by the ultrasonographic findings of gallbladder distension and wall thickening with intramural sonolucency, pericholecystic fluid, cholelithiasis or gallbladder sludge (or both), and a sonographic Murphy's sign.[125] Ultrasonography may also provide valuable information about the status of the pancreas and biliary tree.[4] It is important to recognize, however, that the presence of gallbladder wall thickening or fluid around the gallbladder may not be specific for acute cholecystitis.[126,127] A review by Shea et al.[128] reported the sensitivity and specificity of ultrasonography for acute cholecystitis as 94% and 78%, respectively.

Cholescintigraphy is also useful in the diagnosis of acute cholecystitis. Visualization of the gallbladder typically occurs within half an hour of the administration of tracer.[128] If the gallblader fails to visualize after 45 minutes, an intravenous dose of morphine may facilitate visualization by promoting sphincter of Oddi contraction, thereby diverting flow of tracer into the gallbladder,[182] assuming that the cystic duct is patent. Nonvisualization of the gallbladder indicates obstruction of the cystic duct, a finding that is highly suggestive of acute cholecystitis.[119] The sensitivity and specificity of cholescintigraphy for acute cholecystitis are 93% and 91%, respectively.[128]

The mainstay of treatment for acute cholecystitis in patients of any age is the combination of cholecystectomy and appropriate antibiotic therapy.[4] In the elderly, however, the need for emergency cholecystectomy has significant implications. Cholecystectomy is performed more frequently as an emergency procedure in the elderly than the young. In those older than age 65 having cholecystectomy, the proportion done as an emergency was 37.6% compared to only 3.3% in younger patients.[184] Although the mortality rate is higher for emergency than elective cholecystectomy in all age groups, the risk associated with emergency cholecystectomy is greatly magnified in the elderly, resulting in a mortality rate of nearly 10%.[141] This considerably poorer outcome may be related to the greater likelihood of elderly patients to present with complications of acute cholecystitis, such as gangrenous cholecystitis, empyema, and perforation of the gallbladder.[116] Postoperative morbidity, particularly cardiovascular and pulmonary complications, is also significantly greater after emergent cholecystectomy for acute cholecystitis than after elective cholecystectomy in elderly patients.[183–185]

As mentioned previously, laparoscopic cholecystectomy is now considered the new gold standard treatment for elective management of chronic cholecystitis.[148] The additional role of laparoscopic cholecystectomy in the treatment of acute cholecystitis, however, has only recently come into consideration.[186] Several studies have attempted to assess the suitability of this approach in patients with acute cholecystitis,[186–188] with a few focusing specifically on its appropriateness in elderly patients.[160,161,189]

In 1993, Zucker et al.[187] reported promising results in 83 patients who underwent laparoscopic cholecystectomy for acute cholecystitis. The morbidity and mortality rates were 16.8% and 0%, respectively, comparable to those for laparoscopic cholecystectomy performed for chronic cholecystitis.[187] The conversion rate to open cholecystectomy was 27%, expectedly higher than for elective laparascopic cholecystectomy. Conversion to an open procedure was most commonly required to allow safe dissection in the presence of severe inflammation and adhesions. Common bile duct stones were present in 8.4% of patients.[187] Studies of other investigators have yielded similar results,[186,188] indicating that morbidity and mortality rates compare favorably with those of open cholecystectomy for acute cholecystitis.[190]

The results of laparoscopic cholecystectomy in elderly patients with acute cholecystitis have been equally encouraging. Lo et al.[189] reported morbidity and mortality rates of 26.7% and 0%, respectively, in their study of elderly patients undergoing laparoscopic cholecystectomy for acute cholecystitis. The conversion rate to open cholecystectomy was comparable to that for the general population. Common bile duct stones were present in 4 of 10 elderly patients evaluated by endoscopic retrograde cholangiopancreatography (ERCP).[189] Elderly patients, however, had a longer hospital stay than those under age 65, owing to greater delays in resumption of regular diet and return to ambulatory status.[189]

Although cholecystectomy is the treatment of choice for acute cholecystitis, patients for whom the risk of immediate definitive surgery is considered too high may benefit from several forms of limited intervention. These methods are frequently used as temporizing procedures in critically ill patients who later can tolerate cholecystectomy.[191] Traditionally, decompression of the gallbladder by placing a tube that drained externally (cholecystostomy) was the operative alternative to cholecystectomy. The surgical approach to cholecystostomy has even been reported to be effective as a curative procedure in patients unable to tolerate a more extensive operation.[192] Percutaneous cholecystostomy may be performed under ultasound guidance at a patient's bedside.[193] Van Steenbergen et al. assessed the outcomes of elderly patients treated with cholecystostomy for complicated acute cholecystitis and demonstrated rapid improvement in all patients after percutaneous decompression of the gallbladder. Half of the patients studied underwent elective cholecystectomy 1–12 weeks after cholecystostomy.[194] Mortality rates for cholecystostomy are typically about 10% and relate largely to the severity of illness in patients requiring this procedure.[195] Morbidity is also acceptably low for this procedure.[196] Cholecystostomy tubes may be removed 4 weeks after resolution in elderly or debilitated patients who are not surgical candidates.[134] Endoscopic drainage has also been reported in patients with acute cholecystitis who are unable to tolerate surgery.[197]

### *Gallbladder Perforation*

Elderly patients are more likely than the young to suffer complications of acute cholecystitis, such as gangrenous cholecystitis, gallbladder perforation, and emphysematous cholecystitis.[4] Rates of gallbladder perforation in acute cholecystitis are reportedly as high as 8% in some series,[198] with associated mortality rates approaching 40% for acute rupture.[199] Perforation of the gallbladder may be categorized using the Niemeier classification as acute (type I) with associated bile peritonitis, subacute (type II) with abscess formation in the area of the gallbladder, or chronic (type III) with perforation and fistula formation between the gallbladder and either the skin, bile duct, or digestive tract.[200] Perforation typically occurs at the site of the gallbladder fundus, the area of least blood supply.[201] A study by Roslyn and Busutill demonstrated that this condition occurs more commonly in elderly patients, probably relating to gallbladder wall ischemia associated with atherosclerotic splanchnic vessels and limitations in cardiac output.[202] The mechanisms implicated in the development of gallbladder perforation involve obstruction of the cystic duct leading to gallbladder distension with subsequent vascular impairment resulting in ischemia, necrosis, and perforation of the wall.[203] It has also been noted that acute perforation is more common in young patients, whereas elderly patients are more likely to develop chronic perforation with fistula formation.[204] Complications of chronic perforation arise when gallstones traverse the fistulous tract and cause obstruction in areas of the gastrointestinal tract. Gallstone ileus accounts for nearly one-fourth of all cases of intestinal obstruction in aged patients.[205]

The clinical presentation of acute gallbladder perforation is similar to that of acute cholecystitis. Patients frequently present with abdominal pain, nausea, and fever. Laboratory findings typically include polymorphonuclear leukocytosis and elevations in transaminases as well as in alkaline phosphatase, $\gamma$-glutamyl transpeptidase, and bilirubin.[202] The diagnosis of gallbladder perforation can be aided by several diagnostic modalities, including plain abdominal films, ultrasonography, computed tomography (CT), cholangiography, and radionuclide scanning. Radiographic findings may include calculi within the right upper quadrant (representing spilled gallstones) or soft tissue masses within the area (suggesting the presence of a pericholecystic abscess).[206] Typical findings in gallstone ileus include evidence of a small bowel obstruction, air in the biliary tree, and a radiopaque density in the right lower quadrant.[4] Ultrasonographic findings of pericholecystic fluid collections with free peritoneal fluid, disappearance of the gallbladder wall, and findings consistent with emphysematous cholecystitis are highly suggestive of gallbladder perforation.[207] CT scanning has been shown to be superior to ultrasonography for diagnosing gallbladder perforation, using criteria of pericholecystic fluid collection, streaky omentum, and a gallbladder wall defect on CT.[208] Radionuclide scanning may reveal the characteristic "rim sign" of increased hepatic activity in the pericholecystic area with subacute perforation,[206] but it is less helpful for diagnosing gallbladder perforation in the setting of acute cholecystitis, as cystic duct obstruction prevents the flow of material into the gallbladder.[209]

The treatment of gallbladder perforation relates mainly to the acuteness of the problem and the presence of associated disease. Acute perforation is often not diagnosed preoperatively in patients undergoing cholecystectomy for acute cholecystitis.[201] One should have a high index of suspicion for acute perforation in any patient with a history of immune suppression or vascular disease who presents with abdominal tenderness localized to the right upper quadrant.[203] Initial management in patients with suspected acute perforation consists of intravenous hydration, nasogastric decompression, and antibiotic coverage followed by emergent cholecystectomy.[201] Morbidity and mortality rates following surgery approach 60% and 17%, respectively.[201] Chronic perforation tends to occur in older individuals with a history of longstanding cholelithiasis.[203] The presence of a perforated gallbladder with cholecystoenteric fistula is often recognized only when patients present with small bowel obstruction related to the gallstone.[204] Patients with this condition are treated by removal of the offending stone at laparotomy to relieve the obstruction. Cholecystectomy with fistula repair at the time of laparotomy is not recommended in these patients in the absence of acute biliary tract disease.[210]

### *Emphysematous Cholecystitis*

Another complication of acute cholecystitis that occurs with greater frequency in the elderly population is emphysematous cholecystitis,[211] which is a peculiar variant of acute cholecystitis caused by gas-forming bacteria.[212] It is characterized by the appearance of gas in the gallbladder lumen or wall on abdominal radiographs[213] and has an overall mortality rate approaching 15%.[12] It occurs more frequently in diabetic patients and is less likely to be associated with stones than is the usual form of acute cholecystitis.[212] It is believed to be caused by bacterial invasion of the gallbladder wall, most frequently by bacteria of the *Clostridium* species with *Escherichia coli* often found as a co-pathogen.[212] *Clostridium welchii* is the most common pathogen implicated in emphysematous cholecystitis.[214] This form of acute cholecystitis often progresses to gallbladder gangrene and perforation.[212]

Patients with emphysematous cholecystitis present with signs and symptoms consistent with acute cholecystitis and few added features.[212] In fact, patients are less likely to be febrile and often do not exhibit severe localized abdominal tenderness.[213] Laboratory findings may reveal leukocytosis of less than 16,000/mm.[3,213] The most distinguishing characteristic in these patients is the presence of air within the gallbladder lumen or wall.[211] Three

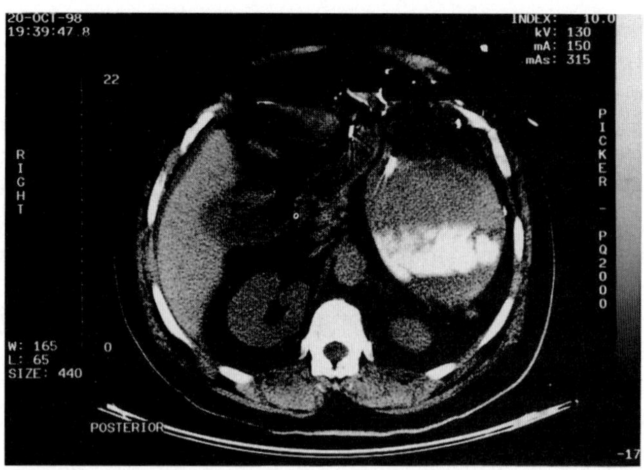


FIGURE 49.2. Computed tomography scan showing air within the gallbladder wall consistent with emphysematous cholecystitis.

stages of emphysematous cholecystitis have been described radiographically and relate to the progression of disease, including findings of gas in the gallbladder lumen, the gallbladder wall, and finally the pericholecystic space.[215] The latter two stages are pathognomonic for emphysematous cholecystitis.[214] Ultrasonography has limited application in the diagnosis of emphysematous cholecystitis, as air within the tissues may lead to nonvisualization of the gallbladder.[216] CT scan findings include visualization of gas within the gallbladder or gallbladder wall (Fig. 49.2).[211]

Treatment of emphysematous cholecystitis is surgery after the patient has been adequately stabilized. Delays in surgical treatment of this condition can be devastating.[214] Appropriate antibiotic coverage both pre- and postoperatively is imperative and should include coverage for anaerobes and gram-negative pathogens as well as for *Clostridium* organisms.[214] Although there is some controversy regarding timing of laparotomy, all agree that rapid clinical deterioration with a palpable mass in the right upper quadrant sanctions immediate cholecystectomy.[217] Reports suggest that a laparoscopic approach is feasible in these patients, but only in the hands of an experienced surgeon, as the gallbladder is often gangrenous and friable.[217]

## Choledocholithiasis

Common duct stones are classified as primary or secondary depending on their site of origin. Primary duct stones, or stones that form within the common bile duct, are rare and account for a small fraction of cases of choledocholithiasis. This subtype of common duct stone is typically associated with infection.[5] Most cases of choledocholithiasis are due to the presence of secondary stones that arise in the gallbladder and later migrate into the common bile duct. The composition of these stones is similar to that of stones found primarily in the gallbladder, consisting of cholesterol and varying degrees of calcium bilirubinate.[16]

The incidence of choledocholithiasis increases considerably with age. Common duct stones are reported to occur in 10% of the general population undergoing cholecystectomy[134] and in up to 50% of patients in their seventies requiring surgery for symptomatic cholelithiasis.[5] Additionally, elderly patients with common bile duct stones are more likely to have positive bile cultures.[218] The reasons for this discrepancy have yet to be elucidated. Untreated common duct stones may lead to complications of cholangitis, pancreatitis, and obstructive jaundice.[134]

The clinical presentation of patients with choledocholithiasis varies depending on the degree of ductal obstruction and the severity of associated complications. The range of symptoms is broad, as patients may be completely asymptomatic or may present with symptoms typical of life-threatening conditions such as ascending cholangitis.[119] Choledocholithiasis should certainly be suspected in any patient who presents with cholelithiasis and associated jaundice. This presentation is common in patients with common duct stones, however 10–20% of patients present with symptoms of cholangitis or pancreatitis.[219] Patients who present with cholangitis may exhibit the classic triad of fever, right upper quadrant abdominal pain, and jaundice; but it is important to recognize that more than half of the patients who present with cholangitis do not exhibit all three of these findings.[16] Laboratory values commonly reveal significant elevations in alkaline phosphatase, bilirubin, and $\gamma$-glutamyl transpeptidase,[220] with elevations in the leukocyte count, amylase, and lipase in patients presenting with complications of choledocholithiasis.[5] Abnormal liver function tests, however, are absent in some individuals with documented common duct stones.[120]

Several studies have attempted to identify predictors of choledocholithiasis. Factors that may lead one to suspect the presence of common duct stones include common bile duct dilation on ultrasonography, age exceeding 60 years, serum bilirubin higher than 2.5 mg/dl,[221] and the presence of acute or chronic cholecystitis.[222] The sensitivity of ultrasonography in the evaluation of choledocholithiasis is fairly low, however, with highest estimates around 60%.[223] CT may reveal biliary ductal dilatation but is typically used to evaluate malignant rather than benign common duct obstruction. ERCP and percutaneous transhepatic cholangiography (PTC) provide the most accurate means of diagnosing choledocholithiasis.[5] Intraoperative cholangiography is useful for this diagnosis in patients undergoing cholecystectomy.[224] Technologic advances in magnetic resonance imaging (MRI) allow rapid acquisition of images with breath-holding to eliminate motion artifacts. Using these new techniques, the sensitivity and specificity of MR cholangiography compare favorably with ERCP.[132] As sophisticated MR cholangiography becomes more widely available, its application in the elderly patient with gallstone disease is certain to be attractive, particularly if high quality noninvasive imaging of the common bile duct can be attained while evaluating acute or chronic cholecystitis (Fig. 49.3).

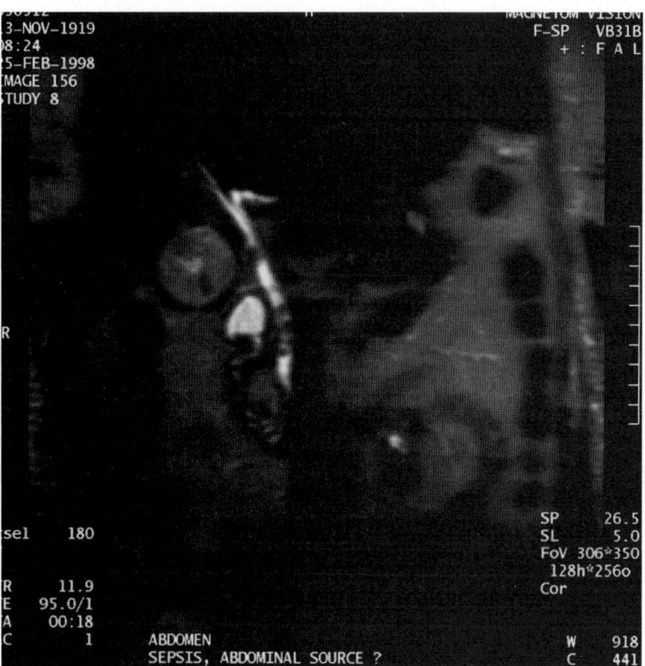


FIGURE 49.3. Magnetic resonance image demonstrating acute cholecystitis and common bile duct stones.

When considering treatment for patients with choledocholithiasis, one must consider the specific conditions under which they occur as well as the advantages and disadvantages of the various forms of treatment. Various endoscopic, radiologic, and surgical methods are available for the treatment of common duct stones. The presence of choledocholithiasis has a major impact on patient outcome in those undergoing cholecystectomy for symptomatic gallstone disease and therefore must be carefully assessed preoperatively.[225]

Most agree that patients who are suspected of harboring common duct stones prior to elective or emergent cholecystectomy should submit to ERCP. Patients who are found to have stones at this time may then undergo endoscopic sphincterotomy (ES) with possible stone extraction.[226] ES has been shown to be the treatment of choice for patients with acute cholangitis[227] or acute pancreatitis[228] before cholecystectomy is performed. Successful stone clearance is possible in more than 90% of patients undergoing ES.[229] Mortality and complication rates for ES are reported to be 0.3% and 4.0%, respectively, for patients under 65 years of age. These rates increase to 0.4% and 6.5% in patients age 65 years or older.[230]

Complication rates are noted to be higher when ES is performed in the absence of common duct dilation.[231]

Choledochotomy at the time of open cholecystectomy was the treatment of choice for choledocholithiasis before the advent of laparoscopic cholecystectomy, endoscopic sphincterotomy and other nonsurgical methods.[232] When open cholecystectomy is performed, common bile duct exploration (CBDE) is effective in clearing the duct of stones in 98% of cases.[233] Unfortunately, this procedure is associated with a significant increase in operative morbidity and mortality, particularly in elderly patients.[139] Because of this additional risk, intraoperative cholangiography is used to avoid unnecessary CBDE.[234] In the critically ill patient, management of choledocholithiasis during open cholecystectomy may be restricted to placement of a T-tube. Subsequent clearance of common bile duct stones can be achieved by ES or radiologic manipulation via the T-tube tract, which is successful in more than 70% of patients.[235]

The presence of associated choledocholithiasis complicates laparoscopic treatment of symptomatic gallstone disease. Ideally, patients with common duct stones are identified preoperatively and undergo ES with stone removal. Roughly 2–3% of patients with choledocholithiasis, however, do not have any associated laboratory or ultrasonographic evidence of common duct pathology.[236] The routine use of intraoperative cholangiography (IOC) may identify these patients and prevent the occurrence of retained common duct stones.[234] Patients in whom common duct stones have been identified have traditionally undergone either conversion to open cholecystectomy with CBDE or completion of the cholecystectomy laparoscopically followed by ES in 1–2 weeks.[134] More recently, laparoscopic CBDE has become part of the armamentarium against choledocholithiasis. Although still not widely used, this method has been shown to be effective in clearing more than 90% of common bile duct stones.[237] Choledocholithiasis discovered after cholecystectomy is best treated by ES.[134]

There are several nonsurgical treatment modalities for treating choledocholithiasis in elderly and debilitated patients who also have cholelithiasis, but who are poor surgical candidates. ES has become the treatment of choice for common bile duct stones in this situation.[238] There has been some concern that ES may predispose these patients to the development of acute cholecystitis. Siegel et al.[239] reported an 8.6% complication rate of acute cholecystitis over 13 years in their study of 1208 patients with calculous gallbladders in situ in whom ES was performed for choledocholithiasis, a rate comparable to that previously described for individuals with mildly symptomatic cholelithiasis.[94] Patients who present with cholangitis, however, are likely to require cholecystectomy.[240] Adjunctive therapies to ES in the case of unretrievable common duct stones include the use of both intra- and extracorporeal lithotripsy,[241] temporary biliary stenting,[242] and the administration of contact dissolution agents through a nasobiliary catheter.[243] Cumulative success rates for these methods in conjunction with ES approach 98–99%.[225] Mortality rates approach 3% in those who initially fail these forms of treatment.[244] Permanent biliary stenting is associated with a high incidence of late complications and should be reserved for elderly patients with a short life expectancy.[242]

Endoscopic sphincterotomy can be challenging in elderly patients. In their study of 182 patients, Deenitchin et al.[245] reported that elderly patients had a higher frequency of periampullary diverticula and were much more likely to require lithotripsy, nasobiliary drainage, and biliary stenting than younger patients. Elderly patients typically had larger and more abundant stones. Significantly higher rates of morbidity, mortality, and cholangitis were demonstrated in elderly patients,[245] which has led some to argue that these patients are better treated via a surgical approach.[246]

## Acalculous Cholecystitis

Symptoms of gallstone disease may arise in the absence of documented cholelithiasis. Patients with chronic acalculous cholecystitis typically describe pain identical to that noted by patients with calculous biliary disease and often tell of extrabiliary symptoms of nausea, vomiting, and fatty food intolerance.[247] Although ultrasonography reveals no abnormalities, cholecystokinin-stimulated cholescintigraphy (CSC) characteristically reveals pain after CCK injection associated with a low gallbladder ejection fraction (<35%), nonvisualization of the gallbladder, or an absence of gallbladder emptying.[248] The treatment of chronic acalculous cholecystitis is identical to that for chronic cholecystitis secondary to cholelithiasis, which is either laparoscopic or open cholecystectomy.[249] Histologic examination of gallbladders following cholecystectomy for chronic acalculous cholecystitis often reveals evidence of chronic inflammation, cholesterolosis, and microscopic cholesterol crystallization.[247] Predictors of symptom relief following cholecystectomy include a convincing history of true biliary colic in conjunction with cholescintigraphic evidence of gallbladder dysfunction.[248]

About 5–10% of patients undergoing cholecystectomy for acute cholecystitis have no demonstrable gallbladder stones.[191] Acute acalculous cholecystitis is a grave complication of critical illness and trauma[250] that has also been associated with extensive surgical procedures,[251] total parenteral nutrition,[252] and the acquired immunodeficiency syndrome (AIDS).[253] An increasing number of patients, however, are presenting with acute acalculous cholecystitis as outpatients.[251] Unlike the chronic form of acalculous cholecystitis, which affects middle-aged women, the acute form is most likely to occur in elderly men.[248] This form of cholecystitis is also associated with high rates of gangrene and perforation.[251] Mortality rates for acute acalculous cholecystitis are high, reaching 50% in some reports.[254]

Factors thought to be implicated in the pathogenesis of acute acalculous cholecystitis involve bile stasis, hyperalimentation, gallbladder ischemia, and systemic infection.[255] Bile stasis in critically ill individuals may be related to prolonged narcotic use[255] or mechanical ventilation,[256] resulting in increased biliary concentration of lysophosphatydil choline, which may in turn lead to inflammatory changes in the gallbladder wall.[257] Total parenteral nutrition has also been implicated in the pathogenesis of acalculous cholecystitis, with gallbladder sludge occurring in 100% of patients after 6 weeks of hyperalimentation.[74] Low-flow states may contribute to gallbladder ischemia,[258] and endotoxemia has been shown to result in acute acalculous cholecystitis in animal models.[259]

The clinical presentation of acute acalculous cholecystitis is similar to that of acute cholecystitis due to calculous gallbladder disease.[191] Shapiro et al.[260] reported that the most common clinical findings in patients with acute acalculous cholecystitis were right upper quadrant pain and tenderness (82% and 71%, respectively), temperature exceeding 101.5°F (55%), and abdominal distension (27%). Laboratory examination most often revealed leukocytosis (82%) and elevated levels of lactate dehydrogenase (86%), total bilirubin (77%), aspartate aminotransferase (64%), alkaline phosphatase (64%), blood urea nitrogen (55%), creatinine (50%), and serum amylase (29%).[260] Acute acalculous cholecystitis provides a diagnostic challenge to clinicians, as many patients who suffer this condition cannot provide an accurate history. It has been suggested that this diagnosis be entertained in any critically ill septic patient with no apparent source of their sepsis.[255]

Ultrasonography, cholescintigraphy, and CT are useful for supporting a diagnosis of acute acalculous cholecystitis (AAC). Cholescintigraphy yielded the highest sensitivity of the diagnostic modalities followed by CT scan and ultrasonography in the study by Shapiro et al.[260] Cholecystitis is suspected when the gallbladder fails to visualize on cholescintigraphy, although false-negative results sometimes occur in the absence of cystic duct obstruction (as in AAC),[261] and false-positive results may occur in patients on hyperalimentation or with intrinsic liver disease.[262] Ultrasonographic findings supportive of a diagnosis of AAC include gallbladder wall thickness exceeding 3.5 mm,[263] the presence of sludge within the gallbladder, pericholecystic fluid, or the presence of gas within the gallbladder wall.[264] These criteria also apply to the diagnosis of AAC by CT scan.[265]

Acute acalculous cholecystitis is treated optimally with cholecystectomy.[266] Improvements in anesthesia and critical care medicine have lowered the mortality rates for these patients.[255] Several options exist, nonetheless, for patients who are too ill to tolerate general anesthesia. Cholecystostomy performed through an open[267] or percutaneous[268] approach, offers a viable alternative to cholecystectomy in patients who are poor surgical candidates. In fact, there are some who suggest that percutaneous cholecystostomy may obviate the need for cholecystectomy in patients with acalculous cholecystitis.[269] Van Sonnenberg et al.[270] reported successful percutaneous cholecystostomy in more than 98% of patients, with a complication rate of roughly 9%. Mortality rates of roughly 10% can be expected for cholecystostomy, relating largely to the acuity of patients requiring this procedure.[195] Endoscopic procedures for the treatment of acalculous cholecystitis have also been described.[271]

## Conclusions

Gallstone disease remains a major issue worldwide, particularly in the elderly population. Its varied presentation in these patients clearly contributes to the increased morbidity and mortality so characteristic of this group. Advances in the diagnosis and therapy of gallstone disease are likely to contribute to improvements in the care of elderly patients with cholelithiasis, but it is only with an astute understanding of the pathophysiology and treatment of gallstone disease that one can best manage this condition in the elderly patient.

## References


1. National Institutes of Health. Consensus statement on gallstones and laparoscopic cholecystectomy. Am J Surg 1993;165:390–393.
2. Sanson TG, O'Keefe KP. Evaluation of abdominal pain in the elderly. Emerg Med Clin North Am 1996;14:615–627.
3. Harness JK, Strodel WE, Talsma SE. Symptomatic biliary tract disease in the elderly patient. Am J Surg 1986;52:442–446.
4. Kahng KU, Roslyn JJ. Surgical Issues for the elderly patient with hepatobiliary disease. Surg Clin North Am 1994;74:345–373.
5. Krasman ML, Gracie WA, Strasius SR. Biliary tract disease in the aged. Clin Geriatr Med 1991;7:347–370.
6. Rosenthal RA, Andersen DK. Surgery in the elderly: observations on the pathophysiology and treatment of cholelithiasis. Exp Gerontol 1993;28:459–472.
7. Cooper GS, Shlaes DM, Salata RA. Intraabdominal infection: differences in presentation and outcome between younger patients and the elderly. Clin Infect Dis 1994;19:146–148.
8. Ingber S, Jacobson IM. Biliary and pancreatic disease in the elderly. Gastroenterol Clin North Am 1990;19:433–457.
9. Sampliner RE, Bennett PH, et al. Gallbladder disease in Pima Indians: demonstrations of high prevalence and

early onset by cholecystography. N Engl J Med 1970;283: 1358–1364.
10. Johnston DE, Kaplan MM. Pathogenesis and treatment of gallstones. N Engl J Med 1993;328:412–421.
11. Bowen JC, Brenner HI, Ferrante WA, et al. Gallstone disease: pathophysiology, epidemiology, natural history, and treatment options. Med Clin North Am 1992;76:1143–1157.
12. Henriksson P, Einarsson K, Eriksson A, et al. Estrogen-induced gallstone formation in males: relation to changes in serum and biliary lipids during hormonal treatment of prostate carcinoma. J Clin Invest 1989;84:811–816.
13. Everson GT, McKinley C, Kern F Jr. Mechanisms of gallstone formation in women: effects of exogenous estrogen (Premarin) and dietary cholesterol on hepatic lipid metabolism. J Clin Invest 1991;87:237–246.
14. Tierney S, Pitt HA, Lillemoe KD. Physiology and pathophysiology of gallbladder motility. Surg Clin North Am 1993;73:1267–1290.
15. Ratner J, Lisbona A, Rosenbloom M, et al. The prevalence of gallstone disease in very old institutionalized persons. JAMA 1991;265:902–903.
16. Giurgiu DI, Roslyn JJ. Treatment of gallstones in the 1990s. Prim Care Clin North Am 1996;23:497–513.
17. Trotman BW, Sotoway RD. Pigment vs cholesterol cholelithiasis: clinical epidemiological aspects. Dig Dis 1975;20:735–740.
18. Pazzi P, Morsiani E, Sighinolfi D, et al. Pigment vs. cholesterol cholelithiasis: clinical and epidemiological aspects. Ital J Gastroenterol 1989;21:310.
19. Apstein MD, Carey MC. Pathogenesis of cholesterol gallstones: a parsimonious hypothesis. Eur J Clin Invest 1996;26:343–352.
20. Portincasa P, Stolk MF, Van Erpecum KJ, et al. Cholesterol gallstone formation in man and potential treatments of the gallbladder motility defect. Scand J Gastroenterol 1995; 30:63S–78S.
21. Nilsell K, Angelin B, Liljeqvist L, et al. Biliary lipid output and bile acid kinetics in cholesterol gallstone disease: evidence for an increased hepatic secretion of cholesterol in Swedish patients. Gastroenterology 1985;89:287–293.
22. Hofmann AF. Bile acid secretion, bile flow and biliary lipid secretion in humans. Hepatology 1990;12:17S–22S.
23. Carey MC, Duane WC. Enterohepatic circulation. In: Arias IM, Boyer JL. Fausto N, Jakoby WB, Schacter D, Shafritz DA (eds) The Liver, Biology and Pathobiology, 3rd ed. New York: Raven, 1994:719–767.
24. LaMont JT, Carey MC. Cholesterol gallstone formation. 2. Pathobiology and pathomechanics. Prog Liver Dis 1992; 10:165–191.
25. Smith JL, Hardie JR, Pillay SP, et al. Hepatic acylcoenzyme A: cholesterol acyltransferase activity is decreased in patients with cholesterol gallstones. J Lipid Res 1990; 31:1993–2000.
26. Einarsson K, Nilsell K, Leijd B, et al. Influence of age on secretion of cholesterol and synthesis of bile acids by the liver. N Engl J Med 1985;313:277–282.
27. Thijs C, Knipschild P, Brombacher P. Serum lipids and gallstones: a case-control study. Gastroenterology 1990;98: 739–746.
28. Admirand WH, Small DM. The physicochemical basis of cholesterol gallstone formation in man. J Clin Invest 1968;47:1043–1052.
29. Holzbach RT, Marsh M, Olszewski M, et al. Cholesterol solubility in bile: evidence that supersaturated bile is frequent in healthy man. J Clin Invest 1973;52:1467–1479.
30. Holan KR, Holzbach RT, Hermann RE, et al. Nucleation time: a key factor in the pathogenesis of cholesterol gallstone disease. Gastroenterology 1979;77:611–617.
31. Burnstein MJ, Ilson RG, Petrunka CN, et al. Evidence of a potent nucleating factor in the gallbladder bile of patients with cholesterol stones. Gastroenterology 1983;85:801–807.
32. Sewell RB, Mao SJT, Kawamoto T, et al. Apolipoproteins of high, low and very low density lipoproteins in human bile. J Lipid Res 1983;24:391–401.
33. Carey MC, Cahalane MJ. Whither biliary sludge? Gastroenterology 1988;95:508–523.
34. Levy PR, Smith BF, LaMont JT. Human gallbladder mucin accelerates in vitro nucleation of cholesterol in artificial bile. Gastroenterology 1984;87:270–275.
35. Lee SP, LaMont JT, Carey MC. Role of gallbladder mucin hypersecretion in the evolution of cholesterol gallstones: studies in the prairie dog. J Clin Invest 1981;67:1712–1723.
36. O'Leary DP, Murray FE, Turner BS, et al. Bile salts stimulate glycoprotein release by guinea pig gallbladder in vitro. Hepatology 1991;13:957–961.
37. Strichartz SD, Abedin MZ, Abdou MS, et al. The effects of extracellular calcium on prairie dog gallbladder ion transport. J Lab Clin Med 1988;155:131–137.
38. Moser AJ, Abedin MZ, Roslyn JJ. Increased biliary protein precedes gallstone formation. Dig Dis Sci 1993;39:1313–1320.
39. Shiffman ML, Sucermart HJ, Kellum JM, et al. Calcium in human gallbladder bile. J Lab Clin Med 1992:875–884.
40. Kaufman HS, Magnuson TH, Pitt HA, et al. The distribution of calcium salt precipitates in the core, periphery and shell of cholesterol, black pigment and brown pigment gallstones. Hepatology 1994;19:1124–1132.
41. Neithercut WD. Effect of calcium, magnesium and sodium ions on in vitro nucleation of human bile. Gut 1989; 30:665–670.
42. Kibe A, Dudley MA, Halpern Z, et al. Factors affecting cholesterol monohydrate crystal nucleation time in model systems of supersaturated bile. J Lipid Res 1985;26:1102–1111.
43. Malet PF, Locke CL, Trotman BW, et al. The calcium ionophore A23187 stimulates glucoprotein secretion by the guinea-pig gallbladder. Hepatology 1986;6:569–573.
44. Plevris JN, Bouchier AD. Defective acid base regulation by the gallbladder epithelium and its significance for gallstone formation. Gut 1995;37:127–131.
45. Moser AJ, Abedin MZ, Cates JA, et al. Converting gallbladder absorption to secretion: the role of intracellular calcium. Surgery 1996;119:410–416.
46. Friedman GD, Kannel WB, Dawber TR. The epidemiology of gallbladder disease: observations in the Framingham study. J Chronic Dis 1996;19:273–292.
47. Roslyn JJ, Pitt HA, Mann LL, Ament ME, DenBesten L. Gallbladder disease in patients on long-term parenteral nutrition. Gastroenterology 1993;84:148–154.

48. Ho KY, Weissberger AJ, Marbach P, Lazarus L. Therapeutic efficacy of the somatostatin analog SMS 201-995 (octreotide) in acromegaly. Ann Intern Med 1990;112:173–181.
49. Shaw SJ, Hajnal F, Lebovitz Y, et al. Gallbladder dysfunction in diabetes mellitus. Dig Dis Sci 1993;38:490–496.
50. Everson GT, Nemeth A, Kourourian S, et al. Gallbladder function is altered in sickle cell hemoglobinopathy. Gastroenterology 1989;96:1307–1316.
51. Nino Murchia M, Burton D, et al. Gallbladder contractility in patients with spinal cord injuries: a sonographic investigation. AJR 1990;154:521–524.
52. Masclee AA, Jansen JB, Dreissen WM, et al. Effect of truncal vagotomy on cholecystokinin release, gallbladder contraction, and gallbladder sensitivity to cholecystokinin in humans. Gastroenterology 1990;98:1338–1344.
53. Patankar R, Ozmen MM, Bailey IS, et al. Gallbladder motility, gallstones, and the surgeon. Dig Dis Sci 1995;40:2323–2335.
54. Howard PJ, Murphy GM, Dowling RH. Gallbladder emptying patterns in response to a normal meal in healthy subjects and patients with gallstones: ultrasound study. Gut 1991;32:1406–1411.
55. Fisher RS, Rock E, Levin G, et al. Effects of somatostatin on gallbladder emptying. Gastroenterology 1987;92:885–890.
56. Cameron AJ, Phillips SF, Summerskill WH. Effect of cholecystokinin, gastrin, secretin, and glucagon on human gallbladder in vitro. Proc Soc Exp Biol 1968;131:149.
57. Kalfin R, Milenov K. The effect of vasoactive intestinal polypeptide (VIP) on the canine gallbladder motility. Comp Biochem Physiol 1991;100:513–517.
58. Conter R, Roslyn JJ, Muller EL, et al. Effect of pancreatic polypeptide on gallbladder filling. J Surg Res 1985;38:461–467.
59. Conter R, Roslyn JJ, Taylor IL. Effects of peptide YY on gallbladder motility. Am J Physiol 1987;252:G736–G741.
60. Lillimoe KD, Webb TH, Pitt HA. Neuropeptide Y: a candidate neurotransmitter for biliary motility. J Surg Res 1988;45:254–260.
61. Jebbink MC, Masclee AA, Van der Klej FG, Schipper J, Rorati LC, Lamers CBHW. Effect of loxiglumide and atropine on erythromycin induced reduction in gallbladder volume in human subjects. Hepatology 1992;16:937–942.
62. Matte L, Sakamoto T, Greely GH, Thompson JC. Effect of substance P on contractions of the gallbladder. Surg Gynecol Obstet 1986;163:163–166.
63. Hildebrand P, Werth B, Beglinger C, et al. Human gastrin releasing peptide: biological potency in humans. Regul Peptides 1991;36:423–433.
64. Kotwall CA, Clanachan AS, Baie HP. Effect of prostaglandins on motility of gallbladders removed from patients with gallstones. Arch Surg 1984;119:709–712.
65. McKirdy ML, McKirdy HC, Johnson CD. Non-adrenergic non-cholinergic inhibitory innervation shown by electric field stimulation of isolated strips of human gallbladder muscle. Gut 1994;35:412–416.
66. Pellegrini C, Ryan T, Broderick W, Way LW. Gallbladder filling and emptying during cholesterol gallstone formation in the prairie dog. Gastroenterology 1986;90:143–149.
67. Behar J, Lee KY, Thompson WR, et al. Gallbladder contraction in patients with pigment and cholesterol stones. Gastroenterology 1989;97:1479–1484.
68. Tilvis RS, Aro J, Stranberg TE, et al. Lipid composition of bile and gallbladder mucosa in patients with acalculous cholesterolosis. Gastroenterology 1982;82:607–615.
69. Yu PR, Chen Q, Biancani P, et al. Membrane cholesterol alters gallbladder muscle contractility in prairie dogs. Am J Physiol 1996;271:G56–61.
70. Behar J, Rhim BY, Thompson WR, et al. Inositol triphosphate restores impaired human gallbladder motility associated with cholesterol stones. Gastroenterology 1993;104:563–568.
71. O'Donnell LJD, Fairclough PD. Gallstones and gallbladder motility. Gut 1993;34:440–443.
72. Jazrawi RP, Pazzi P, Petroni ML, et al. Postprandial gallbladder motor dysfunction: refilling and turnover of bile in health and cholelithiasis. Gastroenterology 1995;109:582–591.
73. Shaffer EA, Lax H, Bomzon A, et al. Hydrophobic bile salts may directly impair gallbladder contractility to cholecystokinin. Gastroenterology 1990;98:A262.
74. Maringhini A, Ciambra M, Baccelliere P, et al. Biliary sludge and gallstones in pregnancy: incidence, risk factors, and natural history. Ann Intern Med 1993;119:116–120.
75. Messing B, Bories C, Kunstlinger F, et al. Does total parenteral nutrition induce gallbladder sludge formation and lithiasis? Gastroenterology 1983;84:1012–1019.
76. Poston GJ, Singh P, Maclellan D, et al. Age related contractility and gallbladder cholecystokinin receptor population in the guinea pig. Mech Ageing Dev 1988;46:225–236.
77. Poston GJ, Draviam EJ, Yao CZ, et al. Effect of age and sensitivity to cholecystokinin on gallstone formation in the guinea pig. Gastroenterology 1990;98:939–999.
78. Khalil T, Walker PJ, Wiener I, et al. Effects of aging on gallbladder contraction and release of cholecystokinin-33 in humans. Surgery 1985;98:423–429.
79. Berger D, Crowther RC, Floyd JC Jr, et al. Effect of age on fasting plasma levels of pancreatic hormones in man. Am J Surg 1978;47:1183–1189.
80. Moser AJ, Abedin MZ, Roslyn JJ. The pathogenesis of gallstone formation. Adv Surg 1993;26:357–386.
81. Cahalane MJ, Neubrand MW, Carey MC. Physical-chemical pathogenesis of pigment stones. Semin Liver Dis 1988;8:317–328.
82. Trotman BW, Bernstein SE, Bove KE, et al. Studies on the pathogenesis of pigment gallstones in hemolytic anemia. J Clin Invest 1980;65:1301–1308.
83. Ostrow JD. The etiology of pigment gallstones. Hepatology 1984;4:215S–222S.
84. Carey MC. Pathogenesis of gallstones. Am J Surg 1993;165:410–419.
85. Cetta F. The role of bacteria in pigment gallstone formation. Am Surg 1991;213:315–326.
86. Nagase M, Hikaro Y, Soloway RD, et al. Gallstones in western Japan: features affecting the prevalence of intrahepatic gallstones. Gastroenterology 1980;78:684–690.
87. Ho KJ. Biliary electrolytes and enzymes in patients with and without gallstones. Dig Dis Sci 1996;41:2409–2416.

88. Apstein MD, Carey MC. Biliary tract stones and associated diseases. In: Stein JH (ed) Internal Medicine, 4th ed. St. Louis: Mosby Yearbook, 1993.
89. Cucchiaro G, Rossitch JC, Bowie J, et al. Clinical significance of ultrasonographically detected coincidental gallstones. Dig Dis Sci 1990;35:417–421.
90. Gibney EJ. Asymptomatic gallstones. Br J Surg 1990; 77:368–372.
91. Comfort MW, Gray HK, Wilson JM. The silent gallstone: a ten to twenty year follow-up study of 112 cases. Ann Surg 1948;128:931–937.
92. Gracie WA, Ransohoff DF. The natural history of silent gallstones: the innocent gallstone is not a myth. N Engl J Med 1982;307:798–800.
93. Attili AF, DeSantis A, Capri R, Repice AM, Maselli S, GREPCO group. The natural history of gallstones: the GREPCO experience. Hepatology 1995;21:656–660.
94. McSherry CK, Ferstenberg H, Calhoun WF, et al. The natural history of diagnosed gallstone disease in symptomatic and asymptomatic patients. Ann Surg 1985;202:59–63.
95. Friedman GD. Natural history of asymptomatic and symptomatic gallstones. Am J Surg 1993;165:399–404.
96. Fendrick AM, Gleeson SP, Cabana MD, Schwartz JS. Asymptomatic gallstones revisited: is there a role for laparoscopic cholecystectomy? Arch Fam Med 1993;2:959–968.
97. Wenckhert A, Robertson B. The natural course of gallstone disease. Gastroenterology 1966;50:376–381.
98. Cucchiaro G, Walters CR, Rossitch JC, et al. Deaths from gallstones: incidence and associated clinical factors. Ann Surg 1989;209:149–151.
99. Lieber MM. The incidence of gallstones and their correlation with other diseases. Ann Surg 1952;135:394–405.
100. Mundth ED. Cholecystitis and diabetes mellitus. N Engl J Med 1962;267:642–646.
101. Turill FL, McCarron MM, Mikkelsen WP. Gallstones and diabetics: an ominous association. Am J Surg 1961;102:184–190.
102. Ransohoff DF, Miller GL, Forsythe SB, et al. Outcome of acute cholecystitis in patients with diabetes mellitus. Ann Intern Med 1987;106:829–832.
103. Friedman LS, Roberts MS, Brett AS, et al. Management of asymptomatic gallstones in the diabetic patient: a decision analysis. Ann Intern Med 1988;109:913–919.
104. Walsh DB, Eckhauser FE, Ramsburgh SR, Burney RB. Risks associated with diabetes mellitus in patients undergoing gallbladder surgery. Surgery 1982;91:254–257.
105. Sandler RS, Maule WF, Baltus ME. Factors associated with postoperative complications in diabetics after biliary tract surgery. Gastroenterology 1986;91:157–162.
106. Hjortrup A, Sorensen C, Dyremose E, et al. Influence of diabetes mellitus on operative risk. Br J Surg 1985;72:783–785.
107. Ikard RW. Gallstones, cholecystitis and diabetes. Surg Gynecol Obstet 1990;171:528–532.
108. Del Favero G, Caroli A, Meggiato T, et al. Natural history of gallstones in non-insulin-dependent diabetes mellitus: a prospective 5 year follow-up. Dig Dis Sci 1994;39:1704–1707.
109. Schreiber H, Macon WL, Pories WJ. Incidental cholecystectomy during major abdominal surgery in the elderly. Am J Surg 1978;135:196.
110. Ouriel K, Ricotta JJ, Adams JT, et al. Management of cholelithiasis in patients with abdominal aortic aneurysm. Ann Surg 1983;198:717–719.
111. Green JD, Birkhead G, Herbert J, et al. Increased morbidity in surgical patients undergoing secondary (incidental) cholecystectomy. Ann Surg 1990;211:50–54.
112. Thistle JL, Cleary PA, Lachin JM, et al. The natural history of cholelithiasis: the National Cooperative Gallstone Study. Ann Intern Med 1984;101:171–175.
113. Friedman GD, Raviola CA, Fireman B. Prognosis of gallstones with mild or no symptoms: 25 years of follow-up in a health maintenance organization. J Clin Epidemiol 1989;42:127–136.
114. Ransohoff DF, Gracie WA. Treatment of gallstones. Ann Intern Med 1993;119:606–619.
115. Pigott JP, Williams GB. Cholecystectomy in the elderly. Am J Surg 1988;155:408–410.
116. Morrow DJ, Thompson J, Wilson SE. Acute cholecystitis in the elderly: a surgical emergency. Arch Surg 1978;113:1149–1152.
117. Diehl AK, Sugarek NJ, Todd KH. Clinical evaluation for gallstone disease: usefulness of symptoms and signs in diagnosis. Am J Med 1990;89:29–33.
118. Rigas B, Torosis J, McDougall CJ, et al. The circadian rhythm of biliary colic. J Clin Gastroenterol 1990;12:409–414.
119. Moscati RM. Cholelithiasis, cholecystitis, and pancreatitis. Emerg Med Clin North Am 1996;14:719–736.
120. Goldman DE, Gholson CF. Choledocholithiasis in patients with normal serum liver enzymes. Dig Dis Sci 1995;40:1065–1068.
121. Zollinger RM. Observations following distension of the gallbladder and common duct in man. Proc Soc Expl Biol Med 1933;30:1260–1261.
122. Fenster LF, Lonborg R, Thirlby RC, et al. What symptoms does cholecystectomy cure? Insights from an outcomes measurement project and review of the literature. Am J Surg 1995;169:535–538.
123. Gilliland TM, Traverso W. Cholecystectomy provides long-term symptom relief in patients with acalculous cholecystitis. Am J Surg 1990;159:489–492.
124. Cobden I, Venables CW, Lendrum R, et al. Gallstones presenting as mental and physical disability in the elderly. Lancet 1984;(May 12):1062–1064.
125. Zeman RK, Garra BS. Gallbladder imaging: the state of the art. Gastroenterol Clin North Am 1991;20:127–156.
126. Jennings WC, Drabek GA, Miller KA. Significance of sludge and thickened wall in ultrasound evaluation of the gallbladder. Surg Gynecol Obstet 1992;174:394–398.
127. Shlaer WJ, Leopold GR, Scheible FW. Sonography of the thickened gallbladder wall: a nonspecific finding. Am J Radiol 1981;136:337–339.
128. Shea JA, Berlin JA, Escarce JJ, et al. Revised estimates of diagnostic test sensitivity and specificity in suspected biliary tract disease. Arch Intern Med 1994;154:2573–2581.
129. Ros E, Valderrama R, Bru C, et al. Symptomatic versus silent gallstones: radiographic features and eligibility for nonsurgical treatment. Dig Dis Sci 1994;39:1697–1703.

130. Baron RL, Rohrmann CA, Lee SP, et al. CT evaluation of gallstones in vitro: correlation with chemical analysis. Am J Radiol 1988;151:1123–1128.
131. Tierneys, Pitt HA, Lillemoe KD. Physiology and Pathophysiology of gallbladder motility. Surg Clin Worth Am 1993;73:1267–1290.
132. Holzknecht N, Gauger J, Sackmann M, et al. Breath-hold MR cholangiography with snapshot techniques: prospective comparison with endoscopic retrograde cholangiography. Radiology 1998;206:657–664.
133. Watkins JL, Blatt CF, Layden TJ. Gallstones: choosing the right therapy despite vague clinical cues. Geriatrics 1993; 48(8):48–54.
134. Wetter LA, Way LW. Surgical therapy for gallstone disease. Gastroenterol Clin North Am 1991;20:157–169.
135. Roslyn JJ, Binns GS, Hughes EFX, et al. Open cholecystectomy: a contemporary analysis of 42,474 patients. Ann Surg 1993;218:129–137.
136. Glenn F. The incidence and causes of death following surgery for nonmalignant biliary tract disease. Ann Surg 1980;191:271–275.
137. Margiotta SJ, Horwitz JR, Willis IH, et al. Cholecystectomy in the elderly. Am J Surg 1988;156:509–512.
138. Pigott JP, Williams GB. Choleystectomy in the elderly. Am J Surg 1988;155:408–410.
139. Escarce JJ, Shea JA, Chen W, et al. Outcomes of open cholecystectomy in the elderly: a longitudinal analysis of 21,000 cases in the prelaparoscopic era. Surgery 1995;117:156–164.
140. Morrow DJ, Thompson J, Wilson SE. Acute Cholecystitis in the elderly: a surgical emergency. Arch Surg 1978; 113–1149–1152.
141. Ransohoff DF, Gracie WA, Wolfenson LB, et al. Prophylactic cholecystectomy or expectant management for persons with silent gallstones: a decision analysis to assess survival. Ann Intern Med 1983;99:199–204.
142. Lygidakis NJ. Operative risk factors of cholecystectomy-choledochotomy in the elderly. Surg Gynecol Obstet 1983; 157:15–19.
143. Gadacz TR, Talamini MA, Lillemoe KD, et al. Laparoscopic cholecystectomy. Surg Clin North Am 1990;70:1249–1262.
144. Dubois F, Icard P, Barthelot G, et al. Coelioscopic cholecystectomy: preliminary report of 36 cases. Ann Surg 1990;211:60–62.
145. Reddick EJ, Olsen DO. Laparoscopic laser cholecystectomy: a comparison with mini-lap cholecystectomy. Surg Endosc 1989;3:131–133.
146. Orlando R, Russell JC, Mattie A, Connecticut Laparoscopic Cholecystectomy Registry. Laparoscopic cholecystectomy: a statewide experience. Arch Surg 1993;128:494–499.
147. Perissat J. Laparoscopic cholecystectomy: the European experience. Am J Surg 1993;165:444–449.
148. Soper NJ, Stockmann PT, Dunnegan DL, et al. Laparoscopic cholecystectomy: the new "gold standard"? Arch Surg 1992;127:917–921.
149. Bass EB, Pitt HA, Lillemoe KD. Cost-effectiveness of laparoscopic cholecystectomy versus open cholecystectomy. Am J Surg 1993;165:466–471.
150. McMahon AJ, Russell IT, Ramsay G, et al. Laparoscopic and minilaparotomy cholecystectomy: a randomized trial comparing postoperative pain and pulmonary function. Surgery 1994;115:533–539.
151. Gadacz TR. U.S. experience with laparoscopic cholecystectomy. Am J Surg 1993;165:450–454.
152. Southern Surgeons Club. A prospective analysis of 1518 laparoscopic cholecystectomies. N Engl J Med 1991;324: 1073–1078.
153. Deziel DJ, Milikan KW, Economou SG, et al. Complications of laparoscopic cholecystectomy: a national survey of 4292 hospitals and an analysis of 77,604 cases. Am J Surg 1996; 165:9–14.
154. Nenner RP, Imperato PJ, Alcorn CM. Serious complications of laparoscopic cholecystectomy in New York State. NY State J Med 1992;92:179–181.
155. Southern Surgeons Club, Moore MJ, Bennett CL. The learning curve for laparoscopic cholecystectomy. Am J Surg 1995;170:55–59.
156. Williams LF, Chapman WC, Bonau RA, et al. Comparison of laparoscopic cholecystectomy with open cholecystectomy in a single center. Am J Surg 1993;165:459–465.
157. Lee VS, Chari RS, Cucchiaro G, et al. Complications of laparoscopic cholecystectomy. Am J Surg 1993;165:527–532.
158. Fried GM, Barkum JS, Sigman HH, et al. Factors determining conversion to laparotomy in patients undergoing laparoscopic cholecystectomy. Am J Surg 1994;167:35–41.
159. Massie MT, Massie LB, Marrangoni AG, et al. Advantages of laparoscopic cholecystectomy in the elderly and in patients with high ASA classifications. J Laparoendosc Surg 1993;3:467–476.
160. Fried GM, Clas D, Meakins JL. Minimally invasive surgery in the elderly patient. Surg Clin North Am 1994;74:375–387.
161. Askew AR. Surgery for gallstones in the elderly. Aust NZ J Surg 1995;65:312–315.
162. Ido K, Suzuki T, Kimura K, et al. Laparoscopic cholecystectomy in the elderly: analysis of pre-operative risk factors and postoperative complications. J Gastroenterol Hepatol 1995;10:517–522.
163. Milheiro A, Sousa FC, Oliveira L, et al. Pulmonary function after laparoscopic cholecystectomy in the elderly. Br J Surg 1996;83:1059–1061.
164. Soper NJ. Effect of nonbiliary problems on laparoscopic cholecystectomy. Am J Surg 1993;165:522–526.
165. Salen G, Tint GS, Shefer S. Treatment of cholesterol gallstones with litholytic bile acids. Gastroenterol Clin North Am 1991;20:171–181.
166. Danzinger RG, Hofmann AF, Schoenfield LJ, et al. Dissolution of cholesterol gallstones by chenodeoxycholic acid. N Engl J Med 1972;286:1–8.
167. Bachrach WH, Hofmann AF. Ursodeoxycholic acid in the treatment of cholesterol lithiasis. Dig Dis Sci 1982;27:333–356.
168. Salen G. Clinical perspective on the treatment of gallstones with ursodeoxycholic acid. J Clin Gastroenterol 1991;10: S12–S17.
169. Walker JW. The removal of gallstones by ether solution. Lancet 1891;1:874–875.
170. Langenbuch C. Ein fall von exstirpation der gallenblase wegen chronischer cholelithiasis: Heilung. Berl Klin Wochenschr 1882;19:725–727.
171. Admirand WH, Way LW. Medical treatment of retained gallstones. Trans Assoc Am Phys 1972;85:382–387.

172. Thistle JL, May GR, Bender CE, et al. Dissolution of cholesterol gallbladder stones by methyl tert-butyl ether administered by percutaneous transhepatic catheter. N Engl J Med 1989;320:633–635.
173. Pauletzki J, Holl J, Sackman M, et al. Gallstone recurrence after direct contact dissolution with methyltert-butyl ether. Dig Dis Sci 1995;40:1775–1781.
174. Albert MB, Fromm H, Borstelmann R, et al. Successful outpatient treatment of gallstones with piezoelectric lithotripsy. Ann Intern Med 1990;113:164–166.
175. Garcia G, Young HS. Biliary extracorporeal shock-wave lithotripsy. Gastroenterol Clin North Am 1991;20:201–207.
176. Sackmann M, Ippisch E, Sauerbruch T, et al. Early gallstone recurrence rate after successful shock-wave therapy. Gastroenterology 1990;98:392–395.
177. Bass EB, Steinberg EP, Pitt HA, et al. Cost-effectiveness of extracorporeal shock-wave lithotripsy versus cholecystectomy for symptomatic gallstones. Gastroenterology 1991;101:189–199.
178. Svanvik J, Pellegrini CA, Allen B, et al. Transport of fluid and biliary lipids in the canine gallbladder in experimental cholecystitis. J Surg Res 1986;41:425–431.
179. Norman DC, Yoshikawa TT. Intraabdominal infections in the elderly. J Am Geriatr Soc 1983;31:677–684.
180. Hafif A, Gutman M, Kaplan O, et al. The management of acute cholecystitis in elderly patients. Am Surg 1991;57: 648–652.
181. De Dombal FT. Acute abdominal pain in the elderly. J Clin Gastroenterol 1994;19:331–335.
182. Kim EE, Pjura G, Lowry P, et al. Morphine augmented cholescintigraphy in the diagnosis of acute cholecystitis. Am J Radiol 1986;147:1177–1179.
183. Margiotta SJ, Willis IH, Wallack MK. Cholecystectomy in the elderly. Am Surg 1988;54:34–39.
184. Glenn F. Acute cholecystitis. Surg Gynecol Obstet 1976;143: 56–60.
185. Ratner JT, Rosenberg CM. Management of gallstones in the aged. J Am Geriatr Soc 1975;23:258–264.
186. Peters JH, Miller J, Nichols KE, et al. Laparoscopic cholecystectomy in patients admitted with acute biliary symptoms. Am J Surg 1993;166:300–303.
187. Zucker KA, Flowers JL, Bailey RW, et al. Laparoscopic management of acute cholecystitis. Am J Surg 1993;165: 508–514.
188. Flowers JA, Bailey RW, Graham SM, et al. Laparoscopic management of acute cholecystitis: the Baltimore experience. Am J Surg 1991;161:388–392.
189. Lo CM, Lai ECS, Fan ST, et al. Laparoscopic cholecystectomy for acute cholecystitis in the elderly. World J Surg 1996;20:983–987.
190. Glenn F. Surgical management of acute cholecystitis in patients of 65 years of age and older. Am J Surg 1981;193: 56–59.
191. Cohen SA, Siegel JH. Biliary tract emergencies: endoscopic and medical management. Crit Care Clin 1995;11:273–294.
192. Kaufman M, Weissberg D, Schwartz I, et al. Cholecystostomy as a definitive operation. Surg Gynecol Obstet 1990;170:533–537.
193. Goodachre B, van Sonnenberg E, D'Agostino H, et al. Interventional radiology in gallstone disease. Gastroenterol Clin North Am 1991;20:209–227.
194. Van Steenbergen W, Rigauts H, Ponette E, et al. Percutaneous cholecystostomy for acute complicated calculous cholecystitis in elderly patients. J Am Geriatr Soc 1993; 41:157–162.
195. Browning PD, McGahan JP, Gerscovich EO. Percutaneous cholecystostomy for suspected acute cholecystitis in the hospitalized patient. J Vasc Int Radiol 1993;4:531–538.
196. Hamy A, Visset J, Likholatnikov D, et al. Percutaneous cholecystostomy for acute cholecystitis in critically ill patients. Surgery 1997;121:398–401.
197. Feretis CB, Manouras AJ, Apostolidis NS, et al. Endoscopic transpapillary drainage of gallbladder empyema. Gastrointest Endosc 1990;36:523–525.
198. Strohl EL, Diffenbaugh WG, Baker JH, et al. Collective reviews: gangrene and perforation of the gallbladder. Int Abstr Surg 1962;114:1–7.
199. Felice PR, Trowbridge PE, Ferrara JJ. Evolving changes in the pathogenesis and treatment of the perforated gallbladder: a combined hospital study. Am J Surg 1984;149: 466–473.
200. Niemeier OW. Acute free perforation of the gallbladder. Ann Surg 1934;99:922–924.
201. Abu-Dalu J, Urca I. Acute cholecystitis with perforation into the peritoneal cavity. Arch Surg 1971;102:108–111.
202. Roslyn JJ, Busutill RW. Perforation of the gallbladder: a frequently mismanaged condition. Am J Surg 1979;137: 307–312.
203. Madrazo BL, Francis I, Hricak H, et al. Sonographic findings in perforation of the gallbladder. AJR 1982;139:491–496.
204. Roslyn JJ, Thompson JE Jr, Darvin H, et al. Risk factors for gallbladder perforation. Am J Gastroenterol 1987;82:636–640.
205. Cooperman AM, Dickson ER, ReMine WH. Changing concepts in the surgical treatment of gallstone ileus. Ann Surg 1968;167:377–383.
206. Siskind BN, Hawkins HB, Cinti DC, et al. Gallbladder perforation: an imaging analysis. J Clin Gastroenterol 1987; 9:670–678.
207. Soiva M, Pamilo M, Paivansalo M, et al. Ultrasonography in acute gallbladder perforation. Acta Radiol 1988;29:41–44.
208. Kim PN, Lee KS, Kim IY, et al. Gallbladder perforation: comparison of US findings with CT. Abdom Imaging 1994;19:239–242.
209. Simmons TC, Miller C, Weaver R. Spontaneous gallbladder perforation. Am Surg 1989;55:311–313.
210. Heuman R, Sjodahl R, Wetterfors J. Gallstone ileus: an analysis of 20 patients. World J Surg 1980;4:595–600.
211. Andreu J, Perez C, Caceres J, et al. Computed tomography as the method of choice in the diagnosis of emphysematous cholecystitis. Gastrointest Radiol 1987;12:315–318.
212. Mentzer RM, Golden GT, Chandler JG, et al. A comparative appraisal of emphysematous cholecystitis. Am J Surg 1975;129:10–15.
213. Yeatman TJ. Emphysematous cholecystitis: an insidious variant of acute cholecystitis. Am J Emerg Med 1986;4: 163–166.
214. Jolly BT, Love JN. Emphysematous cholecystitis in an elderly woman: case report and review of the literature. J Emerg Med 1993;11:593–597.

215. Jacob H, Appelman R, Stein HD. Emphysematous cholecystitis. Am Coll Gastroenterol 1979;71:325–330.
216. Parulekar SG. Sonographic findings in acute emphsematous cholecystitis. Radiology 1982;145:117–119.
217. Banwell PE, Hill ADK, Menzies-Gow N, et al. Laparoscopic cholecystectomy: safe and feasible in emphysematous cholecystitis. Surg Laparosc Endosc 1994; 4:189–191.
218. Csendes A, Burdiles P, Maluenda F, et al. Simultaneous bacteriologic assessment of bile from gallbladder and common bile duct in control subjects and patients with gallstones and common duct stones. Arch Surg 1996;131:389–394.
219. Bernhoft RA, Pelligrini CA, Moston RW, et al. Composition and morphologic and clinical features of common duct stones. Am J Surg 1984;148:77–79.
220. Anciaux ML, Pelletier G, Attali P, et al. Prospective study of clinical and biochemical features of symptomatic choledocholithiasis. Dig Dis Sci 1986;31:449–451.
221. Hauer-Jensen M, Karesen R, Nygaard K, et al. Prospective randomized study of routine intraoperative cholangiography during open cholecystectomy: long-term follow-up and predictors of choledocholithiasis. Surgery 1993;113: 318–323.
222. Hunguier M, Bornet P, Charpak Y, et al. Selective contraindication based on multivariate analysis for operative cholangiography in biliary lithiasis. Surg Gynecol Obstet 1991;172:470–474.
223. Cronan JJ. US diagnosis of choledocholithiasis: a reappraisal. Radiology 1986;161:133–134.
224. Phillips EH. Routine versus selective intraoperative cholangiography. Am J Surg 1993;165:505–507.
225. Perissat J, Huibregtse K, Keane FBV, et al. Management of bile duct stones in the era of laparoscopic cholecystectomy. Br J Surg 1994;81:799–810.
226. Boulay J, Schellenberg R, Brady PG. Role of ERCP and therapeutic biliary endoscopy in association with laparoscopic cholecystectomy. Am J Gastroenterol 1992;87:837–842.
227. Lai ECS, Mok FPT, Tan ESY, et al. Endoscopic biliary drainage for severe acute cholangitis. N Engl J Med 1992;326:1582–1586.
228. Fan ST, Lai ECS, Mok FPT, et al. Early treatment of acute biliary pancreatitis by endoscopic papillotomy. N Engl J Med 1993;328:228–232.
229. Lezoche E, Paganini AM, Carlei F, et al. Laparoscopic treatment of gallbladder and common bile duct stones: a prospective study. World J Surg 1996;20:535–542.
230. Vaira D, D'Anna L, Ainley C, et al. Endoscopic sphincterotomy in 1000 consecutive patients. Lancet 1989;2: 431–434.
231. Sherman S, Ruffolo TA, Hawes RH, et al. Complications of endoscopic sphincterotomy: a prospective series with emphasis on the increased risk associated with sphincter of Oddi dysfunction and nondilated bile ducts. Gastroenterology 1991;101:1068–1075.
232. Pitt HA. Role of open choledochotomy in the treatment of choledocholithiasis. Am J Surg 1993;165:483–486.
233. Moston RW, Wetter LA. Operative choledochoscopy: common bile duct exploration is incomplete without it. Br J Surg 1990;77:975–979.
234. Phillips EH. Routine versus selective intraoperative cholangiography. Am J Surg 1993;165:505–507.
235. Burhenne HJ. Percutaneous extraction of retained biliary tract stones: 661 patients. Am J Radiol 1980;134: 888–891.
236. Levine SB, Lerner SJ, Leifer ED, et al. Intraoperative cholangiography: a review of indications and analysis of age-sex groups. Ann Surg 1983;198:692–697.
237. Petelin JB. Laparoscopic approach to common duct pathology. Ann J Surg 1993;165:487–491.
238. May GR, Shaffer EH. Should elective endoscopic sphincterotomy replace cholecystectomy for the treatment of high-risk patients with gallstone pancreatitis? J Clin Gastroenterol 1991;13:125–128.
239. Siegel JH, Safrany L, Ben-Zvi JS, et al. Duodenoscopic sphincterotomy in patients with gallbladders in situ: report of a series of 1272 patients. Am J Gastroenterol 1998; 83:1255–1258.
240. Himal HS. Role of endoscopic sphincterotomy alone in patients with choledocholithiasis and cholelithiasis. Can J Surg 1996;39:225–228.
241. Adamek HE, Maier M, Jakobs R, et al. Management of retained bile duct stones: a prospective open trial comparing extracorporeal and intracorporeal lithotripsy. Gastrointest Endosc 1996;44:40–47.
242. Bergman JJGHM, Rauws EAJ, Tijssen JGP, et al. Biliary endoprostheses in elderly patients with endoscopically irretrievable common bile duct stones: report on 117 patients. Gastrointest Endosc 1995;42:195–201.
243. Palmer KR, Hofmann AF. Intraductal mono-octanoin for the direct dissolution of bile duct stones: experience in 343 patients. Gut 1986;27:196–200.
244. Cairns SR, Dias L, Cotton PB, et al. Additional endoscopic procedures instead of urgent surgery for retained common bile duct stones. Gut 1989;30:535–540.
245. Deenitchin GP, Konomi H, Kimura H, et al. Reappraisal of safety of endoscopic sphincterotomy for common bile duct stones in the elderly. Am J Surg 1995;170:51–54.
246. Hammarstrom LE, Holmin T, Stridbeck H, et al. Long-term follow-up of prospective randomized study of endoscopic versus surgical treatment of bile duct calculi in patients with gallbladder in situ. Br J Surg 1995;82:1516–1521.
247. Jones DB, Soper NJ, Brewer JD, et al. Chronic acalculous cholecystitis: laparoscopic treatment. Surg Laparosc Endosc 1996;6:114–122.
248. Barron LG, Rubio PA. Importance of accurate preoperative diagnosis and role of advanced laparoscopic cholecystectomy in relieving chronic acalculous cholecystitis. J Laparoendosc Surg 1995;5:357–361.
249. Gilliland TM, Traverso LW. Cholecystectomy provides long-term symptom relief in patients with acalculous gallbladders. Am J Surg 1990;159:489–492.
250. Raunest J, Imhof M, Rauen U, et al. Acute choecystitis: a complication in severely injured intensive care patients. J Trauma 1992;32:443–440.
251. Savoca P, Longo W, Zucker K, et al. The increasing prevalence of acalculous cholecystitis in outpatients: results of a 7-year study. Ann Surg 1990;211:433–437.
252. Peterson SR, Sheldon GF. Acute acalculous cholecystitis: a complication of hyperalimentation. Arch Surg 1984;119: 1389–1392.

253. Kavin H, Jonas RB, Chowdury L, et al. Acalculous cholecystitis and cytomegalovirus infection in the acquired immunodeficiency syndrome. Ann Intern Med 1986;104: 53–54.
254. Scher KS, Sarap D, Jaggers RL. Acute acalculous cholecystitis complicating aortic aneurysm repair. Surg Gynecol Obstet 1986;163:475–478.
255. Barie PS, Fischer E. Acute acalculous cholecystitis. J Am Coll Surg 1995;180:232–244.
256. Orlando R, Gleason E, Drezner AD. Acute acalculous cholecystitis in the critically ill patient. Am J Surg 1983; 145:472–476.
257. Niderheiser DH. Acute acalculous cholecystitis induced by lysophosphatidyl choline. Am J Pathol 1986;124:559–563.
258. Taoka H. Experimental study on the pathogenesis of acute acalculous cholecystitis, with special reference to the roles of microcirculatory disturbances, free radicals and membrane-bound phospholipase A2. Gastroenterol Jpn 1991;26:633–644.
259. Becker CG, Dubin T, Glenn F. Induction of acute cholecystitis by activation of factor XII. J Exp Med 1980;151:81–90.
260. Shapiro MJ, Luchtefeld WB, Kurzweil S, et al. Acute acalculous cholecystitis in the critically ill. Am Surg 1994; 60:335–339.
261. Schneider PB. Acalculous cholecystitis: a case with variable cholescintigram. J Nucl Med 1984;25:64–65.
262. Shuman WP, Roger JV, Rudd TG, et al. Low sensitivity of sonography and cholescintigraphy in acalculous cholecystitis. Am J Radiol 1984;142:531–534.
263. Deitch EA, Engel JM. Ultrasound in elective biliary tract surgery. Am J Surg 1988;140:277–283.
264. Becker CD, Burckhardt B, Terrier F. Ultrasound in postoperative acalculous cholecystitis. Gastrointest Radiol 1986; 11:47–50.
265. Cornwell EEI, Rodriguez A, Mirvis SE, et al. Acute acalculous cholecystitis in critically injured patients: preoperative diagnostic imaging. Ann Surg 1989;210:52–55.
266. Glenn F, Becker CG. Acute acalculous cholecystitis: an increasing entity. Ann Surg 1982;195:131–136.
267. Flancbaum L, Majerus TC, Cox EF. Acute posttraumatic acalculous cholecystitis. Am J Surg 1985;150:252–256.
268. Melin MM, Sarr MG, Bender CE, et al. Percutaneous cholecystostomy: a valuable technique in high-risk patients with presumed acute cholecystitis. Br J Surg 1995; 82:1274–1277.
269. Vauthey JN, Lerut J, Martini M, et al. Indications and limitations of percutaneous cholecystectomy for acute cholecystitis. Surg Gynecol Obstet 1993;176:49–54.
270. Van Sonnenberg E, D'Agostino HB, Goodachre BW, et al. Percutaneous gallbladder puncture and cholecystostomy: results, complications, and caveats for safety. Radiology 1992;183:167–170.
271. Johlin FC, Neil GA. Drainage of the gallbladder in patients with acute acalculous cholecystitis by transpapillary endoscopic cholecystostomy. Gastrointest Endosc 1993;39: 645–651.

# 50
# Malignant Diseases of the Gallbladder and Bile Ducts

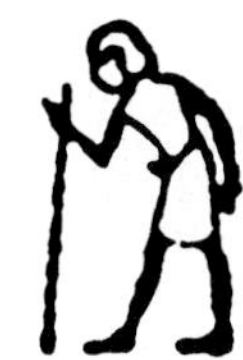

Steven A. Ahrendt and Thomas H. Magnuson

Gallbladder and bile duct cancers are relatively uncommon malignancies and tend to occur primarily in elderly patients. Although the overall prognosis of these malignancies remains poor, recent advances in hepatobiliary surgery, perioperative care, and adjuvant therapy have helped to improve overall survival and quality of life. A multidisciplinary approach in the management of these patients, including surgery, medical oncology, radiation oncology, and invasive radiology, is critical to achieving favorable results.

## Gallbladder Cancer

Cancer of the gallbladder is an aggressive malignancy that occurs predominantly in elderly patients. It is strongly associated with gallstones but is also linked with other geographic and genetic factors. With the exception of early-stage cases detected incidentally at the time of cholecystectomy for gallstone disease, the prognosis is poor. Most patients present with unresectable tumors, and most can be managed nonoperatively. Recently, an aggressive surgical approach for patients with gallbladder cancer has produced encouraging results at several centers with acceptable morbidity and mortality in the predominantly elderly patient population.

### Incidence

Gallbladder cancer is the fifth most common gastrointestinal malignancy following cancer of the colon, pancreas, stomach, and esophagus.[1,2] Cancer of the gallbladder is two to three times more common in women that men, in part due to the higher incidence of gallstones in women.[1–3] With the increase in age of the American population, the incidence of gallbladder cancer has gradually increased, with approximately 5000 new cases diagnosed annually.[4] The overall incidence of gallbladder cancer in the United States is 2.5 cases per 100,000 residents,[1] with the incidence varying considerably with both ethnic background and geographic location.[5,6] In the United States, gallbladder cancer is more common in American Indians than in the non-Indian populations.[6] The annual incidence of gallbladder cancer in American Indian women with gallstones approaches 75 cases per 100,000.[6] Similarly, in Chile, where more than 50% of women over age 50 have gallstones, adenocarcinoma of the gallbladder is the leading cause of cancer deaths among women.[7,8]

Cancer of the gallbladder is a disease of the elderly. More than 75% of patients with this malignancy are over age 65.[3] The peak incidence of gallbladder cancer occurs within the 75- to 79-year age group. The median age for patients with gallbladder cancer (73 years) is older than the median age for patients with pancreatic (67 years) or extrahepatic bile duct (69 years) cancer.

### Etiology

Several factors have been associated with an increased risk of developing gallbladder cancer. Mayo was the first who recognized an association between gallstones and gallbladder cancer.[9] More recently, an anomalous pancreatobiliary duct junction (APBDJ) and other biliary disorders, such as choledochal cysts and primary sclerosing cholangitis, have been associated with gallbladder cancer.

A strong association has long been noted between gallbladder cancer and cholelithiasis, which is present in 75–90% of cases.[3] The incidence of gallstones increases with age, and by age 75 about 35% of women and 20% of men in the United States have developed gallstones.[4] The incidence of gallbladder cancer is approximately seven times more common in the presence of cholelithiasis and chronic cholecystitis than in people without gallstones.[6] Approximately 1% of all patients with elective cholecystectomies performed for chronic cholecystitis and cholelithiasis harbor an occult gallbladder cancer.[1,10] In the elderly patient population, this percentage is certainly higher.[11]

The risk of developing gallbladder cancer is higher in patients with symptomatic gallstones than in those with asymptomatic gallstones.[4] In a review, Ransohoff and Gracie estimated the risk of developing gallbladder cancer in patients with symptomatic or asymptomatic gallstones.[4] The risk of developing gallbladder cancer (0.08% per year) was fourfold higher in patients with symptomatic gallstones over age 50 years than in those who were asymptomatic. Similar results have been observed in a multicenter study evaluating 196 patients with gallbladder cancer.[12] Twenty-eight percent of patients developing gallbladder cancer had undergone a medical evaluation for gallbladder disease in the past. A history of symptoms suggestive of gallbladder disease occurred significantly less frequently in control subjects without cancer.

## Pathology and Staging

Ninety percent of cancers of the gallbladder are classified as adenocarcinoma.[3] Six percent of gallbladder cancers demonstrate papillary features on histologic examination. These tumors are commonly diagnosed while localized to the gallbladder and are also associated with an improved overall survival.[3] At diagnosis, 25% of cancers are localized to the gallbladder wall, 35% have associated metastases to regional lymph nodes or extension into adjacent organs, and 40% have already metastasized to distant sites.[3]

Lymphatic drainage from the gallbladder occurs in a reproducible, predictable fashion and correlates with the pattern of lymph node metastases seen with gallbladder cancer.[13,14] Lymph flow from the gallbladder initially drains to the cystic duct node and then descends along the common bile duct to the pericholedochal lymph nodes. Flow then proceeds to nodes posterior to the head of the pancreas and then to the interaortocaval lymph nodes. Secondary routes of lymphatic drainage include the retroportal and right celiac lymph nodes.[14]

Hepatic involvement with gallbladder cancer can occur by direct invasion through the gallbladder bed, angiolymphatic portal tract invasion, or distant hematogenous spread.[15] Spread via the angiolymphatic portal tracts is the predominant mode of hepatic metastases; it may extend more than 1 cm from the main tumor mass and correlates well with the depth of direct invasion of the liver. Distant spread beyond the region of the gallbladder is associated with hematogenous metastases elsewhere.

The current TNM classification of the American Joint Committee on Cancer is shown in Table 50.1.[16] Stage I tumors are confined to the gallbladder mucosa, submucosa, or muscularis. Stage II tumors extend into the perimuscular connective tissue without penetrating the gallbladder serosa. Stage III tumors penetrate the serosa, extend less than 2 cm into the liver or into another adjacent organ, or involve the cystic duct or pericholedochal lymph nodes. Stage IV tumors have extensive liver invasion, metastatic spread to second-order lymph nodes, or distant metastases.

TABLE 50.1. TNM Staging for Gallbladder Cancer[16]

| | |
|---|---|
| T1 | Tumor invades mucosa (T1a) or muscular (T1b) layer |
| T2 | Tumor invades perimuscular connective tissue, no extension beyond serosa or into liver |
| T3 | Tumor perforates the serosa or directly invades one adjacent organ or both (extension 2 cm or less into liver) |
| T4 | Tumor extends more than 2 cm into liver and/or into two adjacent organs (stomach, duodenum, colon, pancreas, omentum, extrahepatic bile ducts, any involvement of liver) |
| N0 | No lymph node metastases |
| N1 | Metastases in cystic duct, pericholedochal and/or hilar lymph nodes |
| N2 | Metastases in pancreatoduodenal, portal, celiac, or superior mesenteric nodes |
| M0 | No distant metastases |
| M1 | Distant metastases |
| **Stage grouping** | |
| I | T1 N0 M0 |
| II | T2 N0 M0 |
| III | T1 N1 M0 |
| | T2 N1 M0 |
| | T3 N0 M0 |
| | T3 N1 M0 |
| IVa | T4 N0 M0 |
| | T4 N1 M0 |
| IVb | Any T N2 M0 |
| | Any T any N M1 |

*Source:* American Joint Committee on Cancer,[16] with permission.

## Diagnosis

### Clinical Presentation

Gallbladder cancer most often presents with right upper quadrant abdominal pain often mimicking other, more common biliary and nonbiliary disorders.[1] Weight loss, jaundice, and an abdominal mass are less common presenting symptoms. Piehler and Crichlow described five presenting clinical syndromes occurring in a review of more than 1000 patients with gallbladder cancer.[2] Altogether, 16% of patients presented with symptoms of acute cholecystitis with a short duration of pain associated with vomiting, fever, and tenderness; 43% presented with symptoms of chronic cholecystitis often with a recent change in the quality or frequency of the painful episodes; and 34% had signs and symptoms of malignant biliary obstruction with jaundice, weight loss, and right upper quadrant pain. An additional 29% of patients had symptoms of nonbiliary malignancies with anorexia and weight loss in the absence of jaundice, and a small percentage of patients had signs of gastrointestinal bleeding or obstruction.

The preoperative diagnosis of gallbladder cancer is difficult, particularly in the elderly population. In one series only 8% of 53 patients with carcinoma of the gallbladder were diagnosed correctly preoperatively.[17] The most common misdiagnoses included chronic cholecystitis (28%), pancreatic cancer (13%), acute cholecystitis (9%), choledocholithiasis (8%), and gallbladder hydrops (8%).

## *Radiologic Evaluation*

Ultrasonography is often the first diagnostic modality used for evaluating patients with right upper quadrant abdominal pain. Ultrasonographic features of advanced gallbladder cancer include a heterogeneous mass replacing the gallbladder lumen (40–65% of cases) or thickening of the gallbladder wall (20–30% of cases).[18] Most patients have coexistent gallstones, gallbladder wall thickening, or both, suggesting benign biliary disease. Ultrasonography can determine the level of obstruction in patients with biliary ductal involvement. Overall, the sensitivity of ultrasonography for detecting gallbladder cancer ranges from 70% to 100%.[18,19]

Computed tomography (CT) has also improved the detection rate for gallbladder cancer with a sensitivity in the range of 55–100% (Fig. 50.1).[18] CT scanning can demonstrate extension into the liver parenchyma but can overestimate hepatic involvement because of large perfusion defects. CT is less accurate for determining peritoneal seeding or lymph node involvement.

Magnetic resonance imaging (MRI) is also sensitive for detecting gallbladder cancer, but its exact role in preoperative staging remains unclear (Fig. 50.2).[9,18] Hepatic artery and portal vein encasement may also be identified by MRI. Dilatation of the biliary tract that may occur with direct extension of gallbladder cancer into the biliary tree

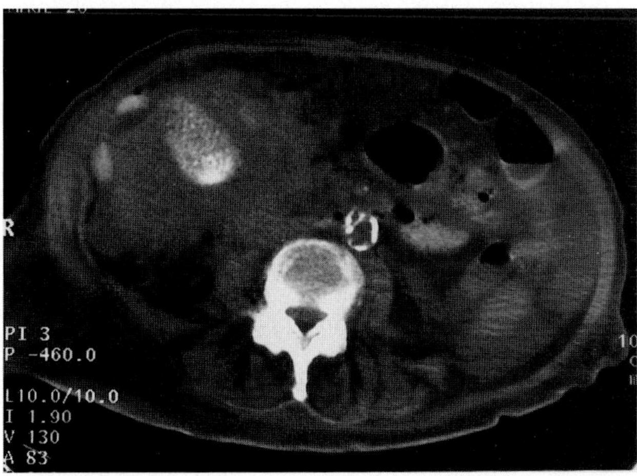

FIGURE 50.1. Computed tomography (CT) scan demonstrates large gallbladder cancer with extension into the duodenum. Gallstones (calcifications) are present within the mass.

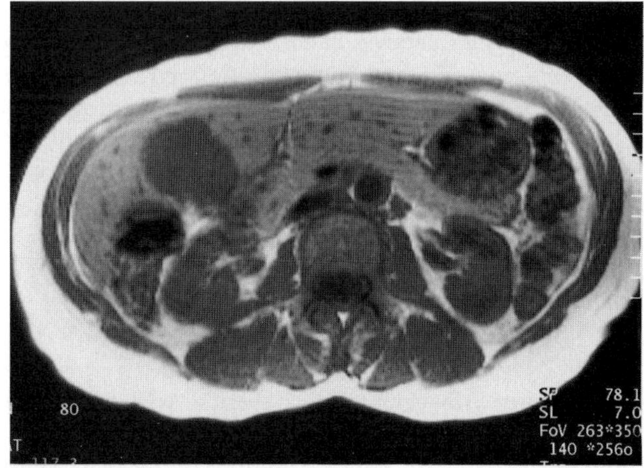

A

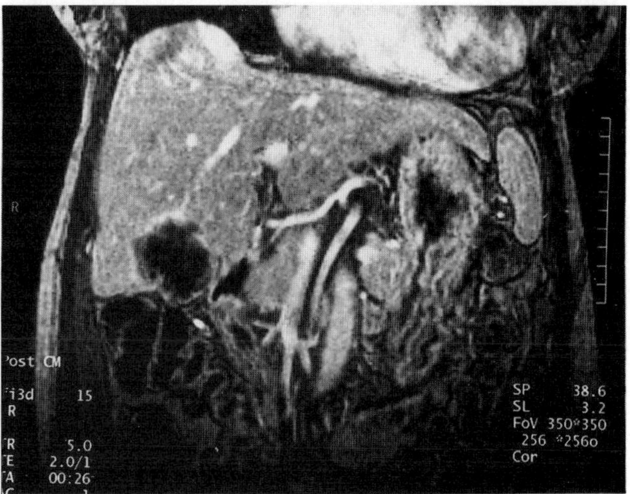

B

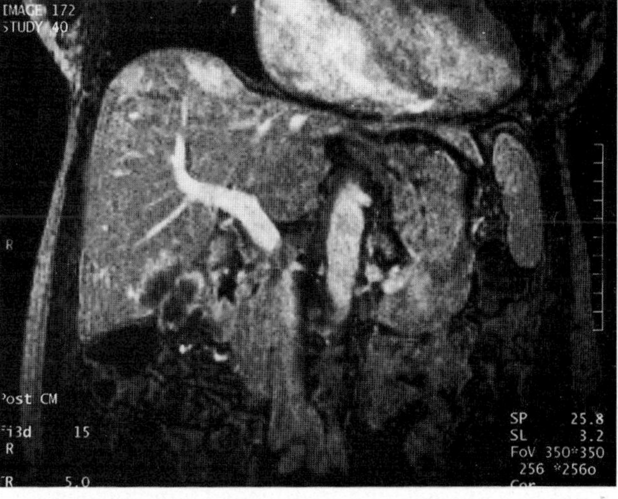

C

FIGURE 50.2. A. Magnetic resonance imaging (MRI) scan demonstrating a mass arising within the gallbladder with extension into the hepatic parenchyma. B. MR angiogram from the same patient demonstrating the relation between the hepatic artery and the mass. C. MR angiogram from the same patient showing the relation between the main and right portal vein and the mass.

can be detected by standard MRI. In the elderly jaundiced patient with gallbladder cancer, the extent of biliary tract involvement should be further defined with cholangiography.[9] Percutaneous transhepatic cholangiography, endoscopic retrograde pancreatography, or magnetic resonance cholangiography are all helpful for the preoperative staging. A typical finding in the jaundiced patient with gallbladder cancer is a long stricture of the common hepatic duct.[9]

## Resection

The primary treatment of patients with localized gallbladder cancer is resection of the primary tumor along with areas of regional lymphatic involvement. After preoperative staging, patients with clinical stage I–IVa tumors warrant exploration if they are otherwise suitable operative candidates. Most of these patients are elderly, but the patient's general medical condition is more important than age when determining operative risk. Preexisting cirrhosis may dramatically increase the risk of surgery particularly if liver resection is contemplated.[9]

### *Simple Cholecystectomy*

The appropriate operative procedure for the patient with localized gallbladder cancer is determined by the pathologic stage. Patients with tumors confined to the gallbladder mucosa or submucosa (stage Ia) have a negligible incidence of lymph node metastases and an overall 5-year survival approaching 100%.[20–22] These early-stage tumors are usually identified postoperatively by the pathologist and following open cholecystectomy, have had an excellent prognosis. More recently, with widespread use of the laparoscopic approach, recurrent cancer at port sites and peritoneal carcinomatosis have been reported following cholecystectomy even for patients with in situ disease.[10] The correct management of patients undergoing laparoscopic cholecystectomy with or without bile spillage for an incidental gallbladder cancer remains unclear.

### *Extended Cholecystectomy*

Cancer of the gallbladder with invasion into or beyond the gallbladder muscularis is associated with an increasing incidence of regional lymph node metastases and should be managed with an extended lymphadenectomy as part of the operative procedure.[22–26] In addition, local extension into the hepatic parenchyma, colon, or duodenum requires en bloc resection of these structures to achieve an adequate resection margin.

The extent of the lymphadenectomy is based on the operative findings and knowledge of the patterns of lymphatic spread in patients with gallbladder cancer.[13,14] This dissection should include the cystic duct, pericholedochal, portal, right celiac, and posterior pancreatoduodenal lymph nodes. In patients without grossly involved lymph nodes, the common bile duct, hepatic artery, and portal vein are skeletonized from the porta hepatis to the pancreas and celiac axis, respectively.[24] Following an extensive Kocher maneuver, the posterior pancreatoduodenal lymph nodes are included with the specimen. In the presence of any grossly enlarged pericholedochal lymph nodes, consideration should be given to resecting the common bile duct to avoid leaving a positive margin.[24] Biliary enteric continuity is restored with a Roux-en-Y hepaticojejunostomy. Several authors have advocated a pancreatoduodenectomy in the setting of pancreatoduodenal lymph node metastases, but this approach increases the operative mortality substantially in the elderly and should be considered in only the good risk patient with no evidence of metastasis to the liver, celiac, or interaortocaval lymph nodes.[24,25,27]

Extension of more advanced staged lesions into the hepatic parenchyma is common, and extended cholecystectomy should incorporate at least a 2 cm margin beyond the palpable or sonographic extent of the tumor to include any angiolymphatic extension from the main tumor mass.[15] For smaller tumors this can be incorporated into a wedge resection of the liver.

### *Extended Resections*

For stage IV tumors invading more than 2 cm into the liver, an anatomic liver resection may be required to achieve a histologically negative margin. Cancers originating in the gallbladder fundus can usually be adequately treated with resection of segments IVb and V (Fig. 50.3).[28] Tumor extension into the right hepatic artery

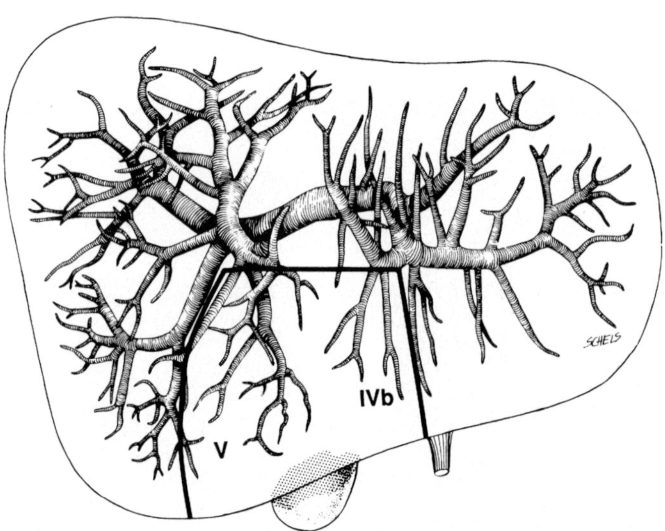


FIGURE 50.3. Extent of bisegmentectomy (segments IVb and V) in patients with T4 gallbladder cancer. (From Gall et al.,[28] with permission.)

or portal vein may be resectable only with a right hepatic lobectomy or trisegmentectomy.[24,29,30]

Locally advanced lesions can also extend into adjacent structures. In the absence of distant lymph node, peritoneal, or hepatic metastases, these lesions may still be resectable for cure. Extension into the right colon should be managed with segmental colectomy, whereas duodenal invasion may require a pancreatoduodenectomy.

## Palliative Therapy

Adequate palliation of the symptoms of advanced gallbladder cancer is eventually required in most elderly patients with this disease.[9,31] Pain, jaundice, and gastric outlet obstruction are the common symptoms requiring palliation and can be managed nonoperatively or operatively. Survival in patients with unresectable gallbladder cancer is just 2–6 months, and therefore operative exploration should be avoided in patients with unresectable disease.[1,17,22] Narcotics should be given when necessary. Percutaneous celiac ganglion block may be helpful in reducing the need for narcotics. Chemical splanchnicectomy can be performed in patients whose lesions are found to be unresectable at the time of operative exploration.[9]

The presence of jaundice is a poor prognostic sign in patients with gallbladder cancer and usually signifies involvement of at least the common hepatic duct or hepatic duct bifurcation (or both). More than 70% of gallbladder cancers that present with jaundice and are explored with an intent to resect are unresectable for cure.[29,32] Nonoperative biliary decompression to relieve jaundice and pruritus can be achieved percutaneously or endoscopically by placing metallic or nonmetallic stents.[9] In patients with hilar or intrahepatic ductal involvement, the percutaneous route is preferred. Relief of gastric outlet obstruction is difficult to achieve nonoperatively and usually requires gastrojejunostomy.

## Survival

Extended cholecystectomy is reasonably well tolerated in the elderly patient population with gallbladder cancer. Operative mortality in several series was 0–1%.[24,29] Common postoperative complications include wound or intraabdominal infection, hemorrhage, or delayed gastric emptying. Mortality increases with the magnitude of the operative procedure. Extended cholecystectomy, combined with a major hepatectomy or pancreatoduodenectomy, has a mortality rate of 10–15% and adds the risks of biliary or pancreatic anastomotic leaks to the procedure.[25]

Survival in elderly patients with gallbladder cancer is strongly influenced by the pathologic stage at presentation. Patients with gallbladder cancer limited to the gallbladder mucosa and submucosa (stage Ia) have a uniformly excellent prognosis[20–22]; 35 patients with incidentally discovered stage Ia gallbladder cancer reported by Shirai et al., had an overall 5-year survival of 100%.[20] Invasion into the muscular wall of the gallbladder increases the risk of recurrent cancer after curative resection. The reported 5-year survival for patients with stage Ib gallbladder cancer varies widely, ranging from 20% to 100% (Table 50.2).[20–22] In a survey of 172 major hospitals in Japan, the 5-year survival for patients with stage Ib tumors was 72%, with many patients undergoing simple cholecystectomy, suggesting that this procedure is inadequate therapy once muscular invasion is present.

Invasion into the muscularis or the subserosa, increases the risk of regional lymph node metastases to 15% and 50%, respectively. Tsukada et al. reported a 5-year overall survival of 80% for patients with stage II disease with extended cholecystectomy.[24] Similar results have been reported with an aggressive surgical approach at Memorial Sloan-Kettering.[29] In patients with tumors confined to the gallbladder wall or with local extension into the liver or other adjacent organs (stages III and IV), long-term survival with extended cholecystectomy is possible.[24,29]

TABLE 50.2. Actuarial Survival with Stage I Gallbladder Cancer

| Study | Year | No. | T stage | 5-Year survival (%) | Cholecystectomy (%) | Extended cholecystectomy (%) |
|---|---|---|---|---|---|---|
| Cubertafond[22] | 1994 | 23 | T1a | 93 | 100 | 0 |
| | | 20 | T1b | 20 | 100 | 0 |
| Donohue[21] | 1990 | 6 | T1 | 100 | 83 | 17 |
| Gall[28] | 1991 | 7 | T1a | 80 | 100 | 0 |
| Ogura[25] | 1991 | 201 | T1a | 83 | 71 | 29 |
| | | 165 | T1b | 72 | 54 | 46 |
| Ouchi[26] | 1994 | 5 | T1a | 80 | 100 | 0 |
| | | 5 | T1b | 40 | 100 | 0 |
| Shirai[20] | 1991 | 35 | T1a | 100 | 100 | 0 |
| | | 4 | T1b | 100 | 100 | 0 |

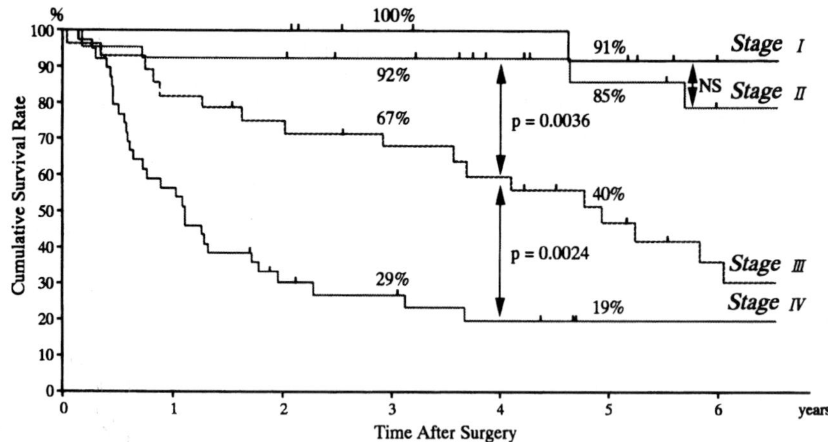


FIGURE 50.4. Actuarial survival for patients with gallbladder cancer by pathologic stage (see Table 50.1). Survival of patients with stage I and stage II tumors was significantly better than that of patients with stage III tumors. In addition, stage III patients survived significantly longer than patients with stage IV disease. (From Tsukada et al.,[24] with permission.)

Several groups have reported 5-year overall survival for patients with stage III and stage IV gallbladder cancer of 40–63% and 19–25%, respectively (Fig. 50.4).[24,29]

Tsukada et al. identified curative, margin-negative resection as the most significant factor in predicting prognosis.[24] Their 5-year survival of 52% in patients undergoing resection with microscopically negative margins was significantly higher than the 5-year survival (5%) in patients with a microscopically positive margin (Fig. 50.5). In the Memorial Sloan-Kettering series, the presence of lymph node metastases was a significant predictor of treatment failure.[29] Eighty-one percent of patients without lymph node metastases were alive 5 years after radical resection, whereas all of the patients with lymph node metastases died within 18 months. In the Japanese series 11 of the 35 five-year survivors had lymph node metastases.[24] Age was not predictive of survival following surgery for gallbladder cancer.[29]

## Adjuvant Therapy

The results of chemotherapy in patients with gallbladder cancer have been poor owing to the limited responsiveness to these agents. Partial response rates to oral 5-fluorouracil (5-FU) alone or in combination with methyl-CCNU or streptozotocin, range from 5% to 13% with a median survival of 10–21 weeks in patients receiving treatment.[33] The combination of intravenous 5-FU, high-dose levofolinic acid, and oral hydroxyurea has achieved a partial response rate of 30% with a median survival of 8 months in patients with unresectable gallbladder cancer.[34] Toxicity was limited, and the regimen was well tolerated in this group of patients (median age 60).

External beam and intraoperative radiation therapy have both been used for management of patients with gallbladder cancer. In the postoperative adjuvant setting, no randomized data have demonstrated improved survival with external beam radiation alone.[9] In a retrospective review of 38 patients with gallbladder cancer managed with postoperative adjuvant therapy, overall survival was improved in patients receiving more than 4000 cGy compared to patients receiving less than 4000 cGy.[35] However, the response to the radiation therapy in this series was difficult to differentiate from the effect of resection alone. Overall survival was not

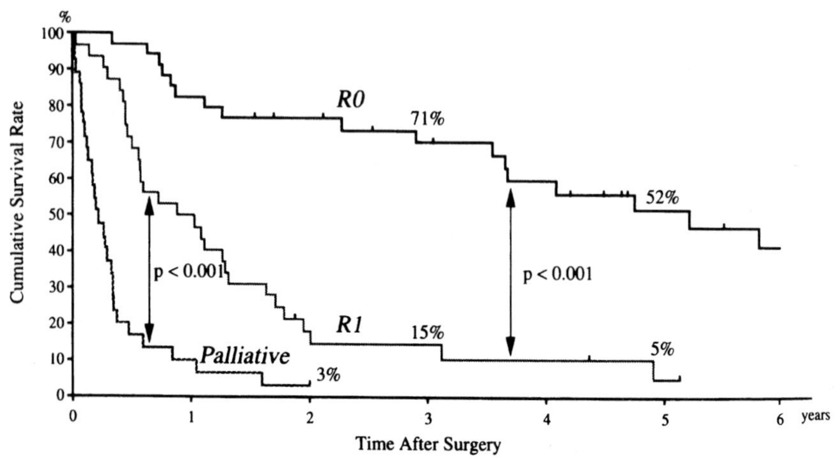


FIGURE 50.5. Actuarial survival for patients with stage III and stage IV gallbladder cancer by resection margin status. Results are shown for patients managed with curative (negative margins) resection (R0), noncurative (microscopically positive margin) resections (R1), and palliative (grossly positive margin) resections (R2). Patients managed with R0 resection survived significantly longer than patients undergoing R1 resection. In addition, patients with extensive tumor resected with palliative intent survived a significantly shorter time than patients with microscopic positive margins. (From Tsukada et al.,[24] with permission.)

influenced by patient age in this series. The use of intraoperative radiation therapy (IORT) in one Japanese series, has been reported to provide a slight survival benefit in patients with locally advanced gallbladder cancer.[36] In a collective review of unresectable gallbladder cancers, patients undergoing IORT had a longer survival (11.0 vs. 6.3 months) than patients with standard external beam radiotherapy.[37]

## Cholangiocarcinoma

Cholangiocarcinomas may occur anywhere along the intrahepatic or extrahepatic biliary tree. The hepatic duct bifurcation is the most frequently involved site, and approximately 60–80% of cholangiocarcinomas encountered at tertiary referral centers are found in the perihilar region.[9,38–41] Cholangiocarcinoma is an uncommon tumor and occurs in conditions in which bile is stagnant, infected, or both. These clinical situations include primary sclerosing cholangitis, choledochal cysts, and hepatolithiasis. Cholangiocarcinoma usually presents with painless jaundice, so this diagnosis should be considered in every case of obstructive jaundice. Perihilar cholangiocarcinomas involve the region of the hepatic duct bifurcation and frequently also involve major portal vascular structures, making resection difficult. When possible, surgical resection offers a chance for long-term disease-free survival. Many patients, however, are candidates only for palliative bypass or operative or nonoperative intubation aimed at providing biliary drainage and preventing cholangitis and hepatic failure.

### Incidence

Approximately 15,000 new cases of liver and biliary tract cancer are diagnosed annually in the United States, and they account for more than 12,000 deaths per year. About 15–25% of these cancers are bile duct tumors or cholangiocarcinomas. The incidence of cholangiocarcinoma increases with age, and these tumors occur with similar frequency in men and women. Approximately two-thirds of patients diagnosed with cholangiocarcinoma are age 50–70 years.[42,43] Overall, the incidence of cholangiocarcinoma in the United States is approximately 1 per 100,000 people per year.[9,44]

### Etiology and Associated Diseases

A number of diseases and environmental agents have been linked to cholangiocarcinoma including primary sclerosing cholangitis, choledochal cysts, and hepatolithiasis. Factors common to a number of these etiologic factors include stones, biliary stasis, and infection.[9] Bile duct cancers in patients with primary sclerosing cholangitis are most often extrahepatic, commonly occur near the hepatic duct bifurcation, and are difficult to differentiate from the multiple, benign strictures associated with this disease.[45] The mean age at presentation in patients with cholangiocarcinoma and primary sclerosing cholangitis is the fifth decade of life, and these tumors occur only rarely in the elderly population. Similarly, choledochal cysts are usually diagnosed during childhood or early adult life. However, choledochal cysts are occasionally diagnosed in the elderly, and the risk of cholangiocarcinoma increases steadily with patient age.[46] Hepatolithiasis occurs in the elderly population and is a known risk factor for cholangiocarcinoma. Cholangiocarcinoma develops in 5–10% of patients with hepatolithiasis.[9,47–49] Cholangiocarcinoma has been reported to develop a mean 8 years following treatment for hepatolithiasis and may occur despite complete stone clearance from the intrahepatic biliary tree.[49]

### Staging and Classification

Cholangiocarcinoma is best classified into three broad groups: (1) intrahepatic; (2) perihilar; and (3) distal (Fig. 50.6). This classification correlates with the anatomic distribution and implies the preferred treatment for each site. Intrahepatic tumors are treated like liver lesions, with hepatectomy when possible. Distal tumors are managed in a fashion similar to that for other periampullary malignancies, with pancreatoduodenectomy. The perihilar tumors make up the largest group and are managed with local resection of the bile duct with or without hepatic resection.

Cancers of the hepatic duct bifurcation were further classified by Bismuth et al. according to their anatomic location.[50] With this system, type I tumors are confined to the common hepatic duct; type II tumors involve the right

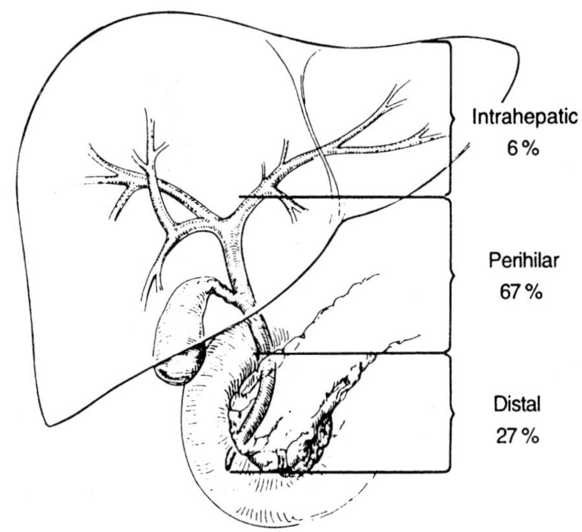


FIGURE 50.6. Distribution of 294 cholangiocarcinoms in intrahepatic, perihilar, and distal subgroups. (From Nakeeb et al.,[39] with permission.)

Table 50.3. TNM Staging for Tumors of the Extrahepatic Bile Duct

| | |
|---|---|
| T1 | Tumor invades mucosa or muscle layer |
| T2 | Tumor invades periductular tissue |
| T3 | Tumor invades adjacent structures (liver, pancreas, duodenum, gallbladder, colon, stomach) |
| N0 | No regional lymph node metastasis |
| N1 | Metastasis in cystic duct, pericholedochal and/or hilar lymph nodes |
| N2 | Metastases in the peripancreatic (head only), periduodenal, periportal, celiac, superior mesenteric, and/or posterior pancreaticoduodenal lymph nodes |
| M0 | No distant metastasis |
| M1 | Distant metastasis |
| **Stage grouping** | |
| I | T1 N0 M0 |
| II | T2 N0 M0 |
| III | T1 N1 M0 |
| | T1 N2 M0 |
| | T2 N1 M0 |
| | T2 N2 M0 |
| IVA | T3 any N M0 |
| IVB | AnyT any N M1 |

*Source:* American Joint Committee on Cancer,[16] with permission.

and left hepatic ducts; type IIIa and IIIb tumors extend into the right or left secondary intrahepatic ducts, respectively; and type IV tumors involve the secondary intrahepatic ducts on both sides.

Cholangiocarcinoma is also staged according to the tumor, node, metastasis (TNM) classification of the American Joint Commission on Cancer (Table 50.3).[16] Using this system, stage I tumors are limited to the bile duct mucosa or muscular layer; stage II tumors invade periductal tissues; stage III tumors have regional lymph node metastases; and stage IV tumors invade adjacent structures (IVa) or have distant metastases (IVb).

## Diagnosis

### *Clinical Presentation*

More than 90% of patients with perihilar or distal tumors present with jaundice. Patients with intrahepatic cholangiocarcinoma are rarely jaundiced until late in the course of the disease. Less common presenting clinical features include pruritus, fever, mild abdominal pain, fatigue, anorexia, and weight loss.[9] Cholangitis is not a frequent presentation but most commonly develops after biliary manipulation by endoscopic or percutaneous techniques.

### *Laboratory Data*

At the time of presentation most patients with perihilar or distal cholangiocarcinoma have a total serum bilirubin level higher than 10 mg/dl.[9] Marked elevations are also observed in serum alkaline phosphatase and $\gamma$-glutamyl transferase levels. Patients with long-standing biliary obstruction may also have a low serum albumin or prolonged prothrombin time. The serum tumor markers carcinoembryonic antigen (CEA) and $\alpha$-fetoprotein (AFP) are typically normal. Serum CA 19-9 and CA 50 may be elevated in patients with cholangiocarcinoma and may be useful for screening patients in high risk groups for developing cholangiocarcinoma.[51]

### *Radiologic Evaluation*

The goals of radiologic evaluation in patients with cholangiocarcinoma include delineation of the overall extent of the tumor, including involvement of the bile ducts, liver, portal vessels, and distant metastases. An ordered sequence of tests can usually achieve these goals. The initial radiographic studies consist of either abdominal ultrasonography or CT scanning. Intrahepatic cholangiocarcinomas are easily visualized on CT scans. A hilar cholangiocarcinoma gives a picture of a dilated intrahepatic biliary tree, a normal or collapsed gallbladder and extrahepatic biliary tree, and a normal pancreas. Distal tumors lead to dilation of the gallbladder and intra- and extrahepatic biliary tree.

Perihilar tumors are often difficult to visualize on ultrasonography and standard CT scans.[52] Duplex ultrasonography has been reported to visualize the primary tumor in more than 85% of patients, whereas bolus contrast-enhanced CT scans were able to define the primary tumor in only 59% of patients.[53,54] Duplex sonography has also been able to determine accurately the extent of bile duct involvement in 87% of patients and the presence or absence of portal vein involvement in 86%.[55] A study comparing enhanced CT scans and MRI in 15 patients with perihilar cholangiocarcinoma managed at Johns Hopkins suggested that MRI is more sensitive than CT scans for detecting these small tumors.[56] However, newer spiral CT techniques are better at detecting the parenchymal extent of the tumor.

After documentation of bile duct dilation, biliary anatomy traditionally has been defined cholangiographically through the percutaneous transhepatic or endoscopic retrograde routes. The most proximal extent of the tumor is the most important feature when determining resectability in patients with perihilar tumors. Percutaneous transhepatic cholangiography is favored in these patients because it defines the proximal extent of tumor involvement most reliably.[9] This approach also allows preoperative placement of percutaneous transhepatic catheters. Recently, magnetic resonance cholangiopancreatography (MRCP) has been documented to have a diagnostic accuracy comparable to those of percutaneous and endoscopic cholangiography. In a series of 14 patients with cholangiocarcinoma, diagnostic quality MRCP images were better at visualizing intrahepatic biliary anatomy than endoscopic retrograde cholangiopancreatography (ERCP).[57] MRCP also has the advantage of obtaining two-dimensional images to define an obstructing lesion. The sensitivity, specificity, and overall accuracy of MRCP at determining the level of biliary obstruction and the presence of a benign or malignant lesion is similar to those for ERCP.

The advantages of transhepatic catheter placement include (1) assistance in the technical aspects of hilar dissection by allowing palpation of the catheter within the biliary tree at the time of exploration and (2) facilitation of intraoperative Silastic transhepatic stent placement. Currently available randomized studies do not support the practice of placing preoperative transhepatic catheters in an effort to reduce operative mortality.[58–60] However, if a liver resection is contemplated, preoperative drainage may be justified.

### *Biopsy/Cytology*

Efforts to establish a tissue diagnosis including percutaneous fine-needle aspiration (FNA) biopsy, brush and scrape biopsy, and cytologic examination of bile have been used.[61–64] Prolonged efforts to obtain a preoperative tissue diagnosis are not indicated unless the patient is not an operative candidate. Bile obtained from a percutaneous catheter demonstrates malignant cells in approximately 30% of cases.[62] This yield may be improved to approximately 40% by brush cytologic techniques through transhepatic stents or at the time of endoscopic procedures and to 67% by percutaneous FNA. Even with these efforts, up to one-third of patients with cholangiocarcinoma have negative biopsy and cytologic results.

## Assessment of Resectability

A careful evaluation of the overall general medical condition of the elderly patient and an accurate staging evaluation are necessary prior to selecting the appropriate management for the patient with cholangiocarcinoma. The preoperative assessment should include the usual evaluation of cardiac risk factors, respiratory status, and renal function, as well as overall performance status. Patients with obstructive jaundice often have decreased hepatic protein synthesis and altered hemostatic mechanisms, and they are at increased risk for infectious complications.

Several studies have defined preoperative risk factors associated with an increase in morbidity and mortality in patients undergoing treatment for malignant biliary obstruction.[39,60,65,66] In 1981, Pitt and colleagues identified eight risk factors predictive of mortality, including serum albumin less than 3.0 g/dl.[65] Little also defined a mortality index predictive of procedure-related mortality in a prospective analysis of patients with obstructive jaundice.[60] The mortality index was derived from the preoperative serum creatinine and albumin levels and the severity of the cholangitis. Several large series of patients undergoing resection for perihilar cholangiocarcinoma have also identified low preoperative serum albumin concentration and perioperative sepsis as factors contributing to operative mortality.[65,66] Control of sepsis and intensive nutritional support should be undertaken preoperatively in the malnourished elderly patient with cholangiocarcinoma.

The preoperative evaluation also includes careful staging to determine the extent of the cholangiocarcinoma.[38,53–55,67–69] In the past, the combination of an abdominal CT scan, cholangiography, and visceral angiography was useful for determining the extent of disease. CT or MRI scan findings signifying unresectable disease include peripheral hepatic metastases or extrahepatic disease. Findings on traditional or MRI cholangiography suggestive of unresectable disease in patients with perihilar cholangiocarcinoma include proximal extension of tumor into second-order bile ducts in both hepatic lobes. The angiographic or MRI findings of tumor encasement or occlusion of the proper hepatic artery, main portal vein, or both right and left portal venous branches or hepatic arterial branches are also considered contraindications to resection by most.

The combination of angiography and cholangiography provides better data than cholangiography alone for staging the elderly patient with perihilar cholangiocarcinoma.[70] More recently, MRI has provided all the data previously obtained by these two studies and CT scanning.[71,72] For patients with distal cholangiocarcinoma, a good quality spiral CT scan can provide sufficient information to predict resectability.

## Palliative Therapy

Palliative therapy in elderly patients with perihilar and distal cholangiocarcinoma is directed at relieving obstructive jaundice and pruritus, preventing recurrent cholangitis, and avoiding hepatic failure secondary to unrelieved biliary obstruction. In addition, palliative therapy in patients with distal cholangiocarcinoma is aimed at preventing or relieving gastric outlet obstruction. Palliation can be achieved nonoperatively with percutaneous or endoscopic techniques or by using an operative approach.

### *Nonoperative Palliation*

Patients with unequivocal evidence of unresectable cholangiocarcinoma at initial evaluation are palliated nonoperatively. Tumor extension into the secondary biliary radicals of both right and left hepatic lobes, the main portal vein, or the main hepatic artery or the presence of distant metastases excludes patients from curative resection. In addition, elderly patients in poor general medical condition may also not be operative candidates. Nonoperative palliation can be achieved endoscopically and percutaneously. A significant proportion of the functioning hepatic parenchyma should be decompressed, and this philosophy may require two or three percutaneously or endoscopically placed catheters in patients with hilar cholangiocarcinoma.[70,73,74]

Percutaneous biliary drainage has several advantages over endoscopic management in patients with perihilar cholangiocarcinoma. Stent placement is more reliably achieved percutaneously than via endoscopic means.[75] In addition, occluded percutaneous stents are easily changed over a guidewire on an outpatient basis, whereas replacement of an endoprosthesis requires an additional invasive procedure. In contrast, endoscopic palliation is the preferred approach in patients with distal cholangiocarcinoma. Placement of an endoprosthesis in experienced centers has been technically successful in approximately 95% of patients with advanced periampullary cancer, with relief of jaundice and pruritus in 80%. More recently, percutaneous or endoscopically placed metallic stents have been used to palliate patients with malignant biliary obstruction.[76–78] Metallic stents remain patent longer than plastic stents and require fewer subsequent manipulations in patients with distal malignant biliary obstruction.[79] Self-expanding metallic stents have also been effective in patients with unresectable perihilar tumors, with median stent patency rates of up to 1 year.[77]

### *Operative Palliation*

In good-risk patients without preoperative evidence of unresectable cholangiocarcinoma, operative exploration is undertaken in an attempt to resect the primary tumor. At Johns Hopkins, approximately 45% of patients with perihilar cholangiocarcinoma were found at exploration to have intraperitoneal or liver metastases (15%) or extensive tumor involvement of the porta hepatis (30%), precluding resection.[38,42,70,80–82] Ten percent of patients with distal cholangiocarcinoma have unresectable lesions at operative exploration. Patients with peritoneal carcinomatosis undergo minimal operative intervention. Cholecystectomy is performed to prevent the subsequent development of acute cholecystitis from cystic duct obstruction related to the percutaneous catheter.[83] Postoperatively, the preoperatively placed transhepatic catheters are replaced with larger, softer transhepatic stents.[84]

In patients with locally advanced unresectable perihilar tumors, several operative approaches are available for palliation, including Roux-en-Y choledochojejunostomy with intraoperative placement of Silastic biliary catheters or a segment III cholangiojejunostomy. The operative procedure for placing transhepatic Silastic catheters begins with obtaining a tissue diagnosis of cholangiocarcinoma. A tissue diagnosis is required prior to initiating postoperative irradiation or chemotherapy.

The gallbladder is then mobilized, and the distal common bile duct is divided and oversewn. Next, the Ring catheters are exchanged for larger Silastic biliary catheters. A hepaticojejunostomy is then performed to a Roux-en-Y limb of jejunum (Fig. 50.7). The advantages of this approach over nonoperative palliation include (1) removal of the gallbladder[83]; (2) placement of larger, softer Silastic stents with a lower risk of hemobilia and improved patient comfort; and (3) positioning the stent into a defunctionalized Roux-en-Y jejunal limb to reduce the incidence of subsequent cholangitis.

In patients with locally unresectable or metastatic distal cholangiocarcinoma, operative palliation is directed at relieving both biliary and gastric outlet obstruction. Symptomatic gastroduodenal obstruction occurs prior to death in approximately 30% of patients with periampullary malignancies. Gastrojejunostomy at the time of initial presentation prevents this complication without increasing the operative morbidity or mortality. Biliary-enteric continuity is restored most often with a hepaticojejunostomy or a choledochojejunostomy.

## Surgical Resection

Curative treatment of patients with cholangiocarcinoma is possible only with complete resection. For patients with anatomically resectable intrahepatic cholangiocarcinoma and without advanced cirrhosis, partial hepatectomy is the procedure of choice. After careful exploration of the peritoneal surfaces and regional lymph nodes for metastatic disease, the liver is mobilized and examined with intraoperative ultrasonography. Approximately 40% of resectable intrahepatic cholangiocarcinomas are multiple or involve both hepatic lobes. Hepatic resection is planned to remove completely all tumor with an adequate margin. Most commonly it involves a formal lobectomy or trisegmentectomy.

Elderly patients with tumors involving the hepatic hilum or proximal common hepatic duct (Bismuth types I or II) that have no vascular invasion are candidates for local tumor excision.[38] Preoperatively, bilateral transhepatic Ring catheters are placed to aid in the intraoperative identification of the right and left hepatic ducts.[38,81,82,84] After excluding the presence of metastatic disease, the common bile duct (CBD) is dissected free and encircled just proximal to the suprapancreatic portion. The CBD is then divided, and the distal end is oversewn. It is then reflected cephalad, skeletonizing the portal vein and proper hepatic artery. Once the entire common hepatic duct has been elevated off the portal vasculature, the left and right hepatic ducts can be identified by palpating the diverging Ring catheters. The left and right hepatic ducts are then divided above the extent of palpable tumor.

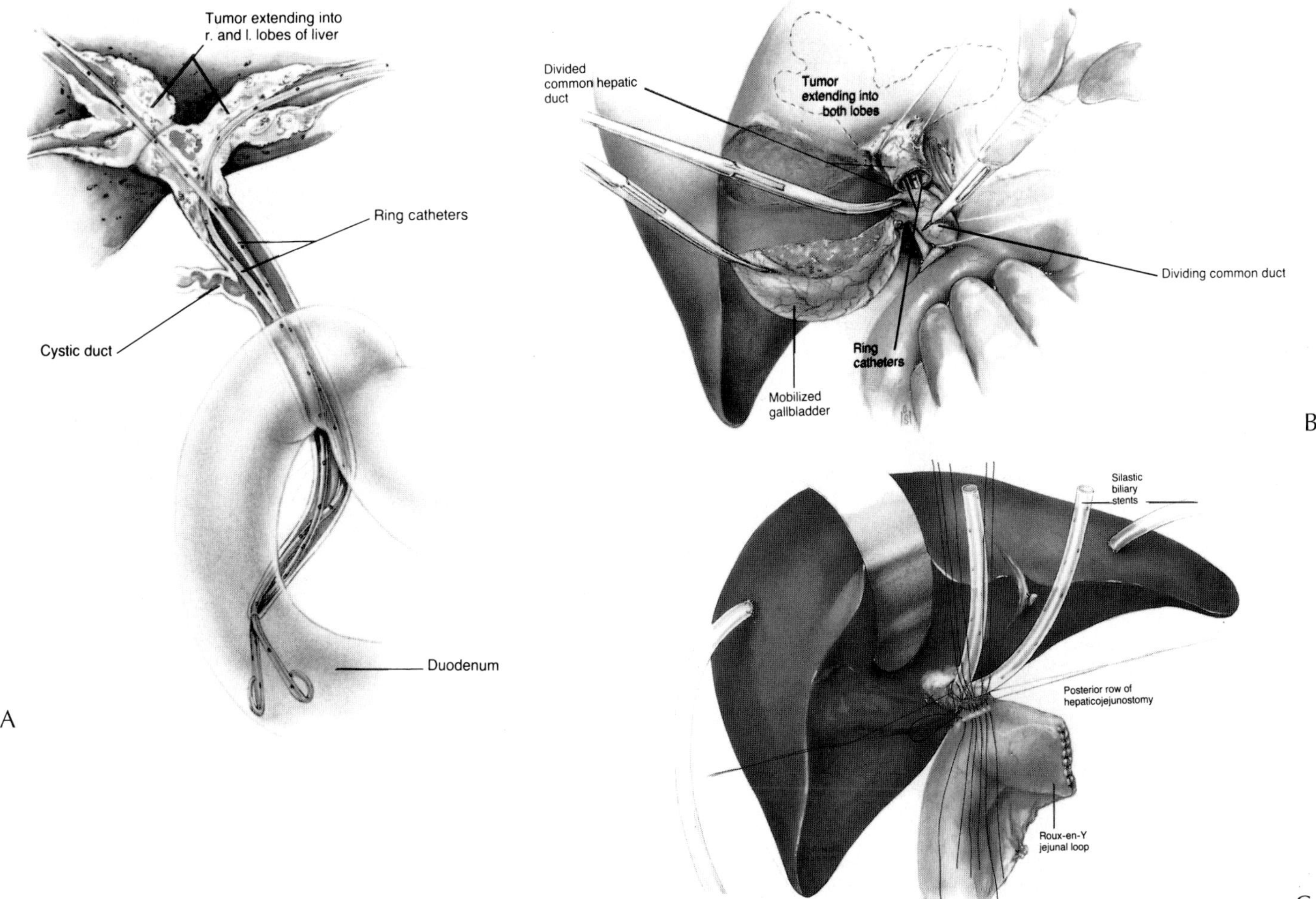


FIGURE 50.7. A. Palliative intubation of Bismuth type IV unresectable perihilar cholangiocarcinoma with preoperatively placed transhepatic stents changed over guidewires. B. Common bile duct is divided distal to the tumor and a cholecystectomy is performed. C. Roux-en-Y choledochojejunostomy is constructed over Silastic transhepatic stents distal to the tumor. (From Cameron,[110] with permission.)

Frozen section examination is used to determine the adequacy of the surgical margin. The percutaneous transhepatic catheters are then exchanged for 16F Silastic catheters. A 60 cm retrocolic Roux-en-Y limb is then constructed, and bilateral hepaticojejunostomies are performed over the Silastic stents.

Proximal extension of a hilar cholangiocarcinoma into either the intrahepatic segments of the right or left hepatic duct renders these tumors incurable by local tumor resection. Complete resection in these patients is achievable only with combined resection of the extrahepatic biliary tree and major liver resection. Improvements in operative morbidity and mortality and in long-term survival when negative surgical margins are achieved, support the use of this approach when complete tumor resection is possible.[38,41,50,52,85–99]

The need for hepatic resection can usually be predicted on the basis of preoperative angiography, cholangiography, or MRI. When unilateral neoplastic involvement of the right or left portal vein or hepatic ducts is visualized radiographically, the initial hilar dissection is performed as described previously with division of the uninvolved hepatic duct. A frozen section should be examined to confirm a negative hepatic duct margin on the uninvolved side. Next, the extrahepatic segments of the hepatic vein, portal vein, and hepatic artery to the involved lobe are divided or occluded with vascular clamps. The hepatic parenchyma is then divided using the ultrasonic dissector or cautery. Extension of the tumor into the caudate lobe frequently necessitates caudate lobectomy to achieve negative tumor margins. Biliary enteric continuity is restored to a Roux-en-Y limb of jejunum, as described above (Fig. 50.8).

Elderly patients with resectable distal cholangiocarcinoma are managed similarly to patients with other periampullary malignancies with pancreatoduodenectomy. More than 85% of these patients are suitable for the pylorus-preserving modification, and gastrointestinal

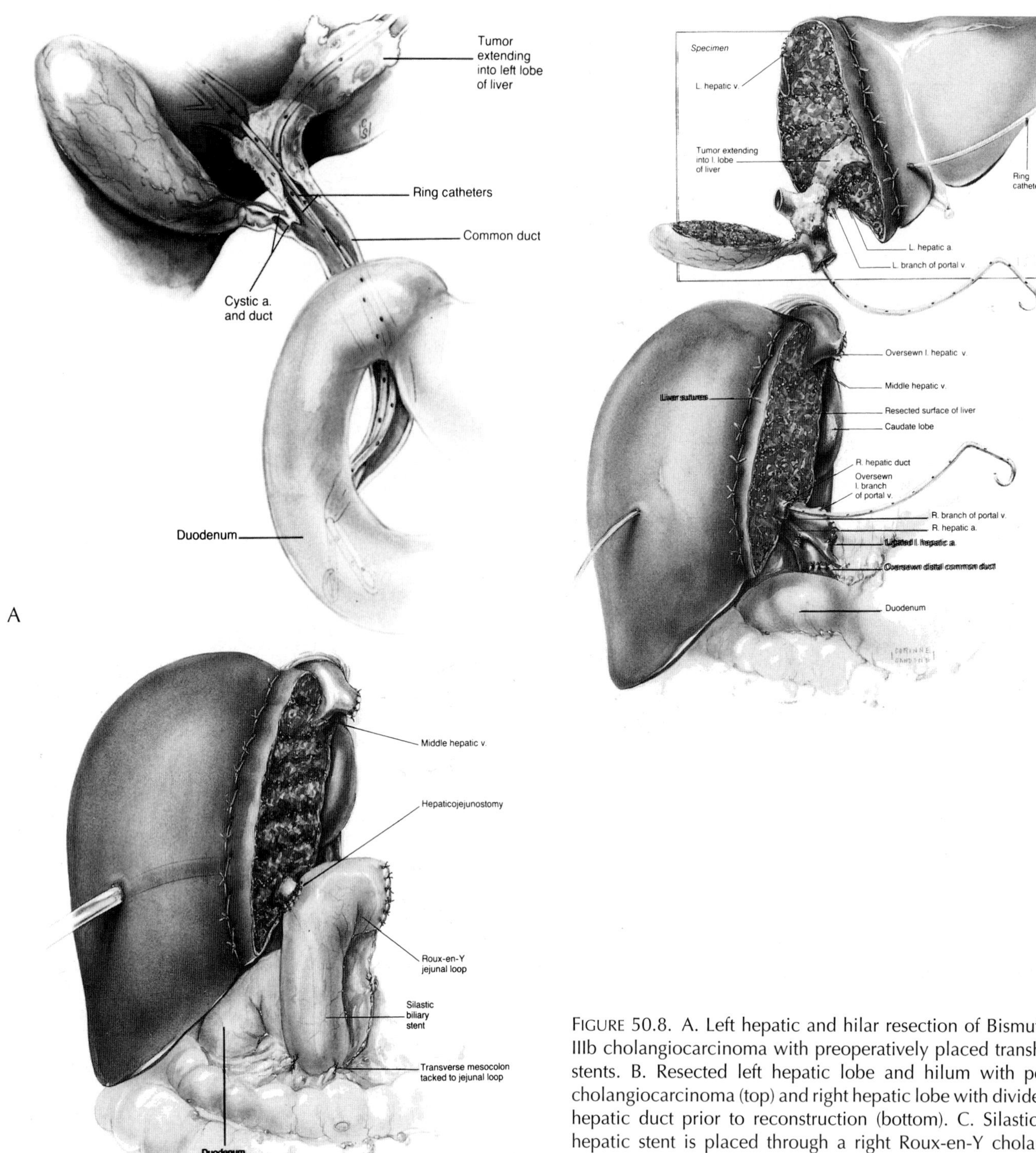


FIGURE 50.8. A. Left hepatic and hilar resection of Bismuth type IIIb cholangiocarcinoma with preoperatively placed transhepatic stents. B. Resected left hepatic lobe and hilum with perihilar cholangiocarcinoma (top) and right hepatic lobe with divided right hepatic duct prior to reconstruction (bottom). C. Silastic transhepatic stent is placed through a right Roux-en-Y cholangiojejunostomy after left hepatic lobectomy. (From Cameron,[100] with permission.)

continuity is restored with an end-to-end pancreatojejunostomy, an end-to-side hepaticojejunostomy, and an end-to-side duodenojejunostomy. The hepaticojejunostomy is usually stented with a T-tube to decompress the system in the event of a biliary or pancreatic leak.

## Survival

Procedure-related morbidity and mortality, quality of survival, and long-term survival are highly dependent on the stage of disease at presentation and on whether the patient is treated by a palliative procedure or complete tumor resection.

### Palliative Therapy

Between 1973 and 1989, a group of 65 patients with unresectable hilar cholangiocarcinoma underwent nonoperative percutaneous stenting or operative palliation at The Johns Hopkins Hospital.[38,70] Altogether, 21 patients were managed with percutaneous biliary stents; 44 patients underwent laparotomy, with placement of large-bore Silastic transhepatic stents in 33. The procedure-related morbidity was similar for patients undergoing nonoperative palliation and those undergoing laparotomy. Hospital mortality was 14% in the nonoperatively palliated group and 7% in those managed operatively. Mean survival was 8 months for the patients managed with operative palliation and 5 months for those managed with percutaneous stenting ($p < 0.05$).

Quality of survival measured by the number of readmissions per month of survival, hospital days per month of survival, and episodes of cholangitis was better in the patients undergoing operative palliation. In addition, patients managed nonoperatively required more frequent stent changes than patients managed operatively. On the other hand, eight patients (15%) managed operatively required late operations. These procedures were most frequently for small bowel or duodenal obstruction. None of the patients managed nonoperatively required laparotomy during the follow-up period.

Several additional studies have examined the results of palliative therapy for hilar cholangiocarcinoma.[74,97,99,101] In a French report, the operative mortality and long-term survival were similar for patients managed with operatively placed biliary stents and those managed with palliative biliary-enteric anastomosis.[97] Guthrie et al. demonstrated more effective palliation with a segment III cholangiojejunostomy than with endoscopic or percutaneous stenting.[101] The operatively managed patients had a lower incidence of cholangitis and jaundice than the patients managed with nonoperative stenting. Lai et al. demonstrated lower procedure-related mortality among patients managed operatively than among those palliated with endoscopic stenting.[74] Overall survival and quality of survival assessed by frequency of cholangitis attacks, episodes of jaundice, and days in the hospital were similar for the two groups. Patients managed with endoscopic stents had a higher incidence of catheter-related problems than patients managed with cholangioenteric bypass. In contrast, Washburn et al. demonstrated better survival in patients palliated nonoperatively than in surgically palliated patients.[99] All of these retrospective analyses are limited, however, by biases in selecting patients for each treatment group.

Several randomized, prospective trials have compared operative versus nonoperative palliation in patients with periampullary cancer.[102] In general, these trials demonstrated lower procedure-related morbidity and mortality rates for the nonoperatively managed patients. However, the procedure-related mortality in the operatively managed patients ranged from 15% to 24%. In addition, a higher rate of recurrent jaundice or gastric outlet obstruction occurred in the nonoperatively managed patients. Survival was similar among the two treatment groups in each study (mean survival 12–22 weeks).

Between 1987 and 1991, a series of 118 patients with unresectable periampullary tumors were explored at The Johns Hopkins Hospital.[102] Seventy percent of the patients were over age 60. The most common operative procedure was choledochojejunostomy and hepaticojejunostomy, which were performed in 67% of patients. Perioperative mortality was 2.5%, and gastric outlet obstruction or recurrent jaundice developed prior to death in only 4.0% and 2.5% of patients, respectively.

### Surgical Resection

A series of 34 patients with intrahepatic cholangiocarcinoma managed with surgical resection was recently reported by Casavilla et al.[103]; 53% of these patients were over age 60. Multiple tumors were present in 44% of the patients, and 41% had involvement of both hepatic lobes. Histologically negative surgical margins were obtained in 71% of patients. Operative mortality was 6%. Overall patient survival was 60% at 1 year, 37% at 3 years, and 31% at 5 years after resection. Significant predictors of postoperative treatment failure were positive surgical margins, multiple tumors, and metastatic disease in regional lymph nodes. Age was not predictive of operative or long-term mortality.

A group of 109 patients with perihilar cholangiocarcinoma was managed with resection at The Johns Hopkins Hospital between 1973 and 1995.[39] Following resection, 36 patients had obvious gross tumor remaining, and 81 patients had a positive microscopic surgical margin. Of the 109 patients, 94 underwent local hilar excision, and 15 were managed with hepatic lobectomy with resection of the extrahepatic biliary tree. Four operative deaths (3.6%) occurred among these 109 patients, including

TABLE 50.4. Operative Mortality of Hilar Versus Hepatic Resection for Perihilar Cholangiocarcinoma (1989 to Present)

| | | Age (years) | | Hilar resection | | Hepatic resection[a] | |
|---|---|---|---|---|---|---|---|
| Study | Year | Mean | Range | No. | Operative mortality (%) | No. | Operative mortality (%) |
| Baer[92] (Berne, Switzerland) | 1993 | 62 | 34–85 | 12 | 0 | 9 | 11 |
| Bismuth[50] (Paris, France) | 1992 | 50 | 22–82 | 10 | 0 | 13 | 0 |
| Fortner[88] (Memorial Sloan-Kettering) | 1989 | 60 | 33–81 | 7 | 0 | 7 | 0 |
| Hadjis[90] (London, England) | 1990 | 55 | 33–74 | 11 | 0 | 16 | 12 |
| Kawasaki[94] (Matsumoto, Japan) | 1994 | 58 | 39–72 | — | — | 9 | 0 |
| Klempnauer[104] (Hanover, Germany) | 1997 | 57 | 25–79 | 31 | 6 | 77 | 8 |
| Nagino[95] (Nagoya, Japan) | 1995 | 55 | 44–64 | — | — | 4 | 0 |
| Nakeeb[39] (Johns Hopkins) | 1996 | 62 | 23–84 | 94 | 3 | 15 | 7 |
| Nimura[96] (Nagoya, Japan) | 1991 | 60 | 33–76 | — | — | 45 | 2 |
| Reding[97] (French Surgical Association) | 1991 | 64 | | 47 | 17 | 50 | 14 |
| Su[66] (Taipei, Taiwan) | 1996 | 62 | 32–74 | 21 | 5 | 28 | 14 |
| Sugiura[98] (Tokyo, Japan) | 1994 | 60 | 33–78 | — | — | 61 | 7 |
| Washburn[99] (Boston) | 1995 | 60 | 25–86 | — | — | 18 | 11 |
| *Total* | | 60 | 22–86 | 233 | 6 | 352 | 8 |

[a] Does not include patients also undergoing portal vein or hepatic artery resection and reconstruction.

one death (6.6%) among the 15 managed with hepatic lobectomy. Actuarial survival among the 109 patients undergoing resection was 68% at 1 year, 30% at 3 years, and 11% after 5 years of follow-up. Survival was significantly prolonged in patients without residual microscopic tumor at the surgical margin. In the 28 patients with a negative margin, the actuarial survival was 68% at 1 year, 56% at 3 years, and 19% after 5 years. Patient age did not influence operative morbidity or mortality or the long-term survival. Fifty-three percent of these patients also received a combination of external beam radiotherapy, a boost of internal irradiation utilizing iridium 192, or both.

In recent years, the trend around the world has been to perform more hepatic resections for perihilar cholangiocarcinoma. More than 580 patients with perihilar cholangiocarcinoma have been reported in the literature since 1989 (Table 50.4).[39,50,66,88,90,92,94–99,104] For 233 patients undergoing local hilar resection, the operative mortality rate was 6%; and for 352 patients managed with combined hilar and hepatic resection, the operative mortality was 8%. The mean age of these 585 patients undergoing aggressive surgical resection for perihilar cholangiocarcinoma was 60 years, with half of them in their seventh, eighth, or ninth decade of life. The mean survival rate in the locally resected patients ranged from 19 to 36 months. Similarly, the mean survival of patients undergoing combined hilar and hepatic resection ranged from 16 to 32 months.

Several factors may be important when determining long-term prognosis following curative resection for hilar cholangiocarcinoma. Achieving negative histologic margins is important for determining overall long-term survival.[41,87,92,99] Bengmark et al. initially reported several 10-year survivors following hepatic resection with negative histologic margins for hilar cholangiocarcinoma.[87] In two large series of patients managed with attempted curative resection for perihilar cholangiocarcinoma, both Klempnauer et al. and Sugiura et al. reported a 33% overall 5-year survival for patients with negative histologic margins, whereas no patient with microscopic cancer at the surgical margins survived 5 years (Fig. 50.9).[98,99,102–104] Among patients with negative histologic margins, the addition of a caudate lobectomy significantly prolonged the 5-year survival (46% vs. 12%). In addition, the presence of regional lymph node metastases adversely affected survival. In several large series, multivariate analysis found that patient age did not influence overall survival.

Seventy-three patients with distal cholangiocarcinoma undergoing pancreatoduodenectomy have been reported from The Johns Hopkins Hospital.[39] The 1-, 3-, and 5-year survival rates were 70%, 31%, and 28%, respectively. Factors associated with prolonged survival of these patients include tumor differentiation and lymph node status. Negative nodes increased the median survival from 17 months to 27 months, whereas poorly differentiated tumors had a lower median survival (10 vs. 22 months).

## Adjuvant Therapy

Radiation therapy has been evaluated in patients with perihilar cholangiocarcinoma using a variety of methods

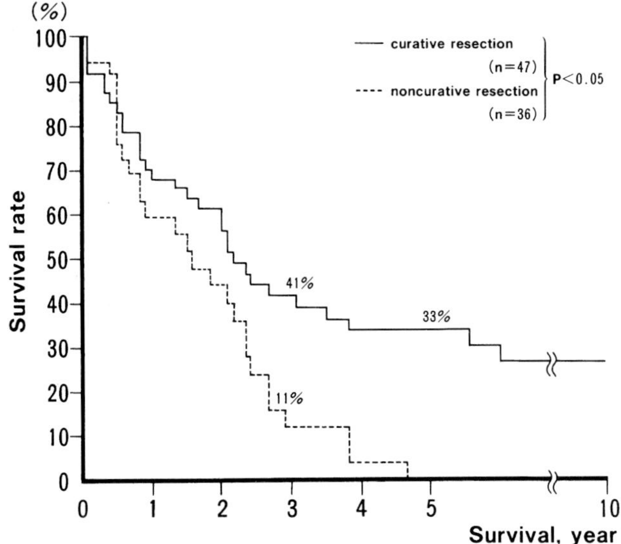


FIGURE 50.9. Actuarial Kaplan-Meier survival of patients with perihilar cholangiocarcinoma undergoing curative or noncurative resection (microscopic tumor at surgical margin). Survival was improved ($p < 0.05$) in the curatively resected patients. (From Sugiura et al.,[98] with permission.)

including external beam radiotherapy, intraoperative radiotherapy, internal radiotherapy, radioimmunotherapy, and charged particle radiation. External beam radiotherapy has been the most commonly used modality and is typically administered to a total dose of 45–60 Gy.[38,105–107] Internal radiotherapy is normally delivered through percutaneous or endoscopically placed biliary stents using iridium 192 as the radiation source.[38,108,109] Multiple retrospective analyses have suggested that radiation therapy may provide some benefit in patients with perihilar cholangiocarcinoma administered via one of these techniques.

In a prospective analysis from The Johns Hopkins Hospital, 23 patients underwent irradiation and 27 did not.[110] The radiation dose ranged from 45 to 63 Gy and consisted of external beam plus iridium 192 seeds. None of the patients underwent adjuvant chemotherapy. Patients undergoing curative resection survived significantly longer than patients undergoing operative palliation. Among those with resection, irradiation had no effect on the mean (24 vs. 24 months), median, or actuarial survival. Similarly, among palliated patients irradiation had no effect on the mean (10 vs. 13 months), median, or actuarial survival. Multivariate analysis identified resection as the only positive predictive factor for prolonged survival.

The use of chemotherapy along (with 5-FU, mitomycin C, or cisplatin) has not been shown to improve survival in patients with resected or unresected cholangiocarcinoma. Response rates using multidrug chemotherapeutic regimens also remain low. Given the potential radiosensitization effect of 5-FU, the combination of irradiation and chemotherapy may be more effective than either agent alone. Preliminary data in relatively small numbers of patients have been reported, but no randomized data are available.[111–115]

## Conclusions

Despite overall advances in the ability to diagnose and treat elderly patients with malignant tumors of the gallbladder and biliary tract, the prognosis for patients with these malignancies remains poor. Improvements in diagnostic CT scanning, duplex ultrasonography, and MRI will improve our ability to diagnose noninvasively and stage gallbladder cancer or cholangiocarcinoma in the elderly patient. Complete surgical resection remains the only curative treatment for malignancy of the biliary tract. Aggressive surgical approaches are likely to continue, and the challenge remains in being able to perform these procedures safely in jaundiced and sometimes septic elderly patients. Unfortunately, for most patients with malignant tumors of the biliary tract, curative resection is not possible, and optimal palliation remains the goal of therapy. Finally, advances in adjuvant chemotherapy and radiotherapy are required to improve the overall prognosis of patients with gallbladder cancer or cholangiocarcinoma.

## References

1. Jones RS. Carcinoma of the gallbladder. Surg Clin North Am 1990;70:1419–1428.
2. Piehler JM, Crichlow RW. Primary carcinoma of the gallbladder. Surg Gynecol Obstet 1978;147:929–939.
3. Carriaga MT, Henson DE. Liver, gallbladder, extrahepatic bile ducts, and pancreas. Cancer 1995;75:171–190.
4. Ransohoff DF, Gracie WA. Treatment of gallstones. Ann Intern Med 1993;119:606–619.
5. Strom BL, Soloway RD, Rios-Dalenz JL, et al. Risk factors for gallbladder cancer: an international collaborative case-control study. Cancer 1995;76:1747–1756.
6. Lowenfels AB, Lindstrom CG, Conway MJ, et al. Gallstones and risk of gallbladder cancer. J Natl Cancer Inst 1985;75:77–80.
7. De Aretxabala X, Roa I, Burgos L, et al. Gallbladder cancer in Chile: a report on 43 potentially resectable tumors. Cancer 1992;69:60–65.
8. Nervi F, Duarte I, Gomez G, et al. Frequency of gallbladder cancer in Chile: a high-risk area. Int J Cancer 1988; 41:657–660.
9. Pitt HA, Dooley WC, Yeo CJ, et al. Malignancies of the biliary tree. Curr Probl Surg 1995;32:1–90.
10. Wibbenmeyer LA, Wade TP, Chen RC, et al. Laparoscopic cholecystectomy can disseminate in situ carcinoma of the gallbladder. J Am Coll Surg 1995;181:504–510.

11. Liu KJM, Richter HM, Cho MJ, et al. Carcinoma involving the gallbladder in elderly patients presenting with acute cholecystitis. Surgery 1997;122:748–756.
12. Zatonski WA, Lowenfels AB, Boyle P, et al. Epidemiologic aspects of gallbladder cancer: a case-control study of the SEARCH program of the international agency for research on cancer. J Natl Cancer Inst 1997;89:1132–1138.
13. Fahim RB, McDonald JR, Richards JC, et al. Carcinoma of the gallbladder: a study of its modes of spread. Ann Surg 1962;156:114–123.
14. Shirai Y, Yoshida K, Tsukada K, et al. Identification of the regional lymphatic system of the gallbladder by vital staining. Br J Surg 1992;79:659–662.
15. Shirai Y, Tsukada K, Ohtani T, et al. Hepatic metastases from carcinoma of the gallbladder. Cancer 1995;75:2063–2068.
16. American Joint Committee on Cancer. Gallbladder and extrahepatic bile ducts. In: Beahrs OH, Henson DE, Hutter RVP et al. (eds) Manual for the Staging of Cancer. Philadelphia: Lippincott, 1993:111–120.
17. White K, Kraybill WG, Lopez MJ: Primary carcinoma of the gallbladder: TNM staging and prognosis. J Surg Oncol 1988;39:251–255.
18. Soyer P, Gouhiri M, Boudiaf M, et al. Carcinoma of the gallbladder: imaging features with surgical correlation. Am J Radiol 1997;169:781–785.
19. Mizuguchi M, Kudo S, Fukahori T, et al. Endoscopic ultrasonography for demonstrating loss of multiple-layer pattern of the thickened gallbladder wall in the preoperative diagnosis of gallbladder cancer. Eur Radiol 1997;7:1323–1327.
20. Shirai Y, Yoshida K, Tsukada K, et al. Inapparent carcinoma of the gallbladder: an appraisal of a radical second operation after simple cholecystectomy. Ann Surg 1992;215:326–331.
21. Donohue JH, Nagorney DM, Grant CS, et al. Carcinoma of the gallbladder: does radical resection improve outcome? Arch Surg 1990;125:237–241.
22. Cubertafond P, Gainant A, Cucchiaro G. Surgical treatment of 724 carcinomas of the gallbladder: results of the French Surgical Association survey. Ann Surg 1994;219:275–280.
23. Tsukada K, Kurosaki I, Uchida K, et al. Lymph node spread from carcinoma of the gallbladder. Cancer 1997;80:661–667.
24. Tsukada K, Hatakeyama K, Kurosaki I, et al. Outcome of radical surgery for carcinoma of the gallbladder according to the TNM stage. Surgery 1996;120:816–822.
25. Ogura Y, Mizumoto R, Isaji S, et al. Radical operations for carcinoma of the gallbladder: present status in Japan. World J Surg 1991;15:337–343.
26. Ouchi K, Suzuki M, Tominaga T, et al. Survival after surgery for cancer of the gallbladder. Br J Surg 1994;81:1655–1657.
27. Nakamura S, Nishiyama R, Yokoi Y, et al. Hepatopancreatoduodenectomy for advanced gallbladder carcinoma. Arch Surg 1994;129:625–629.
28. Gall FP, Kockerling F, Scheele J, et al. Radical operations for carcinoma of the gallbladder: present status in Germany. World J Surg 1991;15:328–336.
29. Bartlett DL, Fong Y, Fortner JG, et al. Long-term results after resection for gallbladder cancer: implications for staging and management. Ann Surg 1996;224:639–646.
30. Bloechle C, Izbicki JR, Passlick B, et al. Is radical surgery in locally advanced gallbladder carcinoma justified? Am J Gastroenterol 1995;90:2195–2200.
31. Jones RS. Palliative operative procedures for carcinoma of the gallbladder. World J Surg 1991;15:348–351.
32. Miyazaki M, Itoh H, Ambiru S, et al. Radical surgery for advanced gallbladder carcinoma. Br J Surg 1996;83:478–481.
33. Falkson G, MacIntyre JM, Moertel CG. Eastern Cooperative Oncology Group experience with chemotherapy for inoperable gallbladder and bile duct cancer. Cancer 1984;54:965–969.
34. Gebbia V, Majello E, Testa A, et al. Treatment of advanced adenocarcinomas of the exocrine pancreas and the gallbladder with 5-fluorouracil, high dose levofolinic acid and oral hydroxyurea on a weekly schedule. Cancer 1996;78:1300–1307.
35. Kraybill WG, Lee H, Picus J, et al. Multidisciplinary treatment of biliary tract cancers. J Surg Oncol 1994;55:239–245.
36. Todoroki T, Iwasaki Y, Orii K, et al. Resection combined with intraoperative radiation therapy (IORT) for stage IV (TNM) gallbladder carcinoma. World J Surg 1991;15:357–366.
37. Todoroki T. Radiation therapy for primary gallbladder cancer. Hepatogastroenterology 1997;44:1229–1239.
38. Gameron JL, Pitt HA, Zinner MJ, et al. Management of proximal cholangiocarcinoma by surgical resection and radiotherapy. Am J Surg 1990;159:91–98.
39. Nakeeb A, Pitt HA, Sohn TA, et al. Cholangiocarcinoma: a spectrum of intrahepatic, perihilar, and distal tumors. Ann Surg 1996;224:463–475.
40. Tompkins RK, Saunders K, Roslyn JJ, et al. Changing patterns in diagnosis and management of bile duct cancer. Ann Surg 1990;211:614–621.
41. Nagorney DM, Donohue JH, Farnell MB, et al. Outcomes after curative resections of cholangiocarcinoma. Arch Surg 1993;128:871–877.
42. Broe PJ, Cameron JL. The management of proximal biliary tract tumors. Adv Surg 1981;15:47–62.
43. Sons HU, Borchard F. Carcinoma of the extrahepatic bile ducts: a postmortem study of 65 cases and review of the literature. J Surg Oncol 1987;34:6–12.
44. Miller BA, Ries LAG, Hankey BF, et al. SEER Cancer Statistics Review: 1973–1990. NIH Publ No. 93-2789. Bethesda: National Cancer Institute, 1993.
45. Ahrendt SA, Pitt HA, Kalloo AN, et al. Primary sclerosing cholangitis: resect, dilate, or transplant? Ann Surg 1998;227:412–423.
46. Lipsett PA, Pitt HA, et al. Choledochal cyst disease: a changing pattern of presentation. Ann Surg 1994;220:644–652.
47. Sheen-Chen SM, Chou FF, Eng HL. Intrahepatic cholangiocarcinoma in hepatolithiasis: a frequently overlooked disease. J Surg Oncol 1991;47:131–135.
48. Fan ST, Lai EC, Wong J. Hepatic resection for hepatolithiasis. Arch Surg 1993;128:1070–1074.
49. Chijiiwa K, Ichimiya H, Kuroki S, et al. Late development of cholangiocarcinoma after the treatment of hepatolithiasis: immunohistochemical study of mucin carbohydrates and core proteins in hepatolithiasis and cholangiocarcinoma. Int J Cancer 1993;55:82–91.

50. Bismuth H, Nakache R, Diamond T. Management strategies in resection for hilar cholangiocarcinoma. Ann Surg 1992;215:31–38.
51. Ramage JK, Donaghy A, Farrant JM. Serum tumor markers for the diagnosis of cholangiocarcinoma in primary sclerosing cholangitis. Gastroenterology 1995;108:865–869.
52. Langer JC, Langer B, Taylor BR, et al. Carcinoma of the extrahepatic bile ducts: results of an aggressive surgical approach. Surgery 1985;98:752–759.
53. Looser CH, Stain SC, Baer HU, et al. Staging of hilar cholangiocarcinoma by ultrasound and duplex sonography: a comparison with angiography and preoperative findings. Br J Radiol 1992;65:871–877.
54. Yamashita Y, Takahashi M, Kanazawa S, et al. Parenchymal changes of the liver in cholangiocarcinoma: CT evaluation. Gastrointest Radiol 1992;17:161–166.
55. Hann LE, Graetrex KV, Bach AM, et al. Cholangiocarcinoma at the hepatic hilus: sonographic findings. Am J Radiol 1997;168:985–989.
56. Saeki M, Pitt HA, Tempany CM. Magnetic resonance imaging of hilar cholangiocarcinoma [abstract]. In: Proceedings of the International Hepatobiliary Pancreatic Association, 1992:100A.
57. Lomanto D, Pavone P, Laghi A, et al. Magnetic resonance-cholangiopancreatography in the diagnosis of biliopancreatic disease. Am J Surg 1997;174:33–38.
58. Pitt HA, Gomes AS, Lois JF, et al. Does preoperative percutaneous biliary drainage reduce operative risk or increase hospital cost? Ann Surg 1985;201:545–553.
59. Nakeeb A, Pitt HA. The role of preoperative biliary decompression in obstructive jaundice. Hepatogastroenterology 1995;42:332–339.
60. Little JM. A prospective evaluation of computerized estimates of risk in the management of obstructive jaundice. Surgery 1987;102:473–476.
61. Cope C, Marinelli DL, Weinstein JK. Transcatheter biopsy of lesions obstructing the bile ducts. Radiology 1988;169:555–560.
62. Desa LA, Akosa AB, Lazzara S, et al. Cytodiagnosis in the management of extrahepatic biliary stricture. Gut 1991;32:1188–1191.
63. Ferrucci JT, Chuttani R. Magnetic resonance cholangiopancreatography (MRCP): comparison to invasive cholangiopancreatography. Hepatology 1995;22:107A.
64. Foutch PG, Kerr DM, Horlan JR, et al. Endoscopic retrograde wire-guided brush cytology for diagnosis of patients with malignant obstruction of the bile duct. Am J Gastroenterol 1990;85:791–795.
65. Pitt HA, Cameron JL, Postier RG, et al. Factors influencing mortality in biliary tract surgery. Am J Surg 1981;141:66–72.
66. Su CH, Tsay SH, Wu CC, et al. Factors influencing postoperative morbidity, mortality, and survival after resection for hilar cholangiocarcinoma. Ann Surg 1996;223:384–394.
67. Lynn RB, Wilson JAP, Cho KJ. Cholangiocarcinoma: role of percutaneous transhepatic cholangiography in determination of resectability. Dig Dis Sci 1988;33:587–592.
68. Dooley WC, Pitt HA, Venbrux AD, et al. Is angiography useful in patients with perihilar cholangiocarcinoma [abstract]. In: Proceedings of the International Hepatobiliary Pancreatic Association, 1992:32A.
69. Dooley WC, Cameron JL, Pitt HA, et al. Is preoperative angiography useful in patients with periampullary tumors? Ann Surg 1990;211:649–655.
70. Nordback IH, Pitt HA, Coleman JA, et al. Unresectable hilar cholangiocarcinoma: percutaneous versus operative palliation. Surgery 1994;115:5977–603.
71. Soto JA, Carish MA, Yucel EK, et al. Magnetic resonance cholangiography: comparison with endoscopic retrograde cholangiopancreatography. Gastroenterology 1996;110:589–597.
72. Lee MG, Lee HJ, Kim MH, et al. Extrahepatic biliary diseases: 2D MR cholangiography compared with endoscopic retrograde cholangiopancreatography. Radiology 1997;202:663–669.
73. Hausegger KA, Kleinert R, Lammer J, et al. Malignant biliary obstruction: histologic findings after treatment with self-expandable stents. Radiology 1992;185:461–464.
74. Lai EC, Chu KM, Lo CY, et al. Choice of palliation for malignant hilar obstruction. Am J Surg 1992;163:208–212.
75. Lamere JS, Stoker J, Dees J, et al. Non-surgical palliative treatment of patients with malignant biliary obstruction: the place of endoscopic and percutaneous drainage. Clin Radiol 1987;38:603–608.
76. Schima W, Prokesch R, Osterreicher C, et al. Biliary wallstent endoprosthesis in malignant hilar obstruction: long-term results with regard to the type of obstruction. Clin Radiol 1997;52:213–219.
77. Peters RA, Williams SG, Lombard M, et al. The management of high-grade hilar structures by endoscopic insertion of self-expanding metal endoprosthesis. Endoscopy 1997;29:10–16.
78. O'Brien S, Hatfield AR, Craig PI, et al. A three year follow up of self-expanding metal stents in the endoscopic palliation of long-term survivors with malignant biliary obstruction. Gut 1995;36:618–621.
79. Becker CD, Glattie A, Mailbach R, et al. Percutaneous palliation of malignant obstructive jaundice with wall stent endoprosthesis: follow-up and reintervention in patients with hilar and non-hilar obstruction. J Vasc Intervent Radiol 1993;4:597–604.
80. Pitt HA. Proximal bile duct: resection and palliation. In: Daly JM, Cady B (eds) Atlas of Surgical Oncology. St. Louis: Mosby-Year Book, 1993:417–437.
81. Yeo CJ, Pitt HA, Cameron JL. Cholangiocarcinoma. Surg Clin North Am 1990;70:1429–1447.
82. Ahrendt SA, Pitt HA. Cholangiocarcinoma. In: Niederhuber JE (ed) Curent Therapy in Oncology. St. Louis: Mosby-Year Book, 1993:410–414.
83. Lillemoe KD, Pitt HA, Kaufmann SL, et al. Acute cholecystitis occurring as a complication of percutaneous transhepatic drainage. Surg Gynecol Obstet 1989;168:348–352.
84. Crist DW, Kadir S, Cameron JL. Proximal biliary tract reconstruction: the value of preoperatively placed percutaneous biliary catheters. Surg Gynecol Obstet 1987;165:421–426.
85. Stain SC, Baer HU, Dennison AR, et al. Current management of hilar cholangiocarcinoma. Surg Gynecol Obstet 1992;175:579–588.

86. Ouchi K, Matsuno S, Sato T. Long-term survival in carcinoma of the biliary tract. Arch Surg 1989;124:248–252.
87. Bengmark S, Ekberg H, Evander A, et al. Major liver resection for hilar cholangiocarcinoma. Ann Surg 1988;207:120–128.
88. Fortner JG, Vitelli CE, Maclean BJ. Proximal extrahepatic bile duct tumors: analysis of a series of 52 consecutive patients treated over a period of 13 years. Arch Surg 1989;124:1275–1282.
89. Lai ECS, Tompkins RK, Roslyn JJ, et al. Proximal bile duct cancer: quality of survival. Ann Surg 1987;205:111–118.
90. Hadjis NS, Blenkhard JI, Alexander N, et al. Outcome of radical surgery in hilar cholangiocarcinoma. Surgery 1990;107:597–604.
91. Boerma EJ. Research into the results of resection of hilar bile duct cancer. Surgery 1990;108:572–580.
92. Baer HU, Stain SC, Dennison AR, et al. Improvements in survival by aggressive resections of hilar cholangiocarcinoma. Ann Surg 1993;217:20–27.
93. Vauthey JN, Baer HU, Guastella T, et al. Comparison of outcome between extended and nonextended liver resections for neoplasms. Surgery 1993;114:968–975.
94. Kawasaki S, Makuuchi M, Miyagawa S, et al. Radical operation after portal embolization for tumor of hilar bile duct. J Am Coll Surg 1994;178:480–486.
95. Nagino M, Nimura Y, Kamiya J, et al. Right or left trisegmental portal vein embolization before hepatic trisegmentectomy for hilar bile duct carcinoma. Surgery 1995; 117:677–681.
96. Nimura Y, Hayakawa N, Kamiya J, et al. Combined portal vein and liver resection for carcinoma of the biliary tract. Br J Surg 1991;78:727–731.
97. Reding R, Buard JL, Lebeau G, et al. Surgical management of 552 carcinomas of the extrahepatic bile ducts: results of the French Surgical Association survey. Ann Surg 1991;213:236–241.
98. Sugiura Y, Nakamura S, Iida S, et al. Extensive resection of the bile ducts combined with liver resection for cancer of the main hepatic duct junction: a cooperative study of the Keio Bile Duct Cancer Study Group. Surgery 1994;115: 445–451.
99. Washburn WK, Lewis DW, Jenkins RL. Aggressive surgical resection for cholangiocarcinoma. Arch Surg 1995;130: 270–276.
100. Cameron JC. Atlas of Surgery, vol 1. Philadelphia: B.C. Decker, 1990.
101. Guthrie CM, Haddock G, de Beaux AC, et al. Changing trends in the management of extrahepatic cholangiocarcinoma. Br J Surg 1993;80:1434–1439.
102. Lillemoe KD, Sauter PK, Pitt HA, et al. Current status of surgical palliation of periampullary carcinoma. Surg Gynecol Obstet 1993;176:1–10.
103. Casavilla FA, Marsh JW, Iwatsuki S, et al. Hepatic resection and transplantation for peripheral cholangiocarcinoma. J Am Coll Surg 1997;195:429–436.
104. Klempnauer J, Ridder GJ, von Wasielewski R, et al. Resectional surgery of hilar cholangiocarcinoma: a multivariate analysis of prognostic factors. J Clin Oncol 1997;15:947–954.
105. Hayes JK Jr, Sapozink MD, Miller FJ. Definitive radiation therapy in bile duct carcinoma. Int J Radiat Oncol Biol Phys 1988;15:735–740.
106. Verbeek PC, van Leeuwen DJ, van der Heyde MN, et al. Does additive radiotherapy after hilar resection improve survival of cholangiocarcinoma: an analysis in sixty-four patients. Ann Chir 1991;45:350–354.
107. Shiina T, Mikuriya S, Uno T, et al. Radiotherapy of cholangiocarcinoma: the roles for primary and adjuvant therapies. Cancer Chemother Pharmacol 1992;31(suppl):S115–S118.
108. Ede RJ, Williams SJ, Hatfield ARW, et al. Endoscopic management of inoperable cholangiocarcinoma using iridium-192. Br J Surg 1989;76:867–871.
109. Koyama K, Tanaka J, Sato S, et al. New strategy for treatment of carcinoma of the hilar bile duct. Surg Gynecol Obstet 1989;168:523–529.
110. Pitt HA, Nakeeb A, Abrams RA, et al. Perihilar cholangiocarcinoma: postoperative radiotherapy does not improve survival. Ann Surg 1995;221:788–798.
111. Minsky BD, Kemeny N, Armstrong JG, et al. Extrahepatic biliary system cancer: an update of a combined modality approach. Am J Clin Oncol 1991;14:433–439.
112. Koyama K, Tanaka J, Sato Y, et al. Experience in twenty patients with carcinoma of hilar bile duct treated by resection, targeting chemotherapy and intercavitary irradiation. Surg Gynecol Obstet 1993;176:239–245.
113. Robertson JM, Lawrence TD, Dworzanin LM, et al. Treatment of primary hepatobiliary cancer with conformal radiation therapy and regional chemotherapy. J Clin Oncol 1993;11:1286–1292.
114. Kraybill WG, Lee H, Picus J, et al. Multidisciplinary treatment of biliary tract cancers. J Surg Oncol 1994;55:239–245.
115. Whittington R, Neuberg D, Teste WJ, et al. Protracted intravenous fluorouracil infusion with radiation therapy in the management of localized pancreaticobiliary carcinoma: a phase I Eastern Cooperative Oncology Group trial. J Clin Oncol 1995;13:227–234.

# 51
# Benign and Malignant Tumors of the Liver

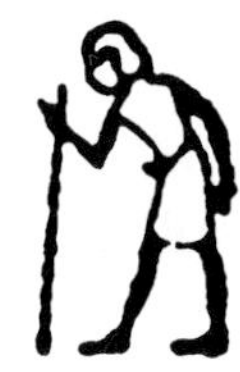

Emery A. Minnard and Yuman Fong

One-eighth of the population of the United States is over the age of 65, and this small portion suffers one-half of all cancers diagnosed. It was estimated that by the year 2005, more than one-fifth of the U.S. population would be over the age of 65.[1] This demographic change alone will increase the number of cancers in America by approximately 30%,[2,3] making no other single factor as important as age for cancer incidence.

Advanced age has also long been associated with higher risk during surgical therapy. Brooks in 1937 reported operative results of 287 patients over the age of 70 years who underwent surgical procedures that today would be considered minor.[4,5] The mortality rate was remarkably high (19%), with approximately one-third of the patients who had undergone abdominal operations having in-hospital deaths. Brooks foretold that with a rapid increase of the elderly population, surgeons would increasingly be confronted with surgical problems among the elderly and should strive to improve their results by becoming more accustomed to the physiologic changes associated with aging. It has been approximately six decades since his paper, and with improvements in anesthetic and surgical technique, there has been substantial improvement in surgical outcomes of elderly patients after routine surgical procedures.[5] Even now, however, debate continues as to the appropriateness of subjecting the elderly population to high risk procedures such as cardiac procedures and liver resections because of the magnitude of these operations.

Surgical extirpation, however, is the only curative therapy for malignant disease of the liver. In approximately 50,000 cases of hepatic colorectal metastasis encountered annually in the United States, and the more than 1 million cases of primary hepatocellular carcinoma seen worldwide, surgical excision has been shown to result in long-term survival for more than one-third of patients.[6] Because the number of elderly persons in the United States is growing and the incidence of many liver tumors increases with age, increasing numbers of patients are presenting for consideration for resection of primary or secondary liver cancers. This chapter summarizes the current data on morbidity and mortality after liver resection in the elderly and the pathophysiology that may underlie the increased risk of complications after resection in this age group. The current approaches for the most common tumors seen in the elderly are then summarized.

## Perioperative Outcome after Liver Resection in the Elderly

The past three decades have seen a dramatic decline in mortality rates after liver resection.[7–9] Major liver resections can now be routinely performed at major centers with perioperative mortality rates less than 5%. In the past, elderly patients were thought to be at particularly high risk for perioperative complications (Table 51.1). Studies published during the late 1980s were still reporting mortality rates of 11–41%.[10–12] Extensive resections consisting of trisegmentectomy were associated with operative mortality of more than 30%.[12] The higher operative mortality and morbidity rates in elderly patients can be explained partly by associated conditions in elderly patients such as diabetes mellitus, cardiopulmonary disease, and renal disease.[18] A more important factor for such high complication and mortality rates in these series, is the high incidence of the concomitant hepatic disorders of hepatitis and cirrhosis.[5,10,14,15,19] Several studies suggest that if these factors were excluded, there would be no difference in morbidity and mortality between old and young patients.[14] In more recent studies, in predominantly noncirrhotic elderly patients, the perioperative mortality mirrored that expected in a younger population.[5,13–17]

We have reported two large series where resections in the elderly were performed with an operative mortality less than 4% and a complication rate less than 35%.[5,17] The major cause of mortality continues to be postoperative hepatic insufficiency; therefore, elderly patients with

TABLE 51.1. Clinical Studies of Liver Resection in the Elderly

| Study | Year | No. | Years of study | Age[a] | Cancer type | No. with cirrhosis | Operative mortality (%) | 5-Year survival (%) | LOS (days) | Cause of death |
|---|---|---|---|---|---|---|---|---|---|---|
| Ezaki[10] | 1987 | 37 | 6 | ≥66 | HCC | 25/37 (68%) | 5 | 18 | NS | Liver failure, infection |
| Yanaga[11] | 1988 | 27 | 13 | ≥65 | HCC | 17/27 (63%) | 41 | NS | NS | Liver failure (3), sepsis (8) |
| Fortner[12] | 1989 | 90 | 18 | ≥65 | Mixed | NS | 11.1 | NS | 15 ± 9[b] | Liver failure (6), MI, infection (2), hemorrhage (1) |
| Mentha[13] | 1992 | 52 | 23 | ≥65 | Mixed | 4/52 (8%) | 6 | NS | 21[c] | Liver failure (2), MI |
| Nagasue[14] | 1993 | 32 | 10 | ≥70 | HCC | 31/32 (97%) | 19 | 18 | NS | Hemorrhage (2), pneumonia, abscess |
| Takenaka[15] | 1994 | 39 | 14 | ≥70 | HCC | 31/39 (79%) | 5 | 76 | NS | Liver failure (2) |
| Karl[16] | 1994 | 16 | 6 | ≥70 | Mixed | NS | 0 | NS | NS | None |
| Fong[5] | 1995 | 128 | 10 | ≥70 | CR mets | 7/128 | 4 | 35 | 13[c] | Liver failure (3), sepsis (2) |
| Fong[17] | 1998 | 133 | 3 | ≥65 | Mixed | 8/133 (6%) | 4 | NS | 11[c] | Liver failure (3), infection, hemorrhage |

HCC, hepatocellular carcinoma; CR mets, colorectal metastasis; LOS, length of hospital stay; MI, myocardial infarction; NS, not stated.
[a] criterion for being elderly (age in years).
[b] Mean.
[c] Median.

cirrhosis should be scrutinized closely before an operation is performed. Chronologic age alone should not be considered a contraindication to liver resection. However, because associated medical conditions are more frequently encountered in patients with advanced age, we routinely refer patients age 65 and over for cardiopulmonary evaluation prior to liver resection. Contrary to recommendations of others,[12,16] we do not believe that trisegmentectomies carry prohibitive risk in the elderly, and routinely offer such extensive resections to medically fit patients of advanced age. Postoperative medical monitoring is based on objective evaluation of medical fitness and not on age alone. In a series of 128 patients undergoing liver resection for metastatic colorectal cancer, only 7% required intensive care unit (ICU) admission at any time during the hospitalization, and the median hospital stay was only 13 days.[5] Liver resection in the elderly can therefore be performed with low mortality and morbidity and with expenditure of health care resources similar to that for resections performed in a younger age group.

## Pathophysiologic Basis of Liver Complications in the Elderly

The liver undergoes physiologic changes during aging, such as a decrease in size and blood flow.[1,2,20] There is an observed increase in mean cellular and mitochondrial volume and a decrease in cell number. There is also a decrease in mitochondrial DNA.[21] Under normal conditions, these changes do not seem to be clinically significant, as hepatocyte functions such as in detoxification, demethylization, conjugation, and hepatic extraction remain normal. However, during periods that require increased hepatocyte function, the liver of an old patient may not be able to respond by increasing synthetic or metabolic function, and so hepatic insufficiency may result.[1,3,22] One clinically important scenario requiring increased hepatocyte function is the immediate postresection period, when a reduced hepatocyte mass must perform the physiologic tasks of the preoperative liver until such time as regeneration may restore the liver to preoperative capacities. The reduced hepatocyte protein synthesis in the elderly may be a factor contributing to postoperative hepatic insufficiency.[23,24] This may help explain the higher incidence of liver failure, particularly in cirrhotic elderly patients after liver resection.[11,14] Elderly patients with cirrhosis should therefore be considered discriminantly for surgical resection.

Postoperative liver insufficiency may also be explained by a reduced "regenerative" capacity in the aged. The basis for major liver resection is the potential for the liver to undergo compensatory hypertrophy and hyperplasia, or "regeneration," as it is more often termed. Resection of up to 80% of the hepatic mass is followed by liver regeneration, such that within a 3-week period a liver of approximately the same size as the preresection liver can be expected, with normalization of liver functions usually within 6 weeks. This regeneration, however, may be altered by the processes of aging. Numerous animal studies have demonstrated retarded liver regeneration in aged animals, as measured by mitotic index, tritiated thymidine uptake, and restoration of liver mass.[25,26] Such alterations in liver regeneration and function in aged animals are particularly dependent on the nutritional status of the animal,[24] making nutritional support particularly important in this age group. One possible mechanism of such retardation of regeneration is a reduction of thymidine kinase expression in the aged animals.[26] In addition, levels of DNA polymerase-α, a key enzyme for DNA synthesis, are diminished in aged animals.[27] These and other enzymes are necessary for maintenance of DNA synthesis in animals. There is also decreased fidelity of DNA synthesis by DNA polymerase-α,[28] which may very well be related to the alterations in histone function that has long been recognized.[29,30] Whether such cellular changes are seen in human regenerating livers is not known, as studies evaluating cellular alterations during liver regeneration in the elderly patient are sparse. For the noncirrhotic patient, the alterations in liver regeneration seen in animals cannot be clinically relevant in humans, as most reports suggest that there is little difference in the hepatic regeneration rate measured by size when the old patient is compared to young individuals. In patients with cirrhosis, it is this parenchymal abnormality that has the greatest influence over the regenerative capacity.

## Treatment of Liver Tumors

In the following section we discuss the most commonly encountered liver tumors in the elderly patient, beginning with benign tumors. The latter usually do not require therapy but are discussed because patients of advancing age are more likely to be subjected to the wide variety of imaging modalities now available. Benign liver tumors are often discovered incidentally and lead to emotional distress and diagnostic confusion. Our discussion then concentrates on the two malignant tumors most commonly encountered: metastatic colorectal cancer and hepatocellular carcinoma.

### Benign Liver Tumors

Most benign liver tumors are asymptomatic and are discovered incidentally at the time of laparotomy or detected on an imaging examination done for other indications. When a patient presents with an incidentally discovered liver mass, a workup should begin as always with a thorough history and physical examination. A history of previous cancers are elicited, as are any symptoms suggestive of gastrointestinal malignancy. Patients should be questioned for a history of hepatitis, alcohol abuse, and familial history of liver disease. Most patients are asymptomatic. It is a highly unusual situation when a patient presents with definable symptoms from a benign tumor, which are usually related to encroachment on adjacent structures or the stretching of Glisson's capsule by a large tumor. On physical examination, signs of portal hypertension such as caput medusal and ascites are sought; and a stool guaiac test is done for occult blood. Serum transaminase levels are sometimes elevated as a consequence of tissue necrosis in hepatic cell adenomas. Alkaline phosphatase levels may be elevated because of impingement of tumor on the biliary tree. Most liver function tests, however, are normal in patients with benign tumors. Hepatitis screen—hepatitis B surface antigen (HBsAg) and hepatitis C antibody—are assayed along with α-fetoprotein (AFP) and carcinoembryonic antigen (CEA). The most common imaging test employed is computed tomography (CT) scanning because it is the most commonly available and most uniform in quality. Ultrasonography is performed if cystic lesions are suspected, but for most other lesions it is not specific enough for a confident diagnosis.[31] Magnetic resonance imaging (MRI) is currently the most accurate noninvasive diagnostic tool used for differentiating various benign lesions including adenomas, fibronodular hyperplasia (FNH), and hemangiomas; and with the recent addition of MR cholangiography, MR techniques have proven to be even more powerful for evaluating liver tumors.[32] Occasionally, angiography is still called on to diagnose a hemangioma, adenoma, or FNH more confidently.

#### *Bile Duct Adenomas*

Bile duct adenomas are sometimes referred to as bile duct harmatomas and are presumed to be developmental defects. They are usually small lesions that rarely exceed 1 cm in diameter. Often discovered at the time of laparotomy and confused with metastatic cancers, they are grayish white and firm to palpation. Microscopically, they are composed of fibrous stroma surrounding bile ducts. It is estimated that approximately one-third of the population have these lesions.[33] Bile duct harmatomas are universally asymptomatic and require no therapy.

#### *Hepatocellular Adenomas*

Hepatocellular adenomas are soft and fleshy with a yellowish-tan color. They are sometimes quite vascular and can grow to an enormous size. These rare tumors have been associated with the use of oral contraceptives. Liver enzyme abnormalities are nonspecific, and tumor markers are usually negative. On CT scan the adenoma is typically a low density solid mass. Even with imaging by MR and angiogram, and occasionally even after biopsy, these lesions are still not distinguishable from a well-differentiated hepatocellular cancer.

Management of the asymptomatic patient presents an interesting and slightly controversial conundrum. There are growing concerns about leaving adenomas in situ, with recent reports suggesting that adenomas are premalignant lesions.[34] Adenomas may also rupture, and the resultant hemorrhage is associated with high mortality.[34] In young individuals, we almost always resect adenomas for fear of rupture and malignant transformation. Oral contraceptives should also be discontinued. In the elderly individual, enthusiasm for resection must be moderated by the medical risks of surgery. Certainly if the tumor was symptomatic, the decision would be easier. Asymptomatic tumors in a patient with significant associated medical illnesses may warrant observation.

### Hemangiomas

Hemangioma is the most common benign tumor of the liver. Cavernous hemangiomas in most autopsy series have a reported incidence of approximately 7%.[35] The age range associated with hemangiomas is usually 55 years or above in most clinical series, although it is probably due to the higher chance for abdominal imaging in patients with advanced age.

Hemangiomas usually present as a solitary lesion but are multiple in about 10% of cases. They usually measure less than 2 cm in diameter but occasionally grow to enormous size and in some cases even replace an entire lobe of the liver. Most of the lesions remain asymptomatic, and hemangiomas <4 cm in diameter rarely become clinically relevant. Sixty percent of the patients with large tumors present with abdominal pain or discomfort, digestive problems, and the sensation of an abdominal mass or distension.[36] Rarely, platelet trapping in the large tumors results in thrombocytopenia, which may manifest as ecchymoses and purpura.

Liver function is almost always normal, and tumor markers are consistently negative. On CT scans hemangiomas present as low-density areas within the liver parenchyma, which upon intravenous injection of contrast, show early peripheral opacification followed by variable degrees of enhancement of the central portion. Even though ultrasonography and CT scanning are usually the first imaging tests used in the investigation of hemangiomas, MRI scans have been shown to improve specificity. A combination of T1-weighted, T2-weighted, and gadolinium-enhanced dynamic scans provide the diagnosis of hemangioma with an accuracy of more than 95% (Fig. 51.1).[32] MRI has replaced the tagged red blood cell (RBC) scan as the modality of choice for evaluating patients with suspected hemangiomas. MRI can provide information for diagnosis of other liver lesions and provide anatomic details not possible on tagged-RBC scans. Percutaneous needle biopsy should be avoided, as it is associated with severe, sometimes fatal hemorrhage.

In the elderly, asymptomatic hemangiomas require no treatment. Indications for treatment include pain, discomfort, early satiety, rapid increase in size, thrombocytopenia, or evidence of bleeding intraperitoneally or intraparenchymally.[37,38] There are a few documented reports of significant reduction in tumor size with the use of external beam radiation, but those results are inconsistent.[39,40] Hepatic artery embolization has also been attempted but has only occasionally been successful.[41] Symptomatic lesions should be resected. Because hemangiomas are usually surrounded by compressed hepatic parenchyma, lesions are often amenable to enucleation, though deep lesions are usually best treated with a formal resection along anatomic planes.

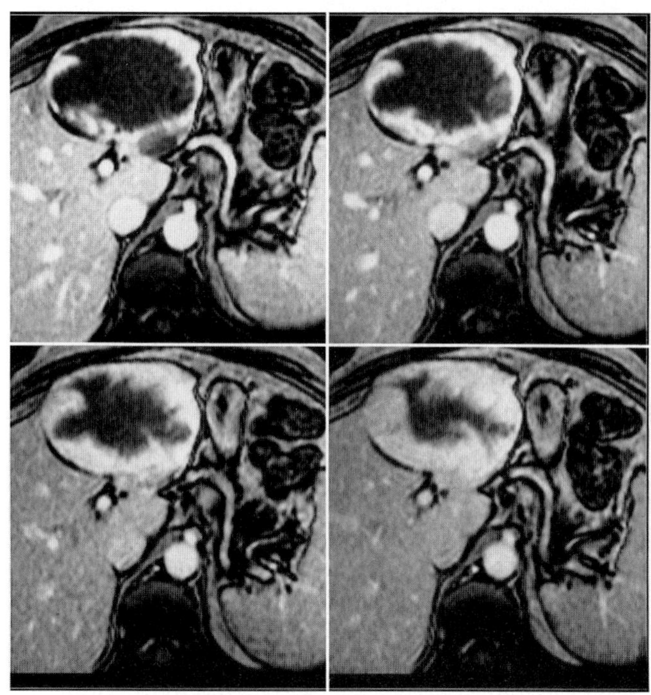

FIGURE 51.1. Gadolinium-enhanced magnetic resonance imaging (MRI) scans of a hemangioma. The peripheral nodular enhancement pattern seen is diagnostic of a hemangioma.

## Malignant Liver Tumors

Hepatic cancers may be subdivided into primary and metastatic cancers. Primary hepatic cancers arise within the liver and include hepatocellular carcinoma (HCC) and cholangiocarcinoma. Metastatic cancers are derived from a variety of primary sites, with metastatic colorectal cancer being predominant and few other types being appropriate for surgical therapy. The challenges of treating elderly patients with HCC or with metastatic colorectal cancer are discussed.

### Hepatocellular Carcinoma

Hepatocellular carcinoma is the most common solid organ tumor worldwide and comprises approximately 90% of all primary liver cancers in the elderly population. Most of these tumors are associated with chronic liver disease, such as viral hepatitis or alcoholic cirrhosis. HCCs may be unifocal or multifocal. Most patients are relatively asymptomatic until the tumor reaches an advanced stage when it causes symptoms, usually right upper quadrant pain. It is then found as a highly vascular, large tumor that is susceptible to rupture and intraperitoneal hemorrhage. The most common physical finding is hepatomegaly with tenderness. Bile duct

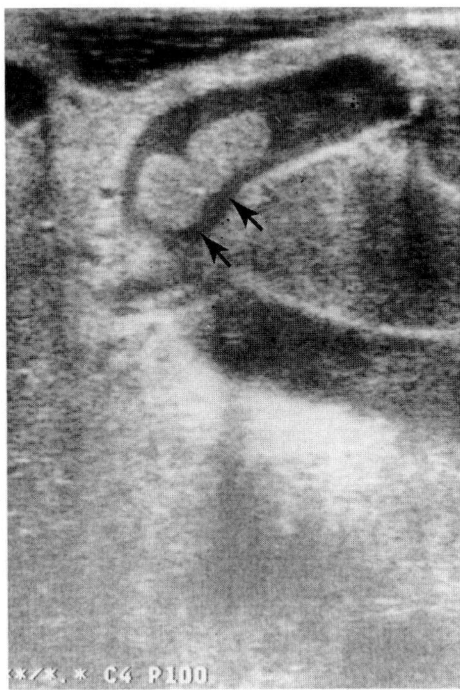


FIGURE 51.2. Portal vein invasion and intraportal extension by hepatocellular carcinoma (HCC) as demonstrated by intraoperative ultrasonography (arrows). HCC has a great propensity for intraluminal growth and extension along major blood vessels and bile ducts.

obstruction and invasion with tumor embolus may cause jaundice. At an advanced stage, these tumors cause a host of other symptoms, including abdominal distension, weight loss, fatigue, anorexia, and fever. Occasionally, hepatic decompensation, ascites, Budd-Chiari syndrome, variceal bleeding, severe jaundice, or encephalopathy is the presentation of HCC in a previously well-compensated cirrhotic patient.[42] Not infrequently the cause of such decompensation is portal vein invasion and thromboocclusion by the tumor (Fig. 51.2).

## Diagnosis

The triad diagnostic of HCC consists of hepatic mass by imaging, positive serologic markers for hepatitis B or C, and a strongly positive AFP level.[42] At presentation, patients should be evaluated for a history of chronic liver disease or a familial history of liver disease. Questions and the examination should be directed at uncovering signs and symptoms of hepatic insufficiency. Blood tests should include liver function tests, renal functions, hepatitis screen, AFP, and CEA. An AFP > 500 ng/dl is diagnostic of HCC.

The goals of diagnostic imaging are to distinguish primary liver cancer, metastatic cancers, and benign liver tumors; to assess the extent of spread of the tumor; and to define local resectability. The patient has usually already been evaluated by CT scan before referral. CT scanning is a widely available test that allows examination of hepatic and tumor anatomy, as well as the presence of cirrhosis or fatty infiltration in uninvolved segments of the liver.[43] Of note, a noncontrast CT is essential for evaluating HCC in addition to the contrast-enhanced scans. This is because an HCC often is isodense to the liver parenchyma on contrast-enhanced images and requires noncontrast scans for imaging.

If the portal veins and hepatic veins are well visualized, a CT scan alone may be sufficient for evaluating the liver tumor. Most often, though, an ultrasound examination or MRI should be performed because of the propensity for HCCs to invade and grow along major vasculature, even when they are small tumors. We prefer abdominal ultrasonography for this evaluation because of the lower cost and the accuracy of this test in experienced hands, acknowledging that the results are highly dependent on the skill of the ultrasonographer. In general practice, MRI is of more uniform quality and should be the test performed. MRI with magnetic resonance angiography (MRA) and magnetic resonance cholangiopancreatography (MRCP),[44] allows not only characterization of various tumors, assessment of the tumor extent, and proximity to vascular structures but also proximity to biliary structures. Hepatic angiography is now rarely used because of the quality of current noninvasive imaging studies; it is reserved largely for patients requiring embolization as treatment of the HCC.

## Surgical Treatment

Surgical resection is the only potentially curative treatment for patients with HCC. However, because small HCCs are usually asymptomatic, most patients do not present until the disease is far advanced, and only 30% of patients with suspected HCC are candidates for surgical exploration. In the elderly, surgical therapy is further restricted because liver transplantation is not an available option. In the general population, liver transplantation is considered for those patients with small tumors but with liver reserve considered too risky for partial hepatectomy. However, most transplant centers do not give liver transplants to patients aged 65 or more, and therefore, total hepatectomy and liver transplantation is not an option for this age group.

Technical aspects of partial hepatectomy are largely as for patients of a younger age group, and the reader is referred to textbooks of liver surgery for a general discussion.[45] The differences are modifications to suit not only elderly patients but also cirrhotic patients who usually comprise the population undergoing HCC resection. Bilateral subcostal incisions are usually employed with a xiphoid extension. This high incision and the likelihood of a right pleural effusion after liver resection, are the main reasons elderly patients should be evaluated carefully for pulmonary status. Respiratory compromise and pneumonia are frequent complications in patients undergoing liver resection, compounded in the elderly patient by the normal loss of pulmonary reserve with advancing age. At exploration the entire liver should be mobilized from its ligamentous attachments to evaluate resectability. Exposure is constantly maintained with a retractor fixed to the table, enabling excellent exposure and decreasing the chances of needing to enter the chest. Intraoperative ultrasonography is performed to determine the relation of the tumor to the major vascular structures and to identify additional sites of disease in the liver not appreciated by conventional preoperative imaging.[46] Inflow and outflow vasculature to the section of liver to be removed is usually controlled. We avoid total vascular exclusion (TVE) in general, but are even more adamant about it in the elderly. The hemodynamic changes often associated with TVE are particularly poorly tolerated in elderly patients, who may have cardiopulmonary disease. The porta hepatis is controlled to allow application of the Pringle maneuver. A Pringle maneuver is performed to decrease bleeding when dividing the liver parenchyma.[47] We prefer use of the Pringle maneuver intermittently, releasing the Pringle every 5 minutes to allow reperfusion of the liver.

Operative mortality in cirrhotic patients of any age undergoing liver resection in a major center, continues to be in the 10% range.[48] In elderly cirrhotic patients, the mortality rate has been reported to be as high as 19–41%[11,14] and as low as 5%.[10,15] Most of the complications following liver resections are usually cardiopulmonary (angina, arrhythmia, myocardial infarction, transient ischemic attacks, pneumothorax, pulmonary embolism).[2] Patient selection is key to a favorable outcome. Although many sophisticated tests have been proposed for preoperative evaluation of liver function, none has been demonstrated to be better than Child's criteria. We routinely consider Child's A patients for surgical resection. Patients with Child's B liver functional status are considered for resection only if the lesion is peripheral and requires resection of little functional liver. Elderly Child's C patients are offered only supportive care, as transplantation is generally not an option in the elderly, and even ablative therapies are associated with prohibitive risk in patients with such little liver functional reserve.[49]

Unfortunately, only 30% of patients explored have resectable lesions. Among patients who undergo resection, long-term survival is achieved in up to 76% (Table 51.1), though most series of HCC resections report long-term survival in one-third of patients.

Cryosurgery has recently increased in popularity among surgeons as therapy for HCC. It involves intraoperative placement of a cryoprobe under ultrasound guidance into the liver tumor and freezing the region two or three times for ablation. There are, of course, limitations to the use of cryosurgery: Biliary damage can result from freezing tumors too close to the major bile ducts, and tumors >5 cm are technically difficult to freeze completely. This technique has great potential for managing high risk elderly patients with concomitant medical problems or cirrhosis (or both), who might not tolerate a resection. Several preliminary reports suggest that cryosurgery may be as effective as liver resection for small tumors,[50] though cryoablation has not been formally compared to other therapies. When a patient clearly has an unresectable tumor, we prefer nonsurgical ablative approaches that do not require anesthesia, abdominal incisions, and the associated risks. In patients who exhaust other ablative options, we offer cryoablation. When patients are explored for resection we usually have the cryoablation instrument prepared in case more tumor than is resectable is encountered, because in such cases the risks of general anesthesia and laparotomy have already been incurred.

## Nonsurgical Treatment

Many ablative therapies have been developed for the treatment of nonresectable HCC. Transarterial embolization or chemoembolization has had the most extensive record. It involves use of a foam, gelatin particles, thrombin-soaked foam, plastic particles, or metallic coils injected into the hepatic artery to selectively occlude blood flow to the tumor (Fig. 51.3).[51] Others have also attempted to increase antitumor efficacy by soaking the various particles in a chemotherapeutic drug,[52] though such chemoembolizations have not been demonstrated objectively to have improved efficacy over plain particle embolization. Embolization is associated with low morbidity and mortality and with 2- to 3-year survival rates of up to 30%.[53] Although this compares favorably with resection results, enthusiasm to supplant potentially curative resection in otherwise healthy patients of advanced age should be tempered. To date, there has not been a prospective randomized trial to compare these modalities with surgical resection.

Percutaneous ethanol injection ablates tumor by using CT- or ultrasound-guided direct injection of ethanol into the tumor. This technique is limited by the size and number of tumors that can be treated. Few investigators treat tumors >4 cm and more than four in number. For small tumors, however, such ablation can be highly effective.[54] The morbidity associated with such treatment includes pain, fever, and infection of the dead tumor. Mortality rates are low. Approximately 40% of these lesions are not detectable on CT scan at 6–12 months. Although this treatment is effective, there is a significant recurrence rate associated with the technique. Recent efforts have combined this technique with transarterial embolization, a combination that appears to be complementary in action. These ablative techniques should be

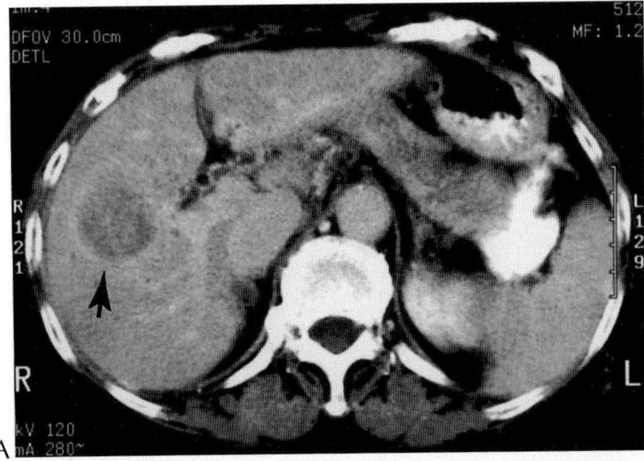


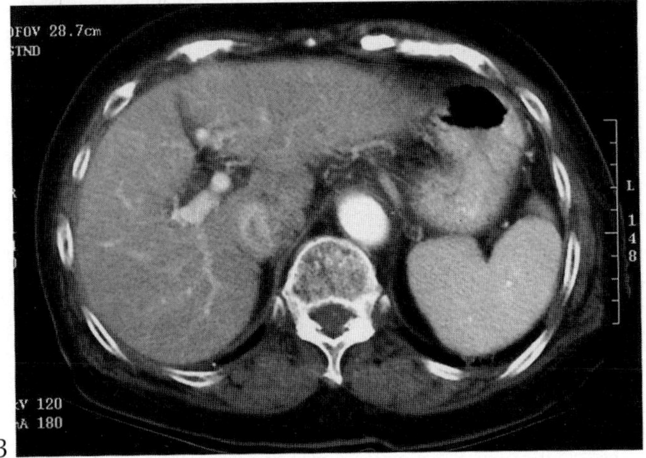


FIGURE 51.3. Embolization as ablative treatment for hepatocellular carcinoma. A large solitary right lobe HCC in a 91-year-old woman is seen on CT before (A) and 3 months after (B) embolization.

considered for patients who are medically unfit or anatomically unsuitable for partial hepatectomy. Irradiation and systemic chemotherapy are of limited value for treating HCCs.[55]

## Metastatic Colorectal Cancer

There are an estimated 150,000 new cases of colorectal cancer diagnosed annually.[6] Of these patients, 25% are over the age of 70, and 6% are over 80 years old. It is believed that 40–45% experience recurrence within 5 years. About 75–80% of these patients have the liver as one of the involved sites of recurrence and 15–20% have the liver as the first or only site of recurrence.[56] Advances in liver surgery and an increasing proportion of elderly patients have encouraged hepatic resection in this ever-growing segment of the population. Early studies on hepatic resection in the elderly reported significant mortality rates, with cirrhosis and concomitant medical problems being the most commonly identified associated factors.[12] Later studies in predominantly noncirrhotic patients, however, reported mortality rates in the elderly population similar to those reported in younger patients.[5] There is little doubt now that liver resection is a potentially curative option for treating metastatic colorectal cancer of the liver, and that such resections can be performed safely in the elderly and with good long-term results.

### Natural History

Several studies have analyzed in a retrospective fashion patients who were not treated for metastatic colon cancer to the liver.[57] In most of these series even when patients had liver metastases that were solitary and clearly resectable by radiologic criteria, fewer than 40% of untreated patients were alive at 3 years and nearly all of the patients were dead at 5 years. Chemotherapy, whether based on 5-fluorouracil[58,59] or irinotecan (CPT-11),[60,61] improves survival but is not curative. The demonstration that resection can provide 10-year disease-free survivors for this disease[62] has led to acceptance of surgical resection as the treatment of choice for liver metastases.

### Preoperative Evaluation

Preoperative evaluation of the elderly patient with colorectal metastases to the liver should address several concerns. As with any major operation, a comprehensive initial examination is paramount. Particular attention should be directed to the cardiopulmonary status of the patient, as nearly 50% of all postoperative deaths that occur in the elderly are related to cardiovasular or pulmonary disease. There have been several predictive risk indices and functional assessments reported that can identify with fairly accurate certainty which of these elderly patients is at increased risk for cardiopulmonary complications.[63] As stated above, the elderly patient undergoing liver resection is at particularly high risk for pulmonary complications because of decreased pulmonary reserve with aging, a high abdominal incision and increased discomfort with the respiratory effort, and postoperative pleural effusion. In series that have examined liver resection for metastatic colorectal cancer, the risk of pneumonia is 2–8%.[64,65]

Generally, patients undergoing evaluation for resection of hepatic colorectal metastases do not have associated cirrhosis. In the noncirrhotic patient there is enormous liver reserve, and resections of up to 80% of liver parenchyma can be performed with confidence of full recovery. In patients with associated liver parenchymal disease such as from alcohol abuse or viral hepatitis, thorough evaluation with a physical examination, liver function tests, coagulation studies, and nutritional assessment for degree of baseline hepatic insufficiency may identify patients intolerant of a liver resection. No test of greater sophistication than these have proved to be clinically useful for distinguishing patients at high risk for liver failure. Tests such as bromosulfophthalein retention, indocyanine green retention, and hepatic wedge pressure[66] have advocates but are not accepted universally.

Selection of patients is also based on clinical details of the colorectal cancer. Risk factors for recurrence after liver resection include regional lymph node involvement by the primary tumor,[56,67,68] symptomatic liver tumors,[56,57] synchronous presentation of liver metastases with the primary tumor,[8,67,69] large numbers of tumors,[8,67] the presence of satellite nodules,[8,69] high preoperative CEA level,[69] and the extent of liver involvement of more than 50%.[68,70] Whereas none of these criteria alone is a complete contraindication for resection, increasing numbers of these criteria, particularly in a patient with medical problems, should lead one to be circumspect when recommending resection. The two criteria considered by most liver surgeons to be absolute contraindications to resection are the presence of extrahepatic disease or the technical inability to clear all liver tumor. The preoperative evaluation must therefore include adequately imaging areas with the highest likelihood of disease spread and adequate imaging for the distribution of tumors within the liver. The radiologic techniques available are the same used for evaluating primary liver cancer. Before surgery, the extent of disease workup should include chest radiography, abdominal and pelvic CT scans, and colonoscopy. CT portography is also highly recommended as the most sensitive test for imaging metastatic tumors within the liver. MRI or sonography is used occasionally if proximity to the vena cava or hepatic veins is a major concern. Routine use of angiography has declined with the increasing use of MRI technology.

## Surgical Treatment

The technical concerns are as for resection of HCCs, except liver failure is less of a concern in this predominantly noncirrhotic population, and up to 80% of the liver can be resected with confidence for recovery. Following entry of the abdomen with bilateral subcostal incisions with xiphoid extension, a complete abdominal exploration is performed. If extrahepatic disease is identified, resection is not justified by the data. Intraoperative ultrasonography is performed to identify lesions missed on preoperative scans and to confirm the relations of known lesions to vascular structures. Resection is then performed using standard inflow and outflow vascular control and low central venous pressure as previously described.[71] In a series of 128 consecutive resections in patients over age 70 with metastatic colorectal cancer, the operative mortality was 4%.[5] This was no different from a cohort of patients less than age 70 operated on during the same time period. Of particular note, long-term survival was also no different between the two groups (Fig. 51.4). In fact, among six series of patients analyzing long-term outcome after liver resection for metastatic colorectal cancer,[9,62,64,68,69,72] only one demonstrated a more adverse outcome for elderly patients.[9] Thus resection of metastatic colorectal cancer in the elderly is safe and can result in long-term survival.

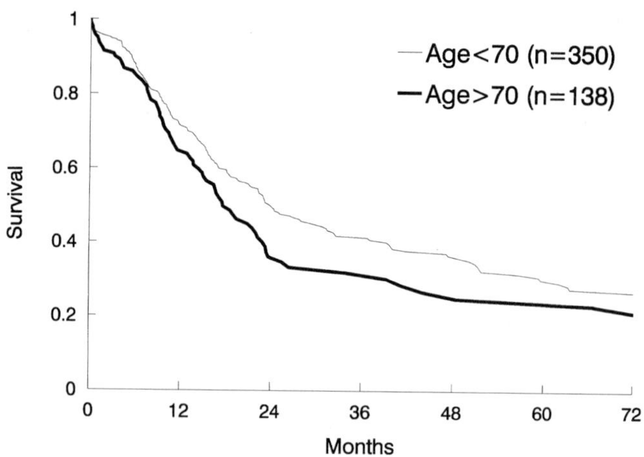


FIGURE 51.4. Survival of patients age 70 or more undergoing liver resection for metastatic colorectal cancer compared to those less than age 70. (From Fong et al.,[64] with permission.)

For metastatic colorectal cancer, large resections can be undertaken with safety and potential eradication of the tumor. Thus unlike the situation with HCCs, where enthusiasm for resection is tempered by the risks of such resections, ablative techniques do not have established roles in metastatic colorectal cancer. Cryoablation has been performed with safety but has not been shown to have an advantage. We reserve cryoablation for the rare patient with widely scattered disease isolated to the liver that is not resectable or for the patient with an unresectable recurrence. In otherwise fit patients regardless of age, we routinely resect up to 10 tumors even if they are bilateral. Medically fit patients who can have complete extirpation of disease are offered potentially curative resections.

## Nonsurgical Treatment

Standard nonsurgical treatment of hepatic colorectal metastases is systemic chemotherapy. As stated previously in this chapter, nonsurgical treatment of hepatic tumors is sometimes the best option in extremely high risk, elderly patients. The most successful chemotherapeutic regimens for metastatic colorectal cancer have been based on 5-fluorouracil (5-FU),[73–75] and the current standard therapy for nonresectable disease is the combination of 5-FU and leucovorin. Tumor response is expected to be 25–30%[73,76–78]; complete response is rare; and median survival is reported to be generally a year or less. Recently, the topoisomerase I inhibitor irinotecan

(CPT-11) was approved as a second-line chemotherapy for patients with nonresectable disease failing 5-FU therapy.[60,61,79] Significant antitumor activity of this agent is expected in only 25–40% of cases. Chemotherapy does not offer potential for cure and therefore is not a substitute for potentially curative resection.

## Conclusions

The aging process generally does not lead to clinically evident compromised liver function under normal conditions, and age alone is not a contraindication for most surgical procedures. For liver resections, clinicians have long feared that the physiologic decrease in liver function with age and a decrease in regenerative capacity would compromise recovery. In clinical practice, these fears have not been substantiated except in the cirrhotic patient. Liver resection remains the only potentially curative therapy for liver tumors of any type. In the noncirrhotic patient, associated medical conditions, measured physiologic function, and clinical case history should be the criteria for patient selection for surgery, not simply chronologic age. A much more cautious approach is recommended in the cirrhotic patient, and ablative therapies are often chosen for physically resectable liver tumors.

### References


1. Adkins RB Jr, Scott HW Jr (eds). Surgical Care for the Elderly. Baltimore: Williams & Wilkins, 1988.
2. Koruda MJ, Sheldon GF. Surgery in the aged. Curr Surg 1992:293–331.
3. Greenfield LJ. Surgery of the Aged. Philadelphia: Saunders, 1975.
4. Brooks B. Surgery in patients of advanced age. Ann Surg 1937;105:481–501.
5. Fong Y, Blumgart LH, Fortner JG, Brennan MF. Pancreatic or liver resection for malignancy is safe and effective for the elderly. Ann Surg 1995;222:426–437.
6. Parker SL. Cancer statistics, 1996. CA Cancer J Clin 1996;65:5–27.
7. Fortner JG, Silva JS, Cox EB, et al. Multivariate analysis of a personal series of 247 consecutive patients with liver metastases from colorectal cancer. Ann Surg 1984;199: 306–316.
8. Rosen CB, Nagorney DM, Taswell HF, et al. Perioperative blood transfusion and determinants of survival after liver resection for metastatic colorectal carcinoma. Ann Surg 1992;216:492–505.
9. Gayowski TJ, Iwatsuki S, Madariaga JR, et al. Experience in hepatic resection for metastatic colorectal cancer: analysis of clinical and pathologic risk factors. Surgery 1994;116:703–711.
10. Ezaki T, Yukaya H, Ogawa Y. Evaluation of hepatic resection for hepatocellular carcinoma in the elderly. Br J Surg 1987;74:471–473.
11. Yanaga K, Kanematsu T, Takenaka K, Matsumata T, Yoshida Y, Sugimachi K. Hepatic resection for hepatocellular carcinoma in elderly patients. Am J Surg 1988;155: 238–241.
12. Fortner JG, Lincer RM. Hepatic resection in the elderly. Ann Surg 1990;211:141–145.
13. Mentha G, Huber O, Robert J, Klopfenstein C, Egeli R, Rohner A. Elective hepatic resection in the elderly. Br J Surg 1992;79:557–559.
14. Nagasue N, Chang YC, Takemoto Y, Taniura H, Kohno H, Nakamura T. Liver resection in the aged (seventy years or older) with hepatocellular carcinoma. Surgery 1993;113: 148–154.
15. Takenaka K, Shimada M, Higahi H, et al. Liver resection for hepatocellular carcinoma in the elderly. Arch Surg 1994; 129:846–850.
16. Karl RC, Smith SK, Fabri PJ. Validity of major cancer operations in elderly patients. Ann Surg Oncol 1995;2:107–113.
17. Fong Y, Brennan MF, Cohen AE, Heffernan N, Freiman A, Blumgart LH. Liver resection in the elderly. Br J Surg 1997;84:1386–1390.
18. Fong Y, Blumgart LH, Cohen A, Fortner J, Brennan MF. Repeat hepatic resections for metastatic colorectal cancer. Ann Surg 1994;220:657–662.
19. Schwartz SI. Biliary tract surgery and cirrhosis: a critical combination. Surgery 1981;90:577–583.
20. Wynne HA, Cope LH, Mutch E, Rawlins MD, Woodhouse KW, James OFW. The effect of age upon liver volume and apparent blood flow in healthy man. Hepatology 1989; 9:297–301.
21. Asano K, Nakamura M, Asano A, Sato T, Tauchi H. Quantitation of changes in mitochondrial DNA during aging and regeneration of rat liver using non-radioactive DNA probes. Mech Ageing Dev 1992;62:85–98.
22. Mooney H, Roberts R, Cooksley WGE, Halliday JW, Powell LW. Alterations in the liver with ageing. Clin Gastroenterol 1985;14:757–771.
23. Yamamoto K, Takenaka K, Matsumata T, et al. Right hepatic lobectomy in elderly patients with hepatocellular carcinoma. Hepatogastroenterology 1997;44:514–518.
24. Carrillo MC, Carnovale CE, Favre C, Monti JA, Scapini C. Hepatic protein synthesis and serum amino acid levels during liver regeneration in young and old malnourished rats. Mech Ageing Dev 1996;91:55–64.
25. Schapiro H, Hotta SS, Outten WE, Klein AW. The effect of aging on rat liver regeneration. Experientia 1982;38: 1075–1076.
26. Beyer HS, Sherman R, Zieve L. Aging is associated with reduced liver regeneration and diminished thymidine kinase mRNA content and enzyme activity in the rat. J Lab Clin Med 1991;117:101–108.
27. Fry M, Silber J, Loeb LA, Martin GM. Delayed and reduced cell replication and diminishing levels of DNA polymerase-alpha in regenerating liver of aging mice. J Cell Physiol 1984;118:225–232.
28. Taguchi T, Ohashi M. Age-associated changes in the template-reading fidelity of DNA polymerase alpha from regerating rat liver. Mech Ageing Dev 1996;92:143–157.
29. Piantanelli L, Ermini M, Ricciotti R. Histone phosphorylation after partial hepatectomy in young and old rats. Experientia 1974;30:210–211.

30. Oh YH, Conard RA. Effect of aging on histone acetylation of the normal and regenerating rat liver. Life Sci 1972;11: 1207–1214.
31. Ferrucci JT. Liver tumor imaging. Cancer 1991;67:1189–1195.
32. Larson RE, Semelka RC. Magnetic resonance imaging of the liver. Top Magn Reson Imaging 1995;7(2):71–81.
33. Nichols FC, Van Heerden JA, Weiland LA. Benign liver tumors. Surg Clin North Am 1989;69:290–313.
34. Leese T, Farges O, Bismuth H. Liver cell adenomas: a 12 year surgical experience from a specialist hepatobiliary unit. Ann Surg 1988;208:558–564.
35. Schwartz SI, Husser WC. Cavernous hemangioma of the liver. Ann Surg 1987;205:456.
36. Kuo PC, Lewis WD, Jenkins RL. Treatment of giant hemangiomas of the liver by enucleation. J Am Coll Surg 1994; 178:49.
37. Trastek VF, Van Heerden JA, Sheedy PFI, Adson MA. Cavernous hemangiomas of the liver: resect or observe? Am J Surg 1983;145:49.
38. Yamagata M, Kanematsu T, Matsumata T, et al. Management of hemangioma of the liver: comparison between surgery and observation. Br J Surg 1991;78:1223.
39. Gaspar L, Mascarenhas F, de Costa MS, Dias JS, Alfonso JG, Silvestre ME. Radiation therapy in the unresectable cavernous hemangioma of the liver. Radiother Oncol 1993; 29:45–50.
40. Biswal BM, Sandhu M, Lal P, Bal CS. Role of radiotherapy in cavernous hemangioma of liver. Indian J Gastroenterol 1995;14:95–98.
41. Yamamoto T, Kawarda Y, Yano T, Noguichi T, Mizumoto R. Spontaneous rupture of hemangioma of the liver: treatment with transcatheter hepatic arterial embolization. Am J Gastroenterol 1991;86:1645–1649.
42. McKenna RJ Sr, Murphy GP. Cancer Surgery. Philadelphia: Lippincott, 1994.
43. Farmer DG, Rosove MH, Shaked A, Busuttil RW. Treatment of hepatocellular carcinoma. Ann Surg 1994;219:236–247.
44. Takayasu K, Moriyama N, Muramatsu Y, et al. The diagnosis of small carcinomas: efficacy of various imaging procedures in 100 patients. Am J Radiol 1990;155:49–54.
45. Blumgart LH. Liver resection: liver and biliary tumours. In: Blumgart LH (ed) Surgery of the Liver and Biliary Tract, 1st ed. New York: Churchill Livingstone, 1988:97:1251–1280.
46. Parker GA, Lawrence W Jr, Horsley JS III, et al. Intraoperative ultrasound of the liver affects operative decision making. Ann Surg 1989;209:569–577.
47. Iwatsuki S, Starzl TE. Personal experience with 411 hepatic resections. Ann Surg 1988;4:421–434.
48. Fong Y, Blumgart LH, Zakim D, Boyer TD (eds) Surgical therapy of liver cancer. In: Hepatology, 3rd ed. Philadelphia: Saunders, 1996;51:1548–1564.
49. Iwatsuki S, Gordon RD, Shaw BW Jr, et al. Role of liver transplantation in cancer therapy. Ann Surg 1985;202: 401–407.
50. Ravikumar TS, Kane R, Cady B, Jenkins R, Clouse M, Steele G Jr. A 5-year study of cryosurgery in the treatment of liver tumors. Arch Surg 1991;126:1520–1523.
51. Bismuth H, Morino M, Sherlock D, et al. Primary treatment of hepatocellular carcinoma by arterial chemoembolization. Am J Surg 1992;163:387–394.
52. Raoul JL, Heresbach D, Bretagne JF, et al. Chemoembolization of hepatocellular carcinomas. Cancer 1992;70:585–589.
53. Brown K, Nevins AB, Getradjman G, et al. Particle embolization of hepatocellular carcinoma. J Vasc Int Radiol 1998;9:822–828.
54. Livraghi T, Bolondi L, Lazzaroni S, et al. Percutaneous ethanol injection in the treatment of hepatocellular carcinoma in cirrhosis: a study of 207 patients. Cancer 1992; 69:925–929.
55. Sitzman JV, Abrams R. Improved survival for hepatocellular cancer with combination surgery and multimodal treatment. Ann Surg 1993;217:149–154.
56. Hughes KS, Simons R, Songhorabodi S, et al. Resection of the liver for colorectal carcinoma metastases: a multiinstitutional study of patterns of recurrence. Surgery 1986;100: 278–284.
57. Wood CB, Gillis CR, Blumgart LH. A retrospective study of the natural history of patients with liver metastases from colorectal cancer. Clin Oncol 1976;2:285–288.
58. Doroshow JH, Multhauf P, Leong L, et al. Prospective randomized comparison of fluorouracil versus fluorouracil and high-dose continuous infusion leucovorin calcium for the treatment of advanced measurable colorectal cancer in patients previously unexposed to chemotherapy. J Clin Oncol 1990;8:491–501.
59. Colucci G, Maiello E, Giuliani F, et al. Biochemical modulation of 5-fluorouracil (FU) and liver metastases of colorectal cancer patients. Ann Oncol 1994;5:53.
60. Kunimoto T, Nitta K, Tanaka T, et al. Antitumor activity of 7-ethyl-10-[4-(1-piperidino)-1-piperidino]carbonyloxy-camptothecin, a novel water-soluble derivative of camptothecin, against murine tumors. Cancer Res 1987;47: 5944–5947.
61. Tsuruo T, Matsuzaki T, Matsushita M, Saito H, Yokokura T. Antitumor effect of CPT-11, a new derivative of camptothecin, against pleiotropic drug-resistant tumors in vitro and in vivo. Cancer Chemother Pharmacol 1988;21:71–74.
62. Scheele J, Stang R, Altendorf-Hofmann A, Paul M. Resection of colorectal liver metastases. World J Surg 1995; 19:59–71.
63. Van de Velde CJH, Sugarbaker PH. Liver Metastases. Amsterdam: Martinus Nijhoff, 1984.
64. Fong Y, Cohen AM, Fortner JG, et al. Liver resection for colorectal metastases. J Clin Oncol 1997;15:938–946.
65. Schlag P, Hohenberger P, Herfarth C. Resection of liver metastases in colorectal cancer: competitive analysis of treatment results in synchronous versus metachronous metastases. Eur J Surg Oncol 1990;16:360–365.
66. Haberkorn U, Bellemann ME, Altmann A, et al. PET 2-fluoro-2-deoxyglucose uptake in rat prostate adenocarcinoma during chemotherapy with gemcitabine. J Nucl Med 1997;38:1215–1221.
67. Hughes KS, Simons R, Songhorabodi S, et al. Resection of the liver for colorectal carcinoma metastases: a multi-institutional study of indications for resection. Surgery 1988;103:278–288.
68. Doci R, Gennari L, Bignami P, Montalto F, Morabito A, Bozetti F. One hundred patients with hepatic metastases from colorectal cancer treated by resection: analysis of prognostic determinants. Br J Surg 1991;78:797–801.

69. Scheele J, Stangl R, Altendorf-Hofmann A, Gall FP. Indicators of prognosis after hepatic resection for colorectal secondaries. Surgery 1991;110:13–29.
70. Ekberg H, Tranberg KG, Andersson R, et al. Pattern of recurrence in liver resection for colorectal secondaries. World J Surg 1987;11:541–547.
71. Cunningham JD, Fong Y, Shriver C, Melendez J, Marx WL, Blumgart LH. One hundred consecutive hepatic resection: blood loss, transfusion, and operative technique. Arch Surg 1994;129:1050–1056.
72. Jamison RL, Donohue JH, Nagorney DM, Rosen CB, Harmsen WS, Ilstrup DM. Hepatic resection for metastatic colorectal cancer results in cure for some patients. Arch Surg 1997;132:505–511.
73. Baker LH, Talley RW, Matter R, et al. Phase III comparison of the treatment of advanced gastrointestinal cancer with bolus weekly 5-FU vs. methyl-CCNU plus bolus weekly 5-FU. Cancer 1976;38:1–7.
74. Ehrlichman C, Fine S, Wong A, Elhakim T. Randomized trial of fluorouracil and folinic acid in patients with metastatic colorectal carcinoma. J Clin Oncol 1988;6:469–475.
75. Petrelli N, Douglas HO, Herrera L, et al. The modulation of fluorouracil with leucovorin in metastatic colorectal carcinoma: a prospective randomized phase III trial. J Clin Oncol 1989;7:1419–1426.
76. Grage TB, Vasilopoulos PP, Shingleton WW, et al. Results of a prospective randomized study of hepatic artery infusion with 5-fluorouracil versus intravenous 5-fluorouracil in patients with hepatic metastases from colorectal cancer: a Central Oncology Group study. Surgery 1979;86:550–555.
77. Macdonald JS, Kisner DF, Smythe T, Woolley PV, Smith L, Schein PS. 5-Fluorouracil (5-FU), methyl-CCNU, and vincristine in the treatment of advanced colorectal cancer: phase II study utilizing weekly 5-FU. Cancer Treat Rep 1976;60:1597–1600.
78. Buroker T, Kim PN, Groppe C, et al. 5-FU infusion with mitomycin-C versus 5-FU infusion with methyl-CCNU in the treatment of advanced colon cancer. Cancer 1978;42:1228–1233.
79. Conti JA, Kemeny NE, Saltz LB, et al. Irinotecan is an active agent in untreated patients with metastatic colorectal cancer. J Clin Oncol 1996;14:709–715.

# 52
# Pancreatitis in the Elderly

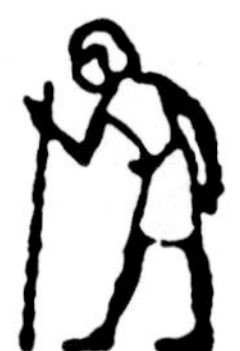

Peter D. Zdankiewicz and Dana K. Andersen

The anatomy of the pancreas changes with normal aging. Atrophy of the pancreas occurs with age, and its weight may fall from a normal 60–100 g to 40 g or less by 85 years of age.[1] This may actually facilitate detection of a small or subtle pancreatic mass, which may appear more prominent on imaging studies relative to the atrophied gland. The head of the pancreas and duodenal C loop may be displaced inferiorly, with the ampulla of Vater found as low as the third or fourth lumbar vertebra; and in one case it was reported at the level of the second sacral vertebra.[2] This inferior displacement of the pancreas can potentially cause difficulty interpreting radiographic studies.

Although clinical observations of pancreatic duct width have not disclosed consistent increases with age, duct ectasia has been described at autopsy.[3,4] One study of postmortem retrograde pancreatography found that duct width increased proportionally along the length of the duct at an average of 8% per decade, although retaining a tapered, smooth appearance[2] (Fig. 52.1). The main duct in the head of an otherwise normal, aged pancreas may reach 1 cm in width without evidence of mechanical obstruction. Small cysts are also found frequently on postmortem study, usually associated with increasing duct width. Other nonpathologic findings associated with age include calcification of splenic and superior mesenteric arteries, which produces calcific densities around the pancreas, narrowed ducts not due to stricture, and displacement of pancreatic parenchyma resulting from osteophyte formation, compression by the aorta or superior mesenteric artery, or enlarged lymph nodes.[2,4]

Ductal changes associated with aging may mimic the effects of chronic pancreatitis. In a study of pancreatograms performed at autopsy in patients with and without chronic pancreatitis, experienced endoscopists reviewed the films in a blinded fashion and were able to diagnose correctly those specimens that had histologic evidence of chronic pancreatitis. However, ductograms of older patients without pancreatitis were often misidentified as showing chronic pancreatitis (Fig. 52.2). Eighty-one percent of pancreatograms from patients who did not have pancreatitis were interpreted as showing chronic pancreatitis, with 37% rated as minimal, 33% as moderate, and 11% as severe chronic pancreatitis.[5] When the pancreatograms were compared to gross and histologic findings, irregularities in the ducts were frequently related instead to perilobular fibrosis. Moreover, perilobular fibrosis and the resultant ductular changes were noted with increasing frequency in older patients, as was ductal epithelial hyperplasia. Although autopsy pancreatograms cannot be directly compared to findings on endoscopic retrograde cholangiopancreatography (ERCP), these findings emphasize the need to interpret radiologic studies of the aging pancreas with caution.

Changes in pancreatic histology can be found in most elderly patients. Proliferation of ductal epithelial cells is frequently found, with stratified squamous epithelium replacing the normal ductal epithelium. Fatty infiltration is found in up to 80% of elderly patients, with small remnants of lobules sometimes completely surrounded by adipose tissue. Fibrosis, found in 60% of elderly patients, appears fine and patchy but is not related to destruction of exocrine tissue as is found in patients with chronic pancreatitis[1,5] (Fig. 52.3).

Functionally, reduced levels of pancreatic enzymes have been noted in the duodenal aspirates of elderly patients.[6] Initial bicarbonate and amylase outputs in response to secretin do not appear to change with age.[7] However, a phenomenon described as exhaustion or fatigue, has been described in pancreatic exocrine function of elderly subjects with diminished secretion of bicarbonate and total fluid volume on repeated stimulation. Similarly, amylase secretion is comparable for young and elderly subjects after initial stimulation but decreases after repeated stimulation.[7] The clinical significance of this diminished exocrine reserve remains speculative.

Endocrine function also decreases with age and plays a better-defined role in altered metabolism. A significant defect in beta cell insulin secretory capacity has been

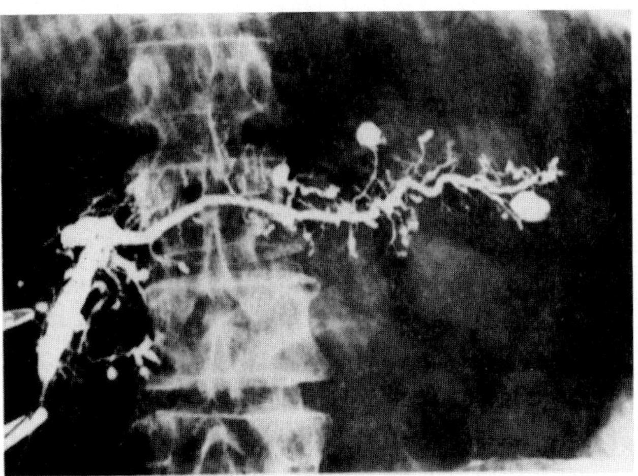

FIGURE 52.1. Necropsy retrograde pancreatography showing moderate dilation with a caliber of 7 mm in the proximal duct and multiple cystic spaces in a patient aged 71 years. (From Kreel and Sandin,[2] with permission.)

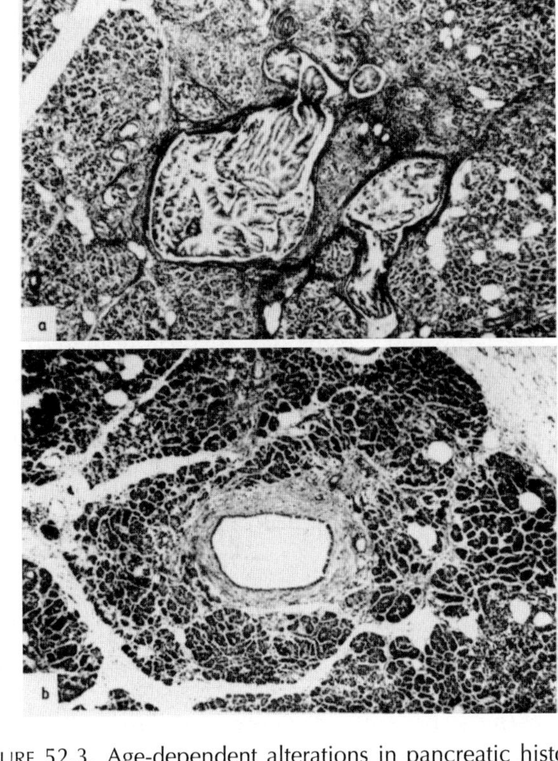

FIGURE 52.3. Age-dependent alterations in pancreatic histology. a. Intraductal epithelial proliferation and slight intralobular fibrosis. b. Periductal fibrosis encroaching on the adjacent parenchyma. (From Schmitz-Moormann et al.,[5] with permission.)

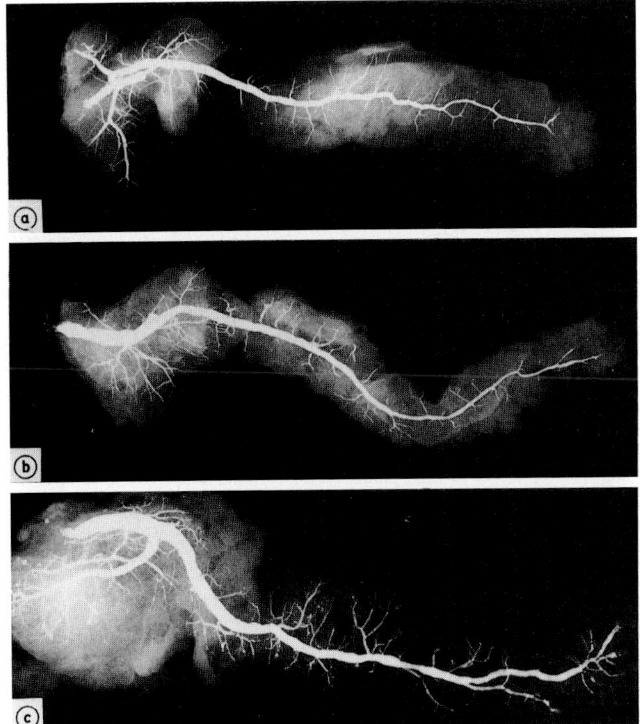

FIGURE 52.2. Postmortem ductograms of pancreases without histologic evidence of chronic pancreatitis. Six experienced endoscopists rated each as showing (a) mild, (b) mild, and (c) moderate degrees of chronic pancreatitis. Pancreases b and c were from patients age 67 and 72 years. (From Schmitz-Moormann et al.,[5] with permission.)

demonstrated in the elderly, with diminished capacity for continued insulin release compared to that in younger subjects.[8] In addition, insulin resistance is common in the elderly, probably as a result of an age-related replacement of lean body mass with adipose tissue and altered post-receptor events.[9] Together, decreased beta cell secretion and decreased sensitivity to insulin contribute to an age-related decline in glucose tolerance (Table 52.1).

TABLE 52.1. Oral Glucose Tolerance Test Results of the National Health and Nutrition Examination Survey II (1976–1980)

| | Percent, by age | | | |
|---|---|---|---|---|
| Parameter | 20–44 | 45–54 | 55–64 | 65–74 |
| Diabetes known prior to testing | 1.1 | 4.3 | 6.6 | 9.3 |
| Diabetes revealed through testing | 1.0 | 4.4 | 6.5 | 8.6 |
| Total prevalence of diabetes | 2.1 | 8.7 | 13.1 | 17.9 |
| Impaired glucose tolerance | 6.5 | 14.9 | 15.2 | 22.9 |
| Total diabetes and impaired glucose tolerance | 8.6 | 23.6 | 28.3 | 40.8 |

*Source:* Goldberg et al.,[10] with permission.

Interpretation of standard tests of glucose tolerance should be corrected for age. Elevated plasma glucose values are especially common in old patients with acute pancreatitis.[10]

## Acute Pancreatitis

### Etiology

The frequency of the various causes of acute pancreatitis in the elderly differs from that in the population as a whole. Gallstones are the most common cause of acute pancreatitis in the elderly and account for at least half of all cases.[11–14] Alcohol abuse is the second most common etiology, causing 20–25% of cases.[11] Of the remaining cases, 10–15% are termed idiopathic; and other causes, including trauma, infection, cancer, and side effects of medications, together make up the remaining 5–10%. Forty percent of patients experiencing their first attack of gallstone pancreatitis are more than 60 years old,[15] which parallels the age-related incidence of cholelithiasis and choledocholithiasis.

Idiopathic pancreatitis is reported at higher rates in the elderly than in the general population and is responsible for 23–40% of acute cases.[12–14,16] A large proportion of these patients is found to have biliary sludge identified by microscopic analysis of duodenal drainage fluid. One study found that in 67% of patients recovering from acute "idiopathic" pancreatitis, clusters of cholesterol monohydrate crystals, calcium bilirubinate granules, or calcium carbonate microspheroliths could be demonstrated in duodenal bile.[17] Furthermore, 73% of patients with unexplained pancreatitis, had biliary sludge or microlithiasis found within 12 months at cholecystectomy or by ultrasonography. Conversely, patients with alcoholic pancreatitis had no evidence of biliary microlithiasis. Ultrasonography revealed biliary sludge only half as often as did microscopic bile analysis, which suggests that biliary pancreatitis is underdiagnosed as a cause of acute pancreatitis in older patients. An indication of the presence of occult choledocholithiasis during an attack of "idiopathic" pancreatitis is frequently obtained from measurement of elevated levels of serum γ-glutamyl transpeptidase (GGTP) and alanine aminotransferase (ALT) during the acute episode (Fig. 52.4). Appropriate therapy such as dissolution therapy of microlithiasis by ursodeoxycholic acid, sphincterotomy, or cholecystectomy may therefore prevent recurrent episodes of "idiopathic" pancreatitis.[17–19]

Alcohol abuse is a less common cause of acute pancreatitis among patients over age 60 than in the general population. In one study, alcohol abuse was the cause of only 20% of cases of acute pancreatitis in an elderly population,[13] and only 8% of patients who experience acute alcoholic pancreatitis have their first attack after age 60.[15,20]

Among old patients, ischemia or hypoperfusion is a frequent cause of pancreatitis, which is rarely seen in a young population. Ischemic pancreatitis is particularly

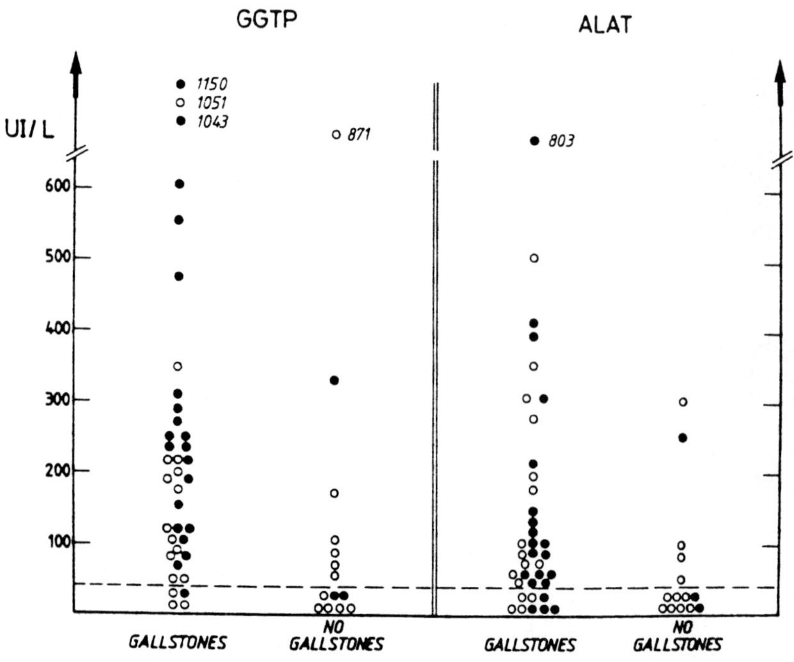


FIGURE 52.4. Serum levels of γ-glutamyl transpeptidase (GGTP) and alanine aminotransferase (ALT) during an episode of acute "idiopathic" pancreatitis in patients with and without a subsequent diagnosis of gallstones. Horizontal broken line, upper normal levels of both enzymes; open circles, patients with a single episode of acute pancreatitis; closed circles, patients with prior relapsing attacks. (From Ros et al.,[17] with permission.)

common following cardiopulmonary bypass. In studies of patients undergoing cardiac surgery, up to one-fourth of patients demonstrate postoperative hyperamylasemia, and 2–5% demonstrate acute pancreatitis.[20,21] Other factors may contribute to the development of pancreatitis in these patients, including preoperative renal insufficiency and perioperative administration of high doses of calcium chloride or potassium.[21]

Trauma as a cause of acute pancreatitis in the elderly usually results from surgery rather than violence or accidents. Acute pancreatitis was an unanticipated complication of major surgery in 12.5% of patients in one review, but it was uncertain whether patients developed pancreatitis as a result of perioperative hypotension or iatrogenic injury to the pancreas.[11] Nonetheless, pancreatitis can result from inadvertent injury during any abdominal operation. It most commonly occurs after biliary surgery, gastric operations, splenectomy, or aortic reconstruction. Similarly, although ERCP is frequently associated with an elevated serum amylase level, it causes clinical pancreatitis in only about 5% of cases.[22]

Pancreatic duct adenomas and carcinoma can cause acute pancreatitis secondary to duct obstruction; they present as some form of pancreatitis 5–10% of the time, which can delay diagnosis. Ten percent of patients with pancreatic or ampullary carcinoma have histologically demonstrated pancreatitis,[23] and 8% of patients age 60 or over who were diagnosed with pancreatic pseudocysts harbored a pancreatic malignancy[24] (Fig. 52.5). Moreover, 31% of patients with malignancy-associated pancreatitis describe recent previous attacks of pain that suggest acute pancreatitis.[23] Fewer than 1% of cases of acute pancreatitis overall are caused by carcinoma of the pancreas, but the diagnosis must be considered in elderly patients without other apparent causes for acute inflammation.[11,23]

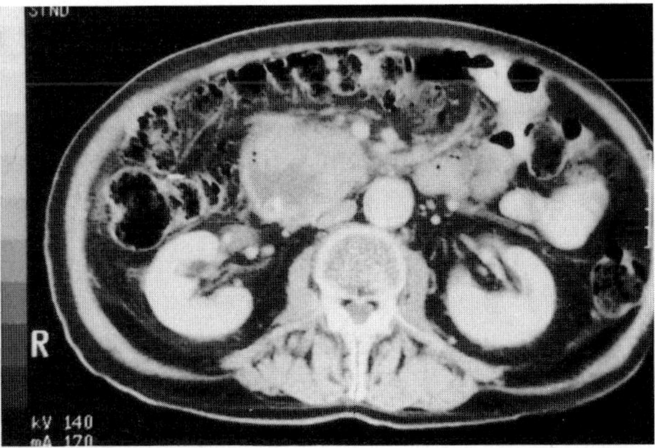


FIGURE 52.5. Computed tomography (CT) scan of a 72-year-old patient with acute pancreatitis, showing a cystic lesion of the pancreatic head. Papillary adenocarcinoma of the proximal pancreatic duct was resected with a pylorus-sparing Whipple procedure.

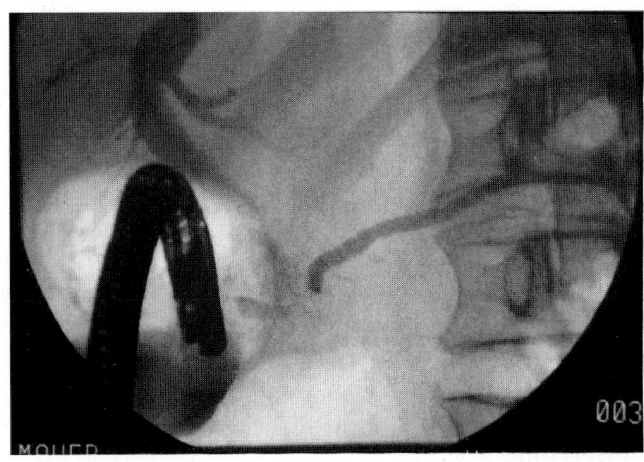


FIGURE 52.6. Endoscopic retrograde cholangiopancreatography (ERCP) of a 77-year-old patient with recurrent pancreatitis. Segmental ductal obstruction in the pancreatic head was due to adenocarcinoma.

Drug-induced pancreatitis has been reported in elderly patients, with cases known to result from tetracycline, diuretics, and steroids. The incidence and severity are similar when compared to the population as a whole.[11,12] Reported infectious causes of pancreatitis among elderly patients include tuberculosis and fungal infections.[15,22] Other factors to be considered are hypertriglyceridemia, hypercalcemia, and penetrating peptic ulcer disease.[12]

If the history and physical examination do not reveal the cause of acute pancreatitis, laboratory evaluation should include serum calcium, bilirubin, alkaline phosphatase, aminotransferases, and triglycerides. A plain roentgenogram of the abdomen may show calcifications, and ultrasonography is indicated to look for gallstones. A computed tomography (CT) scan of the abdomen is indicated when the episode represents recurrent disease, when moderately severe pancreatitis (three or more Ranson's criteria) is present, or when the initial response to treatment is indefinite. Finally, acute pancreatitis should not be labeled idiopathic unless or until ERCP has been performed to rule out periampullary tumors, ductal strictures or other lesions, congenital anomalies such as pancreas divisum, or gallstones that were missed on a previous study (Fig. 52.6). At the same time, manometry of the sphincter of Oddi can be performed to exclude the relatively uncommon cause of sphincter dysfunction. The finding of mucus being extruded from the papilla of Vater during ERCP suggests the presence of a mucin-secreting neoplasm or the premalignant condition of mucinous ductal ectasia. Evaluation of aspirated bile permits exclusion of microlithiasis of the common bile duct. Endoscopic ultrasonography (EUS) is a less invasive method to rule out pancreatic and ampullary tumors, calculi or sludge in the common duct, or pancreatic ductular lesions.

## Clinical Course

The most common symptom of acute pancreatitis at the time of presentation is pain. Typically, it is felt in the epigastrium and may radiate to the back or left shoulder. Involvement of gallstones may also produce pain in the right upper quadrant. The onset of the pain may be gradual or sudden, and it may be associated with nausea and vomiting early in the course of the disease. Acute pancreatitis in elderly patients may present in an atypical fashion, however, and it is not uncommon for the diagnosis to go unsuspected. For example, in reports of patients over 60 years of age in whom pancreatitis was diagnosed at autopsy, pancreatitis was not considered as a premortem diagnosis in 30–40% of patients.[16,25] Only 8% of the patients dying with undiagnosed pancreatitis complained of pain. This may have been confounded by analgesics given for other diagnoses or by sedation given for mechanical ventilation, particularly in the postoperative patient. More commonly, shock, organ failure, hyperglycemia, and hypothermia manifest pancreatitis in these patients. Given the frequently occult nature of the diagnosis, acute pancreatitis must be considered in elderly patients experiencing systemic complications of unclear cause. This is particularly true among postoperative patients, who account for 20–40% of the deaths from undetected acute pancreatitis.[15,16,20]

The importance of advancing age in the severity of acute pancreatitis was recognized by Ranson et al., who determined that age over 55 years correlated with a worse prognosis.[26] Recent data confirm a mortality rate of 6% for patients age less than 50, and 21% for those over 75. A recent examination shows that the increase in mortality appears to be related to concomitant disease, particularly cardiopulmonary and biliary tract diseases.[14] The mortality due to pancreatitis per se did not appear to differ between the young and the elderly. Furthermore, pancreatitis severity at the time of admission and the complication rate did not differ with age. The pattern of complications did differ with age, however. Young patients were more likely to experience local complications such as necrotizing pancreatitis, pseudocyst, or abscess, whereas the elderly were more likely to suffer from systemic complications such as gastrointestinal bleeding, renal failure, or pulmonary failure, which are associated with a higher risk of death.

Although co-morbid diseases may partially explain a higher mortality rate among the elderly with acute pancreatitis, patients with idiopathic acute pancreatitis have more severe disease at the time of presentation than do patients of the same age with either biliary or alcoholic pancreatitis[13] (Table 52.2). Moreover, those with idiopathic acute pancreatitis tend to have longer stays in the intensive care unit (ICU) and are more likely to suffer compromise of other organ function. Dysfunction of other organ systems, in turn, correlates with increased mortality.

TABLE 52.2. Clinical Outcome of Acute Pancreatitis in the Elderly

| Parameter[a] | Unknown etiology | Known etiology[b] |
|---|---|---|
| No. of patients | 21 | 72 |
| Mean age (years) | 71.5 | 71.1 |
| Male/female | 11/10 | 35/37 |
| Coexisting illnesses[c] (no.) | 8 (38%) | 29 (40%) |
| Ranson's criteria | 3.5 ± 0.4* | 2.4 ± 1.8 |
| Morbidity[d] (%) | 48* | 22 |
| Mortality (%) | 24* | 8.3 |
| Mean hospital stay (days) | 14.8 ± 3.5 | 12.9 ± 1.4 |
| SICU stay | 4.4 ± 1.3* | 1.6 ± 0.4 |

*Source:* Browder et al.,[13] with permission.
SICU, surgical intensive care unit.
[a] Presentation characteristics and outcome of 93 patients over age 60 with acute pancreatitis.
[b] Biliary tract disease, alcohol, and medications.
[c] Coexisting illnesses included cardiac, pulmonary, and renal disease.
[d] Most common causes of morbidity were pulmonary failure and congestive heart failure.
* $p < 0.05$ vs. known etiology group.

An increased severity of pancreatitis is associated with the presence of a pseudocyst, sterile pancreatic necrosis, infected necrosis, or abscess. Patients who avoid these additional complications have a low mortality, and patients with sterile necrosis have a death rate of about 10%; this increases to at least a 30% mortality rate if the necrotic tissue is infected.[21]

Clinical series traditionally have noted pancreatic infection to be the most common mortality risk, causing approximately three of every four deaths due to acute pancreatitis. However, a large autopsy study of patients with acute pancreatitis found that most deaths (60%) occurred within the first week of admission, and that for these early deaths respiratory failure was more common than pancreatic infection. Forty percent of deaths occurred after the first week; and among these patients, sepsis was the most common cause.[11]

## Treatment

In general, treatment of elderly patients with acute pancreatitis is the same as for younger patients. Elderly patients with moderately severe disease are best treated in an intensive care setting because pain is frequently absent or reduced, and evidence of recrudescence of inflammation may be subtle. Careful attention to serum amylase and lipase levels is necessary upon resumption of feeding. CT or ultrasonographic evidence of ongoing phlegmon formation should also elicit caution, even in the "asymptomatic" patient.

One therapeutic approach that may differ for elderly patients is the treatment of severe gallstone pancreatitis. A decrease in morbidity and mortality has been shown in elderly patients when urgent ERCP and sphincterotomy are performed on patients with stones in the common bile duct.[19,27] Prompt relief of the biliary obstruction corresponds with a decrease in the severity of the pancreatitis, presumably due to relief of biliary sepsis. Patients with biliary pancreatitis may retain an impacted stone in the ampulla, but more commonly the obstruction resolves spontaneously within 12–24 hours. Patients who do not show improvement in serum aminotransferases, amylase, and lipase levels within this time frame should undergo imaging studies to detect persistent obstruction. Noncontrast helical CT scanning (Fig. 52.7) or EUS may be helpful for identifying those patients who are candidates for urgent endoscopic sphincterotomy.

Biliary pancreatitis may be the only clinical presentation of gallstones, but it should not prevent the appropriate management of symptomatic cholelithiasis. Because gallstone pancreatitis tends to be recur, cholecystectomy is indicated once the patient's overall condition allows.[26,28] Cholecystectomy greatly decreases the likelihood of recurrence as well as future morbidity and mortality, regardless of whether endoscopic sphincterotomy has been performed. Laparoscopic removal of the gallbladder is, in general, as well tolerated in the elderly as in young patients, but the conversion rate to open cholecystectomy is higher in elderly patients with complicated gallstone disease.[29] The presence of periportal inflammation from recent biliary pancreatitis should prompt early conversion to open cholecystectomy when present.

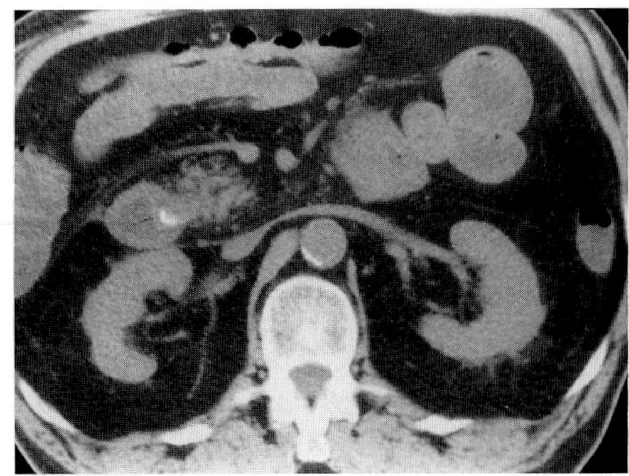

FIGURE 52.7. Helical CT scan (without contrast) demonstrating a gallstone impacted in the ampulla of Vater of a patient with acute biliary pancreatitis.

## Chronic Pancreatitis

Chronic pancreatitis in the elderly can result from ethanolism, the most common cause of the disorder in the young patient, but it can also result from obstruction, usually as the result of carcinoma of the pancreas or the ampulla. Histologically, obstructive chronic pancreatitis differs from chronic pancreatitis of other etiologies. In patients with chronic pancreatitis from either alcohol abuse or of idiopathic origin, inflammation is usually found in a patchy, lobular distribution. However, with chronic pancreatitis of obstructive origin, fibrosis tends to occur uniformly throughout the gland, with nonsegmental ductal dilatation distal to the obstruction.[30] Calcification and protein plugs are not found with chronic pancreatitis of obstructive origin but are frequently found with alcoholic and idiopathic chronic pancreatitis. Dilata-

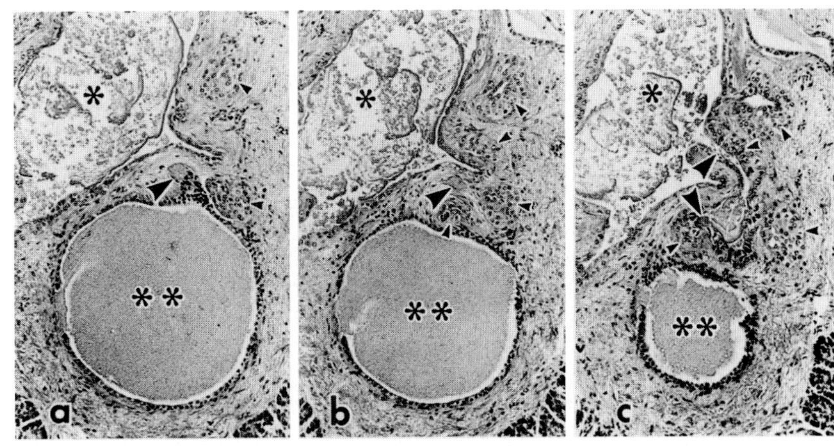


FIGURE 52.8. Pancreatic lithiasis in the elderly. A stricture of the pancreatic duct (large arrows) is demonstrated adjacent to a stone (*) in serial sections (a,b,c) of an autopsy specimen from an elderly patient without a history of pancreatitis. The stone-filled upper duct is connected to the contrast-filled lower duct (**) by a stricture which is surrounded by foci of squamous metaplasia (small arrows). (From Nagai and Ohtsuto,[31] with permission.)

tion of interlobular ducts is found in nearly all cases of alcoholic or idiopathic chronic pancreatitis but rarely in cases of obstructive pancreatitis. In contrast, diffuse dilatation of the main duct is usually found with obstructive disease but is uncommon with alcoholic or idiopathic pancreatitis.

Isolated stones have been found within the pancreatic ducts in elderly patients. The prevalence appears to increase with increasing age, from a frequency of less than 5% in patients in their seventies to 17% among patients over 90 years of age.[30] Typically, these stones are found at autopsy above areas of squamous metaplasia, which causes duct narrowing (Fig. 52.8). They are associated with fibrosis and atrophy of the pancreatic parenchyma in the surrounding area, the findings of which are consistent with chronic pancreatitis. Typically, however, these patients have not experienced signs or symptoms of chronic pancreatitis, so the etiology and significance of pancreaticolithiasis in the elderly is unclear.[15,31]

Some cases of chronic pancreatitis remain idiopathic in etiology, and this entity is more common in men. A bimodal distribution of age at the time of presentation exists with idiopathic pancreatitis, where patients tend to develop the disease either before 20 years of age or after age 65.[25,32] Among old patients, idiopathic chronic pancreatitis is usually painless or nearly so compared to that seen in the young population. Endocrine or exocrine sufficiency develops only very late if at all. Because of the slowly progressive nature of the disease in the elderly, intervention for complications of idiopathic chronic pancreatitis is rarely necessary.

## References


1. Lillemoe KD. Pancreatic disease in the elderly patient. Surg Clin North Am 1994;74:317–344.
2. Kreel L, Sandin B. Changes in pancreatic morphology associated with aging. Gut 1973;14:962–970.
3. Milbourne E. Caliber and appearance of the pancreatic ducts and relevant clinical problems. Acta Chir Scand 1960;118:286–303.
4. Sandin B, Kreel L, Slavin G. The pancreas: radiographic demonstration of pancreatic morphology at autopsy. Radiography 1973;39:151–157.
5. Schmitz-Moormann P, Himmelmann GW, Brandes J-W, et al. Comparative radiological and morphological study of human pancreas: pancreatitis-like changes in postmortem ductograms and their morphological pattern; possible implication for ERCP. Gut 1985;26:406–414.
6. Rosenberg IR, Friedland N, et al. The effect of age and sex upon human pancreatic secretion of fluid and bicarbonate. Gastroenterology 1966;50:191–194.
7. Bartos V, Groh J. The effect of repeated stimulation of the pancreas on the pancreatic secretion in young and aged men. Gerontol Clin 1969;11:56–62.
8. Elahi D, Andersen DK, Muller DC, Tobin JD, Brown JC, Andres R. The enteric enhancement of glucose-stimulated insulin release: the role of GIP in aging, obesity, and non-insulin dependent diabetes mellitus. Diabetes 1984;33: 950–957.
9. Chen M, Bergman RN, Pacini G, Porte D Jr, et al. Pathogenesis of age-related glucose intolerance in man: insulin resistance and decreased β-cell function. J Clin Endocrinol Metab 1985;60:13–20.
10. Goldberg AP, Andres R, Bierman EL. Diabetes mellitus in the elderly. In: Hazzard WR, Andres R, Bierman EL, Blass JP (eds) Principles of Geriatric Medicine and Gerontology, 2nd ed. New York: McGraw-Hill, 1990:739–758.
11. Park J, Fromkes J, Cooperman M, et al. Acute pancreatitis in the elderly: pathogenesis and outcome. Am J Surg 1986;152:638–642.
12. Steinberg WM. Acute pancreatitis: never leave a stone unturned. N Engl J Med 1992;326:635.
13. Browder W, Patterson MD, Thompson JL, Walters DN. Acute pancreatitis of unknown etiology in the elderly. Ann Surg 1993;217:469–475.
14. Fan ST, Choi TK, Lai CS, Wong J. Influence of age on the mortality from acute pancreatitis. Br J Surg 1988;75:463–466.
15. Banks PA. Pancreatic disease in the elderly. Semin Gastrointest Dis 1994;5:189–196.
16. Lankisch PG. Undetected fatal acute pancreatitis: why is the disease so frequently overlooked? Am J Gastroenterol 1991;86:322–326.
17. Ros E, Navarro S, Bru C, et al. Occult microlithiasis in "idiopathic" acute pancreatitis: prevention of relapses by cholecystectomy or ursodeoxycholic acid therapy. Gastroenterology 1991;101:1701–1709.
18. Lee SP, Nicholls JF, Park HZ. Biliary sludge as a cause of acute pancreatitis. N Engl J Med 1992;326:589–593.
19. Williamson RCN. Endoscopic sphincterotomy in the early treatment of acute pancreatitis. N Engl J Med 1993;328:279–280.
20. Hanks JB, Curtis SE, Hanks BB, Andersen DK, Cox JL, Jones RS. Gastrointestinal complications after cardiopulmonary bypass. Surgery 1982;92:394–400.
21. Banks PA. Predictors of severity in acute pancreatitis. Pancreas 1991;6(suppl 1):s7–s12.
22. Steinberg W, Tenner S. Acute pancreatitis. N Engl J Med 1994;330:1198–1207.
23. Gambill EE. Pancreatitis associated with pancreatic carcinoma: a study of 26 cases. Mayo Clin Proc 1971;46:174–177.
24. Itai Y, Moss AA, Goldberg HI. Pancreatic cysts caused by carcinoma of the pancreas: a pitfall in the diagnosis of pancreatic carcinoma. J Comput Assist Tomogr 1982;6:772–776.
25. Gullo L, Sipahi HM, Pezzilli R. Pancreatitis in the elderly. J Clin Gastroenterol 1994;19:64–68.
26. Ranson JHC, Rifkind KM, Roses DF, Fink SD, Eng K, Spencer FC. Prognostic signs and the role of operative management in acute pancreatitis. Surg Gynecol Obstet 1974;139:69–81.
27. Fan ST, Lai ECS, Mok FP, Lo CM, Zheng SS, Wong J. Early treatment of acute biliary pancreatitis by endoscopic papillotomy. N Engl J Med 1993;328:228–232.
28. Büchler M, Uhl W, Beger HG. Surgical strategies in acute pancreatitis. Hepatogastroenterology 1993;40:563–568.

29. Magnuson TH, Ratner LE, Zenilman ME, Bender JS. Laparoscopic cholecystectomy: applicability in the geriatric population. Am Surg 1997;63:91–96.
30. De Angelis C, Valente G, Spaccapietra M, et al. Histological study of alcoholic, nonalcoholic, and obstructive chronic pancreatitis. Pancreas 1992;7:193–196.
31. Nagai H, Ohtsuto K. Pancreatic lithiasis in the aged: its clinicopathology and pathogenesis. Gastroenterology 1984;86: 331–338.
32. Ammann RW. Chronic pancreatitis in the elderly. Gastroenterol Clin North Am 1990;19:905–914.

# 53 Pancreatic Tumors: Pathophysiology and Treatment

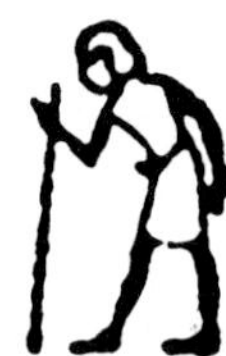

Keith D. Lillemoe

The entire spectrum of benign and malignant pancreatic neoplasms can be seen in the elderly. Adenocarcinoma of the pancreas is by far the most important of these conditions, reflecting the frequency and lethality of the disease and the complexity of treatment. The incidence of pancreatic cancer rose dramatically from the 1930s until the mid-1970s, nearly doubling during this time period. Since 1973, the incidence in the United States has remained stable at 8–9 per 100,000 population, with over 28,000 new cases diagnosed yearly.[1] Carcinoma of the pancreas is an extremely lethal disease with an overall estimated cure rate of less than 5%. Although it represents only 2–3% of all cancers, it results in more than 6% of cancer deaths. As the population ages, it can be expected that increasing numbers of elderly patients will be diagnosed and require treatment for pancreatic cancer.

## Risk Factors

Age is one of the principal risk factors for pancreatic cancer. The annual incidence in the age range of 40–44 years is about 2 per 100,000, increasing thereafter to 100 per 100,000 in the age range of 80–84 years, a 50-fold increase.[2] Nearly 80% of the patients with pancreatic carcinoma are 60 years of age or older. A male/female ratio of 1.7:1.0 is noted in the overall number, but older patients have an equal sex ratio. In the United States, the incidence and mortality rates from pancreatic cancer are higher in Blacks than in Whites.[3]

A number of other possible risk factors often present in elderly patients have been associated with pancreatic cancer. The most important association is with diabetes and pancreatic cancer. Although the data are somewhat inconsistent, most data indicate no association of diabetes with cancer of the pancreas, except when the diabetes was diagnosed within 1–5 years before the cancer diagnosis. The available data suggest that diabetes is most commonly an early symptom of pancreatic cancer rather than a causative influence. The relation between chronic pancreatitis and pancreatic cancer has also been investigated. Chronic pancreatitis is most frequently associated with alcohol abuse. The increased risk appears to exist only for pancreatitis that occurs less than 10 years before the diagnosis of pancreatic cancer. This finding suggests that there is a common risk factor for both diseases or that some forms of pancreatitis represent an indolent manifestation of pancreatic cancer.

The most significant environmental risk factor in pancreatic cancer is cigarette smoking.[3] Data from animal studies suggests that nitrosamines and tobacco smoke are carcinogenic for the pancreas. Hyperplastic changes in pancreatic ductal cells, with atypical nuclear patterns, have been observed in smokers at autopsy, with some relation to the amount of tobacco smoked. Numerous prospective studies have also shown a positive association of smoking with pancreatic cancer. The risk ratios for pancreatic cancer deaths in prospective studies of current cigarette-only smokers compared with nonsmokers ranges from 1.6 to 3.1.[3] Most studies have shown increasing pancreatic cancer risk with increased numbers of cigarettes smoked. There appears to be no association between nutrition or diet with pancreatic cancer including use of alcohol and coffee. A number of occupations are believed to be at increased risk for pancreatic cancer including chemists, coal gas workers, and workers in the metals and textile industries.

## Pathology

The site or origin of a periampullary malignancy is often difficult to determine. Frequently, the clinical presentation, preoperative imaging studies, and findings at laparotomy do not allow differentiation of the specific site of origin. Pathologic examination of resected specimens shows that adenocarcinoma of the head of the pancreas (50–70%) is by far the most common site followed by

TABLE 53.1. Relative Frequency of Periampullary Neoplasms

| Location | Frequency (%) |
|---|---|
| Pancreas | 83 |
| Head | 70 |
| Body and tail | 30 |
| Ampulla of Vater | 10 |
| Duodenum | 4 |
| Common bile duct | 3 |

the ampulla of Vater (20–30%), distal common bile duct (10%), and duodenum (10%). Because these data are from resected specimens, the incidence of ampullary, distal bile duct, and duodenal carcinoma is somewhat higher owing to a greater rate of resection than tumors arising in the head of the pancreas. Therefore overall carcinoma of the pancreas is the likely site of origin in up to 85% of cases (Table 53.1).

Adenocarcinoma of the pancreas arises from the pancreatic ductal tissue. The most common location for the tumor is the head of the pancreas (65–70%). Tumors of the head of the pancreas tend to be smaller than tumors in the body or tail, as they are more apt to be diagnosed earlier by presentation with obstructive jaundice. Nevertheless, most cancers of the pancreas tend to present at an advanced stage. Fewer than 5% of resected pancreatic cancers are classified as stage 1 with the tumor confined to the pancreas or the adjacent duodenum, bile duct, or peripancreatic soft tissues.[4] Furthermore, only 40% of tumors are less than 2cm in size (stage 1), underscoring the virulence of pancreatic cancer. Adenocarcinomas originating from the distal bile duct and ampulla of Vater usually present with obstructive jaundice earlier in their course, resulting in more localized disease and thus a better chance for cure. Duodenal cancers, although often large at the time of diagnosis, also have a better prognosis than pancreatic cancer.

## Clinical Presentation

Carcinoma of the pancreas often presents in an insidious manner. Screening techniques are not available, and the early symptoms of pancreatic cancer are often vague, nonspecific, and similar to functional gastrointestinal disorders. Obstructive jaundice is often the first and only specific symptom leading to the diagnosis. Seventy-five percent of patients with carcinoma of the head of the pancreas develop jaundice that is usually progressive, unremitting, and associated with abdominal pain. The development of jaundice in an elderly patient should lead to prompt attempts at diagnosis with a high index of suspicion of an underlying malignancy. In a report of 80 elderly jaundiced patients with a mean age of 75.7 years, malignant obstruction was the most common cause, with pancreatic cancer being the most common neoplasm.[5] Tumors of the ampulla of Vater, distal bile duct, and periampullary duodenum tend to cause biliary obstruction and jaundice at an earlier stage owing to their location. Ampullary tumors have been described to cause intermittent jaundice due to transient biliary obstruction.

Abdominal pain occurs in most patients and is the presenting symptom in up to two-thirds. The pain is most frequently in the mid-epigastrium or radiating through to the back. Typically, the pain is a dull, boring ache that becomes progressively worse and may be aggravated by food ingestion. Weight loss and anorexia therefore occurs in many patients.

A variety of other symptoms, including change in bowel habit and abdominal distension, may occur but add little to an early diagnosis. Early satiety progressing to complete gastric outlet obstruction with nausea and vomiting may occur from duodenal involvement by the tumor, but it is usually a late occurrence. Duodenal or ampullary carcinomas may also bleed, resulting in melena or symptoms of anemia. An important historic point that may suggest pancreatic carcinoma in an elderly patient, is the new onset of diabetes mellitus. Islet cell injury can result from obstruction of the pancreatic duct with resultant chronic pancreatitis. Therefore, pancreatic carcinoma should be considered in all such patients. Finally, an unexplained attack of pancreatitis in an old patient must be thoroughly investigated once the acute attack has subsided, because this presentation may be the first manifestation of a periampullary tumor.

Cancers arising in the body and tail of the pancreas have a more insidious presentation than periampullary tumors, with abdominal pain and weight loss. By the time these symptoms have occurred, the disease is almost always locally unresectable or metastatic. The duration of symptoms typically precedes the diagnosis by 3–6 months, and survival from the time of diagnosis to death is usually less than 6 months.

## Diagnosis

There is no screening test available at this time for pancreatic or periampullary carcinoma. Virtually all patients with a periampullary carcinoma present with liver function test abnormalities, including increased levels of total bilirubin, alkaline phosphatase, and transaminases. To make an early diagnosis, the physician must have a high index of suspicion. The evaluation of any patient with jaundice regardless of age, should begin with noninvasive imaging studies of the pancreas and biliary tract. Computed tomography (CT) and ultrasonography of the pancreas and biliary tree are the most sensitive and specific for pancreatic disease. CT is probably the better of the two studies in that it not only demonstrates the

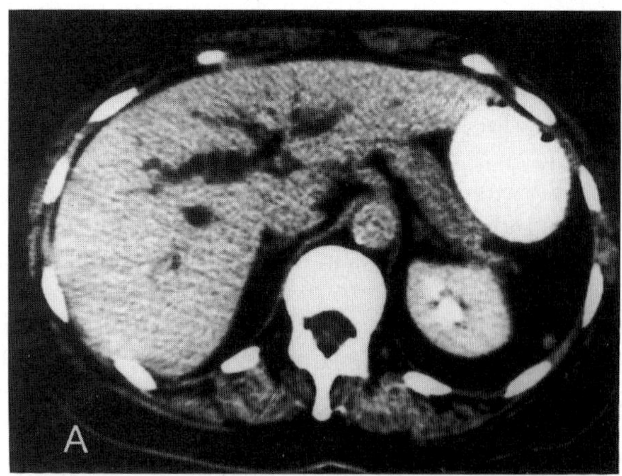


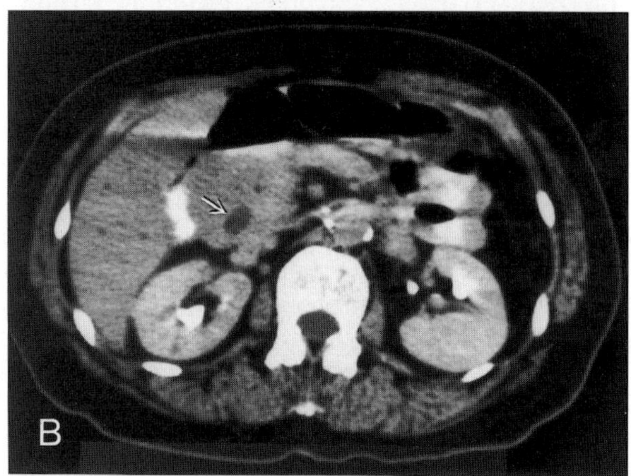


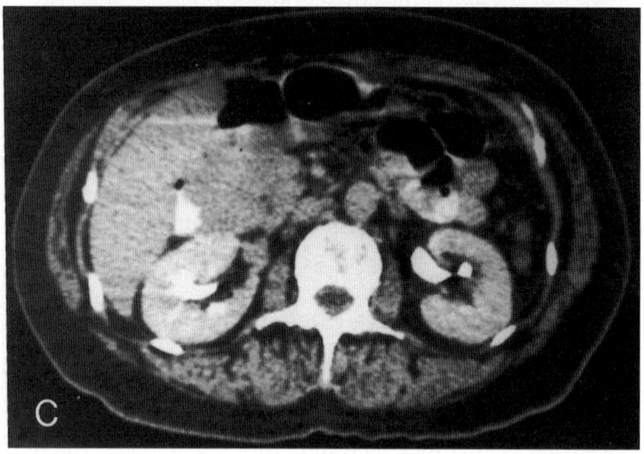


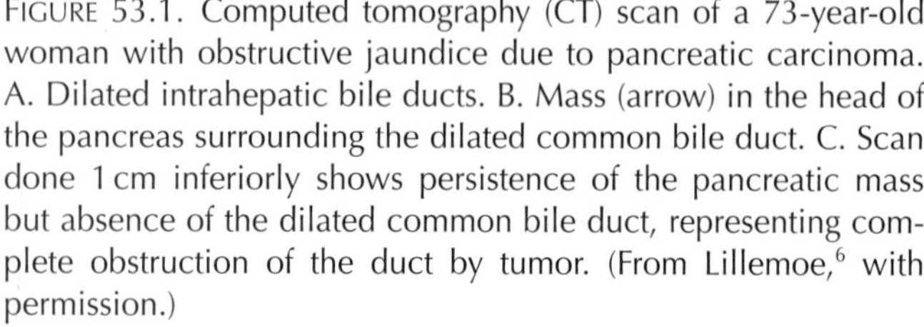

FIGURE 53.1. Computed tomography (CT) scan of a 73-year-old woman with obstructive jaundice due to pancreatic carcinoma. A. Dilated intrahepatic bile ducts. B. Mass (arrow) in the head of the pancreas surrounding the dilated common bile duct. C. Scan done 1 cm inferiorly shows persistence of the pancreatic mass but absence of the dilated common bile duct, representing complete obstruction of the duct by tumor. (From Lillemoe,[6] with permission.)

presence of biliary duct dilatation but defines the presence of a pancreatic mass, pancreatic ductal enlargement, local invasion, and liver metastasis (Fig. 53.1).

If imaging studies demonstrate the presence of biliary obstruction, more invasive techniques to image the biliary system may be indicated. Endoscopic retrograde cholangiopancreatography (ERCP) provides an endoscopic view of the ampulla and visualizes the biliary and pancreatic ductal systems (Fig. 53.2). Endoscopic biopsies can be performed on any masses present in the ampulla or periampullary duodenum. An alternative to ERCP is percutaneous transhepatic cholangiography (PTC). The classic cholangiographic finding associated with a

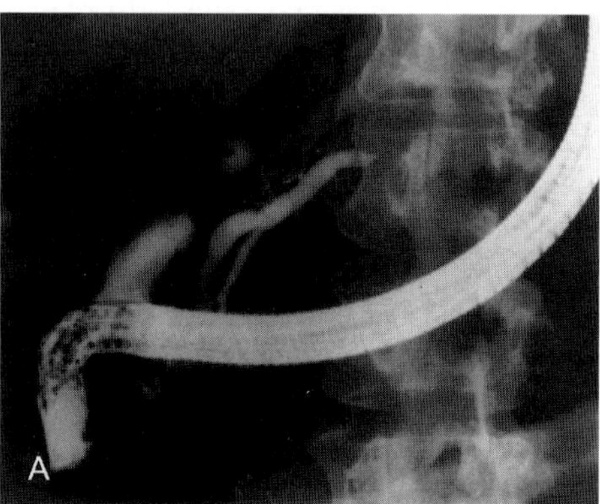


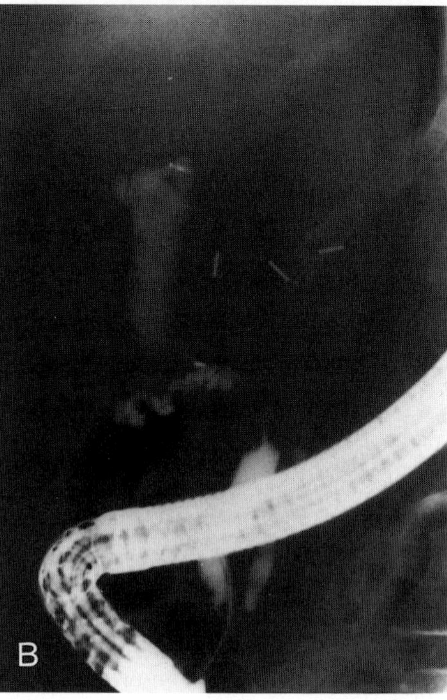


FIGURE 53.2. A. Endoscopic retrograde pancreatogram demonstrating abrupt tapering of the pancreatic duct at the pancreatic body due to pancreatic carcinoma in a 72-year-old woman. B. Endoscopic retrograde cholangiopancreatography (ERCP) of a 71-year-old woman with obstructive jaundice due to pancreatic cancer. The cholangiogram demonstrates a long stricture of the common bile duct just distal to the cystic duct. Dilatation of the proximal bile duct is also seen. (From Lillemoe,[6] with permission.)

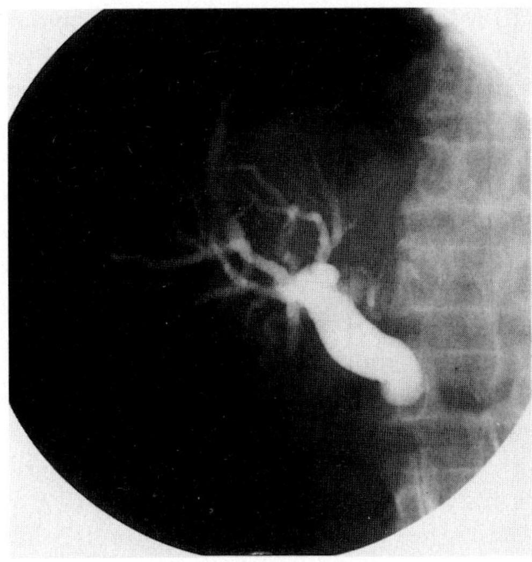

FIGURE 53.3. Percutaneous transhepatic cholangiogram demonstrating obstruction of the common bile duct due to pancreatic cancer in a 76-year-old woman. The area of obstruction is at the "knee" of the common bile duct where it enters the glandular substance of the pancreas. (From Lillemoe,[6] with permission.)

pancreatic neoplasm is the tumor meniscus with complete obstruction of the common bile duct at the knee of the biliary tree as it enters the glandular substance of the pancreas (Fig. 53.3). A biliary stent can be placed through the obstructing lesion in the bile duct by the endoscopic or percutaneous approach to alleviate jaundice.

A tissue diagnosis can be confirmed by several methods preoperatively. Duodenal or ampullary cancers can be easily biopsied by endoscopy and cytologic brushings obtained. A biopsy of a periampullary mass showing invasive adenocarcinoma is diagnostic in virtually all cases. However, the histologic finding of a benign villous adenoma with or without dysplasia may not reliably rule out malignancy. A number of clinical reports have documented a false-negative rate approaching 50% in this scenario. If a pancreatic tumor can be demonstrated by CT, fine-needle aspiration (FNA) can be performed percutaneously to gain material for cytologic diagnosis. Although this technique is highly accurate, with a sensitivity of more than 90% and a specificity of virtually 100%, it is of limited use in patients in whom surgical exploration for attempted resection or palliation is planned. There are two reasons for not using FNA for potentially resectable lesions. First, even after repeated sampling, a negative result cannot exclude malignancy; in fact, it is the small, more likely curable tumors that are most likely to be missed by this technique. A second concern is seeding the tumor along the needle tract or with intraperitoneal spread. The primary indication for percutaneous biopsy is therefore in patients with periampullary or pancreatic carcinoma who do not appear to be surgical candidates because of extent of disease or medical contraindications.

The tumor-associated antigen CA 19-9 has been employed in making the diagnosis of pancreatic carcinoma. CA 19-9 has sensitivity and specificity approaching 90% for tumors arising in the pancreas.[7] CA 19-9 levels are frequently normal during the early stages of pancreatic cancer and with other periampullary neoplasms. Therefore CA 19-9 is not considered suitable as a screening technique. The finding of an elevated CA 19-9 level may be useful for differentiating benign from malignant conditions. Furthermore, after resection, if the CA 19-9 level falls, the antigen may be useful for prognosis and follow-up surveillance.

## Preoperative Staging

The goal of preoperative staging of pancreatic or periampullary carcinoma is to determine the feasibility of surgery and the optimal treatment for each patient. In general, preoperative staging is more useful for pancreatic tumors than for other forms of periampullary cancer because the resectability of the latter lesions is usually significantly higher at the time of presentation than for pancreatic cancer. In many patients, dynamic spiral CT with oral and intravenous contrast provides all the information necessary by demonstrating liver metastases or major vascular invasion (Fig. 53.4). The extent of further staging to be performed depends on the patient and the preference of the surgeon. If the surgeon's philosophy is to pursue surgical treatment for all patients, either to attempt resection or to provide palliation, further staging is unnecessary. However, if the findings at staging could preclude an operation, particularly in an

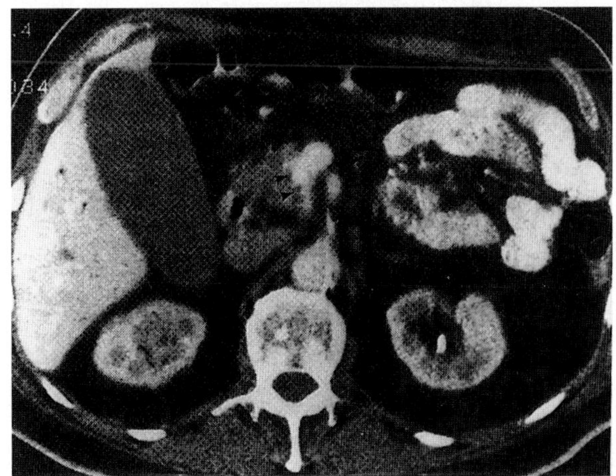

FIGURE 53.4. Spiral CT scan demonstrating superior mesenteric vein involvement with tumor–vessel contiguity. Abnormal enhancement of the medial border of head and uncinate process of the pancreas is seen (arrowheads).

elderly patient, and lead to nonoperative palliation, these efforts are worthwhile.

Local invasion of adjacent visceral vessels precludes resection in a significant number of patients explored for periampullary carcinoma. Of the periampullary malignancies, major vessel involvement is far more common in tumors originating in the head of the pancreas. Preoperative visceral angiography with arterial injection of the celiac and superior mesenteric arteries with venous phase studies provides the best demonstration of vascular anatomy and major vessel encasement or inclusion (Fig. 53.5). In a review of this technique in patients with periampullary carcinomas identified by CT scan at The Johns Hopkins Hospital,[8] if a patient was found by angiography to have major vascular occlusion the chance of resection was nil. If major vessel encasement was seen, 35% of patients had resectable lesions. If, however, there was no evidence of tumor involvement, 77% of the lesions were resectable. Angiography is also useful for detecting anatomic variations, such as a replaced right hepatic artery or celiac stenosis or occlusion, which may alter operative management. The role of angiography has diminished, as contrast-enhanced spiral CT has been demonstrated to have similar sensitivity for evaluating patients for resectability.

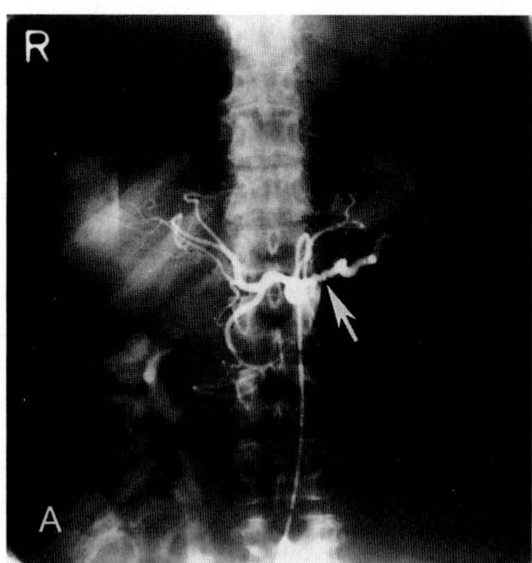


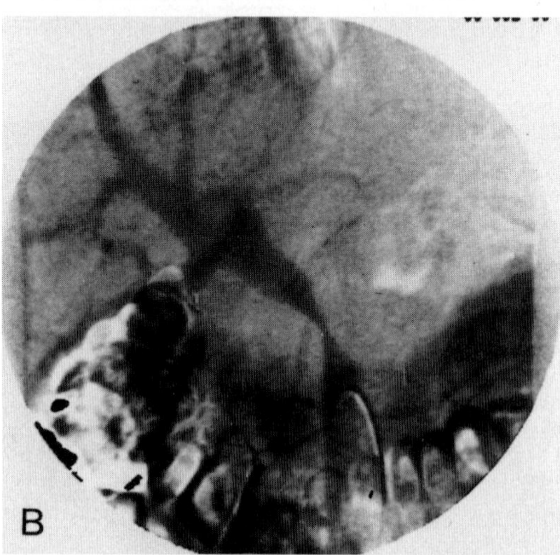


FIGURE 53.5. A. Selective arteriogram of celiac artery demonstrating encasement of the splenic artery (arrow) in a 72-year-old woman with pancreatic carcinoma. B. Venous phase of a selective superior mesenteric arteriogram demonstrating encasement and narrowing of the portal vein at the junction of the superior mesenteric vein. (From Lillemoe,[6] with permission.)

Endoscopic ultrasonography, a minimally invasive technique using high-frequency transducers placed in the gastric and duodenal lumen in close proximity to the pancreas and adjacent organs, has been used for the diagnosis and staging of patients with ampullary and pancreatic neoplasms. This technique is particularly useful during evaluation of ampullary tumors with respect to invasion of the duodenal wall and pancreas. One study in preoperative patients suggested that endoscopic ultrasound examination was superior to conventional sonography, CT, and angiography for assessing resectability.[9] In addition, ultrasound-directed FNA for diagnosis of a pancreatic mass is also possible. Experience with this technique, which is operator-dependent, is still somewhat limited, precluding its widespread use.

Liver metastases and peritoneal implants are the most common site of spread of periampullary carcinoma. Once distant metastases are present, survival is so limited that a conservative approach is indicated. Liver metastases >2 cm can generally be detected by CT, but approximately 30% of metastases are smaller and therefore not routinely detected. Furthermore, peritoneal and omental metastases are usually only 1–2 mm and frequently can be detected only by direct visualization. The technique of diagnostic laparoscopy, before the patient is subjected to laparotomy, has been used by several groups as an additional staging modality for evaluating patients with pancreatic and periampullary malignancies. In one such series, 40% of patients without demonstrable extrapancreatic involvement on the basis of CT scans were found at laparoscopy to have small liver or peritoneal metastases, precluding resection.[10] In addition, at the time of laparoscopy, irrigation of the peritoneal cavity can be performed with washings to analyze cytologically for evidence of shed cells.

The information gained from preoperative staging provides the basis for planning for each individual patient. If preoperative staging with CT, angiography, and laparoscopy is normal, resectability rates may approach 90% for tumors of the head of the pancreas.[11] Preoperative staging therefore, results in considerable improvement from the previous resectability rates of 25% and thus eliminates the need for unnecessary operations in a large number of patients. Because of the added potential risks in elderly patients, careful preoperative staging appears to play a valuable role in determining the need for laparotomy versus nonoperative palliation.

## Management of Periampullary Carcinoma

A number of important risk factors must be considered in the management of carcinoma of the pancreas. Such risk factors include the age and life expectancy of the patient, associated medical conditions, extent of the tumor, and the need for palliation of symptoms. It must be stressed, however, that surgical resection offers the only chance for cure with this disease. Although age cannot be an absolute contraindication for surgical management of any patient, it has been in the past considered to be a factor when predicting surgical morbidity and mortality.

### Preparation for Operation

If the decision is to proceed with an operation for periampullary carcinoma in an elderly patient, proper preoperative preparation is required. Thorough assessment of cardiopulmonary status, renal and hepatic function, the state of hydration, nutrition, anemia, and coagulation abnormalities is necessary. All efforts should be made to optimize the patient's overall health prior to proceeding with operation for resection or palliation.

A major question is the value of preoperative biliary decompression in these patients. Biliary decompression can be performed by percutaneous transhepatic drainage or placement of an endoscopic stent. Although initially uncontrolled studies showed a benefit for such drainage by decreasing operative morbidity and mortality, a subsequent prospective controlled randomized trial performed by Pitt and colleagues at UCLA, showed there was no benefit.[12] The length of hospital stay and hospital costs were significantly increased by preoperative biliary decompression. With both benign and malignant obstruction, there was no difference in the results based on the nature of the obstruction, advanced age, bilirubin level, or other potential risk factors. In contrast, Lyaidakis and his group in Amsterdam, using preoperative endoscopic drainage in patients with cancer of the head of the pancreas, significantly reduced perioperative morbidity and mortality.[13] It has been suggested that internal drainage of biliary secretions provides an immunologic basis for decreased perioperative septic complications. More recently, retrospective series have suggested that the use of preoperative stenting increases the incidence of perioperative complications, specifically wound infection.[14] It appears therefore, that preoperative biliary drainage is not indicated routinely, although in selected elderly patients with advanced malnutrition, sepsis, or correctable medical conditions, preoperative drainage is useful to improve the patient's overall health status.

### Pancreatic Resection

Several decades ago, the operative mortality for pancreaticoduodenectomy for periampullary carcinoma was in the range of 15–25% for all patients. This rate has fallen significantly in a number of recent series, with mortality rates now 5% or less.[15–19] Historically, advanced age was considered a major factor associated with perioperative mortality. Herter et al., noting that major morbidity remained constant in all groups, observed that operative deaths rose from 7.7% in patients in the 41- to 50-year age group to 25% in patients 61–70 years of age.[20] Lerut and colleagues also noted a significant increase in mortality, 41% versus 5% ($p < 0.001$), and morbidity, 58.8% versus 16.3% ($p < 0.01$), in patients undergoing pancreaticoduodenectomy over the age of 65 when compared to that in younger patients.[21] Finally, Obertop et al. reported 33% mortality following pancreaticoduodenectomy in patients over age 70 compared to 4% in patients younger than age 70. For patients undergoing palliative bypass procedures, there were no deaths among 20 patients under 70 years of age, although two of nine patients over age 70 (22%) died postoperatively.[22]

The view that pancreaticoduodenectomy may be contraindicated in elderly patients has been challenged by data from a number of centers. In a report of 145 consecutive pancreaticoduodenectomies performed without a death at our institution, advanced age was not a factor in predicting either morbidity or mortality.[17] In this series, the subgroup of patients 70 years of age or older ($n = 37$) were compared with patients 69 years of age and younger ($n = 108$). No statistically significant differences in preoperative risk factors such as prior myocardial infarction, hypertension, diabetes, chronic obstructive pulmonary disease, peripheral vascular disease, or alcohol use were present in the two groups. No deaths occurred in either age group, nor was there a significant difference in the incidence of postoperative complications. No specific complication was significantly more frequent in the older group; and for many serious complications including intraabdominal abscess, pancreatitis, and biliary anastomotic leak, patients over the age of 70 had a lower incidence (Table 53.2). The hospital courses of the two groups were similar. Operating time, estimated blood loss, number of transfusions per patient, and the length of hospital stay were not significantly different. This experience suggests that age is no longer even a relative contraindication to consideration for pancreaticoduodenectomy of carcinoma of the head of the pancreas.

Similar excellent overall results have been reported from other centers. Delcore and colleagues reported a series of 42 patients undergoing pancreaticoduodenectomy between the ages of 70 and 80 years.[23] The incidence of major complications was 14%, with two operative deaths (5%). Hannoun and colleagues in Paris, reported perioperative morbidity and mortality in 223 patients

TABLE 53.2. Postoperative Complications Following Pancreaticoduodenectomy

| Postoperative complication | Incidence (%) | |
|---|---|---|
| | Age < 69 ($n$ = 108) | Age > 70 ($n$ = 37) |
| Delayed gastric emptying | 32 | 46 |
| Pancreatic fistula | 19 | 22 |
| Intraabdominal abscess | 10 | 5 |
| Wound infection | 6 | 11 |
| Pancreatitis | 7 | 3 |
| Biliary leak | 6 | 3 |
| Cholangitis | 5 | 5 |
| None | 52 | 38 |

*Source:* Modified from Cameron et al.,[16] with permission.

undergoing pancreaticoduodenectomy for periampullary neoplasms.[24] Forty-four patients were 70 years of age or older. The perioperative morbidity was similar in the two groups (35%). The operative mortality was 4.5% in the old patients versus 10% in those under 70 years of age.

Fong and colleagues at the Memorial Sloan-Kettering Cancer Center, analyzed the results at that center for patients undergoing major pancreatic or liver resection.[25] Pancreatic resection was performed in 138 patients 70 years or age or older. The perioperative mortality was 6% and the complication rate 45%. The median stay was 20 days, and only 19% required admission to their intensive care unit. These results were similar to those for a younger cohort of patients undergoing pancreatic resection during the same period (Table 53.3). Analysis of these complications identified that a history of cardiopulmonary disease, an abnormal preoperative electrocardiogram or chest radiograph, and operative blood loss in excess of 2000 ml, were the most powerful predictors or a complication. Operative mortality in 24 patients 80 years of age and older was 0% versus 7% in those patients 70–79 years with a similar incidence of complications.

The experience with pancreaticoduodenectomy in octogenarians at The Johns Hopkins Hospital has been reported.[26] In this series, 46 patients age 80 or older underwent pancreaticoduodenectomy over a 10-year period. The mean age of the 46 patients was 82.9 ± 2.7 years with the oldest patient being 90 years of age. Periampullary cancer was the indication for resection in 91% of patients. These 46 patients were compared with 681 concurrent patients less than 80 years of age undergoing pancreaticoduodenectomy during the same period. The two groups were similar with respect to gender, race, intraoperative blood loss, units of blood transfused, and the type of resection performed. The older patients had a shorter mean operative time (6.3 ± 1.3 vs. 7.1 ± 4.0 hours, $p < 0.05$), but a longer postoperative length of stay (median 15.0 vs. 13.0 days, $p < 0.05$) than their younger counterparts. A higher incidence of complications was seen in the older patients (57% vs. 41%, $p = 0.05$). The perioperative mortality was not statistically different, being 4.3% in the octogenarians compared to 1.6% in the younger patients.

A number of factors have contributed to the reduction in perioperative morbidity and mortality following resection of periampullary cancer. The most likely reason lies in the concentration of more patients in the hands of surgeons in major centers with extensive experience with the procedure.[27,28] If an elderly patient is thought to be a candidate for surgical resection, referral to such a center should be considered.

## Palliation

Unfortunately, by the time the diagnosis is made, many carcinomas of the pancreas are surgically unresectable. Thus optimal palliation of symptoms to maximize the quality of life is of primary importance. The three primary symptoms warranting palliation are obstructive jaundice, gastric outlet obstruction, and pain. Palliation in patients with unresectable pancreatic carcinoma has evolved significantly in recent years with the introduction of nonoperative palliation of jaundice. Four prospective studies have been completed where surgical bypass has been compared with nonoperative biliary stenting for malignant obstructive jaundice[25–28] (Table 53.4). The conclusions of these studies are similar: that the two techniques are equally effective for relieving jaundice. Nonoperative palliation, however, seems to be accompanied by lower complication rates, lower procedure-related mortality rates, and a shorter initial period of hospitalization. As a result of these studies, enthusiasm has been generated for the nonoperative palliation of periampullary carcinoma especially in older patients. Advocates of surgical palliation, however, criticize these studies on two counts. First, 30-day mortality rates in the surgical arms of these studies range from 15% to 24%, which is much higher than in many surgical series.

TABLE 53.3. Perioperative and Long-Term Outcome after Pancreatic Resection

| Parameter | Results, by age | |
|---|---|---|
| | <70 Years | >70 Years |
| No. of patients | 350 | 138 |
| Age (years), median and range | 60 (12–69) | 75 (70–87) |
| LOS (days), median and range | 20 (1–146) | 20 (5–82) |
| Complications (%) | 39 | 45 |
| Mortality (%) | 4 | 6 |
| ICU admittance (%) | 19 | 19 |
| Median survival (months) | 24 | 18 |
| 1-Year survival (%) | 71 | 64 |
| 3-Year survival (%) | 41 | 30 |
| 5-Year survival (%) | 29 | 21 |

*Source:* Modified from Fong et al.,[25] with permission.
LOS, length of stay; ICU, intensive care unit; NS, nonsignificant.

TABLE 53.4. Results of Randomized Comparison of Nonoperative Versus Surgical Bypass for Palliation of Obstructive Jaundice

| | Bronman[29] | | Shepard[30] | | Andersen[31] | | Smith[32] | |
|---|---|---|---|---|---|---|---|---|
| Parameter | Stent | Op | Stent | Op | Stent | Op | Stent | Op |
| Success (%) | 84 | 76 | 82 | 92 | 96 | 88 | 95 | 94 |
| Complication (%) | 28 | 32 | 30 | 56 | 36 | 20 | 11 | 29 |
| 30-Day mortality (days) | 8 | 20 | 9 | 20 | 20 | 24 | 3 | 14 |
| Hospital stay (days) | 18 | 24 | 5 | 13 | 26 | 27 | 20 | 26 |
| Late complications (no.) | | | | | | | | |
| Jaundice/cholangitis | 38 | 16 | 30 | 0 | 0 | 0 | 35 | 2 |
| Gastric outlet obstruction | 14 | 0 | 9 | 4 | 0 | 0 | 17 | 7 |
| Survival (weeks) | 19 | 15 | 22 | 18 | 12 | 14 | 21 | 26 |

Op, operation.

Second, nonoperative palliation is frequently associated with late complications of recurrent jaundice and gastric outlet obstruction. Newly designed self-expanding endoprostheses (wall stents) may be associated with a lower incidence of late jaundice.

In a review from The Johns Hopkins Hospital, 118 consecutive patients underwent surgical palliation for unresectable periampullary adenocarcinoma.[33] The most common operative procedure was a combined biliary bypass and gastrojejunostomy, being performed in 75% of the patients. A gastrojejunostomy with biliary bypass or alone was performed in 107 of the 118 patients (91%). The hospital mortality rate was 2.5%. Postoperative complications occurred in 37% of the patients but were seldom life-threatening. During late follow-up only 4% of the patients had gastric outlet obstruction and 2% had recurrent jaundice. The mean survival time postoperatively was 7.7 months. This series did not compare results of morbidity and mortality based on subgroups of age. However, 70% of the patients were 60 years of age or older, 35% were 70 years or older, and 4% were 80 years or over. The three deaths all occurred in patients 60 years of age or older. Only one death occurred in a patient over age 70. This series concluded that surgical palliation of unresectable periampullary carcinoma can be completed with minimal perioperative mortality and acceptable morbidity, and it provides good palliation.

The role of prophylactic gastrojejunostomy for palliation in patients with unresectable pancreatic carcinoma is controversial. A review of more than 8000 patients reported in the English literature from 1965 to 1970, determined that creation of a gastrojejunostomy did not increase the operative mortality rate.[34] Moreover, if a gastrojejunostomy was not performed, 13% of patients had subsequent duodenal obstruction requiring a gastrojejunostomy before death, and nearly 20% of the remaining patients died with symptoms of gastroduodenal outlet obstruction. A recent prospective randomized trial evaluated this question and found that the performance of a prophylactic gastrojejunostomy did not increase perioperative morbidity or length of hospital stay. Nineteen percent of patients. Who did not receive an initial gastrojejunostomy, required a subsequent gastric by pass prior to death versus none of the patients who received such a procedure at their initial operation ($p < 0.05$).[35]

Pain is the last feature of pancreatic carcinoma that requires palliation. Epigastric and back pain can become the most incapacitating and disabling of symptoms a patient can experience. The incidence of severe unrelenting pain due to pancreatic carcinoma is probably in the range of 30–35% but increases significantly during the advanced stages of disease. In a randomized prospective double-blind study completed at The Johns Hopkins Hospital, intraoperative chemical splanchnicectomy with 50% alcohol was compared with a placebo injection of saline in patients with histologically proven unresectable pancreatic carcinoma.[36] The two groups were similar by all preoperative criteria, with a mean age of patients in both groups being 64 years. Patients were assessed preoperatively and after hospital discharge using a visual analogue scale for pain, mood, and disability. The results of this study showed no difference in hospital mortality or complications, time to return to oral intake, or length of hospital stay between the two groups. Mean pain scores were significantly lower in the alcohol-treated group at the 2-, 4-, and 6-month follow-ups and at the final assessment before the patient's death. Patients were stratified into those who had significant pain preoperatively versus those without preexisting pain. In patients without preoperative pain, alcohol treatment significantly delayed or prevented the subsequent onset of pain. In patients with significant preoperative pain, alcohol treatment significantly reduced it. Finally, a surprising observation was that in patients with significant preoperative pain who received alcohol celiac axis injection, a significant improvement in survival was observed compared to the controls. Celiac axis chemical splanchnicectomy should therefore be performed in all patients found to have unresectable pancreatic carcinoma undergoing laparotomy. In patients not undergoing laparotomy, percutaneous celiac axis injection, using either fluoroscopic or CT guidance, can effectively control pain in most patients.

In conclusion, management of an elderly patient with suspected periampullary carcinoma must be individualized. If the patient's overall health status does not preclude major surgery and the spiral CT scan shows no evidence of liver metastases or carcinomatosis, the patient should be considered a surgical candidate. Visceral angiography or diagnostic laparoscopy may be completed for further staging. If there is no evidence that precludes resection, the patient should undergo exploration with an excellent chance for pancreaticoduodenectomy. If operative findings preclude resection, a palliative biliary bypass, gastrojejunostomy, and chemical splanchnicectomy should be performed.

In patients with preoperative evidence of unresectability based on CT scans, visceral angiography, or laparoscopy, the decision to utilize operative versus nonoperative palliation of obstructive jaundice must also be individualized. Overall medical state, extent of disease with predicted life expectancy, and the presence of symptoms of impending duodenal obstruction are factors to consider. Age alone should not be a primary factor, although in the elderly patient with advanced pancreatic cancer, nonoperative palliation offers an attractive option.

## Postoperative Care and Complications

Adequate fluid and electrolyte maintenance, glucose regulation, pulmonary care, nutritional support, and provision of perioperative antibiotic prophylaxis are routine. Biliary contrast examination via the preoperatively placed biliary stent or operatively placed T-tube may be done at postoperative day 4 or 5 to demonstrate the biliary anastomosis. A gastrografin upper gastrointestinal (GI) series may follow to determine the status of the gastro- or duodenojejunostomy as well as the return of gastric emptying. If all studies are satisfactory, perioperative drains from the area of the biliary and pancreatic anastomosis can be removed, and oral intake can be initiated slowly, watching for potential delays in gastric emptying.

A number of complications can occur following pancreaticoduodenectomy. The leading complication in the recent Johns Hopkins experience with octogenarians was delayed gastric emptying.[26] In that series, delayed emptying was the only specific complication that occurred at a higher incidence in old patients than in young patients (33% vs. 18%, $p < 0.05$). A randomized prospective study from our institution has found a decrease in this overall complication when using perioperative intravenous erythromycin as a prokinetic agent for gastric motility.[37] Leakage at the pancreatic anastomosis has been a particularly disastrous complication in the past. More recent experience suggests that although the incidence of anastomotic leak remains at 10–20%, adequate placement of perianastomotic drains and improved postoperative management have lessened the severity of this complication.[15,17,38] A prospective study at Johns Hopkins compared the results following the operative techniques of pancreaticojejunostomy and pancreaticogastrostomy.[38] The incidence of anastomotic leak was similar with the two techniques (12%). Multivariate analysis revealed that the experience of the surgeon and the texture of the pancreas determined the likelihood of a pancreatic fistula. Age was not a significant factor when predicting anastomotic leak. Although the occurrence of a pancreatic leak significantly prolonged the hospital stay, there were no deaths observed among those patients. In the Johns Hopkins series of pancreaticoduodenectomy in octogenarians, the incidence of pancreatic leak was similar (15% vs. 14%).[26]

Although the incidence of complications following pancreaticoduodenectomy and palliative operations for pancreatic carcinoma continues to be high (35% or more), most are not life-threatening. In general, improvement in the management of these complications has resulted in reports of reduced operative mortality. The elderly patient frequently lacks the reserve to handle such complications, however, and failure to avoid them may be disastrous with ensuing multisystem organ failure and eventual death.

## Survival

Despite improvements in surgical management, the results for long-term survival remain less than optimal. The best results seems to come from series in which a 5-year survival of 20% has been achieved for pancreatic carcinoma.[15–17,39] Ampullary, distal bile duct, and duodenal carcinoma appear to be associated with a better 5-year survival, in the range of 40–60%. A number of factors have been identified as prognostic indicators for long-term survival following pancreaticoduodenectomy for pancreatic cancer[39]: tumor size <3 cm, diploid tumor DNA content, negative surgical margins and negative lymph node status. Age was not a predictor of survival. Analysis of survival in the series from Memorial Sloan-Kettering, revealed that age slightly influenced survival (Table 53.3).[25] Despite this overall difference, the actuarial 5-year survival was still in excess of 20%.

The recent series of octogenarians undergoing pancreaticoduodenectomy for periampullary cancer reported from Johns Hopkins, showed no difference from a younger cohort in long-term survival (Fig. 53.6).[26] The older cohort had a median survival of 32 months with 1-, 2-, and 5-year survival rates of 71%, 63%, and 19%, respectively, compared to a median survival of 20 months and 1-, 2-, and 5-year survival rates of 73%, 47%, and 27% in the younger patients. Similarly, there was no significant difference in survival when the subset of

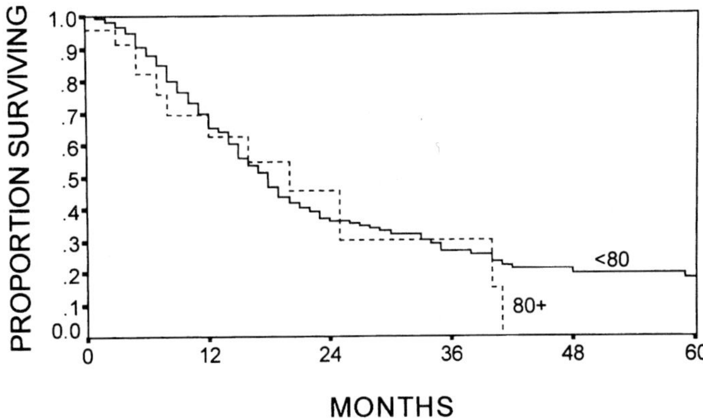


FIGURE 53.6. Actuarial survival curves comparing patients ≥80 years old undergoing pancreaticoduodenectomy for periampullary adenocarcinoma ($n = 41$; median survival 32 months; 5-year survival 27%; $p = 0.077$). (From Sohn et al.,[26] with permission.)

patients with pancreatic adenocarcinomas was analyzed (Fig. 53.7). The older group had a median survival of 17 months compared to 18 months for the younger group.

Survival among patients with unresectable periampullary cancer is based primarily on the extent of disease. Cancers found to be unresectable owing to local extension of the tumor, generally survive longer (9–12 months) than patients with liver metastases or carcinomatosis (less than 6 months). In the Johns Hopkins series of 118 patients undergoing surgical palliation, the mean survival was 7.7 months.[33] The percentage of the patients surviving more than 1 year was approximately 20%.

## Cancer of the Body and Tail of the Pancreas

Survival of patients with carcinoma of the body and tail of the pancreas is even more dismal than that of those with cancer of the pancreatic head. The silent asymptomatic nature of these tumors leads to late presentation, usually long past the time for considering resection. A tissue diagnosis of these tumors can frequently be made by percutaneous techniques because of their advanced size at the time of diagnosis. Often such tumors are not associated with obstructive jaundice, so there is little benefit to proceeding with laparotomy for diagnosis. If the tumor appears resectable on routine CT scan, one should consider preoperative arteriography to demonstrate major vessel encasement or occlusion (or possibly diagnostic laparoscopy) before proceeding to exploratory laparotomy. In patients with significant pain associated with their tumor, percutaneous celiac axis block can provide excellent long-term palliation.

## Chemotherapy Radiation Therapy

Because of the modest results following resection in patients with pancreatic carcinoma, attention has turned to adjuvant chemotherapy or irradiation for this disease. Two prospective randomized studies have demonstrated significant improvement with the addition of postoperative radiation therapy and single-agent chemotherapy with 5-fluorouracil.[40,41] This protocol is reasonably well tolerated by the patients and should be recommended for those undergoing resection of a pancreatic carcinoma regardless of age, if their overall postoperative health status allows such therapy.

The role of radiotherapy and chemotherapy for unresectable pancreatic carcinoma is limited primarily to palliation and likely offers little benefit to elderly patients with unresectable pancreatic carcinoma in which palliation for pain and jaundice can be managed by other means.

## Cystadenoma and Cystadenocarcinoma

Cystadenoma and cystadenocarcinoma are neoplastic cystic lesions of the pancreas. Cystadenomas account for about 10% of nonmalignant cystic lesions of the pancreas, and cystadenocarcinomas represent 1% of the primary pancreatic malignant lesions. Cystadenoma appears primarily in middle-aged women, although reports of patients in their seventies and eighties have appeared. Cystadenocarcinoma occurs at about the same age as pancreatic exocrine cancers, between 50 and 70 years of age. There is no sex predilection in this group.

The symptoms of cystadenoma and cystadenocarcinoma are virtually identical. Patients usually present

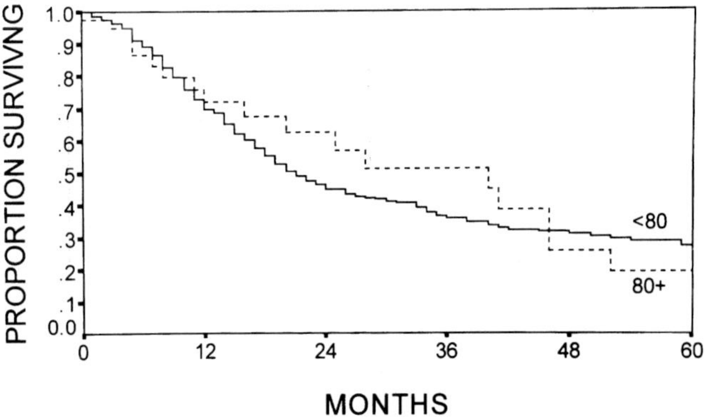


FIGURE 53.7. Actuarial curves comparing patients ≥80 years old undergoing pancreaticoduodenectomy for pancreatic adenocarcinoma ($n = 25$; median survival 18 months; 2-year survival 46%) to those <80 years old ($n = 282$; median survival 17 months; 2-year survival 36%; $p = 0.57$). (From Sohn et al.,[26] with permission.)

with abdominal pain, weight loss, nausea, vomiting, anorexia, weakness, or an enlarging abdominal mass. Jaundice is uncommon with the benign cystadenoma but occurs in up to one-fourth of patients with cystadenocarcinomas.[42]

Management of these lesions is surgical excision. Complete excision of the lesion for pathologic examination is important because needle biopsy is not suitable for detecting malignant potential. Cystadenomas are classified as serous or mucin-producing. The serous cystadenomas, or microcystic adenomas, are benign and are thought to have little or no malignant potential. The mucinous cystadenomas are often filled with a mucinous material and are thought to have malignant potential, with the ability to progress to a cystadenocarcinoma. Surgical resection of either benign lesion is generally considered curable. Cystadenocarcinomas are more often resectable than ductal adenocarcinoma. In the recent experience at Johns Hopkins, two-thirds of these tumors were resectable at the time of surgical exploration.[42] The 5-year survival for resectable cystadenocarcinoma is also better than for ductal carcinoma, ranging from 50% to 76%.[42,43]

## Conclusions

Periampullary neoplasms in the elderly are a common problem surgeons will encounter with increasing frequency as our population ages. The clinical presentation, diagnosis, and staging are not dissimilar from those in young patients. Patients whose tumor appears to be resectable should undergo exploration and an attempt at surgical resection based not on age but on the presence of co-morbid conditions. Ample evidence suggests that pancreatic resection can be performed in elderly patients with the low perioperative morbidity and mortality achieved in other age groups. Furthermore, the long-term survival of older patients is similar to that seen in younger patients.

### References


1. Steele GD Jr, Osteen RT, Winchester DP, et al. Clinical highlights from the National Cancer Data Base. CA Cancer J Clin 1994;44:71.
2. MacMahon B. Risk factors for cancer of the pancreas. Cancer 1982;50:2676–2680.
3. Gold EG, Golden SB. Epidemiology of and risk factors for pancreatic cancer. Surg Oncol Clin North Am 1998;7: 67–91.
4. Wilentz RE, Hruban RH. Pathology of cancer of the pancreas. Surg Oncol North Am 1998;7:43–65.
5. Doll R, Muir M, Waterhous J (eds). Cancer Incidence in Five Continents, vol 2. Geneva: Internationalia Contre le Cancer, 1970.
6. Lillemoe KD. Pancreatic disease in the elderly. Surg Clin North Am 1994;74:317–344.
7. Steinberg W. The clinical utility of the CA-19-9 tumor associated antigen. Am J Gastroenterol 1990;85:350–355.
8. Dooley WC, Cameron JL, Pitt HA, et al. Is preoperative angiography useful in patients with periampullary tumors? Ann Surg 1992;211:649–655.
9. Rösch T, Braig C, Gain T, et al. Stayging of pancreatic and ampullary carcinoma by endoscopic ultrasonography: comparison with conventional sonography, computed tomography, and angiography. Gastroenterology 1992;102:188–199.
10. Warshaw AL, Tepper JE, Shipley WU. Laparoscopy in the staging and planning for pancreatic cancer. Am J Surg 1986;151:76–80.
11. Warshaw AL, Gu ZY, Wittenberg J, Waltman AC. Preoperative staging and assessment of resectability of pancreatic cancer. Arch Surg 1990;125:230–233.
12. Pitt HA, Gomes AS, Louis JF, et al. Does preoperative percutaneous biliary drainage reduce operative risk or increase hospital cost? Ann Surg 1985;201:545–553.
13. Lyaidakis NJ, Van der Heyde MN, Lubler MJ. An evaluation of preoperative biliary drainage in the surgical management of pancreatic head carcinoma. Acta Chir Scand 1987;153:665.
14. Povoski SP, Karpen MS, Conlon KC, et al. Positive intraoperative bile cultures at the time of pancreaticoduodenectomy are associated with preoperative biliary drainage and subsequent development of postoperative infectious complications and mortality. Gastroenterology 1998;114: A537.
15. Crist DW, Sitzmann JV, Cameron JL. Improved hospital morbidity, mortality and survival after the Whipple procedure. Ann Surg 1987;206:358–365.
16. Trede M, Schwall G, Saeger H. Survival after pancreaticoduodenectomy. Ann Surg 1990;211:447–458.
17. Cameron JL, Pitt HA, Yeo CJ, et al. One hundred and forty-five consecutive pancreaticoduodenectomies without mortality. Ann Surg 1993;217:430–438.
18. Castillo CF, Rattner DW, Warshaw AL. Standards for pancreatic resection in the 1990s. Arch Surg 1995;130:295.
19. Yeo CJ, Cameron JL, Sohn TA, et al. Six hundred fifty consecutive pancreaticoduodenectomies in the 1990's: pathology, complications, outcomes. Ann Surg 1997;226: 248–260.
20. Herter FP, Cooperman AM, Ahlborn TN, Antinori C. Surgical experience with pancreatic and periampullary cancer. Ann Surg 1982;195:274–281.
21. Lerut JP, Gianello PR, Otte JB, Kestens PJ. Pancreaticoduodenal resection: surgical experience and evaluation of risk factors in 103 patients. Ann Surg 1984;199:432–437.
22. Obertop H, Bruining HA, Schattenkerk ME, et al. Operative approach to cancer of the head of the pancreas and the periampullary region. Br J Surg 1982;69:573–576.
23. Delcore R, Thomas JH, Hermreck AS. Pancreaticoduodenectomy for malignant pancreatic and periampullary neoplasms in elderly patients. Am J Surg 1991;162:532–536.
24. Hannoun L, Christophe M, Ribeiro J, et al. A report of forty-four instances of pancreaticoduodenal resection in patients more than seventy years of age. Surg Gynecol Obstet 1993; 177:556–560.

25. Fong Y, Blumgart LH, Fortner JG, Brennan MF. Pancreatic or liver resection for malignancy is safe and effective for the elderly. Ann Surg 1995;222:426–437.
26. Sohn TA, Yeo CJ, Cameron JL, et al. Should pancreaticoduodenectomy be performed in octogenarians? J Gastrointest Surg 1998;2:207–216.
27. Gordon TA, Burleyson GP, Tielsch JM, Cameron JL. The effects of regionalization on cost and outcome for one general high-risk surgical procedure. Ann Surg 1995;221: 43–49.
28. Lieberman MD, Kilburn H, Lindsey M, Brennan MF. Relation of perioperative deaths to hospital volume among patients undergoing pancreatic resection for malignancy. Ann Surg 1995;222:638–645.
29. Bronman PC, Harries-Jones EP, Tobias R, et al. Prospective controlled trial of transhepatic incurable carcinoma of the head of the pancreas. Lancet 1986;1:69–71.
30. Shepard HA, Royle G, Ross APR, et al. Endoscopic biliary endoprosthesis in the palliation of malignant obstruction of the distal common bile duct: a randomized trial. Br J Surg 1988;75:1166–1168.
31. Andersen JR, Sorensen SM, Kruse A, et al. Randomized trial of endoscopic prosthesis versus operative bypass in malignant obstructive jaundice. Gut 1989;30:1132–1135.
32. Smith AC, Dowsett JF, Russell RCG, Hatfield ARW, Cotton PB. Randomised trial of endoscopic stenting versus surgical bypass in malignant low bile duct obstruction. Lancet 1994;344:1655–1660.
33. Lillemoe KD, Sauter PK, Pitt HA, et al. Current status of surgical palliation of periampullary carcinoma. Surg Gynecol Obstet 1993;176:1–10.
34. Sarr MG, Cameron JL. Surgical management of unresectable carcinoma of the pancreas. Surgery 1982;91:123–133.
35. Lillemoe KD, Cameron JL, Hardacre JM, et al. Is prophylactic gastrojejunostomy indicated for unresectable pancreatic cancer? Ann Surg 1999;230:322–330.
36. Lillemoe KD, Cameron JL, Kaufman HS, et al. Chemical splanchnicectomy in patients with unresectable pancreatic cancer: a prospective randomized trial. Ann Surg 1993;217: 447–457.
37. Yeo CJ, Barry MK, Sauter PK, et al. Erythromycin accelerates gastric emptying following pancreaticoduodenectomy. Ann Surg 1993;218:229–238.
38. Yeo CJ, Cameron JL, Maher MM, et al. A prospective randomized trial of pancreaticogastrostomy versus pancreaticojejunostomy after pancreaticoduodenectomy. Ann Surg 1995;222:580.
39. Yeo CJ, Cameron JL, Lillemoe KD, et al. Pancreaticoduodenectomy for cancer of the head of the pancreas: 201 patients. Ann Surg 1995;221:721–733.
40. Kalser MH, Ellenberg SS. Pancreatic cancer: adjuvant combined radiation and chemotherapy following curative resection. Arch Surg 1985;97:28–35.
41. Gastrointestinal Tumor Study Group. Further evidence of effective adjuvant combined radiation and chemotherapy following curative resection of pancreatic cancer. Cancer 1987;59:2006–2101.
42. Talamini MA, Pitt HA, Hruban RH, et al. Spectrum of cystic tumors of the pancreas. Am J Surg 1992;10:117–124.
43. Warshaw AL, Comptom CC, Lewandrowski K, et al. Cystic tumors of the pancreas: new clinical, radiologic, and pathologic observations in 67 patients. Ann Surg 1990;212:432–445.

# *Part II*
# *Specific Issues in Geriatric Surgery*

## Section 8
## Urogenital System

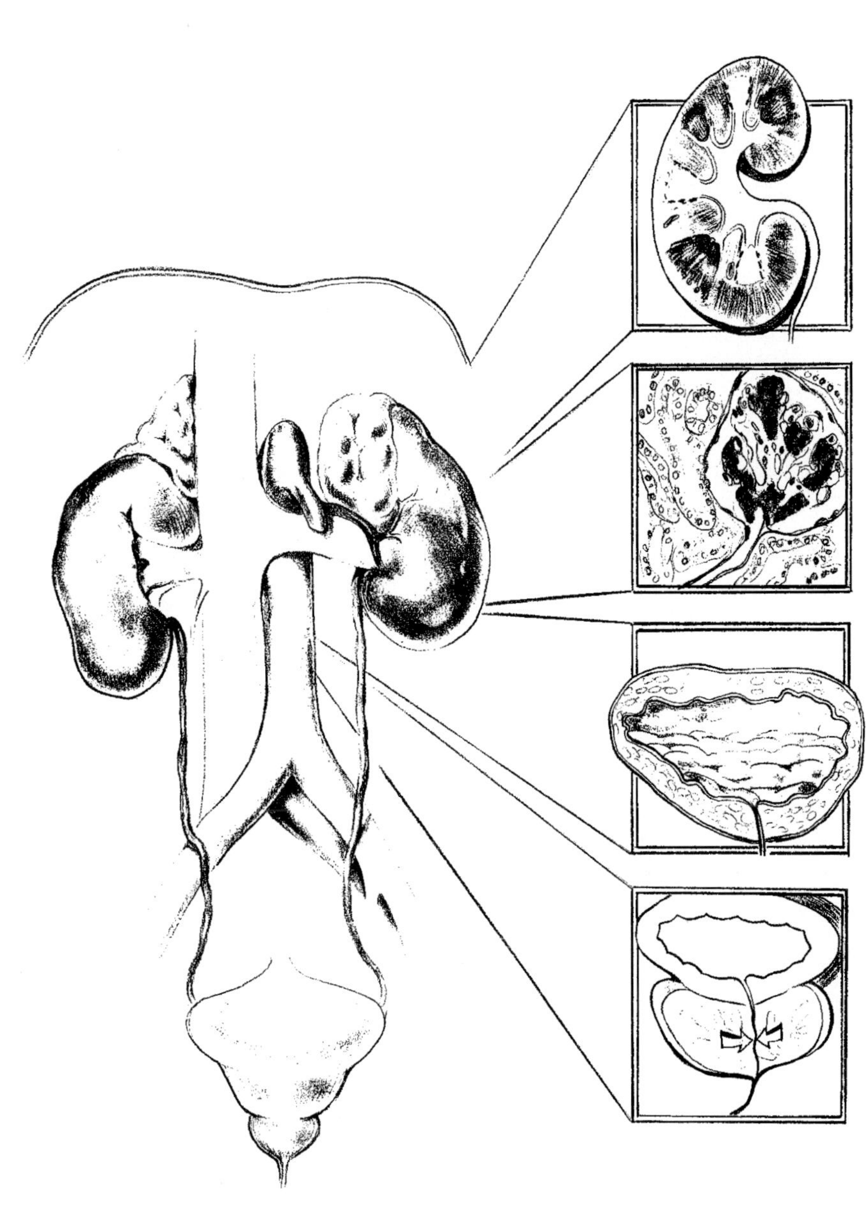

# Invited Commentary

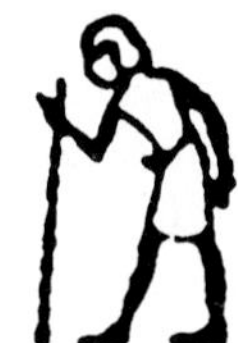

Bernard Lytton

Life expectancy for the average man has risen from 62.0 years in 1940 to 73.5 years today. During this period the population of the United States has more than doubled to over 260 million people, and about 13% of the population is now over 65. The ailments that afflict them are amplified and distorted by the effects of the aging process, creating many problems that are particular to the elderly. At the same time, the improvements in our understanding of the pathophysiology of disease, the psychological and social changes that occur in old people, and the advances that have taken place in technology make it possible to provide better care to the geriatric patient.

The treatments in current use today were not available or not invented when I graduated from medical school. Chain and Florey had recently completed the synthesis of penicillin that made possible clinical application of Fleming's original observations on the effects of *Penicillium* on bacteria and ushered in the golden age of antibiotic therapy. It is the control of infectious diseases and improvement in living conditions that are primarily responsible for the increased life expectancy. Anesthesiologists were abandoning ether and chloroform and began to use analgesic gases, narcotics, soporifics, and muscle relaxants, which allowed longer, more complex surgical procedures to be performed on sicker patients. Clarification of the concepts of fluid and electrolyte balance and their disorders in patients after major surgery together with correction of serious metabolic problems paved the way for more successful postoperative care and a reduction in morbidity and mortality. As a surgeon living through these exciting and changing times, I realized that sound training in the basic sciences and the pathophysiology of disease made it possible to absorb, process, and make use of all these conceptual changes and technologic advances in the treatment of patients.

Care of the elderly is particularly taxing for the surgeon, and humanitarian and scientific skills play an equally important role in their management. A radical surgical procedure that may have cured a cancer in a 75-year-old cannot be considered a success if the patient remains incontinent and chronically depressed as a result. Quality of life is a crucial issue, and prolongation of survival alone is no longer an acceptable goal of treatment.

One of the attractions of urology is the ability to make a fairly definitive diagnosis prior to surgery so exploratory procedures are at a minimum. Since Moses Swick first described the use of intravenously injected iodinated hippuran to visualize the renal collecting system in 1930, the progress in methods of diagnostic imaging has been spectacular. Arteriography was used extensively during the 1950s and 1960s for the diagnosis of kidney tumors. Ultrasound imaging and computed tomography (CT) scanning have largely replaced intravenous pyelography and arteriography, resulting in the early diagnosis of many renal tumors. Today more than 40% of renal tumors being treated surgically are asymptomatic, having been diagnosed serendipitously by ultrasonography or CT scanning performed for other reasons. CT scanning has made it possible to manage elderly, poor risk patients with small tumors, those under 4 cm in diameter, conservatively and to monitor accurately any progression of the lesion by scanning every 6 months. Magnetic resonance imaging (MRI), introduced during the 1980s, obviates the need to use ionizing radiation or potentially toxic contrast materials to image any part of the genitourinary system. It has proved particularly useful for assessing involvement of the renal veins and inferior vena cava by tumor.

Improvements in surgical technique have led to nephrectomy through an anterior subcostal incision in elderly patients to avoid the less well-tolerated flexed lateral position used for the flank approach. Manually assisted endoscopic nephrectomy is becoming the method of choice for removing a kidney with a tumor of less than 6–8 cm. In this procedure, a hand is inserted into the abdomen through a small midline incision, 10–12 cm long, with a sleeve to make the opening airtight. This hand helps mobilize the kidney and assist in exposing the vessels. Endoscopic instruments to be used by the other hand are inserted through the usual ports to dissect the kidney and divide the vessels and ureter. The kidney and tumor can then be removed whole by the intraabdominally placed hand.

The development of a semirigid fiberoptic system 30 years ago enhanced the capability of the cystoscope and led to the design of small instruments to visualize the inside of the ureter and renal collecting system. Subsequently, flexible fiberoptic instruments became available, greatly improving the ability to diagnose and treat stones and tumors in the kidney and ureters endoscopically by percutaneous puncture or transurethrally. Stones are disintegrated by shock waves, lithoclasts, or lasers. The major advance is undoubtedly the extracorporeal shock wave lithotriptor, first made by the Dornier aircraft company based on the work of a group of German urologists and engineers who devised a method of generating and focusing an electrohydraulic shock wave powerful enough to break a calculus. Lithotriptors are now an effective noninvasive method of disintegrating most stones in the kidney or ureter by an external shock wave focused under ultrasound or radiographic guidance with the patient under a local anesthetic or mild sedation. Stone disease, which once accounted for 20–30% of the surgery performed by urologists, is now rarely treated by operation.

The increase in the number of elderly have made the problems of urinary incontinence and obstruction major issues in health care. Fortunately, there has been significant progress in our understanding of the neurophysiology and function of the bladder smooth muscle, which has led to the development of specific pharmacologic agents that influence its activity.

The demonstration that the smooth muscle at the bladder is separately innervated by α-adrenergic nerve fibers coupled with the revised concepts of "prostatism," the symptoms of which are now considered to represent the elements of obstruction and loss of bladder compliance and capacity related to aging, has revolutionized the treatment. Until 10–15 years ago, most of these patients were treated by some form of prostatectomy, usually transurethral resection. Now most are managed by administration of α-adrenergic blocking agents, which reduce bladder outlet resistance and modify detrusor function, providing considerable relief of symptoms and improved bladder emptying. The 5α-reductase inhibitor finasteride, which prevents intracellular conversion of testosterone to the dihydro form, has proved disappointing for relieving prostatic obstruction, as did orchiectomy, widely practiced at the end of the nineteenth century. Although there is significant reduction in prostatic mass that might be helpful in patients with large glands, most patients with prostatic obstruction seen today have little enlargement of the prostate but have anatomic and functional changes at the bladder neck often associated with hypertrophy in the midzone that obstructs the urinary outflow. Finasteride has proved useful for controlling bleeding from the prostate by reducing the size and thus the vascularity of the gland. Pharmacologic therapy has reduced the number of transurethral prostatectomies performed by about 90% over the past 10 years.

Urodynamic testing, combined with simultaneous fluoroscopic visualization of the anatomic changes during voiding, has led to more accurate diagnoses, which in turn indicate specific modes of therapy. Female incontinence due to anatomic changes at the bladder neck can be differentiated from that due to uninhibited detrusor contractions. The latter are usually controlled by administration of medication to inhibit detrusor function, such as oxybutynin and tolterodine. Correction of the bladder neck abnormality by perivesical injection of collagen or by vesicourethral suspension is now more successful, as it is possible to exclude patients with a detrusor abnormality or urethral failure due to fibrosis or loss of intrinsic sphincter function, the latter being best corrected by a urethral sling. Patients who have primarily detrusor instability or in whom it complicates stress urinary incontinence can be treated with anticholinergics. Those with intractable detrusor instability may require an augmentation cystoplasty. A common cause of wetting in the elderly is impaired bladder sensation often associated with forgetfulness. Teaching these patients to void by the clock, every 2–3 hours, is often helpful.

The diagnosis and treatment of bladder cancer has undergone major revisions over the past 40 years. Cytologic examination of the urine is useful for early diagnosis and follow-up after any initial conservative treatment, particularly for more poorly differentiated lesions such as cancer in situ. CT scanning is helpful for evaluating the extent of a bladder tumor, and this is important that it be done prior to resection, as it often produces an extravesical reaction that confuses the interpretation. Superficial tumors have been treated by intravesical instillation of a variety of chemical agents, such as thiotepa, doxyrubicin, and mitomycin C, with a 20–30% success rate in controlling tumor recurrence. More recently, the use of intravesical BCG (bacillle Calmette–Guérin), an attenuated tubercle bacillus used for immunizing against tuberculosis, has proved successful in controlling cancer in situ and the recurrence of superficial tumors in 50–60% of cases. It represents one of the few successful forms of immunotherapy, as it probably exerts its effect by activation of nonspecific killer cells that bind to fibronectin on the tumor cells.

Urinary diversion after cystectomy has been a continual challenge for the urologist. Ureterosigmoidostomy was the first solution to the problem and was introduced at the beginning of the twentieth century, being used initially for patients with extrophy of the bladder and subsequently in patients undergoing cystectomy for cancer. Although some patients survived as long as 50 years after ure-terosigmoidostomy, about 50% died of renal failure after several years as a result of ureteral obstruction, recurrent urinary infections, and stone disease. Moreover, some of the long-term survivors developed colon cancers in the region of the ureterocolonic anastomosis, probably due to elaboration of a carcinogen from the feces being in contact with the urine.

In 1950 Eugene Bricker devised the ileal conduit as an effective way to bring the urine from the posteriorly placed ureters to the anterior abdominal wall and obviated the problem of stomal stenosis that occurred with cutaneous ureterostomies. The urinary stream was now separated from fecal contamination, and recurrent infections were no longer a serious problem. The ileal conduit nearly failed as a form of urinary diversion, as there was no satisfactory method for collecting the urine and patients were constantly wet. A few years later, a suitable skin adhesive was invented so that a watertight rubber collecting device could be glued over the stoma, and the Bricker procedure became the standard urinary diversion for the next 40 years.

The concept of an orthotopic neobladder is not new, and attempts to anastomose loops of bowel directly to the urethra were made by Gil-Vernet and Camay at about the same time the ileal conduit became popular. These procedures did not gain favor, as many of the patients were incontinent, especially at night. Many patients at that time were treated by preoperative irradiation, which made them more susceptible to poor healing at the anastomotic site and fistula formation. Twenty years ago, Koch devised an intraabdominal reservoir fashioned from detubularized loops of intestine with a continent stoma that the patient catheterized. Detubularization of the bowel provides for an increase in capacity and a marked reduction in intraluminal pressure, to less than 30 cm $H_2O$ when filled. The ability to create a low-pressure reservoir of adequate capacity led to a renewed interest in fashioning an orthotopic neobladder. Many techniques were described, but the most popular became the W pouch devised by Hauptmann. More recently, this has been used in women as well as in men. In women, care must be taken to preserve the ligamentous supports of the proximal urethra and to ensure that the bladder neck is completely removed to avoid postoperative retention. Patients void by straining and can empty completely by repeating this maneuver several times. Continence can be achieved with this low-pressure system in 95% by day and in 90% at night, provided the patient awakens once or twice at night to void. This is now regarded as the standard of care in most patients undergoing cystectomy.

Prostate cancer is today one of the major geriatric problems in men. The doubling of the population over the past 50 years and the increase in life expectancy from 62 to 73 years, has resulted in a major increase in the number of men at risk for developing prostate cancer, as 80% of cases are diagnosed between 60 and 80 years of age. Although the mortality rate from prostatic cancer has risen only from 18 to 26 per 100,000 over the past 25 years, the incidence rose from 50,000 to 80,000 between 1973 and 1989, and by 1993 had risen to a peak of 230,000. This sudden increase is ascribed to the introduction of a biochemical marker, prostatic-specific antigen (PSA). It can be measured in the serum by an immunoassay that has allowed early detection of the disease, even before there are any clinical manifestations. Transrectal ultrasound-guided biopsies of the prostate are performed in patients with an elevated PSA to establish the diagnosis.

The increase in incidence has occurred primarily in men with early-stage disease of intermediate grade and has led to a large number being treated for cure by radical surgery or some form of irradiation. Prior to PSA testing, fewer than 20% of patients presenting with prostate cancer were eligible for curative treatment, whereas this figure is now about 70–80%.

Although there is some evidence that deaths from prostate cancer have diminished, there is no doubt that many patients could be spared aggressive treatment if there were a reliable method to evaluate the biologic potential of an individual tumor to predict outcome. It is well established that at least half of the patients over age 65 with intermediate or low grade tumors, die of a cause unrelated to their cancer. The most recent data suggest that the incidence of prostate cancer is now decreasing; in 1995, it was estimated to be only 140,000. It remains to be seen if it falls to pre-PSA levels once the pool of early cases has been diagnosed or if there has been a real increase in the incidence. Any decrease in mortality must be assessed over the next 10 years to determine whether radical treatment of early disease has a significant impact on survival.

The mainstay of treatment for late stage disease or recurrence after radical therapy is ablation or blockage of androgenic steroid hormones. The concept of castration for prostate cancer was introduced by Charles Huggins in 1941, for which he received the Nobel Prize. Presently, orchiectomy has largely been replaced by injection of long-acting luteinizing hormone-releasing hormone (LHRH) agonists that block the LH receptors in the anterior pituitary so the interstitial cells in the testis are no longer stimulated to produce testosterone. A number of antiandrogens are available that block the cancer cell receptors; they are used in conjunction with testosterone ablation to block extra gunadal androgens, or as a substitute in patients who are particularly concerned about their sexual function, as the antiandrogens do not lower testosterone levels, thereby preserving libido. Specific genes associated with prostatic cancer are being identified so that in the future genetic markers may provide a method to determine prognosis and perhaps eventually result in new treatments.

As we extend life expectancy, prostatic cancer will become a progressively more important problem. The new era of molecular medicine should have much to offer patients to improve comfort and quality of life in their later years.

# 54 Renal Function and Fluid and Electrolyte Balance

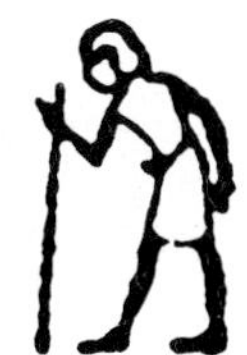

John J. Ryan and Edward T. Zawada, Jr.

Seminal changes in the demographic structure of the Western world over the past 40 years include a falling birth rate and a significant increase in life expectancy of women and men. An ever-increasing proportion of gross national product is being devoted to the health care sector, which reflects advancement in medical technology and in the larger number of patients living longer lives, in part because of this technology. In fact, we are witnessing a demographic revolution evidenced by the mushrooming leisure industry and "retirement" housing and resort developments. These changes reflect the huge demand generated by the needs of an ever-increasing number of active, vital senior citizens. In parallel, significant changes are occurring in health care. Geriatric medicine and surgery have developed to such a degree that the management of complex problems in the elderly is now well established, and the expectations are that patients in their eighth and ninth decades can expect aggressive therapy, including major surgery with, for the most part, good outcomes.[1–4] The concept of wellness is supported by the perceived benefit of a healthy life style with special emphasis on nutrition, exercise, and the avoidance of risk factors, thus postponing or even eliminating the onset of ill health with its associated costs and demands. All these changes have resulted in a crisis in developed countries with reference to the great budget demands of this demographic change.

In this chapter, we describe the structural and functional changes that occur in the kidney with aging. Successful management of the elderly patient perioperatively and of the patient in established renal failure, be it chronic or end-stage, requires a knowledgeable appreciation of the changes occurring in the senescent kidney that result in: (1) decreased ability to tolerate dehydration; (2) decreased ability to tolerate a volume load; (3) increased propensity to accumulate potassium; (4) increased sensitivity to lower levels of potassium; and (5) blunted physiologic response to the effects of aldosterone, antidiuretic hormone, and the production of renin. It is important that physicians involved in the care of these patients are familiar with these changes, so complications in this vulnerable group are minimized, as tolerance of such complications in this patient population is limited. We review the senescent kidney's mechanisms for handling fluid, electrolyte, and acid–base derangements, especially during the perioperative period. Also we discuss the surgical management of patients with established renal diseases. Reviewed are both the older kidney donor and the older recipient for renal transplantation. We review the factors contributing to acute renal failure in the elderly and, in particular, management of this entity in the elderly postoperative patient. Finally we briefly discuss urologic problems and renal vascular diseases.

## Histopathology of the Aging Kidney

Autopsy material, biopsy material from kidney donation, and nephrectomy for tumor and trauma have led to a careful series of measurements, called morphometrics, of the aged glomerulus and tubules.[5] The glomerular changes have been called sclerosis. On light microscopy (Fig. 54.1), sclerosis is an acellular obliteration of glomerular capillary architecture with resultant loss of functional tissue available to perform ultrafiltration of plasma. The difference between the "Swiss cheese" open capillary loops (Fig. 54.2) in normal kidneys and the sclerosis of aged kidneys is readily apparent.

The cause of sclerosis of the aged glomerulus is uncertain, although several theories have been postulated. It is difficult to distinguish change due to age alone from that due to common diseases of late middle life, such as hypertension, diabetes, and atherosclerosis. It appears that even in the absence of these diseases such changes occur. The consequence of reduced filtration area due to obliterative sclerosis is a reduced glomerular filtration rate (GFR). The glomerular changes and functional loss of GFR are responsible for many complications of perioperative management of the elderly patient.

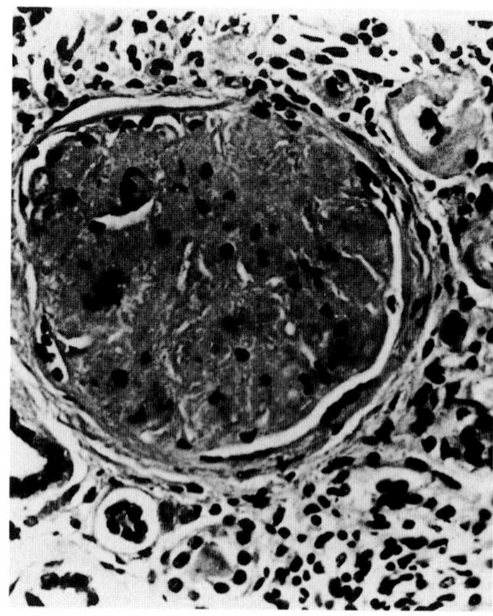

FIGURE 54.1. Light microscopy showing glomerular sclerosis, the glomerular "lesion" of senescence.

The most widely accepted theory to explain the development of this glomerular problem has been summarized as the "hyperfiltration" theory. It was originally described in an animal model of reduced renal mass prepared to study the syndrome of chronic renal insufficiency. The remnant tissue did not remain normal but deteriorated with the development of glomerulosclerosis. Further studies revealed that the glomerulosclerosis resulted from intraglomerular hypertension, which was an attempt to increase the GFR per nephron as an adaptation to compensate for the reduced total GFR.[6] In addition, these studies showed that the intraglomerular hypertension was worse with a normal protein diet, which obligated the kidney to attempt to excrete nitrogenous wastes with reduced excretory units. The efferent arteriole appeared to increase its resistance to accomplish the pathologic adaptation. These glomerular pressures and pathologic anatomy did not occur on reduced protein intake. In individuals with renal diseases that reduce renal mass, continuation of normal protein intake can result in this deterioration of the GFR. Elderly individuals who have hypertension or diabetes may have more deterioration of renal function than elderly people who do not have these underlying medical problems; however, in the absence of diseases affecting the kidney, such intraglomerular hypertension occurs daily after every episode of protein intake. After decades of episodic glomerular hyperfiltration, such glomerulosclerosis develops and eventually causes deterioration of renal function by this same pathophysiology. It appears that renal glomerular senescence begins during the fourth decade of life and progresses linearly with age, reducing the GFR by 1 ml/min for every year over 40 years of age.[7] This predictable reduction of the GFR is one of the main factors responsible for morbidity in the elderly surgical patient. The decreased filtration reserve makes acute renal failure more likely with any nephrotoxic or ischemic renal insult, and fluid and electrolyte and acid–base problems are a challenge to avoid. Reduced filtration of sodium, water, acid, and base loads predisposes to fluid and electrolyte disorders in the perioperative setting. Reduction of glomerular filtration due to aging is inapparent in the day-to-day observation of aged patients. The serum creatinine, which is our usual marker of the GFR, is often normal despite marked reductions of filtration in the elderly. The explanation is that in addition to reduced excretion of creatinine there is a simultaneous reduction of creatinine production in the elderly. Despite reduced GFR, serum creatinine remains in the normal range because of a parallel reduction of muscle mass in the elderly, which leads to reduced creatinine production. It is the normal serum creatinine level that makes glomerular senescence occult to the clinician in the superficial surveillance of renal function solely by the chemistry panel. The serum creatinine is often in the normal range even when glomerular filtration is markedly decreased.

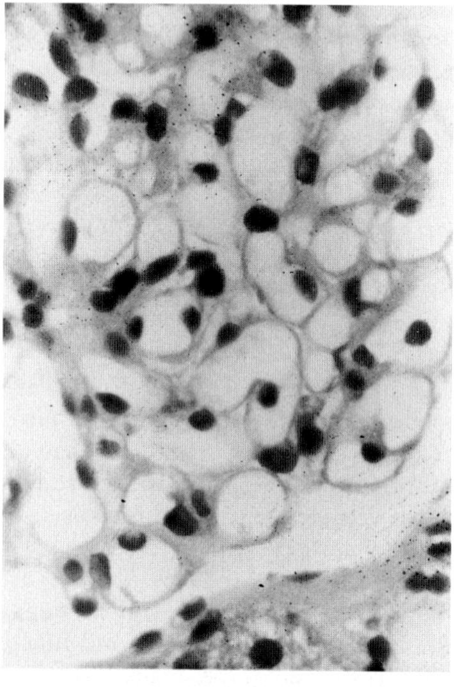

FIGURE 54.2. Normal glomerulus by light microscopy.

In addition to glomerular change, there is tubular senescence with advancing age.[8] Tubular length decreases, interstitial fibrosis between tubules occurs, and tubular basement membrane constitution and anatomy change. Atherosclerosis of nutrient peritubular capillaries contributes in part to these changes. The consequence of tubular senescence is reduced tubular function (i.e., reduced tubular flexibility to reabsorb or secrete an electrolyte load). For example, there is reduced tubular reabsorption of glucose in the elderly tubules. Again, the clinician is usually unaware of this tubular insufficiency because such tubular function is not routinely evaluated preoperatively to assess potential surgical risks. Such tubular dysfunction is hidden because reduced tubular reabsorption of glucose is not manifested by glycosuria: the parallel reduction of GFR leads to a reduced filtered glucose load, with less glucose presenting to the senescent tubule. The clinician is likely to overestimate renal function by failure to appreciate such tubular insufficiency preoperatively.

## Renal Physiology in the Elderly

Beginning at around age 40, the kidney gradually but progressively reduces its ability to clear the plasma. In addition, the renal tubule has decreased capacity to conserve sodium. These changes are not necessarily reflected by measurement of the plasma creatinine and blood urea nitrogen (BUN). A significant reduction in creatinine clearance may obtain in the presence of normal serum creatinine. Reduced cardiac compliance, as seen in the senescent heart, may also result in decreased renal preload and in a reduction in the potency of the cardiorenal endocrine axis. It is clear, therefore, that any substance whose excretion is dependent in part on filtration is affected by aging, and that the body experiences a fundamental reduction in its ability to correct any derangement in fluid and electrolyte balance. Tubular senescence results in disordered reabsorption and secretion of solutes.[9] In addition to reduced ability to reabsorb sodium, there is impaired secretory capacity for potassium and hydrogen ion.

## Clinical Assessment of Renal Function in the Elderly

Data exist strongly suggesting that patients who have preoperative renal insufficiency are prone to postoperative renal failure.[10] As previously mentioned, normal serum creatinine and BUN levels do not necessarily reflect normal renal function. An upper normal level of serum creatinine in a frail, elderly patient with small muscle mass may be indicative of a greatly reduced capacity of the kidney to clear the plasma. It is obvious, therefore, that optimal management of the elderly patient during the perioperative period is facilitated by an appreciation of the clearing capacity of a particular individual patient. The quantity of the 24-hour urine production should reflect not only the minimal obligatory volume (600–700 ml) but the appropriate facultative volume that reflects a normal state of hydration. It is important to elicit any symptoms or signs of obstructive uropathy in the male patient, as postrenal obstruction is a common cause of renal insufficiency in elderly men.

We can assume that the GFR is reduced at a rate of 1 ml/min for every year after age 40. We can take 100 ml/min as normal. Therefore a simple strategy to predict the reduction of renal function in the elderly surgical candidate is to reduce the GFR by 1 ml/min for every year of age over 40 and to compare the resultant filtration rate to a normal of 100 ml/min as a percentage of normal. For example, in the 80-year-old patient, the probable percent GFR is [100 – (age – 40)]/100 = 60% of normal.

A second strategy is to use a urine-free formula to calculate the GFR. These formulas utilize the fact that urine creatinine excretion remains constant under conditions of reduced renal function at the expense of a rise in serum creatinine. The urine creatinine excretion can be estimated from the age and weight of the patient quite accurately, which predicts the muscle mass of the patient from which the urine creatinine is produced and excreted as a constant amount under steady-state conditions. The 24-hour urinary creatinine excretion is approximated by the formula $U_{creat}V$ = [(140 – age) × weight (kg)]/72. The creatinine clearance can then be estimated by using the above urinary creatinine excretion divided by the serum creatinine of the patient, which should be measured preoperatively in the elderly patient. The final formula,[11] which does not require collection of the 24-hour urine, is: Creatinine clearance = [(140 – age) × weight (kg)]/(72 × serum creatinine). For women the above calculation should be multiplied by 0.85 because they have less muscle mass and therefore less creatinine generation and urinary excretion at any age and weight.

Two examples can be used to illustrate these formulas. If a 68-year-old woman weighs 40 kg and has a serum creatinine of 2 mg/dl, it may seem that the patient has mild renal insufficiency because the serum creatinine level is elevated. Using the formula:

$$\begin{aligned}\text{Creatinine clearance} &= [(140-68)\times 40]/(72\times 2)\times 0.85\\ &= (72\times 40)/(72\times 2)\times 0.85\\ &= (40/2)\times 0.85 = 20\times 0.85\\ &= 17\,\text{ml/min}\end{aligned}$$

Thus in an older woman with little muscle mass (40 kg), a serum creatinine level as high as 2 mg/dl reflects a reduction of filtration to 17% of normal.

The second case involves a "healthy," athletic 68-year-old man who weighs 110 kg and has a serum creatinine of 2 mg/dl. It appears that such a patient has mild renal insufficiency, as the serum creatinine is abnormally elevated. Using the formula:

$$\begin{aligned}\text{Creatinine clearance} &= [(140-68)\times 110]/(72\times 2)\\ &= (72\times 110)/(72\times 2)\\ &= 110/2\\ &= 55\,\text{ml/min}\end{aligned}$$

In this case, there is only mild renal insufficiency. In the first case, the filtration reduction was somewhat occult because the serum creatinine was not markedly elevated owing to concomitant muscle loss in an elderly, slightly built woman.

## Drug Dose Modification in the Elderly

Drugs that are eliminated from the body by renal excretion require dose modifications in the aged. Usually these dose modifications require calculation of less frequent doses by a mathematic calculation involving the serum creatinine. Because the serum creatinine does not accurately reflect reduced renal functioning in the elderly, the doses of toxic drugs, such as the aminoglycosides, require adjustments based on creatinine clearance and calculated by the 24-hour urine collection or by the estimate of creatinine clearance using the urine-free formula described above. The dose interval (DI) can be calculated from the following:

$$\text{DI} = (100/\text{estimated creatinine clearance}) \times \text{usual interval}$$

If the 68-year-old woman described above required a course of gentamicin, a loading dose would be given at the usual 2 mg/kg. Then 1 mg/kg would be given every (100/17) × 8 hours. Thus the interval would be every 47 hours. This regimen would lessen the likelihood that the trough level would be elevated, which has been associated with aminoglycoside toxicity in several studies.[12]

## Survey of Renal Diseases of the Elderly

A prospective study was conducted in the United Kingdom on the causes of chronic progressive renal disease leading to admission to a renal unit for initiation of end-stage renal disease (ESRD) management.[13] It revealed that the leading causes in patients over 60 years of age were pyelonephritis (20%), nephrosclerosis (16%), postrenal causes (15%), glomerulonephritis (11%), urolithiasis (6%), polycystic disease (2%), and diabetes (2%). Postrenal causes ranked high on the list.

In the surgical setting, it behooves the clinician to search for obstructive symptoms and signs in the elderly patient with chronic azotemia. Rectal examination of the prostate, postvoid residual volume of urine in the bladder, and renal ultrasonography are quite helpful and minimally invasive. Bladder catheterization may necessitate early consideration of antibiotics for endocarditis prophylaxis in patients with replaced heart valves or prosthetic joints. The choice of antibiotics to cover genitourinary organisms should cover *Enterococcus* as well as gram-negative organisms. Diabetics may have genitourinary colonization with gram-positive organisms. Broad-spectrum prophylaxis is thus likely to be necessary.

Surveillance for occult obstructive uropathy should be considered preoperatively in elderly patients. The etiology of chronic azotemia might become apparent from these tests, and postoperative oliguria might be avoided by routine bladder catheterization prior to surgery in the patient with borderline compensation for benign prostatic hypertrophy (i.e., residual volume 25–150 ml). It can also be seen that parenteral management of hypertension might be necessary in the elderly patient who undergoes surgery, as nephrosclerosis due to hypertension is a common cause of chronic renal disease in this age group.

Common glomerular diseases in the elderly include an idiopathic, rapidly progressive glomerulonephritis.[14] Light microscopy here reveals crescents in Bowman's space (Fig. 54.3), and an indolent glomerular disease, so-called idiopathic membranous nephropathy. The former is nephritic in its clinical presentation, which means that the patient has fever, myalgia, fatigue, and other severe systemic symptoms. The glomerular inflammation results in marked reduction of the GFR. The latter

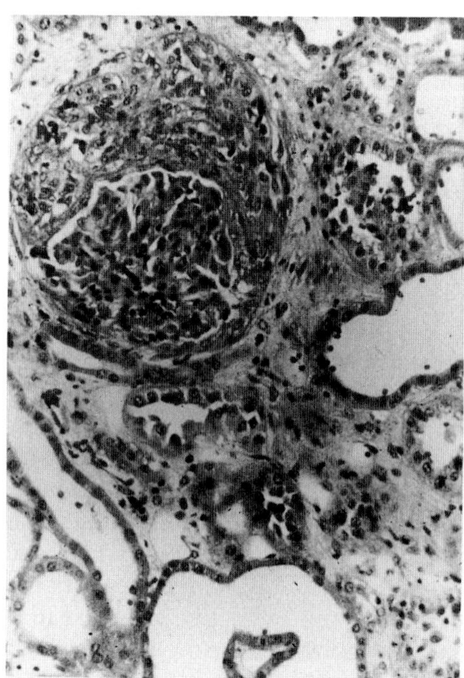

FIGURE 54.3. Crescentic glomerulonephritis, the most common cause of nephritic syndrome in the elderly. The crescent in Bowman's space is rapidly reducing the glomerular filtration rate.

glomerular disease presents as nephrotic syndrome. There is little active inflammation and thus no systemic symptoms. The glomerular pathology reveals thickened capillary loops that are wide open (Fig. 54.4), and so the GFR is not reduced. The pathologic changes in the glomerular capillary wall are caused by immune complex deposition, which alters wall permeability and causes a urinary protein leak into the final urine of more than 3g per 24 hours. The resultant hypoalbuminemia accounts for the clinical findings and the complaint of edema.

In the authors' experience, another common category of chronic renal diseases in the elderly is vascular disease, such as renovascular hypertension due to atherosclerotic renal artery stenosis, renal thromboemboli from clots released from the heart during episodes of cardiac arrhythmias, and atheroemboli that develop spontaneously from severe generalized vascular atherosclerosis or are caused by manipulation of the aorta during diagnostic radiologic procedures or aortic surgery.

At the University of South Dakota Hospitals and Clinics, in a series of 43 patients over the age of 60 with chronic renal failure, 50% had type II diabetes, by far the leading cause of chronic renal failure in this population of patients. Another 25% had renovascular hypertension as the cause of their chronic renal failure. Thus vascular disease made up the second largest group of patients with chronic renal failure in this series. The remaining causes of renal failure included essential hypertension, tubulointerstitial disease, and glomerulonephritis.

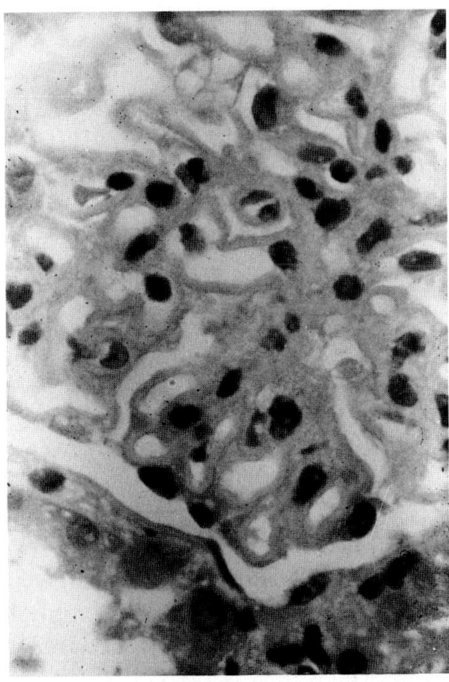

FIGURE 54.4. Membranous nephropathy, the most common cause of nephrotic syndrome in the elderly. The immune complexes are deposited in the basement membrane, causing thickness and altered permeability to albumin.

Other common diseases in the elderly that can lead to chronic renal failure are amyloidosis and multiple myeloma.[15] Multiple myeloma is the plasma cell malignancy that causes lytic lesions of bones and produces high levels of monoclonal immunoglobulins or their subunits. There is an increased incidence of multiple myeloma with advancing years. Multiple myeloma can affect the kidneys by five distinct mechanisms of injury: (1) "Myeloma kidney" refers to direct parenchymal injury due to the immunoglobulins that are tubular cell toxins. (2) Plasma cells can directly infiltrate the kidney, disturbing organ function much like any infiltrating tumor. (3) Hypercalcemia resulting from bone dissolution due to the lytic lesions can lead to calcium deposits in the kidneys or stones. (4) Uric acid crystals can deposit in the kidney during chemotherapy, which destroys the plasma cells, leading to release of nuclear material, such as purines and pyrimidines, which are then metabolized to uric acid. (5) The immunoglobulins or their fragments can be woven into amyloid fibrils, which deposit in the glomeruli and tubules, causing heavy proteinuria, glomerular obliteration, tubular dysfunction, and tubulointerstitial failure.

Amyloidosis can result from multiple myeloma as just described, or it may develop in several other ways. The most treatable form of amyloidosis is that secondary to chronic inflammation in which a serum-reactive protein or complement component is woven into the fibril. In these conditions, such as chronic osteomyelitis, more aggressive therapy of the underlying condition stabilizes the renal deterioration by controlling the degree of amyloid fibril formation. One form of amyloidosis is not secondary to any other disturbance but is idiopathic, and is called primary amyloidosis. It may involve the heart or the kidneys, can be an important cause of morbidity and mortality, and usually has a poor prognosis.[16]

## Fluid and Electrolyte Disorders of the Elderly Undergoing Surgery

It is convenient to consider the particular vulnerability in these patients from the renal standpoint during the perioperative phase in terms of (1) changes in the glomerular filtration rate and (2) changes in tubular function.

The aging kidney is subject to impaired free-water clearance secondary to an impaired GFR. Thus the elderly patient has difficulty excreting a salt and water load. Vigorous saline administration may lead to intravascular and extracellular volume expansion, which results in edema and congestive heart failure with less total fluid administration than in the young surgical patient. Hypotonic intravenous solutions result in decreased plasma osmolarity if administered in excess. A dextrose-containing solution, because of its propensity to cross the blood–brain barrier easily, may potentiate the tendency, in the presence of renal insufficiency, toward cerebral edema. On the other hand, if an elderly patient is put on a low-salt diet with fluid restriction, the aging kidney is less able to conserve sodium[17] and water[18] than the younger kidney. In the elderly patients who receive inadequate oral and intravenous fluid administration, and who are undergoing diagnostic or surgical procedures, there is a net loss of sodium and water with a resultant negative fluid balance and volume contraction. This situation leads to hypotension, predisposing to acute renal failure, and a greater risk of insufficient coronary or cerebral blood flow. It is evident, therefore, that in the elderly patient there is greater risk for, and less ability to compensate for, relative dehydration and fluid overload.

There is also a reduction in renal tubular function in the aging kidney, which results in reduced secretory capacity. Potassium is excreted into the urine by tubular secretion in exchange for sodium under the influence of aldosterone. Tubular dysfunction in the old kidney may impair potassium secretion. Aldosterone is released from the adrenal cortex when an increase in plasma renin levels causes an increase in circulating angiotensin. Renin production by the juxtaglomerular apparatus is reduced in the elderly[19] as a consequence of renal tubular and vascular aging. This leads to impaired aldosterone responses in the elderly. All of these circumstances put the elderly patient at risk for hyperkalemia after too rapid administration of potassium-containing intravenous solutions. Diseases such as diabetes, which commonly affects the elderly, have tubular injury as their predominant renal involvement, which can predispose them to an inability to excrete potassium as described above. These patients are also at risk for hyperkalemia because of potassium release from tissues injured during surgery and the use of maintenance intravenous solutions containing potassium.

The perioperative phase may also place the elderly patient in particular risk for hypokalemia. Nasogastric suction, inadequate potassium replacement, diuretic administration and vomiting, if occurring at this time, exaggerate the physiologic tendency toward potassium loss secondary to sodium conservation. Sodium conservation resulting from increased levels of aldosterone obligate potassium excretion in the urine. Additionally, diarrhea encountered during the perioperative phase further exacerbates the hypokalemia. The tendency toward hypokalemia in these circumstances exists in all age groups as does the kidney's limited ability to conserve potassium under low intake. The elderly kidney is particularly limited (compared to that in younger subjects) in its ability to conserve potassium under low intake. From the above discussion, it is therefore clear that meticulous attention to fluid and electrolyte balance is critical for optimizing operative outcomes in the geriatric patient. If there is renal insufficiency and the GFR is severely reduced, accumulation of potassium may quickly lead to dangerous hyperkalemia. On the other hand, the "normal" senescent kidney has significant limitations in terms of conserving potassium, in particular, during the perioperative phase, when the stress response to surgery obligates sodium conservation.

## Metabolic Acid–Base Disturbances in the Elderly Surgical Patient

### Alkalosis

The reduced GFR in the geriatric patient reduces the body's ability to excrete an alkaline load.[20] Renal tubular damage during the perioperative period resulting, for example, from hypotension or drug injury, may further damage the kidney's ability to excrete bicarbonate. Metabolic alkalosis during the perioperative period is most commonly a result of prolonged nasogastric suctioning or vomiting. In patients with prolonged vomiting, secondary to gastric outlet obstruction, the resultant acid–base disturbance is a hypokalemic hypochloremic metabolic alkalosis. The kidney compensates for the chloride loss by excreting bicarbonate in the urine. Initially, sodium is the cation accompanying the bicarbonate, but as fluid loss increases, the body excretes potassium and hydrogen as the cation in preference to sodium in order to preserve intravascular volume. This results in a paradoxical acidic urine in the presence of a metabolic alkalosis.

The elderly patient is less well able to tolerate metabolic alkalosis and may, in this setting, experience the development of rapid, dangerous hypokalemia, as the body preferentially conserves sodium (under the influence of aldosterone) and hydrogen, which in this setting is titrated by the extra bicarbonate to carbon dioxide and excreted through the lungs. The resultant hypokalemic alkalosis is a risk for cardiac dysrhythmias in the elderly surgical patient, especially in those with coronary artery disease, those taking digitalis, or those who may be taking long-term potassium-losing diuretics.

Lactated Ringer's solution is commonly administered as the maintenance intravenous fluid intraoperatively. This lactate is metabolized to bicarbonate. Because of the impaired renal excretion of alkali in the elderly, the serum bicarbonate may accumulate to an unacceptable level. In this particular scenario, it is preferable that a balanced salt solution such as normal saline be used. Potassium chloride can be added to this solution as needed and the plasma level followed by intraoperative monitoring of potassium levels.

## Acidosis

The elderly are prone to metabolic acidosis. From metabolism of the Western potash diet, 1 mEq of hydrogen ion per kilogram of body weight is created daily. The immediate buffering is accomplished by the bicarbonate ion, which accepts the proton, forming $CO_2$, which is then excreted through the lungs. As shown in Figure 54.5, to regenerate the lost bicarbonate the distal tubule takes $CO_2$ and, under the influence of aldosterone and carbonic anhydrase, delivers regenerated bicarbonate to the circulation. This makes hydrogen ion available to be pumped into the urine, where it lowers the urinary pH. To enhance hydrogen ion excretion, ammonia, filtered phosphate, and filtered sulfate accept hydrogen ions in the urine to reduce the concentration gradient of free hydrogen ions and thus lower the energy necessary for active transport of hydrogen ions against a concentration and charge gradient. Ammonia is produced in the renal tubular cell from glutamine, and phosphate and sulfate are generated during metabolism of the potash diet. This releases sulfate and phosphate as sulfuric and phosphoric acids, which promptly release their hydrogen ion, leaving the phosphate and sulfate to be filtered into the urine. In the elderly, these tubular processes are less efficient. Moreover, the lower aldosterone levels lead to decreased ability to excrete an acid load and to regenerate bicarbonate. The ability of the kidney to compensate for metabolic acidosis is thus diminished.

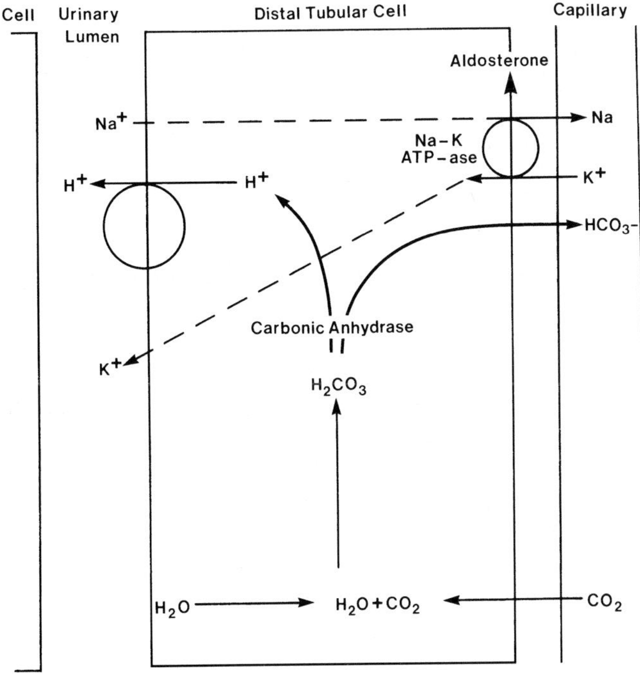


FIGURE 54.5. Distal tubular cell functions. Under the influence of aldosterone, which drives the sodium-potassium-ATPase pump on the basal membrane, a favorable environment is created for sodium entry into the cell at the luminal surface. This allows passive potassium transfer into the urine at the luminal surface, causing potassium to be pumped into the urine at the luminal surface. Bicarbonate is then regenerated and returned to the peritubular capillary.

Metabolic acidosis in the surgical setting results from accumulation of fixed acids (e.g., lactic acid) or from loss of bicarbonate (e.g., through diarrhea, pancreatic or small bowel fistulas, or renal tubular damage). Any significant period of circulatory failure results in the accumulation of lactic acid, reflecting anaerobic metabolism. In the geriatric patient, the impaired GFR leads to less direct filtration of lactic acids. In addition, the reduced tubular function and lower aldosterone levels lead to less regeneration of bicarbonate.[3] Thus the elderly patient is more at risk to develop perioperative disturbances of acid–base balance and, compared with the younger patient, has decreased mechanisms of compensation.

## Suggestions for Fluid and Electrolyte Management in the Elderly Surgical Patient

Before instituting intravenous fluid replacement therapy for the elderly patient undergoing a major surgical procedure, it is necessary to perform a detailed history and clinical examination so problems of relative dehydration and impaired renal perfusion or fluid overload are avoided. Particular attention should be paid to the patient's size and weight, cardiac and renal status, the presence or absence of medications that may have resulted in an altered volume status, and the patient's underlying pathology, which may or may not have significant bearing on the state of hydration at the time of presentation for surgery.

Depending on the nature of the proposed surgery and the possibilities of significant fluid shifts in a high risk setting and a proposed length of surgery exceeding 2 hours, it is prudent to place a Foley catheter so adequate urine output can be measured and maintained. In addition, in high risk patients, where fluid status and replacement may be difficult to assess under anesthesia (or indeed even clinically), a central venous monitor or a pulmonary artery catheter can be valuable. Intraoperatively, lactated Ringer's solution is preferred as a maintenance fluid so the tendency toward metabolic acidosis is avoided. Urine output should reflect a volume greater than the minimal obligate volume. During the postoperative period a maintenance fluid, such as a balanced salt solution containing dextrose 5% and 0.5 N saline, with 20 mEq potassium chloride per liter added, given at a rate of 100 ml/hr should ensure adequate hydration and good urine output in a patient who is not relatively dehydrated. Development of hypovolemia can be corrected by administration of bolus volumes of normal saline. Failure to produce an increased urine output after adequate fluid replenishment in this setting may be an early indicator of renal failure. At this stage, simple dehydration is reflected in a low urine sodium concentration (less than 20 mEq/L). Tubular dysfunction may be demonstrated in this setting by high urine sodium concentration in the presence of low urine output. The administration of furosemide of course, invalidates these values in the diagnostic sense.

The finding of hyponatremia postoperatively should alert the clinician to the presence of free water overload. This may result from excessive fluid replacement with a hypotonic solution (e.g., dextrose 5%, 0.45% saline, or 0.2% saline) or from hypotension leading to decreased renal perfusion, thus aggravating the impaired free water clearance in the geriatric patient. In these older patients, this situation may lead to cerebral edema, with resultant confusion, seizures, and even respiratory arrest.[21]

## Acute Renal Failure and Its Prevention in the Elderly Surgical Patient

Acute renal failure is a disastrous complication of surgery in the elderly patient. In one series, major surgery was the second most common cause of acute renal failure in the elderly.[22] The mortality rate was 57.3% in this group of 122 patients. The causes of death were pneumonia, myocardial infarction and cardiac arrest, pulmonary embolus, and septicemia in decreasing order of frequency. Taken together, bronchopneumonia and septicemia led the authors to conclude that infectious complications were the single greatest mortality risk in the elderly patient with acute renal failure.

There are several types of acute renal failure in the elderly, but the most common (as in other age groups) is acute tubular necrosis (ATN). The tubular necrosis results from ischemia or nephrotoxicity, the latter most commonly due to aminoglycoside antibiotics, chemotherapy drugs, or intravenous contrast agents. It is diagnosed by microscopic analysis of the urinary sediment in which desquamated tubular cells or their degenerative products are observed. The cells degenerate into pigmented granular casts, often called "dirty brown" casts. In addition, there is evidence of tubular dysfunction in the form of impaired sodium conservation. The latter is proven by finding a high fractional excretion of sodium ($FE_{Na}$). The formula for calculating the $FE_{Na}$ is:

$$
\begin{aligned}
FE_{Na}\,(\text{as a }\%) &= \text{excreted sodium/filtered sodium} \times 100 \\
&= U_{Na}V/(P_{Na} \times GFR) \times 100 \\
&= U_{Na}V/[P_{Na} \times (U_{creat}V/P_{creat})] \times 100 \\
&= (U_{Na}/P_{Na})(U_{creat}/P_{creat}) \times 100
\end{aligned}
$$

This calculated test asks the question: What are the tubules doing to influence the final urinary sodium excretion per amount delivered to the tubules in the first place? If there is tubular health, there should be sodium conservation (low $FE_{Na}$, with a value <1%). During tubular necrosis there is failure to conserve sodium (high $FE_{Na}$, with a value >1%). In a typical case of volume contraction with reduced urine output but no tubular necrosis, the urine sodium is typically <20 mEq/L, and the urine creatinine is more than 40 mg/dl. Take, for example, a urine sodium of 15 mEq/L, a serum sodium of 140 mEq/L, a slightly elevated serum creatinine of 1.5 mg/dl, and a urine creatinine of 140 mg/dl (a not uncommon value in concentrated urine). Placing these values into the formula for $FE_{Na}$, the following is derived:

$$
\begin{aligned}
FE_{Na} &= (15/140)/(140/1.5) \times 100 \\
&= 0.107/93.3 \times 100 \\
&= 0.11\%
\end{aligned}
$$

This value is less than 1%, reflecting healthy tubules that are effectively conserving sodium.

In the case of tubular necrosis, common values are likely to be:

$$
\begin{aligned}
U_{Na} &= 140\,\text{mEq/L} \\
P_{Na} &= 140\,\text{mEq/L} \\
U_{creat} &= 15\,\text{mg/dl} \\
\text{Serum creatinine} &= 1.5\,\text{mg/dl}
\end{aligned}
$$

Using the formula:

$$
\begin{aligned}
FE_{Na} &= (140/140)/(15/1.5) \times 100 \\
&= 1/10 \times 100 \\
&= 10\%
\end{aligned}
$$

This high fractional excretion of sodium indicates tubular dysfunction as evidenced by "salt wasting" instead of conservation.

A modification of the fractional excretion expression that is even simpler to apply is called the renal failure index (RFI). With this formula, plasma sodium is thought to be a constant near 100, which cancels the multiplication by 100 to achieve a percent. Thus the formula can be simplified:

$$
\begin{aligned}
FE_{Na} &= (U_{Na}/P_{Na})/(U_{creat}/P_{creat}) \times 100 \\
RFI &= U_{Na}/(U_{creat}/P_{creat})
\end{aligned}
$$

Again, the value 1 is the cutoff between prerenal and tubular necrosis causes of oliguria.

Using the numbers from the examples above in the RFI formula:

$$\text{Example 1: } RFI = 15/(140/1.5) = 0.16$$

Because this is less than 1, it suggests renal conservation of sodium and normal tubular function.

Example 2: RFI = 140/(15/1.5) = 14

This value is much larger than 1, suggesting tubular necrosis and failure to conserve sodium.

This discussion of acute renal failure in the elderly has concentrated on the diagnosis of ATN. If the analysis described above and the bedside evaluation, weight, orthostatic changes in vital signs, low central venous pressure, low pulmonary artery pressures, or low pulmonary capillary wedge pressures point to volume contraction as the cause of decreasing urine output and rising creatinine and BUN, the correct therapy is to restore plasma volume with normal saline. If hemorrhage is the cause of volume contraction, treatment should include colloid, such as packed red blood cells (RBCs) or albumin.

Several theories are used to explain the fall in GFR with ATN. One theory is that tubular necrosis leads to sodium wasting, which triggers excess renin release from the juxtaglomerular apparatus. The renin creates more angiotensin, which leads to afferent arteriolar constriction and reduced GFR and oliguria until tubular cell regeneration reverses the sodium wasting and renin stimulation. Measures that enhance renal vasoconstriction, such as prostaglandin inhibition by nonsteroidal antiinflammatory drugs (NSAIDs) or renin-angiotensin stimulation by volume contraction increase the risk of a reduced GFR. Intratubular obstruction by necrotic tubular cells and debris can reduce the net hydrostatic force of the GFR. These "casts" can be preventively eliminated from causing obstruction by measures that enhance urine flow, such as volume expansion, low-dose dopamine infusion, osmotic diuretics, or loop diuretics (e.g., furosemide). Low-dose dopamine also counteracts the renal vasoconstriction of a stimulated renin-angiotensin axis.

In summary, from these theories it can be seen that prevention of the filtration failure in advance of a renal insult that might cause tubular cell necrosis is accomplished by avoiding NSAIDs and by hydrating to prevent volume contraction and to suppress the renin-angiotensin axis. At the time of the insult and if the volume status of the patient permits it, mannitol and furosemide should be given. If the volume status does not permit use of these drugs, low-dose dopamine (<3 mg/kg/min) and an intravenous furosemide drip at 5–30 mg/hr should be started. When these measures are utilized, the filtration failure often is lessened in the setting of tubular necrosis. The patient frequently is not oliguric and may have a rise of creatinine that stabilizes at a level that does not require dialysis. Nonoliguric ATN has an improved prognosis with less morbidity and mortality.

Other types of acute renal failure that must be ruled out in the elderly include glomerular, vascular, and allergic interstitial causes. The glomerular cause of acute renal failure that occurs in the elderly is crescentic glomerulonephritis (Fig. 54.3). These patients may have systemic symptoms, such as fever and hypertension. The diagnosis requires finding RBC casts during microscopic analysis of the urine sediment. Thus it is strongly recommended that any patient with acute renal failure have the sediment reviewed by the clinician for the presence of these casts. Failure to do so may result in failure to recognize this form of acute renal failure, which can be stabilized with high-dose corticosteroids. Failure to treat these patients with corticosteroids can result in permanent renal failure. It is recommended that such steroid treatment be carried out in consultation with an internist or nephrologist whenever possible.

Vascular causes of acute renal failure are suspected when acute renal failure develops in certain high risk situations. For example, thromboemboli may develop in the elderly surgical patient who has a cardiac arrhythmia. Clots may form in the heart and be expelled into the systemic circulation. Hematuria, flank pain, and hypertension heighten the suspicion. Renal flow scans show reduced flow in the areas of infarct on the static images. Renal lactic dehydrogenase (LDH) isoenzymes may be elevated. Atheroemboli may also occur in the setting of aortic manipulation (i.e., during surgery or angiography). An atherosclerotic plaque is dislodged and travels downstream into the renal arteries, occluding afferent arterioles. Mottling of the skin or ischemic toes (blue-toe syndrome) are clues that atheroemboli may be the cause of a rising serum creatinine level.

Finally, allergic renal interstitial nephritis occurs in response to therapy with certain classes of drugs. Filtration failure is induced by mechanisms similar to that of tubular necrosis. The difference is that fever, rash, eosinophilia, and occasionally eosinophiluria are evidence of the allergic nature of this renal injury. In addition to stopping the offending drug, steroid therapy is often necessary to minimize the course of acute renal failure in these patients. Drug classes associated with allergic interstitial nephritis are penicillins, anticonvulsants, antituberculous drugs, sulfa antibiotics, and sulfa-like diuretics (thiazide, furosemide, metolazone).

Once reduced glomerular filtration has occurred in ATN, it cannot be reversed until the tubular cells regenerate, which usually takes about 2 weeks. Hyperalimentation and aggressive dialysis, when necessary, have been proved to shorten the duration of the acute renal failure when compared to intravenous fluid therapy.[23]

## Management of Hypertension in the Elderly Surgical Patient

Loss of control of hypertension in the elderly surgical patient can cause a great deal of morbidity. Poor control of blood pressure may result in exacerbation of angina due to increased afterload; it may precipitate congestive heart failure in the patient with borderline compensated contractility; finally, it may worsen postoperative bleeding. Exacerbation of hypertension may rarely cause a cerebrovascular accident in the perioperative setting, as the aged individual is at higher risk for this vascular complication of hypertension as well.

If any of the above complications occur or if the hypertension is severe (more than 115 mmHg diastolic), the usual forms of emergency management of hypertension should be employed as in any age group: intravenous nitroprusside by pump infusion or intravenous boluses of labetalol, intravenous boluses of hydralazine, drip infusion of labetalol, drip infusion of nitroglycerine, or drip infusion of fenoldopam, a new dopamine agonist that safely and quickly lowers blood pressure.[24] The latter agent affords promise but has not had wide usage as yet.

Sublingual nifedipine once was the initial treatment of choice for hypertensive emergencies. It is no longer used because of adverse cardiac events related to increased heart work due to reflex tachycardia while coronary perfusion is being lowered resulting in myocardial ischemia. Nitroprusside is used in the following way: Two ampules are dissolved in 250 ml of normal saline or 5% dextrose, and the drip infusion is used to titrate the blood pressure to diastolic blood pressure levels of 95–100 mmHg at the lowest. An arterial line should be in place to monitor the blood pressure reduction if possible. If not possible, a number of excellent accurate electronic blood pressure recording devices that use an arm cuff are routinely available in most hospitals. They allow frequent measurements and are an acceptable alternative to intraarterial blood pressure monitoring.

It is important not to lower the diastolic pressure to normal (i.e., 80 mmHg), as frank cerebral insufficiency may result from decreased perfusion pressure through vessels with extensive atherosclerotic narrowing. Both nitroprusside and nitroglycerine drips have favorable hemodynamic patterns for supply and demand of oxygenated blood to heart muscle and do not exacerbate angina or heart failure as blood pressure is lowered. Because nitroprusside has a cyanide moiety, thiocyanate may accumulate rapidly in the elderly because of their reduced GFR. Thiocyanate blood levels should be measured regularly. Intravenous labetalol is often started as 10 mg boluses every 8 hours. If necessary, the dose can be titrated to as much as 100 mg every 8 hours. Drip infusions are given at 10–20 mg/hr.

Intravenous fenoldopam is used *without* a bolus infusion, ampules of 1 ml, 2 ml, or 4 ml (10 mg/ml) are diluted in normal saline (250 ml, 500 ml, or 1000 ml, respectively) and infused at a dose of 0.01–1.6 μg/kg/min.

Other parenteral antihypertensive therapies that can be used for "maintenance therapy" in the perioperative setting include intravenous methyldopa, intravenous hydralazine, transdermal clonidine, and the newest addition, intravenous labetalol. Drugs to be avoided in the elderly surgical patient with hypertension are intravenous diazoxide, intramuscular hydralazine, and intravenous ganglionic blockers. The lack of dependable controls and the side effect profile make these drugs less desirable.

Intravenous hydralazine can be used in doses of 5–75 mg three times daily. Reflex tachycardia is a potential problem that can exacerbate angina. Cardiac conduction system senescence often makes this problem less common in the elderly patient than in middle-aged patients with coronary artery disease. Intravenous methyldopa is accompanied by somnolence but is otherwise effective and safe. Transdermal clonidine is administered as a patch in small, medium, and large sizes and is applied to the skin once weekly. It is an easy way to prevent exacerbation of hypertension in the mild hypertensive who goes to surgery.[25] The patch should be applied 1–2 days preoperatively. When it effectively controls blood pressure, it is left on throughout the surgery and during the postoperative period.

## Surgery in the Elderly Patient with Advanced Renal Failure

Major surgery no longer is associated with a prohibitive mortality rate in patients with advanced or even end-stage renal failure. Low mortality rates can be achieved with proper preoperative assessment and preparation and perioperative management often involving cooperation between internist/nephrologist and surgeon. This is true even in patients in whom renal failure is associated with other serious morbidities including diabetes mellitus and coronary artery disease. Obviously, optimal preoperative preparation may include dialysis, the correction of bleeding tendencies, and meticulous attention to detail with regard to the correction or near-normalization of all physiologic derangements. The good outcome of dialysis patients undergoing coronary artery bypass surgery has been reported.[26] Consultation with the anesthesia service optimizes the intraoperative management of these patients, and early postoperative hemodialysis may be necessary to correct postoperative derangements of fluid balance, acid–base balance, and electrolyte imbalance during the early postoperative phase. Unexpected bleeding may occur in the uremic patient secondary to platelet dysfunction, and a bleeding time test should be performed preoperatively. Arginine vasopressin may be useful for correcting this problem. Alternatively, it may be necessary to infuse platelets immediately preoperatively to correct a prohibitively prolonged bleeding time. It is not unusual in the uremic patient to have a subclinical pericardial effusion, which may manifest acutely during the perioperative period, leading to possible tamponade and cardiac arrest. Knowledge of the patient's myocardial ejection fraction allows more accurate appreciation of the pumping ability of the heart. Thus echocardiography may be valuable for assessing these patients preoperatively. Constant vigilance for drug toxicity is maintained, as the rate of clearance varies with dialysis of different medications. Conversely, certain medications may best be given at the end of dialysis so adequate blood levels are maintained. Postoperative nasogastric drainage or fistulous losses from the gastrointestinal tract may further complicate fluid and electrolyte derangement and may require alterations in the dialysis formula.

## Renal Vascular Surgery in the Elderly

Renal vascular disease and renal vascular hypertension are common causes of blood pressure disturbances and renal insufficiency in the elderly. Even in the presence of new and powerful antihypertensive medications, many patients benefit by surgical correction of renal vascular hypertension. It is recognized that more than 40% of medically treated patients with renal vascular hypertension, although controlled, continue to experience deterioration in renal function and reduction in renal size.[27] At the University of South Dakota, magnetic resonance angiography (MRA) has become the imaging method of choice with minimum morbidity for investigating these patients. Spiral CT is reported to have high sensitivity and specificity for assessing renal artery stenosis.[28] Patients who are most likely to benefit from surgical correction of this lesion are those with uncontrolled hypertension, especially a diastolic blood pressure higher than 105 mmHg, patients whose onset of hypertension is acute and severe, and particularly those who demonstrate azotemia attributable to renal vascular lesions. Fibromuscular dysplasia is typically not a disease of the elderly. More often than not, the elderly patient with renal vascular hypertension due to atherosclerosis has associated significant atherosclerotic disease of the abdominal aorta, peripheral vascular tree, and cerebrovascular circulation, in addition to coronary artery disease. Nevertheless, several series attest to the excellent early and late results of surgical revascularization for renal vascular hypertension and renal insufficiency.[29–33]

In properly selected patients, hypertension is cured or improved in more than 75% of cases; and in patients with chronic renal insufficiency, improved renal function can be expected in more than 70% of cases. Most of these patients can avoid early or late dialysis. The technical reconstruction is determined by the site and extent of the atherosclerotic lesion(s) and whether simultaneous aortoiliac reconstruction is necessary. These lesions are mostly ostial and thus are not readily amenable to angioplasty. It may be necessary to perform unilateral nephrectomy for a markedly shrunken kidney that is demonstrated to be the culprit in poorly controlled renal vascular hypertension. In the very high-risk patient, however, angioplasty and stent placement may afford an alternative for blood pressure reduction and renal preservation in the short term when major reconstructive surgery cannot be undertaken. It is important to keep in mind that excellent results can be achieved over the long term in patients with renal vascular hypertension surgically corrected from the point of view of both blood pressure control and renal preservation.

## Surgical Considerations for Obstructive Renal Disease in the Elderly

Obstruction of the urinary tract is a common cause of renal failure in the elderly. In elderly men benign prostatic hypertrophy (BPA) is the commonest cause of postrenal obstruction. Typically, there is a long history of increasing difficulty including urinary hesitancy, urgency, and frequency. This picture contrasts with that of cancer of the prostate, which typically is accompanied by a relatively short duration of symptoms. Both diseases are common with advancing age. In the classic study by Franks, microscopic evidence of prostate cancer was ubiquitous in men reaching the age of 90.[34] Screening for prostate cancer by serial digital rectal examinations and detection of elevated plasma PSA levels is now commonplace.

Debate is ongoing regarding the choice of therapy for early lesions. New modalities of therapy allow more options for treatment of benign and malignant obstructive prostatic disease. In the case of invasive carcinoma of the prostate, no increase in survival is obtained by radical prostatectomy over radiation therapy during the first 10 years after definitive treatment. Therefore, if life expectancy is 10 years or less, radiation therapy may be preferred so the morbidity associated with radical prostatectomy can be avoided. Mild to moderate symptoms of BPH may be ameliorated by medical means including selective $\alpha$-adrenergic blocking agents (terazosin, doxazosin, transulosin) or by 5 $\alpha$-reductase enzyme inhibition (finasteride). Many patients, however, require prostatectomy, either transurethrally (TURP) or in the case of very large lesions, open resection. The mortality rate in patients over 65 undergoing these urologic procedures ranges from 0.5% for TURP to 17% for procedures such as radical prostatectomy and cystectomy.[35]

Obstruction of the urinary tract leading to acute retention is uncommon in women, but when it occurs it may be secondary to neurogenic factors or bladder outlet or urethral obstruction secondary to genitourinary carcinoma, benign lesions of the vagina or uterine cervix, or rarely, cystocele. Neurogenic bladder dysfunction with urinary retention may be secondary to spinal cord disease or injury, or it may represent the effects of demyelinating disease. On the other hand, acute retention on a neurogenic basis may follow trauma, pelvic surgery, administration of general anesthetics, spinal anesthesia, or administration of certain drugs that influence enervation of the bladder, bladder neck, proximal urethra, or external sphincter.[36]

Other causes of obstructive uropathy in the elderly include stone disease, retroperitoneal tumors, inflammatory abdominal aortic aneurysm, and retroperitoneal fibrosis. The most common causes of stone disease in the elderly are hypercalcemia due to malignancy, hyperuricemia due to chemotherapy for cancer, and hyperparathyroidism. Additionally, stones arise in patients who had idiopathic hypercalciuria at an earlier age and have survived to the later decades. Magnesium ammonium phosphate stones arise in the presence of urinary tract infection with urea-splitting organisms. The infections are commonly related to inadequate bladder emptying due to prostate disease, spinal cord injury, and detrusor insufficiency from diabetes. Significant progress has been made in the management of urinary tract stone disease over the past 15 years. Approximately 95% of all renal and ureteral calculi can be removed successfully using percutaneous stone techniques, ureterorenoscopy, extracorporeal shock wave lithotripsy, or a combination of these therapeutic modalities.[38]

## Renal Transplantation in the Elderly

Prior to the introduction of cyclosporine it was unusual to consider renal transplantation in individuals over 55 years of age. With improved immune suppression, it is now possible to offer kidney transplantation to patients in the seventh and even eighth decades of life. The patient's physiologic age, rather than chronologic age, is used to make decisions about transplantation. Indeed it is suggested by some that transplantation represents the most satisfactory solution to end-stage renal failure, even in the elderly patient; and several series[36,37] have reported satisfactory results in old patients. At the University of South Dakota, the use of second-line immunesuppressant drugs (monoclonal or polyclonal antibodies) is avoided wherever possible in the elderly transplant recipient. It is considered prudent to optimize cytomegalovirus prophylaxis in these patients. It is not unusual for the elderly transplant recipient to succumb to other pathology in time, rather than to failure of the allograft; indeed many of these patients die with a functioning graft in place.

Additionally, it is now realized that the "older" donor may be a valuable resource of organ availability for transplantation. Donor grafts from those in their sixth and seventh decades of life may be suitable for kidney transplantation, especially in the absence of significant renal artery atherosclerosis and in whom pretransplant biopsy demonstrates an absence of significant (<25%) glomerulosclerosis. The ever-increasing shortage of grafts for transplantation has mandated widening the donor pool and increased utilization of kidneys previously considered to be of marginal suitability. Suitability of the old kidney for transplant should be determined by the donor's history and gross and microscopic evidence of the absence of significant pathologic change.

## Conclusions

The elderly surgical patient represents a management challenge owing to reduced renal reserve, the result of glomerulosclerosis and senescence of tubules. Fluids and electrolytes must be administered carefully. Delay in their institution or too rapid administration of fluids can lead to morbidity. Acute renal failure is best prevented with preoperative hydration. Perioperative hypertension must also be managed definitively but carefully, avoiding "total normalization" of blood pressure. More surgery is being performed in the elderly, such as renal revascularization and renal transplantation. Surgical risks are higher in elderly patients than in young patients, but the risk/benefit ratios are acceptable in most patients.

### References


1. Greenburg AG, Saik RP, Coyle JJ, Peskin GW. Mortality and gastrointestinal surgery in the aged. Arch Surg 1981;116: 788–791.
2. Rorbaek-Madsen M, Dupont G, Kristensen K, et al. General surgery in patients aged 80 years and older. Br J Surg 1992;79:1216–1218.
3. Hosking MP, Warner MA, Lobdell CM, et al. Outcomes of surgery in patients 90 years of age and older. JAMA 1989; 261:1909–1915.
4. Adkins RB Jr, Scott HW. Surgical procedures in patients aged 90 years and older. South Med J 1984;11:1357– 1364.
5. Tauchi H, Tsuboi K, Okutoni J. Age changes in the human kidney of the different races. Gerontology 1971;17: 87–97.
6. Brenner BM, Meyer GW, Hostetter TH. Dietary protein intake and the progresive nature of kidney disease: the role of hemodynamically mediated glomerular injury in the pathogenesis of progressive glomerular sclerosis in aging, renal ablation, and intrinsic renal disease. N Engl J Med 1982;307:652–659.
7. Adler S, Lindeman RD, Yiengst MJ, Beard E, Shock NW. Effect of acute acid loading on urinary acid excretion by the aging human kidney. J Lab Clin Med 1968;72:278–279.
8. Darmady EM, Offer J, Woodhouse MA. The parameters of the aging kidney. J Pathol 1973;109:195–209.
9. Epstein M. Renal physiologic changes with age. In: Zawada ET Jr, Sica DA (eds) Geriatric Nephrology and Urology. Littleton, MA: PSG Publishing, 1985:1–14.

10. Kashyap VS, Cambria RP, Davison JK, L'Italien GJ. Renal failure after thoracoabdominal aortic surgery. J Vasc Surg 1997;26:949–957.
11. Cockroft DW, Gault MN. Prediction of creatinine clearance from serum creatinine. Nephron 1976;16:31–41.
12. Duchin KL. Parmocodynamics and pharmacokinetics of drugs in the elderly. In: Zawada ET Jr, Sica DA (eds) Geriatric Nephrology and Urology. Littleton, MA: PSG Publishing, 1985:215–229.
13. McGeown MG. Chronic renal failure in Northern Ireland, 1968–70 (a prospective survey). Lancet 1972;1:307–310.
14. Moorthy AV, Zimmerman SW. Renal disease in the elderly: clinicopathologic analysis of renal disease in 115 elderly patients. Clin Nephrol 1980;14:223–229.
15. Frocht A, Fillit H. Renal disease in the geriatric patient. J Am Geriatr Soc 1984;32:28–43.
16. Zawada ET Jr, Jensen R, Hicks D, Putnam WD, Ramirez G. An elderly male with deterioration of renal function and heavy proteinuria. Am J Nephrol 1987;7:482–489.
17. Epstein M, Hollenberg NK. Age as a determinant of renal sodium conservation in normal man. J Lab Clin Med 1976;87:411–417.
18. Dontas AS, Marketos SG, Papanayiotou P. Mechanisms of renal tubular defects in old age. Postgrad Med J 1972;48: 295–303.
19. Weidmann P, De Myttenaere-Bursztein S, Maxwell MH, de Lima J. Effect of aging on plasma renin and aldosterone in normal man. Kidney Int 1975;8:325–333.
20. Sica DA, Centor RM. Tests of glomerular and tubular function in the elderly. In: Zawada ET Jr, Sica DA (eds) Geriatric Nephrology and Urology. Littleton, MA: PSG Publishing, 1985:33–47.
21. Arieff AI, Llack F, Massry SG. Neurologic manifestations and morbidity of hyponatremia: correlation with brain water and electrolytes. Medicine 1976;55:121–141.
22. Kumar R, Hill CM, McGeown MG. Acute renal failure in the elderly. Lancet 1973;1:90–91.
23. Abel RM, Beck CH Jr, Abbott WM, Ryan JA Jr, Barnett GO, Fischer JE. Improved survival from acute renal failure after treatment with intravenous essential L-amino acids and glucose. N Engl J Med 1973;288:695–699.
24. White WB, Radford MJ, Gonzalez FM, Weed SG, McCabe EJ, Katz AM. Selective dopamine-1 agonist therapy in severe hypertension: effects of intravenous fenoldopam. J Am Coll Cardiol 1988;11:1118–1123.
25. Horning JR, Zawada ET Jr, Simmons JL, Williams L, McNulty R. Efficacy and safety of two years of antihypertensive therapy with transdermal clonidine. Chest 1988; 93:941–945.
26. Zawada ET Jr, Stinson JB, Done G. New perspectives on coronary artery disease in hemodialysis patients. South Med J 1982;75:694–697.
27. Hallett JW Jr, Fowl R, O'Brien PC, et al. Renovascular operations in patients with chronic renal insufficiency; do the benefits justify the risks? J Vasc Surg 1987;5:622–627.
28. Albrecht A, Blomley MJK. Spiral computed tomography: principles and clinical use. Hosp Med 1998;59:120–125.
29. Dean RH, Krueger TC, Whiteneck JM, et al. Operative management of renovascular hypertension. J Vasc Surg 1984;1:234–242.
30. Hunt JC, Sheps SG, Harrison EG, et al. Renal and renovascular hypertension. Arch Intern Med 1974;133:988–999.
31. Stewart MT, Smith RB, Fuldenwider JT, et al. Concomitant renal revascularization in patients undergoing aortic surgery. J Vasc Surg 1985;2:400–405.
32. Tarazi RY, Hertzer NR, Bevan EG, et al. Simultaneous aortic reconstruction and renal revascularization: risk factors and late results in 89 patients. J Vasc Surg 1987;5:707–714.
33. Dean RH, Keyser JE III, Dupont WD, et al. Aortic and renal vascular disease: factors affecting the value of combined procedures. Am J Surg 1985;200:336–344.
34. Franks LM. Latent carcinoma of the prostate. J Pathol Bacteriol 1954;68:603–616.
35. Stults B. Surgical considerations in the elderly. In: Zawada ET Jr, Sica DA (eds) Geriatric Nephrology and Urology. Littleton, MA: PSG Publishing, 1985:397–428.
36. Baquero A, Goldman MH. Renal transplantation in the elderly. In: Zawada ET Jr, Sica DA (eds) Geriatric Nephrology and Urology. Littleton, MA: PSG Publishing, 1985:253–263.
37. Wedel N, Brynger H, Blohme I. Kidney transplantation in patients 60 years and older. Scand J Urol Nephrol 1980;54:106–108.
38. Peters PC, Boone TB, Irwin NF, et al. Urology. In: Schwartz SI (ed) Principles of Surgery. New York: McGraw-Hill, 1994:1725–1793.

# 55
# Urinary Incontinence in the Elderly

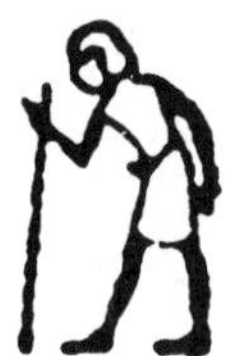

Pat O'Donnell

Urinary incontinence (UI) is one of the most personally devastating diseases of the elderly. It has humiliating social consequences that touch every facet of the quality of life of the old person. One of the most debilitating consequences of UI in the elderly is a loss of self-esteem, which results in self-imposed social isolation. Elderly incontinent persons become prisoners in their own home owing to the behavioral changes that occur from the personal fears and shame of UI. Many elderly people believe they are a victim of a disease without having any control over the personal and social consequences. As a result, they suffer in silence because of the shame and lack of awareness of successful treatment options. Because of the loss of self-esteem, treatment of UI in old people is usually deferred until the disease has become severe and the progressive symptoms have compromised many years of the life of the individual. Personal decisions about treatment of UI often derive from feelings of desperation and shame rather than a careful consideration of the treatment options that meet the quality-of-life needs of the patient. Many elderly people have a strong reluctance to seek treatment or participate in treatment for incontinence because of personal feelings.

Most treatment programs for UI in the elderly require patient involvement and participation, which is important for long-term success of therapy of UI in old people. The requirement to be personally involved in both surgical and nonsurgical treatment programs gives elderly people a feeling of control over their own lives and control over the devastating personal consequences of UI they experience.

Elderly people experience a feeling of loss of control in all areas of their environment and loss of importance to family and society as they become older. They are no longer essential for "the job to get done" in their occupation or essential to "the existence of the family" as they once were when they were younger. The personal feelings of self-esteem and value to society they once experienced in their occupation are no longer present and they no longer feel important or needed. Their importance to the family is different because their role has changed drastically, and it does not provide the same feeling of being needed by the family. The many personal and social changes associated with aging have a collective effect of lowering self-esteem. The ultimate loss of self-esteem for the elderly person is the humiliation of loss of bladder control.

Loss of bladder control is the most profound reminder to elderly persons that they are not able to control even the most basic body functions of normal life. Particularly in the elderly population who have lost a personal feeling of value within themselves and in society, UI has an unusual capacity as a disease to render the individual emotionally paralyzed to seek treatment. The greatest obstacle to successful treatment of UI in the elderly is getting the individual to consult a physician and subsequently to become involved in a treatment program. Successful treatment of UI can restore to the patient essential control over a basic normal body function necessary to restore self-esteem, which has an enormous impact in all other areas of their life.

Although UI is not a life-threatening disease, it is one of the most serious "quality of life" threatening diseases of elderly people. The economic, social, medical, and psychological impact on the lives of elderly people who have UI is immense.[1] Among the elderly people who are community dwelling and live independently, approximately 38% of women and 19% of men experience UI. Of the old people who live in chronic care facilities, approximately 55% experience UI. The total direct health care cost of UI in the United States during 1987, was approximately $10.3 billion and is estimated to be more than $15 billion at the present time. The annual cost of managing UI in old people is more than the combined annual cost of all coronary artery bypass surgery and all renal dialysis in the United States. Although the economic cost to old people and to society is enormous, the greatest cost by far is the personal distress of the elderly person through self-imposed social isolation and loss in self-esteem resulting from UI.

## Urinary Incontinence in Elderly Women

### Clinical Assessment

Elderly women are twice as likely to be incontinent as elderly men in a similar age group. The assessment of incontinence in an elderly patient is essential to ensure that any therapeutic program is based on an accurate diagnosis of urinary bladder and urethral dysfunction. UI in the elderly is much more complex than UI in younger people; and clinical trial and error treatment programs that are not based on a complete diagnostic evaluation of the patient are unlikely to be successful and can be potentially harmful to the patient. The immense importance of the impact of UI on quality of life of the older person must be a factor in every decision including the complexity of the clinical management of UI. Therefore the incontinence assessment is important and involves many aspects of the pathophysiology of incontinence and the life style of the individual.

#### *Incontinence History*

Many elderly women believe that UI is a normal consequence of aging or of being female. Sometimes the patient has been told by a physician that UI is a normal condition associated with becoming older and that nothing should be done about it. The reluctance by the patient to see a physician about the symptoms of UI may be due to personal embarrassment, lack of knowledge of treatment options, fear of surgery, a sense of hopelessness about UI, and low expectations of treatment success. Therefore, the clinical history of old women with UI should always include direct questions about the occurrence of incontinence episodes, the symptomatic characteristics of urinary incontinence, and the severity of urinary incontinence. Typically, incontinence severity can be estimated by a clinician by asking patients how many times they change pads each day. It is important for the clinician to know if the major component of incontinence is urge urinary incontinence or stress urinary incontinence. Typically, stress urinary incontinence (SUI) is associated with involuntary loss of urine with coughing, straining, and movement.[2] Urge urinary incontinence usually is associated with an intense desire to void with an inability to prevent urine loss voluntarily because the patient cannot physically get to the bathroom in time to prevent an incontinence episode.[3]

A urinary diary is an essential part of the initial clinical evaluation of urinary incontinence in old women.[4] The diary helps document the severity of incontinence, determine if associated irritative symptoms are present, establish if there is a pattern to the incontinence, identify precipitating events, and assist in planning the treatment approach. The assessment of symptom distress and quality of life are increasingly important when evaluating the severity of health conditions, such as UI and the impact of the disease on the daily life of the individual.

Although UI in the elderly is a personally devastating disease, it is not a fatal disease for most patients. Successful treatment of UI in elderly women does not prolong survival, so the goal of treatment of UI is to make the life of the person better. Therefore, quality of life assessment is important when determining the success of treatment. Finally, it is essential to determine the functional status of the older patient. Both mental status and physical status of the patient are important when planning treatment so it is specific to the needs of a particular old person. In addition, co-morbid medical conditions may have a significant impact on treatment decisions of UI in older patients.

#### *Physical Examination*

The physical examination of the incontinent elderly woman requires more attention to nuances than in the younger woman. For example, atrophic changes in the vaginal epithelium may indicate that similar changes are present in the urethral mucosa.[5] The general body habitus of the elderly woman is important, as is her agility when planning therapy. A pelvic examination is always performed when possible, including an assessment of the perineal skin, the pelvic floor, and the vaginal wall. It is important for the clinician to identify evidence of anatomic incontinence due to prolapse of the bladder and urethra in old patients. In addition to anatomic changes in the urethra, atrophy of the vaginal epithelium may be associated with poor urethral function, which can contribute to intrinsic sphincter deficiency (ISD) being an etiology of the incontinence. ISD is characterized by failure of the urethra to function properly regardless of the anatomic position of the urethra.[6] ISD can exist in old women who have stress incontinence with an associated anatomic abnormality as well as those who have no evidence of anatomic changes or prolapse. Clinically, it is essential to identify elderly women who have ISD as an etiology of SUI so as to counsel the patient about specific therapy for it. ISD is intrinsic failure of the urethra to function normally and requires a therapeutic approach different from that for anatomic SUI.

#### *Urodynamic Studies*

Urodynamic studies of bladder function in elderly patients are necessary for the diagnosis and treatment of UI. Such studies consist of a sequence of bladder and urethral function measurements that often seem confusing to elderly patients and to the referring physician. Because UI in elderly women is considerably more complex than that in young women, the value of complete urodynamic studies is especially important in the old patient. Complete urodynamic studies can be performed in elderly patients with minimal discomfort, and the studies provide invaluable clinical information essential to the diagnosis and treatment of incontinence in this group of patients.

The urinary flow rate is usually the initial bladder function measurement, and it can be performed in the physician's office without significant inconvenience or discomfort to the patient. To perform a urinary flow study, the patient is positioned on a specially designed commode chair, and she voids into a urinary flow unit. The urinary flow rate is inexpensive, relatively easy to interpret, and provides valuable clinical information about bladder function. The uroflow parameters include the voiding time, peak urinary flow, mean urinary flow, and voided volume of urine. Usually the residual urine volume is measured after the patient voids for the urinary flow rate. The residual urine volume can be measured with an ultrasound scan of the bladder or with a catheterized residual volume determination. Although the uroflow studies are valuable clinically, they alone do not provide the necessary information to establish the presence of such disorders as bladder outlet obstruction; further urodynamic evaluation is required here, including a pressure-flow study.

Cystometrography is one of the most important studies of bladder function in elderly women. It is performed by continuous filling of the urinary bladder using a catheter through the urethra to measure the total capacity of the bladder, the sensation of filling experienced by the patient, the pressure–volume relation of the bladder, and the contractility of the bladder. In many elderly women the capacity of the bladder is small, the bladder may contract involuntarily causing urinary incontinence, or the bladder may not stretch properly, resulting in an abnormal increase in resting pressure during filling. These abnormalities of bladder function are just some of those that occur in elderly patients with UI that can be found on routine cystometric bladder studies, and they must be identified and treated according to the diagnosis provided by routine cystometry.

Pressure-flow studies measure the pressure inside the bladder during voluntary voiding and simultaneously measure the resulting urinary flow rate. This study is essential for assessing the voiding dynamics of the patient who has a low peak flow rate on routine uroflow studies. The clinician must determine if the cause is a low detrusor pressure or a bladder outlet obstruction. Elderly women who have bladder outlet obstruction or low detrusor pressure during voiding also may have incomplete emptying of the bladder. Either of these problems that result in an elevated postvoiding residual urine volume can cause bladder hyperactivity and may be associated with urinary incontinence. A high detrusor pressure during voluntary voiding with an associated low urinary flow rate is diagnostic of bladder outlet obstruction.

Bladder outlet obstruction in elderly women can have a functional or anatomic etiology; it is usually associated with previous surgical procedures that resulted in obstruction of the urethra. Urethral obstruction that results from previous surgery may produce a fixed outlet obstruction without correcting the etiology of the SUI. In these patients, SUI due to sphincteric dysfunction can coexist with bladder outlet obstruction, as the urethral obstruction is enough to produce bladder obstruction but not enough to produce continence. This is because urethral resistance is a static resistance instead of the normal dynamic functional resistance of the urethra. Bladder outlet obstruction due to fixed resistance within the urethra cannot be identified unless combined bladder pressure and urinary flow rate studies are done simultaneously. The pressure-flow studies represent the most important assessment available to determine the dynamics of bladder and urethral function of elderly women who have UI.

Another critical part of the evaluation of elderly women with UI is measurement of urethral function.[7] Measuring the pressure of the urethra throughout the functional length is a study called the urethral pressure profile (UPP). The UPP is an important measurement of urethral function, but it is not necessarily a measure of the continence function of the urethra. Simultaneous measurement of urethral pressure and intravesical pressure during coughing provides a differential pressure between the bladder and urethra. This has been called the stress urethral pressure profile and has added significantly to the clinical applications of the UPP. With the introduction of the concept of ISD, the abdominal leak point pressure measurement has been used much more commonly as a clinical assessment of the continence function of the urethra.

The abdominal leak point pressure (ALPP) is a measurement of the intraabdominal pressure required to produce leakage of urine from the bladder through the urethra.[8] This study requires fluoroscopic evaluation of the patient during a straining maneuver. Although this study is highly accurate and predictive of the outcome of surgical procedures for SUI in elderly women, the requirement of simultaneous use of fluoroscopy during the study precludes routine use of the test in many clinical environments. ALPP does remain the most clinically important study when evaluating urethral function in elderly women with symptoms of SUI and is essential for diagnosing intrinsic ISD. In patients who have a low ALPP, a urethral sling procedure is required to correct the symptoms of SUI if a surgical procedure is being considered. The long-term failure rate of any of the numerous bladder suspension procedures in these patients is high, and a urethral sling procedure is the only operative procedure that has a high long-term success rate in these patients. If the ALPP is more than 60 $cmH_2O$, then ISD is not likely to be a significant factor in the etiology of UI;

hence a routine bladder suspension procedure is usually successful in correcting the problem of anatomic incontinence and alleviating the symptoms of SUI in the elderly woman.

Electromyography (EMG) of the striated sphincteric muscles is one of the more difficult clinical diagnostic studies.[9] Among elderly women it is especially important for patients in whom neurologic disease is the etiology of the UI or a contributing factor. Neurologic disease in the elderly as a cause of urinary incontinence may originate in the central nervous system (CNS) in those who have such diseases as a previous stroke. Neurologic disease as a cause of UI also may originate in the spinal cord in old patients who have diseases such as intervertebral disc disease, or a neurologic disease that causes UI may originate peripherally with such diseases as diabetes. EMG is especially important in patients with UI who may not be suspected to have associated neurologic disease but have a history of degenerative disc disease of the spine or multiple previous operative procedures for disc disease of the back.

## Pathophysiology of UI in Elderly Women

Urinary incontinence is usually considerably more complex in elderly women than in young women. In general, incontinence in old women can be caused by abnormalities of bladder function, abnormalities of urethral function, or combinations of bladder and urethral dysfunction.[10] Close attention to the clinical characteristics of the symptoms of UI in old women from their incontinence history can be helpful for identifying the etiology of the UI. However, a precise description by the elderly patient of her symptoms usually is not nearly as helpful in the diagnosis as is a description of the characteristics of symptoms in young women. For this reason, urodynamic studies along with endoscopic and fluoroscopic studies have a significance in the diagnosis and treatment of UI in old women. Even with extreme attention to every detail of the assessment by the clinician, there is a greater degree of imprecision when determining the pathophysiology of UI in old women compared with young women.

### *Urge Urinary Incontinence*

A common cause of incontinence in elderly women is an overactive bladder, which is characterized by symptoms of urgency, frequency, nocturia, and episodes of urge UI. Elderly women who have symptoms of urinary urgency usually have associated nocturia.

A significant clinical difference between elderly women and young women regarding the symptom of urge UI is that older women frequently complain that they have no warning of the event.[11] Young women usually describe intense urgency with an inability to control the episode of urgency voluntarily. In contrast, the elderly woman often describes the incontinence event as occurring with little or no warning at all. Although the sensation of urgency exists in elderly women, the duration of the sensation prior to the onset of incontinence is often only a few seconds. The etiology of this clinical observation is unclear, but it appears to be associated with aging. The effects of aging on the lower urinary tract function somehow result in bladder overactivity in many elderly women.

### *Hyperreflexic Contractility*

Incontinence associated with true detrusor hyperreflexia is, by definition, caused by some type of associated neurologic disease.[12] Most commonly in the elderly, detrusor hyperreflexia occurs after a stroke or some other CNS disease, such as parkinsonism. Detrusor hyperreflexia may result from spinal cord disease related to herniated disc disease or previous back surgery in old people. Urinary symptoms due to neurologic detrusor hyperreflexia in elderly patients usually occur both day and at night with a smaller than normal urine volume in the bladder. The cystometrogram almost always shows a reflex detrusor contractile response associated with filling of the bladder to a relatively small volume. In elderly patients with spinal cord disease, the EMG often shows simultaneous contraction of the external urethral sphincter and contraction of the urinary bladder, resulting in extremely high bladder pressures with failure to empty. It is due to the high outlet resistance of the contracted external urethral sphincter and is called detrusor-sphincter dyssynergia. In most of these patients, neurologic disease that affects urinary bladder function also affects other areas of the body; and the associated functional deficits are usually clinically apparent.

### *Bladder Compliance*

Urinary incontinence associated with abnormal bladder compliance is a critical diagnosis that must be excluded in every elderly woman who has symptoms of an overactive bladder. In a normal person, the increase in volume in the bladder is not associated with a significant increase in pressure within the bladder. However, in patients with abnormal compliance, the pressure within the bladder increases as the volume in the bladder increases. This is a serious intrinsic problem of the urinary bladder, as it can result in obstruction of the kidneys due to a high resting pressure within the bladder that does not allow the ureters from the kidneys to drain properly. Abnormal bladder compliance can result from an injury to the bladder; it can occur following radiation therapy or chemotherapy to the bladder; or it can be associated with systemic diseases such as diabetes. A common clinical etiology of abnormal bladder compliance resulting from injury is due to bladder decentralization caused by peripheral neural injury that occurs at the time of a radical hysterectomy or an abdominoperineal resection. Abnormal bladder compliance can also be induced by prolonged treatment with a Foley catheter or an indwelling suprapubic catheter. Abnormal bladder compliance is diagnosed by cystometrography. Urodynamic studies are essential to the diagnosis and treatment of the elderly woman with UI.

### Stress Urinary Incontinence

In a normal person the pressure within the urethra increases reflexly with increases in intraabdominal pressure. During episodes of coughing or sneezing the pressure within the abdomen sharply increases to a high pressure. However, through neurologically mediated reflex mechanisms, the normal resting pressure within the urethra quickly increases to a level higher than the pressure within the abdomen to prevent leakage of urine from the bladder through the urethra.[7] When this normal compensatory reflex mechanism of the urethra fails to function properly, urine leaks through the urethra from the bladder during episodes of increased intraabdominal pressure. This condition is called stress urinary incontinence (SUI).

In the elderly woman, there is a gradual decrease in the resting pressure within the urethra with advancing age. Part of the change in pressure is due to a loss in the vascularity of the submucosa of the urethra. This soft submucosa in young women serves as a "gasket" by providing a seal within the urethra when changes in abdominal pressure occur. Estrogen-deficient elderly women usually have a large loss of vascularity in the urethral submucosa, resulting in loss of the gasket effect within the urethra. Loss of the gasket effect of the submucosal seal of the urethra results in failure of the compensatory pressure mechanism within the urethra to be effective in containing the urine within the bladder during episodes of increased intraabdominal pressure. Clinically, this condition results in SUI.

Another effect of aging in women is loss of the normal support of the bladder and urethra. Many elderly women are often told by their physician that their bladder has "fallen down." With increases in intraabdominal pressure such as coughing and straining, there is often rotation of the base of the bladder and proximal urethra into the vagina. Such prolapse is associated with loss of the reflex compensatory pressure mechanism of the urethra. This type of SUI is called anatomic SUI. When an anatomic abnormality or prolapse of the base of the bladder and urethra is associated with urinary incontinence, a surgical procedure is usually required to correct the abnormality and so prevent the persistent symptoms of SUI.

### Intrinsic Sphincter Deficiency

When the compensatory reflex pressure mechanism within the urethra is inadequate because of abnormal function of the intrinsic properties of the urethra itself, it is called intrinsic sphincter deficiency (ISD). In many cases, the cause of ISD is unclear. It is much more common in elderly women owing to loss of the intrinsic function of the urethra associated with the vascular submucosa that provides the gasket seal of the urethra. ISD is diagnosed by the abdominal leak point pressure test.[6] Currently, an abdominal leak point pressure less than 60 cm$H_2O$ is considered to reflect abnormal intrinsic urethral sphincter function. It is more complicated to manage elderly women with ISD clinically than those who do not have ISD.

When ISD coexists with anatomic incontinence or prolapse, a pubovaginal sling procedure is usually the only treatment for successful long-term management of these patients. The short-term postoperative morbidity associated with a pubovaginal sling procedure for treatment of UI in elderly women is significant in some patients. If an anatomic abnormality does not exist, intraurethral bulking agents such as collagen may be used successfully in some cases.

### Mixed Incontinence

Mixed incontinence in elderly women refers to an etiology of UI within the same patient that consists of both an overactive bladder and SUI due to urethral dysfunction.[13] Mixed incontinence is considerably more complex to treat than either SUI or urge urinary incontinence (UUI). Usually both components must be treated, and they are usually treated separately. There appears to be some interaction between SUI and UUI. For example, successful treatment of SUI usually results in improvement or resolution of UUI. Often successful treatment of UUI alleviates the symptoms of SUI. Generally, successful treatment of mixed incontinence requires combination therapy that manages both components.

## Nonsurgical Treatment of UI in Elderly Women

### Pharmacologic Therapy

Although pharmacologic therapy has been effective in many young women with urinary incontinence, the efficacy and side effects have limited its use in elderly women. For patients with UUI symptoms, cholinolytic drugs such as oxybutynin (Ditropan) are among the most common agents used. In general, cholinolytic drugs have not been as effective in the elderly patient with symptoms of an overactive bladder as in the younger woman. Side effects of a dry mouth and dryness of the eyes in the elderly have frequently limited the use of oxybutynin, but the occasional elderly patient who experiences confusion associated with that drug causes major concern about the use of this drug in old people.

The first of a group of new drugs available for clinical use for treatment of the overactive bladder in the elderly is tolterodine (Detrol). Tolterodine is more highly selective for the bladder than for the salivary glands and has been better tolerated in the elderly. In addition, it does not appear that the problem of confusion is as prevalent with tolterodine as it has been with oxybutynin. Tolterodine appears to be a more effective drug for the treatment of bladder overactivity in elderly patients with considerably fewer side effects than are seen with oxybutynin.

α-Adrenergic drugs have produced clinical improvement in young women with mild SUI. One of the most common drugs used is phenylpropanolamine, usually in doses of 75–150 mg daily. Again, the problem of side effects of this class of drugs in the elderly precludes its routine use for SUI. Cardiac problems, including hypertension, are among the many contraindications for use of α-adrenergic medications in elderly women.

### *Behavioral Therapy*

The most common behavioral therapy used for both SUI and UUI in elderly women is some modification of the Kegel exercises. The original technique of pelvic muscle exercises (PMEs) described by Kegel was a form of biofeedback therapy. However, since the original description by Kegel, multiple modifications of PME have occurred that do not involve any type of feedback. In fact, PME taught by verbal instruction alone is inadequate for the elderly woman to learn to perform the desired muscle contractions for the training program. Pelvic muscle exercises work primarily by a reflex inhibition of bladder contraction when the muscles are contracted.

### *Biofeedback Therapy*

Of the behavioral therapies, the most effective form of training is biofeedback, which is a precise technique for teaching patients to do the PMEs. It provides feedback regarding the performance of PMEs to the patient.[14] The performance is usually displayed to the patient by both visual and auditory feedback signals. The patient learns quickly to perform precise muscle contraction activities that allow maximum return of bladder control. PME therapy is useful for both UUI and SUI, although the efficacy of biofeedback for SUI appears to be less than that for UUI. For the elderly woman with UUI, biofeedback is considered by many to be the therapy of choice. It has the advantages of being effective with no potential side effects.

### *Timed Voiding*

It has been shown that the inability to prevent an involuntary bladder contraction is only part of the aging process affecting bladder function. Another significant symptom is the inability to voluntarily initiate voiding. It is common for elderly women who have UUI to be unable to initiate voiding voluntarily even though a significant amount of urine is present in the bladder. Shortly after an unsuccessful attempt to empty the bladder, the elderly woman may experience an episode of UUI. Although it is unclear that prompted voiding addresses this specific problem associated with aging, a timed voiding schedule usually improves continence in this group. The treatment program is relatively simple. The patient voluntarily voids at fixed time intervals while awake. The interval is usually 2 hours during waking hours. This regimen teaches the patient to inhibit the bladder voluntarily during the 2-hour interval and to initiate voiding upon command. A timed voiding schedule can be combined with biofeedback therapy as a part of a comprehensive behavioral therapy program.

## Surgical Treatment of UI in Elderly Women

Surgical treatment of UI is usually much more complex in elderly women than in young women, primarily because of a component of mixed incontinence exists in many elderly women who have SUI and the unusual complexity of the mixed incontinence that often occurs with aging. The approach to surgical treatment of the elderly woman also depends on the general health of the patient and existing co-morbid conditions.

There is no question that UI is a debilitating disease in elderly women, but it is rarely a cause of death. For this reason, it must be recognized that surgical treatment of UI in elderly women has improvement in quality of life as the major goal of treatment. Therefore it is not reasonable to risk survival or existing quality of life with a surgical approach to treatment of UI in these women without reasonable assurance of successful improvement in quality of life resulting from the operative procedure. In properly selected elderly patients, the long-term success of surgery is excellent, but the marked improvement in quality of life resulting from surgery is often denied the older patient on the basis of age alone.[15]

Conventional urethral suspension procedures can be used routinely in the elderly woman with uncomplicated SUI.[16] An uncomplicated patient is one who has not failed previous operative procedures for SUI, does not have intrinsic sphincter deficiency, does not have significant coexisting UUI, and does not have serious co-morbid conditions. In addition, urodynamic studies should demonstrate normal bladder function on cystometry and pressure-flow studies. Transvaginal procedures such as the Raz procedure or the modified Pereyra procedure, are often used in the elderly woman because of the low risk of mortality from the surgery. Other considerations for the surgical treatment of uncomplicated SUI in the elderly woman, include modifications of the Burch operative technique. However, no operative procedure should be considered in the elderly woman with SUI until a complete evaluation of bladder and urethral function has been accomplished.

For elderly women with ISD and any degree of prolapse of the bladder and urethra, a pubovaginal sling procedure is the only operative technique likely to be successful. This operative technique is slightly more difficult to perform than a urethral suspension procedure and has a slightly higher incidence of associated postoperative morbidity. A pubovaginal sling procedure should not be considered in the elderly woman with SUI unless a complete evaluation is done to determine the status of urethral and bladder function. Assessment of the urethra and bladder allows appropriate selection of the operative procedure and the ability to predict the outcome of the operation.

In the elderly woman with ISD without evidence of bladder or urethral prolapse, intraurethral bulking agents such as collagen can be used,[17] which typically works well in these patients. It is common for patients after intraurethral collagen to develop recurrent SUI over a long time, however, requiring repeat intraurethral injections of the collagen material. This problem is usually not significant because the injections can be done in the office with local anesthesia, and the procedure is completed within a few minutes. Complications associated with intraurethral injections are minimal, and the success rate has been particularly good in the elderly woman with SUI due to ISD without an anatomic defect.

## Urinary Incontinence in Elderly Men

### Clinical Assessment

The assessment of UI in elderly men consists of a precise, complete characterization of the symptoms experienced by the patient. A voiding diary is an important part of the assessment of community dwelling elderly men with UI. Also the American Urological Association symptom score for benign prostate hyperplasia (BPH) can be useful for identifying patients with bladder outlet obstruction.[18] In the chronic care environment, assessment of the severity of incontinence is more difficult. Usually the number of times each day absorbent pads must be changed is an indicator of the severity of incontinence in both community dwelling and chronic care elderly men. The severity of incontinence includes the frequency of episodes and the volume of involuntary urine loss. Unlike elderly women, SUI caused by sphincteric incompetence is rare in men who have not undergone previous prostate or pelvic surgery. Therefore incontinence in elderly men is almost always associated with involuntary detrusor contractions, which means that bladder contractions occur without the patient being able to prevent the occurrence of the episodes voluntarily.[19] Elderly men with symptoms of UUI almost always experience involuntary detrusor contractions, which are the cause of the UI. In fact, it is reasonable to assume clinically that the etiology of UUI in elderly men is involuntary detrusor contractions even though the cystometrogram may show a stable bladder during filling.

The initial clinically useful study in elderly men with UI is usually measurement of the urinary flow rate by office ultrasonography or catheterized residual urine measurement. A peak urinary flow rate of less than 15 ml/s is usually associated with bladder outlet obstruction. An elevated residual urine volume of more than 50 ml also is usually associated with bladder outlet obstruction.

A common characteristic of the aging bladder function in men is the inability to initiate voiding voluntarily. Therefore the elderly man may be unable to void for a urinary flow rate test, and ultrasonography may show that the bladder contains more than 100 ml of urine. The elderly man with UI often experiences an episode of UI shortly after being unable to void voluntarily even when the bladder contains an adequate amount of urine for voluntary voiding. When the elderly man is unable to void, a catheterized urine volume at that time does not represent a postvoiding residual urine volume. An accurately performed postvoid residual urine volume may show variation from one voiding episode to another within the same elderly male patient and may need to be repeated for accuracy when possible. The postvoid residual volume can be obtained only after the patient has voided. Also, the postvoid residual volume is useful only if the patient has voided a significant urine volume, usually considered to be 100 ml or more.

Cystometrography is important in elderly men who have UI to determine if bladder compliance is normal. That is, the resting pressure in the bladder should not show a significant rise during filling to the capacity at which the patient feels the urge to void. Unstable detrusor contractions are considered to be a significant finding on filling cystometry studies, although detrusor instability is not necessarily diagnostic of an underlying bladder disorder in elderly men, as the instability is seen in otherwise normal elderly men as well. The most significant finding with filling cystometry is determining the capacity of the bladder and establishing that bladder compliance is normal.

The simultaneous measurement of bladder pressure and urinary flow rate during voluntary voiding is the most important study when evaluating bladder outlet obstruction in elderly men due to BPH. A pressure–flow study in an elderly man that shows a high detrusor pressure and low urinary flow rate during voluntary voiding is diagnostic of bladder outlet obstruction. Therefore, pressure–flow is one of the most important studies in the urodynamic evaluation of the elderly man with UI. Elderly men who have UI and bladder outlet obstruction should be considered for surgical correction of the obstruction. It usually involves transurethral resection of the prostate (TURP). In many elderly men with significant bladder outlet obstruction and associated UUI, the latter resolves within a few weeks to months following surgical correction of the obstruction. If UUI persists after the bladder outlet obstruction has been surgically corrected, cholinolytic drugs such as tolterodine (Detrol) may be used to treat clinical bladder overactivity.

It is clinically necessary to determine if bladder outlet obstruction is present before using a cholinolytic drug in elderly men with UUI. Cholinolytic medications decrease detrusor contractility, which is contraindicated in patients with existing outlet obstruction of the bladder. Elderly men with bladder outlet obstruction due to BPH usually have high bladder pressure during voiding to empty the bladder considering the degree of bladder outlet resistance. If the bladder pressure is decreased by the cholinolytic medications used to treat overactive bladder symptoms, acute urinary retention may result because of a decrease in bladder pressure resulting from the medication. Therefore, surgical correction of bladder outlet obstruction is necessary before implementing cholinolytic drug therapy for bladder overactivity in elderly men who have UI and coexisting bladder outlet obstruction due to BPH.

## Pathophysiology of UI in Elderly Men

Although most continent elderly men experience nocturia, those with UI have a higher number of nocturia episodes than continent men. Most old men awaken completely during these events of nocturia and may complain about having difficulty returning to sleep. Poor-quality sleep in old men is common and may contribute significantly to decreased mental alertness during the daytime. Like elderly women, many elderly men who experience episodes of UUI describe the episode as one in which involuntary voiding occurs with little or no warning of an impending incontinence episode.

The ordered biologic systems regulating micturition in normal young men appears to be impaired in elderly incontinent men, and the normal physiology of voiding is disordered. It may be associated with aging or possible localized CNS deficits. Studies have been performed that carefully measured the exact time of an incontinence episode and the exact volume of involuntary urine loss in elderly incontinent men. It was found that within patients the volume of involuntary urine loss had a wide variation, with no predictability regarding volume of urine loss for any given incontinence episode. In addition, the interval between episodes was measured, and it was found that a wide range of variation in interval between episodes occurred with no predictability of the interval. Also, the residual urine was measured following an incontinence episode. The volumes of the urine loss during the incontinence episode and the residual urine were measured. The total volume at the time of the incontinence episode also showed wide variation within patients. It was apparent from these studies that the occurrence of an incontinence episode in elderly incontinent men was independent of the accumulated volume of urine in the bladder at the time of the incontinence episode.

The same group of patients who demonstrated such irregular bladder activity also demonstrated voluntary voiding without incontinence on a routine basis. These clinical observations suggest that elderly men with UUI have random detrusor contractions resulting in urinary incontinence, whereas the neural pathways required for normal voluntary voiding remain intact. This finding suggests that UI may represent abnormal bladder contractions originating from a neurologic mechanism different from the normal bladder contraction that occurs under voluntary control.

This type of UUI is the most common type of incontinence seen in elderly men. As described previously, SUI is rare in men who have not had previous prostate or pelvic surgery. Elderly men who have undergone radical prostatectomy for adenocarcinoma of the prostate may have SUI resulting from sphincteric incompetence. Failure of the urethral sphincter mechanism following radical prostatectomy is usually due to ISD. Urinary incontinence in elderly men due to an abnormality of the urethral sphincter mechanism following a TURP is uncommon. Patients who have persistent UI after a TURP usually have detrusor dysfunction as the etiology of the UI, with the urethral sphincteric mechanism intact. Elderly men with UI following abdominoperineal resections for colon carcinoma rarely experience SUI due to sphincteric incompetence. The etiology of sphincteric incompetence following abdominoperineal resection is unclear. Voiding disorders following such a resection are uncommon and are likely due to a problem with the bladder, possibly to partial denervation of the bladder during the operative procedure. These patients may also experience UI due to abnormal bladder compliance. Therefore all patients who experienced UI following previous pelvic surgery should have complete urodynamic assessment of both bladder and urethral function before considering therapy.

## Nonsurgical Treatment of UI in Elderly Men

If bladder outlet obstruction has clearly been excluded as an etiology of UUI in elderly men, nonsurgical therapies can be implemented. They include pharmacologic and behavioral therapies.

### *Pharmacologic Therapy*

Medical management of the overactive bladder in elderly men is similar to that in elderly women. Oxybutynin (Ditropan) has been used to treat the overactive bladder in elderly men for years, but the side effects are poorly tolerated in this patient population. The side effect of most serious concern is confusion, which is of particular concern in those who operate automobiles. For this reason, oxybutynin has not been routinely used in elderly men with UUI.

Tolterodine (Detrol) is a newer drug used to treat the overactive bladder in elderly men. It is highly effective and well tolerated in this group. Because of the ease of administration and the low incidence of side effects, tolteradine is considered the drug of choice for initial therapy of the overactive bladder in elderly men. Before initiation therapy with tolterodine, the clinician must be certain that there is no bladder outlet obstruction due to BPH.

### *Behavioral Therapy*

Pelvic muscle exercises can be used in men with UUI that are similar to those used by women. Pelvic muscle exercise (PME) programs are typically variations of the original Kegel exercises. It is important to remember that the original Kegel exercises were done by women using a perineometer, which provided visual feedback of performance to the patient. Over a period of time, modifications of the Kegel exercises became various forms of pelvic muscle exercises. The major problem with PME programs is the instruction of the patient. It is difficult to instruct an elderly man in the PMEs. For this reason more precise techniques (e.g., biofeedback) are considered more efficacious.

Biofeedback is not commonly used for behavioral therapy in elderly men because it requires complex equipment and trained personnel. However, it is extremely effective for treating those with symptoms of an overactive bladder.[14] It is important to select the proper signal source, which is usually perianal EMG activity displayed as visual and auditory feedback of performance.

Biofeedback therapy depends on the functional status of the patient to some extent. It is important that the patient has adequate mental function and reasonable physical function. Because biofeedback is a training program, it requires a level of mental function that allows training to take place; and enough physical function is required to allow contraction of the appropriate muscle groups. Although biofeedback therapy has been used in chronic care patients, it is generally more suitable for community dwelling patients because of the higher level of functional status usually associated with the latter.

A timed voiding schedule is excellent therapy for elderly men with UUI. In general, the patient is required to void every 2 hours while awake. He then attempts to prevent voiding during the 2-hour interval and voluntarily initiates voiding on command at the end of the 2 hours. This regimen teaches the patient to inhibit the bladder voluntarily and to initiate voiding voluntarily, which improves bladder control. As with women, a PME program (which may be biofeedback-based) can be combined with a timed voiding schedule to improve the efficacy of behavioral therapy.

## Surgical Treatment of UI in Elderly Men

Surgical treatment of UI in men depends on the etiology of the UI. In patients who have detrusor hyperactivity and bladder outlet obstruction, the bladder outlet obstruction is treated surgically if possible with a TURP. The patient is then observed for resolution of the symptoms of the overactive bladder, which usually occurs in 2–3 months. If urge UI continues, a cholinolytic drug such as tolteradine should be considered. Behavioral therapeutic treatments may also be considered.

With postprostatectomy incontinence following radical prostatectomy for prostate cancer, the damage to the sphincteric mechanism is something that usually cannot be surgically repaired. Intraurethral injections of a bulking agent such as collagen, may be used as an initial therapy. Collagen has typically been beneficial in patients having relatively mild SUI. The overall long-term results of intraurethral collagen for severe postradical prostatectomy incontinence have been disappointing. In most patients who have severe SUI following radical prostatectomy, an artificial urinary sphincter is the best surgical treatment. Results with an artificial sphincter are good overall, but in the elderly patient manual dexterity is an important part of the functional status of the patient that is required for satisfactory results. The artificial urinary sphincter has a silicone pump located within the scrotum and requires manual pumping of the device through the scrotal skin. This activity requires a reasonable level of both mental function and manual dexterity.

Urinary incontinence following TURP is uncommon even in elderly patients. When it does occur, the etiology is likely detrusor hyperactivity. Rarely, sphincteric incompetence due to ISD is the etiology, and in these cases an artificial urinary sphincter is required to achieve continence.

# Conclusions

Urinary incontinence in elderly women and elderly men has a devastating impact on the quality of life of the individual. Because UI is rarely fatal in old people and because quality of life issues are profound, treatment of UI must improve quality of life without compromising survival or the existing quality of life.

Urinary incontinence in elderly women and men may have an etiology related to dysfunction of the bladder or of the urethra. In elderly men and women, the age-related abnormalities associated with changes in bladder activity are similar. In elderly women, SUI due to abnormal sphincter function is a common cause of incontinence in this group. ISD is much more common in elderly women than in young women. A combination of urethral function and bladder dysfunction may occur in elderly women and is referred to as mixed incontinence. Mixed incontinence is especially complex and usually much more difficult to treat successfully.

The overactive bladder in elderly men is similar to the overactive bladder in elderly women. Bladder outlet obstruction due to BPH is common in elderly men and can be a cause of bladder overactivity and UUI. If bladder outlet obstruction coexists with UUI in elderly men, surgical management of the obstruction should be considered if feasible. Following surgical management of bladder outlet obstruction, significant symptoms of overactive bladder usually appear but resolve over 2–3 months. If significant symptoms continue, cholinolytic drugs such as tolterodine may be used to control them. These drugs are contraindicated in the presence of existing bladder outlet obstruction due to BPH.

Elderly men who have ISD following radical prostatectomy for treatment of prostate cancer can be treated with intraurethral bulking agents such as collagen. Intraurethral collagen is usually more successful with patients who experience mild incontinence. An artificial urinary sphincter is usually required for postprostatectomy incontinence that is more severe.

Often elderly patients do not complain about the problem of incontinence because they are embarrassed about it and have lost their self-esteem. It is only after the problem is corrected that patients recover their self-esteem and are released from their self-imposed social isolation. Such isolation seriously compromises quality of life. For this reason, every reasonable treatment option for managing incontinence in elderly patients should be utilized to achieve maximum improvement in their quality of life.

## References


1. O'Donnell PD. Geriatric issues in female incontinence. In: Walters MD, Karram MM (eds) Clinical Urogynecology. St. Louis: Mosby-Year book, 1993:409.
2. Baldwin DD, Hadley R. Stress urinary incontinence. In: O'Donnell PD (ed) Urinary Incontinence. St. Louis: Mosby-Year Book, 1997:190.
3. Awad SA, Gajewski JB. Urge incontinence. In: O'Donnell PD (ed) Urinary Incontinence. St. Louis: Mosby-Year Book, 1997:202.
4. Wyman JF, Colling J, O'Donnell PD. Incontinence assessment. In: O'Donnell PD (ed) Urinary Incontinence. St. Louis: Mosby-Year Book, 1997:399.
5. Ganabathi K, Zimmern P, Leach GE. Evaluation of voiding dysfunctions. In: O'Donnell PD (ed) Geriatric Urology. Boston: Little Brown, 1994:203.
6. Kennelly MJ, McGuire EJ. Intrinsic sphincter deficiency. In: O'Donnell PD (ed) Urinary Incontinence. St. Louis: Mosby-Year Book, 1997:207.
7. O'Donnell PD. Surgical goals and mechanism of continence in treatment of stress incontinence. In: McGuire EJ, Kursh E (eds) Female Urology. Philadelphia: Lippincott, 1993:175.
8. O'Connell HE, McGuire EJ. Leak point pressure. In: O'Donnell PD (ed) Urinary Incontinence. St. Louis: Mosby-Year Book, 1997:93.
9. O'Donnell PD. Electromyography. In: Nitti VW (ed) Practical Urodynamics. Philadelphia: Saunders, 1998.
10. McGuire EJ. Pathophysiology of incontinence in elderly women. In: O'Donnell PD (ed) Geriatric Urology, Boston: Little Brown, 1994:221.
11. O'Donnell PD. The pathophysiology of urinary incontinence in the elderly. In: McGuire EJ (ed) Advances in Urology, vol 4. Chicago: Year Book, 1991:129–142.
12. Karram MM. Detrusor instability and hyperreflexia. In: Walters MD, Karram MM (eds) Clinical Urogynecology. St. Louis: Mosby-Year Book, 1993:263.
13. O'Donnell PD. Mixed incontinence. In: O'Donnell PD (ed) Urinary Incontinence. St. Louis: Mosby-Year Book, 1997:93.
14. O'Donnell PD. Biofeedback therapy of urinary incontinence. In: Raz S (ed) Female Urology. Philadelphia: Saunders, 1996.
15. O'Donnell PD. Urology in the elderly. In: Atkins RB (ed) Surgical Care for the Elderly, Philadelphia: Lippincott, 1997.
16. Nitti VW, Bregg KW, Raz S. Surgical management of incontinence in elderly women. In: O'Donnell PD (ed) Geriatric Urology. Boston: Little Brown, 1994:239.
17. Appell RA, Winters JC. Intraurethral injections. In: O'Donnell PD (ed) Urinary Incontinence. St. Louis: Mosby-Year Book, 1997:228.
18. American Urological Association Symptom Index. In: O'Donnell PD (ed) Urinary Incontinence. St. Louis: Mosby-Year Book, 1997:449.
19. O'Donnell PD. Pathophysiology of incontinence in elderly men. In: O'Donnell PD (ed) Geriatric Urology, Boston: Little Brown, 1994:229.

# 56
# Renal and Bladder Neoplasms in the Elderly

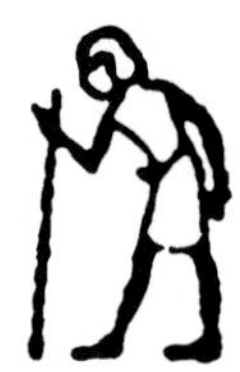

Daniel B. Rukstalis, David M. Hoenig, and Bruce J. Giantonio

One of the most profound events facing medicine today is the aging of the world's population. A triumph for the industrialized societies' efforts in nutrition, sanitation, and disease control, the "graying" of the population also represents a significant challenge for the effective utilization of medical resources. As preventive and therapeutic interventions succeed in reducing mortality from cardiovascular disorders, various other age-related disorders, such as cancer, are expected to increase in incidence. This phenomenon is associated with the observation that morbidity is compressed, or concentrated, in a reduced number of years late in life.[1] As a result, patients and their physicians will be increasingly faced with one of two possible scenarios. One clinical circumstance involves the appearance of a malignancy in an elderly individual in otherwise good health. In this circumstance an age bias against curative therapy may be unwarranted. In the alternative scenario the malignancy manifests in an individual already troubled with a complex set of medical problems such that any approach to therapy, curative or otherwise, would be costly and prone to failure.

Neoplastic diseases are the second most common cause of death in individuals over 65 years of age.[2] Perhaps more importantly, the manifestation of cancer as a chronic disease in elderly patients requires that treatment algorithms incorporate concerns about life expectancy, incidence of treatment complications, and the effect of therapy on the individual's quality of life. In this patient group, life expectancy is determined by age, comorbidity, activity level, and cancer stage.[3] Despite the potential risk of death from cancer, the extent of comorbid disease may be of greater significance than cancer status.[4] Therefore both standard and novel therapeutic approaches to the management of cancer should be evaluated for their impact on functional quality of life and treatment tolerance and their curative efficacy.

Approximately 58,000 men and 26,700 women developed a malignancy of the kidney or bladder in 1996.[5] Most of these individuals were older than 60 years of age and therefore likely to fall into one of the two clinical scenarios described above. Certainly the application of therapeutic technology to these patients requires an understanding of the natural history of the disease relative to the life expectancy of the individual. Importantly, the emerging treatment paradigms that incorporate quality of life considerations have resulted in focusing on the individual patient's point of view. As a result, a wide array of curative and noncurative approaches to renal and bladder cancer care have been developed. The remainder of this chapter discusses the spectrum of options and the rationale behind those options now available to the elderly person with these cancers.

## Renal Cell Carcinoma

### Epidemiology and Etiology

Neoplastic lesions within the renal parenchyma include an array of benign and malignant lesions. The predominant pathologic disorder is renal cell carcinoma, which comprises approximately 90% of all renal tumors. Because only the uncommon benign tumor, angiomyolipoma, can be distinguished from other solid lesions of the kidney by pretreatment radiologic evaluation, therapy is usually directed by the clinical expectation that a solid renal lesion is a renal cell carcinoma (RCC). This malignancy is most common in patients age 50–60 years, although in a review of 735 patients from The Netherlands, the highest incidence was for the age group 75–79 years.[6]

Clinical and basic science investigations have identified several putative etiologic factors for RCC. The increased incidence of this cancer in men relative to women implicates a hormonal factor. Although estrogen has been found to cause renal tumors in hamsters, no causal link has been established in humans.[7] Various chemical carcinogens, such as lead acetate and nitrosamines, also cause tumors in experimental animals but without clear correlates in human biology.[8] Perhaps the most significant etiologic finding has been provided by molecular investigations into genetic alterations associated with RCC. Cytogenetic analysis of chromosomal patterns within RCCs from patients with a hereditary form of the disease revealed a common deletion, or loss of DNA, on the short arm of chromosome 3 at the site of 3p14.2.[9] Subsequent molecular analysis has identified a specific gene, the *VHL* gene, which is inactivated through mutation in most RCCs in patients with an inherited syndrome called von Hippel-Lindau disease.[10] Although the subject of ongoing molecular study, it is likely that the *VHL* gene plays a specific role in the oncogenesis of the more common sporadic RCC, as 88% of these lesions harbor chromosome 3p deletions.[11] Although DNA alterations accumulate over time as individuals age, there is no evidence yet to implicate chromosome 3 deletions in the carcinogenesis of RCC in the elderly. Research in this area is likely to be fruitful.

## Natural History

Oncologic therapy in the geriatric population requires individualized treatment decisions that incorporate life expectancy of the host relative to the tumor biology of the disease. Therefore it becomes imperative to understand the natural history of RCC within the elderly population. Unfortunately, most reports do not specifically address the relation of renal cancer biology to age. Despite this limitation, several concepts can be elucidated. Primarily, the natural history of RCC in an individual patient is highly variable. The clinical presentation of RCC may vary from incidental identification of a small renal lesion to rapid progression of a large-volume cancer. Prior to the advent of computed tomography (CT) and ultrasonography (US), most renal cancers were detected upon clinical presentation with an abdominal mass, flank pain, or hematuria. Often these lesions were large, and up to 25% were associated with metastases.[12] Additionally, as many as 50% of patients manifest asynchronous metastatic spread following an attempt at curative surgical extirpation. RCC appears preferentially to spread to the lungs, lymph nodes, and bone, although metastatic lesions may be found in unusual sites, such as brain, gallbladder, epididymis, and skin. Individuals with distant disease have a median survival of 6–9 months with a 2-year survival of only 10–20% even with aggressive therapy.[13] These figures contrast with the anecdotal reports of 3- and 5-year survivals of 4.4% and 2.7%, respectively, for untreated RCC.[12] Accordingly, the choice of treatment for an elderly individual with a locally advanced or metastatic RCC must include considerations of treatment intensity and toxicity relative to expected survival.

Renal parenchymal neoplasms are now increasingly detected as incidental lesions during a US or CT examination for renal-related and non-renal-related indications.[14] The incidence of asymptomatic RCCs detected by autopsy has been reported to be 0.47%.[15] Another report of 16,294 autopsies performed over a 12-year period in an Italian population with an autopsy rate of almost 90%, demonstrated 350 cases of RCC. Importantly, 235 were unrecognized during the lifetime of the patients, and 80% of the individuals died of causes unrelated to RCC.[16] One plausible conclusion that may be drawn from this observation suggests that most renal cancers detected incidentally during radiologic evaluation do not limit the life expectancy of an elderly patient. However, more detailed information regarding the growth rate and metastatic characteristics of RCC is needed before therapeutic decisions can confidently include noncurative approaches. Bosniak and coworkers examined the growth rate of 40 solid renal masses <3.5 cm at the time of diagnosis in 37 patients.[17] The overall rate of growth was 0.36 cm/year with a mean follow-up of 3.25 years (range 1.8–8.5 years). The growth rate did not appear to correlate with tumor size but was positively correlated with calculated tumor volume. Tumor grade was associated with the size of the renal lesion as each of the four grade 2 cancers were >4.5 cm. There were no grade 3 lesions in this population. Importantly, none of the 37 patients developed evidence of metastatic disease during the period of this study. Alternatively, when a population of 54 patients treated with radical nephrectomy for stage 1 RCC were analyzed for the relation of tumor size to survival outcome, there was no difference in progression or survival between tumor size categories.[18] Interestingly, the median time to progression was 153 months for tumors <5 cm in diameter.

Despite the apparently protracted clinical course of incidentally discovered renal lesions, this cancer represents a significant health risk to an elderly individual. Damhuis and Blom investigated the relation of treatment outcome to patient age in 735 patients with RCC.[6] The overall 5-year survival for all stages was 37%, with both age and stage identified as prognostic factors. The patients over the age of 70 years were statistically less likely to be treated with curative resection (63% vs. 82%). This most likely represents a clinical bias toward noncurative treatments in the elderly, which could be supported with clinical data suggesting a protracted natural history for clinically localized RCC. However, the 5-year disease-specific survival of patients with an RCC localized to the renal unit (stage 1) was only 48% in the group over 70 years of age.

It appears that the natural history of even small renal cancers may be variable and difficult to predict for an individual patient based on size and clinical stage alone. Additional prognostic factors are necessary before treatment decisions can be made prior to surgical extirpation. Percutaneous aspiration biopsy techniques could potentially provide information about tumor grade, but the false-negative rate of this approach has been estimated to be 8%.[19] If adequate tissue could be obtained from a needle core biopsy sample to assess histology, further analysis is possible. One group of clinical investigators found an 88% (seven of eight cases) ability to obtain diagnostic information with a coaxial core biopsy needle in solid renal lesions.[20] Other investigators have demonstrated that the prognosis of RCCs treated with radical nephrectomy is closely correlated with tumor grade and DNA ploidy.[21,22] Therefore one clinical hypothesis suggests that incidentally discovered renal lesions could be evaluated by core biopsy in an effort to identify the poorly differentiated cancers with increased risk of progression. Well to moderately well-differentiated cancers could be considered for observational therapy in elderly individuals, and combination therapy could be focused on patients with more aggressive lesions. This potential approach may be offset by the fact that a percutaneous biopsy does present some risk of false-positive or false-negative results, as well as a reported risk for tumor seeding of the needle tract.[23] Nevertheless, although a percutaneous biopsy is unlikely to contribute useful information in a healthy patient with a solid renal mass, this approach may be useful in an elderly patient in whom conservative therapy is an appropriate option.

## Management

The foundation of surgical therapy for renal cancer is removal or destruction of the putatively localized neoplastic lesion along with adjacent normal parenchyma. In the elderly individual this must be accomplished in the setting of renal function, which diminishes with age. Many investigators have demonstrated a gradual decline in renal mass and creatinine clearance with age, which appears to be secondary to a loss of cortical tissue with sparing of the renal medulla.[24] Importantly, these age-related changes may be clinically silent unless associated with co-morbid conditions, such as hypertension or the use of pharmacologic agents.[25] Despite the clinical relevance, the deleterious effects of surgical extirpation on renal function have not been fully characterized in the elderly population. However, chronic renal insufficiency is a reported complication of both nephrectomy and partial nephrectomy in patients of any age.[26,27] Therefore treatment decisions must incorporate concerns about efficacy, co-morbid illness, and physiologic effects on renal function.

### *Radiologic Evaluation*

Because benign renal parenchymal alterations such as renal cysts are present in up to 50% of patients older than 50 years of age, sensitive and specific imaging techniques are needed to identify renal cancers.[28] The radiologic armamentarium includes the intravenous pyelogram (IVP), renal US, CT, and magnetic resonance imaging (MRI), each of which may be useful for diagnosing and staging a renal cancer. In general, the increased application of US and CT imaging for various medical indications has resulted in a severalfold increase in the diagnosis of RCC and other small renal lesions. Renal US examination is approximately 90% accurate in distinguishing a benign cyst from a solid mass but is unable to provide accurate staging information. The most valuable imaging technique appears to be MRI with intravenous gadopentetate dimeglumine. In a series of 108 patients, MRI identified 58 of 61 renal masses and correctly staged 29 of 31 lesions treated with surgical extirpation.[29] Performance of MRI is particularly important in an elderly individual because of the reduced risk of contrast-induced renal insufficiency with gadopentetate.

### *Radical Nephrectomy*

The performance of a radical nephrectomy as described by Robson et al. to include en bloc removal of the renal unit, perinephric fat within Gerota's fascia, and the ipsilateral adrenal gland is considered the standard treatment for clinically localized renal cancer.[30] Additionally, lymphatic tissue should be removed from around the renal vessels in an effort to identify the presence of lymphatic metastases. The identification of regional lymphatic involvement in up to 14% of individuals portends a poor outcome, as only 11–21% survive 5 years.[31] The extent of the retroperitoneal lymph node dissection, and by association the extent of surgical therapy, in each patient is controversial. It appears that an extensive lymphadenectomy may reduce the local recurrence rate following radical nephrectomy but has not been shown to augment survival.[16] Therefore the choice of curative therapy with radical nephrectomy in an elderly patient may be made with an attempt to minimize morbidity through the choice of surgical incision and without the need for an extended regional node dissection.

The disease-related outcome following this procedure is closely related to pathologic stage. Approximately 67–84% of patients with stage 1 RCC are alive without disease at 5 years.[32] Further information is detailed in Table 56.1. Importantly, the absence of effective systemic chemotherapeutic agents for RCC increases the need for complete surgical extirpation if cure is to be achieved. Of particular interest are the approximately 30% of patients

TABLE 56.1. Survival Following Surgical Therapy for Renal Cell Carcinoma

| Stage (TMN/Robson) | 5-Year survival (%) |
|---|---|
| T1–2 N0 M0/stage 1 | 48–90 |
| T3a N0 M0/stage 2 | 45–80 |
| T3b–3c N0–3 M0/stage 3 | 0–51 |
| T4 N0–3 M0–1/stage 4 | 0–10 |

TABLE 56.2. Complications of Radical Nephrectomy and Partial Nephrectomy

| |
|---|
| Radical nephrectomy |
| Death (0–4%) |
| Local cancer recurrence (<%) |
| Renal insufficiency (1.5–100%)[a] |
| Postoperative hemorrhage (0–2%) |
| Splenic injury (0–12%) |
| Prolonged ileus |
| Acute urinary retention |
| Wound infection |
| Partial nephrectomy |
| Death (0–2%) |
| Local cancer recurrence (4–10%) |
| Renal insufficiency (10–44%) |
| Postoperative hemorrhage (0–4%) |
| Splenic injury (0–5%) |
| Urinary fistula (0–17%) |
| Ureteropelvic junction (UPJ) obstruction (0–1%) |
| Wound infection |

[a] Renal insufficiency must be evaluated relative to the amount of remaining renal parenchyma. A radical nephrectomy for a solitary renal unit would produce renal failure in 100% of cases. A partial nephrectomy in the setting of a normal contralateral renal unit is unlikely to cause renal failure.

with otherwise clinically localized RCCs extending into the renal vein. Further extension into the inferior vena cava (IVC) and ultimately to the right atrium occurs in 0.5–5.0% of cases.[33] Surgical extirpation of these cancers often requires advanced surgical techniques such as IVC reconstruction and cardiopulmonary bypass with hypothermic arrest.[34,35] Although individual patients can be cured of their disease with this surgical approach the complication rate is high, with operative mortality rates of 1.4–13.0%. The choice of this treatment for an elderly patient with RCC is problematic because the associated morbidity and mortality relative to the age of the patient has not been determined.

Removal of a renal unit may be approached through one of several surgical incisions. Although no prospective clinical trials have assessed the morbidity of each approach, surgeons often feel strongly about the choice of incision. The options include a flank incision with or without removal of a portion of the 11th or 12th rib, a subcostal transperitoneal incision, and a thoracoabdominal incision. The latter approach involves resection of a rib and incision through the diaphragm. Exposure of the renal unit is optimized with the thoracoabdominal incision but, anecdotally, so is the postoperative morbidity. Most patients require placement of a tube thoracostomy for management of the consequent pneumothorax. Therefore large renal cancers may be removed expeditiously via this incision, but its application should be limited to patients with adequate pulmonary function.

### *Laparoscopic Radical Nephrectomy*

The first laparoscopic nephrectomy in a patient was reported in 1991 by Clayman and coworkers in an 85-year-old woman with a right renal cancer.[36] Since that initial report, laparoscopic nephrectomy for both benign and malignant disease has become common. Favorable outcomes demonstrating less morbidity than comparable open techniques are the rule. Preliminary data even suggest increased disease-free survival in the laparoscopic radical nephrectomy group compared to historical controls on a stage-to-stage basis.[37]

It appears that laparoscopy affords substantial benefits compared to the standard open radical nephrectomy. Patients experience reduced postoperative pain with diminished requirement for narcotic analgesics. This has been demonstrated to result in improved pulmonary function among patients treated by laparoscopic nephrectomy compared to that after open procedures,[38] suggesting that the minimally invasive laparoscopic approach may be particularly suitable to patients with poor pulmonary reserve.

### *Nephron-Sparing Surgical Therapy*

Considerations regarding postoperative morbidity including renal dysfunction after a radical nephrectomy (Table 56.2), have led surgeons to investigate alternative approaches for surgical ablation of RCCs. Additionally, renal cancer may manifest in an individual with a solitary renal unit, impaired renal function, or synchronous bilateral disease. The current indications for a parenchymal-sparing partial nephrectomy are depicted in Table 56.3. In these situations an attempt may be made to preserve a critical mass of normal renal parenchyma. The 5-year cancer-specific survival rates following performance of a partial nephrectomy for RCC have been reported to be 84–100%.[39,40] In fact, the success of this approach in patients who require a parenchymal-sparing treatment to avoid dialysis has encouraged application of partial nephrectomy in the setting of a normal contralateral kidney.[41] An elderly individual, even if in good health, is still at risk for age-related loss of renal function and is therefore a candidate for partial nephrectomy.

TABLE 56.3. Current Indications for Partial Nephrectomy

| |
|---|
| Mandatory indications |
| Renal cell carcinoma (RCC) in a solitary kidney |
| Bilateral RCC |
| von Hipple-Lindau disease |
| Renal insufficiency |
| Elective indications |
| Medical conditions at risk for renal insufficiency |
| Age-related decline in renal function |
| Small, incidental and peripheral RCCs |

The choice of a partial nephrectomy in an elderly patient with RCC may be viewed as an attempt to preserve adequate renal function while eradicating the malignancy. Further support for this approach is provided by the increased detection rate of small incidental lesions for which a radical nephrectomy may seem excessive. However, advocates of radical nephrectomy point out the 4–9% local recurrence rate of RCC after a partial nephrectomy.[42] Additionally, the surgical complications from a partial nephrectomy include retroperitoneal bleeding, urinary fistula, and nonfunction of the renal unit. Therefore the potential to preserve renal function in an elderly patient through performance of a partial nephrectomy must be weighed against the risk, albeit small, of unique complications. Butler and coinvestigators attempted to address the issue of comparative efficacy and morbidity of the radical and partial nephrectomy procedures in a group of 88 patients with small RCCs.[43] In this series the local recurrence rate and 5-year cancer-specific survival data were statistically similar for the two groups. Each group demonstrated a comparable incidence of postoperative complications, although the partial nephrectomy group did exhibit the expected urinary fistulas (3 of 46) and retroperitoneal hemorrhage (1 of 46). Hence the value of the more technically demanding partial nephrectomy for an elderly patient with RCC is uncertain. Further investigations are warranted, given the frequently emotional desire to preserve renal function.

### Cryoablation

The application of nephron-sparing techniques to patients with RCC have clearly demonstrated the ability to eradicate the malignancy while maximally preserving renal function. However, the performance of partial resection is technically demanding and associated with specific complications. Alternative methods for tissue destruction (e.g., application of cold or heat energy) may provide an opportunity to ablate renal cancer while avoiding the morbidity of surgical resection. Cozzi and coworkers demonstrated the tissue-destructive effects of cryoablation in a sheep model.[44] Importantly, there was no evidence of significant bleeding or urinary extravasation in any animal. An open renal cryotherapy procedure has been reported in two patients with renal lesions.[45] Neither patient required a blood transfusion, and each demonstrated stable renal function after the procedure. Postprocedure radiologic evaluation demonstrated the apparent infarction and resorption of the RCC in one patient. The second individual underwent cryotherapy for a 7 × 10 cm angiomyolipoma with an apparent 10% increase in the size of the lesion after 3 months.

The destruction of RCC by cryoablation is a novel and potentially beneficial therapeutic approach. This procedure is still experimental and should be approached with caution. Elderly individuals with small renal cancers and committed to preservation of normal renal parenchyma would be candidates for this approach.

### Management of Advanced RCC

Individuals with advanced RCC associated with lymphatic or distant metastases are unlikely to benefit from surgical therapy unless a radical nephrectomy is performed with palliative intent. Therefore systemic agents offer the most rational treatment options for old patients with this disease. Recommendations for or against administration of systemic therapy are often based on the age of the patient, although categorical recommendations for the therapy of cancers based on chronologic age are neither appropriate nor feasible. Variability among aging individuals with regard to physiologic senescence and co-morbid illness suggest that a more practical approach for the clinician is the use of guidelines to assess the elderly patient's functional and physiologic tolerability for potentially toxic therapy.

To begin, it is important to define those who are considered elderly. Without readily usable markers of physiologic age, Balducci recommended that the clinician begin to consider those individuals over 75 years of age as elderly.[46] These individuals have an increased occurrence of the following and, if documented, should be considered frail elderly and carefully evaluated: decreased musculoskeletal mass, functional limitations, geriatric syndromes (dementia, malnutrition, polypharmacy, incontinence, delirium), and multiple co-morbidities. Minimizing the risk of side effects from chemotherapeutic drugs in the elderly requires careful clinical assessment for functional ability and preexisting neuropathy, cardiac/hepatic/renal function, bone marrow reserve, nutrition, polypharmacy, and cognitive function. Interventions should include adjusted doses of renally excretable agents, use of support agents such as growth factors and cytoprotective agents when indicated, and appropriate nutritional support.

Treatment of advanced or metastatic RCC with chemotherapy or hormonal therapy has been ineffective. In an extensive review of 83 chemotherapy and hormone therapy trials that included more than 4000 patients, only 6% of patients had an objective response. The most activity, albeit marginal, was reported for 5-fluorouracil and floxuridine as single agents, with response rates of 10.0% and 14.6%, respectively.[47]

Building on observations that spontaneous remission occurred infrequently in individuals with metastatic disease who underwent nephrectomy, modulation of the immune system has become the major focus of therapeutic strategies for RCC. Immunotherapy with interleukin-2 (IL-2), interferon-α (IFN-α), or both are the most effective therapies yet identified for treating metastatic RCC. In the report of a 6-year experience using immunotherapy in 134 patients with RCC, the group at UCLA reported an 11% complete response rate and a 17% partial response rate. The widely varying and potentially lethal toxicity of these agents, particularly that of IL-2, demands that care be exercised when deciding to use these drugs in the elderly population.

Interleukin-2 was approved for use in metastatic RCC by the U.S. Food and Drug Administration (FDA) in 1992 based on data from trials using high dose intravenous infusions. The recommended dose is 600,000 international units (IU)/kg every 8 hours for up to 14 doses. The toxicity of the agent is dose- and schedule-dependent and at the high dose, is dominated by the capillary leak syndrome. Extravasation of intravascular fluids due to increased capillary permeability can occur during IL-2 therapy.[48] This shift can result in pulmonary edema, ascites, oliguria and azotemia, decreased peripheral resistance, peripheral edema, weight gain, and hypotension. Lethal complications include respiratory or renal insufficiency, myocardial infarction, and septic shock-like high output cardiac failure with approximately 4% of patients dying because of adverse events related to therapy.[49,50] This outcome may be avoided by excluding patients with documented cardiac disease by thallium stress testing and echocardiography.

Additional side effects of high-dose IL-2 therapy include fever, chills, malaise, myelosuppression, sepsis, nausea, diarrhea, mucositis, colonic distension, agitation, disorientation, coma, decreased cognitive function, impaired memory, serum bilirubin and transaminase elevations, pruritus, and vitiligo. Most of these effects are transient and resolve with discontinuation of the agent.[51] Fortunately, subcutaneously administered lower-dose IL-2 has demonstrated response rates similar to the high-dose bolus schedules with a much better tolerated toxicity profile. The rationale for using lower-dose IL-2 is based on the variable affinity-effector activation of the components of the IL-2 receptor. In vitro evidence suggests that low-dose IL-2 stimulates expansion of natural killer (NK) cells and antigen-stimulated T lymphocytes, whereas high dose therapy can promote programmed T cell death. Additionally, repeated low-dose immunotherapy may overcome tumor induced anergy.[52] A review of nine studies that included 190 patients treated with subcutaneously administered IL-2, suggested an overall response rate of 18%.[51] Capillary leak syndrome, hypotension, renal toxicity, and infection are infrequent. More commonly, patients experience fever, chills, nausea, and nodule formation at injection sites that are painful and hemorrhagic if the individual is anticoagulated.

The interferons were the first cytokines to be used clinically and have been found to have antiproliferative, immunomodulatory, and antiviral activity. IFN-α, which is available in recombinant form, has significant anticancer activity likely due to its pleiotrophic immunomodulatory effects that include monocyte and macrophage activation, induction of antigen and HLA expression, and induction of cytotoxic lymphocytes and NK cell activity, as well as a direct effect on protein synthesis and gene regulation.[51] As a single agent, IFN-α has reported response rates of 15–20% with less toxicity than IL-2.[53] In a review of more than 400 patients treated during phase II trials, 4 patients experienced a complete response and 57 exhibited a partial remission for an overall response rate of 15%.[54]

The rationale for combining IFN-α and IL-2 includes enhanced cytotoxic lymphocyte-mediated tumor lysis as a result of augmented tumor immunogenicity from increased histocompatibility and tumor antigen expression. Preclinical models have demonstrated synergistic activity for the two agents, and overall reported response rates for the combination are 20–30%.[51] In a study of 20 patients treated with low doses of subcutaneously administered IL-2 and INF-α, there was one complete response and three partial responses for an overall response rate of 20%. The toxicity of the combination was limited to World Health Organization (WHO) grades 1 and 2 and consisted chiefly of fever, chills, fatigue, and malaise.[55]

The use of immunotherapy for advanced RCC in the aged must be approached cautiously. Considerations for high-dose intravenous therapy should be restricted to the setting of a clinical trial and performed by those familiar with these agents. Several reviews have demonstrated that performance status is significant for prognosis and response to therapy. Patients with good performance status are more likely to respond to immunotherapy and have prolonged survival.[56] The relative tolerability of subcutaneously administered immunotherapy, although more attractive for use in the elderly, comes with a low likelihood of benefit, and its use must be carefully evaluated. Metastatic RCC is incurable for most patients, and therefore observation and palliation must also be considered as appropriate therapeutic choices.

## Transitional Cell Carcinoma of the Bladder

Neoplastic disease of the urinary bladder, the eleventh most common form of cancer in the world, represents a broad spectrum of pathologic processes, extending from indolent low grade papillomas to rapidly progressive poorly differentiated malignancies. The predominant pathologic entity is transitional cell carcinoma (TCC), which comprises approximately 90% of bladder lesions and is the focus of this discussion. The incidence of TCC is directly related to patient age, with a peak incidence during the seventh decade of life.[57] Interestingly, although bladder cancer is a common cause of death in men over age 75, an autopsy study of 267 individuals over age 95 discovered only two cases of TCC.[58] Neither of these cancers was responsible for the demise of the

TABLE 56.4. Potential Etiologic Agents for Transitional Cell Carcinoma

| |
|---|
| Established risk factors |
| Cigarette smoking (black tobacco higher than blond tobacco) |
| Phenacetin-containing analgesics |
| Aromatic amines (benzidine, 2-naphthylamine) |
| Leather workers (unknown agent) |
| Cyclophosphamide |
| Ionizing radiation |
| Potential risk factors |
| Age |
| Coffee drinking |
| Saccharin |
| Dietary fats |
| Chlorinated water |

patient, suggesting that the clinical incidence and impact of TCC of the bladder may diminish with advancing age. Therefore successful management of bladder TCC in the elderly patient requires an understanding of the natural history of TCC and the quality of life implications of each therapeutic approach.

## Diagnosis

Bladder cancer represents an important consideration in the differential diagnosis of voiding symptoms in the elderly individual. The presence of a neoplastic lesion within the bladder is often heralded by irritative symptoms such as urinary urgency, frequency, or dysuria. Approximately 12.0–38.8% of older men and women complain of such voiding symptoms, resulting in a large population of patients for whom a diagnostic evaluation may be warranted.[59]

Hematuria, microscopic or grossly visible, may also announce the existence of malignant bladder lesions. The data regarding the incidence of hematuria suggests that a large number of old people may be found with blood in the urine on routine examination. If the definition of clinically significant hematuria includes all urine samples with more than two red blood cells per high power microscopic field, approximately 9–18% of adult individuals exhibit hematuria.[60] It has been estimated that 5–15% of patients, predominantly men, with hematuria harbor unsuspected bladder cancer.[61] The accepted urologic evaluation for TCC includes urinalysis, urine cytology, and cystourethroscopy. Additionally, a radiographic evaluation of the upper urinary tract is also indicated, most commonly with an IVP in patients with normal renal function. The cost implications of this approach, given the incidence of voiding symptoms and hematuria, is obvious. At the present time it is difficult to identify a subpopulation of patients for whom a cancer evaluation is unnecessary. Individuals over the age of 60 with a history of cigarette smoking and any degree of hematuria should be evaluated. New-onset irritative voiding symptoms in the absence of a clear etiology such as infection also deserve consideration for evaluation.

## Natural History

Transitional cell carcinoma of the bladder has been causally linked to many environmental agents, listed in Table 56.4. The reason for the increasing incidence seen with advancing age is uncertain. Molecular biologic evidence suggests that various DNA alterations, such as the *p53* tumor-suppressor gene, are responsible for the initiation and promotion of TCC.[62] It is reasonable to speculate that particular regions of the human genome are more susceptible to age-related DNA damage and that important genes within those regions may be altered, resulting in a bladder cancer.

It is difficult to derive a clear understanding of the natural history of TCC from the literature because of the plethora of clinical presentations. Despite this limitation, a workable architecture can be developed based on the distinction between superficial and invasive carcinoma. Importantly, because superficial TCC exhibits an overall low risk of progression to a life-threatening cancer, this entity may be treated as a chronic illness in an elderly patient. A retrospective review of 761 patients with superficial bladder cancer treated with surgical extirpation alone, found that only 7% died of bladder cancer, and 15% expired owing to other causes.[63] Interestingly, age was not found to correlate with disease-free survival, suggesting that the biologic behavior of superficial TCC is similar in patients of all ages. Therefore a clear understanding of the distinction between a superficial and invasive lesion is central to the treatment of a geriatric patient with bladder cancer. The staging system for the primary bladder TCC is presented in Table 56.5.

## Superficial Transitional Cell Carcinoma

Approximately 75–80% of bladder TCCs present initially as a superficial lesion confined to the mucosa or submucosa of the bladder without evidence of muscle invasion.

TABLE 56.5. TMN Staging System for Carcinoma of the Urinary Bladder: Primary Cancer (T)

| | |
|---|---|
| Tx | Unable to assess primary tumor |
| T0 | No evidence intravesical cancer |
| Ta | Noninvasive papillary cancer |
| Tis | Flat carcinoma in situ |
| T1 | Cancer invades into lamina propria |
| T2 | Cancer invades into superficial one half of bladder muscle |
| T3 | Cancer invades into outer one half of muscle or through wall |
| T3a | Cancer into deep muscle |
| T3b | Penetrates through bladder wall into perivesical fat |
| T4 | Cancer involves adjacent structures |
| T4a | Involves prostate, uterus or vagina |
| T4b | Invades into pelvic or abdominal wall |

This category of lesions encompasses indolent neoplasms confined to the bladder mucosa (stage Ta) and lesions of greater concern that have invaded the lamina propria of the bladder wall (stage T1). Clinically situated between these two stages is the poorly differentiated flat cancer called carcinoma in situ (stage Tis). Given the markedly different natural history of these neoplasms, the traditional category of superficial TCC should be dropped in favor of the specific TMN stage designation. Therefore the remainder of this discussion refers to individual lesions as Ta, Tis, or T1.

The biologic behavior of superficial TCC is difficult to elucidate because most lesions are treated at the time of initial presentation with an endoscopic resection. In fact, the mainstay of conservative therapy for this cancer is performance of a complete transurethral resection which also provides information about cancer stage and grade. This procedure may be performed under inhalational or spinal anesthesia, which can be tailored to the medical condition of the patient. Furthermore, if the concomitant medical condition of the patient precludes general anesthesia, superficial lesions may be destroyed in situ using laser ablation or electrocoagulation with minimal sedation.[64] Information regarding the recurrence and possible progression of a TCC is available predominantly in patients initially treated with resection. Therefore this sequence is considered in the following discussion to represent the natural history of TCC in elderly patients.

The disease-specific outcome for superficial TCC is closely related to stage (Ta vs. T1) and histologic grade.[65] In general, stage Ta lesions exhibit a 50–90% recurrence rate at 5 years with an overall 2–25% rate of progression to muscle-invasive disease.[66,67] The established risk factors for both recurrence and progression include high grade (scale of 1 to 3), tumor size (>5 cm), number of lesions, and association with dysplasia or carcinoma in situ.[68] This is illustrated by the finding that stage Ta grade 1 and 2 cancers exhibit a recurrence rate of approximately 30%, whereas grade 3 lesions manifest a 70% recurrence rate. Importantly, stage Ta lesions rarely progress to a higher stage. Only 2–6% of Ta grade 1 or 2 lesions progress to deeper invasion, suggesting that most Ta lesions may be managed conservatively in geriatric patients with other health issues. In that context, patients who do not develop another tumor within 3 months of the initial resection of a TCC have an 80% probability of never demonstrating another cancer in the bladder.[66] A thorough cystoscopic evaluation of the bladder, coupled with complete resection of all visible Ta lesions, can differentiate an individual with a low risk of recurrence and progression from a patient at risk for progression to a life-threatening muscle-invasive cancer. Individuals with favorable cancers may be managed successfully with intermittent resection or even fulguration of recurrent lesions without additional treatments. However, patients who experience 10 or more recurrences exhibit a high rate of progression and death from TCC.[69] Therefore the paradigm of conservative therapy for stage Ta TCC with endoscopic resection alone should be modified if the patient demonstrates evidence of persistently recurrent disease.

Carcinoma in situ manifests as a flat collection of poorly differentiated cells that are limited to the mucosal surface of the bladder. Clinically, Tis lesions may present as a primary lesion of the bladder urothelium without other papillary lesions or concomitantly with another form of TCC. Interestingly, the natural history of stage Tis TCC is variable, suggesting that the biology is influenced negatively by the high grade and perhaps ameliorated by the lack of invasion. It has been suggested that the behavior of primary Tis lesions is more protracted than that of carcinoma in situ associated with stage Ta or T1 cancers.[70] The primary lesion may diffusely involve the bladder mucosa and extend into the distal ureters or prostatic ducts. Patients often present with severe irritative voiding symptoms and hematuria, or they may be relatively asymptomatic with only a cytologic abnormality visible on cystoscopy or urine cytology. The literature suggests that this lesion has a high recurrence rate (63–92%) despite therapy with both resection and intravesical chemotherapy.[71] Furthermore, Tis lesions maintain the ability to progress to invasive lesions in at least 50% of cases following endoscopic resection alone.[72] Therefore despite the age of the patient with primary or concomitant Tis, surgical therapy alone must be considered inadequate. In this setting, conservative therapy is defined as multimodality therapy involving endoscopic resection or biopsy in conjunction with intravesical chemotherapy. In patients with persistent or recurrent Tis, curative extirpation with a radical cystectomy should be considered.

The category of superficial TCC also includes an invasive lesion, stage T1, in which cells have demonstrated the ability to penetrate the lamina propria of the bladder wall but not the muscularis propria. These lesions exhibit a high likelihood of recurrence (67–81%) and progression (12–49%), with approximately 17–71% of patients dying of TCC following an initial presentation with stage T1 disease.[71] A stage T1 lesion of high grade or with lymphatic invasion within the lamina propria is an indication that more than simple endosurgical resection is required. Similar to stage Tis lesions, conservative therapy for T1 TCC is currently defined as endoscopic ablation in combination with instillation of intravesical chemotherapeutic or immunotherapeutic agents. In a retrospective review of 1205 patients with T1 TCC treated with intravesical agents following resection, only 17% developed muscle invasive disease.[73] In another series of 86 patients with T1 tumors a complete response rate of 91% was demonstrated for the combination of resection and intravesical bacillus Calmette–Guérin (BCG).[74] Alternatively, several published reports have advocated applica-

TABLE 56.6. Characteristics of Candidates for Intravesical Therapy

| |
|---|
| Indications |
| Tumor multiplicity |
| Recurrent Ta, T1 lesions |
| Grade 3 Ta, T1 lesions |
| Stage Tis |
| Size > 4–5 cm |
| Surgically uncontrollable Ta disease |
| Stage Ta with Tis |
| Prostatic urethral disease |
| Relative contraindications |
| Immunocompromised patient |
| Hypersensitivity to bacillus Calmette-Guerin (BCG) |
| Severe irritative voiding symptoms |
| Solitary Ta lesion |

tion of endoscopic resection alone for stage T1 TCC, particularly grades 1 and 2, with up to 40% of patients being cured with a single resection. A closer inspection of the patient series identifies a favorable subgroup of patients with a solitary T1 cancer if complete resection of the lesion is confirmed on a repeat bladder biopsy.[75] Therefore surgical resection alone may be appropriate therapy for the elderly individual with a solitary T1 cancer and other co-morbid illness. Nevertheless, there is a 10–30% difference in survival between patients who present with Ta TCC and those with T1 disease, suggesting that the T1 category of patients may require a more aggressive therapeutic approach.[76] Certainly individuals who manifest a recurrent T1 cancer following initial combination therapy are at high risk of progression to muscle-invasive disease and should be considered for radical cystectomy. Furthermore, at least one study has compared the disease-free survival of patients treated with immediate cystectomy for T1 TCC versus cystectomy for a recurrent T1 lesion after initial conservative treatment. The 5-year recurrence-free survival was 90% in the former group and 62% in the latter group, suggesting that immediate cystectomy at the time of initial diagnosis of a T1 cancer can improve survival.[77] The best therapy for T1 TCC in an elderly patient must be predicated on considerations of performance status, co-morbid illness, and quality of life issues, as either an initial conservative approach or an aggressive approach would be reasonable.

## Intravesical Therapy

The application of chemotherapeutic or immunotherapeutic agents into the urinary bladder has demonstrated efficacy in the eradication of existing disease, inhibition of tumor recurrence, and prevention of cancer progression. Conceptually, this application is provided as specific therapy or prophylaxis against recurrence or progression. Each indication is associated with risks and benefits and therefore should be carefully analyzed for individual patients. Characteristics of the optimal candidates for intravesical therapy are listed in Table 56.6. Table 56.7 identifies the current agents employed for intravesical therapy. Despite many prospective clinical trials designed to identify the best drug for intravesical chemotherapy of TCC, the ideal agent not yet been identified. In fact, at least one meta-analysis found that intravesical chemotherapeutic agents are unable to modify the natural history of stage Ta/T1 TCC.[78] It is apparent that the optimal course of therapy, the best drug, and the best combination of drugs have not yet been established for treatment or prophylaxis of TCC. The remainder of this discussion focuses on the application of BCG as intravesical immunotherapy for Ta, Tis, and T1 TCC.

Bacillus Calmette–Guérin is a live attenuated mycobacterium that has been found to incite an immune response within the bladder, which appears to be responsible for its therapeutic efficacy against TCC. Administration of intravesical BCG as prophylaxis has been found to reduce tumor recurrence by approximately 42% compared to transurethral resection alone. This effect is also associated with diminution in the incidence of tumor progression.[79] BCG has demonstrated effectiveness when administered as therapy for carcinoma in situ of the bladder, with complete response rates of 60–79%.[80] Although still controversial, the optimal strategy for instillation of BCG includes a 6-week course of induction therapy followed by maintenance therapy in the event of a successful response.[81]

Administration of BCG to a patient as therapy or prophylaxis is associated with toxicity that includes fever, chills, irritative voiding symptoms, bone and joint pain, nausea, and fatigue. Importantly, immune-compromised individuals are at risk for systemic BCG sepsis, which has been seen in approximately 0.4% of patients with potentially fatal consequences.[82] Therefore elderly patients with TCC requiring intravesical BCG therapy should be evaluated for factors such as diabetes and poor nutritional state, which could predispose them to severe BCG toxicity. They must be monitored closely during therapy. Nevertheless, for many older individuals the use of intravesical immunotherapy may represent a more desirable therapeutic choice than radical cystectomy with urinary diversion.

TABLE 56.7. Current Medications for Intravesical Chemotherapy and Immunotherapy

| |
|---|
| Chemotherapeutic drugs |
| Doxorubicin (Adriamycin) |
| Epirubicin |
| Mitomycin C |
| Thiotepa |
| Immunotherapeutic agents |
| Bacillus Calmette-Guerin (BCG) |
| Bropiramine |
| Keyhole limpet haemocyanin |
| Interferon-α |

In summary, superficial TCC presents frequently in old individuals often with a protracted natural history and a low risk of progression to a life-threatening malignancy. Most stage Ta lesions may be managed with endoscopic resection alone with subsequent outpatient follow-up with cystourethroscopy and urine cytology. Surveillance protocols for such patients often involve cystoscopy every 3 months for 2 years, every 6 months for 2 years, and then every year thereafter. The intensity of this approach may be reduced for individuals in ill health or with favorable lesions at low risk for recurrence. Patients who present with Tis or T1 cancers should also receive a course of intravesical immunotherapy with BCG following surgical resection. Again, these patients should be carefully observed with an organized surveillance protocol. Individuals with recurrent or refractory Tis or T1 lesions should be considered for curative radical cystectomy.

Several new urine-based assay systems for tumor markers associated with TCC may make the surveillance of patients with TCC even less intensive. These markers, such as NMP 22 (nuclear matrix protein 22) and the bladder tumor antigen (BTA) test, exhibit sensitivities for TCC in the range of 60–83%.[83,84] A positive result with these assays subsequent to a transurethral resection may warrant a more thorough investigation for rapidly recurrent or persistent TCC. Perhaps more significantly, a negative assay result may identify an individual at low risk for recurrence who may then be spared the cost and inconvenience of a surveillance procedure. The exact role of these assays in the management of older individuals with TCC remains to be established.

## Muscle-Invasive TCC of the Bladder

The concept of muscle-invasive or locally advanced TCC of the bladder, concerns lesions that have invaded beyond the lamina propria into the muscular bladder wall. The histologic demonstration of muscularis propria invasion is a particularly ominous sign, as approximately 50% of individuals who present with stage T2–T4 TCC develop distant metastases within 2 years.[85] Most patients who develop locally advanced TCC of the bladder present initially with a muscle-invasive lesion rather than a previous superficial cancer.

Conventional wisdom suggests that there are at least two oncogenic pathways for TCC of the bladder. The first pathway results in a papillary stage Ta/T1 TCC that only occasionally progresses to deeper involvement of the bladder wall. A second pathway involves rapid progression from carcinoma in situ to a solid invasive cancer. Molecular evidence for this wisdom is provided by the statistically significant survival differences, stage by stage, of TCC associated with alterations in the *p53* gene.[86] Spontaneous mutations in the *p53* gene (or other as yet unidentified genes) are likely to initiate a pathway in which neoplastic cells rapidly progress to muscle invasion and metastases. If this is indeed the case, there may then be a selection process for the second pathway with advancing age. It appears that the proportion of patients with localized disease declines with age. Approximately 82% of patients aged 40–44 years have localized disease at presentation, whereas only 61% of patients over the age of 84 years harbor localized cancers.[87] As such, a life-threatening but potentially curable bladder cancer often presents in an old individual with other co-morbidities and overall natural life expectancy, thereby complicating the choice of therapy.

# Locally Advanced Transitional Cell Carcinoma of the Bladder

## Radiologic Evaluation

Once the diagnosis of a stage T2–T4 TCC has been established through transurethral biopsy or resection, the patient should be thoroughly examined for evidence of lymphatic or hematogenous spread. The primary sites for disseminated TCC include the pelvic lymph nodes within the obturator and hypogastric regions, lung, liver, and bone. Pertinent studies include a chest radiograph with abdominal and pelvic CT or MRI scans. Consideration may be given to a thoracic CT scan, but this examination exhibits high sensitivity for small pulmonary nodules but with low specificity. The resultant false-positive findings, particularly in an elderly individual with other benign pulmonary disease, may confuse the treatment algorithm. A bone evaluation with skeletal scintigraphy is indicated in individuals with complaints of musculoskeletal pain or an elevated alkaline phosphatase level.[88] Approximately 5–15% of patients with invasive TCC harbor metastatic bone lesions, which obviate an attempt at curative therapy.

Although clinicians have attempted to apply imaging techniques such as US, CT, and MRI in the evaluation of the depth of invasion into the bladder wall, these efforts have been largely unsuccessful. Both CT and MRI are useful for evaluating the pelvic lymphatic system, soft tissues, and bone. Several reports suggest an increase in both sensitivity and specificity of MRI over CT, and therefore MRI may be the preferred study in the older patient with T2–T4 TCC.[89]

## Treatment

Therapeutic approaches to muscle-invasive TCC of the bladder are determined by the presence or absence of clinically detectable lymphatic or hematogenous metastases. Multimodality curative therapy should be applied only in individuals whose cancers are confined to the bladder wall or associated with minimal-volume regional lymphatic disease. Questions regarding treatment efficacy, toxicity, and expected patient longevity must be answered individually for each patient with this cancer.

## Surgical Therapy

An attempt at complete endoscopic resection of a solid muscle infiltrating lesion within the bladder represents the most conservative surgical treatment approach. Published 5-year survival rates for patients treated with resection alone reveal 56–70% survival for those with stage T2 lesions and 43–57% survival for those with T3a–T3b cancers.[90,91] One retrospective series of 114 patients compared transurethral resection alone to other, more involved protocols and reported that the 5-year cancer-specific survival rate was 63% for those with T2 lesions and 38% for those with T3a cancers.[92] Importantly, these authors concluded that endoscopic treatment alone was as efficacious as radical cystectomy. Although encouraging for the elderly patient with T2–T3a TCC, these data are likely optimistic because only 10% of bladder specimens removed during a radical cystectomy are found to be free of residual cancer after the staging transurethral resection. Nevertheless, an aggressive resection with the possible addition of electrical vaporization or fulguration can eradicate muscle-invasive TCC and so represents a viable treatment option for the patient with significant medical illness.

Complete surgical extirpation with radical cystectomy remains the treatment of choice for locally advanced TCC in patients of all ages. The contemporary surgical approach includes thorough pelvic lymph node dissection followed by complete removal of the bladder, uterus, and anterior vaginal wall in women or bladder with the prostate and seminal vesicles in men. A urinary diversion with either an incontinent ileal conduit or a reconstructed continent reservoir is established following the cystectomy. Skinner and Lieskovsky reported a series of 197 patients in 1984 who had 5-year survival rates of 75% with pT2–T3a disease, 44% with pT3b, and 36% with stage pT4 or positive pelvic lymph nodes.[93] Importantly, the postoperative survival was not affected by application of preoperative radiation therapy; therefore radical cystectomy alone has become established as satisfactory monotherapy for most patients with locally advanced TCC of the bladder. The impact of pathologic stage on survival following radical cystectomy has been corroborated by other clinical investigators. Survival of patients with pT2–T3a cancers in more recent series has been 75–80% but only 42–58% for those with stage pT3b–T4 lesions.[94–96] A further diminution of survival is experienced among patients with lymphatic metastases. Therefore therapy for patients with pT3b–T4 lesions and or lymphatic spread should now be considered multimodality with the addition of systemic chemotherapeutic agents.

It is clear that curative therapy for muscle-invasive TCC is an intensive, costly experience for any individual, perhaps more so for the old person with other life and medical concerns. It should not be surprising, then, that fewer individuals over the age of 70 with T2–T4 TCCs are treated by radical extirpation.[97] This clinical bias is not supported by the reports of outcomes following radical cystectomy in patients over age 70. In one report of 42 individuals the postoperative mortality rate was 9.5% (4 of 42) which was similar to that of a younger group of patients.[98] Given the similarity in morbidity and mortality statistics, the authors concluded that it was not justified to withhold this potentially curative therapy on the basis of age.

The elderly patient with muscle-invasive TCC is often faced with the conundrum of dealing with a significant life-threatening cancer and considerations of natural life expectancy and quality of life concerns. Anecdotally, many individuals are willing to undergo intensive therapy and endure the potential morbidity if the likelihood of cure is high. As already discussed, the ability to eradicate bladder cancer is directly related to the stage at presentation, particularly the presence or absence of lymphatic metastases. Most reports demonstrate that the identification of lymphatic spread at the time of radical cystectomy is associated with 6–23% five-year survival.[99] For many old people with an otherwise asymptomatic, stage T2–T4 bladder cancer, accurate identification of lymphatic disease could dissuade them from undergoing radical cystectomy and point them toward more conservative palliative approaches. In this regard, minimally invasive laparoscopic techniques can be employed for staging the pelvic lymph nodes.

Laparoscopic pelvic lymph node dissection has been used in patients with bladder cancer to provide a less invasive method of cancer staging.[100] Complications have been few, but there has been a report of tumor implantation at a laparoscopic port site in a patient who underwent a laparoscopic biopsy of a TCC of the bladder.[101] Therefore the current recommendations include use of an organ entrapment sac for removing lymph node specimens. Patients found to harbor metastatic deposits within the regional lymphatics may then choose alternative approaches for their treatment in an effort to avoid the morbidity of the radical cystectomy for a cancer with a poor prognosis.

Laparoscopy can also be used as a means of applying destructive energy to bladder tumors while avoiding injury to adjacent structures. Such a protocol has been reported by Gerber and coworkers using transurethral neodymium:yttrium-aluminum-garnet (Nd:YAG) laser fulguration of the base of invasive cancers in an effort to control the malignancy while preserving the bladder in patients unsuited for radical cystectomy.[102] In this series five patients with invasive bladder cancer underwent transurethral laser treatment of the lesion with concomitant laparoscopic mobilization of the bowel away from the bladder wall. Additionally, in two cases the laser energy was directed against the serosal surface of the bladder via the laparoscopic instruments. The initial results were disappointing with respect to disease control, but the potential advantages of laparoscopy may warrant further studies.

Finally, laparoscopic surgical approaches to both bladder and prostatic cancer include the palliative procedure of laparoscopic cutaneous ureterostomy in the case of an advanced and obstructing cancer.[103] The relief of ureteral obstruction with this procedure may offer advantages over standard indwelling ureteral stents or percutaneous nephrostomy tube drainage for some patients.

## Multimodality Therapy for Advanced TCC of the Bladder

Chemotherapy is widely used for therapy of advanced or metastatic bladder cancer and remains an area of active research as adjuvant or neoadjuvant treatment with definitive local therapy. Further applications of systemic chemotherapy include the development of multimodality treatment protocols for curative therapy with bladder preservation. Since Sternberg et al.'s original report of a 72% response rate in metastatic bladder cancer patients using methotrexate/vinblastine/doxorubicin/cisplatin (M-VAC), various other agents and combinations of agents have been evaluated.[104,105] In a randomized trial conducted by the Eastern Cooperative Oncology Group, M-VAC was shown to be superior to single-agent cisplatin in patients with metastatic urothelial carcinomas, with an overall response rate of 39%.[106] Rather unique to this study, 46% of the 246 patients were older than 65 years of age. Poor performance status rather than advanced age predicted poor response and survival. Toxicity for those treated with M-VAC was more severe than with cisplatin alone, with statistically significant differences most notable for leukopenia (24%), granulocytopenic fever (10%), sepsis (6%), and mucositis (17%). Rather strikingly, fewer than one-fourth of the patients treated with M-VAC received chemotherapeutic doses without modification. Although toxicity risk based on age was not analyzed, the regimen employs agents whose excretion and distribution can be affected by age-related physiologic changes. Age alone should not preclude the use of M-VAC; careful evaluation of nutritional state, cardiac and renal function, and screening for underlying neuropathy is paramount to the safe delivery of this combination of drugs.

Promising less toxic agents and combinations for urothelial cancers have been identified. In an early study of a phase I/II trial, carboplatin and paclitaxel were reported to have a 50% response rate in previously treated patients with advanced disease.[107] These two agents demonstrated reduced toxicity relative to M-VAC. Carboplatin dosing utilizes calculation of the glomerular filtration rate, thereby accounting for individual variation in renal function. Paclitaxel is not excreted renally. Neuropathy can be a significant complication that affects mobility and requires careful monitoring during therapy. Gemcitabine as a single agent was reported to have a 28% response rate in a phase II trial of previously untreated patients with metastatic disease. The median age of the patients was 69.5 years, and toxicity was moderate. Altogether, 25% of patients experienced a rapidly reversible grade 3 neutropenia or thrombocytopenia with only a single case of grade 4 neutropenia.[108] At present, several new or established agents and combinations of agents exhibit activity against TCC of the bladder. The efficacy of these systemic agents have stimulated investigations into neoadjuvant or adjuvant protocols for locally advanced TCC associated with such poor prognostic factors as stage T3b–T4 or nodal metastases.[109,110] At the present time such multimodality treatment strategies must be considered experimental with uncertain benefits for the elderly individual.

The clinical response of metastatic TCC to systemic chemotherapeutic agents has stimulated the design of investigational protocols with the intention to eradicate locally advanced TCC while preserving bladder function. These bladder-sparing approaches combine the efficacy of an aggressive transurethral resection with external beam radiation therapy and systemic chemotherapy. Although irradiation has demonstrated only modest efficacy as monotherapy, several investigators have advocated its role in a multimodality approach.[111] One study of 94 patients with T2–T4 TCC treated with endoscopic resection followed by two or three cycles of M-VAC or CMV with subsequent 6480 cCy radiation to the bladder was reported in 1995. The 5-year relapse-free survival was 84% for T2, 53% for T3, and 11% for T4 cancers. Importantly, only 18% of the surviving patients had an intact bladder.[112] Bladder preservation is an admirable goal for the healthy individual with an early invasive T2 lesion within the bladder, but it appears that most patients who are cured by this approach ultimately require a radical cystectomy. The old patient must be prepared to submit to the toxicity of the combined therapy while maintaining the potential requirement of a radical cystectomy. Therefore multimodality therapy for TCC must be considered experimental for patients of all ages, particularly for the person over 70 years of age.

## Conclusions

Improvements in diagnostic imaging, surgical techniques, and systemic chemotherapy have combined to offer old individuals a wide array of treatment options for renal and bladder malignancies. However, the myriad issues confronting these people serve only to complicate the choice of therapy. Elderly persons with a bladder or renal cancer must consider the potential benefit of curative therapy relative to the deleterious impact of the therapy on their quality of life. Commonly, an exact or rational estimate of co-morbid illness and natural life expectancy is unavailable, and patients must rely on the wisdom and experience of their physicians. These clinicians must in turn avoid the unconscious bias against curative treatment for an elderly individual and thoroughly address all potential options with an eye toward quality of life from the patient's point of view. Age-specific investigations are needed before the best treatment options for geriatric patients are identified.

## References

1. Roush W. Live long and prosper? Science 1996;273:42–46.
2. Balducci L, Lyman GH. Cancer in the elderly. Clin Geriatr Med 1997;13(1):1–14.
3. Bennahum DA, Forman WB, Vellas B, Albarede JL. Life expectancy, comorbidity and quality of life. Clin Geriatr Med 1997;13:33–53.
4. Wolinsky FD, Johnson RL, Stump TE. The risk of mortality among older adults over an eight year period. Gerontologist 1995;35:150–161.
5. Cancer Facts & Figures. Washington, DC: American Cancer Society, 1996.
6. Damhuis RAM, Blom JHM. The influence of age on treatment choice and survival in 735 patients with renal carcinoma. Br J Urol 1995;75:143–147.
7. Horning ES. Observations on hormone dependent renal tumors in the golden hamster. Br J Cancer 1956;10:678–687.
8. Outzen HC, Maguire HC. The etiology of renal cell carcinoma. Semin Oncol 1983;10:378–384.
9. Cohen AJ, Li FP, Berg S, et al. Hereditary renal cell carcinoma associated with a chromosomal translocation. N Engl J Med 1979;301:592–595.
10. Tory K, Brauch H, Linehan M, et al. Specific genetic change in tumors associated with von Hippel-Lindau disease. J Natl Cancer Inst 1989;81:1097–1101.
11. Anglard P, Tory K, Brauch H, et al. Molecular analysis of genetic changes in the origin and development of renal cell carcinoma. Cancer Res 1991;51:1071–1077.
12. Ritchie AWS, Chisholm GD. The natural history of renal carcinoma. Semin Oncol 1983;10:390–400.
13. Figlin RA, Pierce WC, Kaboo R, et al. Treatment of metastatic renal cell carcinoma with nephrectomy, interleukin-2 and cytokine-primed or CD8 (+) selected tumor infiltrating lymphocytes from primary tumor. J Urol 1997; 158:740–745.
14. Sweeney JP, Thornhill JA, Grainger R, McDermott TED, Butler MR. Incidentally detected renal cell carcinoma: pathological features, survival trends and implications for treatment. Br J Urol 1996;78:351–353.
15. Carini M, Selli C, Barbanti G, Lapini A, Turini D, Constantini A. Conservative surgical treatment of renal cell carcinoma: clinical experience and reappraisal of indications. J Urol 1988;140:725–731.
16. Hellsten S, Johnsen J, Berge T, Linell F. Clinically unrecognized renal cell carcinoma. Eur Urol 1990;18:2–3.
17. Bosniak MA, Birnbaum BA, Krinsky GA, Waisman J. Small renal parenchymal neoplasms: further observations on growth. Radiology 1995;197:589–597.
18. Nativ O, Sabo E, Raviv G, Madjar S, Halachmi S, Moskovitz B. The impact of tumor size on clinical outcome in patients with localized renal cell carcinoma treated by radical nephrectomy. J Urol 1997;158:729–732.
19. Juul N, Torp-Pedersen S, Gronvall S, Holm HH, Koch F, Larsen S. Ultrasonically guided fine needle aspiration biopsy of renal masses. J Urol 1986;133:579–581.
20. Moulton JS, Moore PT. Coaxial percutaneous biopsy technique with automated biopsy devices: value in improving accuracy and negative predictive value. Radiology 1993; 186:515–522.
21. Roosen JU, Engel U, Jensen RH, Kvist E, Schou G. Renal cell carcinoma: prognostic factors. Br J Urol 1994;74:160–164.
22. Raviv G, Leibovich I, Mor Y, et al. Localized renal cell carcinoma treated by radical nephrectomy. Cancer 1993;72: 2207–2212.
23. Wehle MJ, Grabstald H. Contraindications to needle aspiration of a solid renal mass: tumor dissemination by renal needle aspiration. J Urol 1986;136:446–448.
24. Lichtman SM. Physiological aspects of aging. Drugs Aging 1995;7:212–225.
25. Epstein M. Aging and the kidney. J Am Soc Nephrol 1996;7:1106–1122.
26. Provert J, Tessler A, Brown J, Golimbu M, Bosniak M, Morales P. Partial nephrectomy for renal cell carcinoma: indications, results and implications. J Urol 1991;145:472–476.
27. Hakim RM, Goldszer RC, Brenner BM. Hypertension and proteinuria: long-term sequelae of uninephrectomy in humans. Kidney Int 1984;25:930–936.
28. Mulholland SG, Stefanelli N. Genitourinary cancer in the elderly. Am J Kidney Dis 1990;16:324–328.
29. Semelka RC, Shoenut JP, Magro CM, Kroeker MA, MacMahon R, Greenberg HM. Renal cancer staging: comparison of contrast enhanced CT and gadolinium enhanced fat-suppressed spin-echo and gradient-echo MR imaging. J Magn Reson Imaging 1993;3:597–602.
30. Robson CJ, Churchill BM, Anderson W. The results of radical nephrectomy for renal cell carcinoma. J Urol 1969;101:297–301.
31. Phillips E, Messing EM. Role of lymphadenectomy in the treatment of renal cell carcinoma. Urology 1993;41:9–15.
32. Ramon J, Goldwasser B, Raviv G, Jonas P, Many M. Long term results of simple and radical nephrectomy for renal cell carcinoma. Cancer 1991;10:2506–2511.
33. Montie JE. Inferior vena cava tumor thrombectomy. In: Montie JE, Pontes JE, Bukowski RM (eds) Clinical Man-

agement of Renal Cell Carcinoma. Chicago: Year Book, 1990:121–152.
34. Skinner DG, Pritchett TR, Lieskovsky G, Boyd SD, Stiles QR. Vena caval involvement by renal cell carcinoma: surgical resection provides meaningful long-term survival. Ann Surg 1989;210:387–394.
35. Marshall FF, Dietrick DD, Baumgartner WA, Reitz BA. Surgical management of renal cell carcinoma into the vena cava: clinical review and surgical approach. J Urol 1988; 139:1166–1172.
36. Clayman RV, Kavoussi LR, Soper J, et al. Laparoscopic nephrectomy: initial case report. J Urol 1991;146:278.
37. Ono Y, Kinukawa T, Hattutori R, Yamada S, Ohshima S. Laparoscopic radical nephrectomy: Nagoya experience. J Endourol 1997;11(S1):S127.
38. Eden CG, Haigh AC, Carter PG, Copcoat MJ. Laparoscopic nephrectomy results in better postoperative pulmonary function. J Endourol 1994;8:419.
39. Novick ACI, Streem S, Montie JE, et al. Conservative surgery for renal cell carcinoma: a single-center experience with 100 patients. J Urol 1989;141:835–839.
40. Thrasher JB, Robertson JE, Paulson DF. Expanding indications for conservative renal surgery in renal cell carcinoma. Urology 1994;43:160–168.
41. Herr HW. Partial nephrectomy for renal cell carcinoma with a normal opposite kidney. Cancer 1994;73:150–162.
42. Morgan WR, Zincke H. Progression and survival after renal conserving surgery for renal cell carcinoma: experience in 104 patients and extended follow-up. J Urol 1990; 144:852–858.
43. Butler BP, Novick AC, Miller DP, Campbell SA, Licht MR. Management of small unilateral renal cell carcinomas: radical versus nephron-sparing surgery. Urology 1995;45: 34–41.
44. Cozzi PJ, Lynch WJ, Collins S, Vonthehoff L, Morris DL. Renal cryotherapy in a sheep model: a feasibility study. J Urol 1997;157:710–712.
45. Delworth MG, Pisters LL, Fornage BD, von Eschenbach AC. Cryotherapy for renal cell carcinoma and angiomyolipoma. J Urol 1996;155:252–255.
46. Balducci L, Extermann M. Cancer chemotherapy in the older patient: what the medical oncologist needs to know. Cancer 1997;80:1317–1322.
47. Yagoda A, Abi-Rached B, Petrylak D. Chemotherapy for advanced renal cell carcinoma: 1983–1993. Semin Oncol 1995;22:42–60.
48. Rosenstein M, Ettinghausen SE, Rosenberg SA. Extravasation of intravascular fluid mediated by the systemic administration of recombinant interleukin-2. J Immunol 1986;137:1735–1742.
49. Taneja S, Pierce W, Figlin R, Belldegrun A. Immunotherapy for renal cell carcinoma: the era of interleukin-2 based treatment. Urology 1995;45:911–924.
50. Fyfe G, Fisher RI, Rosenberg SA, Sznol M, Parkinson DR, Louie AC. Results of treatment of 255 patients with metastatic renal cell carcinoma who received high-dose recombinant interleukin-2 therapy. J Clin Oncol 1995;13: 688–696.
51. Bukowski RM. Natural history and therapy of metastatic renal cell carcinoma: the role of interleukin-2. Cancer 1997;80:1198–1220.
52. Caligiuri MA. Low-dose recombinant interleukin-2 therapy: rationale and potential clinical implications. Semin Oncol 1993;18(suppl 7):108–112.
53. Umeda T, Niijima T. A phase II study of alpha interferon on renal cell carcinoma: summary of three collaborative trials. Cancer 1986;58:1231–1235.
54. Choudhury M, Efros M, Mitteman A. Interferons and interleukins in metastatic RCC. Urology 1993;41:67–72.
55. Buzio C, DePalma G, Passalacqua R, et al. Effectiveness of very low doses of immunotherapy in advanced renal cell cancer. Br J Cancer 1997;76:541–544.
56. Fossa SD, Kramar A, Droz JP. Prognostic factors and survival in patients with metastatic renal cell carcinoma treated with chemotherapy or interferon alpha. Eur J Cancer 1994;30A:1310–1314.
57. Dreicer R, Cooper CS, Williams RD. Management of prostate and bladder cancer in the elderly. Urol Clin North Am 1996;23:87–97.
58. Stanta G, Campagner L, Cavallieri F, Giarelli L. Cancer of the oldest old. Clin Geriatr Med 1997;13:55–68.
59. Fultz NH, Herzog AR. Epidemiology of urinary symptoms in the geriatric population. Urol Clin North Am 1996;23:1–10.
60. Mariani AJ, Mariani MC, Macchioni C, Stams UK, Hariharan A, Moriera A. The significance of adult hematuria: 1000 hematuria evaluations including a risk-benefit and cost-effectiveness analysis. J Urol 1989;141: 350–355.
61. Messing EM, Young TB, Hunt VB, et al. Hematuria home screening: repeat testing results. J Urol 1995;154:57–61.
62. Sidransky D, von Eschenbach A, Tsai YC, et al. Identification of p53 mutations in bladder cancers and urine samples. Science 1991;252:706–709.
63. Koch M, Hill GB, McPhee MS. Factors affecting recurrence rates in superficial bladder cancer. J Natl Cancer Inst 1986;76(6):1025–1029.
64. Itoku KA, Stein BS. Superficial bladder cancer. Hematol Oncol Clin North Am 1992;6:99–116.
65. Ro JY, Staerkel GA, Ayala AG. Cytologic and histologic features of superficial bladder cancer. Urol Clin North Am 1992;19:435–453.
66. Fitzpatrick JM, West AB, Butler MR, Lane V, O'Flynn JD. Superficial bladder tumors (stage pTa, grades 1 and 2): the importance of recurrence pattern following initial resection. J Urol 1986;135:920–922.
67. Torti FM, Lum BL, Aston D, et al. Superficial bladder cancer: the primacy of grade in the development of invasive disease. J Clin Oncol 1987;5:125–130.
68. Heney NM, Ahmed S, Managan MJ, et al. Superficial bladder cancer: progression and recurrence. J Urol 1983;130:1083–1086.
69. Holmang S, Hedelin H, Anderstrom C, Johansson SL. The relationship among multiple recurrences, progression and prognosis of patients with stages Ta and T1 transitional cell cancer of the bladder followed for at least 20 years. J Urol 1995;153:1823–1827.
70. Farrow GM. Pathology of carcinoma in situ of the urinary bladder and related lesions. J Cell Biochem 1992; 161(suppl):39–43.
71. Bostwick DG. Natural history of early bladder cancer. J Cell Biochem 1992;161(suppl):31–38.

72. Prout GR, Griffin PP, Daly JJ. The outcome of conservative treatment of carcinoma in situ of the bladder. J Urol 1987;138:766–770.
73. Herr HW, Jakse G, Sheinfeld J. The T1 bladder tumor. Semin Urol 1990;8:254.
74. Cookson MS, Sarosdy MF. Management of stage T1 superficial bladder cancer with intravesical bacillus Calmette-Guerin therapy. J Urol 1992;148:797–801.
75. Herr HW. High-risk superficial bladder cancer: transurethral resection alone in selected patients with T1 tumor. Semin Urol Oncol 1997;15:142–146.
76. Kurfh K. Natural history and prognosis of untreated and treated superficial bladder cancer. In: Agano F, Fair WR (eds) Superficial Bladder Cancer. Oxford: ISIS Medical Media, 1997;42–56.
77. Esrig D, Freeman JA, Stein JP, Skinner DG. Early cystectomy for clinical stage T1 transitional cell carcinoma of the bladder. Semin Urol Oncol 1997;15:154–160.
78. Lamm DL, Riggs DR, Traynelis CL, Nseyo UO. Apparent failure of current intravesical chemotherapy prophylaxis to influence the long-term course of superficial transitional cell carcinoma of the bladder. J Urol 1995;153:1450.
79. Witjes JA, Mulders PFA, Debruyne FMJ. Intravesical therapy in superficial bladder cancer. Urology 1994; 43(suppl 2):2–6.
80. Lamm DL. Comparison of BCG with other intravesical agents. Urology 1991;37(5):30–32.
81. Lamm DL. Carcinoma in situ. In: Pagano F, Fair WR (eds) Superficial Bladder Cancer. Oxford: ISIS Medical Media, 1997:193–202.
82. Lamm DL. Complications of bacillus Calmette-Guerin immunotherapy. Urol Clin North Am 1992;19:565–572.
83. Soloway MS, Briggman V, Carpinito GA, et al. Use of a new tumor marker, urinary NMPf22, in the detection of occult or rapidly recurring transitional cell carcinoma of the urinary tract following surgical treatment. J Urol 1996;156:363–367.
84. Leyh H, Hall R, Mazeman E, Blumstein BA. Comparison of the Bard BTA test with voided urine and bladder wash cytology in the diagnosis and management of cancer of the bladder. Urology 1997;50:49–53.
85. Droller MJ. Treatment of regionally advanced bladder cancer: an overview. Urol Clin North Am 1992;19:685–693.
86. Bochner BH, Esrig D, Groshen S, et al. Relationship of tumor angiogenesis and nuclear p53 accumulation in invasive bladder cancer. Clin Cancer Res 1997;3:1615–1622.
87. Silvennan DT, Hartge P, Morrison AS, Deveas SS. Epidemiology of bladder cancer. Hematol Oncol Clin North Am 1992;6:1–30.
88. Thrasher JB, Crawford ED. Current management of invasive and metastatic transitional cell carcinoma of the bladder. J Urol 1993;149:957–972.
89. See WA, Fuller JR. Staging of advanced bladder cancer. Urol Clin North Am 1992;19:663–683.
90. Flocks RH. Treatment of patients with carcinoma of the bladder. JAMA 1951;145:295.
91. Herr HW. Conservative management of muscle-infiltrating bladder cancer: prospective experience. J Urol 1987;138:1162–1163.
92. Henry K, Miller J, Mori M, Loening S, Fallon B. Comparison of transurethral resection to radical therapies for stage B bladder tumors. J Urol 1988;140:964–967.
93. Skinner DG, Lieskovsky G. Contemporary cystectomy with pelvic lymph node dissection compared to preoperative radiation therapy plus cystectomy in management of invasive bladder cancer. J Urol 1984;131:1069–1072.
94. Wishnow KI, Levinson AK, Johnson DE, et al. Stage B (p2/3a/N0) transitional cell carcinoma of bladder highly curable by radical cystectomy. Urology 1992;39: 12–16.
95. Malkowitz SB, Nichols P, Lieskovsky G, Boyd SD, Huffman J, Skinner DG. The role of radical cystectomy in the management of high grade superficial bladder cancer (PA, P1, PIS, P2). J Urol 1990;144:641–645.
96. Soloway MS, Lopez AE, Patel J, Lu Y. Resuls of radical cystectomy for transitional cell carcinoma of the bladder and the effect of chemotherapy. Cancer 1994;73:1926–1931.
97. Holmang S, Hedelin H, Anderstrom C, Johansson SL. Long-term follow-up of all patients with muscle-invasive (stages T2, T3 and T4) bladder carcinoma in a geographical region. J Urol 1997;158:389–392.
98. Leibovitch I, Avigad I, Ben-Chaim J, Nativ O, Goldwasser B. Is it justified to avoid radical cystoprostatectomy in elderly patients with invasive transitional cell carcinoma of the bladder? Cancer 1993;71:3098–3101.
99. Roehrborn CG, Sagalowsky AI, Peters PC. Long-term patient survival after cystectomy for regional metastatic transitional cell carcinoma of the bladder. J Urol 1991;146: 36–39.
100. Bowsher WG, Clarke A, Clarke DG, Costello AJ. Laparoscopic pelvic lymph node dissection for carcinoma of the prostate and bladder. Aust NZ J Surg 1992;62:634–637.
101. Anderson JR, Steven K. Implantation metastasis after laparoscopic biopsy of bladder cancer. J Urol 1995;153: 1047–1048.
102. Gerber GS, Chodak GW, Rukstalis DB. Combined laparoscopic and transurethral neodymium: yttrium-aluminum-garnet laser treatment of invasive bladder cancer. Urology 1995;45:230–233.
103. Puppo P, Perachino M, Ricciotti G, Bozzo W. Laparoscopic bilateral cutaneous ureterostomy for palliation of ureteral obstruction caused by advanced pelvic cancer. J Endourol 1994;8:425–428.
104. Sternberg CN, Yagoda A, Scher HI, et al. Methotrexate, vinblastine, doxorubicin and cisplatin for advanced transitional cell carcinoma of the urothelium. Cancer 1989;64: 2448–2458.
105. Sternberg CN. The treatment of advanced bladder cancer. Ann Oncol 1995;6:113–126.
106. Loehrer PJ, Einhorn LH, Elson PJ, et al. A randomized trial of cisplatin alone or in combination with methotrexate, vinblastine and doxorubicin in patients with metastatic urothelial carcinoma: a cooperative group study. J Clin Oncol 1992;10:1066–1073.
107. Vaughn DJ, Malkowicz SB, Zotlick B, et al. Paclitaxel plus carboplatin in advanced carcinoma of the urothelium: a

well tolerated outpatient regimen. Proc Am Soc Clin Oncol 1996;15:597A.

108. Stadler WM, Kuzel T, Roth B, Raghavan D, Dorr FA. Phase II study of single agent gemcitabine in previously untreated patients with metastatic urothelial cancer. J Clin Oncol 1997;15:3394–3398.

109. Herr HW, Whitmore WF, Morse MJ, Sogani PC, Russo P, Fair WR. Neoadjuvant chemotherapy in invasive bladder cancer: the evolving role of surgery. J Urol 1990;144: 1083–1088.

110. Seidman AD, Scher HI. The evolving role of chemotherapy for muscle infiltrating bladder cancer. Semin Oncol 1991; 18:585–595.

111. Saiminen E. Recurrence and treatment of urinary bladder cancer after failure in radiotherapy. Cancer 1990;66:2341–2345.

112. Given RW, Parsons JT, McCarley D, Wajsman Z. Bladder sparing multimodality treatment of muscle invasive bladder cancer: a 5 year follow-up. Urology 1995;46: 499–505.

# 57 Benign and Malignant Diseases of the Prostate

Peter C. Albertsen

Benign prostatic hyperplasia (BPH) and prostate cancer are two of the most common neoplastic growths that occur in elderly men. Both of these conditions are rare before age 50 years, but by age 80 more than 80% of men have evidence of BP hyperplasia histology and more than 50% have at least microscopic foci of prostate cancer.[1,2] This chapter reviews the incidence of these two diseases of the prostate, the appropriate evaluation of elderly men, surgical alternatives available to the geriatric patient, and the risks associated with these treatment alternatives.

## Epidemiology

### Benign Prostatic Hyperplasia

The prostate is small at birth. With the onset of puberty it enlarges rapidly and then remains at a constant size during the next several decades of life. After age 50 years the average weight of the prostate slowly increases, accompanied by an increase in the incidence of symptomatic BP hyperplasia (Fig. 57.1). Between age 55 and 75 years, the number of men with symptoms related to BP hyperplasia increases linearly from approximately 25% to 50%. Fortunately, because of successful medical therapies, only a small number of men require surgery for this condition.

Although the development of BP hyperplasia is almost a universal phenomenon in aging men, the cause and pathogenesis of this disorder are poorly understood. Several risk factors have been proposed, but to date there is no evidence to suggest that BP hyperplasia can be attributed to any specific factor.[3] Researchers have investigated several sociocultural variables, including celibacy, specific blood groups, the use of alcohol or tobacco, and diseases commonly found among geriatric men such as coronary artery disease, peripheral vascular disease, hypertension, and diabetes. Several researchers have suggested that estrogen may contribute to the pathogenesis of BP hyperplasia, but the alterations in estrogen and androgen production that occur with aging appear to be minor and occur after the onset of this disease.

### Prostate Cancer

Prostate cancer is now the second most common cancer diagnosed in men. The incidence of this disease increased dramatically following the introduction of testing for prostate-specific antigen (PSA), but it now appears to be declining to rates similar to those seen earlier (Fig. 57.2).[4] Researchers estimated that in 2000, approximately 180,400 men would be diagnosed with this disease and 31,900 men would die from prostate cancer.[5] Prostate cancer is primarily a disease of old men. In 1990 the Surveillance Epidemiology and End Results (SEER) age-adjusted incidence rate was 45.2 per 100,000 men age 50–54 years. The rate for men over age 65 years exceeded 1000 per 100,000 men. Prostate cancer occurs much more frequently among African American men than in white Americans. Although the incidence rates are parallel for Whites and African Americans, the mortality from this disease is almost twice as high for African American men as for white men.

Despite the significant mortality from prostate cancer, many men never experience symptoms from their disease. Many prostate cancers are indolent. Autopsy data from several countries have confirmed a high incidence of prostate cancer histology, suggesting that fewer than 1% of men with histologically identifiable cancer die from this disease.[6] There is little geographic or ethnic variability in the rate of small latent carcinomas even when comparing populations with markedly different clinical prostate cancer incidences and mortalities.[7,8] Numerous studies have demonstrated that as many as 50% of men over the age of 50 years dying of causes other than prostate cancer have microscopic evidence of disease. These studies also demonstrated that the presence of these cancers increases with age. By age 75 years, more than 80% of men have microscopic evidence of prostate cancer at autopsy. Most of these tumors are

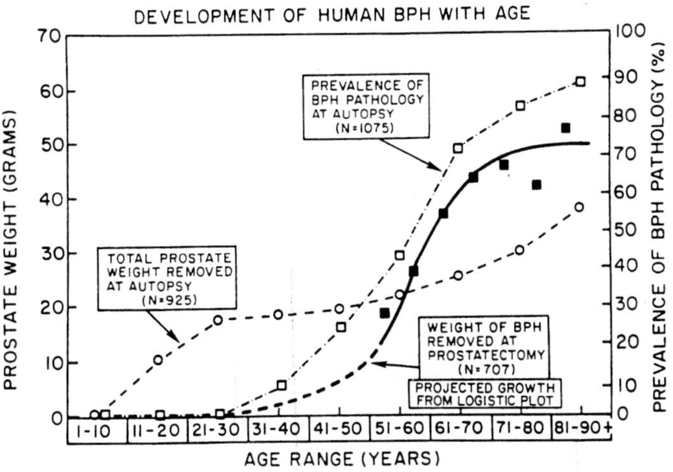


FIGURE 57.1. Development of human benign prostatic hyperplasia (BPH) with age: age-related changes in the weight of the prostate removed at autopsy in 925 men, prevalence of BP hyperplasia at autopsy in 1075 men, and the weight of the adenoma removed at simple perineal prostatectomy in 707 men. Long dashed line indicates the mathematically extrapolated range in this group. (From Berry et al.,[1] with permission.)

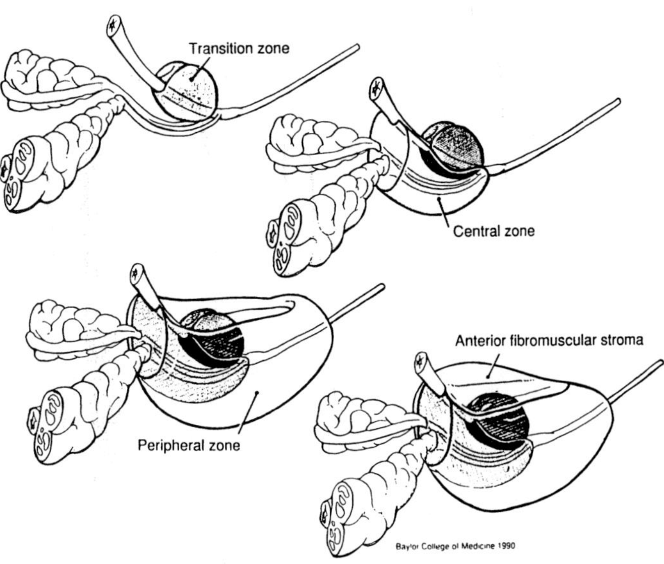


FIGURE 57.3. Zonal anatomy of the prostate as described by McNeal. (From McNeal, McNeal JE. Normal histology of the prostate. Am J Surg Pathol 1988;12:619–633 with permission.)

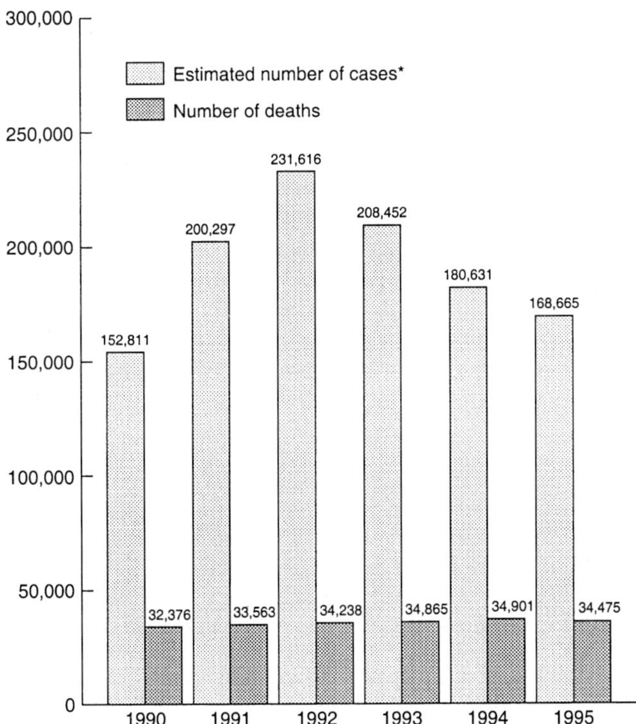


FIGURE 57.2. Prostate cancer incidence and mortality in the USA, 1990–1995. Estimates were obtained by multiplying the age-specific incidence rates for the 11 SEER registries in the U.S. population for each year. (From Stanford et al.,[4] with permission.)

microscopic foci fulfilling the criterion for prostate cancer, but it is not unusual for an 80-year-old American man dying of heart disease to have an intraprostatic tumor measuring 2–4 cm.[9]

The etiology of prostate cancer is unknown. The similar prevalence of latent disease among racial and ethnic groups at autopsy and the vast difference in the incidence of clinically significant disease suggest that the initiation of prostate cancer occurs frequently, but only some groups are susceptible to prostate cancer promoters. Known risk factors include familial inheritance. Several families have been identified with an apparent mendelian pattern of inheritance, and recently a prostate oncogene has been isolated.[10] A man with one first-degree relative with prostate cancer has a two- to threefold risk of being diagnosed with prostate cancer compared with the general population. A man with a first-degree and a second-degree relative may have a sixfold risk of developing prostate cancer.[11]

## Pathophysiology

The adult prostate can be divided into four distinct zones: (1) anterior fibromuscular stroma; (2) peripheral zone; (3) central zone; and (4) transition zone (Fig. 57.3).[12] Prostate cancer can occur in any of the four zones but most commonly arises in the peripheral zone. BP hyperplasia is exclusively restricted to the transition zone. The main ducts of the transition zone arise on the lateral aspects of the urethral wall at the point of urethral angulation near the verumontanum. Proximal to the origin of the transition zone ducts are the glands of the periurethral zone. All BP hyperplasia nodules occur in these two regions.

## Benign Prostatic Hyperplasia

The pathophysiology of BP hyperplasia is complex. Prostatic hyperplasia increases urethral resistance, resulting in compensatory changes in bladder function. Age-related changes also occur in both bladder and nervous system function. These changes lead to the bothersome complaints of urinary frequency, urgency, and nocturia that are commonly associated with symptomatic BP hyperplasia. One of the unique features of the human prostate is the presence of a capsule around the prostate, which plays an important role in the development of urinary symptoms.[13] Presumably the capsule transmits the pressure of tissue expansion to the urethra, which leads to an increase in urethral resistance. Transurethral incision of the prostate capsule results in significant alleviation of the outflow obstruction, despite the fact that the volume of the prostate remains the same. The size of the prostate does not correlate with the degree of obstruction. Other factors, including dynamic urethral resistance, the prostatic capsule, and changes in the function of the bladder muscle, contribute to the symptoms associated with BP hyperplasia.

Benign prostatic hypertrophy is a true hyperplastic process. Histology studies demonstrate an increase in cell numbers throughout the gland. Hyperplasia occurs in the form of nodules that consist of stromal elements and epithelial elements. In addition, many nodules contain smooth muscle. How the smooth muscle tissue contributes to symptomatic BP hyperplasia is unknown, but the muscle fibers are regulated by the adrenergic nervous system. Receptor binding studies indicate that α receptors are the most abundant type of receptor in the human prostate and explain the ability of α-blocking medications to relieve symptoms related to BP hyperplasia.

## Prostate Cancer

Adenocarcinoma of the prostate is frequently diagnosed as a result of an elevation in PSA. In many cases tumors cannot be palpated on rectal examination. Among men with clinically localized prostate cancer, most of the tumor mass is usually located in a peripheral location near the posterior edge of the prostate. In most cases the tumor is multifocal.[14]

As prostate cancer grows, cancer cells invade the soft tissue surrounding the prostate directly and along the perineural pathways. Penetration of the capsule usually occurs posteriorly and posterolaterally, which may lead to extension into the seminal vesicles. The most frequent sites of metastatic spread are the pelvic lymph nodes and bone, especially the pelvis and vertebral bodies.

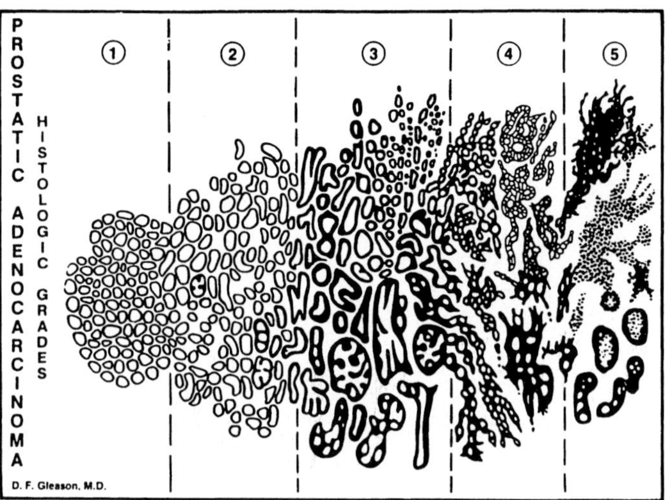


FIGURE 57.4. Gleason grading system. (From Walsh PC, Retik AM, Vaughan ED JR, Wein AJ, eds, Campbell's Urology, 7th ed. Philadelphia: Saunders, 1998, with permission.)

In general the size of a prostate cancer correlates with its extent.[15] Tumors <0.5 ml are usually incidental findings. Capsular penetration is uncommon in tumors <4 ml, whereas larger tumors usually have metastatic elements. The likelihood of developing metastatic prostate cancer depends on the grade of the tumor. The Gleason scoring system is the most common method of estimating malignant potential.[16] The Gleason system is based on the glandular pattern of the tumor as identified at relatively low magnification (Fig. 57.4). The primary (most predominant) and secondary (second most prevalent) architectural patterns are assigned a grade from 1 to 5, with 1 representing the most well differentiated and 5 the most poorly differentiated. A Gleason score is determined by summing the primary and secondary patterns. Men with high grade disease (Gleason score 7–10) generally have a poor prognosis, whereas men with low grade disease (Gleason score 2–5) have an excellent prognosis. Men with Gleason score 6 tumors have a prognosis between these two extremes.

# Diagnosis and Evaluation of Prostate Disease

## Benign Prostatic Hyperplasia

Physicians evaluating men for obstructive urinary symptoms should begin with a detailed history that focuses on the urinary tract, previous surgical procedures, general health issues, and fitness for possible surgical procedures. Specific areas to discuss include a history of hematuria, urinary tract infection, diabetes, neurologic disorders such as Parkinson's disease or pre-

TABLE 57.1. International Prostate Symptom Score (I-PSS)

| Criterion | Not at all | Less than 1 time in 5 | Less than half the time | About half the time | More than half the time | Almost always | Your score |
|---|---|---|---|---|---|---|---|
| **Incomplete emptying**: Over the past month, how often have you had a sensation of not emptying your bladder completely after you finished urinating? | 0 | 1 | 2 | 3 | 4 | 5 | |
| **Frequency**: Over the past month, how often have you had to urinate again less than 2 hours after you finished urinating? | 0 | 1 | 2 | 3 | 4 | 5 | |
| **Intermittency**: Over the past month, how often have you found you stopped and started again several times when you urinated? | 0 | 1 | 2 | 3 | 4 | 5 | |
| **Urgency**: Over the past month, how often have you found it difficult to postpone urination? | 0 | 1 | 2 | 3 | 4 | 5 | |
| **Weak stream**: Over the past month, how often have you had a weak urinary stream? | 0 | 1 | 2 | 3 | 4 | 5 | |
| **Straining**: Over the past month, how often have you had to push or strain to begin urination? | 0 | 1 | 2 | 3 | 4 | 5 | |
| **Nocturia**: Over the past month, how many times did you most typically get up to urinate from the time you went to bed at night until the time you got up in the morning? | 0 | 1 | 2 | 3 | 4 | 5 | |
| *Total I-PSS score* | | | | | | | |

vious stroke, urethral stricture disease, urinary retention, and aggravation of symptoms by cold or sinus medications. Physicians should check all current prescription medications to determine if the patient is taking any anticholinergic drugs (which impair bladder contractility) or $\alpha$-sympathomimetics (which increase outflow resistance). A history of lower urinary tract surgery suggests the possibility of urethral or bladder neck stricture. Use of a voiding diary may help identify patients with polyuria or other nonprostatic disorders.

Symptom assessment is best accomplished using the International Prostate Symptom Score (IPSS)[17] (Table 57.1). This instrument consists of a series of seven questions that have five graded responses. Symptoms are classified as mild when patients score between 0 and 7, moderate when they score between 8 and 19 and severe when they score between 20 and 35. The IPSS should not be used to diagnose BP hyperplasia but, rather, to evaluate treatment response or disease progression. Symptom scores alone do not capture the morbidity of a prostate problem as perceived by the patient. The impact of symptoms on a patient's life style must be considered as well. Intervening with medical or surgical therapy may make more sense in a patient with moderate symptoms he finds relatively troublesome compared with a patient with severe symptoms who is able to manage them fairly well.

The physical examination should include a digital rectal examination and a focused neurologic examination. The rectal examination establishes the approximate size of the gland and helps the urologist determine the most appropriate surgical approach should surgery be warranted. Because prostate size does not correlate with symptom severity or treatment outcomes, size should not be used to make a diagnosis and proceed with treatment. The digital rectal examination is helpful for guiding management. A focused neurologic examination can be used to exclude neurologic problems that may cause the presenting symptoms and should include an assessment of rectal sphincter tone.

Diagnostic tools that should be considered when assessing men with moderate or severe urinary symptoms include urinalysis, measurement of serum creatinine, and possibly a PSA assay. Urinary cytology should be considered in men with severe irritable symptoms, especially if they have a history of smoking. Patients with renal insufficiency have an increased risk for postoperative complications: 25% versus 17% for patients without renal insufficiency.[18] More important, patients with renal insufficiency have a sixfold increase in mortality when undergoing surgical treatment for their disease.[19] Because prostate cancer can produce urethral obstruction and commonly coexists with BP hyperplasia, physicians may wish to consider assessing the serum PSA level should a diagnosis of prostate cancer alter the proposed management.

Most men with moderate to severe symptoms of BP hyperplasia are advised to undergo medical therapy.

Those failing medical treatments are then usually offered surgery. Absolute indications for surgery include refractory urinary retention, recurrent urinary infections, recurrent gross hematuria, bladder stones, renal insufficiency caused by obstruction, and a large bladder diverticulum. Many patients advised to undergo surgical treatment for BP hyperplasia usually undergo cystoscopy. This examination is not recommended to determine the need for surgery but, rather, to help the surgeon determine the most appropriate technical approach.

### Prostate Cancer

Unlike BP hyperplasia, prostate cancer rarely causes symptoms early in the course of the disease because most prostate cancers arise in the periphery of the gland distant from the urethra. Symptoms in men with prostate cancer suggest locally advanced or metastatic disease. Growth of prostate cancer into the urethra or bladder neck can result in obstructive or irritating voiding symptoms. Metastatic disease that involves the bones can cause pain and anemia.

Most men diagnosed with prostate cancer are initially suspected of having the disease based on an abnormality noted on digital rectal examination or because of an elevated PSA test. Aggressive screening efforts have reduced the proportion of men with prostate cancer detected because of symptoms suggestive of advanced disease.[20] Because of the significant risk of prostate cancer, transrectal ultrasonography and prostate biopsy are recommended for all men who have an abnormality on digital rectal examination regardless of the serum PSA level. Unfortunately, in both screened and nonscreened populations, digital rectal examination misses 23–45% of prostate cancers that are subsequently found following prostate biopsy because of elevated serum PSA.[21] Routine use of the serum PSA assay increases the detection of prostate cancer over that achieved by a digital rectal examination alone. The use of serum PSA testing increases the lead time for prostate cancer diagnosis and the likelihood of detecting prostate cancers confined to the prostate. Recognizing that PSA elevations are common in aging men because of the high prevalence of BP hyperplasia, investigators have focused on methods of improving the ability of the PSA test to distinguish between men with BP hyperplasia and men with cancer. Recommendations include adjusting serum PSA levels for patient age, prostate volume, and the rate of change of PSA values.[22–24] With the advent of specific assays quantifying PSA molecular forms, the measurement of free, unbound PSA has been evaluated as a method of distinguishing between BP hyperplasia and cancer.[25]

Imaging studies are frequently employed to evaluate the extent of prostate cancer progression. Bone scans and computed tomography (CT) scans are the most common, but other studies include pelvic magnetic resonance imaging (MRI) and endorectal coil MRI. Unfortunately, most of these studies are insufficiently sensitive to identify microscopic metastases. A prospective analysis of more than 3600 men demonstrated that imaging studies are positive in fewer than 10% of cases when the serum PSA level is less than 20 ng/ml or the Gleason score is less than 8.[26] Only men with serum PSA levels higher than 50 ng/ml are likely to have evidence of metastatic disease that can be identified on bone scan, CT scan, or MRI. Unfortunately, more than half of the men with newly diagnosed prostate cancer who have a serum PSA level over 10 ng/ml already have disease extension beyond the confines of the prostate.[27] Men with serum PSA levels over 20 ng/ml are usually poor candidates for surgical therapy because of the high rate of tumor recurrence within 5 years of surgical therapy.

## Surgical Treatment of Prostatic Disease

### Benign Prostatic Hyperplasia

#### *Transurethral Resection of the Prostate*

Urologists have developed several surgical procedures to manage BP hyperplasia. Open surgical excision, known as a simple prostatectomy, was developed more than 100 years ago. Although surgeons still utilize this approach to remove large glands, most urologists now favor transurethral resection of the prostate (TURP). In 1986 it was reported that 96% of the more than 350,000 men requiring surgical therapy for BP hyperplasia had a TURP. The advent of medical therapies and less invasive office-based procedures to treat BP hyperplasia have decreased the frequency of this procedure, so fewer than 200,000 men in the Medicare age group now undergo TURP annually.

The procedure is usually performed under a spinal or general anesthetic. The patient is generally placed in the lithotomy position with the buttocks located just at the edge of the table. Because urinary tract infections are found in 8–24% of men with BP hyperplasia, many are initially treated with antibiotics and most receive a prophylactic dose of antibiotics prior to initiating surgery. The resection is normally conducted in a fluid medium. Water can be used, but it increases the risk of hemolysis; hence nonhemolytic solutions are more commonly employed, such as 1.5% glycine, sorbitol, or mannitol.

The resection technique varies according to the size and configuration of the prostate. The ventral tissue is usually resected first, so the adenomatous tissue drops into the field of resection. If the patient has a large median lobe, this tissue is usually resected first. The amount of intraoperative bleeding depends on the size of the prostate, the length of time required to resect the hyperplastic tissue, and the skill of the surgeon. Arterial bleeding is controlled by electrocoagulation. Venous bleeding may be apparent at the end of the procedure, when on irrigating the catheter the returning fluid initially clears but then turns dark red. Venous bleeding can be controlled by inserting a catheter and placing it on traction for several minutes. Extravasation occurs in approximately 2% of patients, usually following capsular penetration. The symptoms associated with extravasation and fluid absorption include nausea, vomiting, and abdominal pain. Most of these patients can be managed simply by terminating the procedure and placing a urethral catheter. Patients who absorb large amounts of fluid can become severely hyponatremic and may require treatment with hypertonic saline and diuretics.

Over the past 50 years there has been a steady decline in postoperative complications and mortality associated with transurethral resection. These improvements can be attributed to several factors, including better medical management, better anesthesia, and better surgical equipment including improvements in optics and light sources. Wasson et al. reported that 91% of men undergoing TURP in the Veterans Affairs health care system experienced no complication during the first 30 days after surgery.[28] The mortality rate due to surgery was less than 1%. The most frequent complications reported included the need for catheter exchange (4%), perforation of the prostatic capsule (2%), and hemorrhage requiring transfusion (1%). Long-term complications at 3 years associated with TURP include vesicle neck contracture requiring endoscopic surgery (3%), urethral stricture requiring dilation (3%), and secondary transurethral resection (3%).

### Simple Prostatectomy

Open prostatectomy is usually considered when the prostate gland is approximately 70g or larger. This procedure should also be considered when other concomitant bladder conditions are present, such as a large diverticulum or a large, hard bladder calculus. The advantage of open prostatectomy is complete removal of the adenomatous tissue under direct vision without the risk of dilutional hyponatremia, which is often associated with a prolonged transurethral resection. The disadvantages include the need for a lower midline incision, a longer hospitalization, and an extended convalescence period. In addition there may be an increased potential for intraoperative hemorrhage from the prostate fossa. Contraindications to this operation include a small prostate gland, a previous prostatectomy, previous pelvic surgery, and prostate cancer.

An open prostatectomy can be accomplished using one of two approaches: a retropubic approach or a suprapubic approach. With the retropubic approach, the anterior prostatic capsule is incised and the hyperplastic adenoma enucleated. The advantages of this approach are excellent anatomic exposure of the adenoma, precise transection of the urethra distally to preserve urinary continence, clear and immediate visualization of the prostate fossa to control hemorrhage, and minimal trauma to the urinary bladder. The disadvantages of this approach include the inability to access the bladder and difficulty dealing with a large median lobe.

A suprapubic prostatectomy is accomplished by enucleating the prostate through an extraperitoneal incision in the lower anterior bladder wall. The major advantage of this procedure over the retropubic approach is that it allows better visualization of the bladder neck and bladder. As a result, this operation is ideally suited for patients with a large median lobe protruding into the bladder, a concomitant symptomatic bladder diverticulum, or a large bladder calculus. It also may be the preferred approach in obese men when it is difficult to gain direct access to the prostate capsule and the dorsal vein complex. The major disadvantage of this approach is the inability to visualize the apical portion of the prostate directly. As a result, the apical enucleation is less precise along with hemostasis.

### Minimally Invasive Surgical Techniques

Although TURP is considered the standard surgical procedure for treatment of BP hyperplasia, the associated morbidity and related costs of hospitalization have prompted the development of several alternative surgical procedures. Most of these procedures involve some type of heating of the adenomatous tissue to achieve a reduction in urinary symptoms.

High-intensity focused ultrasound or microwave heating techniques have been used to achieve thermal ablation of adenomatous tissue. Most of these procedures involve delivery of energy through a catheter placed transurethrally. A urologist creates a series of focal lesions in the adenoma by firing a focused ultrasound beam through a cystoscope or placing microwave antennae directly into the adenomatous tissue. The treatment area can be as long as 40mm, as wide as 10mm, and as deep as 10mm. These treated areas develop coagulation necrosis and slough after several days to weeks.

Thermotherapy can alleviate voiding symptoms by utilizing a wide range of temperatures. As the intraprostatic temperature rises with the use of higher power devices, more tissue is destroyed, cavities are produced, and more sedation and analgesia are required. Up to 80% of patients experience urinary retention after thermotherapy at high temperature settings. Usually a catheter is placed and may be needed for up to 3 weeks. Patients undergoing these procedures appear to have some reduction in their voiding symptoms, but results are usually less dramatic than are achieved by transurethral resection. Greater symptom improvement usually occurs following treatment with devices delivering higher temperatures. Unfortunately, long-term results are unavailable for many of these procedures. Their role in the treatment of geriatric patients with BP hyperplasia remain to be defined.

## Prostate Cancer

The appropriate treatment of prostate cancer among old men remains controversial. Studies concerning the long-term outcomes of men treated conservatively for their disease have documented the relatively modest disease-specific mortality among men with low and moderate grade tumors.[29–31] A recently published competing risk analysis of men aged 55–74 years at diagnosis demonstrated that men with Gleason score 2–4 and 5 tumors have a 4–7% and 6–11% chance, respectively, of dying from prostate cancer.[32] Older patients had a much greater chance of dying from competing medical hazards (Fig. 57.5). Conversely, men with Gleason score 7 and 8–10 tumors have a 42–70% and 60–87% chance, respectively,

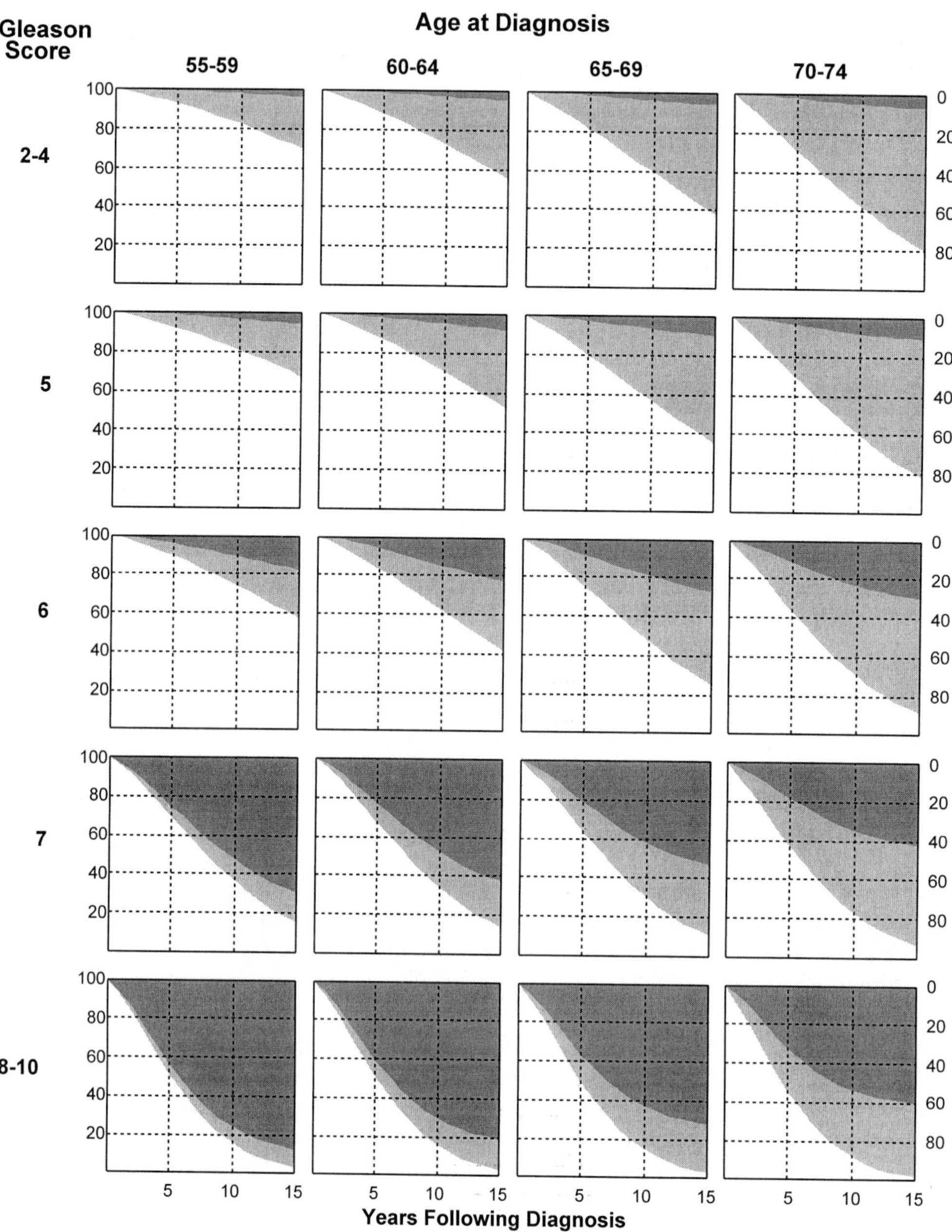


FIGURE 57.5. Survival (white lower band) and cumulative mortality from prostate cancer (dark gray upper band) and other causes (light gray middle band) up to 15 years after diagnosis stratified by age at diagnosis and Gleason score. Percentage of men alive can be read from the left-hand scale, and percentage of men who have died from prostate cancer or from other causes during this interval can be read from the right-hand scale. (From Albertsen et al.,[32] with permission.)

of dying from prostate cancer if it is treated with hormone therapy alone. Men with Gleason score 6 tumors face an intermediate risk (18–30%) of dying from prostate cancer within 15 years if the tumors are treated with hormone therapy alone. Based on these results it appears that men over age 70 years at diagnosis with Gleason score 2–5 disease face a minimal risk of dying from prostate cancer and therefore may not be good candidates for surgical therapy. Men whose biopsy specimens show Gleason score 7–10 disease face a high risk of death from prostate cancer when treated with hormone therapy alone, even when cancer is diagnosed as late as age 74 years. These men may wish to consider surgical treatment in an attempt to cure their disease. Alternatives to surgery include external beam radiation therapy and implantation of radioactive seeds, often referred to as brachytherapy.

When choosing therapy for an individual patient with clinically localized prostate cancer, the age and general health of the patient remain critically important because of the indolent progression of many prostate cancers. Death from a localized cancer left untreated is not likely to occur for 8–10 years, yet the risk of death from prostate cancer continues to increase for at least 15 years (Fig. 57.5). In 1989 the average life expectancy of a man age 70 years was 12.1 years, and for a 75-year-old man it was less than 10 years (Table 57.2). Thus the potential benefits of surgical intervention decreases rapidly as men age.

Chronologic age is only one factor that influences life expectancy. Prostate cancer occurs frequently in elderly men who have associated co-morbid conditions. Conversely, some old patients are in excellent physical condition and have a life expectancy longer than average for their age group. The impact of co-morbid conditions on long-term outcomes among men with localized prostate cancer has been assessed.[33] Men with significant co-morbid disease, measured using one of several instruments, have a much higher probability of dying from causes other than prostate cancer compared with those men with no or relatively few competing medical hazards (Fig. 57.6). Elderly patients must carefully assess the risks and benefits of surgical management compared with those of conservative management before making a decision concerning which therapy is the appropriate management for their localized prostate cancer.

TABLE 57.2. Life Expectancy at Single Years of Age for Men, All Races

| Age (years) | Life expectancy (years) |
|---|---|
| 65 | 14.6 |
| 66 | 13.9 |
| 67 | 13.3 |
| 68 | 12.7 |
| 69 | 12.1 |
| 70 | 11.6 |
| 71 | 11.0 |
| 72 | 10.5 |
| 73 | 10.0 |
| 74 | 9.5 |
| 75 | 9.0 |
| 76 | 8.6 |
| 77 | 8.1 |
| 78 | 7.7 |
| 79 | 7.3 |
| 80 | 6.9 |
| 81 | 6.5 |
| 82 | 6.1 |
| 83 | 5.8 |
| 84 | 5.5 |
| 85 | 5.2 |

### *Radical Prostatectomy*

Surgical excision of prostate cancer can be accomplished using one of two surgical approaches: a retropubic approach or a perineal approach. Each approach has its advantages and disadvantages, but both appear to offer the same probability of controlling spread of disease. In the United States approximately 93% of all radical prostatectomies are accomplished using the retropubic approach, and 7% are completed using the perineal technique.[34]

Radical retropubic prostatectomy is performed with the patient in a supine position with the table hyperextended to increase exposure to the prevesicle space. The procedure is usually performed under general anesthesia, although regional techniques using an epidural catheter are popular because they decrease the need for narcotics during the procedure and the postoperative period. Usually a pelvic lymph node dissection is performed as the first step. The lymphadenectomy is not therapeutic but does provide additional pathology to stage the cancer accurately. The procedure is performed by incising the endopelvic fascia, controlling the dorsal vein complex, and then dividing the urethra at the level of the prostate apex. In young men care is taken to preserve the neurovascular bundles that lie on either side of the prostate apex. Unfortunately, among most old men there is a high probability of impotence associated with this procedure. Once the prostate and seminal vesicles have been removed, the bladder neck is repaired and secured to the stump of the urethra. Careful dissection around the apex of the prostate to avoid injury to the pelvic floor musculature should minimize the chance of incontinence.

Radical perineal prostatectomy was first described by Young more than 90 years ago.[35] Although utilized infrequently for many decades, this operation has attracted renewed interest because of the rapid recovery and short hospitalization associated with it. Major advantages of this approach include a relatively painless incision anterior to the rectum compared with a lower midline

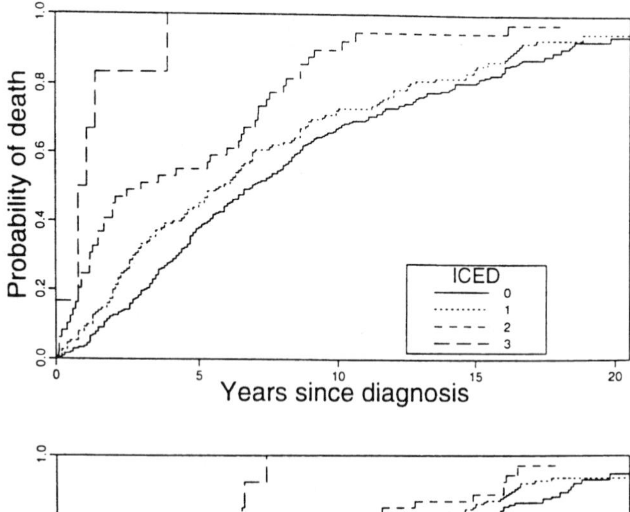


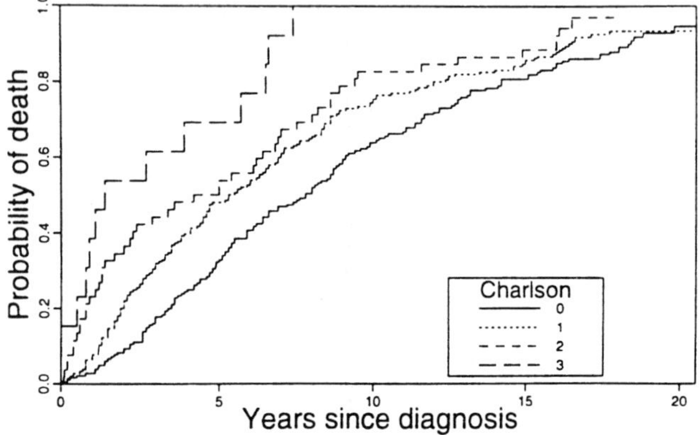


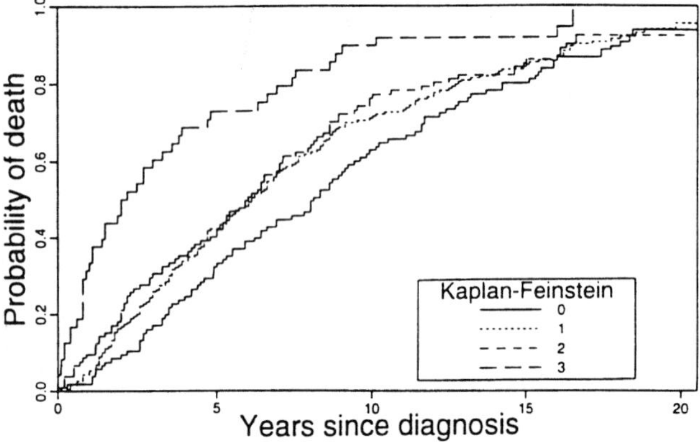


FIGURE 57.6. Cumulative mortality from all causes of death stratified by severity of co-morbidities at diagnosis as measured by each of three instruments tested. Data are not adjusted for patient age or Gleason score, ICED. index of coexistent disease. (From Albertsen et al.,[32] with permission.)

approach and generally less blood loss because the dorsal vein complex is not transected. Its major disadvantage is the inability to assess the pelvic lymph nodes as part of the procedure.

Radical perineal prostatectomy is performed with the patient in an exaggerated lithotomy position. The procedure is often performed under general anesthesia or using a regional technique such as spinal or epidural anesthesia. An incision is made anterior to the rectum in the floor of the perineum. The central tendon is divided; and using blunt and sharp dissection, the rectourethralis muscle is divided and the plane underneath Denonvillier's fascia is developed. The posterior membranous urethra is divided just distal to the apex of the prostate. A special retractor is placed in the bladder to facilitate dissection of the anterior surface of the prostate and guide the surgeon to the proper location to incise the bladder neck. The bladder neck is then separated from the prostate and closed by approximating the tissue posteriorly. The bladder is attached to the urethra, and the incision is closed.

Both radical retropubic prostatectomy and radical perineal prostatectomy are associated with complications, which increase with the patient's age. An analysis of more than 100,000 Medicare claims has demonstrated that approximately one in four patients suffers a major or minor complication associated with these procedures.[34] The radical retropubic approach had higher risks of respiratory complications and miscellaneous medical complications and a lower risk of miscellaneous surgical complications. The perineal approach resulted in a 1–2% incidence of rectal injury, but this appears to be offset by the medical complications of the gastrointestinal tract with the retropubic approach. Short-term mortality following radical prostatectomy is low; approximately 0.5% for men under age 70 years and about 1.0% for men aged 75 years and older. Table 57.3 demonstrates that the risk of mortality increases sharply with age.

Long-term complications associated with radical prostatectomy include impotence and incontinence. Although modern surgical techniques have decreased the incidence of postsurgical incontinence, reported rates of this complication vary widely. Patient reports of incontinence have been as high as 31%, whereas reports from tertiary medical centers suggest rates under 10%.[36,37] The age of the patient and whether an anastomotic stricture develops influence the recovery of continence. Patients over age 65 years have a greater risk of incontinence compared to men under age 65 years.

Return of erectile function has also been correlated with patient age. Quinlan and colleagues evaluated 503 potent men between the ages of 34 and 72 years who

TABLE 57.3. Thirty-Day Mortality Following Radical Prostatectomy by Age and Surgical Approach

| | 30-Day mortality, by surgical approach (%) | |
|---|---|---|
| Age (years) | Retropubic approach | Perineal approach |
| 65–69 | 0.45 | 0.22 |
| 70–74 | 0.60 | 0.36 |
| 75+ | 1.04 | 0.95 |
| Overall | 0.56 | 0.37 |

underwent radical retropubic prostatectomy.[38] Among men under the age of 50, about 90% were potent if one or both neurovascular bundles were preserved.[39] Among men age 65–69 years, only 27% recovered sexual function. Recovery of sexual function is likely to be even lower among men 70 years and older.

## Conclusions

Prostate diseases cause significant morbidity and mortality among elderly men. Both BP hyperplasia and prostate cancer are relatively rare before age 50 years but become increasingly common as men age into their sixties and seventies. For many patients with mild or moderate symptoms of bladder outlet obstruction, watchful waiting or various medical therapies may be sufficient therapy. As symptoms worsen, however, surgical treatment may offer the best chance of relieving symptoms of urinary frequency, hesitancy, and slow stream. Most patients with symptomatic BP hyperplasia should be offered therapy with an α-blocker or a 5α-reductase inhibitor before proceeding to transurethral prostatectomy. Only patients with large prostates should be considered for open prostatectomy.

Prostate cancer poses a much more difficult problem for old men, especially men with well or moderately differentiated tumors. Prostate cancer in these men is frequently a slow-growing tumor, and other medical hazards may become the dominant medical problem long before the cancer metastasizes.

Patients must carefully assess the relative risks and benefits of a surgical approach compared with other less invasive options, such as delayed hormone therapy or irradiation before proceeding with radical prostatectomy. Men with high grade prostate cancers (Gleason scores 7–10) face a significant risk of dying from their disease even when it is diagnosed as a localized disease as late as age 74 years. These men may want to consider radical prostatectomy as the preferred treatment option. Fortunately, in 2001, the primary risk associated with radical prostatectomy is impotence. Incontinence is less common, while mortality from surgery is a relatively rare event.

## References


1. Berry SJ, Coffey DS, Walsh PC, Ewing LL. The development of human benign prostatic hyperplasia with age. J Urol 1984;132:474.
2. Gaynor EP. Zur frage des prostatakrebes. Virchows Arch Pathol Anat 1938;301:602–652.
3. Arrighi HM, Guess HA, Metter EJ, et al. Symptoms and signs of prostatism as risk factors for prostatectomy. Prostate 1990;16:253.
4. Stanford JL, Stephenson RA, Coyle LM, et al. Prostate cancer trends 1973–1995, SEER program, NIH Pub No. 99-4543. Bethesda: National Cancer Institute, 1999.
5. Greenlee RT, Murray T, Bolden S, Wingo PA. Cancer statistics, 1999. CA Cancer J Clin 2000;50:7–33.
6. Edwards CN, Steinthorsson E, Nicholson D. An autopsy study of latent prostatic cancer. Cancer 1953;32:498–506.
7. Halpert B, Sheehan EE, Schmalhorst WR, Scott R. Carcinoma of the prostate: a survey of 5000 autopsies. Cancer 1963;16:737–742.
8. Shimizu H, Ross RK, Bernstein L, Yatani R, Henderson BE, Mack TM. Cancers of the prostate and breast among Japanese and white immigrants in Los Angeles County. Br J Cancer 1991;63:963–966.
9. Yatani R, Chigusa I, Akazaki K, Stemmermann GN, Welsh RA. Geographic pathology of latent prostatic carcinoma. Int J Cancer 1982;29:611–616.
10. Smith JR, Freije D, Carpten JD, et al. Major susceptibility locus for prostate cancer on chromosome 1 suggested by a genome-wide search. Science 1996;274:1371–1374.
11. Steinberg GS, Carter BS, Beaty TH, Childs B, Walsh PC. Family history and the risk of prostate cancer. Prostate 1990;17:337–340.
12. McNeal JE. Origin and evolution of benign prostatic enlargement. Invest Urol 1978;15:340.
13. Caine M, Schuger L. The "Capsule" in Benign Prostatic Hypertrophy. NIH Publ No. 87-2881. Bethesda: US Department of Health and Human Services, 1987:221.
14. Byar DP, Mostofi FK. Veterans Administration Cooperative Urologic Research Groups: carcinoma of the prostate: prognostic evaluation of certain pathologic features in 208 radical prostatectomies. Cancer 1972;30:5–13.
15. McNeal JE. Cancer volume and site of origin of adenocarcinoma of the prostate: relationship to local and distant spread. Hum Pathol 1992;23:258–266.
16. Gleason DF, Mellinger GT. Veterans Administration Cooperative Urological Research Group: prediction of prognosis for prostatic adenocarcinoma by combined histologic grading and clinical staging. J Urol 1974;111:58–64.
17. McConnell JD, Barry MJ, Bruskewitz RC, et al. Benign Prostatic Hyperplasia: Diagnosis and Treatment. Clinical Practice Guideline Number 8. AHCPR Publ No. 94-0582. Rockville, MD: Agency for Health Care Policy & Research, Public Health Service, US Department of Health and Human Services, 1994.
18. Mebust WK, Holtgrewe HL, Cockette ATK, Peters PC, Writing Committee. Transurethral prostatectomy: immediate and postoperative complications: a cooperative study of 13 participating institutions evaluating 3885 patients. J Urol 1989;141:243–247.
19. Melchoir J, Valk WL, Foret JD, Mebust MK. Transurethral prostatectomy in the azotemic patient. J Urol 1974;112:643–646.
20. Gilliland F, Becker TM, Smith A, et al. Trends in prostate cancer incidence and mortality in New Mexico are consistent with an increase in effective screening. Cancer Epidemiol Biol Prev 1994;3:105–111.
21. Ellis WJ, Chetner MP, Preston SD, Brawer MK. Diagnosis of prostatic carcinoma: the yield of serum prostate specific antigen, digital rectal examination and transrectal ultrasonography. J Urol 1994;52:1520–1525.
22. Oesterling JE, Jacobsen SJ, Chute CG, et al. Serum prostate-specific antigen in a community-based population of

healthy men: establishment of age-specific reference ranges. JAMA 1993;270:860–864.
23. Benson MC, Whang IS, Olsson CA, et al. Use of prostate specific antigen density to enhance predictive value of intermediate levels of serum prostate specific antigen. J Urol 1992;147:817–821.
24. Carter HB, Pearson JD, Metter JE, et al. Longitudinal evaluation of prostate specific antigen levels in men with and without prostate disease. JAMA 1992;267:2215–2220.
25. Catalona WJ, Simth DS, Wolfert RL, et al. Evaluation of percentage of free serum prostate-specific antigen to improve specificity of prostate cancer screening. JAMA 1995;274: 1214–1220.
26. Albertsen PC, Hanley JA, Harlan JC, et al. The positive yield of imaging studies in the evaluation of men with newly diagnosed prostate cancer: a population-based analysis. J Urology 2000;163:1138–1143.
27. Catalona WJ, Smith DS, Ratliff TL, Basler JW. Detection of organ-confined prostate cancer is increased through prostate-specific antigen-based testing. JAMA 1993;270: 948–954.
28. Wasson JH, Reda DJ, Bruskewitz RC, et al. A comparison of transurethral surgery with watchful waiting for moderate symptoms of benign prostatic hyperplasia. N Engl J Med 1995;332:75–79.
29. Johansson JE, Homberg L, Johansson S, Bergstrom R, Adami HO. Fifteen year survival in prostate cancer: a prospective, population-based study in Sweden. JAMA 1997;277: 467–471.
30. Chodak GW, Thisted RA, Gerber GS, et al. Results of conservative management of clinically localized prostate cancer. N Engl J Med 1994;330:242–248.
31. Albertsen PC, Fryback DG, Storer BE, Kolon TF, Fine J. Long term survival among men with conservatively treated localized prostate cancer. JAMA 1995;274:626–631.
32. Albertsen PC, Hanley JA, Gleason DF, Barry MJ. Competing risk analysis of men aged 55 to 74 years at diagnosis managed conservatively for clinically localized prostate cancer. JAMA 1998;280:975–980.
33. Albertsen PC, Fryback DG, Storer BE, Kolon TF, Fine J. The impact of co-morbidity on life expectancy among men with localized prostate cancer. J Urol 1996;156:127–132.
34. Lu-Yao GL, Albertsen PC, Warren J, Yao SL. Effect of age and surgical approach on complications and short-term mortality after radical prostatectomy: a population-based study. Urology 1999;54:301–307.
35. Young HH. The early diagnosis and radical cure of carcinoma of the prostate: being a study of 40 cases and presentation of a radical operation which was carried out in four cases. Johns Hopkins Hosp Bull 1905;16:315–321.
36. Fowler FJ, Barry MJ, Lu-Yao G, et al. Patient-reported complications and follow-up treatment after radical prostatectomy. J Urol 1993;149:622–629.
37. Eastham JA, Kattan MW, Rogers E, et al. Risk factors for urinary incontinence after radical retropubic prostatectomy. J Urol 1996;156:1707–1713.
38. Quinlan DM, Epstein JI, Carter BS, Walsh PC. Sexual function following radical prostatectomy: influence of reservation of neurovascular bundles. J Urol 1991;145:998–1002.
39. Murphy GP, Mettlin C, Menck H, et al. National patterns of prostate cancer treatment by radical prostatectomy: results of a survey by the American College of Surgeons Committee on Cancer. J Urol 1994;152:1817–1819.

# 58
# Benign Gynecologic Disorders in the Elderly

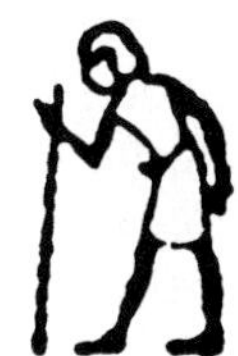

Richard J. Scotti, Juana Hutchinson-Colas, Lauri Ellen Budnick,
George Lazarou, and Wilma Markus Greston

As the American population ages, the demand from the health care system for postreproductive, postmenopausal, and geriatric gynecology increases. A 65-year-old woman can expect to live for another 24 years; a 75-year-old woman can expect to live another 14 years; and an 85-year-old woman will live another 8 years.[1] The striking increase in life expectancy in developed countries over the past century has led to remarkable changes in the spectrum of diseases and is likely to impel major advances in gynecologic technology. Disorders of aging have become common because, for the first time, large numbers of people are living long enough to develop these disorders.

## Menopause

A review of gynecologic conditions in the elderly would not be complete without considering menopause and the physiologic changes that ensue. Menopause is a direct result of the cessation of ovarian function and marks the beginning of a series of changes in the physical, mental, and social aspects of a woman's life. The last menstrual period, the menopause, is a single point in time, but it heralds the beginning of a continuum of declining ovarian function, the postmenopausal period. The average age of menopause is 51 years. A transitional period occurs prior to menopause, when the ovaries become resistant to gonadotropic stimulation. With time, ovulation becomes infrequent, and eventually the ovarian follicles become exhausted; the ovary then produces insignificant amounts of estrogen. Estradiol, the most potent estrogen, falls to $\leq$15 pg/ml with the onset of menopause. With loss of the negative feedback of estrogen on the posterior pituitary, gonadotropin levels rise dramatically.

The primary production of estradiol in postmenopausal women is by peripheral conversion of adrenal androstenedione to estrone, mediated by the aromatase enzyme in fat cells of the body. Small amounts of estradiol are also produced, but, in general, estrone is the principal estrogen produced in postmenopausal women. The natural process of aging results in increased fat body mass and decreased lean body mass. Thus the effect of obesity on estrogen production is biologically important. Not surprisingly, obese postmenopausal women often manifest estrogen excess, such as endometrial hyperplasia and carcinoma.

One of the common physical changes seen with menopause is vasomotor instability characterized by hot flashes. About 75% of postmenopausal women complain of hot flashes, but only one-third seek medical help. Hot flashes decrease in intensity with time. About 80% of affected women have hot flashes for more than 1 year and a significant number have them for at least 5 years. The neural mechanisms controlling hot flashes are not well understood. It has been hypothesized that the neural events that activate pulsatile gonadotropin-releasing hormone (GnRH) secretion may also affect the thalamic centers that regulate body temperature.[2] Estrogen therapy has been clearly demonstrated to be effective treatment for hot flashes.[3] Progestin can relieve hot flashes in postmenopausal women as well.[4]

The process of aging results in cutaneous, mucosal, and genitourinary atrophy. Some of this atrophy can be explained by the fact that connective tissue in general is sex-hormone-sensitive (e.g., collagen, bone). Some of these changes are directly related to estrogen deprivation. Menopause greatly affects the estrogen-sensitive tissues of the urogenital tract. Because the müllerian and mesonephric structures arise in close embryologic proximity, it is not surprising that derivatives of both may be similarly affected by estrogen. In fact, the vagina, cervix, uterus, fallopian tubes, urethra, bladder trigone, pelvic floor, and rectum all have estrogen receptors and are sensitive to a decrease in available estrogen.

Connective tissue in general is sex-hormone-sensitive. Postmenopausal women who are given a combination of estrogen and testosterone have been reported to have greater skin collagen content and greater skin thickness than do untreated women.[5] In untreated women, skin collagen content is inversely proportional to the amount of time since menopause. It also has been shown that oral or transdermal estrogen given together with medroxyprogesterone acetate significantly increases skin collagen content in postmenopausal women.[5]

During the postmenopausal years the natural decline of estrogen production of the ovaries results in atrophic changes of the vulva and vagina. These gradual alterations are physiologic, and many predispose certain women to structural and pathologic conditions. Many of these changes may become chronic if left untreated or worse, if ignored. Physicians who care for the elderly should be aware of the conditions that occur most commonly in this age group so the appropriate diagnostic procedures and treatments may be carried out.

## Lower Genital Tract

### Vulva

The external genitalia of a woman include the mons pubis, labia majora, labia minora, prepuce, frenulum, clitoris, and vestibule. Skene, Bartholin's and minor vestibular glands and the urethral meatus open into the vestibule. The vulva is covered by keratinized stratified squamous epithelium except for the vestibule. The mucosa of the vestibule is glycogenated in women of reproductive age and in those on estrogen supplementation; it resembles vaginal mucosa.

During the postmenopausal years the vulva undergoes progressive changes in appearance as ovarian estrogen production diminishes and aging ensues. There is loss of skin turgor in the vulva as well as in all skin throughout the body. Pubic hair becomes less robust and more sparse. There is loss of labial fat, causing the size of the labia to be reduced. Retraction and thinning of the skin around the introitus may lead to uncomfortable fissures of the epithelium with subsequent dyspareunia and pain with urination.

Benign epithelial disorders of the vulva are divided into neoplastic and nonneoplastic conditions. Invasive lesions of the urogenital tract are reviewed elsewhere in this book (see Chapter 59). Nonneoplastic conditions include the vulvar dystrophies and other dermatoses. It is difficult to distinguish between neoplastic and nonneoplastic conditions of the vulva on the basis of inspection alone. The best approach for establishing a diagnosis is to have a high index of suspicion and to biopsy early.

#### *Neoplastic Conditions*

##### Squamous Papilloma

Squamous papilloma is a benign epithelial neoplasm of concern in the aging woman. It appears as a warty or verrucous exophytic tumor of variable size, arising from the labia. Malignant transformation is rare.

##### Vulvar Intraepithelial Neoplasia

Vulvar intraepithelial neoplasia (VIN) is frequently asymptomatic, although patients may complain of pruritus. This lesion presents clinically with a raised surface that is often pigmented. VIN III has been reported by Friedrich[6] to be the second most common cause of pigmented vulvar lesions. The lesions may be single or multiple. Histologically, there is proliferation of the epithelial layer, with degrees of cellular atypia. There is high mitotic activity, a high nuclear/cytoplasmic ratio, and the absence of cytoplasmic differentiation in the upper epithelial layers. VIN often involves skin appendages, which may be confused with early invasion, especially in hair-bearing areas. Invasion, if present, is most commonly seen in postmenopausal women.

#### *Nonneoplastic Disorders*

In 1987 the International Society for the Study of Vulvar Vaginal Diseases, in collaboration with the International Society of Gynecologic Pathologists, proposed the following classification of nonneoplastic epithelial disorders: (1) lichen sclerosus; (2) squamous cell hyperplasia; (3) other dermatoses.[7]

##### Lichen Sclerosus

Lichen sclerosus is a benign epithelial disorder of unknown etiology that can occur at any age. It is noted most commonly in the extremes of life, particularly in postmenopausal caucasian women. The majority of the afffected women are over age 50. The vulva is the site most commonly involved. Lichen sclerosus is characterized by thinning of the epithelium, with edema and fibrosis of the dermis, resulting in the associated shrinkage and agglutination of the labia with introital stenosis. It accounts for approximately 10% of outpatient visits related to vulvar symptoms. Lichen sclerosus typically does not involve the vagina or urethra. Patients most often experience pruritus in the affected areas. Sexually active women may experience external or entry dyspareunia related to the labial changes and introital shrinkage. In addition, shrinkage of the labia, prepuce, and frenulum may occur with agglutination of the labia minora and the prepuce. This also may lead to severe introital stenosis, with the clitoris buried underneath the agglutinated labia minora. The condition occasionally presents with perianal stenosis. The diagnosis is confirmed by biopsy. Characteristic histologic features include thinning of the epithelium with loss of rete ridges (pegs).

Management is primarily medical, and current treatment for lichen sclerosus includes high-potency topical corticosteroids, such as 0.05% clobetasol propionate or a 0.05% preparation of halobetasol propionate applied twice daily for 2–3 weeks and then decreasing to once daily, usually at night, until symptoms and findings begin to subside. In the past, topical progesterone and topical testosterone were commonly used for lichen sclerosus with varying results. These agents may be no more effective than topical corticosteroids. Simple emollients such as lanolin or hydrogenated vegetable oil often give relief and may improve the involved skin. Antipruritic compounds and antibiotic ointments should be avoided because they may cause irritation. Preventive measures for vulvar lichen sclerosus include maintaining good personal hygiene, keeping the vulva dry, and protecting the skin from injury or local irritants.

After treatment, vaginal dilators may help reduce introital stenosis, provided the lichen sclerosus is not fissured, ulcered, or ecchymotic.[7] Some women with vulvar lichen sclerosus develop vulvar squamous cell carcinoma; therefore if symptoms do not resolve after appropriate treatment, rebiopsy is essential.

### Squamous Cell Hyperplasia

Squamous cell hyperplasia is a benign epithelial disorder that may be indistinguishable clinically from lichen simplex chronicus, discussed below. These patients typically present with vulvar pruritus and have localized, nonspecific thickening of the vulvar skin. The involved skin color may range from white to gray, primarily as the result of epithelial edema. The diagnosis is one of exclusion and is confirmed by biopsy. Microscopic examination of the epithelium reveals broadened, deepened rete pegs without significant dermal inflammation, fibrosis, or thickening.

Treatment is based on limiting or preventing exposure of the vulva to irritants. Topical corticosteroids and antipruritics are also used. It is essential that squamous cell hyperplasia be distinguished from condyloma acuminata. Squamous cell hyperplasia is managed by application of topical medium-strength corticosteroids, such as 0.1% betamethasone valerate, twice daily, decreased to once daily when symptoms resolve. Most patients respond to treatment with resolution of symptoms and clinical improvement within 2–3 weeks. Avoidance of contact with local irritants and good personal hygiene is prudent. Treatment is generally curative.

### Lichen Simplex Chronicus

Lichen simplex chronicus appears to be similar to squamous cell hyperplasia, but there is histologic evidence of chronic inflammatory cells within the superficial dermis, as well as fibrosis and collagenization. The differentiation is based on the histologic specimens. Multiple biopsy specimens should be obtained if the lesions are heterogeneous in appearance. Biopsies sufficient for a histologic diagnosis are easily obtained in the office under local anesthesia with a Keyes punch biopsy. It is important to include the full thickness of the epithelium when obtaining the biopsy. A small margin of normal-appearing skin should be included in the biopsy specimen to minimize interpretation error because of excessive inflammation or necrosis. Silver nitrate or a single stitch is usually adequate to achieve hemostasis.

Proper vulvar hygiene is extremely important, and women with vulvar dysplasia should avoid irritants such as perfumes, soaps, and strong laundry detergents. Corticosteroids initially may help decrease inflammation and provide some comfort and relief from itching.

### Lichen Planus

Lichen planus is another dermatosis seen in women over 40 years of age. Vulvar pruritus and burning are common symptoms, although some patients are asymptomatic. The clinical appearance is highly variable and therefore can be confused with many other vulvar conditions. A biopsy should be performed early. Microscopic features are also variable depending on the age and location of the lesion. Two important features are reported: (1) a band-like chronic inflammatory infiltrate composed predominantly of lymphocytes with rare plasma cells; and (2) liquefactive necrosis of basal epithelial cells admixed with chronic inflammatory cells. Degenerated keratinocytes result in colloidal body formation.

It is important to biopsy all elevated or white lesions of the vulva, as many look alike or their appearance may be altered by excoriation or inflammation. Importantly, vulvar carcinoma can be diagnosed early, if present, and treated appropriately.

### Bartholin's Cyst and Abscess

Bartholin's cyst and abscess is an uncommon lesion in the elderly. In the postmenopausal woman, recurrent cysts or palpable masses after cyst drainage should be excised surgically because of the higher frequency of associated carcinoma of the Bartholin gland in the elderly.[8]

### Necrotizing Fasciitis

Necrotizing fasciitis is a life-threatening condition that is usually secondary to a polymicrobial infection of the skin and subcutaneous fat. This disease may present as an innocuous-appearing labial pustule, with inflammation of the vulva that is rapidly progressive. It may initially appear as mild cellulitis or edema with inflammation. This superficial appearance may mask the underlying pathology. Patients with diabetes are at increased risk of having this condition. A delay in diagnosis results in approximately 50% mortality. Necrotizing fasciitis of the vulva is a surgical emergency. Radical excision and use of broad-spectrum antibiotic therapy offers the only chance for cure.[9]

## Urethra

### Urethral Prolapse

The urethral orifice is within the vestibule, and abnormalities may present as a vulvar mass. Urethral prolapse may occur at any age but is more commonly seen during the extremes of life. A relative lack of estrogen may explain the laxity of the supporting periurethral fascia, which contributes to the formation of urethral prolapse in the elderly woman. The prolapsing urethra may present as a large red polypoid mass covered with urethral mucosa and edematous vascular submucosa protruding from the orifice and mimicking a urethral neoplasm. Histologically, inflammatory infiltrates are seen in the underlying connective tissue.

Treatment consists of hot sitz baths and antibiotics to reduce inflammation and infection. If conservative management fails, surgical treatment is necessary. Cryosurgery is an effective method of treatment. Excision of the mass is preferable and provides tissue for histopathologic diagnosis. Topical estrogen may be applied after surgical intervention to hasten healing.

### Urethral Caruncles

Urethral caruncles are tender polypoid masses that arise at the urethral meatus in postmenopausal women. They are a result of estrogen deprivation and may present as localized areas of prolapse; they are by far the most common lesions of the urethra. Caruncles are often asymptomatic but may cause bleeding or dysuria. Clinical differentiation from the rare condition of urethral carcinoma may be difficult; therefore, biopsy is often helpful for making the diagnosis. They are best treated by the use of systemic and local estrogens.

## Vagina

The vagina is a flattened but distensible muscular and membranous canal that extends from the external genitalia to the cervix. The lining is composed of stratified squamous epithelium and is under the influence of estrogen.

One of the earliest manifestations of the withdrawal of estrogenic effect on the vagina is the change in the vaginal cytologic maturation index. The well-estrogenized vagina normally sheds cells of the most superficial layer. With decreased estrogen, the number of superficial cells shed is reduced, and as the vagina atrophies, parabasal cells alone may be seen cytologically.

Histologically, the epithelium and muscular layer become thin, resulting in the loss of vaginal rugae. There is also a decrease in the vascularity of the lamina propria that results in a pale appearance of the epithelium. These changes result in both shortening of and a decrease in the distensibility of the vagina. The introitus narrows, and the pelvic examination and sexual intercourse may become uncomfortable. Vaginal dryness also occurs, making intercourse difficult without adding lubricants.

Physiologic changes seen during the postmenopausal period include a decrease in vaginal blood flow accompanied by a decrease in vaginal fluid production.[10] The vaginal pH also rises to 5.0–5.5, which is significantly higher than the norm of 3.4–4.5. The associated increase in vaginal pH may result in increased colonization of the vagina by pathogenic bacteria as the number of the naturally protective *Lactobacillus* species decreases.

Relief of symptoms of vaginal atrophy is accomplished in most cases with local estrogen therapy in the form of estrogen creams or an estrogen-impregnated ring. Oral therapy or patch therapy with estrogen should also be initiated or continued. Patients whose uteri remain intact must also be given progestogens to prevent endometrial hyperplasia or frank carcinoma from unopposed estrogen therapy. Estrogen therapy also leads to decreases in vaginal pH to the normal range. Vaginal blood flow and transudation of fluid increases. These changes begin within a matter of days; progressive improvement can take place in the ensuing 2–3 months after therapy has begun.[11]

### Vaginal Intraepithelial Neoplasia

Vaginal intraepithelial neoplasia (VAIN) is a rare condition, detected most often in postmenopausal women. VAIN is graded from I to III. Most cases are found on biopsy to be VAIN III, or carcinoma in situ; and they are associated with previous or concurrent vulvar or cervical neoplasia. There is also an association with human papilloma virus.

VAIN is asymptomatic and is detected on cytologic screening. Colposcopy or application of Lugol's iodine solution aids in localizing the lesions. They are most often present at the vaginal apex.

Treatment modalities include excision, irradiation, laser vaporization, and local application of 5% 5-fluorouracil cream. Women diagnosed and treated for VAIN are at risk for recurrence or for the development of cancer involving the vulva, vagina, and cervix; hence, they require regular gynecologic follow-up indefinitely.

## Cervix

The cervix contains two types of epithelium: stratified squamous and glandular columnar. Stratified squamous epithelium lines the portio and extends to the external os.

Nonciliated glandular columnar epithelium lines the endocervical canal. The transformation zone is the area that marks the dividing line between these two types of epithelium. Active metaplasia is seen in this zone, and these metaplastic cells are most vulnerable to neoplastic change. The transformation zone in the postmenopausal patient is found high in the endocervical canal compared to that in premenopausal patients. With cervical screening, care most be exercised to sample this deep transformation zone. Common cervical causes of postmenopausal bleeding include cervicitis, ulcers, polyps, and possible cancer.

### *Cervicitis*

Cervicitis is most commonly due to postmenopausal atrophic changes, similar to those in the vulva and vagina. This inflammation may also be associated with infection. The cervix may also shrink and become flush with the vaginal vault; additionally, the cervical canal may become stenosed, making endocervical sampling and biopsies difficult.

### *Cervical Intraepithelial Neoplasia*

Cervical intraepithelial neoplasia (CIN) can be detected on a Papanicolaou (Pap) smear. The prevalence of abnormal Pap smears in patients over 65 is somewhat high.[12] These abnormalities in Pap smears are a result of hypoestrogenism rather than neoplasia, which is much less common in this age group. The current American College of Obstetricians and Gynecologists guidelines[13] for cervical cancer screening suggest an annual Pap smear for all women who are sexually active or have reached 18 years of age. The Pap test may be performed less frequently after three consecutive satisfactory cytologic examinations. Screening women over the age of 65 appears to be beneficial if they have not undergone prior regular screening. The primary goal of cervical screening is to detect occult cancer and precancerous lesions that may progress to invasive cancer.

A Pap smear is performed by first visualizing the cervix, usually with the use of a speculum. Synthetic lubricants should not be used on the speculum because they may result in cellular distortion. Both the endocervix and the exocervix must be sampled for the Pap smear to reflect all possible sites of abnormal pathology. A cotton swab or cytologic sampling brush is used to obtain the endocervical sample. The ectocervix is sampled using an Ayre spatula. Both samples are placed on a slide and immediately fixed. A new sampling technique, the Thin Prep, has recently been introduced. This method places the sample in a fluid medium that separates the cells, allowing easier screening by a cytotechnician or a computer reader. Any abnormal or suspicious areas visualized must be biopsied. The interpretation of a cervical smear is reported according to the Bethesda system (Table 58.1).[14]

A patient with a normal Pap smear is followed by repeat screening at 12 months. Any patient with atypical squamous cells on a Pap smear should be examined for lower genital tract infection and treated prior to repeating the Pap test. Colposcopic examination is indicated for persistent atypia. It is also indicated for any degree of dysplasia seen on a Pap smear. If a postmenopausal woman has low grade squamous intraepithelial lesion (SIL) or atypical squamous cells of undetermined significance (ASCUS), it may be a result of estrogen deficiency. Treatment with intravaginal estrogen prior to colposcopy aids in the evaluation of these patients. The goal of colposcopy is to help identify dysplastic area(s) so directed cervical biopsies may be performed. Endocervical curettage is helpful for excluding invasive cancer and ruling out extension of the lesion into the endocervical canal.

Management of CIN depends on the size, location, and distribution of the lesion. Any involvement of the endocervical canal requires cervical conization. A diagnostic cone biopsy is also performed to diagnose any microinvasive cancer, if present. With this procedure a small cone of tissue is excised by incision (cold knife cone), electrocautery, or laser. The cone should include any suspicious areas on the exocervix (the largest diameter of the cone) and part or all of the cervical canal (the smallest diameter) depending on the clinician's relative suspicion of the depth of involvement.

Treatment of CIN includes $CO_2$ laser ablation with or without therapeutic conization,[15] electrocoagulation,[16] loop electroexcision of the transformation zone (LEEP),[17] and cryosurgery.[18] Other procedures such as needle-and-ball radical diathermy, cold knife cone biopsy, and hysterectomy require general anesthesia. Posttherapy surveillance includes a Pap smear and colposcopic examination at 3 months, 6 months, 1 year, 18 months, and 2 years. If these examinations are normal, the patient may return to routine screening thereafter.

## Upper Genital Tract

### Uterus

The postmenopausal uterus undergoes retrogressive changes and gradually becomes smaller with age. Leiomyomas (fibroids) tend to atrophy, although they may still be present. Any abnormality of the uterus may result in postmenopausal bleeding, but endometrial cancer must be ruled out when it occurs in this age group. Causes of postmenopausal bleeding include vaginal atrophy with friability, endometrial atrophy, hyperplasia, polyps, and cancer.

TABLE 58.1. Bethesda System for Reporting Cervical/Vaginal Cytologic Diagnoses

Format of the report
- Statement on adequacy of the specimen for evaluation
- General categorization: may be used to assist with clerical triage (optional)
- Descriptive diagnosis

Adequacy of the specimen
- Satisfactory for evaluation
- Satisfactory for evaluation but limited by [*specify reason*]

Unsatisfactory for evaluation [*specify reason*]

General categorization (optional)
- Within normal limits
- Benign cellular changes (see Descriptive diagnoses, below)
- Epithelial cell abnormality (see Descriptive diagnoses, below)

Descriptive diagnoses
- Benign cellular changes
  - Infection
    - *Trichomonas vaginalis*
    - Fungal organisms morphologically consistent with *Candida* spp.
    - Predominance of coccobacilli consistent with shift in vaginal flora
    - Bacteria morphologically consistent with *Actinomyces* spp.
    - Cellular changes associated with herpes simplex virus
    - Other
- Reactive changes
  - Reactive cellular changes associated with
    - Inflammation (includes typical repair)
    - Atrophy with inflammation ("atrophic vaginitis")
    - Radiation
    - Intrauterine contraceptive device (IUD)
  - Other
- Epithelial cell abnormalities
  - Squamous cell
    - Atypical squamous cells of undetermined significance [*qualify*][a]
    - Low-grade squamous intraepithelial lesion encompassing
      - HPV[b]
      - Mild dysplasia/CIN 1
    - High-grade squamous intraepithelial lesion encompassing
      - Moderate and severe dysplasia
      - CIS/CIN 2 and CIN 3
    - Squamous cell carcinoma
  - Glandular cell
    - Endometrial cells, cytologically benign, in a postmenopausal woman
    - Atypical glandular cells of undetermined significance [*qualify*][a]
    - Endocervical adenocarcinoma
    - Endometrial adenocarcinoma
    - Extrauterine adenocarcinoma
    - Adenocarcinoma, not otherwise specified
- Other malignant neoplasms [*specify*]
- Hormonal evaluation (applied to vaginal smears only)
  - Hormonal pattern compatible with age and history
  - Hormonal pattern incompatible with age and history [*specify*]
  - Hormonal evaluation not possible due to [*specify*]

*Source:* American College of Obstetricians and Gynecologists,[14] with permission.

CIS, cancer in situ; CIN, cervical intraepithelial neoplasia.

[a] Atypical squamous or glandular cells of undetermined significance should be further qualified as to whether a reactive or a premalignant/malignant process is favored.

[b] Cellular changes of human papillomavirus (HPV)—previously termed koilocytosis atypia or condylomatous atypia—are included in the category of low-grade squamous intraepithelial lesion.

### *Endometrial Atrophy*

Endometrial atrophy is a frequent cause of postmenopausal uterine bleeding and may result from trauma of the thin endometrium or myometrial atherosclerosis.[19] The diagnosis is confirmed by endometrial biopsy. Hormone replacement may be therapeutic.

### *Endometrial Hyperplasia*

Endometrial hyperplasia is found in fewer than 10% of patients with postmenopausal bleeding. It is caused by stimulation of the endometrial lining from excess estrogen, endogenous or exogenous. Exogenous stimulation is usually from estrogen use without benefit of concomitant progesterone or progestogen replacement. Endogenous estrogen excess is seen in women who are obese or in those with estrogen-secreting ovarian tumors. When hyperplasia is associated with nuclear atypia, the risk of developing cancer is increased. The progression from hyperplasia to carcinoma occurs in fewer than 3% of patients with lesions without cytologic atypia, whereas 8% of patients with simple atypical hyperplasia and 23% of those with complex atypical hyperplasia are found to develop carcinoma.[20]

### *Endometrial Polyps*

Endometrial polyps develop from the endometrial basalis layer and may be the result of estrogenic stimulation. They may be solitary or multiple and are usually pedunculated. They are usually benign and asymptomatic but account for up to 25% of cases of postmenopausal bleeding.[21] Treatment is removal by dilatation and curettage (D&C) or hysteroscopically guided polypectomy. Excision is essential to rule out carcinoma.

### *Endometrial Cancer*

Endometrial cancer is the most frequent invasive cancer of the female genital tract, and is discussed in Chapter 59. In all cases of postmenopausal bleeding it is necessary to exclude endometrial cancer and other genital malignancy.

Diagnostic evaluations of postmenopausal bleeding include (1) endometrial sampling by aspiration techniques or D&C; (2) hysteroscopy with or without D&C; and (3) transvaginal ultrasonography (TVS), which evaluates the thickness of the endometrial echo.

An endometrial sample is the only means of obtaining a tissue diagnosis. The Pipelle (Prodimed, Neuilly-en-Thelle, France) is a common, effective method of endometrial aspiration. It consists of a short plastic tube, 2 mm in diameter, with a plunger for applying gentle suction to aspirate a small sample of endometrium. This method is reported to have the sensitivity of 97.5% for the diagnosis of endometrial cancer.[22,23] Hysteroscopy allows direct visualization of the endometrial cavity, thereby improving the diagnostic yield. This procedure may be performed in the office with local anesthesia or in the operating room under general anesthesia or intravenous sedation. Hysteroscopy in a postmenopausal woman is considered negative when (1) the entire endometrial cavity is visualized; (2) the uterine lining is smooth, thin, and pale with an easily discernible vascular network; and (3) no structural abnormalities are noted.[24]

Transvaginal ultrasonography has been used to evaluate postmenopausal bleeding. An endometrial thickness of 5 mm is considered to be an appropriate cutoff level for conservative management of patients with postmenopausal bleeding or when screening for endometrial cancer. Thickness of more than 10 mm requires a biopsy.[25]

### Ovary

The incidence of ovarian neoplasms in the postmenopausal patient rises rapidly, plateaus, and then declines. In the elderly population, the incidence is stable until age 70 and then rapidly declines.

As with all of the genital organs, postmenopausal ovaries also atrophy, are smaller than those of the premenopausal woman, and are usually not palpable. The diagnosis of an ovarian neoplasm may be suspected during bimanual examination of the pelvic organs. In the elderly woman, a rectovaginal examination and a guaiac test of the stool is also performed. Benign ovarian enlargement or benign cysts are rarely found in this age group, as the ovary is inactive. Benign teratomas missed at an earlier age are sometimes found, but in general most ovarian masses are suspect for malignancy. Ovarian tumors are discussed in Chapter 59.

## Pelvic Organ Prolapse

Pelvic organ prolapse is commonly encountered in postmenopausal women. Prolapse is abnormal descent or herniation of the pelvic organs from their normal attachment sites. Prolapse presents clinically as partial or complete eversion of the vagina, with the uterus, when present, in the most dependent position. To understand the pathology of prolapse, knowledge of anatomy is essential.

### Primer in Anatomy

Knowledge of the anatomy of the pelvis is essential to understanding pelvic organ prolapse. With the exception of the brain and cranial base, the anatomy of the pelvis is perhaps the most complicated in the body because lying within it, passing through it, attaching to it, and bifurcating or synapsing within it are multiple muscles, nerves, vessels, and organs that support the important functions of ambulation, reproduction, sexuality, and elimination of liquid and solid waste. An explanation of three basic anatomic and functional concepts aid in our understanding of pelvic organ prolapse: (1) the overall structure and function of the pelvic floor; (2) the vaginal-uterine axis; and (3) the circumferential attachment of the vagina and uterus.

#### *Structure and Function of the Pelvic Floor*

The assumption of the upright posture brought with it certain adaptive anatomic and functional evolutionary changes.[26] Let us consider for a moment the anatomy of animals that walk on all fours (quadripeds). They have no pelvic floor. The muscle groups that comprise the pelvic floor in primates are present in these lower mammals but turn backward to wag the tail. The abdominal contents in these animals are supported by the abdominal wall, which during most of their functional activities is parallel to the ground, bearing the effects of gravity.

The pelvic floor evolved in primates, particularly humans, who as bipeds, spend most of their waking hours in the upright position. As the name suggests, the "floor" of the pelvis is its lowermost boundary on which all the pelvic and abdominal contents rest. It is basically a sling of several muscle groups and ligaments connected at the perimeter to the 360 degree ovoid bony pelvis (Fig. 58.1A). The pelvic floor supports the abdominal and pelvic organs, preventing them from descending out of the pelvic and abdominal cavities (Fig. 58.1B). It is slightly concave, funneling in a downward direction. The muscles of the pelvic floor are also in a tonic state of contraction, but coordinated activity can cause the muscles to contract and shorten, reducing the degree of concavity of the pelvic floor.

The pelvic floor contains three principal perforations that allow the urethra, vagina, and rectum to pass through it (Fig. 58.1B). Other smaller perforations of insignificant pathologic importance allow vessels and nerves to pass through and around the pelvic floor.

The largest of the openings in the pelvic floor, the so-called genital hiatus, is of tantamount importance, as it is the site of pelvic organ prolapse. The vagina passes through this opening, which enlarges and stretches during childbirth. The muscles of the pelvic floor can also become partially denervated during labor and childbirth, losing tone, and thereby allowing an increase in the size of the genital hiatus and in the concavity of the downward funneling of the pelvic floor. Because the genital hiatus is the weakest point in the pelvic floor support mechanism, it is the most frequent site of pelvic organ prolapse. The additive effects of aging, declining quality of connective tissue and collagen, estrogen withdrawal, and constipation with straining at stool contribute to the development of pelvic floor prolapse. Furthermore, detachment of the vagina and uterus from lateral and

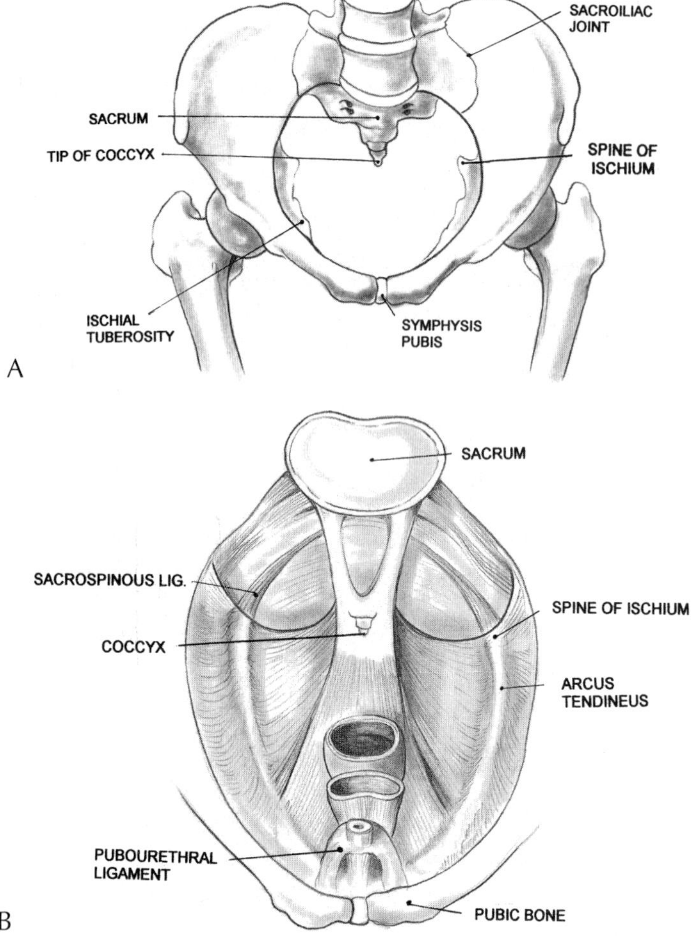


FIGURE 58.1. A. Female bony pelvis. Note the oval opening, which forms the framework for the pelvic floor. B. Pelvic floor, with anterior and posterior triangles of the pelvic floor muscles. Anterior triangles are perforated in the midline by the urethra, vagina, and rectum. (Modified from Retzky et al.,[27] with permission.)

posterior support structures favor downward descent and eversion of the vagina.

## Vaginal-Uterine Axis

Many anatomy texts are based on dissections done on fixed cadavers in the supine position, and for many years no attention was paid to the vaginal axis. The vagina was thought to be more or less parallel to the long axis of the body. Knowledge of the biaxial orientation of the vagina and uterus is critical to our understanding of anatomic and functional relations and to proper surgical restoration of pelvic support. In the supine position, the vagina may appear to be uniaxial, conforming to the long (vertical) axis of the body. However, when a person stands, the axis appears to change: The lower third of the vagina remains parallel to the long axis of the body, yet the upper two-thirds of the vagina and the uterus dip backward, becoming more nearly perpendicular to the long axis (Fig. 58.2A). When the woman is asked to strain, this change becomes more marked as the angle of the upper vagina more closely approaches the perpendicular plane in respect to the long axis of the body, and the upper vagina rests on the pelvic floor (Fig. 58.2B). Barium mold radiographic studies of Nichols et al.[29] and Funt et al.[30] were key milestones in our understanding of this important functional anatomic relation. As we review the anatomy of vaginal and uterine attachment points, we can understand why the concept of the vaginal axis, or "axes" (as the vagina is really biaxial), is functionally so important.

As the upper vagina becomes more nearly parallel to the pelvic floor, it provides a second barrier (in addition to the muscles of the pelvic floor, pelvic diaphragm, and ligaments), which serves to prevent further downward descent or herniation of pelvic and visceral organs through the genital hiatus. This additional barrier, the upper vagina, tends to close the opening in the levator plate, acting like a flap valve. The upper vagina fits snugly against the levator plate during straining, preventing abdominal and pelvic contents from prolapsing through the stretched genital hiatus.

## Circumferential Support of the Vagina and Uterus

The vagina and uterus are attached circumferentially to the bony pelvis by bridges of intervening connective tissue, just as the hub of a wheel (vagina and uterus) is attached to the rim (bony pelvis) by intervening spokes (connective tissue bridges), as figuratively illustrated in Figure 58.3. The anterior supports of the vagina and uterus are perhaps the weakest and least defined. Only the lower third of the vagina is supported anteriorly by the pubourethral ligaments (Fig. 58.3). These ligaments run from the posterior pubic bone and fuse laterally to the urethra and anterior vagina. They are of variable strength, containing elastin, collagen, and

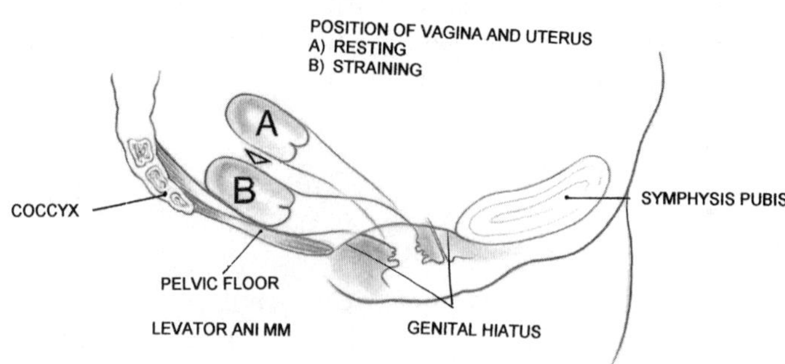


FIGURE 58.2. (A) Barium mold of the vagina in the standing position (at rest). Note the almost horizontal orientation of the upper vagina. A, at rest; B, straining. (B) The vagina in the standing position (straining). The vagina becomes "more" horizontal as it sits on and becomes parallel to the pelvic floor. (Adapted from Nichols and Randall,[28] with permission.)

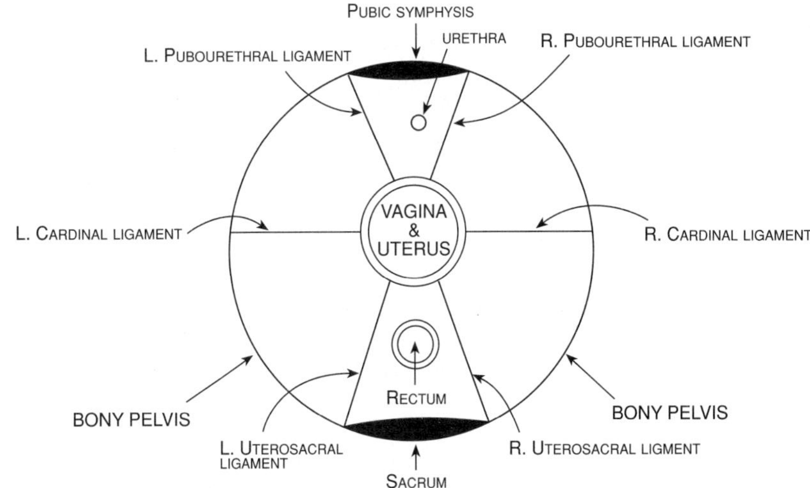


FIGURE 58.3. Figurative illustration of a wheel with a hub (vagina and uterus), spokes (pelvic support structures), and rim (bony pelvis). (From Foundation for Health Education, Research and Care, with permission.)

varying amounts of smooth muscle.[31] Although they have never been tested biomechanically, they probably alone could not support the entire lower vagina because of their small size and the variable amount of muscle contained within them, which has a tendency to stretch. Fortunately, the entire length of the vagina, including the lower third, is also supported laterally by fascial sheets connected to the fibromuscular coat of the vagina (part of the endopelvic fascial circular investment of vagina and cervix). These sheets attach laterally to the arcus tendineus fascia pelvis, a thick fibrous band attached to the underlying obturator internus muscle, running obliquely from the pubic bone to the ischial spine. The arcus tendineus also is the attachment point for the anterior muscles of the pelvic floor. The attachment of the vagina to the arcus tendineus also serves to support the anterior vagina and the lateral vagina.

The anatomic design of the arcus tendineus is functionally nearly perfect. When intact, not only does it support the lateral vagina, but because of its oblique orientation it allows the upper vagina to turn posteriorly such that during standing and straining the upper vagina and uterus become parallel to and sit on the levator plate (the pelvic floor). Moreover, the vaginal fascial attachments to the arcus have a certain degree of mobility that during straining or coughing allow the vagina, particularly the upper two-thirds, to maintain its orientation parallel to the pelvic floor (and perpendicular to the long axis of the body). In addition to the arcus tendineus, the upper vagina and uterus are supported laterally to the cardinal (Mackenrodt's) ligament (Fig. 58.3). The cardinal ligament is also the principal lateral support of the uterus to the pelvic sidewall.

The principal posterior supports of the vagina and uterus are the uterosacral ligaments. They tend to pull the cervix and upper vagina posteriorly, toward the sacrum, helping to maintain the inclination of the upper vagina (Fig. 58.3). Mengert, in his classic studies, was able to demonstrate the strong holding power of the lateral (cardinal ligaments) and posterior (uterosacral ligaments) supports of the vagina and uterus.[32] When any of these supports are stretched, denervated, or detached, the patient may present with varying degrees of prolapse.

## Clinical Presentation

A patient with symptomatic prolapse presents with a bulge, or "ball," in one of the walls of her vagina (anterior, posterior, lateral, or apical). These walls or segments are often referred to as "compartments." To understand which "compartment" is detached, stretched, descended, or prolapsed, we use a conceptual model based on a cubicle.

We developed this model after asking the straightforward question: "What in most persons' experience best depicts the vagina and the various defects in a simple fashion?" We arrived at the idea of a three-dimensional rectangular model, a cubicle, with one wall missing (the introitus). This cubicle can be perceived by patients, students, and clinicians as a simple room or a three-level structure. We then characterized the various compartments in relation to this cubicle: the floor (posterior wall), ceiling (anterior wall), apex (back wall), and side walls (lateral walls). Over time we began to portray the relations of the vault to other anatomic structures in the prolapse. The bladder is above the ceiling (in the attic or the next story); the rectum is below the floor (in the basement or lower story); the remainder of the small and large bowel can be depicted as the bulging behind the back wall (apex) and in the back portion of the floor. Thus one can understand anterior compartment defects (cystocele), posterior compartment defects (rectocele), lateral wall defects ("lateral wall detachment or lateral cystocele"), and apical defects (vaginal vault or uterine prolapse).

## Evaluation

When a patient complains of pelvic pressure or symptoms of prolapse, important steps in her evaluation and eventual treatment are a detailed history and a site-specific assessment of all pelvic floor defects if present. A detailed inventory of the patient's complaints is the cornerstone of the initial evaluation. Often patients are referred for a prolapse that is not symptomatic. Shull quoted an axiom that "the asymptomatic patient cannot be made to feel better by medical or surgical therapy."[33]

It is important to ascertain medical complications (e.g., asthma or obesity) that may have contributed to the problem. It may be prudent to attempt to control some of these problems, if possible, prior to any surgical intervention. If they are not controlled, recurrence may be an unwanted complication.

A detailed sexual history is essential. Often patients discontinue coital activity because of symptomatic or unsightly prolapse. The sexual history should include questions about the erectile function of the patient's partner. With the popularity of erectile altering devices and drugs, many women may have sexually adept partners who previously could not sustain erections, but these women may be too uncomfortable or embarrassed by pelvic organ prolapse symptoms to participate in sexual activity. Many women do not volunteer sexual information and must be queried with the same objectivity as other questions about their medical history.

It is important to ask the patient if she has trouble initiating voiding, if she must replace the prolapse to void, or if she is incontinent of urine or feces. Incontinence is discussed elsewhere in this text (see Chapter 55). Symptoms are often worse in the afternoon and evening and better in the morning. Back pain may also be a concomitant complaint. A generalized feeling of pressure is common. Urinary retention is also common in patients with anterior vaginal wall prolapse. As the anterior walls of the vagina and the bladder descend, they tend to kink the relatively fixed urethra, causing obstructive voiding and urinary retention.

It is imperative to understand the patient's own goals to devise a management plan. Some patients want little to no intervention, whereas others desire reconstructive surgery.

A site-specific physical evaluation is mandatory. There are many methods for pelvic floor evaluation, such as the Baden halfway system,[34] the POPQ system,[35] and the New York classification system.[36] We use the New York classification system because it gives the most information, and we find it simple to use. We assess the anterior (ceiling), posterior (floor), lateral (sidewalls), and apical (back wall) segments of the vagina. The cubicle model analogy aids in understanding. The questions about each of these surfaces that need to be answered are: "How large is the bulge during maximal straining?" "How far does each wall descend during maximal straining?" A checklist and grading form are shown in Figure 58.4. These forms are completed at each visit to monitor changes over time or to report recurrences after surgical procedures.

The ordinal staging of Baden and Walker and the ICS (called POPQ) system is also preserved in the New York classification system. Stage I is descent not reaching the hymen; stage II, to the hymen; stage III, beyond the hymen; and stage IV, total eversion or procidentia. These stages are recorded for each wall of the vagina.

The patient is evaluated initially in the lithotomy position. If this position does not reproduce the patient's account of the severity of her symptoms, she is reevaluated in the standing position. To perform the evaluation, a standard double-bladed speculum is placed in the vaginal vault to examine the vagina and cervix for surface defects, hypoestrogenism, and other problems. Then the speculum is removed and taken apart, leaving only the posterior blade, which is then replaced into the posterior vagina, allowing visualization of the anterior wall. The patient is asked to strain maximally. Anterior wall defects can be seen during this portion of the examination. The point of maximal descent of the anterior, lateral, and apical walls in relation to the ischial spines, hymen, or other landmark is noted in the reporting form (Fig. 58.4). Proper evaluation is best achieved by not grasping the speculum too tightly while allowing the prolapsed segments to descend, carefully observing the size of the bulge and the level of descent.

It is important to differentiate between a lateral wall detachment causing an apparent anterior wall bulge and a true central anterior bulge. A central defect, or "pulsion cystocele," is caused by a tear in the midline pubocervical fascia and may be repaired by standard anterior colporrhaphy. Often the vaginal mucosa overlying the bulge is smooth and devoid of rugae. A lateral wall detachment, or paravaginal fascial defect, is loss of attachment of the pubocervical segment of the endopelvic fascia lateral to the vagina at or near its attachment to the arcus tendineus fascia pelvis (white line). Frequently, there is loss of the lateral sulci of the vagina but preservation of rugae. The rule of rugae is true only in young patients and should not be used as a sole determinant of the location of the defect.

To assess the posterior wall of the vagina, the single-bladed speculum is removed and replaced in the opposite orientation, exposing the posterior wall. The point of maximal descent (in centimeters) from the ischial spines is noted, as is the size of any isolated bulge. The vaginal length and distance from the introitus to the ischial spine are also recorded.

Next, the examiner places his or her two index fingers into the vagina such that each finger opposes the ipsilateral vaginal wall. The patient is then asked to bear down. If the examiner's fingers converge in the midline, it is assumed that there is a loss of lateral vaginal support, which is best corrected surgically with a paravaginal repair (i.e., reattachment of the lateral vagina to the arcus tendineus). This test also is useful to determine if an

| **LOCATION (by vaginal zone)** | **SIZE** (✓ **largest diameter straining)** | | | | **DEGREE** (✓ **the lowest level of descent of <u>each</u> vaginal zone,** i.e., **low, mid, high; if beyond hymen, indicate # of cm)** | | | | | | | | | | | |
|---|---|---|---|---|---|---|---|---|---|---|---|---|---|---|---|---|
| **Low** = hymen to urethrovesical junction<br>**Mid** = urethrovesical junction to ischial spines<br>**High** = above ischial spines | No Defect | Small < 3 cm | Moderate 3-6 cm | Large > 6 cm | Ischial Spines -4 | -3 | -2 | -1 | 0 | +1 | +2 | +3 | +4 | Urethro-vesical Junction | Hymen | Beyond Hymen |
| **ANTERIOR WALL ("Central Cystocele")** | | | | | | | | | | | | | | | | |
| Low | | | | | | | | | | | | | | | | cm |
| Mid | | | | | | | | | | | | | | | | cm |
| High | | | | | | | | | | | | | | | | cm |
| **LEFT LATERAL WALL ("Lateral Cystocele")** | | | | | | | | | | | | | | | | |
| Low | | | | | | | | | | | | | | | | cm |
| Mid | | | | | | | | | | | | | | | | cm |
| High | | | | | | | | | | | | | | | | cm |
| **RIGHT LATERAL WALL ("Lateral Cystocele")** | | | | | | | | | | | | | | | | |
| Low | | | | | | | | | | | | | | | | cm |
| Mid | | | | | | | | | | | | | | | | cm |
| High | | | | | | | | | | | | | | | | cm |
| **POSTERIOR WALL ("Rectocele")** | | | | | | | | | | | | | | | | |
| Low | | | | | | | | | | | | | | | | cm |
| Mid | | | | | | | | | | | | | | | | cm |
| High | | | | | | | | | | | | | | | | cm |
| **APICAL WALL** | | | | | | | | | | | | | | | | |
| Anterior fornix | | | | | | | | | | | | | | | | cm |
| Posterior fornix | | | | | | | | | | | | | | | | cm |
| Cervix | Not Applicable | | | | | | | | | | | | | | | cm |

| | |
|---|---|
| **Urethral Axis: Resting:** ______ ° **Straining:** ______ ° | **Perineal Body Length (PB):** ______ cm |
| **Perineal Descent from Ischial Tuberosities:** ______ cm | **Introital diameter (ID):** ______ cm |
| **Surgical Conjugates (Distances): Hymen to Ischial Spines:** ______ cm | **Hymen to Sacral Promentory:** ______ cm |
| **Total Vaginal Length (TVL):** ______ cm | **Cervical Length (CL):** ______ cm |
| **COMMENTS**: | |

FIGURE 58.4. Grading of genitourinary/visceral prolapse: reporting form. (From Foundation for Medical Education, Research, and Care, with permission.)

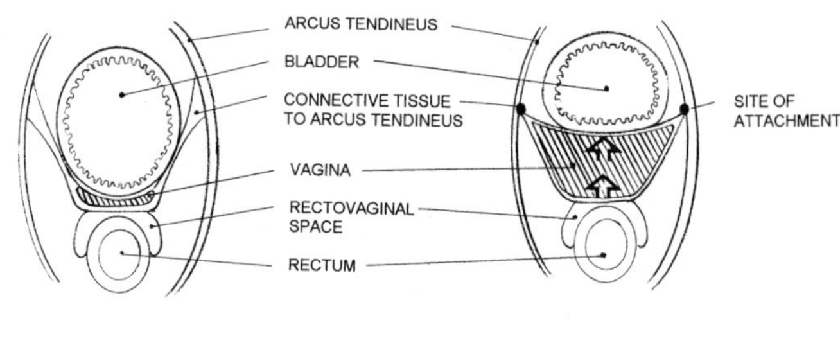


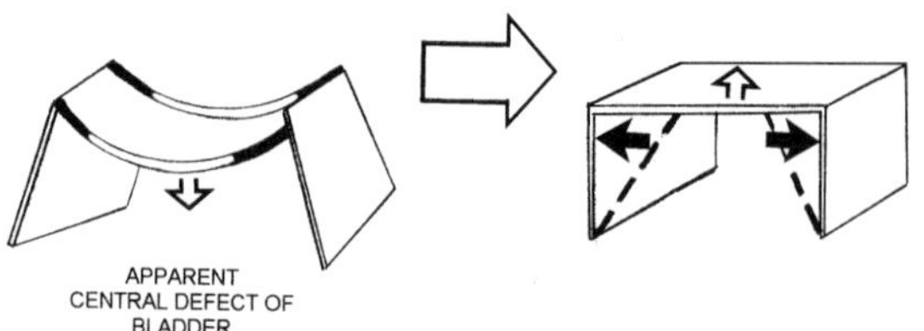


FIGURE 58.5. Principles of lateral wall vaginal detachment. The downward bowing in the ceiling (anterior vaginal wall) can be corrected by straightening the bowed lateral support poles (lateral wall defect). This maneuver (paravaginal repair or fixation) corrects the problem.

apparent central bulge ("ceiling" defect) can be made to disappear by replacing the lateral walls to their attachment points. Two analogies serve to illustrate this point. In Figure 58.5 the center of the canopy is bowing because of the poles supporting it are converging toward the midline. The approach to getting rid of the central ceiling bulge is to straighten the poles at the perimeter (as for paravaginal fixation), not to cut material from the center and resew the cut edges together (as for standard anterior colporrhaphy) (Fig. 58.5). A military bed illustrates this same point. When the sheets and blanket are tucked in at the sides, the center of the bed becomes flat so the proverbial quarter can bounce off the center of the bed like a trampoline. Therefore, if central anterior wall (ceiling) defects flatten while the fingers replace the lateral vaginal walls to the pelvic side wall, the patient is considered to have a lateral defect and is a candidate for a paravaginal fixation of the lateral vaginal wall to the arcus tendineus.

Finally the apex (cervix or vaginal cuff) is assessed. The patient is again asked to strain maximally, and the point of maximal descent is measured (in centimeters) with respect to the ischial spines, hymen, or other point noted in the reporting forms (Fig. 58.4). It is important to remember to ask the patient if the degree of prolapse noted during the examination is consistent with her complaints. It may be necessary to examine the patient in the standing position to allow the prolapse to descend completely. Rectovaginal exam may identify an enterocele which often accompanies apical descent. Occasionally the patient's symptoms can be reproduced only after she walks around to allow sufficient time for the effects of gravity to produce maximum descent.

In addition to a site-specific anatomic inventory, the degree of mobility of the bladder neck is assessed by urethral axis determination (cotton swab or Q-tip test) (Fig. 58.6). This test is performed by placing a cotton swab lubricated with anesthetic gel into the urethra up to the bladder neck. The angle of the wooden portion of the cotton swab is measured with respect to the long axis of the body. At rest, the swab usually rests parallel to the long axis of the body or the examination table and is considered to be, by convention, at 0 degrees (Fig. 58.6A). The patient is then asked to strain maximally. Upward (positive) deflection from the horizontal plane is measured and recorded. Deflections more than 30 degrees are considered to be consistent with "urethral hypermobility," which implies a loss of paraurethral support (Fig. 58.6B). Some patients who have had incontinence procedures with overcorrection of urethral hypermobility have "negative" Q-tip tests (Fig. 58.6C).[37]

The external genitalia are then assessed, noting the width of the introitus and perineal body. A bulge in the region of the urethra may be a urethral diverticulum, especially in a patient who presents with recurrent urinary tract infections, dribbling, or dyspareunia. A urethrogram may aid in the diagnosis of a diverticulum. This must be differentiated from a central cystourethrocele.

If the patient has significant anterior vaginal wall prolapse, it is imperative to rule out potential incontinence. Potential incontinence is, by definition, the development of incontinence only when the anterior vaginal wall prolapse is reduced. This "unmasking" of urinary incontinence is a result of unkinking the urethra by reducing the anterior wall. To test for potential incontinence, the bladder is filled with 300 ml of sterile water, or until the patient feels full, replacing and elevating the prolapse digitally or with the posterior blade of a Graves specu-

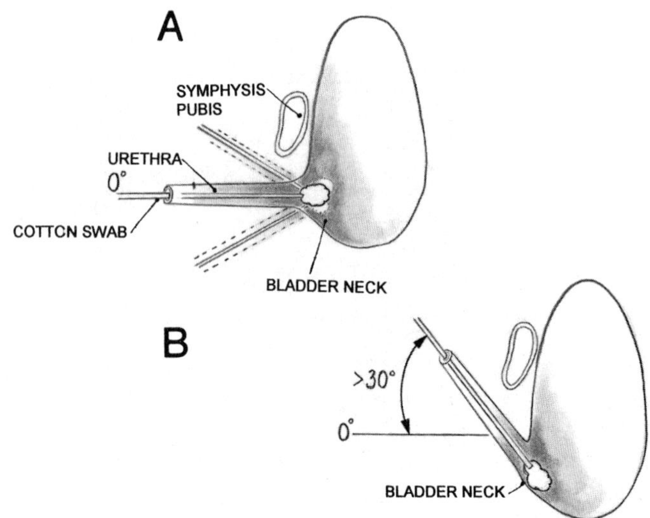


FIGURE 58.6. A. Q-tip test. Cotton swab in the urethra at rest. B. Q-tip test straining. C. Overcorrected bladder neck (negative Q-tip test). (From Scotti,[37] with permission.)

lum, and asking the patient to cough. If the patient leaks urine, further testing is probably necessary. The diagnosis is best made by performing urethral cough pressure profiles with a symptomatically full bladder with the prolapse reduced and extended. If the patient leaks urine or has a positive cough profile (pressure equalization), she is considered to have potential incontinence. If potential incontinence is not addressed at the time of prolapse surgery, the patient may become incontinent after even the best of surgical repairs. If the patient is treated with a pessary, she may also develop urinary incontinence after pessary insertion by the same mechanism of unkinking the urethra.

The patient with potential, "unmarked" or "latent" incontinence may also have unmasked intrinsic sphincter deficiency (ISD) or a low resting urethral pressure when the anterior wall is reduced.[37] Patients with ISD or urethral insufficiency may require treatment for their potential incontinence different from that for patients with normal-pressure urethra (see Chapter 55).

The postvoid residual urine volume should always be determined to rule out obstruction secondary to urethral kinking or incomplete emptying secondary to poor bladder contractility. Complete preoperative assessment can prevent or predict many unwanted postoperative complications.

## Treatment

### *Conservative Treatment*

When queried, many patients initially opt for conservative treatment. Patients who prefer conservative management, who are poor surgical candidates, or who do not want surgical intervention, are offered a pessary, an excellent method of symptom relief. There are few contraindications to pessary use, although a patient with acute pelvic inflammation is not a candidate for a pessary. Any pessary associated with pain after insertion should not be used. Recurrent vaginitis is also a relative contraindication.

There are many types of pessaries, and pessary fitting is far from an exact science. Trial and error is the rule. We initially try the two most common types, the ring pessary and the doughnut pessary. Either may be used in the posthysterectomy patient. Other types are the inflatable ball pessary, cube (bee cell), and Gehrung. The Gelhorn pessary is used most often for massive prolapse in patients with a large introital diameter who have failed a trial of other pessaries. The Gelhorn pessary resembles a large collar button and has a small drainage canal down the center of the stem. These pessaries are associated with greater amounts of leukorrhea and vaginal odor, as they have large surface areas. The Smith-Hodge and Risser pessaries allow for retrodisplacement of the uterus. The Smith-Hodge pessary should be used for the patient with a well-defined pubic notch and the Risser for the patient with greater vaginal width. The patient should be instructed to remove and clean the pessary or douche weekly with a weak vinegar solution (or both) to lessen the chance of developing vaginal discharge.

Prior to insertion, a complete pelvic examination should be performed. One should assess the condition of the vagina, vaginal length, strength of the levator musculature, amount of outlet relaxation, and cytology. After the pessary is placed, the examiner should be able to sweep a fingertip painlessly between each edge of the pessary and the vaginal wall. The patient should then be able to sit and ambulate comfortably and to urinate and defecate without difficulty. A follow-up examination should be performed at 1 week to assess the inflammatory response, ulceration, or urinary or rectal complaints. If the patient is not able to clean and replace the pessary satisfactorily, the provider should clean and replace it every 8–12 weeks.

There are occasional complications after pessary use: vaginitis, vaginal discharge, bleeding, ulceration, abscess formation (rare), urinary obstruction, fistula formation, and erosion into the bladder or rectum. Most complications are from the long-forgotten pessary.[38] Rarely, carcinoma at the site of contact has been reported.[39]

Topical estrogen is an important adjunct in the conservative management of patients with prolapse. Transvaginal cream can be applied to the everted vaginal mucosa or inserted into the vagina with the pessary in situ. We have also found that an estrogen-containing ring (estradiol vaginal ring: Estring; Pharmacia, Kalamazoo, MI) can be placed behind the pessary to provide estrogen to the deficient vaginal tissue. If the patient is receiving oral estrogen replacement therapy, vaginal supplementation may be added, particularly if the target organs (vagina, urethra) still show signs of hypoestrogenism.

### *Surgical Treatment*

If a decision for surgery is made, a surgical plan must be formulated. One must take into account operative surgical risk, coital activity, and the anatomy of the vaginal canal. The correct operation must be tailored to the individual patient.

There are many decisions to be made before surgery is planned. Variables to be taken into consideration are enumerated in Table 58.2. Other questions to be answered are: "Will the operation be performed abdominally or vaginally?" "Is a hysterectomy to be performed?" A hysterectomy is not necessarily a mandatory part of the surgical repair for prolapse, as a uterine suspension can be performed by the abdominal or vaginal route during prolapse surgery; but for practical reasons the uterus is often removed to provide better access to the surgical reattachment points.

TABLE 58.2. Important Considerations for Surgical or Nonsurgical Decision-Making

| |
|---|
| Medical condition and age |
| Severity of symptoms |
| Patient's choice: no surgery or surgery |
| Patient's suitability for surgery |
| Presence of other pelvic conditions including urinary or fecal incontinence necessitating simultaneous treatment |
| Presence or absence of urethral hypermobility |
| Presence or absence of urethrovesical funneling |
| Presence or absence of pelvic floor neuropathy |
| History of previous surgery |

Certain anatomic considerations may make the decision easier. For example, if the patient has genuine stress or potential incontinence and the best chance for cure of incontinence is the abdominal route (e.g., Burch procedure), we generally perform prolapse repair abdominally as well.

### Apical Defects: Abdominal Approach

Apical defects my be repaired abdominally or vaginally, depending on many conditions including the surgical approach for incontinence and the preoperative vaginal length. If an abdominal approach is selected for apical descent (uterovaginal or posthysterectomy vaginal vault prolapse), an abdominal sacral colpopexy or sacral uteropexy allows the upper vagina to regain its normal anatomic axis by securing the vagina or the uterus to the sacrum with sutures through the presacral fascia at the promontary or S2 or S3. The abdominal approach allows higher fixation in the pelvis and is preferable for women with a total vaginal length of more than 10cm. During this procedure a patch of harvested abdominal fascia, fascia lata,[40] dura mater,[41] Marlex, Prolene, Mersiline,[42] or cadaveric fascia is often placed from the vaginal cuff, the amputated cervical stump, or the uterine corpus to the presacral fascia. If the uterus is too bulky, it is removed to facilitate the repair. Permanent suture is used, and the peritoneum is closed over the patch to prevent bowel entrapment.

A culdocleisis should also be performed. This procedure simply involves closing the cul-de-sac by suturing the peritoneal surfaces together, usually incorporating the uterosacral ligaments in the repair. Sacral colpopexy offers the additional advantage of supporting both the anterior vaginal and posterior walls as the graft material is attached to both anterior and posterior aspects of the vagina (cervix and uterus). Not infrequently, by providing adequate anterior and posterior vaginal support, sacral colpopexy substantially reduces what appears to be a large cystocele or rectocele, particularly in the upper vagina. Addison et al.[42] recommended extending the posterior graft material as far down the rectovaginal septum as possible to help elevate the perineum. Long-term studies are not available to test the durability or complication rate of Addison's procedure.

The most serious complication of sacral colpopexy is bleeding.[43] It is possible to injure presacral venous plexi, the middle sacral artery, or the hypogastric vessels while operating in the presacral space. Other complications are ureteral injury, infection, graft rejection, and suture pull-out causing recurrence of the prolapse.

### Apical Defects: Vaginal Approach

Vaginal surgery is often the preferred route, as the patient may have a faster recovery. It is selected when a vaginal surgical approach for incontinence, such as a suburethral sling is indicated, or when concomitant reconstructive procedures favoring the vaginal approach are indicated (e.g., anterior or posterior colporrhaphy). The vaginal route is also preferable in patients whose distance from the hymen to the sacrospinous ligament is relatively equal to the total vaginal length (usually <8 cm). They are ideal candidates for sacrospinous ligament fixation of apical vault prolapse. The apex can be sutured to the ligament without leaving any length of prolapsed vagina, thereby preventing intersusception of redundant vagina postoperatively. The apex is attached to the sacrospinous ligament usually by a pulley stitch (Fig. 58.7). Alternatively, the uterosacral ligaments can be shortened and the apex attached to the ends of the uterosacral ligament. (McCall culdoplasty).

The sacrospinous ligament fixation is usually performed on the patient's right side to avoid the sigmoid colon and rectum. The vaginal apex is sutured to the sacrospinous ligament using permanent sutures. The ligament is located at the posterior border of the coccygeus muscle. It is attached proximally to the posteroinferior surface of the ischial spine and distally to the sacrum. Surgeons performing this (and other reconstructive procedures) must pay meticulous attention to anatomy to avoid complications. The pudendal nerve and vessels exit the pelvis through the greater sciatic foramen and then reenter through the lesser sciatic foramen, passing under (posterior to) the sacrospinous ligament near the ischial spine (Fig. 58.7). Care must be taken to place the suture 1–2 cm medial to the ischial spine to avoid these structures and the inferior gluteal vessels, which lie posterior to the sacrospinous ligament. In young women the ligament is well covered by muscle fibers; but as women age the ligament becomes progressively thicker and more prominent as dense connective tissue replaces muscle at the coccygeal posterior border.[44] It is also somewhat easier to identify. The suture should be placed through the ligament, rather than around it, to avoid injury to the pudendal neurovascular bundle.

Vaginal vault fixation is usually performed after repair of any enterocele. Enteroceles are true hernias. They are

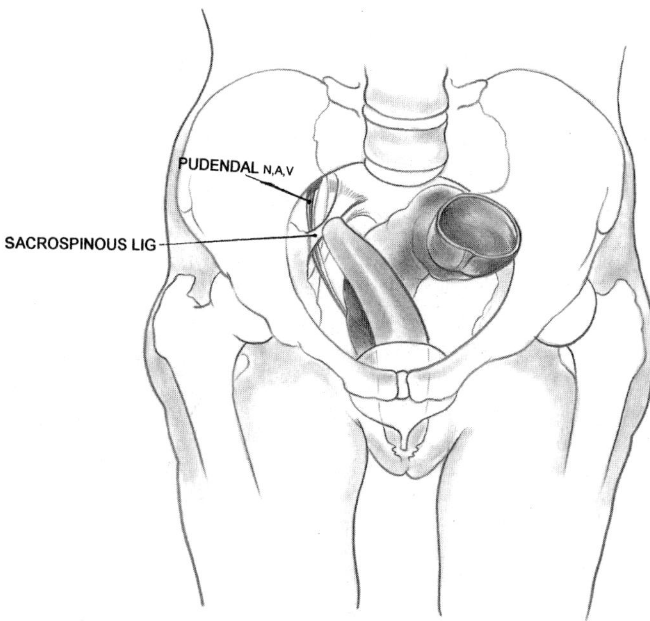


FIGURE 58.7. Sacrospinous vaginal fixation. The vagina is attached to the right sacrospinous ligament. (From Nichols and Randall,[28] with permission.)

formed by the downward descent of small or large bowel with intervening peritoneum into the cul-de-sac of Douglas behind the prolapsed vagina. They must be separated from the vagina and pushed upward during vaginal surgery. The redundant "hernia sac" is ligated and removed. Care must be taken to avoid loops of small bowel which may also prolapse into the cul-de-sac between the vagina and the rectum.

The McCall transvaginal culdoplasty[45] may be used for apical descent or as prophylaxis against future prolapse if the uterosacral ligaments are strong. The ligaments here are shortened and reattached to the vaginal cuff while simultaneously closing the cul-de-sac. A complication of this procedure is ureteral injury; therefore cystoscopy following the procedure is recommended.

### Lateral Wall Defects

If a lateral detachment is present, paravaginal repair may be performed abdominally as described by Scotti et al.,[46] Shull and Baden,[47] Richardson et al.,[48] and others. This repair reapproximates the torn vaginal supports to the arcus tendineus fascia pelvis (or white line of the pelvis). The prolapsed detached lateral vagina may also be attached to the ileococcygeus fascia as the point of its attachment to the pubocervical fascia. We have described attaching the vagina through all of the structures of the pelvic side wall, firmly anchoring the suture to the ischial periosteum.[46]

Complications include injury to the obturator nerve and vessels, bladder, or ureters. If there is any suspicion of bladder perforation, a dye can be infused retrogradely into the bladder to test its integrity.

We also often suspend the lower anterior vagina to Cooper's ligament during abdominal repairs. This technique corrects urethrovesical hypermobility and potential or stress incontinence. It also preserves the biaxial orientation of the vagina.

A paravaginal repair can be performed vaginally for repair of lateral wall detachment. The pubocervical fascia in the region of the lateral vaginal sulcus is attached to the white line as described by Shull and colleagues,[49] with a 93% cure rate at 1.6 years. The lateral vagina can also be attached to the ileococcygeus fascia or ischial periosteum as described for the abdominal route.

### Anterior Wall Defects

Central anterior defects may be easily repaired via the vaginal approach. A variety of techniques exist, but most involve opening the anterior wall and reapproximating the pubocervical fascia in the midline. Sutures should be no closer than 1–2 cm from the urethrovesical junction. This procedure may be combined with antiincontinence operations, such as a suburethral sling (see Chapter 55).

### Posterior Defects

The posterior compartment must be carefully evaluated for the possibility of a concomitant enterocele or rectocele. If an enterocele is discovered, it should be surgically corrected and the cul-de-sac closed. The rectocele should be repaired by opening the posterior vaginal mucosa and dissecting off the underlying rectum and fascia, both sharply and bluntly, from the posterovaginal wall until the medial margins of the pubococcygeus muscle are seen. Several approaches are used. Separate breaks or tears in this fascia are repaired separately. If the fascia is thin, plication and reinforcement of the fascia by sutures or a patch of fascia or mesh can be used. Care must be taken to not constrict the vaginal caliber during this repair such that three or more fingers can be inserted easily into the vagina. Compromising the vaginal caliber may cause dyspareunia, resulting in an unhappy patient and her sexual partner.

The repair should be performed in two layers to eliminate deadspace and prevent fistula formation. Some surgeons also plicate the medial portion of the pubococcygeus muscle across the midline, although this step may create a transverse ridge in the posterior vaginal wall and lead to dyspareunia.[50] The perineal body should be repaired by placing multiple sutures deeply into the bulbocavernosus and superficial transverse perinei muscles to build up the perineal body. The perineal body is then attached to the more proximal rectovaginal fascia by sutures to ensure integrity and continuity of the rectovaginal fascia (of Denonvilliers). The vaginal mucosa is closed, and again attention is given to ensuring adequate vaginal caliber. The patient should be placed on stool softeners for approximately 4 weeks to allow the tissue time to heal.

### *Colpocleisis*

For patients who cannot undergo long surgical procedures and who are not contemplating sexual activity, a partial colpocleisis (Le Forte operation) or vaginectomy are viable options. With these procedures the vagina is obliterated. There are four problems specific to these operations: (1) they limit or destroy vaginal coital function; (2) because the operation is extraperitoneal, colpocleisis or colpectomy does not remove any enterocele; (3) there is a 25% incidence of postoperative urinary stress incontinence caused by induced fusion of the anterior rectal wall to the base of the bladder and flattening the posterior urethrovesical angle; and (4) if the uterus is retained, the patient can bleed in the future from a number of causes including carcinoma.[4]

Prior to colpocleisis, a Pap smear and an endometrial biopsy should be performed to rule out cervical and/or endometrial pathology, as evaluation after colpocleisis is not possible.

With colpocleisis, a patch of anterior and posterior vaginal mucosa is removed. The cut edge of the anterior vaginal wall is sewn to its counterpart on the posterior side. This approximation is continued down each side of the vagina, and the most dependent portion of the mass is progressively inverted. This creates an epithelium-lined tunnel on each lateral side that allows egress of secretions. A tight perineorrhaphy is performed to aid in supporting the inverted vagina and preventing recurrence of the prolapse.

## Conclusions

Geriatric patients are indeed a challenge to the gynecologist, urogynecologist, and reconstructive pelvic surgeon. Close and repeated communication with the patient, her family members, and her primary care physician is essential for an optimal outcome. Treatment is patient-driven, and conservative treatment should be offered as a first option. When surgical intervention is undertaken, assessment of risks and communication of these risks are important elements of the decision-making process. Age alone should not be a factor in the decision, as the patient's desire for mobility and activity are important guidelines. Hopefully, we can improve the quality of life of our patients by listening carefully to them and their families and helping them choose the treatment best suited to their life situation.

## References

1. Walz TH, Blum NS. The coming of the 21st century: probable policy trends in aging. Gerontol Rev 1989;2:1–9.
2. Meldrum DR. The pathophysiology of post-menopausal symptoms. Semin Reprod Endocrinol 1983;1:11.
3. Cooper J. Double blind cross-over study of estrogen replacement therapy. In: Campbell S (ed) Management of Menopause and Post-menopausal Years. Lancaster, UK: MTP, 1976:167.
4. Schiff I, Tulchinsky D, Cramer D, et al. Oral medroxyprogesterone in the treatment of postmenopausal symptoms. JAMA 1980;244:1443–1445.
5. Brincat M, Moniz CJ, Studd WW. Long-term effects of the menopause and sex hormones on skin thickness. Br J Obstet Gynaecol 1985;92:256–259.
6. Friedrich EG Jr. Vulvar Disease, 2nd ed. Philadelphia: Saunders, 1983.
7. American College of Obstetricians and Gynecologists. Vulvar Nonneoplastic Epithelial Disorders. Educational bulletin 241. Washington, DC: ACOG, October 1997.
8. Scotti RJ. Infections of the urethra and Bartholin and Skene glands. In: Pastorek JG II (ed) Obstetric and Gynecologic Infectious Disease. New York: Raven, 1994:89–103.
9. Stephenson H, Dotters DJ, Katz V, et al. Necrotizing fasciitis of the vulva. Am J Obstet Gynecol 1992;166:1324–1327.
10. Semmens JP, Wagner G. Estrogen deprivation and vaginal function in postmenopausal women. JAMA 1982;248:445–448.
11. Semmens JP, Tsai CC, Semmens EC, et al. Effects of estrogen therapy on vaginal physiology during menopause. Obstet Gynecol 1985;66:15–18.
12. Mandelblatt J, Gopaul I, Wistreich M. Gynecological care of elderly women. JAMA 1986;256:367–371.
13. American College of Obstetricians and Gynecologists. Routine Cancer Screening. Educational bulletin 185. Washington, DC: ACOG, September 1997.
14. American College of Obstetricians and Gynecologists. Cervical Cytology: Evaluation and Management of Abnormalities. Technical bulletin 183. Washington. DC: ACOG, August 1993.
15. Baggish MS. High-power-density carbon dioxide laser therapy for early cervical neoplasia. Am J Obstet Gynecol 1980;136:117–125.
16. Richart RM, Sciarra JJ. Treatment of cervical dysplasia by outpatient electrocauterization. Am J Obstet Gynecol 1968;101:200–205.
17. Wright TC Jr, Gagnon S, Richart RM, et al. Treatment of cervical intraepithelial neoplasia using the loop electrosurgical excision procedure. Obstet Gynecol 1992;79:173–178.
18. Creasman WT, Hinshaw WM, Clarke-Pearson DL. Cryosurgery in the management of cervical intraepithelial neoplasia. Obstet Gynecol 1984;64:145–149.
19. Meyer WC, Malkasian GD, Dockerty MB, et al. Postmenopausal bleeding from atrophic endometrium. Obstet Gynecol 1971;38:731–738.
20. Kurman RJ, Kaminski PF, Norris HJ. The behavior of endometrial hyperplasia: a long-term study of "untreated" hyperplasia in 170 patients. Cancer 1985;56:403–412.
21. Van Bogaert LJ. Clinicopathologic findings in endometrial polyps. Obstet Gynecol 1988;71:771–773.
22. Stovall TG, Photopulos GJ, Poston WM, et al. Pipelle endometrial sampling in patients with known endometrial carcinoma. Obstet Gynecol 1991;77:954–956.

23. Grimes DA. Diagnostic dilation and curettage: a reappraisal. Am J Obstet Gynecol 1982;142:1–6.
24. Loffer FD. Hysteroscopy with selective endometrial sampling compared with D&C for abnormal uterine bleeding: the value of a negative hysteroscopic view. Obstet Gynecol 1989;73:16–20.
25. Nasri MN, Shepherd JH, Setchell ME, et al. The role of vaginal scan in measurement of endometrial thickness in postmenopausal women. Br J Obstet Gynaecol 1991;98: 470–475.
26. Davies JW. Man's assumption of the erect posture: its effect on the position of the pelvis. Am J Obstet Gynecol 1955; 70:1012–1020.
27. Retzky SS, Rogers RM Jr, Richardson AC. Anatomy of female pelvic support. In: Brubaker LT, Saclarides TJ (eds) The Female Pelvic Floor. Philadelphia: Davis, 1996;8:11.
28. Nichols DH, Randall CL, Vaginal surgery, 4th ed. Baltimore: Williams & Wilkins, 1996:4–5.
29. Nichols DH, Milley PS, Randall CL. Significance of restoration of normal vaginal depth and axis. Obstet Gynecol 1970;36:251–256.
30. Funt MI, Thompson JD, Birch H. Normal vaginal axis. South Med J 1978;71:1534–1535, 1552.
31. Delancey JOL. Pubovesical ligament: a separate structure from urethral supports (pubo-urethral ligaments). Neurourol Urodyn 1989;8:53–62.
32. Mengert WF. Mechanics of uterine support and position. Am J Obstet Gynecol 1936;31:775.
33. Shull BL. Clinical evaluation of women with pelvic support defects. Clin Obstet Gynecol 1993;36:939–951.
34. Baden WF, Walter TA. Genesis of the vaginal profile: a correlated classification of vaginal relaxation. Clin Obstet Gynecol 1972;15:1048–1054.
35. Bump RC, Mattiasson A, Bo K, et al. The standardization of terminology of female pelvic organ prolapse and pelvic floor dysfunction. Am J Obstet Gynecol 1996;175:10–17.
36. Scotti RJ, Flora RF, Greston WM, et al. Characterizing and reporting pelvic floor defects: the revised New York classification system. Int Urogynecol J 1999;11:48–60.
37. Scotti RJ. Investigating the elderly incontinent woman. In: Grody MHT (ed) Benign Postreproductive Gynecologic Surgery. New York: McGraw-Hill, 1995:114.
38. Scotti RJ, Vargas I, Lippman L. Perforation and fistulization from a vaginal ring pessary. J Gynecol Surg 1994;10:93–96.
39. Schraub S, Sun XS, Maingon P, et al. Cervical and vaginal cancer associated with pessary use. Cancer 1992;69:2505–2509.
40. Ridley JH, A composite vaginal vault suspension using fascia lata. Am J Obstet Gynecol 1976;126:590–596.
41. Lansman HH. Posthysterectomy vault prolapse: sacral colpopexy with dura mater graft. Obstet Gynecol 1984;63: 577–582.
42. Addison WA, Livengood CH III, Sutton GP, et al. Abdominal sacral colpopexy with Mersilene mesh in the retroperitoneal position in the management of posthysterectomy vaginal vault prolapse and enterocele. Am J Obstet Gynecol 1985;153:140–146.
43. Sutton GP, Addison WA, Livengood CH III, et al. Life-threatening hemorrhage complicating sacral colpopexy. Am J Obstet Gynecol 1981;140:836–837.
44. Grody MHT. Posterior pelvis. II. Deep pelvic reconstruction-enterocele repair and sacrospinous fixation. In: Grody MHT (ed) Benign Postreproductive Gynecologic Surgery. New York: McGraw-Hill, 1995:219–245.
45. McCall LM. Posterior culdeplasty. Am J Obstet Gynecol 1957;6:595–602.
46. Scotti RJ, Garely AD, Greston WM, et al. Paravaginal repair of lateral vaginal wall defects by fixation to the ischial periosteum and obturator membrane. Am J Obstet Gynecol 1998;179:1436–1445.
47. Shull BL, Baden WF. A six-year experience with paravaginal defect repair for stress urinary incontinence. Am J Obstet Gynecol 1989;160:1432–1440.
48. Richardson AC, Edmonds PB, Williams NL. Treatment of stress urinary incontinence due to paravaginal fascial defect. Obstet Gynecol 1981;57:357–362.
49. Shull BL, Capen CV, Riggs MW, et al. Bilateral attachment of the vaginal cuff to iliococcygeus fascia: an effective method of cuff suspension. Am J Obstet Gynecol 1993; 168:1669–1677.
50. Nichols DH, Randall CL. Posterior colporrhaphy and perineorrhaphy. In: Nichols DH, Randall CL (eds) Vaginal Surgery, 4th ed. Baltimore: Williams & Wilkins, 1996: 257–289.

# 59
# Gynecologic Malignancies in the Elderly

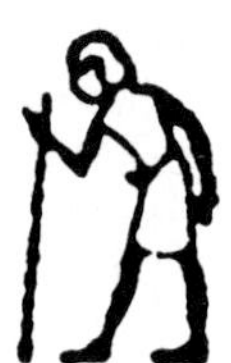

Peter E. Schwartz and Thomas L. Rutherford

Pelvic reproductive organ cancers include those that arise in the vulva, vagina, cervix, uterus, fallopian tubes, and ovaries. In the United States uterine cancer is the fourth most common cancer women develop,[1] ovarian cancer is the fifth most common, and cervical cancer is the ninth most common. Cervical cancer is the second most common cancer in women worldwide.[2] The reason for the disparity between the worldwide and American figures is believed to be the lack of adequate Papanicolaou (Pap) smear screening in many underdeveloped countries of the world. Data from the Connecticut Tumor Registry, the oldest population-based registry in the United States, reveals that 20% of female pelvic reproductive organ cancers in Connecticut occur in women age 70 years or more (Table 59.1).[3] Thus cancers of the pelvic reproductive tract can and do occur in elderly women, and their management must be adjusted for the individual's physical and mental status.

This chapter focuses on the standard treatments for women with pelvic reproductive organ cancers. It also notes the modifications in standard care that are applied to the elderly when they are unable to tolerate standard treatment due to associated medical disabilities.

## Vulvar Cancer

The vulvar skin can present with a variety of premalignant and malignant changes. Premalignant changes vary from mild dysplasia through carcinoma in situ. Invasive cancers range from superficially invasive through extremely aggressive malignancies that involve other pelvic organs or distant metastasis. The Connecticut Tumor Registry reported 1024 vulvar cancers over a 45-year period. The median patient age was 69 years, with 47.3% of the cases occurring in women age 70 years or more (Table 59.1).[3] Premalignant changes of the vulva may be unifocal or multifocal.[4] The disease tends to be unifocal in the elderly population, whereas in younger age women it tends to be multifocal. Elderly patients, particularly those over 70 years of age, are less likely to have an associated human papilloma virus (HPV) infection.[5] Premalignant and malignant squamous cell changes are the dominant histologic patterns seen in vulvar neoplasias.[6] The second most common malignancy is melanoma, and the third most common is adenocarcinoma arising in Bartholin's gland or in skin appendices. Premalignant changes in the vulva in addition to squamous cell changes, include extramammary Paget's disease of the vulva, a premalignant change that at times is associated with an underlying vulvar carcinoma.[7]

The etiology of vulvar carcinoma is unknown. Factors associated with the development of vulvar carcinoma include venereal disease, especially syphilis, exposure to heavy metals, and HPV infection.[4,5,8] HPV subtypes associated with oncogenic potential include HPV-16, which is frequently found in association with invasive vulvar cancers in women of relatively young age.[5]

The diagnosis of vulvar cancer starts with inspection. It is important to distinguish atrophy from premalignant disease. Elderly patients often have atrophic changes of the vulva. Those lesions that are symmetric in distribution, white, and generally nonraised are usually atrophic in nature. Premalignant disease and malignancies tend to be asymmetric in distribution and may be friable. The International Society for Vulvar Studies has classified vulvar changes into three major categories: (1) hyperplastic dystrophy without or with atypia; (2) lichen sclerosis; and (3) mixed dystrophy (lichen sclerosis with hyperplastic dystrophy) without or with atypia.[9] Atypical changes are characterized as mild, moderate, or severe and are premalignant in nature. Lesions lacking atypia are considered benign. Staging of vulvar malignancies is surgical in nature and depends on the extent of the local disease and the presence or absence of inguinal lymph node metastases (Table 59.2).

Treatment for vulvar premalignant changes is a wide local excision. In the elderly it may be done under local anesthesia. Generally a 1 cm margin is sufficient for premalignant changes of the vulva; for extramammary

TABLE 59.1. Newly Diagnosed Cases of Gynecologic Cancer in Connecticut (1935–1979)

| Site | No. of cases | Median age (years) | No. of cases ≥70 years |
|---|---|---|---|
| Vulva | 1024 | 69 | 485 (47.3%) |
| Vagina | 307 | 64 | 105 (34.2%) |
| Cervix | 8615 | 53 | 1125 (13.1%) |
| Uterus | 9914 | 61 | 2161 (21.8%) |
| Fallopian tube | 180 | 58 | 28 (15.6%) |
| Ovaries | 8085 | 58 | 1715 (21.2%) |
| *Total* | 28,125 | 61 | 5619 (20.0%) |

*Source:* Heston et al.,[3] with permission.

Paget's disease of the vulva, however, even 2 cm margins are often insufficient. We have attempted to use frozen section techniques to establish appropriate surgical margins for resections.[7] Unfortunately, this technique has not proved effective, as the same number of lesions recurred after negative frozen section margins as did those that were treated based on clinical judgment alone. For extramammary Paget's disease of the vulva it is sometimes necessary to perform extremely wide local excisions with skin grafts to cover the defect.

The standard surgical management of women with invasive carcinomas of the vulva is a radical vulvectomy with bilateral inguinal-femoral lymphadenectomies.[10] The inguinal lymph nodes are the primary lymphatic drainage for the vulva and lower one-third of the vagina. This treatment can be modified if the tumor is unilateral, in which case a modified radical vulvectomy, effectively a unilateral radical excision of the labia, in association with ipsilateral lymphadenectomy, is performed.[11] Data suggest that a woman with a unilateral vulvar cancer having negative ipsilateral inguinal lymph nodes, is highly unlikely to have contralateral inguinal lymph node involvement.[10,12] If the lesion is less than 2 cm in diameter and is associated with minimal invasion (usually <2 mm), the chance of inguinal lymph node metastases being present is virtually nil. For a medically compromised elderly woman with a superficial lesion (<2 mm invasion), wide local excision may be adequate management. Such surgery can be accomplished under local anesthesia if the patient is not a candidate for general or regional anesthesia.

Further modifications in the management of vulvar cancer include inguinal lymph node sampling, rather than a formal inguinal-femoral lymphadenectomy. Inguinal lymph node sampling reduces the likelihood of the postoperative complication of a lymphocyst.[13] The sampling is done by removing an ellipse of skin in continuity with the underlying fat pad above the cruciform fascia present in the inguinal-femoral subcutaneous tissue. However, the cruciform fascia is difficult to identify in some women or may not be anatomically intact. Use of an injection of isosulfan blue to identify the sentinel inguinal lymph node is now being evaluated.[14] The sentinel inguinal lymph node is the node most likely to be involved if metastatic disease is present from the vulvar lesion. If the sentinel lymph node is free of disease, it is unlikely that other lymph nodes would be involved. This technique may reduce the extent of lymphadenectomy, particularly in an elderly patient.

If an elderly woman is not a surgical candidate because of her medical condition, radiation therapy can be used to palliate a vulvar cancer. In the past, irradiation was

TABLE 59.2. Staging of Vulvar Malignancies

| | |
|---|---|
| Stage 0 | |
| TIS | Carcinoma in situ; intraepithelial carcinoma |
| Stage I | |
| T1N0M0 | Tumor confined to the vulva and/or perineum, 2 cm or less in greatest dimension; nodes are negative |
| Stage IA | Stromal invasion no more than 1.0 μm |
| Stage IB | |
| T2N0M0 | Tumor confined to the vulva and/or perineum, more than 2 cm in greatest dimension; nodes are negative |
| Stage II | |
| T2NOMO | Tumor confined to the vulva and/or perineum, more than 2 cm in greatest dimension; nodes are negative |
| Stage III | |
| T3N0M0<br>T3N1M0<br>T1N1M0<br>T2N1M0 | Tumor of any size with (1) adjacent spread to the lower urethra and/or the vagina or the anus; and/or (2) unilateral regional lymph node metastasis |
| Stage IVA | |
| T1N2M0<br>T2N2M0<br>T3N2M0<br>T4 any N<br>M0 | Tumor invades any of the following: upper urethra, bladder mucosa, rectal mucosa, pelvic bone, bilateral regional node metastasis |
| Stage IVB | |
| Any T<br>Any N, M1 | Any distant metastasis including pelvic lymph nodes |
| TNM classification of carcinoma of the vulva (FIGO) | |
| T | Primary tumor |
| Tis | Preinvasive carcinoma (carcinoma in situ) |
| T1 | Tumor confined to the vulva and/or perineum, ≤2 cm in greatest dimension |
| T2 | Tumor confined to the vulva and/or perineum, >2 cm in greatest dimension |
| T3 | Tumor of any size with adjacent spread to the urethra and/or vagina and/or to the anus |
| T4 | Tumor of any size infiltrating the bladder mucosa and/or rectal mucosa, including the upper part of the urethral mucosa and/or fixed to the bone |
| N | Regional lymph nodes |
| N0 | No lymph node metastasis |
| N1 | Unilateral regional lymph node metastasis |
| N2 | Bilateral regional lymph node metastasis |
| M | Distant metastasis |
| M0 | No clinical metastasis |
| M1 | Distant metastasis (including pelvic lymph node metastasis) |

*Source:* Pettersson,[6] with permission.

reserved for treating extensive vulvar cancer, often used preoperatively to reduce the radicality of the surgery or as a method of avoiding surgery.[15] The vulvar tissue is supplied with an end-arterial blood supply. The skin and subcutaneous tissue are quite sensitive to radiation effect. Dry desquamation followed by moist desquamation are routine problems associated with irradiating the vulva. Nevertheless, relatively low-dose fractions of radiation therapy combined with 5-fluorouracil and mitomycin C have been employed for managing advanced vulvar cancer and cancer in elderly patients who are unable to tolerate a radical vulvectomy.[16,17]

Survival of women with vulvar cancer is related to the presence of lymph node metastases.[18] Patients with no lymph node metastasis have approximately an 80% five-year survival. Those with evidence of lymph node metastasis have a 54% five-year survival.[19] Patients with unilateral lymph node metastases have a 60% five-year survival, whereas those with bilateral lymph node metastases have a 23% five-year survival.[19] The combination of postoperative irradiation with or without chemotherapy is now becoming routine for managing women with vulvar cancer following a radical vulvectomy and inguinal-femoral lymphadenectomy when more than one lymph node with metastatic cancer is identified.

## Vaginal Cancer

Primary cancer arising in the vagina is rare. Over a 45-year period only 307 women were diagnosed to have vaginal carcinoma in Connecticut.[3] Their median age was 64 years, with 34.2% of the women being over age 70. The histology of these lesions is overwhelmingly squamous cell cancer, although adenocarcinoma can arise within the vagina itself. Less common histologies include melanoma and the rare paravaginal sarcoma. The etiology for vaginal cancer is associated with that of cervical cancer. Indeed many of the precancerous changes of the vagina occur after patients have been treated for squamous cell carcinoma in situ of the cervix or invasive cancer of the cervix,[20] although primary vaginal cancers do occur in elderly women without cervical involvement. By convention, if a cancer is present in the vagina and reaches the cervix, the cancer is considered a cervical cancer because cervical cancer is overwhelmingly more common than vaginal cancer.

Vaginal cancer is associated with HPV infection.[20,21] Women with vaginal cancers often present with pelvic pain and vaginal discharge. The discharge may be bloody or purulent, as the lesion can become secondarily infected by vaginal flora. The diagnosis is made by inspection, palpation, and biopsy. Premalignant changes of the vagina may be confined to the vaginal apex, particularly in women with a history of cervical premalignant or malignant disease. However, multifocal premalignant changes of the vagina do occur, usually in association with HPV infection. The diagnosis is confirmed by biopsy.

TABLE 59.3. FIGO Staging for Carcinoma of the Vagina

| Stage | Criteria |
|---|---|
| 0 | Carcinoma in situ, intraepithelial carcinoma |
| I | Carcinoma is limited to the vaginal wall |
| II | Carcinoma has involved the subvaginal tissue but has not extended onto the pelvic wall |
| III | Carcinoma has extended onto the pelvic wall |
| IV | Carcinoma has extended beyond the true pelvis or has clinically involved the mucosa of the bladder or rectum. Bullous edema as such does not permit a case to be allotted to stage IV |
| IVA | Spread to adjacent organs and/or direct extension beyond the true pelvis |
| IVB | Spread to distant organs |

*Source:* Pettersson,[22] with permission.

Staging of vaginal cancer is presented in Table 59.3. Management of vaginal cancer is based on the stage of disease, the volume of tumor present, and its location within the vagina. Vaginal cancers that involve the upper one-third of the vagina and are limited in extent (i.e., stage I or stage II), can be treated with a radical hysterectomy in continuity with a radical vaginectomy.[23] Tumors involving the lower third of the vagina can be treated surgically in the form of a wide local excision that includes the adjacent vulvar tissue or by a vulvectomy in continuity with a partial vaginectomy.[23] Most vaginal cancers, however, occur in older age women and the treatment of choice is radiation therapy.[24] The combination of brachytherapy and external beam therapy is often employed for successful management of vaginal cancer, thereby avoiding aggressive surgery. Complications of radiation therapy include radiation mucositis and subsequent vaginal stenosis. Vaginal necrosis may lead to vesicovaginal or rectovaginal fistulas, the treatment of which are urinary or colon diversions, respectively.

The survival of women with vaginal cancer is based on the stage of the disease at presentation. Overall, the 5-year survival for stage I disease is 60.1%, stage II 47.8%, stage III 22.9%, and stage IV 7.4%.[22] Management of recurrent disease is similar to that for cervical cancer (i.e., exenterative surgery for a centrally localized tumor and chemotherapy for disseminated disease).[23]

## Cervical Cancer

Cervical carcinoma represents the second most common cancer that develops in the female reproductive organs. The Connecticut Tumor Registry recorded 8615 patients with cervical cancer over a 45-year period.[3] The median age for cervix cancer is 53 years, which is the lowest median age for all pelvic reproductive organ cancers. Cervical cancer is predominantly a disease of younger age women; nevertheless, 13.1% of all cervical cancers present in women 70 years or older. In a study of cervical cancer in Connecticut occurring between 1985 and 1990, about 12.5% of all women who developed cervical cancer and never had a Pap smear were 64.5 years of age or older.[25]

The most common histology for premalignant and invasive cervical cancers is the squamous cell variety.[26] A spectrum of changes occur in the cervix, from mild dysplasia through carcinoma in situ, all of which may be treated in the office using simple treatments that mechanically destroy the surface epithelium and allow healthy tissue to grow in. However, when a women goes through menopause, the site at which most cervical cancers begin, the transformation zone (i.e., the junction of the exocervical squamous epithelium with that of the endocervical columnar epithelium) recedes into the endocervical canal. Premalignant changes often cannot be seen within the endocervical canal, although they become evident in elderly women, in whom often there is an associated invasive cancer. Other premalignant and invasive cancers that occur in the cervix are adenocarcinomas arising in the glandular epithelium of the endocervix. Invasive adenocarcinomas represent up to one-third of all of the cancers now being seen in Connecticut. Adenosquamous carcinomas, a combination of malignant glandular and squamous elements, also arise in the cervix but to a much lessor extent than squamous cell carcinoma and adenocarcinoma.

A variety of risk factors have been associated with the development of cervical cancer. They include having multiple sexual partners, sexual intercourse at a young age, cigarette smoking, HPV infections or other sexually transmitted disease infections, immune suppression, genital warts, and multiparity.[27] The most recent studies have concentrated on HPV infection as being the etiologic agent in the development of cervical neoplasia.[28] At least 90% of invasive cervical cancers have evidence of HPV infection.

The diagnosis of premalignant changes of the cervix is based on a biopsy of the cervix. It must be remembered that in the elderly patient, the transformation zone is within the canal, so if the elderly patient has an abnormal Pap smear, the endocervical canal must always be biopsied. An office endocervical curetting of the endocervical canal is extremely useful for determining the nature and extent of the premalignant change. If such a change is present in the endocervical canal, it is the authors' recommendation that the patient should undergo a cone biopsy. A cone biopsy removes a large segment of the cervix and allows the pathologist to determine more accurately the extent and margins of the premalignant or malignant change present. Loop electrical excision of the transformation zone (LEETZ) is an alternative method for evaluating the cervix. Unfortunately, in the elderly, with the transformation zone in the endocervical canal, the LEETZ procedure often causes cautery artifacts so the endocervical and ectocervical margins cannot be interpreted.

Once the pathology reveals the presence of a premalignant change in an elderly patient, it is wisest to consider a hysterectomy. If the patient is medically unfit for surgery, a large cone biopsy can be curative. The FIGO (International Federation of Gynecology and Obstetrics) staging system for invasive cervical cancer is presented in Table 59.4. Management of invasive cancer of the cervix is by radiation therapy or surgery. Surgery is performed in women with early-stage disease who are medically fit and can tolerate a radical hysterectomy with bilateral deep pelvic lymphadenectomies.[29] Patients with microinvasive cancer (<3mm) can undergo a type II radical hysterectomy in which the tissue that is removed includes the parametrial medial to the ureters and the proximal one-third of the vagina.[29] However, if a frankly

TABLE 59.4. FIGO Staging for Carcinoma of the Cervix Uteri

| | |
|---|---|
| Stage 0 | Carcinoma in situ, intraepithelial carcinoma. |
| Stage I | Carcinoma is strictly confined to the cervix (extension to the corpus should be disregarded). |
| IA | Invasive cancer identified only microscopically. All gross lesions even with superficial invasion are stage IB cancers. Invasion is limited to measured stromal invasion with maximum depth of 5.0mm and no wider than 7.0mm. |
| IA1 | Measured invasion of stroma no greater than 3.0mm in depth and no wider than 7.0mm. |
| IA2 | Measured invasion of stroma greater than 3.0mm and no greater than 5.0mm in depth and no wider than 7.0mm. |
| Stage IB | Clinical lesions confined to the cervix or preclinical lesions greater than for stage IA. |
| IB1 | Clinical lesions no greater than 4.0cm in size. |
| IB2 | Clinical lesions greater than 4.0cm in size. |
| Stage II | Carcinoma extends beyond the cervix but has not extended to the pelvic wall. Carcinoma involves the vagina but not as far as the lower third. |
| IIA | No obvious parametrial involvement. |
| IIB | Obvious parametrial involvement. |
| Stage III | Carcinoma has extended to the pelvic wall. On rectal examination there is no cancer-free space between the tumor and the pelvic wall. The tumor involves the lower third of the vagina. All cases with a hydronephrosis or nonfunctioning kidney are included unless they are known to be due to other causes. |
| IIIA | No extension to the pelvic wall. |
| IIIB | Extension to the pelvic wall and/or hydronephrosis or nonfunctioning kidney. |
| Stage IV | Carcinoma has extended beyond the true pelvis or has clinically involved the mucosa of the bladder or rectum. A bullous edema as such does not permit a case to be allotted to stage IV. |
| IVA | Spread of the growth to adjacent organs. |
| IVB | Spread to distant organs. |

*Source:* Pettersson,[26] with permission.

invasive cancer is present, one must perform a type III or a Meigs-Wertheim radical hysterectomy, which removes the parametrial tissue lateral to the ureter and removes approximately one-half of the vagina in continuity with the cervix and uterine corpus.[29]

For the elderly patient who is unable to tolerate a hysterectomy or for whom a radical hysterectomy is inappropriate, standard radiation therapy using intracavitary and external beam techniques is effective for managing invasive cancer of the cervix.[30,31] The efficacy of the treatment depends on the stage of the cancer and the tumor volume. At the Yale-New Haven Medical Center, women who are over age 55 years, have better locoregional control of their cancer using radiation therapy as the method of management than those who are under age 55.[32] This suggests that cancers may be more sensitive to radiation in the older population, although the overall survival is worse for the elderly, as they die of intercurrent disease.

The overall survival for women with cervical cancers correlates with the stage of the disease. Stage I patients have an 81.6% five-year survival, stage II 61.3%, stage III 36.7%, and stage IV 12.1%.[26]

Treatment of recurrent cervical cancer is based on the extent of the disease present. Patients who fail centrally (i.e., at the vaginal apex) with cancer that does not extend to or reach the pelvic side wall may be treated with exenterative surgery.[33–35] In the past we have used 70 years of age as a cutoff for those eligible for exenterative surgery. As improvements in postoperative care evolved, we are now able to offer exenterative surgery to women over age 70 years if they are in good health. Exenterative surgery includes anterior pelvic exenteration, which removes the uterus in continuity with the bladder via a radical hysterectomy, radical cystectomy, and urinary diversion. Posterior pelvic exenteration involves a radical hysterectomy in continuity with resection of the sigmoid colon and rectum; it requires a colostomy. Total pelvic exenteration removes the bladder, uterus, and rectum and sigmoid colon in continuity. Efforts have now been made to try to avoid a colostomy using surgical stapling techniques for low anterior anastomoses.[36] Continent pouches have been developed to avoid the need for continuous collection of urine in an ostomy bag. However, experience at the Yale-New Haven Medical Center suggests that patients who have been heavily pretreated with radiation and are over 65 years of age do poorly with continent pouches and probably are best served by an ileal conduit.

Patients who have extensive recurrent disease not limited to the center of the pelvis are offered experimental chemotherapy. Currently a National Cancer Institute vaccine trial directed against HPV for women with recurrent cervical cancer is available. Chemotherapy and vaccine approaches to the management of recurrent cervical cancer must be considered palliative.

## Uterine Cancer

The uterine corpus is the most common site for cancer in the female reproductive tract. The Connecticut Tumor Registry recorded 9914 women with uterine malignancies over a 45-year period.[3] The median age for these women was 61 years. Uterine cancers in 21.8% of the women were diagnosed at age 70 years or older. The most common histologic types of uterine cancer arise from the endometrium and are endometrioid in appearance.[37] Other subtypes that appear are adenosquamous, clear-cell carcinomas, and uterine serous and adenosquamous cancers. The latter tend to have a much more aggressive behavior and require more than a hysterectomy to achieve cure. In addition, sarcomas can develop within the uterus, including leiomyosarcomas, mixed mesodermal tumors, and endometrial stromal sarcomas.[38–42]

Uterine cancers usually present with an obvious early signal, postmenopausal bleeding. Women must be informed that whenever vaginal bleeding occurs during the postmenopausal era they must be promptly evaluated. If the vulva, vagina, and cervix appear unremarkable on inspection, a Pap smear and endocervical and endometrial biopsies should be obtained. Rarely, women are found to have endometrial cells on a routine Pap smear. The presence of such cells from postmenopausal women may be associated with premalignant or malignant changes of the endometrium. This cytologic finding is another indication to perform an endometrial biopsy. An endometrial biopsy can usually diagnose the presence of premalignant changes of the endometrium and invasive cancer. Endometrial hyperplasias are categorized into two forms: simple hyperplasia, previously known as cystic hyperplasia, and complex hyperplasia, previously known as glandular hyperplasia.[43] The hyperplasias are further subdivided into those with or without atypia. It is extremely unusual for simple hyperplasia to be associated with cytologic atypia, whereas complex hyperplastic changes are often associated with cytologic atypia. Simple hyperplasia rarely progresses to invasive cancer.[43] Complex hyperplasia without atypia progressed to invasive cancer in approximately 2% of patients over a 12-year period, whereas complex hyperplasia with atypia was associated with an up to 30% chance of developing invasive cancer over an 8-year observation period.[43]

Management of simple hyperplasia in the elderly consists of observation. The management of complex hyperplasia without atypia is to treat the patient with progestin therapy (medroxyprogesterone acetate, megestrol acetate). If after 3 months the hyperplasia persists, hysterectomy and bilateral salpingo-oophorectomy is recommended. Atypical hyperplasia in an elderly woman should be treated with hysterectomy. If the patient is unfit to tolerate surgery, progestin therapy in the form of oral medroxyprogesterone acetate or megestrol acetate may

TABLE 59.5. FIGO Staging for Carcinoma of the Corpus Uteri

| | |
|---|---|
| Stage IA | Grade 1, 2, 3; tumor limited to endometrium |
| Stage IB | Grade 1, 2, 3; invasion to less than one-half the myometrium |
| Stage IC | Grade 1, 2, 3; invasion to more than one-half the myometrium |
| Stage IIA | Grade 1, 2, 3; endocervical glandular involvement only |
| Stage IIB | Grade 1, 2, 3; cervical stromal invasion |
| Stage IIIA | Grade 1, 2, 3; tumor invades serosa and/or adnexa and/or positive peritoneal cytology |
| Stage IIIB | Grade 1, 2, 3; vaginal metastases |
| Stage IIIC | Grade 1, 2, 3; metastases to pelvic and/or paraaortic lymph nodes |
| Stage IVA | Grade 1, 2, 3; tumor invasion of bladder and/or bowel mucosa |
| Stage IVB | Distant metastases including intraabdominal and/or inguinal lymph nodes |

Grade 1: 5% or less of a nonsquamous or nonmorular solid growth pattern
Grade 2: 6–50% of a nonsquamous or nonmorular solid growth pattern
Grade 3: more than 50% of a nonsquamous or nonmorular solid growth pattern

*Source:* Pettersson,[44] with permission.

be used on a daily basis to revert the endometrium back to an atrophic state.

Uterine cancer is staged surgically (Table 59.5). Patients should routinely undergo total abdominal hysterectomy, bilateral salpingo-oophorectomy, and pelvic and paraaortic lymph node sampling. Additional therapy is based on the findings of the surgical staging.

Patients with histologically low grade endometrial cancers that do not deeply infiltrate the myometrium require no additional therapy. Patients with high grade endometrial cancers without deep penetration are usually treated at the Yale-New Haven Medical Center with vaginal apex irradiation alone. Patients who have deep penetration of the wall of the uterus with no lymph nodes involved may be considered for vaginal apex radiation therapy. Patients with disease that has extended to the pelvic lymph nodes are also treated with whole pelvic radiation therapy, whereas those whose disease has spread beyond the pelvis are usually offered chemotherapy in combination with vaginal apex radiation. The Gynecologic Oncology Group has reported 40% five-year survivals in the latter circumstance when patients receive pelvic and paraaortic radiation.[45] Extensive radiation therapy, such as pelvic and paraaortic fields, is often poorly tolerated by the elderly and may be difficult to administer.

The 5-year survival of women with uterine cancer confined to the uterine corpus is approximately 85%.[44] Those who have only superficial invasion without any other prognostic factors have survivals of 95–100%. Those patients with deep penetration of the uterine wall (i.e., stage IC) have survivals of 70–80%. As the stage of the cancer increases, the likelihood of cure decreases. The 5-year survival for women with stage II disease is 70%, stage III disease 49%, and stage IV disease 19%.[44]

Elderly patients often are found to have more aggressive histologic types of endometrial cancer and may be in poor medical condition in terms of tolerating surgery. Many centers have reported data showing that elderly women with uterine cancers who have severe medical problems can have their cancers controlled with radiation therapy given by the intracavitary route with or without external beam radiation, particularly if the disease is confined to the uterus.[46] Experience at the Yale-New Haven Medical Center, suggests that this approach is effective, as these patients often die from their underlying disease rather than from their cancer. Fifty-four patients treated at Yale deemed medically inoperable had a significantly shorter overall survival than the 108 control patients with stage I or II disease ($p < 0.0001$).[46] Deaths in the inoperable group were more likely to be due to intercurrent disease (28 of 32 cases) compared to the controls (3 of 15) ($p < 0.0001$). Inoperable patients who did not die of intercurrent disease had a median 5-year survival approaching that of the operable patients. The average age of the stage I patients was 72.0 years (range 44–93 years) and stage II patients 70.0 years (range 51–82 years).

Patients with more advanced disease, particularly with extrapelvic disease, may be treated with the neoadjuvant chemotherapy. The latter treatment must be considered palliative in nature. We have begun to use neoadjuvant chemotherapy in such women (i.e., administering chemotherapy prior to surgery). Using this approach, uterine malignancies can shrink; and when the surgical procedure is performed it is simpler and easier. We have also found that women tend to stop bleeding promptly after the initiation of chemotherapy. In the past, for the medically compromised elderly woman, we usually used pelvic irradiation to stop the bleeding and provide locoregional control. However, radiation therapy is a regional technique that has no significant impact on overall survival for women with advanced-stage endometrial cancers. In contrast, neoadjuvant chemotherapy may potentially have an impact on overall survival and accomplish the same control of bleeding as that offered by radiation therapy.

The management of recurrent uterine cancers is based on the cancer's histology and the extent of disease. Patients with well-differentiated endometrial cancers may respond to progestin therapy. We have used progestin therapy to control recurrent endometrial cancer for prolonged periods of time, although most, but not all, women who have recurrent disease treated with progestin therapy have further recurrences. Figure 59.1 shows a chest radiograph of a 70-year-old woman with a well-differentiated endometrial cancer that had metastasized to the lungs. She had a complete response to progestin therapy for 35 months. Patients with the less

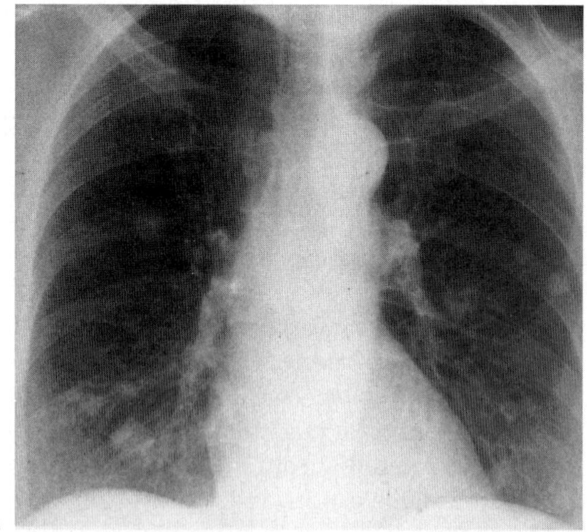

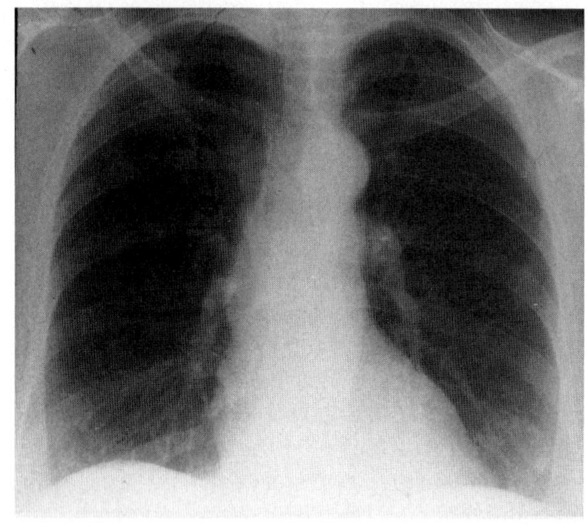

FIGURE 59.1. A. Multiple pulmonary metastases diagnosed 5 years after a total abdominal hysterectomy and bilateral salpingo-oophorectomy for a well-differentiated adenocarcinoma of the endometrium. B. Complete response to medroxyprogesterone acetate 8 months later. The patient remained clinically free of disease for 35 months after starting progestin therapy.

well-differentiated or more aggressive histologic subtypes typical in elderly, are usually treated with chemotherapy to control advanced and recurrent disease.

Three forms of sarcoma involve the uterus: leiomyosarcomas, mixed mesodermal tumors, and endometrial stromal sarcomas. Uterine leiomyosarcomas are treated with hysterectomy. Sarcomas arising within the center of fibroids that are well encapsulated and have not penetrated the capsule of the fibroid often are cured with hysterectomy alone.[38,39] Leiomyosarcomas arising de novo in the muscular wall of the uterus tend to be more aggressive, and surgery alone is insufficient. Currently, a debate remains as to whether such patients should receive chemotherapy at the time of diagnosis or the treatment should be delayed until the leiomyosarcoma recurs.[38] The infrequent occurrence of uterine leiomyosarcomas has limited the opportunity for a prospective randomized trial to address this issue.

Mixed mesodermal tumors of the uterus histologically contain carcinomatous and sarcomatous elements.[40,41] The carcinomatous element of a mixed mesodermal tumor is often uterine serous cancer, although one can also find a poorly differentiated endometrioid carcinoma, and rarely, a squamous cell carcinoma as the carcinomatous element of the mixed mesodermal tumor. The sarcomatous elements have been categorized as homologous elements (normally found in the uterus) and heterologous elements (not normally found in the uterus). An example of a homologous element is a leiomyosarcoma. Heterologous elements include rhabdomyosarcoma, chondrosarcoma, and osteosarcoma.

The management of mixed mesodermal tumors of the uterus is surgical staging, including a total abdominal hysterectomy, bilateral salpingo-oophorectomy, omentectomy, and pelvic and paraaortic lymphadenectomies, followed by combination chemotherapy and irradiation of the vaginal apex. This approach has been most effective for early-stage disease, but it has not been effective when the disease has spread outside the uterus (i.e., stage III or IV disease).

Endometrial stromal sarcomas can be divided into low grade and high grade malignancies.[42] Low grade stromal sarcomas, endolymphatic stromal myosis, tend to push into lymphatic spaces. Endolymphatic stromal myosis is extremely sensitive to progestin therapy. Following a hysterectomy for a low grade endometrial stromal sarcoma, patients should be placed on an oral progestin, either megestrol acetate or medroxyprogesterone acetate. High grade endometrial stromal sarcomas are often found to be at an advanced stage at the time of diagnosis. Their management is cytoreductive surgery, including a total abdominal hysterectomy, bilateral salpingo-oophorectomy, and postoperative combination chemotherapy.

## Fallopian Tube Cancer

The fallopian tube is the least common site for primary cancers to develop in the female reproductive tract. The Connecticut Tumor Registry recorded only 180 cases of primary fallopian tube carcinomas over a 45-year period.[3] The median age for women with fallopian tube carcinomas was 58 years, but 15.6% of the women were age 70 or over at the time of diagnosis. Fallopian tube carcinomas are adenocarcinomas and have the histologic appearance of serous ovarian carcinomas.[47] If the fallopian tube carcinoma involves the ovary, by convention it is considered to be an ovarian cancer, as ovarian cancer occurs more frequently than fallopian tube carcinoma.

The etiology of fallopian tube carcinoma is completely unknown. Symptoms associated with fallopian tube carcinoma include lower abdominal pain and pressure and a profuse, clear vaginal discharge (hydrops tubae profluens).[48] Physical examination often confirms the presence of a mass. Imaging studies may be performed using ultrasonography or computed tomography (CT) scans to identify an adnexal mass. Most fallopian tube carcinomas are not suspected until patients undergo surgery for a pelvic mass.

The current surgical staging system for fallopian tube carcinomas is shown in Table 59.6. The management of fallopian tube carcinomas in the elderly is primarily surgical. Patients undergo an exploratory laparotomy to identify the nature of the pelvic mass. The mass is resected along with the uterus, contralateral ovary, and any other metastatic disease. The goal of the surgery is to remove virtually all visible and palpable cancer (i.e., cytoreductive surgery).

Postoperative treatment for fallopian tube carcinoma is combination chemotherapy using platinum-based protocols.[48,49] The overall survival after fallopian tube cancer is based on the surgical stage. Early-stage disease has a 5-year survival of approximately 70%, whereas with advanced disease the 5-year survival is approximately 20%. Whole abdominal irradiation with a pelvic boost may also be used for treating early-stage fallopian tube cancer.[48,49] Late recurrences of fallopian tube carcinoma (i.e., after 5 years of being free of disease) have been observed.[49] CA 125 determinations are used for routine postoperative follow-up of patients with fallopian tube cancers.[50] Recurrent disease is managed with combination chemotherapy. Surgery may be employed to diagnose recurrent disease and to remove recurrent cancer if the cancer is limited rather than diffuse in nature.

TABLE 59.6. FIGO Staging for Carcinoma of the Fallopian Tube

| | |
|---|---|
| Stage 0 | Carcinoma in situ (limited to tubal mucosa). |
| Stage I | Growth limited to fallopian tubes. |
| IA | Growth limited to one tube with extension into submucosa and/or muscularis but not penetrating serosal surface; no ascites. |
| IB | Growth limited to both tubes with extension into submucosa and/or muscularis but not penetrating serosal surface; no ascites. |
| IC | Tumor either stage IA or stage IB but with extension through or onto tubal serosa or with ascites containing malignant cells or with positive peritoneal washings. |
| Stage II | Growth involving one or both fallopian tubes with pelvic extension. |
| IIA | Extension and/or metastasis to uterus and/or ovaries. |
| IIB | Extension to other pelvic tissues. |
| IIC | Tumor either stage IIA or IIB and with ascites containing malignant cells or with positive peritoneal washings. |
| Stage III | Tumor involving one or both fallopian tubes with peritoneal implants outside the pelvis and/or positive retroperitoneal or inguinal nodes. Superficial liver metastasis equals stage III. Tumor appears limited to true pelvis but with historically proven malignant extension to small bowel or omentum. |
| IIIA | Tumor grossly limited to true pelvis with negative nodes but with histologically confirmed microscopic seeding of abdominal peritoneal surfaces. |
| IIIB | Tumor involving one or both tubes with histologically confirmed implants of abdominal peritoneal surfaces, none exceeding 2 cm in diameter. Lymph nodes are negative. |
| IIIC | Abdominal implants more than 2 cm in diameter and/or positive retroperitoneal or inguinal nodes. |
| Stage IV | Growth involving one or both fallopian tubes with distant metastases. If pleural effusion is present, cytologic fluid must be positive for malignant cells to be stage IV. Parenchymal liver metastasis equals stage IV. |

*Source:* Pettersson, Pettersson F. Staging rules for gestational trophoblastic tumors and fallopian tube cancer. Acta Obstet Gynecol Scand 1992;71:224, with permission.

## Ovarian Cancer

Ovarian cancer is the third most common cancer to develop in the female reproductive tract. The Connecticut Tumor Registry reported 8085 women with ovarian cancer diagnosed during a 45-year period.[3] The median age for these women was 58 years. Ovarian cancer was diagnosed in 21.2% of women age 70 years or older (Table 59.1). Ovarian cancer lacks early warning symptoms and is not usually diagnosed until it spreads beyond the ovary and the pelvis (i.e., stage III or IV disease). Approximately 70% of women present with advanced disease (stage III or IV) (Table 59.7).[51] The most common presenting symptoms are abdominal bloating and distension often in association with vague nonspecific abdominal complaints. Gastrointestinal dysfunction is seen in about 20% of women with ovarian cancers, and less commonly, postmenopausal bleeding is observed. The diagnosis is based on the physical examination and diagnostic imaging, which reveals a pelvic mass compatible with an ovarian malignancy. The staging of ovarian cancer is surgical (Table 59.7). Women able to tolerate surgery should undergo aggressive exploration to establish the diagnosis and remove as much cancer as possible (i.e., cytoreductive surgery).

The ovary forms cancers from a variety of structures. The most common cancer, representing approximately 90% of all ovarian cancers, arises from the surface epithelial cells.[51] These cells give rise to the common epithelial cancers of the ovary, including the serous, mucinous, clear-cell, endometrioid, Brenner, transitional, and undifferentiated cancers. Mixed epithelial cancers also occur. The germ cell is the second most common source for ovarian cancer and represents approximately 5% of all ovarian malignancies.[53] These malignancies include the dysgerminoma, immature teratoma, endodermal sinus tumor, embryonal carcinoma, choriocarcinoma, and polyembryoma. Mixed germ cell tumors containing any of the above elements may also occur. The most common elements in a mixed germ cell tumor are the dysgerminoma and the endodermal sinus tumor. Ovarian germ cell malignancies occur most frequently in teenagers and

TABLE 59.7. FIGO Staging for Carcinoma of the Ovary

| | |
|---|---|
| Stage I | Growth limited to the ovaries. |
| IA | Growth limited to one ovary; no ascites present containing malignant cells. No tumor on the external surface; capsule intact. |
| IB | Growth limited to both ovaries; no ascites present containing malignant cells. No tumor on the external surfaces; capsules intact. |
| IC | Tumor classified as either stage IA or IB but with tumor on the surface of one or both ovaries; or with ruptured capsule(s); or with ascites containing malignant cells; or with positive peritoneal washings. |
| Stage II | Growth involving one or both ovaries, with pelvic extension. |
| IIA | Extension and/or metastases to the uterus and/or tubes. |
| IIB | Extension to other pelvic tissues. |
| IIC | Tumor either stage IIA of IIB but with tumor on the surface of one or both ovaries; or with capsules(s) ruptured; or with ascites containing malignant cells present; or with positive peritoneal washings. |
| Stage III | Tumor involving one or both ovaries with peritoneal implants outside the pelvis and/or positive retroperitoneal or inguinal nodes. Superficial liver metastasis equals stage III. Tumor is limited to the true pelvis but with histologically proven malignant extension to small bowel or omentum. |
| IIIA | Tumor grossly limited to the true pelvis with negative nodes but with histologically confirmed microscopic seeding of abdominal peritoneal surfaces. |
| IIIB | Tumor of one or both ovaries with histologically confirmed implants of abdominal peritoneal surfaces, none exceeding 2 cm in diameter; nodes are negative. |
| IIIC | Abdominal implants greater than 2 cm in diameter and/or positive retroperitoneal or inguinal nodes. |
| Stage IV | Growth involving one or both ovaries, with distant metastases. If pleural effusion is present, there must be positive cytologic findings to allot a case to stage IV. Parenchymal liver metastasis equals stage IV. |

*Source:* Pettersson,[52] with permission.

women in their twenties. They are not found after menopause.

Sex cord-stromal tumors are the third most common cancers developing in the ovary.[54] They may be functional in nature (i.e., produce hormones). The most common functional tumor is the granulosa cell tumor, which produces estrogen. The Sertoli-Leydig cell tumor produces androgens. Mixed tumors and sex cord-stromal tumors are rare and are called gynandroblastomas. Occasionally one finds pure Sertoli cell or pure Leydig cell tumors, particularly in elderly patients. These tumors are benign and may be associated with symptoms related to hormone production; they are treated by removing the involved ovary. Nonfunctioning tumors include fibromas, fibrosarcomas, leiomyomas, leiomyosarcomas, and mixed mesodermal tumors involving both carcinomatous elements and sarcomatous elements. Mixed mesodermal tumors often occur in women over age 70. They are a particularly virulent form of ovarian cancer and are usually diagnosed as stage III or IV disease.[55]

The ovary is a frequent site of metastasis particularly from breast and colon cancer. When evaluating women with intraabdominal carcinomas involving the ovaries preoperatively, it is always wise to make certain the patient does not have an abnormal breast examination or mammogram, and that there are no gastrointestinal symptoms consistent with a primary colon carcinoma.

The conventional treatment for ovarian cancer is aggressive cytoreductive surgery followed by aggressive platinum-based chemotherapy.[56] Survival is directly related to the stage of the cancer; and for women with advanced disease, survival is correlated with the amount of residual tumor left at the time of the initial therapy.[57] The actuarial 5-year survival reported by FIGO for stage IA disease is 82.3%, stage IB 83.9%, and stage IC 67.7%.[52] Stage IIA patients have 60.6% five-year survivals, stage IIB and IIC 53.8%, stage IIIA 49.0%, stage IIIB 32.9%, stage IIIC 18.5%, and stage IV 8.0%.[52]

Conventional wisdom is that all women suspected of having ovarian cancer should be treated with aggressive surgery followed by aggressive chemotherapy. Recently, we have found that patients with extremely advanced ovarian cancer or who are medically unable to tolerate surgery for what appears to be an advanced ovarian cancer, do extremely well with neoadjuvant chemotherapy (i.e., giving the chemotherapy traditionally used for managing ovarian cancer prior to surgery).[58] To be eligible for such an approach at the Yale-New Haven Medical Center, we require that the patient has a CT scan compatible with advanced ovarian cancer and cytologic evidence or needle biopsy compatible with an epithelial cancer of the ovary.[59] In such circumstances, if the CT scan suggests that the disease is nonresectable or the woman is unable to tolerate a surgical approach, we administer platinum-based chemotherapy.

Patients treated with neoadjuvant chemotherapy have the same survival rates as those treated in a conventional fashion for stage IIIC or IV disease.[60] A retrospective review of 59 women treated in this fashion compared to 206 women with stage IIIC or IV ovarian cancer treated by a conventional surgical approach, showed no difference in survival.[60] Of the 59 patients, 38 had disease spread beyond the abdominal cavity. The survival of patients with neoadjuvant therapy was exactly the same as those who had stage IV disease and underwent conventional therapy. Patients who received chemotherapy first had a much quicker return to their normal status than those women who underwent conventional surgery followed by chemotherapy. The rapid improvement in performance status among the women who underwent neoadjuvant chemotherapy was impressive despite the fact that their performance status was statistically worse than that of the women who underwent conventional treatment. In addition, the median age of the women who received neoadjuvant chemotherapy was significantly older than those who received conventional treatment.

Two-thirds of the women who underwent neoadjuvant chemotherapy for ovarian cancer management also underwent cytoreductive surgery. The survival of the women who underwent cytoreductive surgery was statistically better than the survival of those who did not. Most of the women who underwent cytoreductive surgery were optimally cytoreduced; that is, there was no residual tumor at the surgery. A larger proportion of the lesions treated with neoadjuvant chemotherapy were cytoreduced compared to those that underwent conventional therapy. One-third of the neoadjuvant-treated patients were unable to undergo surgery. Chemotherapy alone can be used to palliate women who are elderly and medically unfit to undergo surgery. Patients treated with neoadjuvant chemotherapy who do not have a complete response or who remain unfit to undergo cytoreductive surgery, can receive alternative chemotherapy or observation. Patients who do not have a complete response to neoadjuvant chemotherapy invariably die of ovarian cancer or intercurrent disease.

Most women with advanced ovarian cancer at the time of the initial diagnosis develop recurrent cancer. Treatment is based on whether the cancer recurs locally or appears diffusely throughout the abdominal cavity. Isolated recurrent cancers are usually treated by secondary cytoreductive surgery followed by combination chemotherapy. Patients whose lesions are optimally cytoreduced at the time of secondary cytoreductive surgery appear to have a longer survival than those whose lesions could not be optimally cytoreduced.[61] Once ovarian cancer recurs, it acts like a chronic disease that invariably leads to the patient's demise unless she has intercurrent disease.

## References


1. Parker SL, Tong T, Bolden S, Wingo P. Cancer statistics, 1997. CA Cancer J Clin 1997;47:5–27.
2. Boffetta P, Parkin DM. Cancer in developing countries. CA Cancer J Clin 1994;44:81–90.
3. Heston JF, Kelly JAB, Meigs JW, Flannery JT. Forty-five years of cancer incidence in Connecticut: 1935–1979. Natl Cancer Inst Monogr 1986;70:359–398.
4. Van Beurden M, ten Kate FJ, Smits HL, et al. Multifocal vulvar intraepithelial neoplasia grade III and multicentric lower genital tract neoplasia is associated with transcriptionally active human papilloma virus. Cancer 1995;75: 2879–2884.
5. Monk BJ, Burger RA, Lin F, Parham G, Vasilev SA, Wilczynski SP. Prognostic significance of human papilloma virus DNA in vulvar carcinoma. Obstet Gynecol 1995;85: 709–715.
6. Pettersson F. Annual report on the results of treatment in gynecological cancer. Int J Gynecol Obstet 1991;36(suppl): 278–285.
7. Fishman DA, Chambers SK, Kohorn EI, Chambers JT. Extramammary Paget's disease of the vulva. Gynecol Oncol 1995; 56:266–270.
8. Edwards CL, Tortolero-Luna G, Linares AC, et al. Vulvar intraepithelial neoplasia and vulvar cancer. Obstet Gynecol Clin North Am 1996;23:295–324.
9. International Society for the Study of Vulvar Disease: New nomenclature for vulvar disease. Obstet Gynecol 1976;47: 122.
10. Homesley HD. Management of vulvar cancer. Cancer 1995;76(suppl):2159–2170.
11. Stehman FB, Bundy BW, Dvoretsky PM, Creasman WT. Early stage I carcinoma of the vulva treated with ipsilateral superficial inguinal lymphadenectomy and modified radical hemivulvectomy: a prospective study of the Gynecologic Oncology Group. Obstet Gynecol 1992;79:490–197.
12. Morris JM. A formula for selective lymphadenectomy: its application to cancer of the vulva. Obstet Gynecol 1977;50: 152–158.
13. Hoffman MS, Mark JE, Cavanagh D. A management scheme for postoperative groin lymphocysts. Gynecol Oncol 1995; 56:262–265.
14. Levenback C, Burke TW, Gershenson DM, Morris M, Malpica A, Ross MI. Intraoperative lymphatic mapping for vulvar cancer. Obstet Gynecol 1994;84:163–167.
15. Boronow RC, Hickman BT, Reagan MT, Steadham RE. Combined therapy as an alternative to exenteration for locally advanced vulvovaginal cancer. II. Results, complications and dosimetric and surgical considerations. Am J Clin Oncol 1987;10:171–181.
16. Landoni F, Maneo A, Zanetta G, et al. Concurrent preoperative chemotherapy with 5-fluorouracil and mitomycin C and radiotherapy (FUMIR) followed by limited surgery in locally advanced and recurrent vulva carcinoma. Gynecol Oncol 1996;61:321–327.
17. Cunningham MJ, Goyer RP, Gibbons SK, Kredentser SC, Malfetano JH, Keys H. Primary radiation, cisplatin and 5-fluorouracil for advanced squamous carcinoma of the vulva. Gynecol Oncol 1997;66:258–261.
18. Homesley HD, Bundy BN, Sedlis A, Adcock L. Radiation therapy versus pelvic node resection for carcinoma of the vulva with positive groin nodes. Obstet Gynecol 1986;68: 733–740.
19. Burger MPM, Hollema H, Emanuels AG, Kraws M, Pras E, Bouma J. The importance of the groin node status for the survival of $T_1$ and $T_2$ vulvar carcinoma patients. Gynecol Oncol 1995;57:377–334.
20. Sugase M, Matsukura T. Distinct manifestations of human papilloma viruses in the vagina. Int J Cancer 1997;72:412–415.
21. Minucci D, Cinel A, Insacco E, Oselladore M. Epidemiological aspects of vaginal intraepithelial neoplasia (VAIN). Clin Exp Obstet Gynecol 1995;22:36–42.
22. Pettersson F. Annual report on the results of treatment in gynecological cancer. Int J Gynecol Obstet 1991;36(suppl): 302–308.
23. Stock RG, Chen AS, Seski J. A 30 year experience in the management of primary carcinoma of the vagina: analysis of prognostic factors and treatment modalities. Gynecol Oncol 1995;56:45–52.
24. Chyle V, Zagars GK, Wheeler JA, Wharton JT, Delclos L. Definitive radiotherapy for carcinoma of the vagina: outcome and prognostic factors. Int J Radiat Oncol Biol Phys 1996;35:891–905.

25. Janerich DT, Hajimichael O, Schwartz PE, et al. Cervical cancer, Connecticut. Am J Public Health 1995;85:791–794.
26. Pettersson F. Annual report on the results of treatment in gynecological cancer. Int J Gynecol Obstet 1991;36(suppl): 27–43.
27. Brinton LA, Fraumeni JF. Epidemiology of uterine cervical carcinoma. J Chronic Dis 1986;31:1051.
28. Holly EA. Cervical intraepithelial neoplasia, cervical cancer and HPV. Annu Rev Public Health 1996;17:69–84.
29. Piver MS, Rutledge F, Smith JP. Five classes of extended hysterectomy for women with cervical cancer. Obstet Gynecol 1974;44:265–272.
30. Perez CA. Radiation therapy in the management of cancer of the cervix. Oncology 1993;7:89–96.
31. Keys H, Gibbons SK. Optimal management of locally advanced cervical carcinoma. J Natl Cancer Inst Monogr 1996;21:89–92.
32. Kapp DS, Fischer D, Gutierrez E, Kohorn EI, Schwartz PE. Pretreatment prognostic factors in carcinoma of the uterine cervix: a multivariate analysis of the effect of age, stage, histology and blood counts on survival. Int J Radiat Oncol Biol Phys 1983;9:445–455.
33. Magrina HF, Stanhope CR, Weaver AL. Pelvic exenterations: supralevator, infralevator and with vulvectomy. Gynecol Oncol 1997;64:130–135.
34. Penalven MA, Barreau G, Sevin BU, Averette HE. Surgery for the treatment of locally recurrent disease. J Natl Cancer Inst Mongr 1996;21:117–122.
35. Vergote IB. Exenterative surgery. Curr Opin Obstet Gynecol 1997;9:25–28.
36. Burke TW, Weiser EB, Hoskins WJ, Heller PB, Nash JD, Park RC. End colostomy using the end-to-end anastomosis instrument. Obstet Gynecol 1987;156–159.
37. Rose PG. Endometrial carcinoma. N Engl J Med 1997;335: 640–649.
38. Hannigan EV, Gomez LG. Uterine leiomyosarcoma. Am J Obstet Gynecol 1979;134:557–564.
39. Resnik E, Chambers SK, Carcangiu ML, Kohorn EI, Schwartz PE, Chambers JT. Malignant uterine smooth muscle tumors: role of etoposide, cisplatin and doxorubicin (EPA) chemotherapy. J Surg Oncol 1996;63:145–147.
40. Olah KS, Dunn JA, Gee H. Leiomyosarcomas have a poorer prognosis than mixed mesodermal tumors when adjusting for known prognostic factors: the results of a retrospective study of 432 cases of uterine sarcoma. Br J Obstet Gynaecol 1992;99:590–594.
41. Resnik E, Chambers SK, Carcangiu ML, Kohorn EI, Schwartz PE, Chambers JT. A phase II study of etoposide, cisplatin and doxorubicin chemotherapy in mixed mullerian tumors (MMT) of the uterus. Gynecol Oncol 1995;56:370–375.
42. Katz L, Merino MJ, Sakamoto J, Schwartz PE. Endometrial stromal sarcoma: estrogen and progestin receptor levels and their significance in hormone treatment. Gynecol Oncol 1987;26:87–97.
43. Kurman RK, Kaminski PF, Norris HJ. The behavior of endometrial hyperplasia: a long-term study of "untreated" hyperplasia in 170 patients. Cancer 1985;56:403–412.
44. Pettersson F. Annual report on the results of treatment in gynecological cancer. Int J Gynecol Obstet 1991;36(suppl): 132–155.
45. Morrow CP, Bundy BW, Kurman RJ, et al. Relationship between surgical-pathological risk factors and outcomes in clinical stage I and II carcinoma of the endometrium: a Gynecologic Oncology Group study. Gynecol Oncol 1991; 40:50–65.
46. Fishman DA, Roberts KB, Chambers JT, Kohorn EI, Schwartz PE, Chambers SK. Radiation therapy as exclusive treatment for medically inoperable patients with stage I and II endometrioid carcinoma of the endometrium. Gynecol Oncol 1996;61:189–196.
47. Cormio G, Maneo A, Gabriele A, Rota SM, Lisson A, Zanetta G. Primary carcinoma of the fallopian tube: a retrospective analysis of 47 patients. Ann Oncol 1996;7:271–275.
48. Baekelandt M, Kockx M, Wesling F, Gerris J. Primary adenocarcinoma of the fallopian tube: review of the literature. Int J Gynecol Cancer 1993;3:65–71.
49. Brown MD, Kohorn EI, Kapp DS, Schwartz PE, Merino M. Fallopian tube carcinoma. Int J Radiat Oncol Biol Phys 1985;11:583–590.
50. Rosen AC, Klein M, Rosen HR, et al. Preoperative and postoperative CA 125 serum levels in primary fallopian tube carcinoma. Arch Gynecol Obstet 1994;255:65–68l.
51. Cannistra SA. Cancer of the ovary. N Engl J Med 1993;329:1550–1559.
52. Pettersson F. Annual report on the results of treatment in gynecological cancer. Int J Gynecol Obstet 1991;36(suppl): 238–257.
53. Fishman DA, Schwartz PE. Current approaches to the diagnosis and treatment of ovarian germ cell malignancies. Curr Opin Obstet Gynecol 1994;6:98–104.
54. Price FV, Schwartz PE. Management of ovarian stromal tumors. In: Rubin SC, Sutton GP (eds) Ovarian Cancer. New York: McGraw Hill, 1993:405–423.
55. Cass I, Chambers JT, Chambers SK, Carcangiu ML, Kohorn EI, Schwartz PE. Combination chemotherapy with etoposide, cisplatin and doxorubicin in mixed mullerian tumors of the adnexa. Gynecol Oncol 1996;61:309–314.
56. Schwartz PE. Surgical management of ovarian cancer. Arch Surg 1981;116:99–106.
57. Hoskins WJ, Bundy BN, Thigpen JT, Omura GA. The influence of cytoreductive surgery on recurrence-free interval and survival in small-volume stage III epithelial ovarian cancer: a Gynecologic Oncology Group study. Gynecol Oncol 1992;47:159–166.
58. Schwartz PE. Neoadjuvant chemotherapy for advanced ovarian cancer. J Gynecol Techniques 1995;1:175–180.
59. Nelson BE, Rosenfield AT, Schwartz PE. Preoperative abdominopelvic computed tomographic prediction of optimal cytoreduction in epithelial ovarian carcinoma. J Clin Oncol 1993;11:166–172.
60. Schwartz PE, Rutherford TJ, Chambers JT, Kohorn EI, Thiel RP. Neoadjuvant chemotherapy for advanced ovarian cancer: long-term survival (Gynecol Oncol 1999;72:93–99).
61. Segna RA, Dottino PR, Mandeli JP, Konsker K, Cohen CJ. Secondary cytoreduction for ovarian cancer following cisplatin therapy. J Clin Oncol 1993;11:434–439.

# *Part II*
# *Specific Issues in Geriatric Surgery*

## Section 9
## Soft Tissue and Musculoskeletal System

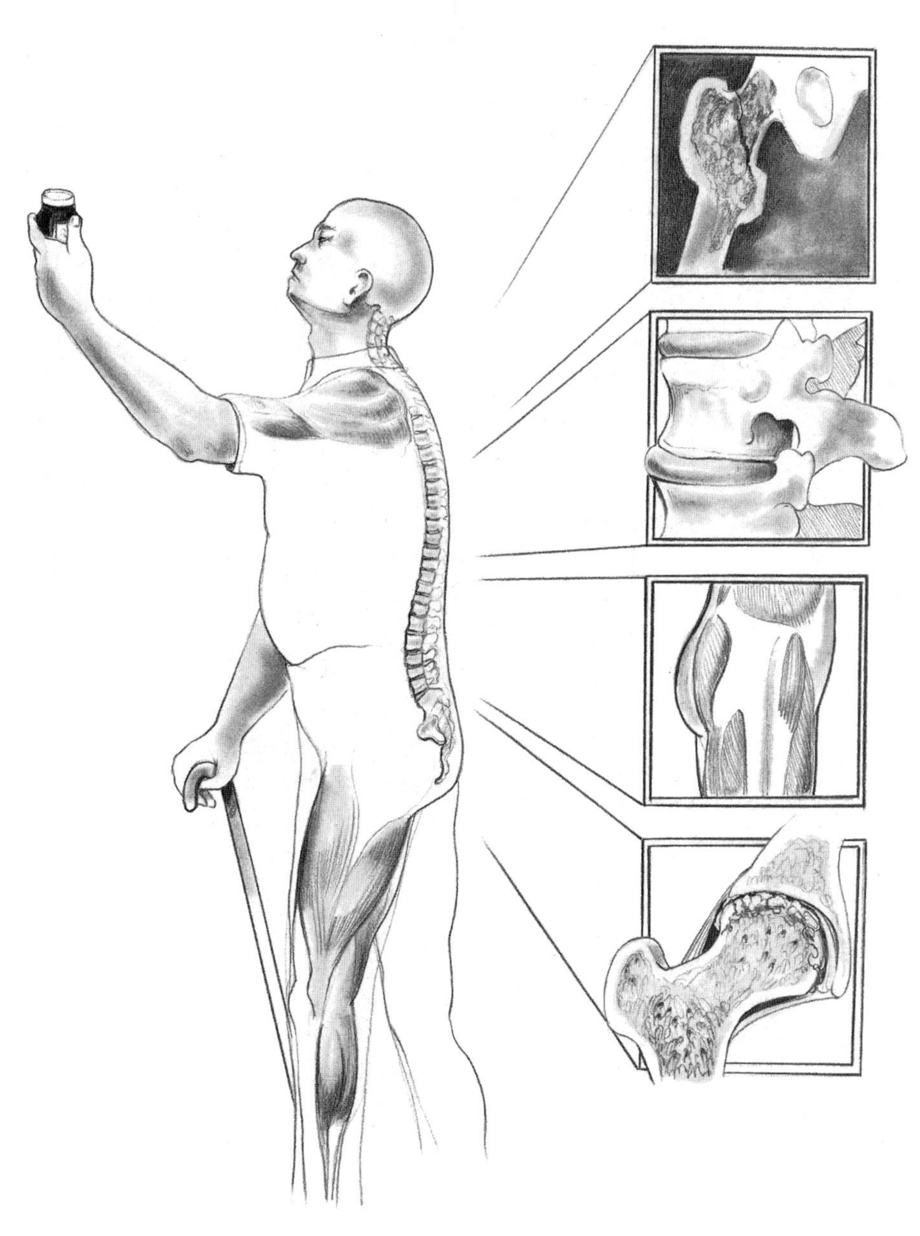

# Invited Commentary

Roby C. Thompson, Jr.

During the past 35 years the ability to provide expanded care for geriatric patients with soft tissue and musculoskeletal disease and injury has expanded exponentially. As I reflect on the changes experienced in my practice as an orthopedic surgeon from 1963 to now, I am struck by a wide range of opportunities related to advances in either technology or our understanding of the biology of the connective tissues. These advances have fed off each other; in some circumstances they have been largely dependent on their own merit, whereas in others they are intimately linked. I have divded this introduction into advances dependent on one or the other—basic biology or technology—and interdependent fields.

## Biologic Advances

During the early 1960s the field of wound healing was just beginning to emerge from the histologic understanding of soft tissue repair and fracture healing to more quantitative understanding of the role of foreign bodies and the cellular response to injury. The advances that have occurred in our understanding of soft tissue healing of tendons and ligaments are responsible for much-improved outcomes for patients of all ages with tendon lacerations or ligament tears. We have learned that the temporal relations of repair and reaction to injury dictate the appropriate rehabilitation of these injuries. As a result, rather than external immobilization in a cast for 3–6 weeks to protect a torn ligament or lacerated tendon, those injuries are now treated by early surgical intervention and early controlled motion to enhance the healing and the mobility of the injured part. Likewise, the role of surgical intervention in fracture healing during the 1960s was considered heretical by some because of the complications of fixation failure and infection. Much of this was due to a lack of appreciation of the concomitant soft tissue injury associated with the fracture and the need for managing the fracture based on the magnitude of the soft tissue injury. This point is best exemplified by the expanded classification systems of "open fractures" to three of four strata depending on the author who has studied these injuries. This has been a great leap forward in managing what were previously described as "compound fractures." It has allowed expanded opportunities for return to function by patients who were previously subjected to prolonged immobilization in casts or traction and for what the great fracture surgeons of the 1960s, such as Harrison L. McLaughlin, Preston Wade, and Reginald Watson-Jones, called "fracture disease."

As a result of our better understanding of the relations between soft tissue injury and fractures, we have been able to modify our treatments to capitalize on early limb function using a variety of techniques. These have spanned "functional bracing," early ambulation in casts for femoral and tibial fractures, and early hand motion for "Colle's fractures," among others. From our expanded understanding of open fractures based on the early classification of Gustilo and Anderson, we learned that a type 1 open fracture with minimal soft tissue injury (e.g., a low-velocity gunshot wound) could be managed with local irrigation and débridement, with conventional fracture management for that fracture. This is in contrast to proceeding to an operating room environment for a type 3 fracture with massive soft tissue damage with or without comminution that demanded meticulous, thorough débridement on an as-necessary basis to provide healthy tissue for wound healing and resistance to infection.

Concomitant with our understanding of fracture repair and bone formation was an expanded understanding of the use of bone grafts largely based on the work of Marshall Urist, C. Andrew Bassett, and others. They pointed out that bone grafts could be osteoproductive, osteoconductive, or even osteoinductive, depending on the characteristic of the graft and how it was applied. We now know that when osteoproduction is required from a bone graft it can occur only with autogenous cancellous bone that is carefully handled to protect the transplanted osteoblasts. Moreover, the graft must be in a viable, receptive environment with adequate well-oxygenated blood supply. In a similar manner we can rationally expect cancellous allogeneic bone prepared in a way that removes primary cellular antigens and decreases the transplant antigenicity of the residual protein matrix to be comparable to autogenous bone for filling a cavity that requires primary conduction of bone, such as a benign cyst of bone. We have also learned that massive allogeneic bone grafts can be used for reconstructing major skeletal defects, including osteoarticular defects with expectations of 75–80% long-term function in limbs that were potentially doomed to amputation during the 1960s.

The expanded understanding of tumor biology and the role of surgery of those primary tumors of the musculoskeletal system is a product of the past 35 years. We now know that as sarcomas spread in tissue planes associated with bone and muscle compartments, amputating the limb with a sarcoma is not necessarily the best or the only way to remove the tumor for the best outcome of local control. Thus with a soft tissue sarcoma of the vastus lateralis muscle in the geriatric patient it would be unusual today to recommend amputation. Rather, resection of the involved muscle with a fascial envelope surrounding the muscle and reconstruction with muscle transfers and rehabilitation are recommended, following the principles described above for soft tissue healing.

Much of what the surgeon caring for the musculoskeletal system can provide to the geriatric patients of the 2000s is based on generic advances in medicine and on our better understanding of pharmacotherapy. With the advances in antibiotics, chemotherapy, and hormone replacement, we are better able to control the aging process, which is pathologic in certain individuals. The classic example is osteoporosis and the discoveries of the estrogen dependence of the osteoblast-osteoclast relation for maintenance of skeletal mass. Through the development of a class of drugs called bisphosphonates, we now have the ability to block bone resorption, which holds out major opportunities for better control of osteoporosis. Additional therapies in tumor-related bone resorption are available as well.

Similar advances in the use of blood products and anesthesia have allowed the orthopedic surgeon reasonably to consider surgical intervention in an aging population that would have been unthinkable 35 years ago. For example, it is common today for elective joint replacements to be recommended in octogenarians in reasonably good general health. We are confident that the ability of anesthesiologists to monitor vital signs, oxygenation, and visceral functions allows most unexpected conditions to be corrected quickly, just as we have become accustomed to correcting coagulopathies in our pre- and postoperative patients by defining the problem and replacing the deficit component of the coagulation system.

## Technologic Advances

The advancing experience with biomaterials and giant leaps in our understanding of the fundamentals of the biomechanics of the skeletal system have been products of the past 35 years. These 35 years of practice have seen many technologic changes; they have not all been advances, and many have subsequently been abandoned. Even those advances that have proved successful have been subject to misapplication as we grope for the appropriate application. If there is one lesson for the future, it would be to enhance our scrutiny of new technology and demand accurate, well-done outcome studies before we embrace the new technology.

With that editorial comment out of the way, I offer the following technologic advances as the most important of the past 35 years for the orthopedic patient. First is our understanding of biomaterials and the biomaterial interface with the biologic and mechanical environment. Biocompatibility was a science well on its way during the 1960s, but it has become virtual cookbook science during the past few years. Hence we rarely concern ourselves with the new material and its relation to the biologic environment when it is accepted for market by the U.S. Food and Drug Administration (FDA). In the field of musculoskeletal diseases we have seen silicone and Teflon arthroplasty wreak havoc at the local level owing to wear product debris in the absence of reaction to an inert material product. Today the biggest challenge in the field of joint replacement is defining the interface between artificial articulations that have minimal and tolerable wear and yet do not transmit unacceptable forces to the implant–bone interface that is the link for long-term fixation of the implant. During the past 30 years we have gone from catastrophic failures with total hips of stainless steel and Teflon articulation, or acrylic replacements of femoral heads, to more successful stainless steel or cobalt-chrome alloy replacements that rely on a press-fit interface with bone, yet frequently there were only one or two options in size for this interface with articular sizing based on 0.25-inch increments. Today we have a more than 20-year record of successful experience with the use of polymethylmethacrylate as a bone cement for implant fixation. We have learned new implant skills over the past 30 years that promise a more than 85% twenty-year survival of the implants currently in use. Implant manufacturers have responded to competition and demand; and as a result, our patients can expect a large inventory of sizes and shapes for accommodating the individual idiosyncrasies of their anatomy.

The field of internal fixation for fracture care has paralleled the implant development for joint disease. The linked technology of low-exposure intraoperative fluoroscopy and our better understanding of infection control and fracture healing has led to a change in the management of most displaced fractures, which allows early return to function, diminished hospitalization, and lower complication rates with a superior functional outcome.

The mid-shaft femoral fracture is a good example. If one looks at the standard of care during the 1960s, it was skeletal traction for 6–8 weeks followed by a spica cast for a similar time period, frequently associated limb length discrepancy and, commonly, a stiff knee. This practice was measured against an open reduction and internal fixation with an intramedullary nail or plates and screws that even in skilled hands carried a 10% infection rate. Today those fractures are most commonly treated with closed intramedullary fixation. Commonly there is a 3- to 5-day hospital stay with return to full unrestricted weight-bearing in 4 months, with expectations of a normal knee joint in most cases. The common expectation for any intraarticular fracture in the current environment is anatomic restoration of the joint surface through open or semiopen techniques, with early joint motion providing maximum functional return.

Another major technologic advancement of the past 35 years has been the ability to perform semiopen surgery via endoscopic techniques. Arthroscopy was the forerunner of much of the endoscopic surgery that is now common in all fields. Introduction of the Watanabe arthroscope during the 1960s, was a major opportunity for orthopedists to see the pathology in the joint; but until the fiberoptic light and hand-held video camera made the arthroscope a practical tool for correcting pathology and removing loose bodies or torn meniscii, the potential went unrecognized. Once again, the 3- to 5-day hospital stay with an open arthrotomy for a meniscus injury has become same-day surgery, with athletes returning to their performance in weeks rather than months.

The other technologic advance with dramatic effect in bone and soft tissue surgery, has been the ability to perform free vascularized tissue transfers as a result of the introduction of intraoperative microscopy and magnification for microvascular anastomosis. The biologic understanding of the rheology of microvascular flow and reflow has been essential to the successful application of this technology.

The future for soft tissue and skeletal injury and disease management is exciting. Looking back over the past 35 years makes one realize how unpredictable that future may be. The emerging science of biologic manipulation of tissue growth and reconstitution seems real and potentially achievable over the next 30 years. One might eventually resurface a joint with genetically engineered tissue to replace injured or diseased tissue or use a series of linked cytokines or growth factors to reverse a fracture nonunion or reconstitute a skeletal defect.

# 60 Physiologic Changes in Soft Tissue and Bone as a Function of Age

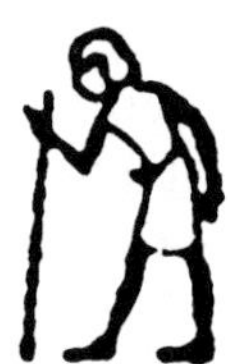

Neal S. Fedarko and Jay R. Shapiro

Changes in the musculoskeletal system give visible and functional evidence that the aging process has left its imprint on our bodies. In contrast to the vigorous youngster, the elderly appear to have lost height, their posture is bent in part due to the development of kyphosis, and a cane provides the support and security that are required because of weakened musculature and peripheral nerve degeneration. These characteristics reflect the fact that significant changes have occurred in all the components of the extracellular matrix: ligaments and tendons, muscle fiber composition, and the structure and quantity of bone mass. As a result, the elderly typically display thinned skin (which is more susceptible to injury), diminished muscle bulk (which results in weakness that magnifies the effects of neurologic degeneration on gait and posture), and diminished bone mass (which increases the risk of fracture).

This chapter discusses atrophic changes in connective tissues and bone that accompany the aging process. We include the effect of aging on type I and III collagens, matrix proteoglycan and glycoproteins, and the noncollagenous proteins of bone. Bone remodeling changes with age in women and men toward increased bone resorption and decreased bone formation, which eventually permits fractures of cancellous and cortical bone following even minimal trauma. Critical to age-related alterations in bone remodeling are the effects of hormones, locally acting growth factors, and cytokines that modulate osteoclastic bone resorption and osteoblastic bone formation. Finally, we discuss physical and pharmacologic methods by which these aging effects can be retarded or reversed.

## Bone Remodeling and Age

### Organization of Skeletal Tissues

Skeletal tissues develop via two distinct processes: intramembranous and endochondral bone formation.[1] Intramembranous bone formation involves the growth of mesenchymal cells in a highly vascularized area of embryonic primordium that differentiate into preosteoblasts and osteoblasts. Embryonic bone containing irregularly oriented collagen fibrils (termed woven bone) is formed, which following remodeling is replaced by mature trabecular (lamellar) bone. Examples of intramembranous bone include the calvarium, scapula, and ilium. Endochondral bone formation involves mesenchymal cells that undergo differentiation into prechondroblasts and mature chondroblasts. These cells secrete a cartilaginous matrix that forms the template in which matrix calcification occurs. Calcification of the matrix in the periosteal layer and at the growth plate (epiphysis) follows hypertrophy and apoptosis of chondrocytes with the appearance of osteoblastic stromal cells derived from intramembranous bone formation that occurs in a perichondral (periosteal) zone of apposition. Vascular ingrowth into this periosteal zone of woven bone facilitates the development of hematogenous marrow and the movement of osteoprogenitor cells from the developing periosteum into the marrow space. Endochondral bone formation at the growth plate follows cartilage deposition, hypertrophy of chondrocytes, vascularization, removal of the cartilaginous matrix by osteoclasts, and subsequent replacement of cartilaginous lamellae by mature bone formed by now-differentiated osteoblasts.[1]

A significant advance has emerged with the recognition of several gene transcription factors that modulate osteoblast differentiation. Recent studies indicate that the transcription factor Osf2 (osteoblast specific transcription factor 2)/Cbfa1 (core binding factor activity 1) regulates osteoblast-specific gene expression.[2,3] The gene is expressed only in cells of the osteoblast lineage. When expressed in nonskeletal cells, the cells assume many of the characteristics of an osteoblast. In knockout experiments designed to assess the importance of the gene in osteogenesis, no evidence of bone formation could be observed in animals homozygous for the deletion.

Studies of the heterozygote indicate that osteoblast function is compromised: There is severe reduction in the number of bone cells, the tissue is deficient in bone proteins, and the activity of the enzyme alkaline phosphatase is low. It was noted that the heterozygote displays abnormalities that are remarkably similar to those exhibited by cleidocranial dysplastic individuals. Cleidocranial dysplasia (CCD) is a dominantly inherited disorder characterized by patent fontanelles, wide cranial sutures, hypoplasia of the clavicles, short stature, supernumerary teeth, and other skeletal anomalies. Mutations in the transcription factor CBFA1, on chromosome 6p21, are associated with CCD.[4]

Members of the hedgehog gene family, initially viewed as patterning factors in embryonic limb and vertebral development, have been shown to regulate skeletal development in vertebrates.[5] Mutations in human and murine sonic hedgehog (SHH) cause midline patterning defects that manifest in the head as holoprosencephaly and cyclopia. Thus the loss of SHH signaling during early stages of neural plate patterning has a profound influence on craniofacial morphogenesis.[6] In contrast, excess SHH leads to a mediolateral widening of the frontonasal plate (FNP) and widening between the eyes (hypertelorism).

## Cortical and Cancellous (Trabecular) Bone: Effect of Aging on Bone Mass

### *Measurement of Bone Mass*

Bone mass is measured by several techniques. At the tissue level, histomorphometric analysis of static and dynamic parameters is conducted on an iliac crest bone biopsy following a tetracycline double labeling.[7] The clinical standard is the areal measurement of bone mineral density expressed as per square centimeter (gs/cm$^2$) by dual energy x-ray absorptiometry (DEXA), or the volumetric measurement (gs/cm$^3$) by quantitative computed tomography (CT). Areal DEXA measurements are widely available and form the database against which gender-, race-, and age-related standards have been developed. The use of CT is preferable where differences in size (i.e., the areal measure) may distort the analysis of bone mineral content, which does not occur with volumetric-based determinations.[8] There has been extensive clinical interest in the measurement of bone density using ultrasonography (US). US has been applied using different methods that examine sound transmission characteristics in the calcaneus or the tibia.[9] Calcaneal US measurements have value when predicting fracture risk in the hip but are less predictive of fracture risk in the lumbar spine.[10]

### *Organization of Cortical Bone*

Cortical bone is found mainly in the appendicular skeleton; it surrounds cancellous bone, as in vertebral bodies and in the calcaneus. Cortical bone is composed of concentric lamellae of densely packed, mineralized collagen fibers. The mass of cortical bone is approximately four times greater than that of cancellous bone. Cortical bone has two surfaces: The endosteal surface faces the marrow cavity; and the outer surface, the periosteum, which is related to neurovascular supply, is integrated with muscle and tendon attachment points. Sharpy's fibers are dense collagenous bands that penetrate through the periosteum into the cortex. The periosteum has a rich "cellular component, which responds to alterations of mechanical strain and injury.[11] The basic structural unit of cortical bone is the haversian system, which is composed of branching neurovascular channels enclosed in cortical bone lamellae and oriented to the long axis of the bone. The "osteon" refers to the bone surrounding that vascular channel defined by cement lines within which are the osteoblasts and osteoclasts of the basic multicellular unit. Osteons are connected to each other by Volkmann's canals.

## Patterns of Bone Remodeling Associated with Increasing Age

The remodeling process in bone is the result of resorption of older packets of mineralized tissue and their replacement with newly synthesized, mineralized bone matrix. It is a continuous process throughout life, one that is influenced by genetic and environmental factors including race, gender, pubertal status, physical activity, drugs, and diet.[12]

Mechanical strain related to the effects of gravity and muscle pull on bone has a dominant impact of bone remodeling. Bone remodeling has been observed to be high when mechanical loading is low and again when it is excessively high. Conversely, low bone remodeling is associated with the administration of antiresorptive drugs such as estrogens or bisphosphonates, used for treatment of osteoporosis.

Because of constant remodeling, progressive growth and change in the shape of the skeleton occurs during childhood and adolescence, achieving their maximum at that chronologic age at which peak bone mass is achieved. During pubertal years bone mineral density increases by four- to sixfold over a 3-year period in girls (11–14 years) and over a 4-year period in boys (13–17 years).[13] Young adult peak bone mass is achieved at approximately 25–35 years of age. Constant remodeling leads to net bone deposition during the early years and net bone loss as a consequence of a relative excess of bone resorption during later life. Research during the past decade has focused on the myriad factors, local and hormonal, that alter rates of remodeling during health and as a consequence of disease. The occurrence of age-dependent bone loss, or osteoporosis, can therefore occur by two mechanisms: (1) failure to achieve adequate peak bone mass as a young adult; and

(2) an increased rate of bone loss during mid- or late adulthood leading to a negative balance and the occurrence of fractures with minimal trauma. It is now appreciated that bone remodeling may remain increased during old age in women and men.

Bone remodeling rates determined by histomorphometry tend to show increased remodeling rates in patients who develop osteoporosis. Increased remodeling is associated with decreased bone mineral density and increased levels of serum and urine biomarkers of bone turnover, reflecting: (1) increased bone formation (e.g., serum alkaline phosphatase, osteocalcin, and procollagen type I-C terminal propeptide, or PICP); and (2) increased bone resorption measured as urinary excretion of collagen-derived cross-links (e.g., *N*-telopeptide fraction or deoxypyridinoline cross-link excretion).[14] Serum and urine biomarkers also have been used clinically to estimate rates of bone turnover and their alteration by aging, drugs, or disease.[15] Increased markers of bone resorption have been associated with faster rates of bone loss and increased fracture risk.[16]

## Cellular Elements Determining Bone Remodeling

Bone mass changes constantly throughout our lifetimes, albeit more slowly than is typical for other organs and in a manner that is nonuniform from site to site. Although this is evident as we watch children develop from infancy through adolescence to adulthood, we tend to underestimate the dynamic state of skeletal tissue in older individuals. Normally, bone formation and bone resorption are tightly coupled: an increase in bone resorption is followed by an increase in bone formation. The common disorders associated with abnormal bone remodeling in the geriatric population are all too familiar: osteoporosis, osteomalacia associated with vitamin D deficiency, and the bone loss associated with malignancy. In each instance, rates of bone formation are depressed *relative* to the rate of bone resorption. Thus net bone loss occurs, weakening the skeleton and increasing the risk of fracture. Paget's disease of bone (osteitis deformans) is characterized by large increases in bone formation and resorption, with the result that bone mass is increased. Formation and resorption remain coupled in Paget's disease, which accounts for the marked cellular hyperactivity characteristic of the disorder.[17] The *quality* of bone is defective, however, because of the irregular manner in which bone deposition occurs.[18]

Bone remodeling represents the coordinated interaction of a series of hormones, growth factors, and locally acting cytokines operating on different cell populations in a highly regulated manner.[19] The cellular elements in bone responsible for bone formation and resorption have been recognized to form a functional unit termed the basic multicellular unit (BMU).[19,20] The BMU is composed of preosteoclastic mononuclear cells that fuse into osteoclasts; the latter then become activated and initiate bone resorption. Preosteoblastic cells differentiate into mature osteoblasts that lay down osteoid matrix in areas of resorption, demonstrating the phenomenon of coupling. Osteoblasts differentiate into flat lining cells that cover the endosteal surface pending activation of the next BMU remodeling front.

The remodeling process, as defined by histomorphometry, involves four major sequential steps: (1) *activation*, which signals the start of BMU remodeling at a specific site and by which lining cells expose underlying matrix and osteoclast precursor cells are recruited; (2) a *resorption* phase, which is dependent on osteoclast activity; (3) a *reversal* stage, during which mononuclear cells are present on the bone surface to complete resorption and signal the initiation of bone formation; and (4) *formation*, which is dependent on the differentiation of osteoblasts, their migration to the bottom of the resorption cavity, and the synthesis of osteoid and its mineralization in the resorption cavities.

The retraction of endosteal lining cells exposing underlying osteoid indicates the site of the resorption event. The resorption phase of bone remodeling involves excavation of a resorption cavity by the osteoclast in a specific region of cortical or trabecular bone. Resorption cavities average 50 μm deep. Adhesion protein receptors and integrin receptors on the osteoclast cell surface also are important for directing the osteoclast to a resorption site, which include integrin receptors for vitronectin ($\alpha_v\beta_3$), collagen ($\alpha_2\beta_3$), and the $\alpha_v\beta_1$ integrin.[21] The factor(s) responsible for signaling recruitment of osteoclasts to the resorption cavity are unknown, although several factors responsible for the differentiation of bone marrow and peripheral blood mononuclear/macrophage osteoclast precursor cells have been identified (see Osteoclasts, below). Osteoblasts recruited to the resorption site synthesize organic matrix (osteoid) to replace the resorbed bone; however, the extent of replacement of the cavity by new bone determines whether net loss of bone has occurred during that remodeling cycle. Aging is one factor that diminishes net osteoblastic replacement of the resorption cavity.

### *Osteoprogenitor Cells*

Also termed bone marrow stromal fibroblast cells, osteoprogenitor cells are pluripotential cells that differentiate into the preosteoblastic and mature osteoblastic cells lining the endosteal surfaces of bone.[22] Under appropriate conditions, these cells also differentiate into adipocytes, fibroblasts, myocytes, and chondroblasts. Normally quiescent until recruitment is initiated, osteoprogenitor cells isolated from marrow and grown in tissue culture are induced to differentiate when dexamethasone is added to the culture medium. Multiple growth factors [platelet-derived growth factor, epidermal growth factor, fibroblastic growth factor, and transforming growth factor-β (TGF-β)] and mechanical strains promote differentiation of these cells in vivo.[23] The cells secrete several matrix proteins and form mineralized nodules in tissue culture.[24–26]

### Osteoblasts

Osteoblasts are bone-forming cells, the differentiated product of the marrow stromal (osteoprogenitor) cell. Osteoblasts direct the deposition of bone matrix and its subsequent calcification in trabecular and cortical bone. Osteoblasts are recognized as plump cells lined up in clusters on unmineralized osteoid at sites of bone formation. Distant from sites of matrix deposition, the osteoblasts flatten into lining cells on the quiescent trabecular surface. An osteocyte is an osteoblast that has been incorporated into skeletal matrix. The osteoblast is responsible for the synthesis of collagen, proteoglycans, and other matrix proteins essential for the structural integrity of bone (see below). These differentiated functions are under the control of a series of regulatory factors, including hormones, growth factors, cytokines, gene transcription factors, and tissue-specific factors.[27] In addition, osteoblasts produce locally active factors that indirectly influence osteoclast activity, as exemplified by the requirement for osteoblasts to induce the osteoclast response to parathyroid hormone (PTH).[28]

### Osteoclasts

The osteoclast is the major bone-resorbing cell. They differentiate from early hematopoietic precursors [granulocyte/macrophage colony-forming units (GM-CFU)] that differentiate into mononuclear precursor cells (preosteoclasts), which form mature osteoclasts under the influence of several differentiating factors including interleukin-1 (IL-1), tumor necrosis factor (TNF), PTH, and 1,25-dihydroxy [1,25(OH)$_2$] vitamin D. The mature osteoclast is a multinucleated cell with a characteristic ruffled border that overlies the endosteal surface, forming a bone-resorbing compartment. The attachment is dependent on specific cell-surface integrin receptors that bind to specific matrix protein sequences. The osteoclast synthesizes lysosomal enzymes, including tartrate-resistant acid phosphatase (TRAP) and collagenases that are secreted via the ruffled border into this extracellular space. Osteoclasts synthesize carbonic anhydrase and $H^+$ exchangers ($Na^+K^+$-ATPase, $HCO_3^-/Cl^-$, and $Na^+/H^+$ exchangers), which facilitate secretion of acid across the ruffled border into the sealed zone.

A series of newly described factors have been found to promote osteoclast differentiation. RANK, a receptor activator of NFκB, is a type I transmembrane receptor of the TNF receptor superfamily. Rank ligand (RANKL) acts to promote activation of osteoclast precursor cells.[29] RANKL or TRANCE, originally described as dendritic cell survival factor, is identical to the osteoclast differentiation factor (ODF), which is expressed by stromal cells and osteoblasts. Its receptor, RANKL, acts via RANK expressed on osteoclast hemopoietic precursors to promote their differentiation to bone-resorbing osteoclasts. RANKL acts on mature osteoclasts to promote survival and bone-resorbing activity.[30]

Studies suggest that peripheral blood mononuclear cells may also contribute to bone resorption, but the extent of this remains undetermined. Schilling et al.[30] cultured mononuclear cells isolated from marrow and peripheral blood in the presence of macrophage colony-stimulating factor (M-CSF) and osteoclast differentiation factor (TRANCE/RANKL/OPGL).[31] No difference was seen in the expression of osteoclast vitronectin receptor and TRAP on these cells, nor was the resorptive activity different between these cell populations. The results suggested that osteoclastic-inducing factors are capable of inducing osteoclastic action in cells from the periphery, which supports the hypothesis that these cell populations are important in modulating bone resorption.

### Osteocytes

The osteocyte is the final differentiation stage for the osteoblast. During the process of bone formation, osteoblasts on the endosteal surface are incorporated into bone matrix where they form osteocytes. Mature osteocytes are stellate-shaped cells enclosed in the lacunar-canalicular system of mineralized bone matrix. The dendritic processes of individual osteocytes are in contact with other cells though the canalicular system, providing a syncytial meshwork of cells that communicate with each other through gap junctions. Osteocytes have low metabolic activity, but they probably serve several functions including regulation of calcium diffusion from bone and as mechanosensor cells sensitive to mechanical loading. Osteocytes are extremely sensitive to mechanical stress, a quality that is probably linked to the process of mechanical adaptation (Wolff's law). The in vivo operating cell stress derived from bone loading is likely flow of an interstitial fluid along the surface of the osteocytes and lining cells.

### Lining Cells

Lining cells are present as a layer of flattened cells on the trabecular surfaces, where they may function in the process of remodeling by influencing the organization or orientation of the basic multicellular unit. Derived from the osteoblast lineage, the lining cell may contribute metabolically during calcium transport or by synthesis of specific proteins, but their role is undefined at present. Lining cells may also function in transducing mechanical strain signals to other bone cells.[32]

## Hormonal Regulation of Matrix Synthesis and Bone Remodeling

### *Growth Hormone/Insulin-Like Growth Factors 1 and 2*

Growth hormone and insulin-like growth factors 1 and 2 (IGF-1, IGF-2) have been intensively studied during the past decade because of their anabolic action on bone.[33] Growth hormone induces the synthesis and secretion of IGF-1 from the liver. It is hepatic IGF-1 that forms the bulk of plasma IGF-1. IGF-2 is largely produced during fetal bone development. Human osteoblasts secrete primarily IGF-2 but also lesser amounts of IGF-1, which acts locally in a paracrine or autocrine manner to regulate cell growth and the synthesis of matrix proteins. IGF-1 also supports osteoclast differentiation.[34] Bone serves as a major reservoir for IGF-1, which is liberated to act locally as bone resorption occurs.[35]

Local IGF-1 secretion in bone is stimulated by growth hormone and other hormones (PTH, estrogen, prostaglandin $E_2$) that also regulate its production by osteoblasts. IGF receptors on bone cells also serve to regulate the cell response to IGF-1. IGF-1 increases osteoblast DNA synthesis and the replication of osteoblast progenitors. Glucocorticoids, human fibroblast growth factor, and platelet-derived growth factor (PDGF) decrease osteoblast IGF-1 secretion. The metabolic activity of IGF-1 is regulated by binding proteins (IGFBPs), which are synthesized by osteoblastic bone cells, six of which have been reported to date. IGFBPs exert both stimulatory and inhibitory effects on IGF function. IGFBP3 is the main circulating protein that limits IGF activity and inhibits bone cell growth because it binds the IGF-1 peptide. However, when endogenous IGFBP3 accumulates it has been associated with enhanced IGF function.[36] IGBP5 is preferentially stored in extracellular matrix, where it acts to inhibit IGF-1-stimulated bone cell activity.[37] However, recombinant IGFBP-5 protein administered to mice increases osteocalcin and alkaline phosphatase levels, suggesting increased osteoblastic activity.[38]

Adults who specifically are growth hormone (GH)-deficient have decreased bone mass. However, pituitary growth hormone secretion normally declines with increasing age to the point that elderly individuals may be considered functionally GH-deficient. IGF-1 levels decline in parallel with the decrease in GH secretion. However, administration of GH to deficient individuals increases bone mass only after a delay of up to 21 months, and GH or IGF-1 administration to normal elderly is associated with increased bone turnover without a significant increase in bone mass before the onset of significant side effects such as edema and peripheral nerve compression.[39,40]

### *Adrenal Glucocorticoids*

Decreased bone mass is a major complication of the chronic administration of adrenal glucocorticoids for pulmonary, dermatologic, and immune disorders.[24,41] Glucocorticoids impose a negative effect at each step in the synthesis and mineralization of bone matrix. Glucocorticoids suppress transcription of type I collagen mRNA. Adrenal glucocorticoids decrease the differentiation of bone marrow osteoprogenitor cells. Gonadotropin secretion from the pituitary decreases, serum testosterone is decreased in the presence of cortisol use, and ovarian steroid secretion falls. Serum osteocalcin levels are depressed. Transport of calcium across the intestinal epithelium is decreased, while at the same time urinary calcium excretion increases. Glucocorticoid administration can be viewed as inducing secondary hyperparathyroidism. Although serum PTH levels are not increased, the sensitivity of osteoclast cells to the action of PTH is increased.

### *Parathyroid Hormone*

Parathyroid hormone acts at three sites: the kidney, the gastrointestinal (GI) tract, and bone. PTH acts directly on the skeleton to release calcium, on the kidney to increase calcium reabsorption, and indirectly via $1,25(OH)_2$ vitamin D on the GI tract to increase calcium absorption. PTH increases renal phosphorus excretion and stimulates osteoclast-directed bone resorption. However, the osteoclast does not have receptors for PTH, although they are present on osteoblasts. PTH decreases type I collagen synthesis, reduces alkaline phosphatase activity, and increases collagenase synthesis by the osteoblast.[42] The factor(s) responsible for activation of the osteoclast by PTH via osteoblasts is not known.[28] PTH has complex effects on bone, as seen in the osteoblastic response of bone when human PTH (hPTH) is administered intermittently in low dose as treatment for osteoporosis.[43]

Levels of PTH increase with increasing age as a consequence of the progressive decline in GI calcium absorption, mediated in turn by a decline in the $1,25(OH)_2$ vitamin D level that occurs with increasing age. Low-dose intermittent administration of human 1–34 PTH stimulates bone formation,[43] an effect that may in part be mediated by IGF-1. However, as seen in patients with hyperparathyroidism, sustained high plasma levels of PTH lead to bone resorption.

### *PTH-Related Protein*

Parathyroid hormone-related protein (PTHrP) was first identified as a cause of hypercalcemia in patients with a variety of malignant solid tumors (squamous, renal and breast tumors, islet cell tumors, pheochromocytoma, and adult T cell leukemia syndrome).[44] PTH levels were found to be suppressed in these individuals, suggesting the presence of a hypercalcemic factor mimicking the effects of PTH.[45] In fact, PTH and PTHrP bind to a common receptor. The circulating levels of PTHrP are considerably lower than those of PTH. Tissue distribution of PTHrP is wide, with expression found in the central nervous system (CNS), placenta, uterus, breast, and vascular smooth muscle. PTHrP probably does not play a role in skeletal homeostasis in the adult, but it does play a role in fetal tissues where it may regulate placental calcium transport. PTHrP secretion in breast milk is regulated by prolactin. PTHrP acts to relax smooth muscle. PTHrP is widely distributed in fetal tissues, where it may play a role in the development of normal skeletal tissue. Wide tissue distribution suggests that PTHrP is a cellular cytokine involved in cell growth and differentiation.[46]

The PTHrP knockout mice have multiple defects in cartilage and endochondral bone development. Long bones are shorter, thicker, and irregular in shape; and there is advanced mineralization.[47] Chondrocytes in growth columns are disorganized, and the proliferating columns are shorter than normal. Overexpression of PTHrP in mouse chondrocytes induces a form of chondrodysplasia that displays short-limbed dwarfism and a delay in endochondral ossification.[48]

### Calcitonin

Calcitonin (CTn), primarily secreted by C-cells of the thyroid, acts to decrease osteoclastic bone resorption. Calcitonin has also been identified in several other tissues including lung, thymus, liver, small intestine, and bladder.[49] The CTn gene family consists of four genes: *CALC I* produces mature calcitonin. *CALC I* and *CALC II* genes produce calcitonin gene-related peptide (CGRP). *CALC III* gene procures neither CTn nor CGRP. The *CALC IV* gene produces the peptide amylin in pancreatic beta cells, which in common with GCRP, has significant effects on carbohydrate metabolism in addition to acting on skeletal tissues via increasing cyclic adenosine monophosphate (cAMP) synthesis. Amylin and CGRP inhibit glycogen synthesis and stimulated glycogenolysis. CGRP decreases bone resorption by acting on osteoclasts. Amylin's effects on bone resorption parallel those of CGRP, but it is less potent than mature CTn.

Administration of CTn acutely lowers serum calcium and serum phosphorus in a parallel manner. CTn has immediate effects on bone osteoclasts, decreasing their mobility and smoothing the ruffled border, producing a small, rounded, nonmotile cell. CTn has actions in other organs: It increases renal sodium and chloride excretion, decreases the frequency and amplitude of GH pulses from the pituitary, affects calcium transport by pulmonary cells, and increases gastric acid and pepsin secretion by the GI tract. CTn decreases pancreatic amylase and pancreatic polypeptide secretion. The levels of mature CTn in postmenopausal or elderly women has been reported as either decreased compared to premenopausal women or within normal values.[50,51] High levels in postmenopausal women have also been reported.[52]

### Vitamin D

The major vitamin D metabolites in serum are 25-hydroxy vitamin D (25OHD), 24,25$(OH)_2$D, and calcitriol [1,25$(OH)_2$D]. Circulating vitamin D metabolites are almost completely bound by vitamin D binding protein (DBP) and albumin. Receptors for vitamin D are found in multiple tissues including the parathyroids, epidermis, bone, kidney, pancreas, breast, and placenta. The antirachitic activity of 1,25$(OH)_2$D is probably based on increased intestinal absorption of calcium and phosphorus. 1,25$(OH)_2$D increases differentiation of osteoclast precursors via a mechanism involving osteoblast release of differentiating factors.[28] Vitamin D regulates expression of several matrix-associated genes, including those for osteocalcin, osteopontin, and calbindin.[53] In addition to its action in skeletal tissues, vitamin D has been under investigation for its role in modulating cellular immune function.[54] Effects include inhibition of T cell proliferation and regulation of IL-1, IL-2, IL-3, and IL-6, regulation of interferon-$\gamma$ (INF-$\gamma$), tumor necrosis factor (TNF), and GM-CSF. The use of 1,25$(OH)_2$D for skin diseases such as psoriasis is related to its effect on increasing differentiation and decreasing proliferation of keratinocytes.[55] 1,25$(OH)_2$D has found application in the treatment of various malignancies, including prostate and colon cancers.[56]

Aging decreases the amount of 7-dehydrocholesterol in the epidermis. Although uncommon in younger subjects, deficiency of vitamin D is not rare among the elderly, particularly those in nursing homes and those who are house-bound with little sunlight exposure. In addition to the decreased serum levels, the responsivity of individual tissues may change with increasing age.

### Gonadal Hormones

Gonadal hormones exert a major influence on bone remodeling throughout the life-span. Achievement of peak bone mass is dependent on normal levels of gonadal hormone during puberty and early adulthood. It is during later years that alterations in these hormones exert a negative effect on bone mass, as evidenced by the development of osteoporosis due to estrogen deficiency in postmenopausal women and in men whose testosterone levels decline with increasing age.

Estrogen receptors (ER) $\alpha$ and $\beta$ have been found in multiple tissues where variation in receptor levels may influence hormone responsiveness.[57] Osteoblasts have been found to express both of the currently recognized estrogen receptors: ER-α and ER-β.[58] Variability in estrogen response may in part be the results of variable expression of these receptors. Estrogen acts directly on osteoblasts to increase cell proliferation, the synthesis of bone matrix proteins, transcription factors, growth factors such as IGF-1 and IGF-binding proteins, and TGF-β. Estrogen inhibits osteoclastic bone resorption[59] and formation of the bone resorbing cytokines IL-1, IL-6, and TNF.[60] Evidence for osteoclast receptor expression is equivocal, with one study indicating that ER-α is present[61] and another failing to identify any ER expression or responsiveness.[62]

The important role estrogen plays in the development of bone mass in men was illustrated by two clinical reports. In each case estrogen action was compromised, in one case by a mutation involving ER-α and in the second by a deficiency in the aromatase essential for normal estrogen synthesis.[63] Each case was associated with osteoporosis, which was correctable in the case of aromatase deficiency by administration of estrogen to the affected man.[64] Hypogonadal men with low serum-free testosterone levels also develop osteoporosis.[65]

## Growth Factors: Matrix Synthesis and Bone Remodeling

### *TGF-β Superfamily*

A multigene family, the TGF-β superfamily, includes the TGF-β isoforms, activins, inhibins, müllerian inhibitory substance, growth differentiation factors, and several bone morphogenic proteins (BMPs).[66]

### *TGF-β*

Four proteins comprise the TGF-β isoforms: TGF-β1–3 and 5. TGF-β is a multifunctional cytokine whose major functions include regulation of cell growth, stimulation of extracellular matrix production, and inhibition of the immune system. TGF-β produces new bone when injected in proximity to bone; but unlike BMPs, it does not produce bone when injected into an ectopic site. In tissue culture, TGF-β stimulates the recruitment and differentiation of osteogenic cells and the synthesis of several matrix proteins, including collagen, osteonectin, and osteopontin. It inhibits synthesis of osteocalcin and the in vitro mineralization of chondrocytes and calvarial cells. TGF-β inhibits osteoclastic bone resorption by inhibiting osteoclast formation.[67]

### *Bone Morphogenic Proteins*

Bone morphogenic proteins are part of a large family: the TGF-β superfamily. Although members of this group share certain sequence similarities, they have diverse functions. BMPs 2, 4–7, and 9 have been shown to have bone-inducing properties.[68] BMPs appear to initiate the sequence of events leading to endochondral bone formation, starting with differentiation of osteoprogenitor cells followed by the laying down of a cartilaginous matrix that is then resorbed and replaced by mature bone. BMPs are important in the processes of embryonic cell differentiation and limb bud development. BMP receptors are of the serine/threonine receptor kinase group.

The BMP-1 has been found to be identical with the N-terminal collagen propeptidase.[69] BMP-2 and BMP-4 have been localized to healing fracture sites by immunohistochemical methods.[70] Healing of skeletal defects has been promoted by inclusion of BMP-2 and BMP-7 in the cell mix used to fill these defects.[71]

### *Cytokines*

The discovery of several locally acting peptides that modulate bone resorption and formation has been of signal importance in furthering our understanding of bone physiology. Current studies involve the measurement of cytokines in serum and supernatants from monocytes.[71–73] The members of the interleukin family (IL-1, IL6, IL-11), TNFs, M-CSF, and prostaglandins $E_2$ and $F_2$ play important roles in modulating osteoblast and osteoclast activity. IL-1ra (IL-1 receptor antagonist) decreases the activity of IL-1, which is one of the most powerful bone-resorbing agents known.

## Effects of Aging on the Composition of Connective Tissue

### Collagenous and Noncollagenous Protein Components of Musculoskeletal Tissues

Currently, 19 distinct collagen types are recognized, representing 30 genes dispersed among 12 chromosomes. This bewildering array of proteins, which is further diversified through mechanisms of alternative splicing of segments of the transcribed gene or through the use of alternative promoters that transcribe a separate ribonucleic acid (RNA), makes it difficult to relate each gene to its corresponding clinical disease.

Collagens, the main structural proteins of skin, tendon, and bone, are a family of proteins that have in common one or more regions containing a characteristic triple helix configuration (Fig. 60.1). This configuration in the collagen peptide chains is based on the repeating triplet (Gly-X-Y), where X and Y are proline and hydroxyproline. The collagen genes have been grouped into several classes: fibrillar collagens (types I, II, III, V, and XI), interstitial collagens, collagens forming sheets (types IV and VIII), and the fibril-associated collagens (FACIT) (types IX, XII, XIV, XVI, and XIX). The reader may find it helpful to group the individual collagens into families of extra-

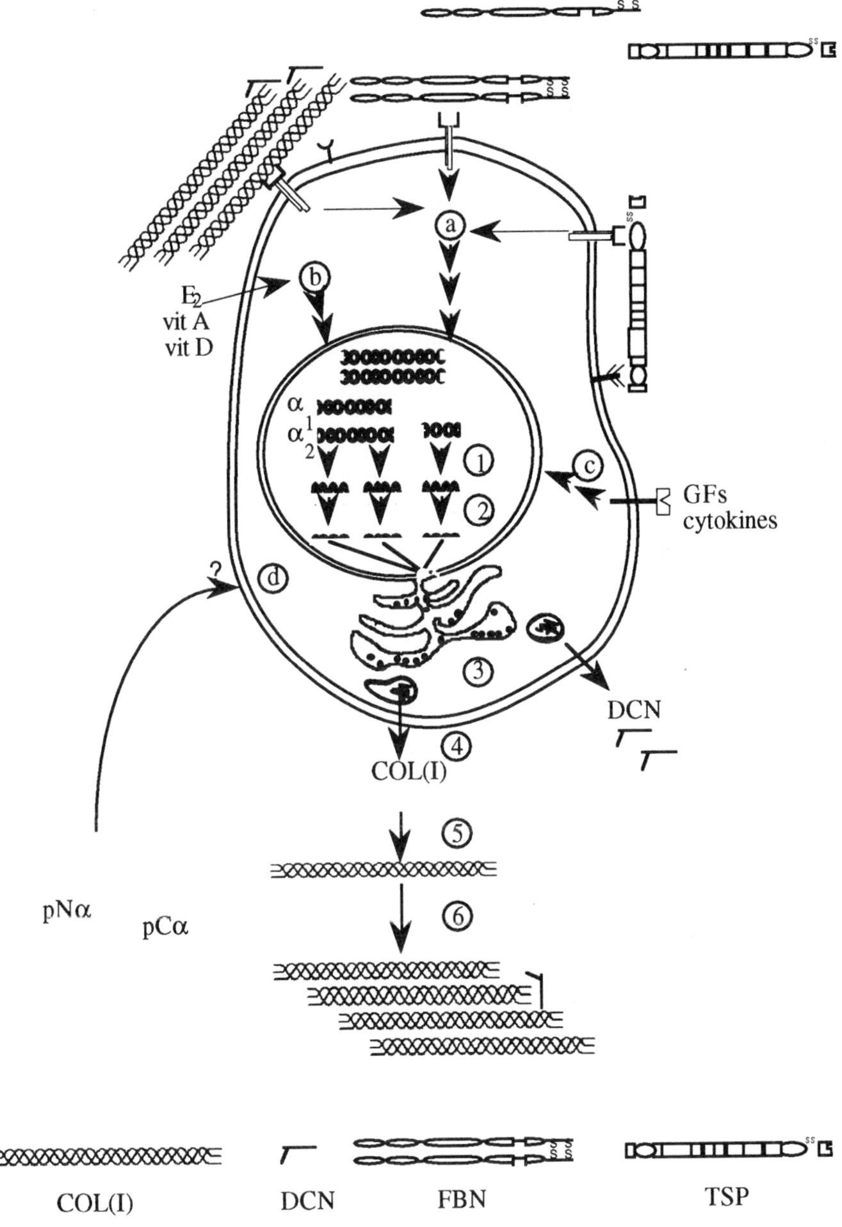


FIGURE 60.1. Extracellular matrix and collagen metabolism. Following transcription (1) and processing (2) of type I collagen mRNA, export of mRNA into the endoplasmic reticulum and golgi apparatus (3) occurs, and nascent procollagen chains are made. Secretion of pro-α chains (4) is followed by cleavage of the propeptide domains (5) and assembly of a mature fibril array (6). Cellular–matrix feedback systems that are operative include collagen (COL), fibronectin (FBN), and thrombospondin (TSP) interactions with integrins (a); hormone, vitamin and cytokine sequestration and presentation by extracellular matrix components (b, c); and procollagen peptide binding, modulation of collagen, and perhaps other noncollagenous protein metabolism (d). DCN, decorin.

cellular matrix proteins that provide a specific connective tissue function: tensile strength, resistance to compressive forces, and barrier-filtration (Table 60.1). To meet these structural requirements, the properties of the major collagen protein within the family are modified by the presence of minor collagens and noncollagenous proteins. This concept, that the primary protein is modified by specialized or minor collagens, portrays the connective tissue as an alloy of a number of components that are added or varied to meet the specialized demands of specific connective tissues (Table 60.2).

Type I collagen, the major structural protein of bone, is composed of two pro-α1(I) and one pro-α2(I) polypeptide chains coiled in a helical configuration. The polypeptide chains assemble intracellularly. They are posttransactionally modified during intracellular processing, including glycoslyation reactions and hydroxylation of proline residues and the formation of lysyl aldehyde-based cross-links. The C- and N-terminal ends contain propeptide extensions that are cleaved following extrusion of the pro-α chains into the extracellular matrix. Self-assembly of triple helical molecules into fibrils and then collagen fibers occurs in the extracellular space. In its role as the major structural component, the collagenous network is stabilized by covalent cross-links within and between the α chains by the formation of somewhat bone-specific deoxypyridinoline cross-links. The importance of type I collagen structure in bone matrix metabolism is reflected in observations of the pathophysiologic consequences of mutations in the genes that code for it that are the cause of the brittle bone disorder, osteogenesis imperfecta.

TABLE 60.1. Collagen Types Grouped into Families of Proteins with Common Structural Properties

| Functional component | Type I family (compressive CT) | Type II family (compressive CT) | Type IV family (barrier CT) |
|---|---|---|---|
| Primary collagen | I (2) | II (1, as) | IV (5) |
| Integral with primary protein | V (3) | XI (3) | |
| Surrounding the primary protein | XII (1) | IX (2, ap) | |
| Anchoring | VI (3, as) | VI (as) | VII (1) |
| Specialized tissue distribution | III (1) in viscera and blood vessels Elastin (as)-microfibrilin | X (1) in hypertrophic chondrocytes | VIII (1) in blood vessels, neural tissue |
| Uncertain | XIII (as) | | Short chain |

The numbers in the parentheses are the numbers of genetically distinct chains in the collagen molecule.
as, messenger RNA is alternatively spliced; ap, alternative promoter; CT, connective tissue.

Type III collagen, which consists of a homotrimer with a triple helical domain of a size (about 1000 amino acids) similar to that of type I collagen, has also been found in bone, though its role in bone matrix metabolism is unclear. It is likely associated with type I collagen in the matrix produced by preosteogenic cells that have not yet dedicated themselves to the synthesis and deposition of copious amounts of osteoid. In tissues other than bone, data support the hypothesis that the heterotypic interaction of different collagens, specifically types I and III, plays a role in regulating fibril size.[74]

With increasing age, changes in collagen manifest as stiffening joints and decreased compliance of the vascular system (including renal and retinal capillaries). These changes are due primarily to alterations in the normal intermolecular cross-linking of collagen molecules.[75] Cross-linking of collagen molecules involves two independent mechanisms: The enzymatic mechanism involves oxidation of lysyl and hydroxylysyl residues to aldehydes with the formation of divalent cross-links. A second mechanism, termed glycation, is nonenzymatic and involves reaction with glucose and oxidation of the complex to form Amadori condensation products including furosine. These cross-links alter the surface charge on collagen fibrils and lead to increased stiffness.[76]

## Extracellular Matrix

### *Proteoglycans and Glycosaminoglycans*

Proteoglycans are a family of molecules that possess a core protein to which one or more glycosaminoglycan chains are covalently attached. Decorin and biglycan are

TABLE 60.2. Principal Proteins of Bone

| Protein | Gene | Size (kDa) | Function |
|---|---|---|---|
| ***Collagen*** | | | |
| Type I | 17q21.3–22, 7q21.3–22 | 300 | Major structural protein in all connective tissues; binds to noncollagenous proteins; may orient nucleators of matrix mineralization |
| Type III | 2q31 | 300 | Regulates fibril size |
| ***Proteoglycans/glycosaminoglycans*** | | | |
| Biglycan | Xq27 | 270 | May bind to collagen and TGF-β; involved in morphogenesis |
| Decorin | 12q21–23 | 130 | Binds to collagen and TGF-β; inhibits cell attachment to fibronectin |
| Hyaluronan | — | $>10^6$ | Captures space |
| Versican | 5q12–14 | $10^6$ | Captures space that becomes bone |
| ***Glycoproteins*** | | | |
| Bone sialoprotein | 4q13–21 | 46–85 | Binds to cells, may initiate mineralization |
| Fibronectin | 2p14–16 1q34–36 | 400 | Binds to cells, fibrin, heparin, gelatin, collagen |
| Osteonectin | 5q31–33 | 35–45 | May mediate hydroxyapatite deposition; binds to growth factors; influences cell cycle |
| Osteopontin | 4q13–21 | 44–75 | Binds to cells; may regulate mineralization and proliferation; inhibits nitrous oxide synthase; regulates resistance to viral infections |
| Thrombospondins | 15q15 6q27 1q21–24 | 450 | Cell attachment properties; binds to heparin, platelets, types I and V collagens, thrombin, fibrinogen, laminin, plasminogen and its inhibitor, histidine-rich glycoprotein |
| ***Gla proteins*** | | | |
| Matrix Gla protein | 12p | 15 | May function in cartilage metabolism |
| Osteocalcin | 1.2 kb | 5 | One disulfide bond; may regulate activity of osteoclasts and their precursors; may mark the turning point between bone formation and resorption |

TGF-α, transforming growth factor-α.

interstitial proteoglycans found in many connective tissues, including bone.[77,78] Decorin binds to ("decorates") the collagen fibrils,[79] and biglycan is found in pericellular areas, including that of osteoblasts and osteocytes.[80] The small proteoglycans may be acting as matrix organizers, orienting and ordering the collagen fibrils, with the protein portion binding to collagen fibrils at specific sites and the glycosaminoglycans chains aggregating to hold the proteins and hence the collagen fibrils at defined distances from each other.[81] Targeted disruption of the decorin gene in mice yields an abnormal collagen morphology with coarser and irregular fiber outlines in skin and tendon, suggesting that control of collagen fibril growth and diameter involves decorin.[82] In contrast to decorin, targeted disruption of the biglycan gene yields a mouse phenotype that has a reduced growth rate and failure to achieve peak bone mass, with the low bone mass becoming more pronounced with increasing age.[83] This phenotype suggests that biglycan may be a genetic determinant that contributes to peak bone mass.

Hyaluronan (or hyaluronic acid) is comprised of a repeating disaccharide that forms a large glycosaminoglycan chain (>1000 kDa) that lacks a covalently attached core protein. Found in bone,[84] hyaluronan is synthesized by bone cells in culture and has been proposed to "capture space" for subsequent matrix deposition.[77,85,86] Within this context, hyaluronan is a component of "immature" bone matrix; and its increased levels in bone matrix is consistent with the early, "immature" bone matrix being less structurally rigid compared to mature, highly collagenous matrices.

Although the exact function of bone versican is not known, it has been proposed to act as a space filler in fetal and young bone, to be replaced by osteoid during later growth.[85] The paradigm for proteoglycan–hyaluronan interaction is cartilage, where the hydrated array of hyaluronan with the proteoglycan aggrecan bound via the link protein provide structural integrity and tissue resilience.

### Glycoproteins

Bone sialoprotein (along with osteocalcin) is considered a defining noncollagenous protein marker of the mature osteoblast phenotype. Bone sialoprotein is expressed at late stages of osteoblastic differentiation and is found to mark cells in the secretory but not the proliferative compartment. It has been localized to the earliest sites of mineral deposition.[87–90]

Osteopontin has an acidic amino terminal with a polyaspartic acid sequence. Immune localization of osteopontin revealed the highest density of gold particles associated with electron-dense organic material found at the mineralization front and in "cement lines."[91] Osteopontin is a potent inhibitor of hydroxyapatite formation[92]; and reduced mRNA and protein expression levels in $Src^{-/-}$ mice is associated with the inability of osteoclasts to adhere to bone.[93]

Because of their inherent polyanionic nature the sialoproteins can bind calcium and hydroxyapatite, coating the mineral phase of bone; then, via their arginine-glycine-aspartate (RGD) moieties, they enable cellular adherence to specific sites. Mice lacking a functional osteopontin gene exhibit a phenotype of altered wound healing.[94] The disorganized matrix and altered collagen fibrillogenesis (small-diameter collagen fibrils) suggest that osteopontin affects the synthesis or turnover of matrix components involved in regulating fibril formation. Targeted disruption of the bone sialoprotein gene has yet to reveal an apparent phenotype.

Osteonectin (also termed SPARC, culture shock protein, or BM40) is a 32-kDa $Ca^{2+}$-binding glycoprotein found in many connective tissues, though relatively high concentrations are present in bone.[95] Osteonectin inhibits hydroxyapatite crystal growth,[96] and binds to collagens type I, II, and IV, as well as to thrombospondin.[97–99] Targeted disruption of osteonectin/SPARC in mice yields normal development, a phenotype of severe cataract formation and low bone mass with increasing age.[100]

Fibronectin and thrombospondins exemplify proteins found in bone that are composed of various combinations and content of modular structures. In addition, they contain the arginine-glycine-aspartate (RGD) cell attachment consensus sequence and are believed to play a role in cell-matrix adhesion via binding to integrin receptors on the cell surface.[101] Thrombospondins have distinct domains that modulate matrix protein interactions, cell attachment, migration, and proliferation. Fibronectin is a multifunctional dimeric protein [relative moleculular mass ($M_r$) 450 kDa] that has the capacity to modulate cell migration, cell attachment, and matrix organization. It contains binding domains for fibrin/heparin, gelatin/collagen, and cell surfaces.

Matrix gla protein (MGP) has an expression pattern that begins early during development in many tissues, including lung, kidney, heart, and bone[102]; but the highest levels are found in smooth muscle and cartilage.[103] Transgenic mouse devoid of MGP expression exhibited arterial calcification and early calcification of the growth, pointing to MGP as a major inhibitor of calcification in soft tissues.

Osteocalcin comprises 10–20% of the noncollagenous proteins in bone, depending on the developmental age and the species. Osteocalcin levels are low at early stages of bone formation and increase with increasing age. The function of osteocalcin may be to inhibit mineralization (because osteocalcin inhibits hydroxyapatite crystal growth in solution) until the appropriate temporal and spatial conditions are met.[104] It has also been suggested that osteocalcin may function in bone resorption rather than formation.[105] Targeted disruption of the osteocalcin gene in mice yielded a phenotype of increased bone mass and strength, suggesting that this small protein normally inhibits bone growth and promotes bone resorption.[106]

## Aging Effects on Dermal Matrix

The clinically relevant morphologic changes of the skin during aging include diminished thickness of the epidermis with a reduced mitosis rate of epidermal basal cells, shortened and attenuated rete ridges, reduction of epidermal appendages, and decreased number of fibroblasts and capillaries in the dermis. Skin thickness declines with aging and parallels the thinning of the bony skeleton. Both skin and bone are composed of more than 70% type I collagen. It may be hypothesized that the pathophysiologic processes involved in chronologic atrophy of both tissues may overlap.[107] The content of type I and III collagen in skin from subjects of different ages was studied by means of a new high-performance liquid chromatography (HPLC) method and by sodium dodecyl sulfate (SDS)-polyacrylamide gel electrophoresis and scanning electron microscopy (SEM). Whereas the ratio of type I and III collagen in covered normal human skin remained constant throughout childhood and young adult life, in the elderly the proportion of type III collagen in the dermis increased.[108] SEM examination showed a decrease in the number of collagen fiber bundles and greater average bundle width variation with age. The data have been interpreted to indicate impaired synthesis of type I collagen in aged skin, though a separate study concluded that age had no effect on collagen synthesis.[109] In women, skin collagen content decreases significantly with age after the fourth decade and after menopause, and changes in bone mass are closely related to those detected in collagen.[110,111] A study of donor age and the modification of skin collagen showed that the glycoxidation products, *N*ε-(carboxymethyl)lysine (CML) and pentosidine increased, correlating strongly with age.[112] Increased glycated extracellular matrix has been associated with an impaired ability of fibroblasts to remodel and coincides with decreased matrix metalloproteinase production.[113] Other skin extracellular matrix components also change in abundance with aging. In skin, versican associates with elastic fibers and decorin with collagen fibers; increased versican but decreased decorin expression is associated with aging.[114] Decreases in fibrillin-1 in the microfibrillar network of the upper dermis has been correlated with age-related skin loss of elasticity.[115]

## Aging Effects on Cartilage

The loss of structural integrity of the cartilaginous matrix has been well described for decades. The large proteoglycan aggrecan, which forms a compressive hydration gel by binding to hyaluronan via link protein, changes in structure with increasing age. With advanced age, the ability of aggrecan to form multimeric complexes on hyaluronan decreases, as does the content of chondroitin sulfate chains (Fig. 60.2). Link protein becomes fragmented, and hyaluronan chains are smaller.[116] A biomechanical failure of the collagen network is postulated in many hypotheses of the development of osteoarthritis with advancing age. The advanced glycation end-product pentosidine exhibited levels that were low up to age 20 years but increased linearly after this age. Consistently higher pentosidine levels were associated with a stiffer collagen network. A stiffer, more cross-linked collagen network may become more brittle and more prone to fatigue.[117] The age-related increase in collagen glycation also correlates negatively with the rate of cartilage proteoglycan synthesis.[118] Thus the major components of the cartilage matrix alter dramatically with aging.

## Intervertebral Disc: Effects of Aging

In aging spines the collagen content of the annuli increases both outward in the disc and downward along the spinal levels. Proteoglycan content was higher in the nucleus, and the keratan/chondroitin sulfate ratio increases with age, as does the hyaluronate content. It is concluded that differences in mechanical function may be reflected by differences in chemical composition of the discs, and that mechanical failure could result from local variations in chemical composition.[119] With age or scoliosis, some cells from the inner annulus or nucleus of the disc differentiate to the hypertrophic chondrocyte phenotype. This might be the initiating event for the abnormal calcification described in aged and scoliotic discs in other studies.[120] The presence of CML, a biomarker for oxidative stress modification of extracellular matrix proteins, mainly collagen, increases significantly with age.[121] Forty-two postmortem lumbar intervertebral discs were harvested from nine individuals whose ages were 24, 44, 47, 52, 67, 72, 75, 82, and 89 years. The findings indicated a decrease in pyridinoline and an increase in pentosidine cross-link levels with disc aging.[122] The levels and structural integrity of two noncollagenous components of the discs' extracellular matrix, fibromodulin and lumican, decreased with increasing age.[123] Fibromodulin and lumican are thought to interact with collagen fibrils and contribute to the mechanical properties of intervertebral discs.

## Changes in Skeletal Matrix Proteins with Age

In general, bone matrix composition changes with aging such that the levels of collagen cross-links increase with increasing age, and the ability to extract intact collagen decreases. Aside from type I collagen, noncollagenous components such as the cell attachment proteins fibronectin, thrombospondin, and osteopontin are also degraded to lower-molecular-weight fragments with advancing age (Fig. 60.3). It is not known whether the

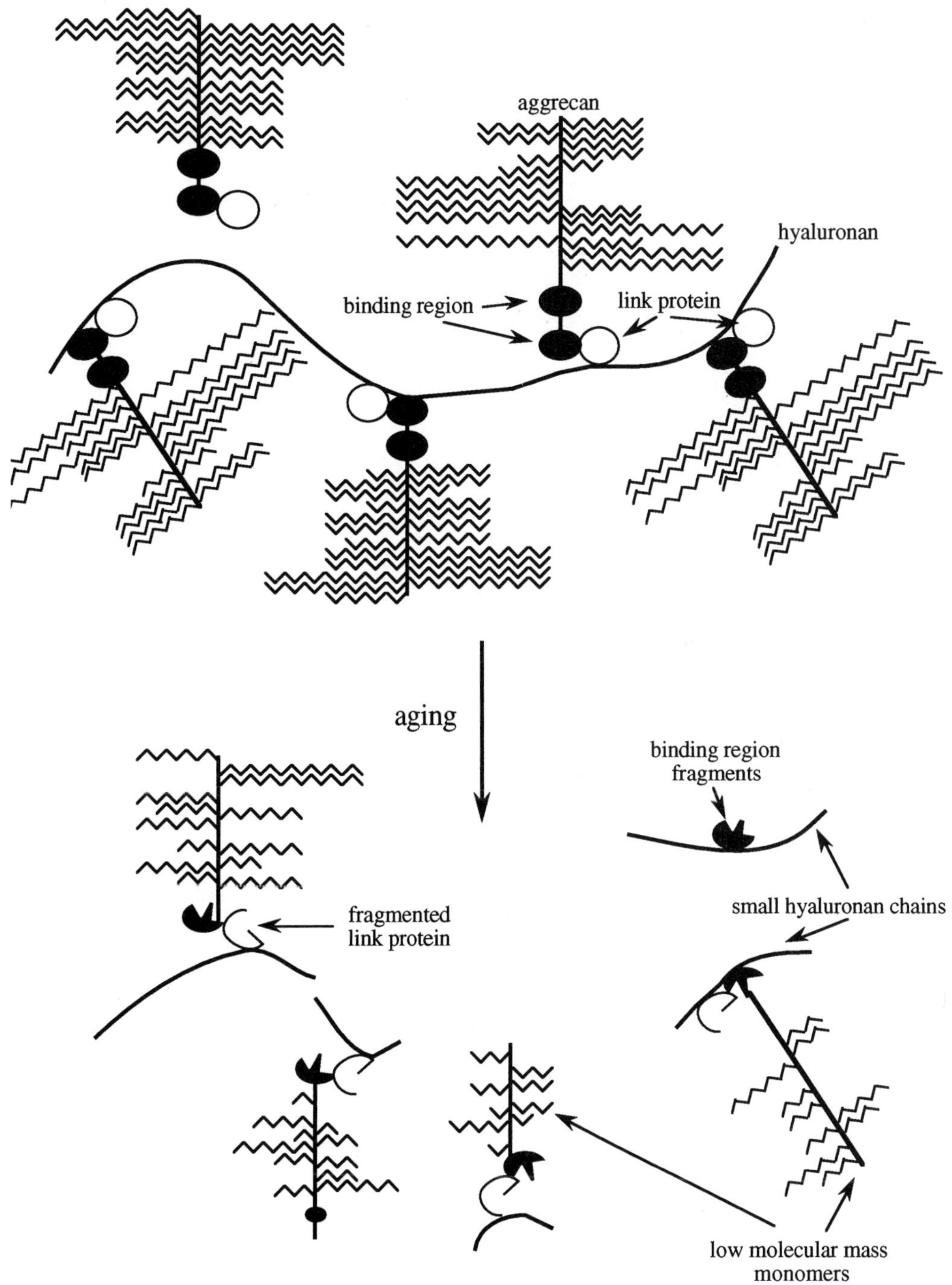


FIGURE 60.2. Major age-related changes in human cartilage structural components. With increasing age, the molecular integrity of the cartilage extracellular matrix is lost, as there is a reduction in proteoglycan size, glycosaminoglycan chain length, and proteolytic fragmentation of hyaluronan chains and link proteins. The ability to form the resilient macromolecular scaffolding involving aggrecan and hyaluronan decreases.

age-related degradation of these proteins affects bone cell function in aged individuals.[124] A study of age-related changes in the composition of bone showed that the amounts of $\alpha_2$HS-glycoprotein, albumin, sialoprotein, soluble collagen, and EDTA-soluble protein were all higher in bone from children than in bone from adults.[125] In the rat bone matrix, the sialic acid and hexose contents increase with age, the uronic acid value decreases, and hydroxyproline does not change. In the EDTA extracts, the collagen extractability decreases markedly with age, the sialic acid content increases, and the hexose and uronic acid contents do not vary.[126] In human bone, the nonenzymatic glycation product pentosidine exhibited an age-related increase.[127]

Human bone cells grown in culture produced less collagen, osteonectin, fibronectin, thrombospondin hyaluronan, versican, decorin, and biglycan with increasing donor age.[86,128] The responsiveness of osteoblasts derived from older donors to IGF-1 and estradiol were significantly reduced when compared to the responsiveness of cells derived from younger donors.[129] The rate and quantity of ectopic bone formation in response to BMP are

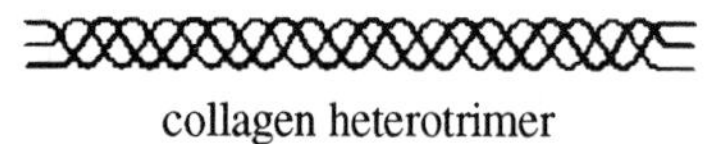


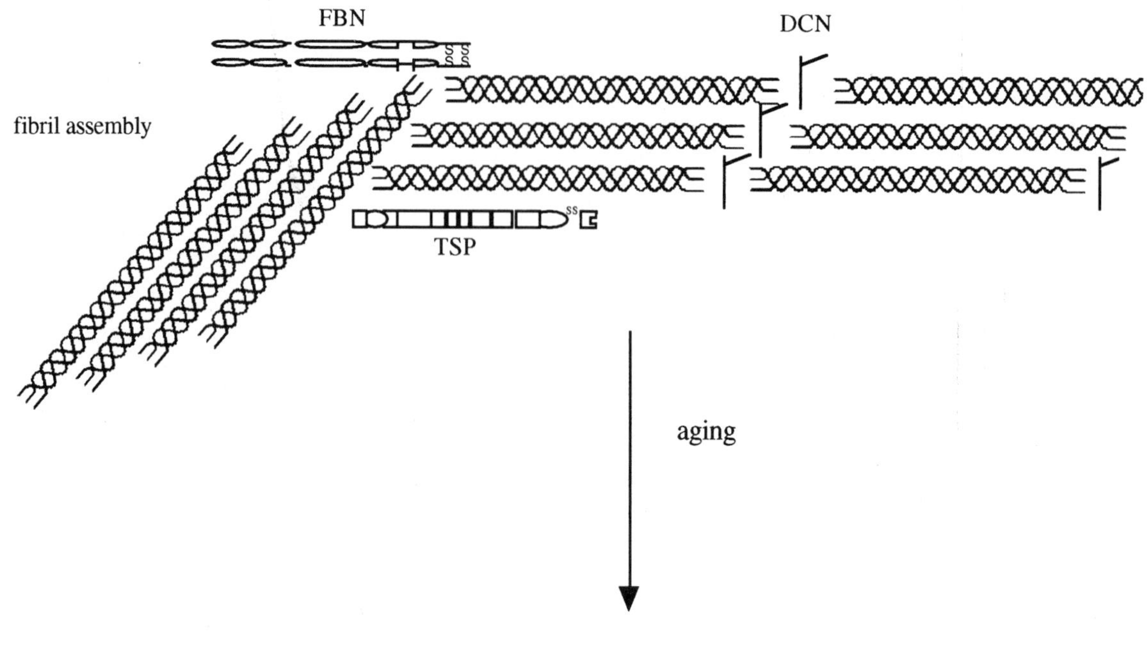


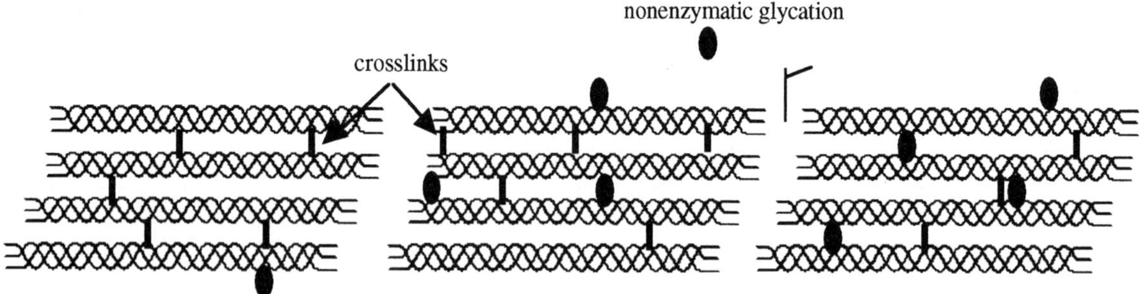


FIGURE 60.3. Major age-related changes in human bone structural components. The bone matrix array of an ordered collagen framework becomes less elastic through the increase in intermolecular cross-links. Pyridinoline–deoxypyridinoline and nonenzymatic glycation cross-links increase. At the same time the content of the noncollagenous proteins that modify the bone matrix decreases with increasing age.

reduced in aged rats and suggest that the difference in blood vessel distribution is related to this reduction in ectopic bone formation.[130]

## Conclusions

Similar to aging skin, cartilage and bone exhibit changes not only in their major component collagen but in other extracellular matrix components that are known to modify and elaborate the collagenous scaffolding. In general, there are increases in cross-links (enzymatic and nonenzymatic) that alter compressibility and decreases in the composition of proteoglycans/glycosaminoglycans, which alter tissue hydration and supramolecular organization. Thus loss of elasticity in skin and increased brittleness in bone are the result of complex alterations in multiple extracellular matrix components. The altered stoichiometry of the extracellular matrix invokes a cascade of events influencing not only organ structural integrity but also cellular functioning.

## References

1. Marks S Jr, Hermey DC. The structure and development of bone. In: Belezikian J, Raisz LC, Rodan GA (eds) Principles of Bone Biology. San Diego: Academic, 1996:3–14.
2. Konori T, Yagi H, Nomura S. Targeted disruption of CBFA 1 results in a complete lack of bone formation owing to maturational arrest of osteoblasts. Cell 1997;89:755–764.

3. Shapiro IM. Discovery: Osf2/Cbfa1, a master gene of bone formation. Clin Orthodontal Res 1999;2:42–46.
4. Quack I, Vonderstrass B, Stock M, et al. Mutation analysis of core binding factor A1 in patients with cleidocranial dysplasia. Am J Hum Genet 1999;65:1268–1278.
5. Iwamoto M, Enomoto-Iwamoto M, Kurisu K. Actions of hedgehog proteins on skeletal cells. Crit Rev Oral Biol Med 1999;10:477–486.
6. Hu D, Helms JA. The role of sonic hedgehog in normal and abnormal craniofacial morphogenesis. Development 1999;126:873–884.
7. Parfitt AM, Drezner MK, Glorieux FH, et al. Histomorphometry: standardization of nomenclature, symbols and units. J Bone Miner Res 1987;2:595–610.
8. Johnston C Jr, Slemenda CW, Melton LJ. Bone density measurements and the management of osteoporosis. In: Favus M (ed) Primer on the Metabolic Bone Diseases and Disorders of Mineral Metabolism. Philadelphia: Lippincott-Raven, 1996:152–164.
9. Bouxein ML, Coan BS, Lee SC. Prediction of the strength of elderly proximal femur by bone mineral density and quantitative ultrasound measurements on heel and tibia. Bone 1999;25:49–54.
10. Sone T, Imai Y, Tomonitsu T, Fukunaga M. Calcaneus as a site for the assessment of bone mass. Bone 1998;22:155S–157S.
11. Matsumoto T, Nakayama K, Kodama Y, Fuse H, Nakamura T, Fukumoto S. Effect of mechanical unloading and reloading on periosteal bone formation and gene expression in tail-suspended rapidly growiing rats. Bone 1998;22:89S–93S.
12. Raisz LG. Physiology and pathophysiology of bone remodeling. Clin Chem 1999;45:1353–1358.
13. Theintz G, Buchs B, Rizzoli R, et al. Longitudinal monitoring of bone mass accumulation in healthy adolescents: evidence for marked reduction after 16 years of age at the levels of lumbar spine and femoral neck in female subjects. J Clin Endocrinol Metab 1992;75:1060–1065.
14. Eastell R, Peel NF, Hannon RA, et al. The effect of age on bone collagen turnover as assessed by pyridinium crosslinks and procollagen I C-terminal peptide. Osteoporos Int 1993;3(suppl 1):100–101.
15. Miller PD, Baran DT, Bilezikian JP, et al. Practical clinical application of biochemical markers of bone turnover: consensus of an expert panel. J Clin Densitom 1999;2:323–324.
16. Garnero P, Sornay-Rendu E, Duboeuf F, Delmas PD. Markers of bone turnover predict postmenopausal forearm bone loss over 4 years: the OFELY study. J Bone Miner Res 1999;14:1614–1621.
17. Meunier P, Coindre JM, Edouard CM, Arlot ME. Bone histomorphometry in Paget's disease: quantitative and dynamic analysis of pagetic and non-pagetic bone tissue. Arthritis Rheum 1980;23:1095–1103.
18. Ankrom M, Shapiro JR. Paget's disease. J Am Geriatr Soc 1997;46:1025–1033.
19. Ott SM. Theoretical and methodological approach. In: Belezikian J, Raisz LG, Rodan GA (eds) Principles of Bone Biology. San Diego: Academic, 1996:231–241.
20. Frost HM. Tetracycline-based histological analysis of bone remodeling. Calcif Tissue Res 1969;3:211–237.
21. Nesbitt S, Nesbitt A, Helfrich M, Horton M. Biochemical characterization of human osteoclast integrins: osteoclasts express alpha v beta 3, alpha 2 beta 1 and alpha v beta 1 integrins. J Biol Chem 1993;268:16737–16745.
22. Aubin JE, Turksen K, Heersche JNM. Osteoblastic cell lineage. In: Noda M (ed) Cellular and Molecular Biology of Bone. San Diego: Academic, 1993:1–49.
23. Triffitt JT. The stem cell of the osteoblast. In: Belezikian J, Raisz LC, Rodan GA (eds) Principles of Bone Biology. San Diego: Academic, 1996:39–50.
24. Reid I, Veale AG, France JT. Glucocorticoid osteoporosis. J Asthma 1994;31:7–18.
25. Grzesik WJ, Gehron Robey P. Bone matrix RGD glycoproteins: immunolocalization and interaction with human primary osteoblastic cells in vitro. J Bone Miner Res 1994;9:487–496.
26. Berresford JN, Graves SE, Smoothey CA. Formation of mineralized nodules by bone derived cells in vitro: a model of bone formation. Am J Med Genet 1993;45:163–178.
27. Pusaz E. Osteoblast cell biology. In: Favus M (ed) Primer on the Metabolic Bone Diseases and Disorders of Mineral Metabolism. Philadelphia: Lippincott-Raven; 1996:11–16.
28. McSheehy PMJ, Chambers TJ. Osteoblastic cells mediate osteoclastic responsiveness to parathyroid hormone. Endocrinology 1986;118:824–828.
29. Takahashi N, Udagawa N, Suda T. A new member of tumor necrosis factor ligand family, ODF/OPGL/TRANCE/RANKL, regulates osteoclast differentiation and function. Biochem Biophys Res Commun 1999;256:449–455.
30. Myers DEMF, Minkin C, Holloway WR, Wang H, Malakellis M, Nicholson GC. The expression and activation of RANK on mature osteoclasts. J Bone Miner Res 1999;14(suppl 1):S483.
31. Schilling AF, Briem D, Rueger JM, Amling M. Human bone marrow cells and peripheral blood cells have the same capacity to differentiate into functional active osteoclast-like cells (OCLs). J Bone Miner Res 1999;14(suppl 1):S487.
32. Chow JW, Wilson AJ, Chambers TJ, Fox SW. Mechanical loading stimulates bone formation by reactivation of bone lining cells in 13-week-old rats. J Bone Miner Res 1998;13:1760–1767.
33. Canalis E. Insulin-like growth factors and the local regulation of bone formation. Bone 1993;14:273–276.
34. Mochizuki H, Hakeda Y, Wakatsuki N, et al. Insulin-like growth factor-I supports formation and activation of osteoclasts. Endocrinology 1992:1075–1080.
35. Benedict MR, Ayres DC, Calore JD, Richman RA. Differential distribution of insulin-like growth factors and their binding proteins within bone: relationship to bone mineral density. J Bone Miner Res 1994;9:1803–1811.
36. Ernst M, Rodan GA. Increased activity of insulin-like growth factor (IGF) in osteoblastic cells in the presence of growth hormone (GH): positive correlation with the presence of the GH-induced IGF-binding protein BP-3w. Endocrinology 1990;127:807–814.
37. Kalus W, Zweckstetter M, Renner C, et al. Structure of the IGF-binding domain of the insulin-like growth factor-binding protein-5 (IGFBP-5): implications for IGF and IGF-I receptor interactions. EMBO J 1998;17:6558–6572.

38. Richman C, Baylink DJ, Lang K, Dony C, Mohan S. Recombinant human insulin-like growth factor-binding protein-5 stimulates bone formation parameters in vitro and in vivo. Endocrinology 1999;40:4699–4705.
39. Thompson J, Halloway L, Hoffman A, Butterfield E, Ghiron L, Marcus R. Effects of rGH amnd IGF-I on bone turnover in elderly women. J Bone Miner Res 1994;9:S238.
40. Marcus R, Butterfield L, Holloway L, et al. Effects of short term administration of rhGH to elderly people. J Clin Endocrinol Metab 1990;70:519–525.
41. Eastell R. Management of corticosteroid-induced osteoporosis. J Intern Med 1995;237:439–447.
42. Fitzpatrick LA, Belezikian JP. Actions of parathyroid hormone. In: Belezikian J, Raisz LC, Rodan GA (eds) Principles of Bone Biology. San Diego: Academic, 1996: 339–346.
43. Fujita T, Inoue T, Morii H, et al. Effect of an intermittent weekly dose of human parathyroid hormone (1–34) on osteoporosis: a randomized double-masked prospective study using three dose levels. Osteoporos Int 1999;9: 296–306.
44. Stewart AF, Horst R, Deftos LJ, Cadman EC, Lang R, Broadus AE. Biochemical evaluation of patients with cancer-associated hypercalcemia: evidence for humoral and nonhumoral groups. N Engl J Med 1980;303:1377–1383.
45. Henderson JE, Shustik C, Kremer R, Rabban SA, Hendy G, Goltzman D. Circulating concentrations of parathyroid hormone-like peptide in malignancy and hyperparathyroidism. J Bone Miner Res 1990;5:105–112.
46. Moseley JM, Martin TJ. Parathyroid hormone-related protein: physiological actions. In: Belezikian J, Raisz LC, Rodan GA (eds) Principles of Bone Biology. San Diego: Academic, 1996:363–376.
47. Lanske B, Amling M, Neff L, Guiducci J, Baron R, Kronenberg HM. Ablation of the PTHrP gene or the PTH/PTHrP receptor gene leads to distinct abnormalities in bone development. J Clin Invest 1999;104:399–407.
48. Wier E, Phillbrick W, Neff L, Amling M, Baron R, Broadus A. Targeted overexpression of parathyroid-related peptide in chondrocytes causes skeletal dysplasia and delayed osteogenesis. J Bone Miner Res 1995;10(suppl 1):S157.
49. Becker KL, Nylen ES, Cohen R, Snider RHJ. Calcitonin: structure, molecular biology, and actions. In: Belezikian J, Raisz LC, Rodan GA (eds) Principles of Bone Biology. San Diego: Academic, 1996:476–494.
50. Seth R, Motte P, Kehely A, et al. The development of a two-site enzuyme immunometric assay (EIA) for calcitonin and its application in the measurement of the hormone in normal subjects, MCT patients and post-menopausal women. Horm Metab Res 1989;21:3–5.
51. Stevenson JC, Hillyard CJ, MacIntyre I, Cooper H, Whitehead MI. Calcitonin and calcium regulating hormones in post-menopausal women. Lancet 1981;1:693–695.
52. Tiegs RD, Brody JJ, Wahner HW, Barta J, Riggs BL. Calcitonin secretion in post-menopausal osteoporosis. N Engl J Med 1985;312:1097–1100.
53. Jones G, Strugnell SA, DeLuca HF. Current understanding of the molecular actions of vitamin D. Physiol Rev 1998;78:1193–1231.
54. Willheim M, Thien R, Schrattbauer K, et al. Regulatory effects of 1 alpha,25-dihydroxyvitamin D3 on the cytokine production of human peripheral blood lymphocytes. J Clin Endocrinol Metab 1999;84:3739–3744.
55. Holick MF. Noncalcemic actions of 1,25-dihydroxyvitamin $D_3$ and clinical applications. Bone 1995;17:107S–111S.
56. Tong WM, Hofer H, Ellinger A, Peterlik M, Cross HS. Mechanism of antimitogenic action of vitamin D in human colon carcinoma cells: relevance for suppression of epidermal growth factor-stimulated cell growth. Oncol Res 1999;11:77–84.
57. Kuiper GG, Carlsson B, Grandien K, Enmark E, Haggblad J, Nilsson S, Gustafsson JA. Comparison of the ligand binding specificity and transcript tissue distribution of estrogen receptors alpha and beta. Endocrinology 1997; 138:863–870.
58. Kuiper GG, Shughrue PJ, Merchenthaler I, Gustafsson A Jr. The estrogen receptor beta subtype: a novel mediator of estrogen action in neuroendocrine systems. Front Neuroendocrinol 1998;19:253–286.
59. Qu Q, Harkonen PL, Monkkonen J, Vaananen HK. Conditioned medium of estrogen-treated osteoblasts inhibits osteoclast maturation and function in vitro. Bone 1999;25: 211–215.
60. Spelsberg TC, Subramanian M, Riggs L, Khosla S. The actions and interactions of sex steroids and growth factors/cytokines on the skeleton. Mol Endocrinol 1999; 1999:819–828.
61. Oreffo RO, Kusec V, Virdi AS, et al. Expression of estrogen receptor-alpha in cells of the osteoclastic lineage. Histochem Cell Biol 1999;111:125–133.
62. Collier FM, Huang WH, Holloway WR, et al. Osteoclasts from human giant cell tumors of bone lack estrogen receptors. Endocrinology 1998;139:1258–1267.
63. Smith EP, Boyd J, Frank GR, et al. Estrogen resistance caused by a mutation in the estrogen-receptor gene in a man. N Engl J Med 1995;331:1056–1061.
64. Belezikian JP, Morishima A, Bell J, Grumbach MM. Increased bone mass as a result of estrogen therapy in man with aromatase deficiency. N Engl J Med 1998;339: 599–603.
65. Ebeling PR. Osteoporosis in men: new insights into aetiology, pathogenesis, prevention and management. Drugs Aging 1998;13:421–434.
66. Bonewald LF. Transforming growth factor-β. In: Belezikian J, Raisz L, Rodan G (eds) Principles of Bone Biology. San Diego: Academic, 1996:647–659.
67. Bonewald LF, Dallas SL. Role of active and latent transforming growth factor beta in bone formation. J Cell Biochem 1994;55:350–357.
68. Groeneveld EH, Burger EH. Bone morphogenetic proteins in human bone regeneration. Eur J Endocrinol 2000;142: 9–21.
69. Prockop DJ, Sieron AL, Li SW. Procollagen N-proteinase and procollagen C-proteinase: two unusual metalloproteinases that are essential for procollagen processing probably have important roles in development and cell signaling. Matrix Biol 1998;16:399–408.
70. Bostrom MP, Saleh KJ, Einhorn TA. Osteoinductive growth factors in preclinical fracture and long bone defects models. Orthop Clin North Am 1999;30:647–658.
71. Bax BE, Wozney JM, Ashhurst D. Bone morphogenetic protein-2 increases the rate of callus formation after fracture of the rabbit tibia. Calcif Tissue Int 1999;65:83–89.

72. Pacifici R. Aging and cytokine production. Calcif Tissue Int 1999;65:345–351.
73. Pratelli L, Cenni E, Granchi D, Tarabusi C, Ciapetti G, Pizzoferrato A. Cytokines of bone turnover in post-menopause and old age. Minerva Med 1999;90:101–109.
74. Birk DE, Mayne R. Localization of collagen types I, III and V during tendon development: changes in collagen types I and III are correlated with changes in fibril diameter. Eur J Cell Biol 1997;72:352–361.
75. Bailey AJ, Paul RG, Knott L. Mechanisms of maturation and aging of collagen. Mech Ageing Dev 1998;106:1–56.
76. Hadley JC, Meek KM, Malik NS. Glycation changes the charge distribution of type I collagen fibrils. Glycoconj J 1998;15:835–840.
77. Fisher LW, Termine JD. Noncollagenous proteins influencing the local mechanisms of calcification. Clin Orthop 1985;200:362–385.
78. Fisher LW, Termine JD, Young MF. Deduced protein sequence of bone small proteoglycan I (biglycan) shows homology with proteoglycan II (decorin) and several non-connective tissue proteins in a variety of species. J Biol Chem 1989;264:4571–4576.
79. Fleischmajer R, Fisher LW, MacDonald ED, Jacobs L Jr, Perlish JS, Termine JD. Decorin interacts with fibrillar collagen of embryonic and adult human skin. J Struct Biol 1991;106:82–90.
80. Bianco P, Fisher LW, Young MF, Termine JD, Robey PG. Expression and localization of the two small proteoglycans biglycan and decorin in developing human skeletal and non-skeletal tissues. J Histochem Cytochem 1990;38:1549–1563.
81. Scott JE. Extracellular matrix, supramolecular organisation and shape. J Anat 1995;187:259–269.
82. Danielson KG, Baribault H, Holmes DF, Graham H, Kadler KE, Iozzo RV. Targeted disruption of decorin leads to abnormal collagen fibril morphology and skin fragility. J Cell Biol 1997;136:729–743.
83. Xu T, Bianco P, Fisher LW, et al. Targeted disruption of the biglycan gene leads to an osteoporosis-like phenotype in mice. Nat Genet 1998;20:78–82.
84. Oohira A, Nogami H. Elevated accumulation of hyaluronate in the tubular bones of osteogenesis imperfecta. Bone 1989;10:409–413.
85. Fedarko NS, Termine JD, Robey PG. High-performance liquid chromatographic separation of hyaluronan and four proteoglycans produced by human bone cell cultures. Anal Biochem 1990;188:398–407.
86. Fedarko NS, Vetter UK, Weinstein S, Robey PG. Age-related changes in hyaluronan, proteoglycan, collagen, and osteonectin synthesis by human bone cells. J Cell Physiol 1992;151:215–227.
87. Bianco P, Fisher LW, Young MF, Termine JD, Robey PG. Expression of bone sialoprotein (BSP) in developing human tissues. Calcif Tissue Int 1991;49:421–426.
88. Bianco P, Riminucci M, Bonucci E, Termine JD, Robey PG. Bone sialoprotein (BSP) secretion and osteoblast differentiation: relationship to bromodeoxyuridine incorporation, alkaline phosphatase, and matrix deposition. J Histochem Cytochem 1993;41:183–191.
89. Riminucci M, Silvestrini G, Bonucci E, Fisher LW, Gehron Robey P, Bianco P. The anatomy of bone sialoprotein immunoreactive sites in bone as revealed by combined ultrastructural histochemistry and immunohistochemistry. Calcif Tissue Int 1995;57:277–284.
90. Riminucci M, Bradbeer JN, Corsi A, et al. Vis-a-vis cells and the priming of bone formation. J Bone Miner Res 1998;13:1852–1861.
91. Chen J, McKee MD, Nanci A, Sodek J. Bone sialoprotein mRNA expression and ultrastructural localization in fetal porcine calvarial bone: comparisons with osteopontin. Histochem J 1994;26:67–78.
92. Hunter GK, Kyle CL, Goldberg HA. Modulation of crystal formation by bone phosphoproteins: structural specificity of the osteopontin-mediated inhibition of hydroxyapatite formation. Biochem J 1994;300:723–728.
93. Chackalaparampil I, Peri A, Nemir M, et al. Cells in vivo and in vitro from osteopetrotic mice homozygous for c-src disruption show suppression of synthesis of osteopontin, a multifunctional extracellular matrix protein. Oncogene 1996;12:1457–1467.
94. Liaw L, Birk DE, Ballas CB, Whitsitt JS, Davidson JM, Hogan BL. Altered wound healing in mice lacking a functional osteopontin gene (sppl 1). J Clin Invest 1998;101: 1468–1478.
95. Termine JD, Kleinman HK, Whitson SW, Conn KM, McGarvey ML, Martin GR. Osteonectin, a bone-specific protein linking mineral to collagen. Cell 1981;26:99–105.
96. Romberg RW, Werness PG, Riggs BL, Mann KG. Inhibition of hydroxyapatite crystal growth by bone-specific and other calcium-binding proteins. Biochemistry 1986;25: 1176–1180.
97. Clezardin P, Malaval L, Ehrensperger AS, Delmas PD, Dechavanne M, McGregor JL. Complex formation of human thrombospondin with osteonectin. Eur J Biochem 1988;175:275–284.
98. Kelm RJ Jr, Mann KG. The collagen binding specificity of bone and platelet osteonectin is related to differences in glycosylation. J Biol Chem 1991;266:9632–9639.
99. Sage H, Vernon RB, Decker J, Funk S, Iruela-Arispe ML. Distribution of the calcium-binding protein SPARC in tissues of embryonic and adult mice. J Histochem Cytochem 1989;37:819–829.
100. Gilmour DT, Lyon GJ, Carlton MB, et al. Mice deficient for the secreted glycoprotein SPARC/osteonectin/BM40 develop normally but show severe age-onset cataract formation and disruption of the lens. EMBO J 1998;17:1860–1870.
101. D'Souza SE, Ginsberg MH, Plow EF. Arginyl-glycyl-aspartic acid (RGD): a cell adhesion motif. Trends Biochem Sci 1991;16:246–250.
102. Hale JE, Fraser JD, Price PA. The identification of matrix Gla protein in cartilage. J Biol Chem 1988;263:5820–5824.
103. Luo G, D'Souza R, Hogue D, Karsenty G. The matrix Gla protein gene is a marker of the chondrogenesis cell lineage during mouse development. J Bone Miner Res 1995;10: 325–334.
104. Price PA, Williamson MK, Haba T, Dell RB, Jee WS. Excessive mineralization with growth plate closure in rats on chronic warfarin treatment. Proc Natl Acad Sci USA 1982;79:7734–7738.
105. Lian JB, Dunn K, Key LL Jr. In vitro degradation of bone particles by human monocytes is decreased with the depletion of the vitamin K-dependent bone protein from the matrix. Endocrinology 1986;118:1636–1642.

106. Ducy P, Desbois C, Boyce B, et al. Increased bone formation in osteocalcin-deficient mice. Nature 1996;382:448–452.
107. Whitmore SE, Levine MA. Risk factors for reduced skin thickness and bone density: possible clues regarding pathophysiology, prevention, and treatment. J Am Acad Dermatol 1998;38:248–255.
108. Lovell CR, Smolenski KA, Duance VC, Light ND, Young S, Dyson M. Type I and III collagen content and fibre distribution in normal human skin during ageing. Br J Dermatol 1987;117:419–428.
109. Holt DR, Kirk SJ, Regan MC, Hurson M, Lindblad WJ, Barbul A. Effect of age on wound healing in healthy human beings. Surgery 1992;112:293–297; discussion 297–298.
110. Castelo-Branco C, Duran M, Gonzalez-Merlo J. Skin collagen changes related to age and hormone replacement therapy. Maturitas 1992;15:113–119.
111. Castelo-Branco C, Pons F, Gratacos E, Fortuny A, Vanrell JA, Gonzalez-Merlo J. Relationship between skin collagen and bone changes during aging. Maturitas 1994;18:199–206.
112. Dyer DG, Dunn JA, Thorpe SR, et al. Accumulation of Maillard reaction products in skin collagen in diabetes and aging. J Clin Invest 1993;91:2463–2469.
113. Rittie L, Berton A, Monboisse JC, Hornebeck W, Gillery P. Decreased contraction of glycated collagen lattices coincides with impaired matrix metalloproteinase production. Biochem Biophys Res Commun 1999;264:488–492.
114. Bernstein EF, Fisher LW, Li K, LeBaron RG, Tan EM, Uitto J. Differential expression of the versican and decorin genes in photoaged and sun-protected skin. Comparison by immunohistochemical and Northern analyses. Lab Invest 1995;72:662–669.
115. Watson RE, Griffiths CE, Craven NM, Shuttleworth CA, Kielty CM. Fibrillin-rich microfibrils are reduced in photoaged skin: distribution at the dermal-epidermal junction. J Invest Dermatol 1999;112:782–787.
116. Bayliss MT. Proteoglycan structure and metabolism during maturation and ageing of human articular cartilage. Biochem Soc Trans 1990;18:799–802.
117. Bank RA, Bayliss MT, Lafeber FP, Maroudas A, Tekoppele JM. Ageing and zonal variation in post-translational modification of collagen in normal human articular cartilage: the age-related increase in non-enzymatic glycation affects biomechanical properties of cartilage. Biochem J 1998;330:345–351.
118. DeGroot J, Verzijl N, Bank RA, Lafeber FP, Bijlsma JW, TeKoppele JM. Age-related decrease in proteoglycan synthesis of human articular chondrocytes: the role of nonenzymatic glycation. Arthritis Rheum 1999;42:1003–1009.
119. Adams P, Eyre DR, Muir H. Biochemical aspects of development and ageing of human lumbar intervertebral discs. Rheumatol Rehabil 1977;16:22–29.
120. Aigner T, Gresk-Otter KR, Fairbank JC, von der Mark K, Urban JP. Variation with age in the pattern of type X collagen expression in normal and scoliotic human intervertebral discs. Calcif Tissue Int 1998;63:263–268.
121. Nerlich AG, Schleicher ED, Boos N. 1997 Volvo Award winner in basic science studies: immunohistologic markers for age-related changes of human lumbar intervertebral discs. Spine 1997;22:2781–2795.
122. Pokharna HK, Phillips FM. Collagen crosslinks in human lumbar intervertebral disc aging. Spine 1998;23:1645–1648.
123. Sztrolovics R, Alini M, Mort JS, Roughley PJ. Age-related changes in fibromodulin and lumican in human intervertebral discs. Spine 1999;24:1765–1771.
124. Termine JD. Cellular activity, matrix proteins, and aging bone. Exp Gerontol 1990;25:217–221.
125. Dickson IR, Bagga MK. Changes with age in the noncollagenous proteins of human bone. Connect Tissue Res 1985;14:77–85.
126. Mbuyi-Muamba JM, Dequeker J. Age and sex variations of bone matrix proteins in Wistar rats. Growth 1983;47:301–315.
127. Duance VC, Crean JK, Sims TJ, et al. Changes in collagen cross-linking in degenerative disc disease and scoliosis. Spine 1998;23:2545–2551.
128. Fedarko NS, Vetter UK, Robey PG. Age-related changes in bone matrix structure in vitro. Calcif Tissue Int 1995;56(suppl 1):S41–S43.
129. D'Avis PY, Frazier CR, Shapiro JR, Fedarko NS. Age-related changes in effects of insulin-like growth factor I on human osteoblast-like cells. Biochem J 1997;324:753–760.
130. Nagai N, Qin CL, Nagatsuka H, Inoue M, Ishiwari Y. Age effects on ectopic bone formation induced by purified bone morphogenetic protein. Int J Oral Maxillofac Surg 1999;28:143–150.

# 61
# Common Benign and Malignant Skin Lesions

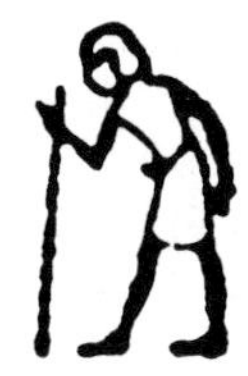

Maryam M. Asgari and David J. Leffell

The elderly patient presents us with a variety of benign and malignant skin lesions. The ability to differentiate various cutaneous neoplasms is especially important in the geriatric population because of the higher incidence of malignant skin tumors that arise in aging skin. The aim of this chapter is to acquaint the surgeon with normal skin anatomy, with changes in skin anatomy during aging, and with the pathophysiology, diagnosis, and treatment of common benign and malignant skin tumors of the elderly.

## Basic Skin Anatomy

The skin is composed of two layers: a stratified squamous epithelial layer, or epidermis, and an underlying connective tissue layer, or dermis. The interface between these two layers is termed the dermal–epidermal junction and is characterized by downward folds of the epidermis into the dermis. These folds, called rete ridges, provide mechanical support against shearing forces. Embryologic downgrowths of epithelium into the dermis give rise to epidermal appendages such as hair follicles, sweat glands, and sebaceous glands. Underneath the dermis lies a fatty layer of subcutaneous tissue that serves to insulate and protect the underlying structures.

### Epidermis

The ectoderm-derived epidermis is comprised of four cell types: keratinocytes, melanocytes, Langerhans' cells, and Merkel cells. Keratinocytes are specialized stratified squamous epithelial cells that make up most of the epidermis. As keratinocytes migrate upward from their origin at the dermal–epidermal junction, they differentiate, forming four morphologically distinct layers. The innermost layer, which contains the germinative keratinocytes, is called the stratum basale. Immediately above the stratum basale, keratinocytes enlarge to form the stratum spinosum, or prickle cell layer. Progressive maturation leads to the accumulation of intracellular keratohyalin granules, giving rise to the next cell layer called the stratum granulosum.

Keratinocytes at the outermost portion of the stratum granulosum lose their nuclei and fuse to form a cornified layer or stratum corneum. These dead keratinocytes function to protect the underlying cells and prevent dehydration. They are eventually exfoliated at a rate that matches the production of cells at the basal layer.

Neuroectoderm-derived melanocytes, which comprise 1% of epidermal cells, are located in the basal layer of the epidermis. They synthesize melanin, which is taken up by nearby keratinocytes and serves to protect the skin from penetration of ultraviolet light, which can damage underlying epidermal and dermal cells. Langerhans' cells make up 3–5% of the epidermal cell population. They are derived from cells of the monocyte/macrophage lineage and act as antigen-presenting cells in the skin. Merkel cells are the least abundant cells of the epidermis, comprising less than 1% of all epidermal cells. They are thought to be of neuroendocrine origin from the amine precursor uptake and decarboxylation (APUD) group of cells. Like melanocytes, they are also located in the basal layer of the epidermis. They function as a slowly adapting sensory receptor for touch.

### Dermis

The mesoderm-derived dermis sits just below the avascular epidermis, supplying it with a rich neurovascular system. Histologically the dermis can be divided into two layers. Occupying the space around the rete ridges is the superficial papillary dermis, which is composed of a loosely woven arrangement of connective tissue bundles. Underneath it lies the reticular dermis, so named for its denser, interwoven pattern of connective tissue fibers. The resident cells of the dermis are mostly fibroblasts, which secrete collagen, elastin, and ground substance. Collagen and elastin give the skin its toughness, dispensability, and flexibility. Ground substance, which is comprised of polysaccharides and proteins, provides a supportive matrix for the connective tissue fibers. The overall structure accommodates the network of vascular, lymphatic, and nerve plexi that supply the skin. Other cellular constituents of the dermis include mast cells, macrophages, lymphocytes, and other leukocytes.

### Epidermal Appendages

During embryologic development, epidermal cells bud down into the dermis, forming adnexal structures such as hair follicles, sebaceous glands, and eccrine and apocrine sweat glands collectively termed epidermal appendages. Hair follicles are composed of modified keratinocytes that form a tubular structure enclosed by a collagenous sheath. Each hair follicle is associated with one or more sebaceous glands, which secrete an oily substance called sebum. Sebum functions to help moisturize and waterproof skin. Like sebaceous glands, apocrine sweat glands secrete their product into the follicular lumen. Apocrine glands are modified sweat glands located in the axillae and groin and are thought to be remnants of scent glands in animals. With the exception of the groin and axillae, the remainder of skin is covered by eccrine sweat glands. These glands, which are responsible for thermoregulation, are independent of the hair follicle, having ducts that open directly onto the surface of skin.

## Changes in the Skin Associated with Aging

The intrinsic changes that occur in aging skin are important for understanding the pathophysiology of benign and malignant lesions that affect senescent skin.

### Epidermis

Between the third and seventh decades the turnover rate of keratinocytes is reduced by 50%.[1] The slower epidermal turnover rate increases the length of keratinocyte exposure to carcinogens such as solar radiation, making the epidermis more susceptible to the development of keratinocyte-derived neoplasms. Decreased proliferative capacity of keratinocytes also prolongs wound healing, which can affect the choice of treatment employed for cutaneous lesions in the elderly.

The aging epidermis also undergoes structural alterations. The rete pegs at the dermal–epidermal junction retract, making elderly skin more susceptible to shearing forces. Keratinocytes in the basal layer become increasingly heterogeneic, displaying variations in size, shape, and staining pattern.[2] Xerosis, or dry skin, becomes increasingly problematic as the moisture content of stratum corneum diminishes with age.[3]

Melanocytes also undergo age-related changes, most notably decreasing in number over time. After age 30, the surviving population of melanocytes drops by 8–20% each decade.[4] As a result, less melanin is produced, allowing greater penetration of ultraviolet (UV) radiation, which can increase the risk of developing skin neoplasms. Like melanocytes, Langerhans' cells also diminish in number with age. Langerhans' cells are especially sensitive to UV radiation and are further functionally impaired by the decrease in protective melanin with aging. This compromises the cell-mediated immune response in elderly skin, thereby more readily permitting the development of tumors.

### Dermis

The dermis thins and becomes less vascular with age. Collagen fibers become thickened and less resilient, making the dermis more susceptible to tear-type injuries. Elastin fibers display structural degradative changes resulting in skin laxity and wrinkle formation.[2] The amount of ground substance decreases, reducing the supportive dermal matrix, so structures such as blood vessels become more susceptible to damage. This manifests clinically as easy bruising in the elderly. Thinning of vessel walls may also contribute to the increased susceptibility to ecchymoses. Other changes in cutaneous vasculature include a decrease in the density of vessels. Diminished cutaneous circulation can lead to reduced clearance of foreign material, delayed wound healing, and poorer thermoregulatory capacity. The aging skin also loses its ability to mount an inflammatory response, leading to muted clinical presentations of cutaneous disease.

### Epidermal Appendages

Marked age-related changes also occur in the epidermal appendages. There is an overall reduction in the number and function of eccrine sweat glands, leading to a decrease in thermoregulatory capacity. Apocrine glands attenuate and accumulate lipofuscin with a resultant reduction in secretory function.[3] Sebaceous glands enlarge with age, but their sebum production is paradoxically reduced. These changes in sebaceous glands manifest clinically as sebaceous hyperplasia and xerosis.

## Benign Lesions

### Epidermal Lesions

#### *Seborrheic Keratoses*

Seborrheic keratoses are common, benign, flat-topped papules or plaques that are composed of hyperprolifer-

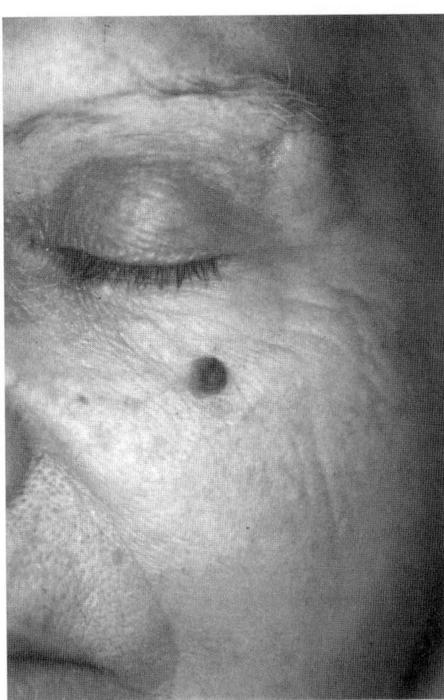

FIGURE 61.1. Seborrheic keratoses, the most common benign cutaneous tumor in the elderly. Its significance lies in its potential to mimic malignant melanoma. Although treatment is not normally indicated, the lesion, which may appear rough or greasy, may be irritated necessitating removal. Alternatively, if there is suspicion about melanoma, biopsy is indicated.

ating keratinocytes. They typically appear during the fifth decade, though early lesions can present as early as the fourth decade. Early lesions manifest as discrete 1- to 3-cm skin-colored to dark brown patches that progress to form slightly elevated, warty, greasy plaques. Their exophytic growth pattern makes them appear "stuck on."[5] Although seborrheic keratoses can be found on any part of the body, they are most prevalent on the face and upper trunk (Fig. 61.1). Males and females are equally affected; the lesions occur more frequently in whites and are uncommon in blacks and native Americans.

The number of lesions on any given individual can vary from one or two up to hundreds,[5] often increasing in number as the patient ages. Once formed, seborrheic keratoses are permanent, remaining in place unchanged for the lifetime of the individual. Seborrheic keratoses are benign and have no malignant potential. However, the eruption of multiple lesions in a short duration of time, known as the sign of Leser-Trelat, had been thought to point to internal malignancy. Alternatively, multiple seborrheic keratoses may also occur as a familial trait with autosomal dominant inheritance or may be precipitated by an inflammatory dermatosis.

Histologically, seborrheic keratoses show accumulation of immature keratinocytes with papillomatosis between the basal layer and stratum corneum. Focal keratinization may occur, leading to the formation of horn cysts within the lesion. Melanocytes usually proliferate in the lesion and transfer melanin to immature keratinocytes, accounting for the wide spectrum of color the lesions can acquire.

The diagnosis of seborrheic keratoses is made clinically. Some early lesions may be confused with solar lentigos or pigmented actinic keratoses. Differentiation may be made upon closer inspection with a hand lens, which can reveal a characteristic verrucous appearance and at times the presence of horn cysts. Late lesions may resemble a pigmented basal cell carcinoma or malignant melanoma. If a lesion is thought to be a basal cell carcinoma, a shave biopsy is recommended. For lesions suspicious for malignant melanoma, an excisional biopsy should be performed.

Although seborrheic keratoses require no therapy, some patients prefer to have them removed for cosmetic reasons. Treatment should be rapid and nonscarring. This can be accomplished with light curettage, which destroys the superficial layer of the epidermis and minimizes the risk of scarring. The potential for regrowth exists. Should this occur, retreatment may be performed as necessary. Electrodesiccation should be avoided, as it may cause excessive scarring.[6] If the clinical diagnosis is unclear, a shave biopsy should be performed.

### *Solar Lentigo (Senile Lentigo, Actinic Lentigo)*

Chronic sun exposure can induce melanocytes to proliferate locally forming small brown macules known as solar lentigos, or "liver spots." Their presence in more than 90% of individuals over the age of 70 has led to the unflattering descriptive term "senile lentigo." These lesions are localized to sun-exposed areas, such as the cheek, forehead, nose, dorsa of hands and forearms, upper back, and chest (Fig. 61.2). They affect males and females equally and are more commonly seen in Caucasians than in Asians.

Solar lentigos can be confused with other benign lesions, such as early seborrheic keratoses, and premalignant lesions such as pigmented actinic keratoses and lentigo maligna. To differentiate solar lentigos from seborrheic keratoses and pigmented actinic keratoses, the lesion must be examined with a hand lens in oblique light. Seborrheic keratoses and pigmented actinic keratoses generally display features of epidermal change, whereas solar lentigos are completely flat. Lentigo maligna, like solar lentigo, may not show epidermal changes. However, it has distinct variations in color from light brown to dark brown with flecks of black. If any lentigo has an irregular border, change in pigment, or focal thickening, a biopsy should be performed to exclude lentigo maligna.

Histologically, solar lentigos display elongated, club-shaped rete ridges containing numerous melanocytes and increased melanin production without cellular atypia

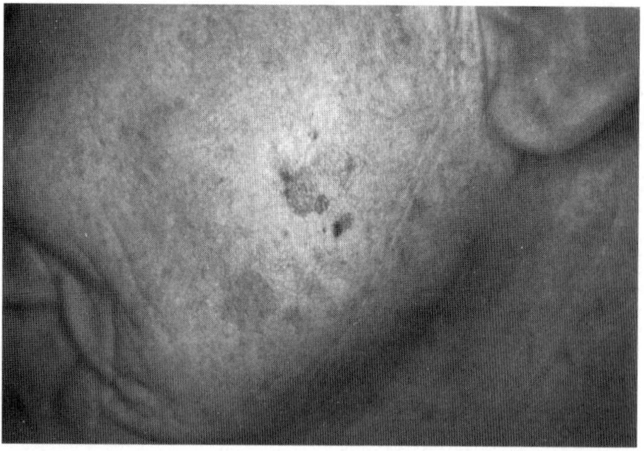

FIGURE 61.2. Solar lentigo, seen mostly on the face and dorsa of the hands, have tan to brown pigmentation and are flat. They may be of cosmetic concern and occasionally must be biopsied to rule out lentigo maligna.

or nest formation. Most solar lentigos have virtually no malignant potential. Rarely, a small proportion of lesions occurring on the face slowly develop into lentigo maligna.[5] The incidence of malignant transformation is so rare, however, that most lesions require no treatment. If the patient finds these "age spots" cosmetically unacceptable, treatment can be accomplished in several ways. Application of bleaching agents may decrease the pigment, but ongoing treatment is necessary. Laser methods[7] that emit light at wavelengths better absorbed by melanin than other skin components allow selective damage. The Q-switched ruby laser is now the treatment of choice.[8] For those seeking treatment, the use of sunscreen for preventing new lesions should be emphasized.

### Melanocytic Nevocellular Nevi (Moles)

Benign nevocellular nevi, or moles, are small, well-circumscribed macules and papules that vary in color from skin-colored to tan and brown (Fig. 61.3). They are composed of nests of melanocytes located in the epidermis, dermis, and rarely subcutaneous tissue. If the cluster of melanocytes is localized to the dermal–epidermal junction, the nevus is classified as a junctional nevus; if the cells are in the dermis, it is called a dermal nevus; and if there are features of both, the lesion is referred to as a compound nevus. Dermal nevi can lack pigment.

Nevocellular lesions are acquired during childhood and early adulthood. They typically increase in number up to the age of 40, following which they begin to involute. With the exception of dermal nevi, most nevocellular nevi disappear by the age of 60. If new nevocellular lesions are acquired after mid-adulthood, they should be regarded with a high degree of suspicion and closely followed to rule out the development of malignancy.[9]

## Benign Dermal Lesions

### Acrochordons (Skin Tags)

Skin tags are soft, pliable, skin-colored to tan-brown pedunculated polyps that occur in intertriginous areas such as the neck and axillae. They are common in middle-aged and elderly individuals, with at least 50% of individuals above the age of 50 having at least one.[10] Over time, they can become larger and more numerous. Skin tags are especially prevalent in postmenopausal women, pregnant women,[11] and obese individuals, suggesting a hormonal influence on their development. The exact etiology of skin tags is unknown, though some familial groupings have been noted. Early studies suggested that skin tags could potentially serve as cutaneous markers for colonic polyps,[12] but more recently that association has been largely disproved.[13]

Histologically, skin tags consist of protruding loose fibrous tissue covered by a thin epidermis attached to the skin by a narrow stalk. Upon visual inspection they are easily recognized, though they are rarely misdiagnosed as pedunculated seborrheic keratoses, pedunculated melanocytic nevus, neurofibroma, or molluscum contagiosum. Their size offers a clue to their diagnosis: Skin tags tend to be smaller than the average pedunculated melanocytic nevus or neurofibroma.

Skin tags have no malignant potential but tend to be a cosmetic nuisance, especially if they occur in areas exposed to friction such as the belt line. Treatment consists of simple excision requiring no local anesthetic. Lesions can be severed at their base by grasping them

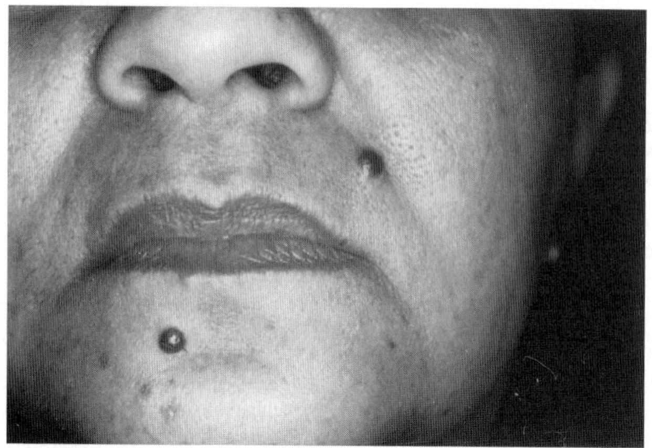

FIGURE 61.3. Nevi of medical significance are uncommon in the elderly but new pigmented lesions that are not seborrheic keratoses should be evaluated.

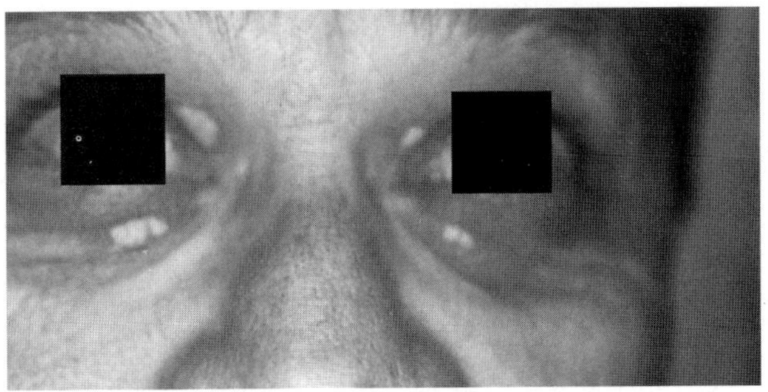

FIGURE 61.4. Xanthelasma. These cholesterol deposits occur on the upper and lower lids and can best be removed surgically. They are yellowish with a smooth surface.

with forceps and cutting them with scissors, razors, or scalpels. Skin tags may also be electrodesiccated.

### *Xanthelasma Palpebrarum (Eyelid Xanthomas)*

Xanthelasma palpebrarum is seen mostly in adults in their fourth to fifth decade. They present as yellow velvety plaques confined to the eyelids. The lesions often begin as small yellow spots that initially may be confused with milia or senile closed comedones. They grow over a span of months to form coalescing plaques on the upper eyelids and around the inner canthus (Fig. 61.4). Once their growth stabilizes, these plaques remain permanently.

Histologically, xanthelasma palpebrarum is characterized by lipid-laden macrophages in the superficial dermis. Approximately 50% of patients who present with these lesions have an underlying disorder of lipid metabolism, such as familial hypercholesterolemia or familial dysproteinemia. Patients with these disorders typically have elevated low density lipoprotein (LDL) and apoprotein E levels and are prone to atherosclerotic cardiovascular disease. Patients who present for the first time with xanthelasma palpebrarum should have their serum lipoproteins and apolipoproteins checked. If the levels are within normal limits, no further testing need be pursued, as nearly half of the patients who present with the lesion have no lipid disturbances. The etiology of xanthelasma palprebrarum in patients with no lipid disorder is unknown.

Systemic therapy with lipid-lowering agents rarely affects the appearance of these lesions. Prior to the advent of $CO_2$ lasers, excision, cryotherapy, and topical application of 30% trichloracetic acid were the preferred methods of treatment. With most of these treatments, however, recurrences are common. Excision with primary closure is effective in only 60% of patients and is limited by the location of the lesions.[14] Some authors have advocated excision with secondary intention healing, thereby minimizing the risk of ectropion and complications with skin grafting.[15] Although healing by secondary intention may allow greater margins of resection and therefore minimize the rate of recurrence (7% in a recent study),[15] the risk of scarring and infection may make this procedure risky in the hands of the untrained. Recently, there have been case reports of complete eradication of xanthelasma using an ultrapulse $CO_2$ laser requiring only one treatment session without complications or recurrences at follow-up of up to 1 year.[16] Though promising, the efficacy of this new modality must be further studied in controlled clinical trials.

### *Sebaceous Hyperplasia*

Sebaceous hyperplasia is a benign lesion that is often found on the face of older patients. It typically presents as a cream to yellow umbilicated papule on the forehead, cheeks, eyelids, and nose of individuals over the age of 30 (Fig. 61.5). The incidence of sebaceous hyperplasia increases with age such that about 25% of patients over the age of 65 carry these lesions. Its etiology is unknown, but genetic factors most likely play a role in its pathogenesis as most lesions arise in patients of northern European heritage and occur independent of sun exposure.

Sebaceous hyperplasia often begins as a small, 2- to 3-mm papule with a central depression. This depression represents the opening of a wide sebaceous duct that is surrounded by several enlarged sebaceous gland lobules, lending the lesion its characteristic lobular configuration.

Some lesions of sebaceous hyperplasia contain central telangectasias. This feature, combined with the papule's

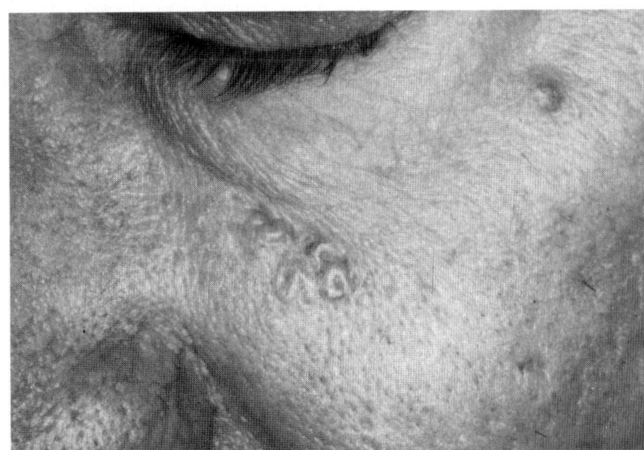

FIGURE 61.5. Sebaceous hyperplasia. These lesions represent benign hypertrophy of the sebaceous glands. With their central umbilication and rounded edge, they are occasionally confused with basal cell carcinoma.

translucent appearance, often leads clinicians to confuse sebaceous hyperplasia with basal cell carcinoma. A clue to the correct diagnosis can be obtained with diascopy (applying pressure on the lesion with a glass slide), which reveals the yellow-white color of sebaceous hyperplasia. Relying on diascopy for diagnosis is not perfect: the yellow-white color sometimes leads to the incorrect diagnosis of xanthomas. Xanthomas can usually be differentiated by their larger size and absence of umbilication.[17]

When the clinical diagnosis is uncertain, a biopsy should be performed. In general, no treatment is necessary unless cosmetically desirable. Cryotherapy, in a single freeze-thaw cycle or shave excisions of the elevated portion of the lesion, has been variably succesful. Electrodesiccation and curettage should be avoided, as it may result in scarring. The ultrapulse $CO_2$ laser has proven helpful.

### *Chondrodermatitis Nodularis Helicis*

Chondrodermatitis nodularis helicis (CNH) typically presents as a painful, erythematous nodule on the helices of men over the age of 40. Approximately 30% of cases of CNH occur in young individuals and in women, but the location varies to include the antihelix, tragus, antitragus, and concha.[18] The nodule, which often displays central crusting and ulceration, is typically surrounded by hyperemic skin. It enlarges to reach its maximum size of 0.5–2.0 cm within a few months and then remains unchanged indefinitely without evolution to malignancy (Fig. 61.6).

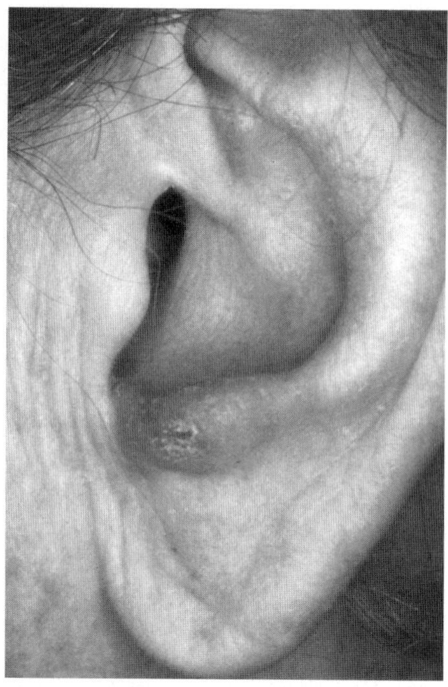

FIGURE 61.6. Chondrodermatitis nodularis helicis. This benign condition of the ear is painful and may present with eroded epidermis. It can be confused with squamous cell cancer of the ear, which usually is not painful.

This disorder is thought to be due to compromised local blood supply as a result of pressure or cold temperatures. It often arises in individuals who habitually sleep on one side. Aggravating factors include cold temperatures, pressure from head gear, and trauma. Despite the characteristic exquisite tenderness of these lesions, CNH is often mistaken for squamous cell carcinoma. Biopsy, which is indicated only if there is a degree of suspicion for squamous cell carcinoma, characteristically reveals degenerated homogeneous collagen surrounded by vascular granulation tissue with acanthotic overlying epidermis containing a central ulcer. The perichondrium is thickened and shows a lymphocytic infiltrate.

Treatment of CNH may be medical or surgical. Medical therapies include intralesional injection of steroids and collagen[18] and cryotherapy. Intralesional steroids, such as Kenalog administered in a 5–10 mg/ml dose, are generally reserved for first-line treatment of early lesions, as it is successful in only 25% of cases.[19] Higher cure rates, approaching 85%,[20] are achieved with surgical approaches, including excision. Electrodesiccation and curettage can be easily performed with adequate margins by allowing the curette to be the guide. Necrotic cartilage, which tends to be soft, is removed easily. Curettage is stopped when healthy, firm cartilage is reached.[21] Techniques for excision vary widely: Some advocate removal of abnormal auricular cartilage only,[19] whereas others recommend removal of involved cartilage as well as overlying skin.[1] Leaving the overlying skin intact has the advantage of decreasing the deformity of the ear, resulting in a better cosmetic result.[22] A cure rate approaching 100% over a 2-year follow-up period has been reported using $CO_2$ laser surgery,[23,24] but data from large-scale comparative trials are not yet available. To prevent recurrences, the patient should be instructed to minimize pressure and trauma to the ear.

### *Cherry Hemangioma (Campbell de Morgan Spots)*

Cherry angiomas are small, benign, bright red to violaceous, dome-shaped papules that are commonly found in middle-age and older adults. They become more numerous with age. They are distributed over the trunk and proximal extremities and can vary from 2 to 8 mm in diameter (Fig. 61.7). Their etiology is unknown.

Histologically, cherry angiomas are characterized by the presence of numerous dilated capillaries lined by flattened endothelial cells with edematous surrounding stroma and collagen homogenization. The overlying epidermis is frequently thinned with fenestrations.

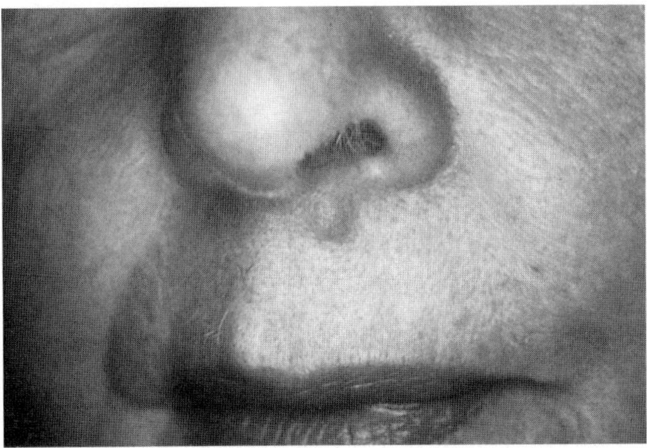

FIGURE 61.7. Hemangioma. This deep-seated hemangioma on the upper lip is benign, but in the absence of the ability to blanch on compression it should be biopsied to rule out other tumors.

Cherry angiomas are diagnosed clinically and require no treatment. Occasionally, they are mimicked by angiokeratomas, venous lakes, nodular melanomas, or metastatic carcinomas. If nodular melanoma or metastatic carcinoma is suspected, an excisional biopsy should be performed. If a cherry angioma is at a site of recurrent trauma and therefore prone to ulceration or if it is at a site that is cosmetically unacceptable to the patient, it can be treated by shave excision, cryotherapy, electrodesiccation, or laser ablation.

### *Venous Lakes*

Venous lakes are angiomatous dilations of venules occurring on the face, lips, and ears of patients who are usually above the age of 50. They manifest clinically as dark-blue to violaceous papules with an irregular, cobblestone appearance. After an initial growth phase these lesions stabilize and do not regress. The cause of venous lake formation is unknown. It occurs with equal incidence in both sexes. Microscopically, the lesion reveals small, single-layered interconnected vessels (or one large dilated space) in the upper dermis surrounded by a thin wall of fibrous tissue. A venous lake can resemble a pyogenic granuloma, which should be removed or biopsied, or a nodular melanoma, which requires an excisional biopsy. In most instances, however, venous lakes can be easily distinguished clinically by applying prolonged pressure to the lesion, which causes it to lose its violaceous hue as the venous bed empties.

Treatment of venous lakes is only indicated cosmetically. They can be obliterated with electocoagulation or laser; alternatively, they can be surgically excised although it may leave a cosmetically unacceptable scar.

## Premalignant Lesions

### Actinic Keratoses (Solar Keratoses)

Actinic keratoses (AKs) are discrete, scaly, pink to red lesions that are found on chronically sun-exposed skin of the face, ears, neck, forearms, and dorsal hands. They have a rough quality, allowing them to be more easily felt than seen. Typically, they arise in middle-age individuals, though they may occur earlier in people living in sunny climates. AKs are precancerous lesions with a conversion rate to squamous cell carcinoma ranging between 0.24% and 25%,[20] although a rate of 1% is frequently cited in the literature.[25] The squamous cell carcinomas that arise from AKs have been considered to be less aggressive than ones arising de novo, with a metastatic rate of only 1.6%,[26] although there is some doubt about this association.

There are three clinical subtypes types of AKs: hypertrophic, pigmented and lichenoid (Fig. 61.8). The hypertrophic variety develops as a thickened papule which may border on early squamous cell cancer. Pigmented AKs can resemble solar lentigo, seborrheic keratoses, nevi, or in situ melanoma. Lichenoid AK may mimic lichen planus. In general, AKs are relatively easy to recognize clinically and do not require a biopsy unless there is suspicion of malignant transformation. Biopsy

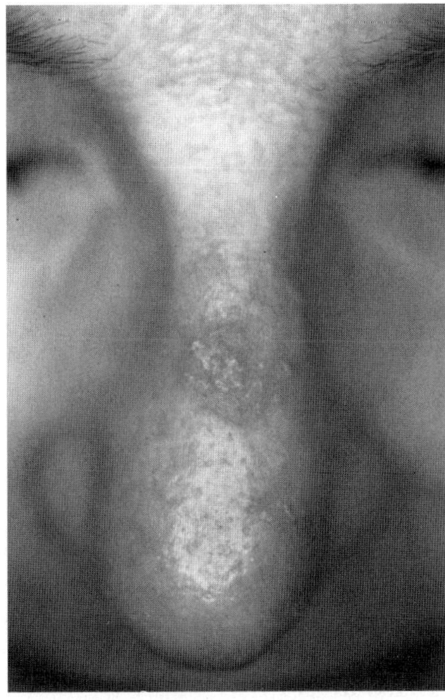

FIGURE 61.8. Actinic keratoses. This is one of the most common sun-related lesions in the elderly. It is biologically and clinically premalignant and should be treated because of the risk of malignant transformation. The lesions can vary in size from 1 to 2 mm up to more than 1 cm and have a rough surface overlying a reddened background.

typically reveals large, bright staining keratinocytes with mild to moderate basal layer pleomorphism that spares follicular units. The abnormal keratinocytes do not invade the dermis.

Because AKs are considered premalignant, treatment is ablative and is determined by the number and location of lesions. If a patient presents with fewer than 10 AKs, cryotherapy is the method of choice. Flat to slightly raised lesions are treated with liquid nitrogen until frosted. For lesions that are thick and hyperkeratotic, 3–5 seconds of freezing may be necessary. With this technique, cure rates as high as 98% have been reported.[27] Light electrodesiccation and curettage and $CO_2$ lasers are other effective methods for scattered lesions, but they have the disadvantages of requiring local anesthesia and may increase the risk of scarring.

For numerous lesions, topical fluorouracil (5-FU), which selectively targets abnormal keratinocytes, is one treatment option. It is applied as a 1%, 2%, or 5% cream or solution one or two times daily until the AKs become inflamed and ulcerate. The treatment period can last 2–6 weeks and can cause significant discomfort, which may hamper patient compliance. Inflammation can be minimized with mid-potency topical steroids during the healing phase without affecting the efficacy of the treatment. The recurrence rate with 5-FU is high.

Other exfoliative methods include chemical peels with trichloroacetic acid and dermabrasion (by laser or with diamond fraize). Chemexfoliation with 35% tricholoracetic acid, on a repeated basis, can decrease the number of AKs. The advantage of these methods is that their efficacy is not dependent on patient compliance, and they have the added benefit of improving cosmetic appearance.

Patients presenting with AKs usually have a history of chronic sun exposure, which places them at increased risk for developing other skin cancers. Therefore it is important to follow these patients at regular intervals and to emphasize preventive care by recommending sun protection strategies.

## Actinic Cheilitis

Actinic cheilitis is a premalignant disorder of the lip. It usually localizes to the labial surface of the lower lip where sunlight exposure is greatest but occasionally occurs on the upper lip (Fig. 61.9). The lesion initially presents as an edematous patch of erythema that proceeds to become an indurated, scaly plaque with a whitish-gray to brown discoloration. Vertical fissuring and crusting can occur and become painful. Vesicles may arise and burst, giving rise to superficial ulcerations which may then become secondarily infected. Eventually, warty nodules may form that can undergo malignant change to squamous cell carcinoma.

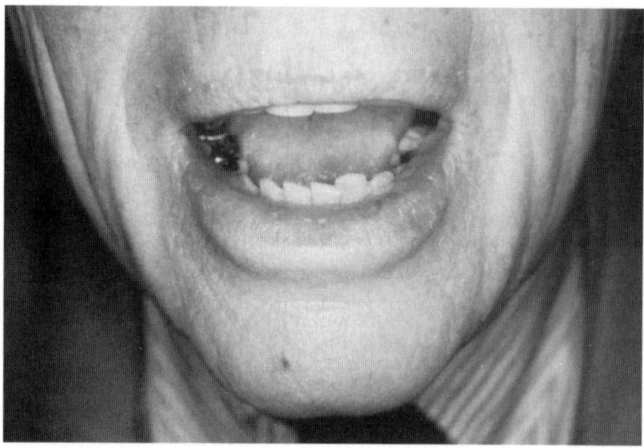

FIGURE 61.9. Actinic cheilitis. This confluent, hyperkeratotic tumor of the lip is sun-induced. It can be asymptomatic or develop painful fissures. It is premalignant and biologically analogous to actinic keratoses on nonmucosal skin.

The main risk factor for developing actinic cheilitis is chronic sun exposure, as evidenced by a higher incidence of the lesions in people living in sunny regions, outdoor workers, and light-skinned individuals. Its decreased incidence in women may be due to the protective effects of lipstick.[1]

Histologically, actinic cheilitis displays regions of flattened, atrophic epithelium adjacent to acanthotic areas. The epidermis may also show disordered maturation without evidence of nuclear atypia. Lymphocytes and plasma cells infiltrate the dermis, which frequently shows signs of solar elastosis such as basophilic degeneration of collagen and elastic fibers.

Actinic cheilitis is often confused with other forms of cheilitis, including lupus erythematosus, lichen planus, and eczematous cheilitis secondary to contact allergies. The occasional blistering may lead to the diagnosis of sunlight-induced herpes simplex virus infection. The propensity for these lesions to develop into squamous cell carcinomas should alert the clinician to look for features associated with malignancy such as ulceration, persistent flaking or crusting, generalized atrophy with focal areas of leukoplakia, and a red and white blotchy appearance with an ill-defined vermilion border. Any lesion with suspicious features should be biopsied.

If the lesion is not indurated, a trial of conservative therapy with opaque zinc oxide or titanium dioxide containing sunscreens and topical steroids may be initiated.[28] If after 1 month the lesion persists, a more aggressive mode of therapy, such as laser ablation, is indicated. $CO_2$ laser ablation, with a cure rate approaching 100%, is the preferred treatment.[32,33] Topical 5% fluorouracil applied three times daily for 9–15 days results in brisk ulceration followed by a 2- to 3-week period of healing.[20] Even with good compliance, recurrence rates range from 17% at 22 months to 60% at 50 months.[29,30] The most aggressive form of therapy is vermilionectomy which involves excision of the vermilion border down to orbicularis oris muscle with subsequent advancement of a labial mucosal flap.[20] This procedure should be reserved for cases of actinic cheilitis that do not respond to laser or other therapy.

## Cutaneous Horn

Cutaneous horn is a clinical term used to describe a hard, yellowish-brown, conical outgrowth of skin resembling an animal's horn. Cutaneous horns develop on sun-exposed areas such as the scalp, upper part of the face, tips of the ears, and dorsum of hands; they may grow as long as 20 cm.[31] They can arise from benign, premalignant, or malignant epidermis. A clue to malignancy can be obtained from close examination of the surrounding epidermis: If the skin surrounding the lesion is normal looking or slightly acanthotic, the lesion is more likely to be benign, whereas inflammation or induration of the surrounding skin suggests malignancy. More than 60% of cutaneous horns are derived from benign lesions of epithelial hyperplasia, such as warts, skin tags, seborrheic keratoses, and nevi: 23% arise from premalignant lesions including actinic keratoses, and the remaining 16% arise from mostly squamous cell cancer. Horns arising from basal cell cancer and metastatic and sebaceous carcinomas have been reported.[31,32] Therefore, all horns should be biopsied with care to preserve their base by performing a deep tangential biopsy.

## Bowen's Disease (Squamous Cell Carcinoma In Situ)

Squamous cell carcinoma in situ that localizes to the epidermis is referred to as Bowen's disease. It typically arises in individuals over the age of 60 and has a slow, indolent course. It is listed as a premalignant lesion because it is so early in development; however, it must be considered a noninvasive squamous cell cancer. Approximately 5% of the lesions progress to invasive squamous cell carcinomas.[25] Bowen's disease initially presents as a slowly enlarging, solitary, erythematous macule with a sharp border that can evolve into a scaling, crusting plaque usually 2–6 cm in diameter (Fig. 61.10). When this lesion develops on the penis, it is known as erythroplasia of Queyrat. Its etiology has been associated with chronic exposure to solar radiation, psoralin ultraviolet A-range (PUVA) radiation and environmental toxins such as arsenic, mustard gas, pesticides, and herbicides.

The clinical differential diagnosis for Bowen's disease includes other papulosquamous diseases such as psoriasis and lichen simplex, superficial basal cell carcinoma, actinic keratoses, and dermatitis. If a lesion looks suspicious for Bowen's disease, a punch or shave biopsy should be performed.

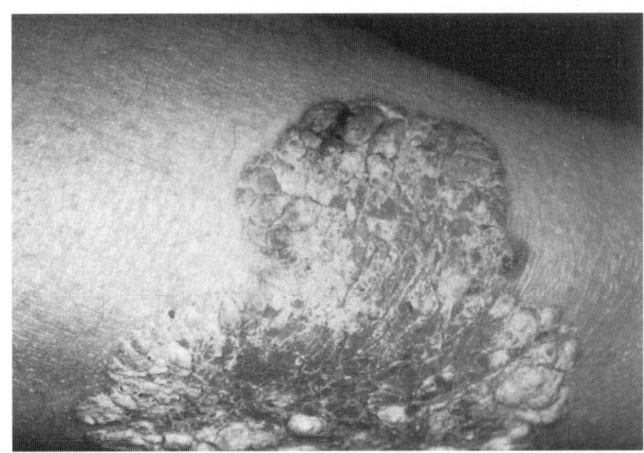

FIGURE 61.10. Bowen's disease. This large plaque is an extreme example of squamous cell carcinoma in situ, or Bowen's disease. This noninvasive cancer does extend down the hair follicles, so failure to eradicate cells at this level, surgically or otherwise, may result in recurrence of the tumor.

Microscopically, the keratinocytes in Bowen's disease demonstrate full-thickness atypia with hyperchromatic nuclei, loss of polarity, and decreased intracellular adhesions. Giant cells and mitotic figures may be frequent. By definition, tumor cells do not invade the dermis, although the upper dermis may be infiltrated by mononuclear inflammatory cells.

Bowen's disease can be treated with excision, Mohs microscopically-controlled surgery, or with destructive therapies such as cryotherapy, electrodesiccation and curettage, topical 5-FU, and photodynamic therapy. Histologic confirmation should be obtained before using one of the destructive modalities. Cryotherapy has had reported cure rates of 90–97%.[27,33] A recently emerging treatment modality, called photodynamic therapy, uses a photosensitive drug (e.g., 5-aminolevulinic acid) that is activated by visible light to target tumor cells selectively. Two independent studies, both involving a small series of patients, cited highly variable recurrence rates with photodynamic therapy, ranging from 0% to 50%.[33,34] This rather large discrepancy highlights the need for further evaluation of this new treatment. The disadvantage with topically applied treatments such as photodynamic therapy and 5-FU is that the vehicle often cannot penetrate the epidermal appendages. If the tumor involves the appendages, it may not be fully eradicated. Excision, where feasible, remains the therapeutic method of choice for Bowen's disease. Because of indistinct borders, Mohs surgery is often the treatment of choice.

## Lentigo Maligna (Hutchinson's Freckle)

Lentigo maligna is a noninvasive disorder of atypical melanocytes that is limited to the epidermis. This flat, pigmented lesion, which occurs on sun-exposed skin of elderly fair-skinned individuals, develops into invasive melanoma in about 1 of 750 cases per year.[35] As a result of its malignant potential, most authors view lentigo maligna as a melanoma in situ.[36] The major risk factors for developing lentigo maligna are chronic cumulative sun exposure and light skin color. Additional risk factors include a history of severe sunburn, radiation exposure, estrogen and progesterone therapy, and use of nonpermanent hair dyes.[37] The incidence of lentigo maligna, which is slightly higher in women, peaks during the seventh and eighth decades, with the average age of onset around 65 years.

Clinically, lentigo maligna presents as a uniformly flat macule ranging in size from 3 to 20 cm with intralesional variations in color (Fig. 61.11). The color often appears as a disorganized array of dark browns and black on a background of light browns, pinks, and white. The borders of the lesion tend to be irregular with a notched, "geographic" shape.

Biopsy of lentigo maligna reveals cytologically atypical melanocytes proliferating in distinct units throughout the basal layer. These atypical melanocytes can extend far beyond the clinical margin, leading to a high recurrence rate. The black areas of the lesion often display the most advanced histologic changes, whereas the white areas show signs of regression. Regions with surface irregularity may signify invasion.

Several lesions can simulate lentigo maligna, including seborrheic keratoses, solar lentigos, pigmented actinic keratoses, pigmented Bowen's disease, and pigmented basal cell carcinoma. However, these lesions tend to be more uniform in color and rarely contain black pigment. Seborrheic keratoses can usually be distinguished based on their characteristic verrucous surface. Solar lentigos do not exhibit variations in color as seen with lentigo maligna. Pigmented carcinomas tend to be raised. To confirm the diagnosis an incisional punch or shave biopsy that includes the most darkly pigmented area is recommended.

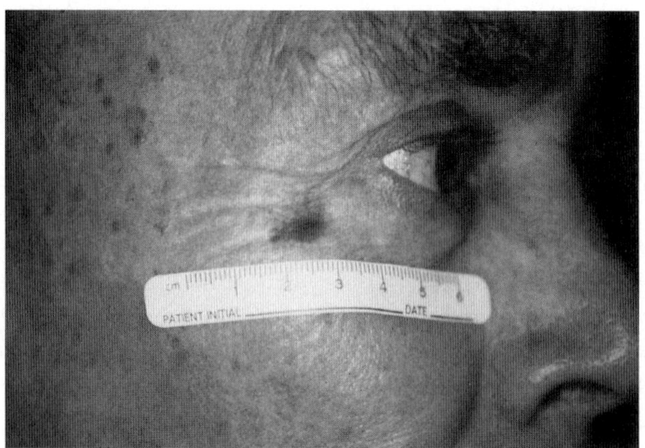


FIGURE 61.11. Lentigo maligna. Lentigo meligna is melanoma in situ on sun-exposed skin. Although this lesion is small and easy to excise, these lesions are often long-standing in the elderly and can reach sizes that make excision unfeasible.

Complete excision is the treatment of choice for lentigo maligna. Conventional surgery, which provides a 91% cure rate[38] should be performed with 0.5 cm margins.[40] Although Mohs surgery is recommended by some, this treatment for lentigo maligna is still controversial.

Some lesions of lentigo maligna do not lend themselves to excision because of their size, location, or the patient's co-morbid conditions. In such cases, destructive therapies such as $CO_2$, ruby laser, electrodesiccation and curettage, x-ray therapy, cryotherapy, and topical azelaic acid have been attempted. The major disadvantages of these methods is that they do not provide a specimen to rule out melanoma, and they may fail to treat the adnexal melanocytes, which cause recurrence. This is suggested by the high recurrence rate of lentigo maligna for these modalities, which is 20–25% for electrodesiccation and curettage, 38% for irradiation, 6–36% for cryotherapy, and up to 100% for azelaic acid.[37] Q-switched ruby lasers may be more efficacious because the laser can penetrate the reticular layer of the dermis so adnexal melanocytes can be destroyed. Success has been reported with ruby lasers,[39] but the long-term recurrence rate with this method remains to be determined. Cryosurgery may leave scar tissue that can mask recurrence, especially the development of an invasive desmoplastic melanoma. This is the greatest risk of incomplete treatment of melanoma in situ, and the patient must be aware of this potential problem.

## Malignant Lesions

### Epidermis

#### *Squamous Cell Carcinoma*

Squamous cell carcinoma (SCC) is a malignant tumor of keratinocytes that arises on sun-damaged skin and on mucous membranes. The incidence is higher in men but occurs more frequently on the extremities in women. Individuals over the age of 55 are most frequently affected, with the mean age of onset at 60 years.

The biggest risk factor for SCC is chronic sun exposure. This is evidenced by the fact that SCC occurs most frequently in geographic areas that have sunny weather, such as California and Florida. Also, the incidence of SCC is higher in people who work outdoors. Other predisposing factors include prior trauma, frostbite, ionizing radiation, PUVA therapy, chemical carcinogens (arsenic, topical hydrocarbons, nitrogen mustards), viruses (human papilloma virus 16, 18, 31, 33, and 35), and chronic immune suppression. These tumors may also arise from preexisting pathology, such as chronic inflammation, discoid lupus, burn scars (Marjolin's ulcer), osteomyelitis sinuses, lichen planus, and chronic stasis dermatitis.[28] Squamous cell carcinoma of the lip may additionally be provoked by tobacco use.

Squamous cell carcinomas may arise from a premalignant lesion such as actinic keratosis or Bowen's disease. A clue to malignant transformation in these lesions is increased induration and inflammation. Patients often notice that the lesion is growing or changing. Well-differentiated SCC typically presents as an indurated papule, plaque, or nodules with overlying adherent hyperkeratosis. It may become ulcerated or bleed with formation of a crust in the center of the lesion, which becomes surrounded by a firm, scaly margin. If the carcinoma is undifferentiated, it may appear as a fleshy, granulating nodule with central ulceration and a necrotic base surrounded by a soft, fleshy margin.

Clinically, squamous cell carcinomas may resemble actinic keratoses, amelanotic melanoma, granulomatous disease, or adnexal tumors. If a lesion appears suspicious for malignancy, it must be biopsied (Fig. 61.12).

Dermatopathologic examination typically reveals masses, strands, or buds of atypical keratinocytes that proliferate downward into the dermis. In well-differentiated tumors, keratin pearls may be present within or on the surface of the tumor. Undifferentiated types display multiple mitoses and little evidence of keratinization.

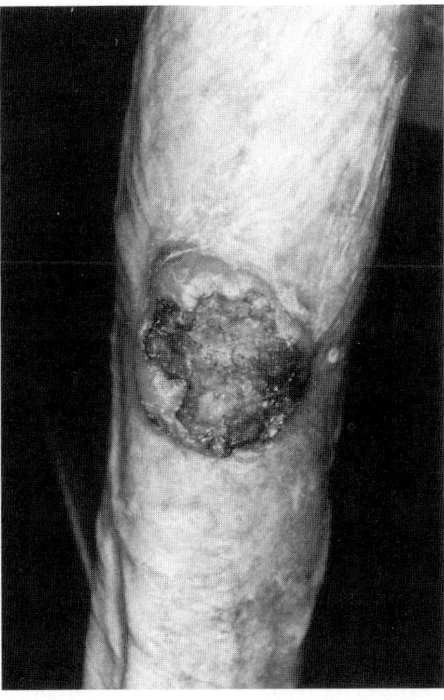

FIGURE 61.12. Squamous cell cancer. This large lesion was present for many months. Occasionally, when the lesion arises over a 6-week period, keratoacanthoma, a variant of squamous cell cancer, must be considered.

Squamous cell carcinoma has the capacity to metastasize. The metastatic potential depends on the location and size. For SCCs arising from actinic keratoses, the metastatic propensity reportedly is low (approximately 0.5%),[41] whereas for those developing de novo the risk is 7.7–13.7%. Tumors arising from preexisting pathology, such as a burn scar, have a much higher rate of metastasis, estimated to be 20–40%. Patients presenting with an SCC should have regional lymph nodes examined clinically as regional lymphadenopathy is often the first sign of metastasis. The prognosis for tumors that have spread is poor, with an estimated 5-year survival rate of 26% if the metastases is localized to regional lymph nodes and 23% if it has spread systemically.[42]

The most widely used method for treating SCC is excision. Simple excision with clinically normal appearing margins is often satisfactory for most lesions up to 0.5 cm. For tumors that are large, deep, recurrent, have aggressive histology, or are located in areas with high metastatic potential (e.g., lips or ears), the Mohs microscopically-controlled technique should be performed. This is a tissue-sparing, office-based method that involves the sequential excision and mapping of the cancer. The final defect can be repaired immediately or allowed to heal by second intention. The Mohs technique has a 3% recurrence rate compared to an 8% recurrence rate with simple excision. As an alternative to excision, small, superficial tumors (<0.5 cm) can be destroyed by electrodesiccation and curettage, which yields a 5-year cure rate of approximately 90%.[43] Radiotherapy can also be effective but is typically reserved for patients who cannot undergo surgery. It is extremely expensive. The treatment regimen can take as much as 4 to 6 weeks. This method relies on patient compliance; but if used properly it has a 5-year cure rate similar to that of electrodesiccation and curettage.[43] Topical retinoids have also been shown to be effective for some inoperable lesions.[44] Lymph node dissection is not indicated unless nodes are clinically involved.

## Squamous Cell Carcinoma

### *Keratoacanthoma*

Keratoacanthomas (KAs) are well-differentiated squamous cell carcinomas. Interestingly, in some cases they have a tendency to resolve spontaneously. KAs most often appear as isolated lesions on sun-exposed areas of middle-age or older individuals. The lesion begins as a small papule that rapidly enlarges over 4–8 weeks to form a painless nodule often containing a central keratin-filled crater. KAs occur twice as often in men as in women and are most commonly found in Caucasians.

The cause of this lesion is unknown. Human papilloma virus has been extracted from some lesions. Others have been associated with carcinogens including UV light, pitch and tar, and other factors such as trauma and immune suppression.[45] Keratoacanthomas are usually solitary, but multiple lesions may arise as part of a syndrome such as Ferguson Smith-type KAs or generalized eruptive KAs of Grybowski.[46]

Clinically, KAs appear as well-differentiated SCCs. Unlike most other SCCs, KAs have a history of rapid onset and are not usually associated with regional adenopathy. The history of rapid onset (4–6 weeks) is key to making the diagnosis and distinguishing the KA from other types of SCC. Biopsy of a suspicious lesion is required because KAs can behave like aggressive SCCs, especially when located in the central face. Biopsy can be incisional or excisional so long as it is inclusive of the full depth of the tumor down to the subcutaneous fat. Typically, a biopsy shows a large central crater filled with keratin surrounded by buttressing epidermis. The keratinocytes often display nuclear atypia, mitotic figures, and dyskeratoses. KA-type SCCs can be differentiated from other SCCs histologically based on the presence of epithelial "lips," which surround a central crater, and intradermal abscesses with an accompanying inflammatory infiltrate—both of which are rare features of SCCs.

There remains legitimate controversy regarding the true nature of KAs. Some authorities classify the lesion as a benign epithelial neoplasm,[47] whereas others view it as an aborted malignancy[46] or a well-differentiated subtype of SCC.[5,48] We consider KAs a form of SCC. Unlike other malignancies, KAs can spontaneously regress; but they have also been shown to metastasize and ultimately be fatal.[48] Therefore the question of identity becomes more than an academic exercise. KAs should be definitively treated.

Currently, most experts favor early intervention to minimize local tissue destruction because localized scarring can occur with spontaneous healing. Those who favor excision recommend Mohs micrographic surgery because it allows resection with tumor-free margins while maximizing the preservation of normal skin. In a study examining 42 KAs treated by Mohs surgery, the rate of recurrence after 2 years was less than 3%.[49] Other treatment modalities include curettage and desiccation, which has a recurrence rate of 8%[46]; cryosurgery, which is beneficial for small early KAs; radiation therapy; topical and intralesional 5% 5-FU; interferon-α2a; podophyllin; intralesional steroids; systemic retinoids; methotrexate; and bleomycin.[45] Any lesion that does not respond promptly to the above nonsurgical treatments by involuting at least 60% should be excised.[20]

### *Basal Cell Carcinoma*

Basal cell carcinoma (BCC) is the most common type of malignant cutaneous neoplasm, constituting 75% of all nonmelanoma skin cancers. BCCs are not thought to be associated with a premalignant lesion. Though they are slow-growing tumors that rarely metastasize, they can be locally invasive and destructive. BCCs most commonly present on habitually sun-exposed skin of the head and neck in fair-skinned individuals over the age of 40. Aside from chronic sun exposure, race, and age, other predisposing factors include genetic defects (basal cell nevus syndrome, xeroderma pigmentosa), radiation exposure, immune suppression, and prolonged contact with chemical carcinogens such as arsenic. The incidence of BCC in the United States has been estimated at approximately 150 cases per 100,000 per year, with men more frequently affected. One exception to this trend is in the lower extremities where the lesion arises three times more commonly in women.

The exact cell of origin of the BCC is unclear. It is thought to be derived from either the pleuripotent stem cells of the epidermis or the matrix cells of epidermal appendages. The tumor celis histologically resemble cells in the stratum basale with compact, basophilic nuclei and scant cytoplasm. However, in support of the epidermal appendage derivation, tumor development occurs only in areas of the skin that have the capacity to develop hair follicles. The tumor cells grow in strands or nests into the dermis, displaying little anaplasia and infrequent mitosis. In the more aggressive variants, finger-like strands can extend far into dermal stroma, inducing significant fibrosis. A lymphocytic dermal infiltrate is usually present.

Morphologically, BCCs can be classified into at least five subtypes: noduloulcerative, cystic, pigmented, superficial, and morpheaform. The most common is the noduloulcerative variant, which usually starts as a small papule that slowly enlarges, appearing translucent and pearly with a rolled border and overlying telangiectasias (Fig. 61.13). As the tumor continues to grow, it eventually exceeds its own blood supply and becomes necrotic and centrally ulcerated ("rodent ulcer"). Most lesions are asymptomatic, though some are pruritic. Noduloulcerative BCC may resemble melanocytic nevi, sebaceous hyperplasia, molluscum contagiosum, SCC, verruca vulgaris, keratoacanthoma, amelanotic melanoma, atypical fibroxanthoma, or an adnexal tumor.

Cystic BCC presents as a smooth, pearly, erythematous nodule that rarely ulcerates. The cystic cavity may contain necrotic debris or mucin. This BCC variant can mimic other cystic lesions, such as epidermal inclusion cysts and hidrocystomas.

Excess melanin from epidermal melanocytes can cause BCCs to become pigmented. Pigmented BCCs often occur in dark-skin individuals and can be clinically confused with melanoma. Unlike melanoma, the border of this BCC variant is often rolled, and the color is more brown in contrast to the black-brown hue of malignant melanomas.

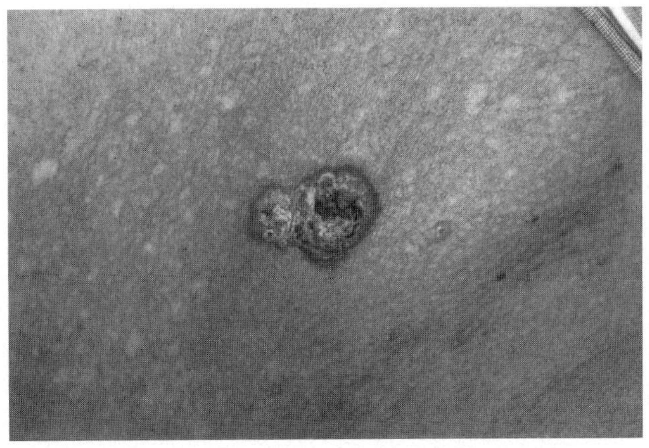

FIGURE 61.13. Basal cell cancer. The large nodule on the chest is a neglected basal cell cancer. Actinic keratoses and severe solar damage are noted on the rest of the chest.

The superficial variety of BCC appears as erythematous, scaling, raised plaques with irregular borders. This tumor does not invade beyond the superficial dermis. It is often confused clinically with benign processes (e.g., localized eczema or psoriasis). Superficial BCCs can be differentiated by biopsy.

The most aggressive BCC subtype is the morpheaform, or infiltrative, variety. This locally destructive lesion typically appears as a whitish, sclerotic patch with ill-defined borders. It is firm upon palpation due to the extensive fibrous stroma associated with the tumor. The strands of tumor cells can travel well beyond the clinical margin, making these tumors notoriously difficult to treat without the Mohs technique. Their differential includes morphea and scar.

Knowledge of the pathology of these five BCC subtypes is important when choosing the appropriate method of treatment. In addition to taking the morphologic type into account, the proper treatment modality also depends on the size and location of the tumor, the age and co-morbid conditions of the patient, and patient preference. For patients who can undergo surgical procedures, electrodesiccation and curettage, simple excision, and Mohs surgery are the methods of choice. With the exception of the morpheaform subtype, most small, nonrecurrent varieties of BCC can be treated with electrodesiceation and curettage (ED&C) or simple excision, achieving a cure rate exceeding 95%.[50] The disadvantage of ED&C is that it may cause hypopigmentation and scarring, especially when used for deeply invasive tumors. Similarly, it is not possible to know if the margins were negative. For large tumors (>1–2cm), recurrent cancer, infiltrative subtypes, or cancer in the central face, which may invade deeply, Mohs surgery is recommended. It has the added benefit of being tissue-sparing and offers a cure rate approaching 99% for nonrecurrent lesions.[51]

Nonsurgical treatment methods include radiotherapy and topical chemotherapy with agents such as 5-FU. Topical 5-FU is reserved for the superficial type of BCC because the drug cannot readily penetrate beyond the dermis. The treatment course lasts up to 6 weeks, thus requiring high patient compliance. Radiotherapy can also be used to eradicate BCCs but is best reserved for patients who cannot undergo therapy with other destructive modalities. Cutaneous atrophy at the treatment site is a common side effect. The overall cure rate approaches 90%.

For patients presenting with a BCC, regular follow-up is essential because a patient with one BCC has a 36% chance of developing a second lesion within 5 years.[51] The protective use of sunscreen should be emphasized.

### Melanoma

Melanoma is a malignant tumor of epidermal melanocytes. It is the eighth most prevalent cancer in the United States and its incidence is rising faster than any other cancer.[52] The current lifetime risk of developing melanoma is estimated 1 in 75. Age-specific incidence rates are highest in elderly patients, who have a worse prognosis than their younger counterparts. Elderly patients have different incidences of melanoma subtypes than younger patients. Men and women are equally affected, though women have a better overall survival rate.

The main risk factor for melanoma is high exposure to UV radiation, as evidenced by the rise in incidence

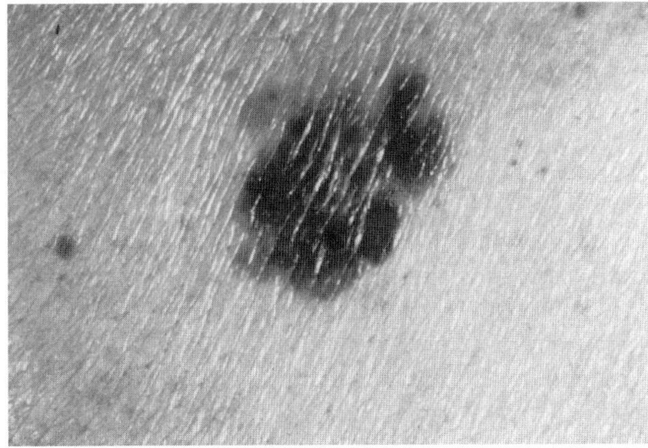

FIGURE 61.14. Melanoma. This example of superficial spreading melanoma has irregular edges and variable coloration. The elderly have an increased incidence of melanoma relative to other age groups, and early diagnosis is the key to cure.

of the tumor in areas close to the equator. Other predisposing factors include fair skin, blond or red hair, a family history of melanoma, congenital or atypical nevi, an inability to tan, and an antecedent blistering sunburn. Pigment is a protective factor, as evidenced by the relative rarity of this tumor in dark-skinned individuals.

Melanoma is traditionally classified into four clinicopathologic variants: superficial spreading melanoma, nodular melanoma, lentigo maligna melanoma, and acral lentiginous melanoma. Superficial spreading melanoma is the most common subtype, comprising 40–50% of all cases in patients over age 65[53] (Fig. 61.14). It typically presents on the trunk in men and on the legs in women in their fourth to fifth decade. The tumor often begins as a small pigmented lesion that develops irregular features such as marked variations in color involving reds, whites, blues, and blacks, as well as notched borders. The tumor is characterized by a radial growth phase, where malignant cells are localized to epidermis, followed by a vertical growth phase, which signifies dermal invasion. The vertical phase is often heralded by elevation, bleeding, and ulceration of the lesion.

The second most common type of melanoma in the elderly is the nodular melanoma. These lesions present as elevated, dome-shaped, reddish brown nodules most commonly localized on the legs or trunk; they arise more frequently in men. They have a short radial growth phase and therefore rarely grow to more than 2cm in diameter. As they quickly enter their vertical growth phase, nodular melanomas can easily bleed and ulcerate and develop satellite lesions with surrounding inflammation. The tumors begin to develop during the fifth to sixth decade and peak in incidence during the eighth decade, with men more frequently affected than women. Nodular melanomas must be differentiated from seborrheic keratoses, pyogenic granulomas, and pigmented BCCs. Amelanotic melanoma, considered a subtype of nodular melanoma, displays a similar rapid vertical growth phase. These lesions may lack pigment and prove difficult to diagnose.

Lentigo maligna melanoma develops in preexisting lentigo maligna lesions. Although lentigo maligna melanoma represents only 5% of all malignant melanoma cases, it accounts for 10% of melanoma cases in the elderly. Lentigo maligna is, in essence, an in situ melanoma that is in a horizontal growth phase that can last for decades before proceeding to a vertical growth phase. Transformation to lentigo maligna melanoma is defined as invasion of malignant melanocytes into the dermis and is heralded by the formation of an elevated nodule.

Like lentigo maligna melanoma, acral lentiginous melanoma also occurs with a disproportionately greater frequency in the geriatric population. Unlike all other subtypes, these melanomas most commonly affect Blacks, Asians, and Hispanics. Acral lentiginous melanoma appears as a macular, hyperpigmented area with irregular borders and a blue to black color; it arises on the plantar or palmar surfaces of the hands and feet, on mucous membranes, and in the subungual areas of nails. Its location often leads to the mistaken diagnosis of traumatic hematoma. These tumors are therefore often diagnosed at an advance stage. When the tumor becomes invasive, it may appear nodular, ulcerate, and bleed.

Any pigmented lesion that has undergone changes in size, shape, or color or is inflamed, oozing, bleeding, or itching, or is larger than 5mm in diameter should be considered malignant until proven otherwise by biopsy. The most frequently occurring colors in melanomas are shades of brown, red, white, or blue and black. Pinks and reds signify inflammation. A blue color arises from light scattering from pigment deep within the dermis (Tyndal effect) and is a bad prognostic indicator.

Lesions suspicious for malignant melanoma should undergo elliptical or tangential excisional biopsy. Shave biopsies are inadvisable because they may prevent accurate determination of lesion thickness. For large tumors or those that cannot be completely excised because of their anatomic location, an incision biopsy, such as a punch or elliptical biopsy, is recommended.

Although prognosis depends on the type of lesion and the presence or absence of lymphatic invasion, the single strongest prognostic factor is the depth of the melanoma measured in millimeters (Breslow depth) (Table 61.1). Clark's level is no longer used as reliably as the Breslow depth. Clinical subtypes of melanoma vary in aggressiveness. For example, lentigo maligna melanoma has a long horizontal growth phase and

TABLE 61.1. Clark and Breslow Classification of Malignant Melanoma

| Clark level | | |
|---|---|---|
| I | Tumor does not invade dermis | |
| II | Tumor invades only papillary dermis | |
| III | Tumor expands into papillary dermis but spares reticular dermis | |
| IV | Tumor invades reticular dermis | |
| V | Tumor invades subcutaneous tissue | |
| **Breslow level (mm)** | **Excision margin** | **Sentinel node studies** |
| 1 | 1 cm | No |
| 1.0–1.5 | 1–2 cm | +/– |
| 1.5–4.0 | 2–3 cm | + |
| 4 | 3 cm | No |

Breslow depth does not correspond precisely to Clark level. It is used for prognostic purposes and to direct therapy.

TABLE 61.2. American Joint Committee on Cancer Classification for Malignant Melanomas

| Stage | Classification | Clinical criteria |
|---|---|---|
| IA | T1N0 | Breslow I or Clark I or II |
| IB | T2N0 | Breslow II or Clark III |
| IIA | T3N0 | Breslow III or Clark IV |
| IIB | T4N0 | Breslow IV or Clark V |
| III | Any T, N1 | Invasion of tumor to one set of regional nodes positive |
| IV | Any T, N2 | Invasion of tumor to more than one set of regional nodes |
| | *or* M1 | Secondary cutaneous metastases |
| | *or* M2 | Visceral metastases |

is usually recognized prior to the development of metastases.

The American Joint Committee on Cancer has devised a classification system for melanomas that not only takes depth into account but also the extent of regional or distant metastasis. This clinical staging system is designated the TNM classification and is described in Table 61.2. Stage I and II represent localized disease, stage III advances to regional disease, and stage IV involves distant metastases.

Elderly patients tend to present with poor prognostic features and therefore have increased mortality rates. Malignant melanoma in the elderly tend to be thicker upon presentation than those occurring in younger patients. A recent study found that malignant melanoma occurring in patients over the age of 60 were almost double the thickness of those in individuals under the age of 50 (2.4 vs. 1.3 mm).

Patients presenting with malignant melanoma should be thoroughly evaluated. This includes a complete physical examination with special attention to a total body skin examination and lymph node palpation; laboratory studies including a complete blood count with differential, liver function tests, and chest radiography. Treatment of malignant melanoma depends on the depth and stage of the tumor. Though most authorities agree that excision of the primary lesion is the mainstay of treatment for all stages of malignant melanoma, there is controversy surrounding the size of the excisional margin and the method with which the margins are obtained.

In situ lesions (Clark's level I) are by definition noninvasive. The goal for treatment of these lesions is to remove all tumor cells locally. If standard excision is the method of choice, usually 0.5 cm margins are adequate for in situ lesions. However, if the tumor is clinically ill-defined, wider margins may be advisable. The tumor margins should be assessed with a Wood's lamp and marked prior to administration of anesthesia. Lesions that have invaded the dermis and are up to 1 cm in depth require excisional margins of 1 cm. Margins of 2 cm are recommended for lesions with a Breslow depth of 2–3 mm. Any lesion more than 4 mm thick should undergo wide excision with margins up to 3- to 5-cm.

The role of lymphadenectomy in malignant melanoma is controversial. Prophylactic lymphadenectomy is not indicated for in situ lesions, as they do not show evidence of metastasis. For superficially invasive melanomas, most authorities deem it necessary only if regional lymph node involvement is clinically apparent. Patients with intermediate thickness melanoma without palpable lymph nodes can undergo selective lymphadenectomy involving the sentinel node. The sentinel node is the first node that drains a regional lymphatic plexus and is thought to be representative of all nodes in that region. Sampling the sentinel node may be a good method for selecting patients who could benefit from more extensive lymphadenectomy.

Lymph node involvement carries a poorer prognosis, with the 5-year survival dropping to 40%. Treatment for Breslow depth >3 mm or regional disease involves excision with appropriate margins and consideration of lymph node dissection. Isolated limb perfusion is sometimes used to administer chemotherapeutic agents for regional disease. Because malignant melanoma is considered a radioresistant tumor, the role of irradiation in metastatic disease is mostly palliative.

Patients who have been diagnosed with melanoma need close follow-up because they can be prone to developing a second primary tumor. Most recurrences arise within the first 18 months but can be delayed for many years. Follow-up should occur four times a year for the first year and at least twice a year thereafter.[52] Early recognition of local or regional disease or new primary melanoma lesions in this population can significantly alter the mortality rate from malignant melanoma.

## *Atypical Fibroxanthoma*

Atypical fibroxanthoma is a spindle cell neoplasm of mesenchymal origin that develops on the head and neck of elderly, light-skinned individuals. The tumor clinically presents as an asymptotic, solitary, firm nodule less than 2 cm in diameter that may go on to ulcerate or hemorrhage. Grossly, the lesion can resemble a SCC, BCC, epidermoid cyst, or pyogenic granuloma. Risk factors for tumor development include chronic sun exposure, radiation, local trauma, and male gender.

One of the unique features of this tumor is its malignant-appearing histology. Aside from the well-defined tumor margins and absence of deep tissue invasion, the tumor appears histologically indistinguishable from malignant fibrous histiocytoma.[54] It is composed of sheets of polymorphous cells, including spindle cells, large polyhedral cells, and giant multinucleated cells with marked nuclear atypia and numerous mitoses.

Despite its malignant histology, atypical fibroxanthoma has a relatively benign course. Metastases, however, have been reported.[55] This has led some to classify the tumor as a superficial form of malignant fibrous histiocytoma,[54] therefore requiring treatment.

Mohs surgery is the treatment for atypical fibroxanthoma. Electrodesiccation and curettage is not considered adequate treatment because it does not remove the deep tissue, which may be invaded by tumor cells. The recurrence rate with tumors treated by wide excision is estimated to be approximately 10%.[56] Mohs surgery, which has the added advantage of conserving more normal tissue than wide excision, is currently the preferred method of treatment.

### *Merkel Cell Carcinoma*

Merkel cell carcinoma is a rare malignant tumor of the neuroendocrine-derived Merkel cell. This tumor of unknown etiology typically affects persons over the age of 65, though cases of Merkel cell carcinoma developing in individuals as young as 7 years of age have been reported.[57] There have been no documented differences in incidence between men and women.

Merkel cell carcinoma manifests as rapidly growing, solitary, pink to violet nodules on sun-exposed skin. These firm, dome-shaped nodules are most commonly distributed on the head and neck (50% of cases), extremities (40% of cases), and trunk (10% of cases) of elderly Caucasians. Most tumors are less than 2 cm in diameter but can grow to become as large as 15 cm. The overlying epidermis may be shiny and intact with fine telangiectasias, or it may be ulcerated. Because of its nonspecific presentation, Merkel cell carcinoma is often not recognized prior to biopsy. It is often misdiagnosed as an SCC or BCC, a desmoplastic or amelanotic melanoma, a pyogenic granuloma, or a cutaneous metastasis of an oat cell carcinoma. Light microscopy may not be diagnostic because the tumor mimics other poorly differentiated small-cell tumors. The tumor is typically comprised of clusters of small, undifferentiated cells possessing scant cytoplasm that form trabeculae separated by strands of connective tissue. The trabeculae may extend down to the subcutaneous fat but do not invade the epidermis. Frequent mitoses and necrotic cells may be present. Confirmation of the diagnosis requires electron microscopy, which shows the characteristic secretory granules and paranuclear fibrous bodies.

Once the diagnosis of Merkel cell carcinoma is confirmed, a complete physical examination with attention to regional lymphadenopathy and organomegaly and a thorough workup including chest radiography and baseline laboratory tests, with liver function tests, should be performed. Merkel cell carcinoma is an aggressive tumor with a high rate of local recurrence and early lymphatic spread. The treatment protocol for Merkel cell carcinoma is stage-dependent. Stage I, or localized disease that has no evidence of lymph node metastases, is treated by wide local excision with 2.5- to 3.0-cm margins. For localized tumors, adjuvant therapy with irradiation of the primary site is frequently employed, especially if there is angiolymphatic invasion. The role of prophylactic lymph node dissection is controversial, but most recent literature advocates its use because of the high incidence of lymph node metastases in early disease.[58,59]

About 55–65% of stage I lesions progress to stage II or locally recurrent disease.[60] Stage II disease is defined by metastases to regional lymph nodes. Treatment involves wide excision of the primary tumor in combination with irradiation and lymph node dissection. Despite aggressive therapy, which may also involve chemotherapy, the mortality rate of stage II disease approaches 66%.

One-third of all patients with Merkel cell carcinoma progress to stage III, or systemic disease involving distant metastases. Stage III disease is managed primarily with chemotherapy. Chemotherapeutic agents similar to those used for treating oat cell carcinoma have been shown to be the most efficacious. The prognosis for stage III disease is grim, with an expected survival of less than 12 months. The average length of survival may increase with the use of in vitro assays that test a tumor's specific drug sensitivities, allowing optimization of the chemotherapeutic regimen.[60] Due to the high recurrence rate of this tumor, patients who initially present should be followed monthly for the first 2 months, every 2–3 months for the next 2 years, and every 6 months thereafter.

## Dermis

### *Angiosarcoma*

Angiosarcoma is a rare malignant tumor arising from vascular or lymphatic endothelium. The lesion often starts as a dusky erythematous, painless, "bruise-like" macule with poorly differentiated margins that proceeds to ulcerate and hemorrhage as the cancer progresses to involve subcutaneous tissue. This aggressive vascular tumor, which affects men more commonly than women, has a predilection for the scalp and face of patients over the age of 60. Its etiology is unknown, although human herpes virus 8[61] and environmental toxins such as Thorotrast, vinyl chloride, and insecticides have been implicated.[62] Chronic lymphedema and chronic radiodermatitis are predisposing factors.

Histologically, the early stages of the tumor show endothelial cell-lined intercommunicating vascular channels that appear to dissect through collagen bundles.[63] During the latter stages, the tumor loses its organized vascular pattern and develops into large cell aggregates. There is subsequent formation of solid nodules of tumor followed by invasion of vascular channels.

The clinical appearance of this purple, flat, indistinctly bordered tumor often leads to its misdiagnosis as a bruise, hemangioma, infection such as chronic cellulitis, localized lymphedema, or scarring alopecia.[63] The persistence of a bruise-like lesion, especially in an elderly individual, should warrant a biopsy. Angiosarcomas are frequently recognized late in their course, which partially accounts for their poor prognosis, with an estimated 5-year survival 12–27%.[62] They tend to recur locally and metastasize early in their course. Important prognostic factors include size, grade, and location of the tumor. High-grade tumors >5 cm located on the face tend to carry the worst prognosis.[62,63] The mainstay of treatment is local excision combined with radiotherapy. Other forms of treatment, such as chemotherapy, have not been shown to alter survival significantly.[61]

## Conclusions

Common cutaneous neoplasms that afflict the elderly arise from the epidermis or dermis and can be benign, premalignant, or malignant. Recognizing these lesions is important for providing care to a growing geriatric population. A regular, thorough skin examination enables physicians to monitor the elderly patient closely for the development of precancerous and cancerous lesions, which can ultimately be life-threatening. Minimizing the risk of malignant tumor development by avoiding precipitating factors such as UV radiation should be emphasized in this population.

## References


1. Champion RH, Burton JL, Ebling FJG. Rook/Wilkinson/Ebling Textbook of Dermatology, 5th ed. Oxford: Blackwell Scientific, 1992.
2. Lavker RM, Zheng PS, Dong G. Aged skin: a study by light, transmission electron, and scanning electron microscope. J Invest Dermatol 1987;88:44s–51s.
3. Richey ML, Richey HK, Fenske NA. Age-related skin changes: development and clinical meaning. Geriatrics 1988;43:49–64.
4. Gilchrest BA, Blog FB, Szabo G. Effects of aging and chronic sun exposure on melanocytes in human skin. J Invest Dermatol 1979;73:141–143.
5. Lynch PJ. Dermatology, 3rd ed. Baltimore: Williams & Wilkins, 1994.
6. Epstein E. Treatment of basal cell papillomas. Br J Dermatol 1995;133:492.
7. Grekin RC, Shelton RM, Geisse JK, et al. 510-nm Pigmented lesion dye laser: its characteristics and clinical uses. J Dermatol Surg Oncol 1993;19:380–387.
8. Kopera D, Hohenleutner U, Landthaler M. Q-switched ruby laser application is safe and effective for the management of actinic lentigo (topical glycolic acid is not). Acta Dermatol Venerol 1996;76:461–463.
9. Beacham BE. Common skin tumors in the elderly. Am Fam Physician 1992;46:138–163.
10. Banik R, Lubach D. Skin tags: localization and frequencies according to sex and age. Dermatologica 1987;174:180–183.
11. Beitler M, Eng A, Kilgour AB, et al. Association between acrochordons and colonic polyps. J Am Acad Dermatol 1986;14:1042–1044.
12. Leavitt J, Klein I, Kendricks BS, et al. Skin tags: a cutaneous marker for colonic polyps. Ann Intern Med 1983;98:928–930.
13. Gould BE, Ellison C, Greene HL, et al. Lack of association between skin tags and colonic polyps in a primary care setting. Arch Intern Med 1988;148:1799–1800.
14. Mendelson BC, Masson JK. Xanthelasma: follow-up on results after surgical excision. Plast Reconstr Surg 1976;58:535–538.
15. Eedy DJ. Treatment of xanthelasma by excision with secondary intention healing. Clin Exp Dermatol 1996;21:273–275.
16. Alster TS, West TB. Ultrapulse $CO_2$ laser ablation of xanthelasma. J Am Acad Dermatol 1996;24:848–849.
17. Liu HH, Perry HO. Identifying a common—and benign—geriatric lesion. Geriatrics 1986;41(7):71–76.
18. Greenbaum SS. The treatment of chondrodermatitis nodularis chronica helicis with injectable collagen. Int J Dermatol 1991;30:291–294.
19. Lawrence CM. The treatment of chondrodermatitis nodularis with cartilage removal alone. Arch Dermatol 1991;127:530–535.
20. Morganroth GS, Leffell DJ. Nonexcisional treatment of benign and premalignant cutaneous lesions. Clin Plast Surg 1993;20:91–104.
21. Coldiron BM. The surgical management of chondrodermatitis nodularis chronica helicis. J Dermatol Surg Oncol 1991;17:902–904.
22. Long D, Maloney ME. Surgical pearl: surgical planning in the treatment of chondrodermatitis nodularis chronica helicis of the antihelix. J Am Acad Dermatol 1996;35:761–762.
23. Taylor MB. Chondrodermatitis nodularis chronica helicis: successful treatment with the carbon dioxide laser. J Dermatol Surg Oncol 1991;17:862–864.
24. Taylor MB. Chondrodermatitis nodularis chronica helicis. J Dermatol Surg Oncol 1992;18:641.
25. Sober AJ, Burstein JM. Precursors to skin cancer. Cancer 1995;75:645–650.
26. Marks R, Rennie G, Selwood T. The relationship of basal cell carcinomas and squamous cell carcinomas to solar keratoses. Archives of Dermatology 1988;124(7):1039–1042.
27. Graham G. Advances in cryosurgery during the past decade. Cutis 1993;12:365–372.
28. Ries WR, Aly A, Vrabec J. Common skin lesions of the elderly. Otolaryngol Clin North Am 1990;23:1121–1139.
29. Robinson JK. Actinic cheilitis: a prospective study comparing four treatment methods. Arch Otolaryngol Head Neck Surg 1989;115:848–852.
30. Picascia DD, Robinson JK. Actinic cheilitis: a review of the etiology, differential diagnosis and treatment. J Am Acad Dermatol 1987;17:255–264.
31. Thappa DM, Garg BR, Tahduea J, et al. Cutanous horn: a brief review and report of a case. J Dermatol 1997;24:34–37.

32. Yu RC, Pryce DW, MacFarlane AW, et al. A histopathological study of 643 cutaneous horns. Br J Dermatol 1991; 124:449–452.
33. Morton CA, Whitehurst C, Moseley H, et al. Comparison of photodynamic therapy with cryotherapy in the treatment of Bowen's disease. Br J Dermatol 1996;135:766–771.
34. Fijan S, Honigsmann H, Ortel B. Photodynamic therapy of epithelial skin tumors using delta-aminolaevulinic acid and desferrioxamine. Br J Dermatol 1995;133:282–288.
35. Weinstock MA, Sober AJ. The risk of progression of lentigo maligna to lentigo maligna melanoma. Br J Dermatol 1987; 116:303–310.
36. Somach SC, Taira JW, Pitha JV, et al. Pigmented lesions in actinically damaged skin. Arch Dermatol 1996;132: 1297–1302.
37. Cohen LM. Lentigo maligna and lentigo maligna melanoma. J Am Acad Dermatol 1995;33:923–936.
38. Coleman WP, Davis RS, Reed RI, et al. Treatment of lentigo maligna and lentigo maligna melanoma. J Dermatol Surg Oncol 1980;6:476–479.
39. Thissen M, Westerhof W. Lentigo maligna treated with ruby laser. Acta Derm Venereol 1997;722:163.
40. National Institutes of Health Consensus Conference. Diagnosis and treatment of early melanoma. JAMA 1992; 268:1314–1319.
41. Silverberg N, Silverberg L. Aging and the skin. Postgrad Med 1989;86:131–144.
42. Kwa RE, Campana K, Moy RL. Biology of cutaneous squamous cell carcinoma. J Am Acad Dermatol 1992; 26:1–20.
43. Proper SA, Rose PT, Fenske NA. Non-melanomatous skin cancer in the elderly: diagnosis and management. Geriatrics 1990;45:57–65.
44. Lippman SM, Meyskens FL. Treatment of advanced squamous cell carcinoma of the skin with isotretinoin. Ann Intern Med 1987;107:494–501.
45. Warner DM, Flowers F, Ramos-Caro FA. Solitary keratoacanthoma (squamous cell carcinoma): surgical management. Int J Dermatol 1995;34:17–19.
46. Schwartz RA. Keratoacanthoma. J Am Acad Dermatol 1994;30:1–19.
47. Fitzpatrick TB, Johnson RA, Palano MK, et al. Color Atlas and Synopsis of Clinical Dermatology: Common and Serious Diseases, 2nd ed. New York: McGraw-Hill, 1992.
48. Hodak E, Jones RE, Akerman AB. Solitary keratoacanthoma is a squamous cell carcinoma: three examples with metastases. Am J Dermatopathol 1993;15:332–342.
49. Larson PO. Keratoacanthomas treated with Mohs' micrographic surgery (chemosurgery). J Am Acad Dermatol 1987;16:1040–1044.
50. Gloster HM, Brodland DF. The epidemiology of skin cancer. Dermatol Surg 1996;22:217–226.
51. Keller KL, Fenske NA, Glass LF. Cancer in the older patient. Clin Geriatr Med 1997;13:339–361.
52. Bernstein SC, Brodland DG. Melanoma in the geriatric patient. J Geriatr Dermatol 1995;3:271–279.
53. Mackie RM, Young D. Human malignant melanoma. Int J Dermatol 1984;23:433–443.
54. Fish FS. Soft tissue sarcomas in dermatology. Dermatol Surg 1996;22:268–273.
55. Helwig EB, May D. Atypical fibroxanthoma of the skin with metastases. Cancer 1986;57:368.
56. Davis JL, Randle HW, Zalla MJ, et al. A comparison of Mohs micrographic surgery and wide excision for the treatment of atypical fibroxanthoma. Dermatol Surg 1997;23:105–110.
57. Ratner D, Nelson BR, Brown MD, et al. Merkel cell carcinoma. J Am Acad Dermatol 1993;29:143–156.
58. Smith DE, Bielamowicz S, Kagan AR, et al. Cutaneous neuroendocrine (Merkel cell) carcinoma: a report of 35 cases. Am J Clin Oncol 1995;18:199–203.
59. Victor NS, Morton B, Smith JW. Merkel cell cancer: is prophylactic lymph node dissection indicated? Am Surg 1996;62:879–822.
60. Krasagakis K, Almond-Roesler B, Zouboulis CC, et al. Merkel cell carcinoma: report of ten cases with emphasis on clinical course, treatment, and in vitro drug sensitivity. J Am Acad Dermatol 1997;36:727–732.
61. McDonagh DP, Liu J, Gaffey MJ, et al. Detection of Kaposi's sarcoma-associated herpesvirus-like DNA sequence in angiosarcoma. Am J Pathol 1996;149:1363–1368.
62. Marc RJ, Poen JC, Tran LM, et al. Angiosarcoma: a report of 67 patients and a review of the literature. Cancer 1996; 77:2400–2406.
63. Jones WE. Some special skin tumors in the elderly. Br J Dermatol 1990;122(suppl 35):71–75.

# 62 Orthopedic Injuries

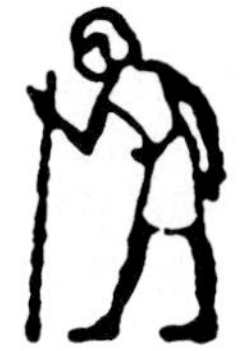

Jeffrey H. Richmond, Kenneth J. Koval, and Joseph D. Zuckerman

Orthopedic injuries in the elderly are a major challenge in geriatric medicine. This rapidly growing segment of the population sustains a disproportionate number of fractures and, more than other age groups, requires treatment tailored to the needs of the entire patient, not just the fracture itself. As with all orthopedic care, the goal of treatment in the elderly is to restore or improve on their preinjury level of function. However, a fracture superimposed on the combination of preexisting physical infirmities and systemic medical problems often makes for a tenuous ability to maintain independent living status. Immobilization of an extremity or dependence, even temporarily, on a walker or crutches can render a patient unable to manage independently and so require institutional care. Consideration of this point is mandatory when planning the treatment of any orthopedic injury in the elderly.

This chapter reviews general concepts in orthopedic injury management in the elderly. It gives specific consideration to the more common fractures seen in this age group: femoral neck, intertrochanteric and subtrochanteric hip fractures, ankle fractures, proximal humerus fractures, distal radius fractures, vertebral compression fractures, and pathologic fractures.

## Preinjury Status

The goal of treatment is to restore, or in some cases improve on, the preinjury level of patient function. This requires a detailed history of the functional status of the patient prior to injury and any medical and cognitive history that would affect the surgical options and potential for rehabilitation. For example, a community ambulator who sustains an intertrochanteric hip fracture requires urgent operative fracture fixation followed by aggressive rehabilitation, whereas a nonambulator or someone without the potential for rehabilitation due to cognitive or other physical infirmities may benefit more from nonoperative treatment consisting of pain control and early mobilization to a wheelchair. In either case, full evaluation of the entire patient is necessary to make the appropriate management decision.

## Systemic Disease

Elderly individuals often have systemic medical problems that affect injury management. Preexisting cardiac or pulmonary disease, common in the elderly population, diminishes a patient's ability to tolerate prolonged recumbency, surgery, and rehabilitation. The American Society of Anesthesiologists (ASA) classification of surgical risk is an excellent tool for assessing this preoperative risk. The ASA rating classifies patients as: I, normal and healthy; II, mild systemic disease; III, severe systemic disease, not incapacitating; IV, severe incapacitating disease, constant threat to life; and V, moribund. Diabetes, in addition to complicating cardiac disease, increases the risk of wound complication and infection; and it can cause delayed fracture union, particularly in surgically treated patients.[1] Peripheral vascular disease, either arterial or venous, also complicates wound healing and fracture union in operative cases; skin breakdown is problematic with closed treatment even in a well-padded cast. Thromboembolic disease is a significant complication after lower extremity injury, particularly following surgery. Because of concomitant medical problems, the elderly have a lower tolerance for pulmonary emboli than do younger, healthier individuals.

Medical problems have an impact on intraoperative patient care. Factors such as intraoperative hypotension, sometimes associated with cemented hip arthroplasty, or pulmonary complications from intubation must be considered in each individual patient. Most orthopedic procedures can be performed under general or regional anesthesia; recent studies of hip fracture patients have reported no difference in long- or short-term mortality or functional outcome after spinal or general anesthesia.[2,3]

The cognitive status of the patient is a critical factor in the success of orthopedic treatment. Unlike many other areas of surgery, active participation of the patient in rehabilitation following injury often determines his or her ultimate functional outcome. Alzheimer's disease, mental deficits from cerebrovascular accident, Parkinson's disease, and other forms of senile dementia, may render a patient unable to participate actively in the rehabilitation necessary in virtually all fracture cases, both operative and nonoperative. Careful consideration of these factors is necessary when determining the optimum management for a given patient's injury. For example, a patient with severe dementia who sustains an unstable displaced distal radius fracture may not be a good operative candidate because of an inability to be cooperative with the therapy necessary to achieve a good functional outcome; the same functional outcome may be achieved in this patient with closed treatment and acceptance of a suboptimal-appearing radiograph.

However, a patient with mild deficits may rely on optimum motor performance to compensate for cognitive deficiencies; this patient should be treated aggressively.

In addition, previous functional limitations must be considered when planning treatment to allow a patient to maintain as much function as possible. For example, a patient with a hemiplegia secondary to stroke may not tolerate immobilization of the functional extremity to treat a humeral shaft fracture. Though these injuries are usually treated closed, surgery may be considered to permit more rapid restoration of function of the patient's only usable arm.

Given the complexity of a patient's preinjury functional, medical, and cognitive status, determining the appropriate management of a geriatric fracture patient is difficult. Many factors must be taken into consideration, and the decision should be made by the surgeon after discussion with the patient and family members, and with consulting geriatricians, anesthesiologists, physiatrists, and other appropriate specialists.

## Osteopenia

Osteopenia, or decreased bone mass, is frequently encountered in the elderly. It is caused by either osteoporosis (decreased bone density with normal bone mineralization) or osteomalacia (decreased bone matrix mineralization with or without a change in bone density). Although some degree of osteopenia is found in nearly all healthy elderly patients ("senile osteoporosis"), treatable causes must be investigated in severe cases. These include nutritional deficiency such as low calcium and high phosphate intake, malabsorption syndromes, metabolic derangements such as hyperparathyroidism, Cushing's disease or renal pathology, and local causes such as tumors.[4] Risk factors for significant osteopenia include female sex, northern European ancestry, multiparity, sedentary life style, and excessive alcohol intake.

Osteopenia undoubtedly complicates fracture treatment and healing, although its incidence in patients with common geriatric injuries such as femoral neck fractures remains controversial.[5–7] The major complication is difficulty obtaining stable internal fixation of hardware in osteopenic bone. Stable internal fixation is the fundamental principle behind modern operative fracture care, as it permits early range of motion and weight-bearing on the operated extremity while maintaining fracture reduction. Osteopenia results in poor screw purchase and increased risk of screw pullout from the bone, leading to fixation failure. The risk of fixation failure often leads to prolonged immobilization despite operative treatment, which in turn can cause "disuse osteopenia," further complicating fracture treatment. Adjunctive use of methylmethacrylate (bone cement) can augment screw fixation in osteopenic bone.

In addition, experience has shown that osteopenic patients are at increased risk for nonunion. This is because the fracture callus formed is not as dense or as well organized as is fracture callus formed by nonosteopenic bone. Bone grafting is often necessary at the time of surgery to augment natural bone stock in osteopenic patients. Frequently it must be of allograft or synthetic origin, as the iliac crest in osteopenic patients is a poor source of cancellous bone.

## Hip Fractures

Hip fractures are devastating injuries that have a significant impact on the patient's functional, medical, and psychological status. They also have a significant financial impact on society. The number of these fractures doubled from the mid-1960s through the 1980s to approximately 250,000 in the United States alone, costing approximately $8.7 billion annually. The number of hip fractures is predicted to double today's levels by the year 2050.[8–10]

The incidence of hip fracture increases after age 50, possibly doubling each decade. These fractures occur more commonly in women than in men by a ratio of at least 2:1. Along racial lines, they are most common in white women, followed by white men, black women, and black men. This is thought to be due to differences in bone density between whites and blacks.[11–13] Institutionalized patients are at increased risk for hip fracture, probably secondary to a higher prevalence of dementia, associated medical conditions, and the use of psychotropic medications.[14–16]

Hip fractures in the elderly are predominantly low energy injuries sustained during a simple fall. They are grouped according to anatomic location: intracapsular (femoral neck) or extracapsular (intertrochanteric or subtrochanteric). In our experience, 95% of hip fractures in patients over age 65 are either of the femoral neck or intertrochanteric type. These two fracture patterns occur with almost equal frequency.[17]

Patients typically present to a medical facility shortly after the injury complaining of hip or groin pain and an inability to bear weight on the affected extremity. With displaced fracture patterns, the affected leg is often shortened relative to the noninjured side. In addition, the leg is often held with the hip in some degree of flexion and external rotation. This is the position of maximum capsular volume, and hence maximal comfort, when there is a capsular hematoma. Initial orthopedic evaluation includes a careful neurovascular survey of the involved extremity, an assessment of skin integrity, and a complete examination to rule out other associated trauma, particularly to the head. Medical consultation is obtained, anticipating probable surgical treatment; at the Hospital For Joint Diseases we usually obtain a baseline arterial blood gas determination at the time of hospital admission.

Radiographic evaluation consists of an anteroposterion (AP) view of the pelvis and AP and cross-table lateral views of the affected hip. Frog lateral views are avoided because of the discomfort involved and the risk of displacing a nondisplaced fracture. Plain radiographs are usually sufficient for evaluating hip fractures. However, there are cases where a fracture is suspected based on the mechanism of injury and the symptoms, but it cannot be seen on plain radiographs. In the case of femoral neck fractures, an internal rotation view may reveal an otherwise unrecognized fracture. Technetium bone scanning is a sensitive indicator of occult hip fracture, though it may require 2–3 days to become positive. Magnetic resonance imaging (MRI) has been shown to be as accurate as bone scanning and can be reliably performed within 24 hours of injury.[18]

Ideal management of a patient who sustains a fracture of the proximal femur is prompt operative stabilization followed by early mobilization. Surgical treatment is preferred owing to the prolonged period of non-weightbearing required of nonoperative treatment along with the unacceptable rates of mortality, medical morbidity, and fracture nonunion or malunion. In addition, it has been shown that operative treatment is the most economic management.[19] Regardless of the treatment selected, deep venous thrombosis (DVT) and subsequent pulmonary embolism is a cause of significant morbidity and mortality following hip fracture and surgery. Warfasin (Coumadin) has been the standard means of prophylaxis in the past, but it requires close monitoring of coagulation profiles and takes 24–48 hours before it becomes effective. Subcutaneous unfractionated heparin has been shown to be inadequate for DVT prophylaxis following orthopedic surgery. More recently, low-molecular-weight heparin preparations have been used successfully for DVT prophylaxis in orthopedic patients.[20] At the Hospital For Joint Diseases, we treat nearly every hip fracture patient postoperatively and up to 12 hours preoperatively, with subcutaneous low-molecular-weight heparin and have had satisfactory results. If anticoagulation is contraindicated, inferior vena cava filter placement may be considered.

## Outcome Following Hip Fracture

Results after fracture care are divided into two categories. Fracture-related outcomes refer to healing characteristics of the fracture, such as union versus nonunion and the quality of the reduction. Functional outcomes address patient satisfaction, the level of pain, and the ability of the patient to use the injured extremity and perform activities of daily living. Restoration of the preinjury level of functioning is the goal of all surgery. A recent prospective study performed at the Hospital For Joint Diseases of 336 hip fracture patients who were community dwelling and ambulatory at the time of injury demonstrated that at the 1-year follow-up, 41% had regained their preinjury level of ambulatory function, 40% remained community or household ambulators but were now dependent on assistive devices, 12% became exclusively household ambulators, and 8% became nonfunctional ambulators. Statistical analysis demonstrated that patients younger than age 85, those with preoperative ASA ratings of I or II, and those who sustained intertrochanteric fractures were the most likely to regain their ambulatory status. Male sex and the absence of preexisting dementia have also been shown to correlate with better functional recovery.[21]

Mortality following hip fracture remains a significant problem. Studies of elderly patients with operatively treated hip fractures demonstrated a 1-year mortality of approximately 25%.[22,23] The highest mortality rate is within the first 6 months following fracture; and after 1 year mortality rates return to that of age-matched controls. Lowest 1-year mortality was seen among patients who were community dwelling and cognitively intact prior to injury (12.6%).[24] In this patient population, age >85 years, preinjury dependence for basic activities of daily living, a history of malignancy other than skin cancer, an ASA rating of operative risk of III or IV, and the development of one or more in-hospital complications was associated with increased mortality at the 1-year follow-up.

The timing of surgery for stabilization of a hip fracture is controversial. Studies have demonstrated both increased and decreased mortality associated with delaying surgery anywhere from 1 day to several days following injury to allow medical stabilization.[25–27] These conflicting studies were based on heterogeneous patient populations and were not well controlled for confounding variables. At the Hospital For Joint Diseases, 367 hip fracture patients who were cognitively intact, home-dwelling, and ambulatory prior to injury were studied prospectively with regard to 1-year mortality based on the number of calendar days between the injury and surgery. Age, sex, and number and severity of comorbidities were controlled. In this controlled population, surgical delay of more than two calendar days doubled the risk of 1-year mortality.[28] Although the issue of surgical delay has yet to be completely resolved, it seems reasonable to say that operative fixation should be performed within two calendar days of the injury; if surgery is to be delayed beyond two calendar days, the physicians involved must address how much improvement can be expected in the patient's medical condition by delaying surgery and weigh it against the risks of prolonging the period of recumbency.

Postoperatively, the goal of treatment is to mobilize the patient as soon as possible to avoid the morbidity associated with bed rest. Some have recommended restricted weight-bearing until there are radiographic signs of fracture healing, but biomechanical data have shown that non-weight-bearing places significant stress across the hip owing to muscular contraction at the hip and knee. A simple activity such as moving onto a bedpan places forces up to four times body weight across the hip joint.[29] Furthermore, elderly patients may have difficulty complying with partial or non-weight-bearing status because of the demands it places on their upper extremities and balance. Therefore attempting to protect the hip from stress is unrealistic. Studies have shown that patients allowed to bear weight as tolerated initially tend to limit the load on the operative extremity voluntarily. Over time, they gradually increase the weight on the affected limb.[30,31] Therefore we allow almost all geriatric hip fracture patients to bear weight as tolerated immediately following surgery.

## Femoral Neck Fractures

Femoral neck fractures are intracapsular fractures that occur between the base of the femoral head and the intertrochanteric line. The intracapsular location of the fractures has significant bearing on treatment and fracture healing. The blood supply to the femoral head arises distal to the femoral neck from the medial and lateral femoral circumflex arteries. These vessels anastomose to form an extracapsular ring at the base of the femoral neck, which then gives rise to ascending arterial branches that traverse the neck and form a ring at the base of the femoral head. This is the predominant blood supply to the femoral head. These arteries are at risk for disruption following an intracapsular fracture. Additional blood supply comes from the artery of the ligamentum teres through the acetabulum, but this blood supply may be insufficient to maintain viability of the femoral head if the other blood supply is disrupted.

Various classification systems have been proposed for femoral neck fractures. A useful classification system is one that is simple and conveys information pertinent to the treatment and prognosis of the fracture. Given the treatment options and potential complications discussed below, the most useful classification of femoral neck fractures is either nondisplaced/impacted (Fig. 62.1A) or displaced (Fig. 62.1B).

There is general agreement that nondisplaced/impacted femoral neck fractures should be treated by internal fixation using multiple screws or pins placed in parallel across the femoral neck (Fig. 62.1C). This is accomplished under radiographic guidance and can be done through a small (3–4 cm) incision laterally over the greater trochanter or percutaneously with small stab incisions. Impacted fractures have some degree of inherent stability and have been treated nonoperatively. However, a disimpaction rate of 8–15% has been reported in patients treated nonoperatively.[32] Therefore it is generally recommended that all nondisplaced and impacted femoral neck fractures be treated by internal fixation. Nonunion occurs in fewer than 5% of these fractures and osteonecrosis in approximately 8%.[33] Following surgery, these patients are allowed to bear weight as tolerated with assistive devices.

Displaced femoral neck fractures pose a greater problem in surgical planning than do nondisplaced fractures. The two operative treatment options are closed reduction/internal fixation or prosthetic replacement of the proximal femur (Fig. 62.1D). The decision whether to preserve or replace the femoral head must be individualized and depends on multiple factors. Preservation of the native femoral head is generally preferred, provided that there is not significant degenerative joint disease prior to injury. As such, we attempt to treat displaced fractures by reduction/internal fixation in most patients under age 75, provided anatomic reduction can be achieved in a timely manner. This is done after counseling the patient and family that reoperation may be required if there is failure of fixation, nonunion, or symptomatic avascular necrosis. Primary prosthetic replacement in the form of hemiarthroplasty is generally performed in: (1) patients whose chronologic age is more than 75 years regardless of preinjury activity level or health; (2) patients under age 75 with a low preinjury level of functioning or poor general health; and (3) fractures with a significant degree of comminution. Total hip arthroplasty may be performed if there is preexisting degenerative hip disease.

Internal fixation of displaced fractures is performed the same way as for nondisplaced fractures but after a closed or open reduction. A closed reduction is preferred owing to less soft tissue disruption; open reduction is generally reserved for young patients in whom preservation of the femoral head is preferred to prosthetic replacement. The risk of nonunion or avascular necrosis of the femoral head following reduction/internal

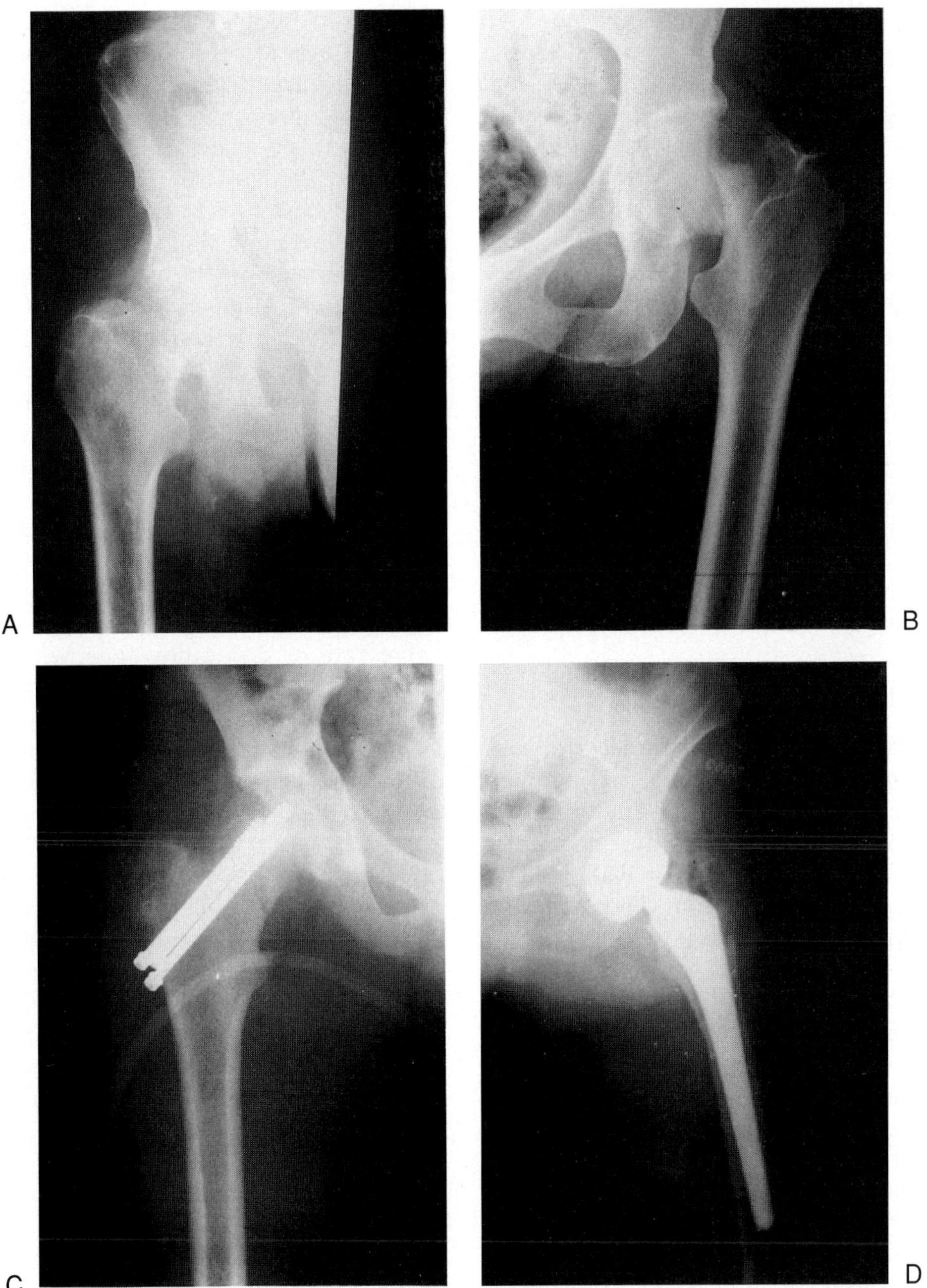


FIGURE 62.1. A. Anteroposterior (AP) view of a nondisplaced/impacted femoral neck fracture. B. AP view of a displaced femoral neck fracture. C. Three screws transfixing a nondisplaced/impacted femoral neck fracture. D. Unipolar hemiarthroplasty.

fixation following displaced fractures ranges up to 30%.[34] Nonunion requires reoperation 75% of the time, and approximately 30% of cases of avascular necrosis require further surgery.

Prosthetic replacement, consisting of a hemiarthroplasty (replacement of only the proximal femur) or total hip arthroplasty (replacement of the proximal femur and insertion of an acetabular component), can also be performed. Hemiarthroplasty can be unipolar (where the prosthesis has a single articulation with the native acetabulum) or bipolar (where the head of the femoral prosthesis articulates with a polyethylene liner surrounded by a metal shell, which in turn articulates with the native acetabulum, allowing motion at two sites). Results of unipolar versus bipolar hemiarthroplasty have been shown to be equivalent.[35] Prosthetic replacement is generally accomplished via a posterolateral incision and is a more extensive surgical procedure than simple internal fixation, involving more operating time and more blood loss. It can be performed under general or spinal anesthesia.

Hemiarthroplasty can lead to acetabular erosion and subsequent groin pain. Primary total hip replacement is associated with more surgical morbidity than hemiarthroplasty. Additionally, there is a greater risk of postoperative dislocation following primary total hip arthroplasty when performed for fracture rather than for degenerative disease.

Most femoral neck fractures should be treated operatively, although there are cases when nonoperative treatment is indicated, particularly for a demented, nonambulatory patient or one with an incapacitating illness prior to injury. The treatment goal in these patients, as with all fracture patients, is to return them to their preinjury level of function. This may be accomplished without surgery by early mobilization to a wheelchair with adequate analgesia, thereby avoiding the morbidity of prolonged recumbency and acceptance of the resulting malunion or nonunion.

## Intertrochanteric Fractures

Intertrochanteric fractures are extracapsular fractures occurring in the region distal to the femoral neck between the greater and lesser trochanters. The bone in this region is dense trabecular bone that transmits and distributes the large forces borne by the hip. A vertical wall of dense bone, the calcar femorale, extends from the posteromedial aspect of the femoral shaft to the posterior aspect of the femoral neck. The calcar functions as an internal strut, transmitting significant amounts of stress. The greater trochanter is the site of insertion of the abductor and short external rotator muscles, both important for gait. The iliopsoas, the primary flexor of the hip, inserts on the lesser trochanter. The bone in the intertrochanteric region is well vascularized; hence the healing problems seen with intracapsular fractures are rarely encountered with extracapsular fractures.

Numerous classification systems have been described for intertrochanteric hip fractures. The key to treatment of these fractures is the ability to obtain a stable reduction. A stable reduction is dependent on posteromedial cortical continuity (the region of the calcar femorale).[36] As such, the simplest, most useful way to classify intertrochanteric fractures is stable versus unstable. Stability can be predicted, on plain radiographs, if the lesser trochanter is intact (Fig. 62.2A). With an unstable fracture pattern, the lesser trochanter is usually detached (Fig. 62.2B).

Intertrochanteric fractures are usually treated surgically, most often under general or spinal anesthesia. After induction of anesthesia, reduction is achieved in a closed fashion. If adequate closed reduction cannot be achieved, an open reduction is performed. This operation is usually done through a lateral thigh incision. The implant of choice is a sliding hip screw (Fig. 62.2C). The hip screw is inserted through the femoral neck into the femoral head under radiographic guidance. The lateral unthreaded portion of the screw inserts into a barrel attached to a sideplate, which is fixed to the femoral shaft by screws. The hip screw may then "telescope," or slide, within the barrel when the patient bears weight, allowing controlled impaction of the fracture. The ability of the screw to slide within the barrel is what prevents the screw from migrating superiorly in the femoral head and "cutting out" when the fracture "settles." This is particularly important if the fracture pattern is unstable. If the greater trochanter is fractured, it is advantageous to reduce the fragment and stabilize it using wires. A fractured lesser trochanter generally does not need to be reduced unless it is large.

Primary prosthetic replacement of the proximal femur may be considered if there is a significant degree of fracture comminution. However, this procedure is associated with a longer operating time, increased blood loss, and a higher rate of dislocation than with elective total hip arthroplasty. Nonoperative treatment may be considered if the patient was a nonambulator prior to injury or is deemed a high surgical risk. These patients are mobilized to a chair as soon as possible with appropriate analgesia, with acceptance of the resulting malunion or nonunion.

## Subtrochanteric Fractures

Subtrochanteric fractures begin at or below the level of the lesser trochanter and involve the proximal femoral shaft (Fig. 62.3). Typically, these fractures are high-energy injuries that occur in young patients, but they can be sustained during a minor fall in an older patient with osteopenic bone. They are far less common in the elderly than femoral neck or intertrochanteric fractures.

As with intertrochanteric fractures, the simplest classification system is based on the stability of the fracture pattern, which in this case is also dependent on the degree of comminution of the posteromedial cortex. Regardless of the fracture pattern, these injuries can almost always be treated with an intramedullary nail, with locking screws that may or may not traverse the femoral neck. High rates of union have been achieved with these devices. A plate and screws can also be used, particularly if the fracture extends into the greater trochanter, which makes insertion of the intramedullary nail technically difficult.

# Ankle Fractures

Ankle fractures are a common injury in the elderly. The ankle is a modified hinge joint consisting of the talus, medial malleolus, and lateral malleolus. The medial and lateral malleoli are the distal ends of the tibia and fibula,

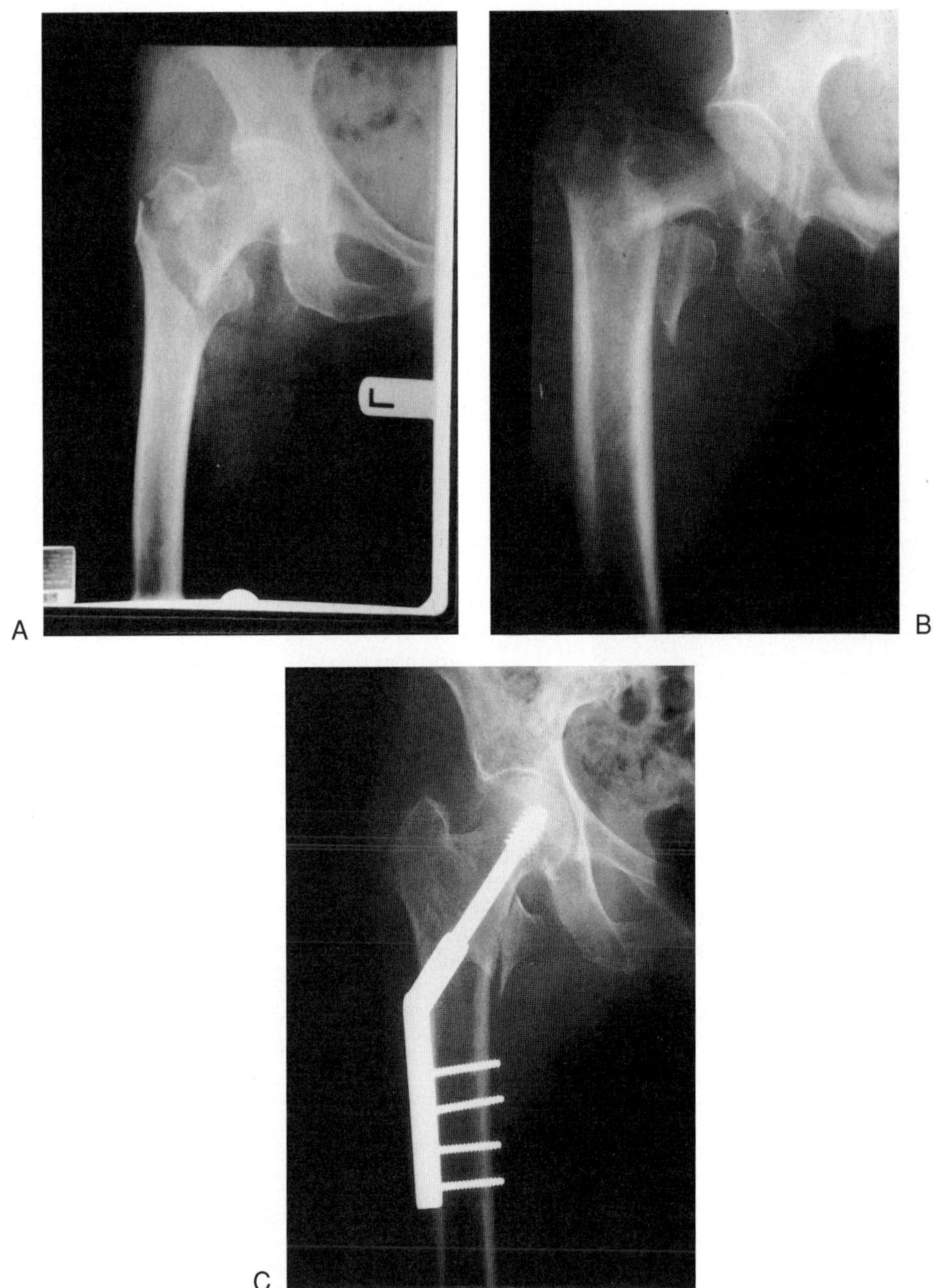


FIGURE 62.2. A. AP view of a stable intertrochanteric hip fracture. Note that the lesser trochanter is intact. B. AP view of an unstable intertrochanteric hip fracture. The lesser trochanter is fractured. C. Sliding hip screw and side plate transfixing an unstable intertrochanteric fracture.

respectively. The superficial and deep layers of the deltoid ligament form a thick triangular structure that connects the medial malleolus with the navicular, calcaneus, and talus bones. The distal tibia and fibula are attached via four ligaments that together form a complex called the syndesmosis. Laterally, the fibula is joined to the talus and calcaneus by a complex of three ligaments.

Ankle fractures generally occur when a patient twists or rotates the foot relative to the lower leg, often after a misstep or fall. The fracture pattern reflects the relative strength of the ligaments compared to bone in the elderly, osteopenic patient. Fractures typically occur as avulsions caused by a tensioned ligament pulling on weak bone or by impact between bone and bone. Pure ligamentous injuries are also encountered and have the same effect on ankle stability as a corresponding fracture.

Patients presenting with an acute ankle fracture are usually unable to bear weight on the affected side. There is frequently edema and ecchymosis, and with displaced fractures there is obvious deformity. A careful examina-

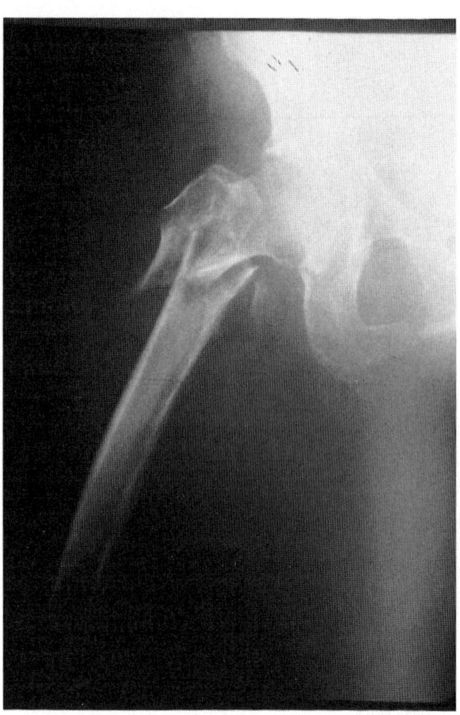

FIGURE 62.3. AP view of a displaced subtrochanteric hip fracture.

tion must be performed, and associated injuries ruled out, particularly to the hip, wrist, and head. Standard radiographic evaluation includes AP, lateral, and oblique views of the ankle. An oblique view taken in 10–15 degrees of internal rotation reveals the ankle mortise, the continuous clear space medial, lateral, and superior to the talus. The entire length of the fibula must be examined radiographically if there is medial ankle tenderness or injury without associated fibular injury apparent on the ankle views.

The specific fracture pattern varies depending on the mechanism of injury. Multiple classification systems have been described, such as the Lauge-Hansen and Danis-Weber systems; but they are beyond the scope of this chapter. Treatment of these fractures is aimed at restoring normal congruity to the ankle mortise. The specific treatment depends on the stability of the fracture and patient considerations. Stable injuries are defined as those that can withstand physiologic stress without displacement.

An isolated nondisplaced malleolar fracture without evidence of disruption of the syndesmotic ligaments (as evidenced by widening of the medial clear space, loss of the normal 10mm tibia/fibula overlap on the AP view, or a more proximal fibular fracture) can be treated by immobilization in a short leg cast once swelling subsides. These patients may be allowed to bear weight on the extremity.

Unstable fracture patterns are those with bimalleolar involvement, disruption of the syndesmosis, or a unimalleolar fracture with displacement of the talus. These fractures must be reduced because even slight displacement of the talus from under the tibia may result in degenerative changes within the ankle joint.[37] Reduction may be achieved via closed methods, and the patient must then be treated in a long leg cast for 6–8 weeks. A short leg cast is insufficient because it does not control rotation. However, a long leg cast imposes significant burdens on the elderly patient. Operative treatment of reducible unstable fractures, as described below, may be preferable to closed treatment owing to the difficulty many geriatric patients have managing routine activities in a long leg cast.

If adequate closed reduction of an unstable or displaced fracture cannot be achieved, open reduction/internal fixation is required. It can be done under general or regional anesthesia. The skin over the ankle is thin and has a poor blood supply, putting this area at risk for wound complications such as dehiscence and infection. Operative treatment must be delayed until postinjury edema is reduced sufficiently to allow tension-free skin closure, and any fracture blisters must be allowed to re-epithelialize. Incisions are made laterally and medially as necessary, and reduction is achieved and confirmed under direct visualization or radiographic guidance (or both). The lateral malleolar fracture is generally fixed with a plate and screws; the syndesmosis is stabilized with a horizontally placed screw if necessary; and the medial fracture is stabilized with screws (Fig. 62.4).

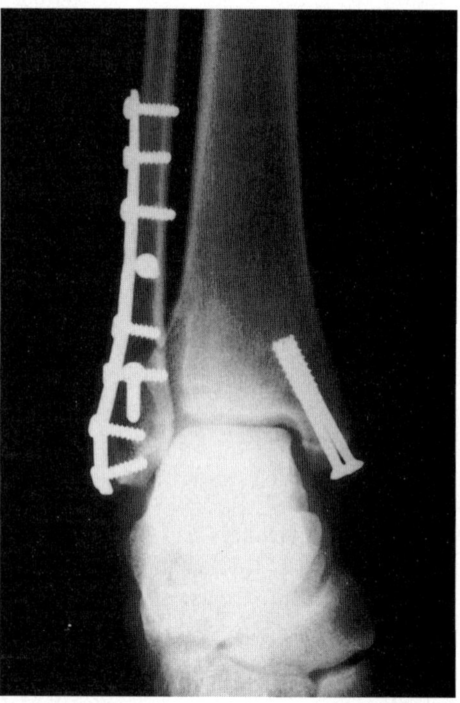

FIGURE 62.4. Mortise view of an ankle. The lateral malleolar fracture is stabilized by two small lag screws and a plate and screws. The medial malleolar fracture is fixed by two cancellous lag screws.

Fixation may be suboptimal owing to osteopenia. It is imperative that the ankle be kept elevated pre- and postoperatively to avoid wound complications. We generally treat these patients in a short leg cast after edema has resolved sufficiently and the patient is allowed partial weight-bearing for 6–8 weeks.

Two studies have reported the results of treatment after unstable ankle fractures in the elderly. Comparing operative versus nonoperative treatment of displaced fractures, operative treatment achieved better fracture position, but there was a high complication rate in women due to loss of fixation, mostly because of osteoporosis. Two years after injury there was no difference in function between the two groups.[38] Another study showed that, in patients who had a satisfactory reduction, the satisfaction with regard to pain, deformity and stability were higher in the operative group.[39]

We prefer operative treatment whenever possible in patients with unstable or displaced ankle fractures. Although both operative and nonoperative treatment require up to 2 months of immobilization, it is much easier to function independently with crutches or a walker wearing a short leg cast than a long leg cast. Despite undergoing surgery, preinjury functional status is likely to be achieved earlier.

## Proximal Humerus Fractures

Proximal humerus fracture is a common injury in the geriatric population, reaching a peak incidence of 112 and 439 fractures per 100,000 person-years in men and women, respectively.[40] These fractures are usually the result of low-energy trauma, such as a fall from a standing height. These fractures have a significant effect on independent living owing to a necessary period of immobilization of the upper extremity, particularly if the dominant arm is involved. Therefore, as with all fractures, treatment is aimed at rapidly restoring pain-free function of the shoulder. Full range of motion is often not achievable.

The proximal humerus articulates with the glenoid portion of the scapula to form the shoulder joint. The proximal humerus includes the humeral head, the greater and lesser tuberosities, and the humeral shaft. The anatomic neck is at the base of the head, and the surgical neck marks the beginning of the shaft. A complex combination of bony, muscular, capsular, and ligamentous structures maintains the stability of the humerus in the glenoid. The most significant are the four muscles that make up the rotator cuff: The subscapularis inserts on the lesser tuberosity, and the supraspinatous, infraspinatous, and teres minor all insert on the greater tuberosity. The pull of the rotator cuff muscles contributes to displacement of bony structures following proximal humerus fracture. Additionally, tears in the rotator cuff often compromise functional outcomes following fracture if not repaired.

The most useful classification of proximal humerus fractures was developed by Neer.[41] This system divides the proximal humerus into four anatomic segments, or "parts": the humeral head, the great tuberosity, the lesser tuberosity, and the humeral shaft. A fracture is described by the number of "parts" that have fractured and are displaced more than 1 cm or angulated more than 45 degrees from their anatomic position. A minimally displaced fracture is described as a one-part fracture and displaced fractures as two-, three-, and four-part fractures. Additional fracture patterns are described as involving the articular surface or involving dislocation of the humeral head.

Patients who have sustained a proximal humerus fracture typically present with shoulder pain and an inability to move the involved arm. The skin must be carefully examined, along with a complete neurovascular examination of the involved extremity. Associated injuries that may have been sustained in a fall must be ruled out. A full radiographic survey includes AP, scapular Y lateral, and axillary views. Though uncomfortable for the patient, the axillary view is mandatory because it may be impossible to rule out a fracture/dislocation without it (Fig. 62.5).

Treatment of proximal humerus fractures aims at achieving pain-free maximal range of motion. It consists of either closed management, open reduction/internal fixation, or prosthetic replacement. These procedures can be performed under general or regional anesthesia.

Minimally displaced (one-part) fractures, which account for 80–85% of proximal humerus fractures, are usually stabilized by the surrounding soft tissue and periosteum, or they are impacted. After a brief period of immobilization, gentle range-of-motion exercises are instituted. These exercises initially consist of pendulum motion of the arm and then progress to active/assisted exercises as union becomes apparent on the radiographs, usually at around 4 weeks. Long-term results following closed treatment of these injuries are excellent. In a study of 104 minimally displaced proximal humerus fractures, 91% of patients had either no pain or mild pain.[42]

Displaced anatomic neck fractures are uncommon. They have a high rate of osteonecrosis of the humeral head, so prosthetic replacement is indicated. Isolated lesser tuberosity fractures require operative fixation only if the fragment contains a large articular piece or limits internal rotation. Isolated displaced greater tuberosity fractures are often associated with longitudinal rotator cuff tears and require open reduction and fixation. Displaced surgical neck fractures, which are separated, comminuted, or impacted and angulated, can be treated by closed reduction under appropriate anesthesia with radiographic guidance. If a stable, satisfactory reduction is achieved, the shoulder and arm are immobilized for approximately 3 weeks followed by progressive

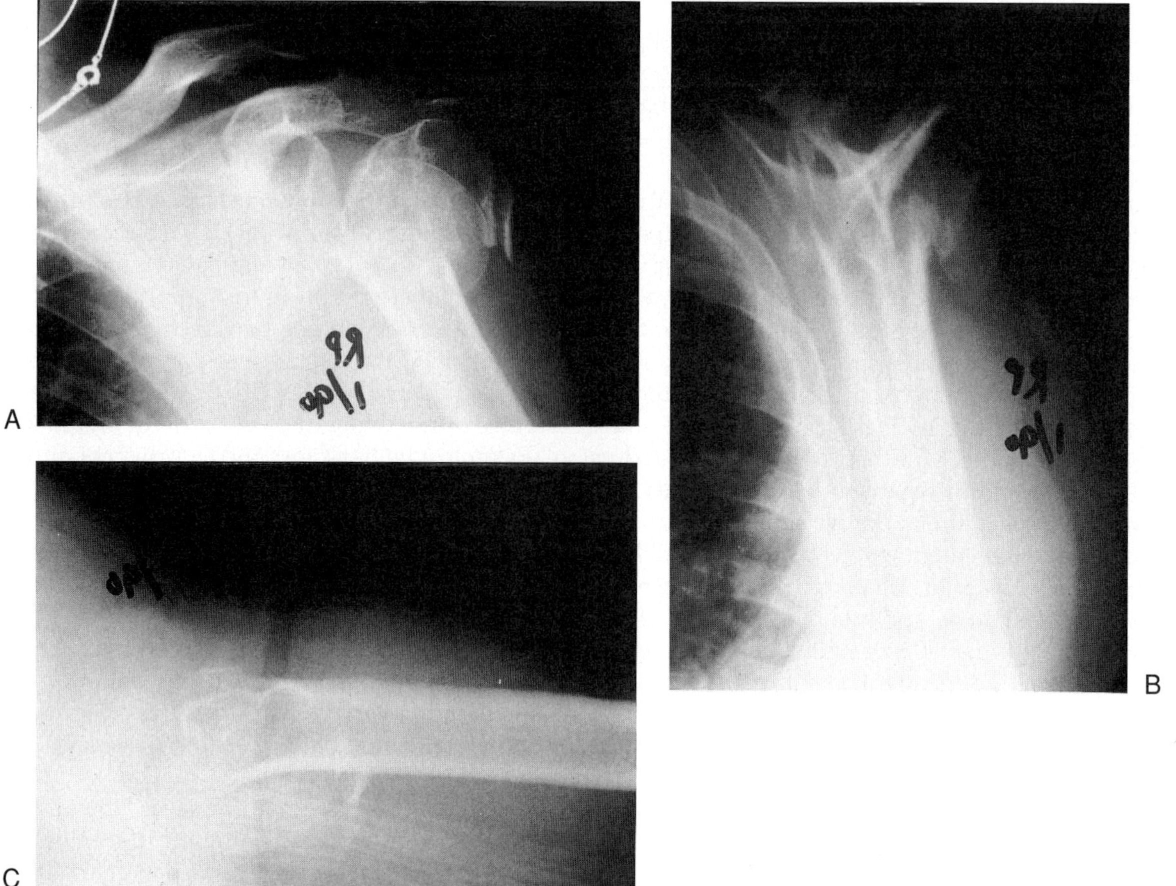

FIGURE 62.5. AP A. and scapular B. Y views of the shoulder showing a displaced proximal humerus fracture. The associated glenohumeral dislocation was initially missed because the axillary view C. was not obtained.

range-of-motion exercises. If an acceptable reduction is not obtained, operative treatment is indicated.

Closed treatment of three- and four-part fractures has yielded poor results.[43] For three-part fractures in young patients with good quality bone, open reduction/internal fixation with wire or nonabsorbable suture is recommended, sometimes in combination with intramedullary fixation. Fixation failure is a problem in osteopenic bone, so prosthetic replacement of the proximal humerus is recommended (Fig. 62.6). It is also the treatment of choice for four-part fractures, where the risk of fixation failure or osteonecrosis is high. Prosthetic replacement is in the form of hemiarthroplasty, but it can include glenoid resurfacing if there is preexisting degenerative disease. Prosthetic replacement is also used for head-splitting fractures, fracture/dislocation, and fractures that involve more than 40% of the articular surface.

Regardless of the method of treatment, following proximal humerus fractures, patients require prolonged, supervised rehabilitation. Minimally displaced fractures generally have a good functional outcome, as do adequately reduced two-part injuries. Poor results may be related to associated rotator cuff injuries, malunion, or nonunion. Patients undergoing prosthetic replacement following three- and four-part fractures can be expected to have relatively pain-free shoulders. However, recovery of function and range of motion, particularly overhead motion, is variable.[44]

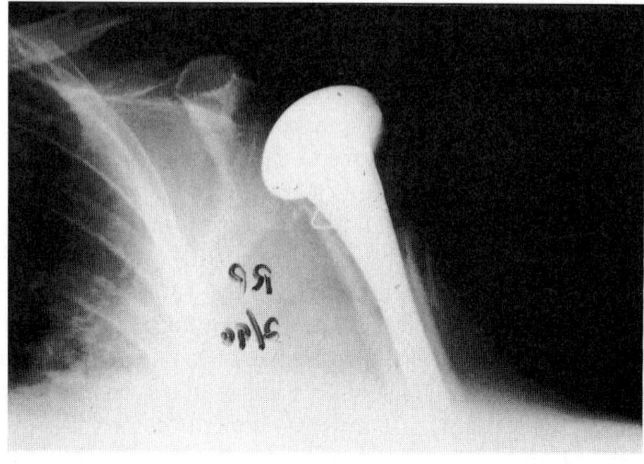

FIGURE 62.6. Hemiarthroplasty of the proximal humerus.

## Distal Radius Fractures

Fractures of the distal radius are a common injury in the elderly, usually occurring after a simple fall onto an outstretched hand. Studies have shown that the incidence of these fractures increases dramatically with age, particularly in women.[45] This age-related increase parallels that seen for fractures of the hip and proximal humerus and is related to osteoporosis. As with all other extremity fractures, factors associated with an increased risk of falls such as dementia, poor eyesight and decreased coordination contribute to the high incidence of these injuries.

The distal radius and distal ulna articulate with each other and the carpal bones of the wrist. These complex articulations are stabilized by numerous ligamentous structures. Many classification systems have been described for these fractures, most of which are based on the geometry of the fracture, degree of displacement and comminution, and involvement of the articular surface.[46]

Patients with acute distal radius fractures typically present after a fall, complaining of pain and inability to move the affected wrist. There is typically marked edema and, with displaced fractures, obvious deformity. A careful neurovascular assessment of the wrist and hand is performed, and the skin integrity is evaluated. Associated injuries to the head and other extremities must be ruled out. Radiographic evaluation consists of PA, lateral, and oblique views of the wrist. The contralateral wrist is frequently imaged to define any variations in the patient's individual anatomy. The history (including hand dominance, occupation, and functional needs) is essential for determining appropriate management.

The injury described by Colles is a shortened distal radius fracture with dorsal tilting of the articular surface and apex-volar angulation (Fig. 62.7).[47] Other fracture patterns include volar tilting of the articular surface with apex-dorsal angulation (Smith's fracture), shear fractures (Barton's fracture), nondisplaced fractures, and fractures involving the distal ulna. There may also be varied amounts of comminution and intraarticular extension of fracture lines. Treatment of these fractures is aimed at restoring normal anatomy to allow smooth, painless motion of the wrist.

Nondisplaced fractures may be immobilized in a short arm cast for approximately 6–8 weeks or until there is evidence of healing. It is imperative that motion of the metacarpal-phalangeal and interphalangeal joints be encouraged.

Displaced fractures should be reduced, with restoration of radial length and the normal volar tilt of the distal radial articular surface.[48] A stable reduction is more easily obtained if there is minimal comminution and displacement. This is usually accomplished by manipulation combined with longitudinal traction under local (hematoma block) or regional anesthesia. If a satisfactory reduction is obtained, the arm is splinted and, when edema permits, placed in a long or short arm cast. Initially, weekly radiographic evaluation is mandatory, as the reduction may be lost and remanipulation may be required at 1–2 weeks.

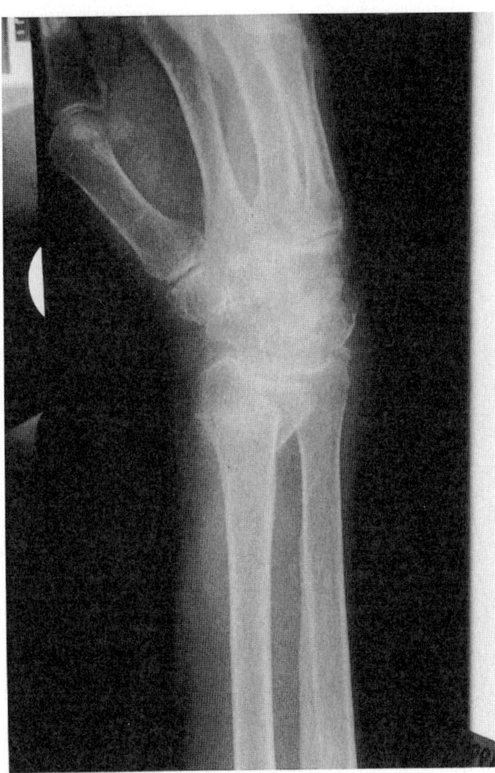

FIGURE 62.7. Oblique view of the wrist showing a distal radius fracture with dorsal tilt and loss of the radial height, along with an ulnar styloid fracture.

If anatomic reduction cannot be obtained and maintained, operative intervention is required to restore pain-free range of motion and strength of the wrist. Various methods can be used, including open reduction/internal fixation followed by casting, external fixation, or percutaneous pinning. Bone grafting may be necessary. At the Hospital For Joint Diseases, we frequently employ external fixation, sometimes in combination with limited internal fixation and bone grafting (Fig. 62.8). These operations can be performed under general or regional anesthesia and involve minimal blood loss. Motion of the fingers must be encouraged immediately to prevent postoperative stiffness.

The results of distal radius fracture treatment are variable and depend on the fracture type, amount of comminution, articular involvement, and reduction achieved. Minimally displaced fractures and displaced fractures in which stable anatomic reduction is achieved have a good functional outcome without surgery. Displaced fractures treated surgically with internal and external fixation techniques are reported to produce good to excellent results

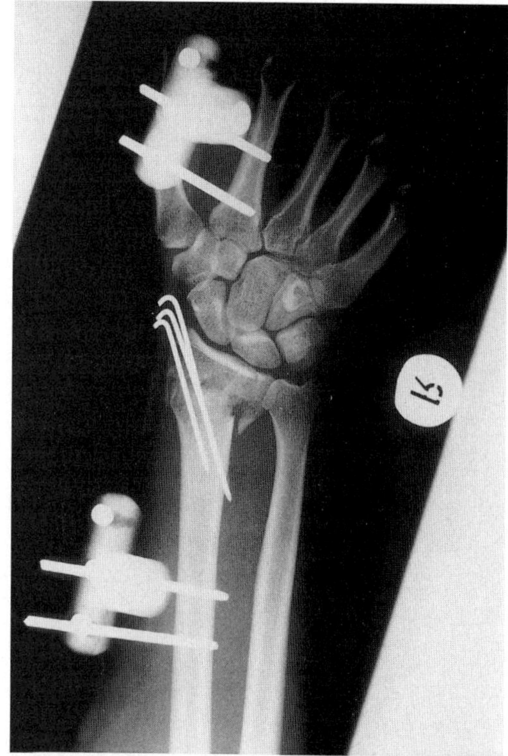

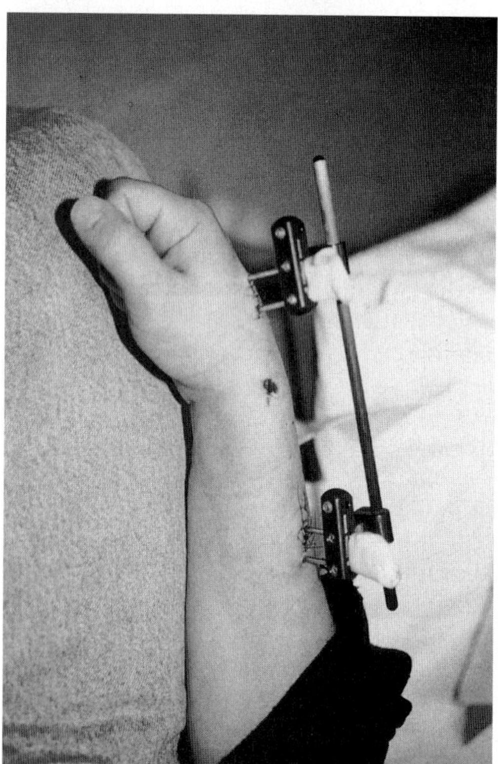

FIGURE 62.8. A. PA view of the wrist showing limited internal fixation with pins and stabilization with an external fixator. B. External fixator stabilizes a distal radius fracture.

in 70–90% of patients.[49] Functional limitations include pain, wrist stiffness, and decreased grip strength.

## Vertebral Compression Fractures

The vertebral compression fracture, usually the result of a relatively atraumatic event such as rising from a chair or lifting a light object, is virtually synonymous with osteoporosis. Nearly all postmenopausal women are at risk. It is estimated that 44% of women over age 70 have sustained a vertebral compression fracture.[50] These fractures usually occur in the thoracolumbar spine between T8 and L2. If there are compression fractures at several segments, a kyphosis or scoliosis, which are markers for osteoporosis,[51] may develop.

Three patterns of compression fractures are described. The first is a biconcave central compression fracture, which occurs primarily in the upper lumbar spine where axial forces predominate. Anterior wedge-type fractures typically occur in the thoracic spine, where the normal kyphosis transmits most of the axial loading onto the anterior portion of the vertebrae. They are usually the result of a flexion mechanism. Lastly, a symmetric compression fracture represents complete collapse of the vertebral body, resulting in a flattened appearance of the vertebral body. It most often occurs at the thoracolumbar junction.

The patient presenting with an acute vertebral compression fracture typically complains of pain in the lower thoracic or upper lumbar region, but these fractures can present as incidental radiographic findings. On physical examination the spinal range of motion is decreased, and there may be tenderness or deep palpation. Scoliotic or kyphotic deformity may be present if multiple segments are involved. Neurologic deficit following these fractures is rare.

Radiographic evaluation includes standing AP and lateral (Fig. 62.9) plain radiographs. If the height of a symptomatic vertebra is one-third less than the adjacent vertebrae, a fracture is present. Fractures above T6 are unusual, and other diagnoses must be considered. A bone scan may be helpful for distinguishing an old fracture from an acute one.

Simple osteoporotic vertebral compression fractures are treated nonoperatively and symptomatically. A short period of bed rest may be required because of pain, but prolonged bed rest should be avoided owing to the potential for increased bone loss and stiffness. Necessary analgesia and muscle relaxants may be used, and heat frequently provides symptomatic relief. Progressive ambulation should be started early, and a program of back exercises should be instituted after a few weeks. A corset may be helpful for patient comfort. Most of these fractures heal uneventfully.

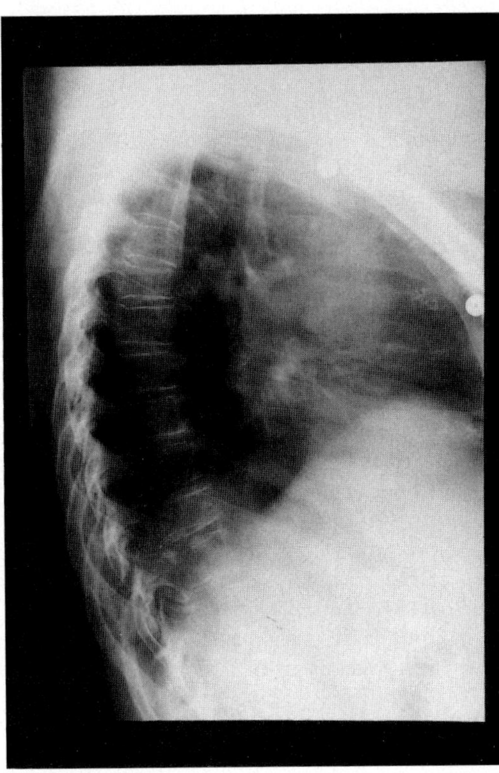

FIGURE 62.9. Lateral view of the lumbosacral spine with an L2 compression fracture.

## Pathologic Fractures

Pathologic or impending pathologic fractures are common in the elderly, reflecting the prevalence of neoplastic disease in this population. Improved survival rates for cancer patients have resulted in a higher incidence of skeletal metastases. Neoplastic processes occurring primarily in bone also contribute to the incidence of pathologic fracture.

Common malignancies that metastasize to bone include prostate, breast, lung, kidney, thyroid, and stomach cancer. Several other tumors are capable of affecting bone.[52] Neoplasms that occur primarily in bone are lymphomas and multiple myeloma. Lesions involving bone are described radiographically as osteoblastic, osteolytic, or mixed; most metastatic lesions are osteolytic or mixed. Metastases from prostate adenocarcinoma, Hodgkin's disease, and carcinoid tumors tend to be purely osteoblastic. Although radiodense, these lesions predispose bone to fracture nearly as often as osteolytic processes by disrupting the normal architecture and stress transmission of bone.[53] Metastases most commonly affect the axial skeleton and proximal region of long bones. The proximal femur is the most commonly affected long bone. Other common locations of lesions are the femoral shaft, acetabulum, and proximal humerus.

Patients with long-bone metastases typically present with pain, frequently before the lesion is apparent radiographically. Bony lesions may also be associated with hypercalcemia secondary to bone destruction by tumor. It may be treated with calcium-wasting diuretics or chemotherapeutic agents.[54] Large lesions, those with significant cortical involvement, or lesions in areas that transmit significant stress can lead to fracture.

Treatment of a pathologic fracture is aimed at relieving symptoms and restoring function. Resection for cure is rarely indicated except in the rare case of a solitary metastasis from a primary thyroid or renal carcinoma.[55] Irradiation is sometimes used to treat painful lesions. This option is problematic, however, because radiation causes a hyperemic response that weakens bone. It peaks at 10–14 days, making the bone more susceptible to fracture. It also disrupts the normal healing process of callus formation.[56]

Nonoperative management involves immobilization in the form of casting or traction. Problems associated with this option in the elderly include the usual risks of pneumonia, decubiti, and thromboembolic disease. Nonunion is also common. In patients with metastatic malignancy, disseminated intravascular coagulation and malignant hypercalcemia are also of concern. Additionally, nonoperative treatment of a lower extremity fracture often involves prolonged hospitalization, which should be avoided as long as possible in patients with metastatic cancer.

Operative treatment of pathologic fractures in the lower extremity is preferred in patients medically able to tolerate the surgery and whose life expectancy exceeds 1 month. Fixation of upper extremity fractures is also considered to enable the patient to carry out activities of daily living. Surgical treatment is palliative in that stabilization of the fracture relieves pain, particularly in conjunction with radiotherapy. Internal fixation is usually in the form of intramedullary devices. Preoperatively, the patient should be carefully evaluated for unrecognized pathologic lesions by whole-body bone scanning to avoid iatrogenic fractures when positioning the patient.

Results following operative treatment of pathologic fractures are generally good. Studies have reported that 85% of patients had adequate pain relief and 94% who could ambulate before fracture regained their ability to walk following internal fixation.[57]

Prophylactic internal fixation of impending pathologic fracture remains controversial. Currently accepted indications for prophylactic fixation of impending femoral fractures include (1) a destructive lesion involving more than 50% of the cortical bone circumference; (2) a lytic lesion of the proximal femur >2.5 cm; (3) a lesion of the proximal femur associated with avulsion of the lesser trochanter; and (4) a lesion of any size with persisting pain despite adequate radiotherapy.[58] Prophylactic internal fixation of humeral metastases is generally not recommended owing to the relatively low risk of fracture, except in patients who are reliant on assistive devices such as a cane, crutch, or walker.

## Conclusions

Orthopedic injuries in the elderly cause considerable morbidity and mortality. As the population ages, the absolute number of orthopedic injuries is predicted to increase, compounding the already significant financial cost of treatment. The ideal treatment of these injuries is prevention, mostly by preventing falls and treating osteoporosis. When an orthopedic injury does occur, attention must be paid to the entire patient, not just the injured bone or joint. Elderly patients have unique needs pertaining to treatment and rehabilitation, and these needs must be considered to maximize both fracture and functional outcomes.

### References


1. Loder RT. The influence of diabetes on the healing of closed fractures. Clin Orthop 1988;232:210–216.
2. Davis FM, Woolner DF, Frampton C, et al. Prospective, multi-centre trial of mortality following general or spinal anaesthesia for hip fracture surgery in the elderly. Br J Anaesth 1987;59:1080–1088.
3. Valentin N, Lomholt B, Jensen JS, Hejgaard N, Kreiner S. Spinal or general anaesthesia for surgery of the fractured hip? Br J Anaesth 1986;58:284–291.
4. Lane JM, Vigorita VJ. Osteoporosis. J Bone Joint Surg Am 1983;65:274–278.
5. Aaron JE, Gallagher JC, Anderson J, et al. Frequency of osteomalacia and osteoporosis in fractures of the proximal femur. Lancet 1974;1:229–233.
6. Jenkins DHR, Roberts JG, Webster D, Williams EO. Osteomalacia in elderly patients with fracture of the femoral neck: a clinico-pathological study. J Bone Joint Surg Br 1973; 55:575–580.
7. Wilton TJ, Hosking DJ, Pawley E, Stevens A, Harvey L. Osteomalacia and femoral neck fractures in the elderly. J Bone Joint Surg Br 1987;69:388–390.
8. Frandsen PA, Kruse T. Hip fractures in the county of Funen, Denmark: Implications of demographic aging and changes in incidence rates. Acta Orthop Scand 1983;54:681–686.
9. Praemer A, Furner S, Rice DP (eds). Musculoskeletal Conditions in the United States 1992. Rosemont, IL: American Academy of Orthopaedic Surgeons.
10. Brody JA. Commentary: prospects for an ageing population. Nature 1985;315:463–466.
11. Greenspan SL, Meyers ER, et al. Fall severity and bone mineral density as risk factors for hip fractures in ambulatory elderly. JAMA 1994;271:128–133.
12. Hinton RY, Smith GS. The association of age, race, and sex with the location of proximal femoral fractures in the elderly. J Bone Joint Surg Am 1993;75:752–759.
13. Hinton RY, Lennox DW, et al. Relative rates of fracture of the hip in the United States. J Bone Joint Surg Am 1995; 77:695–702.
14. Garraway WM, Stauffer RN, Kurland LT, O'Falba WM. Limb fractures in a defined population. I. Frequency and distribution. Mayo Clin Proc 1979;54:701–707.
15. Johnell O, Sernbo I. Health and social status in patients with hip fractures and controls. Age Ageing 1986;15: 285–291.
16. Uden G, Nilsson B. Hip fracture frequency in hospital. Acta Orthop Scand 1986;57:428–430.
17. Gallagher JC, Melton LJ, Riggs BL, Bergtrath E. Epidemiology of fractures of the proximal femur in Rochester, Minnesota. Clin Orthop 1980;150:163–167.
18. Rizzo PF, Gould ES, Lyden JP, Asnis SE. Diagnosis of occult fractures about the hip: magnetic resonance imaging compared with bone-scanning. J Bone Joint Surg Am 1993;75: 395–401.
19. Parker MJ, Myles JW, Anand JK, Drewatt R. Cost-benefit analysis of hip fracture treatment. J Bone Joint Surg Br 1992;74:261–264.
20. Merli GJ. Update: deep venous thrombosis and pulmonary embolism prophylaxis in orthopaedic surgery. Med Clin North Am 1993;77:397–412.
21. Koval KJ, Skovron ML, Aharonoff GB, Meadows SE, Zuckerman JD. Ambulatory ability after hip fracture: a prospective study in geriatric patients. Clin Orthop 1995;310: 150–159.
22. Sexson SB, Lehner JT. Factors affecting hip fracture mortality. J Orthop Trauma 1988;1:298–305.
23. White BL, Fischer WD, Lauren C. Rates of mortality for elderly patients after fracture of the hip in the 1980s. J Bone Joint Surg Am 1987;69:1335–1340.
24. Aharonoff GB, Koval KJ, Skovron ML, Zuckerman JD. Hip fractures in the elderly: predictors of one year mortality. J Orthop Trauma 1997;11:162–165.
25. Kenzora JE, McCarthy RE, Lowell JD, Sledge CB. Hip fracture mortality: relation to age, treatment, preoperative illness, time of surgery and complications. Clin Orthop 1984;186:45–56.
26. Sexson SB, Lehner JT. Factors affecting hip fracture mortality. J Orthop Trauma 1988;1:298–305.
27. White BL, Fischer WD, Lauren C. Rates of mortality for elderly patients after fracture of the hip in the 1980s. J Bone Joint Surg Am 1987;69:1335–1340.
28. Zuckerman JD, Skovron ML, Koval KJ, Aharanoff GB, Frankel VH. Postoperative complications and mortality associated with operative delay in older patients who have a fracture of the hip. J Bone Joint Surg Am 1995;77: 1551–1556.
29. Frankel VH, Burstein AH, Lygre L, Brown RH. The telltale nail. J Bone Joint Surg Am 1971;53:1232.
30. Koval K, Sala DA, Kummer FJ, Zuckerman JD. Postoperative weightbearing after hip fracture. J Bone Joint Surg 1998;80(3)A:352–356.
31. Koval K, Friend KD, Aharanoff GB, Zuckerman JD. Weightbearing after hip fracture: a prospective series of 596 geriatric hip fracture patients. J Orthop Trauma 1996; 10(8):526–530.
32. Bentley G. Treatment of non-displaced fractures of the femoral neck. Clin Orthop 1980;152:93–101.

33. Barnes R, Brown JT, Garden RS, Nicoll EA. Subcapital fractures of the femur: a prospective review. J Bone Joint Surg Br 1976;58:2–24.
34. Koval K, Sala DA, Kummer FJ, Zuckerman JD. Postoperative weightbearing after hip fracture. J Bone Joint Surg 1998;80(3)A:352–356.
35. Calder SJ, Anderson GH, Jagger C, Harper WM, Gregg PJ. Unipolar or bipolar prosthesis for displaced intracapsular hip fractures in octogenarians. J Bone Joint Surg Br 1996; 78:391–394.
36. Evans EM. The treatment of trochanteric fractures of the femur. J Bone Joint Surg Br 1949;31:190–203.
37. Ramsey PL, Hamilton W. Changes in tibitalar area of contact caused by lateral talar shift. J Bone Joint Surg Am 1976;58:356–357.
38. Beauchamp CG, Clay NR, Thexton PW. Displaced ankle fractures in patients over 50 years of age. J Bone Joint Surg Br 1983;63:329–332.
39. Ali MS, McLaren AN, Routholamin E, O'Connor BT. Ankle fractures in the elderly: nonoperative or operative treatment. J Orthop Trauma 1987;1:275–280.
40. Horak J, Nilsson BE. Epidemiology of fractures of the upper end of the humerus. Clin Orthop 1975;112:250–253.
41. Neer CS. Displaced proximal humeral fractures. Part I. Classification and evaluation. J Bone Joint Surg Am 1970;52: 1077–1089.
42. Koval K, Gallagher MA, Marsicano JG, Cuomo F, McShinway A, Zuckerman JD. Functional outcome after minimally displaced fracture of the proximal part of the humerus. J Bone Joint Surg Am 1997;79:203–207.
43. Neer CS. Displaced proximal humerus fractures. Part II. Treatment of three-part and four-part displacement. J Bone Joint Surg Am 1970;52:1090–1103.
44. Goldman R, Koval KJ, Guomo F, Gallagher MA, Zuckerman JD. Functional outcome after humeral head replacement for acute three- and four-part proximal humeral fractures. J Shoulder Elbow Surg 1995;4(2):81–86.
45. Alffram P, Bauer G. Epidemiology of fractures of the forearm. J Bone Joint Surg Am 1962;44:105–114.
46. Fryckman G. Fractures of the distal radius including sequelae. Acta Orthop Scand Suppl 1967;180:1–153.
47. Colles A. On the fracture of the carpal extremity of the radius. Edinb Med Surg J 1814;10:182–186.
48. Villar RN, Marsh D, Righton N, Greatorex RA. Three years after Colles' fracture: a prospective review. J Bone Joint Surg Br 1987;69:635–638.
49. Cooney WP, Linscheid RL, Dobyns JH. External pin fixation for unstable Colle's fractures. J Bone Joint Surg Am 1979;61: 840–845.
50. Jensen GF, Christiansen C, Boesen J, et al. Epidemiology of postmenopausal spinal and long bone fractures. Clin Orthop 1982;166:75–81.
51. Healey JH, Lane JM. Structural scoliosis in osteoporotic women. Clin Orthop 1985;95:216–223.
52. Bhardwaj S, Holland JF. Chemotherapy of metastatic cancer in bone. Clin Orthop 1982;169:34.
53. Harrington KD. Impending pathological fractures from metastatic malignancy: evaluation and management. CV Mosby St. Louis, MO: AAOS Instruct Course Lect 1986;35: 357–381.
54. Galasko CSB. Skeletal metastases. Clin Orthop 1986;210: 18–30.
55. Bhardwaj S, Holland JF. Chemotherapy of metastatic cancer in bone. Clin Orthop 1982;169:34.
56. Bonarigo BC, Rubin P. Nonunion of pathological fracture after radiation therapy. Radiology 1967;88:889–898.
57. Harrington KD, Sim FH, Enis JE, et al. Methylmethacrylate as an adjunct in internal fixation of pathological fractures. J Bone Joint Surg Am 1976;58:1047–1055.
58. Harrington KD. Impending pathological fractures from metastatic malignancy: evaluation and management. AAOS Instruct Course Lect 1986;35:357–381.

# 63
# Joint Replacement in the Elderly Patient

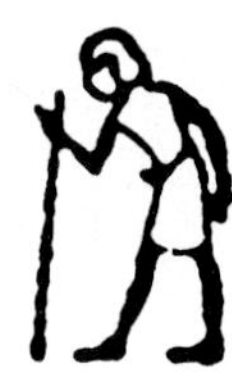

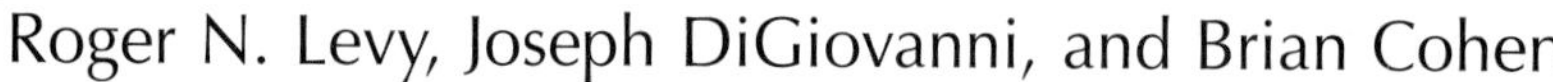

Roger N. Levy, Joseph DiGiovanni, and Brian Cohen

The goal of orthopedic surgery in the geriatric population is to preserve independence. The ability to get around and cognitive ability are the most important factors in maintaining independence. Despite the medical problems with which the elderly are sometimes faced, the musculoskeletal system is frequently the sole cause of loss of independence. Disabling arthritis, failed treatment of fractures, and secondary avascular necrosis are common conditions affecting the hip in the elderly and can threaten independence as well as contribute to a deterioration in quality of life. Joint replacement can restore independence and improve quality of life by eliminating pain and disability.

Previously, geriatrics has been an integral part of medical practice more so than a surgical practice; but in contemporary practice, surgical care is increasing in the elderly. In a study in Canada, the rate of coronary artery bypass surgery increased 700% during the period 1981–1989.[1] The rate of total hip replacement more than doubled in people age 65 years or older. This progression is expected to continue in the coming years, so surgical care of the elderly will become a significant part of any health care delivery system. The emergence of geriatrics as an increasingly important part of medicine and surgery in society has stressed the importance of the orthopedic surgeon as a member of a multidisciplinary team in maintaining the independence and quality of life of the elderly.

The use of total joint replacement has increased because of the documented efficacy and safety of the procedures. Longer life expectancy and better control of many serious illnesses have led to increased demand for quality-enhancing procedures. Because of these factors there has been a change in the demographics of total hip recipients over time. There has been an upward shift in the age distribution of patients receiving total joint replacements, more than can be simply attributed to the aging of the population. One to three percent of the population over age 65 requires a joint replacement for the relief of arthritic pain and disability. It can be assumed that this figure increases during the eighth, ninth, and tenth decades. In addition to the upward shift in the age of patients receiving total joint replacements, increased proportions of patients have serious co-morbidities. The safety of the procedures has improved in terms of documented decreased mortality.[2]

Total joint replacement is one of the most costly hospital inpatient procedures, both per case and in total Medicare dollars. The demand for expensive, elective procedures has been increasing for patients previously regarded as too old or impaired to benefit sufficiently.[3] This process leads to continuing increases in real health care expenses, even without the invention and introduction of new technologies. The safety and efficacy with which total joint replacements can be performed are making them common surgical procedures in the octogenarian and nonagenarian despite the increased health care cost. Joint replacement is actually cost-effective because it maintains personal independence for the patient and relieves the family and community of the financial burden that would have to be borne if institutionalization became necessary owing to increasing disability.

Evidence suggests that elderly patients are weaker, have less endurance, and have smaller muscle fibers than do younger patients.[4] It is known that the elderly do have fewer anterior horn cells,[5] but part of their weakness is due to a lower level of conditioning. Elderly patients can increase both strength and endurance with training programs,[6,7] and fitness can be increased after joint replacements.[8]

Joint range of motion is diminished in the elderly. The tendons, ligaments, and capsules surrounding joints lose elasticity as evidenced by the decrease in the joint range of motion and a sense of stiffness.[9] Stiffness following sleep, prolonged sitting, or exercise is more common and prolonged in old patients.

Rehabilitation is crucial after orhthopedic surgery, and the physiatrists must take into consideration the special needs of the geriatric patient, as discussed above. The presence of osteoporosis should be determined before prescribing exercises that load the spine. Range of motion should be initiated slowly and gently. In principle, the rehabilitation goals are to return each patient to the premorbid functional level of mobility and self-care, teach exercises that are to be performed after hospital discharge, reduce the risk of falls, and ensure that the patient is discharged to a safe environment.[10]

## Common Diagnoses Requiring Total Joint Replacement

Total joint replacement is necessary in the elderly when articular degeneration leads to discomfort and disability that is unresponsive to nonsurgical treatment. Osteoarthrosis, secondary traumatic arthritis (postfracture), rheumatoid arthritis, and avascular necrosis of the femoral head commonly affect old patients and often are the first signs of aging in an otherwise healthy elderly individual. The pain of arthritic joints tends to be chronic in nature and forces the elderly to accept a more sedentary life style. When severe, loss of independence occurs. Degenerative joint disease (osteoarthrosis) is by far the most common affliction of the knees and hips in the geriatric population. Knee and hip osteoarthrosis are more likely to result in disability than osteoarthrosis of any other joint. Osteoarthrosis therefore is the most common cause of total joint replacement in the elderly. Others are rheumatoid arthritis, fractures, and avascular necrosis of the affected joint.

Osteoarthrosis is due to wearing away of the articular cartilage over time. Cartilage has little ability to heal itself, and injury to the cartilage is cumulative over time. Also, damaged areas of cartilage are less able to bear weight; adjacent areas of cartilage must then bear more load, and the stress or load per unit area increases in this remaining cartilage. Such increased stress prematurely destroys the cartilage. Lubrication deteriorates as the joint surface degenerates; therefore any irreversible damage to the cartilaginous surface of a joint proceeds to osteoarthrosis if the joint continues to bear a load.

During the early stages of osteoarthrosis the disease often can be treated nonsurgically. Treatments are aimed at pain control and maintaining motion. Nonsteroidal antiinflammatory drugs (NSAIDs) are used to decrease the pain associated with osteoarthrosis. Although they are effective in reducing joint inflammation, it is the analgesic effect that matters. Acetaminophen should be used first because of the lower potential for complications in the aged. The most important way to mitigate the effects of osteoarthrosis is to reduce the force transmitted across the joint. Decreasing body weight can have a substantial effect on symptoms. However, weight reduction is difficult to obtain especially in the elderly. A cane is the other way to decrease force transmission across a joint and does so rather effectively when used properly. Many patients refuse to use a cane because of its stigma as a sign of old age and fragility. Nevertheless, a cane used in the hand opposite from the affected side can be a mainstay of nonsurgical treatment.

Surgical treatment for osteoarthrosis can involve débridement of loose areas of cartilage that are symptomatic, osteotomies to redirect the load-bearing to areas of the joint that are not involved, and joint replacement. Arthroscopic débridement is done in the knee.[11–15] It is not typically done in the hip. Osteotomies are more common in Europe; they have limited value in the elderly because typically the entire or large portions of the head are involved, and results are not predictable.

Total joint replacement is the procedure of choice for osteoarthrosis of the hip in the elderly. The results, even in the octogenarian and nonagenarian, can approach those for young patients. There is a suitable improvement in the parameters of pain, walking ability, and range of motion. Also, the elderly record a high degree of satisfaction with the results of the operation. This coincides closely with the high patient satisfaction usually observed in young patients who undergo the same procedure.[16] In addition to the subjective satisfaction with the results of surgery, expressions of hopelessness, helplessness, and depression that are common with the elderly with chronic illnesses are alleviated after surgery.[17] Total joint replacement can be an effective way to maintain an independent quality of life.

Rheumatoid arthritis is the most common form of inflammatory arthritis, affecting 3% of women and 1% of men. It is also a common cause of total hip replacement in the elderly. Inflammatory rheumatoid arthritis has a spike of peak incidence in the geriatric age group. The etiology of rheumatoid arthritis is unclear, but it is probably related to a cell-mediated immune reaction that incites an inflammatory response initially against soft tissues and later against cartilage (chondrolysis) and bone (periarticular bone resorption). Rheumatoid arthritis usually presents as an insidious onset of morning stiffness and polyarthritis. Most commonly the hands and feet are affected early; but involvement of the knees, elbows, hips, shoulders, ankles, and neck is also common. Synovium and soft tissues are affected first, and only later are joints significantly involved. Pannus ingrowth denudes articular cartilage and leads to chondrocyte death. Radiographs typically demonstrate periarticular erosions and osteopenia.

The treatment for rheumatoid arthritis includes control of synovitis and pain, maintenance of joint function, and prevention of deformities. A multidisciplinary approach involving therapeutic drugs, physical therapy, and sometimes surgery, is necessary to achieve these goals. A pyramid approach to drug therapy for patients with rheumatoid arthritis, beginning with NSAIDs and slowly progressing to disease-modifying antirheumatic drugs, steroids, and cytotoxic drugs, is used to try to control the disease. Surgery includes synovectomy (rarely indicated—only if aggressive drug therapy fails), soft tissue realignment procedures, especially in the hand, and various reconstructive procedures, including total joint replacements. Chemical and radiation synovectomy can be successful if done early. Athroscopic synovectomy, especially in the knee, has proven efficacy. Following all forms of synovectomy, the synovium initially regenerates normally, but with time it demonstrates rheumatoid synovial tissue. Evaluation of the cervical spine with preoperative radiographs is important.

## Hip Replacement

Problems due to fractures of the hip are a reason for total hip replacement. If the hip fracture occurs in the femoral neck and the fracture is displaced, the blood supply to the remaining femoral head may be disrupted. This results in a femoral head that becomes avascular and unable to bear weight without mechanical failure. Therefore the femoral head is replaced. If the patient already has osteoarthrosis of the hip, total hip replacement is considered.[18,19]

Avascular necrosis of the hip can occur without a fracture as well. Avascular necrosis is associated with alcohol intake and steroid use. Patients with geriatric-onset inflammatory bowel disease or polymyalgia may be at risk. Idiopathic avascular necrosis occurs in patients without risk factors. Avascular necrosis of the hip results in a femoral head that is unable to bear weight because the subchondral bone, which is the bone under the cartilage, collapses. The spherical geometry of the femoral head is lost, and the cartilage unsupported by the bone collapses. The load per unit area increases in the surrounding areas of cartilage, and secondary degeneration ensues. Eventually the entire joint is affected and destroyed. The only treatment for pain due to advanced avascular necrosis is to replace the joint.

### Indications

The indications for total hip replacement include pain with weight-bearing, pain at rest, pain that awakens the patient from sleep, limited walking ability, and limited standing ability. Loss of ability to perform standard activities of daily living, inability to ascend or descend stairs, inability to perform routine dress and hygiene, and problems getting in and out of a car result in loss of independence. The old person is quite prepared to have an operation if the results can significantly improve his or her quality of life.

When the decision has been made to replace a joint, a careful medical and orthopedic evaluation is necessary that is specific to the geriatric patient. From a purely orthopedic standpoint, the joints to be replaced must be considered. If a patient has an involved hip and knee it is wise to do one at a time, usually with the more symptomatic joint being done first. If an ipsilateral hip and knee are involved, we recommend that the hip be replaced first. Some of the apparent knee symptoms may be referred from the hip.

A complete medical evaluation is performed, and special tests are performed as necessary. Medical problems such as hypertension, coronary artery disease, and pulmonary disease are optimized, and all medications are reviewed. The family practitioner, internist, or geriatrician follows the patient postoperatively to ensure that the stress of surgery does not adversely affect any medical problems and potentially jeopardize the results of surgery.

The patient is usually admitted the day of surgery and given preoperative antibiotics 1 hour prior to incising the skin. A first-generation cephalosporin is generally used unless an allergy is present. Special attention is given to sterility because of insertion of a foreign body. Sterile hoods with dual exhaust fans are used by most total joint surgeons. Deep vein thrombosis (DVT) and pulmonary embolism are relatively common in orthopedic procedures and can be devastating and life-threatening complications. Prevention of thromboembolic disease remains one of the most controversial issues in orthopedics. The prevention of proximal DVT and pulmonary embolism are the goals of prophylactic intervention. If prophylaxis is not used, DVT develops in 40–60% of patients undergoing total hip or knee arthroplasty. Asymptomatic pulmonary embolism occurs in 10–15% of patients and fatal pulmonary embolism in 1–3% of patients. Various prophylactic regimens against DVT include warfarin prior to the operation, which is afterward adjusted based on the patient's INR, compression stockings, external pneumatic compression devices, aspirin, dextran, intravenous heparin given intraoperatively at the time of canal preparation, and low-molecular-weight heparins. In general, we have found a predictive relation between American Society of Anesthesiology (ASA) classes I and II preoperatively and an absence of postoperative problems.

### Surgery

Total hip replacement involves removing the arthritic femoral head and acetabular surface and replacing them with prosthetic components (Fig. 63.1). The acetabulum is resurfaced by placing a metal cup within the prepared bony acetabulum. An ultra-high-molecular-weight polyethylene liner is locked within the metal-backed acetabulum (Fig. 63.2). The femoral component is typically modular, containing a stem with a neck and a head. Ideally, the stem has a range of size and shape combinations to accommodate differences in femoral canal anatomy. Femoral heads are available in a range of diam-

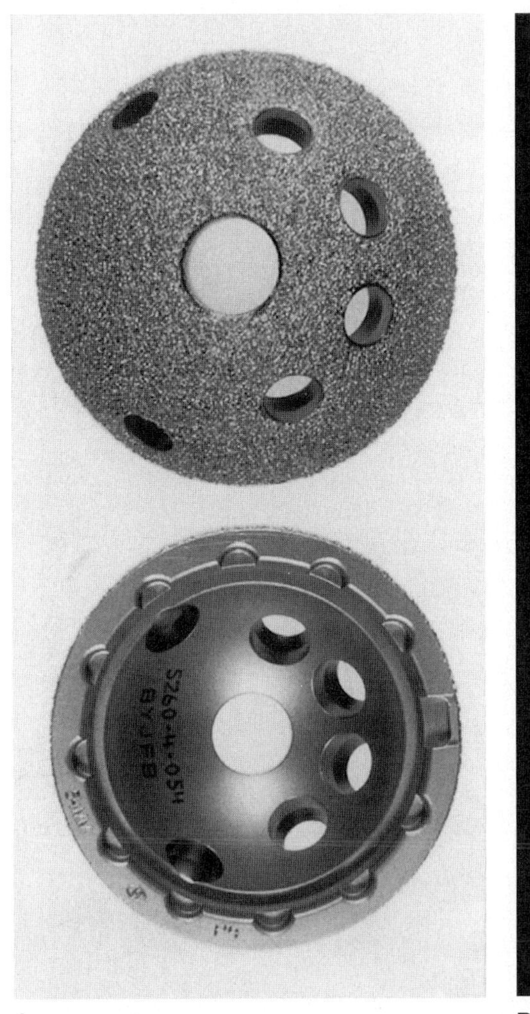
A

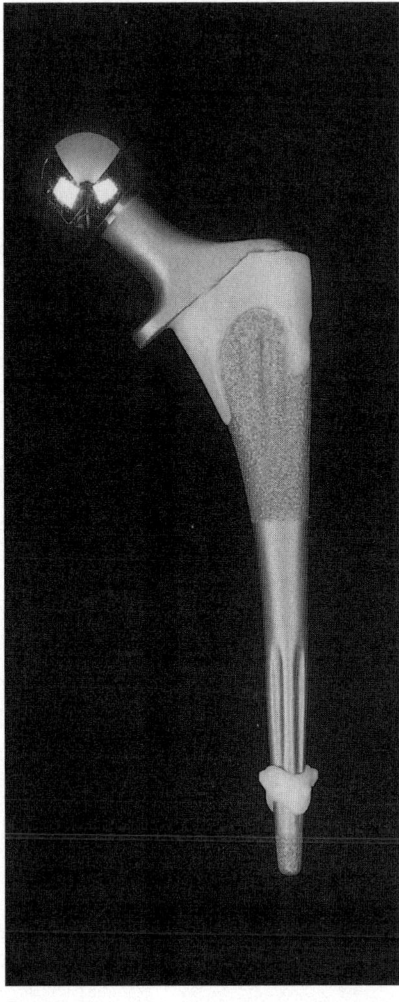
B

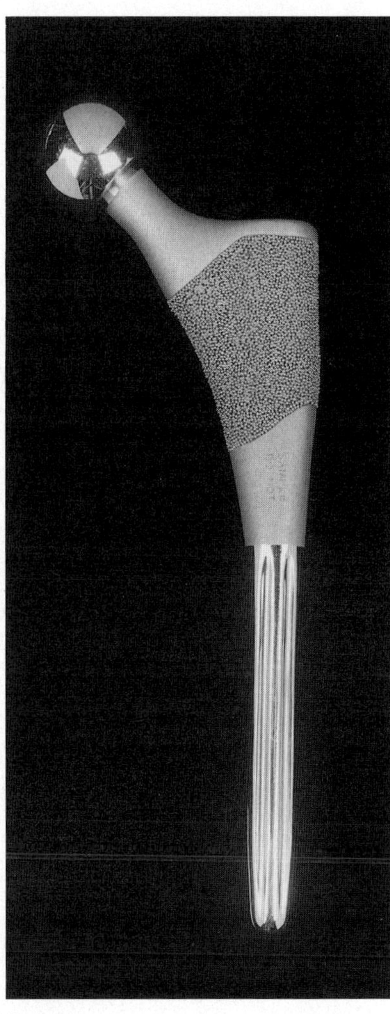
C

FIGURE 63.1. A. Metal acetabulum which is placed in the prepared bony acetabulum. B. Metal stem which is placed in the prepared femoral canal. This stem is cemented into the femur. It contains a preformed cement mantle (white portion proximally) and a plastic distal centralizer to position the stem in the midddle of the canal. The femoral head is applied separately to the stem. Both the stem and head come in varying sizes. C. Metal stem which is press-fit into the femoral canal after preparation. This stem contains a proximally coated beaded surface to allow bony ingrowth. The distal part of the stem is slotted to allow reduction of the stiffness in the stem. This allows bony ingrowth to occur proximally in the stem.

eters, most commonly 26 or 28 mm to match the polyethylene liner. The morse tapers of the head and neck allow for a variation in length. The prosthesis should be made of forged high-strength metal alloy and is fashioned according to whether it is cemented into the femur or press-fit into the femur to allow bony ingrowth. Ingrowth stems contain a porous coating with a pore size of roughly 400 μm, the size of bony trabeculae, to allow bony ingrowth onto prioritized zones of the stem. Other ingrowth stems contain a bioactive hydroxyapatite coating to allow molecular bonding to the hydroxyapatite in bone. Cemented stems are made to allow a cement mantle within the femoral canal and to form a bone–cement interface and a metal–cement interface. The metal cup to replace the acetabulum can be press-fit, requiring some bony deformation to allow a tight fit, or it can be cemented into the bony acetabulum. This is a matter of the surgeon's preference. Most acetabulum replacements inserted in the United States are press-fit. Then a polyethylene liner is snapped into the metal shell and articulates with a head placed on the femoral prosthesis. This articulation is a source of wear and debris formation, which can induce a macrophage-mediated response. This inflammatory response can cause bony destruction if the rate of wear is rapid. As a cost-saving step, polyethylene sockets without a metal shell are commonly used when the cup is cemented owing to lack of proven superiority of the more expensive metal-backed shell. The improved results with the press-fit bone ingrowth sockets explain the general preference for this type.

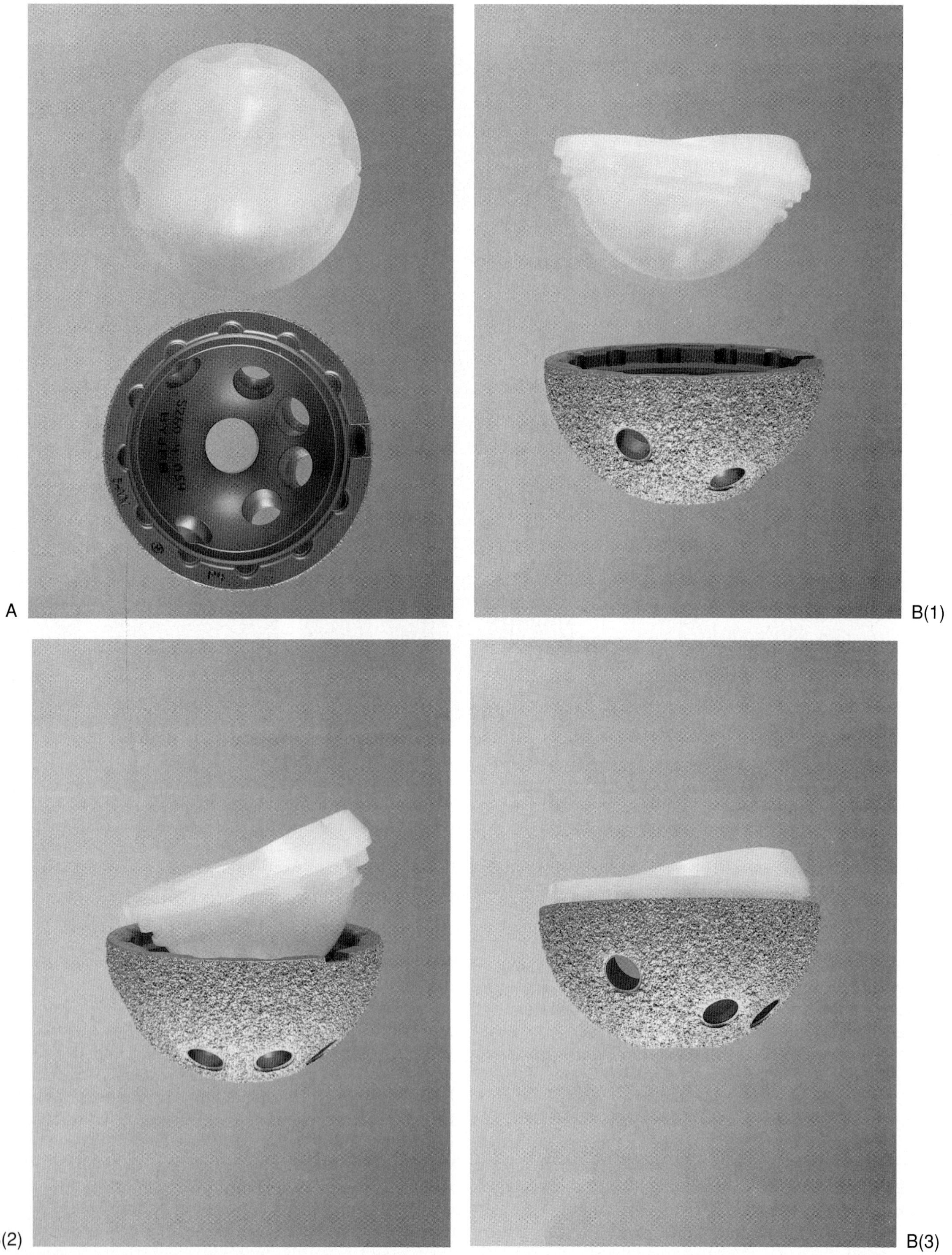


FIGURE 63.2. A. Metal acetabulum with high-molecular-weight polyethylene. B. Locking of the polyethylene into the metal acetabulum.

An elective total hip replacement is performed by exposing the hip joint through a posterior, lateral, or anterolateral approach to the hip. The posterior or posterolateral approach is more commonly performed. The hip capsule is exposed by incising the skin over the greater trochanter. The fascia lata is incised, and the muscle fibers of the gluteus maximus are split for a few centimeters. The greater trochanter is now visible. The leg is rotated internally to expose the external rotators of the hip, which lie superficial to the hip capsule. The external rotators are removed from their insertion and are reflected back to expose the hip capsule. The capsule is then opened to expose the femoral head and neck. The hip is dislocated posteriorly to allow visualization of the acetabulum. The pathologic femoral head is removed. The diseased acetabulum is prepared by contouring it with hemisheric reaming instruments to allow proper fitting of the metal part of the actebular component. The femoral canal is prepared to accommodate the prosthesis. The metal femoral head articulates with the polyethylene, creating a new joint. The external rotators are then reattached to their insertion site. The fascia lata is closed along with the subcutaneous tissue and skin. The patient starts physical therapy on the first postoperative day.

The prosthesis in total hip replacements can be secured by cementing techniques or by a press-fit technique that attempts to allow bony ingrowth into the prosthesis. The most common, and possibly preferred, method at present is a hybrid total hip replacement. It is a technique by which the femoral component is cemented and the acetabulum is press-fit. A cemented femoral component can be ideal for the elderly patient because it accommodates for age-related changes in the bone of the femoral canal, and the patient can immediately bear full weight on the lower extremity. The issue of longevity of hip arthroplasty is not of as much concern in the elderly as in patients less than 60 years of age. Cementing the femoral prosthesis is currently the method of choice of in the elderly. Cemented total hips have lasted as long as 20–25 years. Hopefully, with modern prostheses and advanced cementing techniques, the hip replacements done today will last at least as long in a larger percentage of patients; but long-term follow-up studies are not yet available.

Other total hip arthroplasty methods have been used in the past and are now being tried again but with contemporary designs, including total hip replacements with metal-on-metal articulation. In a current study by Hilton et al., 74 patients received total hip replacements with metal-on-metal articulation with an average of 2.2 years of follow-up.[20] The patients are doing well, but the follow-up is too short to draw any conclusions, especially for this age group.

Ceramic femoral head components can be used for total hip replacements. Femoral heads made of highly polished ceramic are used in the articulation with polyethylene in an attempt to reduce polyethylene wear. The ceramic heads have a lower coefficient of friction. There are reports, however, of fractures of these ceramic heads. At present, the need for this improvement is remote in aged individuals.

## Postoperative Course and Rehabilitation

The general rehabilitation goals for patients who undergo elective total hip replacement are to attempt to return each patient to his or her premorbid functional level of mobility and self-care, demonstrate the exercises that should be performed after hospital discharge, reduce the risk of falls, and ensure that the patient is discharged to a safe environment. Before elective surgery, the elderly orthopedic patient should be instructed to perform breathing exercises to prevent pulmonary complications and active lower extremity exercises to maintain adequate circulation and joint mobility. In addition, functional activities for mobilization in and out of bed are demonstrated. Postoperatively, the interdisciplinary rehabilitation team must facilitate early resumption of active exercises and self-care tasks and discourage prolonged bed rest and dependence on nursing staff and family members. Physical and occupational therapy should be provided to restore mobility and self-care functions. The discharge planning should include assessment of the home environment, with recommendations for modifications to reduce the risk of falls and facilitate independent functioning as much as possible.

The patient who has had a total hip replacement should be encouraged to get out of bed on the first postoperative day. The day after the operation, the patient is encouraged to ambulate with assistance and sit in a high chair for a specified amount of time. Epidural anesthesia, urinary catheters, and drains are not contraindications to ambulation. Postoperative rehabilitation revolves around the surgical approach used to insert the prosthesis and the type of fixation. For example, no abduction of the hip is allowed if a trochanteric osteotomy with reattachment of the greater trochanter was performed. The gluteus medius muscle, which is an abductor of the hip, is attached to the greater trochanter. The greater trochanter is osteotomized at times to enhance exposure of the hip joint. In the elderly, most total hip replacements are cemented, rather than press-fit, which allows immediate and unrestricted weight-bearing. The press-fit prosthesis relies on bony ingrowth for fixation, which can take up to 6 weeks to occur. During this time some surgeons recommend only partial weight-bearing.

Hip stability governs successful postoperative hip function. For the hip to function properly, the femoral head must remain within the acetabulum. During the procedure, the capsular tissue must be incised or partially excised to expose the hip. Capsular tissue can regenerate in 6–8 weeks. It is during this time that the hip is most susceptible to postoperative dislocation, and there is an increased incidence of postoperative dislocations in the elderly.[21–23]

The basic factors governing hip stability include component positioning, soft tissue tension, and possible impingement of structures. The most common positions of impingement leading to dislocation are (1) 60 degrees of hip flexion, adduction, and internal rotation past neutral—posterior dislocation; (2) 90 degrees or more flexion, adduction, and internal rotation—posterior dislocation; (3) full extension, adduction, and external rotation—anterior dislocation. These positions may be noted in the following situations: (1) rising from bed or chair while moving to the contralateral side with the leg adducted and internally rotated; (2) toilet activities in a low seat with feet apart and knees together, or managing foot care in the same position; (3) turning away from the operated hip in extension while lying in bed or standing. All of these instabilities have adduction of the hip in common and should be avoided postoperatively. An abduction pillow to keep the legs apart is usually placed in the operating room and used while the patient is in bed or seated.

In general, later rehabilitative efforts progress toward obtaining full range of motion, strengthening the periarticular musculature (particularly the hip abductors and extensors), and gait training. Range of motion exercises also avoid contractures about the hip. Flexion and extension contractures are the most common. Unfortunately, the gluteus medius and minimus, the hip abductors, are likely atrophied owing to the joint disease. Restoration of normal leverage to the abductors is frequently an inherent part of total hip replacement. Muscle strengthening is important postoperatively to regain confidence in the ability to walk and to avoid an abductor lurch. Exercises that strengthen the abductors avoid the abductor lurch. These exercises are always performed with the positions of hip stability in mind, thereby guiding the extent of motion that can be performed in each patient. Gait training is begun the first postoperative day as well. Assistive walking devices are often required by the elderly for up to 2 months postoperatively. In debilitated elderly patients or those with poor conditioning, walking devices may be used indefinitely. Levy et al. found that most octogenarian and nonagenarian individuals continued to use assistive walking devices even after successful total hip replacement and complete pain relief.[17] The emphasis during gait training is to utilize full extension of the hip, avoid "breaking the knee" during the late stance phase, and maintain symmetrical stride length. Finally, stair-climbing is emphasized by ascending with the nonoperated limb and descending with the operated limb. Concomitantly, the patient should be instructed on modifications necessary to accommodate all activities of daily living by the occupational therapist. Most patients go home with an elevated toilet seat as well, to avoid using the common positions of instability for the first 6 weeks. After 6 weeks a gradual return to normal is anticipated.

## Results

Most total hip replacements are done because of degenerative disease in patients older than 60 years of age. Total hip replacement has been documented to be one of the most successful procedures in contemporary medicine and surgery. In terms of cost versus quality of life-years, it is many times more cost-effective than almost every other major intervention performed. Pain is relieved, walking ability is restored, and enough motion is restored to recuperate all or much of the lost ability to perform activities of daily living.

Results of total hip replacements are usually divided among the 60- to 80-year-olds and those over 80 years of age. In large series the incidence of infection and dislocation, the two most common complications, is 1–2%. These series usually do not separate the two age groups. The operation is highly successful with regard to patient satisfaction in the younger age group. Even in the octogenarian and nonagenarian, total hip replacement is a successful operation in terms of achieving pain relief and subjective satisfaction. Utilizing the Charnley hip score system, a standard scale for measuring the surgical results of total hip replacement, octogenarians and nonagenarians demonstrate suitable improvement in the parameters of pain relief, improved walking ability, and range of motion. These findings are consistent with the improvement found in arthritic patients in younger age groups following surgery.[24] There is, however, an increased rate of complications in the elderly undergoing elective total hip replacement, especially during the early postoperative period. Newington et al. reported a perioperative mortality in the oldest-old as twice that for younger patients.[21] Phillips et al. reported two deaths (2/100) and a 10% incidence of life-threatening medical complications, including one fatal myocardial infarction, one fatal pulmonary embolism, and two other myocardial infarctions in the oldest-old.[22] Levy et al. reported no postoperative mortality within the first 6 months in a group of 100 octogenarians and nonagenarians undergoing elective total hip replacement.[17]

Studies utilizing a proportional hazards model have quantified that the excess mortality that affects elderly patients who require endoprosthetic femoral head replacement for hip fractures is limited to the first 4–6 months after surgery,[19] after which the expected survival for such patients is identical to the standard age group population: 8.2 years for women and 6.4 years for men at 80 years of age. In patients undergoing elective total hip replacement for degenerative diseases, the mortality rate, which ranges from 1% to 3%, is confined to the 3 months after operation.[25] Mortality early on is 2.0- to 4.0-fold higher than during the rest of the first postoperative year.[21,25] Mortality increases with age and with coexistent or co-morbid diseases.[2]

Care of the elderly patient with an orthopedic complaint is stimulating and requires a multidisciplinary team to ensure a good result. Although it is more labor-intensive to perform elective total hip replacements on the elderly because of the co-morbid conditions and specialized therapy required, the surgery should never be denied when it can restore a satisfactory quality of life. In a study by Levy et al. in octogenarian and nonagenerian patients, 98% recorded a high degree of satisfaction with the results of the operation.[17] This coincides closely with 97% patient satisfaction recorded by Nevitt et al. in 1000 patients of younger age who underwent the same procedure. In addition to the subjective satisfaction with the results of surgery, expressions of hopelessness, helplessness, and depression noted before surgery were greatly relieved after surgery.[17] Hip replacement surgery has also been shown to be effective in maintaining an independent quality of life.[17] In the study by Levy et al., 96% of patients were able to continue to either live alone or with the help of a family member or aide.[17] Prior to surgery, it was this relative level of independence that was typically in jeopardy due to the problems imposed by the hip disability. This confers an excellent degree of cost-effectiveness in the oldest-old.

## Complications

Complications with total hip replacement include dislocations, mechanical loosening, infection, and intraoperative complications such as femoral fracture and injury to the sciatic nerve. The geriatric patient is also susceptible to postoperative complications consisting of mental confusion, pulmonary disorders, DVT, pulmonary embolism, urinary tract infections, and skin breakdown. Although not unique to the elderly patient, the complications are more common and can be more problematic in this age group. The complications can dramatically slow recovery from the surgery and prolong the hospital stay. Hospitals are not ideal locations for the aged, and it is imperative that the stay be carefully planned so that as soon as sufficient mobility and independence is regained, the patient may leave.

Mechanical loosening is currently considered the primary problem following hip replacement. The rate of aseptic loosening of the femoral component, the main shortcoming of total hip replacement, has been reduced in general series to as low as 1.5% at 5 years.[26,27] Peterson et al. reported one case of acetabular cup loosening and two cases of 5mm settling of femoral components of total hip replacements in patients more than 80 years of age.[23] Levy et al. found no instances of mechanical loosening in a series of 100 patients over age 80 who were followed an average of 5 years and individual observation for as long as 12 years.[17] The results of these two studies in patients over age 80 correspond to those reported by Sutherland et al., who found a lower rate of loosening of the femoral component in the older age group, probably due to a lower level of activity, than in the younger age group.[28] Three factors have been related to mechanical loosening: patient selection, surgical technique, and component design. With regard to patient selection, it is likely that the general level of physical activity of elderly patients places them in a low risk category for late loosening. The component designs for hip replacement currently available are improved compared to those used in the past. It remains to be seen, however, whether these new designs produce a lower rate of long-term loosening.

Osteolysis is a form of loosening mediated by an immune response. Particulate debris from the polyethylene can induce a macrophage response that causes osteoclast activation and resorption of bone. Such resorption around the femoral and acetabular components can produce loosening of the components and loss of bone stock. Osteolysis is a difficult problem because of the loss of bone, which makes revision surgery more difficult. Osteolysis can be even more problematic in the elderly, where the remaining bone is not strong enough to allow fixation of the prosthesis.

Infection is another complication seen after total hip replacement. Various forms of infection can occur. Postoperative hematomas require attention to prevent the possibility of infection. Two types of deep infection involve the prosthesis: primary (within 12 weeks of the operation) and secondary (any time thereafter, sometimes up to 2 years later). The latter may be due to hidden infection at the cement–bone interface, which takes a long time to develop, or seeding of the prosthesis from an occult bacteremia or frank illness, such as pneumonia, urinary tract infection, or sepsis. The presence of a large foreign body is conducive to infection, especially in debilitated patients such as those with rheumatoid disease or other chronic illness, and many elderly fall into the latter category. These patients should be given antibiotics if they have a total hip replacement and there is suspicion of infection or transient bacteremia. Current recommendations are to offer the same antibiotic prophylaxis for dental procedures as are offered to patients with cardiac valvular disease. Usually, this protocol is recommended for the first 2 years following surgery. Particular emphasis must be paid to preventing infection in the elderly, who may be more prone to it and who have less resistance than the younger adult. Late infection of the prosthesis can present as pain or as loosening of the prosthesis, and it is most important to remember the possibility. Levy et al. reported a 1% incidence of infection with total hip replacements performed in the elderly.[17] The rate of infection in similar series has been reported to range from 1% to 3%,[29] which is identical to that seen in younger patients.

Treatment of an infected prosthesis varies according to the time and type of bacteria involved in the infection. Early infections can be treated with a primary exchange of the prosthesis. This procedure includes excising the infected components, surgical débridement, and immediate reconstruction with a cemented total hip arthroplasty. The basis of this procedure is the addition of antibiotics in powdered form to polymethylmethacrylate (acrylic bone cement). The success of this technique may be influenced by the ability of the organism to elaborate a glycocalyx. A two-stage technique has been the treatment of choice in the United States for the past two decades. The components and all the cement are removed, and an antibiotic-impregnated cement spacer is placed within the hip joint, followed by 6 weeks of intravenous antibiotics. An interval of time is allowed to elapse for the infectious process to be arrested before reconstruction with components is attempted. The ideal timing of the second stage remains to be defined and may again depend on the virulence of the organism.

The incidence of deep postoperative wound infections complicating total hip arthroplasty has decreased significantly with improvements in operating room discipline, including clean-air rooms and body exhaust suits, surgical technique, more assiduous preoperative assessment of the patient, and prophylactic administration of antimicrobial agents. It remains the most difficult complication of total hip replacement to treat and is the most dangerous for the patient. It threatens not only the survival of the prosthesis but in the elderly, can prove to be life-threatening.

The other major complication of total hip replacement is dislocation of the prosthesis. As mentioned earlier, this complication is of special concern in the elderly population because the factors that predispose to dislocation are more prevalent. Weak musculature surrounding the hip, lax capsular structures, component malposition, mental confusion, and forgetfulness are all factors than can contribute to dislocation. Postoperatively, patients must use an abduction pillow for 6 weeks to maintain an abducted position, the safe position for hip replacements done through a posterior approach. At times, elderly patients forget the importance of avoiding movements that lead to dislocation: extreme adduction, flexion, and internal rotation of the hip. It is also not rare for an elderly patient to experience a period of confusion immediately postoperatively. The rate of such confusion in the geriatric population varies from 6% to 26% in patients aged 80 years or older.[17,22] Such postoperative confusion may increase the incidence of dislocation in the elderly.

The incidence of dislocation among elderly patients ranges from 4% to 15%.[17,21,22,23,30] This dislocation rate is two to seven times higher than that reported in younger patients.[24,31–33] Thus dislocation is a special concern in the geriatric patient and requires more vigorous intervention. Preoperative teaching, postoperative reinforcement by the in-hospital physical therapist, and maintenance by the home care staff are crucial adjuncts to preventing later dislocations. Appropriate dosages of postoperative pain medications and limiting large amounts of narcotics during general anesthesia may be helpful for minimizing confusion during the early postoperative period.

Deep vein thrombosis and pulmonary embolism remain serious, life-threatening complications after total hip replacement. Clinical findings such as swelling, pain in the calf, palpable cord, and pain on passive dorsiflexion (Homan's sign) are notoriously poor indicators of DVT. Pulmonary embolism is unfortunately many times the first clinical sign of thromboembolic disease. The treatment for proximal DVT is heparinization concurrent with warfarin therapy until the INR is in the therapeutic range. Heparin therapy should be continued for 5 days. The current recommendation is to maintain the INR between 2.0 and 3.0. The treatment of calf DVT remains controversial. Treatment for symptomatic calf vein DVT and proximal DVT has traditionally been 3 months of warfarin. Patients with documented pulmonary embolism should be treated initially with intravenous heparin for 5 days and concurrent oral warfarin until the INR is in the therapeutic range. Duration of anticoagulation for documented pulmonary embolism is not well established in the literature, but, a minimum of 6 months is recommended. The INR should be kept between 2.0 and 3.0. If the patient cannot tolerate anticoagulation therapy, a vena caval filter is recommended. For these reasons, efforts at DVT prevention are paramount.

During an era when the hospital stay allowance was more liberal, the average length of stay for patients aged 80 years and older after total hip replacement was 14–30 days.[17,21,23,34,35] Elderly patients may be delayed in their successful progression through physical therapy regimens and often have more associated complications than younger patients, which inevitably prolongs their hospital stay.

In terms of the primary goal of relieving pain in the elderly, total hip replacement is extremely successful, thereby markedly improving quality of life. In a study evaluating the benefit of total hip replacement to the community, Taylor estimated that for patients less than 60 years of age, a 10:1 monetary benefit exists after total hip replacement; and for those after retirement age there is a 2:1 monetary benefit.[36] These estimates were based on the recapture of lost earnings before retirement. Even better cost-effectiveness is present when consideration is given to the preservation of independence in the elderly. The average cost for voluntary or religious-affiliated nursing home care is estimated to be $50,000 per year. Thus for every individual who can avoid institutionalization because of total hip replacement the cost-effectiveness is high. This is especially the case in elderly patients who are operated on electively for arthritic conditions of the hip.[17,37]

## Conclusions

A satisfactory health outcome can be expected after total hip replacement even in the oldest-old. Standard hip scores are comparable to those in younger patients. Independence and thus patient contentment can be achieved. The procedure is cost-effective. Mechanical loosening and early dislocation are avoidable problems with appropriate care. Prudent preoperative medical evaluation and well-administered anesthesia help avert postoperative mental confusion and complications, ensuring a smooth postoperative course. The elderly individual should not be excluded from the potential benefits of total hip replacement when the procedure is indicated. The predictable improvement in quality of life to the person and the long-term cost savings to society are worthwhile.

## Total Knee Arthroplasty

### Historical Review

"Total knee arthroplasty is a safe and reliable procedure in the very aged patient for the management of pain and deformity secondary to arthritis of the knee."[38] This statement by Tankersley and Hungerford is the result of more than 135 years of research and development related to biomechanical concepts, prosthetic materials and designs, and surgical techniques utilized on the knee that have evolved for total knee arthroplasty. The history of knee replacement surgery is extensive and is only briefly outlined to document the progression of events that have unfolded to reach the successful designs and techniques of today.

Knee replacement surgery is a resurfacing procedure and is most effective when the principal cause of knee pain is related to pathologic bone contact. Based on this concept, resection arthroplasty is seen as an early attempt to treat these disease processes. Ferguson in 1861 documented the first results of resection knee arthroplasty and reported "satisfactory" function at 5 years of follow-up.[39] Verneuil went a step further and performed what is believed to be the first interpositional knee arthroplasty in 1863. He used flaps of joint capsule to cover the resected articular surfaces. Other tissues (including fat and fascia lata, bursal tissue, skin) and other materials (including cellophane and nylon) were also utilized for interpositional arthroplasty.[40] No material proved to be effective in relieving pain in the diseased knee, and all proved to be less successful than knee arthrodesis, which relieved pain and provided stability.

Metal was first used as a resurfacing material in the knee by Campbell in 1938. He performed two hemiarthroplasties with replacement of the distal femur using an inert metallic alloy mold designed by Boyd.[41] Campbell concluded that "the use of vitallium (an alloy of Co-Cr-Mb) in the reconstruction of a new joint is in the experimental stage, and the ultimate outcome of these cases is at present doubtful."[41] Variations of the distal femoral mold were created and expanded to include a medullary stem, which improved fixation. Hemiarthroplasty eventually crossed the knee joint in the form of a tibial plateau replacement. Overall, the general consensus was that hemiarthroplasty of the knee was not successful and frequently failed secondary to loosening and continued pain in the unreplaced joint surfaces.[40]

The first total knee replacement prostheses were a hinged design and replaced both the femoral and tibial surfaces. One of the first hinged replacements was performed by Magoni in 1949. Indications for this procedure were limited to patients who suffered from advanced degenerative joint disease and rheumatoid arthritis and who required reconstruction following tumor resection or after trauma. The hinged prosthesis dictated the amount of flexion and extension of the knee while providing stability. It was these advances that made it a viable alternative to knee fusion.[40]

The advancements in total knee arthroplasty were directly related to the success obtained with hip replacement surgery. Major gains were made with the use of polymethylmethacrylate (bone cement) for prosthetic fixation, and with the research and development of a variety of materials for prosthetic use including stainless steel, cobalt-chrome, and ultra-high-molecular-weight polyethylene.

The first nonhinged prosthesis was designed by Gunston in 1968. It included a metal femoral component and a tibial component designed from high-density polyethylene fixed to the tibia with polymethylmethacrylate. This design was the first to allow near-physiologic knee motion. It also was the first prosthesis that relied on the patient's own ligaments for stability.

In 1978 Scott et al. reported on the use of patella replacements and found a decrease in patients' patellofemoral pain and overall improvement in the quality of the arthroplasty.[42] Now with the patellofemoral joint accounted for, present-day advances in knee replacement surgery focus on stability, prosthetic fixation, and the materials used.

Stability ranges from the constrained prosthesis (e.g., the hinged prosthesis), to the semiconstrained (e.g., the posterior stabilized prosthesis), to the unconstrained, which relies exclusively on the patient's own ligamentous restraints for stability (Fig. 63.3). Prosthetic fixation can be accomplished with bone cement or by press-fit bone for growth fixation.

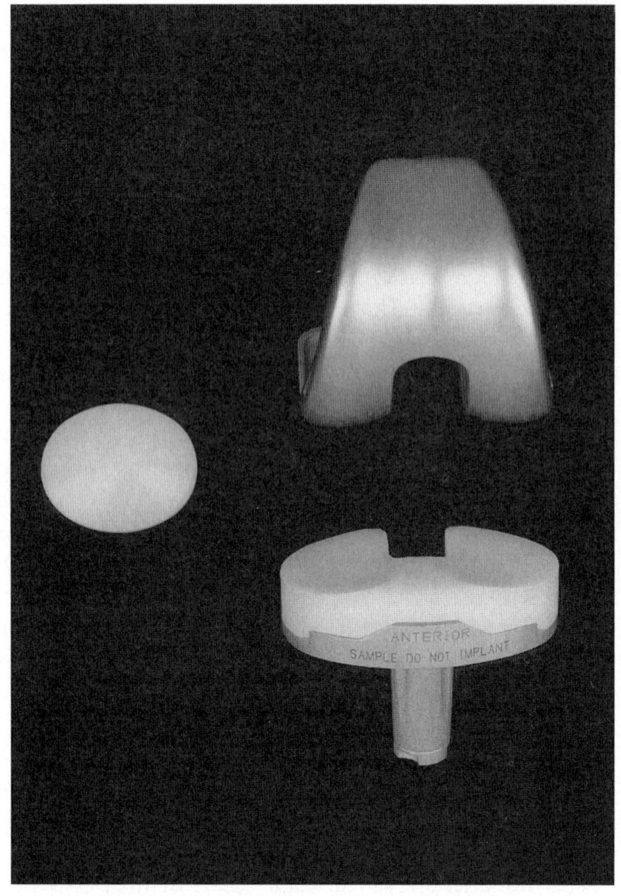


FIGURE 63.3. A. Unconstrained metal and polyethylene sample total knee components. This polyethylene does not contain a central peg. Ligamentous stability must be preserved when inserting these components. B. Semiconstrained components. This polyethylene contains a central peg that articulates with a groove in the femoral component, providing posterior as well as some medial and lateral stability.

The history of knee replacement surgery documents a stepwise progression to the development of today's prostheses. The energies and efforts required has made total knee arthroplasty a successful treatment option for patients with proper indications.

## Disabling Disease Processes about the Knee

Similar to the hip joint, the knee joint is subject to pathologic changes and traumatic events that can severely alter its normal biomechanical function and immobilize the patient with a painfully compromised lower extremity. "Processes" occur that have the potential to compromise the knee joint of the elderly patient to the point where total knee arthroplasty is the most effective therapeutic option available to treat the problem.

Osteoarthrosis is by far the leading cause of knee pain in the geriatric population. An estimated 18 million to 20 million North Americans suffer from symptoms related to osteoarthrosis of the knee.[43] The prevalence of this disease increases with age, affects nearly 10% of the population over 60 years of age, and is second only to cardiovascular disease in producing functional disability.[44] Osteoarthrosis is believed to develop as a result of two possible mechanisms. The first involves abnormal loading of normal cartilage, leading to cartilage destruction. The second occurs when abnormal cartilage is unable to accommodate normal loads. In either situation a potentially compromised knee joint may develop.

Clinically, patients present at different stages of the disease process, and their complaints accordingly vary. In all patients, knee pain is the chief complaint, with diminished walking ability, followed by a decrease in knee motion. Physical findings include joint line tenderness, possibly joint effusion, crepitus, a decrease in motion, and possibly a lower limb deformity including genu varum or valgum.

Osteoarthrosis is confirmed by proper radiologic examinations. Radiographic studies should include anteroposterior (AP), lateral, and patellofemoral views of the knee. The single most useful examination, though, is a weight-bearing AP study.[45] Characteristic findings on radiologic assessment include joint space narrowing, subchondral sclerosis, subchondral cysts, osteophyte formation, flattening or irregularity of the joint surface, and an abnormal varus or valgus alignment ("bow-legged" or "knock-kneed"). Posttraumatic arthritis is a pathologic entity that can mimic osteoarthrosis but has an identifiable insult. Although it is not as prevalent as osteoarthrosis, it is still a cause of debilitating knee pain in the elderly.

The knee in the elderly patient is also a target for destruction in those with rheumatoid arthritis. Rheumatoid arthritis has a prevalence of about 1% in the adult Western population, and two-thirds of these patients are female.[43] Ninety percent of patients with long-standing rheumatoid arthritis have some type of disease manifestations involving the knee joint.[46] The presentation is usually bilateral and relates to the severity of the patient's knee pathology. Early findings may be limited to pain and swelling. With advancing stages of the disease process, the joint space narrows and correlates with the amount of destruction of the articular cartilage and the menisci. Patients develop loss of knee motion with an extensor lag. Ligamentous laxity can develop and predisposes the patient to subluxation of the knee joint. Evaluation of synovial fluid may reveal a total white blood cell (WBC) count of 3000–7000 cells/ml, with 70–80% polymorphonuclear leukocytes, an increase in protein concentration, and a decrease in viscosity. Radiologic findings on complete knee films may include joint effusion, joint space narrowing, osteopenia, erosion of subchondral bone, and a deformity related to the severity of the disease.

Osteonecrosis of the knee, although less common than in the hip, is a well-recognized cause of debilitating knee pain in the geriatric population. It usually occurs in elderly women, with greater involvement of the medial femoral condyle.[47] The exact etiology is unknown but is believe to be related to stress fractures of weakened bone or the result of compromised blood supply. Presentation is with a sudden onset of medial-side knee pain. The pain is severe, persistent, and usually worse at night.[47] The pain may be associated with swelling and a loss of both flexion and extension. Physical examination may reveal a mild effusion and moderate synovitis, but the major clinical finding is tenderness over the medial femoral condyle.

Findings on radiographic examination may range from a normal study to an examination that reveals complete involvement of the medial femoral condyle. Technetium 99m bone scan shows focal uptake in the area of the lesion within a few days of the onset of symptoms. Magnetic resonance imaging (MRI) examination becomes more helpful later in the disease process and shows changes in the marrow consistent with osteonecrosis in the area of the lesion. Lotke and Malcolm developed a classification system of osteonecrosis-like syndromes about the knee that predicted patient prognosis based on the size of the femoral lesion. Their findings indicated that patients with 50% or more of femoral condyle involvement would progress to degenerative changes within 6–12 months and ultimately require surgical intervention.[47]

When differentiating among osteoarthrosis, rheumatoid arthritis, and osteonecrosis in a painful swollen knee, one needs to rule out septic arthritis as a possible diagnosis. A complete evaluation should include a history and physical examination, laboratory studies, and evaluation of joint fluid.

Trauma about the knee is not uncommon in the geriatric population. Supracondylar and intercondylar femoral fractures occur in the elderly population with an increasing incidence and can be related to their osteoporotic bone quality. Nonoperative and operative fixation are treatment options that have been extensively explored; each has associated inherent complications. Bell et al. studied the utilization of primary knee arthroplasty for the treatment of supracondylar and intercondylar femoral fractures in elderly patients. Their results indicate good to excellent results, with most of their patients returning to their preinjury level of independence.[48] Although it is not the definitive answer for treating these fractures in the elderly, it is a treatment option that needs to be explored when the surgeon is faced with a complex femoral fracture about the knee in this patient population.

## Indications

Total knee arthroplasty has proven to be effective in reducing knee deformities, improving patient function, and relieving pain in patients with degenerative and rheumatologic changes about the knee. For this procedure to be successful in the geriatric patient, certain indicative criteria must be met with regard to the patient's physical findings, disability, and overall medical condition. Patients who can benefit from total knee arthroplasty must be properly identified because salvage procedures for failed knee replacements are challenging and usually have limited patient and physician satisfaction.

Disabling knee pain is usually the main reason total knee arthroplasty is performed in the elderly patient,[38,49] but pain should not be the only indication for surgery. A complete history is important to document a patient's disease course. Patients should be carefully questioned about the pain: The duration and location of the pain are noted and whether the pain is related to activity. Do they experience rest or night pain (or both)? What relieves the pain, and what exacerbates it? What medications are required to alleviate the pain? How has the pain affected their lives? Do they require a cane or walker for ambulation? Is their ability to perform activities of daily living impaired? These questions can paint a picture for the physician about how the pain has affected their patients' lives. The individual who states that he or she has "pain" but leads a normal, active life is not the ideal candidate for a reconstructive procedure such as a knee replacement. The history should also explore successful and failed treatments the patient has experienced.

The physical examination must be complete, always beginning with observation. A great deal of information can be gained by watching the patient walk into the office. Speed of ambulation and the ability to sit and stand relates important information about how patients are affected by their disability. When examining a patient with complaints of lower extremity pathology, the complete examination includes spine and neurologic evaluation. It is common for patients with lumbar or sacral spine pathology to present with complaints of lower extremity pain. When knee pain is the chief complaint, it is important to examine the ipsilateral hip for abnormalities. Hip pathology is commonly referred to the knee. It is also important to evaluate the patient's vascular status because, like neurologic disease, vascular disease can present with lower extremity complaints.

The degree of deformity and the condition of the skin of the knee are important observations that must be documented. Palpation should be utilized to localize areas of tenderness and to assess the degree of crepitus. Active and passive range of motion should be recorded as well as the integrity of the muscle.

Weight-bearing films are needed to document the deformity and the bone pathology. Total knee arthroplasty is a surface replacement procedure. Radiologic examinations include weight-bearing studies to document joint space narrowing, flattening or irregular joint surfaces, and bone-on-bone contact. Failure to see these problems indicate to the physician that there may be another cause of the patient's pain, which should be explored with further investigative studies. As previously discussed, spine and hip pathology are distant sources of referred knee pain. Synovitis, bursitis, meniscal pathology, and pathologic fractures are a few of many local etiologic factors that can cause knee pain.

The destruction of multiple joints by various disease processes is not uncommon. It is important to assess the functional status of the other joints involved before performing knee replacement surgery. Compromise of the upper extremities can adversely affect a patient's ability to rehabilitate their surgically replaced knee. In these situations preoperative consultation with a physiatrist may help the patient utilize assisstive devices and rehabilitative therapies, which may better prepare the patient for postoperative rehabilitation. When the patient's ipsilateral hip is also affected, regardless of the etiology, the general consensus is to perform hip replacement surgery first. Inital hip surgery may relieve referred knee pain. It is also easier for patients to rehabilitate the hip with a painful knee than vice versa.[50] When both knees require replacement surgery in an elderly patient, the possibility of bilateral total knee replacements at one operation should be considered. This relates to the advantages of the supine position and the protective effect of the tourniquet.[51] Patients who have had both knees replaced at one operation or within approximately 3 months tend to have better results than patients in whom the total knee replacements were delayed for a longer time. However, in the oldest-old the risks of the bilateral procedure must be addressed.

Total knee arthroplasty is always an elective procedure. The surgeon must always consider the general health of the patient first and how the surgery can adversely affect their lives. The elderly patient is frequently subject to a multitude of illnesses and has a higher incidence of cardiovascular and neoplastic diseases, as well as Alzheimer's-type dementia.[50] Although studies have shown no increased perioperative morbidity in the geriatric patient undergoing total knee arthroplasty, they have shown an increase in medical morbidity, postoperative complications, and perioperative mortality.[49,52]

Absolute contraindications for total knee arthroplasty focus on two major factors: the quality of the skin and a history of infection. A patient whose skin around the knee would compromise the surgical exposure or the success of wound healing may not be a candidate for this procedure. Patients who are combating an acute infection or who have a history of a knee infection or osteomyelitis around the knee may not be acceptable knee replacement candidates.[43]

When contemplating knee replacement surgery in the elderly, it is important to incorporate all of the findings of the history and physical examination and then discuss with the patient and their medical physicians the risks, benefits, expectations, and treatment goals. When properly indicated, total knee arthroplasty in the elderly has relieved pain and in most cases improved the quality of life.[38,50–53]

## Treatment Options

Prior to surgical intervention, patients with disabling knee pain have a variety of conservative treatment options available that should be carefully explored. The proper diagnosis is the cornerstone for effective treatment. Pain relief is the initial goal; it allows patients to regain some independence and to begin to rehabilitate themselves. Pain control for osteoarthrosis, rheumatoid arthritis, and osteonecrosis can begin with the use of extra-strength acetaminophen and can progress to a well-monitored regimen using NSAIDs. Prior to prescribing any medication, one must be aware of the patient's comorbidities and the medications already being taken. Potential drug interactions must be identified and high risk side effects avoided.

Conservative therapy may include judicious use of intraarticular steroid injections. Steroid injections remain an area of controversy, although they have a proved efficacy in rheumatoid patients who have an inflammatory component as part of the disease process. Unique to rheumatoid patients is the utilization of specific rheumatologic medications prescribed by their rheumatologist.

Unloading the knee joint by either weight loss or use of an ambulatory assistive device is highly effective but may be poorly received by the patient. Physical therapy to maintain knee motion and build muscle strength is important for both nonsurgical and surgical candidates. Unloading braces or shoe wedges occasionally have some limited benefit for pain relief in patients with unicompartmental disease.

When conservative therapy fails, surgical options are explored. Surgical intervention is stratified from conservative to more complex procedures. Each operation has specific pathologic entities it can treat. Operative treatment is not necessarily an ordered continuum of procedures that one can progress through to treat a patient.

### *Arthroscopy*

The least invasive procedure available is arthroscopy. Arthroscopy is highly effective in relieving knee pain in patients with meniscal pathology and early-stage degenerative joint disease. Arthroscopic lavage and débridement have produced inconsistent results in patients with grade III and IV chondromalacia, with only 50–70% of patients showing some improvement for several months to 5 years.[54] This procedure has also had "limited effect" on the clinical course of patients with osteonecrosis.[47]

### *Osteotomy*

The objective of osteotomies around the knee is to shift the joint forces passing through the knee from the diseased compartment closer to the healthy compartment. These procedures have specific indications and are more appropriate for the young, active patient with primarily unicompartmental disease. In the elderly population knee replacement surgery has been more successful for treating these patients, especially as prosthetic survival is rarely an issue.

### *Arthrodesis*

Arthrodesis (fusion) is effective for pain relief, correction of deformity, and providing stability. It is an operation that is more appropriate as a salvage procedure and should not be thought of as a primary treatment option for most cases of disabling knee pain due to the complete loss of knee motion.

### *Total Knee Replacement Arthroplasty*

Total knee arthroplasty is an effective surgical option for geriatric patients who suffer from degenerative changes about the knee and have failed conservative treatment. Even elderly patients with isolated degenerative patellofemoral disease are being well treated with knee replacement surgery, which in a younger patient is treated with less radical surgical procedures. The recent literature has shown comparable results of knee arthroplasty with regard to patient satisfaction, pain relief, stability, and range of motion for the elderly and younger patient populations.[38,53] One difference pertaining to function is the continued use of ambulatory aids postoperatively in the elderly population, which may be indicative of a lower baseline level of functioning.[53] A functional outcome study of the geriatric patient after knee replacement surgery reported 90% patient improvement, 89% patient satisfaction, and a 92% subjective response that the right treatment choice was made.[54–55] In-hospital costs and length of stay were also found to be equivalent for elderly and younger population groups undergoing knee replacement surgery, whereas postoperative costs were found to be higher for the elderly population.[53] Total knee arthroplasty is a successful treatment option for geriatric patients experiencing disabling knee pain where the normal anatomy of the knee has been altered and degeneration of the knee joint has developed.

#### Preoperative Evaluation

Once knee replacement surgery is indicated, it is important that the patient's overall medical condition is evaluated and optimized. Potential risk factors must be identified, and when possible this risk is reduced. The risk of surgery increases with age and is primarily due to a loss of cardiac and pulmonary reserve and to the increased incidence of co-morbidities.[56] However, the effects of aging are not uniform, which makes each patient unique; therefore each requires an individualized workup. The preoperative evaluation targets patients' cardiopulmonary and renal systems, their immune function, and their nutritional status, as all can be compromised in the geriatric patient and all can adversely affect the postoperative recovery.

Surgical disease in the elderly has a significant impact on the health care system. Although they comprise approximately 11% of the population, the elderly undergo 40% of all surgical procedures and account for 75% of the postoperative deaths.[57]

Ergina and Meakins recommended a three-step strategy for perioperative management of the geriatric patient: (1) estimation of the predicted risk of complications with surgery based on history and physical examination; (2) prediction of the most likely complications during the postoperative period, permitting early detection and prophylaxis to minimize the risk; and (3) use of perioperative, intraoperative, and postoperative management strategies to optimize outcome.[56]

Total knee arthroplasty and surgical risks in the elderly overlap in three distinct areas: cardiopulmonary function, thromboembolic disease and prophylaxis, and infection. Even though knee replacement surgery is performed in the supine position and with tourniquet control, fluid shifts secondary to operative and postoperative blood loss can occur. It is well known that elderly patients do not tolerate blood loss as well as younger patients.[58] This is a major reason for undertaking a preoperative cardiac evaluation prior to total knee arthroplasty.

Extended bed rest has been shown to increase the risk of cardiopulmonary complications and functional losses.[58] It is important that a clearly established postoperative regimen is outlined for patients preoperatively. It enables them to better prepare for the postsurgical challenges. It is important to focus on what will be expected of them on each postoperative day. Emphasis is placed on their being out of bed and in a chair on the first postoperative day.

Immune function is known to decline with age, making the elderly more susceptible to infection.[58] Regardless of the reason, they have an increased incidence of pulmonary, urologic, and wound infections. The goal is to be aware of, and implement the necessary precautions to avoid these complications. Pulmonary disease can be decreased by mobilizing the patient early and by utilizing chest physical therapy and an incentive spirometer following surgery, which have been shown to open airways and keep them free of congestion. It is important that patients be taught preoperatively to use the incentive spirometer because many are not alert enough following surgery to understand how to use it correctly.

Urologic infections can be decreased by removing indwelling catheters as soon after surgery as possible and by avoiding unnecessary repeat catheterizations. Prompt recognition and treatment of urinary tract infections is essential to avoid potential wound problems. With regard to wound infections, perioperative antibiotics with a cephalosporin is required prior to skin incision, and thorough irrigation and mechanical débridement of the wound are important to reduce the risk of this *devastating* complication. Elderly patients may also be at increased risk of malnutrition, which can affect overall healing; hence there must be complete optimization of their nutritional status preoperatively.

The incidence of DVT is increased in patients following knee replacement surgery and can lead to a fatal pulmonary embolism. Prophylaxis for DVT is essential during the postoperative period to avoid a pulmonary embolus. Regardless of the pharmacologic regimen chosen, close attention must be paid to the anticoagulation status in the geriatric patient. It has been shown that elderly patients have a change in both the pharmacokinetics and response to drugs.[50] For example, geriatric patients have an increased sensitivity to warfarin. Physicians utilizing this treatment protocol must be aware of this possibility and avoid excessive anticoagulation of their patients.[59] Elderly patients have an increased risk for gastritis and an increased incidence of falling. In both instances, anticoagulation therapy and especially overanticoagulation can prove to be fatal by allowing gastrointestinal hemorrhage or traumatic intracranial bleeding. In either case, careful assessment of the risk factors and avoidance management must be appropriately planned.

The choice of anesthesia for knee replacement surgery can be general or regional. In the past it was believed that general anesthesia had an increased risk of inducing postoperative mental changes in the geriatric population and had a direct correlation with mental deterioration.[51,60] Recent studies have contradicted these findings and indicated that general anesthesia does not induce iatrogenic sequelae among elderly patients undergoing knee arthroplasty.[61] They further concluded that general anesthesia poses no more risk to long-term mental function than regional anesthesia, which also was a common fear regarding utilization of general anesthesia in the elderly.[61] The American Academy of Orthopaedic Surgeons recommends epidural anesthesia for lower extremity surgery whenever possible. The choice of anesthetic must be a joint decision between the patient's physician, the orthopedic surgeon, and the anesthesiologist. Any potential risk factors must be identified and conveyed to the anesthesia team well in advance of surgery so the appropriate risk reduction measures can be explored and implemented.

## Surgical Procedure

Total knee arthroplasty is performed in the supine position with tourniquet control. The knee is approached, in general, through a midline skin incision centered over the patella. The skin incision may need to be adjusted in patients who have had prior knee surgery. Although it is usually safe to cross prior transverse incisions utilized for previous surgeries, it is recommended to avoid parallel incisions and the creation of isolated skin islands.[62] When parallel skin incisions must be used, it is important to create an adequate skin bridge to avoid potential wound healing problems. Also essential for proper wound healing is meticulous soft tissue care and creation of thick skin flaps when obtaining exposure.

The knee joint is approached through a paramedial capsular arthrotomy that extends the length of the skin incision. Exposure is gained by subperiosteal release of the medial capsule and to a lesser extent the lateral capsule. More extensive release of the medial structures may be required in a varus knee, whereas a valgus knee requires more extensive lateral release. Further exposure is gained by removal or release of soft tissue structures, such as the medial and lateral menisci; fat pad; anterior cruciate ligament; lateral patellofemoral ligament; for a posterior cruciate prosthesis, the posterior cruciate ligament; and the posterior capsule in flexed contracted knees.

Prior to bone cuts the patella is everted and the knee is flexed to 90 degrees. This part of the surgery places the patella tendon at risk for avulsion. Close monitoring of the patella tendon insertion is required. In patients with "tight" knees, where the patella tendon is at increased risk, additional procedures can be performed to reduce stress on the tendon (e.g., quadriceps snip, quadriceps turndown, and tibial tubercle osteotomy).

Once the patella tendon is deemed safe and the patella is everted with the knee flexed, the bone pathology can be assessed. Special attention is paid to the compartment most affected by the disease process, as it is generally the area of the greatest bone loss. It essentially dictates the amount of bone to be resected, as it can become a reference point from which the bone cuts are made. It is important that the correct amount of bone is resected.

As discussed previously, knee replacement surgery is a resurfacing procedure that requires resection of the bone ends of the femur, tibia, and patella using specialized cutting guides. The goal is to restore the knee joint to match up with the patient's mechanical axis or their anatomic axis; it is achieved by use of intramedullary or extramedullary cutting guides or with a combination of the two.

Prior to and after the components are inserted, the soft tissues are balanced in both flexion and extension. Tightened structures are released to obtain appropriate range of motion. Patellar tracking also is examined; and when necessary, lateral release of the retinaculum can be performed to improve patellar motion.

Once the components are inserted and stable, the tourniquet can be released and hemostasis obtained. Prior to closure, the wound should be irrigated aggressively and all necrotic tissue excised. A drain is usually placed in the knee joint to evacuate postsurgical blood loss. It is removed from the patient in most cases by postoperative day 2. The arthrotomy is closed with interrupted figure-of-eight sutures. The knee is once again evaluated for range of motion and patellar tracking prior to closure of the skin. A sterile dressing is applied, and the patient is transferred to the recovery room with the knee immobilized in extension.

## Prosthetic Design

Total knee prostheses can be divided into three categories based on the relative freedom of movement allowed by a particular design. They include constrained, semiconstrained, and unconstrained prostheses.

A constrained prosthesis is a stemmed component with a uniaxial hinge. The stability and motion of the knee is dictated by the implant. Constrained replacements have a high incidence of mechanical loosening and are recommended only for low-demand patients, following tumor reconstruction, and in patients with severely compromised soft tissue restraints. Bell et al. recommended their use when treating elderly patients with traumatic supracondylar or intercondylar femoral fractures[48] based on the fact that the collateral and cruciate ligaments are generally removed with the distal femur, thereby eliminating the patient's static restraints.

A semiconstrained prosthesis is defined as one that has sufficient design features to provide stability during weight-bearing. An example is the posterior stabilized implant. In many patients, especially those with fixed flexion contractures or rheumatoid arthritis, the posterior cruciate ligament (PCL) is likely to be compromised by the disease process. The posterior stabilized design depends on excision of the incompetent PCL. This prosthesic design is intended to sustitute for the PCL by a cam action of the tibial post against a femoral base, which allows more flexion to occur by providing increased rollback of the femoral component on the tibial component.

Unconstrained designs are replacements that rely on the integrity of the patient's own ligaments to provide stability. In the elderly patient whose ligaments may be attenuated with age, this prosthesis may have less overall success but can be equally successful depending on the pathologic anatomy.

The components can be fixed to bone by press-fit fixation or cement fixation. With press-fit implants, the quality of the bone plays a major role in the stability of the components. In the geriatric patient, who has an increased incidence of osteopenia, the chance of success of a press-fit replacement is reduced. Patients with press-fit prostheses may require a period of limited weight-bearing, which is not practical in the elderly patient.[51] As a result, cement fixation is generally recommended in this population.

The initial unconstrained total knee replacements utilized a tibial component of ultra-high-molecular-weight polyethylene cemented directly to the tibia. During the early 1980s, the tibial design was modified to a metal-backed component that proved to be biomechanically more sound. It had a more even distribution of load to the proximal tibia and a reduced possibility of deformation of the plastic when being loaded. This change in design was accompanied by an increase in the cost for the components. L'insalata et al. compared two elderly population groups who underwent total knee arthroplasty and found no difference in tibial implant survival between metal-backed or cemented polyethylene.[63] They attributed their results to their geriatric patient population being less active and therefore placing less stress on the prosthesis. They concluded that the use of all-polyethylene tibial components can be a cost-saving option in this patient population.

## Postoperative Care and Rehabilitation

A smooth postoperative course is dictated by an efficient, concise preoperative outline of the goals and expectations of what is required following surgery. This is especially true for elderly patients, who may have a decline in independence following an injury or surgical procedure.[10] The geriatric patient is subject to a number of age-related co-morbidities that can adversely affect their rehabilitation.

It is essential that preoperative teaching includes basic instruction on the use of the incentive spirometer, deep-breathing exercises, and utilization of a "good" cough to keep airways open and free of congestion. They should be taught isometric exercises for the quadriceps and gluteus muscles to minimize loss of muscle bulk. They should undergo strengthening of the upper extremities, which helps them with ambulation following surgery and enables them to turn in bed and perform transfers more efficiently. The more that is covered prior to surgery the better prepared the patient will be to perform these functions and regain independence.

Following surgery, patients who undergo uncomplicated procedures are placed in a continuous passive motion machine early during the postoperative period. Motion typically begins at 0–30 degrees and is advanced by 15 degrees as tolerated by the patient to a flexion goal of 90 degrees. Continuous passive motion is utilized as much as practically possible by the patient throughout the day. Patients may continue use of the machine at home. Although not without controversy, continuous passive motion has been shown to increase short-term flexion with little effect on ultimate knee flexion.[64,65] It is believed to be favored by patients, who feel that normal motion is returning to their surgically replaced knee. It is not a substitute for active range-of-motion exercise but an addition to it. It should be noted that Medicare does not usually pay for continuous passive motion machines at home.

Patients are encouraged to be up and in a chair on post-surgical day 1. On day 1, they are visited by the physical therapist for a general assessment and prepared once again for their postoperative therapy routine. Therapy should continue on day 2 in uncomplicated cases. Physical therapy exercises that were taught preoperatively are begun. Patients need to develop good quadriceps control, which is indicated by their ability to perform a strong straight-leg raise. This ability facilitates transfers and enables safe gait training. Additional active exercises are implemented to enhance the redevelopment of quadriceps function.

When the patient is "safe," gait training is begun with use of a walker, with the knee splinted in extension. Extension splinting is continued until the patient exhibits the quadriceps strength to prevent buckling with weight-bearing. General goals prior to discharge are range of motion from 0 to 90 degrees, safe ambulation with a walker for 150–200 feet, and comfort climbing up and down stairs. Failure to meet these criteria at discharge usually results in a patient being transferred to a rehabilitation facility or discharged with home physical therapy prescribed. It is important to note that some surgeons delay any range of motion exercises for as long as 5 days to encourage early wound healing.

As outlined by Flanagan et al., the general rehabilitation treatment goals in the elderly are to return patients to their preoperative functional level of independence, educate them in the exercises that are to be performed after hospital discharge, reduce their risk of falls, and guarantee that they are discharged to a safe environment.[10] If all the above criteria are met, a successful outcome can be expected.

Appropriate postoperative pain control is important with knee replacement surgery. Patients should be comfortable enough to participate actively in their rehabilitation and not overly medicated so they are predisposed to complications of oversedation, such as pulmonary compromise. Patient-controlled analgesia is supported by the literature as an effective pain control option in elderly patients following surgery. It has been shown to provide effective postsurgical pain control and to have a decreased sedative effect, decreased incidence of confusion, and decreased risk of pulmonary complications compared to patients receiving intramuscular injections for pain control.[66]

The incidence of DVT is increased following total knee arthroplasty, so active prophylaxis is required. Two types of prophylaxis are available: mechanical and pharmacologic. Mechanical prophylaxis includes static and dynamic devices, and pharmocologic prophylaxis can be achieved with a variety of medications. In general, mechanical and pharmocologic prophylaxis can be used in tandem. The choice is dictated primarily by the patient's medical status, including co-morbidities and potential drug interactions that may occur, and secondarily by the surgeon's preferred regimen. Regardless of the protocol, close monitoring of the patient's anticoagulation status is required. Clinical suspicion for the signs and symptoms of DVT is important to avoid anticoagulation complications and potentially fatal pulmonary embolism. A major concern in the geriatric patient is the threat of overanticoagulation with conventional dosing schedules.

## Complications

Elderly patients are at increased risk for operative and postoperative complications following all surgical procedures. It is related to changes in their health and the existence of co-morbidities.[56] A number of specific complications can occur in geriatric patients following total knee arthroplasty.

The cardiovascular system is at increased risk secondary to fluid shifts following postsurgical blood loss. Close monitoring of the patient's hemoglobin/hematocrit and appropriate fluid resuscitation can decrease the morbidity associated with postoperative blood loss.

Prolonged bed rest can adversely affect the pulmonary system and lead to complicating bed sores. Aggressive mobilization can effectively decrease the risk of either of these problems.

Elderly patients have an increased risk for urinary tract infections, which can be the source of seeding a knee replacement. Indwelling catheters should be removed as early as possible; and urinary tract infections, when contracted, must be diagnosed and treated immediately.

The elderly also have a high incidence of postoperative confusion: a 34% occurrence following knee replacement surgery in one study.[49] Although there are numerous possible causes, including pharmacologic and intraoperative embolization, the key is close monitoring and a return to normalcy for the patient as rapidly as possible.

There is a high risk of DVT following total knee arthroplasty. Treatment is by a combination of mechanical and pharmacologic measures. The appropriate protocol is dictated by the patient's overall medical status accompanied by a clinical suspicion for the signs and symptoms of DVT. Diagnostic tools available when a DVT is suspected include duplex Doppler and venography examinations.

Complications of knee replacement surgery can be divided into three categories: intraoperative, early postoperative, and late postoperative. Although these complications can occur following any total knee arthroplasty, there is some indication that the effects of aging on the body may predispose the geriatric patient to some of them. It is important that the risks of the procedure are indicated to patients so they may be better prepared for all possible outcomes.

Intraoperatively, two main complications can occur and may have an increased incidence in the elderly: neurovascular injuries and fractures. The popliteal artery and vein and the tibial and common peroneal nerves are closely approximated to the posterior aspect of the distal femur and proximal tibia. These structures are at risk of direct injury with posteriorly directed bone cuts or dissection and indirect injuries from excessive knee motion, possibly including anterior subluxation of the tibia for exposure. Elderly patients have an increased incidence of atherosclerosis, which makes their vessels less compliant, further jeopardizing these structures. Although not routinely practiced, it is recommended that the tourniquet be released at some point during the surgery to look for excessive bleeding and obtain hemostasis. If at any time during the procedure a major arterial or nerve injury is documented, direct repair or a graft procedure should be performed immediately by the appropriate surgical team. It should be noted that use of a pneumatic tourniquet facilitates knee surgery but is not mandatory. In our experience, total blood loss from the procedure is the same with or without the use of a tourniquet.

Elderly patients are known to have poorer bone quality, which puts them at increased risk for fractures of the femur, tibia, and patella and for avulsion of their patellar tendon during bone preparation and prosthesis insertion. It is important that these complications are recognized when they occur, as it enables one to make the necessary adjustments to improve fixation. In general, fracture stability can be obtained using basic internal fixation techniques or by bypassing the fracture with a longer-stemmed implant.

During the early postoperative period, a number of complications may occur and require close monitoring so appropriate treatment can be implemented upon diagnosis. Postoperative hemorrhage is not easily diagnosed because there are no concrete parameters that define "excessive" bleeding. Blood loss of 1–2 units during the first 2 hours of surgery may prove to be acceptable, whereas blood loss of 100–200 ml/hr at 10 hours after operation may be reason for concern.[62] Postoperative blood loss in general is poorly tolerated by the elderly and is potentially fatal. When hemostasis is obtained prior to wound closure, one can be more confident that the source of bleeding is from the cut bone surface. Initial treatment is a compressive dressing, cessation of continuous passive motion, and clamping of suction drains. Monitoring the patient's vital signs and hemoglobin can indicate how the patient's body is responding to the blood loss. Fluid resuscitation should be approached in a cautious but aggressive fashion in an effort to maintain but not overload the cardiovascular system. If a vascular injury is suspected, emergent angiography is performed. If it is positive, surgical exploration and vascular repair are undertaken. The possibility of postoperative coagulopathy should also be investigated.

Wound healing is always a potential problem following surgery in the elderly. The knee joint is basically subcutaneous and can be exposed easily to the environment following wound breakdown. When wound complications arise, they should be treated aggressively. If wound breakdown occurs and components are exposed, thorough irrigation and débridement are required, and a soft tissue coverage procedure is necessary. To avoid wound problems it is recommended that (1) the patient's nutritional status be optimized and (2) meticulous soft tissue care be practiced.

Loss of motion is a diagnosis that is patient-specific. It is closely related to the amount of motion that could be achieved on the operating room table at the end of surgery. A general indication for manipulation of the knee is loss of 50 degrees of knee motion postoperatively. It is important to monitor their physical therapy closely to be able to recognize a loss of milestones early and treat it appropriately.

There are two rare physical conditions that can occur postoperatively resulting in decreased knee motion. Arthrofibrosis is a complication of excessive scarring reaction and results in limited motion. Reflex sympathetic dystrophy is a neurologic abnormality of the sympathetic nervous system that severely compromises knee motion. Arthrofibrosis can be treated with closed manipulation and operative débridement, whereas reflex sympathetic dystrophy is treated with aggressive physical therapy or, in unresponsive cases, sympathetic blockade.

Deep infection following total knee arthroplasty has an incidence of 0.5–5.0%.[67] Infection can result from direct colonization or indirect hematogenous dissemination at any time after surgery. Regardless of the reason, infected knee replacements are potentially devastating complications that require the use of multiple resources for successful treatment. A variety of treatment options are available, including antibiotic suppression, surgical irrigation and débridement without removing the components, removing components with staged reimplantation, resection arthroplasty, arthrodesis, and amputation. The goal of total knee arthroplasty is a functioning, pain-free knee, which is also the goal following treatment of an infected knee replacement; here, though, it is much more difficult to achieve. Failure of treatment is directly related to retention of the original prosthesis. The most successful surgical outcomes are the result of staged reimplantation procedures following an appropriate course of antibiotic therapy.[68] Treatment options may be dictated by the patient's medical condition. High risk surgical candidates are best managed with chronic antibiotic suppression. Patients who present acutely during the early postoperative period and have documentation of an organism with low virulence may respond successfully to aggressive surgical irrigation and débridement, with replacement of the tibial insert and retention of the implant plus appropriate intravenous antibiotic therapy. Knee arthrodesis is a salvage procedure that may be severely compromised in patients with excessive bone loss. Patients who are markedly septic from the infection may require an above-knee amputation for survival, a rare event. Regardless of the situation, infected knee replacements must be diagnosed early and treated aggressively.

Late postoperative complications relate more to implant stability, which can be compromised by trauma or aseptic loosening. Elderly patients are at an increased risk of falling and have a high incidence of fractures secondary to their poorer bone quality.[10] Treatment of periprosthetic fractures in the geriatric patient should consist of closed management in a cast or brace when there is minimal displacement and acceptable alignment. Usually there is unacceptable alignment or displacement, and the patient is a surgical candidate; stabilization can then be afforded by internal fixation or prosthetic revision.

Aseptic loosening can be attributed to increased polyethylene wear but has a lower incidence in the elderly because of their more sedentary life style. As the knee replacement population ages, aseptic loosening may become more of a problem. The goal of revision surgery is to relieve pain while maintaining function. Revision procedures are generally more extensive procedures with an increased risk of surgical and postsurgical complications. Selection of geriatric patients for these procedures must be closely scrutinized with a clear focus on the risk/benefit relation.

### Conclusion

Total knee arthroplasty is a safe, reliable procedure in the elderly population; it can relieve pain and maintain independence in patients afflicted by degenerative knee pain. It is a procedure that has been shown to be as effective in the geriatric population as it is in younger patients, with the exception of the continued use of ambulatory assistive devices by the elderly.[38] The procedure is cost-efficient to society and of predictable benefit to the patient.

Knee replacement surgery is a reconstructive procedure and should be utilized following an inadequate response to nonsurgical treatment. For success it requires carefully selected patients. Preoperative patient and physician communication is essential and should focus on expectations, rehabilitation goals, and potential complications. Close presurgical consultation between the medical doctor, the anesthesiologist, and the surgeon are essential to identify potential risk factors and adjust treatments accordingly.

Total knee arthroplasty, although successful, has a number of complications that are potentially crippling and may have an increased incidence in the geriatric population. Treatment focuses on clinical awareness first, followed by early diagnosis and swift, aggressive treatment. Prophylactic treatment to avoid potential postoperative complications is also important.

With the elderly population forming a larger proportion of the U.S. population, it is important that procedures are available that effectively treat pathology that can compromise their autonomy. Total knee arthroplasty is such a procedure. It has proven to be both cost-effective and successful in providing elderly patients with a second chance at independence. Surgery should be timed so relative independence can be maintained.

## References

1. Durand PJ, Verreault R, Dugas M, Morin J, Paradis C. The use of diagnostic and surgical procedures in the elderly persons in Quebec. Un Med Can 1994;123:226–236.

2. Greenfield S, Apolone G, McNeil BJ, Clearly PD. The importance of coexistent disease in the occurrence of postoperative complications and one-year recovery in patients undergoing total hip replacement: comorbidity and outcomes after hip replacement. Med Care 1993;31:141–154.
3. Friedman B, Elixhauser A. Increased use of an expensive procedure: total hip replacement in the 1980s. Med Care 1993;31:581–599.
4. Shepard RJ. Physiology and Biochemistry of Exercise. New York: Praeger, 1982.
5. Howard JE, McGill KC, Dorfman LJ. Age effects on properties of motor units action potentials: ADEMG analysis. Ann Neurol 1988;24:207–212.
6. Fiatrone MA, Marks EC, Ryan ND, Meridith CN, Lipsitz LA, Evans WJ. High intensity strength training in nonagenarians, effects of skeletal muscle. JAMA 1990;263:3029–3034.
7. Sidney KH, Shepard RT. Frequency and intensity of exercise training for elderly subjects. Med Sci Sports 1978;10: 125–131.
8. Patterson AJ, Murphy NM, Nugent AM, et al. The effect of minimal excercise on fitness in elderly women after hip surgery. Ulster Med J 1995;64:118–125.
9. Swanborg A. Practical and functional consequence of aging. Gerontology 1988;34(suppl 1):11–15.
10. Flanagan SR, Ragnarsson KT, Rosss MK, Wong DK. Rehabilitation of the geriatric orthopaedic patient. Clin Orthop 1995;316:80–92.
11. Altman RD, Gray R. Diagnostic and therapeutic uses of the arthroscope in rheumatoid arthritis and osteoarthritis. Am J Med 1983;31:50–55.
12. Burks RT. Arthroscopy and degenerative arthritis of the knee: a review of the literature. Arthroscopy 1990;6:43–47.
13. Casscells SW. What, if any, are the indications for arthroscopic debridement of the osteoarthritic knee? Arthroscopy 1990;6:169–170.
14. Chang RW, Falconer J, Stulberg SD, et al. A randomized, controlled trial of arthroscopic surgery versus closed-needle joint lavage for patients with osteoarthritis of the knee. Arthritis Rheum 1993;36:289–296.
15. Yang SS, Nisonson B. Arthroscopic surgery of the knee in the geriatric patient. Clin Orthop 1995;316:50–58.
16. Kay A, Davison B, Bradley E, Wagstaff S. Hip arthroplasty patient satisfaction. Br J Rheum 1983;22:243.
17. Levy RN, Levy CM, Snyder J, DiGiovanni J. Outcome and long-term results following total hip replacement in elderly patients. Clin Orthop 1995;316:25–30.
18. Sim FH, Stauffer RN. Management of hip fractures by total hip arthroplasty. Clin Orthop 1980;152:191–197.
19. Coates RL, Armour P. Treatment of subcapital femoral fractures by primary total hip replacement. Injury 1980;11: 132–135.
20. Hilton KR, Dorr LD, Wan Z, McPherson EJ. Contemporary total hip replacement with metal on metal articulation. Clin Orthop 1996;329(suppl):99–105.
21. Newington DP, Bannister GC, Fordyce M. Primary total hip replacement in patients over 80 years of age. J Bone Joint Surg Br 1990;72:450–452.
22. Phillips TW, Grainger RW, Cameron HS, Bruce L. Risks and benefits of elective hip replacement in the octogenarian. Can Med Assoc J 1987;137:497–500.
23. Peterson VS, Solgard S, Simonsen B. Total hip replacement in patients aged 80 years and older. J Am Geriatr Soc 1989;37:219–222.
24. Charnley J. The long-term results of low-friction arthroplasty of the hip performed as a primary intervention. J Bone Joint Surg Br 1972;54:61–76.
25. Seagroatt V, Tan HS, Goldcare M, Bulstrode C, Nugent I, Gill L. Elective total hip incidence, emergency readmission rate, and postoperative mortality. BMJ 1991;303:1431–1435.
26. Harris WH, Sledge CB. Total hip and knee replacement. Part 1. N Engl J Med 1990;323:725–731.
27. Harris WH, Sledge CB. Total hip and knee replacement. Part 2. N Engl J Med 1990;323:801–807.
28. Sutherland CJ, Wilde, Borden LS. A ten year follow-up of one-hundred consecutive Muller curved stem total hip arthroplasties. J Bone Joint Surg Am 1981;64:970–982.
29. Zuckerman JD, Sledge CB. Total joint replacement: latest developments for the geriatric patient. Geriatrics 1985;40: 71–92.
30. Ekelund A, Rydell N, Nilsson OS. Total hip arthroplasty in patients 80 years of age and older. Clin Orthop 1990; 281:101–106.
31. Lewinnek GE, Lewis JL, Tarr R, Compere CL, Zimmerman JR. Dislocations after total hip-replacement arthroplasties. J Bone Joint Surg Am 1978;60:217–220.
32. Coventry MB, Beckenbaugh RD, Nolan DR, Ilstrup DM. 2,012 Total hip arthroplasties: a study of postoperative course and early complications. J Bone Joint Surg Am 1974;56:273–284.
33. Khan MA, Brakenbury PH, Reynolds ISR. Dislocation following total hip replacement. J Bone Joint Surg Br 1981; 63:214–218.
34. Wilcock GK. Economic aspects of the demand for total hip replacement in the elderly. Age Ageing 1979;8:32–35.
35. Wilcock GK. Benefits of total hip replacement to the older patient and to the community. Br Med J 1978;2:37–39.
36. Taylor DG. The costs of arthritis and the benefits of joint replacement surgery. Proc R Soc Lond B 1976;192:145–155.
37. Wigley FM. Osteoarthritis: practical management in older patients. Geriatrics 1984;39:101–120.
38. Tankersley WS, Hungerford DS. Total knee arthroplasty in the very aged. Clin Orthop 1995;316:45–49.
39. Ferguson M. Excision of the knee joint: recovery with a false joint and useful limb. Med Times Gaz 1861;1: 601.
40. Hungerford DS, Krackow KA, Kenna RV. Total Knee Arthroplasty: A Comprehensive Approach. Baltimore: Williams & Wilkins, 1984.
41. Campbell WC. Interposition of vitallium plates in arthroplasties of the knee: preliminary report. Am J Surg 1940;47: 639–641.
42. Scott WN, Rosbruch JD, Otis JS, Insall J, Ranawat CS, Burstein AH. Clinical and biomechanical evaluation of patella replacement in total knee arthroplasty. Orthop Trans 1978;2:203.
43. Lewis CB, Knort KA. Orthopedic Assessment and Treatment of the Geriatric Patient. St. Louis: Mosby-Year Book, 1993.
44. Peyron JG. Osteoarthritis: the epidemiologic view point. Clin Orthop 1986;213:13.

45. Leach RE, Gregg T, Siber FJ. Weight bearing radiography in osteoarthritis of the knee. Radiology 1970;97:265–268.
46. Sculco TP. Surgical Treatment of Rheumatoid Arthritis. St. Louis: Mosby-Year Book, 1992.
47. Lotke PA, Malcolm EI. Osteonecrosis of the knee. Orthop Clini North Am 1985;16:797–808.
48. Bell KM, Johnstone AJ, Court-Brown CM, Hughes SPF. Primary knee arthroplasty for distal femoral fractures in elderly patients. J Bone Joint Surg Br 1992;74:400–402.
49. Hosick WB, Lotke PA, Baldwin A. Total knee arthroplasty in patients 80 years of age and older. Clin Orthop 1994;299:77–80.
50. Newman RJ. Orthogeriatrics: Comprehensive Orthopaedic Care for the Elderly Patient. Oxford: Butterworth-Heinemann, 1992.
51. Sculco TP, Powell SE. Joint replacement in the elderly. Bull NY Acad Sci 1987;63:199–208.
52. Adam RF, Noble J. Primary total knee arthroplasty in the elderly. J Arthroplasty 1994;9:495–497.
53. Zicat B, Rorabeck CH, Bourne RB, Devane PA, Nott L. Total knee arthroplasty in the octogenarian. J Arthroplasty 1993;8:395–400.
54. Larson RI, Grana WA. The Knee: Form, Function, Pathology, and Treatment. Philadelphia: Saunders, 1993.
55. Anderson JG, Wixson RI, Tsai D, Stulber SD, Chang RW. Functional outcome and patient satisfaction in total knee patients over the age of 75. J Arthroplasty 1996;11:831–840.
56. Ergina PI, Meakins JI. Perioperative care of the elderly patient. World J Surg 1993;17:192–198.
57. Vowles KJD. Surgical Problems In The Aged. Bristol: John Wright, 1979.
58. Manning FC. Preoperative evaluation of the elderly patient. Am Family Phys 1989;39:123–128.
59. Gladman JR, Dolan G. Effect of age upon the induction and maintenance of anticoagulation with warfarin. Postgrad Med J 1995;71;153–155.
60. Bedford PD. Adverse cerebral effects of anesthesia in old people. Lancet 1955;2:259.
61. Nielson WR, Gelb AW, Casey JE, Penny FJ, Merchant RN, Manninen PH. Long-term cognitive and social sequelae of general versus regional anesthesia during arthroplasty in the elderly. Anesthesiology 1990;73:1103–1109.
62. Krackow KA. The Technique of Total Knee Arthroplasty. St. Louis: Mosby, 1990.
63. L'insalata JI, Stern SH, Insall JN. Total knee arthroplasty in the elderly: comparison of tibial component designs. J Arthroplasty 1992;7:261–266.
64. Ververeli PA, Sutton DC, Hearn SI, Booth Re Jr, Hozack WJ, Rothman RR. Continuous passive motion after total knee arthroplasty: analysis of cost and benefits. Clin Orthop 1995;321:208–215.
65. Wasilewski SA, Woods LC, Torerson WR Jr, Healy WI. Value of continuous passive motion in total knee arthroplasty. Orthopedics 1990;13:291–295.
66. Egbert AM, Parks LH, Short LM, Burnett MI. Randomized trial of postoperative pain-controlled analgesia vs intramuscular narcotics in frail elderly men. Arch Intern Med 1990;150:1897–1903.
67. Rand JA. Alternatives to reimplantation for salvage of the total knee arthroplasty complicated by infection. J Bone Joint Surg Am 1993;75:282–289.
68. McLauren AC, Spooner CE. Salvage of infected total knee components. Clini Orthop 1993;331:146–150.

# *Part II*
# *Specific Issues in Geriatric Surgery*

## Section 10
## Nervous System

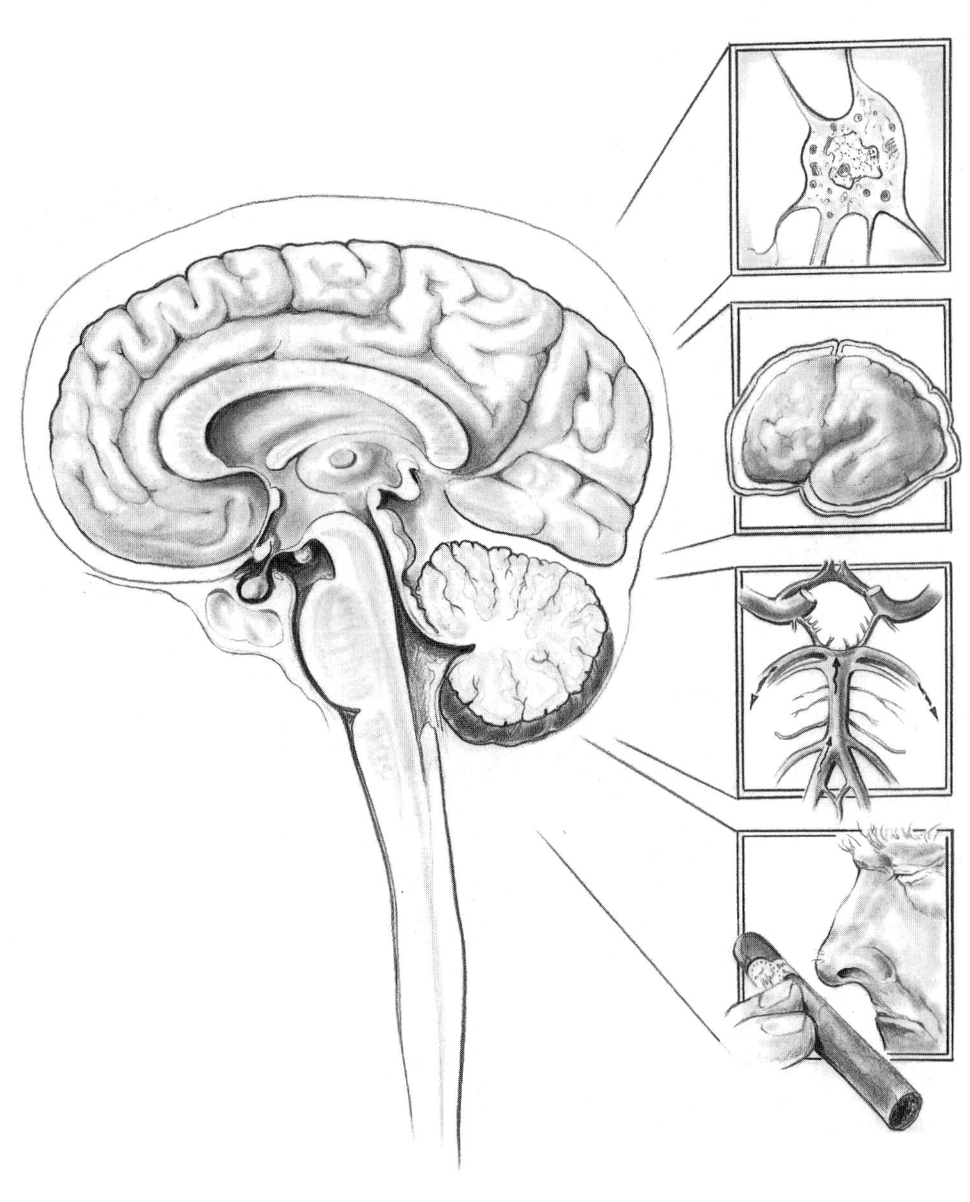

# Invited Commentary

William F. Collins

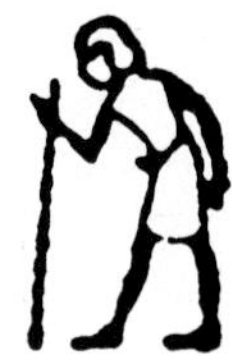

Although the development of modern neurosurgery has been a continuum since the end of the nineteenth century, the changes that have occurred during the past three to four decades have been notedly different. During the first half of the twentieth century, improvements in the diagnostic and surgical techniques of the first few decades were the primary direction taken, whereas during the past 40 years development focused on perioperative care and diagnostic imaging. There also were improvements in operative techniques with the use of the operating microscope, the development of microsurgical instruments, and new approaches to the cranium and the spine; but most of the advances that have resulted in improvement in mortality, morbidity, and functional outcome, have been related to or based more on basic physiology and technical diagnostic innovations than on general surgical skills. This improvement in the risk/benefit ratio for neurosurgical procedures has allowed neurosurgeons to apply curative and palliative operative techniques to a significantly increased number of conditions, even to high risk and geriatric patients with a relatively short life expectancy.

One of the first effective perioperative changes occurred in 1961 when Galicich et al. reported that the steroid dexamethasone could control the brain edema caused by tumors.[1] This decreased the morbidity and mortality of brain tumor surgery by allowing increased intracranial pressure to be brought under control before surgery, so the surgeon could take the time necessary to prepare the patient and plan for surgery without the risk of brain herniation. In addition, the steroid helped control postoperative brain reaction so postoperative courses were smoother with decreased morbidity.

Although the concept of cerebrovascular autoregulation had been proposed by Forbes and Wolff as early as 1928[2] and the reaction of pial vessels to altered blood pressure had been described by Fog in 1938,[3] it was not until the mid-1960s that the principles of cerebrovascular autoregulation were used to control intracranial blood volume and, secondarily, intracranial pressure. The concept that intracranial pressure related to the volume of intracranial blood, extra- and intracellular fluid, and intracranial tissue, helped focus on intraoperative means to control intracranial pressure. The finding that intracranial blood volume was directly related to the $PaCO_2$ resulted in the use of controlled respiration of the anesthetized patient so the $PaCO_2$ could be kept at approximately 30 mmHg. This markedly decreased intracranial pressure compared to the intracranial blood volume and the pressure of the self-respiring anesthetized patient with approximately a $PaCO_2$ of 60–70 mmHg.

The use of intravenous solute diuretics, first urea and then mannitol, enhanced the $PaCO_2$ effect on intracranial pressure. Although ventricular aspiration of cerebrospinal fluid (CSF) had been used for some time to relieve increase intracranial pressure, it was relatively ineffective, except when the ventricles were large. In contrast, circulating hyperosmolar blood was capable of decreasing intracranial water volume regardless of the size of the ventricles. With control of edema around a tumor, minimizing cerebral blood volume with assisted respiration and decreasing the volume of intracranial water with vascular hyperosmolarity, the operating neurosurgeon was able to assess the situation without initial internal decompression of the "noneloquent" brain to control intracranial pressure and could intraoperatively plan approaches to the pathology because there was time and space. The need for accurate intraoperative control of respiration, blood pressure, and fluids was instrumental in the development of the subspecialty of neuroanesthesia.

During the first half of the twentieth century, improvement in the technical and interpretive aspects of pneumoencephalography and ventriculography made each a basic tool for diagnosis of intracranial pathology. As the 1960s came to a close, a major change occurred when the British engineer Godfrey Hounsfield, decided that x-ray film was an inexact way to measure the number of photons that were absorbed when x-rays passed through a structure. He devised an imaging system whereby the output of a focused x-ray beam was accurately controlled and the unabsorbed photons of x-rays sent in fine beams through 180 degrees of a structure could be accurately measured by detectors. With computerized matrix mathematics, the findings were used to reconstruct the internal structure of the object radiographed. For example, when examining a skull, the resulting photon absorption measurements were fed to a computer, and with matrix technology, a three-dimensional picture of the cranial and intracranial contents was plotted and axial tomographic slices were obtained. By 1979 the procedure known as computerized axial tomographic scanning (CAT scan), later called a CT scan, was available clinically. The advances in pneumoencephalography and ventriculography were dismissed as the CT scanner was improved, allowing accurate localization of intracranial pathology without invasive procedures to outline the ventricles and subarachnoid space.

The phenomenon of nuclear magnetic resonance (NMR) had been known since Block and Purcell discovered it in 1946. It had been used mainly for NMR spectrometry during structural and analytic investigations of liquids and solids in experimental laboratories and industry. The development of sensitive radiowave detectors and computerized matrix mathematics made NMR imaging available to medicine during the mid-1970s. It was modified and developed until a magnetic resonance (MR) image was as graphic as a CT scan. Because it most commonly measured the concentration of protons of hydrogen in the central nervous system (CNS), rather than the absorption of photons, it complemented the CT scan.

During this same period the subspecialty of neuroradiology was developing; and instead of having busy neurosurgeons doing diagnostic procedures that were a sideline to the practice of surgery, radiologists specializing in imaging the nervous system began to develop techniques to improve and make diagnostic imaging safer. Arteriography of the nervous system progressed rapidly; and along with intravascular techniques for visualizing the arterial supply of various lesions in the cranium and spinal canal, the ability to occlude or open a vessel was developed and became part of the preoperative treatment of neurosurgery. The ability to control the blood supply of vascular tumors and to partially occlude large arteriovenous malformations before a surgical procedure decreased morbidity and mortality. Thus, along with improved arteriography that had fewer complications, it allowed neurovascular surgery to develop rapidly.

During the 1950s, with the recognition that a considerable portion of the intracranial vascular problems related to cervical vessel disease, cervical carotid endarterectomy became part of the neurosurgeon's armamentarium, and procedures for correction of cervical carotid defects were developed. Surgery for ruptured and unruptured intracranial aneurysms improved with the control of intraoperative blood and intracranial pressure, surgery with magnification, and the use of graded spring-closing clips that could obliterate or temporarily occlude intracranial vessels. The operative mortality that, during the first few decades of the twentieth century had stood at close to 50%, now was reduced to almost one-tenth of that.

The clinical and pathologic entity of hydrocephalus has been known for centuries.[4] During the second and third decades of the twentieth century, Dandy and Blackfan[5] proposed that the cause of hydrocephalus was usually lack of absorption and not overproduction of CSF. They divided the entity into obstructive and nonobstructive hydrocephalus on the basis of whether the block in absorption was in the aqueduct of Sylvius (obstructive) or the subarachnoid space (nonobstructive). Dandy and Blackfan proposed to treat the obstructive condition with a third ventriculostomy and the nonobstructive condition with a choroid plexectomy. Although both therapies worked, the mortality was high (25–30%) and the success rate relatively low (35–40%). During the mid-1950s, Holter designed a one-way pressure-controlled valve that allowed drainage of spinal fluid into the venous system. Pudenz at about the same time devised a similar valve, and the treatment of hydrocephalus changed. Both of these shunts could be tested for patency while in place and in a short time were used not only for ventriculovenous drainage but also for ventriculopleural or ventriculoperitoneal shunting. Controlled ventricular pressure was relatively simple to produce with a Holter or a Pudenz valve. Although there were and continue to be problems with complications of infection, blockage, and overdrainage, in general their correction has been simple and the patients have done well.

The pressure-controlled shunt technique affected geriatric neurosurgery when in 1961 Hakim and Adams[6] presented the results of shunting CSF in four cases of normal-pressure hydrocephalus (NPH). The syndrome they described and treated consisted in the adult of progressive dementia, apraxic gait, and incontinence, with imaging evidence of hydrocephalus and a block in the absorption of CSF in the ventricles or the subarchnoid space. The results of shunting NPH were almost miraculous and opened an entirely new therapy for one type of adult-onset dementia.

Another concept that has made a difference in neurosurgical mortality and morbidity, has been the idea that spinal cord compression should be relieved by direct removal of the compressing force. Until the early 1950s, the major approach to the spinal cord had been laminectomy; decompression of the spinal cord consisted of removing the spinal column lamina from the posterior approach, no matter the direction of the compression. Although this measure released circumferential compression of the cord, it often caused further displacement of the spinal cord and compromise of the blood supply, with an increase in neurologic deficit. It is difficult to assign the development of the various approaches to the spinal cord to one neurosurgeon or even a group of neurosurgeons, but probably it was the popularization of the anterior approach to the cervical spine by Cloward[7] that gave the impetus to develop the various approaches. With his anterior cervical diskectomy procedure, neurosurgeons were able to remove compressing tissue from the anterior spinal canal without displacing the spinal cord. Soon approaches to the spinal canal other than laminectomy, including anterior and anterolateral cervical, transoral, transthoracic, costotransverse, and retroperitoneal procedures, were developed to treat cervical spondylosis, ruptured thoracic discs, tumors of the vertebral body, and any lesion that was causing myelopathy from pressure on the spinal cord in a direction other than posteriorly. These procedures and the ability to stabilize the postoperative spinal column, allowed operative intervention for compressive myelopathy, with minimal risk of increasing the neurologic deficit, and with a more rapid recovery, especially for traumatic and malignant lesions of the spinal column.

At the turn of the century, operative intervention for dyskinesias focused on relief from adventitious motor movements such as athetosis. Horsley proposed and performed perfrontal cortical resections for hemiathetosis. During the 1930s Bucy and his associates expanded the procedure of cortical resection for control of Parkinson's tremor, choreothetosis, and hemiballismus. A major deficit of the procedure was paresis (proportional to the movement control) and spasticity (proportional to the paresis). It was Meyers' observation during the 1940s that a lesion in the globus pallidus or its outflow, the ansa lenticularis, controlled dyskinesias without significant paresis.[8] The relatively high mortality of the craniotomy approach led to the development of stereotactic procedures to produce focal lesions. In 1947 Spiegal et al.[9] reported the development of a stereotactic instrument that could be used in human operations that was based on the 1908 Horsley-Clark[10] animal experimental stereotactic instrument. It was rapidly accepted, and a number of stereotactic instruments were developed along with refinement in lesion-making and localization control. Cooper[11] popularized stereotactic lesion treatment of Parkinson syndrome, and during the 1950s and 1960s stereotactic surgery flourished. Its popularity declined with the availability of L-dopa during the late 1960s, and it was not until the dyskinesias caused by the drug and its decreasing effectiveness with the passage of time that stereotactic surgery had a resurgence during the 1980s. The resurgence not only included treatment of abnormal motor movements; but with the development of better diagnostic imaging to control lesion localization and to evaluate lesions without invasive procedures, its use was expanded. Because of its low morbidity and its accuracy, stereotactic biopsy of tumors, degenerative diseases of the CNS, and infection processes became common. Techniques with stereotactic control of protons, gamma rays, or photons were developed to produce localized high-energy radiosurgical lesions that could destroy metastatic or primary tumors, obliterate arteriovenous malformations, or be used for focal controlled radiation therapy.

Current developments in neurosurgery appear to be concentrating on the efforts of subspecialist neurosurgeons working with basic neuroscientists and with other surgical and medical subspecialists. This concentration of effort and the widening of the base for neurosurgical investigation should, in the next 40 years, help change neurosurgery even more than it was changed during the past 40 years. The results should give neurosurgical patients an even better chance for a functional life.

## References

1. Galicich JH, French LA, Melby JC. Use of dexamethasone in the treatment of cerebral edema associated with brain tumors. Lancet 1961;81:46–52.
2. Forbes HS, Wolff HG. Cerebral circulation. III. The vasomotor control of cerebral vessels. Arch Neurol Psychiatry 1928;19:1057–1086.
3. Fog M. Relationship between blood pressure and tonic regulation of pial arteries. J Neurol Psychiatry 1938;1:187–197.
4. Scarff JE. Treatment of hydrocephalus: an historical and critical review of methods and results. J Neurol Neurosurg Psychiatry 1963;26:1–27.
5. Dandy WE, Blackfan KD. An experimental and clinical study of internal hydrocephalus. JAMA 1914;61:2216–2217.
6. Hakim S, Adams RD. The special clinical problem of symptomatic hydrocephalus with normal cerebrospinal fluid pressure: observations on cerebrospinal fluid hydrodynamics. J Neurol Sci 1965;2:307–327.
7. Cloward RB. The anterior approach for the removal of ruptured cervical disks. J Neurosurg 1958;15:602–617.
8. Meyers R. The modification of alternating tremor, rigidity, and festination by surgery of the basal ganglion. Res Publ Assoc Res Nerv Ment Dis 1942;21:602–665.
9. Spiegal EA, Wycis HT, Marks M, Lee A. Stereotaxic apparatus for operation on the human brain. Science 1947; 106:349–350.
10. Horsley V, Clark RH. The structure and function of the cerebellum examined by a new method. Brain 1947;31:45–124.
11. Cooper IS. Results of 1000 consecutive basal ganglion operations for parkinsonism. Ann Intern Med 1960;52:483–499.

# 64
# Effects of Aging on the Human Nervous System

J.C. de la Torre and L.A. Fay

Elderly patients are known to represent a major proportion of problems affecting the central nervous system (CNS) and consequently make up a significant percentage of patients requiring elective or emergency surgery of the brain and spinal cord. The significance of this statistic is of great medical and socioeconomic importance.

It is estimated that the number of people over the age of 65 in the world make up about 11% of the general population. In the United States, those over the age of 75 make up 12 million of the population, and this figure is projected to exceed 13 million by the year 2000.[1,10] This rapid growth in increased longevity reflects a better understanding of the aging process and the result of major medical advancements in the past half century. However, the increase in the life-span of these individuals is not without consequences. Epidemiologic studies show that 10% of the noninstitutionalized elderly over age 65 and 20% of those over 75 may suffer substantial intellectual impairment from organic brain causes.[1,2] The concept of aging and intellectual deterioration involves many etiologies and is not well understood by many health care professionals.[3,4] A better understanding of the neurology of aging is essential for managing and improving the prognosis of age-related disorders.

Although the aging phenomenon is the focus of many disciplines, including physiology, anatomy, psychology, and sociology, the purpose of this chapter is to review the physiologic, neuroanatomic, and psychological data on aging that may be useful to the surgeon. The morphologic and physiologic alterations of the challenged CNS will therefore be discussed to provide a profile of how easily this system can become dysfunctional in the elderly individual. The latter portion of this chapter focuses on the clinical concepts of the aging nervous system.

Certain generalizations about the aging process can be made. First, intellectual performance with respect to semantic knowledge peaks at 20–30 years, plateaus until the mid-eighties, and thereafter steadily declines.[5–8] Second, performance on reaction-timed tasks and speed of central processing of information peak at approximately age 20 and steadily decline throughout a life-span. Third, episodic memory changes may be affected, particularly recall and working memory. Fourth, there is evidence that reduced perception of sensory stimuli affects the visual and auditory systems.[9,10] Also, because motor and sensory abilities decline with aging, postural maintenance and balance can be compromised, and gait changes frequently develop. There is some evidence that some presynaptic terminals in the cerebral neocortex and hippocampus are lost during aging. Cerebral hypoperfusion (defined as the inability of cerebral blood flow to meet neuronal energy demands) and cerebral oxygen and glucose utilization are reduced with increased aging.[11–16] Mild but persistent cerebral hypoperfusion may consequently develop during "normal" aging and act as a precursor to many age-related anomalies of the nervous system.[17] Morphologically and biochemically, the individual neurons respond to the neurochemical changes initiated at the molecular level and compensate in various ways. For example, aging neurons can accumulate lipofuscin pigmentation, a degradation of the lipid bilayer of the membrane, and develop enlargements of the cytoplasmic transport organelles. Lipofuscin accumulation may result as a response to repeated stimulation of the neuron with weakened reuptake of neurotransmitters at the synaptic region.[18–21] Neurons may also compensate when physiologically challenged by dendritic lengthening, a reduction in dendritic spines, decreased axoplasmic transport, synaptic enlargements, demyelination, and a host of other changes that contribute to decreased generation of action potentials for transmission.[22–24]

When age-related changes are assessed on a larger scale (e.g., on individual organs that compose an entire functional system within the body), reduced nerve action potentials to vital organs hamper the normal homeostasis of these life-sustaining centers within the body.

# Morphologic Cell Changes Related to Aging

## Nucleus of the Neuron

The nucleus is the functional center of a neuron, regulating the nerve cell's activities (Fig. 64.1). The aging nucleus of a neuron in elderly humans has been shown to contain increased basophilia and an irregularly shaped nucleus.[2] Loss of a clear, regular nuclear outline and sharp demarcation of the nuclear–cytoplasmic border has been observed in aging neurons in old mice and aging humans.[2,25] This change in nuclear morphology in senescent neurons may lead to functional inefficiency or death even when an insult to the brain is mild and otherwise inconsequential.

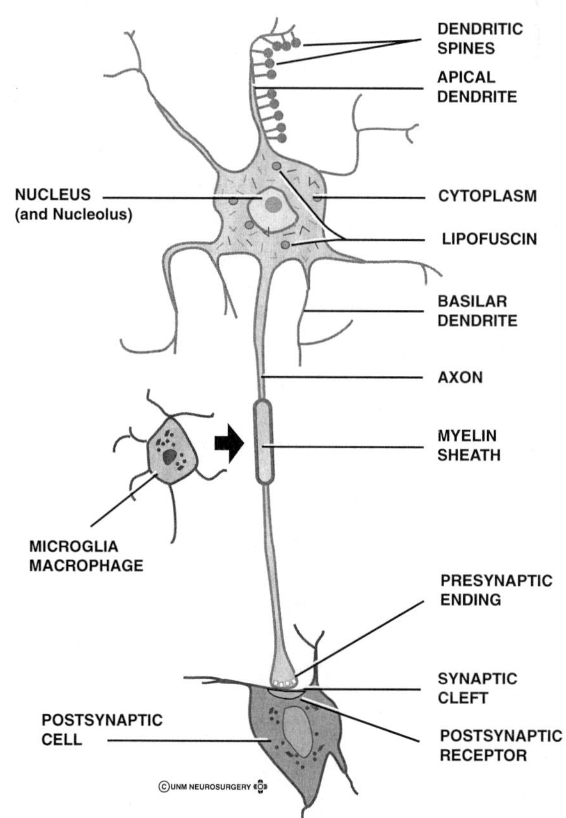


FIGURE 64.1. Main structures of typical aging in the human neuron. The cell body is the metabolic center of the neuron and gives rise to 20–40 dendrites and an axon. Some neurons (e.g., hippocampal) have dendritic spines (which receive synaptic input from other neurons) or a fatty myelin sheath (for high speed conduction of action potentials). The synapse is composed of a terminal ending (presynaptic), synaptic cleft (where the chemical transmitter is released), and postsynaptic receptor (soma, axon, dendrite of another neuron) which is activated by the chemical transmitter. Microglia and macrophages can phagocytize neuronal and myelin debris after injury. Most of the structures below this point are altered negatively during aging (see text for details).

## Neuronal Perikaryon

The perikaryon is the body of the neuron and houses most of its organelles. Among the most prominent organelles is the Golgi apparatus, the subsurface cisternae, and the smooth and rough endoplasmic reticulum, the latter forming part of the Nissl substance.[20] Depletion of Nissl material appears to coincide with increased lipofuscin formation.[20] With respect to the Golgi complex and smooth endoplasmic reticulum, dilation of these structures has been associated with neuronal aging.[2] The mitochondria in these neurons exhibit loss of the outer membrane, accompanied by vesiculation of the cristae and the formation of multivesicular bodies. These alterations of the mitochondrial structure can cripple or kill the neurons by robbing them of their main energy generator, by producing toxic free radicals, and by impairing adrenergic neurotransmitter activation.

## Dendrites

Dendrites are processes concerned with the reception of stimuli from their environment. The size, shape, orientation, and complexity of the dendritic tree and its branching pattern show a direct correlation with the location of the neuron in the CNS and the number of functioning contacts that can be made with other neurons.[26] Structural losses in dendritic branching have been demonstrated in aged rats and elderly humans.[27] A reduction in dendritic lengths up to 50% and a loss of one-third of dendritic spines has been observed in rats, with similar results seen in aging humans.[27,28] Increased dendritic density is observed in the somatosensory cortex but not in the occipital cortex of aging animals. Such specific anatomic sparing of dendrites may be a compensatory reaction by the unaffected neurons relative to those neurons developing a decrease in dendritic population.[29]

In 1976, Diamond and Connor[29] became interested in learning if dendritic changes occurred in vivo when two groups of rats were exposed to an enriched or impoverished environment. Their findings concluded that rats that spent their last 30 days in an enriched environment had longer terminal segments in the most distal portions of their dendritic trees in both the occipital and somatosensory cortex when compared to the impoverished environment group.[29] This was one of the first examples of an environmental effect on the dendritic structure in aging animals. The findings may be interpreted as a growth or elongation of the distal segments of dendrites or as a retraction of dendrites. It is possible to conclude from these data that during aging, hypertrophy of many aspects of the neuron can occur, and therefore an enriched environment may prevent dendritic hypertrophy in aged rats. In terms of human relevance, activities that reduce known risk factors to stroke and hyperlipidemia or that increase cerebral perfusion to the brain, such as intellectual stimuli by way of reading, analyzing problems, using complex oral or written language, and other activities requiring "brain work," have been shown to reduce the risk of dementia and cognitive decline in the aged population.[13,15,30]

## Axons

Neurons have only one axon, and it is this process that transmits information to other neurons by way of the synapse (Fig. 64.1). One of the major functions of axons is to transport proteins, synaptic vesicles (containing neurotransmitters), axolemmal precursors, and mitochondria from the cell cytoplasm to its presynaptic terminal by fast axonal transport. Slow axonal transport *returns* many of these "repackaged" macromolecules back to the cell body, including exogenous trophic substances and growth factors picked up by the distal region of the axon via endocytosis.[31] These factors can later ensure the survival of the challenged neuron and probably modulate neuronal gene expression.

The morphology of the axon, such as its diameter and the presence of myelin, contributes to regulation of the conduction velocity or speed of the neural impulse. Myelin is the spirally wrapped lipid membrane that functions to increase the efficiency of nerve conduction.[32] For normal functioning of axons, fast axonal transport of synaptic vesicles and the neurotransmitter material the vesicles carry are essential for proper interneuronal communication. This transport relies on the microtubules and neurofilaments within the axonal cytoskeleton, which are laterally interconnected by various associated proteins.[33] The lateral bridges connecting the filamentous structures and the microtubules and neurofilaments may function as a three-dimensional sieve with pore sizes comparable to the slightly varying diameters of the vesicles.[34] This suggests that there is organized transport of vesicles to achieve maximum efficiency and speed in neurotransmitter secretion by size filtering. When vesicles travel through the intact axoplasm, there develops an inverse relation between vesicle size and transport speed, with small vesicles being transported faster.[33,35] When vesicle travel is within a single microtubule, the relation between size and speed is lost.

Factors that disrupt vesicle transport can significantly impair neurotransmission and upset axonal homeostasis, leading to compromised cell function or death. The effect of aging on fast axonal transport has been studied in isolated nerve preparations in aged rats.[23,24,34,36] The data have shown that transport rates (anterograde and retrograde) of all vesicles slow down with age, though the larger vesicles undergo greater reductions in transport rate than do the smaller vesicles.[23,36–38]

Slower axonal transport and delayed nerve impulses may result from a breakdown of the microtubule matrix within the axons, contributing to slower vesicle transport. The microtubule structure is analogous to a scaffolding structure used during construction. If a portion of the scaffold is missing, provided it is not a sole supporting structure, the overall function of the system is disrupted and delayed.

Metabolic reasons contribute to age modifications in the axons, such as reduced availability of the main energy substrate adenosine triphosphate (ATP) and cumulative defects in mitochondrial DNA.[34] Nonspecific aging of the microtubules, such as nonenzymatic glycosylation and accumulation of its end-products, could interfere with molecular attachment, thereby slowing transport.[34] Finally, increased diameters of the vesicles, which correlate with enlarged synaptic endings due to repeated stimulation over one's life-span, may also slow vesicle movement along the axon.[34] Microtubule disruption is further enhanced with the incidence of disease, most likely due to metabolic abnormalities.

## Synapses

Synaptic terminal regions are the neuronal compartments where neurotransmitters are released in response to a particular stimulus (Fig. 64.2). The morphology of synapses can be regulated by electrical stimulation, behavioral conditioning, and trophic factors.[39] Thus synaptic modulation is dependent on a constant ongoing physiologic process as well as sensitivity to the environmental stimulation of the CNS.[39] When these factors are disturbed, such as by the normal progression of aging, modifications occur within the synapses.

Synaptic surface density (Sv) is a morphometric parameter that quantifies the total area of the synaptic contact zones present in $1\,\mu m^3$ of tissue.[39] Significant reductions and morphologic degeneration in Sv were observed within the CNS of aged laboratory rats and were also found within the physiologically normal aging human brain.[39]

Understanding the numeric density of synapses per unit volume provides insight into the functioning of the CNS. These measurements are taken as the number of synaptic contact areas related to the numerical density of the neurons in the same zone, and the final calculation is the number of synapses per neuron.[40,41] It is this quantification of synaptic density that has been reported to influence the size of the postsynaptic potential.[42] Consequently, the arrangement and quantity of synaptic connectivity would extensively affect the transmission and processing of the nerve impulses.[40,43–45] With aging, a decrease in synaptic density in the cortex, cerebellum, and hippocampus of laboratory animals has been reported by several investigators.[43,46] There is general agreement that a marked decline of synaptic numerical

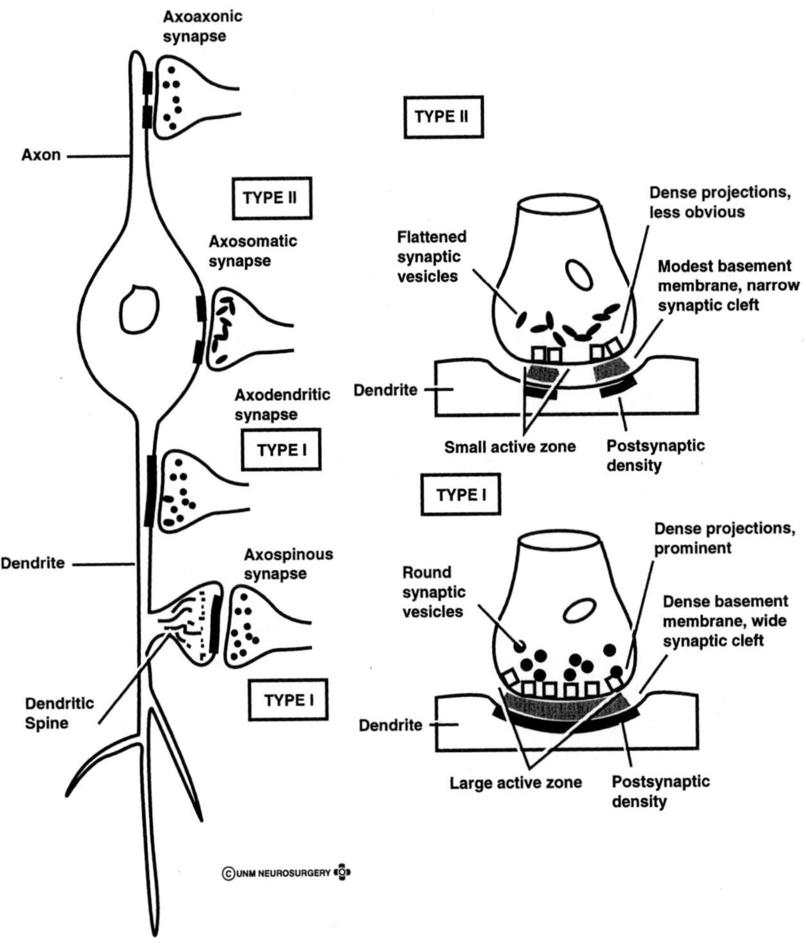


FIGURE 64.2. Synaptic contacts (axosomatic, axoaxonic, axodendritic and axospinous), which can be excitatory (type I) or inhibitory (type II) and are classified according to the presence of a basement membrane, shape of vesicles containing the neurotransmitter, size of the active zone, and width of the synaptic cleft. Possible changes to these structures can occur during aging. (Adapted from Kandel and Schwartz,[32] with permission.)

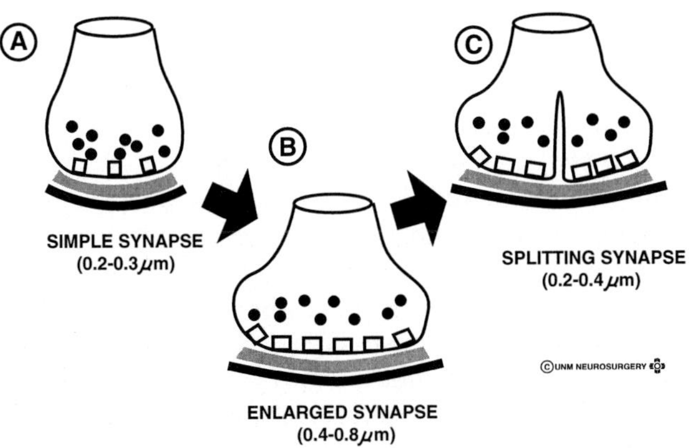


FIGURE 64.3. Phases of synaptic fragmentation. Repeated stimuli cause the synapse to increase in size over time. Eventually, the synapse perforates and splits into separate synapses, a condition known as synaptic fragmentation. The incidence of this fragmentation is higher in young populations and declines with aging (see text for details).

density occurs in the hippocampal region of the aged human brain.[40,43] Recent research on the quantitative assessment of synaptic numerical density and contact surface areas in adult, healthy aged brain and old demented brain, confirm that during physiologic non-pathologic aging, human CNS, synaptic contact areas undergo severe morphologic degeneration with significant reductions in synaptic numeric density.[43] These findings are markedly amplified in the pathologically demented brain.

During a person's life-span, it is a common belief that synaptic morphologic remodeling via fragmentation occurs in response to repeated stimulations at the pre- and postsynaptic sites (Fig. 64.3). As a consequence of sustained stimulation, the synapse enlarges, and a process of perforation and splitting into smaller synapses develops, a condition termed "synaptic fragmentation."[42,47,48] When an undefined limit of synaptic size is attained, an intrinsic mechanism within the synapse is activated to initiate the process of fragementation.[8] This hypothesis is currently under investigation, but there has been physiologic evidence that during post-epileptic discharges, these megasynapses are not seen.[8] In a young healthy adult, these fine fragmentations could contribute to increased synaptic volume density and contact areas, thereby creating extensive amplification of a specific neurotransmitter for efficient signal transmission. Experimental data have documented that a preserved complement of perforated synapses is needed to maintain proper spatial memory in rats.[49] In the elderly, however, there is less fragmentation of synapses, indicating a slowdown of structural synaptic turnover and enlarged synaptic structures.[50]

In old individuals, experimental evidence indicates that there is a decline in synaptic contacts, and the total surface area of synaptic appositions per unit volume of tissue and the average synaptic size increases at a different rate according to the CNS area sampled (Fig. 64.3). Less fragmentation of the synapses at the junctional zones is observed. The result is larger synaptic terminals, which appear to represent unfinished synaptic turnover cycles. It is possible that these morphologic changes play an important function in inadequate nerve impulse transmission. If there is a deficit in nerve impulse transmission, all body functions are affected. Decreases in the surface contact area and numeric density in turn decrease the amount of neurotransmitter released in response to a stimulus and decrease the speed at which the information is transported. Often, spatial memory and cognition are affected by slower neural impulses in the normal aging brain. The sensory and motor systems are greatly influenced by these changes for similar reasons (e.g., slower conduction of the neural impulses). Diminished neural perception and response decrease the efficiency of vital functions in the body and eventually alter the life style and health of the older individual.

## Glial Cells

Glial cells differ from neurons in that they have no synaptic contacts and can divide, proliferate, and in some cases hypertrophy, particularly in response to neuronal stress or injury. They are known to play a role in brain vessel transport of vital molecules and neural tissue repair (astrocytes), phagocytosis (microglia), and produce myelin for neurons (oligodendrocytes). The distribution of microglia and astrocytes following brain ischemia often predicts the extent and subsequent damage to brain tissue,[51] a useful index during aging.

## Neurotransmitters and Receptors

Neurotransmitters are the chemical signals released at the synapse and have a direct effect on the subsynaptic membrane. Their function is to transmit the neural impulse to other sites of the nervous system. Acetylcholine, 5-hydroxytryptamine, dopamine, and norepinephrine are the major chemical transmitters of the nervous system.[52] The terms cholinergic and adrenergic refer to neurons that release either acetylcholine or norepinephrine, and the post-junctional sites where the two transmitters are released, are called cholinoceptive or adrenoceptive, meaning they exert their activity on cholinergic or adrenergic receptors.[20]

Acetylcholine is found in all postganglionic parasympathetic fibers, all preganglionic autonomic fibers, in a few postganglionic sympathetic fibers, and at neuromuscular junctions.[52] Dopamine is stored in large dense-core vesicles in the presynaptic terminal and is an important neurotransmitter in both the CNS and the autonomic nervous system. There are three main types of dopamine receptor ($D_1$, $D_2$, $D_3$), which function antagonistically to acetylcholine by reversing those effects caused by cholinergic release.[52,53] $D_1$ and $D_2$ receptors differ in that the former activates and the latter inhibits adenylyl cyclase, a membrane protein that catalyzes the conversion of adenosine triphosphate (ATP) to cyclic adenosine monophosphate (cAMP). Serotonin, also known as 5-hydroxytryptamine (5-HT), is a neurotransmitter whose neurons are localized to midline regions of the pons and upper brain stem corresponding to distinct nuclear groups.[54] Norepinephrine is the principal transmitter for the postganglionic sympathetic fibers and is characterized by two types of receptor, $\alpha$ and $\beta$. Noradrenergic receptors function in the sympathetic nervous system by responding to adrenoceptive stimuli to contract, relax, inhibit, or activate the target tissue.[52] Norepinephrine- and dopamine-containing neurons are located in anatomically different regions of the brain; and ostensibly each transmitter serves a separate functional role.[55] Noncholinergic and nonadrenergic neurotransmitters also play an important role in nerve impulse conduction and are responsible for the synthesis, storage, and release of purine nucleotides such as ATP.[56]

The ATP is stored and released with other neurotransmitters, but it may also function as a fast, excitatory neurotransmitter in the CNS.[57] Receptors for ATP are of two types: One type is coupled with ion channels, and the other is coupled with guanosine triphosphate (GTP)-binding proteins. It is these GTP-binding proteins that are responsible for the inhibition of $K^+$ channels.[56] Although ATP serves many functions, it is the action of these GTP-binding proteins and the ATP receptors that can make ATP behave as an inhibitory neurotransmitter, decreasing the overall action potential.[58]

The response by specific tissues to various neurotransmitters alters with aging.[59] Many studies have examined the changes neurotransmitters undergo during aging and suggest that there is a decrease in activity or sensitivity to various neurotransmitters and their receptive counterparts. Some exceptions contradict this hypothesis.[60] In the parasympathetic system, the rate of biosynthesis and hydrolysis of acetylcholine has been shown to decrease with age.[52] This reaction involves a decrease in choline acetyltransferase and cholinesterase activity with increased sensitivity of the cholinoceptor protein to acetylcholine.[52] In the sympathetic system, studies have shown that older individuals experience reduced adrenoceptor sensitivity.[61,62] This evidence suggests that a decline in the adrenoceptor sensitivity decreases the amount of neurotransmitter released, reducing the nerve impulse transmission to the sympathetic system. An example of this decline in sensitivity is seen in the cardiac system of the aged person. The reduced sympathetic drive to the heart is reflected in low-renin hypertension in the elderly.[63]

Consistent age-related declines have been observed in the dopamine neurotransmitter owing to decreased densities of the dopaminergic receptors $D_1$ and $D_2$ in both rodents and humans.[64,65] It is this dopaminergic regulation that is responsible for control of motor function. Hence declines in the dopaminergic receptor density and dopamine are associated with declines in a number of motor behavioral tasks necessary for normal daily activities.

Contrary to these findings, studies conducted on the pathologic aging brain, for example, those afflicted with parkinsonism, have shown neurochemical changes involving marked depletion of dopamine and norepinephrine in regions of the brain that are normally rich in catecholamines.[66] This condition significantly contributes to the motor deficits, tremors, and cognitive loss observed with Parkinson's disease.

The serotonin receptors are divided into two subtypes, 5-$HT_1$ and 5-$HT_2$. Decreased numbers of the 5-$HT_1$ and 5-$HT_2$ binding sites have been shown to occur with normal aging. Studies confirming these data have been analyzed from human autopsied brains and from positron emission tomographic (PET) analysis of old living subjects.[67]

γ-Aminobutyric acid (GABA) is a major inhibitory neurotransmitter in the CNS. The major mechanism for its inactivation is reuptake of neurotransmitters at the synapse. Most investigations done on this neurotransmitter have been carried out in rodents, but a few human studies exist. Age-related changes of GABA have been conducted looking at synaptic uptake studies and have shown age-associated decreases in receptor binding in the cortex, mid-brain, and cerebellum in the rodent; but elevated numbers of GABA receptors have been indicated in the temporal cortex of the human brain.[68,69] A 30% *N*-methyl-D-aspartate receptor loss for the glutamate neurotransmitter is reported to be age-related in normal rhesus monkeys.[59] Glutamate is a key neurotransmitter in the modulation of memory and learning.

The available data clearly indicate that CNS neurotransmission declines with normal aging. This is evidenced by a decrease in enzymatic activity that functions to metabolize the neurotransmitters and, in turn, decrease reuptake of the neurotransmitter for reuse, and reduce receptor densities on which the neurotransmitters act. In the normal aging nervous system, the brain may compensate for the loss of neural secretion by increasing the activity or amount of impulse transmission from the remaining neurons. This plasticity lessens with time, and eventually any onset of disease late in life accelerates the neurotransmission degradation process.

## Intracellular Pigment Accumulation

Pigmented bodies, known as lipofuscin age pigments, have been found in all types of nondividing cells after childhood (Fig. 64.1). Laboratory evidence indicates that these pigmentations are by-products of lipoprotein auto-oxidation, particularly of intracellular membranes, which accumulate in gradually increasing amounts during aging and at different rates in different neurons. For example, lipofuscin accumulates at a faster rate in hippocampal neurons, which modulate learning and memory, than in the Purkinje neurons of the cerebellum.[70] They are characterized by a dark brown appearance, and their composition may reflect the level and kinds of circulating and intracellular lipids present, with fluctuations in their specific gravities relative to nutritional conditions.[71] Light microscopic examination and staining of these pigments shows them to consist of either fine individual granules 1–3 μm in diameter or clumped masses of variable size. Each lipofuscin granule is ensheathed in a single limiting membrane.[18] It is known that in neuronal processes where cellular atrophy and degeneration are present, the number and size of lipopigment granules, increases dramatically.[18] This is an indication of catabolic activity at the cellular level. The formation of lipofuscin is dependent on the metabolic demand made on the cell and on a balance between the catabolic and anabolic processes. A continuous increase in the amount of lipofuscin in the nerve and glial cells during aging appear to be the expression of continuous catabolic activity of these cells, leading to increased formation of autophagic residual bodies.[21] However, it has been observed that under conditions of protein malnutrition, enhanced lipofuscin formation may be reversible.[21]

The function of lipofuscin pigments has not been clearly defined. It is postulated that these granules may be insignificant waste material from long-term wear and tear and deposit as debris within the cells. Another theory suggests that it is a physiologic constituent of the cell, reflecting metabolic activity, and is an important mechanism designed to remove accumulating material within the cytoplasm during catabolic breakdown.[19]

Neuromelanins are also age-related pigments found mostly in catecholaminergic neurons located in the locus ceruleus and substantia nigra. Neuromelanins may be products of aminergic metabolism or possibly decomposing cell body RNA, and it is not known whether their accumulation is damaging to the cell.[72] Neuromelanins have become the focus of intensive research since the discovery that $MPP^+$, a neurotoxin product of the synthetic heroin product MPTP, binds to neuromelanin.[73] This binding of $MPP^+$ to neuromelanin kills dopaminergic neurons in the substantia nigra and produces a parkinsonian-type syndrome in humans and monkeys.[66] Because reactive $MPP^+$ is converted from MPTP by monoamine oxidase, investigators speculated that the use of monoamine oxidase inhibitors (MAOIs) might benefit patients with Parkinson's disease. Deprenyl, a specific inhibitor of monoamine oxidase B, is a promising treatment that appears to slow the progression of this disorder, possibly by raising the levels of dopamine in parkinsonian patients.[74]

Fluorescent yellow-brown lipopigments called ceroid pigments are also found to accumulate in cells in an age-dependent manner.[21] Ceroid is a waxy material closely related to lipofuscin; but unlike lipofuscin, its intracellular accumulation can cause neuronal loss and brain atrophy.[72] Progressive encephalopathies described as neuronal ceroid lipofuscinosis (NCL), however, are found to be more prevalent in children than in adults; the exact pathogenesis of this disorder is unknown.[75] NCL is associated with ubiquitous accumulation of ceroid and lipofuscin material in the neuronal perikarya, which can result in significant cortical loss of neurons.[75]

Glycation reactions occur when reducing sugars, such as glucose and fructose, react with amino acids to form stable ketoamine compounds known as Amadori products. Degradation of Amadori products results in unsaturated carbonyls, which can react with amino compounds to produce yellow-brown intracellular accumulations known as advanced glycation end-products (AGE).

Formation of the AGE products is increased during aging owing to elevated levels of oxidative stress-induced protein carbonyls.[76] The age-related increase in the amount of oxidized protein could result from increased production of free radicals, which can damage specific genetic expression that controls the balance of protein oxidation and protein degradation.[76] The search for therapy that can prevent neuronal protein degradation or excessive free radical formation, could diminish age-related neuronal atrophy and loss of these cells in the brain.

## Neuronal Loss

Neurons are postmitotic cells and when they die, they are not replaced. Before the 1980s, a popular scientific tenet held that massive neocortical neuron loss occurred during senescence in healthy individuals.[77] A loss in the density of neurons could certainly account for the failing memory, abstract thinking, reasoning, and language skills commonly associated with pathologic aging. More recent findings, however, have challenged the notion of widespread neuronal loss in aged primates, including humans, unless a neurodegenerative process leading, for example, to dementia is unfolding. Consistent with the idea that little or negligible neuronal loss during normal aging occurs are histologic studies performed on normal brains that have been carefully screened to rule out dementia or other cerebral pathology[78] and in animals that develop human-like cognitive decline, such as rhesus monkeys.[27] Consequently, examination of aging subjects whose health status was known and confirmed at autopsy has revealed that atrophy (shrinkage) of cortical neurons can occur in healthy elderly subjects in the absence of substantial degeneration (death) of these neurons.[79–85] Moreover, accurate stereologic procedures for counting neurons have shown no loss of neurons in nondemented elderly humans in the entorhinal cortex or CA1, the two hippocampal regions most responsible for memory function.[86–88]

Neuronal atrophy does not necessarily equate with neuronal death but may precede neurodegeneration, which is the dying state of nerve cells. In this context, experimental data have shown that neuronal atrophy can be prevented[89] or reversed.[90] For example, cortical neurons lost during aging in rats can induce atrophy in basal nucleus cholinergic neurons that send afferents to the cortex.[89] However, providing basal nucleus neurons with trophic factors that are lost during cortical death can prevent atrophy of the basal nucleus neurons.[89] Similarly, hippocampal neurons that have atrophied because of reduced cerebral blood flow can reverse their atrophy when cerebral blood flow is restored.[90] Cerebral blood flow restoration not only can reverse chronic neuronal atrophy it can restore memory function controlled by these damaged nerve cells.[90] These findings hold great promise for the elderly afflicted with age-related neurodegeneration because prior to neurodegeneration many of these neurons are in a predegenerative stage of atrophy (shrinking nucleus and cytoplasm combined with increased cell membrane permeability), a state that can precede but not necessarily lead to neuronal death.[90]

Opposing the argument of negligible neuron loss during healthy aging are data from nonsymptomatic 60- and 25-year-old volunteers undergoing noninvasive magnetic resonance imaging (MRI). This study concluded that about 10% brain atrophy is found in the older subjects, and that such atrophy reflects or presupposes significant neuron loss.[91] However, in the absence of a neuropathologic examination of these atrophic brains, this finding should be considered with caution, owing to the experimental data described above.

Other neuroimaging studies have indicated that cerebral atrophy in healthy elderly subjects is limited exclusively to white matter, which from the age of 30 to 80 develops 8% shrinkage.[3,92] Indeed, if this finding of white matter atrophy is valid, it suggests that demyelination of white matter axons occurs during aging, a problem that could affect neurotransmission, receptor and nerve cell function, and consequently cognitive ability. Some loss of neurons nonetheless has been reported to be age-related, for example, large neurons in the hypothalamus, hippocampus, locus ceruleus, and substantia nigra,[93,94] although it is unlikely that all aging individuals demonstrate such region-specific loss. There is also the possibility that otherwise nonsymptomatic old subjects examined at postmortem, may be on the threshold of initiating a neurodegenerative disorder (e.g., Alzheimer's, Parkinson's, or Huntington's disease) at the time such neuronal losses are recorded. Neuronal loss during aging is most notable when a disease process affecting the brain is present. This condition has been amply demonstrated in neurodegenerative disorders such as Alzheimer's disease, vascular dementia, stroke, and Parkinson's disease.[79,81,95,96]

As neuroimaging tools improve to study the brain, the issue of neuronal structural and functional changes during aging will be better appreciated, and the design of specific therapy to prolong neuronal health and delay neurodegeneration will more likely be developed.

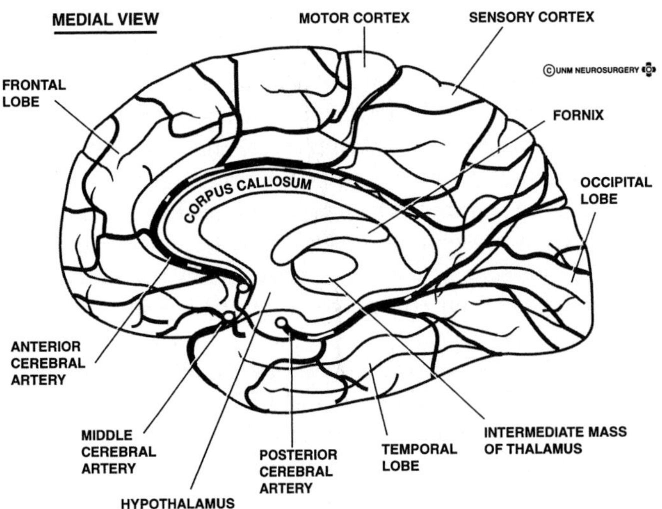


FIGURE 64.4. Major divisions of the human brain showing midsagitally the four cortical lobes, arterial vasculature, and important landmarks. Brain size, cerebral blood flow, metabolism of glucose and oxygen, trauma, sleep, hypothalamic regulation of food, water intake, and pain are only some of the elements affecting the brain regions represented here.

## Brain Size

With respect to changes in brain size, it is safe to conclude that there is no significant decrease observed in brain weight with normal aging. In terms of volume, the overall volume does not decrease significantly.[92] However, the presence of neurodegenerative syndromes can affect brain size significantly as will be seen below.

Gross measurements can be reliably obtained from postmortem brains and, in vivo, from computed tomography (CT) and MRI. Thus, a vast collection of human data regarding brain size is available. Extensive research on brain size has been conducted, and many researchers have shown a 6–11% loss of brain weight in humans more than 80 years of age (Fig. 64.4).[7]

Anatomic changes of the aging brain, particularly macroscopic changes in volume fraction of different regions of the brain anatomy, have been reported by Haug et al.[83] Twelve human brains were macroscopically assessed using a stereologic procedure with point-counting methodology to evaluate overall brain size and the size of the distinct structures within the brain.[83,84] The volume of the total brain for the aged group (70–80 years) was 6% smaller than that of the younger group (20–30 years). Specific structures such as the frontal lobe were found to be diminished 17%, and the basal ganglia was reduced more than 20% in the aged group when compared to their younger counterparts.[83,84] Other gross morphologic changes in the brain accompany aging, including atrophy of ridges (gyri) and crevices (sulci) of the cerebral surface. Ventricular enlargements of the brain are also observed with aging.[97,98]

## Cerebral Blood Flow and Ischemia

Metabolic activity of the brain is measured in terms of oxygen or glucose metabolism and represents the neuronal activity of the brain. Therefore, these parameters provide useful mechanisms for examining changes within the aged brain. Cerebral blood flow (CBF) is a measurement of the amount of blood perfusing the brain to deliver its metabolic needs. In 1955, Kety[99] developed the nitrous oxide technique as the gold standard of measurement for CBF. The technique was invasive, requiring substantial samples of arterial and jugular venous blood, which represented hemispheric rather than local flow. His study consisted of comparing the cerebral metabolism of oxygen ($CMRO_2$) and CBF of an aging and a young population.[99] Analyses showed no measurable difference between the aging population and the young population (mean $CMRO_2$ $3.33 \pm 0.08$ ml/100 g/min, mean CBF $57.9 \pm 2.1$ ml/100 g/min). However, when the aging population was reassessed 11 years later, most of those who had remained cognitively intact had significantly reduced CBF, indicating an increased vulnerability to lowered blood flow during the eighth decade of life. Because these changes occurred in the absence of any age-related diseases, it was concluded that a decrease in CBF is part of the natural evolution that accompanies increased aging. Dastur[100] and Fazekas et al.[101] found no variation in CBF between individuals younger than 40 years of age and in individuals over the age of 50, but found significant reductions in brain blood flow and oxygen consumption in the over 50 group. Lassen et al.[14] found no age-related changes in CBF but did observe significant reductions of $CMRO_2$ (as much as 6%) with increased aging. Subjects with a mean age of 50 or 63 have been reported to have lower cerebral blood flow values when compared to young subjects in their mid-twenties.[102]

Other techniques using xenon 133, single-photon emission tomography (SPECT), and PET have been used to study CBF with relative success and with only minor disadvantages. With the introduction of functional magnetic resonance technology, highly accurate and noninvasive assessment of CBF of the human brain in all stages of life can be performed.

Cerebral ischemia with respect to the aging individual can contribute to other biochemical changes at the cellular and molecular level. Hypoperfusion of the brain initiates cellular changes that lead to irreversible damage if blood flow is not restored rapidly. In the brain, neurons are the cells most sensitive to ischemic insults, followed by oligodendroglia, astrocytes, and endothelial cells.[103] Among neuronal populations, the CA1 pyramidal cells of the hippocampus and cerebellar Purkinje cells appear most vulnerable, followed by medium-sized neurons within the striatum and neocortical neurons in cortical layers 3, 5, and 6.[103,104]

An influx of calcium into the cell is associated with significant ischemia. Lipolysis, derived from phospholipase $A_2$ and phospholipase C activities, disaggregation of microtubules into tubulin subunits, degradation of neurofilaments and other cytoskeletal components using neutral calcium dependent proteases, and protein phosphorylation, can be enhanced by increased influx of calcium into the cell.[105] These degradative processes damage cell membrane integrity and disrupt the neuronal transport mechanisms.

Glutamate, a nonessential amino acid, functions as an excitatory neurotransmitter in several pathways within the CNS. It has been shown that glutamate can exert neurotoxic damage following ischemia, and increased glutamatergic release is reported to cause cell damage and neuronal death.[106] After cerebral ischemia, there is a rise in extracellular glutamate levels and a decreased affinity of glutamate uptake, thereby increasing glutamatergic release, which results in neurotoxicity.[107] Neurons in the cerebral cortex and hippocampus are most susceptible to this cytotoxic reaction.

Cerebral ischemia from stroke can lead to ischemic brain lesions and zones of tissue necrosis. Cerebral infarction has been defined as an area of necrosis with irreversible damage to all cell types within a specific vascular territory of the brain.[108] A distinct transition zone between an infarcted area and normal brain tissue (the penumbral region) is distinguished by partial neuronal damage with surviving astrocytes.[108] Penumbral neurons may be "rescued" from death if appropriate therapy is applied to stroke patients soon after infraction. With this in mind, it is easy to understand the detrimental chain of events that occur to the peripheral and central nervous systems following a decrease in blood flow to the aging brain. The blood nourishes and transports vital nutrients and molecules to every system of the human body; and without proper levels to maintain normal homeostasis, cellular systems degenerate over time causing malfunction of the entire organ system.

## Cerebral Metabolism of Glucose and Oxygen

Cerebral metabolic rates for glucose (CMRGlu) and oxygen ($CMRO_2$) have been mapped out in conscious elderly subjects using PET. Specific brain regions can be studied with PET using markers such as $^{15}O$ for $CMRO_2$ and $^{18}F$-fluoro-2-deoxy-D-glucose ($^{18}F$-FDG) for CMRGlu activites.[11,12,109]

Because glucose is normally the sole substrate for cerebral energy metabolism and oxygen is required for oxidative phosphorylation and the formation of ATP, their metabolism in brain can reflect functional neuronal activity in relation to aging. By carefully screening healthy and asymptomatic elderly subjects to measure $CMRO_2$ and CMRGlu brain activity, comparisons to age-matched individuals with a variety of organic brain disorders can be made. Healthy, elderly subjects, whose range of $CMRO_2$ and CMRGlu activities in brain are known, can also be compared to other population groups for differences in age, sex, race, nutrition, and demographics.

Most studies that have examined $CMRO_2$ during normal aging have concluded that oxygen utilization is reduced in most brain regions of the cerebral cortex.[16,110–113] One study has reported no changes in oxygen metabolism in healthy elderly individuals.[114] $CMRO_2$ reduction in healthy aged subjects may be related to decreased gray and white matter cerebral perfusion, which generally occurs in regions of low oxygen utilization.[113] Consequently, the age-related decline in cerebral blood flow observed in the elderly presumably affect cerebral oxygen transport and eventually neural tissue utilization, a finding that has been amply confirmed using PET. These changes are severely pronounced in the demented patient.[115,116] $CMRO_2$ appears to correlate positively with cerebral blood flow and negatively with blood viscosity. A study of elderly subjects with various types of polycythemia or increased red blood cell production and low $CMRO_2$ accompanied by reduced cerebral blood flow, revealed that following phlebotomy, blood viscosity gradually decreased. The reduction in blood viscosity was sufficient to increase regional cerebral blood flow and $CMRO_2$ in these patients.[117]

There is no general agreement as to whether CMRGlu is affected in healthy, asymptomatic aged persons. Studies have shown either a decrease in regional CMRGlu activity in normal elderly brains[115,118,119] or no changes.[120–122] Because the metabolism of glucose involves countless anaerobic and aerobic pathways with the production of a variety of substrates, its rate of utilization may vary widely among neuronal populations that have different energy requirements. Another factor that may explain the different findings in CMRGlu in normal aged brain as opposed to $CMRO_2$ is the fact that glucose delivery to neurons requires a transporter at the blood–brain barrier level (Glut 1) and another transporter to deliver glucose to neurons (Glut 3), whereas oxygen transport is facilitated by diffusion through the blood–brain barrier.[123,124]

Alavi[125] found a 26% reduction of glucose metabolism in psychometrically normal elderly subjects age 72 years compared to a control group 22 years of age. Overall, it has been shown that there is a reduction in CMRGlu of approximately 25% with normal cerebral aging.[100,126] During hypoxia/ischemia of the brain, the elderly patient almost always suffers more extreme and prolonged changes in $CMRO_2$ and CMRGlu than the younger adult, and this effect results in a worse neurologic outlook with respect to morbidity and mortality.[108] These vascular insults can be in the form of occlusive infarcts, encephalic hemorrhage, and dementia. All three conditions can severely affect the older patient in terms of cerebral blood flow, brain energy metabolism, and neuronoglial homeostasis.[13]

## Sensory Perception

Sensory perception declines with aging.[37,127–130] Deficit can develop from degenerative, morphologic, biochemical, and physiologic changes that occur within the sensory organs themselves. These impairments increase in frequency with age, making it more difficult for the elderly to adapt to their environment, a process that often leads to enhanced frustration and severe depression.

### Vision

Visual abilities deteriorate during normal aging. Many age-related visual problems cannot be solely attributed to optic changes, and hence the retina or central visual pathways must be suspected. Anatomic arrangements within the receptor cells of the retina, rods, and cones have been shown to develop age-related changes[131] (Fig. 64.5). Qualitative studies on the aging human retina reveal disorganization of the outer segments of the rods and cones and an accumulation of lipofuscin in the cone inner segments. Curcio and Drucker[132] estimated that 30% of the rods are

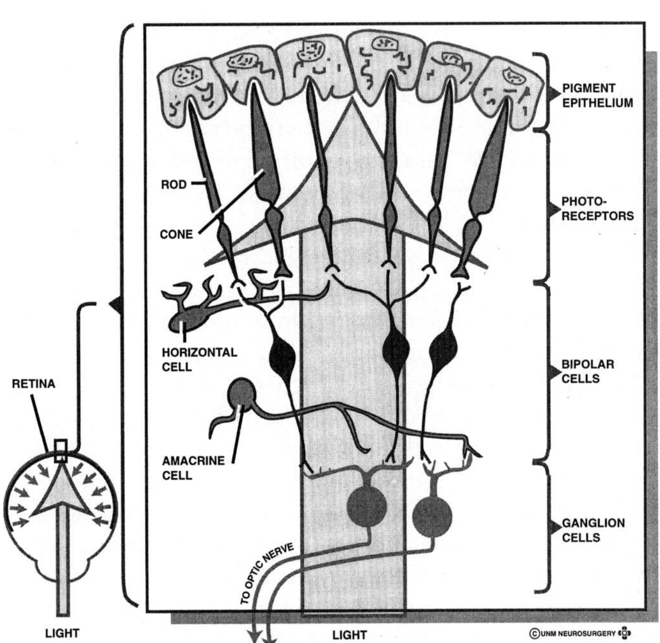


FIGURE 64.5. Anatomic structure of the retina. Light strikes the retina (left inset) and passes through all three cell layers: Ganglion cells form synapses with the optic nerve and bipolar cells, which in turn connect with rods (for black and white perception) and cones (for color perception). The ganglion cell axons traverse the retina to become an optic nerve fiber that terminates in the visual centers of the brain. Aging can affect the perception of colors, visual field size, and depth.

lost from the central visual portion of the retina after age 90 in healthy eyes. Interestingly, this group also observed that despite the large loss of central retinal rods the remaining rods in the inner segments increase in size and fill the void by the dying rods.[132] As a result, the coverage of rods in the retina of the elderly eye is similar to that in the young eye. This appears to be a compensation mechanism for the loss of rods, which are lost at a greater frequency than cones in the older human retina. In contrast, the foveal cones have not been seen to diminish in the human retina until after the age of 90, when there is a slight decrease in the cone population.[133]

The ganglion cells are the projection neurons of the retina that are connected to the receptor cells by a group of interneurons known as bipolar cells. It is the ganglion cells that are responsible for relaying the visual information perceived at the receptor level to the CNS and that have been found to decline with age. There is a relatively mild and variable loss of retinal ganglion cells, approximately 15–20% concentrated within the foveal region of the retina.[132]

Structurally, a variety of changes occur in the eye that affect visual perception in the elderly. These changes include cataract depositions on the lens, increased lens rigidity, modifications in the circumference and shape of the lens, decreases in the size of the pupil and the macula lutea, and alterations of the electrophysiologic response in the retina.[134] The resulting complications of these morphologic ocular changes is decreased sensitivity of the eye to detect and interpret visual stimuli. Visual thresholds, glare, acuity, accommodation, visual field size, and depth perception all undergo degenerative changes with aging and are caused by these structural modifications.[128,134]

Variations in the visual threshold related to aging is the result of a reduction in pupil size, modification of the lens, and retinal metabolism alterations, causing a change in the light/dark adaptation. Aging increases the susceptibility to glare owing to an increased dispersion of light within the ocular media.[134] Reduced visual acuity, which involves a decline in the ability to distinguish the contrast between the background and foreground, follows a downward slope with increased aging.[128] Accommodation, visual field size, and depth perception are also influenced by age. The ability to focus on near objects (due to structural changes in the lens) declines after the age of 40 years.[128] The visual field size decreases after age 55, thus affecting proportionately the amount of peripheral vision of the aged individual. Depth perception affects the ability of the elderly to distinguish properly the overlap of objects or the distance between them.[128]

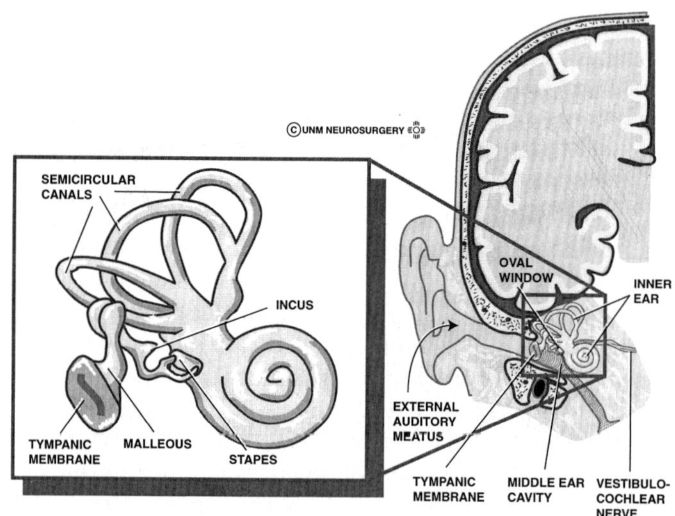


FIGURE 64.6. Normal anatomy of the auditory apparatus. Deficits of the external, middle, and inner ear structure are often observed to cause hearing losses in the elderly subject. Otosclerosis, tinnitus, increase in endolymphatic pressure, and loss of high sounds are some of the problems encountered during normal aging (see text for details).

## Auditory Loss

Similarly, structural changes occur in the auditory system that interfere with proper conduction of the vibrational tones to the inner ear (Fig. 64.6). Several age-related structural and physiologic changes lead to hearing loss. Anatomically, the outer ear enlarges throughout a person's life and can cause a stenosis within the ear canal. With respect to the middle ear, the tympanic membrane stiffens as a result of aging.[134] A stiffened tympanic membrane modifies the mechanics of the transmission of sound from the middle ear to the inner ear. Consequently, different ranges of audible frequencies travel to the inner ear and are processed differently in the brain. The inner ear—that portion of hearing responsible for receiving and transmitting the auditory nerve impulses—undergoes many changes in the normal aging individual. The cochlea of the inner ear manifests sensory losses owing to lowered elasticity of the basilar membrane, initially in the high frequency region of the membrane. This reduces the amplitude and shearing force on the organ of Corti.

Cochlear otosclerosis with stapes disorders are other common pathologies the elderly encounter.[81] The stria vascularis, a specialized region within the cochlea responsible for maintenance of the ionic composition of the endolymph, atrophies with age. These fundamental changes within the auditory system influence the auditory capabilities of the individual and result in hearing loss over time.

The physiologic response to anatomic alterations of the cochlea result in decreased thresholds and sensitivities to sound and in problems with frequency discrimination, especially within the high frequency bandwidths, sound localization deficiencies, and background noise discrimination.[37] Auditory thresholds decline after age 20. It is most dramatic after age 75, but is not unusual to observe an initial loss in sensitivity to pure tones after the second decade of life. Most of the frequency losses are at 1000 Hz and above, and frequencies above 4000 Hz at 30 dB are especially vulnerable. Pitch discrimination declines with age; and with the passage of time there is a decrease in the ability to discriminate among frequencies. The most dramatic changes are seen for the high frequency sounds. The elderly individual also has difficulty localizing sounds, especially in the high frequency range.[128] Increased sensitivity to background noises and loudness recruitment create a masking situation in which the presence of broadband background noise enhances with aging and masks the reception of important narrow signals. Loudness recruitment contributes to noise confusion by amplifying the background noise without filtering the insignificant sounds, which is basically how a hearing aid functions. The loss of concise high frequency sounds results in a decline in the ability to identify consonants (particularly s, z, t, f, and g). Consonants that contribute to the understanding of speech are high frequency sounds (2000–4000 Hz), whereas vowels tend to be low frequency sounds (250–750 Hz). Consequently, perception of tones and comprehension of speech can be lost with aging and create frustration in the elderly individual.[135]

Tinnitus is often a major complaint of sensorineural hearing loss in the aging population.[81,135] Tinnitus is presumed to result from irritation of the nerve endings in the cochlea by degenerative vascular or vasomotor disease, but its exact mechanisms remains obscure. It is defined as the perception of sound in the absence of an acoustic stimulus. At the present time, an effective way to manage tinnitus is to mask it with background music or some other pleasant sound. A hearing aid is useful for suppressing tinnitus when an associated hearing loss is present. A tinnitus masker can be worn much like a hearing aid and emits more pleasant sounds than the tinnitus.

A variety of diseases that afflict the older population may induce changes in the auditory receptors and magnify the degradation of the sensory system. Diabetes and hypertension affect the peripheral tissues of the auditory system and reduce the sensitivity of the receptors. Other pathologic conditions are degenerative and afflict the brain, diminishing the ability to interpret auditory information.[134] Alzheimer's disease and strokes are medical problems that can modify the sensory perception at the central level.

## Touch, Taste, Olfactory Sense

Vibrotactile sensation is mediated by the mechanoreceptors. Studies have shown significant reductions due to aging in mechanoreceptor density and sensitivity, rigidity and elasticity of the dermal structures, and peripheral nerve conductivity, which affect cutaneous reception.[127,129,130] To assess tactile sensitivity in the elderly, vibration is the main stimulus used to understand the physiologic changes in tactile sensation with aging. It is mainly dependent on two mechanoreceptors for tactile stimuli. Below 50 Hz Meissner's corpuscles are activated, and above 50 Hz the Pacinian corpuscles respond.[130] Age-related reductions of the receptor population correlate with increases in tactile thresholds and decreases in tactile sensitivities.[130] This threshold increases in diabetics and in patients with peripheral arteriosclerosis, and has been noted to increase in the affected hemiplegic side after a stroke.[136]

An increase in taste thresholds exist for many substances during aging, and this reflects decreases in taste sensitivity. The decrease in sensitivity to certain foods may be coupled with nutritional problems that have an adverse effect on geriatric health. There tends to be a diminished perception of saltiness and artificial sweeteners during old age that leads to increased preferences for salt and sugar-laden foods.[137,138] These taste preferences have detrimental health consequences, as they can aggravate hypertension from increased salt intake and increase the risk factor for obesity and diabetes mellitus from increased fat and sugar intake; they can also generate a state of nutritional imbalance. Bitterness is often the taste quality most commonly affected with age, but extrinsic factors such as smoking, medications, alcohol abuse, and certain eating habits can affect taste perception with age.[139] Anatomically, the reduction in taste receptors on the tongue within these neighboring key regions is believed to be the culprit to diminished taste perception. Hence, the elderly experience some discrete taste loss, but generally taste intensity is preserved.[140]

The appreciation of smell ties into the sense of taste. The receptor cells within the olfactory epithelium are altered, and there is a decrease in olfactory function with age. After age 65 the olfactory thresholds increase and signal a decrease in olfactory function. The outcome of reduced olfaction is hyposmia, a condition diagnosed in old subjects that can lead to total loss of olfaction, or anosmia.[141,142] Elderly subjects perceive suprathreshold odors as weaker, identify common odors less effectively, and have less ability to discriminate among odors.[141] Odor losses are enhanced by disease, especially in the case of Alzheimer's disease.[142]

## Postural Changes

Postural stability may be thought of as the ability to maintain the body in an upright position during subconsciously controlled movement. To accomplish this task, the CNS must rapidly integrate sensory information from a wide range of sources, mainly the visual, somatosensory, and vestibular apparatus. This information is centrally processed, and motor responses related to the timing, direction, and magnitude of the stimuli are generated.[143,144] Therefore age-related transformations in the sense organs can affect the postural control of the geriatric population. The reduction of visual acuity, depth perception, glare, and contrast sensitivity interfere with the ability to perceive one's surroundings adequately, consequently endangering the aged individual by provoking falls that result in serious injury.[145,146]

The vestibular system detects the position and motion of the head in space and is essential for the coordination of motor responses, eye movement, and posture[32] (Fig. 64.6). Progressive loss of labyrinth hair cells, vestibular ganglion cells, and nerve fibers is age-related and can induce adjustments within the vestibulo-ocular reflex.[144] Reductions in proprioception, defined as the sense of static and dynamic position of the limbs and body in three-dimensional space, have been observed in the elder population.[144] Somatosensation changes with maturation show marked decreases in tactile sensitivity, two-point discrimination, and vibration.[130] All of these factors contribute to significant postural instabilities because of inadequate sensory perception. Thus, a small dip in the sidewalk may not be perceived visually or felt, and it might create imbalance in the individual leading to a fall.

Aging can also create modifications within the CNS that affect posture. Transformations within neurons (e.g., the dendritic spine, reduced dendritic branching, lipofuscin accumulation, synaptic alterations, and altered neurotransmitter metabolism[67,144]) interfere with proper transmission of the sensory input and motor output. It is likely that the sensory, motor, and CNS changes discussed above disrupt mobilization of the complex postural responses and decrease the ability to compensate for the sensory and motor impairments. Slowing of the nerve conductions, which results from the physiologic changes within the neuron, further disrupt the postural responses.

## Changes in Learning and Memory with Aging

Forgetfulness is a frequent complaint of the elderly that can lead to feelings of frustration. The complaint is real for most of the aging population; some degree of impairment of the episodic memory develops and progresses, especially after age 70 years.[147] Memory has been classified into three types: semantic, episodic, and procedural.[147] Semantic memory is defined as one's cumulative knowledge of the world, language, and concepts. Such information is held for various lengths of time and can be stable or even improve with time. This is often expressed in elderly individuals as a form of nostalgic recall, which tends to be embedded deep within the memory. It is the episodic memory that declines with age. Episodic memory relates to personally experienced events contextually bound to time and place. It is most sensitive to aging and has been widely studied. Procedural memory, or implicit memory, refers to enhancement of performance on perceptual-motor skills or cognitive operations by recent experience, without intention or conscious awareness.[10] This type of memory has not been investigated in depth, although some studies have shown that procedural memory does not appear to show age-related differences.[148]

Many studies have shown significant decrements in episodic memory in most older subjects. This has been confirmed by a large number of cross-sectional studies, where old and young subjects were matched according to education.[10] This decrement was observed in tasks that involved nonmeaningful lists of numbers or words. Both young and old remember a list of five to seven digits without difficulty, but when the list is increased to 15 digits the young subjects improve their scores more rapidly on repeated trials than the old subjects. In a test for word recall, a list of 25 words was presented to the two groups; the old group recalled only 55% as many words as the young subjects.[147] Overall, there was difficulty remembering several tasks simultaneously for the older group.[147]

## Memory and Behavior

It is generally well accepted that reasoning, abstraction, language, and memory are severely affected in aged, demented individuals.[81] General intelligence tests can measure these intellectual abilities but only in a complex manner and without assessing all aspects of cognition. Consequently, one can ask: for those of us free of dementia and other organic brain disease, is there a cognitive decline during aging? If so, how does it differ from pathologic aging? Because it is well documented that aging involves biologic decline, is performance of cognition ability in healthy, elderly subjects biologically based?

Healthy elderly subjects show considerable stability in intellectual performance during their lifetime. Some aspects of intelligence appear sensitive to the aging process. For example, primary, or short-term, memory (the ability to store information briefly if actively repeated) has not been found to be significantly affected by age.[149] By contrast, long-term, or secondary, memory (storage of unlimited amounts of information for a long duration) appears to be much more sensitive to increasing age than primary memory.[150] This memory loss is often referred to by physicians as "benign forgetfulness" because it does not progress to dementia and death.[151] What causes secondary memory loss in subjects 75 and over is the focus of intense clinical and basic research. Barring organic brain disease, or depression or dementia, memory decline during aging may be due to changes in neurotransmitter synthesis, synapse formation, neuronal receptor density, and cerebral energy metabolic slowdown. The etiology of memory loss during aging can be summarized by the useful mnemonic DEMENTIA, which stands for drug-intoxication (D), emotional disorders (E), metabolic and endocrine disease (M), eyes and ears affecting perceptual changes (E), neurodegeneration, nutrition, and normal-pressure hydrocephalus (N), tumors, toxins, and trauma (T), infections of organ systems (I), and atherosclerosis (A), a process that can reduce blood flow to the brain.

Behavioral or emotional changes do not occur in the healthy aged subject. They are usually the result of mental, systemic, or organic brain diseases such as psychoses, depression, stroke, diabetes, dementia, or head trauma. Except for mental changes, abundant neurodegeneration accompanies most organic brain disorders and the associated neurologic signs that may be present.[6,108] Because neurodegenerative syndromes can lead to behavioral dysfunction, it is important to evaluate the elderly patient who presents with neurologic abnormalities involving visual, olfactory, and gait disturbances together with an emotional or behavioral disorder in the search for a treatable cause. The prevalence of dementia, specifically Alzheimer's disease in those older than 85 years, is estimated to be 47%.[152] Similarly, the incidence of cerebrovascular disease rises dramatically after the eighth decade of life, and these patients often have a two to three times higher incidence for stroke than the "younger" elderly age 65–74.[153]

## Brain Stress and Aging

It is well known that physical or psychological stress can induce the release of adrenergic neurotransmitters and glucocorticoids. Excessive exposure to glucocorticoids has been shown in animal experiments to damage the hippocampus, a structure vital to memory and learning.[154] Glucocorticoids can also impair the regulation of calcium and glutamate in neurons during cerebral ischemia and posttraumatic seizures, consequently damaging or killing hippocampal dendrites and neurons when glucocorticoid secretion becomes chronic.[154,155] Such continued secretion of glucocorticoids in time can induce damage to the human hippocampus, resulting in depression[156] or in posttraumatic stress disorder.[157] It is only speculative that the outcome of excessive glucocorticoid secretion would be more pronounced or more abundantly expressed in aged subjects owing to the longer duration of glucocorticoid exposure in an elderly individual or that such exposure would anatomically target the hippocampus where most glucocorticoid receptors are found. More studies of the aging brain are needed to clarify this critical issue.

## Clinical Concepts of Aging

### Pain

Pain has been defined as the perception of unpleasant or aversive sensation originating from some specific body region.[158] The prevalence of chronic pain is reported to be higher in the elderly than in the young adult population.[158] Contrary to popular opinion, and despite its higher prevalence, elderly individuals report less pain than younger subjects.[26,159,160] Pain has a direct influence on the psychosocial and physical function of the geriatric patient. Its pharmacological management requires careful and particular attention to pharmacokinetics, as well as awareness of the drug's side effects and interactions with other medicines the older patient is likely taking. Chronic pain in the elderly represents a major economic, psychosocial and medical problem in the United States and is a major cause of sleeplessness, anxiety, and depression.[161] The major goal of the physician should be to eliminate needless drug dependence and establish an appropriate dose of analgesics or psychosocial intervention. In a survey of patients who had undergone five or more major surgeries in their lifetime, the use of analgesics was 3.7 times greater than in a control group that averaged one surgery per person.[162] This study implies that the older we get the more chances a polysurgical experience has developed; and with it, pain medication is the foremost clinical problem. In fact, it is reported that the chronic pain patient is the most serious user and abuser of narcotics and psychoactive medication.[162]

The impact of intellectual dysfunction on pain reveals that even in individuals with a slow decline in cognition, little or no influence on pain thresholds is perceived or felt by the older subject.[163] Acute pain in the elderly differs from chronic pain in that the former is generally an indicator of a physiologic problem that requires treatment. Acute pain often presents with autonomic nervous system signs such as increased heart rate, diaphoresis, and increased blood pressure.[158] By contrast, chronic pain usually lasts longer than the usual duration of an acute disease or than what is generally required for an acute injury to heal. It is rarely associated with autonomic nervous system activity, and workup often fails to reveal the source of pain.[164] This is a particularly difficult situation for the physician and caretaker, as it has been reported that in nursing homes there is a frequency of chronic pain ranging from 71% to 83% in the resident population.[159,165] More intense research is needed to evaluate chronic pain in the elderly and to find better ways to manage this growing problem.

### Pain and Treatment

Pain sensation is mediated by a diffuse bundle of fibers located at the junction of the anterior and lateral funiculi of the spinal cord. These fibers make up the anterolateral spinothalamic tract and consist of thalamic neurons that are activated by two fiber pathways: small myelinated $A\delta$ fibers 2–5 $\mu$m in diameter that conduct at rate of 12–30 m/s and unmyelinated C fibers 0.4–1.2 $\mu$m in diameter conducting at a lower rate of 0.5–2.0 m/s.[20]

All pain sensations are primarily transported to the brain by the dorsal roots, which consist of afferent or sensory fibers. Pain is perceived as acute and "sharp" or chronic and "dull": The quality is dependent on whether "fast" $A\delta$ fibers or "slow" C fibers are activated. The receptors that receive noxious stimuli are basically chemoreceptors with a free nerve ending, but other types of receptors may also pick up noxious signals such as those generated by bradykinin, histamine, and various neurotransmitters, particularly substance P.[134] The spinoreticulothalamic tract is connected to neural systems that integrate signals from most organs associated with vital functions. Signals that ascend via the spinoreticulothalamic tract reach the intralaminar thalamic nuclei after passing through the reticular system; from there they are recruited and synchronized at the level of other thalamic nuclei, cortex, hypothalamus, and septal regions. Intractable pain can be reduced by severing the anterolateral spinothalamic tract (tractotomy) or the anterolateral spinal column (cordotomy). The treatment of pain in the elderly can be summarized by the following approaches: (1) pharmacologic; (2) behavioral; (3) biofeedback; (4) psychological; (5) multiphasic.

Pharmacotherapy presents special problems to the aging patient because of increased susceptibility to drug side effects, metabolic and pharmacokinetic differences in drug clearance,[166] and altered states of nutrition and health. Caution and a history of other medicines being taken can reduce the potential for complications and increase the manageability of geriatric pain.

Behavioral management of pain suggests that this approach may be beneficial to the geriatric patient. The technique consists of abolishing the elderly's propensity to seek attention and sympathy and reinforcing non-pain-related activities.[167] Several studies have suggested that behavioral treatment can reduce the use of pain medication in these subjects,[168] but more extensive clinical trials are needed to fully validate this approach.

The success rate of biofeedback and relaxation methods as an aid to pain therapy are controversial. Conclusions range from little or no benefit,[169] to reduced age-related benefit when elderly and young subjects are compared,[170] to extremely useful in the older population.[171] The difficulty encountered by the elderly when learning or remembering the biofeedback responses to alleviate pain may be countered by increased training and repetition of instructions in the use of these techniques.[172] As stated in another section of this review, short-term memory may be reinforced by constant repetition, even in mildly cognitive-impaired patients.

The benefits of psychological treatment of the elderly may be hampered by the presence of senility, depression, psychosis, reduced ambulation, nutritional deficits, and other age-related health risks.[26,173] Psychological therapy may exert its best influence when used as an adjunct with treatments that can target the age-related deficits mentioned above.[174–177]

A multiphasic approach offering tailor-made treatment at the physical, metabolic, and psychosocial setting may reduce the intensity of pain and medication intake.[178,179] Not all investigators agree that this technique is beneficial to the aged group.[178] Despite this controversy, many patients appear to benefit from multiphasic therapy for different pain experiences. Even those refractory to these techniques could benefit to some extent by identifying subjects taking extensive and numerous analgesics or those not being treated with any pain-reducing therapy.

## Sleep

A normal "sleep pattern" or the time required for effective sleep is not easy to define. Rechschaffen[180] has argued that analysis of need for sleep varies according to type of subject studied and the various methods used to determine normal and abnormal sleep times.

Insomnia is reported to affect 5–10% of the adult population, and the elderly is the group most likely to report disturbed sleep and the use of hypnotics.[181] Increased nocturnal awakenings in the aged have been consistently reported in a number of studies.[182–186] It is important to emphasize that although insomnia is more common in old age *it is not due to old age*. This finding does not necessarily imply a correlation between increased aging and poor sleep but may be consistent with a higher incidence of psychological and health problems encountered during old age.[187] This is demonstrated by the fact that sleep disturbances among the healthy elderly population are not more prevalent than in younger subjects.[188]

Nocturnal delirium, or "sundowning," develops in demented geriatric patients and is characterized by confused, agitated behavior that disrupts nocturnal sleep.[1] Its etiology stems from a variety of problems, including metabolic, nutritional, infectious, or toxic states in the presence or absence of dementia.[189] Treatment for sundowning begins by recognizing the possible underlying cause (e.g., toxin, infection, metabolic problem) with appropriate therapy. In the absence of such reversible conditions, nocturnal agitation can be reduced with haloperidol (0.5–1.0 mg tid) or thioridazine (25 mg tid), taking into consideration the long-term sequelae or worsening of extrapyramidal symptoms and tardive dyskinesia (haloperidol) and the possible orthostatic hypertension and anticholinergic side effects, which may accelerate cholinergic deterioration in Alzheimer's disease (thioridazine). Hypnotics and neuroleptics appear to have minimal effects on sundowning, but β-blockers (e.g., propranolol) or pindolol have been reported to be effective in geriatric patients with organic brain disease.[190–192]

The most recognized age-related sleep disturbance is a reduction of the non-rapid-eye-movement (NREM) cycle, which includes light sleep (stages 1 and 2) and slow wave sleep (stages 3 and 4).[193,194] It is not certain when NREM cycle first begins to decline during aging, but some studies indicate it may start during the early twenties. Slow-wave sleep can disappear completely after the ninth decade.[195] Changes in the rapid-eye-movement (REM) sleep cycle (stage 5) and aging are more controversial, with some studies indicating no changes during aging[196–198] and others showing a significant decline in this sleep cycle.[199–201] Because REM sleep is associated with muscular atony, ocular saccades, intense neuronal activity, and dreaming, increased regional cerebral blood flow is required to maintain this sleep cycle.[202,203] REM sleep can be problematic to the normal elderly subject, who may be unable to meet the higher cerebral blood flow rate needed for this sleep cycle owing to an age-related decline in cerebral perfusion. Thus adequate cerebral perfusion and normal REM sleep appear to be interdependent, although the threshold for cerebral blood flow required to maintain this stage of sleep is unknown. It is important to point out, however, that the depth, duration, and continuity of sleep during normal aging can vary considerably and still remain nonpathologic even though it affects the subjective quality of sleep. Troubled sleep is common in the elderly but can be managed with careful personal attention to the needs of the patient and recognition of the cause or conditions leading to such sleep disturbance. A key aspect of understanding geriatric sleep disturbances is to recognize that elderly patients have a high prevalence of depression, obstructive airway disease, cardiac disease, and pain from a variety of sources. The physician can dramatically improve the quality of sleep in these individuals by treating the primary disorder rather than the sleep complaint itself.

## Food and Water Intake: Pathway to Delirium

Old age tends to change the homeostatic control of the hypothalamus for food and water intake. The ventromedial and lateral hypothalamus appear to regulate the hunger and satiety center. During aging, the satiety center may become hypersensitive and reduce the desire for food intake. This condition can lead to hypophagia and anorexia in the more elderly subjects who typically develop a frail body. Water homeostasis is also under hypothalamic modulation, and controls in this brain center respond to hyperosmolarity changes, by the sensation of thirst, increased water intake, and release of antidiuretic hormone. Studies have indicated that antidiuretic hormone is either preserved or increased in the older person and tends to reduce drinking behavior.[204] Reduced water intake can lead to dehydration and typically less rapid rehydration ability by the elderly, probably because of the loss in thirst drive.

One of the most common causes of acute delirium or confusional state in the elderly patient who has been hospitalized for a minor or major pathologic event is dehydration. It is important to monitor total fluid intake and apply frequent intake and output measurements in these patients for the reasons cited above. Other causes of delirium in the elderly can develop from intoxication with medical drugs (e.g., diuretics, hypoglycemic agents, narcotics, sedative-hypnotics, antihypertensives, antacids, nonsteroidal antiinflammatory agents, lithium, and antiarrhythmic compounds).[1] Many other causes can trigger delirium in old people, and the reader is referred to a comprehensive review of the causes and treatment of this disorder.[189]

## Brain Trauma

Studies of patients over age 65 who have sustained brain trauma show that mortality is twice that of younger patients.[205–207] The reason for this grim statistic is multifactorial. Premorbid and co-morbid diseases may play a critical role in the outcome of brain injury; for example, declining cerebral blood flow associated with normal aging, higher prevalence of coronary heart disease, hypertension, diabetes, poor nutritional state, obesity, reduced physical activity, atherosclerosis, and reduced bone density comprise only part of a major list of risk factors that can increase morbidity and mortality following brain injury in these patients.[208] The Traumatic Coma Data Bank reports that 75% of patients over the age of 55 had systemic medical disorders, in contrast to 5% for 16- to 25-year-old trauma victims.[209] This statistic may explain the outcome of severe head injury in patients over the age of 65, whose mortality is 85%, considerably higher than that of younger adult patients (45%) or pediatric patients (24%).[210] It is estimated that 70% of all the deaths from falls occur among the elderly.[211] Mortality may be even higher among old people who are admitted with severe brain trauma accompanied by extracranial injury, intracranial mass lesions, or hypovolemic shock.[211]

It is not clear whether aggressive treatment of the severely brain injured elder patients can reduce mortality or prevent a vegetative state, although previous experience indicates that old patients with nonsurgical lesions (i.e., intracranial mass) who regain consciousness after trauma may be the best candidates for good prognosis from extracranial complications.[212] Elderly patients with brain trauma are a unique medical challenge, and surgeons trained to recognize their problems may be in a better position to manage and improve their outcome.

## Surgery of CNS

Preparation of the surgical patient for brain or spinal cord surgery must take into account that elderly patients have less reserve capacity than younger individuals in time of stress and therefore may have more difficulty during surgery and recovery.[213] Accurate diagnosis of the chief complaint, evaluation of co-morbid disease, assessment of polypharmacy medications, age of the subject, and the necessity of elective surgery should be major concerns of the surgeon. The ability to differentiate primary illness from age-related physical, social, nutritional, or mental deficiency must be considered. Some form of dementia screening or cognitive testing may be helpful prior to brain surgery of an aged patient to better evaluate postoperative recovery and complications. The choice of premedication and anesthesia for the elderly should be based on the medicines the patient is likely taking or the presence of confusion. Regional analgesia for brain and spinal cord surgery is one of the safest methods and is well tolerated by the elderly patient. When regional analgesia is not possible, light general anesthesia can be considered.

General considerations for surgery of the older patient should recall that the elderly are more likely to develop hypothermia owing to lowering of the basal metabolic rate; other aged patients may be susceptible to local analgesics due to progressive demyelination of pain fibers; and if a confusional state due to a neurodegenerative syndrome is found preoperatively, hypotension or hypoxia can worsen this condition.[214] Many elderly patients are hypertensive because of increased blood vessel resistance due to a variety of causes and surgery of these individuals can lead to an increased tendency to hemorrhage and the development of cerebrovascular or cardiovascular complications due to decreased perfusion of these organs.[215]

## Neuroimaging

Neuroimaging techniques, which include magnetic resonance imaging (MRI), positron emission tomography (PET), spectroscopy (SPECT), and computed tomography (CT), play an increasingly important role in the assessment of dementias of older adults.[109] Currently, no unequivocal diagnostic test is available to assess such disorders as Alzheimer's disease and other dementias during aging. The advent of MRI has enabled physicians to evaluate the brain noninvasively in vivo with faithful resolution. CT, an inexpensive anatomic imaging technology commonly used for the assessment of neurodegenerative diseases, can perform rapid image acquisition but still has a variety of limitations that may not make it the tool of choice. Limited-entry angles and imaging planes, decreased resolution of gray-white matter and bone interfaces, and beam-hardening artifacts lessen the value of image quality.[92]

Imaging of age-related changes are better viewed with continuous scan slicing, volumetric acquisitions, segmentation techniques, and pulse sequences with enhancing features in signal intensity.[92] MRI is more sensitive for detecting small changes related to dementia than CT, PET, or SPECT because of the increased resolution of the system. Whereas MRI can detail changes in cerebral blood flow, cerebral spinal fluid, and structural anatomy, PET and SPECT excel in the assessment of metabolic disorders of the nervous system. The advantage of MRI is that it can be conducted throughout many decades of life for an individual without risk of physical harm.

Quantitative CT and MRI grading systems have been developed to assess the normal aging pattern and the dementia pattern (Fig. 64.7). These techniques have substantially contributed to a better understanding of the aging brain. Brain tissue volume, ventricular size, white matter lesions, and enlargements within the perivascular spaces are entities that have been studied using these

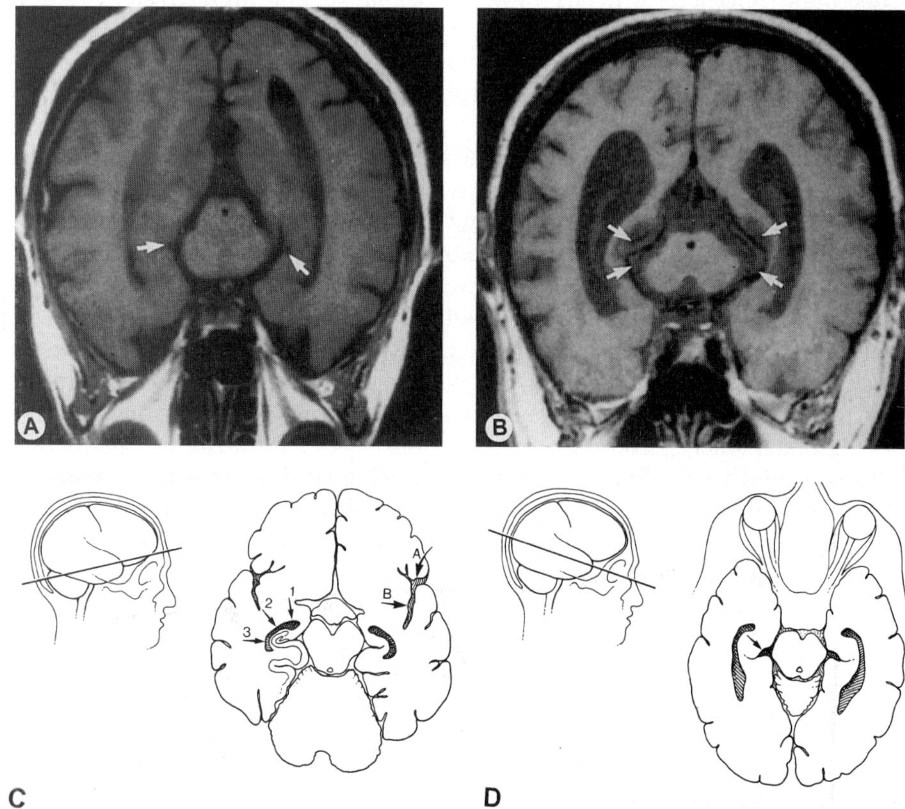


FIGURE 64.7. A. Left magnetic resonance imaging (MRI) scan shows enlargement of the choroid-hippocampal fissures due to hippocampal volume loss in an 80-year-old patient with probable Alzheimer's disease (arrows). B. Right MRI scan of a cognitively intact 86-year-old man shows no hippocampal volume loss and considerably less enlargement of the choroid-hippocampal fissures (arrows). C, D. MRI scans show anatomic landmarks that are useful for discriminating Alzheimer's disease from normal aging. C. Width of the temporal horn at three locations (1,2,3), which, when enlarged more than 3 mm at any of the three locations, can distinguish Alzheimer's from normal aging. D. Enlargement of choroid-hippocampal fissure (arrow), a sensitive marker for Alzheimer's disease. (From Davis et al.,[92] with permission.)

methods in the normal and pathologic aging brain. At present, the most consistent findings in Alzheimer's disease are those reflecting the volume loss in the medial temporal lobes and cerebral hypoperfusion as detected by SPECT.[92,216] This condition is also accompanied by enlargement of the temporal horn, cisternae, and fissures medial to the hippocampus, all detectable with MRI. It is a reliable way to distinguish the normal from the pathologic brain consistently, noninvasively, and over long periods of time. PET and SPECT in conjunction with MRI provide additional metabolic data that can confirm the neuroimaging findings and facilitate early diagnoses of the aging nervous system.

## Conclusions

Many physiologic, mechanic, genetic, and iatrogenic factors can diminish and impair normal aging. There is no medical or social formula that can sidestep the gauntlet of increased aging. Sustained evidence however, indicates that the old cliché "a sound mind in a sound body" may offer the best option to stay mentally alert and physically able during aging; and this process should start during the peak years of one's youth. Consequently, physical activity coupled with mental workouts and abstinence from major risk factors to stroke may offer the best protection presently known for delaying or preventing cognitive decline associated with age-related neurodegenerative syndromes.

### References


1. Lipowski ZJ. Delirium and impaired consciousness. In: Evans JG, Williams TF (eds) Oxford Textbook of Geriatric Medicine. Oxford: Oxford University Press, 1992:490–495.
2. Maletta GJ, Pirozzolo FJ. Introduction to the aging nervous system. In: Maletta GJ, Pirozzolo FJ (eds) The Aging Nervous System. New York: Praeger, 1980:3–9.
3. Albert M. Neuropsychological and neurophysiological changes in healthy adult humans across the age range. Neurobiol Aging 1993;14:623–627.
4. Peters G, Vaughan DW. Central nervous system. In: Johnson JF (ed) Aging and Cell Structure, vol 1. New York: Plenum, 1981:1–34.
5. Blessed G, Tomlinson BE, Roth M. The association between quantiative measures of dementia and of senile change. Br J Psychiatry 1968;114:797.
6. Duckett S. The normal aging human brain. In: Duckett S (ed) The Pathology of the Aging Human Nervous System. Philadelphia: Lea & Febiger, 1991.
7. Hoch-Ligeti C. Effect of aging on the central nervous system. J Am Geriatr Soc 1963;2:403.
8. Petit TL. Synaptic plasticity and the structural basis of learning and memory. In: Petit TL, Ivy GO (eds) Neural Plasticity: A Lifespan Approach, vol 36. New York: Liss, 1988:201–234.
9. Damon A. Discrepancies between findings of longitudinal and cross-sectional studies in adult life: physique and physiology. Hum Dev 1965;8:16–22.
10. Katzman R. Human nervous system. In: Masoro EJ (ed) Handbook of Physiology, Sect 11: Aging. New York: Oxford University Press, 1995:325–344.
11. Baron JC, Marchal G. Vieillessement cérébral et cardiovasculaire et metabolisme énergétique, cérébral. Paris: Presse Med 1992;21:1231–1237.
12. Baron JC, Rougemont D, Soussaline F. Local interrelationships of cerebral oxygen consumption and glucose utilization in normal subjects and in ischemic stroke patients: a positron tomography study. J Cereb Blood Flow Metab 1984;4:140–149.
13. de la Torre JC. Cerebrovascular changes in the aging brain. Adv Cell Aging Gerontol 1997;2:77–107.
14. Lassen NA, Feinberg I, Lane MH. Bilateral studies of cerebral oxygen uptake in young and aged normal subjects and in patients with organic dementia. J Clin Invest 1960;39:491.
15. Meyer JS, Terayama Y, Takashima S. Cerebral circulation in the elderly. Cerebrovasc Brain Metab Rev 1993;5:122–146.
16. Pantano P, Baron JC, Lebrum-Grandie P, Duguesnoy N, Boussen M, Comar G. Regional cerebral blood flow and oxygen consumption in human aging. Stroke 1984;15: 635–641.
17. de la Torre JC. Impaired brain microcirculation may trigger Alzheimer's disease. Neurosci Behav Rev 1994;18:397–401.
18. Brizzee KR, Ordy JM, Knox C, Jirge SK. Morphology and aging in the brain. In: Maletta GJ, Pirozzolo FJ (eds) The Aging Nervous System. New York: Praeger, 1980:10–18.
19. Glees P, Hasan M. Lipofuscin. In: Neuronal Aging and Disease. Stuttgart: Thieme, 1976.
20. Ranson SW. The Anatomy of the Nervous System, 8th ed, revised by Clark SL. Philadelphia: Saunders, 1951.
21. Schlote W, Boellaard JW. Role of lipopigment during aging of nerve and glial cells in the human central nervous system. In: Cervos-Navarro J, Sarkander HI (eds) Brain Aging: Neuropathology and Neuropharmacology, New York: Raven, 1983:27–28.
22. Brizzee KR, Sherwood N, Timiras PS. A comparison of various depth levels: cerebral cortex of young adults and aged Long-Evans rats. J Gerontol 1968;23:289–297.
23. Brunetti M, Miscena A, Salviati A, Gaiti A. Effect of aging on the rate of axonal transport of choline phosphoglycerides. Neurochem Res 1987;12:61–65.
24. Inestrosa NC, Alvarez J. Axons grow in the aging rat but fast transport and acetylcholinesterase content remain unchanged. Brain Res 1988;441:331–338.
25. Anderton BH, Brion JP, Flament Durand J, et al. Changes in the neuronal cytoskeleton in aging and disease. In: Bergener M, Ermini M, Stahelin HB (eds) Dimensions in Aging. San Diego: Academic, 1986:69–90.
26. Ferrell BR, Ferrell BA, Kaiko R. Pain in the elderly. Presented at the American Pain Society, St. Louis, October 1990.
27. Peters A, Rosene D. The effects of aging on area 46 of the frontal cortex of the rhesus monkey. Cereb Cortex 1994;6:621–628.

28. Scheibel ME, Lindsay RD, Tomiyasu U, Scheibel AB. Progressive changes in aging human cortex. Exp Neurol 1975;47:392–403.
29. Diamond MC, Connor JR. Morphological measurements in the aging rat cerebral cortex. In: Scheff SW (ed) Aging and Recovery of Function in the Central Nervous System. New York: Plenum, 1984:47–55.
30. Rogers RL, Meyer JS, Mortel KF. After reaching retirement age, physical activity sustains cerebral perfusion and cognition. J Am Geriatr Soc 1990;38:123–128.
31. Kristersson R. Retrograde transport of macromoelcules in axons. Annu Rev Pharmacol Toxicol 1987;18:97–110.
32. Kandel ER, Schwartz JH. Directly gated transmission at central synapses. In: Kandel ER, Schwartz JH, Jessell TM (eds) Principles of Neural Science, 3rd ed. East Norwalk, CT: McGraw-Hill, 1991:153–172.
33. Vale RD, Schnapp BJ, Reese TS, Sheetz MP. Movement of organelles along filaments dissociated from the axoplasm of the squid giant axon. Cell 1985;40:559–569.
34. Viancour TA, Kreiter NA. Vesicular fast axonal transport in young and old rat axons. Brain Res 1993;628:209–217.
35. Edmonds B, Koenig E. Powering of bulk transport (varicosities) and differential sensitivities of directional transport in growing axons. Brain Res 1987;406:288–293.
36. Stromska DP, Ochs S. Axoplasmic transport in aged rats. Exp Neurol 1982;77:215–224.
37. Strehler BL, Barrows CH. Senescence: cell biological aspects of aging. In: Schjjeide OA, DeVellis J (eds) Cell Differentiation. New York: Van Nostrand Reinhold, 1970.
38. McMartin D, O'Connor JA Jr. Effect of age on axoplasmic transport of cholinesterase in rat sciatic nerves. Mech Ageing Dev 1979;10:241–248.
39. Certoni-Freddari C, Fattoretti P, Paoloni R, Caselli U, Galeazzi L, Meier-Ruge W. Synaptic structural dynamics and aging. In: Meier-Ruge W (ed) Gerontology. New York: Karger, 1996:170–180.
40. deToledo-Morrell L, Geinisman Y, Morrell F. Age-dependent alterations in hippocampal synaptic plasticity: relation to memory disorders. Neurobiol Aging 1988;9: 581–590.
41. Meier-Ruge W. Morphometric methods and their potential value for gerontological research. In: von Hahn HP (ed) Interdisciplinary Topics: Gerontology. Basel: Karger, 1988:90–100.
42. Dyson SE, Jones DG. Synaptic remodelling during development and maturation: junction differentiation and splitting as a mechanism for modifying connectivity. Dev Brain Res 1984;13:125–137.
43. Bertoni-Freddari C, Fattoretti P, Casoli T, Meier-Ruge W, Ulrich J. Morphological adaptive response of the synaptic junctional zones in the human dentate gyrus during aging and Alzheimer's disease. Brain Res 1990;517:69–75.
44. Scheff SW, DeKosky ST, Price DA. Quantitative assessment of cortical synaptic density in Alzheimer's disease. Neurobiol Aging 1990;11:29–37.
45. Scheff SW, Scott SA, DeKosky ST. Quantitation of synaptic density in the septal nuclei of young and aged Fischer 344 rats. Neurobiol Aging 1991;12:3–12.
46. Desmond NL, Levy WB. Changes in the numerical density of synaptic contacts with long-term potentiation in the hippocampal dentate gyrus. J Comp Neurol 1986;253:466–475.
47. Carlin RK, Siekevitz P. Plasticity in the central nervous system: do synapses divide? Proc Natl Acad Sci USA 1983;80:3517–3521.
48. Nieto-Sampedro M, Hoff SF, Cotman CW. Perforated postsynaptic densities: probable intermediates in synapse turnover. Proc Natl Acad Sci USA 1982;79:5718–5722.
49. Geinisman Y, Morrell F, de Toledo-Morrell L. Axospinous synapses with segmented postsynaptic densities: a morphologically distinct synaptic subtype contributing to the number of profiles of perforated synapses visualized in random sections. Brain Res 1987;423:179–188.
50. Wolff JR, Laskawi R, Spatz WB, Missler M. Structural dynamics of synapses and synaptic components. Behav Brain Res 1995;66:13–20.
51. Wakita H, Tomimoto H, Kimura J. Glial activation and white matter changes in rat brain induced by chronic cerebral hypoperfusion. Acta Neuropathol (Berlin) 1994; 87:484–492.
52. Exton-Smith AN, Collins KJ. The autonomic nervous system. In: Pathy MSJ (ed) Principles and Practice of Geriatric Medicine, 2nd ed. New York: Wiley, 1997:817–820.
53. Frolkis VV, Bezrukov VV, Duplenko YP, Shcheglovea IV, Shevtchnk VG, Verkhratsky NS. Acetylcholine metabolism and cholinergic regulation of functions in aging, Gerontologia 1973;19:45–54.
54. Smith CUM. Elements of Molecular Neurobiology, 2nd ed. New York: Wiley, 1996:335–338.
55. de la Torre JC. Dynamics of Brain Monoamines. New York: Plenum, 1972.
56. Nakazawa K, Koizumi S, Inoue D. ATP as a neurotransmitter in the brain: its possibility based upon recent findings. Nohon Shinkei Seishin Yakurigaky Zasshi 1995;15(1):1–11.
57. Strosznajder J, Strosznajder RP. ATP, a potent regulator of inositol phospholipids-phospholipase C and lipid mediators in brain cortex. Acta Neurobiol Exp 1996;56:527–534.
58. Todorov LD, Mihaylova TS, Westfall TD, et al. Neuronal release of soluble nucleotidases and their role in neurotransmitter inactivation. Nature 1997;387:76–79.
59. Gazzaley AH. Circuit-specific alterations of N-methyl-D-aspartate receptor subunit 1 in the dentate gyrus of aged monkeys. Proc Natl Acad Sci USA 1996;93: 3121–3123.
60. Severson JA. Synaptic regulation of neurotransmitter function in aging. In: Rothstein M (ed) Review of Biological Research in Aging, vol 3. New York: Liss, 1987:191–206.
61. Bertel O, Buhler FR, Kiowski W, Lutold BE. Decreased beta adrenoreceptor responsiveness as related to age, blood pressure, and plasma catecholamines in patients with essential hypertension. Hypertension 1980;2:130–138.
62. Vestal RE, Wood AJ, Shand DG. Reduced beta-adrenoreceptor sensitivity in the elderly. Clin Pharmacol Ther 1979;26:181–186.
63. Buhler FR, Burkart F, Lutold BE, Kung M, Marbet G, Pfisterer M. Antihypertensive beta-blocking action as related to renin and age: a pharmacologic tool to identify

pathogenetic mechanisms in essential hypertension. Am J Cardiol 1975;36:653–669.
64. Joseph JA, Bartus RT, Clody D, et al. Psychomotor performance in the senescent rodent: reduction of deficits via striatal dopamine receptor upregulation. Neurobiol Aging 1983;4:313–319.
65. Roberts J, Turner N. Age-related changes in autonomic function of catecholamines. In: Rothstein M (ed) Review of Biological Research in Aging, vol 3. New York: Liss, 1987:257–298.
66. Youdin MBH, Riederer P. Understanding Parkinson's disease. Sci Am 1997;276:52–59.
67. Marcusson JO, Oreland L, Winblad B. Effect of age on human brain serotonin, (S-1) binding sites. J Neurochem 1984;43:1699–1705.
68. Allen SJ, Benton JS, Goodhardt MJ, et al. Biochemical evidence of selective nerve cell changes in the normal aging human and rat brain. J Neurochem 1983;41: 256–265.
69. DeBlasi A, Cotecchia S, Tiziana M. Selective changes of receptor binding in brain regions of aged rats. Life Sci 1982;31:335–340.
70. Mann DM, Yates PO, Stamp JE. The relationship between lipofuscin pigment in aging in the human nervous system. J Neurol Sci 1978;37:83–93.
71. Bjorkerud S. Isolated lipofuscin granules: a survey of a new field. Adv Gerontol Res 1964;1:257–288.
72. Porta EA, Mower HF, Lee C, Palimbo NE. Differential features between lipofuscin (age pigment) and various experimentally produced "ceroid pigments." In: Lipofuscin—1987: State of the Art. Amsterdam: Excepta Medica, 1988:341–374.
73. D'Amato RJ, Alexander GM, Schwartzman RJ, Kitt CA, Price DL, Snyder SH. Evidence for neuromelanin in MPTP-induced neurotoxicity. Nature 1987;327:324–326.
74. Kopin IJ. Features of the dopaminergic neurotoxin MPTP. Ann NY Acad Sci 1992;648:96–104.
75. Zeman W, Donohue S, Dyken P, Green J. The neuronal ceroid lipofuscinoses (Batten-Vogt syndrome). In: Vinken P, Bruyn GW (eds) Handbook of Clinical Neurology, vol 10. Amsterdam: North Holland, 1970:588–679.
76. Stadtman ER. Protein oxidation and aging. Science 1992;257:1220–1224.
77. Brody H. An examination of cerebral cortex and brainstem in aging. In: Terry RD, Gersham S (eds) Neurobiology of Aging. New York: Raven, 1976:177–181.
78. Terry RD, De Teresa R, Hansen LA. Neocortical cell counts in normal human adult aging. Ann Neurol 1987;21: 530–539.
79. Coleman PD, Flood DG. Neuron numbers and dendritic extent in normal aging and Alzheimer's disease. Neurobiol Aging 1987;8:521–545.
80. Finch CE. Neuron atrophy during aging: programmed or sporadic? TINS 1993;16:104–110.
81. Finch CE. Longevity, Senescence and the Genome. Chicago: University of Chicago Press, 1990:188–193.
82. Haug H. The evaluation of cell-densities and of nerve-cell-size distribution by stereological procedures in a layered tissue (cortex cerebri). Microsc Acta 1979;82:147–161.
83. Haug H, Barmwater U, Eggers R, Fischer D, Kuhl S, Sass NL. Anatomical changes in aging brain: morphometric analysis of the human prosencephalon. In: Cervos-Navarro J, Sarkander HI (eds) Brain Aging: Neuropathology and Neuropharmacology. New York: Raven, 1983:1–12.
84. Haug H. Macroscopic and microscopic morphometry of the human brain and cortex: a survey in the light of new results. Brain Pathol 1984;1:123–149.
85. Terry RD. Some morphometric aspects of the brain in senile dementia of the Alzheimer type. Ann Neurol 1981;10:184.
86. de la Torre JC, Cada A, Nelson N, Davis G, Sutherland RJ, Gonzalez Lima F. Reduced cytochrome oxidase and memory dysfunction after chronic brain ischemia in aged rats. Neurosci Lett 1997;223:165–168.
87. Haug H. Nervous tissue. In: Weibel ER (ed) Stereological Methods, vol 1: Practical Methods for Biological Morphometry, London: Academic, 1979:311–322.
88. Morrison JH, Huf PR. Life and death of neurons in the aging brain. Science 1997;278:412–419.
89. Sofroniew MV, Isacson O, Bjorklund A. Corticol grafts prevent atrophy of cholinergic basal nucleus neurons induced by excitotoxic cortical damage. Brain Res 1986;378:409–415.
90. de la Torre JC, Fortin T, Park G, Pappas B, Saunders J, Richard M. Brain blood-flow restoration "rescues" chronically damaged rat CA1 neurons. Brain Res 1993;623:6–15.
91. Murphy DG, Decarli C, Schapiro MB, Rapoport SF, Horwitz B. Age-related differences in volumes of subcortical nuclei, brain matter and cerebral spinal fluid in healthy men as measured with magnetic resonance imaging. Arch Neurol 1992;49:839–845.
92. Davis PC, Mirra SS, Alazraki N. The brain in older persons with and without dementia: findings on MR, PET, and SPECT images. Am J Radiol 1994;162:1267–1278.
93. Flood DG, Coleman PD. Neuron numbers and sizes in aging brain: comparisons of human, monkey and rodent data. Neurobiol Aging 1988;94:453–463.
94. Mervis R. Cytomorphological alterations in the aging animal brain with emphasis on Golgi studies. In: Johnson JE (ed) Aging and Cell Structure. New York: Plenum, 1981:143–186.
95. Meier-Ruge W, Hunziker O, Iwangoff P, Reichmeier K, Sandoz P. Alterations of morphological and neurochemical parameters of the brain due to normal aging. In: Nandy K (ed) Senile Dementia: A Biological Approach. Amsterdam: Elsevier North-Holland, 1987:33–44.
96. Flood DG, Coleman PD. Hippocampal plasticity in normal aging and decreased plasticity in Alzheimer's disease. Prog Brain Res 1990;83:435–443.
97. Kemper T. Neuroanatomical and neuropathological changes in normal aging and in dementia. In: Albert ML (ed) Clinical Neurology of Aging. New York: Oxford University Press, 1984:9–52.
98. Duara R, London ED, Rapoport SI. Changes in structure and energy metabolism of the aging brain. In: Finch CE, Schneider EL (eds) Handbook of the Biology of Aging. New York: Van Nostrand Reinhold, 1985:595–616.
99. Kety SS. Human cerebral blood flow and oxygen consumption as related to aging. In: Moore JE, Merritt HH,

Masselink RJ (eds) The Neurologic and Psychiatric Aspects of the Disorders of Aging. Baltimore: Williams & Wilkins, 1955:31–45.

100. Dastur DK. Cerebral blood flow and metabolism in normal human aging, pathological aging, and senile dementia. J Cereb Blood Flow Metab 1985;5:1–9.
101. Fazekas JF, Alivan RW, Bessman AN. Cerebral physiology of the aged. Am J Med Sci 1952:223–245.
102. Scheinberg P, Blackburn I, Rich M. Effects of aging on cerebral circulation and metabolism. Arch Neurol Psychiatry 1953;70:77.
103. Pulsinelli WA. Selective neuronal vulnerability: morphological and molecular characteristics. Prog Brain Res 1985;63:29.
104. Hossmann KA. Post-ischemic resuscitation of the brain: selective vulnerability versus global resistance. Prog Brain Res 1985;63:3.
105. Tymianski M, Sattler RG. Is calcium involved in excitotoxic or ischemic neuronal damage? In: Welch KMA, Caplan L, Reis DJ, Siesjo BK, Weir B (eds) Primer on Cerebrovascular Diseases. San Diego: Academic, 1997:190–198.
106. Greenmayre JT. The role of glutamate in neurotransmission and in neurologic disease. Arch Neurol 1986;43:1058.
107. Rothman SM, Olney JW. Glutamate and the pathophysiology of hypoxic-ischemic brain damage. Ann Neurol 1988;45:148.
108. Vinters HV. Vascular diseases in the elderly. In: Duckett S, de la Torre J (eds). Pathology of the Aging Human Nervous System. 2nd ed. New York: Oxford University Press, 2000: in press.
109. Grady CL, Horwitz B, Schapiro MB, Rapoport SI. Changes in the integrated activity of the brain with healthy aging and dementia of the Alzheimer type. In: Rapoport SI, Petit H, Leys D, Christe Y (eds) Aging Brain and Dementia: New Trends in Diagnosis and Therapy. New York: Liss, 1990:355–369.
110. Leenders KL, Perani D, Lammertsma AA. Cerebral blood flow, blood volume and oxygen utilization; normal values and effect of age. Brain 1990;113:27–47.
111. Lenzi GL, Frackowiak RSJ, Jones T. $CMRO_2$ and CBF by oxygen-15 inhalation technique. Eur Neurol 1981;20:285–290.
112. Marchal G, Rioux P, Petit-Taboue MC. The effects of optimally healthy aging on cerebral oxygen metabolism, blood flow and blood volume in humans: a PET study. J Cereb Blood Flow Metab 1991;11(suppl 2):S785.
113. Yamaguchi T, Kanno I, Uemura K. Reduction in regional cerebral metabolic rate of oxygen during human aging. Stroke 1986;17:1220–1228.
114. Itoh M, Hatazawa J, Miyazawa H. Stability of cerebral blood flow and oxygen metabolism during normal aging. Gerontology 1990;36:43–48.
115. Frackowiak RSJ, Lenzi GL, Jones T, Heather JD. Quantitative measurement of regional cerebral blood flow and oxygen metabolism in man using $^{15}O$ and positron emission tomography: theory, procedure, and normal values. J Comput Assist Tomogr 1980;4:727–736.
116. Frackowiak RSJ, Pozzilli C, Legg NJ. Regional cerebral oxygen supply and utilization in dementia: a clinical and physiological study with oxygen-15 and positron tomography. Brain 1981;104:753–778.
117. Shirakura T, Kubota K, Tamura K. Blood viscosity and cerebral blood flow in the aged. Jpn J Geriatr 1993;30:174–181.
118. Grady C. Quantitative comparison of measurements of cerebral glucose rate made with two positron cameras. J Cereb Blood Flow Metab 1991;11:A57–A63.
119. Pawlik G, Heiss WD, Beil C, Wienhard K, Herholtz K, Wagner K. PET demonstrates differential age dependence, asymmetry and response to various stimuli of regional brain glucose metabolism in healthy volunteers. J Cereb Blood Flow Metab 1987;7(suppl 1):S376.
120. de Leon M, George AE, Tomanelli J. Positron emission tomography studies of normal aging: a replication of PET III and $^{18}F$ FDG using PET VI and 11-CDG. Neurobiol Aging 1987;8:319–323.
121. Duara R, Grady C, Haxby J. Human brain glucose utilization and cognitive function in relation to age. Ann Neurol 1984;16:702–713.
122. Junck L, Moen JG, Bluemlein I. Cerebral glucose metabolism in normal aging studied with PET. J Cereb Blood Metab 1989;9(suppl 1):S524.
123. Kalaria RN, Harik SI. Reduced glucose transporter at the blood-brain barrier and cerebral cortex in Alzheimer's disease. J Neurochem 1989;53:1083–1088.
124. Stewart RR, Morrazzi CA. Oxygen transport in the human brain: analytical solutions. Adv Exp Med Biol 1973;37: 843–848.
125. Alavi A. Regional cerebral glucose metabolism. Exp Brain Res 1982;5(suppl 5):187–195.
126. Kuhl DE. Effects of human aging on patterns of local cerebral glucose utilization determined by the $^{18}F$ fluorodeoxyglucose method. J Cereb Blood Flow Metabol 1982;2:163.
127. Kenshalo DR. Somesthetic sensitivity in young and elderly humans. J Gerontol 1986;41:732.
128. Meier-Ruge W (ed). The Elderly Patient in General Practice. New York: Karger, 1987:78.
129. Verrillo RT. Age related changes in the sensitivity to vibration. J Gerontol 1980;35:185–193.
130. Verrillo RT, Verrillo V. Sensory and perceptual performance. In: Charness N (ed) Aging and Human Performance. New York: Wiley, 1985:1.
131. Marshall J, Grindle J, Ansell PL, Brewein B. Convolution in human rods: an aging process. Br J Opthalmol 1979;63:181–187.
132. Curcio CA, Drucker DN. Retinal ganglion cells in Alzheimer's disease and aging. Ann Neurol 1993;33:248–257.
133. Gao H, Hollyfield JG. Aging of the human retina differential loss of neurons and retinal pigment epithelial cells. Invest Opthalmol Vis Sci 1992;33:1–17.
134. Skinner HB, Barrack RL, Cook SD. Age-related declines in proprioception. Clin Orthop 1984;184:208.
135. Pickles JO. Sensorineural hearing loss. In: An Introduction to the Physiology of Hearing, 2nd ed. San Diego: Academic, 1988:310–311.
136. Wall PD, Noordenbos W. Sensory functions which remain in man after complete transection of dorsal columns. Brain 1977;100:641–653.
137. Drewnoswki A, Henderson SA, Driscoll A, Rolls BJ. Salt taste perceptions and preferences are unrelated to sodium

consumption in healthy older adults. J Am Diet Assoc 1996;96:471–474.
138. Schiffman SS, Lindley MS, Clark TB, Makino C. Molecular mechanism of sweet taste: relationship of hydrogen bonding to taste sensitivity for both young and elderly. Neurobiol Aging 1981;2:173–185.
139. Murphy C, Gilmore MM. Quality specific effects of aging on the human taste system. J Percept Psychophys 1989;45:121–128.
140. Bartoshuk LM. Taste, robust across the age span? Ann NY Acad Sci 1989;561:65–75.
141. Cain WS, Stevens JC. Uniformity of olfactory loss in aging. Ann NY Acad Sci 1989;561:29–38.
142. Doty RL. Influence of age and age related diseases on olfactory function. Ann NY Acad Sci 1989;561:76–86.
143. Broe GA, Williamson M, Tate PL, Locke M, McFarlane A, Mitchell R. Senescent gait disorder and forgetfulness? Normal ageing or early dementia. In: Fenelon B, Pfister HP (eds) Proceedings of the 1983 Brain Impairment Conference and Workshops. Victoria: Australian Society for the Study of Brain Impairment, 1983:269–277.
144. Paige GD. The aging vestibulo-ocular reflex (VOR) and adaptive plasticity. Acta Otolaryngol Suppl (Stockh) 1991;481:297.
145. Koller WC, Glatt SL, Fox JH. Senile gait: a distinct neurologic entity. Clin Geriatr Med 1985;1:661–668.
146. Scheibel AB. Falls, motor dysfunction, and correlative neurohistologic changes. Clin Geriatr Med 1985;1:671.
147. Drachman DA, Zaks MS. The memory cliff beyond span in immediate recall. Psychol Rep 1967;21:105–112.
148. Baddeley AD, Hitch GJ. Working memory. In: Bower G (ed) Recent Advances in Learning and Motivation. San Diego: Academic, 1974:47–90.
149. Craik FIM. Age differences in human memory. In: Birren JE, Schaie KW (eds) Handbook of the Psychology of Aging. New York: Van Nostrand Rheinhold, 1977.
150. Botwinick J, Storandt M. Memory, Related Functions and Age. Springfield, IL: Charles C Thomas, 1974.
151. Tulving E. How many memory systems are there? Am Psychol 1985;40:385–398.
152. Evans DV. Prevalence of Alzheimer's disease in a community population of older persons. JAMA 1989;262: 2551–2556.
153. Kurtzke JF. Epidemiology of cerebrovascular disease. In: McDowell F, Caplan L (eds) Cerebrovascular Report. Bethesda: NINDS, 1985.
154. McEwen BS. Re-examination of the glucocorticoid hypothesis of stress and aging. Prog Brain Res 1992;93: 365–385.
155. Wooley CS, Gould E, McEwen BS. Exposure to excess glucocorticoids alters dendritic morphology of adult hippocampal pyramidal neurons. Brain Res 1990;531: 225–231.
156. Sheline YI, Wang PW, Gado M, Csernansky JG, Vannier MN. Hippocampal atrophy in major depression. Proc Natl Acad Sci USA 1995;93:3908–3913.
157. Bemner JD, Randall R, Scott TM, Bronen R. MRI-based measurement of hippocampal volume in patients with combat-related post-traumatic stress disorder. Am J Psychriatry 1995;152:973–981.
158. Bonica JJ. The Management of Pain, 2nd ed. Philadelphia: Lea & Febiger, 1989.
159. Ferrell BA, Ferrell BR, Osterweil D. Pain in the nursing home. J Am Geriatr Soc 1990;38:409–414.
160. Sengstaken EA, King SA. The problems of pain and its detection among geriatric nursing home residents. J Am Geriatr Soc 1993;41:541–544.
161. Hendler N. The Diagnosis and Nonsurgical Management of Chronic Pain. New York: Raven, 1981.
162. De Vaul R, Hall R, Faillace L. Drug use by the polysurgical patient. Am J Psychiatry 1978;135:682–685.
163. Fry PS, Wong PTP. Pain management training in the elderly: matching interventions with subjects coping styles. Stress Med 1991;7:93–98.
164. Wall RT. Use of analgesics in the elderly. Clin Pharmacol 1990;6:345–347.
165. Roy R, Thomas M. A survey of chronic pain in the elderly population. Can Fam Physician 1986;32:513–516.
166. McCaffery M, Beebe A. Pain in the elderly: special considerations. In: McCaffery M, Beebe A (eds) Pain: Clinical Manual for Nursing Practice. St. Louis: Mosby, 1989: 308–323.
167. Fordyce WE. Evaluating and managing chronic pain. Geriatrics 1978;33:59–62.
168. Libb JW, Clements CB. Token reinforcement in an exercise program for hospitalized geriatric patients. Percept Mot Skills 1969;28:957–958.
169. Holyrod KA, Penzien DB. Client variables and the behavioral treatment of recurrent tension headache: a meta-analytic review. J Behav Med 1986;9:515–536.
170. Middaugh SJ, Woods E, Kee WG, Harden RN, Peters JR. Biofeedback-assisted relaxation training for the aging chronic pain patient. Biofeedback Self Regul 1991;16:361–377.
171. Jessup BA, Gallegos X. Relaxation and biofeedback. In: Wall PD, Melzack R (eds) Textbook of Pain. Edinburgh: Churchill Livingstone, 1994:1321–1335.
172. Noda HH. An exploratory study of the effects of EMG and temperature biofeedback on rheumatoid arthritis. Diss Abstr Int B 1978;39:3532B.
173. Portenoy RK, Farkash A. Practical management of non-malignant pain in the elderly. Geriatrics 1988;43:29–47.
174. Roche RJ, Forman WB. Pain management for the geriatric patient. Clin Podiatr Med Surg 1994;11:41–53.
175. Sandin KJ. Specialized pain treatment for geriatric patients. Clin J Pain 1993;9:60.
176. Sorkin BA, Rudy TE, Hanlon RB, Turk DC, Steig RL. Chronic pain in old and young patients: differences appear less important than similarities. J Gerontol Psychol Sci 1990;45:64–68.
177. Sorkin BA, Turk DC. Pain management in the elderly. In: Roy R (ed) Chronic Pain in Old Age. Toronto: University of Toronto Press, 1995:56–80.
178. Aronoff GM, Evans WO. The prediction of treatment outcome at a multidisciplinary pain center. Pain 1982;14: 67–73.
179. Middaugh SJ, Levin RB, Kee WG, Barchiesi FD, Robers JM. Chronic pain: its treatment in geriatric and younger patients. Arch Phys Med Rehabil 1988;69: 1021–1025.

180. Rechschaffen A. The function of sleep: methodological issues. In: Drucker-Colin Skurovich M, Sterman MB (eds) The Functions of Sleep. San Diego: Academic, 1979:1–17.
181. Parineu M. Epidemiology of sleep disorders. In: Roth T, Dement WC (eds) Principles and Practice of Sleep Medicine. Philadelphia: Saunders, 1994:437–452.
182. Poelstra PAM. Relationship between physical, psychological, social and environmental variables and subjective sleep quality. Sleep 1984;7:255–260.
183. Bliwise DL. Sleep in normal aging and dementia. Sleep 1993;16:40–81.
184. Ford DE, Kamerow DB. Epidemiologic study of sleep disturbances and psychiatric disorder. JAMA 1989;262: 1479–1484.
185. Gerard P, Collins KJ, Dore C, Exton-Smith AN. Subjective characteristics of sleep in the elderly. Age Ageing 1978;7(suppl):55–63.
186. Hohagen F, Grabhoff U, Ellringmann D, et al. The prevalence of insomnia in different age groups and its treatment modalities in general practice. In: Smirne S, Franceschi M, Ferini-Strambi L (eds) Sleep and Ageing. Milan: Masson, 1991:205–215.
187. Phillips B, Berry D, Schmitt F, Patel R, Cook Y. Sleep quality and pulmonary function in the healthy elderly. Chest 1989;95:60–64.
188. Habte-Gabr E, Wallace RB, Colsher PL, Hulbert JR. Sleep patterns in rural elders: demographic, health and psycho-behavioral correlates. J Clin Epidemiol 1991; 44:5– 13.
189. Lipowski ZJ. Delirium in the elderly patient. N Engl J Med 1989:320:578–582.
190. Greendyke RM, Kanter DR. Therapeutic effects of pindolol on behavioral disturbances associated with organic brain disease: a double-blind study. J Clin Psychiatry 1986:47: 423–426.
191. Jenike MA. Treatment of rage and violence in elderly patients with propranolol. Geriatrics 1983;38:29–34.
192. Jenike MA. Psychoactive drugs in the elderly: antipsychotics and anxiolytics. Geriatrics 1988;43:53–65.
193. Ehlers CL, Kupfer DJ. Effects of age on delta and REM sleep parameters. Electroencephalogr Clin Neurophysiol 1989;72:118–125.
194. Feinberg I. Changes in sleep cycle patterns with age. J Psychiatr Res 1974;10:283–306.
195. Sarajishvili PM, Geladze T, Bibileishvili SE, Shubladze GN, Toidze O. The electroencephalogram sleep patterns of long-lived males. Soobshch Akad Nauk Gruz SSR 1974;75:693–695.
196. Feinberg I, Koresko RL, Heller N. EEG sleep patterns as a function of normal and pathological aging in man. J Psychiatr Res 1967;5:107–144.
197. Gillin JC, Duncan WC, Murphy DL, et al. Age-related changes in sleep in depressed and normal subjects. Psychiatr Res 1981;4:73–78.
198. Spiegel R. Sleep and Sleeplessness in Advanced Age. New York: SP Medical, 1981.
199. Hayashi Y, Endo S. All-night sleep polygraphic recordings of healthy aged persons: REM and slow wave sleep. Sleep 1982;5:277–283.
200. Kales A, Wilson T, Kales JD, et al. Measurements of all-night sleep in normal elderly persons: effects of aging. J Am Geriatr Soc 1967;15:405–414.
201. Williams RL, Karacan I, Hursch CJ. EEG of Human Sleep: Clinical Applications. New York: Wiley, 1974.
202. Hajak G, Klingelhofer J, Schultz-Varszegi M, Ruther E. Blood circulation and energy metabolism of the brain in healthy sleep. Nervenarzt 1993;64:456–467.
203. Maquet P, Peters J, Aerts J, et al. Functional neuroanatomy of human rapid-eye-movement sleep and dreaming. Nature 1996;383:163–166.
204. Rolls BJ, Phillips PA. Aging and disturbances of thirst and fluid balance. Nutr Rev 1990;48:137–144.
205. Conroy C, Kraus JF. Survival after brain injury: cause of death, length of survival, and prognostic variables in a cohort of brain-injured people. Neuroepidemiology 1988;7:13–22.
206. Hernesniemi J. Outcome following head injuries in the aged. Acta Neurol Scand 1970;46:343–348.
207. Luerssen TG, Klauber MR, Marshall LF. Outcome from head injury related to patient's age: a longitudinal prospective study of adult and pediatric head injury. J Neurosurg 1988;68:409–416.
208. Bush TL, Miller SR, Criqui MH, Barrett-Connor E. Risk factors for morbidity and mortality in older population: an epidemiological approach. In: Hazzard WR, Andres R, Bierman EL, Blass JP (eds) Principles of Geriatric Medicine and Gerontology, 2nd ed. New York: McGraw-Hill, 1990:125–137.
209. Jane JA, Francel PC. Age and outcome of head injury. In: Narayan RK, Wilberger JE, Povlishock JT (eds) Neurotrauma. New York: McGraw-Hill, 1996:793–804.
210. Alberico AM, Ward JD, Choi S, Marmarou A, Young JF. Outcome after severe head injury. J Neurosurg 1987;67: 648–656.
211. Vollmer DJ, Torner JC, Jane JA. Age and outcome following traumatic coma: why do older patients fare worse? J Neurosurg 1991;75:537–549.
212. Vollmer DG. Prognosis and outcome of severe head injury. In: Cooper PR (ed) Head Injury. Baltimore: Williams & Wilkins, 1993:553–581.
213. Dujovny M, Charbel F, Berman SK, Diaz FG, Malik G, Ausman JI. Geriatric neurosurgery. Surg Neurol 1987;28: 10–16.
214. Pentland B, Jones PA, Roy CW. Head injury in the elderly. Age Ageing 1986;15:193–202.
215. Savino JA, Del Guercio LRM. Preoperative cardiopulmonary evaluation and postsurgical convalescence. In: Calkins E, Ford AB, Katz PR (eds) Practice of Geriatrics, 2nd ed. Philadelphia: Saunders, 1992:578–587.
216. de la Torre JC. Cerebral hypoperfusion, capillary degeneration and development of Alzheimer's disease. Alzheimer Dis Assoc Dis 2000;14:S72–S81.

# 65
# Benign and Malignant Tumors of the Brain

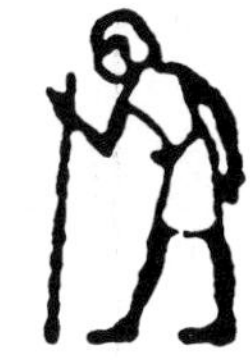

Elizabeth B. Claus and Joseph Piepmeier

Data from the National Cancer Institute (NCI) indicate that approximately 17,600 individuals within the United States were expected to be diagnosed with a first primary cancer of the central nervous system (CNS) in 1997, of whom approximately 15% would be aged 70 years or more.[1] Most of these individuals would die from their disease, with overall 5-year survival rates estimated to be approximately 30%.[1] In addition, up to 100,000 Americans are diagnosed each year with metastatic brain lesions, most of whom are elderly patients. Although improved technology and treatment modalities have led to increased detection of brain lesions and better control of systemic primary malignancies, little progress has been made with respect to survival and identification of risk factors in individuals diagnosed with these lesions. The conflict between these two is particularly important in the elderly, given that Americans over the age of 70 years now make up the fastest growing portion of the U.S. population.[2] This chapter provides a review and discussion of options for the detection, treatment, and outcome of elderly patients diagnosed with tumors of the brain.

## Primary Brain Tumors

### Epidemiology

The incidence of specific histologic subtypes of CNS tumors varies with respect to age. Most primary brain tumors among the elderly consist of a group of lesions defined as astroglial neoplasms. Glial cells make up the supporting cells of the brain and assist neurons with a variety of structural, protective, and metabolic functions. The various clinical presentations of astroglial tumors may represent discrete points along a continuum of malignancy, although the data are not consistent with respect to this point. The grading of brain lesions is complex; grading schemes for this continuum are many and vary by institution and pathologist. For tumors in the astroglial series, most pathologists use a three- or four-tiered grading system to subdivide these cases. A classification scheme proposed by Daumas-Duport has four grades and uses nuclear atypia, mitoses, endothelial proliferation, and necrosis as classification covariates. With the three-tiered systems, tumors are defined by increasing malignancy as astrocytoma, anaplastic astrocytoma, and glioblastoma, respectively. Each of these three tumor grades has a distinct epidemiology and prognosis. Low-grade astrocytomas tend to occur in young adults (median age 35 years), and recent data report survivals of 5–10 years. Anaplastic astrocytomas typically occur in middle-age adults (median age 45 years), and the median survival appears limited to 3–4 years. Glioblastomas are tumors more frequently found in older patients (median age 55 years), and survival is limited to approximately 1 year. Using 1975–1994 data from the Connecticut Tumor Registry (CTR), the oldest tumor registry in the United States (which uses the state of Connecticut as its population base), approximately 15% of primary brain tumors are diagnosed in individuals aged 70 years of age or more. In this age group, 60% of lesions were defined as glioblastomas, 11% as astrocytomas, 9% as gliomas, 3% as meningiomas, and 1% as lymphomas. Within the CTR data, men were less frequently reported to have primary brain tumors than women (46% vs. 54%).

As is true for most cancers, a relation exists between age and incidence rate of primary brain tumors. For brain tumors, there appear to be two peak ages at which these lesions occur: one during the first decade of life and a second during the sixth decade. Specifically, data from the Surveillance, Epidemiology, and End Results (SEER) program of the NCI or cross-sectional data[3–5] report an increase in the age-specific incidence rates of glioblastoma up to age 64 with a decline in rates at older ages. However, birth-cohort analyses[6] suggest that these rates increase in groups of individuals older than 65 years of age. SEER data indicate that age-specific incidence rates for glioblastoma, astrocytoma, and meningioma peak at age groups 70–74, 65–69, and 70–74, respectively,[6] whereas other types of gliomas, medulloblastomas and

TABLE 65.1. Trends in Age-specific Incidence Rates for Brain and CNS Cancers in Connecticut: 1965–1969 to 1985–1988

| Age | Years of diagnosis | No. of cases | Rate per $10^5$ | Cases confirmed by radiography alone (%) | Rate after excluding cases confirmed by radiography alone |
|---|---|---|---|---|---|
| 70–74 years | 1965–1969 | 39 | 10.28 | 5.1 | 9.76[a] |
| | 1970–1974 | 70 | 17.83 | 5.7 | 16.81[b] |
| | 1975–1979 | 71 | 16.34 | 21.1 | 12.88[c] |
| | 1980–1984 | 109 | 22.00 | 25.7 | 16.35[d] |
| | 1985–1988 | 107 | 24.46 | 11.2 | 21.72[e] |
| 75–79 years | 1965–1969 | 22 | 8.32 | 9.1 | 7.56 |
| | 1970–1974 | 38 | 12.95 | 18.4 | 10.56[a] |
| | 1975–1979 | 63 | 20.55 | 20.6 | 16.31[b] |
| | 1980–1984 | 68 | 19.36 | 44.1 | 10.82[c] |
| | 1985–1988 | 70 | 21.96 | 30.0 | 15.37[d] |
| 80–84 years | 1965–1969 | 11 | 7.11 | 18.2 | 5.82 |
| | 1970–1974 | 7 | 3.71 | 14.3 | 3.18 |
| | 1975–1979 | 22 | 10.22 | 36.4 | 6.50[a] |
| | 1980–1984 | 53 | 23.82 | 32.1 | 16.18[b] |
| | 1985–1988 | 31 | 15.55 | 54.8 | 7.02[c] |

*Source:* Polednek,[6] with permission.
The number of cases in the age group 85+ was too small (e.g., one case during 1965–1969) for meaningful analyses.
[a] Cohort born around 1895.
[b] Cohort born around 1900.
[c] Cohort born around 1905.
[d] Cohort born around 1910.
[e] Cohort born around 1915.

ependymomas, are rare among individuals age 70 or more.

In addition to an association between cancer risk and age, there are multiple reports of increasing incidence rates over time within age groups. With respect to the elderly population, reported age-specific incidence rates of primary malignant brain tumors have increased up to fivefold between 1973 and 1985. These increases were similar for men and women. In addition, among individuals age 70 years and above, mortality from brain tumors increased up to eightfold over the 20-year period between 1968 and 1988.[7] The explanation for reported increases in age-specific primary brain cancer incidence and mortality rates among the elderly remains unclear.[8] A number of hypotheses have been proposed, including the presence of a true increase, increased use of radiologic screening methods such as computed tomography (CT) and magnetic resonance imaging (MRI), increased interest in neurologic disorders of elderly patients such as Alzheimer's (and therefore associated biopsies and autopsies), change in disease classification, delayed response to an environmental exposure (i.e., DDT), and change in health care delivery.

Polednek[6] analyzed data from the Connecticut Tumor Registry (Table 65.1) in an effort to examine some of these issues. If one includes cases confirmed by radiology or histology, the age-specific incidence rates can be seen to increase fairly uniformly for all ages over 70 years from 1975 to 1988. When the rates are examined after excluding cases confirmed by radiography alone, the picture is less consistent, especially for the oldest age group (i.e., 80 years of age or more). One confounding issue in these data is the fact that older individuals are more likely to have their disease diagnosed purely by radiography without surgical biopsy, an important issue, given the fact that 11–50% of patients thought to have a primary cancer by radiography, later prove to have either an infectious lesion or a second primary lesion.[9] Of interest is the suggestion of a cohort effect (i.e., an effect seen within a group of individuals born within the same time period). Increases in rates have been observed for cohort groups born between 1910 and 1920 among individuals age 65–79 years, thus providing some evidence that not all of the increased rates are due to the increased use of radiography.

## Environmental Risk Factors

A wide variety of environmental risk factors for primary malignant and benign brain tumors have been proposed.[10] The list of variables includes electromagnetic fields, trauma, occupational and industrial chemicals, medications including anticonvulsants, and viral infections among others. At present, however, no single risk factor has been consistently identified as being associated with cancer risk, particularly within the elderly population.

## Symptoms

The presenting symptoms for intracranial lesions vary by location, rate of growth, type of tumor, and age. In elderly patients the most common presentations are confusion or mental status changes, personality changes, headache, seizure associated with motor and sensory deficits such as paresis of an arm or leg, and dysphasia. Papilledema and nausea/vomiting are less common symptoms in elderly patients. In some cases the symptoms are complicated by or confused with co-morbid conditions such as dementia (i.e., Alzheimer's disease) and cerebrovascular disease. The presenting symptoms may be subtle, particularly if the tumor is located in a "quiet" area of the brain or if it grows slowly (e.g., a meningioma). Tumor symptoms may also present acutely, as with a seizure or hydrocephalus, when the flow of cerebrospinal fluid is suddenly blocked by the tumor.

## Diagnosis

Most brain tumors in the elderly are now identified by CT and MRI. These noninvasive tests are generally well tolerated by the elderly patient, although one must take care to monitor kidney function in individuals receiving dye for these scans, as is generally needed to define a tumor. In addition, angiography may play a role in defining the vascular supply of tumors such as meningiomas, although again in the elderly patient concerns related to the use of contrast dye may outweigh the benefits of any information gained from angiography. In many instances information gained from magnetic resonance angiography (MRA) may be substituted for that obtained from angiography.

The use of diagnostic imaging is of particular interest in the elderly, as its increased use in Western countries has been proposed as one of the reasons for the reported increase in brain tumors among the elderly over the past 20 years. In the United States, the annual increase for brain tumors over age 65 is 3.0% compared to 0.5% in younger groups.[11] For many elderly patients imaging remains the sole mechanism of diagnosis with the associated errors in sensitivity and specificity. A continued examination of the incidence of brain tumors in this age group in relation to the proportion diagnosed solely by means of radiology will be of interest in the coming years.

## Surgery

A variety of surgical options exist for the type of primary brain tumors generally seen in the elderly patient (i.e., astroglial tumors and meningiomas), including gross total resection, partial resection, or stereotactic biopsy. There are, however, few data from studies that specifically examined the survival and quality of life by surgical treatment group and histopathologic classification among the elderly. Furthermore, there are no prospective, randomized data with respect to surgical treatment for this age group. The current literature fairly uniformly reports age as being the most significant variable correlated with survival, with a less favorable prognosis associated with increased age.[12–14] For this chapter we reviewed data from the Connecticut Tumor Registry, which indicated that the overall 1- and 5-year survival rates for individuals over the age of 70 diagnosed with glioblastoma were 20% and 3%, respectively. This age group therefore shows 1- and 5-year death rates that are 1.3- and 1.8-fold higher, respectively, than those of individuals diagnosed prior to 70 years, respectively. Within these CTR data, survival rates for individuals diagnosed with astrocytoma over the age of 70 are somewhat more encouraging, with 59% and 36% of these individuals remaining alive 1 and 5 years, respectively, after diagnosis. These older patients are 1.3 and 2.7 times more likely to succumb to their disease at these time points than are individuals diagnosed prior to age 70, highlighting again the deleterious effect of age on outcome.

Despite the fact that elderly patients do less well, there is some limited evidence that surgery does benefit these patients if they are selected carefully (i.e., if expected lifespan and quality of life with treatment exceeds that without treatment). In the case of elderly patients, the general medical condition must be carefully considered along with the neurologic status. As would be expected, patients with poor Karnofsky performance scores, a measure of functional outcome, do less well with respect to survival.[15] In general, elderly patients undergoing craniotomy for primary brain tumor resection have longer survivals than those undergoing a biopsy, but this benefit is complicated by intraoperative and postoperative mortality and morbidity rates, which exceed those in younger individuals.

Tomika and Raimondi's 1981 study of 61 individuals diagnosed with primary brain cancer reported that approximately 25–30% of patients suffered postoperative complications, with pulmonary complications including pulmonary embolism, pneumonia, atelectasis, and pleural effusion reported most commonly.[16] In their nonrandomized, clinical audit of 80 patients over the age of 60 diagnosed with supratentorial glioma, Whittle et al. reported 30-day surgical morbidity rates for biopsy and cytoreduction of 8% and 61%,[17] respectively, and mortality rates of 33% and 0% for the two procedures. When patients receiving radiation therapy following biopsy or cytoreduction were examined, the mortality and morbidity rates were zero for both groups. Furthermore, although the median hospital stay for these patients ranged from a low of 5 days for patients receiving only steroids to 9 days for patients undergoing only biopsy, up to 19–21 days for patients receiving more extensive treatment, patients having more treatment had significantly increased survival time. A third, more recent study[18] of 128 elderly patients diagnosed with glioblastomas, reported a 4.5% death rate during the first 30 days after surgery in patients undergoing biopsy versus a rate of 2.5% in patients undergoing gross total resection. Although the prevention of pulmonary and other peri-

and postoperative complications has decreased with better care over the years, elderly patients are still at increased risk of death and postoperative complications relative to younger patients.

The specifics of surgical treatment vary according to histologic subtype and by location of the lesion within the CNS. Most primary brain tumors in the elderly are located supratentorially, particularly in the cerebral hemispheres, making a surgical approach feasible.[16] In general, if a tumor is surgically accessible (i.e., not deeply placed in such regions as the brain stem or hypothalamus), surgical resection appears to offer the greatest overall benefit to most patients (both young and old) with respect to survival and quality of life, as measured by the ability to function independently. As would be expected, individuals who are able to undergo gross total resection have increased survival times compared to those who undergo partial resection or biopsy, although the increases are generally modest.[18–20] A study by Kelly and Hunt examined a retrospective, consecutive series of 128 patients diagnosed with glioblastomas at 65–83 years of age (mean age 71 years).[18] The study compared survival rates for individuals undergoing stereotactic biopsy with those undergoing stereotactic gross resection. The two groups did not differ significantly with respect to age, Karnofsky score, or presenting symptoms. As would be expected, individuals with brain stem, callosal, or thalamic tumors were treated primarily by biopsy rather than gross resection. The authors reported that the mean survival in the two groups was 15.4 weeks versus 27.0 weeks ($p = 0.01$), respectively. Of note, approximately 20% of elderly patients undergoing resection survived beyond 1 year. As is noted by the authors, patients were not randomly assigned to treatment groups; hence the relationship between assignment and treatment group and baseline expected survival are likely to be correlated. In addition, because of the small sample size, more sophisticated multivariate analyses were not possible to sort out the interplay between treatment, irradiation, tumor location, and other variables.

In addition to astroglial tumors, elderly patients frequently are found to have meningiomas and lymphomas of the CNS. In fact, the overall reported incidence of CNS lymphomas has increased over the past decade, primarily due to increases in both immune-compromised individuals and the elderly. Lymphomas of the CNS are generally treated with biopsy, chemotherapy, and radiation therapy. Meningiomas, which originate from the arachnoid cap cell of the brain, comprise the most common benign tumors of the brain in the United States, although they occur less frequently in the elderly than in other age groups. The primary treatment for meningioma is surgical, with irradiation an important therapy for lesions that are surgically unmanageable. In addition, although it is well known that a proportion of meningiomas express hormone receptors such as estrogen and progesterone receptors, the relation between the types of hormonal therapy frequently prescribed for elderly patients (particularly postmenopausal women), such as tamoxifen and estrace, remains unknown. In general, there are currently few data specific to individuals over the age of 70 for these two tumor groups.

## Radiation Therapy

Data show that individuals who receive radiation therapy after surgical resection for astroglial tumors have an increased survival time relative to those who undergo surgery (with or without chemotherapy). The extent to which radiation therapy is effective, however, is once again dependent on age, with elderly individuals (defined in most studies as more than age 60 years) faring less well.[14] In the Radiation Therapy Oncology Group and Eastern Cooperative Oncology Group Study joint trial in 1983, patients diagnosed with gliomas at age 60–69 years who were treated with surgery and radiation therapy had a median survival of 5–6 months.[14] More recently, Kelly and Hunt[18] retrospectively examined the effects of radiation therapy in a series of consecutive series of patients over the age of 65 diagnosed with glioblastoma and treated with resection or biopsy. After surgery, radiation therapy was completed in 96 patients; it was not completed in 9 patients, and 23 patients refused radiation therapy. The mean survival in the group receiving radiation was 21.0 weeks versus 7.1 weeks in the nonradiation group ($p < 0.001$). When information on the surgical group is incorporated in the analysis, the mean survival time in 62 of 88 biopsied patients who completed radiation therapy was 17 weeks versus 30 weeks in the 34 of 88 patients who underwent resection ($p = 0.02$).

Data from the Connecticut Tumor Registry indicate that 44% of individuals diagnosed with all types of primary brain tumors over the age of 69 received radiation therapy. For those over age 69 years diagnosed with glioblastoma multiforme or astrocytoma, data from the CTR indicate that there is no benefit from radiation therapy with respect to survival time. Similar findings were reported by Peschel et al.[21] This differs from what is reported for younger individuals within the registry. For example, among patients diagnosed with astrocytoma, those under age 70 years who received radiation therapy had a survival time that was 1.33 times that of individuals who did not receive radiation therapy. Among patients diagnosed with astrocytoma who were 70 years of age or more, those who received radiation were less likely to survive than were those who did not receive such therapy. Although these data are intriguing, the statistics obtained from them must be interpreted with caution because there are insufficient data to explain these results.

The negative influence of age on outcome and survival in glioblastoma patients is so pervasive it has led many clinicians and researchers to adjust treatment protocols for elderly patients in an effort to minimize the time spent in treatment, particularly when survival is estimated to be less than 6 months.[22] For example, standard radiation therapy for a glioma is delivered in 1.8 Gy fractions with five treatments each week for a period of 6 weeks, with a total radiation dose of 55 Gy. Consideration for increasing the dose per fraction to 3 Gy can reduce the time devoted to treatment when this is anticipated to consume half the expected survival. Recent data from the Radiation Therapy Oncology Group indicate that this shortened course of radiation therapy results in survival similar to that seen with a standard radiation therapy regimen.[23]

Newall et al.[22] present an intriguing examination of 18 patients over age 60 years (five over age 70 years) diagnosed with glioblastoma and treated with surgery (total or subtotal resection or biopsy) and a shortened radiation therapy protocol (3000 cGy whole-brain irradiation). Of the 18 patients, 7 lived longer than 1 year, and the median survival for the individuals over age 70 was 306 days. These numbers compare favorably with other studies of elderly patients with glioblastoma. Perhaps even more importantly, all but one were able to return home and function to some degree on a day-to-day basis. Although the number of patients is small, nonrandomized, and without a control group, it is an intriguing concept that one may offer elderly patients decreased treatment times without compromising outcome.

## Chemotherapy

The benefit of chemotherapy to individuals diagnosed with tumors of the CNS remains controversial. Chemotherapeutic agents have been particularly unsuccessful for gliomas, the tumor type most frequently seen in elderly patients. A number of explanations exist for this result, including the presence of enzyme systems within glial cells that may repair injured DNA, the existence of multidrug resistance gene products that transport chemotherapeutic agents out of glioma cells, and the increased intolerance of elderly patients to the side effects of chemotherapy such as nausea, vomiting, and fatigue.

The medications most frequently used in elderly patients include the nitrosoureas, such as carmustine (BCNU) and semustine (CCNU), as well as procarbazine and cisplatin. There is currently no evidence to support the hypothesis that chemotherapy is beneficial in elderly patients. Large trials that have studied the effects of chemotherapy or chemotherapy used in conjunction with radiation therapy have not formally investigated the effect on patients age 70 years or more.

One of the first large cooperative trials to study anaplastic gliomas examined the effect of 1,3-bis(2-chloroethyl)-1-nitrosourea with and without radiotherapy in a randomized series of patients age 6–79 years. A combination of radiotherapy and BCNU provided the best survival rates, and age was an important prognostic factor (although there were too few old patients to examine treatment effect among that age group).[24]

The Brain Tumor Study Group (BTSG) trial of 467 patients diagnosed with glioblastoma and randomized to radiation alone, radiation with BCNU, radiation with semustine, or semustine alone found no significant increase in median survival when chemotherapy was added to treatment regimen.[25] One of the most statistically significant variables in the analysis of survival time was age, with old individuals having the shortest survival time. Although approximately 20% of the patients in the study were aged 65 years or more, there was no discussion of how treatment affected outcome by age (i.e., no examination of an age by treatment group effect within the statistical model).

A third large clinical trial, the 1983 Radiation Therapy Oncology Group and Eastern Cooperative Oncology Group Study (RTOG/ECOG) trial randomized 626 patients into four groups including two radiation groups (usual versus high dose), a radiation with BCNU chemotherapy group, and a radiation with methyl-CCNU/DTIC chemotherapy group.[14] Although no treatment option appeared better than the control (usual-dose radiation therapy), age was the most important prognostic factor with respect to survival time. The authors of this study examined the treatment effects on survival within age groups, noting that a beneficial effect from chemotherapy was identified only among patients age 40–60 years. In this age group, the use of BCNU appears to confer significantly increased survival relative to patients in the control group ($p = 0.02$). Unfortunately, patients more than 70 years of age were not included in the trial.

Similar exclusion of elderly patients is noted in data from the Connecticut Tumor Registry, which lists only 8% of patients over the age of 70 years as having received chemotherapy for treatment of a CNS tumor. This exclusion reflects an underlying belief that chemotherapy is not beneficial in elderly patients, a belief that may be true but remains formally untested.

In general, chemotherapy is administered in an intravenous form. However, because the blood–brain barrier frequently makes effective delivery of chemotherapeutic agents difficult, new protocols exist to examine the effect of delivering chemotherapeutic agents in alternative forms, including supraselective intraarterial delivery, intrathecal delivery, and surgically implanted biodegradable polymer disks such as those that contain carmustine polymers.[26] Most of the results from these attempts remain preliminary, although some initial reports list some improvement in survival but few elderly patients are included. In addition, many of these treatments have been associated with a greater complication rate at least during the initial period after administering the agent.

## Steroid Therapy

Steroid therapy is an extremely useful adjuvant therapy for treatment of CNS tumors in patients of all ages. It may be particularly beneficial in old patients when surgical or additional treatments are deemed unwise.[27] The most frequently used steroid, dexamethasone, may be given intravenously or orally. Typically the initial dose is approximately 10 mg, with maintenance doses of 2–6 mg every 6 hours thereafter. The medication works by reducing edema; clinical response and neurologic improvement are generally seen within 24 hours. Although complications do exist (hyperglycemia, wound dehiscence, gastric/duodenal ulcers), the benefits appear to far outweigh the risks, particularly with respect to quality of life.

## Immunotherapy

At present there are few data with respect to the effectiveness of immunotherapy in elderly patients. In general, this area of research is hampered by the difficulty of delivering the agents to the tumor and avoiding damage to normal brain tissue. Researchers are continuing to explore this field using such methods as interferon therapy, monoclonal antibodies, and injections of interleukin-2.

## Genetics

Most inherited cancers have been associated with an early age at onset. Study of the interrelated roles of inherited genes, family history, and age at onset of primary brain tumors has proved difficult for molecular biologists and genetic epidemiologists for a number of reasons, including the relative rarity of these cases, the difficulty of obtaining tissue samples, and the rapidly fatal course of many brain lesions, making interview of these subjects difficult.

Familial aggregation studies have reported relative risks of primary brain cancer associated with a family history of brain tumors ranging from one to nine times that of individuals without a reported family history of brain tumors. One recent, relatively large case–control study[28] of 462 newly diagnosed adults (including 24 individuals over the age of 69 years) reported that patients diagnosed with glioma were 2.3 times more likely than controls to report a positive family history of brain cancer. One must be careful when interpreting the data, as patients with a confirmed family history were significantly older (rather than younger) than those without a family history; as the authors pointed out, these findings do not point to an obvious role for inheritance of a major susceptibility allele for early-onset glioma. Furthermore, although a number of genetic cancer syndromes, including neurofibromatosis 1 and 2, tuberous sclerosis, and the Li-Fraumeni cancer syndrome, are associated with tumors of the brain and CNS, these syndromes are rarely diagnosed in the elderly patient and, in fact, remain relatively rare in the general population.

In addition to the study of inherited genes, scientists have attempted to elucidate the somatic genetic changes and pathways associated with the development of a number of primary brain tumors, including most prominently, those associated with the development of glioblastomas. Glioblastoma multiforme is considered to be a clinical manifestation of at least two pathways with respect to genetics. One form appears to result from anaplastic transformation of a low-grade astrocytoma. The timing of this transition or progression to a higher grade is variable and it remains controversial whether aggressive therapy for a low grade astrocytoma can prevent or delay the subsequent evolution of a glioblastoma. There is some evidence to suggest that progression of tumor grade is associated with a series of genetic changes, similar to those seen for the progression from polyp to carcinoma in colon cancers, although the evidence is preliminary and much less well defined than for other cancers. The second form of glioblastoma appears to be a tumor that arises de novo in patients with no prior evidence of a low grade glioma. When survival is measured for the two groups, there does not appear to be an advantage for either type. The latter, the de novo form is more commonly seen in the elderly population.

Data indicate that evolution of glioblastoma from a low grade glioma is genetically distinct from the de novo glioblastoma. Tumors that progress from a low grade glioma to glioblastoma are associated with *p53* mutation.[29–31] In contrast, de novo glioblastoma does not appear to manifest evidence of a *p53* mutation; instead, these tumors have been shown to have amplification and mutation of epidermal growth factor receptor (*EGFR*) and amplification of *MDM2*, as well as loss of heterozygosity of chromosome 10.[29–31] Of interest is the fact that epidemiologic data from these studies suggest that advanced age is associated with *EGFR* and *MDM2* amplification, a condition not present in gliomas arising in younger patients.

# Metastatic Brain Tumors

Secondary, or metastatic, brain tumors represent the majority of brain tumors in the elderly, with intracranial metastases occurring in approximately one-third of individuals initially diagnosed with a systemic malignancy. Median survival is poor regardless of treatment protocol and is commonly measured in weeks and months. There are few data to indicate whether survival differs by age group, although in general, elderly patients do less well with respect to survival and quality of life. In the sole randomized trial[9] designed to examine survival time for individuals with radiographic evidence of a single metastatic lesion, the median survival was significantly longer in the group undergoing surgical excision and radiation therapy compared with the comparison group, individuals undergoing needle diagnostic biopsy and radiation therapy (40 vs. 15 weeks). In addition, patients who had their single metastases removed remained functionally independent longer (38 vs. 8 weeks) and had fewer recurrences at the site of the original metastasis (20% vs. 52%).

A more recent study compared whole brain irradiation (WBI), surgical excision with WBI, and stereotactic radiosurgery with WBI in 231 patients with single brain metastases, although the data were not presented by age group.[32] Median survival times for the three groups were 3.8, 10.5, and 9.8 months, respectively ($p < 0.01$). The 2-year survivals for the three groups were 6%, 19%, and 21%, respectively. These findings suggest that radiosurgery offers an alternative to radical surgery in selected patients.

## Conclusions

Much of the reason for the poor prognosis noted in elderly patients diagnosed with primary brain tumors is related to the negative impact that neurologic deficits have on survival and the reduced capacity for recovery and adaptation present in the aged patient. Addition of other co-morbid conditions (i.e., cardiac, pulmonary, renal, or musculoskeletal disease) associated with advanced age increases the risk of surgical intervention and reduces the systemic tolerance to radiation therapy and chemotherapy. As a result, elderly patients as a group are more likely to be functionally impaired by their disease than are younger patients; and they have less capacity to withstand the adverse effects of therapy, potentially limiting their treatment options. The negative influence of age on outcome and survival in glioblastoma patients is so pervasive that some have suggested it is not possible to demonstrate any survival benefit from any treatment in patients over the age of 70 years.

Elderly Americans, however, are probably more healthy and less disabled than they were perceived to be in the past. This is reflected in all aspects of society including the workplace where mandatory retirement restrictions are beginning to fall and more and more senior citizens enter or reenter the workforce. Although as a group elderly patients may do less well, there may be a significant subset of individuals who might benefit from treatment of their CNS tumors. These issues indicate that a clinical trial examining the effect of various treatments for primary and metastatic brain tumors in the elderly is needed, including whether survival can be improved with less toxicity and morbidity. This issue remains controversial with respect to the cost/benefit ratio to society. For primary brain tumors the effort would require a multicenter trial, as reports of outcome are relatively rare. For metastatic lesions, the pool of eligible patients is much greater, allowing one or two centers to organize a study. The ability to mount such a study depends greatly on society's willingness to accommodate the medical needs of its aging population within the framework of stressed medical resources.

## References

1. Parker SL, Tong T, Bolden S, Wingo PA. Cancer statistics, 1997. CA Cancer J Clin 1997;47:5–27.
2. Randall T. Demographers ponder the aging of the aged and await unprecedented looming elder boom. JAMA 1994;269: 2331–2332.
3. Velema JP, Percy CL. Age curves of central nervous system tumors in adults: variation of shape by histologic subtype. J Natl Cancer Inst 1987;79:623–629.
4. Polednak AP, Flannery JT. Brain, other central nervous system, and eye cancer. Cancer 1995;75:330–337.
5. Roush GC, Holford TR, Schymura MJ. Cancer Risk and Incidence Trends: the Connecticut Perspective. New York: Hemisphere, 1987.
6. Polednek AP. Time trends in incidence of brain and central nervous system cancer in Connecticut. J Natl Cancer Inst 1991;83:1679–1681.
7. Modan B, Wagener DK, Feldman JJ, Rosenberg HM, Feinleib BK. Increased mortality from brain tumors: a combined outcome of diagnostic technology and changes in attitude toward the elderly. Am J Epidemiol 1992;135:1349–1357.
8. Grieg NH, Ries LG, Yancik R, Rapoport SI. Increasing annual incidence of primary malignant brain tumors in the elderly. J Natl Cancer Inst 1990;82:1621–1624.
9. Patchell RA, Tibbs PA, Walsh JW, et al. A randomized trial of surgery in the treatment of single metastases to the brain. N Engl J Med 1990;332:494–500.
10. Wrensch M, Bondy M, Wiencke J, Yost M. Environmental risk factors for malignant brain tumors: a review. J Neurooncol 1993;17:47–64.
11. Larsen NS. Brain tumor incidence rising; researchers ask why. J Natl Cancet Inst 1993;88:1024–1025.
12. Kallio M. Therapy and survival of adult patients with intracranial glioma in a defined population. Acta Neurol Scand 1990;81:541–549.
13. Laws ER Jr, Taylor WF, Clifton MB, Okazaki H. Neurosurgical management of low-grade astrocytoma of the cerebral hemispheres. J Neurosurg 1984;61:665–673.
14. Chang CH, Horton J, Schoenfeld, et al. Comparison of postoperative radiotherapy and combined postoperative radiotherapy and chemotherapy in the multidisciplinary management of malignant gliomas. Cancer 1983;52:997–1007.
15. Ampil F, Fowler M, Kim K. Intracranial astrocytoma in elderly patients. J Neurooncol 1992;12:125–130.
16. Tomika T, Raimondi AJ. Brain tumors in the elderly. JAMA 1981;246:53–55.

17. Whittle IR, Denholm SW, Gregor A. Management of patients aged over 60 years with supratentorial glioma: lessons from an audit. Surg Neurol 1991;36:106–111.
18. Kelly PJ, Hunt C. The limited value of cytoreductive surgery in elderly patients with malignant gliomas. Neurosurgery 1994;34:62–67.
19. Winger MJ, Macdonald DR, Cairncross JG. Supratentorial anaplastic gliomas in adults: the prognostic importance of resection and prior low grade glioma. J Neurosurg 1989; 71:487–493.
20. Ammirati M, Vick N, Liao Y, Ciric I, Mikhael M. Effect of the extent of surgical resection on survival and quality of life in patients with supratentorial glioblastomas and anaplastic astrocytomas. Neurosurgery 1987;21:201–206.
21. Peschel RE, Wilson L, Haffty B, Papadopoulos D, Rosenzweig K, Feltes M. The effect of advanced age on the efficacy of radiation therapy for early breast cancer, local prostate cancer and grade III–IV gliomas. Intl J Radiat Oncol 1993;26:539–544.
22. Newall J, Ransohoff J, Kaplan B. Glioblastoma in the older patient: how long a course of radiotherapy is necessary? J Neurooncol 1988;6:325–327.
23. Kleinberg L, Slick T, Enger C, Grossman S, Brem H, Wharam MD Jr. Short course therapy is an appropriate option for most malignant glioma patients. Intl J Radiat Oncol 1997;38:31–36.
24. Walker MD, Alexander E, Hunt WE, MacCarty CS, Mahaley MS Jr, Mealey J Jr. Evaluation of BCNU and/or radiotherapy in the treatment of anaplastic gliomas. J Neurosurg 1978;49:333–343.
25. Walker MD, Green SB, Byar DP, et al. Randomized comparisons of radiotherapy and nitrosoureas for the treatment of malignant glioma after surgery. N Engl J Med 1980;303: 1323–1329.
26. Brem H, Piantadosi S, Burger PC, et al. Placebo-controlled trial of safety and efficacy of intraoperative controlled delivery by biodegradable polymers of chemotherapy for recurrent gliomas. Lancet 1995;345:1008–1012.
27. Graham K, Caird FI. High-dose steroid therapy of intracranial tumour in the elderly. Age Ageing 1978;7:146–150.
28. Wrensch M, Lee M, Miike R, et al. Familial and personal medical history of cancer and nervous system conditions among adults with glioma and controls. Am J Epidemiol 1997;145:581–593.
29. Bello MJ, de Campos JM, Kusak ME, et al. Molecular analysis of genomic abnormalities in human gliomas. Cancer Genet Cytogenet 1994;73:122–129.
30. Watanabe K, Tachibana O, Sata K, Yonekawa Y, Kleihues P, Ohgaki H. Overexpression of the EGF receptor and p53 mutations are mutually exclusive in the evolution of primary and secondary glioblastomas. Brain Pathol 1996;6: 217–223.
31. Von Deimling A, Louis DN, Wiestler OD. Molecular pathways in the formation of gliomas: review. Glia 1995;15:328–338.
32. Hall WA, Cho KH, Lee A, Gerbi BJ, Lee CK. Solitary brain metastases: surgery, stereotactic radiosurgery and/or radiation therapy? Presented at the annual meeting of the Congress of Neurological Surgeons, Montreal 1997.

# 66 Spinal Disorders and Nerve Compression Syndromes

Jonathan D. Lewin and John Olsewski

Spinal disorders and nerve compression syndromes of the elderly are common presenting complaints to both internist and surgeons. In fact, approximately 70% of all patients seeking medical attention have the complaint of back pain at one time in their life. More than 13% have pain lasting more than 2 weeks.[1] A directed history and physical examination and working knowledge of the spinal bony and neural anatomy are key elements for appropriate diagnosis and management. This chapter defines the major disorders affecting the geriatric population and guides the surgeon in the diagnosis and treatment options for each disorder.

## Anatomy

The spinal cord is housed by the vertebral column consisting of 33 bony vertebrae. There are normally 7 cervical, 12 thoracic, 5 lumbar, 5 sacral, and 4 coccygeal vertebrae. The sacral and coccygeal vertebrae are fused. When viewed from the front, the spine is straight unless a preexisting or degenerative scoliosis is present. A lateral projection reveals a concave appearance to the cervical and lumbosacral vertebrae from back to front and a convex appearance to the thoracic vertebrae. This arrangement is referred to as cervical and lumbosacral lordosis and thoracic kyphosis.[2] Any reversal of this arrangement (e.g., cervical kyphosis) can be a clue to underlying pathology. With whiplash injuries in particular, the only abnormality present on examination and radiographs may be straightening of the cervical spine.

The spinal cord rests within the vertebral canal, which is normally triangular. The canal is guarded in front by the vertebral body, from the side by pedicles, and posteriorly by the laminae and spinous processes (Fig. 66.1). The nerve roots leave the cord to become peripheral nerves through the neural foramen bounded by the pedicles above and below and by facet joints posteriorly. In addition, between each vertebral body is a vertebral disc (Fig. 66.2). This fibrocartilaginous structure acts as a shock absorber of the spine.[2] Alterations in any aspect of these structures, be it disc, foramina, or facet joints, can be a cause of pain or nerve compression leading to arm or leg pain depending on where in the spine compression takes place.

## Biomechanics

The healthy spine is responsible for protecting the spinal cord and absorbing the forces of axial loading. Tremendous compressive forces act on the spine during everyday activities such as lifting and carrying. The osteoporotic spine often fails under these stresses, leading to compression fractures. Normally, 6 degrees of freedom are present between each vertebral body and the one below. Flexion, extension, right and left lateral bending, and clockwise and counterclockwise rotations comprise these motions.[3] Processes such as pain, trauma, and previous surgery impede spinal mobility and function.

## Pathophysiology

Cadaver studies have shown that more than 70% of spines show signs of degeneration between 60 and 70 years of age. These findings may be localized to the disc, vertebral bodies, or facets; or they may involve combinations of structures.[4] It is important to note that most patients with such anatomic changes, even when confirmed by radiography, are asymptomatic[5] (Fig. 66.3). The intervertebral disc is believed to be the first structure to undergo both morphologic and biochemical changes in the aging spine. The aging disc loses its ability to maintain water and develops cracks in its substance, leading to protrusion of disc material toward the spinal canal or neural foramina. Further disc injury leads to frank extrusion of disc

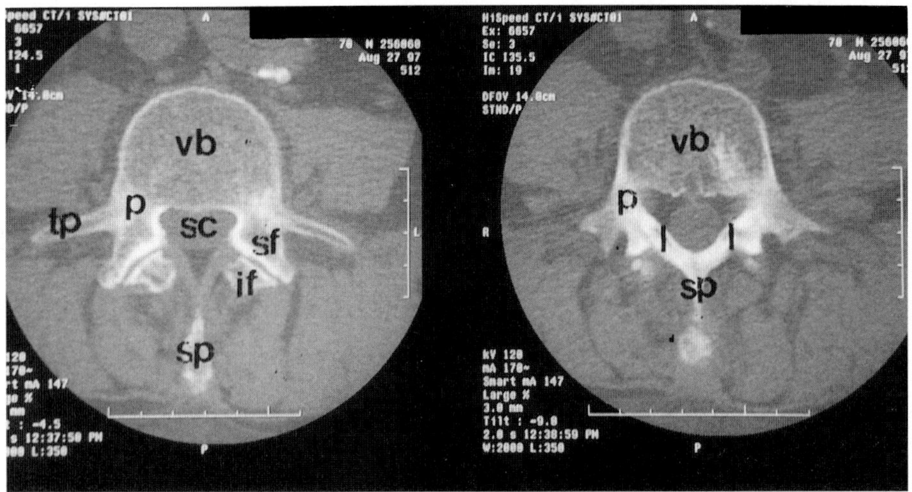


FIGURE 66.1. Bone window axial cuts of a computed tomography (CT) scan of the lumbar spine showing the relation of the bony anatomy in the transverse plane. vb, vertebral body; p, pedicle; tp, transverse process; sc, spinal canal; sf, superior articular facet; if, inferior articular facet; sp, spinous process; l, lamina.

material. When it occurs suddenly, it can lead to acute back or leg pain. More likely, disc generation continues slowly and leads to a more generalized bony incompetence. In particular, the facets become hypertrophied, perhaps because of closer contact due to loss of disc height. This hypertrophy may lead to mechanical symptoms of arthritis or neurologic symptoms. Neurologic symptoms develop when these arthritic spurs encroach on the neural foramina or the spinal canal itself. Furthermore, excessive motion may occur between vertebral bodies, leading to a "slip," or listhesis, of one body on the other. This too can cause bony or neurologic complaints.[3,6,7] The clinician must know how to distinguish among these various processes.

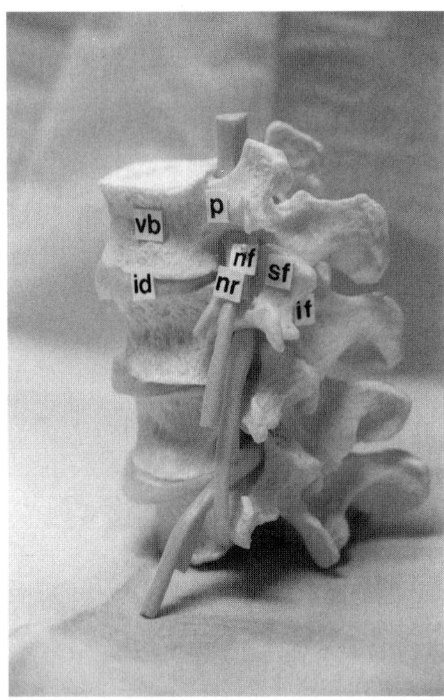


FIGURE 66.2. Model of the motion segment of the lumbosacral spine in the sagittal plane showing the relations of soft tissues and bony elements. vb, vertebral body; id, intervertebral disc; p, pedicle; nf, neuroforamen; nr, nerve root; sf, superior articular facet; if, inferior articular facet.

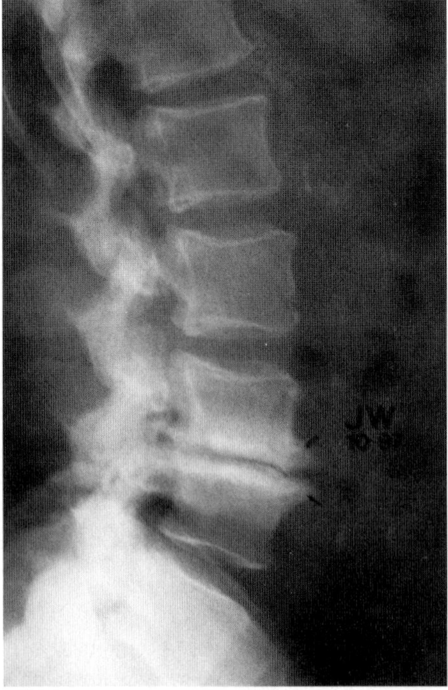


FIGURE 66.3. This 67-year-old man had symptoms of spinal stenosis and degenerative disc disease. This lateral radiograph of the lumbosacral spine shows severe degenerative changes at the L4–5 disc space, including disc space narrowing, vertebral body endplate sclerosis, neuroforaminal narrowing, and traction osteophytes (arrows).

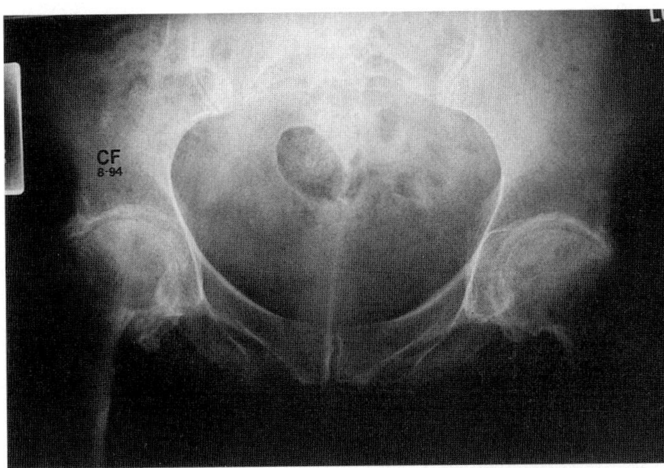


FIGURE 66.4. A 70-year-old woman was referred for back and buttock pain. The clinical examination was consistent with osteoarthritis of the right hip being the cause of her symptoms. Patient was relieved of her back and buttock pain with total hip arthroplasty.

## Mechanisms of Back Pain

As mentioned, back pain can be related to various pathologic elements of the aging architecture. It may also be related to systemic manifestations such as tumor, infection, or ankylosing spondylitis. Patients over age 60 with loss of appetite, fatigue, and night pain must be carefully evaluated for tumor or infection. Although rare, herpes zoster can cause back pain along a unilateral distribution prior to eruption of skin lesions. Back pain may be referred from renal colic, vascular, or splenic pathology. Patients often confuse hip pain and back pain. Assessment of hip range of motion, crepitus, and the nature of the complaint can distinguish between the two. We believe that all geriatric patients who warrant radiographic evaluation of their back pain should also undergo anteroposterior (AP) pelvis radiography to detect concomitant hip disease (Fig. 66.4). Lastly, back pain is known to have a large emotional component. Compensation workers and those involved in litigation cases often present with a back complaint for secondary gain.[8–10] Care must be maintained when labeling back pain as psychogenic. A full history and physical examination is warranted to rule out organic pathology.

## Specific Pathologic Entities of the Elderly Spine

### Cervical Spine Degeneration

Cervical spine degeneration usually begins at age 45–55 and affects men more often than women. Any level of the cervical spine can be involved, but pathologic changes are most often seen at levels C5, C6, and C7. The predominating symptoms depend on the anatomic site of the disease (disc, facet, neural foramina). The three most common presenting complaints are neck pain (mechanical etiology), radicular pain (nerve root compression), and myelopathic symptoms (cord compromise). A combination of the three elements is often evident.[11,12]

### Neck Pain/Mechanical Pain

Patients may present with a complaint of neck pain often exacerbated by motion. Fatigue exacerbates the condition, and rest alleviates it. Pain and discomfort may be localized to the midline neck or radiate to the occiput causing headache. It may also radiate to the interscapular region. Patients may feel worse in cold weather, not unlike arthritis in other body areas. Chronic splinting may lead to overuse of surrounding muscles leading to pain in the sternocleidomastoid or deltoid region. Mechanical neck pain can easily be confused with shoulder pathology. A history and physical examination consistent with discomfort with overhead activities is more likely to be related to rotator cuff pathology than cervical degeneration. The patient with rest or night pain, nonmechanical in nature, must be evaluated for the possibility of neoplasm or infection.[13]

Physical examination can reveal midline tenderness to palpation. Typically, the examiner notes pain with rotation to the right or left. Strength in the upper extremities is preserved, and reflexes are present in the biceps, triceps, and brachioradialis distributions. Appropriate studies for a patient with mechanical symptoms include AP, lateral, and oblique radiographs. We also order flexion and extension views to detect any dynamic instability (Fig. 66.5). Radiographs typically show loss of disc height and possibly some mild loss of cervical lordosis. Arthritic changes in the facet joints may also be evident. It must be emphasized that such changes may be apparent in the completely asymptomatic patient, and that correlation of clinical and radiographic findings is mandatory.

Treatment of mechanical-type neck pain without neurologic involvement is almost always nonsurgical. First-line therapy involves use of a soft or hard collar in conjunction with a trial of nonsteroidal antiinflammatory drugs (NSAIDs) in an attempt to decrease the inflammatory process. Most patients have considerable relief over a 6-week period. Refractory cases can begin a physical therapy regimen with isometric neck and shoulder exercises followed by active strengthening. If 6 months of therapy does not significantly alleviate symptoms, the patient can be considered for surgery. Any patient considered for surgery for mechanical symptoms should receive an additional study such as magnetic resonance imaging (MRI) or computed tomography (CT) of the neck

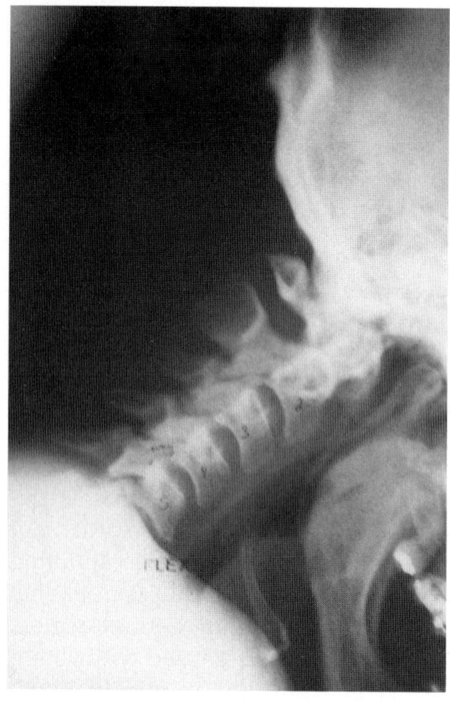

A

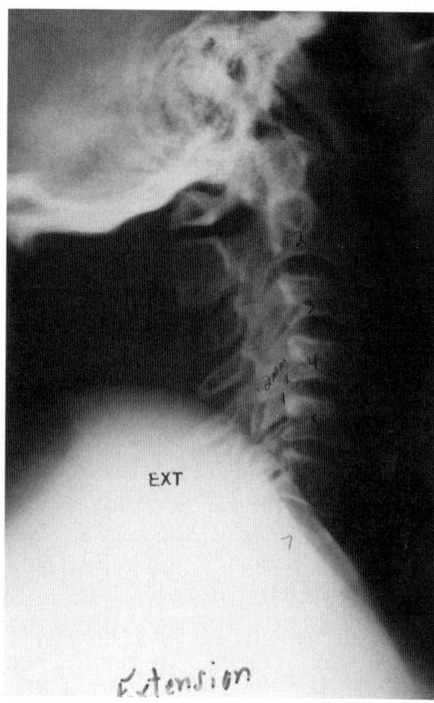


B

FIGURE 66.5. A 66-year-old man had symptoms of cervical myelopathy. Flexion (A) and extension (B) lateral radiographs of the cervical spine show dynamic instability of C4 on C5, with 6 mm of anterior subluxation on flexion, which reduces to 2 mm of anterior subluxation on extension.

to delineate the exact nature of the degenerative process. The mainstay of surgical management is fusion via an anterior or posterior approach. The patient should be cautioned that the results of such surgery for pain relief are variable. In general, surgical management is reserved for all but the most refractory cases.[14]

## Radicular Neck Pain

### *Signs and Symptoms*

Patients with radicular pain (pain secondary to neural compression) initially present with neck pain. This pain may be acute in nature or develop slowly over time. The geriatric population usually presents with the latter, as the neural compression is related to narrowing of the neural canal from osteophyte or generalized loss of disc height rather than an acute disc herniation. In addition, pain often radiates down the shoulder to the arm or hand. The patient often describes it as a burning or tingling sensation.

The area of radiation corresponds to the level of the neural compression. C4 compression affects the back of the neck; C5 the lateral shoulder and arm; C6 the lateral forearm, thumb, and index finger; C7 the middle finger; C8 the ring and little finger; and T1 the medial arm and forearm. These distributions are not exact, and there is a considerable amount of dermatomal overlap between the nerve roots. Patients often complain of exacerbation with particular motions: neck rotation and flexion toward the side of the arm pain and hyperextension of the neck. Furthermore, they may present with motor weakness in the upper extremity. This too, roughly corresponds to the level of neural compression. C5 compression affects deltoid and biceps strength; C6 compression, wrist extension, and biceps; C7 triceps and wrist flexion; C8 finger flexion; T1, grip strength.

Physical examination should assess neck motion, tenderness to palpation along the midline, and the neck muscles. The physician should document the area of burning or tingling down the arm and correlate it with dermatomal distributions. Muscle weakness should be noted in the upper extremity, and this too is correlated with the area of sensory abnormality. Pain in a particular muscle group must also be assessed. Reflex testing with a hammer can reveal diminished reflexes in the biceps, brachioradialis and triceps. Spurling's test (rotation and lateral bend toward the side of arm pain evokes increased symptoms). Holding the head and neck in extension exacerbates symptoms. Placing the affected extremity with the palm of the hand on top of the head relieves the pain by expanding room for the neural elements.[15]

### *Pathophysiology*

As mentioned, radicular pain is secondary to compression of the exiting nerve roots from the neural foramina of the cervical spine. It can be secondary to acute disc herniation, arthritic changes of bony elements, or a combination of the two. Although not fully understood, it is believed that this compression leads to the release of chemical mediators, such as substance P, evoking an inflammatory and painful response.[16]

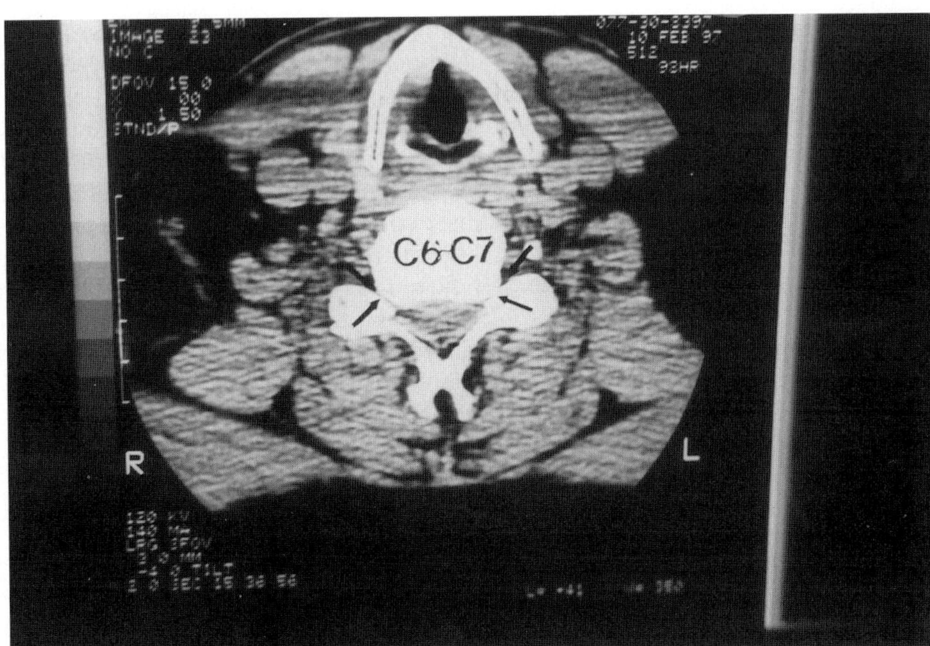


FIGURE 66.6. A 67-year-old man had symptoms of C7 radiculopathy. This soft tissue window axial CT scan cut of the cervical spine shows severe foraminal stenosis at C6–7 (arrows).

### Imaging

As with purely mechanical pain, plain radiographs are the first-line study.

The oblique film should be studied carefully, as it often demonstrates narrowing of a particular neural foramina and significant osteophyte. MRI or electrodiagnostic studies are reserved for surgical candidates. Axial and sagittal cuts at the level of the neuroforamina can be particularly useful (Fig. 66.6).

### Natural History

The natural history of this disease is not as favorable as for purely mechanical neck pain. Despite nonoperative measures it is estimated that 25% of patients with radicular complaints are left with severe symptomatology.[17] These patients may be considerably improved with surgical management.[18]

### Differential Diagnosis

Cervical radiculopathy can be mimicked by many other conditions affecting the elderly population. Compressive neuropathies (carpal tunnel syndrome or cubital tunnel syndrome) may lead to radicular-like symptoms. In addition, thoracic outlet syndrome, which represents compression of the brachial plexus or subclavian vessels from a cervical rib or hypertrophic scalene muscles leading to symptoms in the medial arm and forearm may present similarly to cervical radiculopathy.[15] Rotator cuff pathology may mimic a C5–6 radiculopathy. Multiple sclerosis may present with upper extremity sensory symptoms, such as tingling and weakness not following an anatomic distribution. Amyotrophic lateral sclerosis may appear as an upper extremity weakness with preservation of sensation. Finally, spinal tumors occasionally present with radicular symptoms. A careful history concerning systemic signs and night pain or nonmechanical pain must be sought.[19]

### Nonoperative Management

Nonoperative management of cervical radiculopathy is similar to treatment of mechanical neck pain. Patients are begun on a regimen of NSAIDs, which often decreases the inflammation of affected nerve roots and leads to significant pain relief. A soft collar can be provided for comfort, followed by a course of passive stretching exercises and active strengthening of the neck, shoulder, and arm when symptoms tolerate it. Patients unresponsive to those measures can receive epidural steroid injections or selective nerve root injections at the level of neural compression. Surgery is reserved for patients who have unremitting pain for 3–6 months despite conservative measures or those with progressive neurologic deficit.[20]

### Surgical Management

All patients considered for surgical management should undergo preoperative MRI. This study can confirm the anatomic level of compression based on the location of the patient's radicular symptoms. As mentioned, it is less likely in the geriatric population to have radicular symptoms due to an acute disc herniation than due to slowly evolving nerve root compression from the spondylitic process. Surgery must be aimed at decompression of the affected nerve roots. The most common operation for radiculopathy at a single nerve root level is a diskectomy and fusion from an anterior approach. The affected level of disc degeneration is removed completely, as are any visible osteophytes. Next, a piece of bone graft slightly larger than the original disc height is inserted into the former disc space. This provides further enlargement of the neural foramina via distraction. If the graft is well impacted, no hardware need be placed; otherwise, a cervical plate can be used. The patient is placed in a postoperative collar for about 6 weeks. The goal here is solid bony fusion, which halts further degeneration and eliminates nerve root compression.

Decompression of affected nerve roots can also be accomplished via posterior approaches. With this procedure, small amounts of cervical lamina and facet are removed at the affected level. The surgeon may remove the offending disc material as well. As this procedure is less destabilizing than full diskectomy, no bony fusion is needed.

### Results

The results of surgery for radicular symptoms are encouraging. More than 90% of people can be effectively relieved of pain and discomfort. The best results have been obtained with anterior procedures, making it the recommended choice. Posterior approaches are reserved for foraminal stenosis without a large disc herniation, failed anterior approaches, or for patients unable to undergo anterior procedures for other reasons such as poor skin condition.[19,21]

## Cervical Myelopathy

Cervical myelopathy involves compression of the cervical spinal cord (not exiting nerve roots) leading to classic symptomatology in the geriatric population.

### Signs and Symptoms

Although neck pain may be present, it is not as constant a feature as with mechanical or radicular compression. Patients can complain of an increasing loss of manual dexterity (typically bilateral). They often describe a vague weakness and numbness to the upper extremities. Lower extremity weakness is a frequent complaint; it leads to gait disturbance (wide based) with frequent falling. When advanced, bowel or bladder function may be affected. Physical examination should begin by noting the patient's gait. A wide-based gait is typical. Patients may be unable to open and close a fist rapidly. Spasticity of the upper extremities is not uncommon. An objective weakness of the upper and lower extremities may be evident. Wasting of the upper extremity is possible in long-standing cases. Reflex changes are important in the myelopathic examination. Typically, the upper extremities are hyporeflexive and the lower extremities hyperreflexive. Bilateral Babinski reflexes are often noted. A positive Hoffman reflex (flexion of the thumb or index finger upon flicking the nail of the middle finger) is a classic test for cervical myelopathy. An inverted radial reflex (hyporeflexive brachioradialis with involuntary contraction of the fingers) is another classic sign for C5 myelopathy. Lhermitte's sign (cervical compression and flexion leading to an electric-like sensation in the upper and or lower extremities) is another such sign.[19]

### Pathophysiology

The etiology of the myelopathy is most often spinal cord encroachment secondary to a single or multilevel degenerative process. The arthritic changes of the facets, bodies, uncovertebral joints, and ligamentum flavum impinge centrally, leading to a reduced space available for the spinal cord. This process is usually slow and evolving, occurring over many years. Patients with a congenitally small spinal canal may develop symptoms more rapidly. A midline disc herniation can lead to the development of acute myelopathy, but this is uncommon except in those with congenitally narrow canals.[22]

### Natural History

Cervical myelopathy is a slowly progressive entity. Although most patients' complaints do not warrant surgical intervention, once the onset of myelopathy has begun, episodic deterioration is the most common course. As many as 5% of patients have acute deterioration and require urgent intervention.[23]

### Imaging

Initial studies include AP and lateral plain films of the cervical spine. The presence of disc degeneration should be noted. The space available for the spinal cord can be estimated on the lateral radiograph. A 13 mm distance between the back of the vertebral body and the back of the lamina at any given level is considered the lower limit of normal. Smaller distances are considered congenitally narrowed and may predispose toward myelopathic symptoms. MRI and CT scans of the cervical spine are invaluable for confirming the myelopathy. Axial cuts demonstrate the available room for the spinal cord as well as evidence of disc or osteophytes leading to canal narrowing. Sagittal MRI cuts further demonstrate pathology and allow determination of the total number of cervical vertebrae involved as well as the relative health of the cord (Fig. 66.7).

### Differential Diagnosis

All of the conditions listed for the differential diagnosis for cervical radiculopathy can mimic myelopathy as well.

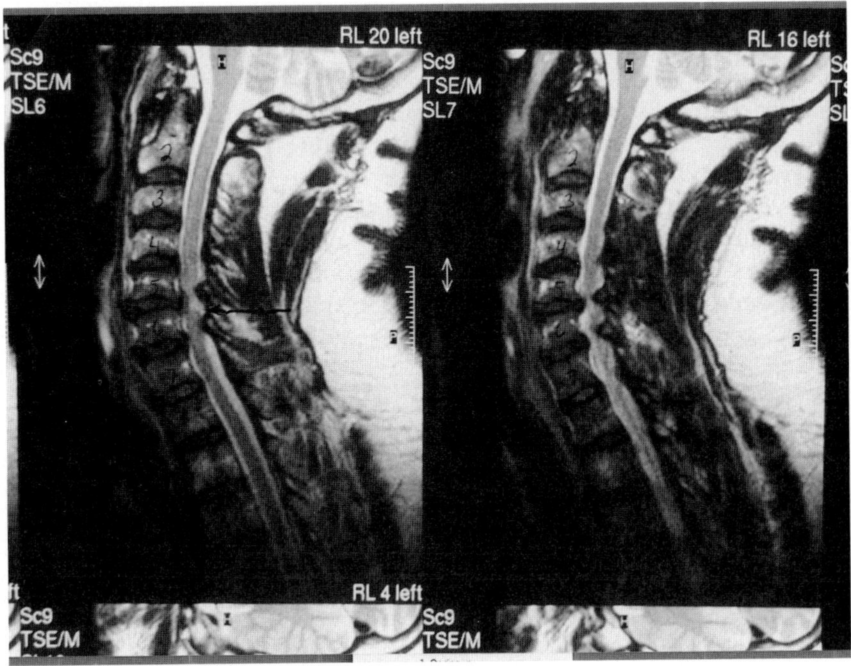


FIGURE 66.7. A 66-year-old man had symptoms of cervical myelopathy. This sagittal T2-weighted MRI scan of the cervical spine shows multilevel cervical stenosis and an area of myelomalacia in the spinal cord at C5–6 (arrow).

In particular, intra- or extradural tumors of the spine can lead to myelopathic symptoms. They are easily detected on the MRI scan. Furthermore, cerebellar pathology can lead to gait disturbance, as in myelopathy. Neurologic consultation should be considered if cerebellar pathology is considered the etiology of the gait disturbance.[24]

### Nonoperative Treatment

Patients can be started on a course of pain medication, physical therapy, and exercise modalities similar to patients with radiculopathic or mechanical symptoms. However, with increasing weakness, gait disturbance, or extremity pain, surgery is indicated. Furthermore, patients with any evidence of bowel or bladder disturbance secondary to cord compression should be considered for emergent decompression.[20]

### Operative Treatment

Operative treatment of myelopathy focuses on decompression of the spinal canal to expand the space for the spinal cord. The procedure or approach depends on the nature and extent of pathology. If myelopathy is secondary to disc herniation or bony encroachment at one or two levels, the recommendation is anterior discectomy, decompression, and fusion. If the constriction is secondary to a congenitally narrow canal or encroachment at three or more levels, the decompression should be performed posteriorly. This can be done via laminectomies, foraminotomies, or "open door" laminoplasty, depending on the clinical indication. Posterior approaches are contraindicated in patients with preexisting cervical kyphosis.

### Results

Results of surgery for myelopathy are often related to the duration and severity of the disease. If it is secondary to single-level disease without major gait disturbance, about 90% of patients are improved surgically. If symptoms are long-standing, with profound weakness or gait abnormality, the degree of recovery is unpredictable. It is for this reason that myelopathic patients should be monitored aggressively and counseled early about the need for surgery with worsening symptoms.[25–27]

## Thoracic Degenerative Disease

Symptomatic disease in the thoracic spine is relatively uncommon in comparison to disease in the cervical and lumbar levels. The attachment of the ribs to thoracic vertebrae convey an additional stability to the thoracic spine, leading to less bony and soft tissue changes to the thoracic spine with aging. When present, thoracic disc disease can be debilitating and on occasion requires emergent intervention. It is also difficult to diagnose.[28]

### Signs and Symptoms

Pain is the most frequent presenting complaint. The pain may be localized to the involved thoracic vertebrae or radiate in a dermatomal band-like fashion unilaterally or bilaterally around the chest wall. Occasionally, the pain radiates to the lower extremity or hip region. Complaints of sensory abnormalities are the second most likely presentation. These may follow chest wall dermatomal patterns or manifest as paresthesias extending to the lower extremities. More concerning is the occasional complaint of weakness, gait disturbance, and loss of bowel and bladder control. These patients must undergo an aggressive workup. The physical examination may be completely normal early in the course of disease. Later, diminished sensation testing to the affected chest wall dermatome may be apparent. Motor weakness, diminished rectal tone, clonus, hyperreflexia, and other upper motor neuron signs may be noted in long-standing cases or with acute large disc herniations.[8]

### Pathophysiology

Degeneration in the thoracic spine is secondary to the same processes as in the cervical spine. Water loss to the disc with aging leads to incompetence of bony elements, including the facets and bodies of affected vertebrae. Osteophytes may form, leading to impingement of nerve roots or if centrally located on the cord itself. The ligamentum flavum may become buckled with age and contribute to central impingement. Acute disc herniations can also occur and often lead to sudden onset of symptomatology.[3,6,28]

### Natural History

The natural history of thoracic disc disease is variable.[28] In the geriatric population a slow, gradual onset of symptoms is the most likely course. When not accompanied by motor signs or bladder or rectal incompetence, most patients respond well to conservative therapy.[29]

### Imaging

Diagnostic imaging should begin with AP and lateral projections of the thoracic spine. These are often difficult to interpret because of overlying structures but may show disc narrowing or calcification within an affected disc space. These radiographs may also show evidence of excessive kyphosis in the thoracic spine, a possible predisposition to symptomatic disease. MRI of the thoracic spine is currently the premier modality for evaluating suspected thoracic disc disease. Sagittal and axial cuts can determine the site of pathology (disc level, central or foraminal) and bony versus disc impingement. It must be stressed that all radiographic findings must be closely correlated to the physical examination and patient complaints because the presence of an asymptomatic radiographic abnormality is quite common.[30]

### Differential Diagnosis

A number of conditions can mimic thoracic disc disease, including neurologic conditions (amyotrophic lateral sclerosis, multiple sclerosis) and infectious causes of back pain (e.g., discitis, osteomyelitis). Spinal tumors or dural arteriovenous malformations can have similar presentations.[28] Herpes zoster often appears as a unilateral dermatomal chest wall pain band prior to the onset of the classic rash.[8] It is especially prevalent in the geriatric population. Cardiac or pulmonary disease refers to the posterior chest wall on occasion.

### Nonoperative Treatment

Avoiding precipitating flexion or extension motions is the first-line therapy. Patients may be begun on NSAIDs for pain relief, which often relieves the occasional pain and discomfort. A trial of brace immobilization can be suggested in more refractory cases. Patients must be monitored for development of motor weakness or bladder/bowel symptoms. These patients should be seriously evaluated for surgical therapy.

### Operative Treatment

Patients manifesting motor weakness, bladder symptoms, and other upper motor neuron signs are candidates for surgical therapy. Patients with pain unresponsive to nonoperative modalities are also appropriate for surgical management. A preoperative MRI scan or myelography is mandatory in all surgical cases. Surgery involves removing the offending disc, ligament, or bony material. The approach and technique depend on the level of pathology and the surgeon's familiarity with the surgery. Approaches include transternal, transpedicular, costotransversectomy, transthoracic,[31] or thoracoscopic.[32] Thoracic spine surgery is among the most challenging operations performed by the orthopedic surgeon. Appropriate intraoperative neural monitoring and consultation with a general or vascular surgeon can ensure a more predictable result.

### Results

Results of surgery are often dependent on the severity and duration of the complaint. Acute-onset weakness secondary to thoracic herniation offers a good chance of restoring neurologic function if dealt with emergently. More than 75% of patients are significantly relieved of their pain and discomfort.[33] Surgery for long-standing weakness or bladder dysfunction may halt the progression of the disease but does not restore full, premorbid function.

## Lumbar Degenerative Disease

Low back pain in the elderly ranks as one of the most frequent presenting complaints to internists and family practitioners. Attention must be paid to the nature of the pain, its duration, and its aggravating and mitigating factors. Conditions with back pain only, such as degenerative disc disease, must be distinguished from conditions affecting the lower extremities such as sciatica and lumbar spinal stenosis. Referred pain to the back from abdominal, retroperitoneal, or vascular pathology is not infrequently found in the elderly population and must be discerned via an accurate history and physical examination.[34]

## Degenerative Disc Disease/Mechanical Back Pain

With aging, the lumbar spine alters its original architecture. The aging disc loses height as its water content decreases. Disc space height between adjacent vertebrae diminishes, most commonly at L4–5.[8] This leads to incompetence of the bony elements of the lumbar spine and increased micromotion between adjacent vertebrae. Osteophytes develop at the facets and along the vertebral body itself[35] (Fig. 66.8). Additionally, the paraspinal musculature becomes affected and may tend toward reflex spasm.

The typical patient with degenerative disc disease offers a history of chronic back pain with pain-free intervals. This point is important for distinguishing this condition from tumor, infection, or other systemic processes. The pain is localized to the lower back with some radiation across the midline or upper buttock, but it does not radiate to the lower extremities. Patients often relate morning stiffness with a decrease in symptoms as the day progresses. Rest or recumbency relieve the pain, and certain activities or motions tend to exacerbate it. Often sitting in a firm chair that tends to stabilize the spine relieves pain, whereas sitting in a soft cushioned seat sags the lumbar spine and increases discomfort. Pain may be present during exercise but often is more pronounced several hours after activity or the next morning.

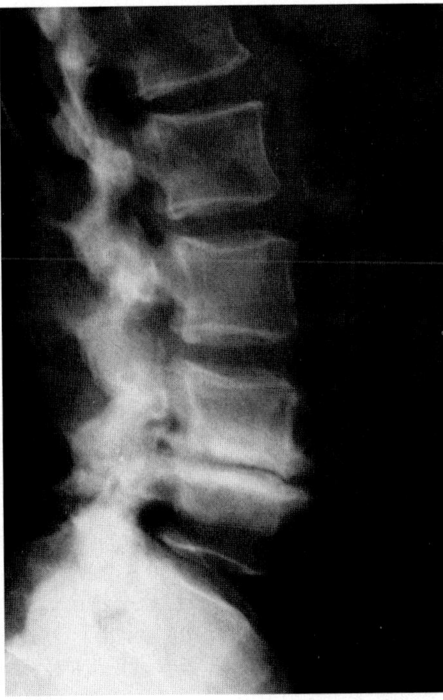

FIGURE 66.8. A 67-year-old man had symptoms of degenerative disc disease and spinal stenosis. This lateral radiograph of the lumbosacral spine shows traction osteophytes (arrows).

The physical examination should note the presence of scoliosis, spinal range of motion in flexion and extension, bending, and lateral rotation. The abdomen should be inspected for muscle tone, which is often diminished, and the presence of an enlarged aorta. Tenderness along the affected region of the spinal column is not uncommon. Asking the patient to maintain a semiflexed position often leads to exacerbation, as does asking the patient to drop down on his or her raised heels. Of note, reflexes are normal, full strength of the lower extremities is present, and no clonus or other upper motor neuron signs exist.

First-line imaging studies are AP and lateral radiographs of the lumbosacral spine and an AP view of the pelvis to help distinguish the presence of coexistent hip disease. If symptoms have been of short duration, less than 6 weeks, radiographs need not be obtained, as management will not differ based on their findings. Furthermore, the degree of symptomatology has limited correlation with the radiographic findings. As mentioned, narrowing at the L4–5 level is most common, but patients may also have extensive evidence of multilevel disease with severe arthrosis and little or no symptomatology.[36]

Treatment for mechanical back pain is predominantly nonsurgical. A short duration of bed rest, 2 days, may be prescribed in conjunction with administration of NSAIDs to decrease the inflammatory component. Exacerbating motions are to be avoided. Next, a physical therapy regimen should be instituted. Strengthening of the abdominal musculature can relieve stress on the paraspinal muscles and vertebral column.

Extension exercises of the lumbar spine are often helpful for pain relief. Flexion exercises in select patients are of benefit but may lead to increased pain. A holistic aerobic reconditioning program should be instituted to ensure a more adequate overall physical profile.

Many patients obtain significant relief from lumbosacral corset or brace wear during symptomatic periods. Other modalities include manipulation, trigger-point injections, and ultrasound therapy. Most patients obtain significant pain control and improved functional abilities through the use of such nonoperative modalities.

Surgery is only rarely indicated for this condition. Patients with unremitting pain unresponsive to other modalities can be considered. A secondary study, such as MRI or discography, should corroborate the patient's symptomatology (Fig. 66.9). Secondary gain factors such as workmen's compensation or other litigation portends a poor surgical result. The clinician must be sure that a concomitant psychological disorder is not present. The

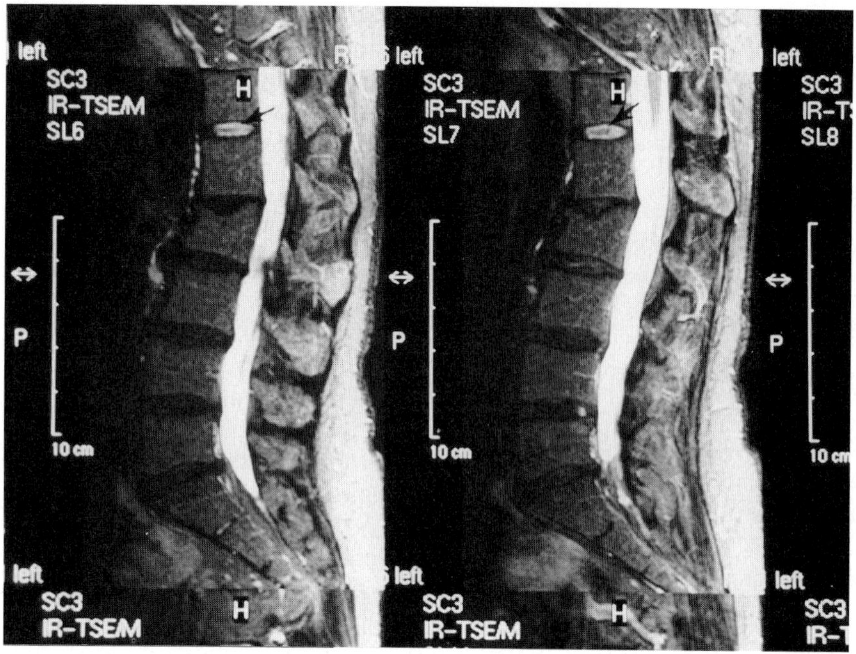


FIGURE 66.9. A 69-year-old woman had symptoms of degenerative disc disease. Sagittal T2-weighted magnetic resonance imaging (MRI) of the lumbosacral spine shows a normally hydrated disc at T12–L1 (arrow) and mutlilevel degenerative changes at the remaining disc spaces.

surgical procedure is a solid arthrodesis of the spine most commonly from a posterior approach. It can be accomplished with or without the use of instrumentation. The theory behind this procedure is to stop motion at the level of the degenerated disc. In the appropriately selected patient, pain relief can be expected 50–80% of the time.[37–39]

## Sciatica

Sciatica is a general term referring to irritation of lumbar or sacral nerve roots (or both) leading to back pain with radiation down the leg. The most common cause is from protrusion, extrusion, or sequestration of an intervertebral disc. The site of pain and numbness depend on the nerve root involved and the site of involvement. Patients are generally 30–50 years old upon presentation, but the elderly can also be affected with this entity.

### *Signs and Symptoms*

If presenting acutely, patients often recall a straining or twisting event to the back, such as lifting a heavy object. Motor vehicle accidents can also lead to acute herniations. The injury leads to intense pain in the back, followed by pain and numbness in the lower extremities. Over the next several days the back pain becomes less intense, and the lower extremity symptoms predominate. Activities such as bending, walking, and exercise exacerbate the symptoms, whereas lying supine tends to relieve the pain. Coughing or sneezing worsens it.

Upon presentation the patient may exhibit "sciatic scoliosis."[39] This refers to a standing posture where the back and trunk tilt away from the side where painful bending occurs. Examination of range of motion to the spine often reveals restriction, especially to forward flexion, which increases the pressure within the disc. Occasionally, no restriction in motion is present. Examination of the lower extremities is most important in the consideration of sciatica. Midline herniations (less common) may lead to bilateral leg involvement, whereas lateral herniations (more common) produce unilateral symptoms.

Signs and symptoms are dependent on the particular disc and nerve root involved, corresponding to particular sensory and motor dermatomal levels. The most common level for herniation is the L4–5 disc affecting the L5 nerve root. Herniation affecting the L2–3 roots leads to numbness and paresthesias to the anterior thigh and weakness in hip flexion. L4 root involvement leads to medial calf symptoms and knee extension and ankle weakness. L5 root involvement affects sensation along the lateral calf and dorsal foot with weakness to ankle or great toe extension. If the S1 root is affected, the numbness predominates along the posterior calf and the lateral and plantar foot, with weakness to ankle plantar flexion. S2–4 nerve root disease manifests as perianal sensation loss and bowel and bladder dysfunction. It must be emphasized that most patients presenting with a history suggestive of sciatica do not have evidence of motor weakness upon presentation. In fact, the only findings may be subjective numbness and pain in a particular anatomic site of the leg with gross sensation still intact. Reflex testing may reveal abnormalities on examination.

Knee jerk is diminished if L4 roots are impinged. Ankle jerk is diminished if S1 is affected. Finally, an absent cremasteric reflex may be present if sacral roots are involved. It must be remembered that symmetric reflex decrease is common in the elderly.

Special nerve root tension signs are helpful for detecting sciatica and nerve root irritation. The femoral stretch test is performed with the patient prone; the affected leg is raised off the table with the knee flexed and the hip extended. Pain or electricity down the anterior thigh or medial calf is suggestive of L2–4 nerve root irritation. The straight leg raise test is performed with the patient supine and the extended knee raised off the table. Pain along the ischial tuberosity radiating down the posterior thigh and lateral foot indicate stretch to the sciatic nerve with irritation to the L5–S1 nerve roots. If pain is present soon after attempting to raise the leg with a tendency toward knee flexion, it is indicative of tight hamstrings and not a positive straight leg raise test. If the pain is accentuated when the foot is quickly dorsiflexed, it is known as a positive Lasegue test. Perhaps the most specific test for sciatica is the contralateral straight leg raise in which the opposite extremity is raised and pain travels down the affected extremity. Digital examination can document rectal tone, and the lower extremity pulses should be noted.[40]

### Pathophysiology

The mechanisms by which herniated disc material leads to pain is a topic of intense research. Mechanical compression of nerve roots by disc material can lead to vascular injury to the nerves and other forms of trauma. However, it does not appear to be enough to induce the syndrome of sciatica. Contents from the nucleus pulposus, such as interleukins and prostaglandins, may induce edema and fibrosis of adjacent nerve roots. In addition, direct channels may form over time between the disc and adherent nerve roots, leading to further inflammatory responses. Hence the most probable explanation for painful sciatica is a combined mechanical and neurotoxic effect of disc material on involved nerve roots.[41,42]

### Natural History

The natural history of sciatica is favorable. More than 50% of patients are relieved of symptoms by 1 month, and in 90% of patients the symptoms resolve by the end of 3 months.[8,43] Hence most patients can be effectively managed without the need for surgery.

### Imaging

Standard AP and lateral lumbosacral radiographs are first-line studies. Most cases fail to reveal anything other than degeneration at various levels. L4–5 is most commonly affected. In fact, acute sciatica is more likely to appear in the setting of normal disc height without narrowing than in one with evidence of degeneration. Hence it is less prevalent in the elderly population. Occasionally, plain films demonstrate a transosseous herniation in which the disc carries with it a small part of the vertebral body into the spinal canal. Patients considered for surgical decompression should undergo MRI studies of the lumbosacral spine to confirm the clinical diagnosis. Keep in mind that 35% of patients older than 40 years have MRI or CT evidence of disk herniation in the absence of symptoms[5,44] (Fig. 66.10). Electromyography (EMG) studies can also be helpful in difficult cases.

### Differential Diagnosis

When an accurate history and physical examination are conducted, sciatica does not present a problem to diagnosis. On occasion, intraspinal tumors present as nerve compression with unremitting pain, which can be easily discerned by MRI. Other neurologic conditions such as multiple sclerosis (MS) or amyotrophic lateral sclerosis (ALS) can be mistaken for sciatica. Vascular claudication can also present with paresthesias to the lower extremities. A good history and neurovascular examination can help discern between the two. One entity that must be immediately recognized is cauda equina syndrome. It presents as a massive midline disc herniation leading to bilateral buttock and leg pain and loss of bladder (urinary retention most common) or bowel control (or both). The patients may also demonstrate diminished rectal tone and decreased perianal sensation. Saddle anesthesia of the buttocks is common. Such patients should undergo urgent MRI to define the site of obstruction and urgent surgery to decompress the neural elements.[8,40,43]

### Nonoperative Treatment

Therapy should begin with a trial of NSAIDs to decrease pain and the inflammatory component of the sciatica. A short course of bed rest, 2 days, can also be helpful. Patients should then be encouraged to ambulate and begin a therapy regimen similar to that for axial back pain. Precipitating activities should be avoided. In particular, flexion exercises may increase symptoms, as they tend to increase pressure within the disc. An aerobic conditioning program must be instituted in the overall therapy scheme. If no relief is achieved after 6 weeks, the patient may benefit from an epidural steroid injection. As mentioned, 90% of patients with sciatica are significantly relieved of symptoms by 3 months.[43]

### Operative Treatment

Only 10% of patients with sciatica warrant surgical consideration. Patients with bowel/bladder symptoms

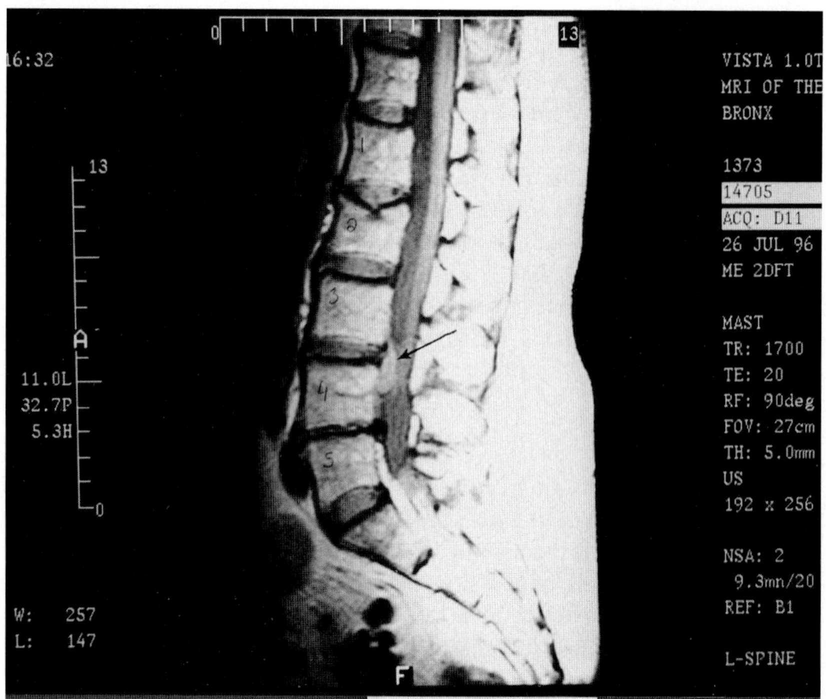


A

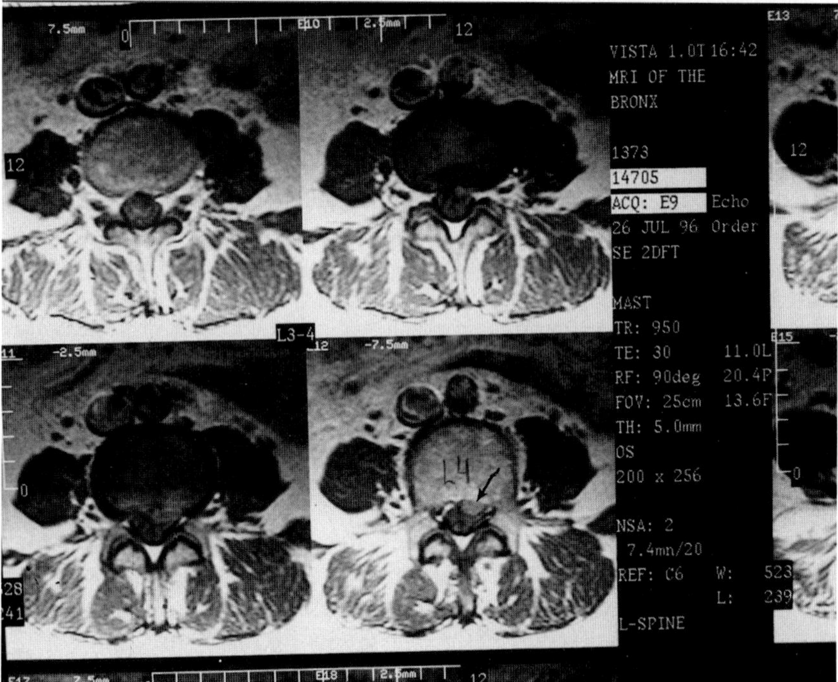


B

FIGURE 66.10. A 66-year-old woman had symptoms of L4 radiculopathy. Sagittal (A) and axial (B) MRI cuts show herniated nucleus pulposis at L3–4 with extrusion of disc material posterior to the vertebral body of L4 (arrow).

should warrant consideration immediately upon onset of symptoms. Those with increasing neurologic deficit, particularly motor weakness, should be considered for early surgery. Lastly, patients without relief from conservative therapy should undergo surgical decompression. The standard procedure for disc herniation leading to sciatica is midline decompression with laminotomy and disc excision. It is usually done without fusion. However, if back pain was a source of pain prior to the onset of leg symptoms, some surgeons opt toward fusion in the same surgical sitting. Also, if considerable bone was removed when decompressing the nerve root and stability is in question, the spine should be fused at that level.[45,46]

Geriatric patients in particular are susceptible to "far lateral herniations." These disc herniations occur outside the spinal canal itself at the level of the neural foramina. Preoperative MRI is helpful for detecting this condition. The surgeon must be careful to ensure that the decompression and disc excision extends laterally into the neural foramina and that the nerve root is free at the end of the procedure. Other surgical procedures available for disk excision include chemonucleolysis and percutaneous discectomy.[43] The indications for these procedures are few, and the results must be weighed against the gold standard of open excision. Recently, arthroscopic spinal procedures have been used in the treatment of disc herniation. More long-term data are needed to assess its usefulness for management of sciatica in the elderly.

### *Results*

If appropriately selected, more than 90% of patients obtain relief from sciatica by surgical disc excision. Patients with long-standing motor weakness may not regain full strength postoperatively. In addition, up to 10% of patients are at risk of having a recurrence of their herniation.[43]

## Degenerative Lumbar Spinal Stenosis

Lumbar spinal stenosis, also known as spinal claudication, represents narrowing of the overall dimension of the lumbar spinal canal leading to a classic symptomatology. Stenosis may be central, in which the central canal has reduced dimension, or lateral, in which individual nerve roots are encroached by a stenotic condition. Patients are generally elderly, most over age 65, so the geriatric clinician must be intimately familiar with the often subtle presentation of this disease entity.

### *Signs and Symptoms*

Elderly patients with central stenosis usually present with a history of chronic back pain that may have recently improved or worsened. A dull ache across the lumbosacral region is often present, but lower extremity symptoms predominate. A vague or heavy feeling in both legs is described. Some patients also have a feeling of the legs giving way. Additionally, the patient states that he or she can only walk several blocks before the pain becomes severe. Sitting relieves the pain, and standing worsens it. Patients often describe relief from leaning forward over a shopping cart, as this tends to widen the overall dimension of the spinal canal. Lying supine with the spine in extension may exacerbate the condition, and as a result night pain is often a feature of this condition. Lateral stenosis patients may present similarly but with unilateral complaints. Physical examination may demonstrate sensory or motor weakness as with sciatica but is most remarkable in most cases for its lack of specific findings. Straight leg testing, strength, and reflex examination usually are normal.[47]

### *Pathophysiology*

The normal young lumbar spinal canal is triangular and has abundant room to house the neural elements. The spinal cord usually ends at approximately the midbody of L1. Below this level the cauda equina nerve roots exit through their respective neural foramina without impingement. The aging process leads to incompetence of the disc, hypertrophy of posterior ligamentous structures (particularly the ligamentum flavum), and osteophytes of the facets. All these factors may lead to medial encroachment into the canal leading to central spinal stenosis. When the absolute area of the lumbar canal is reduced to less than $100\,mm^2$, absolute stenosis exists.[48] Furthermore, some patients have an abnormally narrow, or trefoil-shaped, canal, which makes them even more susceptible to the development of stenosis. An acute disc herniation may also contribute to stenosis of the canal, although it is less commonly seen. Lateral stenosis is similarly the result of osteophtyes of the facets, particularly the superior articular facet, and chronic disc disease leading to stenosis at the level of the neural foramina (Fig. 66.11). A common scenario is spondylolisthesis causing spinal stenosis. Spondylolisthesis refers to the vertebra above slipping in front of the vertebra below. Various causes exist, but the most frequently encountered scenario in the elderly is that of a degenerative spondylolisthesis. Chronic disc degeneration with concomitant arthrosis and incompetence of the facet joints allows vertebral slippage and elongation of the vertebral elements of the upper vertebrae. The slippage most commonly occurs between the L4 and L5 vertebrae. It may lead to signs and symptoms of central stenosis or of L5 nerve root impingement. It may manifest with pain along the lateral calf and with ankle or great toe weakness.[39,43]

### *Natural History*

Spinal stenosis is usually a chronic disease process. Symptoms are often present for many years prior to presentation to a clinician. With continued aging and spinal degeneration, the stenotic spinal canal and neural foramina tend to reduce further in size. Although most patients do not require surgery, 15% have slowly worsening symptoms as the years progress.[49]

### *Imaging*

Standard AP and lateral radiographs are first-line studies. They often reveal chronic disc degeneration, arthrosis, and possibly spondylolisthesis. If spondylolisthesis is present, additional flexion and extension views can demonstrate if the slippage increases with those maneuvers and represents a more dynamic and unstable situation. MRI is invaluable for confirming the diagnosis. Axial cuts can give a true measurement of the cross-

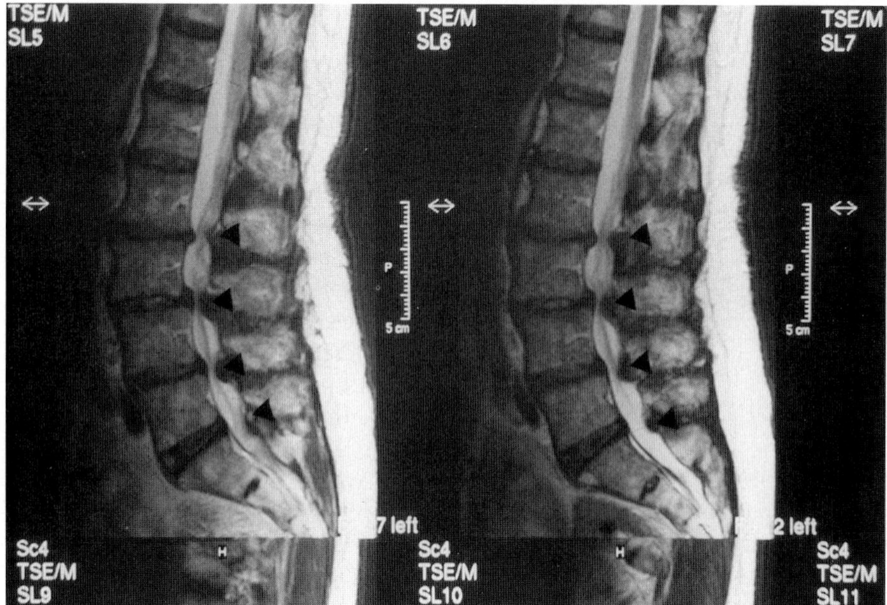


FIGURE 66.11. A 78-year-old woman had symptoms of spinal stenosis. These MRI scans show central stenosis secondary to loss of disc height and inbuckling of the ligamentum flavum posteriorly (arrows).

sectional area of the canal and of stenosis at the foraminal level and lateral recess. CT scans are helpful for determining the contribution of the bony elements and osteophytes to the stenosis. Prior to the advent of MRI, myelographic CT scan had been the gold standard.

### Differential Diagnosis

Vascular claudication is the most common entity entering in the differential diagnosis of lumbar spinal stenosis. An accurate history and physical examination can often discern between the two. First, vascular claudication has more severe distal lower extremity pain, whereas neurogenic claudication typically has a proximal to distal pain pattern. Also, with vascular claudication pain is relieved by ceasing to walk and standing still, whereas neurogenic claudication patients need to sit down to relieve the pain. Lastly, vascular patients have significant relief from lying supine, whereas stenosis in the canal may be increased in the supine position. The physical examination in the vascular claudicant is also noteworthy for the trophic skin changes secondary to arterial disease and the lack of peripheral pulses. Nonetheless, the two conditions can coexist in the elderly population, and consultation with a vascular surgeon should be sought in equivocal cases. Any of the previously mentioned neurologic conditions can also mimic lumbar stenosis. Unilateral or foraminal stenosis can present similar to atypical sciatica.[8,39,47]

### Nonoperative Treatment

Nonoperative treatment includes short courses of bed rest, if helpful, and antiinflammatory medications. Physical therapy with an emphasis on aerobic conditioning and abdominal strengthening should be employed. Weight loss alone can significantly diminish symptoms in the stenotic patients. Flexion exercises are also helpful. Epidural steroid injections can be utilized, especially with acute exacerbations.

### Operative Treatment

Patients unresponsive to conservative measures and those with increasing pain and gait disturbance should be considered for surgical therapy. The cornerstone to surgical management is adequate decompression of all stenotic segments. The preoperative MRI and CT scans must be carefully evaluated for all possible locations of stenosis. Not infrequently the entire length of the lumbar canal must be decompressed to ensure adequate room for the neural elements. The surgeon must be meticulous when addressing the bony, disc, and ligamentous contributions to the narrowed canal. If no more than 50% of any facet level must be removed and the spine is not unstable for other reasons, fusion is not needed to ensure a good postoperative result. If degenerative spondylolisthesis exists, fusing these segments should be strongly considered in light of the findings of numerous long-term studies.[50–52]

### Results

Among appropriately selected patients, more than 75% have significant relief postoperatively.[53,54] Workmen's compensation patients, secondary gain, and smoking are among the predictors of a poor result.[55]

## Adult Scoliosis

The normal adult spine when viewed from the front is straight. Any deviation or curvature in the lateral plane is referred to as scoliosis. In actuality, the curvature represents a three-dimensional deformity with rotation of all the vertebral elements and the rib cage. Scoliosis generally affects adolescent girls, but the elderly population may also present with scoliosis from various causes.

### *Pathophysiology*

The two major categories of adult scoliosis are the idiopathic and degenerative varieties. Idiopathic scoliosis usually represents missed or untreated adolescent scoliosis. As mentioned, young girls present with this condition during adolescence. The curves are usually in the thoracic spine and are not painful during youth. Curves of less than 40–50 degrees tend not to progress once growth has stopped.[56] Larger curves may progress into adult life. Most are thoracic curves in which the convexity of the curve is to the right. The pathophysiology is unknown, although a hereditary pattern seems to exist. The recommended treatment of curves of more than 40–50 degrees are fusion during adolescence; bracing and observation are recommended for lesser curves. Degenerative scoliosis primarily affects the lumbar spine. Disc degeneration, facet arthrosis, osteoporosis, and muscle imbalance contribute to the three-dimensional deformity. Abnormal rotation of the lumbar vertebral elements is also evident. Why certain patients with chronic disc degeneration develop a concomitant lumbar scoliosis and others do not is not known.[57–59]

### *Natural History*

Adult scoliosis arising from adolescent scoliosis generally does not present a problem with curves less than 40–50 degrees. For larger curves, pain is often localized to the concavity of the curve (where the facet joints are excessively loaded).[35] Nerve roots along the concavity may be compressed, and the patients may present with signs of nerve root irritation. Cosmetic concerns such as increasing rib prominence and shoulder asymmetry may be presenting complaints. For extremely large curves (>100 degrees), shortness of breath secondary to diminished lung capacity can be a problem.[60,61] Degenerative scoliosis usually is less a cosmetic concern, as curves tend to be much smaller. Patients present with nonspecific back pain usually along the concavity of the curve, signs of nerve root irritation, or even spinal stenosis.

### *Nonoperative Treatment*

Adult scoliosis should be approached with caution. Nonoperative treatment should be fully exhausted prior to surgical consideration. NSAIDS, bracing, weight reduction, exercise, and epidural steroids may be employed.

### *Operative Treatment*

Patients with refractory pain or signs of neural compression (or both) can be considered for operative treatment. All patients should undergo full-length radiography of the entire spine in the AP and lateral projection. Bending films can help assess the degree of rigidity to the curve. Additionally, patients with symptoms of nerve root compression or spinal stenosis should undergo MRI or myelography of the affected area.

The operative approach to treatment must be highly individualized. If the presenting problem is back pain without nerve root compression or stenosis, a posterior approach with curve correction, instrumentation, and fusion are recommended. If nerve root compression or stenosis are significant, careful decompression of the affected area must be included. Lumbar degenerative curves can often be approached anteriorly. Combined anterior and posterior approaches may be needed for difficult rigid curves.[59] If the only symptom is that of a single nerve root compression, simple posterior decompression without curve correction or fusion is reasonable. For patients with pulmonary compromise due to thoracic curves, curve correction to allow increased pulmonary capacity is of paramount importance.

### *Results*

Surgery for adult scoliosis is associated with a high incidence of complications, including blood loss, infection, pneumonia or atelectasis, inability to achieve fusion, and neurologic injury. Adult curves are stiffer than pediatric curves, and achieving curve correction is limited. Patients must be carefully selected and appraised of these potential complications. Residual back pain may remain despite the presence of a solid fusion.[62,63]

## Trauma

Spinal trauma and spinal cord injury represent significant sources of morbidity and mortality. It is estimated that more than 50,000 spine fractures occur yearly, with neurologic injury occurring one-fifth of the time.[64] Most are secondary to significant energy mechanisms such as motor vehicle accidents, falls from heights, and gunshot wounds. The patients generally are young, 20–40 years old, but the elderly are not immune to these injuries. Patients presenting to emergency rooms or practitioners with a history and mechanism suggestive of spinal injury warrant a full evaluation. The elderly often sustain spinal injuries with lesser degrees of energy because of fragility, osteoporosis, or other predisposing conditions of the spine.

## *Cervical Spine Trauma*

Patients sustaining cervical spine trauma present with the complaint of neck pain and or extremity weakness if spinal cord injury has taken place. The mechanism of injury must be carefully ascertained and preexisting medical conditions and any loss of consciousness delineated. The physical examination must be thorough. The cervical spine is examined for evidence of soft tissue contusion as well as tenderness to palpation. Flexion, extension, and rotation are documented. A careful overview of upper extremity motor power, sensation, and reflexes is undertaken.

Any abnormality on the examination should prompt the treating physician to obtain cervical spine radiographs. The standard trauma protocol for cervical spine injury includes an AP, lateral, and open-mouth odontoid view. The lateral view must demonstrate C1–T1 to be considered adequate. If the mechanism of injury is significant, such as a motor vehicle accident, an AP pelvis and chest radiograph should be obtained.

A variety of injuries can occur in the cervical spine including flexion-type compression injuries, dislocation of one vertebra on another, burst injuries of the vertebral bodies, spinous process fractures, and lamina fractures. Treatment is affected by the degree of instability present and whether a neurologic injury has occurred. In cases presenting with an acute progressive neurologic injury, urgent MRI, CT or myelogram CT, and surgical decompression with stabilization comprise the treatment of choice once the patient is medically stabilized. Urgent decompression offers the best chance of recovery of neurologic function. Injuries with a static neurologic injury can be addressed on a more elective basis. If an injury has occurred without neurologic injury, the degree of instability rendered greatly influences further management. Attempts have been made to define criteria for cervical spine instability.[3] The amount of vertebral body destroyed, the angulation and translation at the injury site, and disc space narrowing contribute to the relative instability of the injury.

Certain injuries do not confer instability to the spine. They include isolated lamina fractures, spinous process avulsions or fractures, and simple compression injuries to isolated vertebral bodies. These injuries can be managed with a hard or soft collar depending on the level of patient discomfort. Other injuries are inherently unstable. All dislocations are unstable. They must be reduced regardless of whether neurologic injury has occurred[65] (Fig. 66.12). Difficulty with reduction warrants an MRI to ensure that an entrapped disc fragment is not present.[66] If present, an anterior disc excision should precede the

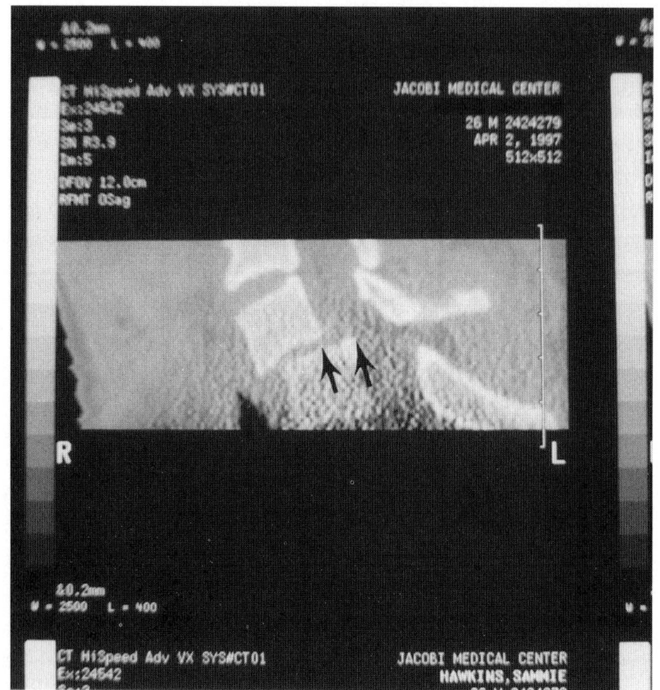

A

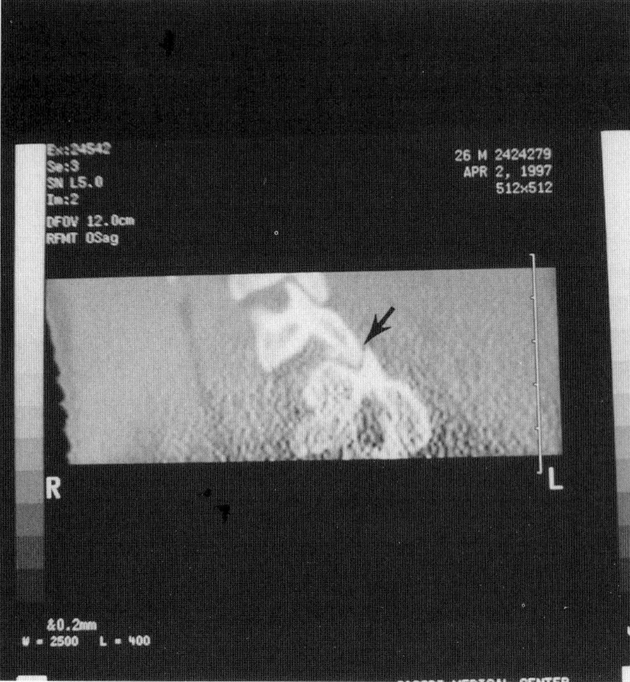

B

FIGURE 66.12. A 60-year-old man sustained a status post flexion injury to the cervical spine during a motor vehicle accident. The patient complained of neck pain and inability to feel his lower extremities. Plain radiographs in the emergency suite were unable to visualize the cervicothoracic junction. These sagittal reconstruction CT scans of C7–T1 show a bilateral perched facet-type dislocation of C7 on T1 (arrows). Patient was relieved of neurologic compromise after urgent reduction.

reduction. Following reduction of dislocations, the spine should be stabilized via posterior fusion. When the posterior ligamentous complex is injured, it should be treated by elective posterior fusion.[65]

Frequently, patients have negative radiographic and MRI findings despite persistent pain. The severity of these whiplash injuries should not be underestimated. The patient should be placed in a hard collar for support and given adequate muscle relaxant and pain medication. A follow-up appointment with an orthopedic surgeon should take place within 2 weeks. If pain persists, the patient should obtain flexion and extension views of the cervical spine to rule out a ligamentous injury.[67]

### *Thoracolumbar/Lumbar Spinal Trauma*

As with cervical spinal trauma, thoracolumbar and lumbar spinal trauma are usually the result of high-energy injuries. Timely and appropriate evaluation are crucial to successful management and outcome of these injuries.

Upon presentation to the emergency room, a thorough history and physical examination must take place. Preexisting medical conditions, mechanism of injury, and loss of consciousness at the scene should be ascertained. If secondary to a motor vehicle accident, questioning as to the use of a seat belt or lap belt is important. Assuming the patient maintains stable vital signs, a thorough examination is undertaken. In particular, the presence of bruising to the flank or back suggests a significant injury to the spinal column or retroperitoneum. A thorough examination of all four extremities for motor, sensation, and reflex responses is vital. A rectal examination should be done to document tone. The presence of any neurologic deficit must be noted. Patients noted to have neurologic deficit should be given intravenous steroids. When administered within 8 hours after injury, steroids have been shown to be helpful in recovering some neurologic function.[68]

Once adequately stabilized, the patient should undergo appropriate radiography. AP and lateral films of the thoracolumbar spine for those with suspected injuries are first-line studies. An AP film of the pelvis, a chest radiograph, and films of the cervical spine complete the trauma series.

There are numerous mechanisms of injury to the thoracolumbar spine leading to various injury patterns, including axial compression, flexion, extension, rotation, and distraction mechanisms. Flexion-distraction injuries are associated with the use of a lap belt without a shoulder strap, which is associated with a high incidence of visceral injuries. They should be suspected in a patient after a motor vehicle accident with abrasions across the abdomen.

Treatment must be individualized to the patient and the injury pattern. Goals of treatment are rapid mobilization of the elderly patient with the avoidance of further neurologic deterioration. Emergency surgery is indicated only in cases of worsening neurologic deficit. Emergent CT or MRI should be performed in these cases to detect the site of neural compression. A canal or foraminal decompression should take place to remove impinging fragments, and the spine should be stabilized with instrumentation and fusion. The decision to approach the spine from an anterior or posterior approach depends on the injury pattern and the site of neural compression. Generally, more thorough decompression is possible from an anterior approach.

In cases of static neurologic deficit, elective surgery to decompress the canal may be beneficial for regaining neurologic function. Timing of surgical decompression is a topic of debate. We tend to intervene during the first week, although recovery of some neurologic function has been noted with late decompression.[69–71]

If no neurologic deficit is present, treatment should be based on the relative stability of the injury and the propensity for satisfactory healing. Certain injuries are stable. Examples include isolated fracture of a spinous process or transverse process secondary to a direct blow. Patients can be managed with a short period of bed rest and pain medication. A brace may be worn for comfort. Compression fractures of the spine are usually secondary to flexion mechanisms (Fig. 66.13). When the height of the

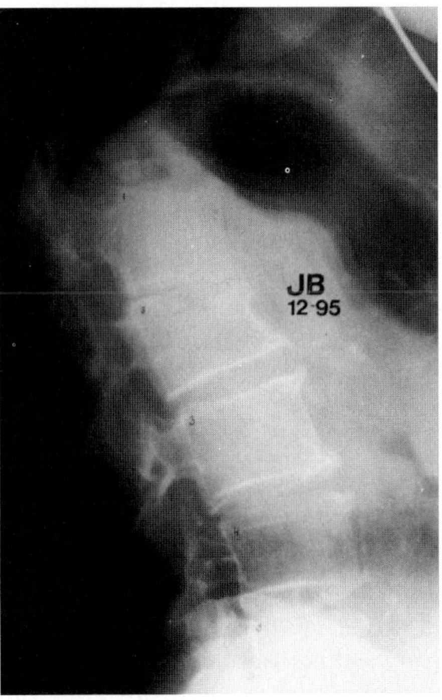


FIGURE 66.13. A 65-year-old woman was involved in a motor vehicle accident and had an onset of lower back pain. The lateral lumbosacral spine shows evidence of a compression fracture of L2.

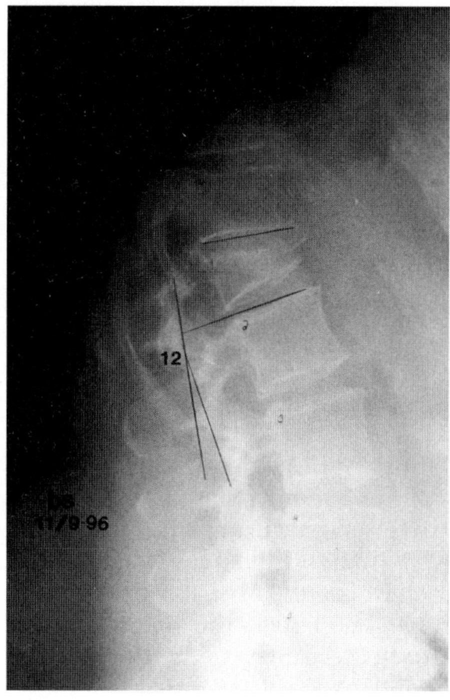


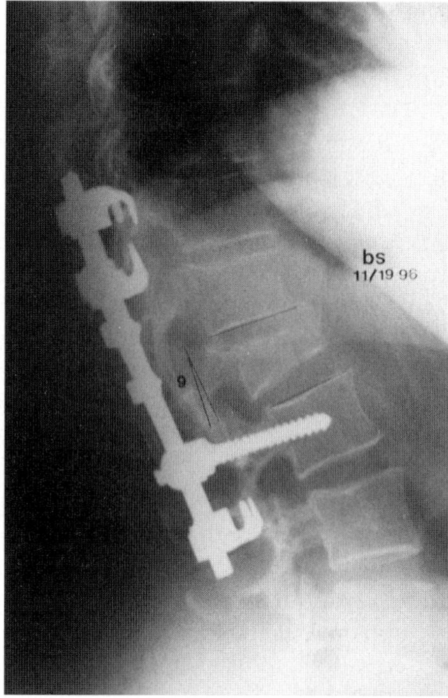


FIGURE 66.14. A 66-year-old woman who had fell from height experienced an onset of lower back pain. A. This lateral radiograph of the lumbosacral spine shows evidence of a burst fracture of L1 with widening of spinous processes posteriorly, consistent with a posterior ligamentous disruption. B. Patient underwent a posterior spinal fusion from T12 to L2 with instrumentation to stabilize this unstable injury.

anterior vertebral body is compressed less than 50% of the posterior aspect of the body and when no reversal of lumbar lordosis is present, the injury is relatively stable. Treatment can be placement in a thoracolumbosacral orthotic molded in extension for several months.

Injuries with anterior compression of more than 50% of the posterior body vertebral height or with reversal of lumbar lordosis are more unstable injuries because they connote injuries to the posterior ligamentous complex of the spine.[3] Surgical stabilization and fusion offer the most predictable healing results (Fig. 66.14). Surgery also allows more predictable restoration of sagittal alignment.

Other injuries further destabilize the spine. They include all fracture-dislocations of the spine and most flexion distraction injuries. To ensure healing, preservation of neurologic function, and avoidance of postinjury deformity, surgical stabilization and fusion should be undertaken. It is usually done from a posterior approach.

## Systemic Disorders of the Spine

Osteoporosis refers to decreased bone mass and increased risk of fracture. The vertebrae are the bones most commonly affected. This condition affects up to 20 million people yearly and represents a significant source of morbidity and cost. This is a condition of the elderly, with postpartum women affected more than twice as frequently as men. An understanding of the pathophysiology and treatment of this entity is essential for the geriatric clinician.[72]

### Pathophysiology

Bone is a living tissue constantly undergoing resorption and formation under the control of osteoblasts and osteoclasts. Peak bone mass is generally achieved during the third decade of life. Adequate daily calcium and vitamin D intake as well as exercise are essential for achieving the highest peak bone mass possible. Once peak mass is attained, resorption of bone exceeds formation, leading to a gradual diminution in bone mass. The rate of resorption is higher for women than it is for men. Rates of resorption further increase with the onset of menopause, probably secondary to the absence of estrogen, which acts to increase calcium absorption. Genetics also plays an important role in the development of osteoporosis. Fair-skinned individuals of northern European descent have the highest risk of disease progression. Other associated factors include early menopause, smoking, sedentary life style, phenytoin use, and excessive alcohol intake.[72]

With advancing age, susceptible individuals may experience fragility fractures. The spine and the hip are most commonly affected. These fractures are often seen after minor trauma such as lifting or tripping.

### Evaluation

Evaluation begins with a thorough history with attention to the aforementioned predisposing factors. The onset of pain and discomfort must be discerned. A history of longstanding pain, night pain, or other systemic signs such as fever or weight loss, should alert the physician to the possibility of tumor or infection rather than an osteoporotic fracture. The presentation is usually of local pain to the affected vertebrae without neurologic deficit or radiation to the lower extremities.

Examination reveals tenderness at the fracture site. Patients with previous vertebral compression fractures may demonstrate increased kyphosis to the thoracic spine. Radiographs of the affected area reveal osteopenia, decreased bone mass, and fracture of the affected vertebrae. In the thoracic spine this usually takes the form of an anterior compression or wedged appearance. In the lumbar spine more generalized flattening of the vertebrae occurs. It is not uncommon for asymptomatic or minimally symptomatic vertebral compression fractures to be discovered incidentally by radiography.

For first time presenters, laboratory tests should be done to rule out the reversible causes of osteoporosis, which include hyperthyroidism and increased cortisol levels. Otherwise, routine blood values are normal including calcium, hemoglobin, phosphorus, and alkaline phosphatase levels.[73]

More sophisticated methods for evaluating osteoporosis include dual energy x-ray absorptiometry (DEXA). This test subjects patients to a low dose of radiation with high accuracy. Bone mass is quantified in terms of density within standard deviations of normal. Individuals with more than 2 SD of normal are considered osteoporotic and are at significantly increased risk of fracture.[8]

#### Treatment

The cornerstone of management is prevention. As mentioned, ensuring adequate calcium and vitamin D intake as well as exercise during youth are the most reliable methods of increasing peak bone mass.[74] Patients older than 65 should maintain a daily intake of 1500 mg of elemental calcium. This is especially important in susceptible individuals. Once fracture has occurred, the goals include pain relief, patient mobilization, and prevention of further bone loss and deformity. Pain relief can be managed with NSAIDs or a short course of a narcotic analgesic. Several days of bed rest may be prescribed, after which the patient is encouraged to mobilize. The letter can be aided with the use of a thoracolumbar orthosis molded in extension, which should be worn until pain is resolved and follow-up radiographs show no increase in the deformity. Usually 6–12 weeks suffices.

Pharmacologic treatment of osteoporosis includes administration of supplemental calcium and vitamin D, which can help avoid further bone loss. The use of estrogen in perimenopausal and postmenopausal women has been shown to reduce vertebral compression fractures. Other agents include biphosphonates (Fosamax),[75] which also decrease osteoclastic activity, and fluoride, which stimulates osteoblastic proliferation. The appropriate pharmacologic protocol should be managed by a knowledgeable internist or rheumatologist.

Most of these injuries heal uneventfully. Surgery is rarely indicated for management of osteoporosis of the spine. One indication is an acute fracture with neurologic deficit, which is a rare occurrence. Loss of bowel/bladder control is another indication for surgical decompression. Other indications for surgery include progressive deformity with unremitting pain. The clinician must also be aware of insidious onset of neurologic deficit in the setting of multiple compression fractures with increasing kyphosis or scoliosis. This situation may represent spinal stenosis due to anterior canal compromise. It can occur months to years after injury. Therefore it is recommended that osteoporotic fractures be followed on a regular basis until increasing deformity has definitively stopped.

These patients are often risky surgical candidates because of their multiple medical problems. Additionally, poor bone quality makes fixation difficult. The surgical approach depends on the deformity and may be anterior, posterior, or combined. Patients must be made aware of the significant risk of these surgeries.[76]

## Infections of the Spine

Infections of the spinal column are common in the elderly or the immune compromised population. Diabetes, rheumatoid disease, concurrent urine infection, skin ulceration, and abscesses predispose to spinal infection. Unfortunately, the diagnosis is often missed early in its course, leading to delay in treatment and increased patient morbidity.[77]

### *Vertebral Osteomyelitis: Pyogenic and Mycobaterial*

#### Presentation

The most common presentation of vertebral osteomyelitis is chronic vague back pain. Hematogenous spread is the most common mode of transmission. The lumbar region is most commonly affected followed by the thoracic and cervical regions. Patients relate that the pain is not activity-related and is not relieved with standard measures. Furthermore, it often wakes the patient at night or prevents sleep. Patients may complain of systemic manifestations such as fever, chills, weight loss, and loss of appetite; but these findings are often absent. The physical examination may reveal local erythema and increased temperature over the affected region. The area may be tender to palpation with surrounding muscle spasm. Range of motion is often restricted owing to pain and spasm. Fewer than 10% of patients have neurologic findings upon presentation, although diabetes and a cephalad level of involvement put the patient at increased risk.[78]

Laboratory results may indicate an elevated white blood cell (WBC) count but are often normal. The erythrocyte sedimentation rate (ESR) is an extremely sensitive but nonspecific test, with elevated values in more than 90% of cases. It is, however, an excellent method for serial monitoring of the response to treatment.

If fever is present, blood cultures should be obtained but are often negative outside of temperature spikes. Radiographs can be entirely normal early in the disease; later they reveal destruction of the anterior vertebral metaphysis, diminished disc space height, and reactive subchondral bone formation. With mycobacterial infections the disc spaces are remarkably well preserved until late in the disease process.[79] Paraspinal shadows may be prominent owing to soft tissue extension of infection. A technetium bone scan with gallium has a more than 90% accuracy record for infection of the spine, but MRI is currently the modality of choice for confirming the diagnosis of infection; it distinctly reveals decreased signal to the disc and vertebrae on T1-weighted scans and increased signal on T2-weighted scans.[80]

#### Treatment

The key to management of osteomyelitis is identification of the offending agent. *Staphylococcus aureus* causes approximately half of all infections but *Escherichia coli, Staphylococcus epidermidis*, and *Pseudomonas* are other common organisms.[77] Recently, *Mycobacterium* tuberculosis has made a resurgence among the immune compromised and the elderly. Hence, suspected patients should undergo PPD testing and chest radiography in a search for pulmonary nodules. Thorough evaluation of the MRI scan to look for anterior and paravertebral masses and anterior bony destruction should be undertaken. These are classic findings associated with spinal tuberculosis. Other granulomatous diseases of the spine are also being seen with increasing frequency in this population.

Blood cultures, if positive, can direct antibiotic therapy. Unfortunately, they are positive only 25% of the time. In the absence of positive cultures, biopsy may be attempted via closed technique, CT- or fluoroscopy-guided. The yield for closed technique is approximately 75%. If the closed technique fails, open biopsy is mandatory to establish organism identification. Tumor and infection can have similar clinical and radiographic appearances, so all tissues should be sent for pathologic study. Gram staining, aerobic and anaerobic, *Mycobacterium*, and fungal testing should take place. Once an organism has been identified and its sensitivities established, antimicrobial therapy can be instituted. Six weeks of intravenous therapy followed by oral antibiotics is standard. Additionally, the spine should be immobilized in a brace. Multidrug therapy consisting of isoniazid, rifampin, ethambutol, and pyrazinamide are recommended for tuberculosis infections. Patients are usually treated for 6–12 months. The course of the disease should be monitored by clinical examination, repeat laboratory tests, and repeat MRI at appropriate intervals. When identified early, most infections can be resolved without the need for major surgical procedures.[81]

#### Surgery

Drug therapy is the treatment of choice for spinal infections. Surgery is indicated in specific instances: inability to establish diagnosis; failure of medical management to relieve pain and sepsis; worsening neurologic deficit; or increasing deformity and bony destruction. Additionally, patients with spinal tuberculosis in the cervical region and a neurologic deficit should be treated with surgical débridement because of the high risk of paralysis without surgical intervention. An attempt should be made to delay surgery for 2 weeks to allow the antibiotics to decrease the inflammation and allow an easier surgical approach.[82]

If surgery is indicated, the approach and procedure are dictated by the location of the infection. Most of the infections are located anteriorly in the vertebral bodies. The approach therefore is usually anterior via removal of infectious material including the involved vertebral bodies and any soft tissue abscess. Iliac crest bone graft or fibular strut graft should replace the removed bodies (Fig. 66.15). If the spine is rendered unstable, an additional posterior fusion can be utilized for further stabilization.[78,83]

### *Epidural Abscess*

Epidural abscesses are foci of infection in the potential space of the spinal canal outside the covering of the cord itself. They occur most commonly in the elderly and are a true medical and surgical emergency. More than 10% of cases are misdiagnosed at the initial visit to a physician. Predisposing factors are similar to those of osteomyelitis of the spine.

Epidural abscesses may arise via hematogenous spread from a distant site or via direct extension from a focus of vertebral osteomyelitis. Most abscesses are in the lumbar and thoracic region and are located dorsally within the canal. Cervical abscesses are less common but usually represent an extension of vertebral osteomyelitis and are located anteriorly.[84]

The most frequent presentation is that of pain localized to the site of the abscess. Patients look and feel ill. More than 50% of patients have increased temperature upon presentation. The examination is otherwise nonspecific and may include spasm, tenderness, and restricted range of motion. Patients may have signs of nerve root irritation. Usually, neurologic deficit is absent during the first 48 hours followed by neurologic dysfunction over the next several days. Frank paresis

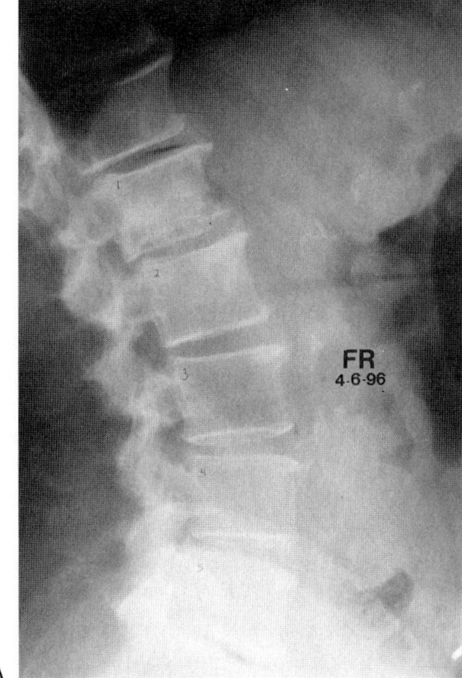


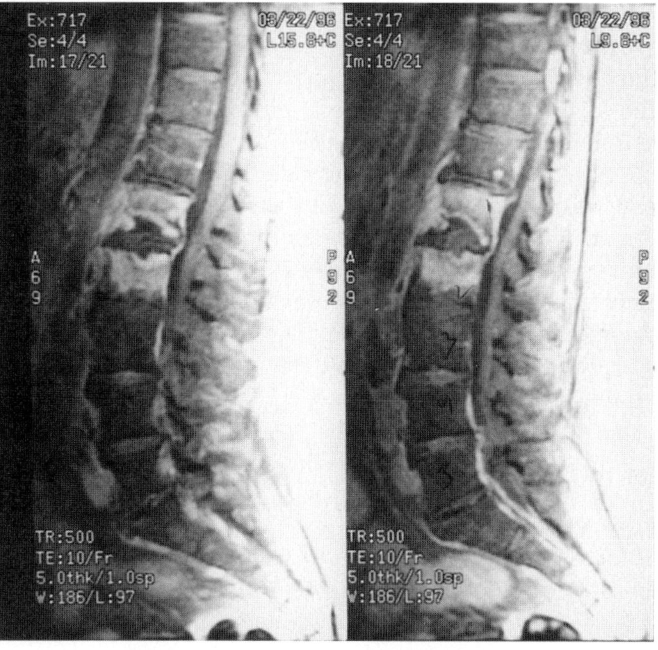


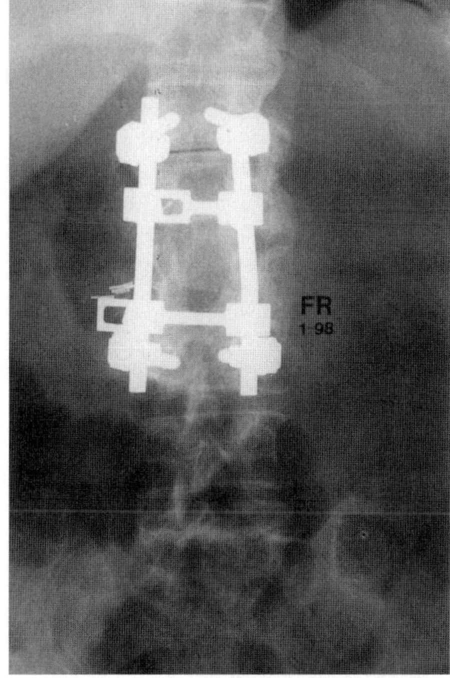


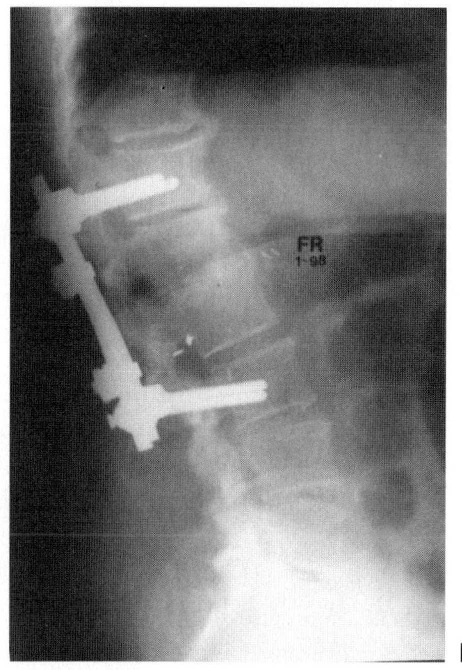


FIGURE 66.15. A 71-year-old woman with diabetes presented with constant back pain and difficulty with ambulation. A. Lateral radiograph of the lumbosacral spine showed evidence of destruction of the disc space and vertebral endplates at L1–2. B. Sagittal T1-weighted MRI scan of the lumbosacral spine confirmed discitis with osteomyelitis and psoas abscess at L1–2 and an impending epidural abscess. C, D. Patient underwent anterior débridement, decompression, and fusion with a vascularized 12th rib graft. She also had posterior stabilization from T12 to L3, with eradication of infection and return of neurologic status.

may evolve if left untreated. Early diagnosis and treatment are essential.

Laboratory values often reveal an increased WBC count and ESR. Radiographs are not usually helpful but may show vertebral endplate erosions or increased soft tissue outlines, especially in the cervical spine. If the diagnosis is suspected, urgent MRI of the affected region is done. The addition of gadolinium further sensitizes the study. Findings are of decreased epidural signal on T1-weighted scans and hyperintensity of the abscess on T2-weighted images.[85]

Once the diagnosis is established, broad-spectrum antibiotics to include coverage of *Staphylococcus*, *Streptococcus*, and *Mycobacterium* when indicated, should be administered without delay, followed by urgent surgical decompression. If located in the lumbar or thoracic region simple drainage with laminectomy may suffice. Cervical abscesses necessitate an anterior approach and removal of vertebral bodies with fusion. If the diagnosis is established early, the prognosis is good; delay may lead to mortality rates in excess of 10%.[84]

## Tumors of the Spine

With the exception of multiple myeloma, primary neoplasms of the spine are rare, especially in the elderly. Metastatic lesions of the spine, however, are common in this population. Other than lung and liver, the spine represents the most frequent site of metastasis and is the most frequent site of skeletal metastasis.[86]

### Presentation

Patients present most frequently with the complaint of back pain localized to the site of metastases. The pain is slowly progressive and does not respond to standard analgesics, rest, or other modalities. Frequently, night pain is present resulting in an inability to fall asleep. Systemic symptoms such as fever, weight loss, and lethargy are often communicated. Neurologic signs and symptoms may be present, suggesting invasion of the spinal cord or nerve roots by the lesion. The patient may present with chronic progressive back pain, with an acute onset of severe pain, which is often the result of a fracture through a pathologic lesion.

### Evaluation

As always, the history and physical examination are the keys to proper evaluation. Back pain in the setting of a current or prior malignancy should alert the physician to the possibility of spinal metastases. Standard laboratory test may reveal anemia, increased alkaline phosphatase, elevated ESR, or in the case of multiple myeloma elevated urine and serum electrophoresis measurements. Standard radiographs of the affected region should be obtained. Close attention should be paid to vertebral body changes and pedicle destruction, as they are the frequent sites of the metastatic deposits (Fig. 66.16). Unfortunately, radiographs are frequently normal, as approximately 50% of marrow replacement must occur to findings on plain films.[87] If clinical suspicion exists, an MRI scan should be obtained. MRI is extremely sensitive for the marrow changes seen with malignancy. Metastases appear hyperintense on T2-weighted images. MRI also enables study of the spinal cord, epidural space, and surrounding soft tissues. This is especially important when evaluating patients with neurologic deficit. Once MRI confirms a lesion, a bone scan is recommended to localize additional bony deposits. Of note, multiple myeloma is frequently cold on bone scans. A chest radiograph may reveal a

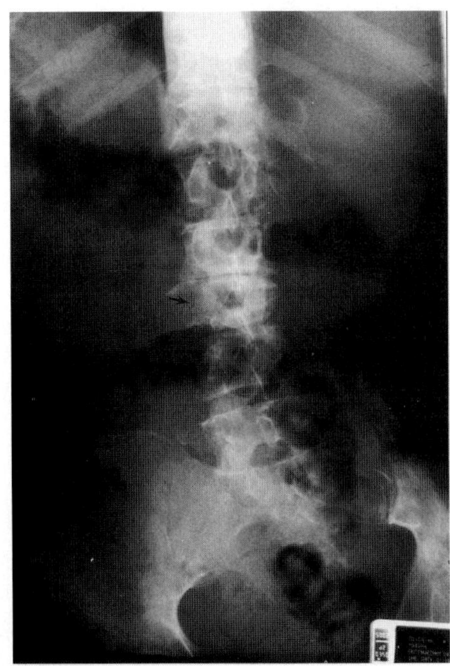
A

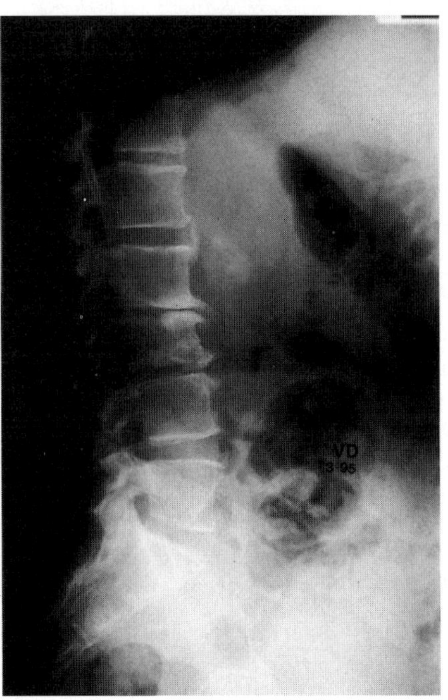
B

FIGURE 66.16. A 75-year-old woman presented with an 8-month history of constant low back pain and night pain. A. Anteroposterior radiograph of the lumbosacral spine shows absence of the left pedicle at L3 (arrow), the "winking owl" sign. B. Lateral radiograph of the lumbosacral spine shows replacement of the pedicle and posterior vertebral body of L3, consistent with metastatic disease. Biopsy confirmed ovarian carcinoma.

module suggesting the lung as the site of the primary malignancy.

### Management

Once a metastatic lesion to the spine has been established, its pathology must be ascertained. This should be done by correlating the remainder of the workup (laboratory results, radiographs, abdominal or pelvic CT, colonoscopy) or if necessary via biopsy of the lesion. This may be done via a closed technique using CT or fluoroscopic guidance. If this is unsuccessful, an open biopsy must be performed. Once a definitive diagnosis is established, further management must emphasize a team approach, including the help of an internist, oncologist, orthopedic surgeon, and neurosurgeon.

The most sensitive prognostic indicator for survival is not the extent of the spinal lesion but the primary diagnosis. Hence, any treatment must take into account the expected lifetime of the patient. Patients with breast cancer and multiple myeloma have a longer life expectancy, often more than 2 years from the diagnosis. Gastrointestinal and lung malignancies involving the spine have a much shorter life expectancy.

Available modalities include analgesics, bracing, radiotherapy, chemotherapy, and surgery. If no neurologic deficit is present or fracture has not occurred, there is no need for emergent surgery. The radiosensitivity of the lesion should be determined and the effectiveness of chemotherapy. For example, multiple myeloma and lymphoma are extremely radiosensitive. If the tumor is radiosensitive, irradiation can be done. If significant pain relief occurs, it may serve as definitive management. Emergent surgery is indicated for patients with progressive neurologic deficit or fracture of a vertebral element with a propensity for instability, further neurologic injury, or both. All additional lesions must be dealt with on an individual basis. Specifically, surgery may be indicated for unremitting pain unresponsive to other modalities and large lesions suspicious of impending fracture or instability. For highly vascular tumors, such as thyroid and renal cell carcinoma, where irradiation and surgery are planned, surgery should take place prior to initiation of radiotherapy. This is to prevent wound healing complications associated with radiation use. The surgery must be highly individualized. Anterior lesions should be approached anteriorly and posterior legions posteriorly. Generally, lesions causing neurologic compromise necessitate an anterior approach. All pathologic tissue should be removed and the spine stabilized with instrumentation. Careful study of the preoperative MRI is necessary. If possible, asymptomatic lesions are included in the stabilization. If life-span is limited, fusion is not mandatory; but if doubt exists as to life expectancy, fusion should be performed.[88]

### Results

The prognosis for spinal metastases is the same as for the primary lesion. Spinal surgery is never curative, only palliative. However, in patients with unremitting pain and neurologic compromise, surgery enables an improved life style and easier mobilization.

## References

1. Deyo R, Tsui-Wu Y. Descriptive epidemiology of low back pain and its related medical care in the United States. Spine 1987;12:264–268.
2. Moore KL. The back. In: Gardner J (ed) Clinically Oriented Anatomy. Baltimore: Williams & Wilkins, 1985:565–625.
3. White AA III, Panjabi MM. Clinical Biomechanics of the Spine, 2nd ed. Philadelphia: Lippincott, 1990.
4. Miller JA, Schwatz C, Schultz AB. Lumbar disc degeneration: correlation with age, sex, spinal level in 600 autopsy specimens. Spine 1988;13:173–178.
5. Boden SD, Davis DO, et al. Abnormal magnetic resonance scans of the lumbar spine in asymptomatic subjects: a prospective investigation. J Bone Joint Surg Am 1990;72: 403–408.
6. Lipson SJ. Aging versus degeneration of the intervertebral disc. In: Weinstein JW, Wiesel JW (eds) The Lumbar Spine. Philadelphia: Saunders, 1990.
7. Pritzker KP. Aging and degeneration in the lumbar intervertebral disc. Orthop Clin North Am 1977;8:65–77.
8. Miller M. Spine: Review of Orthopaedics. Philadelphia: Saunders, 1996:270–291.
9. Rohling ML, Binder LM, Langhinrichsen-Rohling J. Money matters: a meta-analytic review of the association between financial compensation and the experience and treatment of chronic pain. Health Psychol 1995;14:537–547.
10. Gatchel RJ, Rolatin PB, Mayer TG. The dominant role of psychosocial risk factors in the development of chronic low back pain disability. Spine 1995;20:2702–2709.
11. Jahnke RW, Hart BL. Cervical stenosis, spondylosis and herniated disc disease. Radiol Clin North Am 1991;29: 777.
12. MacNab I, McCulloch J. Cervical disc degeneration. In: Passano WM III (ed) Neck Ache and Shoulder Pain. Baltimore: Williams & Wilkins, 1994:53–62.
13. MacNab I, McCulloch J. Classification of shoulder disorders and assessment of shoulder function. In: Passano WM III (ed) Neck Ache and Shoulder Pain. Baltimore: Williams & Wilkins, 1994:275–307.
14. MacNab I, McCulloch J. Treatment of cervical disc disease. In: Passano WM III (ed) Neck Ache and Shoulder Pain. Baltimore: Williams & Wilkins, 1994:79–120.
15. Hoppenfeld S. Physical examination of the cervical spine and temporomandibular joint. In: Physical Examination of the Spine and Extremities. East Norwalk, CT: Appleton-Century-Crofts, 1976:105–132.
16. Cornefjord M, Olmarter K, Farley DB, et al. Neuropeptide changes in compressed spinal nerve roots. Spine 1995;20:670–673.
17. Lees F, Alden Turner JW. Natural history and prognosis of cervical spondylosis. Br Med J 1963;2:1607–1610.

18. Bohlman H, Emery SE, Goodfellow DB, et al. Robinson anterior cervical discectomy and arthrodesis for cervical radiculopathy: long-term follow-up of one hundred and twenty-two patients. J Bone Joint Surg Am 1993;75: 1298–1307.
19. An HS. Clinical presentation of discogenic neck pain, radiculopathy, and myelopathy. In: Clark C (ed) The Cervical Spine, 3rd ed. Philadelphia: Lippincott-Raven, 1998:755–763.
20. Kurz LT. Nonoperative treatment of degenerative disorders of the cervical spine. In: Clark C (ed) The Cervical Spine, 3rd ed. Philadelphia: Lippincott-Raven, 1998:779–783.
21. Herkowitz HN, Kurz LT, Overholt D. Surgical management of cervical soft disc herniation: a comparison between the anterior and posterior approach. Spine 1990;15:1026–1030.
22. Benner B. Etiology, pathogenesis, and natural history of discogenic neck pain, radiculopathy and myelopathy. In: Clark C (ed) The Cervical Spine, 3rd ed. Philadelphia: Lippincott-Raven, 1998:735–740.
23. Clark E, Robinson PK. Cervical myelopathy: a complication of cervical spondylosis. Brain 1956;79:483–570.
24. Sachs BL. Differential diagnosis of neck pain, arm pain, and myelopathy. In: Clark C (ed) The Cervical Spine, 3rd ed. Philadelphia: Lippincott-Raven, 1998:741–753.
25. Bohlman HH. Cervical spondylosis with moderate to severe myelopathy: a report of 17 cases treated by Robinson anterior cervical discectomy and fusion. Spine 1977;2:151.
26. Yonenbou K, Fuji T, Ono K, et al. Choice of surgical treatment for multisegmented cervical spondylotic myelopathy. Spine 1985;10:710.
27. Garvey TA, Eismont FJ. Diagnosis and treatment of cervical radiculopathy and myelopathy. Orthop Rev 1991;20: 595–603.
28. Mirkovic S, Cybulishi GR. Thoracic disc herniations. In: Garfin JR, Vaccaro AR (eds) Orthopaedic Knowledge Update Spine. Rosemont, IL: AAOS, 1997:87–96.
29. Brown CW, Deffer PA Jr, Akmatijian J, et al. The natural history of thoracic disc herniation. Spine 1992;17(suppl 16):S97–S102.
30. Wood KB, Garvey TA, Grundy C. Magnetic resonance imaging of the thoracic spine: evaluation of asymptomatic individuals. J Bone Joint Surg Am 1995;77:631–638.
31. Hoppenfeld S, deBoer P. The spine. In: Hannon BC (ed) Surgical Exposures in Orthopaedics; The Anatomic Approach, 2nd ed. Philadelphia: Lippincott, 1994:216–301.
32. Rosenthal D, Rosenthal R, DeSimone A. Removal of a protruded thoracic disc using microsurgical endoscopy: a new technique. Spine 1994;19:1087–1091.
33. Simpson JM, Siveri CP, Simeone FA. Thoracic disc herniation: reevaluation of the posterior approach using a modified costotranversectomy. Spine 1993;18:1872–1877.
34. MacNab I, McCulloch J. A classification of low back pain. In: Grayson T (ed) Backache, 2nd ed. Baltimore: Williams & Wilkins, 1986:22–25.
35. Seimon LP. Applied anatomy, pathological anatomy, sources of pain. In: Low Back Pain: Clinical Diagnosis and Management. East Norwalk, CT: Appleton-Century-Crofts, 1983:3–30.
36. Turner JA, Ersch M, Herron L. Patient outcomes after lumbar spinal fusions. JAMA 1992;268:907–911.
37. Colhoun E, McCall I, Williams L. Proactive discography as a guide to planning operations on the spine. J Bone Joint Surg Br 1988;70:267–271.
38. MacNab I, McCulloch J. Pain and disability (psychogenic back pain) In: Grayson T (ed) Backache, 2nd ed. Baltimore: Williams & Wilkins, 1986:26–44.
39. Seimon LP. History, examination, special investigations. In: Low Back Pain: Clinical Diagnosis and Management. East Norwalk, CT: Appleton-Century-Crofts, 1976.
40. Hoppenfeld S. Physical Examination of the Spine and Extremities. East Norwalk, CT: Appleton-Century-Crofts, 1976.
41. O'Donnell JL. Prostaglandin $E_2$ content in herniated lumbar disc disease. Paper No. 266. Presented at the 62nd meeting of American Academy of Orthopaedic Surgeons, February 1995.
42. Olmarker K. The experimental basis of sciatica. J Orthop Sci 1996;1:230–242.
43. MacNab I, McCulloch J. Disc degeneration with root irritation. In: Grayson T (ed) Backache, 2nd ed. Baltimore: Williams & Wilkins, 1986:283–334.
44. Wiesel SW, Tsourmas N, Teffer HL, et al. A study of computer assisted tomography: the incidence of positive CAT scans in an asymptomatic group of patients. Spine 1984;9:549–551.
45. Katz JN, Lipson SJ, Larson MG, et al. The outcome of decompressive laminectomy for degenerative lumbar stenosis. J Bone Joint Surg Am 1991;73:809–816.
46. Hanley EN. The surgical treatment of lumbar degenerative disease. In: Garfin JR, Vaccaro AR (eds) Orthopaedic Knowledge Update Spine. Rosemont, IL: AAOS, 1997:127–140.
47. Seimon LP. Subacute and chronic low back pain. In: Low Back Pain: Clinical Diagnosis and Management. East Norwalk, CT: Appleton-Century-Crofts, 1983:89–113.
48. Spengler DM. Current concepts review: degenerative stenosis of the lumbar spine. J Bone Joint Surg 1987;69:305.
49. Johnson KE, Rosen I, Uden A. The natural course of lumbar spinal stenosis. Clin Orthop 1992;279:82–86.
50. Herkowitz HN, Kurz LT. Degenerative lumbar spondylolisthesis with spinal stenosis: a prospective study comparing decompression with decompression and intertransverse process arthrodesis. J Bone Joint Surg 1991;73:802–808.
51. Simmons JC ED, Zheng Y, Munschauer C. Comparative analysis of instrumented and noninstrumented lumbar fusion. Paper No. 454. Presented at the 62nd meeting of American Academy of Orthopaedic Surgeons, February 1995.
52. Bauchard JA, Aletari H. Degenerative lumbar scoliosis and stenosis: comparison of surgical treatment with and without instrumentation. Paper No. 453. Presented at the 62nd meeting of American Academy of Orthopaedic Surgeons, February 1995.
53. Lauerman WC, Frame JC, Cain JE, et al. A randomized prospective study of lumbar fusion with and without transpedicular instrumentation. Paper No. 455. Presented at the 62nd meeting of American Academy of Orthopaedic Surgeons, February 1995.
54. Fischgund JS. Degenerative lumbar spondylolisthesis with spinal stenosis: a prospective randomized study comparing arthrodesis with and without instrumentation. Paper No.

456. Presented at the 62nd meeting of American Academy of Orthopaedic Surgeons, February 1995.
55. MacNab I, McCulloch J. Failure of spinal surgery. In: Grayson T (ed) Backache, 2nd ed. Baltimore: Williams & Wilkins, 1986:392–435.
56. Weinstein SL, Ponseti IV. Curve progression in idiopathic scoliosis. J Bone Joint Surg Am 1983;65:447–455.
57. Perennou D, Marcelli C, Henesson C, et al. Adult lumbar scoliosis: epidemiologic aspects in a low back pain population. Spine 1994;19:123–128.
58. Bradford DS. Adult scoliosis: current concepts of treatment. Clin Orthop 1988;229:70–87.
59. Bradford DS. Adult scoliosis. In: Moe's Textbook of Scoliosis and Other Spinal Deformities, 3rd ed. Philadelphia: Saunders, 1995:369–386.
60. Swank S, Winter RB, Moe JH. Scoliosis and cor pulmonale. Spine 1984;7:343–354.
61. Stagnara P, Fleury D, Pauchet R, et al. Scoliosis majeures de l'adulte superieures a 100–183 cas traites chirurgicalement. Rev Chir Orthop 1975;61:101–122.
62. Kostiuk JP. Current concepts review: operative treatment of idiopathic scoliosis. J Bone Joint Surg Am 1990;72:1108–1113.
63. Kostiuk JP. Recent advances in the treatment of painful adult scoliosis. Clin Orthop 1980;147:238–252.
64. Connolly PJ, Abitbol JJ, Martin RJ, et al. Spine: trauma. In: Garfin JR, Vaccaro AR (eds) Orthopaedic Knowledge Update: Spine. Rosemont, IL: AAOS, 1997:197–217.
65. Bucholz RW. Lower cervical spine injuries. In: Skeletal Trauma: Fractures, Dislocations, Ligamentous Injuries. Philadelphia: Saunders, 1992:699–727.
66. Eismont FJ, Arena MJ, Green BA. Extrusion of an intervertebral disk associated with traumatic subluxation or dislocation of cervical facets. J Bone Joint Surg Am 1991;73:1555–1560.
67. MacNab I, McCulloch J. Whiplash injury of the cervical spine. In: Passano WM (ed) Neck Ache and Shoulder Pain. Baltimore: Williams & Wilkins, 1994:140–159.
68. Bracken MB, Shepard MJ, Collins WF, et al. A randomized, controlled trial of methylprednisone or naloxone in the treatment of acute spinal cord injury: results of the Second National Acute Spinal Cord Injury Study. N Engl J Med 1990;322:1405–1411.
69. Bohlman HH. Treatment of fractures and dislocations of the thoracic and lumbar spine. J Bone Joint Surg Am 1985;67: 165–169.
70. Bohlman HH, Freehafer A, Dejak J. The results of treatment of acute injuries of the upper thoracic spine with paralysis. J Bone Joint Surg Am 1985;67:360–369.
71. Denis F. Thoracolumbar spine trauma. In: Moe's Textbook of Scoliosis and Other Spinal Deformities, 3rd ed. Philadelphia: Saunders, 1995:431–449.
72. Lane JM, Riley EH, Wirganowicz PZ. Osteoporosis: diagnosis and treatment. J Bone Joint Surg Am 1996;78:618– 632.
73. Lane JM, Sandhu HS. Osteoporosis of the spine. In: Garfin JR, Vaccaro AR (eds) Orthopaedic Knowledge Update Spine. Rosemont, IL: AAOS, 1997:227–234.
74. National Institutes of Health. Optimum calcium intake: NIH consensus statement. 1994:12:1–31.
75. Watts NB, Harris ST, Genant HK, et al. Intermittent cyclical etidronate treatment of postmenopausal osteoporosis. N Engl J Med 1990;323:73–79.
76. Kostuik JP, Heggeness MH. Surgery of the osteoporotic spine. In: Frymoyer JW (ed) The Adult Spine: Principles and Practice, 2nd ed. Philadelphia: Lippincott-Raven, 1997:1639–1664.
77. Sapico FL. Microbiology and antimicrobial therapy of spinal infections. Orthop Clin North Am 1996;27:9–13.
78. Eismont FJ, Bohlman HH, Soni PL, et al. Pyogenic and fungal vertebral osteomyelitis with paralysis. J Bone Joint Surg Am 1983;65:19–29.
79. Ho EKW, Leong JCY. Tuberculosis of the spine. In: Weinstein SL (ed) The Pediatric Spine: Principles and Practice. New York: Raven, 1994:837–850.
80. Modic MT, Feigh DH, Pirano DW, et al. Vetebral osteomyelitis: assessment using MR. Radiology 1985;157: 157–166.
81. Keenen TL, Benson DR. Differential diagnosis and conservative treatment of infectious diseases. In: Frymoyer JW (ed) The Adult Spine: Principles and Practice. Philadelphia: Lippincott-Raven, 1997:871–894.
82. Keenen TL, Benson DR. Infectious diseases of the spine; surgical treatment. In: Frymoyer JW (ed) The Adult Spine: Principles and Practice. Philadelphia: Lippincott-Raven, 1997.
83. Hodgson AR, Stock FE, Fang HS, et al. Anterior spinal fusion: the operative and pathological findings in 412 patients with Pott's disease of the spine. Br J Surg 1960;48:172–178.
84. Danner RL, Hartman BJ. Update of spinal epidural abscess: 35 cases and review of the literature. Rev Infect Dis 1987;9:265–274.
85. Angtuaco EJ, McConnell JR, Chadduch WM, et al. MR imaging of spinal epidural sepsis. Am J Radiol 1987;149: 1249–1253.
86. Dahlin DC. Bone Tumors: General Aspects and Data on 6221 Cases, 3rd ed. Springfield, IL: Charles C Thomas, 1978.
87. Boriani S, Weinstein JN. Differential diagnosis and surgical treatment of primary benign and malignant neoplasms. In: Frymoyer JW (ed) The Adult Spine: Principles and Practice, 2nd ed. Philadelphia: Lippincott-Raven, 1997:951–987.
88. Harrington KD. Metastatic disease of the spine. J Bone Joint Surg 1986;68:1110–1115.

# *Part II*
# *Specific Issues in Geriatric Surgey*

## Section 11
## Transplantation

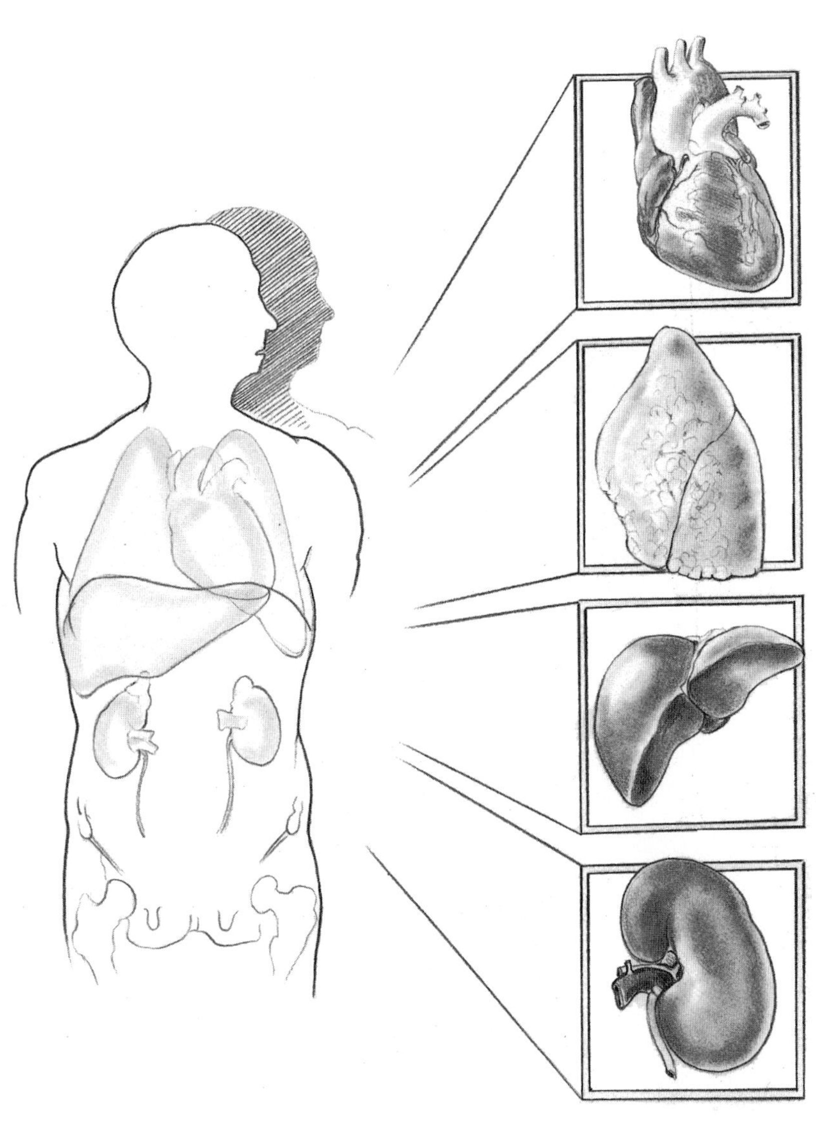

# Invited Commentary

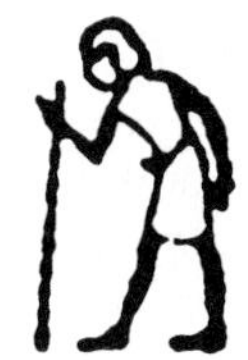

John S. Najarian

During the early years of transplantation, recipients were primarily those with the optimum chance for a successful outcome. Kidney recipients were between the ages of 15 and 45. Similar age ranges existed for liver, pancreas, heart, lung, and heart-lung recipients. As success rates and immunosuppression improved, transplant surgeons began "pushing the envelope," accepting both younger children and older adults as recipients. Given our increasing ability to manage the complications of advancing age and other improvements in medicine, the average age of the overall population—and of transplant recipients—continues to increase. Currently, a 60-year-old person who undergoes a successful transplant can be expected to live 17 years or more; even someone 65–70 has an average of 16 years left.

The highest ages of donors and recipients, by organ, in 1996 were as follows.

| | |
|---|---|
| Kidney donor | 81 |
| Kidney recipient | 84 |
| Kidney–pancreas recipient | 58 |
| Single Pancreas recipient | 62 |
| Liver recipient | 76 |
| Liver donor | 85 |
| Heart recipient | 74 |
| Heart donor | 65 |
| Heart–lung recipient | 59 |
| Single-lung recipient | 68 |
| Double-lung recipient | 66 |
| Bone marrow recipient | 68 |
| Bone marrow donor | 77 |

Our continuing good results warrant this age extension for recipient and donor selection. Here is a summary of our experience with kidney transplantation in older patients at the University of Minnesota.

## Early 1970s

Our initial experience with kidney transplantation for older recipients, especially with cadaver grafts, was dismal. In 1971 our 1-year patient and graft survival rates for primary cadaver graft recipients ≥45 years of age were 40% and 20%, respectively, both considerably worse than for younger recipients.

Other transplant centers had similar experiences. In their initial reports, patient survival rates for older cadaver kidney recipients were worse than for comparable patients treated with dialysis. Patient survival rates for living donor recipients were better. Accordingly, in 1977 we suggested that cadaver transplants should not be offered to patients ≥45 years of age.

## Mid-1980s

With the development of cyclosporine (CsA)-based immunosuppressive protocols, results improved; this improvement was particularly striking in high-risk groups. By 1987 we reported that the outcome for primary cadaver recipients ≥50 years of age was similar to that for those <50 years. Since then, the age limits for transplantation have been extended further.

## Late 1990s

Our current analysis suggests that immunologic graft loss for new patients ≥60 (death with function censored) is no different from for those 18–59 years of age. Long-term patient and graft survival rates are lower for those ≥60, but this is due to increased mortality. Although patients ≥60 have a somewhat longer initial hospitalization, they have significantly fewer readmissions; more of them remain rejection-free. Importantly, quality of life is within the national norms for the age-matched population.

## Current Debate

Should there be an upper age limit for kidney transplantation? The answer is complicated and involves many conflicting issues. First, concurrent with the aging of the American population is the aging of the subgroup with end-stage renal disease (ESRD). By the year 2000, more than 60% of ESRD patients in the United States were projected to be ≥65 years. Currently, 50% of new patients with ESRD are ≥61 years of age.

Second, patients ≥60 years have the potential for many quality years. The average 60-year-old in the United States lives another 17 years or more. Transplantation provides better quality of life than dialysis. Compared with dialysis, it is a more cost-effective treatment for ESRD.

Both of the above factors would support kidney transplantation for patients ≥60, but other considerations also apply. It must be recognized that not all patients ≥60 are equivalent transplant candidates. Physicians generally accept that chronologic age and "biologic" age, although difficult to quantitate, differ considerably. Most of our patients ≥60 had at least one extrarenal system affected by disease, some attributable to the consequences of renal failure. Although cost-effective compared with dialysis, transplantation is expensive. Importantly, unlike dialysis, most transplant costs occur during the first years. Thus if an older transplant candidate's potential for survival is accurately predicted to be severely limited by extrarenal disease, the expense of transplantation may not be justified.

## Ethical Issues

Cadaver kidneys are a scarce resource. As a result, ethical allocation priorities are a topic of ongoing discussion. Should every patient on a waiting list have an equal opportunity to have a transplant? Should kidneys be allocated to the patient with the best chance of long-term success? If long-term success is the major goal, perhaps cadaver kidneys should be allocated to young patients.

The answers are somewhat easier for transplant candidates with living donors because the competing priorities of organ allocation are not a problem. We believe that the donor must be fully aware of the limitations of transplantation. However, rather than set arbitrary age limits, we continue to consider each case individually. If the transplant candidate is otherwise healthy and is not tolerating dialysis (physically, emotionally, or because of limitations on quality of life) and if the donor fully understands the risks and benefits, we consider older patients. Remember, the outcome with living donor transplantation must be compared with alternate treatments for the same patient subgroup. Our data suggest that for patients ≥60 years, the outcome of a primary transplant with a living donor is better than with a cadaver donor and better than dialysis. Currently, our oldest recipient (transplanted when ≥60) of a nonidentical living donor kidney is 84 years old, 21 years posttransplant.

Unfortunately, patients ≥60 years frequently do not have potential living donors. Many of the diseases causing ESRD in old people (e.g., polycystic kidneys, hypertension) are familial. Many siblings are already too old or have renal or extrarenal disease that precludes donation, and the patients are often reluctant to accept kidneys from their children. Thus only 30% of our recipients ≥60 had living donor transplants (versus 51% of those 18–59 years of age).

In our current series, for CsA-immunosuppressed primary cadaver recipients ≥60, the patient survival rate was 91% at 1 year, 81% at 3 years, and 64% at 5 years. At other centers the patient survival at 5 years ranged from 57% to 80%.

In contrast, for dialysis-treated Medicare patients age 60–69, the patient survival rate is only 73% at 1 year and 24% at 5 years; for those age 55–65 it is 35% at 5 years. It is difficult to determine whether these transplant and dialysis patients are comparable. Healthier patients might be more likely to be considered for transplantation, whereas patients with significant extrarenal disease that would limit life-span might be relegated to dialysis. Yet in our series most transplant recipients had significant extrarenal disease pretransplant. Interestingly, the patient survival rate for accepted transplant candidates ≥60 years who were maintained on dialysis while waiting, was reported to be the same as for patients rejected for transplantation: 48% and 44% at 1 year, 29% and 30% at 2 years. Other investigators comparing transplant and dialysis outcome in old patients have suggested that definitive data are not available as to which is superior, but they believe that transplantation should be offered as an option for patients 65–75 years of age.

## Immune Status

Our finding of fewer acute rejection episodes for recipients ≥60 is not new. Immune competence decreases with age, providing a possible explanation. When patient death was censored, other investigators have reported that recipients ≥60 years had significantly better graft survival rates, with no immunologic graft loss after 36 months. In our series, five recipients ≥60 years lost their graft to chronic rejection 24–60 months posttransplant. One difference may be our tendency to use lower dosages of immunosuppression for old recipients. In our early (pre-CsA) experience, infection was a major cause of graft loss for older recipients; consequently, we are now less aggressive when treating acute rejection episodes in these recipients. At the same time, we now tend to use lower immunosuppressive dosages late posttransplant.

Importantly, our lower incidence of rejection in recipients ≥60 years is associated with a lower rate of rehospitalization. More recipients ≥60 years were readmission-free (a statistically significant difference for cadaver recipients). Recipients ≥60 years had fewer posttransplant readmission days.

## Effect of Extrarenal Disease

Few data exist on the relation of extrarenal disease to transplant outcome. Recipients ≥60 years have been subdivided into those free of both diabetes and cardiac disease (low-risk) versus those with pretransplant diabetes or cardiac disease (high-risk). In our series, low-risk recipients had better patient ($p = 0.055$) and graft survival rates. We were surprised to see so little impact of pretransplant cardiac disease: Patient survival rates at 3 years differed by 3% among those with or without identified cardiac disease and at 5 years by 10%. This minor difference suggests that cardiac disease should not be an exclusion criterion for transplantation. Similarly, pretransplant respiratory or gastrointestinal disease had no impact on outcome. Our most striking findings involved recipients with pretransplant peripheral vascular disease (arterial or venous) or liver/biliary tract disease. The numbers in each of these subgroups, however, were small, so it was impossible to identify a specific increase in cause of death or cause of graft loss. Those with liver disease tended to have late failure due to sepsis.

## Quality of Life

In addition, few data exist on the quality of life for old transplant recipients. Our informal questionnaire returned by 151 respondents in 1993 suggested that they are doing reasonably well. All continue to state that they made the correct decision in choosing transplantation. We also received the more rigorous SF-36 Health Survey, designed to measure general health concepts that are "not age, disease, or treatment specific," from these same respondents. The SF-36 survey is meant to be short, practical (with less data collection and analysis costs), and precise. National norms have been developed for various adult age groups, so it is easy to compare any patient group with the U.S. population. We found little difference in SF-36 scores for our recipients ≥60 years and the national norms. Our recipients scored lower on two scales of physical functioning, but the difference was not statistically different. A limitation of our analysis is that it took place at a single time point: the time posttransplant varied from a few months to 8 years. Sequential analyses with larger numbers are necessary to separate out immediate posttransplant issues from those related to age or to the consequences of immunosuppression. Of note, our recipients ≥60 years had scores identical to the national norms on scales of bodily pain, general health, vitality (energy level/fatigue), social functioning, and mental health.

Clearly, transplantation is successful for recipients ≥60 years of age. Outcome is limited by patient survival. Death-censored graft survival for recipients ≥60 years is identical to graft survival for patients age 18–59. Most of our recipients ≥60 years had extrarenal disease at the time of their transplant; but extrarenal disease was not an important predictor of outcome and should not be used as an exclusion criterion. Our recipients ≥60 years have a lower rejection rate and fewer readmissions than those 18–59 years. In addition, quality of life for our recipients ≥60 years is similar to that of the age-matched U.S. population.

The question is often asked: Why are the results as good as they are for the old population? The answer is that immunologic incompetence occurs as we grow older and can be measured. $CD\text{-}4^+$ cells increase slightly and $CD\text{-}8^+$ cells decrease. Thus older recipients are more likely to develop infections or tumors. At the same time, overall results are far better for old, more immunoincompetent recipients. In addition, even the lymphokines that are produced by the increased number of $CD\text{-}4^+$ cells are not of good quality.

## Donors

Finally, what about the age of donors? This issue is important. Old donors are not as desirable as young donors: With advancing age, nephrons are lost. After age 60–65, the quality of the kidney is diminished. Hence we often pass up kidneys from would-be donors ≥65, especially for young recipients, but these kidneys could readily be transplanted into old patients. We prefer to accept kidneys from old donors for our old recipients who are waiting on dialysis.

With living related donors we draw the line for donation at age 65. We do not accept an organ from a spouse (a living unrelated donor) ≥65 years. However, the living related kidneys that we use for our old recipients are most commonly from their children. These kidneys do well and often are as good as HLA-identical grafts. Thus living related donors pose less of an ethical problem. Conversely, the supply of cadaver donors is limited and has remained almost flat for the past 6 years. The main reason for the increased number of kidney transplants in recent years is that more and more centers are using living related and living unrelated donors.

# 67
# Selection of Elderly Patients for Transplantation

John B. Dossetor

Transplanted organs are a precious commodity for which there is increasing demand. There is also an ever-widening gap between the need for organs and our capacity to meet that need. The waiting lists are increasing, and the gap between need and supply is also increasing, as seen in Figure 67.1. The situation is similar in all countries where programs exist for the transplantation of solid organs. The data shown are for kidney failure, but the overall transplant data are similar. In this chapter, the discussion is confined to cadaveric organ transplants, as live donor transplants are seldom used for the elderly.

Not surprisingly, therefore, the allocation of this scarce resource, which Figure 67.1 shows to be associated with an ever-increasing gap between supply and demand, presents considerable ethical problems. Should the organs be given to those with limited mental capacity? Should they be given to foreign nationals with the ability to pay? Should they be given to the elderly? Who is to make these "rationing" decisions? What are the principles that bear on these situations, by the application of which one hopes to make just decisions? Are there alternative sources, such as organs from old donors for old recipients? Could organs be used from those from whom life support is being ethically withheld—if the organs are suitable—such as the non-brain-dead cadaver donor[2] and the non-heart-beating cadaver donor (NHBCD)[3]? Then, of course, there is the xenograft source.

This chapter considers the entitlement of elderly persons to organ transplants by paying special attention to kidney transplants. It is the most common solid organ transplant and therefore the field in which there are more data to examine.

Ethical deliberation should lead to public policies that must be available for public scrutiny in a just society. This should apply to hospitals, even those in the private sector. Transplant teams are therefore ethically obliged to look carefully into the principles or rules or preferences they use to allocate these precious means of saving the lives of those with organ failure.

Before considering the role age plays in organ allocation, as with any ethical dilemma in resource allocation, we must review (1) *the question of entitlement* (what are the reasons for including or excluding individuals in different categories, and do such reasons stand up to our ethical norms); and (2) *the known facts on aspects of efficacy and cost-effectiveness*, in this case in regard to organ transplant outcomes. These two aspects—entitlement and efficacy—determine whether a category of persons should be considered for an organ transplant waiting list in the first place. Once on the waiting list, we should consider the whole question of (3) *allocative principles for those on a waiting list*. Thus, we are faced with three steps: (1) who gets referred for consideration of transplant; (2) who, from among those referred for transplant assessment, goes on the waiting list; and (3) how decisions are then made when allocating a particular cadaveric organ.

Many factors determine who gets on a waiting list. Essentially, it is an interaction between *referring sources* (largely physicians) and *the program gatekeepers* (largely transplant physicians), who then also may play the role of *cadaveric organ allocation decision-makers*. One of the objectives for this chapter is to examine these physician processes for their ethical probity,* but before such aspects are considered, it is necessary to look at the question of health care entitlement.

## Health Care Entitlement

Entitlement is determined by the philosophic and ethical foundations of each health care system. In those that are largely underwritten by a single-payer insurance, based on universal equity of entitlement to health care, every-

*As a former allocative decision-maker, I observed some years ago that the age of acceptance for the transplant waiting list bore a direct relation to the increasing age of the transplant program directors.

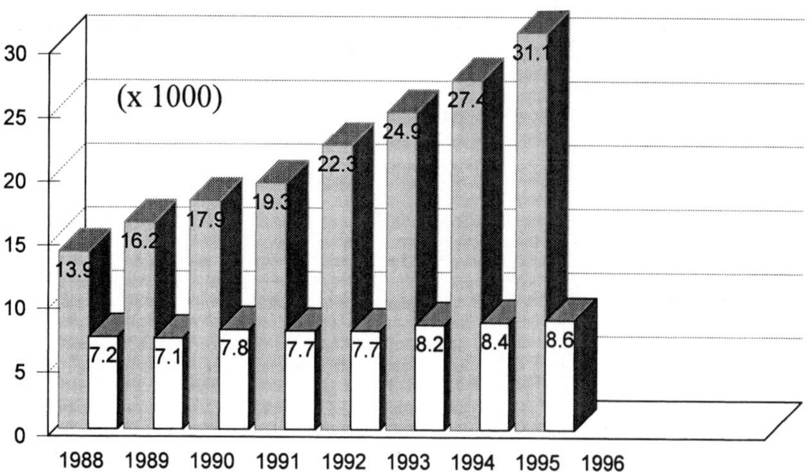


FIGURE 67.1. The widening gap between "supply" of cadaveric kidneys for tranplantation in the United States and the "demand" for the same resource on dialysis programs. (From UNOS,[1] with permission.)

one is entitled regardless of discrimination on the basis of age, sex, race, or social worthiness. Thus, there is universal entitlement* of the elderly in Canada[4] and the United States through the Medicare program. Does this entitlement include all vital organ transplants? In the United States it does not. In Canada, it does include all forms of transplant; but having the entitlement still does not mean that aged recipients will receive transplants, as their needs still must compete with those of younger potential recipients for a scarce, valuable resource. Even with full entitlement, allocative decision-making may exclude the elderly from being placed on the waiting list and from fair opportunity for an organ when on the waiting list. It is these two aspects that must be carefully examined.

There is literature that considers placing certain limits on the entitlement of the elderly to certain forms of "high-tech" medical care. Callahan[5] outlined a philosophic argument based on the natural "biographic narrative" of a life-largely-lived, which as it nears the end, benefits more from *care* measures than *cure* measures, especially in respect to high-tech procedures such as vital organ transplants. He saw acceptance by the elderly of this different philosophic approach as feeding the concept of "intergenerational" justice. However, he did not make clear how the elderly could be led to make these reorientations away from curative interventions; and few can support his tentative suggestion that the elderly should, past a certain age (when they can be considered as having entered the category of the "old, old") must lose high-tech medical entitlement by societal necessity. Although the elderly still have full entitlement to health care and have the most need of it, especially during the last year or so of their lives, there is growing concern that they may not be able to hold on to this entitlement in the future.[6]

## Stages in Access to Transplant Services

Access to transplant services is complicated. The situation is summarized in Figure 67.2. First, what factors determine who is referred for assessment?

There have been instances in the past where the perception ("They surely will never consider anyone of this age or with these co-morbidities") is out of keeping with the contemporary success. This was certainly the case for referral of individuals to nephrologists for dialysis in prior decades, with respect to renal failure caused by diabetes mellitus [7.8% of accepted new end-stage renal disease (ESRD) cases in Canada in 1981 but up to 26.4% of accepted new ESRD cases by 1993[7]] and for those over 65 years of age (23% of accepted new cases in Canada in 1981 but up to 41% by 1993[8]).

There are indications that some dialysis programs, especially those not closely associated with transplant programs, refer fewer patients for transplant assessment than those that are associated. The factors at work here are not known for sure. It has been suggested that some units do not want to lose the patient from the collectivity of the dialysis unit ("trapped in a culture of dialysis"). Some dialysis physicians may believe that they can make as good a judgment of transplant outcome efficacy as those responsible for formal assessment by a transplant team; but they may not be sufficiently informed on transplant outcomes, especially for certain groups such as the elderly.

In the case of kidney transplant, which often involves referral of someone who is doing reasonably well on dialysis, there have been instances where the judgment to refer could be negatively influenced by the fact that the referring physician loses income by so doing. Such failure to refer may not be a conscious decision but, rather, a belief that it is futile and contrary to the individual

*Health care entitlement in Canada is not, in fact, legislated as such. Individuals have entitlement to "medically necessary" insured procedures in hospital under the single-payer insurance system controlled by the Canada Health Act of 1984.

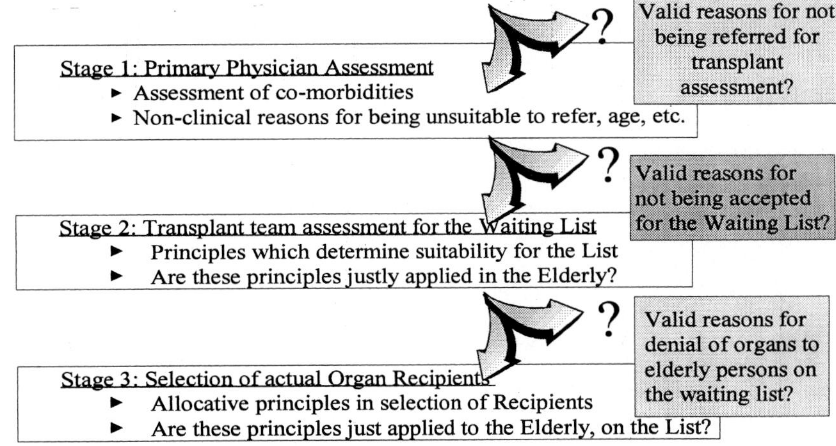


FIGURE 67.2. Three stages of accessing transplantation services.

patient's "best interests" and sometimes ignorance of transplant outcome statistics.

At the second stage—selection for the list after being referred for assessment—there are additional ethical dilemmas; here too, age and co-morbidities play a discriminatory role. The question must be asked: Are these discriminations just? Are people denied opportunity on the basis of the just application of "maximizing the medical outcomes" (efficacy) or the unjust application of "social worth" factors, physician value systems, or ageism?

The ethical safeguard is to offer assessment by a transplant program to everyone in potential need. It is also highly to be desired that the steps outlined in Figure 67.2 are not carried out by separate units but integrated into a process and suitably coordinated, where referral doctors, dialysis physicians, cardiologists, and transplant teams work together. Helderman has reported such a process,[9] illustrated in Figure 67.3. At all stages it is appropriate to ask if the reasons for restricting access of elderly persons to transplantation is based on valid criteria. Even if they are—because such criteria always reflect actual outcomes—they should be reexamined regularly to see if they remain appropriate. The outcome facts may have changed.

Once on the waiting list, the principles listed in Table 67.1 are used to select the recipient for a gifted cadaveric organ, be it a kidney, heart, or liver. Here the selection is made by the members of the transplant team, often the same group who place people on the waiting list.

There is a tendency for kidney transplant teams to wait for the optimal HLA match, and they use HLA compatibility as an important factor in "maximizing the medical benefit" (principle 4 in Table 67.1), though others have described it as an "ethical crutch." For vital organs other than kidney, this criterion is much less used often for several reasons: There is no evidence that it is crucial to intermediate-term survival and there is an absence of the competing benefit dialysis gives to potential kidney recipients, making the urgency of need or rescue (principle 1 of Table 67.1) a much more important factor. All programs may use such factors of "chance" (principle 8 in Table 67.1) as "time on the waiting list" and "distance

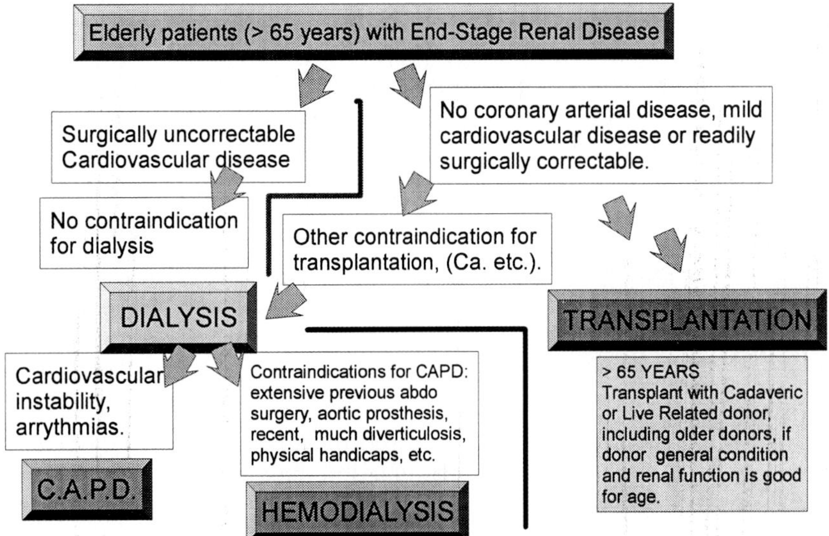


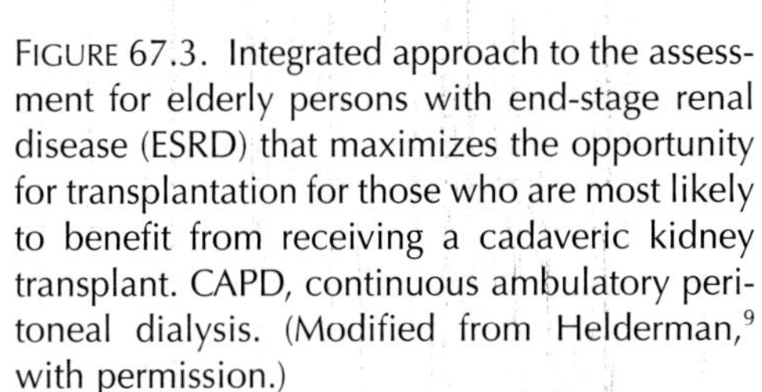
FIGURE 67.3. Integrated approach to the assessment for elderly persons with end-stage renal disease (ESRD) that maximizes the opportunity for transplantation for those who are most likely to benefit from receiving a cadaveric kidney transplant. CAPD, continuous ambulatory peritoneal dialysis. (Modified from Helderman,[9] with permission.)

TABLE 67.1. Principles for Allocation of Resources and the Ethics Theory to Which They Are Related

| Principle applied | Ethics theory |
|---|---|
| 1. Principle of RESCUE | Deontology |
| 2. Fiduciary obligations to others (patients) | |
| 3. Using equity of need—not able to pay | |
| 4. Optimizing the medical outcome | Utilitarianism |
| a. Importance of HLA matching | |
| b. Absence of co-morbidities | |
| 5. Considering the good of the transplant program | |
| 6. Ability to pay, directly or through insurance | Libertarianism |
| 7. Social merit or worth (good life styles, good compliance with regimens | |
| 8. Element of chance ("the lottery of life") | Pragmatic |
| a. Time on the waiting list—"first come, first served" | Egalitarianism |
| 9. Priority based on past injustice | Restorative justice |
| 10. Ethically flawed principles | Ethically unacceptable |
| a. Nepotism, favoritism | |
| b. Inappropriate concept of fiduciary duty | |
| c. "Squeaky wheel" | |
| d. Unfair use of the media | |

from the center" to compensate for injustice which may creep in from such factors as having a rare HLA profile (for those waiting on dialysis) or difficulty meeting the urgency of some situations (for those who live far away). Age is not used as a discriminatory factor in stage 3, as it has usually played a decisive role in stages 1 and 2, though elderly patients on the list are more likely to receive organs from old donors.

## Expecting Clear Answers to Ethical Dilemmas, Leading to Frustration

Allocative dilemmas (except when the flawed principles are applied) depend on a balance (or clash) of perfectly legitimate value systems. It therefore follows that there is no right way to resolve allocation problems. This point must be stressed. It is also the reason, apart from the facts changing (as mentioned above), allocative policies must be reviewed repeatedly and be open to question by those affected by them and by society at large in the hope of reaching consensus by all concerned. It is appropriate to consider old recipients, or representatives of senior groups, among those who are "concerned," as these policy decisions are "societal" as well as "medical."

## Do Transplant Programs Discriminate Against the Elderly?

Transplant programs probably do discriminate against the elderly. However, for the factors noted in the preceding section, there may be defensible reasons for claiming that what seems like discrimination is, in fact, a different balance of ethically valid allocative principles. Instead of regarding the elderly as less worthy from a social point of view (principle 7 in Table 67.1), most would regard selection against the elderly as the use of an arbitrary and convenient surrogate factor for principle 4 in Table 67.1, especially factor 4b (optimization of medical outcome because of co-morbidities).

As difficult selection decisions are inevitable, even among those judged suitable for the waiting list, it may be ethically legitimate to decrease the number of those who have to be individually assessed by using arbitrary methods to "limit the field." One such arbitrary factor is age. It is often used as a surrogate for "significant co-morbidities." Such prejudgments could be defended if the transplant outcome results supported the belief that the elderly have such poor transplant outcomes that principle 4 justifies not offering them transplants. However, the data do not support this conclusion. Much preferable, however, is the sort of triage approach outlined in Figure 67.3; judiciously applied coronary artery bypass surgery, for example, might make an elderly dialysis patient a suitable transplant candidate.

## Kidney Transplant Outcomes in the Elderly

Results of kidney transplants obtained over more than a decade show there is a clear difference in outcomes, which is attributed to the advent of cyclosporin A as an immunosuppressive agent. The results presented in Table 67.2 are derived from a full review and meta-analysis by Ismail et al.[10] They compare graft and patient survival for those under 60 years of age with those over that age. The data provide 3-year actuarial outcomes. Table 67.2 includes three reports from before the cyclosporin era,[11–13] four more from the mid- to late 1980s,[14–17] and five reports from the 1990s.[18–22] It is evident that (1) cyclosporin made a significant difference, and (2) the gap between outcomes in the two age groups has gradually closed (as judged at 3 years).

Examination of results from one particular center—those from Albrechtsen et al.[21] in Norway—are shown (redrawn, with permission, in Figure 67.4 for ease of comparison). The two dark graphed lines represent graft survival and patient survival for those over 70 years of age. Few of those who lost their grafts were successfully reestablished on dialysis; indeed most of those who died had functioning grafts. They died from factors other than graft loss in the main. The two "stepped" graph lines represent patient survival (above) and graft survival (below) for those 55–70 years of age. In the younger group, there may be a tendency for more graft loss during the first 24 months, with some being reestablished on dialysis. There are no significant differences between these four graphs.

TABLE 67.2. Three-year actuarial outcomes, patient and kidney graft survival, for two groups of transplant patients: >60 years of age and <60 years of age. Cyclosporine (CYA) was introduced as an immunosuppressive agent prior to the studies during 1986–1995.

| | 1980 | | | | 1986 | 1988 | 1989 | | 1991 | 1992 | 1994 | 1995 | |
|---|---|---|---|---|---|---|---|---|---|---|---|---|---|
| Survival | 11 | 12 | 13 | CYA | 14 | 15 | 16 | 17 | 18 | 19 | 20 | 21 | 22 |
| Recipients >60 years of age | | | | | | | | | | | | | |
| % Patient survival | 50 | 35 | 60 | C | 65 | 66 | 91 | 61 | 59 | 89 | 86 | 72 | 90 |
| % Graft survival | 50 | 35 | 49 | Y | 56 | 59 | 74 | 54 | 57 | 71 | 68 | 64 | 81 |
| Recipients <60 years of age | | | | | | | | | | | | | |
| % Patient survival | | | | – | 78 | | | | 85 | | 90 | – | 96 |
| % Graft survival | | | | A | 78 | | | | 62 | | 84 | – | 81 |

The numbers under the years are the references from which the data were derived.

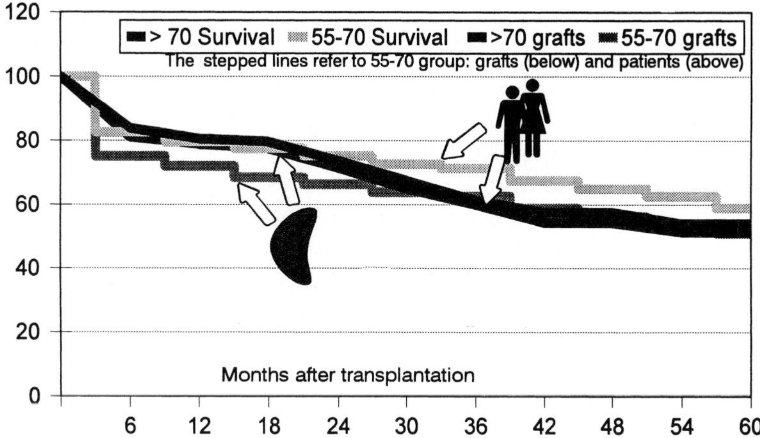


FIGURE 67.4. Comparison of patient and graft survival for 5 years after transplantion of two age groups of patients: those aged 55–70 (stepped lines) compared with those over 70 years of age. (Data from Albrechtsen et al.,[20] with permission)

## What Factors Are Valid for Assessing Outcomes in the Elderly?

There are important aspects when assessing outcomes other than graft and patient survival. Some of these are listed as questions in Table 67.3. Some evidence suggests that the elderly require less immune suppression because their immune systems respond less vigorously to allogeneic grafts. However, it is clear that they are more likely to have co-morbidities, though not necessarily more than a similar age cohort on dialysis. The real question is the most difficult: Is their quality of life improved sufficiently, in comparison with that of a younger group, to justify using a precious and increasingly scarce resource? Many are beginning to say "yes," which calls into question the ethical status of statistics from the United Network for Organ Sharing (UNOS).[1] Their data show that during 1988–1995 only 5.8% of cadaveric kidney in the United States were given to patients 65 years of age or older (who constitute 33.7% of those in ESRD programs[23]), whereas 37% of such kidneys were given to patients 45–64 years of age (who constitute 38% of those in ESRD programs). The 2-year and 3-year patient and graft survivals of the former compare favorably with outcomes with those 45–64 years of age, as shown in Table 67.4.

It is acknowledged that those transplanted in the older group may be a specifically selected subgroup, and the good outcomes reflect this bias. It is equally possible that a few centers have policies that offer patients over 65

TABLE 67.3. Kidney Transplant Outcomes: Assessment of Benefit in the Elderly

The following factors are relevant when assessing benefit:
- Overall quality of life, in comparison to alternative treatment, such as dialysis
- Recipient survival, compared to age-matched cohort of general population
- Recipient survival, compared to a younger cohort with failure of same vital organ
- Recipient survival, in comparison to alternative treatment, such as dialysis
- Graft survival (years), in comparison with a younger cohort
- Requirement for immune-suppressive therapy, compared to a younger cohort
- Complications of immune suppressive therapy, compared with a younger cohort
- Complications due to increased prevalence of co-morbidities in the elderly
- Cost-benefit assessment, compared with a younger cohort
- Cost-benefit assessment, compared with a same-age cohort on dialysis
- Quality adjusted life years (QALYs) provided in comparison with alternative treatment

TABLE 67.4. Comparison of Posttransplant Survival of Patients and Cadaver Kidney Grafts in Two Age Groups of Patients with End Stage Renal Disease

| | | % Survival | | |
|---|---|---|---|---|
| % of ESRD population | Patient and kidney graft | 2 Years after transplantation, | 3 Years after transplantation | % Recipients of cadaver kidneys |
| Patients >65 years of age | | | | |
| 33.7 | Patient | 81 | 74 | **5.8** |
| | Graft | 72 | 65 | |
| Patients 50–64 years of age | | | | |
| 38.0 | Patient | 86 | 82 | **37** |
| | Survival | 75 | 70 | |

*Sources:* UNOS 1996 Annual Report[1] and USRDS.[23]

These posttransplant results are contrasted with (1) the proportion of ESRD patients in these two age-groups, and (2) the proportion of cadaver kidneys given to them.

It is acknowledged that those in the >65 group of graft recipients may be specifically selected, and the outcomes might not be as close to the younger cohort if a proportion of more than 5.8% of cadaver kidneys had been given to them.

years of age an equal opportunity for a graft, but most do not. Can this second type of policy be just, in view of the overall shorter life expectancy of the older group owing to co-morbidities, or is it age discrimination? The question is one that can be answered only at the local level and for each vital organ transplant program individually.

## References


1. UNOS Annual Report. Transplant Data: 1988–1995. Washington, DC: US Department of Health and Human Services, 1996.
2. Truog RD. Is it time to abandon brain death? Hastings Center Rep 1997;27:29–37
3. Arnold RM, Youngner SJ. Time is of the essence: the pressing need for comprehensive non-heart-beating cadaveric donation policies. Transplant Proc 1995;27:2913–2921.
4. Fraser RC. What Has the Law Got to Do with It: Health Care Reform in Canada. Ottawa: Canadian Bar Association Task Force Report, 1994.
5. Callahan D. Setting Limits. Medical Goals in an Aging Society. New York: Simon & Schuster, 1987.
6. Barry RL, Bradley GV. Eds. "Set No Limits: A Rebuttal to Callahan's Proposal to Limit Health Care for the Elderly." Urbana, IL: University of Illinois Press, 1991.
7. Canadian Organ Replacement Register. 1993 Report. March 1995:Table 93.
8. Canadian Organ Replacement Register. 1993 Report. March 1995:Table 28.
9. Helderman JH. Transplantation and the elderly [editorial comments]. Nephrol Dial Transplant 1995;10:773–774.
10. Ismail N, Hakim R, Helderman JH. Renal replacement therapies in the elderly. Part 2. Renal transplantation. Am J Kidney Dis 1994;23:1–15.
11. Kock B, Kuhlback B, Ahonen J. Kidney transplantation in patients over 60 years of age. Scand J Urol Nephrol 1980; 54(suppl):203–205.
12. Wedel N, Brynger H, Blohme I. Kidney transplantation in patients 60 years of age. Scand J Urol Nephrol 1980; 54(suppl):106–108.
13. Ost L, Groth CG, Lindholm B, et al. Cadaveric renal transplantation in patients of 60 years of age. Scand J Urol Nephrol 1980;54(suppl):339–340.
14. Cardella CJ, Harding ME, Abraham G, et al. Renal transplantation in older patients on peritoneal dialysis. Transplant Proc 1986;21:2022–2023.
15. Fauchald P, Albrechtsen D, Leivestad T, et al. Renal replacement therapy in patients over 60 years of age. Transplant Proc 1988;20:432–433.
16. Pirsch JD, Stratta RH, Armbrust NJ, et al. Cadaveric renal transplantation with cyclosporin in patients more than 65 years old or older. Transplantation 1989;47:259–261.
17. Fehrman I, Brattstrom C, Duraj F, et al. Kidney transplantation in patients between 65 and 75 years of age. Transplant Proc 1989;21:1749–1752.
18. Morris GE, Jamieson NV, Small J, et al. Cadaveric renal transplantation in elderly recipients: is it worthwhile? Nephrol Dial Transplant 1991;6:877–892
19. Vivas CA, Hickey DP, Jordan ML, et al. Renal transplantation in patients 65 years old or older. J Urol 1992;147:990–993.
20. Tesi RJ, Elkhammas EA, Davies EA, et al. Renal transplantation in older people. Lancet 1994;343:461–464.
21. Albrechtsen D, Leivestad T, Sodal G, et al. Kidney transplantation in patients older than 70 years of age. Transplant Proc 1995;27:986–988.
22. Mourad G, Cristol JP, Vela C, et al. Cadaveric renal transplantation in patients 60 years of age and older: experience with 58 patients in a single centre. Nephrol Dial Tranplant 1995;10(supple 6):105–107.
23. US Renal Data System (USRDS) 1997 Annual Data Report (Table II-1). Bethesda: National Institute of Diabetes and Digestive and Kidney Diseases.

# 68
# Transplantation in Elderly Patients

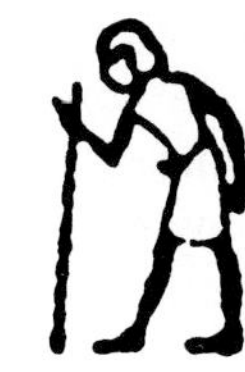

Sandy Feng, Stephen L. Tomlanovich, Fraser Keith, and Nancy L. Ascher

As the United States population ages and as results of transplantation improve, there are increasing numbers of older patients who avail themselves of transplantation. As a consequence, the percentage of older waiting list individuals has been increasing.

In 1988, about 23.5% of the 14,000 kidney waiting list patients were aged 50–64 years and 2.9% were more than 65 years of age. In 1995, there were 31,000 patients awaiting kidney transplantation, and 38.3% were older than 50 years. Similarly, for patients awaiting liver transplantation, the number of all patients increased 10-fold from 1988 to 1995; the percentage of older patients has doubled, so the absolute number of patients over age 50 years awaiting liver transplantation has increased 20-fold. The absolute number of older patients awaiting lung transplantation has increased 40-fold. Only in those patients awaiting heart transplantation has the percentage of older patients not increased. Because the overall number of patients awaiting heart transplantation has increased more than threefold, the absolute number of older patients awaiting heart transplantation has also increased threefold. Similarly, the number and percentage of older patients who undergo solid organ transplantation increased from 1988 to 1995. Both the percentage and absolute number of older patients undergoing liver and lung transplantation has increased significantly. For kidney and heart recipients the percentage of older patients has not increased, but the absolute number of older patients reflect the increased numbers of transplants performed.

Interestingly, although the percentage of older patients who died awaiting solid organ transplantation did not change from 1988 to 1995, the absolute numbers of patients and older patients who die awaiting transplantation has increased. These data indicate that more older patients are availing themselves of solid organ transplantation and that the medical condition of the older patients who are listed for transplantation is similar to that of the younger patient in terms of risk of dying while awaiting transplantation. Given the large number of older patients who undergo transplantation and who are awaiting transplantation, it is appropriate to evaluate results after transplantation for this group of patients to determine whether results are comparable to that of younger patients and what modifications should be made in their treatment to optimize the results.

## Kidney Transplantation

Elderly patients represent the age group with the steepest rising incidence and prevalence of end-stage renal disease (ESRD) from the early 1980s to the present. According to the United States Renal Data System, patients ≥60 years of age represented 39% of the dialysis population in the United States in 1981 and 51% of the dialysis population in 1990.[1] It was estimated that by the year 2000 more than 60% of the dialysis population in the United States would be 60 years or older.[2] In 1990 patients ≥65 years of age represented more than two-thirds of all new patients receiving treatment for ESRD. These trends highlight the importance of determining the relative efficacy of the two main therapeutic modalities, dialysis versus transplantation, to treat ESRD in the elderly population.

Parallel to the rise of ESRD has been the rise of renal transplantation in the elderly population. In the United States, the United Network for Organ Sharing (UNOS) has reported that patients over age 65 years comprised only 2.8% of all patients in 1988 compared to 5.8% in 1995. In Spain, there has been a similarly dramatic increase in the percentage of renal transplants performed in older patients. Patients over 55 years of age comprised 8.0% of the transplant population in 1984 compared to 34.7% in 1995.[3] In Canada, whereas only one kidney transplant was performed in a patient older than 60 years in 1981, there were 116 performed in patients over 60 years in 1991.[4] Although more transplants are being performed in older patients, most older patients with ESRD are still being treated with dialysis. Compared to younger patients with ESRD, older patients have a significantly lower rate of renal transplantation.[5–7] There are multiple reasons for this inequality.

Cadaver donors rather than living donors remain the predominant source of kidneys for transplantation. In 1990 of the kidneys transplanted 77.6% were cadaveric allografts and 22.4% were living allografts.[1] As with all of the solid organ transplants discussed here, there is a marked disparity between the supply of and the demand for kidneys for transplantation. The total incidence and prevalence of ESRD continue to rise, whereas the number of yearly renal allografts has plateaued since the mid-1980s.[1] Therefore the percentage of ESRD patients undergoing transplantation has actually decreased from around 6.0% during the years 1982–1986 to around 4.7% in 1989 and 1990. The disparity between supply and demand is even worse in the elderly population. Few elderly patients undergo living donor transplantation, as they often lack appropriate donors.

In an effort to optimize the use of available cadaveric kidneys, transplantation historically has been somewhat restricted to younger patients, who were considered better able to tolerate both the procedure and the immune suppression and to derive maximal benefit from an improved quality of life. This practice was supported by three reports in 1980 of poor 1-year patient and graft survival in the elderly, averaging 62% and 57%, respectively—significantly worse than that observed in younger patients.[8–10] The introduction of cyclosporine (CYA) use dramatically changed the risk/benefit analysis for transplantation in older patients. During the late 1980s, multiple institutions reported patient and graft survival statistics for elderly patients that were essentially equivalent to those for younger patients.[10–12] Successful programs chose their elderly transplant candidates with care, often establishing protocols for preoperative evaluation and criteria for exclusion. Therefore, by the late 1980s, potential transplant candidates were no longer judged primarily by chronologic age but by biologic age, which the evaluation process was designed to determine.

Simultaneous with the realization that transplantation can be safely performed in carefully selected elderly patients, was the validation of transplantation as an appropriate therapeutic option for elderly patients with ESRD. Kidney transplantation is unique among the solid organ transplants discussed in this chapter in that it is not a life-saving procedure. Dialysis is available as an alternative treatment modality. Several studies have tried to compare the efficacy of transplantation and dialysis with particular regard to mortality for the treatment of ESRD in the elderly. Early reports in 1981 and 1982, indicated inferior survival probability for elderly patients who received transplantation compared to dialysis.[13,14] As results of renal transplantation improved during the early to mid-1980s, studies began to report comparable survivals for transplantation and dialysis.[15–19]

During the 1990s, well-controlled population-based studies indicated that the results of transplantation are superior to that of dialysis in elderly patients. In 1995, the University of Manitoba and University of Toronto using data from the Canadian Organ Replacement Registry, examined the outcome of 6400 patients who registered to initiate treatment for ESRD between 1987 and 1993 and who were 60 years or older at the time. Transplant recipients were matched by age, etiology of renal disease, and number of co-morbid conditions to two randomly selected patients who did not undergo transplantation. Using Cox regression analysis, the time-dependent hazards ratio for kidney transplantation was estimated at 0.47 [95% confidence interval (CI) 0.33–0.67] indicating a statistically significant ($p < 0.001$) decrease in the probability of death among patients who received a renal transplant.[4] A subanalysis was performed where each transplant patient was randomly matched to a dialysis patient as before but with the additional constraint that the dialysis patient had to have at least as much follow-up time as the transplant recipient's waiting time. The calculated 5-year survival probabilities were 81% for transplant recipients compared to 51% for dialysis recipients, another highly statistically significant ($p = 0.001$) survival difference.

Similarly, the Catalan Health Service, using the Renal Patient Registry of Catalonia, examined the results of ESRD therapy in patients between 55 and 70 years of age who initiated treatment between 1984 and 1993.[3] Instead of matching for co-morbidities, this study limited its analysis to patients who fulfilled selection criteria and were accepted for transplantation, comparing those who did or did not undergo transplantation. The mean age of the hemodialysis group was lower ($p = 0.04$) than that of the transplanted group: 60.8 versus 61.6 years. Survival of the transplant patients was superior from the second year onward, although initial mortality was higher in transplant versus dialysis patients as a result of perioperative complications. Finally, analysis of all patients alive on December 31, 1993, revealed that, based on the Karnovsky index modified for renal disease by Gutman, transplant patients had significantly higher functional autonomy than dialysis patients ($p = 0.0002$).

During the past 15 years, transplantation has been validated as a safe, appropriate method to treat ESRD in a selected subset of elderly patients. We discuss in some detail the University of California, San Francisco (UCSF) experience with renal transplantation in patients over 60 years of age in the context of reports from other programs worldwide.

## Patient Selection and Demographics

All patients are evaluated by a complete history, physical examination, and laboratory tests. Baseline age-appropriate screening tests such as breast examination and mammography, gynecologic examination and Papanicolaou smear, prostate examination and prostate-specific antigen (PSA) assay, and stool guiaic testing are mandatory elements of the evaluation process. Serologic studies for cytomegalovirus (CMV), hepatitis B and C viruses (HBV, HCV), human T cell leukemia virus (HTLV-1), and human immunodeficiency virus (HIV) are routine. Patients who are positive for hepatitis B surface antigen (HBsAg) or antibodies to HCV were screened with liver function tests and, in most cases, abdominal ultrasonography. If either of these tests was abnormal, a liver biopsy was obtained. The patients were denied transplantation if the biopsy demonstrated active hepatitis or cirrhosis.

A critical aspect of the evaluation process, particularly for elderly patients, is assessment of cardiac risk. It has been well known for years that cardiovascular disease is a major cause of morbidity and mortality in all patients with ESRD.[20] At UCSF most patients over age 60 years underwent a complete preoperative cardiac evaluation within 2 years of transplantation. Patients were excluded from transplantation only after consultation with a cardiologist regarding significant, uncorrectable ischemic disease or severely diminished left ventricular function. The same algorithm for cardiac evaluation was applied to younger patients with signs or symptoms of cardiac disease and to all patients with diabetes. For all potential transplant candidates, investigation of other organ systems for significant dysfunction was driven by signs or symptoms elucidated by history, physical examination, or mandatory screening tests.

During the 5-year period between January 1, 1992 and December 31, 1996, a total of 888 kidney transplants were performed at UCSF in patients over 18 years of age, excluding those with an additional solid organ transplant such as simultaneous kidney–pancreas, kidney–liver, and kidney–heart transplants. Of these 888 transplants, 94 were performed in 93 patients more than 60 years of age. The UCSF experience represents one of the largest reports on transplantation in an elderly population within a study period of less than 10 years. The demographics for the study and comparison groups are shown in Table 68.1.

The 94 transplants performed in patients over 60 years of age represent 10.6% of the transplants performed in adults at UCSF within the 5-year study period. The percentage of older patients undergoing transplantation remained constant from year to year during the 5-year study period and was remarkably similar to that of other centers within the United States.[21–23] Although the European average of 10.2% is commensurate with that of American centers, there is considerable variability among European countries. The European Dialysis and Transplant Association–European Renal Association (EDTA-ERA) reported in 1992 that the proportion of grafts performed in patients ≥60 years ranged from 2% in Poland and Italy, to 16% in the United Kingdom, to 19% in Switzerland.[24]

TABLE 68.1. Demographics of Patients Undergoing Renal Transplantation at UCSF: January 1, 1992 to December 31, 1996

| Parameter | >60 Years ($n$ = 93) | >18 and <60 Years ($n$ = 795) |
|---|---|---|
| Age (years) | | |
| Median | 64.23 | 40.23 |
| Mean | 64.92 | 39.73 |
| Range | 60.02–77.34 | 18.08–59.64 |
| Sex | | |
| Male | 63 (67.7%) | 440 (55.3%) |
| Female | 30 (32.3%) | 355 (44.7%) |
| Kidney source | | |
| Cadaveric | 77 (81.9%) | 554 (69.7%) |
| Living | 17 (18.1%) | 241 (30.3%) |
| Indication | | |
| Hypertension/ nephrosclerosis | 25 (26.9%) | 67 (8.4%) |
| Diabetes mellitus | 19 (20.4%) | 119 (15.0%) |
| Polycystic kidney disease | 17 (18.3%) | 52 (6.5%) |
| Glomerulonephritides | 16 (17.2%) | 232 (29.2%) |
| Pyelonephritis | 1 (1.1%) | 21 (2.6%) |
| Lupus nephritis | 0 | 50 (6.3%) |
| Congenital urologic disorders | 0 | 33 (4.2%) |
| Hereditary nephritis | 0 | 12 (1.5%) |
| Other/unknown | 15 (16.1%) | 209 (26.3%) |
| Follow-up (months) | | |
| Mean | 28 | 35 |
| Median | 27 | 35 |
| Range | 8–67 | 1–67 |

There are some differences between the study group of older patients and the comparison group of younger patients in the UCSF experience. The older group had a larger proportion of male patients. Older patients had a higher incidence of hypertension/nephrosclerosis, polycystic kidney disease, and diabetes mellitus and a lower incidence of glomerulonephritides and congenital urologic disorders as the etiology of their renal failure. Similar differences were reported by other programs.[22,25] A smaller proportion of older patients received live donor grafts: 18.1% versus 30.3%. There are several reasons for this disparity. Older recipients tend to present with fewer candidates for living donation. Their parents, siblings, spouses, and friends are usually older than those of younger patients, and therefore a higher percentage prove to be medically unsuitable for donation. Parents are frequently reluctant to accept organs from their children. Finally, polycystic kidney disease causes a significant proportion of ESRD in the elderly population, and its familial nature eliminates many family members from

TABLE 68.2. Co-morbidities Identified in Patients >60 Years Undergoing Renal Transplantation at UCSF (1992–1996) ($n$ = 93)

| Co-morbidity | No. |
|---|---|
| Cardiac | |
| S/P CABG | 10 |
| S/P PTCA | 6 |
| S/P AVR | 1 |
| H/O arrhythmias | 6 |
| H/O pericarditis | 3 |
| Decreased left ventricular function (EF < 40%) | 3 |
| H/O cardiac arrest | 1 |
| Vascular | 6 |
| Respiratory | |
| COPD | 2 |
| Asthma | 3 |
| TB/PPD$^+$ | 4 |
| Gastrointestinal | |
| H/O UGIB/PUD | 7 |
| H/O diverticulitis | 5 |
| Hepatitis B (HBsAg$^+$) | 4 |
| Hepatitis C (Hep CAb$^+$) | 7 |
| H/O colon cancer | 1 |
| Crohn's disease | 2 |
| Other | 5 |
| Endocrine (diabetes mellitus) | 22 |
| Neurologic | 9 |
| Oncologic | |
| Skin | 6 |
| Prostate | 2 |
| Breast | 1 |
| Cervical | 1 |
| Rectal | 1 |
| Renal | 1 |

S/P, postoperative status; CABG, coronary artery bypass graft; PTCA, percutaneous transluminal coronary angioplasty; AVR, aortic valve replacement; H/O, history of; EF, ejection fraction; COPD, chronic obstructive pulmonary disease; TB/PPD$^+$, tuberculosis/purified protein derivative-positive; UGIB/PUD, upper gastrointestinal bleed/peptic ulcer disease; HBsAg$^+$, hepatitis B surface antigen-positive; HCV$^+$, hepatitis C virus-positive.

consideration as potential donors. Two other American institutions have reported the breakdown of cadaveric and living donor transplants in their experience and similarly found that older patients received fewer living donor grafts. Whereas Ohio State University reported percentages essentially identical to those of UCSF, the University of Minnesota reported 29.6% compared to 51.9% of living donor grafts for older and younger patients, respectively.[21,22] The EDTA-ERA reported that living donation is rare in Europe with the notable exception of Norway, where 47% of patients >60 years underwent living donor renal transplantation.[24]

Table 68.2 lists the major co-morbidities identified in patients over 60 years of age who underwent renal transplantation at UCSF during the 5-year study period. Of the 93 patients, 25 (26.9%) had the cardiac co-morbidities listed in Table 68.2. Fourteen patients had definite and significant coronary artery disease, as evidenced by a history of coronary bypass or angioplasty. An additional 11 patients had abnormal stress tests and underwent coronary angiography; 10 of the 11 were found to have no, minimal, or mild coronary disease; only one patient was found to have significant coronary disease but intervention was not recommended. Six patients had clearly documented histories of atrial arrhythmias, supraventricular tachycardias, or ventricular arrhythmias; and one patient had an automatic defibrillator implanted. Three patients accepted for transplantation had abnormally depressed ejection fraction ranging from 25% to 40%. Other institutions have described similar algorithms for pretransplant assessment of cardiac risk.[4,22,23,25,26] Most published studies, however, provide no detailed information on the criteria used to decide the suitability of an elderly patient for renal transplantation or the cardiac profile of their elderly transplant patients.

Several co-morbidities identified in noncardiac systems in elderly patients undergoing renal transplantation at UCSF are worthy of note. First, only two elderly patients (2.2%) had significant chronic obstructive pulmonary disease (COPD), showing a moderate obstructive defect on pulmonary function tests. Six patients (6.5%) had significant vascular disease, with three patients having undergone intervention for renal artery stenosis and three having had surgical correction of significant vascular disease including abdominal aortic aneurysm or limb-threatening ischemia. Eleven patients (11.8%) were positive for hepatitis: four were positive for hepatitis B and seven for hepatitis C. Diabetes was the indication for transplantation in 19 patients and was present in only 3 additional patients. Nine patients (9.7%) had a significant neurologic history defined as either seizure disorder or documented cerebrovascular accident.

## Details of Transplantation, Immune Suppression, Infection Prophylaxis, and Rejection Surveillance

All patients undergoing renal transplantation at UCSF received blood group-compatible kidneys with a negative lymphocytotoxic cross-match on current sera. There was no matching for HLA antigens except for the use of the six-antigen match and zero mismatch kidneys, as distributed by UNOS. There were no preoperative donor-specific transfusions.

Immune suppression for 45 of the 94 (47.9%) transplants was initiated with an anti-lymphocytic preparation. Thirty-two patients (34%) received Minnesota anti-lymphocyte globulin (MALG) or anti-thymocyte globulin (ATG) for a mean course of 7.97 days (median 7 days, range 1–17 days). Nine patients (9.6%) received OKT3 for a mean course of 8.56 days (median 7 days, range 6–13 days). Four patients (4.2%) received anti-interleukin-2 (anti-IL2) receptor antibody (daclizumab) as part of the phase 1 or the phase 3 study. The remaining 49 (of the 94) transplants (52.1%) were performed without cytolytic induction therapy. Sequential therapy was the primary strategy for 84% (28/33) of the transplants performed during 1992–1993 compared to 39% (23 of 59) of transplants performed during 1994–1996.

All patients received methylprednisolone intravenously at the beginning of the transplant procedure. Subsequently, prednisone was administered in tapering doses. CYA was a component of the maintenance immune-suppression regimen for 86 of the 94 transplants (91.4%) performed in elderly patients during the study period. Tacrolimus was used for seven transplants (7.4%). Four of the seven patients were enrolled in a range-finding trial of tacrolimus in primary kidney transplantation; one of the seven patients was undergoing a second transplant; one was undergoing a living unrelated transplant; and one was switched to tacrolimus during the immediate perioperative period secondary to an adverse reaction to CYA.

Azathioprine (AZA) was the predominant antimetabolite used from 1992 to 1995. Midway through 1996 there was a switch to mycophenylate mofetil (MMF) as the third agent of maintenance immune suppression. A summary of the maintenance immune suppression initiated for the 94 transplants in elderly patients is shown in Table 68.3.

During the study period and usually in conjunction with treatment of a rejection episode, seven patients were switched from CYA to tacrolimus, and 12 patients were switched from AZA to MMF. Currently, of the 64 patients who have a functioning kidney transplant, 46 (71.9%) remain on triple maintenance therapy, and 18 (28.1%) are stable on double therapy after discontinuation of AZA or, in one case, MMF but remaining on prednisone and CYA or tacrolimus.

The immune suppression regimens used by other institutions that have recently (since 1992) reported their experience with transplantation in elderly patients is somewhat variable. Four programs routinely employed cytolytic induction therapy and maintenance immune suppression with prednisone, CYA, and AZA.[4,20,24,25]

TABLE 68.3. Maintenance Immunosuppression Initiated in Patients >60 Years of Age after Kidney Transplantation at UCSF (1992–1996)

| Regimen | No. |
|---|---|
| Prednisone + CYA + MMF | 26 |
| Prednisone + CYA + AZA | 60 |
| Prednisone + tacrolimus + MMF | 2 |
| Prednisone + tacrolimus + AZA | 4 |
| Prednisone + tacrolimus + cytoxan | 1 |
| Prednisone + MMF | 1 |

CYA, cyclosporine A; MMF, mycophenylate mofetil; AZA, azathioprine.

Another program initiated triple therapy maintenance immune suppression after induction but aimed to discontinue both prednisone and AZA around 2 months after transplant, using CYA monotherapy for long-term maintenance immune suppression.[26] Yet another program followed induction with predominantly double-agent maintenance immune suppression;[25] 97% of their patients >60 years of age and 69% of their patients under 60 years received prednisone and CYA alone, with the remainder receiving prednisone, CYA, and AZA. Four European programs did not use cytolytic induction therapy at all.[27–30] Two of these four programs used triple immune suppression with prednisone, CYA, and AZA for maintenance therapy; the other two programs used CYA monotherapy. Like UCSF, nearly all programs used a coherent strategy of immune suppression for all patients without regard to age at the time of transplantation.

At UCSF, five prophylaxis regimens were initiated routinely at the time of renal transplantation. A first- or second-generation cephalosporin was typically administered for surgical wound prophylaxis. CMV prophylaxis was determined by the immune suppression strategy and the serologic status of the recipient and donor. All recipients of anti-lymphocytic therapy and all CMV-negative recipients of CMV-positive organs were treated with intravenous gancyclovir and converted to oral gancyclovir prior to discharge. All other patients received oral acyclovir. Trimethoprim/sulfamethoxazole, dapsone, or inhaled pentamidine was prescribed for *Pneumocystis carinii* prophylaxis. Weekly fluconazole was administered for thrush prophylaxis. Inhaled amphotericin was given during hospitalization to prevent *Aspergillus* pneumonia. Prophylaxis regimens are infrequently detailed in reports from other institutions.

After renal transplantation and discharge from UCSF, renal function was monitored two or three times a week for 2 weeks, weekly for 10 weeks, and finally monthly. Abnormal or unexplained elevations in the serum creatinine were investigated with ultrasound examination of the transplant kidney and, during the early postoperative period, Doppler examination of the renal vessels for patency. If no anatomic reasons responsible for graft dysfunction were identified, renal biopsy was performed. On occasion, treatment for rejection was initiated on clinical grounds alone while awaiting histologic confirmation or, in some cases, when biopsy could not be safely or expeditiously performed. Therefore, a rejection episode was registered when a course of antirejection therapy was administered based on histologic or clinical evidence of rejection.

## Mortality

The actuarial survival curves for patients more than and less than 60 years of age who have undergone kidney

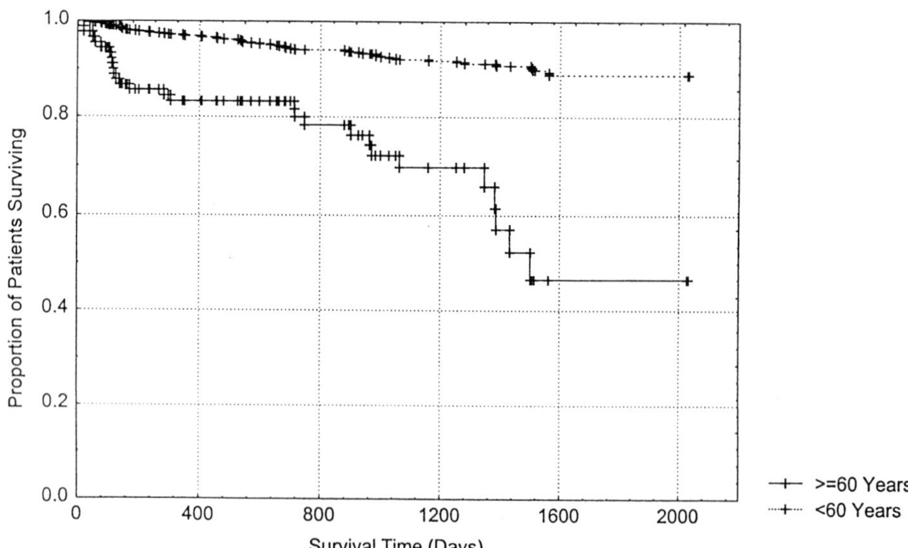


FIGURE 68.1. Patient survival after kidney transplantation, UCSF 1992–1996.

transplantation at UCSF are shown in Figure 68.1. Clearly, the curves diverge early after transplantation, and the actuarial survival for older patients was significantly inferior to that of younger patients. During the study period, 27 of 93 elderly patients (29.0%) died, as did 57 of 795 younger patients (7.2%). Deaths tended to occur somewhat earlier in the older group than in the younger group: 13 of 27 deaths (48.1%) compared to 16 of 57 (28.1%) occurred within 6 months of transplant. At UCSF the 1-, 2-, 3-, and 5-year actuarial survivals for patients older than 60 years were 83.2%, 80.0%, 69.7%, and 46.5%, respectively, compared with 96.9%, 94.1%, 92.1%, and 88.9%, respectively, for patients under 60 years. In the literature, two institutions have reported a significantly lower 1-year survival for older patients,[28,31] whereas several programs reported no significant difference.[21,22,25,26] At the 5-year time point, one program reported comparable survival of older and younger patients (80% and 89%, respectively),[26] while other programs reported significantly lower survival for older patients.[21,22] Their 5-year statistics were nearly identical with survival averaging 66% for older patients and 87% for younger patients. The ESRD-ERA summary of the European experience concurred with decreased survival of older patients at 5 years after transplantation.[24] Finally, a summary of the U.S. experience using data reported to the UNOS Scientific Renal Transplant Registry between October 1987 and March 1995, indicated that the recipient's age at the time of transplant was the most significant factor influencing survival in a multivariate analysis. The relative risk of dying for a patient over age 45 was 3.82 times that of a patient 2–15 years of age ($p < 0.0001$) and about twice that of a patient between 31 and 45 years.[32]

The causes of death for the UCSF transplant experience are shown in Table 68.4. Infectious and cardiac diseases claimed comparable percentages of older and younger transplant recipients. In older patients, deaths from sepsis occurred early: 10 of 12 deaths occurred within 6 months of transplantation. In contrast, deaths from heart disease occurred late: six of nine deaths occurred 30 months or more after transplantation. In younger patients, septic deaths were more evenly distributed in time, whereas cardiac deaths remained predominantly a late event, with 12 of 16 deaths occurring 18 months or more after transplantation. Malignancy and hepatic failure were not responsible for any deaths in transplant patients over 60 years of age. In concordance with the UCSF experience, the recent literature does not indicate any consistent or significant differences in the causes of death between older and younger patients.[22,25,26,28,29,31]

The impact of pretransplant parameters on the risk of death in elderly UCSF patients was considered. The recipient's age, sex, and etiology of renal failure did not affect the risk of death following renal transplantation. Positive cardiac co-morbidity as listed in the previous section, was also not a significant risk factor for

TABLE 68.4. Causes of Death for Patients Over and Under 60 Years after Kidney Transplantation at UCSF (1992–1996)

| Cause of death | >60 Years ($n$ = 27) | <60 Years ($n$ = 57) |
|---|---|---|
| Sepsis | 12 (44.4%) | 23 (40.4%) |
| Cardiac | 9 (33.3%) | 16 (28.1%) |
| Vascular (CVA, PE) | 4 (14.8%) | 3 (5.3%) |
| Cancer | — | 5 (8.8%) |
| Hepatic failure | — | 5 (8.8%) |
| Pulmonary | 1 (3.7%) | — |
| Pancreatitis | — | 1 (1.8%) |
| Other | 1 (3.7%) | 4 (7.0%) |

CVA, cerebrovascular accident; PE, pulmonary embolism.

death. Using the Cox proportional hazards model, the relative risk for death of preexisting cardiac disease in the elderly group was 1.12 (95% CI 0.498–2.508; $p = 0.787$). Of the 25 patients with an identified cardiac risk factor, 8 died (32.0%); of the 68 without an identified cardiac risk factor, 18 died (26.5%). Diabetes mellitus was found to have a relative risk of 0.850 (95% CI 0.308–2.340; $p = 0.752$) and thus also did not increase the risk of death after transplantation. Among diabetics 5 of 22 (22.7%) died, whereas among nondiabetics 22 of 71 (31.0%) died. A positive gastrointestinal history, including a history of hepatitis, did not increase the risk of death following renal transplantation.

The impact of posttransplant parameters on the risk of death in elderly UCSF patients was examined. Induction therapy was associated with a slightly higher incidence of posttransplant death. Of 45 elderly patients who received either MALG/ATG, OKT3, or daclizumab, 17 (37.8%) died compared to 10 (20.4%) of the 49 elderly patients who did not receive an antibody preparation during the perioperative period. All of the 17 deaths occurred in the group of 32 patients who received MALG/ATG; no deaths occurred among patients receiving either OKT3 or daclizumab. Because sequential therapy employing MALG/ATG was the primary strategy for perioperative immune suppression until 1994, MALG/ATG is not simply a marker for poor graft function. There was indeed a higher incidence of mortality among patients with poor graft function, defined as the need for dialysis during the perioperative period. Seven of fifteen patients (46.7%) who required dialysis died compared to 20 of 79 patients (25.3%) who did not require dialysis. Of the seven deaths in patients with poor graft function, five were within 6 months of transplantation. Four patients expired during their transplant hospitalization; three of these patients required continuous dialysis after renal transplantation, never having achieved adequate renal function. Two of the three patients had a complication directly related to the transplant operation: One developed partial thrombosis of the renal vein necessitating reexploration of the transplant kidney, thrombectomy, and anticoagulation, which resulted in further complications culminating in a cardiac arrest; the other suffered a significant perioperative myocardial infarction, and continued ischemia necessitated coronary angiography and bypass grafting. The fourth patient achieved good renal function (creatinine < 2.0 mg/dl) for less than a week but then developed respiratory insufficiency followed by sepsis, which resulted in graft failure and ultimately death during the transplant hospitalization. The Royal Liverpool University Hospital reported a higher probability of death in older patients if there was early graft failure.[27] At 3 months, 6 of 16 patients (37.5%) with graft failure had died, which was significantly higher ($p < 0.001$) than 4 of 97 patients (4.1%) with functioning grafts who had died.

Beyond immediate postoperative graft function, rejection was also found to increase significantly the probability of death in elderly patients after transplantation at UCSF. Univariate and multivariate analysis using the Cox proportional hazards model with rejection as a time-dependent covariate, indicated relative risks of 2.692 (95% CI 1.229–5.873) and 3.011 (95% CI 1.348–6.722), respectively. This was corroborated by data from the program at the Centre Hospitalier et Universitaire de Nantes,[26] one of the only programs providing data in the literature regarding the relation between rejection and the risk of death in elderly patients.

## Graft Survival

The actuarial graft survival curve for patients over and under 60 years who underwent renal transplantation at UCSF between 1992 and 1996 is shown in Figure 68.2. Like patient survival but less dramatically so, graft survival for older patients is inferior to that for younger patients at all times after transplantation. Actuarial 1-, 2-, 3-, and 5-year survivals for patients older and younger than 60 years were 79.9%, 73.5%, 65.4%, and 48.4%, respectively, compared to 88.8%, 82.8%, 79.3%, and 69.4%, respectively. Although there is a strong, consistent tendency in the literature for older patients to have inferior graft survival compared to that in younger patients, all recent studies, including that from the EDTA-ERA Registry, reported that the difference was not statistically significant.[21,22,24–27,29,31] At UCSF over the 5-year study period, 30 (31.9%) of the 94 kidneys transplanted into patients older than 60 years and 169 (21.3%) of the 795 kidneys transplanted into patients younger than 60 years were lost. Of the 30 kidneys in older patients that are no longer functioning, 15 were lost to patient death and 6 more were lost during the acute hospitalization that ended in the patient's death. Of the remaining nine grafts, three kidneys never functioned, one was lost to recurrent disease, one was lost secondary to donor disease, one was lost because of inadequate immune suppression necessitated by the development of Kaposi's sarcoma less than 3 months after transplant, and three were lost to rejection.

Therefore in addition to discussing actuarial graft survival, where death with a functioning graft is considered a graft loss, several reports have emphasized the importance of discussing actuarial graft survival with death censored.[32–34] This point is particularly important when considering the graft survival of older patients, who as a population have a high incidence of death with a functioning graft. As stated above, 50% (15/30) of graft losses in the elderly group at UCSF were secondary to death. Comparable percentages (40–60%) have been reported by many programs.[21,22,25,26,28,31] The EDTA-ERA reported that 65.3% of graft loss in patients older than 60 years is secondary to patient death.[24] In contrast, at UCSF only 30

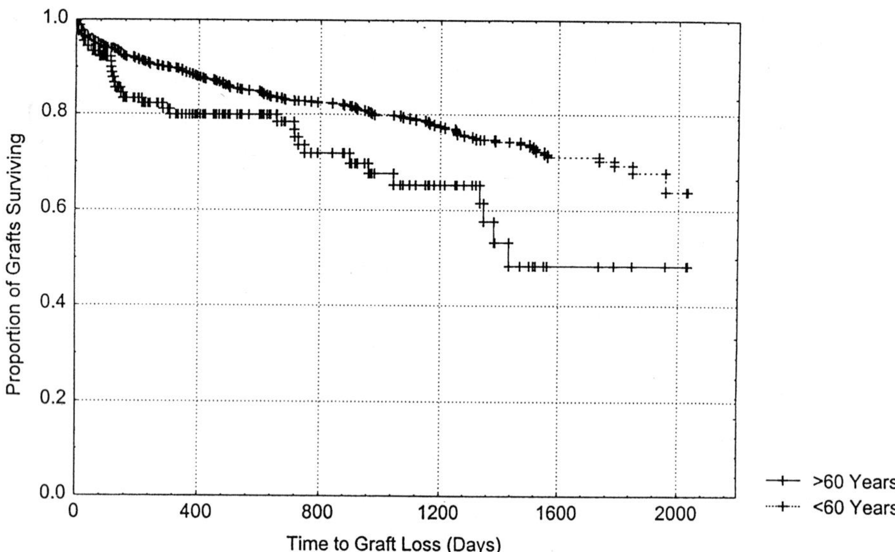


FIGURE 68.2. Kidney graft survival, UCSF 1992–1996.

of 169 grafts lost in younger patients were secondary to death. Figure 68.3 shows actuarial graft survival with death censored in patients over and under 60 years given transplants at UCSF. The curves are similar, suggesting that the increased graft loss seen in older patients is from nonimmunologic causes. Recent reports from two programs indicate that elderly patients, in their experience, had a significantly superior rate of graft survival if deaths with functioning grafts were censored.[21,31] They attributed the improved rate of immunologic graft survival to the lower incidence of graft rejection in older patients.

## Rejection

Figure 68.4 shows the actuarial time to first rejection for patients over age 60 who had undergone renal transplantation at UCSF. There is a dramatic incidence of rejection early after transplantation. The 1-, 2-, 3-, 6-, and 12-month actuarial freedom from rejection values for elderly patients were 76.0%, 69.4%, 62.7%, 58.1%, and 58.1%, respectively. Overall, at the end of the follow-up period, 54 of 94 (57.4%) of kidney transplants in older patients had not a single episode of rejection. This is comparable to the percentage of transplants in elderly patients free of rejection reported by other programs, which ranged from 51.5% to 72.6%.[21,22,26,30,31] Two of these programs compared the percentage of transplants in older and younger patients free of rejection during the observation period. Both programs indicated that a significantly higher percentage of transplants in older patients were free from rejection.[21,31] Of the 40 transplanted kidneys in older patients at UCSF treated for

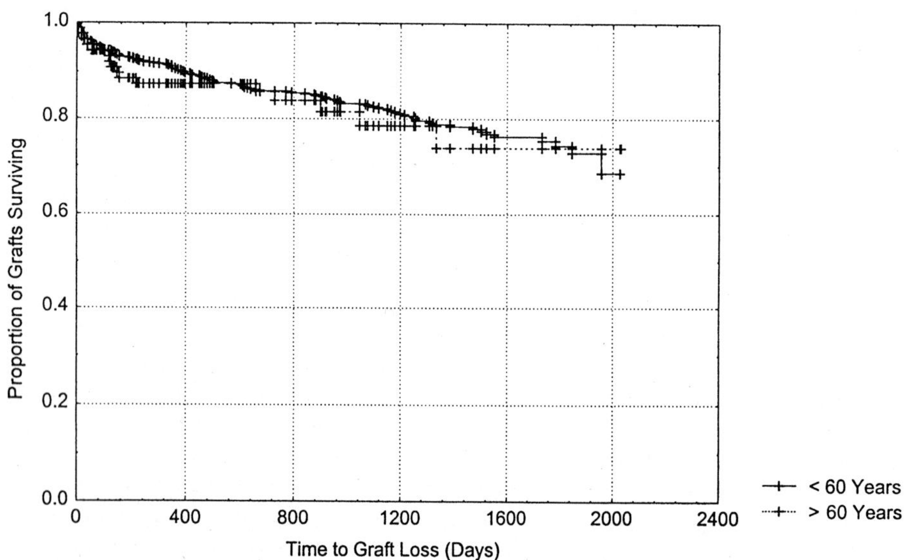


FIGURE 68.3. Kidney graft survival with death censored, UCSF 1992–1996.

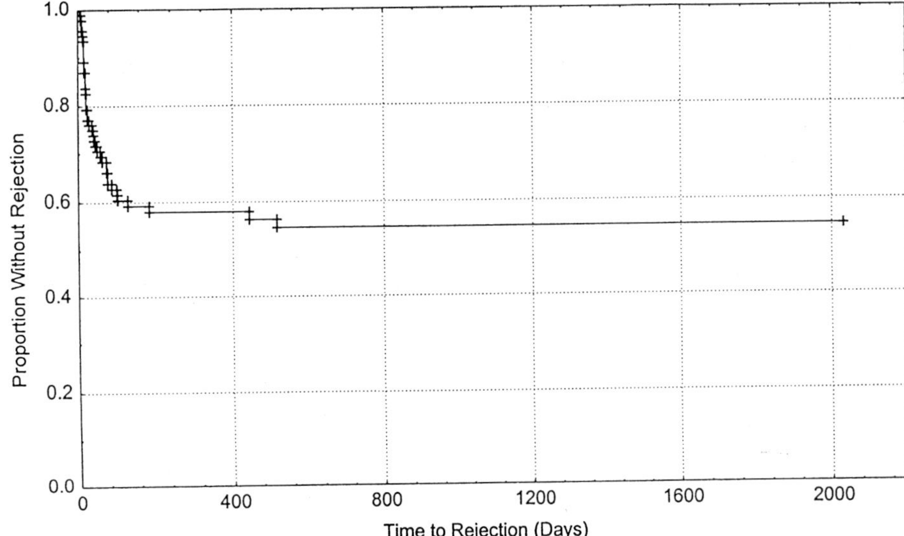


FIGURE 68.4. Kidney transplant rejection for patients >60 years of age, UCSF 1992–1996.

rejection, 31 transplants (77.5%) had a single episode, six transplants (15.0%) had two episodes, and 3 transplants (7.5%) had three episodes of rejection. The same two programs also reported that a significantly lower percentage of transplants in older patients had more than one episode of rejection compared to younger patients.[21,31] At UCSF, the number of rejection episodes per elderly patient who had at least one episode of rejection was 1.30. The University of Minnesota reported 1.36 episodes per elderly patient who had a rejection compared to 1.61 episodes per younger patient who had rejection, a difference nearly reaching statistical significance ($p = 0.07$).[22] Therefore by several measures, there is a consistent theme in the literature that the incidence and prevalence of transplant kidney rejection are lower in older patients than in younger patients.

## Morbidity

Elderly patients at UCSF experienced a significant number of postoperative surgical complications related to kidney transplantation. Among 94 transplants, there were five fascial dehiscences necessitating reoperation for wound reclosure. Two patients developed ureteral stricture and ureteral obstruction that required operative correction. There were four instances of ureteral leak, all of which occurred in male patients. Two were repaired operatively, and two were managed conservatively by Foley catheter drainage with or without nephrostomy drainage. Two patients who had ureteral leak, along with five other patients who had urinary obstruction secondary to benign prostatic hypertrophy, underwent transurethral resection of the prostate gland within 2 months of transplantation. One patient required internal drainage of a lymphocele that was causing ureteral obstruction. Finally, one patient developed partial renal vein thrombosis necessitating thrombectomy.

Multiple cardiac complications occurred in elderly patients after renal transplantation at UCSF. Of the 93 patients, 10 had documented myocardial infarction, seven of which occurred during the perioperative period. Although all these patients had a negative and complete preoperative workup, 6 of the 10 patients had cardiac co-morbidity by history. In three patients, myocardial infarction was the critical event leading ultimately to death. In addition to the 10 patients who suffered myocardial infarction, 16 had other significant cardiac complications requiring hospitalization, intervention, or both, such as atrial arrhythmias, congestive heart failure, coronary disease requiring angioplasty, or pacemaker insertion.

Three studies have presented somewhat conflicting data regarding the sensitivity and specificity of thallium stress tests for detecting ischemic coronary disease in ESRD patients. The Cleveland Clinic Foundation reported 37% sensitivity and 73% specificity for dipyridamole single-photon emission computed tomography (SPECT) thallium.[35] The University of Minnesota reported 86% sensitivity, 79% specificity, and 83% accuracy for the detection of coronary disease for dipyridamole perfusion thallium imaging.[36] Similarly, the Manchester Royal Infirmary reported 88% sensitivity, 70% specificity, and 73% predictive value of a positive test for exercise-graded thallium perfusion myocardial imaging.[37] Although all of the reports studied ESRD patients considered for transplantation, each studied a different subset of the population. Furthermore, although two of the studies used hemodynamically significant lesions detected by coronary angiography as the endpoint, the other used cardiac events during the follow-up period as the endpoint. These differences in study design may have contributed to the differences in results. A more recent paper from the University of Michigan, reported that dobutamine stress echocardiography has 95% sen-

TABLE 68.5. Malignancies in Patients >60 Years after Kidney Transplantation at UCSF (1992–1996)

| Cancer | No. |
|---|---|
| Basal cell skin cancer | 7 |
| Squamous cell skin cancer | 6 |
| Skin cancer, unspecified | 2 |
| Melanoma | 4 |
| Kaposi's sarcoma | 1 |
| Rectal cancer | 1 |

sitivity, 86% specificity, and 90% accuracy for detecting coronary disease.[38] It may be possible to reduce the number of cardiac complications after transplantation when the most appropriate and accurate screening tests for stratifying cardiac risk in older ESRD patients are identified.

There was a significant incidence of predominantly skin malignancies in older patients who received renal transplants at UCSF. Of the 93 patients, 15 were diagnosed with 21 cancers, as listed in Table 68.5; 3 of the 15 patients had a history of basal cell skin cancer prior to transplant and developed additional skin cancers (basal and squamous cell, melanoma) after transplant. Notably, there was a single case of Kaposi's sarcoma in both lower extremities that was diagnosed within 3 months of transplantation. There were no cases of post-transplant lymphoproliferative disorder in this group of elderly patients.

## Liver Transplantation

### Patient Selection and Demographics

Improved results after liver transplantation have established it as optimal therapy for most kinds of chronic liver disease and extended its application over a broad range of recipients. In general, patients with progressive liver insufficiency or compromised quality of life but without significant contraindications are candidates for liver transplantation. Previous criteria that the patient's liver disease be associated with a life expectancy of less than 1 year have relaxed, as survival after transplantation has improved and waiting times have lengthened. Recently, standard criteria have been established to justify registration with UNOS.

At UCSF patients considered for orthotopic liver transplantation (OLT) are evaluated using a standard protocol regardless of age. Biochemical assessment of liver function, indications of portal hypertension, and nutritional status are all evaluated. Ultrasonography is used to determine hepatic vessel size and patency. Occlusion of the hepatic artery or portal vein requires confirmation by angiography. Patients older than 50 years and those with alcoholic liver disease (ALD) routinely undergo cardiac echocardiography and thallium stress testing or dobutamine echocardiography to identify cardiac contraindications. Renal insufficiency is not a contraindication to transplantation, as concomitant liver–kidney transplants may be performed. Exclusion from transplantation candidacy is dictated by nonreversible disease in other organ systems.

At UCSF 872 transplants were performed from the initiation of the program in 1988 through December 1996, with a minimum of 8 months follow-up. A total of 101 liver transplants were performed in 99 patients 60 years or older for an overall rate of transplantation in the older patient population of 11.6%. Table 68.6 demonstrates the range over time (from 4.5% to 17%); in recent years the rate has been approximately 12%. These percentages are similar to those reported elsewhere.[39,40] Two reports from the United Kingdom reported a 10.2% rate in all of England in 1992[41] and 12.0% at King's College.[42] A higher percentage was seen in centers applying for Medicare accreditation, though the numbers are not entirely comparable; 28% of transplants were reported in patients older than 55 years.[43] In our series, 25 patients were 65 years or older, three patients were 70 years or older, and the oldest patient was 72 years.

Table 68.7 depicts the diseases for which liver transplantation was performed at UCSF in patients age 60 years. More than one-third of older patients had chronic active hepatitis C infection (HCV). Alcoholic liver disease was also present in two patients. In seven patients with HCV, the indication for transplantation was evidence of hepatocellular carcinoma (HCC). Twenty percent of patients had primary biliary cirrhosis (PBC), and 10% had ALD. These etiologies reflect the same distribution of disease seen in our younger patients. The King's College experience in older patients was weighted much more to patients with PBC, which represented 60% of their transplant population.[42] In contrast to the U.K. data, the Health Care Financing Administration data and Pittsburgh showed a distribution similar to ours and a similar male-female distribution.[40,43] Among the male

TABLE 68.6. Liver Transplantation in Patients >60 Years at UCSF (1988–1996)

| Year | No. of patients > 60 years | Total transplantations | % |
|---|---|---|---|
| 1988 | 2 | 39 | 5.0 |
| 1989 | 4 | 89 | 4.5 |
| 1990 | 8 | 92 | 8.7 |
| 1991 | 18/17 | 105 | 17.1 |
| 1992 | 11 | 120 | 9.2 |
| 1993 | 18/17 | 112 | 16.0 |
| 1994 | 13 | 106 | 12.2 |
| 1995 | 13 | 106 | 12.2 |
| 1996 | 14 | 103 | 13.6 |

TABLE 68.7. Liver Disease Etiologies in Elderly Patients Undergoing Orthotopic Liver Transplantation at UCSF (1988–1996)

| Disease | Total | Men | Women |
|---|---|---|---|
| Hepatitis C (HCV) | 31 | 17 | 14 |
| Primary biliary cirrhosis (PBC) | 19[a] | 3 | 16 |
| Cryptogenic cirrhosis (CC) | 16 | 8 | 8 |
| Alcoholic liver disease (ALD) | 9[a] | 9[b] | 1[b] |
| Hepatitis C/hepatocellular carcinoma (HCV/HCC) | 7 | 5 | 2 |
| Primary/secondary sclerosing cholangitis (PSC/SSC) | 7 | 3 | 4 |
| Fulminant hepatic failure (FHF) | 4 | 2 | 2 |
| Autoimmune chronic hepatitis (AICH) | 2 | 1 | 1 |
| Hepatitis B (HBV) | 2 | 0 | 2 |
| Miscellaneous | 2 | 1 | 1 |
| Total | 99 | 48 | 51 |

[a] Patient in each group with two transplants.
[b] One patient in each group with ALD/HCV.

patients, half were diagnosed with HCV and 20% with ALD as an etiology. In female patients, HCV and PBC were the most common diagnoses and of equal incidence. ALD was present in only one female patient older than 60 years.

Table 68.8 lists the co-morbid pretransplant conditions identified in the older patient population at UCSF. The three most common conditions were hypertension, cardiac disease, and diabetes mellitus. Though none of these diseases are absolute contraindications to transplantation, they may be associated with significant perioperative morbidity. We have not yet analyzed the specific impact of any of these pretransplantation co-morbid conditions on the survival, posttransplantation complication rate, or length of hospitalization. Clearly this analysis is important for determining the best way to select and manage these patients.

Among the patients with evidence of cardiac or pulmonary disease, three had had a previous myocardial infarction, three had evidence of stress-induced ischemia, two had previous coronary artery bypass or aortic bypass, three had coronary artery disease, and five had a history of rhythm or conduction disturbances without coronary artery disease. Three patients had COPD, two of whom also had cardiac histories. The association of pretransplant cardiac disease with posttransplant cardiac complications is discussed below.

## Details of Transplantation, Immune Suppression, Infection Prophylaxis, and Rejection Surveillance

Standard OLT was performed in this group of older patients. If the patient demonstrated cardiovascular instability or had familial amyloidosis or hemachromatosis, the piggyback technique was used at the time of transplantation with conservation of the intrahepatic vena cava. Continuous venovenous hemofiltration (CVVH) was performed intraoperatively in patients with renal failure in whom renal transplantation was not performed. For patients with portal venous thrombosis, endarterectomy of the portal vein was done, or a bypass was performed to the superior mesenteric vein. One patient in this older group was supported at the time of transplantation with an intraaortic balloon pump because of concern for poor cardiac function. This patient survived the transplant procedure and died at 39 months with colon cancer.

All patients undergoing liver transplantation at UCSF received the same immune suppression that evolved during the study period. Early, patients were treated with MALG, AZA, CYA, and prednisone. Subsequently MALG was eliminated, and patients were treated with either CYA or tacrolimus in combination with AZA and prednisone. Since 1995, MMF has been substituted for AZA. In the setting of pretransplant renal insufficiency, MMF or AZA and prednisone were initiated at the time of surgery, and CYA or tacrolimus was delayed until recovery of adequate renal function.

Protocol biopsies were obtained at weekly intervals following transplantation until two normal biopsies were obtained. Liver biopsy was also performed to evaluate elevated liver function tests or fever following transplantation. Rejection was diagnosed by the presence of a mixed inflammatory infiltrate in the portal regions with bile duct injury. Endothelialitis (inflammation of the endothelium of the central vein) may also be present. The initial rejection was treated with additional steroids. A second rejection was treated with a switch from CYA to tacrolimus (or vice versa) in addition to a second cycle of steroids. Currently, OKT3 is reserved for the third rejection episode, although prior to 1993, it was instituted earlier. Biopsy was used to confirm resolution of the rejection.

TABLE 68.8. Co-morbid Pretransplantation Conditions in Elderly Patients Undergoing Liver Transplantation at UCSF (1988–1996)

| Condition[a] | No. of patients |
|---|---|
| Cardiac disease | 16 |
| Hypertension | 19 |
| Diabetes mellitus | 16 |
| Portal vein thrombosis | 8 |
| Portocaval shunt | 2 |
| Osteoporosis | 7 |
| Renal failure | 3 |
| Previous liver transplant | 3 |
| Obesity | 3 |
| Cancer (other than liver) | 4 |
| Hepatopulmonary syndrome/COPD | 3 |
| Psychiatric problem | 2 |

[a] Many patients had more than one co-morbid condition.

Prophylaxis against CMV infection was 1 week of intravenous gancyclovir followed by 3 weeks of high dose oral acyclovir. *Pneumocystis* prophylaxis was trimethaprim/sulfamethoxazole, given every other day for the entire posttransplant period. Nystatin was administered for 3 months after transplantation. All patients were monitored with twice-weekly laboratory tests for 1 month, weekly blood tests for 1 month, and then with decreasing frequency until monthly intervals were achieved. Patients were seen at the clinic weekly for 1 month, every other week for 2 months, and gradually less frequently as determined by the patient's condition. At 1 year after transplant the patients underwent liver biopsy. Subsequent biopsies were dictated by the patient's course and by the possibility of disease recurrence. Patients with inflammatory bowel disease in association with primary sclerosing cholangitis were advised to have yearly colonoscopy following transplantation.

TABLE 68.9. Causes of Early Death ($n$ = 8, 9%) in Elderly Patients after Liver Transplantation at UCSF (1988–1996)

| Cause of death | No. |
|---|---|
| Sepsis | 3 (aspergillosis 3: post second transplant 2) |
| Myocardial infarction | 1 |
| Angiotrophic lymphoma | 1 |
| Cerebrovascular accident (CVA) | 1 |
| Primary nonfunction (PNF) | 1 |
| Bleeding after biopsy | 1 |

## Mortality

Figure 68.5 demonstrates the actuarial survival in this group of 99 older patients who received 101 liver transplants. A steep curve of early patient loss is seen within 4 months of transplantation. Unlike survival curves seen in younger patient groups, the attrition continues after 4 months in these patients. These patients experienced a 9% perioperative mortality three times that seen in patients less than 60 years old.

Table 68.9 shows the cause of death in the eight older patients who died 7–68 days after transplantation without having been discharged. Sepsis was the etiology in three patients; in all three, *Aspergillus* was cultured, among other organisms.

Table 68.10 categorizes the causes and timing of death after transplantation in the older patients. Cancer, including posttransplantation lymphoproliferative disease (PTLD), was the most common cause of death in these patients. Cancer deaths tended to occur late after transplantation; the one exception was a patient with widespread angiotrophic lymphoma that was not diagnosed prior to transplantation. Three of the remaining cancer deaths were of colonic origin, which was recurrent disease in two patients. PTLD was a common cause of death in these patients; it occurred in five patients 60 years or older and was fatal in four of them. Cardiovascular disease was also a common cause of fatality, with four cardiac deaths and three fatal strokes. Sepsis was the cause of death in a relatively small number of patients; it occurred early after transplantation and was common in patients who died during their initial transplant admission. Recurrent HCV infection was the cause of death in three patients following transplantation and occurred relatively late after transplantation.

## Rejection

Of the 99 older patients who received liver transplants, 91 could be evaluated for rejection. As shown in Table 68.11,

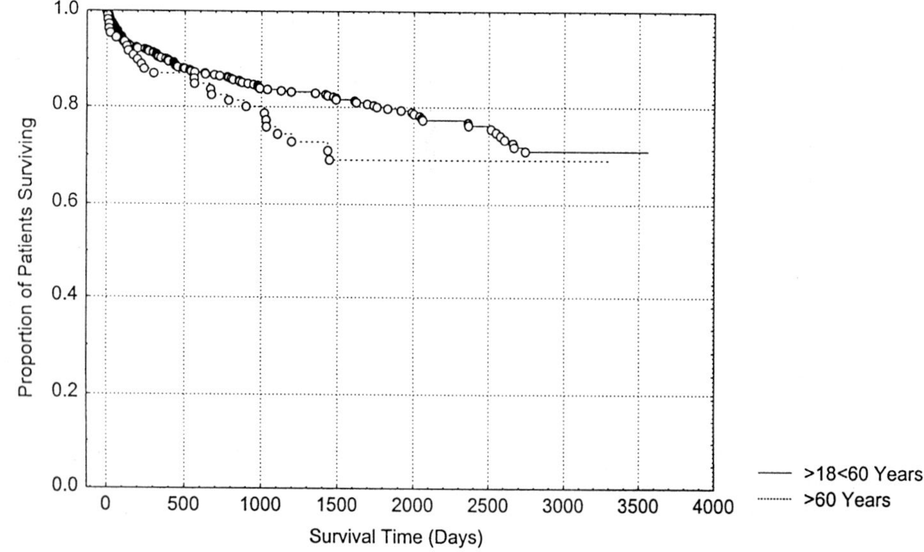


FIGURE 68.5. Patient survival after liver transplantation, UCSF 1988–1996.

TABLE 68.10. Causes of All Deaths in Patients >60 Years after Liver Transplantation at UCSF (1988–1996)

| Cause of death | No. | Time after transplantation (months) |
|---|---|---|
| Cancer | 6 | <1–39 (1[a,b], 19, 22, 34, 36, 39) |
| Posttransplant lymphoproliferative disease (PTLD) | 4 | 5–47 (5, 8, 9, 47) |
| Cardiac | 4 | 2–34 (2[b], 4, 18, 34) |
| Sepsis | 3 | <1–4 (<1[b], <1[b,c], 4[b,c]) |
| Cerebrovascular accident | 3 | <1–8 (<1[b], 4, 8) |
| Recurrent hepatitis C | 3 | 23–34 (23, 26, 34[d]) |
| Biliary complications | 2 | 8[d], 22[d] |
| Rejection | 1 | 26[e] |
| Primary nonfunction | 1 | <1[b,c] |
| Bleed | 1 | <1[b] |

[a] Missed diagnosis of angiotrophic lymphoma.
[b] Death in hospital during Tx admission.
[c] Death following 2nd Tx.
[d] Element of rejection could not be ruled out.
[e] Associated with noncompliance.

TABLE 68.12. Morbidity in Patients >60 Years after Liver Transplantation at UCSF (1988–1996) ($n$ = 99)

| Morbidity | No. | Comment |
|---|---|---|
| Cardiac | 16 | Major events: MI 6, CHF 3, fib/flutter 5, aortic valve replacement 1, cardiac arrest 1 |
| Hypertension | 47 | Including 19 with pretransplantation HTN |
| Diabetes mellitus | 24 | Including 8 patients with pretransplant DM |
| Recurrent HCV | 26 | |
| Osteoporosis | 16 | Including 7 patients with pretransplant osteoporosis |
| Biliary stricture/leak | 19 | |
| New cancer | 8 | |
| Recurrent cancer | 3 | |
| PTLD | 5 | |
| Renal insufficiency | 5 | Required HD |
| Recurrent HBV | 3 | |
| Recurrent PBC | 3 | |
| Portal vein thrombosis | 1 | |

one-third of older patients experienced no rejection, one-third had one rejection episode, and one-third experienced two or more rejection episodes. Eleven percent had four or more episodes of rejection. In no patient did rejection lead to the need for retransplantation. In four patients chronic rejection was associated with, but was not the sole cause of death.

The rate of rejection in the older patient, as defined by protocol biopsy, was similar to that in the younger patient group. However, the number of older patients with no rejection was 10% higher than in younger patients. The 1.4 rejection episodes per patient was higher than that seen in the University of Wisconsin series.[39] This difference may reflect our use of protocol biopsies, which tended to maximize the number of rejection episodes diagnosed.

## Morbidity

Table 68.12 categorizes the major posttransplant complications experienced by patients over 60 years of age. Of the 16 patients who had major cardiac events following transplantation, 8 had pretransplant cardiopulmonary co-morbidity. Five patients had posttransplant congestive heart failure with a known history of cardiac disease. Three of these patients died: one with subsequent myocardial infarction, one with congestive heart failure secondary to progressive amyloidosis, and one with a fatal cardiac arrest 4 months after transplantation. Eight patients with cardiac events following transplantation had no history of preexisting disease. Five of these patients died of cancer of the colon, cerebrovascular accident, angiotrophic lymphoma, myocardial infarct, and arterial fibrillation with pulmonary failure, respectively.

Table 68.13 depicts the rate of disease recurrence after transplantation in the older patient population. Recurrent HCV infection was particularly common, with 80% of patients demonstrating varying degrees of hepatitis after transplantation. Of these 33 patients, 7 died; and in 3 patients the deaths were related to recurrent disease. Among seven patients for whom transplantation was performed for hepatocellular carcinoma (HCC) on the background of chronic hepatitis, three patients demonstrated recurrent HCV infection and one patient died of recurrent HCC. Recurrent primary biliary cirrhosis was seen in four patients; one patient died with primary nonfunction following a second transplant.

Table 68.14 shows the length of stay after liver transplantation in patients without perioperative death. A wide range of posttransplantation hospitalization was observed (7–65 days). The mean and median lengths of stay were not different from those seen in younger patients. It is noteworthy that patients with perioperative death had the same range of hospital stay as discharged patients.

TABLE 68.11. Rejection Rates in Patients >60 Years[a] after Liver Transplantation at UCSF (1988–1996)

| No. of patients | No. of rejections[b] | Rejection rate (%) |
|---|---|---|
| 30 | 0 | 33 |
| 28 | 1 (1 chronic rejection) | 31 |
| 10 | 2 | 11 |
| 13 | 3 (2 chronic rejections) | 14 |
| 10 | ≥4 (3 chronic rejections) | 11 |

[a] There were 91 patients who survived the transplant admission.
[b] There were 1.4 rejections per patient. Four chronic rejections were associated with death.

TABLE 68.13. Recurrent Disease in Patients >60 Years After Liver Transplantation at UCSF (1988–1996)

| Diagnosis | No. | No. with recurrent disease | No. of deaths | No. of deaths from recurrent disease |
|---|---|---|---|---|
| HCV | 33[a] | 28 | 7 | 3 |
| HCV/HCC | 7 | HCV 3, HCC 1 | 3 | 1 |
| PBC | 19 | 4 | 5 | 1 |
| CC | 16 | — | 4 | — |
| PSC | 7 | — | 1 | — |
| ALD | 7 | 1[b] | 3 | — |
| Fulminant hepatic failure (FHF) | 4 | 1 | 1 | — |
| HBV | 2 | 1 | — | — |
| AICH | 2 | — | — | — |
| Miscellaneous | 2 | — | 2 | — |

[a] Includes two patients with ALD/HCV.
[b] FHF.

There are relatively few data regarding retransplantation in the older population. Two patients underwent acute retransplantation. The indications for second transplant were hepatic artery thrombosis in one and primary nonfunction in the other. Both these patients died with sepsis following the second transplant. Three additional patients were less than 60 years at the time of first transplant but required a second transplant 2–8 years later for recurrent disease, at which time they were more than 60 years of age. Two patients had recurrent HCV infection and one had recurrent PBC. The PBC patient died secondary to primary nonfunction; the two HCV infection patients are alive with recurrent HCV disease at 1.5 and 2.5 years after retransplantation.

## Heart Transplantation

Heart transplantation has been a well-established and widely practiced therapy for the treatment of end-stage heart disease for more than a decade. As with other solid-organ transplants, the dramatic increase in heart transplantation was fueled by advancements in surgical technique and immune suppression. In turn, the enhanced success of transplantation therapy encouraged relaxation of both donor and recipient criteria. The volume of heart transplantation has plateaued since 1991, limited predominantly by donor availability.[44]

Parallel to the increased volume of overall transplantation during the last half of the 1980s, was the increased volume of transplantation in elderly patients. Patients over 55 years of age represented fewer than 3% of heart transplant recipients in 1984 but nearly 25% in 1986.[45] By 1992, patients between 50 and 60 years of age represented 33% of the transplant population,[46] and mortality statistics indicate that an additional 25,000 individuals age 56–65 years may be candidates.[47] In the face of such a glaring disparity between supply and demand, which will inevitably worsen as the population ages, the results of transplantation in the elderly continue to receive appropriate careful scrutiny.

TABLE 68.14. Length of Stay after Liver Transplantation in Patients >60 Years[a] at UCSF (1988–1996)

| | |
|---|---|
| Range | 7–65 days |
| Median LOS | 15.5 days |
| Mean LOS | 19.9 days |
| LOS of early deaths | 7–68 days |

[a] The 91 patients who survived transplant admission.

### Patient Selection and Demographics

Heart transplantation is offered to people with an estimated life expectancy of 12 months or less. Older patients at UCSF were not subjected to more rigorous evaluation protocols than their younger cohort. Ultrasound examination of the abdominal aorta and femoral arteries and carotid Doppler studies were routine. Further investigation to identify significant dysfunction of other organ systems was driven by the history, physical examination, and symptomatology.

The demographic characteristics of the UCSF heart transplant experience are shown in Table 68.15. From

TABLE 68.15. Demographics of Patients Undergoing Heart Transplantation at UCSF (1989–1996)

| Parameter | >60 Years | <60 Years |
|---|---|---|
| Transplants (no.) | 25 (26.9%) | 68 (73.1%) |
| Age (years) | | |
| Mean | 63.60 | 48.46 |
| Median | 63.40 | 49.30 |
| Range | 60.20–69.90 | 15.40–59.95 |
| Men | 21/25 (84%) | 52/68 (76.5%) |
| Women | 4/25 (16%) | 16/68 (23.5%) |
| Diagnosis | | |
| Ischemic | 19 (76.0%) | 29 (42.0%) |
| Dilated | 5 (20.0%) | 33 (47.8%) |
| Restrictive | — | 2 (2.9%) |
| Retransplant | — | 1 (1.4%) |
| Other | 1 (4.0%) | 4 (5.8%) |
| Prior cardiac surgery | 14 (56.0%) | 28 (40.6%) |
| Inotropic support | 12 (48.0%) | 29 (42.0%) |
| Follow-up (months) | | |
| Mean | 29.9 | 62.7 |
| Median | 19 | 52 |
| Range | 7–84 | 10–100 |

March 1989 to December 1996, a total of 94 transplants were performed in 93 patients. At the time of transplantation 25 patients (26.9%) were over 60 years of age. Older patients at UCSF were given transplants predominantly for ischemic disease, similar to the experience in other institutions.[45,48–56] Again, similar to most other reports, a higher percentage of older patients had a history of previous cardiac surgery.[48,50,52,56] A comparable percentage of old and young patients in the UCSF experience were dependent on inotropes, mechanical ventilation, or ventricular assist devices, or a combination of these modalities. The follow-up of older patients was shorter than that of younger patients because most older patients were given transplants late in the study period.

## Details of Transplantation, Immune Suppression, Infection Prophylaxis, and Rejection Surveillance

Donors and recipients were matched for ABO blood group compatibility and general body size. Intraoperative immune suppression consisted of methylprednisolone and AZA. Immediately after transplantation, ATG was administered and continued until an adequate blood level of CYA was achieved. Methylprednisolone was continued postoperatively in tapering doses. CYA was usually started, depending on graft, renal, and gastrointestinal function, on the second or third postoperative day and dosed according to the blood level. AZA was continued postoperatively with adjustment for leukocyte count and hepatic function. Within the last 18 months, some patients received MMF instead of AZA. Most reports from other centers indicate reliance on triple therapy (prednisone, CYA, AZA) for immune suppression in the older recipient,[45,48,50–54,56] though some centers report gradual steroid withdrawal.[48,49] The Harefield Hospital program goes further by using only a single dose of methylprednisolone intraoperatively.[55]

As part of infection prophylaxis, 48 hours of cefazolin or vancomycin was administered perioperatively. Intravenous gancyclovir was given during the initial hospitalization for CMV prophylaxis; and upon discharge, patients were converted to oral acyclovir. Trimethoprim/sulfamethoxazole, dapsone, or inhaled pentamidine was prescribed for *Pneumocystis* prophylaxis. Mycelex Troches or, more recently, weekly fluconazole was used for thrush prophylaxis.

The protocol for rejection surveillance at UCSF is intensive. Unlike other solid organ transplants, heart transplantation has no chemical or functional studies capable of signaling rejection. A protocol of endomyocardial biopsies at regular intervals after transplantation was followed. Of the institutions that described their biopsy protocol, many were comparable. The frequency of biopsy affects the detection and reported incidence of rejection.

## Mortality

The 1-year and 5-year actuarial survivals for all heart transplant recipients were 79% and 63%, respectively, according to The Registry of the International Society for Heart and Lung Transplantation (ISHLT).[44] There was a statistically significant decrease in survival with each decade of increasing age starting at 45, although it did not reach statistical significance until age >65 years.[44] Multivariate logistic regression analysis for heart transplant patients indicates odds ratios of 1.3 and 1.92 for 1-year mortality and odds ratios of 1.26 and 1.81 for 5-year mortality for the risk factors of age >60 years and >70 years. Repeat analysis with age as a continuous variable again shows a highly statistically significant increase in risk with increasing age.[44]

The actuarial survival curves for patients more and less than 60 years of age who underwent heart transplantation at UCSF are shown in Figure 68.6. There was no statistically significant difference between older and younger patients. The indication for transplantation did not significantly influence mortality. A history of previous sternotomy did not increase the incidence of death, which is in concordance with other reports.[57,58]

Table 68.16 shows the actuarial survival for UCSF and six other heart transplant programs. Two of the centers reported significantly poorer results in older patients and so merit discussion. The Cardiovascular Hospital in Lyon, France,[53] reported significantly worse short- and long-term survival in older patients. The older patients received hearts from donors whose mean age was 11 years greater than that of the donors for younger patients. The actuarial survival curves for older and younger patients transplanted at the University of Utah, progressively diverged beginning at 6 months after transplant. They reported an increased death rate among elderly patients due to infection and malignancy, predominantly posttransplant lymphoproliferative disease. This may result, at least in part, from their routine use of a 14-day course of OKT3 for induction immune suppression. The remainder of the studies, like the UCSF experience, reported no significant survival difference between older and younger patients.

A striking feature of the actuarial survival curve for older patients in the UCSF experience is the early dropoff in survival. All of the seven deaths occurred within 9 months of transplant, and five of the seven occurred within 1 month of transplant. The other institution with a significant increase in early deaths after transplantation was Papworth Hospital (Cambridgeshire, England), which also used antilymphocyte induction therapy, although only for 3 days.

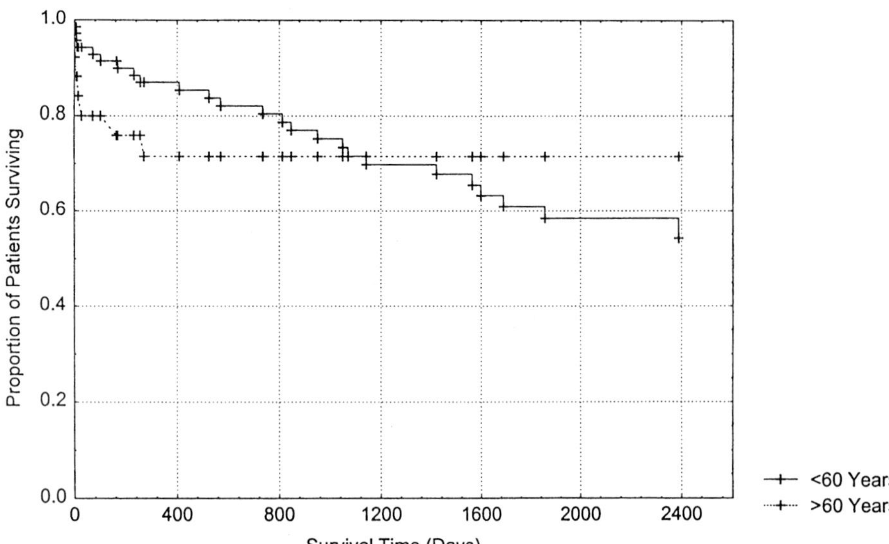


FIGURE 68.6. Patient survival after heart transplantation, UCSF 1989–1996.

The causes of death for both older and younger patients transplanted at UCSF are shown in Table 68.17. There was no correlation between the incidence of death and any pretransplant parameter including the recipient's sex, etiology of heart failure, history of cardiac surgery, and preoperative inotrope requirement. The high incidence of graft dysfunction leading to death in the older patient group at UCSF, has been noted by two other programs.[49,53] Although the comparable incidence of sepsis between older and younger patients was also observed in the Stanford University experience,[48] the University of Utah reported a significantly higher incidence[51] and two other programs reported a tendency toward a higher incidence of septic deaths in their older patients.[45,49] No patients over 60 years of age died from rejection or malignancy at UCSF. A significantly lower incidence of death from rejection in older patients was noted by one program,[51] whereas a tendency toward a lower incidence was noted by several others.[45,48,53] Two programs reported a significantly higher incidence of death from malignancy in older patients,[51,53] whereas one program noted a lower incidence.[49]

TABLE 68.16. Actuarial Survival after Heart Transplantation at UCSF and Other Institutions

| Institution | Age (years) | Survival (%) 1 Year | 3 Years | 5 Years |
|---|---|---|---|---|
| UCSF | >60 | 71.5 | 71.5 | 71.5 |
| | <60 | 86.8 | 71.6 | 60.9 |
| University of Minnesota[50] | >60 | 90.0 | — | 85.0 |
| | <60 | 91.0 | — | 86.0 |
| St. Vincent Medical Center[52] | >60 | 94.0 | — | 82.0 |
| | <60 | 91.0 | — | 76.0 |
| University of Utah[a51] | >60 | 80.0 | 72.0 | 63.0 |
| | <60 | 88.0 | 81.0 | 74.0 |
| Cardiovascular Hospital[a] Lyon, France[53] | >60 | 68.8 | — | 43.5 |
| | <60 | 88.5 | — | 76.4 |
| Stanford University[48] | >54 | 78.0 | — | 52.0 |
| | <54 | 81.0 | — | 66.0 |
| Cedars Sinai[49] | >65 | 86.6 | 72.0 | — |
| | <65 | 93.0 | 81.0 | — |

[a] Centers reporting statistically significant difference in survival between young and old patients.

## Rejection

At UCSF the rejection is graded histologically according to the guidelines of the ISHLT[59] and treated accordingly. A 3-day course of intravenous steroids followed by tapering is typical. Cytolytic therapy (MALG/ATG early and OKT3 later in the study period) was reserved for severe rejection (ISHLT grade IV), rejection resistant to steroids, or rejection resulting in hemodynamic instability. During the entire period of follow-up, 54.5% of the older patients and 80.6% of the younger patients undergoing heart transplantation at UCSF, had one or more episodes of rejection. The actuarial freedom of rejection for both

TABLE 68.17. Causes of Death in Patients Undergoing Heart Transplantation at UCSF (1989–1996) (Total $n$ = 25)

| Cause of death | >60 Years ($n$ = 7) | <60 Years ($n$ = 23) |
|---|---|---|
| Intraoperative death/ primary graft failure | 4 | 3 |
| Graft failure | 1 | 2 |
| Sepsis | 2 | 7 |
| Rejection | — | 3 |
| Malignancy | — | 2 |
| Hepatic failure | — | 2 |
| Other | — | 4[a] |

[a] Includes hemolytic uremic syndrome (1), renal failure (1), recurrent amyloidosis (1), and hemorrhage after liver biopsy (1).

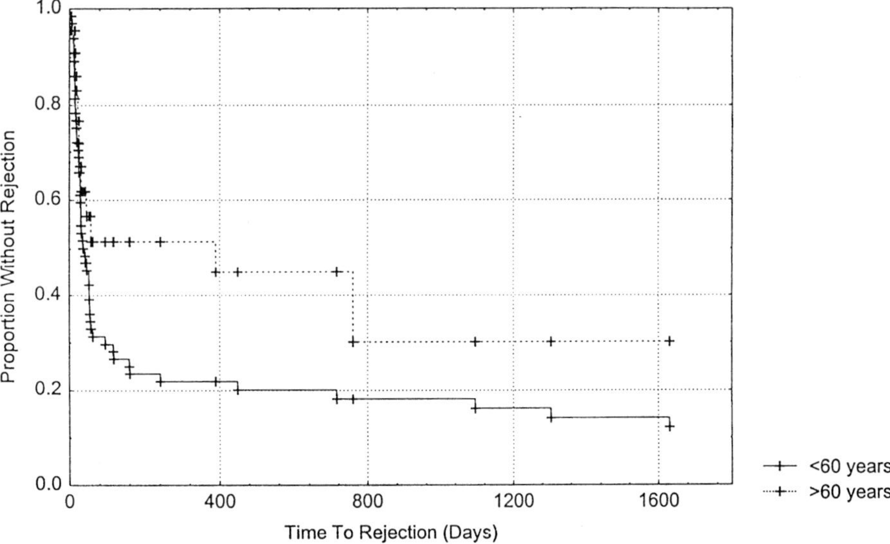


FIGURE 68.7. Heart transplant rejection, UCSF 1989–1996.

patient groups is shown in Figure 68.7. The younger patients clearly had a higher incidence of first rejection, although this did not quite reach statistical significance ($p = 0.071$). The steep dropoff of both curves immediately from the time of transplantation indicates that the first rejection episode tended to occur early, within 1–2 months of transplantation in both groups, despite the use of cytolytic induction therapy. The multiinstitutional study of early rejection, based on the Transplant Cardiologists Research Database, has also found that induction therapy did not appear to delay first rejection episodes or enhance the cumulative freedom from rejection.[60]

The lack of general agreement regarding the protocol for rejection surveillance and the level of histologic abnormality that merits intensified immune suppression renders any comparison of incidence and severity of rejection among various institutions difficult. Several early studies[54,56,61,62] reported that elderly patients experience less rejection after heart transplantation. Both recent reports of statistically significant differences in rejection between older and younger patients are from institutions that administered induction immune suppression. The University of Utah reported significantly fewer rejection episodes per patient in patients older than 60 years compared to those younger than 60 years: $1.9 \pm 1.3$ versus $2.6 \pm 1.8$ ($p = 0.009$).[51] Although Stanford University found no difference in the number of rejection episodes for the first 6 months after transplantation, they reported significantly fewer rejection episodes after the first 6 months for patients older than 54 years compared to those younger than 54 years: $0.5 \pm 0.9$ versus $0.9 \pm 1.0$ ($p < 0.04$).[48]

TABLE 68.18. Length of Stay after Heart Transplantation at UCSF (1989–1996)

| | Length of stay (days) | |
|---|---|---|
| Parameter | >60 Years | <60 Years |
| Mean | 21.3 | 25.7 |
| Median | 14.0 | 20.0 |
| Range | 10–78 | 8–105 |

## Morbidity

Table 68.18 shows the duration of hospital stays for UCSF patients who were successfully discharged after heart transplantation. There was no significant difference in the length of the perioperative hospital stay between older and younger patients. No institution reported a statistically significant difference in the length of hospitalization for their older versus younger patients.[45,48,49,52,54]

Most institutions including UCSF, perform mandatory angiography on a yearly basis after transplantation to monitor the development of accelerated atherosclerosis. At UCSF, 10 of 69 (14.5%) of the younger patients were diagnosed with graft atherosclerosis compared to none of the older patients. Two other centers similarly report increased graft coronary artery disease in younger versus older patients.[49,52] One program reported an equivalent incidence,[48] and one other program reported a tendency toward a higher incidence of graft atherosclerosis in the older patients, which did not reach statistical significance, however.[45]

Over the entire follow-up period, four older patients (16%) and seven younger patients (10%) developed a malignancy. Among the older patients, there were two cases of squamous cell skin cancer and a single case each of basal cell skin cancer and lung cancer. No deaths among the older patients were attributable to malignancy. In contrast, two deaths among the younger patients were attributable to malignancy. In total, there were four cases of PTLD of which one was fatal, one case of leukemia that was fatal, and one case each of melanoma and squamous cell skin cancer. The literature in general concurs that there is a higher incidence of malignancy in elderly patients. Statistically significant differences have been reported by St. Vincent Medical Center[52] and Stanford University,[48] whereas Loyola University[54] reported a comparable incidence. No institution has reported a lower incidence of malignancy in elderly patients. With regard to death from malignancy, three programs reported a significantly higher incidence in their older patients,[48,51,53] and two programs reported a comparable incidence.[52,54]

Five programs reported the posttransplant incidence of infection and osteoporosis in older and younger patients. Four found no statistically significant difference in the incidence of infection,[48,51,52,56] and one found a significantly higher number of infections per patient per month in patients over age 65 compared to patients 55–65 years.[54] All three programs that reported on posttransplant osteoporosis found no statistically significant difference in incidence when comparing older and younger patients.[48,52,54]

Finally, using various measures to assess functional capacity and posttransplant rehabilitation, several institutions have tried to determine and compare quality of life measures between older and younger patients. During the first few months after transplantation, both St. Vincent[52] and Loyola University[54] reported significantly inferior functional capacity scores for the older patients compared to the younger patients, but they achieved parity over time. At 3 months after transplantation, the University of Minnesota[63] reported equivalent rates of achieving a normal life style but a significantly lower rate of return to work for patients over 55 years compared to those under 55 years. St. Louis University Medical Center[61] reported equivalent performance on the Bruce protocol exercise treadmill test at 4–6 months and comparable return to work percentages for patients over and under 55 years of age. Finally, at 18 months after transplantation, Stanford University[48] reported comparable subjective levels of physical ability but superior subjective levels of social functioning, indicating a superior quality of life, for those over 54 years compared to those under 54 years.

## Lung Transplantation

Of the four areas of solid organ transplantation discussed in this chapter, lung transplantation was the last to mature and continues to have the lowest patient and graft survival. Single- and double-lung transplantation has been successful only since 1983 and 1986, respectively, although heart–lung transplantation was available earlier. To minimize complications and optimize results, transplantation efforts have been concentrated in younger patients. The literature contains only a single report from the University of Toronto on transplantation in older patients, defined as those over the age of 50 years.[64] We describe here the UCSF experience with lung transplantation in patients over 60 years of age.

Lung transplantation is a therapy offered to patients whose end-stage lung disease limits their life expectancy to 18 months or less[65] or significantly impairs their quality of life (or both).[64] The etiology of pulmonary failure determines whether single- or double-lung transplantation is more appropriate, with pulmonary fibrosis as the paradigm for single-lung transplantation and pulmonary sepsis (cystic fibrosis and bronchiectasis) as the paradigm for double-lung transplantation.

### Patient Selection and Demographics

Medical evaluation to identify patients with the best opportunity for long-term survival and full rehabilitation is a critical aspect of a successful lung transplant program. Significant dysfunction of any relevant organ system can affect a patient's ability to not only survive the procedure but also tolerate immune suppression. In general, approximately 10% of referred patients are accepted for lung transplantation. Cardiac evaluation is aggressive; at UCSF all patients over the age of 50 undergo noninvasive evaluation with echocardiography and thallium stress testing. Patients with abnormal results undergo coronary angiography. The demographic characteristics, indications for lung transplantation, and length of follow-up for the UCSF experience are shown in Table 68.19. Of the 42 transplants performed between October 1991 and December 1996, seven were performed in patients over 60 years of age; the first older patient received a transplant in 1994. Six of seven older patients received a single-lung transplant. This can be anticipated by the indications for liver transplantation in the older group; obstructive disease was the most common indication, and pulmonary sepsis was distinctly rare at both UCSF and the University of Toronto.[64]

### Details of Transplantation, Immune Suppression, Infection Prophylaxis, and Rejection Surveillance

Donors and recipients for lung transplantation were matched for ABO blood group compatibility and general body size or total lung capacity. Intraoperative immune suppression was with methylprednisolone and AZA. Maintenance immune suppression comprised prednisone in tapering doses, CYA started intravenously and converted to oral therapy, and AZA except for a few patients who received MMF during the last year of the study period.

TABLE 68.19. Demographics of Patients Undergoing Lung Transplantation at UCSF (1991–1996)

| Parameter | >60 Years ($n$ = 7) | <60 Years ($n$ = 35) |
|---|---|---|
| Age (years) | | |
| Mean | 62.16 | 47.10 |
| Median | 62.30 | 47.00 |
| Range | 60.30–65.00 | 29.80–59.40 |
| Sex | | |
| Male | 5 (71.4%) | 14 (40.0%) |
| Female | 2 (28.5%) | 21 (60.0%) |
| Single-lung transplant | 6 (85.7%) | 23 (65.7%) |
| Double-lung transplant | 1 (14.3%) | 12 (34.3%) |
| Diagnosis | | |
| Emphysema | 5 (71.4%) | 11 (31.4%) |
| Pulmonary fibrosis | 1 (14.3%) | 5 (14.3%) |
| Pulmonary HTN | — | 6 (17.1%) |
| $\alpha_1$-Antitrypsin deficiency | — | 6 (17.1%) |
| CF/bronchiectasis | — | 4 (11.4%) |
| Amyloid | 1 (14.3%) | — |
| Other | — | 3 (8.6%) |
| Follow-up (months) | | |
| Mean | 18 | 28 |
| Median | 16 | 23 |
| Range | 9–35 | 8–64 |

Quadruple antibiotics in the form of vancomycin, ceftazidime, metronidazole, and fluconazole were given for 7 days perioperatively for prophylaxis against bacterial and fungal pneumonia. CMV, fungal, and *Pneumocystis* prophylaxis was similar to that for heart transplantation. The protocol for rejection surveillance at UCSF requires bronchoscopy with biopsy, formal pulmonary function tests, and chest computed tomography (CT) at set intervals. Because biopsy has proven to be insensitive to early rejection, patients were requested to report by telephone simple spirometry parameters on a frequent basis. Abnormally low volumes may signal either rejection or infection, prompting further evaluation. Treatment of rejection was determined by the histologic evaluation of biopsy specimens.[66]

## Mortality

The 1-year and 5-year actuarial survivals for all lung transplant recipients was approximately 70% and 45%, respectively, as reported in 1997 by the Registry of the ISHLT.[44] The Registry reported a statistically significant decrease in actuarial survival for patients more than 55 years of age compared to patients less than 55 years. Multivariate logistic regression analysis for the 1-year mortality after lung transplantation identifies odds ratios of 1.15, 1.80, and 3.32 for the risk factors of age >50, >60, and >70 years, respectively.[44]

The actuarial survival curves for patients more than and less than 60 years who have undergone lung transplantation at UCSF are shown in Figure 68.8. All of the three deaths in the seven older patients occurred during the first year after transplantation, resulting in 1- and 2-year actuarial survival of 53.6%. The Toronto experience reported a higher 1-year actuarial survival (72%) for patients over 50 years but a lower 1-year actuarial survival (68%) for patients less than 50 years.[64] The three deaths in the older UCSF group were due to sepsis (two) and sudden death (one).

## Rejection

Kaplan-Meier curves describing first rejection events for patients more and less than 60 years given transplants at UCSF are shown in Figure 68.9. It is striking that only two of the seven older patients had any episodes of acute rejection, leaving 71.4% free of rejection. In contrast, 18 of

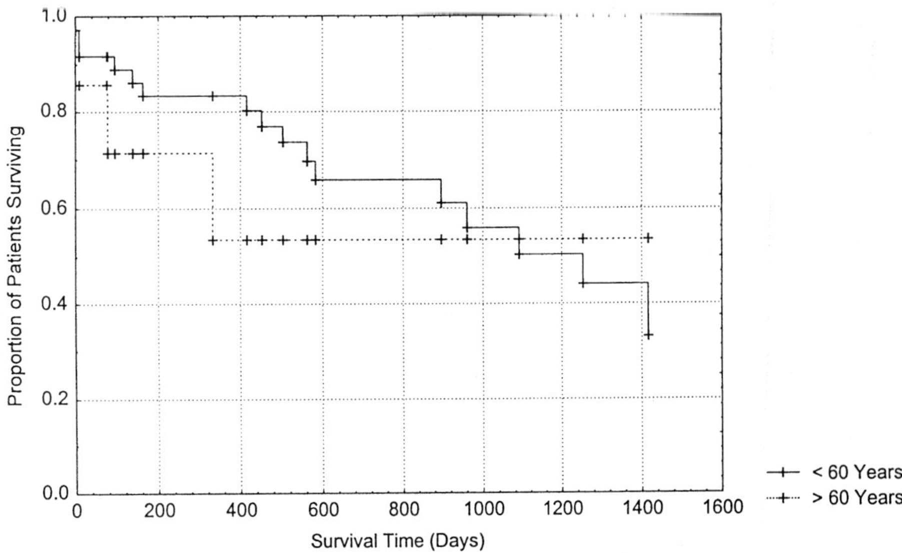


FIGURE 68.8. Patient survival after lung transplantation, UCSF 1991–1996.

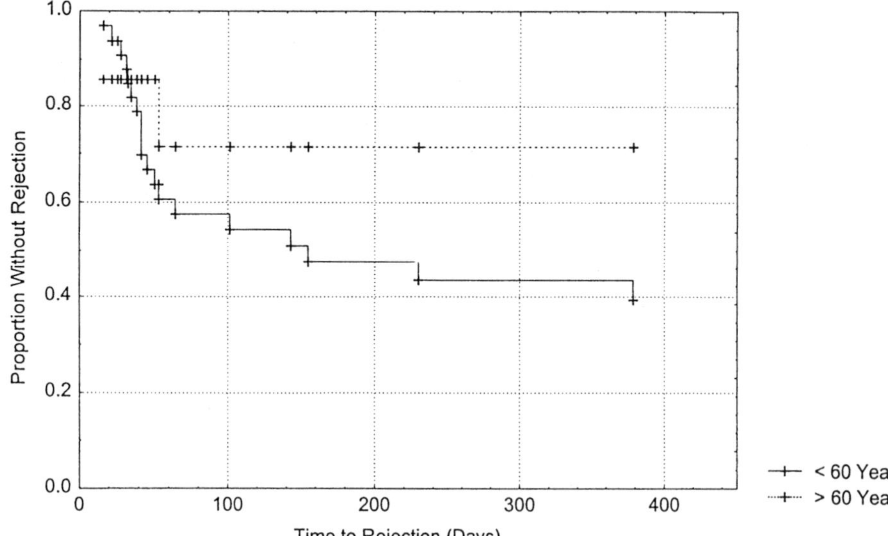


FIGURE 68.9. Lung transplant rejection, UCSF 1991–1996.

the 35 younger patients had rejection, leaving only 48.6% free of rejection. Chronic rejection, or bronchiolitis obliterans, has not been documented in any of the older patients given transplants at UCSF. Nine of the younger patients, however, had documented bronchiolitis obliterans; and as discussed above, three patients died as a result. The University of Toronto also reported a lower incidence of both acute and chronic rejection in their older patients.[64]

## Morbidity

The Toronto group presented data regarding quality of life after lung transplantation for older and younger patients.[63] Of patients who were alive 1 year after transplantation, only 1 of 16 older patients but 8 of 40 younger patients were functionally disabled. All other measures of posttransplant morbidity, including the incidence of CMV pneumonitis and postoperative renal function, did not differ between patients more or less than 50 years of age. Finally, Table 68.20 shows the hospital stays for UCSF patients who were successfully discharged after lung transplantation. There was no significant difference in the length of hospitalization between patients more or less than 60 years of age.

TABLE 68.20. Length of Stay after Lung Transplantation at UCSF (1991–1996)

| | Length of stay (days) | |
|---|---|---|
| Parameter | >60 Years | <60 Years |
| Mean | 17 | 23 |
| Median | 17 | 19 |
| Range | 8–31 | 10–71 |

## Conclusions

As the population continues to age, an increasing number of older patients with end-stage organ failure will compete for the limited supply of available organs. Data from UCSF and other programs presented here, clearly indicate that older patients can undergo kidney, liver, heart, or lung transplantation with excellent results. Several themes that distinguish older and younger transplant patients have emerged that merit discussion.

First, there is strong concordance that the incidence of rejection, both acute and chronic, is lower in older transplant patients. Nevertheless, essentially all transplant programs apply immune suppression protocols in a uniform fashion to all patients without regard to age. We suggest that reduction of immune suppression in older patients may improve both short- and long-term survival. In several areas of transplantation, older patients have a higher incidence of perioperative and early posttransplant mortality resulting in a steep decline in short-term survival. There are already some data from UCSF and other programs in kidney and heart transplantation, suggesting that cytolytic induction therapy may be associated with higher posttransplant mortality. Furthermore, because sepsis is responsible for a significant proportion of early deaths, less immune suppression during the perioperative period may translate into improved short-term survival.

The long-term impact of immune suppression may also contribute to enhanced patient loss over time in the older transplant population. The higher incidence of malignancy, including posttransplant lymphoproliferative disease, among older patients is a recurrent theme in the transplant literature. Unique to liver transplantation, the high rate of recurrent hepatitis C (80%) in patients over 60 years of age underscores the possibility that older patients are simply being overly immune suppressed. It is striking that in all areas of transplantation the incidence of acute rejection in older patients more than 6 months after transplantation is low. Yet transplant programs do not report any efforts to wean immune suppression preferentially in older patients. Although decreased immune suppression may in turn be associated with increased rejection, the correlation between acute rejection and decreased patient survival has not been clearly established in all areas of transplantation.

A substantial percentage of late posttransplant deaths in kidney and liver patients over 60 years of age were attributable to cardiac disease despite thorough pretransplant cardiac evaluation. In addition, many cardiac complications occurred in patients who had no pretransplant evidence of significant cardiac disease. An evaluation of overall left ventricular function in conjunction with an assessment of myocardial perfusion has been widely used to determine cardiac risk prior to surgery. The results in kidney and liver transplant patients over 60 years of age, suggest that such conventional testing regimens are insufficiently sensitive to predict future cardiac events in these patient populations. Other factors that may contribute to increased cardiac risk after transplantation are the side effects of common immune suppressive medications used. Prednisone, tacrolimus, and CYA predispose patients to important cardiac risk factors, such as hypertension, diabetes mellitus, and hyperlipidemia/hypercholesterolemia. Aggressive management of these conditions may substantially reduce posttransplant cardiac morbidity and mortality.

Therefore, although the current results of solid-organ transplantation in patients over 60 years of age are acceptable, our analysis suggests several areas where a change in practice may improve results in the future. It is clear that meticulous and individualized pretransplant evaluation and posttransplant care are critical to successful transplantation in older patients. Past experience has elucidated important differences between older and younger patients that have been highlighted in this chapter. Understanding and exploiting these differences to the advantage of the older patient can optimize the outcome of solid-organ transplantation in this expanding population of patients.

## References

1. Agodoa LY, Eggers PW. Renal replacement therapy in the United States: data from the United States renal data system. Am J Kidney Dis 1995;25:119–133.
2. Inglehart G. The American health care system: the end stage renal disease program. N Engl J Med 1993;328:366.
3. Bonal J, Cleries M, Vela E. Renal Registry Committee. Transplantation versus haemodialysis in elderly patients: Renal Registry Committee. Nephrol Dial Transplant 1997;12: 261–264.
4. Schaubel D, Desmeules M, Mao Y, et al. Survival experience among elderly end-stage renal disease patients. A controlled comparison of transplantation and dialysis. Transplantation 1995;60:1389–1394.
5. Nyberg G, Nilsson B, Hallste G, et al. Renal transplantation in elderly patients: survival and complications. Transplant Proc 1993;25:1062–1063.
6. Albrechtsen D, Leivestad T, Sodal G, et al. Kidney transplantation in patients older than 70 years of age. Transplant Proc 1995;27:986–988.
7. Eggers P. Effect of transplantation on the Medicare end-stage renal disease program. N Engl J Med 1988;1:223.
8. Wedel N, Brynger H, Blohme I. Kidney transplantation in patients 60 years and older. Scand J Urol Nephrol 1980; 54(suppl):106.
9. Kock B, Luhlback B, Ahonen J, et al. Kidney transplantation in patients over 60 years of age. Scand J Urol Nephrol 1980; 54(suppl):103.
10. Ost L, Groth C, Lindholm B, et al. Cadaveric renal transplantation in patients of 60 years and above. Transplantation 1980;30:339–340.
11. Hunsicker L. Impact of cyclosporine on cadaveric renal transplantation: a summary statement. Am J Kidney Dis 1985;6:335.
12. Pirsch JD, Stratta RJ, Armbrust MJ, et al. Cadaveric renal transplantation with cyclosporine in patients more than 60 years of age. Transplantation 1989;47:259–261.
13. Sommer B, Ferguson R, Davin T, et al. Renal transplantation in patients over 50 years of age. Transplant Proc 1981;13: 33–35.
14. Lundgren G, Fehrman I, Gunnarson B, et al. Cadaveric renal transplantation in patients over 55 years of age with special emphasis on immunosuppressive therapy. Transplant Proc 1982;14:601–604.
15. Vollmer W, Wahl P, Blagg C. Survival with dialysis and transplantation in patients with end-stage renal disease. N Engl J Med 1983;308:1553–1558.
16. Taube D, Winder E, Ogg C, et al. Successful treatment of middle aged and elderly patients with end-stage renal failure. Br Med J 1983;286:2018–2020.
17. Hutchinson T, Thomas D, Lemieux J, Harvey C. Prognostically controlled comparison of dialysis and renal transplantation. Kidney Int 1984;26:44–51.
18. Garcia-Garcia G, Deddens J, D'Achiardi-Rey R, et al. Results of treatment in patients with end stage renal disease: a multi-variate analysis of risk factors and survival in 341 successive patients. Am J Kidney Dis 1984;5:10–18.
19. Burton P, Walls J. Selection-adjusted comparison of life-expectancy of patients on continuous ambulatory peritoneal dialysis, haemodialysis, and renal transplantation. Lancet 1987;1:1115–1119.
20. Lindner A, Charre B, Sherrard D, Scribner B. Accelerated atherosclerosis in prolonged maintenance hemodialysis. N Engl J Med 1974;290:697–701.
21. Tesi RJ, Elkhammas EA, Davies EA, et al. Renal transplantation in older people. Lancet 1994;343:461–464.
22. Benedetti E, Matas AJ, Hakim N, et al. Renal transplantation for patients 60 years of older: a single-institution experience. Ann Surg 1994;220:445–458.
23. Abouna GM, Kumar MS, Curfman K, Phillips K. Kidney transplantation in patients older than 60 years of age—is it

worth it? Transplant Proc 1995;27:2567–2568.

24. Berthoux FC, Jones EH, Mehls O, Valderrabano F. Transplantation report. 1. Renal transplantation in recipients aged 60 years or older at time of grafting: the EDTA-ERA Registry, European Dialysis and Transplant Association–European Renal Association. Nephrol Dial Transplant 1996;11(suppl 1):37–40.
25. Hestin D, Frimat L, Hubert J, et al. Renal transplantation in patients over sixty years of age. Clin Nephrol 1994;42: 232–236.
26. Cantarovich D, Baatard R, Baranger T, et al. Cadaveric renal transplantation after 60 years of age: a single center experience. Transpl Int 1994;7:33–38.
27. Sharma AK, Brown M, Connolly J, et al. Analysis of factors affecting the outcome of renal transplantation in older people. Transplant Proc 1997;29:261.
28. Nyberg G, Nilsson B, Norden G, Karlberg I. Outcome of renal transplantation in patients over the age of 60: a case-control study. Nephrol Dial Transplant 1995;10:91–94.
29. Phillips AO, Bewick M, Snowden SA, et al. The influence of recipient and donor age on the outcome of renal transplantation. Clin Nephrol 1993;40:352–354.
30. Andreu J, de la Torre M, Oppenheimer F, et al. Renal transplantation in elderly recipients. Transplant Proc 1992; 24:120–121.
31. Mourad G, Cristol JP, Vela C, et al. Cadaveric renal transplantation in patients 60 years of age and older: experience with 58 patients in a single centre. Nephrol Dial Transplant 1995;10(suppl 6):105–107.
32. Hirata M, Cho Y, Cecka J, Terasaki P. Patient death after renal transplantation: an analysis of its role in graft outcome. Transplantation 1996;61:1479–1483.
33. West M, Sutherland D, Matas A. Kidney transplant recipients who die with functioning grafts. Transplantation 1996; 62:1029–1030.
34. Matas A, Gillingham K, Sutherland D. Half-life and risk factors for kidney transplant outcome: importance of death with function. Transplantation 1993;55:757–761.
35. Marwick T, Steinmuller D, Underwood D, et al. Ineffectiveness of dipyridamole SPECT thallium imaging as a screening technique for coronary artery disease in patients with end-stage renal failure. Transplantation 1990;49:100–103.
36. Boudreau R, Strony J, duCret R, et al. Perfusion thallium imaging of type I diabetes patients with end stage renal disease: comparison of oral and intravenous dipyridamole administration. Radiology 1990;175:103–105.
37. Brown JH, Vites NP, Testa HJ, et al. Value of thallium myocardial imaging in the prediction of future cardiovascular events in patients with end-stage renal failure. Nephrol Dial Transplant 1993;8:433–437.
38. Reis G, Marcovitz PA, Leichtman AB, et al. Usefulness of dobutamine stress echocardiography in detecting coronary artery disease in end-stage renal disease. Am J Cardiol 1995; 75:707–710.
39. Pirsch JD, Kalayoglu M, Am DA, et al. Orthotopic liver transplantation in patients 60 years of age and older. Transplant Proc 1991;51:431–433.
40. Stieber AC, Gordon RD, Todo S, et al. Liver transplantation in patients over sixty years of age. Transplantation 1991; 51:271–273.
41. United Kingdom Transplant Support Service Authority. Annual Report, 1993.
42. Bromley PN, Hilmi I, Tan KC, et al. Orthotopic liver transplantation in patients over 60 years old. Transplantation 1994;58:800–803.
43. Kilpe VE, Krakauer H, Wren RE. An analysis of liver transplant experience from 37 transplant centers as reported to Medicare. Transplantation 1993;56:554–561.
44. Hosenpud JD, Bennett LE, Keck BM, et al. The Registry of the International Society for Heart and Lung Transplantation: fourteenth official report—1997. J Heart Lung Transplant 1997;16:691–712.
45. Fabbri A, Sharples LD, Mullins P, et al. Heart transplantation in patients over 54 years of age with triple-drug therapy immunosuppression. J Heart Lung Transplant 1992;11:929–932.
46. Kaye M. The Registry of the International Society for Heart and Lung Transplantation: ninth official report—1992. J Heart Lung Transplant 1992;11:599–606.
47. O'Connell J, Gunnar R, Evans R, et al. 24th Bethesda conference: task force 1: organization of heart transplantation in the U.S. J Am Coll Cardiol 1993;22:8–14.
48. Rickenbacher PR, Lewis NP, Valantine HA, et al. Heart transplantation in patients over 54 years of age: mortality, morbidity and quality of life. Eur Heart J 1997;18:870–878.
49. Blanche C, Takkenberg JJ, Nessim S, et al. Heart transplantation in patients 65 years of age and older: a comparative analysis of 40 patients. Ann Thorac Surg 1996;62:1442–1446.
50. Everett JE, Djalilian AR, Kubo SH, et al. Heart transplantation for patients over age 60. Clin Transplant 1996;10:478–481.
51. Bull DA, Karwande SV, Hawkins JA, et al. Long-term results of cardiac transplantation in patients older than sixty years: UTAH cardiac transplant program. J Thorac Cardiovasc Surg 1996;111:423–427.
52. Gheissari A, Yokoyama T, Hendel J, Fuentes J. Effect of advanced age on short- and long-term outcome of heart transplantation. Transplant Proc 1995;27:2628–2632.
53. Robin J, Ninet J, Tronc F, et al. Long-term results of heart transplantation deteriorate more rapidly in patients over 60 years of age. Eur J Cardiothorac Surg 1996;10:259–263.
54. Heroux AL, Costanzo-Nordin MR, Je OS, et al. Heart transplantation as a treatment option for end-stage heart disease in patients older than 65 years of age. J Heart Lung Transplant 1993;12:573–578.
55. Aravot DJ, Banner NR, Khaghani A, et al. Cardiac transplantation in the seventh decade of life. Am J Cardiol 1989;63:90–93.
56. Frazier OH, Macris MP, Duncan JM, et al. Cardiac transplantation in patients over 60 years of age. Ann Thorac Surg 1988;45:129–132.
57. Ott GY, Norman DJ, Hosenpud JD, et al. Heart transplantation in patients with previous cardiac operations: excellent clinical results. J Thorac Cardiovasc Surg 1994;107:203–209.
58. Carrel T, Neth J, Mohacsi P, et al. Perioperative risk and long-term results of heart transplantation after previous cardiac operations. Ann Thorac Surg 1997;63:1133–1137.
59. Billingham ME, Cary NR, Hammond ME, et al. A working formulation for the standardization of nomenclature in the diagnosis of heart and lung rejection: Heart Rejection Study

Group, The International Society for Heart Transplantation. J Heart Transplant 1990;9:587–593.

60. Kobashigawa JA, Kirklin JK, Naftel DC, et al. Pretransplantation risk factors for acute rejection after heart transplantation: a multiinstitutional study: the Transplant Cardiologists Research Database Group. J Heart Lung Transplant 1993;12:355–366.
61. Renlund DG, Gilbert EM, Gay WA Jr, et al. Age-associated decline in cardiac allograft rejection. Am J Med 1987;83: 391–398.
62. Miller LW, Vitale-Noedel N, Pennington G, et al. Heart transplantation in patients over age fifty-five years. J Heart Transplant 1988;7:254–257.
63. Olivari MT, Antolick A, Kaye MP, et al. Heart transplantation in elderly patients. J Heart Transplant 1988;7:258–264.
64. Snell GI, De Hoyos A, Winton T, Maurer JR. Lung transplantation in patients over the age of 50. Transplantation 1993;55:562–566.
65. Morrison DL, Maurer JR, Grossman RF. Preoperative assessment for lung transplantation. Clin Chest Med 1990;11:207–215.
66. Berry GJ, Brunt EM, Chamberlain EM, et al. A working formulation for the standardization of nomenclature in the diagnosis of heart and lung rejection: Lung Rejection Study Group, The International Society for Heart Transplantation. J Heart Transplant 1990;9:593–601.

# *Part II*
# *Specific Issues in Geriatric Surgery*

## Section 12
## Applications of Minimal Access Techniques to the Surgical Case of the Elderly

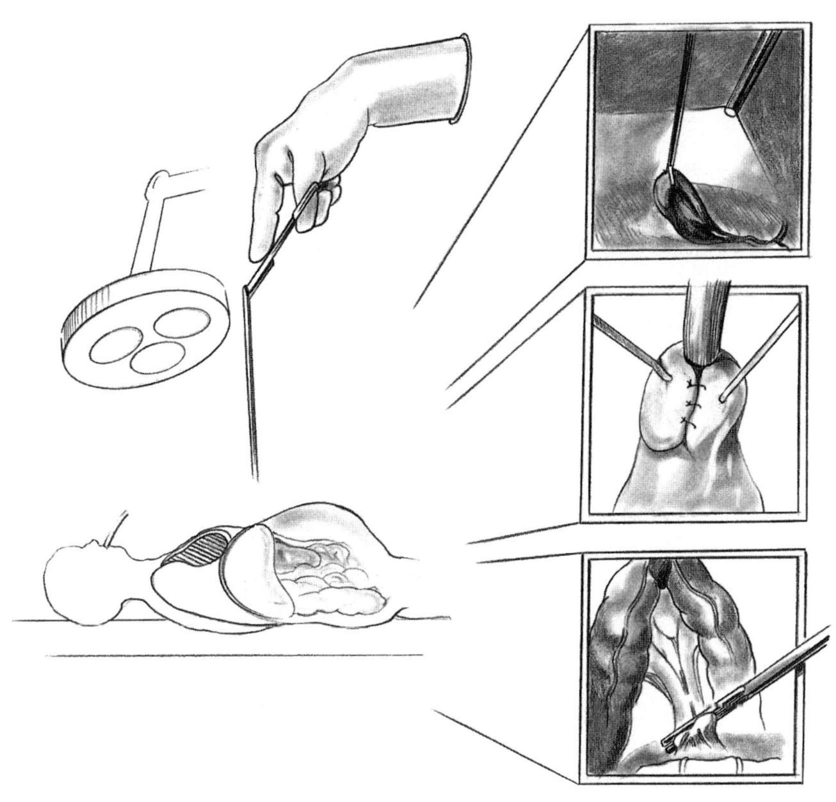

# 69 Physiology of Laparoscopic Surgery

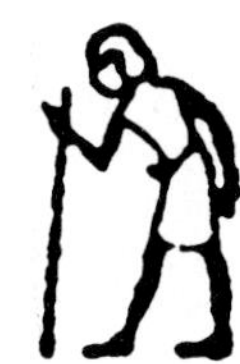

Jeffrey H. Peters and Namir Katkhouda

The basic physiologic alterations associated with controlled surgical trauma have been studied for decades.[1] These cardiovascular, metabolic, and hormonal responses to injury are fundamental to surgical practice and are well known to most practicing surgeons. It is also clear that the host response is proportional to the magnitude of the operative procedure.[2] Minor procedures evoke minimal metabolic and hormonal alterations, and major procedures stress the individual to a greater degree, potentially leading to an increased incidence of perioperative complications.

The emergence of laparoscopic surgery over the past decade has rekindled the study of physiologic alterations associated with surgical access. The shorter hospital stay, less pain, and earlier return to normal activity with laparoscopy is immediately evident to clinicians and has been amply documented by objective studies. Whether laparoscopy results in an amelioration of the traumatic response to elective surgery is a topic of current interest. Differences in hemodynamic and pulmonary function have been described, as have changes in the hormonal stress responses and immunologic consequences. Despite the widespread enthusiasm for laparoscopic procedures, we now are only beginning to understand the real advantages of avoiding an incision.

The rapid expansion of laparoscopy in general surgery has shifted the patient demographics. More often, elderly and debilitated patients with significant co-morbidity are undergoing laparoscopic surgical procedures. Although elderly and disabled patients benefit greatly from the reduction in surgical trauma effected by laparoscopy, they may be at increased risk for perioperative complications due to the hemodynamic and cardiorespiratory changes caused by the pneumoperitoneum.

## Hemodynamic and Cardiovascular Physiology

Most endoscopic surgery is performed in the abdomen or pelvis using insufflation of gas into the peritoneal cavity. Thus the dynamics of the pneumoperitoneum are central to understanding hemodynamic and cardiovascular physiology during endoscopic surgery. The cardiovascular changes associated with the pneumoperitoneum are a complex balance between the mechanical effects of increased intraabdominal pressure and the systemic effects of the absorbed gas. A variety of factors mitigate these two fundamental processes, including control of hypercarbia through augmentation of minute ventilation, intravascular volume status, absolute level of intraabdominal pressure, body positioning, anesthetic technique, degree of surgical or pain stimulus, and cardiovascular co-morbidity (Table 69.1).

### Mechanical Effects of Increased Intraabdominal Pressure

Elevation of intraabdominal pressure via establishment of a pneumoperitoneum results in systemic cardiovascular effects including (1) increased afterload; (2) increased peripheral venous resistance; and (3) increased mean systemic pressure (Fig. 69.1). Isolated elevation of intraabdominal pressure produces compression of the splanchnic circulation, increased afterload, and depressed cardiac function. For example, infusion of saline into the peritoneal cavity results in increased cardiac afterload and changes in the left ventricular func-

TABLE 69.1. Factors Influencing Hemodynamic Changes During Endoscopic Surgery and Pneumoperitoneum

| |
|---|
| Mechanical effects of increased intraabdominal pressure |
| Systemic effects of the absorbed gas |
| Control of hypercarbia/minute ventilation |
| Intravascular volume status |
| Absolute level of intraabdominal pressure |
| Body positioning |
| Anesthetic technique |
| Cardiovascular co-morbidity |

tion curve such that at any given left atrial filling pressure the cardiac output is lower.[3]

Cardiac output is further influenced by the effects of increased intraabdominal pressure on venous return through the inferior vena cava. Venous return is influenced by both mean systemic pressure and venous resistance. The mean systemic pressure is the pressure at the level of capillaries, small veins, and venules. It therefore constitutes the "pump," or pressure head, driving the venous return and reflects "preload" in the broadest sense. It is determined by blood volume, vascular tone, and the pressure of tissues surrounding the capacitance vessels. Its effect as a pump driving the venous return is opposed by venous resistance, or the hydraulic resistance of the veins, between the site of highest mean systemic pressure and the right atrium. In the context of endoscopic surgery employing a pneumoperitoneum, the highest venous resistance is located in the intraabdominal inferior vena cava.

Intraabdominal hypertension therefore results in two opposing factors on venous return: (1) increased mean systemic pressure, which promotes venous return; and (2) increased venous resistance, which impedes venous return (Fig. 69.1). Kashtan et al. demonstrated that in hypovolemic and normovolemic states the relative effect of increased venous resistance predominates over the increased mean systemic pressure.[3] Venous return is diminished with intraabdominal hypertension, and cardiac output is reduced by Starling mechanisms (Fig. 69.2). Conversely, in relatively hypervolemic subjects, the increased mean systemic pressure produces increased hydrostatic pressure within the inferior vena cava, which is minimally compressed. The pump effect of increased mean systemic pressure therefore influences venous return to a greater degree than the increase in venous resistance during hypervolemia. The net effect is increased venous return and increased cardiac output mediated by Starling mechanisms (Fig. 69.2).

Cardiac performance in terms of the mechanical effects of the pneumoperitoneum is therefore most dependent on the volume status of the patient, but it is also influenced by the level of intraabdominal pressure applied. An intraabdominal pressure of 5 mmHg in dogs was associated with increased flow through the inferior vena cava, increased cardiac output, and increased mean arterial pressure.[4] At an intraabdominal pressure of

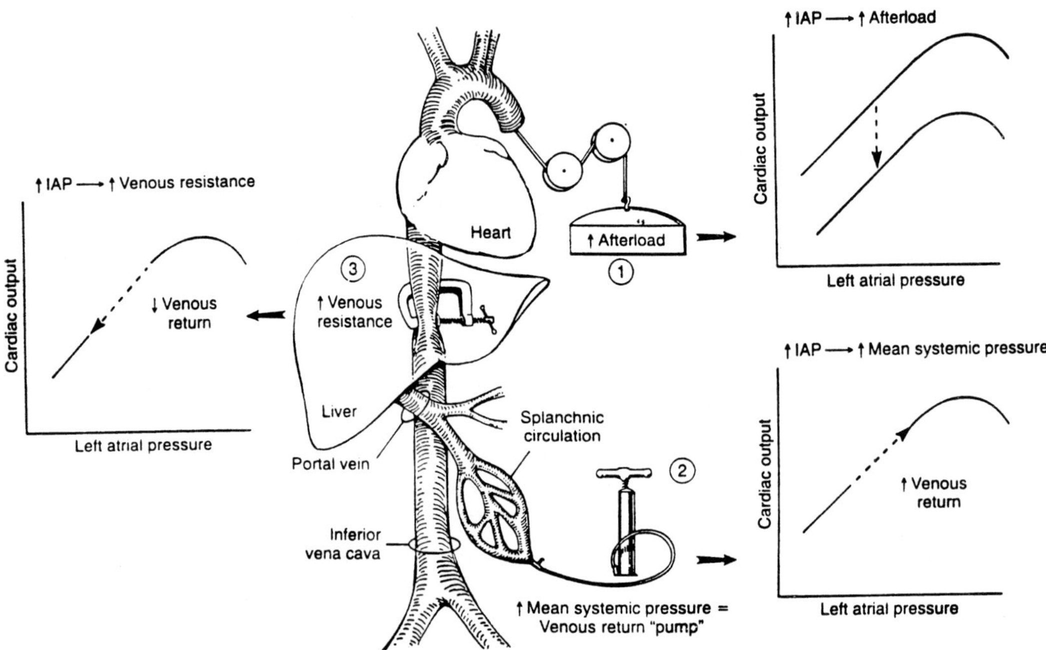


FIGURE 69.1. Hemodynamic effects of increased intraabdominal pressure (IAP). (1) Increased afterload increases the work of the heart and myocardial oxygen consumption. (2) Intraabdominal hypertension increases venous resistance at the level of the intraabdominal inferior vena cava, which impedes venous return. (3) Increasing mean systemic pressure augments the "pump" effect around capacitance vessels, tending to drive the venous return toward the heart. The isolated impact of these effects is depicted in each Starling curve.

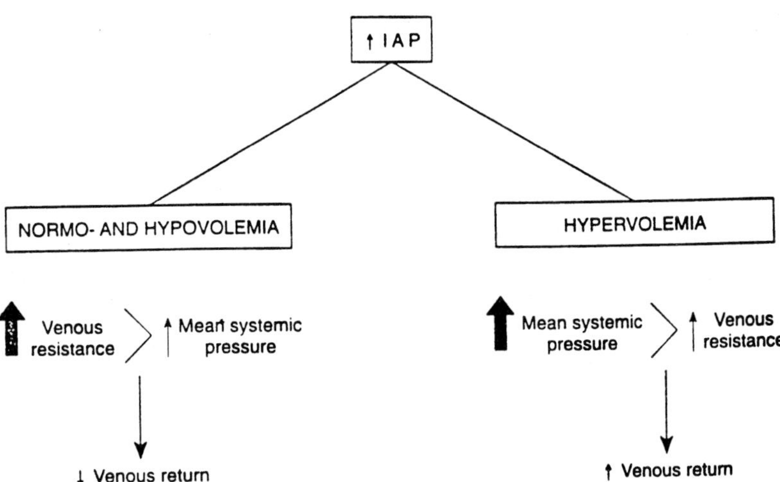


FIGURE 69.2. Hemodynamic effects of increased intraabdominal pressure on venous return (volume dependence). Increased intraabdominal pressure in normovolemic and hypovolemic subjects produces an elevation of venous resistance that is greater than the concomitant increase in mean systemic pressure. The net result is decreased venous return during insufflation in normo- and hypovolemic patients. Conversely, relatively hypervolemic subjects experience an increased mean systemic pressure that is greater than the elevation in venous resistance. Hypervolemic patients experience increased venous return during insufflation.

40 mmHg, caval flow, cardiac output, and mean arterial pressure were diminished. Similarly, Kelman et al. reported that intraabdominal pressures up to 20 mmHg were associated with increased central filling pressures and cardiac output.[5] Elevations of intraabdominal pressures up to 40 mmHg were associated with decreased central venous pressure and cardiac output.

## Physiologic Effects of Gas Absorption with Pneumoperitoneum

Since its inception, laparoscopy has utilized a variety of gases to produce pneumoperitoneum including air, nitrous oxide, carbon dioxide ($CO_2$), and more recently, helium and argon. $CO_2$ has been the gas of choice for decades.[6] Unlike air or nitrous oxide, $CO_2$ does not support combustion. It is clear, colorless, widely available, and rapidly absorbed from the abdominal cavity.

### *Carbon Dioxide Absorption*

The principal determinants of gas absorption from a body cavity are the difference in partial pressures between the two compartments (peritoneum and bloodstream) and the diffusion coefficient of the gas. Absorption from the abdominal cavity of an insufflated gas depends on the diffusion characteristics of the gas employed and the blood flow to the peritoneal surface. Net diffusion can be expressed as a single formula:

$$D = \frac{\Delta P \times A \times S}{d \times \sqrt{MW}}$$

where $D$ is the diffusion rate; $\Delta P$ is the partial pressure difference between the abdominal cavity and the bloodstream; $A$ is the cross-sectional area between the two; $S$ is the solubility of the gas; $d$ is the distance across which diffusion takes place; and $MW$ is the molecular weight of the gas. The two properties unique to each gas are its solubility and its molecular weight. This ratio of $S/\%MW$ is the diffusion coefficient. If oxygen is arbitrarily assigned a diffusion coefficient of 1.0, the *relative diffusion coefficients* of a variety of gases are as follows:

| | |
|---|---|
| Oxygen | 1.00 |
| Carbon dioxide | 20.30 |
| Nitrogen | 0.53 |
| Helium | 0.95 |
| Nitrous oxide | 11.80 |

Thus, the diffusion coefficient of carbon dioxide is 20 times that of oxygen or helium and 40 times that of nitrogen. This is largely due to the increased solubility of $CO_2$. Because of its high solubility, $CO_2$ reaches rapid equilibrium with the blood circulating at the surface of the peritoneal cavity. Because absorption is influenced by the rate of blood flow to the peritoneum, increased cardiac output also increases gas absorption from the peritoneal cavity (Fig. 69.3).

Once absorbed into the bloodstream, only a small fraction of $CO_2$ is carried in solution. Most is bound by hemoglobin and ultimately eliminated by the lungs. Not all $CO_2$ is eliminated by the lungs during periods of hypercarbia. The body responds to hypercarbia by moving $CO_2$ into various storage sites.[7] The total $CO_2$ storage capacity of the body is estimated to be 120 liters. In addition to the hemoglobin-buffering system, other storage facilities for $CO_2$ include bone and visceral stores, such as skeletal muscle. Bone constitutes the largest potential reservoir.

The net effect of $CO_2$ storage is to lower the circulating levels of $CO_2$. Short periods of hypercarbia, such as that produced by a Valsalva maneuver, result in transient increases in alveolar and blood $CO_2$ levels. Longer periods (20–60 minutes), such as those seen during insufflation for endoscopic procedures, may result in recruitment from skeletal muscle and other visceral storage sites. Hypercarbia lasting several weeks or more results in significant storage of $CO_2$ by bone. These storage dynamics explain

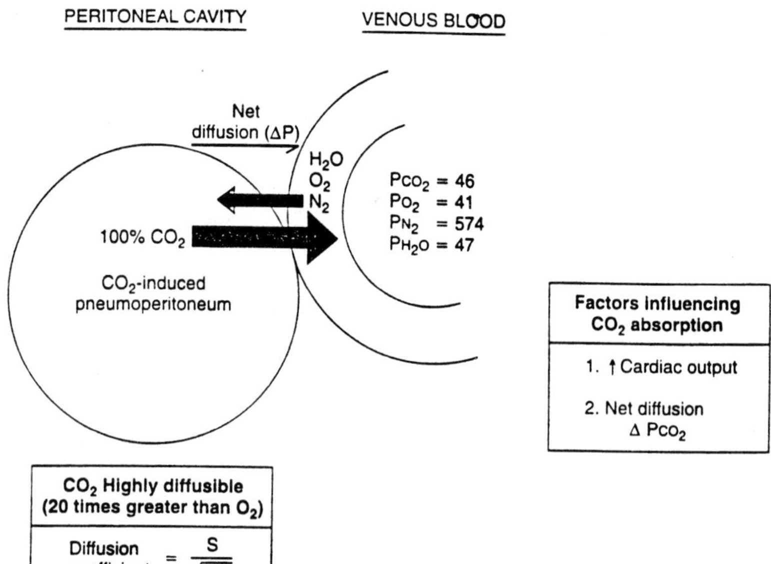


FIGURE 69.3. Systemic absorption of insufflated carbon dioxide. Differences in carbon dioxide pressures in the peritoneal cavity and the bloodstream favor its absorption. This process is rapid for carbon dioxide, given its high solubility in comparison to other gases. Increased cardiac output also favors absorption.

why patients in chronic $CO_2$ retentive states show precipitously increased and exaggerated plasma levels of $CO_2$ and why patients exposed to long periods of insufflation may have elevated arterial carbon dioxide ($PaCO_2$) for extended periods following dessufflation.

Hypercarbia and acidosis are well documented sequelae of the $CO_2$ pneumoperitoneum used for laparoscopic surgery. Liu et al. studied 16 healthy patients undergoing laparoscopic cholecystectomy, observing a 10mmHg rise in both the mean arterial and end-tidal $CO_2$ concentrations.[8] Eighty percent of patients required increased minute ventilation during the procedure to maintain safe levels of $CO_2$. In these otherwise healthy patients, there was excellent correlation between the end-tidal $CO_2$ ($PetCO_2$) and arterial blood gas measurement of carbon dioxide ($PaCO_2$). This may not be so in the elderly, and arterial blood gases should be monitored during the procedure.

The correlation of end-tidal and arterial $CO_2$ diminishes in patients with pulmonary disease and other comorbid conditions. Witgen et al. compared a group of healthy American Society of Anesthesiologists (ASA) class I patients undergoing laparoscopic cholecystectomy with ASA class II and III patients.[9] They observed more pronounced hypercarbia and acidosis in the ASA class II and III patients than in the healthy ASA class I patients. Moreover, in patients with additional co-morbidity, the end-tidal $CO_2$ may differ widely from arterial blood gas analysis of $CO_2$. The discrepancy lies in the fact that end-tidal capnography measures $CO_2$ at the end of expiration and contains both deadspace air and alveolar air. Chronic lung diseases increase the deadspace component of expired air, resulting in an underestimation of the end-tidal $CO_2$ when compared to arterial blood gas measurements.

Comparison of the effects of $CO_2$- and helium-induced pneumoperitoneum on cardiopulmonary function in both animal models and human subjects, suggests that hypercarbia and acidosis are not the results of mechanical impairment of pulmonary function resulting from the pneumoperitoneum. Leighton et al. have shown that although $CO_2$ pneumoperitoneum is associated with a rise in the $PaCO_2$, the arterial $CO_2$ concentration does not change with helium pneumoperitoneum.[10,11] Bongard et al. also noted a significant corresponding acidosis in the $CO_2$ pneumoperitoneum with a mean fall in pH from 7.43 to 7.29.[11]

## Chemical Effects of Hypercarbia

Unlike an inert gas such as helium, $CO_2$ exhibits potent effects on the heart and vasculature. This is in part mediated by acid–base changes but also through the direct effects of soluble $CO_2$ and indirect effects on the sympathetic nervous system (Fig. 69.4).

The direct effects of hypercarbia and acidosis on the myocardium and blood vessels are generally opposite the effects mediated through increased sympathetic activity.[12,13] Hypercarbia and acidosis are direct myocardial depressants. The predominant effect on denervated blood vessels appears to be vasodilation. The relative importance of an increasing $PaCO_2$ versus a decreasing pH is unknown. Moreover, the greatest effect of hypercarbia and acidosis appears to be on the capacitance blood vessels (i.e., the postarteriolar capillaries and veins).

Paradoxically, the aortic and carotid body chemoreceptors are exquisitely sensitive to hypercarbia. Chemoreceptor afferent impulses stimulate the posterior hypothalamus, mesencephalic reticular substance, and respiratory and vasomotor centers to produce hyper-

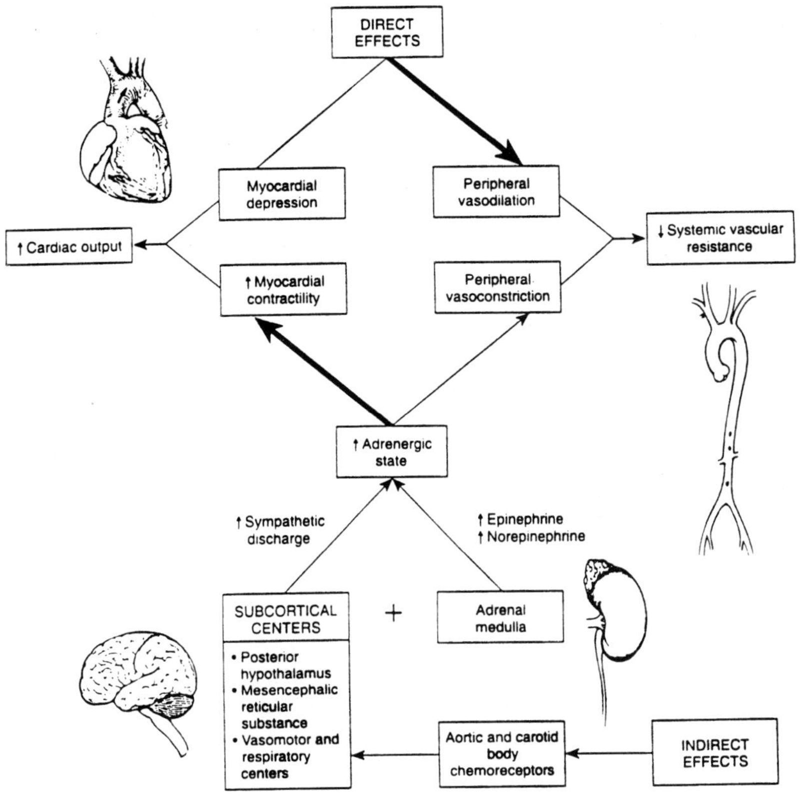


FIGURE 69.4. Hemodynamic effects of hypercarbia. Increased $PaCO_2$ and acidosis produce hemodynamic alterations through their direct actions on the heart and vasculature and indirect effects mediated through the sympathetic nervous system. The direct and indirect effects generally oppose one another. Overall, hypercarbia produces increased cardiac output with diminished systemic vascular resistance.

ventilation, cortical activation, increased sympathetic outflow, and increased skeletal muscular activity. The overall effects of these "centrally mediated" actions of hypercarbia coupled with increased adrenomedullary discharge generally are tachycardia, enhanced myocardial contractility, vasoconstriction, and arterial hypertension. Thus the centrally mediated actions of $CO_2$ antagonize its direct effects on the myocardium and the peripheral vascular system. In healthy, normal subjects breathing $CO_2$-rich air, the net effects include elevation in circulating levels of epinephrine and norepinephrine and hyperventilation. $CO_2$ "breathing" also produces greater increases in cardiac output relative to the arterial hypertension. Overall there is a decrease in systemic vascular resistance because the local vasodilatory effects of $CO_2$ are greater than the neurologically or sympathetically mediated vasoconstriction.[12]

Rasmussen et al. examined the effects of hypercarbia and cardiac function in 12 ASA class II–III patients undergoing carotid endarterectomy.[14] Anesthesia was maintained with a combination of oxygen, nitrous oxide, and methoxyflurane. $CO_2$ insufflation, resulting in elevation of the $PaCO_2$ to 56–65 mmHg (a range not uncommonly seen during endoscopic surgery), produced significant elevations in cardiac output and stroke volume and decreased systemic vascular resistance. Plasma catechols were increased two to three times above their baseline.

Extreme hypercarbia adversely affects myocardial contractility. The attendant acidosis interferes with the ability of sympathetically innervated cells to respond to the chemical stimulus of sympathetic nerves. Moreover, acidosis stimulates parasympathetic nervous activity, potentially manifesting as increased cardiac vagal tone.

## Other Factors Mitigating Hemodynamic Function

An analysis of the literature on hemodynamic function in laparoscopic surgery reveals often confounding and confusing results. Studies reporting increased, decreased, or unchanged cardiac output and every other hemodynamic parameter during insufflation are found in the literature.[5,15–23] These discrepant results suggest that a variety of cardiovascular manifestations are possible and depend on a number of factors. The importance of intravascular volume status and control of hypercarbia have been described. Several other factors may contribute to the net hemodynamic effects observed in any given patient, including body positioning, anesthetic technique, and the presence of underlying cardiopulmonary disease (Fig. 69.5).

Body positioning in the horizontal, Trendelenburg, and reverse Trendelenburg positions, influences venous return and cardiac output. The Trendelenburg position may increase cardiac output by as much as 20%.[24] Kelman

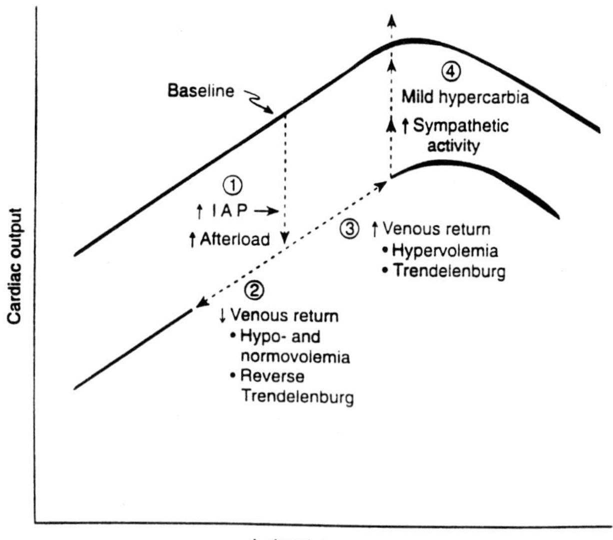


FIGURE 69.5. Summary of cardiac function after carbon dioxide insufflation. (1) Increased intraabdominal pressure (IAP) increases afterload, downshifting the Starling curve. (2) Venous return is diminished in hypo- and normovolemia and in the reverse Trendelenburg position. (3) Relative hypervolemia results in increasing venous return that drives the Starling curve higher. (4) Mild to moderate degrees of hypercarbia shift the Starling curve up via the net effects of enhanced sympathetic activity. Other factors modulating these responses are anesthetic technique and underlying cardiac disease.

et al. studied hemodynamic changes in patients undergoing laparoscopy in the horizontal versus Trendelenburg position.[5] Central filling pressures and cardiac outputs were significantly greater in the patients tilted head-down.

Anesthetic techniques are equally important when determining the net hemodynamic changes associated with laparoscopic surgery. Inhalational agents may variously produce myocardial depression (halothane) or increased myocardial contractility (isoflurane). Narcotic blockade of the sympathetic outflow from surgical/pain stimuli is also important. There are no comparative studies specifically examining the difference in hemodynamic effects during endoscopic surgery using different anesthetic regimens, and these investigations are needed.

Patients, including the elderly, with significant cardiopulmonary co-morbidity deserve special mention. Because of the association of pulmonary disease with cardiovascular disease and vice versa, patients in both disease groups may be at risk for intraoperative hypercarbia and acidosis, with their attendant alterations in hemodynamic function. Sarfan et al. examined the cardiopulmonary responses in 15 high risk cardiac patients (ASA class III–IV) undergoing laparoscopy.[18] They reported significant elevations in central filling pressures, systemic vascular resistance, and mean arterial pressure. On average, cardiac output was reduced. However, the risk class per se was not predictive of the degree of hemodynamic compromise. The authors concluded that pneumoperitoneum induces increased mean arterial pressure and systemic vascular resistance as well as decreased cardiac output in patients with poor cardiac reserve. They suggested that augmentation of preload volume loading may offset the stress of increased afterload and avoid left ventricular decompensation. This approach is counterintuitive to the more common practice of reducing preload in patients with left ventricular failure. It does, however, seem reasonable given the dynamics of increased intraabdominal pressure and its effects on venous return. Sarfan et al.'s study underscores the importance of careful and invasive monitoring of high risk patients during minimally invasive procedures.

## Organ-Specific Perfusion

Organ-specific and regional blood flow may be acutely altered during abdominal insufflation. Hepatic, renal, and mesenteric blood flow have been shown to decrease with pneumoperitoneum. In a canine model, Ishizaki et al. demonstrated that insufflation to 16mmHg diminished flow through the portal vein and superior mesenteric artery.[20,25] Hepatic arterial flow was not significantly altered. Iwase et al. compared urine output and clearance of *p*-aminohippurate (PAH) as indirect measures of renal blood flow in patients undergoing laparoscopic or open cholecystectomy (minilaparotomy).[26] Although there were no significant differences in blood pressure, pulmonary artery pressure, central venous pressure, or cardiac index between the groups, transient oliguria and decreased renal plasma flow calculated from PAH clearance were noted in the laparoscopy group.

The mechanisms responsible for these alterations in organ-specific blood flow remain obscure. One possible explanation invokes Poiseuille's law:

$$\text{Flow} \propto \text{radius}^4$$

Blood flow through any given vessel is proportional to its radius to the fourth power. Minor diminution in vessel diameter may dramatically decrease flow. Other mechanisms invoked include humorally mediated vasoconstriction by $CO_2$ and intrinsic myogenic control of vascular tone produced by increased intraabdominal pressure.

## Pulmonary Function

It has been recognized since the early part of the twentieth century that laparotomy, particularly upper abdominal surgery, results in a self-limited (5–7 days) but significant decrease in pulmonary function following surgery.[27] Standard spirometric pulmonary function is derived from the rate of flow measured by having the patient inspire maximally to total lung capacity and then exhale as forcefully and as rapidly as possible to residual volume. The rate of airflow measured during this period indirectly reflects the flow resistance properties of the airways. Airway obstruction can be detected by calculating flow rates during certain time intervals along the forced vital capacity (FVC) curve, most commonly the volume exhaled during the first second ($FEV_1$). The $FEV_1$ expressed as a percentage of the FVC ($FEV_1$/FVC, termed the FEV%) is an alternative measure of airway obstruction. Normal patients can exhale 75–80% of the FVC during the first second. Obstructive diseases (e.g., asthma) tend to impair expiratory flow rates and cause a decline in $FEV_1$ and the FEV%. Restrictive conditions (e.g., postoperative pain) results in a decreased FVC. The absolute volume of the $FEV_1$ may decline as well, but the $FEV_1$ as a percentage of FVC is usually normal.

The pulmonary consequences of abdominal surgery are complex. Physiologic changes are related to the anesthesia and the magnitude and type of the surgical procedure. Abdominal surgery generally results in a restrictive pattern of pulmonary physiologic change, with reductions in vital capacity and function residual capacity.[28,29] Investigators measured decreases in tidal volume and FVC averaging 40–50% after an upper midline incision.[27] More recently, transcutaneous oxygen saturation monitoring has identified a 30–35% incidence of hypoxemia ($O_2$ saturation < 85%) during the postoperative period after laparotomy.[30]

A number of factors account for these observed changes.[28,31] Pulmonary volumes are markedly altered after upper abdominal surgery as a result of incisional pain, muscular dysfunction, and diaphragmatic alterations. Intercostal nerve blockade and epidural analgesia only partly return pulmonary measurements to their preoperative levels.[32–35] Careful study has found fluid accumulation in the pleural space in a large percentage of patients, which may also account for some of the observed changes.[36]

Investigations into the decrement in pulmonary function after open cholecystectomy have documented declines averaging 50%. Latimer et al. studied 46 patients after upper abdominal surgery and noted a 59% decline in FVC on postoperative day 1, which slowly improved to 27% by postoperative day 7.[28] Similar changes were seen in the measured $FEV_1$. Patel et al., interested in the effects of incisional infiltration of bupivacaine, found a 49% decline in FVC immediately after open cholecystectomy, which improved to 21% with a local anesthetic.[35] Both Frazee et al. and Peters et al. reported that laparoscopic cholecystectomy diminishes pulmonary function by approximately one-fourth.[37,38] Peters et al. compared FVC, FEV, and forced expiratory flow (FEF) between patients undergoing laparoscopic versus open cholecystectomy.[38] The results are depicted in Table 69.2. Because of the small number of open cholecystectomy patients in this study, two of the differences in these parameters did not reach statistical significance, but the trends are suggestive.

Putensen-Himmer et al. reported a prospective randomized trial of 20 healthy (ASA I) patients undergoing elective open versus laparoscopic cholecystectomy.[39] The FVC and FEV were reduced by 57% and 54%, respectively, for the open cholecystectomy patients 24 hours postoperatively. The laparoscopic patients experienced decrements from the preoperative FVC and $FEV_1$ values of 30% and 15%, respectively. When measured at 72 hours postoperatively, these values had improved to nearly normal in the laparoscopic patients but not in those operated by an open technique (FVC 91% vs. 77% and $FEV_1$ 92% vs. 77%).

The adequacy of postoperative pain control certainly influences the magnitude of change observed in postoperative measurements, but is difficult to control and measure. Schauer et al. examined this issue in a comparative study between patients undergoing laparoscopic and open cholecystectomy.[40] They noted 30–38% differences in all areas studied including FVC, $FEV_1$, FEF, mid-expiratory phase, maximum forced expiratory flow, maximum voluntary ventilation total lung capacity, and oxygen saturation. Pulmonary function returned

TABLE 69.2. Pulmonary Function after Open and Laparoscopic Surgery

| Test | Preoperative | Postoperative | % Difference | $p^a$ |
|---|---|---|---|---|
| Forced vital capacity (liters) | | | | |
| Open ($n$ = 9) | 3.52 ± 0.32 | 2.24 ± 0.24 | 35.8 | 0.09 |
| Laparoscopic ($n$ = 31) | 3.56 ± 0.18 | 2.67 ± 0.17 | 22.9 | |
| Forced expiratory volume (liters) | | | | |
| Open ($n$ = 9) | 2.86 ± 0.33 | 1.81 ± 0.21 | 35.0 | 0.15 |
| Laparoscopic ($n$ = 31) | 2.76 ± 0.15 | 2.01 ± 0.12 | 24.3 | |
| Forced expiratory flow (liters) | | | | |
| Open ($n$ = 7) | 3.3 ± 0.47 | 1.98 ± 0.35 | 40.2 | 0.67 |
| Laparoscopic ($n$ = 31) | 2.59 ± 0.21 | 1.83 ± 0.14 | 24.4 | |

*Source:* Peters et al.,[38] with permission.
Results are given as means ± SEM.
[a] Student's *t*-test.

to baseline levels 4–10 days sooner after laparoscopic cholecystectomy. Pulmonary complications including atelectasis and hypoxia are were less frequent in patients following laparoscopic cholecystectomy. Schauer et al. reported an eightfold decrease in postoperative pain medication required [delivered via patient-controlled analgesia (PCA) devices] in those undergoing laparoscopic versus those with open cholecystectomy.

The above studies highlight differences in postoperative pulmonary function between patients undergoing laparoscopic and those with conventional open surgery. Preoperative pulmonary function tests may also play an important role in identifying patients susceptible to extreme hypercarbia and acidosis during abdominal insufflation with $CO_2$. Witgen et al. examined more than 80 demographic, laboratory, and perioperative parameters in 31 patients undergoing laparoscopic cholecystectomy.[41] Preoperative arterial blood gas analysis and pulmonary functions tests were performed in an effort to identify patients at risk for intraoperative acidosis (pH < 7.35). Neither age nor preoperative arterial blood gas analysis was predictive. Preoperative pulmonary function tests demonstrating FEVs less than 70% and diffusion defects less than 80% of predicted values identified patients at risk for intraoperative hypercarbia and acidosis.

## Metabolic and Stress Hormonal Response

Injury and surgery are associated with metabolic and stress hormonal responses. Cuthberson divided the metabolic response to injury into the *ebb* phase and the *flow* phase.[42] The ebb phase corresponds to the immediate response to injury and occurs during the first several hours after injury. The physiologic alterations are usually associated with tissue hypoxia particularly due to systemic or regional hypoperfusion. Volume loss, anxiety, pain, hypothermia, and release of cytokines and inflammatory mediators are the major contributors to the ebb phase.

With restoration of blood flow and with time, the ebb phase evolves into the flow phase. The time required for this transition depends on the magnitude of the injury and the efficacy of resuscitative efforts. For massive injuries, it may last up to 24–48 hours, even with appropriate and aggressive care. The flow phase corresponds to the period of compensation with an increase in metabolic rate, restoration of blood volume, and stimulation of the immune system. Most current management strategies in critically ill patients are designed to support the altered physiology of the flow phase.

Moore later divided the flow phase into the catabolic and anabolic stages.[1] The catabolic stage reflects the early phase of injury. The early metabolic alterations of injury include increased lipolysis, hyperglycemia secondary to gluconeogenesis and insulin resistance, and net proteolysis with negative nitrogen balance. The anabolic stage begins after the correction of volume deficits, control of infection and pain, restoration of oxygenation, and wound healing.

The metabolic responses and other physiologic alterations induced by injury are mediated by complex interactions among a variety of systems. These systems include the hypothalamic-pituitary axis, autonomic nervous system, endocrine system, and inflammatory mediators such as cytokines and vascular endothelial cell products. Table 69.3 lists hormones and hormone-like substances involved in the response to injury.

Immediately after injury, there is a rapid increase in the secretion of catecholamines. Because catecholamines rapidly disappear from blood, increased levels are not readily demonstrated following injury. An increase in urine catecholamines is much more readily apparent. Catecholamines increase lipolysis and promote gluconeogenesis and glycogenolysis.

Plasma cortisol is also transiently elevated usually 24–48 hours following injury. It plays a permissive role

TABLE 69.3. Stress Hormonal Responses to Injury or Surgery

| |
|---|
| **Increased release** |
| Epinephrine |
| Norepinephrine |
| Dopamine |
| Glucagon |
| Renin |
| Angiotensin |
| Arginine vasopressin |
| ACTH |
| Cortisol |
| Aldosterone |
| β-Endorphin |
| Growth hormone |
| Prolactin |
| Somatostatin |
| Eicosanoids |
| Histamine |
| Kinins |
| Serotonin |
| Interleukin-1 |
| Tumor necrosis factor |
| Interleukin-6 |
| **Decreased release** |
| Insulin |
| Estrogen |
| Testosterone |
| Thyroxine |
| Triiodothyronine |
| Thyroid-stimulating hormone |
| Follicle-stimulating hormone |
| Luteinizing hormone |
| Immunoglobulin F |

*Source:* Adapted from Schwartz SI (ed) Principles of Surgery, 6th ed. New York: McGraw Hill, 1994:3–59, with permission.

in the actions of catecholamines. Growth hormone aids in the mobilization of lipids. Glucagon is also involved in glycogenolysis, gluconeogenesis, and lipolysis.

The magnitude of the metabolic and hormonal responses is primarily tailored to the degree of injury,[43–45] and the duration of surgery.[44,45] A variety of other factors mitigate the injury response, including age, pain, nutritional status, and infection. Decreasing or abolishing the metabolic response to surgery may reduce postoperative morbidity.[46,47]

Minimally invasive surgery may present an alternative approach to diminishing metabolic responses by the avoidance of a substantial abdominal incision. Minimally invasive surgery is also associated with less pain, improved postoperative pulmonary function, decreased ileus, shorter convalescence, decreased hospital stay, and more rapid return to productivity.[48–51] Minor surgery causes minimal metabolic and hormonal alteration, whereas major surgery produces a great stress response, leading to an increased incidence of perioperative complications.

Laparoscopic cholecystectomy is a typical example of minimally invasive surgery, characterized by minor access to the body cavities using endoscopic techniques.[52] Laparoscopic cholecystectomy therefore provides a means for determining the normal physiologic responses to surgery.

## Stress Hormonal Response

The earliest response following a major operation is stimulation of the hypothalamic-pituitary-adrenal axis. It involves both afferent nervous signals, which can indicate the presence and status of a wound, and efferent nervous signals, which affect end-organ function.

The pituitary gland is activated when afferent nervous signals from the wound reach the hypothalamus to initiate the stress response, which stimulates the release of cortisol. An increase in sympathetic nervous system activity not only results in release of catecholamines, primarily epinephrine, from the adrenal medulla, it also stimulates the release of glucagon while suppressing the release of insulin.[53] These hormones initiate the acute metabolic response, which causes an increased metabolic rate, hyperglycemia, increased lipolysis, negative nitrogen balance, and insulin resistance.[53] The plasma concentration of growth hormone is elevated for 24 hours after injury.[54] Antidiuretic hormone and aldosterone are also elevated following injury.[55,56] The renin-angiotensin system is activated, and the glucagon level is elevated about 12 hours after major injury.[57,58]

An elevation in plasma catecholamine levels is observed during laparoscopy,[59] with the catechol response normalizing within 24 hours after the surgery (Fig. 69.6).[60] The peak cortisol response to laparoscopic cholecystectomy is lower than after standard cholecystectomy, although the pattern of elevation is similar (Fig. 69.7). Ortega et al. showed that serum cortisol and urinary free cortisol levels were similar for open and laparoscopic cholecystectomy.[60] The serum ACTH and cortisol levels were higher during the first 4 hours postoperatively, then were normal by 24 hours.

There are no differences in thyroid-stimulating hormone (TSH), thyroxine ($T_4$), or triodothyromine ($T_3$) levels for the open and laparoscopic groups during the first 24 hours after surgery.[60] The antidiuretic hormone (ADH) response was higher in patients undergoing laparoscopy, particularly intraoperatively (Fig. 69.8). The rise of ADH is caused by the pneumoperitoneum that alternatively decreases the inferior vena cava blood flow and subsequently activates ADH release.[61,62] The serum level of growth hormone is similar for open and laparoscopic surgery.[60]

## Carbohydrate Metabolism

Hyperglycemia occurs immediately after injury (ebb phase) and persists into the flow phase. The easily established response is initially the result of enhanced glycogenolysis[63] and later a consequence of increased glucose production coupled with reduced peripheral glucose utilization.[64] Increased hepatic gluconeogenesis and impaired peripheral glucose uptake result from increased secretion of catecholamines, cortisol, glucagon, and growth hormone and reduced secretion of insulin following injury.

Glucose production during the flow phase results primarily from hepatic and renal gluconeogenesis mediated through glucagon and insulin using amino acids, lactate, pyruvate, and glycerol substrates. In burn patients, it has been shown that lactate is quantitatively the most important gluconeogenic substrate.[64]

Insulin concentration is decreased following injury owing to a reduction in beta islet cell sensitivity to glucose, which is mediated by catecholamines, cortisol, and increased activity of the sympathetic nervous system.[65] During the flow phase, insulin concentrations increase but hyperglycemia persists owing to insulin resistance.[66]

Minimally invasive surgery demonstrates mild hyperglycemia intraoperatively comparable to open surgery.[60] Postoperatively, serum glucose and insulin levels are lower in patients undergoing laparoscopy than open surgery at 4, 12, and 24 hours (Fig. 69.9).

## Protein Metabolism

Protein degradation is balanced by synthesis in the normal fed condition. This balance is disturbed during starvation, with an initial increase in protein catabolism to provide substrate for gluconeogenesis. As starving progresses, protein degradation falls, sparing the muscle

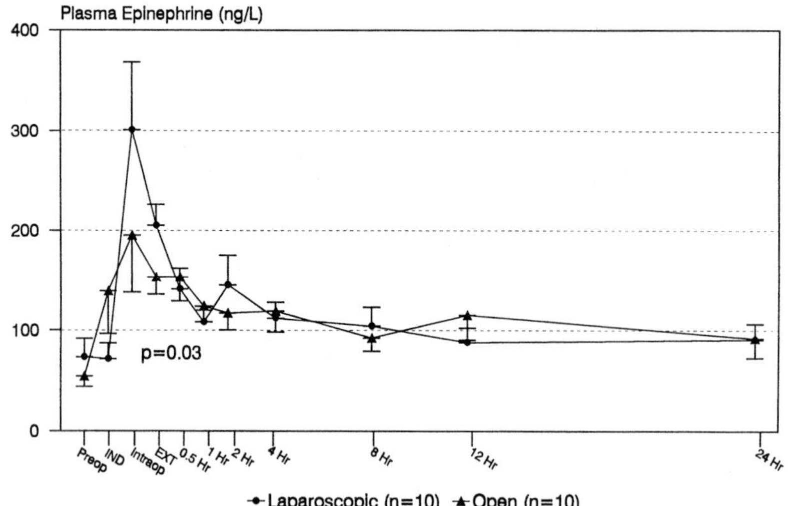


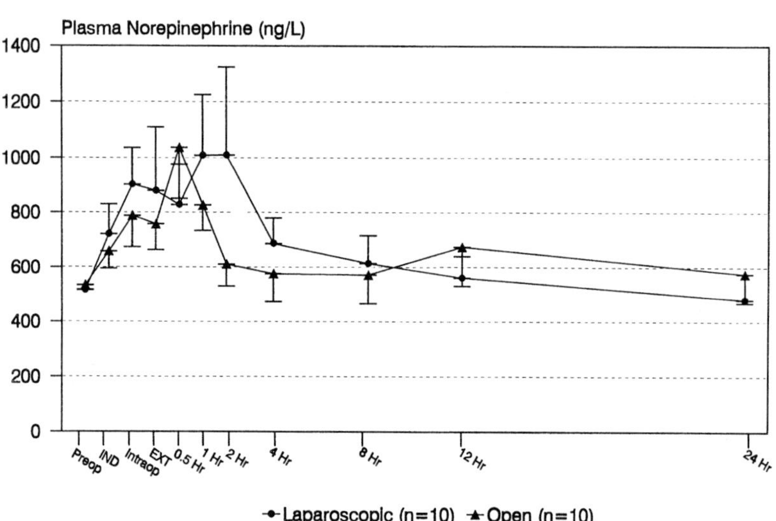


FIGURE 69.6. Adrenomedullary response. A. Plasma epinephrine was higher intraoperatively and immediately following extubation in patients undergoing laparoscopic cholecystectomy. B. Norepinephrine levels were similar in the two groups.

and visceral protein stores.[67,68] Protein-sparing is not observed during trauma or sepsis. Protein breakdown exceeds protein synthesis at a time when nutritional intake is absent and metabolic demands are great. Urinary nitrogen excretion is markedly increased as a result of breakdown of muscle protein, leading to muscle wasting.[69]

The intake of protein for a healthy young adult is approximately 80–120g/day (13–20g of nitrogen/day). Daily urinary excretion of nitrogen is 10–16g. Following injury, daily nitrogen excretion in the urine increases up to 30–50g. These changes are mediated by increased secretion of catecholamines, cortisol, and glucagon.

Elective operation and minor injury result in decreased protein synthesis and normal rates of protein breakdown. Severe trauma, major surgery, burns, and sepsis are associated with increased protein turnover and greatly increased protein catabolism.

The loss of nitrogen following injury is not only related to the extent of the trauma but also to the age, sex and previous nutritional status of the patient, as these factors help determine the muscle mass. Young healthy men lose more protein in response to an injury than do women or the elderly, presumably owing to the smaller body cell mass in the latter two.

Twenty percent of the protein that is broken down is metabolized for generation of energy; the remainder is used by the liver and kidney to produce glucose. Specific proteins, the acute-phase proteins, are synthesized at an accelerated rate during injury and infection. The acute-phase proteins include those involved in immune function, coagulation, and opsonization.

Alanine and glutamine constitute most of the amino acids released from skeletal muscle.[70] Glutamine is a major energy source for lymphocytes, fibroblasts, and the gastrointestinal tract following injury. Souba showed that glutamine is preferentially used as an energy source by the gut during catabolic states.[71] Failure to supply adequate glutamine during these conditions leads to bacterial translocation. Alanine is extracted by the liver

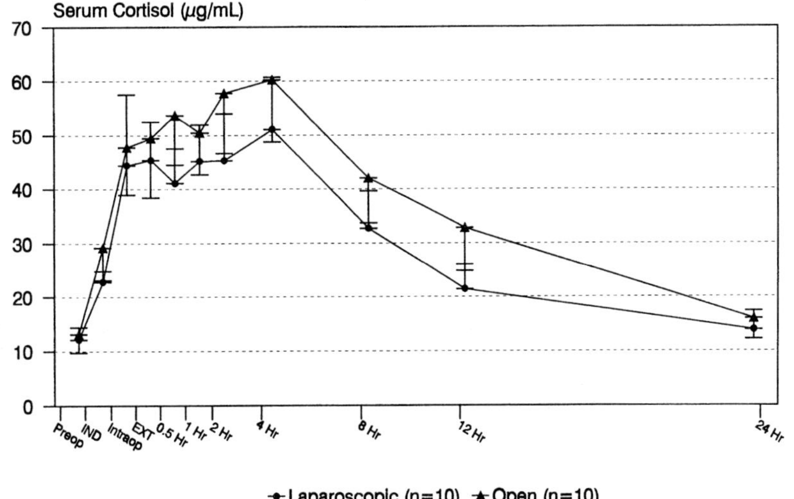


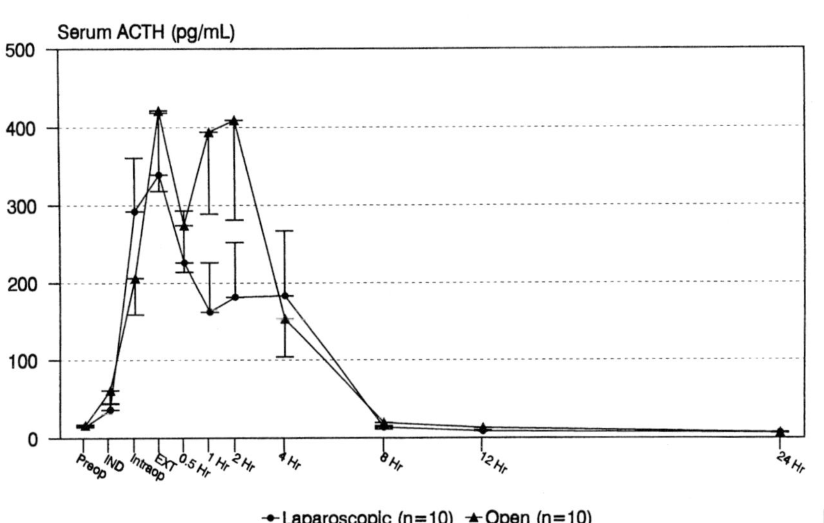


FIGURE 69.7. Adrenocortical axis. A self-limited adrenocortical response returning to baseline within 8–24 hours follows both open and laparoscopic cholecystectomy. Mean ACTH (A), cortisol (B), and urinary free cortisol levels were insignificantly higher in the open cholecystectomy group when examined cross-sectionally for each time point or longitudinally for the 24 hours of the study.

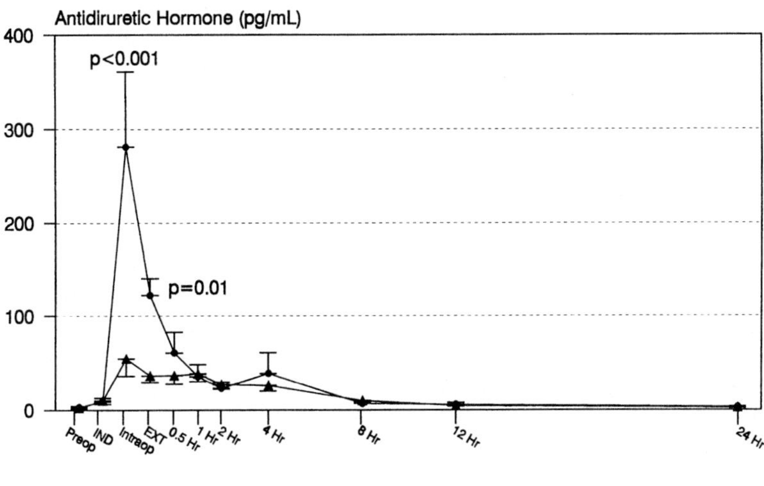


FIGURE 69.8. Precipitous rise in antidiuretic hormone is associated with pneumoperitoneum during laparoscopic cholecystectomy but was not observed in the open surgical group.

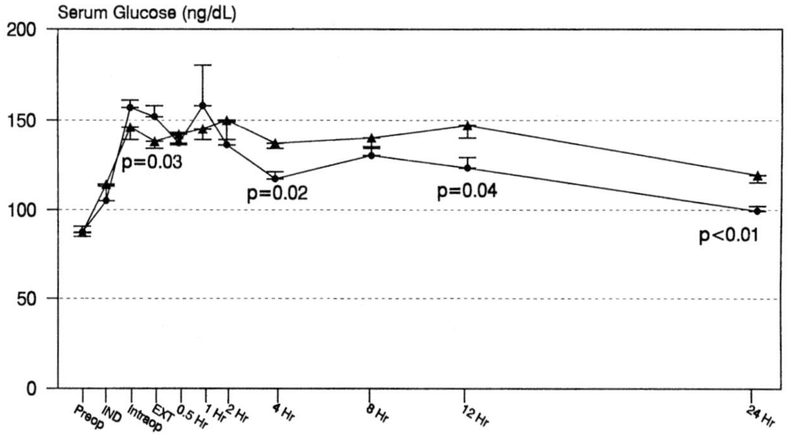


A

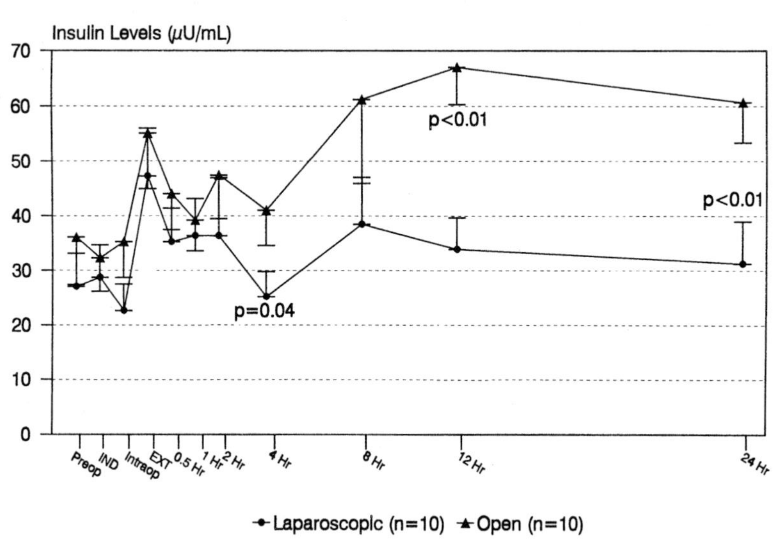


B

FIGURE 69.9. Glucose homeostasis. The postoperative state was associated with mild hyperglycemia (A) and hyperinsulinemia (B). These findings were significantly more pronounced following open cholecystectomy. Glucose levels were higher during the immediate perioperative period of laparoscopic cholecystectomy.

for gluconeogenesis and the synthesis of acute-phase protein.

Glerup et al. reported that laparoscopy results in a much smaller postoperative catabolic response. Laparoscopic cholecystectomy produces a lower increase in nitrogen clearance than does open cholecystectomy.[72]

## Lipid Metabolism

The major metabolic response of injury includes disruption of the normal operation of the glucose–fatty acid cycle, greatly increased fat mobilization, extensive degradation of muscle protein, and an increase in energy expenditure. Adipose tissue is the largest fuel reserve in the body and is an important source of energy during periods of starvation. Lipolysis is enhanced immediately after injury by stimulation of the sympathetic innervation of the adipose tissue by elevated plasma ACTH, cortisol, catecholamines, glucagon, and growth hormone and by a reduction in insulin.[73,74]

Trauma increases glycerol turnover twofold compared with control subjects. Triglyceride is broken down to free fatty acids and glycerol during lipolysis. The free fatty acids are used for oxidation, ketone formation, or resynthesis of triglyceride. Net lipolysis continues during the flow phase despite increased insulin. In the presence of oxygen, the released fatty acids can be oxidized by cardiac and skeletal muscle to produce energy.

Ketogenesis is variable and correlates inversely with the severity of the injury. After minor injury, ketogenesis increases but to a lesser extent than that seen during nonstressed starvation. After major injury and sepsis, ketogenesis is decreased secondary to an increased insulin level.[75]

To date, there is no report on lipolysis associated with laparoscopy. It has been known, however, that laparoscopy is associated with lower catecholamine release than is open surgery.[59] We may therefore expect a lesser lipolytic response with laparoscopy than with open surgery.

## Cytokines

Cytokines are a group of soluble protein cell regulators produced by a number of cells in the body. They act as mediators of the immune and acute-phase responders. Each cytokine mediates a variety of frequently overlapping effects, and their actions can be additive.

Tumor necrosis factor-α (TNF-α), interleukin-1 (IL-1), and IL-6 are major mediators of the acute-phase response in humans. TNF-α and IL-1 are considered to be primarily responsible for the nonhepatic manifestations of the response, such as fever and accelerated catabolism.[76] If the extent of the injury is small, the impact of these mediators is limited and the inflammatory response remains localized. If the injury is more extensive, a systemic inflammatory response involving all body systems is elicited. IL-1, IL-6, and TNF-α also trigger the hypothalamic-pituitary-adrenal axis and increase sympathetic nervous system activity.[77]

Significant lower values of intraoperative and postoperative measured IL-1and IL-6 are seen with laparoscopic cholecystectomy, indicating a minor stress response and tissue trauma in this group of patients.[78] Corresponding changes in the levels of IL-1 and TNF, however, may also occur.[79] Hepatic acute-phase protein production is significant higher with open cholecystectomy than with the laparoscopic procedure, indicating a greater inflammatory response in the open group.[79]

## References

1. Moore FD. Bodily changes in surgical convalescence. Ann Surg 1953;137:289.
2. Udelsman R, Norton JA, Jelenich SE, et al. Responses of the hypothalamic-pituitary-adrenal and renin-angiotensin axes and the sympathetic system during controlled surgical and anesthetic stress. J Clin Endocrinol Metab 1987;64: 986–994.
3. Kashtan J, Green JF, Parsons EQ, Holcroft JW. Hemodynamic effects of increased abdominal pressure. Surg Res 1981;30:249.
4. Diamant M, Benumof JL, Saidman LJ. Hemodynamics of increased intra-abdominal pressure: interaction with hypovolemia and halothane anesthesia. Anesthesiology 1978;48:23.
5. Kelman GR, Swapp GH, Smith I, Benzie RJ, Gordon LM. Cardiac output and arterial blood-gas tension during laparoscopy. Br J Anaesth 1972;44:1155.
6. Nadeau OE, Kampmeier OF. Endoscopy of the abdomen: abdominoscopy; a preliminary study, including a summary of the literature and description of the technique. Surg Gynecol Obstet 1925;41:259.
7. Farhi LE, Rahn H. Gas stores of the body and the unsteady state. J Appl Physiol 1955;7:472.
8. Liu S-Y, Leighton T, Davis I, Klein S, Lippmann M, Bongard F. Prospective analysis of cardiopulmonary responses to laparoscopic cholecystectomy. J Laparoendosc Surg 1991; 1:241.
9. Witgen CM, Andrus CH, Fitzgerald SD, Baudendistel LJ, Dahms TE, Kaminski DL. Analysis of hemodynamic and ventilatory effects of laparoscopic cholecystectomy. Arch Surg 1991;126:997.
10. Leighton TA, Liu S-Y, Bongard FS. Comparative cardiopulmonary effects of carbon dioxide versus helium pneumoperitoneum. Surgery 1993;113:527.
11. Bongard FS, Pianim NA, Leighton TA, et al. Helium insufflation for laparoscopic operation. Surg Gynecol Obstet 1993;177:140.
12. Price HL. Effects of carbon dioxide on the cardiovascular system. Anesthesiology 1960;21:652.
13. Rasmussen JP, Dauchot PJ, DePalma RG, et al. Cardiac function and hypercarbia. Arch Surg 1978;113:1196.
14. Hodgson C, McClellan RMA, Newton JR. Some effects of peritoneal insufflation of carbon dioxide at laparoscopy. Anaesthesia 1970;25:382.
15. Smith I, Benzie RJ, Gordon NLM, Kelman GR, Swapp GH. Cardiovascular effects of peritoneal insufflation of carbon dioxide for laparoscopy. Br Med J 1971;3:410.
16. Lenz RJ, Thomas TA, Wilkins DG. Cardiovascular changes during laparoscopy; studies of stroke and cardiac output using impedance cardiography. Anaesthesia 1976;31:4.
17. Sarfan D, Sgambati S, Orlando R. Laparoscopy in high-risk cardiac patients. Surg Gynecol Obstet 1993;176:548–554.
18. Johannsen G, Anderson H, Juhl B. The effects of general anaesthesia on hemodynamic events during laparoscopy with $CO_2$-insufflation. Acta Anaesthesiol Scand 1989;33:132.
19. Ishizaki Y, Bandai Y, Shimomura K, Abe H, Ohtomo Y, Idezuki Y. Changes in splanchnic blood flow and cardiovascular effects following peritoneal insufflation of carbon dioxide. Surg Endosc 1993;7:420.
20. Westerband A, Van De Water JM, Amzallag M, et al. Cardiovascular changes during laparoscopic cholecystectomy. Surg Gynecol Obstet 1992;175:535.
21. Marshall RL, Jebson DJR, Davie IT, Scott DB. Circulatory effects of carbon dioxide insufflation of the peritoneal cavity for laparoscopy. Br J Anaesth 1972;44:680.
22. Motew M, Ivankovich AD, Bieniarz J, Albrecht R, Zahed B, Scommegna A. Cardiovascular effects and acid-base and blood gas changes during laparoscopy. Am J Obstet Gynecol 1973;115:1002.
23. Pentecost BL, Irving DW, Shillingford JP. The effects of posture on the blood flow in the inferior vena cava. Clin Sci 1963;24:149.
24. Ishizaki Y, Bandai Y, Shimomura K, Abe H, Ohtomo Y, Idezuki Y. Safe intraabdominal pressure of carbon dioxide pneumoperitoneum during laparoscopic surgery. Surgery 1993;114:549.
25. Iwase K, Takenaka H, Oshima S, Ohata T, Ishizaka T, Yagura A. Serial changes in renal function during laparoscopic cholecystectomy: a comparison with minilaparotomy cholecystectomy [abstract]. Presented at the International Society of Surgery, Hong Kong, August 1993.
26. Beecher HK. The measured effect of laparotomy on respiration. J Clin Invest 1993;12:63.
27. Latimer RG, Dickman M, Day WC, Gunn ML, Schmidt CD. Ventilatory patterns and cardiopulmonary complications after upper abdominal surgery determined by preoperative pulmonary spirometry and blood gas analysis. Am J Surg 1971;122:622.

28. Gal TJ. Physiologic basis and rationale for pulmonary function testing in patients undergoing head and neck surgery. Otolaryngol Clin North Am 1982;14:723.
29. Aldren CP, Barr LC, Leech RD. Hypovolemia and postoperative pulmonary complications. Br J Surg 1991;78:1307.
30. Ford GT, Whitelow WA, Rosenal JW, Cruse PJ, Cuenter CA. Diaphragm function after upper abdominal surgery in humans. Am Rev Respir Dis 1983;127:431.
31. VadeBoncouer TR, Riegler FX, Gautt RS, Weinberger GL. A randomized, double-blind comparison of the effects of interpleural bupivacaine and saline on morphine requirements and pulmonary function after cholecystecotmy. Anesthesiology 1989;71:339–343.
32. Hendolin H, Lahtinene J, Tuppurainen T, Partanen K. The effect of thoracic epidural analgesia on respiratory function after cholecystecotmy. Acta Anaesthesiol Scand 1987;31: 645.
33. Ross WB, Tweedie JH, Leong YP, Wyman A, Smithers BM. Intercostal blockage and pulmonary function after cholecystectomy. Surgery 1989;105:166.
34. Patel JM, Lanzofome RJ, Williams JS, Muller BV, Hinshaw JR. The effects of incisional infiltration of bupivacaine hydrochloride upon pulmonary functions, atelectasis and narcotic need following elective cholecystectomy. Surg Gynecol Obstet 1983;157:378.
35. Light RW, George RB. Incidence and significance of pleural effusion after abdominal surgery. Chest 1976;69:621.
36. Frazee RC, Roberts RW, Okeson GC, et al. Open versus laparoscopic cholecystectomy: a comparison of postoperative pulmonary function. Ann Surg 1991;213:651.
37. Peters JH, Ortega A, Lehnerd SL, et al. The physiology of laparoscopic surgery: pulmonary function after laparoscopic cholecystectomy. Surg Laparosc Endosc 1993;3:1.
38. Putensen-Himmer G, Putensen C, Lammer H, Lingnau W, Aigner F, Benzer H. Comparison of postoperative respiratory function after laparoscopy or open laparotomy for cholecystectomy. Anesthesiology 1992;77:675.
39. Schauer PR, Luna J, Ghiatas AA, Glen ME, Warren JM, Sirinek KR. Pulmonary function after laparoscopic cholecystectomy. Surgery 1993;114:389.
40. Witgen CM, Naunheim KS, Andrus CH, Kaminski DL. Preoperative pulmonary function evaluation for laparoscopic cholecystectomy. Arch Surg 1993;128:880.
41. Cuthberson DP. Observations on the disturbance of metabolism by injury to the limb. Q J Med 1932;1:233.
42. Dominioni L, Dionigi R, Cividini F. Determination of C-reactive protein and alpha-1 antitrypsin for quantitative assessment of surgical trauma. Eur Surg Res 1980; 12(suppl):133–136.
43. Cruickshank AM, Fraser WD, Burns HJG, VanDamme J, Shenkin A. Response of serum IL-6 in patients undergoing elective surgery of varying severity. Clin Sci 1990;79: 161–165.
44. Shenkin A, Fraser WD, Series J. The serum IL-6 response to elective surgery. Lymphokine Res 1989;8:123–127.
45. Kehlet H. The modifying effect of general and regional anesthesia on the endocrine response to surgery. Reg Anesth 1982;9(suppl):38–48.
46. Kehlet H. The stress response to surgery: release mechanisms and the modifying effect of pain relief. Acta Chir Scand 1989;550:22–28.
47. Grace PA, Quereshi A, Coleman J. Reduced postoperative hospitalization after laparoscopic cholecystectomy. Br J Surg 1991;78:160–162.
48. Garcia-Caballero M, Vara-Thorbeck C. The evaluation of postoperative ileus after laparoscopic cholecystectomy. Surg Endoscogy 1993;7:416–419.
49. McMahon AJ, Baxter JN, Anderson JR. Assessment of pain after laparoscopic and minor cholecystectomy: a randomized control trial. Br J Surg 1992;79:1224.
50. McMahon AJ, Ross S, Russel IT. Return to normal activity after laparoscopic and minor cholecystectomy: a prospective randomized trial. Gastroenterology 1993;104:A370.
51. Wickham JEA. Minimally invasive surgery. Br J Surg 1990;22:721–722.
52. Wilmore DW. Homeostasis: bodily changes in trauma and surgery. In: Sabiston DC Jr (ed) Textbook of Surgery: The Biological Basis of Modern Surgical Practice, 14th ed., Philadelphia: Saunders, 1991:19–33.
53. Cavey LC, Cloutier CT, Lowery BD. Growth hormone and adrenal cortical response to shock and trauma in the human. Ann Surg 1971;174:451–458.
54. Morgan RJ, Martyn JA, Philbin DM, Coggins CH, Burke JF. Water metabolism and anti-diuretic hormone (ADH) response following thermal injury. J Trauma 1980;20: 468–472.
55. Le Quesna LP, Cochrane JPS, Fieldman NR. Fluid and electrolyte disturbances after trauma: the role of adrenocortical and pituitary hormones. Br Med Bull 1985;41:212–217.
56. Stoner HB. Metabolism after trauma and sepsis. Circ Shock 1986;19:75–87.
57. Meguid MM, Brennan MF, Aoki TT, Muller WA, Moore FD. Hormone–substrate interrelationships following trauma. Arch Surg 1974;109:776–783.
58. Sarfan D, Orlando R III. Physiologic effects of peritoneum. Am J Surg 1994;167:281–286.
59. Ortega AE, Peters JH, Raffaello I, Estrada L, Ehsan A. A prospective randomized comparison of the metabolic and stress hormonal responses of laparoscopic and open cholecystectomy. J Am Coll Surg 1996;183:249–256.
60. Pumonen R, Vinamaki O. Vasopressin release during laparoscopy. Lancet 1982;1:175–176.
61. Melville RJ, Frizis HI, Frosling ML, Lequesne LP. The stimulus for vasopressin release during laparoscopy. Surg Gynecol Obstet 1985;161:253–256.
62. Stoner HB, Frayn KN, Barton RN, Threlfall CJ. The relationship between plasma substrates and hormone and the severity of injury in 277 recently injured patients. Clin Sci 1979;56:563–573.
63. Wolfe RR, Miller HI, Spitzen JJ. Glucose and lactate metabolism in burn and shock. Am J Physiol 1977;232:415–418.
64. Allison SP, Hinton P, Chamberlain MJ. Intravenous glucose tolerance, insulin and free fatty acid level in burned patients. Lancet 1968;2:1113–1116.
65. Wolfe RR, Durkot MJ, Allshop JR, Burke JF. Glucose metabolism in severely burned patients. Metabolism 1979;28: 1031–1039.
66. Kinney JM, Elwyn DH. Protein metabolism in the traumatized patients. Acta Chir Scand Suppl 1985;522:45–46.
67. Millward DJ, Waterlow JC. Effect of nutrition on protein turnover in skeletal muscle. Fed Proc 1978;37:2283–2290.

68. Cuthbertson DP. The disturbance of metabolism produced by bony and non-bony injury, with notes on certain abnormal conditions of bone. Biochem J 1930;24:1244.
69. Ruderman NB, Berger M. The formation of glutamine and alanine in skeletal muscle. J Biol Chem 1974;249:5500–5506.
70. Souba WW. The metabolic role of the gut in the systemic response to injury. Adv Trauma 1987;2:269.
71. Glerup H, Heindorff H, Flyvbjerg A, Jensen SL, Vilstrup H. Elective laparoscopic cholecystectomy nearly abolishes the postoperative hepatic catabolic stress response. Ann Surg 1995;221:214–219.
72. Frayn KN. Substrate turnover after injury. Br Med Bull 1985;41:232–239.
73. Frayn KN, Price DA, Maycock PF, Carroll SM. Plasma somatomedin activity after injury in man and its relationship to other hormonal and metabolic changes. Clin Endocrinol (Oxf) 1984;20:179–187.
74. Neufeld HA, Pace JG, Kaninski ML, et al. A probable endocrine basis for the depression of ketone bodies during infection or inflammatory state in rats. Endocrinology 1980;107:596–601.
75. Dinarello CA. Interleukin-1. Rev Infect Dis 1984;6:51–95.
76. Basedovsky H, del Ray A, Sorkin E, Dinarello CA. Immunoregulatory feedback system between interleukin-1 and glucocorticoid hormones. Science 1986;223:652–654.
77. Glaser F, Sannwald GA, Buhr HJ, Kuntz C, Mayer H, Herfarth C. General stress response to conventional and laparoscopic cholecystectomy. Ann Surg 1995;221:372–380.
78. Mealy K, Gallagher H, Barry M, Lennon F, Traynor O, Hyland J. Physiological and metabolic responses to open and laparoscopic cholecystectomy. Br J Surg 1992;79: 1061–1064.

# 70
# Outcomes of Minimal Access versus Open Surgical Procedures in the Elderly

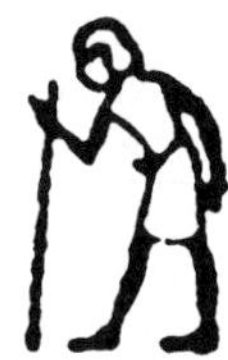

L. Michael Brunt and Nathaniel J. Soper

The progressive aging of the population in Western countries has placed tremendous demands on our health care systems. This increase in the proportion of elderly individuals has occurred as a result of both a prolongation in life expectancy and a decline in fertility rates. In 1978 there were approximately 24 million people age 65 years and older in the United States, representing 11.2% of the population.[1] The elderly are currently the fastest growing segment of our society, and demographic estimates suggest that sometime in the twenty-first century as the "baby boomers" age the proportion of elderly could be as great as 20%.[2] Furthermore, the elderly utilize medical resources at a much higher rate than do younger individuals. From a surgical perspective, the elderly are often more challenging to manage because of decreased functional reserve, the presence of multiple pathologies, and more complex and complicated illnesses. Elderly patients also often present with urgent or emergent clinical problems and are more likely to require emergency surgery, which is associated with much higher morbidity and mortality and greater costs than elective surgery.[3]

The revolution in minimally invasive surgery that has taken place has resulted in unquestionable benefits to patients undergoing a variety of surgical procedures.[4] These benefits include reduced postoperative pain, shortened hospitalization, fewer complications, a more rapid recovery to full activity, and in some cases decreased hospital costs. For elderly patients who may have marginal functional reserve and decreased capacity to recover from the trauma and stress of open abdominal surgery, the advantages of a minimally invasive approach to treatment may be especially important. The purpose of this review, therefore, is to analyze the impact that minimally invasive surgery has had on surgical outcomes in the elderly population. The emphasis is necessarily on laparoscopic treatment of gallstone disease where elderly-specific data are available for consideration. In addition, the potential role for minimally invasive procedures in the management of nonbiliary surgical disorders that affect the elderly is also considered, despite the absence of age-focused studies in these other areas.

## Laparoscopic Cholecystectomy

Gallstones increase in prevalence with advancing age, and cholecystectomy is the most common intraabdominal surgical procedure performed in the elderly population. In 1990 about 150,000 Medicare patients underwent cholecystectomy in the United States.[5] Epidemiologic studies have suggested that the incidence of gallstones in individuals during the eighth decade of life may be as high as 50% overall and up to 61% in white women.[6–9] Minimally invasive techniques have almost totally replaced open cholecystectomy for the treatment of symptomatic gallstone disease. To understand the impact that laparoscopic cholecystectomy has had in elderly patients, one must first consider historical data from the era of open cholecystectomy.

A number of large series have evaluated the results of open cholecystectomy in the elderly (Table 70.1).[10–20] Several common themes emerge from an analysis of these studies. First, elderly patients have a high incidence of presentation to the hospital with acute or emergent biliary problems that often require early therapeutic intervention. Escarce et al.,[20] in a study based on Medicare claims from Pennsylvania, found that only 36.5% of elderly patients who required cholecystectomy presented for elective surgery, whereas 63.5% of these patients had urgent or emergent presentations leading to hospitalization and surgery. The incidence of complicated cholelithiasis is also higher in elderly patients. Elderly patients are more likely to present with common bile duct stones, cholangitis, and jaundice than their younger counterparts.[10,11,15,21] Likewise, gallstone pancreatitis is more prevalent in the elderly, where it comprises 7–19% of patients who present with acute gallstone symptoms.[14,18,20,21] The incidence of acute cholecystitis is approximately two to four times as high in individuals

TABLE 70.1. Morbidity and Mortality of Open Cholecystectomy in Elderly Patients

| Series | Year | No. of patients | % Acute and/or emergent cases | Complications (%) | Mortality (%) |
|---|---|---|---|---|---|
| Sullivan[10] | 1982 | 42 | 40.4 | 62.0 | 9.5 |
| Huber[11] | 1983 | 93 | 46.0 | 28.0 | 7.5 |
| Lygidakis[12] | 1983 | 789 | NA | 30.2 | 4.9 |
| Houghton[13] | 1985 | 151 | 13.9 | 33.0 | 3.4 |
| Harness[14] | 1986 | 118 | 58.4 | 24.6 | 12.7 |
| Sandler[15] | 1987 | 142 | 20.4 | 26.0 | 9.2 |
| Irvin[16] | 1988 | 145 | 40.0 | 11.0 | 2.1 |
| Margiotta[17] | 1988 | 212 | 50.0 | 28.0 | 6.0 |
| Pigott[18] | 1988 | 347 | 53.0 | NA | 1.1 |
| Girard[19] | 1993 | 732 | NA | 13.8 | 2.5 |
| Escarce[20] | 1995 | 21,131 | 63.5 | 18.6 | 2.1 |

NA, not available.

over age 65 than in younger persons and has ranged from 20% to 50% in series of open cholecystectomy[10,15,16] and as high as 60% in patients over age 80.[22] Older patients are also more likely to have empyema, gangrene, or perforation of the gallbladder. Each of these conditions complicates surgical management because of the increased difficulty of surgery, associated sepsis, and the possible need for treatment of bile duct stones. Consequently, elderly patients who present emergently have a higher incidence of complications and deaths after open cholecystectomy than do similar aged patients who undergo elective surgery (Table 70.2).[11,13,17,20] In a large population-based study performed by Roslyn et al.[23] assessing 42,474 patients who underwent open cholecystectomy in the United States in 1989, the overall mortality rate for patients over age 65 was 0.5% compared to 0.03% for younger individuals. Hospital length of stay, charges, and mortality correlated not only with increased age but also with emergency admission status and the presence of acute or complicated cholecystitis; the single most important determinant of mortality was age over 65 years.

Associated co-morbid medical conditions may further increase the possibility of complications and an adverse outcome in the elderly. In a multivariate analysis of the impact of medical risk factors,[23] hypertension, congestive heart failure, and diabetes were the only co-morbid factors that affected mortality independently. Conditions that did not affect mortality included obesity, asthma, previous coronary artery bypass, and hypothyroidism.

Laparoscopic cholecystectomy became firmly established as the gold standard for the treatment of symptomatic cholelithiasis during the 1990s.[24] Retrospective series[25,26] and a few small prospective, randomized trials[27–31] have shown that, when compared to open cholecystectomy, laparoscopic cholecystectomy is associated with less postoperative pain, shorter hospitalization, faster recovery, and decreased hospital costs. Elderly patients may, however, pose an added challenge for laparoscopic surgeons for the reasons alluded to previously, including the presence of complicated cholelithiasis, previous abdominal surgery, and associated co-morbid medical conditions. Despite these potential concerns, most elderly patients should be candidates for a laparoscopic approach unless there are compelling contraindications to surgery or general anesthesia. Several groups,[32–41] including ours, have evaluated the results and impact of laparoscopic cholecystectomy in the elderly as summarized in Table 70.3. Some of the important variables to consider in this analysis include conversion rates to open surgery, operating times, length of hospital stay, complication rates, and mortality.

Laparoscopic cholecystectomy in the elderly has been associated with higher rates of conversion to open cholecystectomy than in younger individuals.[34,39,41] In the combined series shown in Table 70.3,[32–41] the mean rate of conversion was 8.3%. Conversion rates have been highest in patients with complicated cholelithiasis,[39] and the most common reason for conversion has been increased scarring and inflammation around the gallbladder. Other causes for conversion have been bleeding, intraabdominal adhesions, and the presence of common bile duct stones. In uncontrolled series of laparoscopic cholecystectomy that have analyzed risk factors for conversion to open cholecystectomy in large numbers of patients, old age (>65 years) has been associated with higher conversion rates in every report.[42–45] Additional risk factors for conversion to open cholecystectomy, many of which are also common in the elderly, include a past history of acute cholecystitis, multiple (>10) previous attacks of biliary pain, male sex, and a thickened gallbladder wall seen by ultrasonography.

Operating times for laparoscopic cholecystectomy have not been extensively analyzed in elderly patients. Fried et al.[44] found no significant difference in operating room (OR) time between elderly patients over age 65

TABLE 70.2. Results of Elective versus Urgent/Emergent Open Cholecystectomy in Elderly Patients

| Study | Type of case | No. | Complications | Mortality |
|---|---|---|---|---|
| Huber[11] | Elective | 50 (53.8%) | 5 (10%) | 1 (2%) |
| | Emergent | 43 (46.2%) | 14 (33%) | 6 (14%) |
| Houghton[13] | Elective | 130 (86.0%) | 36 (28%) | 1 (2%) |
| | Emergent | 21 (14.0%) | 14 (66%) | 6 (14%) |
| Margiotta[17] | Elective | 119 (56.1%) | 30 (25.2%) | 4 (3.3%) |
| | Emergent | 93 (43.9%) | 53 (57%) | 9 (9.7%) |
| Escarce[20] | Elective | — (36.5%) | NA | — (0.8%) |
| | Emergent | — (63.5%) | NA | — (2.9%) |

NA, not available.

TABLE 70.3. Institutional Series of Laparoscopic Cholecystectomy in Elderly Patients

| Study | No. of patients | Mean age (years) | No. converted | Complications | Mortality |
|---|---|---|---|---|---|
| Nenner[32] | 304 | 72 | 3 (1.0%) | 72 (23.7%) | 2 (0.7%) |
| Saxe[33] | 94 | 72 | 11 (12.0%) | NA | 1 (1.2%) |
| Fried[34] | 337 | NA | 35 (10.4%) | 46 (13.6%) | 2 (0.6%) |
| Askew[35] | 51 | NA | 8 (22.0%) | 5 (9.8%) | 0 |
| Firilas[36] | 217 | 73 | 23 (10.6%) | 42 (18.0%) | 2 (1.0%) |
| Behrman[37] | 144 | 72 | 7 (4.9%) | 21 (15.2%) | 1 (1.4%) |
| Tagle[38] | 90 | 74 | 3 (3.0%) | 5 (5.0%) | 2 (2.0%) |
| Magnuson[39] | 62 | 73 | 21 (35.0%) | 11 (18.0%) | 0 |
| Lujan[40] | 133 | 71 | 11 (8.3%) | 18 (13.5%) | 0 |
| Jones[41] | 113 | 76 | 11 (9.7%) | 18 (15.9%) | 1 (0.9%) |
| *Total* | 1545 | 75.6 | 133 (8.6%) | 238 (15.4%) | 11 (0.7%) |

(mean OR time 74.2 ± 1.9 minutes) compared to younger individuals (mean OR time 72.4 ± 0.9 minutes). Our group[41] found that operating times were similar in elderly and nonelderly patients who had a low American Society of Anesthesiologists (ASA) classification (ASA class 1 or 2) (Table 70.4). However, elderly patients who were ASA class 3 or 4 had longer operating times when compared to patients less than age 70 with a similar ASA class. Magnuson et al.[39] stratified patients by age (>65 years) and the presence of complicated versus uncomplicated cholelithiasis. Their group found that compared to younger patients operating times were longer only in elderly patients who had complicated cholelithiasis but were not prolonged in uncomplicated cases. Behrman et al.[37] compared operating times for open and laparoscopic cholecystectomy in patients with chronic or acute cholecystitis. Operating times were a mean of only 11 minutes longer for the laparoscopic approach in patients with chronic cholelithiasis but averaged 28 minutes longer than the open approach in patients with acute cholecystitis. These data suggest that the adverse local conditions of the gallbladder frequently encountered in elderly patients may account for their longer operating times.

Laparoscopic cholecystectomy is associated with a reduced length of hospital stay compared to open cholecystectomy in both elderly and younger individuals. This holds true for elderly patients who have acute or chronic cholecystitis.[37] Elderly patients do have a slightly longer duration of hospitalization after laparoscopic cholecystectomy than do patients less than age 65 years. Our data show that elderly patients who are ASA class 3 or 4 require an average of 1.1 additional days of hospitalization after laparoscopic cholecystectomy compared to age-matched patients who are ASA class 1 and 2 (Table 70.4). The reduction in length of hospital stay has also resulted in lower direct and indirect costs for laparoscopic cholecystectomy compared to open cholecystectomy.[46] The only study that specifically addressed the issue of cost in elderly patients found that laparoscopic cholecystectomy was less expensive for patients with chronic cholecystitis but cost more than open cholecystectomy

TABLE 70.4. Effect of Age and ASA Classification on Outcome of Laparoscopic Cholecystectomy

| Parameter | Group I | Group II | Group III | Group IV |
|---|---|---|---|---|
| Age (years) | <70 | <70 | ≥70 | ≥70 |
| ASA | 1 + 2 | 3 + 4 | 1 + 2 | 3 + 4 |
| No. of patients | 808 | 119 | 56 | 57 |
| Operative time (minutes) | 101 ± 1 | 104 ± 4 | 101 ± 6 | 115 ± 7 |
| Converted to open | 19 (2%) | 6 (5%) | 5 (9%) | 6 (11%) |
| Length of hospital stay (days) | 1.2 ± 0.3 | 1.4 ± 0.1 | 1.5 ± 0.2 | 2.6 ± 0.3 |
| Biliary injury | 2 | 0 | 2 | 0 |
| Complications | | | | |
| Total | 53 (6.6%) | 13 (10.9%) | 11 (19.6%) | 7 (12.3%) |
| Grade I + II | 48 (6.0%) | 12 (10.0%) | 10 (18.0%) | 6 (11.0%) |
| III + IV | 5 (1.0%) | 1 (1.0%) | 1 (2.0%) | 1 (2.0%) |
| Return to normal activity (days) | 9.4 ± 0.2 | 10.1 ± 0.7 | 9.3 ± 0.7 | 11.4 ± 1.0 |

*Source:* Data from Jones et al.[41]

TABLE 70.5. Profile of Complications from Compiled Series of Laparoscopic or Open Cholecystectomy in Elderly Patients

| Parameter | Open cholecystectomy[a] | Laparoscopic cholecystectomy[b] |
|---|---|---|
| No. of patients | 719 | 1040 |
| Type of complication: | | |
| Wound | 38 (5.3%) | 16 (1.5%) |
| Biliary[c] | 4 (0.56%) | 11 (1.1%) |
| Pulmonary | 67 (9.3%) | 26 (2.5%) |
| Urinary tract | 21 (2.9%) | 36 (3.5%) |
| Pulmonary embolus | 2 (2.8%) | 1 (0.1%) |
| Cardiovascular | 16 (2.2%) | 9 (0.9%) |
| Total morbidity | 188 (26.1%) | 184 (17.7%) |
| Deaths | 43 (6.0%) | 8 (0.8%) |

Data were derived from recent series in which complications were adequately detailed for analysis.
[a] Compiled from references 11, 13, 14, 16, 19.
[b] Compiled from references 32, 34, 36, 38, 39, 47.
[c] Includes bile or cystic duct leaks and comon bile duct injury.

for patients with acute cholecystitis.[37] Factors that accounted for increased costs in elderly patients with acute cholecystitis were longer operating times, a higher rate of conversion to open cholecystectomy, and a higher incidence of complications than in uncomplicated cases.

Laparoscopic cholecystectomy appears to be associated with a lower incidence of complications overall when compared to open cholecystectomy. The data in Table 70.5 were compiled from several series of cholecystectomies reported during the past two decades. These data must be interpreted cautiously because they are derived from uncontrolled series, and additional factors unrelated to the method of cholecystectomy such as the increased use of endoscopic retrograde cholangiopancreatography (ERCP) to treat bile duct stones and cholangitis could have an impact on the results. It appears, however, that laparoscopic cholecystectomy has resulted in a slightly lower incidence of complications and fewer deaths than were seen during the era of open surgery. The pattern of complications also appears to have changed somewhat, with fewer wound and pulmonary complications in the laparoscopic group. Wound dehiscence and incisional hernia are both rare after laparoscopic cholecystectomy. Although not shown in Table 70.5, complications of deep venous thrombosis, pulmonary embolus, and renal failure were occasionally seen in patients after open cholecystectomy but were rare in the laparoscopic series. The incidence of biliary injury, which appears to be higher with laparoscopic cholecystectomy, is addressed below.

The mortality rate for laparoscopic cholecystectomy in the elderly appears to be lower than was observed historically during the prelaparoscopic era. Feldman et al.[48] analyzed mortality rates in a subset of 2865 elderly patients undergoing cholecystectomy for uncomplicated cholelithiasis in the state of Connecticut between 1989 and 1992. A significant reduction in mortality was seen for elderly patients from a death rate of 1.4% in 1989 prior to the introduction of laparoscopic cholecystectomy into practice compared to a mortality rate of 0.5% when laparoscopic cholecystectomy was in use during 1991–1992. For both laparoscopic and open cholecystectomy, most deaths are due to cardiopulmonary causes or biliary sepsis. The decrease in mortality from cholecystectomy during the 1990s, therefore, may be due to better preoperative management of biliary sepsis and fewer cardiopulmonary deaths from the less invasive laparoscopic procedure.

Despite the apparent advantages of laparoscopic cholecystectomy in the elderly, the complication rate for this procedure is still higher than it is for younger patients. In Magnuson et al.'s series,[39] elderly patients had a morbidity rate of 18% compared to 6% in patients under age 65. In both age groups, complications were more common in patients with complicated gallstone disease (21% in elderly, 12% in <65) than in patients with uncomplicated presentations (10% in elderly, 4% in <65). In another study of elderly patients undergoing laparoscopic cholecystectomy, those admitted to the hospital preoperatively had more complications than outpatients undergoing laparoscopic cholecystectomy, probably because of a higher incidence of complicated cholelithiasis and associated co-morbid conditions in the hospitalized group.[36] As shown in Table 70.4, our series[41] shows a higher incidence of minor complications (grades 1 and 2) in the elderly than in individuals under age 70, but for patients who were ASA class 3 or 4, the incidence of minor complications was similar regardless of age. Major complications occurred about twice as often in the elderly groups as in patients under age 70. Therefore, both age and ASA class are important determinants of outcome after laparoscopic cholecystectomy.

A prospective, randomized trial of laparoscopic versus open cholecystectomy in elderly patients has been conducted,[40] the results of which are summarized in Table 70.6. All patients in the study were over age 65, and the only exclusion criterion was the presence of choledocholithiasis. Eleven patients (8.3%) in the laparoscopic group required conversion to open cholecystectomy. Operating times were similar in the two groups, but hospital length of stay was significantly longer after open cholecystectomy. The incidence of postoperative complications was also higher in the open group, which was primarily due to more wound and pulmonary complications following open cholecystectomy. The authors stratified complications by severity (grades I–IV) and found that the open group had a significantly higher incidence of potentially serious grade II complications (7.6% open vs. 2.3% laparoscopic, $p < 0.05$). Laparoscopic cholecystectomy therefore is the preferred method of

TABLE 70.6. Prospective, Randomized Trial of Laparoscopic versus Open Cholecystectomy in Elderly Patients

| Parameter | Open cholecystectomy | Laparoscopic cholecystectomy | p |
|---|---|---|---|
| No. of patients | 131 | 133 | NS |
| Age (years), mean | 72 (65–88) | 71 (65–87) | NS |
| Acute cholecystitis (%) | 29.7 | 32.3 | NS |
| Operative time (minutes) | 70.9 | 75 | NS |
| Hospitalization (days) | 9.9 | 3.7 | <0.05 |
| Complications | 31 (23.6%) | 18 (13.5%) | <0.05 |

*Source:* Lujan et al.,[40] with permission.
NS, not significant.

cholecystectomy in elderly patients with symptomatic gallstones.

## Special Biliary Problems in the Elderly

### Acute Cholecystitis

The combination of advanced age and acute cholecystitis is a significant risk factor for cholecystectomy. Several studies have demonstrated that, on the whole, laparoscopic cholecystectomy can be performed safely in patients with acute cholecystitis despite a higher rate of conversion to open surgery.[49–52] When compared to open cholecystectomy, the laparoscopic procedure also results in fewer complications, shorter hospitalization, more rapid recovery, and reduced costs.[52,53] Only one study has specifically addressed the issue of laparoscopic cholecystectomy for acute cholecystitis in the elderly. Lo et al.[47] evaluated the results of laparoscopic cholecystectomy for acute cholecystitis in 30 elderly patients and compared them to 40 similar patients who were under age 65. Elderly patients were more likely to be female and had a higher incidence of associated medical diseases. No differences were noted in operating times, analgesic requirements, or complications between the two groups. However, elderly patients had a much higher rate of conversion to open cholecystectomy (23.3%), compared to a conversion rate of only 2.5% for the younger group. The elderly patients who did undergo successful laparoscopic cholecystectomy also had a longer delay before return to ambulation and resumption of a regular diet and had a prolonged hospital stay compared to the under 65 group.

The optimal timing of laparoscopic cholecystectomy in the setting of acute cholecystitis is controversial. This is especially problematic in elderly patients, who often present to the hospital several days into an acute attack. During the prelaparoscopic era, open cholecystectomy performed within 7 days of the onset of symptoms was shown to be superior to delayed interval cholecystectomy several weeks later, decreasing the length of hospitalization and recuperation period and lowering hospital costs.[54,55] However, because of the difficulty of performing laparoscopic cholecystectomy in the setting of acute inflammation, the issue of an initial conservative treatment period followed by interval cholecystectomy has been revisited. Data from uncontrolled studies[56,57] suggest that patients with acute cholecystitis who undergo attempted laparoscopic cholecystectomy within 72 hours after the onset of symptoms have a lower rate of conversion to open cholecystectomy, shorter and less difficult operations, and a faster convalescence than do patients operated more than 72–96 hours after becoming symptomatic. To address this issue further, Lo et al.[58] randomized patients with acute cholecystitis to early laparoscopic cholecystectomy within 72 hours of development of symptoms versus delayed interval surgery after initial medical treatment. Although this trial was not limited to elderly patients, the mean age of patients entered in the study was 60 years. Of 41 patients (19.5%) in the delayed group, 8 (19.5%) required urgent operation a median of 63 hours after admission because of disease progression. In the remaining patients, operating times were shorter in the delayed group (105 vs. 135 minutes), but the rate of conversion to open cholecystectomy (23%) and incidence of complications (29%) were both higher than in the early group (conversions 11%, complications 13%). These results suggest that the preferred approach to the patient with acute cholecystitis is early laparoscopic cholecystectomy, provided it can be performed within 72 hours of the onset of symptoms.

Many elderly patients who present with acute cholecystitis are at high risk for emergency surgery because of sepsis and associated co-morbid conditions. An alternative to laparoscopic cholecystectomy in the high risk patient is percutaneous decompression of the gallbladder followed by interval laparoscopic cholecystectomy 6–12 weeks later. The rationale for this approach is that decompression of the acutely inflamed gallbladder allows more rapid resolution of the inflammatory process and decreases the technical difficulty of the subsequent laparoscopic procedure; moreover, it allows the patient to recover from the acute illness prior to surgery.[59] Patterson and associates[59] treated 50 such patients with acute cholecystitis who were at high risk for emergency surgery and general anesthesia due to their critical illness or underlying medical conditions. Symptoms of acute cholecystitis were relieved by percutaneous cholecystostomy in 90% of patients within 48 hours of drainage. Laparoscopic cholecystectomy was attempted subsequently in 13 patients and was successful in 9. Conversion to open cholecystectomy was necessary in four patients (31%) owing to extensive scarring and adhesions around the gallbladder (three patients) or bleeding (one patient). Complications occurred in 23% of patients, and there was no perioperative mortality. Percutaneous cholecystostomy followed by interval laparoscopic cholecystectomy, therefore, may be considered a minimally invasive alternative for this select group of high risk patients with acute cholecystitis.

## Choledocholithiasis

The prevalence of common bile duct stones in patients undergoing cholecystectomy ranges from 7% to 20%[60,61] and is higher in elderly individuals. The principal options available for the management of common bile duct stones are (1) open common bile duct exploration, (2) preoperative ERCP with sphincterotomy and stone extraction followed by laparoscopic cholecystectomy (two-stage treatment), and (3) laparoscopic common bile duct exploration at the time of laparoscopic cholecystectomy (one-stage procedure). Open exploration of the bile duct is rarely indicated today with the availability of minimally invasive alternatives. The success rate for ERCP and extraction of bile duct stones is approximately 90% in experienced hands.[62–64] Likewise, laparoscopic techniques for removal of bile duct stones have been reported to be successful in more than 90% of patients, as shown in Table 70.7.[65–71] An ongoing controversy is whether patients with suspected bile duct stones should undergo preoperative clearance of the duct by ERCP before laparoscopic removal of the gallbladder.

Clearly, patients with ascending cholangitis or severe pancreatitis with ongoing biliary obstruction and those who are at high risk (often elderly) for surgery and anesthesia are best managed with endoscopic decompression and stone clearance. Lai and associates[72] carried out a prospective, randomized trial to compare open surgical decompression of the biliary tree versus endoscopic biliary drainage in 82 patients with severe acute cholangitis, all of whom were elderly (>64 years). Complications (34% vs. 66%) and mortality (10% vs. 32%) were significantly lower in the patients treated endoscopically. Endoscopic stone clearance alone, without subsequent cholecystectomy, may also be adequate therapy for elderly patients who are deemed to be excessively high risks for surgery and general anesthesia. Recurrent gallbladder symptoms have been observed in only 9–15% of patients treated in this manner in whom the gallbladder with stones has been left in situ.[73–75] Patients who have cystic duct obstruction identified at the time of ERCP have the greatest risk of subsequent biliary problems, most commonly acute cholecystitis.[76]

Normal ERCP examinations have been reported in up to two-thirds of patients in whom bile duct stones are suspected preoperatively,[77,78] resulting in many unnecessary procedures and subjecting patients to increased risks and costs. Complications occur in 5–10% of patients; pancreatitis occurs in 2% of cases, but bleeding, which is the most common serious complication, requires surgical intervention in only 0.4% of patients who undergo endoscopic sphincterotomy.[78] With increasing experience and success with laparoscopic techniques for exploration of the bile duct and confidence in the ability of biliary endoscopists to clear the duct postoperatively of stones that cannot be removed laparoscopically, the use of preoperative ERCP has declined in many centers, including our own. Laparoscopic common bile duct exploration can be carried out via a transcystic approach or by choledochotomy. The transcystic approach is simpler, less technically demanding, and associated with fewer complications than choledochotomy but is limited by the size and location of stones that can be extracted. The results of laparoscopic common bile duct exploration from several large series are shown in Table 70.7. Although elderly patients were not specifically considered in these reports, the mean age of patients in every series was over 50 years, indicating that these are predominantly aging populations. The success rate for stone clearance laparoscopically in these reports was 95%; and the incidence of retained stones, most of which were removed by postoperative ERCP, ranged from 0.5% to 9.0%. Of note, Phillips and associates[66] stratified patients by age and found that old patients had a higher complication rate from laparoscopic bile duct exploration (28% vs. 9%) than did young individuals.

To attempt to answer the question of whether a one-stage (laparoscopic) or a two-stage (laparoscopic and

TABLE 70.7. Results of Laparoscopic Common Bile Duct Exploration

| Study | Year | Total no. of Cases | Age (years) | Transcystic technique | Choledochotomy | Total success rate | Retained stones | Complications | Deaths |
|---|---|---|---|---|---|---|---|---|---|
| De Paula[65] | 1994 | 119 | 51.7 (17–82) | 107 | 12 | 108 (91%) | 1 (0.9%) | 6 (5.0%) | 1 (0.84%) |
| Phillips[66] | 1994 | 120 | 56 (11–86) | 111 | 9 | 112 (93%) | 4 (3.6%) | 19 (14.6%) | 1 (0.83%) |
| Stoker[67] | 1995 | 64 | 61 (14–83) | 27 | 33 | 60 (94%) | 3 (5%) | 6 (10%) | 0 (0) |
| Dorman[68] | 1997 | 137 | 53 (21–93) | 3 | 129 | 132 (96%) | 3 (2.2%) | 7 (5.1%) | 1 (0.8%) |
| Petelin[69] | 1996 | 197 | NA | 173 | 24 | 189 (96%) | NA | NA | 1 (0.5%) |
| Berthou[70] | 1998 | 220 | 63 (19–93) | 77 | 108 | 210 (95.5%) | 7 (3.2%) | 20 (9.1%) | 4 (0.9%) |
| Paganini[71] | 1998 | 161 | 57.1 (12–94) | 107 | 50 | 157 (97.5%) | 8 (5%) | 6 (3.8%) | 1 (0.6%) |
| *Total* | | 1018 | — | 605 | 365 | 968 (95.1%) | 26 (3.2%)[a] | 64 (7.8%)[a] | 9 (1.2%) |

NA, not available.

[a] Excludes data from Petelin's series.

ERCP) procedure was preferable for managing patients with suspected bile duct stones, the European Association of Endoscopic Surgeons conducted a prospective, randomized trial that involved 207 patients.[79] Complication rates and the success rate for stone clearance were similar for the two groups, but patients treated by the one-stage approach had a shorter hospital stay. Financial data were not available owing to the multiinstitutional nature of this study. Although the results of this one study do not permit definitive conclusions, what is clear is that almost all patients with bile duct stones can now be managed in a minimally invasive fashion. Whether an individual patient should undergo preoperative ERCP or should proceed directly to laparoscopic surgery is a decision that should be made based on the degree of suspicion that a bile duct stone is present as well as consideration of locally available expertise in laparoscopic and endoscopic techniques.

## Gallstone Pancreatitis

The management of gallstone pancreatitis has evolved considerably over the past two decades with the availability of laparoscopic cholecystectomy and the success of endoscopic treatment of bile duct stones by ERCP and endoscopic sphincterotomy. With the exception of patients with pancreatic necrosis or abscess, who require open operative drainage and débridement, gallstone pancreatitis can be managed effectively in most patients by a combination of laparoscopic and endoscopic techniques, as demonstrated by several groups during the 1990s.[80–84] Although few series have stratified patients by age, it appears that the results for treatment of elderly patients are comparable to those for younger individuals.[85] As most patients with gallstone pancreatitis spontaneously pass the offending stone within a few days,[86] laparoscopic cholecystectomy with intraoperative evaluation of the common bile duct by cholangiography can usually be carried out during the index admission without further delay. Early ERCP has been shown to be beneficial in patients with severe gallstone pancreatitis who have evidence of persistent biliary obstruction.[87–89] ERCP is not indicated routinely to clear the bile duct prior to laparoscopic cholecystectomy in patients with mild pancreatitis that resolves rapidly. Increasingly, laparoscopic exploration of the common bile duct is used to extract bile duct stones found at cholangiography, further limiting the role of preoperative ERCP in this setting.

Elderly patients with biliary pancreatitis who have comorbid conditions that put them at greatly increased risk for surgery and general anesthesia may benefit from ERCP with sphincterotomy as definitive therapy. Welbourne et al.[90] followed 48 patients with gallstone pancreatitis (mean age 78 years) treated by endoscopic sphincterotomy and clearance of all bile duct stones who did not undergo cholecystectomy. No further episodes of pancreatitis were observed during a mean follow-up of 27 months. Similar results were reported by Siegel et al.[91] in 49 elderly patients treated by endoscopic sphincterotomy alone, none of whom had recurrent pancreatitis over 48 months of follow-up.

## Risk of Gallbladder Cancer and Missed Pathology

Elderly individuals have a higher incidence of gallbladder cancer and other intraabdominal malignancies than do younger individuals. The presence of gallbladder cancer, suspected on preoperative imaging studies or at the time of surgery, is a contraindication to a laparoscopic approach. Several groups[92–94] have reported tumor dissemination or implantation of tumor at the umbilicus and other port sites when cancer-containing gallbladders were removed laparoscopically. Both the higher rate of perforation of the gallbladder during laparoscopic cholecystectomy (up to 30% of cases) and the use of $CO_2$ pneumoperitoneum are factors that may contribute to tumor seeding and port implantation. Patients in whom an incidental gallbladder cancer is discovered after laparoscopic removal should be considered for excision of all port sites and definitive resection of the liver bed and portal lymph node dissection.

An additional risk of minimal access surgery is the possibility that the diagnosis is in error and a nonbiliary intraabdominal malignancy will be missed.[95,96] Among 838 laparoscopic cholecystectomies performed in one center,[95] five patients were readmitted 2–28 months (median 14 months) after laparoscopic cholecystectomy with a missed primary malignancy; two additional patients were referred after laparoscopic cholecystectomy at other institutions. The median age of these patients was 72 years; three of the patients were found to have pancreatic cancer, and four had carcinomas of the right colon. In retrospect, each patient was thought to have had atypical biliary pain at the time of laparoscopic cholecystectomy. Although the 0.6% incidence of missed malignancies is low, patients with atypical biliary pain, especially elderly individuals, should undergo careful preoperative assessment prior to laparoscopic cholecystectomy to avoid missing an occult cancer. Likewise, thorough inspection of the peritoneal cavity should be a routine component of laparoscopic cholecystectomy, particularly if there are any atypical or unusual features of the patient's clinical presentation.

## Common Bile Duct Injury

Laparoscopic cholecystectomy has been associated with an increased number of biliary injuries when compared to open cholecystectomy. These injuries are serious and potentially life-threatening; and they are associated with major morbidity, prolonged hospitalization, high costs, and often litigation.[97] The incidence of major bile duct injury in most large series of open cholecystectomy has been 0.3% or less.[97] Bernard and Hartman,[98] in a statewide database study from New York of 4000 patients undergoing open cholecystectomy, found a major bile duct injury rate of 0.075% and an incidence of bile leak or biloma of 0.5%, for a total biliary injury rate of 0.13%. In contrast, the rate of major bile duct injury in New York State for 8000 patients undergoing laparoscopic cholecystectomy was 0.4% and the total biliary injury rate was 0.55%. Orlando et al.,[99] in an analysis of 4000 laparoscopic cholecystectomies performed in Connecticut over 15 months, found a bile duct injury rate of 0.32%. Gouma and Go[100] reviewed biliary injury rates in a survey of 11,712 cholecystectomies performed in The Netherlands. Common bile duct injuries occurred in 32 of 2932 patients (1.1%) undergoing laparoscopic cholecystectomy compared to 45 injuries (0.51%) in 8780 patients who underwent open cholecystectomy ($p < 0.001$). Moreover, common bile duct injuries during laparoscopic cholecystectomy were more likely to consist of transection injuries, which were more complicated and difficult to repair. Overall the estimated injury rate appears to be two to four times higher for laparoscopic cholecystectomy than with an open operation, and the nature of the injuries is more complex.

Although the problem of bile duct injury during laparoscopic cholecystectomy has been analyzed extensively, no studies have specifically addressed this issue in the elderly despite the greater likelihood of complicated gallstone disease and a procedure that is often more difficult in old individuals. In several studies from referral centers where patients with bile duct injuries have been treated,[101–104] the elderly do not appear disproportionately represented. However, bile duct injury in the elderly, when it occurs, does carry a worse prognosis. Gigot et al.,[105] in a Belgian survey of 9959 patients, found an overall mortality rate of 9% among patients who suffered a bile duct injury. Multivariate analysis showed that both increasing age and the presence of biliary peritonitis were independent predictors of mortality. Also, age and postoperative occurrence of biliary complications after the initial biliary repair were independent predictors of late biliary stricture.

Much has been written in regard to various methods for avoiding bile duct injury during laparoscopic cholecystectomy. Strasberg and colleagues[97] have emphasized the importance of clear and precise dissection to define the anatomy and identification of the cystic duct and artery in Calot's triangle. These structures must be conclusively identified in each and every case not only by dissecting in Calot's triangle but also in the reverse view (dorsolateral aspect) of Calot's and by dissecting the base of the gallbladder from the liver bed. These steps provide the surgeon with a "critical view" of the anatomy such that two and only two structures (cystic duct and artery) are seen to enter the gallbladder (Fig. 70.1). No tubular structure should be clipped or cut until these structures have been unequivocally identified and this view obtained.

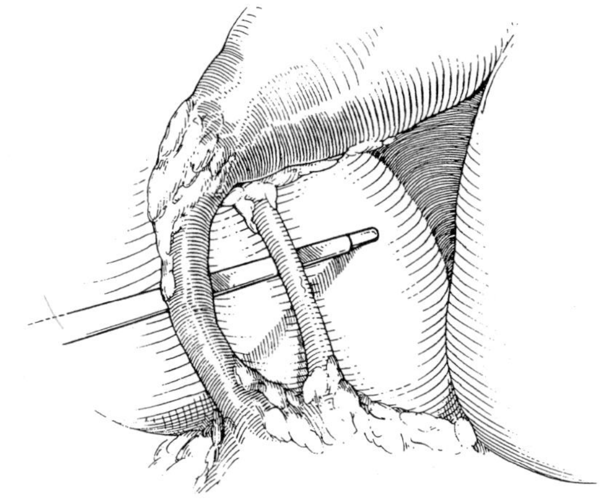

FIGURE 70.1. Critical view during laparoscopic cholecystectomy. Calot's triangle has been dissected to expose the cystic duct and artery as they enter the gallbladder; and the base of the liver bed has been dissected from the gallbladder. When this view has been achieved, the two structures entering the gallbladder can only be the cystic duct and artery. (From Strasberg et al.,[97] with permission.)

## Diagnostic Laparoscopy

### Evaluation of Abdominal Pain

Laparoscopy has been useful for evaluating patients with acute and chronic abdominal pain. It may be especially valuable as a diagnostic aid in the critically ill elderly patient with a suspected acute abdomen. Results from laparoscopic evaluation of the acute abdomen in the critically ill are shown in Table 70.8.[106–109] Although these studies were not limited to the elderly, most of the patients in each of these series was over age 65. In most cases, laparoscopy was performed in the operating room under general anesthesia, but bedside procedures under local anesthesia with sedation have also been described.[106] Overall, 41% of patients in this series had pathology identified by laparoscopy that led to immediate open laparotomy. About 10% of patients had therapeutic procedures (mainly cholecystectomy) carried out laparoscopically, and 48% of patients had either a negative examination or pathology identified that could be managed nonoperatively. There were no deaths attributed to the laparoscopic procedures, although 58% of patients subsequently died from their underlying medical conditions. Laparoscopy therefore appears to be an appropriate consideration for critically ill, elderly patients suspected of having an acute intraab-

TABLE 70.8. Results of Laparoscopy in Critically Ill Patients

| Study | No. of patients | Mean age (years) | Results | | |
|---|---|---|---|---|---|
| | | | Treated laparoscopically | Converted to open laparotomy | Negative or nonsurgical disease |
| Forde[106] | 10 | 67.7 | 0 | 4 | 6 |
| Bender[107] | 7 | 64.3 | 1 | 3 | 3 |
| Brandt[108] | 25 | 61.5 | 0 | 12 | 13 |
| Orlando[109] | 26 | 69 | 6 | 9 | 11 |
| *Total* | 68 | 65.6 | 7 (10.2%) | 28 (41.2%) | 33 (48.5%) |

dominal condition that would otherwise necessitate open exploratory laparotomy.

## Staging of Malignancy

Laparoscopy can also be a useful modality for staging intraabdominal malignancies that have a peak incidence in the elderly, such as gastric and pancreatic cancer. Laparoscopy in this setting may be especially valuable in the elderly to avoid an unnecessary laparotomy in patients with unresectable tumors and a limited life expectancy. In patients with gastric cancer, unsuspected metastases have been found at laparoscopy in 21–40% of cases,[110–112] and laparoscopy has provided an accurate assessment of the depth of invasion for T3 and T4 tumors.[111] Burke and colleagues[112] compared outcomes in 24 patients with gastric cancer who underwent laparoscopy alone with 60 patients subjected to laparotomy without resection. Postoperative length of hospital stay was 1.4 days in the laparoscopy group compared to 6.8 days in the patients who had a laparotomy without resection. For patients with pancreatic cancer, 10–38% of patients with lesions deemed resectable preoperatively by CT scanning, have been found to have unresectable tumor with laparoscopic staging.[113–116] The use of laparoscopic ultrasonography may further enhance the accuracy of tumor staging in these patients.[117,118] Laparoscopy has also been used to diagnoses and stage lymphoma[119,120] and to examine pelvic lymph nodes when staging patients with prostate cancer.[121]

## Laparoscopic Hernia Repair

Inguinal hernia repair is the most common general surgical operation performed in the United States today, with more than 600,000 repairs performed annually.[122] Elderly men are frequently afflicted with groin hernias as a result of deterioration in the inguinal floor due to the aging process, as well as coexisting medical conditions, such as prostatic hypertrophy and constipation that can lead to increased intraabdominal pressure. A variety of methods of hernia repair are available, although prosthetic mesh repairs have begun to replace the more traditional Bassini, McVay, and Shouldice primary tissue repairs. Approximately 15% of hernia repairs in the United States are now performed laparoscopically. Whether laparoscopic hernia repair is appropriate in elderly patients is debatable because the laparoscopic technique is usually done under general anesthesia, whereas open hernia repair is safe and effective and can be carried out under local anesthesia with minimal cardiopulmonary risk to the patient and essentially no risk of postoperative urinary retention. The main potential advantages of laparoscopic hernia repair (i.e., reduced postoperative pain and a faster recovery) are not marked when this approach is compared to open tension-free mesh repairs.

There are no studies that address the specific issue of laparoscopic hernia repair in the elderly, so the results of several prospective, randomized trials of laparoscopic versus open hernia repair in adult patients are presented for review (Table 70.9).[123–135] Most of these series involve small numbers of patients with a short follow-up. In general, laparoscopic hernia repair has been associated with less postoperative pain than open herniorrhaphy and a somewhat more rapid return to full activity and to work, although the differences were not statistically significant in every series. Operative times have been longer for the laparoscopic procedure but have diminished with increasing operative experience. Complication rates and the incidence of recurrent herniation have been similar, although a large multiinstitutional trial of laparoscopic hernia repair showed a recurrence rate of 4.5%,[136] which is considerably higher than the less than 1% incidence of recurrence reported with the open tension-free mesh repairs.[137,138] However, one prospective, randomized trial[139] did show a lower recurrence rate for laparoscopic repair (3%) than with open primary tissue repair (6%). Direct medical costs have also been higher for laparoscopic repairs,[133] owing to longer operating times and the increased cost of the laparoscopic equipment. Laparoscopic hernia repair may also be associated with potentially serious operative complications including injury to the bladder, bowel, and other intraperitoneal organs,[136] which almost never occur with an open

TABLE 70.9. Prospective Randomized Trials of Laparoscopic vs. Open Hernia Repair

| Study | No. of patients | Operative time (min) | Return to normal activity (days) | Return to work (days) | Compl. (%) | Hernia recurrences | Follow-up (months) | Costs |
|---|---|---|---|---|---|---|---|---|
| Stoker[123] | | | | | | | | |
| Lap: TAPP | 75 | 50 | 3[a] | 14[a] | 8 | 0 | 7 | |
| Open: primary | 75 | 35 | 7 | 28 | 21 | 0 | | |
| Payne[124] | | | | | | | | |
| Lap: TAPP | 48 | 68 | | 8.9[a] | 12 | 0 | 10 | 3093 |
| Open: mesh | 52 | 56 | | 17 | 18 | 0 | | 2494 |
| Maddern[125] | | | | | | | | |
| Lap: TAPP | 42 | 35 | NS | 17.5 | 40 | 2 | 8.1 | |
| Open: 1° (Bassini) | 44 | 31 | NS | 30 | 41 | 0 | | |
| Lawrence[126] | | | | | | | | |
| Lap: TAPP | 58 | 72 | 22 | | 12 | 1 | | £850 |
| Open: 1° w/o mesh | 66 | 32 | 28 | | 2 | 0 | | £268 |
| Barkum[127] | | | | | | | | |
| Lap: TAPP/IPOM | 43 | 87 | 9.6 | | 22.5 | 0 | 14 | $1718 |
| Open: Mesh or Shouldice | 49 | 80 | 10.9 | | 11.9 | 1 | | $1223 |
| Vogt[128] | | | | | | | | |
| Lap: IPOM | 30 | 63 | 7.5 | | 16.7 | 1 | 8 | |
| Open: 1° w/o mesh | 31 | 81 | 18.5 | | 16.1 | 2 | | |
| Tschudi[129] | | | | | | | | |
| Lap: TAPP | 44 | 87 | | 25 | 16 | 1 | 6.7 | |
| Open: Shouldice | 43 | 59 | | 48 | 26 | 2 | | |
| Filipi[130] | | | | | | | | |
| Lap: TAPP | 24 | 109 | NS | | 8.3 | 0 | 11 | |
| Open: Mesh | 29 | 87 | | | 6.9 | 2 | | |
| Wright[131] | | | | | | | | |
| Lap: TEP | 60 | 58 | | | | | | |
| Open: Mesh | 60 | 45 | | | | | | |
| Kozol[132] | | | | | | | | |
| Lap: TAPP | 30 | 128 | | | 20 | | | |
| Open: 1° mesh | 32 | 126 | | | 32 | | | |
| Liem[133] | | | | | | | | |
| Lap: TEP | 487 | 45 | 6 | 14 | 15.2 | 3% | | 4916[a] |
| Open: 1° w/o mesh | 507 | 40 | 10 | 21 | 20.3 | 6% | | 4665 |
| Zieren[134] | | | | | | | | |
| Lap: TAPP | 80 | 61 | 3 | 16 | 21 | 0 | 32 | 1211[b] |
| Open: Plug/patch | 80 | 36 | 4 | 18 | 15 | 0 | | 124[b] |
| Open: Shouldice | 80 | 47 | 11[a] | 26[a] | 16 | 0 | | 69[a] |
| Tanphiphat[135] | | | | | | | | |
| Lap: TAPP | 60 | 95 | 8[a] | 14 | 41.7 | 1 | 32 | $400 more |
| Open: Bassini | 60 | 67 | 14 | 15 | 50[c] | 0 | | |

Pain scores were significantly lower for laparoscopic hernia repair in all series evaluated except those of Maddeur, Filipi, and Zieren. Pain scores were not recorded in two of these series (Payne and Vogt).

1°, primary tissue repair without mesh; TAPP, transabdominal preperitoneal; IPOM, intraperitoneal onlay mesh; TEP, total extraperitoneal; NS, not significant; w/o, without.

[a] Difference between laparoscopic and open repair was statistically significant.

[b] Material costs.

[c] Includes paresthesias of groin.

approach. Consequently, it is our belief that laparoscopic hernia repair should be employed judiciously in elderly patients and should be reserved for patients with good performance status who have no increased medical risk factors for general anesthesia. Elderly patients in whom laparoscopic inguinal herniorrhaphy may be particularly beneficial include those with recurrent hernias and bilateral hernias.

## Laparoscopic Antireflux Surgery

Gastroesophageal reflux is a common condition in the United States. For most patients with reflux, life style changes and antisecretory medications provide sufficient control of symptoms. However, for patients with severe gastroesophageal reflux disease (GERD), antireflux surgery is an effective treatment option and may be superior to intensive medical therapy.[140] The most commonly performed antireflux operation has been the Nissen fundoplication (360-degree fundic wrap), which in recent years has been carried out increasingly with laparoscopic techniques. No studies have evaluated results of the laparoscopic Nissen fundoplication in elderly patients. A study of male veterans did demonstrate that the elderly have prevalence rates, disease patterns, and clinical features of GERD that are similar to those of younger patients.[141] Therefore, elderly patients who have complications of GERD or who have symptoms refractory to medical management, should be candidates for a laparoscopic antireflux operation provided they have a good performance status and no medical contraindications to general anesthesia.

Large series of laparoscopic Nissen fundoplications have reported success rates of 93–97% and an acceptably low incidence of postoperative dysphagia and other complications.[142,143] When compared to open Nissen fundoplication, the laparoscopic procedure has been associated with decreased postoperative pain, a shortened hospital stay, and faster recovery.[144–147] Wound complications and incidental splenectomy for bleeding, both well-described complications of open Nissen fundoplication, are rare with the laparoscopic approach. A somewhat higher incidence of pneumothorax (1.0–1.7%) from entering the pleura during the hiatal dissection and pulmonary embolism have been reported laparoscopically.[143,148] These preliminary results suggest that the laparoscopic antireflux operations are safe and will largely replace their open counterparts. Long-term follow-up evaluation and elderly-specific studies are needed to provide definitive validation of this approach.

Paraesophageal hernias account for approximately 5% of hiatal hernias and occur predominantly in old individuals, with a peak incidence between ages 60 and 70 years.[149,150] Because of the risk of incarceration and strangulation, these hernias should be repaired even when asymptomatic. Laparoscopic repair of paraesophageal hernias has been accomplished with good outcome by several groups.[150–152] When compared with historical controls, the traditional benefits of laparoscopic surgery appear to be realized for this procedure. The difference in postoperative length of stay has been especially striking, averaging 2–3 days in the laparoscopic series[150–152] compared to 9–10 days in patients who underwent open repair.[153]

## Laparoscopic Colorectal Surgery

Diseases of the colon and rectum, including cancer, diverticulitis, and other abnormalities, commonly afflict the elderly population. The primary indication for colon resection in the elderly is colon cancer, which is the third most prevalent cancer in the United States and increases in incidence with advancing age. Although laparoscopic colon resection is feasible for many colorectal problems, its role has not been clearly defined for several reasons. Laparoscopic colon resections are technically challenging procedures because of the need to mobilize and resect a bowel segment of variable length and location and to construct a watertight anastomosis and remove an intact specimen for pathologic examination. Laparoscopic colon surgery for cancer, in particular, has been controversial owing to several anecdotal reports of tumor implantation at trocar sites.[154] Nonetheless, elderly patients may stand to benefit the most from a less invasive approach because of the stress and limitations imposed by a conventional open colectomy.[155]

Two retrospective series of laparoscopic colon surgery in elderly patients support this contention.[156,157] Peters and Fleshman[156] attempted laparoscopic colon resection in 103 patients over 65 years of age, 31 of whom were 80 or older. Cancer or large adenomatous polyps were the most common indications for operation. Conversion to open operation was necessary in 20 patients (20%). Hospital length of stay was 5.3 days; and complications, most frequently prolonged ileus, occurred in 20 patients (25%). There were two deaths for a 30-day mortality rate of 2.5%. The authors concluded that these results compared favorably to historical series of open colon resection in elderly patients.

Reissman and associates[157] compared outcomes of laparoscopic colon resection in 36 elderly patients with 36 otherwise comparably matched younger individuals. No significant differences were found between the older and younger patients in terms of conversion rates (11% vs. 8%), duration of postoperative ileus (4.2 vs. 2.8 days), or complications (14% vs. 11%).

Several groups have reported successful resection of colorectal cancers using laparoscopic techniques.[158–165] In most cases the anastomosis is carried out in an extracorporeal fashion, which facilitates the most difficult technical portion of the procedure while providing a mechanism for removing the specimen. Despite concerns regarding tumor implantation, most large series have not reported an increased rate of tumor implantation or recurrence.[158,162,163,165] A prospective, randomized multi-institutional trial by the Clinical Outcomes of Surgical Therapy Study Group (COST) is currently in progress to address this issue. Preliminary data have been reported from 372 patients in the laparoscopic arm of the COST study.[163] Most of these patients have been elderly (mean age 70 years), and about one-half underwent a right hemicolectomy. Conversion to open operation was necessary in 15.6% of patients, and operative mortality was 2%. Local recurrence of tumor was observed in 3.5% of patients, which is not dissimilar from local recurrence rates for open colectomy. Trocar or abdominal wall implants were seen in four patients (1.1%), one of whom had tumor invasion of the pancreas and was con-

TABLE 70.10. Results of Prospective, Randomized Trials of Laparoscopic versus Open Colectomy for Cancer

| | Lacy[166] | | Milsom[167] | |
|---|---|---|---|---|
| Parameter | Open | Laparoscopic | Open | Laparoscopic |
| No. of patients | 26 | 25 | 54 | 55 |
| Conversions | — | 4 (16%) | — | 4 (6.8%) |
| Operative time (minutes) | 111 | 149* | 125 | 200* |
| Blood loss | 218 | 107 | 344 | 252 |
| Time to passage of flatus (days) | 3.0 | 1.5* | 4 | 3* |
| Postoperative length of stay (days) | 8.1 | 5.2* | 7 | 6 |
| Lymph nodes in specimen | 12.5 | 13 | 25 | 19 |
| Complications (%) | 30.8 | 8* | 15 | 15 |

* Significant difference compared to open colectomy.

verted to an open operation. Trocar site recurrences were resected in the remaining three patients, all of whom remain without evidence of disease. Three-year survival rates have been similar to those reported for open colectomy.

Two small institutional prospective, randomized trials, the results of which are summarized in Table 70.10, have been carried out in patients with colorectal neoplasms.[166,167] In both studies, operative times were significantly longer in the laparoscopic group. In the study by Lacy et al.,[166] patients in the laparoscopic group had a more rapid return of bowel function and a shorter hospitalization, whereas Milsom et al.[167] observed no significant differences in these parameters. However, the failure to observe any difference in the latter series may have been due in part to the study design chosen. The complication rate for laparoscopic colectomy was lower in one study[166] but not significantly different in the other.[167] Lymph node harvests were similar for both the laparoscopic and open groups in each study. Interestingly, in Milsom et al.'s series there were two local recurrences of cancer, both in the open group. Definitive conclusions must await the results of the COST trial, but these preliminary results suggest that laparoscopic colon resection for cancer is valid from an oncologic standpoint and may offer advantages over traditional open colectomy.

Beyond the treatment of colon cancer, there are several other potential applications for laparoscopic colorectal surgery in the elderly. Laparoscopic techniques for fecal diversion are relatively simple procedures that require minimal dissection and involve no resection. These procedures can be performed for a variety of indications and have been associated with few complications.[168,169] Laparoscopic approaches have also been described for patients with rectal prolapse using a combination of resection and rectopexy techniques.[170] Some groups[171,172] have also managed patients with acute diverticulitis laparoscopically, although laparoscopic dissection in this setting is more difficult. Consequently, conversion rates have been higher among these patients than with most other colorectal procedures.

## Laparoscopic Adrenalectomy

Laparoscopic adrenalectomy became the preferred method for adrenalectomy during the 1990s. Although no studies have specifically examined the role of this procedure in the elderly, several groups have reported success with the technique in large numbers of patients.[173–176] Furthermore, every study that has compared laparoscopic to open adrenalectomy has shown benefits of decreased pain and a faster recovery in favor of the laparoscopic procedure.[176–182] Laparoscopic adrenalectomy may be carried out via either a transperitoneal[173] or retroperitoneal approach.[183] The retroperitoneal approach may offer advantages in patients with previous upper abdominal surgery or in those who require bilateral adrenalectomy. Regardless of the approach used, most patients with functioning adrenal tumors are candidates for laparoscopic excision. Laparoscopic adrenalectomy is contraindicated, however, in patients with large tumors (>8 cm) or in whom there is suspicion of a primary adrenal malignancy. Patients with isolated adrenal metastases may be considered for laparoscopic excision provided the lesion is small (<6 cm) and without evidence of invasion of adjacent structures. The availability of laparoscopic adrenalectomy does not justify a more liberal approach to removing small (<4 cm), incidentally discovered, nonfunctioning adrenal masses.

## Laparoscopic Splenectomy

Laparoscopic splenectomy has been applied increasingly to treat patients with a wide variety of splenic disorders. The conditions for which elective splenectomy is most commonly indicated—immune thrombocytopenia, spherocytosis, hemolytic anemias—are primarily diseases of young individuals. Lymphomas and leukemias more commonly affect the elderly, but do not often necessitate splenectomy. Therefore, laparoscopic splenectomy probably does not have wide applicability in the elderly population, although it should be considered in appropriate candidates. Laparoscopic splenectomy is most easily accomplished in patients with normal or near-normal size spleens. Contraindications to the laparoscopic approach, which are still being defined, include massive splenomegaly, portal hypertension, and bulky splenic hilar adenopathy. Several groups[184–189] have shown that laparoscopic splenectomy is safe and effective, although conversion rates to open surgery have been somewhat higher than with other laparoscopic procedures, primarily because of the increased difficulty of managing intraoperative bleeding. Data from several large retrospective series have compared laparoscopic to open splenectomy.[184,188–191] Overall, these studies have shown that laparoscopic splenectomy results in longer operative times but less operative blood loss, decreased narcotic use, and a faster recovery. Some series have shown a reduction in hospital costs with the laparoscopic procedure,[188,191] but others have reported higher costs due to the longer operative times and the use of disposable laparoscopic instrumentation.[189,190]

## Conclusions

Laparoscopic surgery has had a major impact on the surgical approach to elderly patients and has resulted in improved clinical outcomes for a variety of surgical procedures. Although elderly patients often present with more complicated disease processes, minimally invasive techniques are still applicable to most of these patients. Additional elderly-specific studies are needed, however, to more clearly define the role of some of the more advanced applications of laparoscopy in this age group. With the progressive aging of society, these studies and the role of minimally invasive surgery in the management of surgical problems in the elderly will be increasingly important in this new millenium.

### References

1. US Bureau of the Census. Social and economic characteristics of the older population. Washington, DC: Government Printing Office, 1978:23.
2. Duplessis P, Spitzer WO. Demography of aging. In: Meakins JL, McClaren JC (eds) Surgical Care of the Elderly. Chicago: Year Book, 1988:3–14.
3. Keller SM, Markovitz LJ, Wilder JR, Aufses AH. Emergency and elective surgery in patients over age 70. Am J Surg 1987;11:636–640.
4. Soper NJ, Brunt LM, Kerbl K. Laparoscopic general surgery. N Engl J Med 1994;330:409–419.
5. US Bureau of the Census. Statistical Abstract of the United States, 111th ed. Washington, DC: GPO, 1991.
6. Newman HF, Northup JD. The autopsy incidence of gallstones [abstract]. Int Abstr Surgery 1959;109:1149.
7. Barbara L, Sama C, Labate AM, et al. A population study on the prevalence of gallstone disease: the Sirmione study. Hepatology 1987;7:913–917.
8. Jorgensen T, Kay L, Schultz-Larsen K. The epidemiology of gallstones in a 70-year old Danish population. Scand J Gastroenterol 1990;25:335–340.
9. Zahor Z, Sternby NH, Kagan A, Uemura K, Vanecek R, Vichert AM. Frequency of cholelithiasis in Prague and Malmo: an autopsy study. Scand J Gastroenterol 1974;9: 3–7.
10. Sullivan D, Ruffin Hood T, Griffen W. Biliary tract surgery in the elderly. Am J Surg 1982;143:218–220.
11. Huber D, Martin E, Cooperman M. Cholecystectomy in elderly patients. Am J Surg 1983;146:719–722.
12. Lygidakis NJ. Operative risk factors of cholecystectomy-choledochotomy in the elderly. Surg Gynecol Obstet 1983;157:15–19.
13. Houghton PWJ, Jenkinson LR, Donaldson LA. Cholecystectomy in the elderly: a prospective study. Br J Surg 1985;72:220–222.
14. Harness JK, Strodel WE, Talsma SE. Symptomatic biliary tract disease in the elderly patient. Am J Surg 1986;52:442–445.
15. Sandler RS, Maule WF, Baltus ME, Holland KL, Kendall MS. Biliary tract surgery in the elderly. J Gen Intern Med 1987;2:149–154.
16. Irvin TT, Arnstein PM. Management of symptomatic gallstones in the elderly. Br J Surg 1988;75:1163–1165.
17. Margiotta SJ, Horwitz JR, Willis IH, Wallack MK. Cholecystectomy in the elderly. Am J Surg 1988;156:509–512.
18. Pigott JP, Williams GB. Cholecystectomy in the elderly. Am J Surg 1988;155:408–410.
19. Girard RM, Morin M. Open cholecystectomy: its morbidity and mortality as a reference standard. Can J Surg 1993;36:75–80.
20. Escarce JJ, Shea JA, Chen W, Qian Z, Schwartz JS. Outcomes of open cholecystectomy in the elderly: a longitudinal analysis of 21,000 cases in the prelaparoscopic era. Surgery 1995;117:156–164.
21. Magnuson TH, Ratner LE, Zenilman ME, Bender JS. Laparoscopic cholecystectomy: applicability in the geriatric population. Am J Surg 1997;63:91–96.
22. Gonzalez JJ, Sanz L, Grana JL, Bermejo G, Navarrete R, Martinez E. Biliary lithiasis in the elderly patient: morbidity and mortality due to biliary surgery. Hepatogastroenterology 1997;44:1565–1568.
23. Roslyn JJ, Bins GS, Hughes EF, Saunders-Kirkwood K, Zinner MJ, Cates JA. Open cholecystectomy: a contemporary analysis of 42,474 patients. Ann Surg 1993;2:129–137.
24. Soper NJ, Stockman PT, Dunnegan DL, Ashley SW. Laparoscopic cholecystectomy: the new "gold standard"? Arch Surg 1992;127:917–921.
25. Reddick EJ, Olsen DO. Laparoscopic laser cholecystectomy: a comparison with mini-lap cholecystectomy. Surg Endosc 1989;3:131–133.
26. Soper NJ, Barteau JA, Clayman RV, Ashley SW, Dunnegan DL. Comparison of early postoperative results for laparoscopic versus standard open cholecystectomy. Surg Gynecol Obstet 1992;174:114–118.
27. Barkun JS, Barkun AN, Sampalis JS, et al. Randomised controlled trial of laparoscopic versus mini cholecystectomy. Lancet 1992;340:1116–1119.
28. McMahon AJ, Russell IT, Baxter JN, et al. Laparoscopic versus minilaparotomy cholecystectomy: a randomised trial. Lancet 1994;343:135–138.
29. McGinn FP, Miles AJG, Uglow M, Ozmen M, Terzi C, Numby M. Randomised trial of laparoscopic cholecystectomy and mini-cholecystectomy. Br J Surg 1995;82:1374–1377.
30. Squirrell DM, Majeed AW, Troy G, Peacock JE, Nicholl JP, Johnson AG. A randomized, prospective, blinded com-

parison of postoperative pain, metabolic response, and perceived health after laparoscopic and small incision cholecystectomy. Surgery 1998;123:485–495.

31. Trondsen E, Reiertsen O, Andersen OK, Kjaersgaard P. Laparoscopic and open cholecystectomy: a prospective, randomized study. Eur J Surg 1993;159:217–221.
32. Nenner RP, Imperato PJ, Alcorn CM. Complications of laparoscopic cholecystectomy in a geriatric population group. NY State J Med 1992;92:518–520.
33. Saxe A, Lawson J, Phillips E. Laparoscopic cholecystectomy in patients aged 65 or older. J Laparoendosc Surg 1993;3:215–219.
34. Fried GM, Clas D, Meakins JL. Minimally invasive surgery in the elderly patient. Surg Clin North Am 1994;74:375–387.
35. Askew AR. Surgery for gallstones in the elderly. Aust NZ J Surg 1995;65:312–315.
36. Firilas A, Duke BE, Max MH. Laparoscopic cholecystectomy in the elderly. Surg Endosc 1996;10:33–35.
37. Behrman SW, Melvin WS, Babb ME, Johnson J, Ellison EC. Laparoscopic cholecystectomy in the geriatric population. Am J Surg 1996;62:386–390.
38. Tagle FM, Lavergne J, Barkin JS, Unge SW. Laparoscopic cholecystectomy in the elderly. Surg Endosc 1997;11:636–638.
39. Magnuson TH, Ratner LE, Zenilman ME, Bender J. Laparoscopic cholecystectomy: applicability in the geriatric population. Am J Surg 1997;63:91–96.
40. Lujan JA, Sachez-Bueno F, Parrilla P, Robles R, Torralba JA, Gonzalez-Costa R. Laparoscopic vs. open cholecystectomy in patients aged 65 and older. Surg Laparosc Endosc 1998;8:208–210.
41. Jones DB, Soper NJ, Brunt LM, Dunnegan DL, Strasberg SM. Effect of age and ASA status on outcome of laparoscopic cholecystectomy [abstract]. Surg Endosc 1996;10: 238.
42. Sanabria JR, Gallinger S, Croxford R, Strasberg S. Risk factors in elective laparoscopic cholecystectomy for conversion to open cholecystectomy. J Am Coll Surg 1994;179:696–704.
43. Liu C, Fan S, Lai E, Lo C, Chu K. Factors affecting conversion of laparoscopic cholecystectomy to open surgery. Arch Surg 1996;131:98–101.
44. Fried GM, Barkun JS, Sigman HH, et al. Factors determining conversion to laparotomy in patients undergoing laparoscopic cholecystectomy. Am J Surg 1994;167:35–41.
45. Wiebke EA, Pruitt AL, Howward TJ, et al. Conversion of laparoscopic to open cholecystectomy. Surg Endosc 1996;10:742–745.
46. Bass EB, Pitt HA, Lillemoe KD. Cost-effectiveness of laparoscopic cholecystectomy versus open cholecystectomy. Am J Surg 1993;165:466–471.
47. Lo C, Lai E, Fan S, Liu C, Wong J. Laparoscopic cholecystectomy for acute cholecystitis in the elderly. World J Surg 1996;20:983–987.
48. Feldman MG, Russell JC, Lynch JT, Mattie A. Comparison of mortality rates for open and closed cholecystectomy in the elderly: Connecticut statewide survey. J Laparoendosc Surg 1994;4:165–172.
49. Cox MR, Wilson TG, Luck AJ, Jeans PL, Padbury TA, Touli J. Laparoscopic cholecystectomy for acute inflammation of the gallbladder. Ann Surg 1993;218:630–634.
50. Miller RE, Kimmelstiel FM. Laparoscopic cholecystectomy for acute cholecystitis. Surg Endosc 1993;7:296–299.
51. Rattner DW, Ferguson C, Warshaw A. Factors associated with successful laparoscopic cholecystectomy for acute cholecystitis. Ann Surg 1993;217:233–236.
52. Unger SW, Rosenbaum G, Unger HM, Edelman DS. A comparison of laparoscopic and open treatment of acute cholecystitis. Surg Endosc 1993;7:408–411.
53. Lujan JA, Parrilla P, Robles R, Marin P, Torralba JA, Garcia-Ayllon J. Laparoscopic cholecystectomy vs. open cholecystectomy in the treatment of acute cholecystitis. Arch Surg 1998;133:173–181.
54. Jarvinen HJ, Hastbacka J. Early cholecystectomy for acute cholecystitis: a prospective randomized study. Ann Surg 1980;191:501–505.
55. Norrby S, Herlin P, Holmin T, Sjodahl R, Tagesson C. Early or delayed cholecystectomy in acute cholecystitis? A clinical trial. Br J Surg 1983;70:163–165.
56. Koo KP, Thirlby RC. Laparoscopic cholecystectomy in acute cholecystitis. Arch Surg 1996;131:540–545.
57. Garber SM, Korman J, Cosgrove JM, Cohen JR. Early laparoscopic cholecystectomy for acute cholecystitis. Surg Endosc 1997;11:347–350.
58. Lo C, Liu C, Fan S, Lai E, Wong J. Prospective randomized study of early versus delayed laparoscopic cholecystectomy for acute cholecystitis. Ann Surg 1998;227:461–467.
59. Patterson EJ, McLoughlin RF, Mathieson JR, Cooperberg PL, MacFarlane JK. An alternative approach to acute cholecystitis: percutaneous cholecystostomy and interval laparoscopic cholecystectomy. Surg Endosc 1996;10:1185–1188.
60. Hermann R. The spectrum of biliary stone disease. Am J Surg 1989;158:171–173.
61. Faris I, Thompson JP, Grundy DJ. Operative cholangiography: a reappraisal based on a review of 400 cholangiograms. Br J Surg 1975;62:966–972.
62. Cotton PB. Endoscopic management of bile duct stones (apples and oranges). Gut 1984;25:587–597.
63. Vaira D, Ainley C, Williams S. Endoscopic sphincterotomy in 1,000 consecutive patients. Lancet 1989;2:431–433.
64. Lambert ME, Betts CD, Faragher EB. Endoscopic sphincterotomy: the whole truth. Br J Surg 1991;78:473–476.
65. DePaula AL, Hashiba K, Bafutto M. Laparoscopic management of choledocholithiasis. Surg Endosc 1994;8:1399–1403.
66. Phillips EH, Rosenthal RJ, Carroll BJ, Fallas MJ. Laparoscopic trans-cystic duct common-bile-duct exploration. Surg Endosc 1994;8:1389–1394.
67. Stoker M. Common bile duct exploration in the era of laparoscopic surgery. Arch Surg 1995;130:265–269.
68. Dorman J, Franklin M. Laparoscopic common bile duct exploration by choledochotomy. Semin Laparosc Surg 1997;4:34–41.
69. Petelin J. Techniques and cost of common bile duct exploration. Semin Laparosc Surg 1997;4:23–33.
70. Berthou J, Drouard F, Charbonneau P, Moussalier K. Evaluation of laparoscopic management of common bile duct stones in 220 patients. Surg Endosc 1998;12:16–22.

71. Paganini AM, Lezoche E. Follow-up of 161 unselected consecutive patients treated laparoscopically for common bile duct stones. Surg Endosc 1998;12:23–29.
72. Lai EC, Mok FP, Tan ES, et al. Endoscopic biliary drainage for severe acute cholangitis. N Engl J Med 1992;326: 1582–1586.
73. Perissat J, Huibregtse K, Keane FB. Management of bile duct stones in the era of laparoscopic cholecystectomy. Br J Surg 1994;81:799–810.
74. Davidson BR, Neoptolemos JP, Carr-Locke DL. Endoscopic sphincterotomy for common bile duct calculi in patients with gallbladder in situ considered unfit for surgery. Gut 1988;29:114–120.
75. Escourrou J, Cordova JA, Lazorthes F. Early and late complications after endoscopic sphincterotomy for biliary lithiasis with and without the gallbadder "in situ." Gut 1984;25:598–602.
76. Worthley CS, Touli J. Gallbladder non-filling: an indication for cholecystectomy after endoscopic sphincterotomy. Br J Surg 1988;75:796–798.
77. Graham SM, Flowers JL, Scott TR. Laparoscopic cholecystectomy and common bile duct stones. Ann Surg 1993;218:61–67.
78. O'Mahoney S, Lintott DJ, Axon A. Endoscopic retrograde cholangiopancreatography. Semin Laparosc Surg 1995;2: 93–101.
79. Cuschieri A, Croce E, Faggioni A, et al. EAES ductal stone study: preliminary findings of multi-center prospective randomized trial comparing two-stage vs. single-stage management. Surg Endosc 1996;10:1130–1135.
80. Soper NJ, Brunt LM, Callery MP, Edmundowicz SA, Aliperti G. Role of laparoscopic cholecystectomy in the management of acute gallstone pancreatitis. Am J Surg 1994;167:42–50.
81. Pellegrini CA. Surgery for gallstone pancreatitis. Am J Surg 1993;165:515–518.
82. Tate JJT, Lau WY, Li AKC. Laparoscopic cholecystectomy for biliary pancreatitis. Br J Surg 1994;81:720–722.
83. Delorio AV Jr, Vitale GC, Reynolds M, Larson GM. Acute biliary pancreatitis: the role of laparoscopic cholecystectomy and endoscopic retrograde cholangiopancreatography. Surg Endosc 1995;9:392–396.
84. Tang E, Stain SC, Tang G. Timing of laparoscopic surgery in gallstone pancreatitis. Arch Surg 1995;130:496–500.
85. McGrath MF, McGrath JC, Gabbay J, Phillips EH, Hiatt JR. Safe laparoendoscopic approach to biliary pancreatitis in older patients. Arch Surg 1996;131:826–833.
86. Acosta JM, Ledesma DL. Gallstone migration as a cause of acute pancreatitis. N Engl J Med 1974;290:484.
87. Neoptolemos JP, Carr-Locke DL, London NJ, et al. Controlled trial of urgent endoscopic retrograde cholangiopancreatography and endoscopic sphincterotomy versus conservative treatment for acute pancreatitis due to gallstones. Lancet 1988;2:979–983.
88. Nowak A, Nowakowska-Duzawa E, Rybicka J. Urgent endoscopic sphincterotomy vs. conservative treatment in acute biliary pancreatitis: a prospective, controlled trial. Hepatogastroenterology 1990;37(suppl II):A5.
89. Fan ST, Lai EC, Mok FP. Early treatment of biliary pancreatitis by endoscopic papillotomy. N Engl J Med 1993;328:228–232.
90. Welbourn C, Beckly DE, Eyre-Brook IA. Endoscopic sphincterotomy for gallstone pancreatits. Gut 1995;37:119–120.
91. Siegel JH, Veerappan A, Cohen SA, Kasmin FE. Endoscopic sphincterotomy for biliary pancreatitis: an alternative to cholecystectomy in high-risk patients. Gastrointest Endosc 1994;40:573–575.
92. Yamaguchi K, Chijiiwa K, Ichimiya H, et al. Gallbladder carcinoma in the era of laparoscopic cholecystectomy. Arch Surg 1996;131:981–984.
93. Wade TP, Comitalo JB, Andrus CH, Goodwin MN, Kaminski DL. Laparoscopic cancer surgery. Surg Endosc 1994;8:698–701.
94. Horvath LZ, Flautner LE, Tihanyi TF, Miklos IJ. Trocar site metastasis of gallbladder cancer after laparoscopic cholecystectomy. Minim Invasive Ther 1996;5:193–196.
95. Slim K, Pezet D, Clark E, Chipponi J. Malignant tumors missed at laparoscopic cholecystectomy. Am J Surg 1996;171:364–365.
96. Gal I, Szivos J, Jaberansari MT, Szabo Z. Laparoscopic cholecystectomy: risk of missed pathology of other organs. Surg Endosc 1998;12:825–827.
97. Strasberg S, Hertl M, Soper NJ. An analysis of the problem of biliary injury during laparoscopic cholecystectomy. J Am Coll Surg 1995;180:101–125.
98. Bernard HR, Hartman TW. Complications after laparoscopic cholecystectomy. Am J Surg 1993;165:533–535.
99. Orlando R III, Russell JC, Lynch J, Mattie A. Laparoscopic cholecystectomy. Arch Surg 1993;128:494–499.
100. Gouma DJ, Go PM. Bile duct injury during laparoscopic and conventional cholecystectomy. J Am Coll Surg 1994;178:229–233.
101. Branum G, Schmitt C, Baillie J, et al. Management of major biliary complications after laparoscopic cholecystectomy. Ann Surg 1993;217:532–541.
102. Stewart L, Way L. Bile duct injuries during laparoscopic cholecystectomy: factors that influence the results of treatment. Arch Surg 1995;130:1123–1129.
103. Lillemoe KD, Martin SA, Cameron JL, et al. Major bile duct injuries during laparoscopic cholecystectomy: follow-up after combined surgical and radiologic management. Ann Surg 1997;225:459–471.
104. Soper NJ, Flye W, Brunt LM, et al. Diagnosis and management of biliary complications of laparoscopic cholecystectomy. Am J Surg 1993;165:663–669.
105. Gigot JF, Etienne J, Aerts R, et al. The dramatic reality of biliary tract injury during laparoscopic cholecystectomy. Surg Endosc 1997;11:1171–1178.
106. Forde KA, Treat MR. The role of peritoneoscopy (laparoscopy) in the evaluation of the acute abdomen in critically ill patients. Surg Endosc 1992;6:219–221.
107. Bender JS, Talamini MA. Diagnostic laparoscopy in critically ill intensive-care-unit patients. Surg Endosc 1992;6:302–304.
108. Brandt CP, Priebe PP, Eckhauser ML. Diagnostic laparoscopy in the intensive care patient: avoiding the nontherapeutic laparotomy. Surg Endosc 1993;7:168–172.
109. Orlando R III, Crowell KL. Laparoscopy in the critically ill. Surg Endosc 1997;11:1072–1074.
110. Ascencio F, Aguilo J, Salvador JL, et al. Video-laparoscopic staging of gastric cancer: a prospective multicenter

comparison with noninvasive techniques. Surg Endosc 1997;11:1153–1158.
111. D'Ugo DM, Persiani R, Caracciolo F, Ronconi P, Coco C, Picciocchi A. Selection of locally advanced gastric carcinoma by preoperative staging laparoscopy. Surg Endosc 1997;11:1159–1162.
112. Burke EC, Karpeh MS, Conlon KC. Laparoscopy in the management of gastric adenocarcinoma. Ann Surg 1997;225:262–267.
113. Friess H, Kleeff J, Silva JC, Sadowski C, Baer HU, Buchler MW. The role of diagnostic laparoscopy in pancreatic and periampullary malignancies. J Am Coll Surg 1998;186:675–682.
114. Warshaw AL, Gu Z, Wittenberg J, Waltman A. Preoperative staging and assessment of resectability of pancreatic cancer. Arch Surg 1990;125:230–233.
115. Conlon KC, Dougherty E, Klimstra DS, Coit DG, Turnbull AD, Brennan MF. The value of minimal access surgery in the staging of patients with potentially resectable peripancreatic malignancy. Ann Surg 1996;223:134–140.
116. Andren-Sandberg A, Lindberg CG, Lundstedt C, Ihse I. Computed tomography and laparoscopy in the assessment of the patient with pancreatic cancer. J Am Coll Surg 1998;186:35–40.
117. John TG, Greig JD, Carter DC, Garden OJ. Carcinoma of the pancreatic head and periampullary region: tumor staging with laparoscopy and laparoscopic ultrasonography. Ann Surg 1995;221:156–164.
118. Callery MP, Strasberg SM, Doherty GM, Soper NJ, Norton JA. Staging laparoscopy with laparoscopic ultrasonography: optimizing resectability in hepatobiliary and pancreatic malignancy. J Am Coll Surg 1997;185:33–39.
119. Lightdale CJ. Clinical applications of laparoscopy in patients with malignant neoplasms. Gastrointest Endosc 1982;28:99–102.
120. Spinelli P, Beretta G, Bajetta E. Laparoscopy and laparotomy combined with bone marrow biopsy in staging Hodgkin's disease. Br Med J 1975;4:554–556.
121. Kerbl K, Clayman RV, Chandhoke PS, Gill IS. Staging pelvic lymphadenectomy for prostate cancer: a comparison of laparoscopic and open techniques. J Urol 1993;150:396–399.
122. Rutkow IM. Open versus laparoscopic groin herniorrhaphy: economic realities. In: Arregui NE, Nagan RF (eds) Inguinal Hernia: Advances or Controversies. Oxford: Radcliffe Medical Press, 1994:145–150.
123. Stoker DL, Spiegelhalter DJ, Singh R, Wellwood JM. Laparoscopic versus open inguinal hernia repair: randomized prospective trial. Lancet 1994;343:1243–1245.
124. Payne JH, Grininger LM, Izawa MT, Podoll EF, Lindahl PJ, Balfour J. Laparoscopic or open inguinal herniorrhaphy? Arch Surg 1994;129:973–981.
125. Maddern GJ, Rudkin G, Bessell JR, Devitt P, Ponte L. A comparison of laparoscopic and open hernia repair as a day surgical procedure. Surg Endosc 1994;8:1404–1408.
126. Lawrence K, McWhinnie D, Goodwin A, et al. Randomised controlled trial of laparoscopic versus open repair of inguinal hernia: early results. Br Med J 1995;311:981–985.
127. Barkun JS, Wexler MJ, Hinchey EJ, Thibeault D, Meakins JL. Laparoscopic versus open inguinal herniorrhaphy: preliminary results of a randomized controlled trial. Surgery 1995;118:703–710.
128. Vogt DM, Curet MJ, Pitcher DE, Martin DT, Zucker KA. Preliminary results of a prospective randomized trial of laparoscopic onlay versus conventional inguinal herniorrhaphy. Am J Surg 1995;169:84–90.
129. Tschudi J, Wagner M, Klaiber C, et al. Controlled multicenter trial of laparoscopic transabdominal preperitoneal hernioplasty vs. Shouldice herniorrhaphy. Surg Endosc 1996;10:845–847.
130. Filipi CJ, Gaston-Johansson F, McBride PJ, et al. An assessment of pain and return to normal activity: laparoscopic herniorrhaphy vs. open tension-free Lichtenstein repair. Surg Endosc 1996;10:983–986.
131. Wright DM, Kennedy A, Baxter JN, et al. Early outcome after open versus extraperitoneal endoscopic tension-free hernioplasty: a randomized clinical trial. Surgery 1996;119:552–557.
132. Kozol R, Lange PM, Kosir M, et al. A prospective, randomized study of open vs. laparoscopic inguinal hernia repair. Arch Surg 1997;132:292–295.
133. Liem MS, Halsema JA, Van Der Graaf Y, Schrijvers AJ, Van Vroonhoven TJ. Cost-effectiveness of extraperitoneal laparoscopic inguinal hernia repair: a randomized comparison with conventional herniorrhaphy. Ann Surg 1997;226:668–676.
134. Zieren J, Zieren HU, Jacobi CA, Wenger FA, Muller JM. Prospective randomized study comparing laparoscopic and open tension-free inguinal hernia repair with Shouldice's operation. Am J Surg 1998;175:330–333.
135. Tanphiphat C, Tanprayoon T, Sangsubhan C, Chatamra K. Laparoscopic vs. open inguinal hernia repair. Surg Endosc 1998;12:846–851.
136. Fitzgibbons RJ, Camps J, Cornet DA, Nguyen NX. Laparoscopic inguinal herniorrhaphy: results of a multicenter trial. Ann Surg 1995;221:3–13.
137. Kark AE, Kurzer MN, Belsham PA. Three thousand one hundred seventy-five primary inguinal hernia repairs: advantages of ambulatory open mesh repair using local anesthesia. J Am Coll Surg 1998;186:447–456.
138. Amid PK, Shulman AG, Lichtenstein IL. Critical scrutiny of the tension-free hernioplasty. Am J Surg 1993;165: 369.
139. Liem MS, Van Der Graaf Y, Van Steensel CJ, et al. Comparison of conventional anterior surgery and laparoscopic surgery for inguinal hernia repair. N Engl J Med 1997;336:1541–1547.
140. Spechler SJ. Comparison of medical and surgical therapy for complicated gastroesophageal reflux disease in veterans. N Engl J Med 1992;326:786–792.
141. Triadafilopoulos G, Sharma R. Features of symptomatic gastroesophageal reflux disease in elderly patients. Am J Gastroenterol 1997;92:2007–2011.
142. Hunter JG, Trus TL, Branum GD, Waring JP, Wood WC. A physiologic approach to laparoscopic fundoplication for gastroesophageal reflux disease. Ann Surg 1996;223:673–687.
143. Hinder RA, Filipi CJ, Wetscher G, Neary P, DeMeester TR, Perdikis G. Laparoscopic Nissen fundoplication is an effective treatment for gastroesophageal relux disease. Ann Surg 1994;220:472–483.

144. Laine S, Rantala A, Gullichsen R, Ovaska J. Laparoscopic vs conventional Nissen fundoplication: a prospective randomized study. Surg Endosc 1997;11:441–444.
145. European Association for Endoscopic Surgery consensus development conference. Laparoscopic antireflux surgery for gastroesophageal reflux disease (GERD). Surg Endosc 1997;11:413–426.
146. Viljakka MT, Luostarinen ME, Isolauri JO. Complications of open and laparoscopic antireflux surgery: 32-year audit at a teaching hospital. J Am Coll Surg 1997;185:446–450.
147. Eshraghi N, Farahmand M, Soot SJ, Rand-Luby L, Deveney CW, Sheppard BC. Comparison of outcomes of open versus laparoscopic Nissen fundoplication performed in a single practice. Am J Surg 1998;175:371–374.
148. McKenzie D, Grayson T, Polk HC. The impact of omeprazole and laparoscopy upon hiatal hernia and reflux esophagitis. J Am Coll Surg 1996;183:413–418.
149. Landrenau RJ, Johnson JA, Marshall JB. Clinical spectrum of paraesophageal herniation. Dig Dis Sci 1992;37:537–544.
150. Willekes CL, Edoga JK, Ermenegildo EF. Laparoscopic repair of paraesophageal hernia. Ann Surg 1997;225:31–38.
151. Perdikis G, Hinder RA, Filipi CJ, et al. Laparoscopic paraesophageal hernia repair. Arch Surg 1997;132:586–590.
152. Wu JS, Dunnegan DL, Soper NJ. Clinical and radiologic assessment of laparoscopic paraesophageal hernia repair. Surg Endosc 1998;13:497–502.
153. Ellis FH, Crozier RE, Shea JA. Paraesophageal hiatus hernia. Arch Surg 1986;121:416–420.
154. Wexner SD, Cohen SM. Port site metastasis after laparoscopic colorectal surgery for cure of malignancy. Br J Surg 1995;82:295–298.
155. Ogunbiyi OA, Fleshman JW. Colorectal cancer and laparoscopic colorectal surgery in the elderly patient. Prob Gen Surg 1997;13:154–162.
156. Peters WR, Fleshman JW. Minimally invasive colectomy in elderly patients. Surg Laparosc Endosc 1995;5:477–479.
157. Reissman P, Agachan F, Wexner SD. Outcome of laparoscopic colorectal surgery in older patients. Am Surg 1996;12:1060–1063.
158. Franklin ME, Rosenthal D, Abrego-Medina D, et al. Prospective comparison of open vs. laparoscopic colon surgery for carcinoma: five-year results. Dis Colon Rectum 1996;39:S35–S46.
159. Zucker KA, Pitcher DE, Martin DT. Laparoscopic-assisted colon resection. Surg Endosc 1994;8:12–17.
160. Hoffman GC, Baker JW, Doxey JB. Minimally invasive surgery for colorectal cancer: initial follow-up. Ann Surg 1996;223:790–796.
161. Kockerling F, Schneidner C, Reymond MA. Early results of a prospective multicenter study on 500 consecutive cases of laparoscopic colorectal surgery. Surg Endosc 1998;12:37–41.
162. Kwok SP, Carey PD, Kelly SB, Leung KL, Li AK. Prospective evaluation of laparoscopic-assisted large bowel excision for cancer. Ann Surg 1996;223:170–176.
163. Fleshman JW, Nelson H, Peters WR, et al. Early results of laparoscopic surgery for colorectal cancer: retrospective analysis of 372 patients treated by clinical outcomes of sugical therapy (COST) study group. Dis Colon Rectum 1996;39:S53–S58.
164. Stage JG, Schulze S, Moller P. Prospective randomized study of laparoscopic versus open colonic resection for adenocarcinoma. Br J Surg 1997;84:391–396.
165. Leung KL, Kwok SPY, Lau WY, et al. Laparoscopic-assisted resection of rectosigmoid carcinoma. Arch Surg 1997;132:761–764.
166. Lacy AM, Garcia-Valdecases JC, Pique JM, et al. Short-term outcome analysis of a randomized study comparing laparoscopic vs. open colectomy for colon cancer. Surg Endosc 1995;9:1101–1105.
167. Milsom JW, Bohm B, Hammerhofer KA, Fazio V, Steiger E. A prospective, randomized trial comparing laparoscopic versus conventional techniques in colorectal cancer surgery: a preliminary report. J Am Coll Surg 1998;187:46–57.
168. Fuhrman GM, Ota DM. Laparoscopic intestinal stomas. Dis Colon Rectum 1994;37:444–449.
169. Ludwig KA, Milsom JW, Garcia-Ruiz A, Fazio VW. Laparoscopic techniques for fecal diversion. Dis Colon Rectum 1996;39:285–288.
170. Stevenson AR, Stitz RW, Lumley JW. Laparoscopic-assisted resection-rectopexy for rectal prolapse: early and medium follow-up. Dis Colon Rectum 1998;41:46–54.
171. Sher ME, Agachan F, Bortul M, Nogueras JJ, Weiss EG, Wexner SD. Laparoscopic surgery for diverticulitis. Surg Endosc 1997;11:264–267.
172. Hoffman GC, Baker JW, Fitchett CW, Vansant JH. Laparoscopic assisted colectomy: initial experience. Ann Surg 1994;219:732–743.
173. Gagner M, Lacroix A, Bolte E, Pomp A. Laparoscopic adrenalectomy: the importance of a flank approach in the lateral position. Surg Endosc 1994;8:135–138.
174. Duh Q-Y, Siperstein AE, Clark OH, et al. Laparoscopic adrenalectomy: comparison of the lateral and posterior approaches. Arch Surg 1996;131:870–876.
175. Rutherford JC, Stowasser M, Tunny TJ, Klemm SA, Gordon RD. Laparoscopic adrenalectomy. World J Surg 1996;20: 758–761.
176. Brunt LM, Doherty GM, Norton JA, Soper NJ, Quasebarth MA, Moley JF. Laparoscopic adrenalectomy compared to open adrenalectomy for benign neoplasms. J Am Coll Surg 1996;183:1–10.
177. Guazzoni G, Montorsi F, Bocciardi A, et al. Transperitoneal laparoscopic versus open adrenalectomy for benign hyperfunctioning adrenal tumors: a comparative study. J Urol 1995;153:1597–1600.
178. Prinz RA. A comparison of laparoscopic and open adrenalectomies. Arch Surg 1995;130:489–494.
179. MacGillivay DC, Shichman SJ, Ferrer FA, Malchoff CD. A comparison of open vs. laparoscopic adrenalectomy. Surg Endosc 1996;10:987–990.
180. Linos DA, Stylopoulos N, Boukis M, Souvatzoglou A, Raptis S, Papadimitriou J. Anterior, posterior, or laparoscopic approach for the management of adrenal diseases? Am J Surg 1997;173:120–125.
181. Thompson GB, Grant CS, van Heerden JA, et al. Laparoscopic versus open posterior adrenalectomy: a case control study of 100 patients. Surgery 1997;122:1132–1136.
182. Ting AC, Lo CY, Lo CM. Posterior or laparoscopic approach for adrenalectomy. Am J Surg 1998;175:488–490.

183. Mercan S, Seven R, Ozarmagan S, Tezelman S. Endoscopic retroperitoneal adrenalectomy. Surgery 1995;118:1071–1076.
184. Brunt LM, Langer JC, Quasebarth MA, Whitman ED. Comparative analysis of laparoscopic versus open splenectomy. Am J Surg 1996;172:596–601.
185. Flowers JL, Lefor AT, Steers J. Laparoscopic splenectomy in patients with hematologic disease. Ann Surg 1996;224: 19–28.
186. Kathouda N, Waldrep DJ, Feinstein D. Unresolved issues in laparoscopic splenectomy. Am J Surg 1996;72:585–590.
187. Park A, Gagner M, Pomp A. The lateral approach to laparoscopic splenectomy. Am J Surg 1997;173:126–130.
188. Friedman RL, Hiatt JR, Korman JL. Laparoscopic or open splenectomy for hematologic disease: which approach is superior? J Am Coll Surg 1997;185:49–54.
189. Yee LF, Carvajal SH, de Lorimier AA, Mulvihill SJ. Laparoscopic splenectomy. Arch Surg 1995;130:874–879.
190. Diaz J, Eisenstat M, Chung R. A case-controlled study of laparoscopic splenectomy. Am J Surg 1997;173:348–350.
191. Watson DI, Coventry BJ, Chin T. Laparoscopic versus open splenectomy for immune thrombocytopenia purpura. Surgery 1997;121:18–22.

# Index

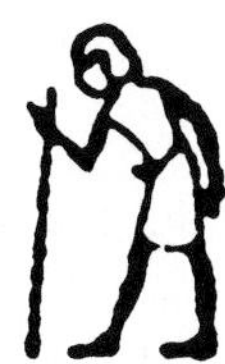

**H**

J



K

**Q**



**R**